Surgical Procedure Videos

Video 1: ...VR Plating

Video 2: ...ion, Percutaneous Pinning

Video 3: ...xation

Video 4: ...merus and Distal Radial Fractures

Video 5: Diaphyseal Radial Ulna Fractures, Intramedullary TENS Fixation

Video 6: ... condylar Humeral Fracture, Open Reduction, Internal Fixation

Video 7: ...Fracture Delayed Union, Open Reduction Internal Fixation with Osseous Screw

Video 8: ...Slipped Capital Femoral Epiphysis, In Situ Epiphysiodesis with Cannulated Screw

Video 9: Supracondylar Humerus Type II Fracture, Closed Reduction, Percutaneous Pinning

Video 10: Supracondylar Humerus Type IV Fracture, Closed Reduction, Percutaneous Pinning

Video 11: ...bial Tubercle Fracture, Open Reduction, Internal Fixation

Video 12: Tillaux Shaft Distal Tibia Fracture, Open Reduction, Internal Fixation

Video 13: ...Wrist Laceration, Nerve and Tendon Repair

Rockwood and Wilkins'
Fractures in Children

NINTH EDITION

Rockwood and Wilkins'
Fractures in Children

NINTH EDITION

EDITORS

Peter M. Waters, MD
Orthopaedic Surgeon-in-Chief
Boston Children's Hospital
John E. Hall Professor of Orthopaedic Surgery
Harvard Medical School
Boston, Massachusetts

David L. Skaggs, MD, MMM
Chief of Orthopaedic Surgery
Children's Endowed Chair of Spine Surgery
Children's Hospital Los Angeles
Professor of Orthopaedic Surgery
Keck School of Medicine, University of Southern California
Los Angeles, California

John M. (Jack) Flynn, MD
Chief, Division of Orthopaedics
Children's Hospital of Philadelphia
Richard M. Armstrong Jr. Endowed Chair in
 Pediatric Orthopaedic Surgery
Perelman School of Medicine at the
 University of Pennsylvania
Philadelphia, Pennsylvania

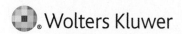 Wolters Kluwer

Philadelphia • Baltimore • New York • London
Buenos Aires • Hong Kong • Sydney • Tokyo

Acquisitions Editor: Brian Brown
Development Editor: Stacey Sebring
Editorial Coordinator: David Murphy
Marketing Manager: Julie Sikora
Production Project Manager: Barton Dudlick
Design Coordinator: Holly McLaughlin
Manufacturing Coordinator: Beth Welsh
Prepress Vendor: Aptara, Inc.

Copyright © 2020 Wolters Kluwer.

9 8 7 6 5 4 3 2 1

Printed in China

Library of Congress Cataloging-in-Publication Data

Names: Waters, Peter M., editor. | Skaggs, David L., editor. | Flynn, John
   M., editor. | Court-Brown, Charles M., editor.
Title: Rockwood and Wilkins' fractures in children / [edited by] Peter M.
   Waters, David L. Skaggs, John M. (Jack) Flynn, Charles Court-Brown.
Other titles: Rockwood & Wilkins' fractures in children | Fractures in
   children
Description: Ninth edition. | Philadelphia : Wolters Kluwer, [2020] |
   Preceded by Rockwood & Wilkins' fractures in children / [edited by] John
   M. Flynn, David L. Skaggs, Peter M. Waters. 8th ed. 2015. | Includes
   bibliographical references and index.
Identifiers: LCCN 2018056468 | ISBN 9781496386540
Subjects: | MESH: Fractures, Bone | Adolescent | Child | Infant | Joint
   Dislocations
Classification: LCC RD101 | NLM WE 180 | DDC 617.1/5083–dc23
LC record available at https://lccn.loc.gov/2018056468

shop.lww.com

I want to acknowledge my wife Mary and children Erin, Colleen, John, and Kelly for patience and understanding while I dedicated many hours to this project. They understand that Dad has homework too. Also, I would like to recognize the injured children, medical students, residents, and fellows who count on this textbook to be the trusted source of information for fracture care; their needs are the inspiration that drive us to create an excellent final product.

Jack Flynn

I wish to thank my wife Janet, expanding family of James, Rebecca, Billy, Izzy, and Elle. They, along with our unique collection of friends, supported me doing the binge work on this book during the hours before the real fun begins. I am indebted to my partners and patients who teach me about fracture care every day.

Peter M. Waters

I want to most of all thank my wife Val for always being there for me. Thanks to my children Kira, Jamie, and Clay for being good friends in every sense of the word and assisting me with the many children who come to our home with injuries. I hope readers will welcome my daughter Kira to the medical profession; she is a first-year medical student at the time of this publication. And thank you to everyone at the Children's Orthopaedic Center at Los Angeles Children's Hospital that make it fun and rewarding to come to work every day.

David L. Skaggs

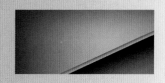

Contributors

Joshua M. Abzug, MD
Associate Professor
Departments of Orthopedics and Pediatrics
University of Maryland School of Medicine
Director
University of Maryland Brachial Plexus Clinic
Director of Pediatric Orthopedics
University of Maryland Medical Center
Deputy Surgeon-in-Chief
University of Maryland Children's Hospital
Baltimore, Maryland

Benjamin A. Alman, MD
James Urbaniak Professor and Chair
Department of Orthopaedic Surgery
Duke University
Durham, North Carolina

Lindsay Andras, MD
Assistant Professor of Orthopaedic Surgery
Keck School of Medicine of USC
Children's Orthopaedic Center
Children's Hospital Los Angeles
Los Angeles, California

Alexandre Arkader, MD
Pediatric Orthopedics and Orthopedic Oncology
Children's Hospital of Philadelphia
Associate Professor of Orthopedic Surgery
Perelman School of Medicine at the University of Pennsylvania
Philadelphia, Pennsylvania

Haleh Badkoobehi, MD, MPH
Pediatric Orthopaedic Fellow
Children's Orthopaedic Center
Children's Hospital Los Angeles
Los Angeles, California

Donald S. Bae, MD
Associate Professor
Department of Orthopaedic Surgery
Harvard Medical School
Boston Children's Hospital
Boston, Massachusetts

Brian K. Brighton, MD, MPH
Associate Professor
Department of Orthopaedic Surgery
Carolinas Healthcare System
Levine Children's Hospital
Charlotte, North Carolina

Haemish Crawford, FRACS
Paediatric Orthopaedic Surgeon
Starship Children's Health
Auckland, New Zealand

Eric W. Edmonds, MD, FAOA
Associated Professor of Clinical Orthopedic Surgery
UC San Diego School of Medicine
Director of Orthopaedic Research
Division of Orthopaedic Surgery and Scoliosis
Rady Children's Hospital San Diego
San Diego, California

Mark A. Erickson, MD, MMM
Professor
University of Colorado Anschutz Medical Campus
Department of Orthopaedic Surgery
Children's Hospital Colorado
Aurora, Colorado

John M. Flynn, MD
Chief, Division of Orthopaedics
Chidlren's Hospital of Philadelphia
Richard M. Armstrong Jr. Endowed Chair in Pediatric
    Orthopaedic Surgery
Perelman School of Medicine at the University of Pennsylvania
Philadelphia, Pennsylvania

Steven L. Frick, MD
Professor and Vice Chair
Department of Orthopaedic Surgery
Stanford Medicine
Stanford Children's Health—Lucile Packard Children's
    Hospital Stanford
Palo Alto, California

Sumeet Garg, MD
Associate Professor
Department of Orthopaedics
University of Colorado School of Medicine
Children's Hospital Colorado
Aurora, Colorado

Michael Glotzbecker, MD
Assistant Professor
Department of Orthopaedic Surgery
Harvard Medical School
Boston Children's Hospital
Boston, Massachusetts

Rachel Y. Goldstein, MD, MPH
Assistant Professor of Orthopaedic Surgery
Keck School of Medicine of USC
Director of the Hip Preservation Program
Director of Orthopaedic Education
Children's Hospital Los Angeles
Los Angeles, California

Matthew A. Halanski, MD
Associate Professor
Department of Orthopaedics and Rehabilitation
University of Wisconsin—Madison
American Family Children's Hospital
Madison, Wisconsin

Daniel J. Hedequist, MD
Associate Professor of Orthopedic Surgery
Boston Children's Hospital
Harvard Medical School
Boston, Massachusetts

William L. Hennrikus, MD
Professor and Associate Dean
Department of Orthopaedic Surgery
PennState College of Medicine
Hershey, Pennsylvania

Martin J. Herman, MD
Professor of Orthopedic Surgery and Pediatrics
Drexel University College of Medicine
Section Chief of Orthopedic Surgery
St. Christopher's Hospital for Children
Philadelphia, Pennsylvania

Benton E. Heyworth, MD
Assistant Professor
Harvard Medical School
Attending Orthopaedic Surgeon
Department of Orthopaedic Surgery
Division of Sports Medicine
Boston Children's Hospital
Boston, Massachusetts

Christine Ann Ho, MD
Associate Professor of Orthopaedic Surgery
Department of Orthopaedic Surgery
UT Southwestern Medical School
Texas Scottish Rite Hospital for Children
Dallas, Texas

Robert M. Kay, MD
Professor of Orthopaedic Surgery
Keck School of Medicine of USC
Vice Chief, Children's Orthopaedic Center
Children's Hospital Los Angeles
Los Angeles, California

Derek M. Kelly, MD
Pediatric Orthopaedic and Spinal Deformity Surgeon
Associate Professor Campbell Clinic
University of Tennessee College of Medicine
Department of Orthopaedic Surgery and Biomechanical
    Engineering
Le Bonheur Children's Hospital
Memphis, Tennessee

Young-Jo Kim, MD, PhD
Professor, Department of Orthopaedic Surgery
Harvard Medical School
Boston Children's Hospital
Boston, Massachusetts

Harry K. W. Kim, MD
Director, Research
Texas Scottish Rite Hospital for Children
Professor, Department of Orthopaedic Surgery
UT Southwestern Medical Center
Dallas, Texas

Mininder S. Kocher, MD, MPH
Professor of Orthopaedic Surgery
Harvard Medical School
Associate Director
Division of Sports Medicine
Boston Children's Hospital
Boston, Massachusetts

Scott H. Kozin, MD
Chief of Staff & Hand/Upper Extremity Surgeon
Clinical Professor of Orthopaedic Surgery
Lewis Katz School of Medicine at Temple University
Clinical Professor of Orthopaedic Surgery
Sidney Kimmel Medical College at Thomas Jefferson University
Philadelphia, Pennsylvania

Dennis E. Kramer, MD
Assistant Professor
Harvard Medical School
Department of Orthopaedic Surgery
Boston Children's Hospital
Boston, Massachusetts

Nina Lightdale-Miric, MD
Assistant Professor
Department of Orthopaedic Surgery
Keck School of Medicine
Director of Upper Extremity Program
Children's Hospital Los Angeles
Los Angeles, California

James J. McCarthy, MD
Alvin H. Crawford Chair in Pediatric Orthopaedics
Professor of Orthopaedic Surgery
University of Cincinnati College of Medicine
Division Director—Orthopaedics
Cincinnati Children's Hospital
Cincinnati, Ohio

Amy L. McIntosh, MD
Associate Professor of Orthopedic Surgery
UT Southwestern Medical School
Texas Scottish Rite Hospital for Children
Dallas, Texas

Charles T. Mehlman, DO, MPH
Professor of Pediatric Orthopaedic Surgery
Cincinnati Children's Hospital Medical Center
Cincinnati, Ohio

Todd Milbrandt, MD, MS
Orthopedic Surgeon
Department of Orthopaedics
Mayo Clinic
Rochester, Minnesota

James F. Mooney, MD
Chief of Staff
Shriners Hospital for Children
Springfield, Massachusetts

Blaise A. Nemeth, MD, MS
Associate Professor (CHS)
Department of Orthopaedics and Rehabilitation
American Family Children's Hospital
University of Wisconsin School of Medicine & Public Health
Madison, Wisconsin

Peter O. Newton, MD
Clinical Professor
Department of Orthopedic Surgery
UC San Diego School of Medicine
Chief of Orthopedic Surgery
Rady Children's Hospital San Diego
San Diego, California

Kenneth J. Noonan, MD
Associate Professor
Department of Orthopedics and Rehabilitation
University of Wisconsin School of Medicine & Public Health
Madison, Wisconsin

Karl E. Rathjen, MD
Professor
Department of Orthopaedic Surgery
UT Southwestern Medical Center
Texas Scottish Rite Hospital for Children
Director of Pediatric Orthopaedic Services Children's Health
Dallas, Texas

Julie Balch Samora, MD, PhD, MPH
Director of Quality Improvement
Department of Orthopaedics
Nationwide Children's Hospital
Clinical Associate Professor
The Ohio State University College of Medicine
Columbus, Ohio

Wudbhav N. Sankar, MD
Associate Professor of Orthopaedic Surgery
Division of Orthopaedics
Chidlren's Hospital of Philadelphia
Perelman School of Medicine at the University of
    Pennsylvania
Philadelphia, Pennsylvania

Jeffrey R. Sawyer, MD
Professor of Orthopaedic Surgery
University of Tennessee—Campbell Clinic and Campbell
    Foundation
Le Bonheur Children's Hospital
Memphis, Tennessee

Susan A. Scherl, MD
Professor, Pediatric Orthopaedic Surgery
UNMC College of Medicine
Children's Hospital and Medical Center Omaha
Omaha, Nebraska

Richard M. Schwend, MD
Professor Orthopaedics and Pediatrics
Division of Orthopaedics
Children's Mercy Hospital
Kansas City, Missouri

Apurva S. Shah, MD, MBA
Assistant Professor
Division of Orthopaedic Surgery
Perelman School of Medicine at the University of Pennsylvania
Children's Hospital of Philadelphia
Philadelphia, Pennsylvania

Kevin G. Shea, MD
Professor of Orthopaedic
Surgery, Department of Orthopaedic Surgery
Stanford School of Medicine
Director of Pediatric Sports Medicine
Lucile Packard Children's Hospital Stanford
Palo Alto, California

Benjamin J. Shore, MD, MPH, FRCSC
Assistant Professor
Department of Orthopedic Surgery
Harvard Medical School
Co-Director
Cerebral Palsy and Spasticity Center
Boston Children's Hospital
Boston, Massachusetts

David L. Skaggs, MD, MMM
Chief of Orthopaedic Surgery
Children's Endowed Chair of Spine Surgery
Children's Hospital Los Angeles
Professor of Orthopaedic Surgery
Keck School of Medicine
University of Southern California
Los Angeles, California

Brian G. Smith, MD
Director of Pediatric Orthopaedics
Professor, Resident Director
Department of Orthopaedics
Yale University School of Medicine
New Haven, Connecticut

Anthony Stans, MD
Surgeon in Chief
Mayo Clinic Children's Center
Department of Orthopaedic Surgery
Mayo Clinic
Rochester, Minnesota

Milan V. Stevanovic, MD
Professor of Orthopaedic Surgery
Keck School of Medicine of University of Southern California
Los Angeles, California

Vidyadhar V. Upasani, MD
Assistant Clinical Professor
Department of Orthopedic Surgery
UC San Diego School of Medicine
Rady Children's Hospital-San Diego
San Diego, California

Michael Vitale, MD, MPH
Ana Lucia Professor of Pediatric Orthopaedic Surgery
Columbia University Irving Medical Center
Co-Director
Division of Pediatric Orthopaedics
Morgan Stanley Children's Hospital of New York—
    Presbyterian Kids
New York City, New York

Carley Vuillermin, MBBS, MPH, FRACS
Instructor of Orthopaedics
Harvard Medical School
Department of Orthopaedic Surgery
Boston Children's Hospital
Boston, Massachusetts

Eric J. Wall, MD
Professor
Department of Orthopaedic Surgery
University of Cincinnati
Director
Orthopaedic Sports Medicine
Cincinnati Children's
Cincinnati, Ohio

William C. Warner, Jr., MD
Professor of Orthopaedics
University of Tennessee—Campbell Clinic and Campbell
    Foundation
Memphis, Tennessee

Peter M. Waters, MD
Orthopaedic Surgeon-in-Chief
Boston Children's Hospital
John E. Hall Professor of Orthopaedic Surgery
Harvard Medical School
Boston, Massachusetts

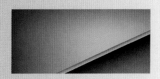

Preface

With all of the information that is now available to physicians, it can be difficult to know what sources to trust. By asking top thought leaders in pediatric orthopedics to critically evaluate the medical literature, we hope the ninth edition of *Rockwood and Wilkins' Fractures in Children* eliminates this problem for our readers. In each chapter, subject matter experts offer their overviews and analyses of existing clinical research and provide the very best evidence-based recommendations possible. The "author's preferred method" at the end of each chapter serves as a concise and practical algorithm for treating children.

We've added a number of new features for the ninth edition, including checklists for preoperative planning and key surgical steps, tables of potential pitfalls and preventative measures, and short lists of key annotated references. We've retained the author's preferred treatment section, which has been popular since its introduction a few editions ago.

This ninth edition also inaugurates a new partnership with the Orthopaedic Trauma Association (OTA). The ninth edition is the official publication of the OTA, and is a foundational component in *OTAOnline*, an electronic knowledge portal that brings together *Rockwood, Green, and Wilkins Fractures in Adults and Children, Journal of Orthopaedic Trauma*, an extensive orthopaedic trauma video library, OTA International (an open access journal), and routine updates.

This project has been a labor of love for its editors. Our collaboration on the ninth edition has both satisfied our never-ending drive to improve patient care and strengthened our already close friendship. We hope our work will be of service to you, the reader, and your young patients whose lives you strive to make better.

Peter M. Waters, MD
David L. Skaggs, MD, MMM
John M. (Jack) Flynn, MD

Contents

Epidemiology of Fractures in Children

Brian K. Brighton and Michael Vitale

INTRODUCTION

Epidemiology is defined as the study of the distribution and determinants of health and disease and the application of this science to the control of diseases and other health problems. As such, epidemiology is the cornerstone of an evidence-based approach to preventing disease and to optimizing treatment strategies. Various epidemiologic methods including surveillance and descriptive studies can be used to investigate the distribution of frequency, pattern, and burden of disease whereas analytical methods can be used to study the determinants of disease. An understanding of the epidemiology of pediatric trauma is a prerequisite for the timely evolution of optimal care strategies, and for the development of effective prevention strategies.

Injuries in children and adolescents represent a major public health challenge facing pediatric patients, families, and health care providers worldwide. Given the wide-reaching impact that pediatric musculoskeletal injury has on public health, an understanding of the epidemiology of pediatric fractures provides an opportunity to maximize efforts aimed at prevention and optimal treatment. Unintentional injuries are the leading cause of death for children in the United States. In 2015, the Centers for Disease Control and Prevention (CDC) reported over 10,000 deaths of children between the ages of 0 and 18 years caused by unintentional injuries (http://webappa.cdc.gov/sasweb/ncipc/mortrate.html). However, fatalities only represent a small portion

1

of the impact unintentional injuries have on children. There were over 7.5 million nonfatal unintentional injuries to children of the same age group in 2015 (http://webappa.cdc.gov/sasweb/ncipc/nfirates.html). Pediatric trauma often results in temporary activity limitation, hospitalization, and sometimes in permanent disability.[1,40] The Center of Disease Control's Web-based Injury Statistics Query and Reporting System (CDC WISQARS™) estimates that nonfatal injuries requiring medical attention affected more than 8.5 million children and adolescents and resulted in $24 billion in medical care and work loss costs (https://wisqars.cdc.gov:8443/costT/). As the leading cause of death and disability in children, pediatric trauma presents one of the largest challenges to the health of children, as well as an important opportunity for positive impact.

INCIDENCE OF FRACTURES IN CHILDREN

"CLASSIFICATION BIAS": DIFFICULTIES DEFINING DISEASE

Descriptive epidemiologic studies demand consistent information about how we define and classify a given disease state. This is a challenge in pediatric trauma, making it difficult to compare studies. An international study group has developed and performed early validation of a standardized classification system of pediatric fractures.[96–99] The authors of an agreement study found that with appropriate training, the AO Pediatric Comprehensive Classification of Long Bone Fractures (PCCF) system could be used by experienced surgeons as a reliable classification system for pediatric fractures for future prospective studies (Fig. 1-1).[96,99] In addition, follow-up studies have provided useful epidemiologic reporting of pediatric long-bone fractures using the AO PCCF.[5,33–35]

The incidence of pediatric fractures differs among published series because of geographical, environmental, gender,

and age differences. Early studies on the incidence of fractures in children formed a knowledge base about fracture healing in children. Landin's 1983 report on 8,682 fractures remains a landmark study on the incidence of fractures in children.[45] He reviewed the data on all fractures in children that occurred in Malmö, Sweden, over 30 years and examined the factors affecting the incidence of children's fractures. By studying two populations, 30 years apart, he determined that fracture patterns were changing and suggested reasons for such changes. His initial goal was to establish data for preventive programs, so he focused on fractures that produced clean, concise, concrete data. Lempesis provided the most recent update from Malmö, Sweden over the years 2005 to 2006 and noted the previously reported declines in overall fracture rate remained unchanged and may have been related to a change in the region's demographics. There was however a decrease in incidence among girls. The pediatric fracture incidence during the period 2005 to 2006 was 1,832 per 10,000 person-years (2,359 in boys and 1,276 in girls), with an age-adjusted boy-to-girl ratio of 1.8 (1.6% to 2.1%).[48]

More recently, studies on the incidence of fractures in Edinburgh, Scotland in 2000, as reviewed by Rennie et al.,[84] was 20.2 per 1,000 children annually. A similar fracture incidence of 201/10,000 among children and adolescents was reported in northern Sweden between 1993 and 2007 with a 13% increase during the years between 1998 and 2007. The authors also reported the accumulated risk of sustaining a fracture before the age of 17 being 34%.[29] In Landin's series from Malmö, Sweden, the chance of a child sustaining a fracture during childhood (birth to age 16) was 42% for boys and 27% for girls.[45] When considered on an annual basis, 2.1% of all the children (2.6% for boys; 1.7% for girls) sustained at least one fracture each year. These figures were for all fracture types and included those treated on an inpatient basis and an outpatient basis. The overall chance of fracture per year was 1.6% for both girls and boys in a study from England of both outpatients and inpatients by Worlock and Stower.[114] The chance of a child sustaining a fracture severe enough to require inpatient treatment during the first 16 years of life is 6.8%.[10] Thus, on an annual basis, 0.43% of the children in an average community will be admitted for a fracture-related problem during the year. The overall incidence and lifetime risk of children's fractures are summarized in Table 1-1.

Early reports of children's fractures grouped the areas fractured together, and fractures were reported only as to the long bone involved (e.g., radius, humerus, femur). More recent reports have split fractures into the more specific areas of the long bone involved (e.g., the distal radius or the distal humerus). In children, fractures in the upper extremity are much more

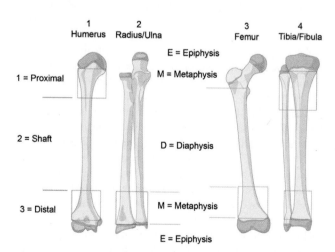

Figure 1-1. The AO PCCF for fracture classification with bone, segment, and subsegment nomenclature. (From Slongo TF, Audige L. Fracture and dislocation classification compendium for children: the AO Pediatric Comprehensive Classification of Long Bone Fractures (PCCF). *J Orthop Trauma.* 2007;21(10 Suppl):S135–S160.)

TABLE 1-1. Overall Frequency of Fractures[16,30,36,46,57,68]

Percentage of children sustaining at least one fracture from 0–16 yrs of age:

    Boys, 42–60%

    Girls, 27–40%

Percentage of children sustaining a fracture in 1 yr: 1.6–2.1%

Annual rate of fracture in childhood: 12–36/1,000 persons

TABLE 1-2. Incidence of Fractures in Long Bones	
Bone	%
Radius/ulna	59
Humerus	21
Tibia/fibula	15
Femur	5

From Joeris A, Lutz N, Wicki B, et al. An epidemiological evaluation of pediatric long bone fractures: a retrospective cohort study of 2716 patients from two Swiss tertiary pediatric hospitals. *BMC Pediatr.* 2014;14:314 © Joeris et al; licensee BioMed Central. 2014.

common than those in the lower extremity.[115] Overall, the radius is the most commonly fractured long bone, followed by the humerus. In the lower extremity, the tibia is more commonly fractured than the femur (Table 1-2).[35]

The individual reports agree that the most common area fractured in children is the distal radius. The next most common area involves the hand (phalanges and metacarpals), clavicle and distal humerus.[46,71,83,84]

Physeal Fractures

The incidence of physeal injuries overall varied from 14.8% to as high as 30% in the literature across various series.[37,60,63,77,84,106]

Open Fractures

The overall reported incidence of open fractures in children has changed over time ranging 1.5% to 2.6% in older series[10,60,114] to 0.7% to 1% in recent reports.[35,84] Regional trauma centers often see patients exposed to more severe trauma, so there may be a higher incidence of open fractures in these patients. The incidence of open fractures was 9% in a report of patients admitted to an urban trauma center.[7]

Despite the importance of understanding the epidemiology of pediatric fractures, there are still significant gaps in our knowledge base, and there is much work to be done. There are several challenges to gathering appropriate data in this area: risk factors for pediatric injury are diverse and heterogeneous, practice patterns vary across countries and even within countries, and the available infrastructure to support data collection for pediatric trauma is far from ideal.

PATIENT FACTORS THAT INFLUENCE FRACTURE INCIDENCE AND FRACTURE PATTERNS

Age

Fracture incidence in children increases with age. Age-specific fracture patterns and locations are influenced by many factors including age-dependent activities and changing intrinsic bone properties. Starting with birth and extending to age 12, all the major series that segregated patients by age have demonstrated a linear increase in the annual incidence of fractures with age (Fig. 1-2). The peak age for fracture occurrence in girls is age 11 to 12 and for boys it is age 13 to 14.[16,28,36,83,84]

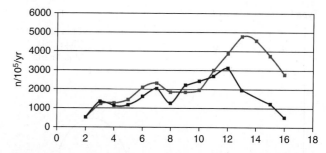

Figure 1-2. Incidence of fractures by age. Boys (*blue*) peak at 13 years whereas girls (*red*) peak earlier, at 12 years, and then decline. (Reprinted from Rennie L, Court-Brown CM, Mok JY, et al. The epidemiology of fractures in children. *Injury.* 2007;38(8):913–922. Copyright © 2007 Elsevier Ltd. With permission.)

Although there is a high incidence of injuries in children of ages 1 to 2, the incidence of fractures is low with most fractures being related to accidental or nonaccidental trauma from others.[14,42] The anatomic areas most often fractured seem to be the same in the major series, but these rates change with age. Rennie et al.[84] demonstrated in their 2000 study from Edinburgh that the incidence of fractures increased and fracture patterns changed as children aged. Fracture incidence curves for each of the most common fractures separated by gender were shown on six basic incidence curves similar to Landin's initial work (Fig. 1-3).[45] When Landin compared these variability patterns with the common etiologies, he found some correlation. For example, late-peak fractures (distal forearm, phalanges, proximal humerus) were closely correlated with sports and equipment etiologies. Bimodal pattern fractures (clavicle, femur, radioulnar, diaphyses) showed an early increase from lower-energy trauma, then a late peak in incidence caused by injury from high- or moderate-energy trauma likely caused by motor vehicle accidents (MVAs), recreational activities, and contact sports in the adolescent population. Early-peak fractures (supracondylar humeral fractures are a classic example) were mainly caused by falls from high levels.

Gender

Gender differences can be seen across the incidence of injures, location of injuries, and etiology of injuries across all age groups. For all age groups, the overall ratio across a number of series of boys to girls which sustains a single fracture is about 1.5:1.[16,29,30,36,46,84]

In some areas, there is little difference in the incidence of fractures between boys and girls. For example, during the first 2 years of life, the overall incidence of injuries and fractures in both genders is nearly equal. During these first 2 years, the injury rates for foreign-body ingestion, poisons, and burns have no significant gender differences. With activities in which there is a male difference in participation, such as with sports equipment and bicycles, there is a marked increase in the incidence of injuries in boys.[9,85] The injury incidence may not be caused by the rate of exposure alone; behavior may be a major factor.[107] For example, one study found that the incidence of auto/pedestrian childhood injuries peaks in both sexes at ages 5 to 8.[86] When the total number of street crossings per day was studied, both sexes did so equally. Despite this equal exposure, boys had a higher number of

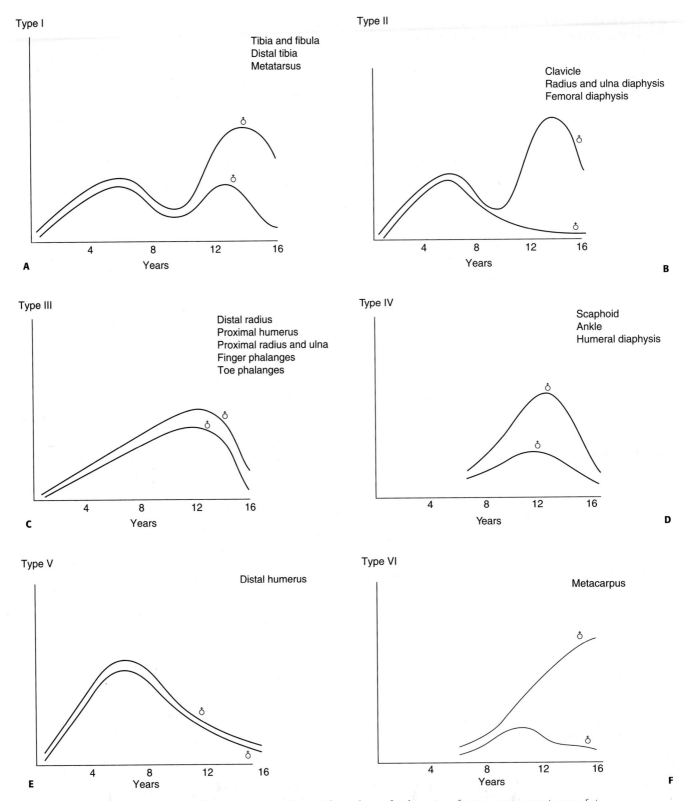

Figure 1-3. Variations of fracture patterns with age. The peak ages for the various fracture types occur in one of six patterns. (Reprinted from Rennie L, Court-Brown CM, Mok JY, et al. The epidemiology of fractures in children. *Injury.* 2007;38(8):913–922. Copyright © 2007 Elsevier Ltd. With permission.)

injuries. Thus, the difference in the rate between the sexes begins to develop a male predominance when behaviors change.

Socioeconomic and Cultural Differences

The incidence of pediatric fracture varies in different geographic settings, socioeconomic climates, and differing ethnicities. Two studies from the United Kingdom looked at the relationship of affluence to the incidence of fractures in children and had differing conclusions. Lyons et al.[56] found no difference in the fracture rates of children in affluent population groups compared to those of children in nonaffluent families. On the other hand, Stark et al.[103] in Scotland found that the fracture rates in children from nonaffluent social groups were significantly higher than those in affluent families. There are also contradictory results in the literature with regard to fracture risk associated with living urban versus rural settings.[21,30] In the United States, the increased rate of pediatric femur fractures was influenced by adverse socioeconomic and sociodemographic fractures.[32] Wren et al.[115] in a large prospective cohort studied the association of race and ethnicity as a risk factor for fracture in children and adolescents. They found that fracture rates were higher, regardless of sex, for white children compared with all other racial and ethnic groups.

Clinical Factors

In recent years there has been an attention to a number of clinically related factors in determining children's fractures, such as obesity, low bone mineral density (BMD), and low calcium and vitamin D intake. Obesity is an increasing health problem in children and adolescents representing a complex interaction of host factors, and is the most prevalent nutritional problem for children in the United States. In a retrospective chart review, Taylor et al.[105] noted that overweight children had a higher-reported incidence of fractures and musculoskeletal complaints. Although Leonard et al.[50] found increased BMD in obese adolescents, the lack of physical activity often seen in obesity may in fact lead to reduced muscle mass, strength, and coordination resulted in impaired proprioception, balance and increased risk of falling and fracture. In a recent study, Valerio et al.[108] confirmed a greater prevalence of overweight/obesity in children and adolescents with a recent fracture when compared to age- and gender-matched fracture-free children, and found obesity rate was increased in girls with upper limb fractures and girls and boys with lower limb fractures.

Low BMD and decreased bone mass are linked to increased fracture risk in the adult population; however, in children, the relationship is less clear with a meta-analysis showing some association between fracture risk and low BMD.[13] In 2006, Clark examined in a prospective fashion the association between bone mass and fracture risk in childhood. Over 6,000 children at 9.9 years of age were followed-up for 2 years and the study showed an 89% increased risk of fracture per standard deviation (SD) decrease in size-adjusted BMD.[11] In a follow-up study of this same cohort, the risk of fracture following slight or moderate to severe trauma was inversely related to bone size relative to body size perhaps reflecting the determinants of volumetric BMD such as cortical thickness on skeletal fragility.[12]

Nutritional factors may also play a role in the incidence of fractures in children.

THE IMPACT OF ENVIRONMENTAL FACTORS ON FRACTURES IN CHILDREN

Seasonal and Climatic Differences

Fractures are more common during the summer, when children are out of school and exposed to more vigorous physical activities. An analysis of seasonal variation in many studies shows an increase in fractures in the warmer months of the year.[9,10,29,45,83,84,95,111,114]

Children in colder climates, with ice and snow, are exposed to risks different from those of children living in warmer climates. The exposure time to outdoor activities may be greater for children who live in dry and warm weather climates.[94] The most consistent climatic factor appears to be the number of hours of sunshine. Masterson et al.,[61] in a study from Ireland, found a strong positive correlation between monthly sunshine hours and monthly fracture admissions. There was also a weak negative correlation with monthly rainfall. Overall, the average number of fractures in the summer was 2.5 times than that in the winter. In days with more sunshine hours than average, the average fracture admission rate was 2.31/day; on days with fewer sunshine hours than average, the admission rate was 1.07/day. Pediatric trauma should be viewed as a disease where there are direct and predictable relationships between exposure and incidence.

Time of Day

The time of day in which children are most active seems to correlate with the peak time for fracture occurrence. Seasonal variation and geographic location seem to play a role as to which time during the day injury occurs (Fig. 1-4).[61] In a Swedish study, the incidence peaked between 2 PM and 3 PM,[83] whereas in a study out of Texas by Shank et al.,[73] the hourly incidence of fractures formed a well-defined bell curve peaking at about 6 PM.

Home Environment

Fractures sustained in the home environment are defined as those that occur in the house and surrounding vicinity. These generally occur in a fairly supervised environment and are mainly caused by falls from furniture, stairs, fences, and trees as well as from injuries sustained from recreational equipment (trampolines and home jungle gyms). Falls can vary in severity from a simple fall while running, to a fall of great magnitude, such as from a third story window. In falling from heights, adults often land on their lower extremities, accounting for the high number of lower-extremity fractures, especially the calcaneus. Children tend to fall head first, using the upper extremities to break the fall. This accounts for the larger number of skull and radial fractures in children. Femoral fractures also are common in children falling from great heights. In contrast to adults, spinal fractures are rare in children who fall from great heights.[90] In one study, children falling three stories or less all survived. Falls from the fifth or sixth floor resulted in a 50% mortality rate.[6,62,93,102]

Interestingly, a Swedish study showed that an increased incidence of fractures in a home environment did not necessarily correlate with the physical attributes or poor safety precautions of the house.[6] Rather, it appears that a disruption of the family

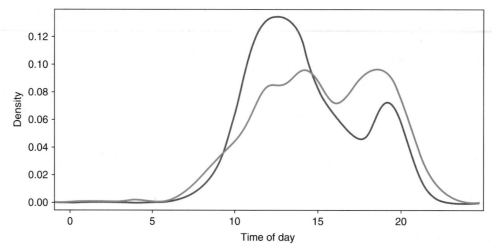

Figure 1-4. Distribution of fractures during time of day by summertime (*green*) and wintertime (*blue*). Density estimates are computed using kernel-smoothing method with normal kernel function and suitable bandwidth. The *x* axis represents the hours in 5-hour intervals throughout the day (i.e., *0*, midnight; *5*, 5 AM; *10*, 10 AM; *15*, 3 PM; and *20*, 8 PM), and the *y* axis represents the probability density that a fracture would occur at any given time of day. (Redrawn from Randsborg PH, Gulbrandsen P, Saltyte Benth J, et al. Fractures in children: epidemiology and activity-specific fracture rates. *J Bone Joint Surg Am.* 2013;95A:e42.)

structure and presence of social handicaps (alcoholism, welfare recipients, etc.) are important risk factors for pediatric fracture.

School Environment

The supervised environments at school are generally safe, and the overall annual rate of injury (total percentage of children injured in a single year) in the school environment ranges from 2.8% to 16.5%.[73] Most injuries occur as a result of use of playground or recreational equipment or participation in athletic activity. True rates may be higher because of inaccurate reporting, especially of mild injuries. The annual fracture rate of school injuries is thought to be low. Of all injuries sustained by children at school in a year, only 5% to 10% involved fractures.[52] In Worlock and Stower's series of children's fractures from England,[24,49,91] only 20% occurred at school. Most injuries (53%) occurring in school are related to athletics and sporting events,[114] and injuries are highest in the middle school children, with one study citing a 20% fracture rate in school-aged children of those injured during physical education class.[49]

ETIOLOGY OF FRACTURES IN CHILDREN

THREE BROAD CAUSES

Broadly, fractures have three main causes: accidental trauma, nonaccidental trauma (child abuse), and pathologic conditions. Accidental trauma forms the largest etiologic group and can occur in a variety of settings, some often overlapping others. Nonaccidental trauma and fractures resulting from pathologic conditions are discussed in later chapters of this book.

SPORTS-RELATED ACTIVITIES

The last two decades have seen an increase in youth participation in organized athletic participation, especially among younger children. Wood et al. studied at the annual incidence of sports-related fractures in children 10 to 19 years presenting to hospitals in Edinburgh. The overall incidence was 5.63/1,000/yr with males accounting for 87% of fractures. Soccer, rugby, and skiing were responsible for nearly two-thirds of the fractures among the 30 sporting activities that adolescents participated in. Upper-extremity fractures were by far the most common injury accounting for 84% of all fractures with most being low-energy injuries and few requiring operative intervention.[74] A retrospective study over a 16-year time period from an emergency department at a level 1 trauma center in the Netherlands examined risk factors for upper-extremity injury in sports-related activities. Most injuries occurred while playing soccer and upper-extremity injuries were most common. Risk factors for injury were young age and playing individual sports, no-contact sports, or no-ball sports. Women were at risk in speed skating, in-line skating, and basketball, whereas men mostly were injured during skiing and snowboarding.[113]

In the United States, football- and basketball-related injuries are common complaints presenting to pediatric emergency departments, with fractures occurring more frequently in football.[22] In a 5-year survey of the NEISS National Electronic Injury Surveillance System (NEISS)-All Injury Program, injury rates ranged from 6.1 to 11 per 1,000 participants/year as age increased, with fractures and dislocations accounting for nearly 30% of all injuries receiving emergency room evaluation.[64]

Recreational Activities and Devices

In addition to increasing participation in sports, new activities and devices[65] have emerged that expose children to increased fracture risk. Traditional activities such as skateboarding, roller skating, alpine sports, and bicycling have taken on a new look in the era of extreme sports where such activities now involve high speeds and stunts. Many of these activities have safety equipment available but that does not assure compliance.

Organizations such as the American Academy of Pediatrics and the American Academy of Orthopaedic Surgeons (AAOS) have issued position statements regarding the proper use and supervision of such devices, but it remains within the duty of the physician to educate and reinforce to patients and families to promote safety around these activities.[54]

Playground Equipment

Play is an essential element of a child's life. It enhances physical development and fosters social interaction. Unfortunately, unsupervised or careless use of some play equipment can endanger life and limb.[44] When Mott et al.[66] studied the incidence and pattern of injuries to children using public playgrounds, they found that approximately 1% of children using playgrounds sustained injuries. Swings, climbers, and slides are the pieces of playground equipment associated with 88% of the playground injuries.[58]

In a study of injuries resulting from playground equipment, Waltzman et al.[110] found that most injuries occurred in boys (56%) with a peak incidence in the summer months. Fractures accounted for 61% of these injuries, 90% of which involved the upper extremity and were sustained in falls from playground equipment such as monkey bars and climbing frames. Younger children (1 to 4 years old) were more likely to sustain fractures than older children.

Lillis and Jaffe[51] made similar observations in a study in which upper-extremity injuries, especially fractures, accounted for most of hospitalizations resulting from injuries on playground equipment. Older children sustained more injuries on climbing apparatus, whereas younger children sustained more injuries on slides.

Loder[53] used the NEISS dataset to explore the demographics of playground equipment injuries in children. Monkey bars were the most common cause of fractures. In another study looking specifically at injuries from monkey bars, the peak age group was the 5- to 12-year-old group, with supracondylar humeral fractures being the most common fracture sustained.[59]

The correlation of the hardness of the playground surface with the risk of injury has been confirmed in numerous studies.[43,53,67,69] Changing playground surfaces from concrete to more impact-absorbing surfaces such as bark reduced the incidence and severity of head injury but increased the tendency for long-bone fractures (40%), bruises, and sprains.

Public playgrounds appear to have a higher risk for injuries than private playgrounds because they usually have harder surfaces and higher pieces of equipment,[78] although playground injury was most likely to occur at school compared to home, public, and other locations.[79]

Bicycle Injuries

Bicycle injuries are a significant cause of mortality and morbidity for children.[82] Bicycle mishaps are the most common causes of serious head injury in children.[112] Boys in the 5- to 14-year age group are at greatest risk for bicycle injury (80%). Puranik et al.[82] studied the profile of pediatric bicycle injuries in a sample of 211 children who were treated for bicycle-related injury at their trauma center over a 4-year period. They found that bicycle injuries accounted for 18% of all pediatric trauma patients. Bicycle/motor vehicle collisions caused 86%

of injuries. Sixty-seven percent had head injuries and 29% sustained fractures. More than half of the incidents occurred on the weekend. Sixteen percent were injured by ejection from a bicycle after losing control, hitting a pothole, or colliding with a fixed object or another bicycle. Fractures mainly involved the lower extremity, upper extremity, skull, ribs, and pelvis in decreasing order of incidence. Over the last decade, youth participation in mountain biking has seen an increase and with that so has the number of injuries related to mountain biking increased with many caused by unpredictable terrain and falls as one rides downhill.[2,3] As public awareness of both the severity and preventability of bicycle-related injuries grows, the goal of safer bicycling practices and lower injury rates can be achieved.[82]

Skateboarding

Skateboarding and in-line skating have experienced a renewed surge in popularity over the past three decades. With the increasing number of participants, high-tech equipment development, and vigorous advertising, skateboard and skating injuries are expected to increase. Since the late 1990s, there has been an increase in the number of skateboard injuries.[41] Because the nature of skateboarding encompasses both high speed and extreme maneuvers, high-energy fractures and other injuries can occur, as highlighted by several published reports.[25,75,80] Studies have shown that skateboarding-related injuries are more severe and have more serious consequences than roller skating or in-line skating injuries.[75] In a study of skateboarding injuries, Fountain et al.[25] found that fractures of the upper or lower extremity accounted for 50% of all skateboarding injuries. Interestingly, more than one-third of those injured sustained injuries within the first week of skateboarding. Most injuries occurred in preadolescent boys (75%) from 10 to 16 years of age; 65% sustained injuries on public roads, footpaths, and parking lots. In a study over a 5-year period of time using data from the National Trauma Data Bank, skateboarding injuries were associated with a higher incidence of closed-head injuries and long-bone fractures with children under age 10 more likely to sustain a femur fracture.[55] Several authors[25] have recommended safety guidelines and precautions such as use of helmets, knee and elbow pads, and wrist guards, but such regulations seldom are enforced.

Trampolines

Trampolines enjoyed increasing popularity in the 1990s and are a significant cause of morbidity in children. Several studies have noted a dramatic increase in the number of pediatric trampoline injuries during the past 10 years, rightfully deeming it as a "national epidemic."[26,100] Using the NEISS data, Smith[100] estimated that there are roughly 40,000 pediatric trampoline injuries per year. Younger children had a higher incidence of upper-extremity fractures and other injuries. Furnival et al.,[26] in a retrospective study over a 7-year period, found that the annual number of pediatric trampoline injuries tripled between 1990 and 1997. In contrast to other recreational activities in which boys constitute the population at risk, patients with pediatric trampoline injuries were predominantly girls, with a median age of 7 years. Nearly a third of the injuries resulted from falling off the trampoline. Fractures of the upper and lower extremities occurred in 45% and were more frequently associated with falls off the trampoline. In a later study, Sandler et al.[87] reported injuries requiring surgery in over 60% of patients with 20% requiring operative fixation for upper-extremity fractures. These researchers, along with others,[26] rightly concluded that use of warning labels, public education, and even direct adult supervision were inadequate in preventing these injuries and have called for a total ban on the recreational, school, and competitive use of trampolines by children.[20,26,87,100,101]

Motor Vehicle Accidents

This category includes injuries sustained by occupants of a motor vehicle and victims of vehicle–pedestrian accidents.

The injury patterns of children involved in MVAs differ from those of adults. In all types of MVAs for all ages, children constitute a little over 10% of the total number of patients injured.[45,89] Of all the persons injured as motor vehicle occupants, only about 17% to 18% are children. Of the victims of vehicle-versus-pedestrian accidents, about 29% are children. Of the total number of children involved in MVAs, 56.4% were vehicle–pedestrian accidents, and 19.6% were vehicle–bicycle accidents.[23]

The fracture rate of children in MVAs is less than that of adults. Of the total number of vehicle–pedestrian accidents, about 22% of the children sustained fractures; 40% of the adults sustained fractures in the same type of accident. This has been attributed to the fact that children are more likely to "bounce" when hit.[23]

Children are twice as likely as adults to sustain a femoral fracture when struck by an automobile; in adults, tibial and knee injuries are more common in the same type of accident. This seems to be related to where the car's bumper strikes the victim.[7,8] MVAs also produce a high proportion of spinal and pelvic injuries.[7]

All-Terrain Vehicles

Recreational all-terrain vehicles (ATVs) have emerged as a new cause of serious pediatric injury. Despite product training and safety education campaigns, ATV accidents continue to cause significant morbidity and mortality in children and adolescents.[28,31,38,39,88,92] In contrast to other etiologies of injury, children who sustained ATV-related fractures had more severe injuries and a higher percentage of significant head trauma, with 1% of these injuries resulting in inhospital death. These statistics point to the failure of voluntary safety efforts to date and argue for much stronger regulatory control.

In a review of 96 children who sustained injuries in ATV-related accidents during a 30-month period, Kellum et al.[38] noted age-related patterns of injury. Younger children (≤12 years) were more likely to sustain an isolated fracture and were more likely to sustain a lower-extremity fracture, specifically a femoral fracture, than older children. Older children were more likely to sustain a pelvic fracture. In a recent review of the Kids' Inpatient Database, Sawyer et al.[88] found that despite the known risks associated with ATV use in children, their use and injury rate continue to increase. The injury rate for children from ATV accidents has increased 240% since 1997, whereas the spinal injury rate has increased 476% over the same time frame. The authors found that injuries to the spinal column occurred in 7.4% of patients with the most common level of fracture was thoracic (39%), followed by lumbar (29%) and cervical (16%). Pelvic fractures were the most common associated fractures, accounting for 44% of all musculoskeletal injuries, followed by forearm/wrist fractures (15%) and femoral fractures (9%). Despite educational and legislative efforts, children account for a disproportionate percentage of morbidity and mortality from ATV-related accidents. The sport of motocross has also been shown to have a high rate of musculoskeletal injuries requiring hospitalization in children.[47]

The etiologic aspects of children's fractures are summarized in Figure 1-5.

Gunshot and Firearm Injuries

Gunshot or missile wounds arise from objects projected into space by an explosive device. Gunshot wounds have become increasingly common in children in the United States. In a reflection of the changing times and pervasive gun culture, firearms are determined to be second only to motor vehicles as the

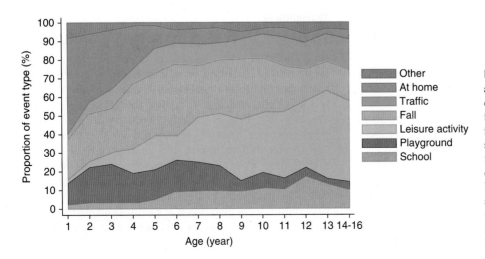

Figure 1-5. Accident types correlated to age. There is a predominance of fractures due to accidents at home throughout the first 4 years of life, whereas leisure activities become the leading cause during school-age and adolescence. (Redrawn from Joeris A, Lutz N, Wicki B, et al. An epidemiological evaluation of pediatric long bone fractures: a retrospective cohort study of 2716 patients from two Swiss tertiary pediatric hospitals. *BMC Pediatr.* 2014;14:314. © Joeris et al.; licensee BioMed Central. 2014.)

leading cause of death in youths. In considering the prevalence of firearms in the United States, it has been estimated that there are about 200 million privately owned guns in the United States and that approximately 40% of US households contain firearms of some type.[17]

Two recent epidemiologic reports from pediatric trauma centers, orthopedic injuries related to firearms, demonstrated varying rates of complications and need for operative intervention (35% and 54%) in gunshot wound–related injuries and complications.[72,76] Perkins et al.[76] found that in 46 patients with 50 injuries, gunshot-related fractures had an increased incidence of permanent neurologic deficits, infection (11%), and fracture non-union rates (9%).

The two most common complications associated with firearm-related injuries are growth arrest and infection. Other complications included delayed union and malunion. The treatment of fractures associated with gunshot wounds in children is never simple. Bone defects, associated peripheral nerve injuries, and involvement of the joint can negatively influence outcomes.[4]

Firearm-related injury and safety have received much attention nationally and internationally in the wake of the events over the last decade. Rather than modifying behavioral or environmental issues, which are more complex, strategies to reduce firearm-related injuries and deaths among the youth include reducing the number of guns in the environment through restrictive legislation, gun buy-back programs, gun taxes, physician counseling, and modifying the design of guns to make them more childproof and prevent unauthorized and unintended use.

EVOLVING EPIDEMIOLOGY OF FRACTURES IN CHILDREN

PREVENTIVE PROGRAMS

While studying the epidemiology of fractures, it is important to focus on the etiology of fractures and the settings in which they occur. Fractures do not occur in a vacuum, and well-researched studies that analyze the physical and social environment in which they occur are extremely valuable. Efforts can be made toward creating a safer environment for play and recreation. It is hoped that by targeting these areas, programs can be designed to decrease the risk factors.

NATIONAL CAMPAIGNS

Several national organizations have developed safety programs. The foremost is the American Academy of Pediatrics, which has committees on injury and poison prevention and sports medicine and fitness that has produced guidelines for athletics,[15] playgrounds, trampolines,[20] ATVs,[18] and skateboards.[19] The AAOS has also produced a program designed to decrease the incidence of playground injuries. These programs offer background data and guidelines for various activities, but their effectiveness has not been fully studied. In addition, the AAOS, the Orthopaedic Trauma Association (OTA), and Pediatric Orthopaedic Society of North America (POSNA) have issued updated position statements regarding the safe use of ATVs, trampolines, skateboards, and in-line skating.

EXPANDED OPPORTUNITIES TO EXAMINE THE EPIDEMIOLOGY OF PEDIATRIC TRAUMA

Several sources of administrative, national, and regional data have recently become available, providing significantly improved investigation into various areas within pediatric trauma. The Healthcare Cost and Utilization Project (HCUP) is a family of databases including the State Inpatient Databases (SID), the Nationwide Inpatient Sample (NIS), and the KID. Although administrative data may lack clinical detail for certain purposes, these datasets provide a comprehensive overview of health care utilization in the United States and are available without purchase (http://www.ahrq.gov/research/data/hcup/index.html).[104] The KID database has been increasingly used to examine the incidence of pediatric trauma as well as practice patterns in pediatric trauma. Data for KIDS are collected and published every 3 years. In 2011 study, using the 2006 HCUP KID dataset, Gao[27] reported on lower-extremity fractures requiring hospitalization and found there were about 11,500 admission records for children aged 0 to 20 with lower-extremity fractures. Urban hospitalizations accounted for 93% of cases and 66% of admissions were to teaching hospitals in Gao's study. There was an increased mortality risk among patients cared for in nonteaching hospitals and hospitals located in a rural region. An additional study using this dataset, Nakaniida et al.[70] found femur and humerus fractures as the most common injuries requiring hospitalization, with pelvic and vertebral fractures largely due to MVAs representing the most costly injuries.

Trauma registries are another source for injury data that document clinical and demographic information regarding acute care delivered to hospitalized patients with injuries at trauma centers. These databases are designed to provide information that can be used to study the effectiveness and quality of trauma care, collect information on rare injuries,[81,109] and identify areas for quality improvement. Although the amount of information available through regional and national databases allowed is immense, the creation and maintenance of these registries require a significant amount of time and financial resources. Several limitations of these databases include the focus on adult over pediatric injuries and the data that do not always reflect population-based samples. Currently, the American College of Surgeons National Trauma Data Bank serves as the largest database, producing annual reports on pediatric injury from trauma centers from the United States and Canada (http://www.ntdb.org). In the future, databases such as these may provide the infrastructure needed to study pediatric musculoskeletal trauma care.

ACKNOWLEDGMENT

With appreciation to Kaye Wilkins for work on previous editions of this chapter.

Annotated References

Reference	Annotation
Clark EM, Ness AR, Bishop NJ, et al. Association between bone mass and fractures in children: a prospective cohort study. *J Bone Miner Res.* 2006;21:1489–1495.	The largest prospective study on bone mass in nearly 6,000 children demonstrated low bone density as a risk factor for fractures in children.
Garay M, Hess J, Armstrong D, et al. Pediatric ATV injuries in a statewide sample: 2004 to 2014. *Pediatrics.* 2017;140(2).	Data over an 11-year period from a statewide trauma database was reviewed to report the incidence of ATV-related injuries, mortality rates, as well as associated fracture patterns.
Hedstrom EM, Waernbaum I. Incidence of fractures among children and adolescents in rural and urban communities: analysis based on 9,965 fracture events. *Inj Epidemiol.* 2014;1:14.	In a study of nearly 10,000 fracture events in children, known risk factors of age and sex were predictive of fracture incidence. The authors also found a lower rate of fractures in rural and less densely populated municipalities.
Joeris A, Lutz N, Wicki B, et al. An epidemiological evaluation of pediatric long bone fractures: a retrospective cohort study of 2716 patients from two Swiss tertiary pediatric hospitals. *BMC Pediatr.* 2014;14:314.	Using the AO Pediatric Comprehensive Classification of Long Bone Fractures (PCCF) the morphologic patterns of over 2,700 upper- and lower-extremity fractures are presented along with age, sex, and injury data.
Lempesis V, Rosengren BE, Nilsson JA, et al. Time trends in pediatric fracture incidence in Sweden during the period 1950–2006. *Acta Orthop.* 2017;88:440–445.	Epidemiologic studies on pediatric fractures have been ongoing in the Swedish city of Malmö since 1950. This most recent report describes the fracture epidemiology including etiology comparing this to historical data and describes changes in age- and sex-adjusted pediatric fracture incidences to identify time trends independent of changing population demographics.
Monteilh C, Patel P, Gaffney J. Musculoskeletal injuries associated with hoverboard use in children. *Clin Pediatr (Phila).* 2017;56:909–911.	Hoverboards, which are self-balancing, elevated motorized scooters, have recently been introduced as recreational devices to children and adolescents. This early report describes the increase in fractures especially of the upper extremity with falls associated with this device.
Naranje SM, Gilbert SR, Stewart MG, et al. Gunshot-associated fractures in children and adolescents treated at two level 1 pediatric trauma centers. *J Pediatr Orthop.* 2016;36:1–5.	A recent retrospective review from two trauma centers reports on 49 patients with 58 gunshot-associated fractures in the pediatric population. While nearly two-thirds of patient's fractures were successfully managed nonoperatively, more than one-third required surgery to manage their fracture or associated complications.
Wren TA, Shepherd JA, Kalkwarf HJ, et al. Racial disparity in fracture risk between white and nonwhite children in the United States. *J Pediatr.* 2012;161:1035–1040.	A longitudinal study of nearly 1,500 children with data collected on diet, activity, ethnicity, and body composition including DXA measures reported on risk factors for fracture. Skeletal age 10–14 and white race along with increased sports participation were some predictors of fracture risk in this population.

REFERENCES

1. Aitken ME, Jaffe KM, DiScala C, et al. Functional outcome in children with multiple trauma without significant head injury. *Arch Phys Med Rehabil.* 1999;80:889–895.
2. Aitken SA, Biant LC, Court-Brown CM. Recreational mountain biking injuries. *Emerg Med J.* 2011;28:274–279.
3. Aleman KB, Meyers MC. Mountain biking injuries in children and adolescents. *Sports Med.* 2010;40:77–90.
4. Arslan H, Subasi M, Kesemenli C, et al. Problem fractures associated with gunshot wounds in children. *Injury.* 2002;33:743–749.
5. Audigé L, Slongo T, Lutz N, et al. The AO Pediatric Comprehensive Classification of Long Bone Fractures (PCCF). *Acta Orthop.* 2017;88:133–139.
6. Barlow B, Niemirska M, Gandhi RP, et al. Ten years of experience with falls from a height in children. *J Pediatr Surg.* 1983;18:509–511.
7. Buckley SL, Gotschall C, Robertson W Jr, et al. The relationships of skeletal injuries with trauma score, injury severity score, length of hospital stay, hospital charges, and mortality in children admitted to a regional pediatric trauma center. *J Pediatr Orthop.* 1994;14:449–453.
8. Centers for Disease Control and Prevention (CDC). Nonfatal motor-vehicle-related backover injuries among children—United States, 2001–2003. *MMWR Morb Mortal Wkly Rep.* 2005;54:144–146.
9. Cheng JC, Ng BK, Ying SY, et al. A 10-year study of the changes in the pattern and treatment of 6,493 fractures. *J Pediatr Orthop.* 1999;19:344–350.
10. Cheng JC, Shen WY. Limb fracture pattern in different pediatric age groups: a study of 3,350 children. *J Orthop Trauma.* 1993;7:15–22.
11. Clark EM, Ness AR, Bishop NJ, et al. Association between bone mass and fractures in children: a prospective cohort study. *J Bone Miner Res.* 2006;21:1489–1495.
12. Clark EM, Ness AR, Tobias JH. Bone fragility contributes to the risk of fracture in children, even after moderate and severe trauma. *J Bone Miner Res.* 2008;23:173–179.
13. Clark EM, Tobias JH, Ness AR. Association between bone density and fractures in children: a systematic review and meta-analysis. *Pediatrics.* 2006;117:e291–e297.
14. Clarke NM, Shelton FR, Taylor CC, et al. The incidence of fractures in children under the age of 24 months—in relation to non-accidental injury. *Injury.* 2012;43:762–765.
15. Committee on Sports Medicine and Fitness and Committee in School Health. Organized sports for children and preadolescents. *Pediatrics.* 2001;107:1459–1462.
16. Cooper C, Dennison EM, Leufkens HG, et al. Epidemiology of childhood fractures in Britain: a study using the general practice research database. *J Bone Miner Res.* 2004;19:1976–1981.
17. Council on Injury, Violence, and Poison Prevention Executive Committee. Firearm-related injuries affecting the pediatric population. *Pediatrics.* 2012;130:e1416–e1423.
18. Council on Injury, Violence, and Poison Prevention Executive Committee. All-terrain vehicle injury prevention: two-, three-, and four-wheeled unlicensed motor vehicles. *Pediatrics.* 2000;105:1352–1354.
19. Council on Injury, Violence, and Poison Prevention Executive Committee. Skateboard and scooter injuries. *Pediatrics.* 2002;109:542–543.
20. Council on Sports Medicine and Fitness. Trampoline safety in childhood and adolescence. *Pediatrics.* 2012;130:774–779.

21. Danseco ER, Miller TR, Spicer RS. Incidence and costs of 1987–1994 childhood injuries: demographic breakdowns. *Pediatrics.* 2000;105:E27.

22. de Putter CE, van Beeck EF, Looman CW, et al. Trends in wrist fractures in children and adolescents, 1997–2009. *J Hand Surg Am.* 2011;36:1810-1815.e1812.

23. Derlet RW, Silva J Jr, Holcroft J. Pedestrian accidents: adult and pediatric injuries. *J Emerg Med.* 1989;7:5–8.

24. Feldman W, Woodward CA, Hodgson C, et al. Prospective study of school injuries: incidence, types, related factors and initial management. *Can Med Assoc J.* 1983;129:1279–1283.

25. Fountain JL, Meyers MC. Skateboarding injuries. *Sports Med.* 1996;22:360–366.

26. Furnival RA, Street KA, Schunk JE. Too many pediatric trampoline injuries. *Pediatrics.* 1999;103:e57.

27. Gao Y. Children hospitalized with lower extremity fractures in the United States in 2006: a population-based approach. *Iowa Orthop J.* 2011;31:173–180.

28. Garay M, Hess J, Armstrong D, et al. Pediatric ATV injuries in a statewide sample: 2004 to 2014. *Pediatrics.* 2017;140(2):pii:e20170945.

29. Hedstrom EM, Svensson O, Bergstrom U, et al. Epidemiology of fractures in children and adolescents. *Acta Orthop.* 2010;81:148–153.

30. Hedstrom EM, Waernbaum I. Incidence of fractures among children and adolescents in rural and urban communities: analysis based on 9,965 fracture events. *Inj Epidemiol.* 2014;1:14.

31. Helmkamp JC, Furbee PM, Coben JH, et al. All-terrain vehicle-related hospitalizations in the United States, 2000–2004. *Am J Prev Med.* 2008;34:39–45.

32. Hinton RY, Lincoln A, Crockett MM, et al. Fractures of the femoral shaft in children. Incidence, mechanisms, and sociodemographic risk factors. *J Bone Joint Surg Am.* 1999;81:500–509.

33. Joeris A, Lutz N, Blumenthal A, et al. The AO Pediatric Comprehensive Classification of Long Bone Fractures (PCCF). Part II: Location and morphology of 548 lower extremity fractures in children and adolescents. *Acta Orthop.* 2017;88:129–132.

34. Joeris A, Lutz N, Blumenthal A, et al. The AO Pediatric Comprehensive Classification of Long Bone Fractures (PCCF). Part I: Location and morphology of 2,292 upper extremity fractures in children and adolescents. *Acta Orthop.* 2017;88:123–128.

35. Joeris A, Lutz N, Wicki B, et al. An epidemiological evaluation of pediatric long bone fractures - a retrospective cohort study of 2716 patients from two Swiss tertiary pediatric hospitals. *BMC Pediatr.* 2014;14:314.

36. Jones IE, Williams SM, Dow N, et al. How many children remain fracture-free during growth? a longitudinal study of children and adolescents participating in the Dunedin Multidisciplinary Health and Development Study. *Osteoporos Int.* 2002;13:990–995.

37. Kawamoto K, Kim WC, Tsuchida Y, et al. Incidence of physeal injuries in Japanese children. *J Pediatr Orthop B.* 2006;15:126–130.

38. Kellum E, Creek A, Dawkins R, et al. Age-related patterns of injury in children involved in all-terrain vehicle accidents. *J Pediatr Orthop.* 2008;28:854–858.

39. Kirkpatrick R, Puffinbarger W, Sullivan JA. All-terrain vehicle injuries in children. *J Pediatr Orthop.* 2007;27:725–728.

40. Kopjar B, Wickizer TM. Fractures among children: incidence and impact on daily activities. *Inj Prev.* 1998;4:194–197.

41. Kyle SB, Nance ML, Rutherford GW Jr, Winston FK. Skateboard-associated injuries: participation-based estimates and injury characteristics. *J Trauma.* 2002;53:686–690.

42. Laffoy M. Childhood accidents at home. *Ir Med J.* 1997;90:26–27.

43. Laforest S, Robitaille Y, Lesage D, et al. Surface characteristics, equipment height, and the occurrence and severity of playground injuries. *Inj Prev.* 2001;7:35–40.

44. Lam KY, Sumanth Kumar G, Mahadev A. Severity of playground-related fractures: more than just playground factors? *J Pediatr Orthop.* 2013;33:221–226.

45. Landin L. Fracture patterns in children. Analysis of 8,682 fractures with special reference to incidence, etiology and secular changes in a Swedish urban population 1950–1979. *Acta Orthop Scand Suppl.* 1983;202:1–109.

46. Landin L. Epidemiology of children's fractures. *J Pediatr Orthop B.* 1997;6:79–83.

47. Larson AN, Stans AA, Shaughnessy WJ, et al. Motocross morbidity: economic cost and injury distribution in children. *J Pediatr Orthop.* 2009;29:847–850.

48. Lempesis V, Rosengren BE, Nilsson JA, et al. Time trends in pediatric fracture incidence in Sweden during the period 1950–2006. *Acta Orthop.* 2017;88:440–445.

49. Lenaway DD, Ambler AG, Beaudoin DE. The epidemiology of school-related injuries: new perspectives. *Am J Prev Med.* 1992;8:193–198.

50. Leonard MB, Shults J, Wilson BA, et al. Obesity during childhood and adolescence augments bone mass and bone dimensions. *Am J Clin Nutr.* 2004;80:514–523.

51. Lillis KA, Jaffe DM. Playground injuries in children. *Pediatr Emerg Care.* 1997;13:149–153.

52. Linakis JG, Amanullah S, Mello MJ. Emergency department visits for injury in school-aged children in the United States: a comparison of nonfatal injuries occurring within and outside of the school environment. *Acad Emerg Med.* 2006;13:567–570.

53. Loder RT. The demographics of playground equipment injuries in children. *J Pediatr Surg.* 2008;43:691–699.

54. Lovejoy S, Weiss JM, Epps HR, et al. Preventable childhood injuries. *J Pediatr Orthop.* 2012;32:741–747.

55. Lustenberger T, Talving P, Barmparas G, et al. Skateboard-related injuries: not to be taken lightly. A National Trauma Databank Analysis. *J Trauma.* 2010;69:924–927.

56. Lyons RA, Delahunty AM, Heaven M, et al. Incidence of childhood fractures in affluent and deprived areas: population based study. *BMJ.* 2000;320(7228):149.

57. Lyons RA, Delahunty AM, Kraus D, et al. Children's fractures: a population based study. *Inj Prev.* 1999;5:129–132.

58. Mack MG, Hudson S, Thompson D. A descriptive analysis of children's playground injuries in the United States 1990–4. *Inj Prev.* 1997;3:100–103.

59. Mahadev A, Soon MY, Lam KS. Monkey bars are for monkeys: a study on playground equipment related extremity fractures in Singapore. *Singapore Med J.* 2004;45:9–13.

60. Mann DC, Rajmaira S. Distribution of physeal and nonphyseal fractures in 2,650 long-bone fractures in children aged 0–16 years. *J Pediatr Orthop.* 1990;10:713–716.

61. Masterson E, Borton D, O'Brien T. Victims of our climate. *Injury.* 1993;24:247–248.

62. Meller JL, Shermeta DW. Falls in urban children: a problem revisited. *Am J Dis Child.* 1987;141:1271–1275.

63. Mizuta T, Benson WM, Foster BK, et al. Statistical analysis of the incidence of physeal injuries. *J Pediatr Orthop.* 1987;7:518–523.

64. Monroe KW, Thrash C, Sorrentino A, et al. Most common sports-related injuries in a pediatric emergency department. *Clin Pediatr (Phila).* 2011;50:17–20.

65. Monteilh C, Patel P, Gaffney J. Musculoskeletal injuries associated with hoverboard use in children. *Clin Pediatr (Phila).* 2017;56:909–911.

66. Mott A, Evans R, Rolfe K, et al. Patterns of injuries to children on public playgrounds. *Arch Dis Child.* 1994;71:328–330.

67. Mott A, Rolfe K, James R, et al. Safety of surfaces and equipment for children in playgrounds. *Lancet.* 1997;349(9069):1874–1876.

68. Moustaki M, Lariou M, Petridou E. Cross country variation of fractures in the childhood population. Is the origin biological or "accidental"? *Inj Prev.* 2001;7:77.

69. Mowat DL, Wang F, Pickett W, et al. A case-control study of risk factors for playground injuries among children in Kingston and area. *Inj Prev.* 1998;4:39–43.

70. Nakaniida A, Sakuraba K, Hurwitz EL. Pediatric orthopaedic injuries requiring hospitalization: epidemiology and economics. *J Orthop Trauma.* 2014;28:167–172.

71. Naranje SM, Erali RA, Warner WC Jr, et al. Epidemiology of pediatric fractures presenting to emergency departments in the United States. *J Pediatr Orthop.* 2016;36:e45–e48.

72. Naranje SM, Gilbert SR, Stewart MG, et al. Gunshot-associated fractures in children and adolescents treated at two Level 1 pediatric trauma centers. *J Pediatr Orthop.* 2016;36:1–5.

73. Nathorst Westfelt JA. Environmental factors in childhood accidents: a prospective study in Goteborg, Sweden. *Acta Paediatr Scand Suppl.* 1982;291:1–75.

74. Nelson NG, Alhajj M, Yard E, et al. Physical education class injuries treated in emergency departments in the US in 1997–2007. *Pediatrics.* 2009;124:918–925.

75. Osberg JS, Schneps SE, Di Scala C, et al. Skateboarding: more dangerous than roller skating or in-line skating. *Arch Pediatr Adolesc Med.* 1998;152:985–991.

76. Perkins C, Scannell B, Brighton B, et al. Orthopaedic firearm injuries in children and adolescents: An eight-year experience at a major urban trauma center. *Injury.* 2016;47:173–177.

77. Peterson HA, Madhok R, Benson JT, et al. Physeal fractures: Part 1. Epidemiology in Olmsted County, Minnesota, 1979–1988. *J Pediatr Orthop.* 1994;14:423–430.

78. Petridou E, Sibert J, Dedoukou X, et al. Injuries in public and private playgrounds: the relative contribution of structural, equipment and human factors. *Acta Paediatr.* 2002;91:691–697.

79. Phelan KJ, Khoury J, Kalkwarf HJ, et al. Trends and patterns of playground injuries in United States children and adolescents. *Ambul Pediatr.* 2001;1:227–233.

80. Powell EC, Tanz RR. In-line skate and rollerskate injuries in childhood. *Pediatr Emerg Care.* 1996;12:259–262.

81. Prentice HA, Paxton EW, Hunt JJ, et al. Pediatric hip fractures in California: results from a community-based hip fracture registry. *Perm J.* 2017;21:pii:16-081.

82. Puranik S, Long J, Coffman S. Profile of pediatric bicycle injuries. *South Med J.* 1998;91:1033–1037.

83. Randsborg PH, Gulbrandsen P, Saltyte Benth J, et al. Fractures in children: epidemiology and activity-specific fracture rates. *J Bone Joint Surg Am.* 2013;95:e42.

84. Rennie L, Court-Brown CM, Mok JY, et al. The epidemiology of fractures in children. *Injury.* 2007;38:913–922.

85. Rivara FP, Bergman AB, LoGerfo JP, et al. Epidemiology of childhood injuries. II. Sex differences in injury rates. *Am J Dis Child.* 1982;136:502–506.

86. Routledge DA, Repetto-Wright R, Howarth CI. The exposure of young children to accident risk as pedestrians. *Inj Prev.* 1996;2:150–161.

87. Sandler G, Nguyen L, Lam L, et al. Trampoline trauma in children: is it preventable? *Pediatr Emerg Care.* 2011;27:1052–1056.

88. Sawyer JR, Bernard MS, Schroeder RJ, et al. Trends in all-terrain vehicle-related spinal injuries in children and adolescents. *J Pediatr Orthop.* 2011;31:623–627.

89. Schalamon J, Sarkola T, Nietosvaara Y. Injuries in children associated with the use of nonmotorized scooters. *J Pediatr Surg.* 2003;38:1612–1615.

90. Shank LP, Bagg RJ, Wagnon J. Etiology of pediatric fractures: the fatigue factors in children's fractures. Presented at Proceedings of the 4th National Conference on Pediatric Trauma; Indianapolis, Indiana; September 24–26, 1992.

91. Sheps SB, Evans GD. Epidemiology of school injuries: a 2-year experience in a municipal health department. *Pediatrics.* 1987;79:69–75.

92. Shults RA, West BA, Rudd RA, et al. All-terrain vehicle-related nonfatal injuries among young riders in the United States, 2001–2010. *Pediatrics.* 2013;132:282–289.

93. Sieben RL, Leavitt JD, French JH. Falls as childhood accidents: an increasing urban risk. *Pediatrics.* 1971;47:886–892.

94. Sinikumpu JJ, Pokka T, Hyvonen H, et al. Supracondylar humerus fractures in children: the effect of weather conditions on their risk. *Eur J Orthop Surg Traumatol.* 2017;27:243–250.

95. Sinikumpu JJ, Pokka T, Sirnio K, et al. Population-based research on the relationship between summer weather and paediatric forearm shaft fractures. *Injury.* 2013;44:1569–1573.

96. Slongo T, Audige L, Clavert JM, et al. The AO comprehensive classification of pediatric long-bone fractures: a web-based multicenter agreement study. *J Pediatr Orthop.* 2007;27:171–180.

97. Slongo T, Audige L, Lutz N, et al. Documentation of fracture severity with the AO classification of pediatric long-bone fractures. *Acta Orthop.* 2007;78:247–253.

98. Slongo T, Audige L, Schlickewei W, et al. Development and validation of the AO pediatric comprehensive classification of long bone fractures by the Pediatric

Expert Group of the AO Foundation in collaboration with AO Clinical Investigation and Documentation and the International Association for Pediatric Traumatology. *J Pediatr Orthop*. 2006;26:43–49.

99. Slongo TF, Audige L. Fracture and dislocation classification compendium for children: the AO pediatric comprehensive classification of long bone fractures (PCCF). *J Orthop Trauma*. 2007;21(10 Suppl):S135–S160.
100. Smith GA. Injuries to children in the United States related to trampolines, 1990–1995: a national epidemic. *Pediatrics*. 1998;101(3 Pt 1):406–412.
101. Smith GA, Shields BJ. Trampoline-related injuries to children. *Arch Pediatr Adolesc Med*. 1998;152:694–699.
102. Smith MD, Burrington JD, Woolf AD. Injuries in children sustained in free falls: an analysis of 66 cases. *J Trauma*. 1975;15:987–991.
103. Stark AD, Bennet GC, Stone DH, et al. Association between childhood fractures and poverty: population based study. *BMJ*. 2002;324(7335):457.
104. Steiner C, Elixhauser A, Schnaier J. The healthcare cost and utilization project: an overview. *Eff Clin Pract*. 2002;5:143–151.
105. Taylor ED, Theim KR, Mirch MC, et al. Orthopedic complications of overweight in children and adolescents. *Pediatrics*. 2006;117:2167–2174.
106. Tiderius CJ, Landin L, Duppe H. Decreasing incidence of fractures in children: an epidemiological analysis of 1,673 fractures in Malmo, Sweden, 1993–1994. *Acta Orthop Scand*. 1999;70:622–626.
107. Valerio G, Galle F, Mancusi C, et al. Pattern of fractures across pediatric age groups: analysis of individual and lifestyle factors. *BMC Public Health*. 2010;10:656.
108. Valerio G, Galle F, Mancusi C, et al. Prevalence of overweight in children with bone fractures: a case control study. *BMC Pediatr*. 2012;12:166.
109. von Heyden J, Hauschild O, Strohm PC, et al. Paediatric acetabular fractures. Data from the German Pelvic Trauma Registry Initiative. *Acta Orthop Belg*. 2012;78:611–618.
110. Waltzman ML, Shannon M, Bowen AP, et al. Monkeybar injuries: complications of play. *Pediatrics*. 1999;103:e58.
111. Wareham K, Johansen A, Stone MD, et al. Seasonal variation in the incidence of wrist and forearm fractures, and its consequences. *Injury*. 2003;34:219–222.
112. Weiss BD. Bicycle-related head injuries. *Clin Sports Med*. 1994;13:99–112.
113. Wood AM, Robertson GA, Rennie L, et al. The epidemiology of sports-related fractures in adolescents. *Injury*. 2010;41:834–838.
114. Worlock P, Stower M. Fracture patterns in Nottingham children. *J Pediatr Orthop*. 1986;6:656–660.
115. Wren TA, Shepherd JA, Kalkwarf HJ, et al. Racial disparity in fracture risk between white and nonwhite children in the United States. *J Pediatr*. 2012;161:1035–1040.

OTHER RESOURCES

ATV Position Statement. Available at: http://www.aaos.org/about/papers/position/1101.asp

Injuries from In-Line Skating and Skateboarding. Available at: http://www.aaos.org/about/papers/position/1127.asp

National Center for Injury Prevention and Control, US Centers for Disease Control and Prevention. Web-based Injury Statistics Query & Reporting System (WISQARS) Injury Mortality Reports, 1999–2010, for National, Regional, and States (September, 2012). Available at: http://www.cdc.gov/injury/wisqars/fatal_injury_reports.html. Accessed September 8, 2012.

Trampolines and Trampoline Safety. Available at: http://www.aaos.org/about/papers/position/1135.asp

2

The Injured Immature Skeleton

Karl E. Rathjen, Harry K. W. Kim, and Benjamin A. Alman

INTRODUCTION

Roughly 20% of children will sustain a fracture, and the incidence of pediatric fractures is increasing over time.[62,93,123] Thus, childhood fractures are not only important from an orthopedic standpoint, but are also an important societal health issue. A child's bones heal quicker, are surrounded by thicker periosteum, and have a substantially greater remodeling potential than adults. These differences change the way fractures are treated. In a growing child, injury can damage the growth plate, which can be the weakest region of bone.[123] Such injury can result in temporary or permanent growth arrest. The growth plate can also remodel less than perfect reductions and there can be tremendous remodeling potential. As an example, the distal radius can correct deformities at a rate of one degree a month in line with the flexion and extension arc of motion of the wrist.[80,97,131]

Children can have underlying disorders that weaken bone or slow healing, such as osteogenesis imperfecta,[82,182] neurofibromatosis,[73] or a bone tumor.[105] The first presentation of such conditions may be a referral to an orthopedist for a fracture. Understanding how the bone normally behaves to an injury can help in the identification of a pathologic bone injury, which may be caused by such an underlying condition. For instance, an avulsion fracture, such as in the ulna, can be the first presentation for a preteen with osteogenesis imperfecta.[149] Identification of unusual fracture patterns can also help in the identification of nonaccidental trauma, and an orthopedist can save a child's life by the early identification of nonaccidental trauma in childhood.[110] For these reasons it is critical to understand the normal response of a child's bone to trauma to know when there is something unusual in the presentation or course of healing, to make these diagnoses.

ANATOMIC CONSIDERATIONS OF THE IMMATURE SKELETON

Five regions characterize long bones: The bulbous, articular cartilage-covered ends (epiphyses) tapering to the funnel-shaped

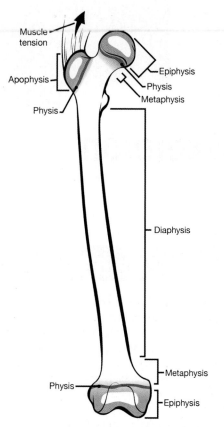

Figure 2-1. A schematic diagram of femur illustrating the terminology used to describe various anatomical regions of a growing bone.

metaphyses, with the central diaphysis interposed between the metaphyses (Fig. 2-1). During growth, the epiphyseal and metaphyseal regions are separated by the organized cartilaginous physis, which is the major contributor to longitudinal growth of the bone. The larger long bones (clavicle, humerus, radius, ulna, femur, tibia, and fibula) have physes at both ends, whereas the smaller tubular bones (metacarpals, metatarsals, and phalanges) usually have a physis at one end only. The relative contribution to longitudinal growth of the proximal and distal physes of the long bones is variable and listed for the upper and lower extremities in Figure 2-2.

EPIPHYSIS

The epiphysis is the region of a long bone between the end of the bone and the growth plate (or physis). At birth, the end of the bones is completely cartilaginous (except for the distal femur and occasionally the proximal tibia), and termed as chondroepiphysis. A secondary center of ossification forms at a specific time for each chondroepiphysis, which gradually enlarges until the cartilaginous area has been almost completely replaced by bone at skeletal maturity. The appearance of the ossification centers differs between different bones (Figs. 2-3 and 2-4), and this needs to be taken into account when diagnosing fractures of these regions.[22,136] As the ossification center matures, there is increased rigidity at the end of the bone, and this increase in rigidity is responsible for changes in the fracture pattern with age. Indeed, injuries that might not result in a fracture in this

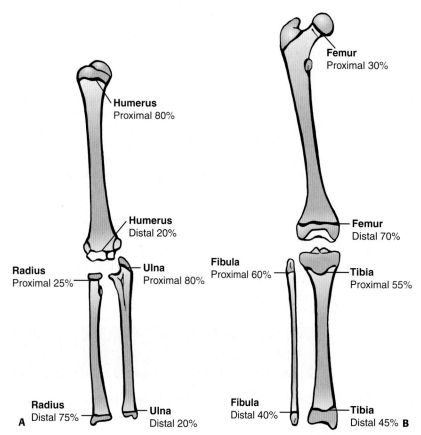

Figure 2-2. Approximate percentage of longitudinal growth provided by the proximal and distal physes for each long bone in the upper (**A**) and lower (**B**) extremities.

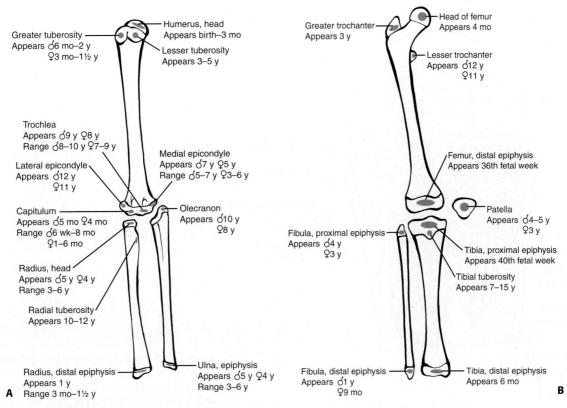

Figure 2-3. Typical age (and range) of development of the secondary ossification centers of the epiphyses in the (**A**) upper extremity and (**B**) lower extremity.

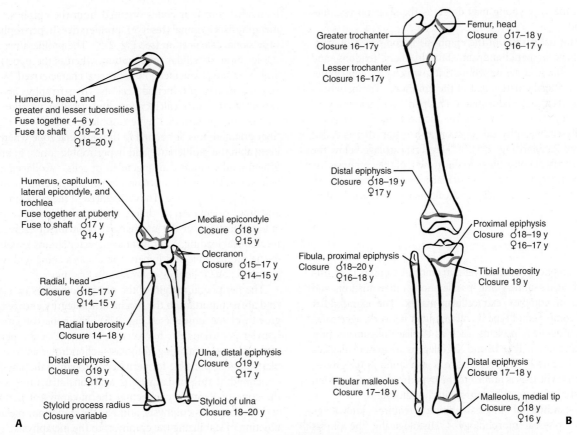

Figure 2-4. Typical age (and range) of closure of physes in the (**A**) upper extremity and (**B**) lower extremity.

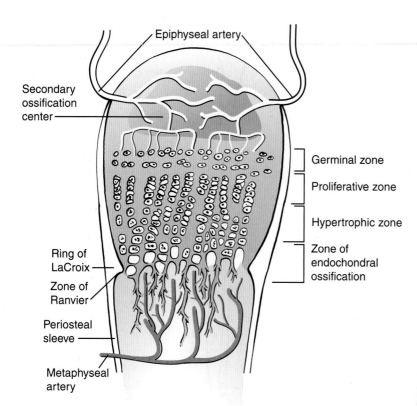

Figure 2-5. Schematic diagram of the organization of the physis. Four zones are illustrated: The germinal, proliferative, hypertrophic, and provisional calcification (or enchondral ossification) layers. Note also the groove of Ranvier and the perichondral ring of LaCroix.

region in the very young may do so as the skeleton becomes more rigid.

The external surface of the epiphysis is composed of articular cartilage or perichondrium. Muscle fibers, tendons, and ligaments attach to the perichondrium, which also contributes to the centrifugal enlargement of the epiphysis. The perichondrium blends into the periosteum. This perichondrial/periosteal tissue continuity contributes to the biomechanical strength of the epiphyseal/metaphyseal junction at a region that is called the zone of Ranvier (Fig. 2-5).[42,190] Hyaline cartilage below the articular cartilage contributes to the growth of the epiphysis. As skeletal maturity is reached, a tidemark develops at the demarcation between the articular and calcified epiphyseal hyaline cartilage.

PHYSIS

Physis is a highly organized, yet dynamic structure that consists of chondrocytes undergoing proliferation, differentiation, and formation of complex extracellular matrix. The extracellular matrix is composed of type II collagen fiber network, aggrecans, and noncollagenous proteins, such as cartilage oligomeric protein and matrilin-3. Type IX and XI collagens are minor collagens found in the physis. Type X collagen is also found in the physis; however, its synthesis is limited to the hypertrophic zone and is a distinguishing feature of hypertrophic chondrocyte.

Understanding of physeal injuries requires knowledge of normal physeal morphology.[179] Histologically, the physis

is divided into four zones oriented from the epiphysis to the metaphysis: Germinal (reserve), proliferative, hypertrophic, and provisional calcification (see Fig. 2-5). The proliferative zone is the location of cellular proliferation, whereas the hypertrophic and provisional calcification zones are characterized by extracellular matrix production, cellular hypertrophy, apoptosis, extracellular matrix calcification, and vascular invasion of the lacunae of the terminal hypertrophic chondrocytes. Collagen fiber orientation is horizontal in the germinal zone whereas it is vertical in the proliferative and hypertrophic zones, in line with growth and columnar arrangement of cells.[11] Collagen content is lower in the proliferative and hypertrophic zones compared with the germinal zone. The differences in the collagen content and fiber orientation of different physeal zones have important implications in the mechanical behavior of each zone to mechanical loading.[12] For instance, greater strains are observed in the proliferative and hypertrophic zones compared with the germinal zone following compression loading.

The peripheral margin of the physis comprises two specialized areas important to the mechanical integrity and peripheral growth of the physis (see Fig. 2-5). The zone (or groove) of Ranvier is a triangular microscopic structure at the periphery of the physis, containing fibroblasts, chondroblasts, and osteoblasts. It is responsible for peripheral growth of the physis. The perichondral ring of LaCroix is a fibrous structure overlying the zone of Ranvier, connecting the metaphyseal periosteum and cartilaginous epiphysis, and has the important mechanical function of stabilizing the epiphysis to the metaphysis.

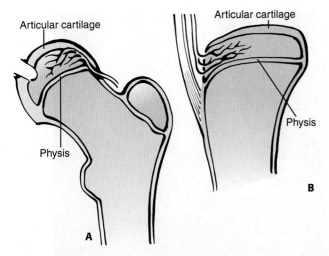

Figure 2-6. Classification of epiphyseal blood supply according to Dale and Harris. **A:** Type A epiphyses are nearly completely covered by articular cartilage. Blood supply must enter via the perichondrium. This blood supply is susceptible to disruption by epiphyseal separation. The proximal femur and proximal humerus are examples of type A epiphyses. **B:** Type B epiphyses are only partially covered by articular cartilage. Such epiphyses are more resistant to blood supply impairment by epiphyseal separation. The distal femur, proximal and distal tibia, and distal radius are clinical examples of type B epiphyses.

The epiphysis and secondary ossific nucleus must receive blood supply for viability.[204] Dale and Harris[63] identified two types of blood supply to the epiphysis (Fig. 2-6). Type A epiphyses (such as the proximal humeral and proximal femoral epiphyses) are nearly completely covered with articular cartilage; therefore, most of the blood supply to the epiphysis must enter from the perichondrium in a distal to proximal direction. The blood supply to these epiphyses may be easily compromised by epiphyseal separation. A complete disruption of the epiphyseal vasculature, however, may not produce an extensive ischemic damage to the physis if the metaphyseal vasculature is intact.[117] The studies using multiphoton microscopy also suggest that growth plate nutrition is not unidirectional from the epiphysis to the metaphysis as traditionally believed but is contributed by the epiphyseal, metaphyseal, and circumferential perichondrial vasculature.[72,209] Type B epiphyses (such as the proximal and distal tibia and the distal radius) have only a portion of their surface covered with articular cartilage and are theoretically less susceptible to devascularization from epiphyseal separation.

In the past decade there has been a substantial increase in research into the control of growth plate chondrocyte function. Such work is the first step in developing approaches to modulate growth plate function, such as using a drug, a cell, or a biologic approach. Such treatments could someday be used to treat a partial growth arrest following an injury. Chondrocytes develop from an undifferentiated mesenchymal precursor cell, sometimes called MSCs, which differentiate into a common osteochondroprogenitor cell. The Wnt/β-catenin signaling pathway plays a key role in determining if these cells become osteoblasts or chondrocytes, as in the absence of β-catenin they develop into chondrocytes.

Several drugs are available that modulate β-catenin, and these could someday be used to modulate growth plate activity.[96,100,120] Once cells become committed to be growth plate chondrocytes, they undergo a coordinated process of differentiation, with expression of various genes (*SOX9, IHH, PTHrP, RUNX2,* and then *type X collagen*)[7,101,215] marking the states of differentiation. Resting cells proliferate, then hypertrophy, before undergoing terminal differentiation, where they express *type X collagen* and become replaced by bone. The resting cells maintain the growth plate cells, and as such these cells located nearest to the epiphysis are critical to normal bone growth, and damage to these cells will permanently disrupt growth.

The hedgehog (Hh) signaling pathway is crucial in the regulation of chondrocyte fate in the growth plate. Prehypertrophic chondrocytes in the growth plate express the Hh ligand Indian Hh (IHH).[28,135,161] IHH serves as a key regulator of endochondral ossification, acting in a negative feedback loop with parathyroid hormone-like hormone (PTHrP), also called parathyroid hormone-related protein (PTHrP). IHH regulates chondrocyte differentiation and induces ossification of the perichondrium in a PTHrP-independent manner.[121] The regulation of PTHrP by IHH involves mediators such as BMPs which also play a role initiating the chondrocyte differentiation cascade.[146] In this way, IHH and PTHrP act in a feedback loop controlling the pace of growth plate chondrocyte differentiation.

METAPHYSIS

The metaphysis is the flared portion of the bone at each end of the diaphysis. It has a decreased cortical thickness and increased volume of trabecular bone in the secondary spongiosa. During growth, endochondral modeling centrally and peripherally initially forms the primary spongiosa, which then is remodeled into the more mature secondary spongiosa by osteoclasts and osteoblasts. For this reason, there is considerable bone turnover in the metaphysis compared to other regions of the bone. The metaphyseal cortex is thinner and is more porous than the diaphysis, and there are cortical fenestrations, which contain fibrovascular soft tissue elements that connect the metaphyseal marrow spaces with the subperiosteal region. The metaphyseal region does not develop extensive secondary and tertiary haversian systems until the late stages of skeletal maturation. These microscopic and anatomic changes correlate with changing fracture patterns, and the ability of bone to deform without breaking in this region is why buckle (or torus) fractures are more likely to occur than complete metaphyseal or epiphyseal/physeal fractures.[115,163,205]

Although the periosteum is attached relatively loosely to the diaphysis, it is firmly fixed to the metaphysis because of the increasingly complex continuity of fibrous tissue through the metaphyseal fenestrations. The periosteum subsequently attaches densely into the peripheral physis, blending into the zone of Ranvier as well as the epiphyseal perichondrium. The zone of Ranvier is a specialized region between bone and cartilage formation, and cells in this zone contribute to growth plate remodeling over time.[42,190] The fenestrated metaphyseal cortex extends to the physis as the thin osseous ring of LaCroix. There are no significant direct muscle attachments to the metaphyseal bone;

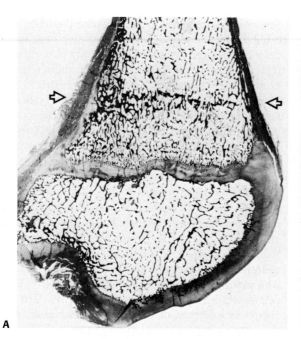
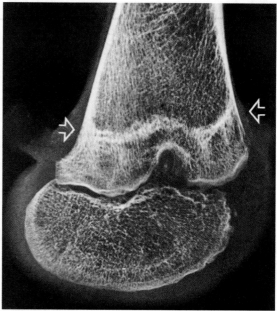

A   **B**

Figure 2-7. Growth lines. Histologic section (**A**) and x-ray study (**B**) of a distal femur showing a typical Harris line (*arrows*). This is formed during an acute illness and chemotherapy for leukemia. The child then resumed a more normal pattern of growth until her death from leukemia about 14 months later.

instead, muscle fibers primarily blend into the periosteum. The medial distal femoral attachment of the adductor muscles is a significant exception.

Growth Lines of Park and Harris

Many bones exhibit transversely oriented, dense trabecular linear bone patterns within the metaphysis. These lines duplicate the contiguous physeal contour, and appear after processes which transiently slow growth or increase mineralization. As such, they are seen after generalized illnesses, treatment with bisphosphonate drugs (which inhibit osteoclasts, and therefore decrease bone resorption and remodeling of the primary spongiosa), or after localized processes within the bone, such as infection or growth plate trauma. The lines are called Harris or Park growth slowdown or arrest lines. Once the normal longitudinal growth rate resumes, longitudinal trabecular[8] orientation is restored. The thickened, transversely oriented osseous plate is left behind, will be gradually remodeled, and with time will disappear (Fig. 2-7).[193]

In a systemic problem slowing bone growth, the lines are distributed relatively symmetrically throughout the skeleton, and are thickest in metaphyses from bones that grow most rapidly. The lines are important in analyzing the effects of a fracture on growth. They can be measured and the sides compared to corroborate femoral overgrowth after diaphyseal fracture and eccentric overgrowth medially after proximal tibial metaphyseal fracture. A line that converges toward a physis suggests localized growth damage that may result in an osseous bridge and the risk of angular deformity (Fig. 2-8).

DIAPHYSIS

The diaphysis constitutes the major portion of each long bone, and is formed from bone remodeled from the metaphysis. Mature, lamellar bone is the dominant feature of the diaphyseal bone, and the developing diaphyseal bone is extremely vascular. When analyzed in cross section, the center is much less dense than the maturing bone of older children, adolescents, and adults. Subsequent growth leads to increased complexity of the haversian (osteonal) systems and the formation of increasing amounts of extracellular matrix, causing a relative decrease in cross-sectional porosity and an increase in hardness. Some bones, such as the tibia, exhibit a decrease in vascularity as the bone matures; this factor affects the rate of healing and risk of nonunion.[40,162] The vascularity of bone is important not only because it brings nutrients to the bone, but also because pericyte cells surrounding blood vessels contribute to new osteoblasts.[19]

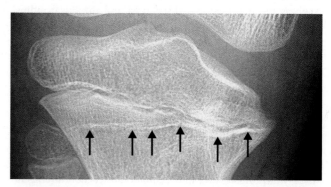

Figure 2-8. Example of a growth arrest line converging toward the area of physeal arrest at the medial proximal tibial physis. (Used with permission from the Children's Orthopedic Center, Los Angeles.)

PERIOSTEUM

A child's periosteum is thicker and more readily elevated from the bone than in adults. It also has a much greater osteogenic potential than that of an adult. Indeed, in young children, one can remove the entire diaphysis of a bone, but leave the periosteum, and the bone will regrow. The thicker and stronger periosteum affects fracture displacement, ease of closed reduction, and the capacity to form new bone. The periosteum usually remains intact on the concave (compression) side of an injury. This intact periosteal hinge or sleeve may lessen the extent of displacement of the fracture fragments, and it also can be used to assist in the reduction, because the intact portion contributes to the intrinsic stability. Thus, accentuating the deformity, unlocks the periosteum, helping with the reduction. Because the periosteum allows tissue continuity across the fracture, the subperiosteal new bone that forms quickly bridges the fracture gap and leads to more rapid long-term stability.[10,20]

The periosteum comprises two tissue layers. An outer fibroblast layer provides fibrous attachment to subcutaneous connective tissue, muscles, tendons, and ligaments, whereas the inner cambium layer contains a pool of cells that support bone formation and repair. The periosteum, rather than the bone itself, serves as the origin for muscle fibers along the metaphysis and diaphysis. This mechanism allows coordinated growth of bone and muscle units; something that would be impossible if all the muscle tissues attached directly to the developing bone or cartilage. Exceptions include the attachment of muscle fibers near the linea aspera and into the medial distal femoral metaphysis. The latter pattern of direct metaphyseal osseous attachment may be associated with significant irregularity of cortical and trabecular bones. Radiographs of this area often are misinterpreted as showing a neoplastic, osteomyelitic, or traumatic response, even though this is actually a variation of skeletal development. The periosteum in the growing child also plays a critical role in remodeling, as the tissues in tension over the concave side of a deformity will produce new bone. The bone on the tension, or convex, side of a deformity will be resorbed over time, ultimately resulting in a straight diaphysis.[10,20,106]

APOPHYSIS

An apophysis is composed of fibrocartilage instead of columnar cartilage and grows primarily in response to tensile forces. They are generally attached to muscular structures. With growth secondary ossification centers can form in the apophysis. Because of the differing histologic composition of these structures, they fail differently than other parts of the bone, and excessive tensile stress may avulse the apophysis, especially during the late stages of closure. Such injuries can generate large amounts of new bone, and may be mistaken for tumors, especially around the pelvis. Healing of a displaced fragment to the underlying undisplaced secondary center creates the symptomatic reactive overgrowth, and in the tibial tuberosity apophysis, this is known as an Osgood–Schlatter lesion.[64,140,181]

MECHANISMS OF FRACTURE HEALING

Fracture healing is a complex regenerative process initiated in response to injury, in which bone can heal by primary or secondary mechanisms. In primary healing, new bone is laid down without any intermediate. This type of healing is rare in a complete bone fracture, except when the fracture is rigidly fixed through certain types of surgery. In the more common secondary healing, immature and disorganized bone forms between the fragments, which is termed the callus.[45,70,142,164] During the fracture repair process, cells progress through stages of differentiation reminiscent of those that cells progress through during normal fetal bone development. In normal development of long bone, undifferentiated mesenchymal cells initially form a template of the bone, which differentiate to chondrocytes. This cartilaginous template is termed the bone's anlage. Following this phase, blood vessels enter the cartilaginous template, and osteoblasts, which differentiate from perivascular and other cells surrounding the bone, form bone.

There are, however, several important differences between bone repair and development. One is that repair does not need to progress through a cartilaginous template. Another is that the liberation of growth factors in the extracellular environment and inflammatory mediators initiates fracture repair, and the activation of these factors does not occur during development. Indeed, this inflammatory initiation of repair processes may be the fundamental difference between development and regeneration. This is one reason that agents that modulate inflammation can affect bone formation. Although some inflammatory pathways can have both positive and negative effects on bone repair, an inhibition of prostaglandin activity inhibits bone formation, and indeed this has been used clinically to prevent bone formation.[29,151,177]

Osseous repair progresses through closely integrated phases. In the *initial* phase of fracture repair, bleeding from the damaged tissues causes a hematoma at the fracture site, stopping blood loss and liberating growth factors and cytokines. Endothelial cells respond by increasing their vascular permeability, allowing leukocytes, monocytes, macrophages, and multipotential mesenchymal cells to reach the fracture site.[159] The blood supply is temporarily disrupted for a few millimeters on either side of the fracture site, producing local necrosis and hypoxia. In the *proliferative* phase, undifferentiated mesenchymal cells aggregate at the site of injury, proliferate, and differentiate presumably in response to growth factors produced by the injured tissues.[45] This process involves both intramembranous and endochondral ossification. Intramembranous ossification involves the formation of bone directly from committed osteoprogenitor cells and undifferentiated mesenchymal cells that reside in the periosteum, resulting in hard callus formation.[68] During endochondral ossification, mesenchymal cells differentiate into chondrocytes, producing cartilaginous matrix, which then undergoes calcification and eventually is replaced by bone. The formation of primary bone is followed by extensive *remodeling* until the damaged skeletal element regains its original shape and size (Fig. 2-9).[68,70,142]

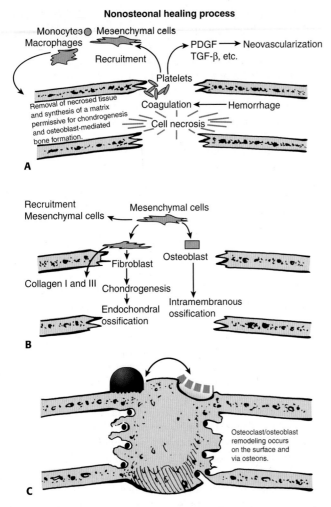

Figure 2-9. Phases of fracture repair. The figure demonstrates the three phases of fracture repair: (**A**) inflammatory phase, (**B**) reparative phase, and (**C**) remodeling phase. The inflammatory cells remove the debris from the fracture site and, together with the fibroblastic cells, develop the site into a matrix that will support the cells that enable new bone to be formed. The mesenchymal cells are recruited by the release of growth factors in the fracture site. The mesenchymal cells may differentiate into osteoblasts that produce bone in a membranous fashion. Alternately the mesenchymal cell may become chondrogenic and produce bone by the endochondral pathway. Remodeling begins with resorption of mechanically unnecessary, inefficient portions of the callus and the subsequent orientation of trabecular bone along the lines of stress.

The strength of bone is a function of the intrinsic mechanical properties of the ossified tissue as well as the way the tissue is organized. When a child's fracture heals, the weaker callous has a larger diameter than the intact bone, but because the weaker material is farther from the center, the moment of inertia is increased, and as a whole unit the bone can be just as strong as if it had not fractured. Children form a larger diameter callous than adults, in part because the stronger periosteum comes off the bone easier and forms a wider barrier to the callous. In addition, during the proliferative phase of fracture repair, children form new bone faster than adults. These factors combine

to make children's bone regain its strength much quicker following a fracture than an adult. Furthermore, these factors are responsible for the observation that the younger the child the quicker a fractured bone will regain its strength.

Several cell signaling pathways are normally activated during fracture repair, and many of these are the same ones that are activated during bone development. Certain BMPs are liberated early in the repair process, and they stimulate undifferentiated mesenchymal cells to achieve an osteoblastic phenotype. Tibial fractures are a high-risk injury for developing a nonunion and clinical studies show that treatment with select BMPs will improve the rate of healing in this situation.[85] Another pathway that plays an important role in bone repair is β-catenin. There is upregulation of β-catenin during the healing process,[21,55,56] and healing is repressed in mice lacking β-catenin. However, β-catenin functions differently at different stages of fracture repair. Because drugs that modulate β-catenin are in development, this is an area in which novel therapies could be used to improve delayed repair.[55,58,198]

The various signaling pathways which play a role in bone repair also interact with each other during the repair process. For instance, the inflammatory process activates prostaglandin synthesis, which regulates BMP expression in mesenchymal progenitors.[18] In a similar manner, prostaglandin activity also regulates β-catenin activity.[118] Furthermore, BMP stimulation requires β-catenin to produce bone.[56] Thus, the various signaling pathways involved in bone repair and regeneration do not act alone but in a coordinated manner to allow for bone regeneration.

UNIQUE ASPECTS OF INJURY IN THE IMMATURE SKELETON

REMODELING OF BONES AFTER A FRACTURE IN CHILDREN

In a growing child, the normal process of bone growth and remodeling may realign initially malunited fragments, making anatomic reduction less important than in an adult. Bone and cartilage generally remodel in response to normal stresses of body weight, muscle action, and joint reaction forces, as well as intrinsic control mechanisms such as the periosteum. The potential for spontaneous, complete correction is greater if the child is younger, the fracture site is closer to the physis, and there is relative alignment of the angulation in the normal plane of motion of the joint (Fig. 2-10).[201] This is particularly evident in fractures involving hinge joints such as the knee, ankle, elbow, or wrist, in which corrections are relatively rapid if the angulation is in the normal plane of motion. As an example, the distal radius can correct deformities at a rate of one degree a month.[80,97,131] However, spontaneous correction of angular deformities is unlikely in other directions, such as a cubitus varus deformity following a supracondylar fracture of the humerus. Similarly, rotational deformities usually do not correct spontaneously.[163,184]

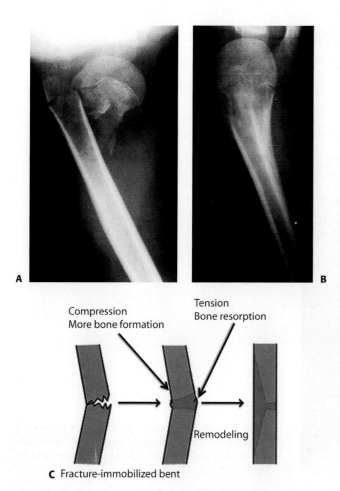

Compression
More bone formation

Tension
Bone resorption

Remodeling

C Fracture-immobilized bent

Figure 2-10. Remodeling of a fracture. **A** and **B** show the initial and follow-up radiographs of a proximal humeral fracture, illustrating an impressive degree of remodeling. **C** shows how bone deposition and resorption result in straightening of the deformity over time. Efficient remodeling requires an open growth plate, and as such is a unique feature of childhood injury.

GROWTH STIMULATION

Fractures may stimulate longitudinal growth by increasing the blood supply to the metaphysis, physis, and epiphysis, and at least on an experimental basis, by disrupting the periosteum and its physiologic restraint on the rates of longitudinal growth of the physes. Such increased growth may make the bone longer than it would have been without an injury. Eccentric overgrowth may also occur; this is particularly evident in tibia valgum following an incomplete fracture of the proximal tibial metaphysis (Fig. 2-11).[201]

PHYSEAL INJURIES

Etiology of Physeal Injuries

Physes can be injured in many ways, both obvious and subtle. Obviously, the most frequent mechanism of injury is fracture. Most commonly, physeal injury is direct, with a fracture involving the physis itself. Occasionally, physeal injury from trauma is associated with a fracture elsewhere in the limb segment, either as a result of ischemia[167] or perhaps compression[1,13,33,103,143,150,206]

(see discussion of Salter–Harris type V physeal fractures below). Other mechanisms of injuries to the physes include infection[26,31,126,165]; disruption by tumor, cysts,[199] and tumor-like disorders; vascular insult[167]; repetitive stress[9,34,49,50,134,213]; irradiation[43,180]; and other rare etiologies.[25,39,48,189,213]

Repetitive Stress Physeal Injuries

Repetitious physical activities in skeletally immature individuals can result in physeal stress–fracture equivalents.[9,49,50] The most common location for such injuries is in the distal radius or ulna, as seen in competitive gymnasts (Fig. 2-12); the proximal tibia, as in running and kicking sports such as soccer (Fig. 2-13); and the proximal humerus, as in baseball pitchers.[49] These injuries should be managed by rest, judicious resumption of activities, and longitudinal observation to monitor for potential physeal growth disturbance.

Classification of Physeal Fractures

Physeal fractures have been recognized as unique since ancient times. Hippocrates is credited with the first written account of this injury. Poland reviewed accounts of physeal injuries in his 1898 book, *Traumatic Separation of the Epiphysis*,[174] and is credited with the first classification of the patterns of physeal fracture. Modifications to Poland's original scheme have been proposed by a number of authors,[2–5,63,66,137,153,155,168,169,172,185] including Aitken,[4] Salter and Harris,[185] Ogden et al.,[143,155] and Peterson.[168,169] Classifications of physeal fractures are important because they alert the practitioner to potentially subtle radiographic fracture patterns, can be of prognostic significance with respect to growth disturbance potential, and guide general treatment principles based on that risk and associated joint disruption. Currently, the Salter–Harris classification, first published in 1963,[185] is firmly entrenched in the literature and most orthopedists' minds. The reader also should be aware of some deficiencies in that classification, as pointed out by Peterson and discussed below.[168–170]

Salter–Harris Classification of Physeal Fractures

Salter–Harris Classification consists of five types of physeal injuries.[185] The first four types were adopted from Poland (types I, II, and III) and Aitken (Aitken type III became Salter–Harris type IV) (Fig. 2-14). Salter and Harris added a fifth type, which they postulated was an unrecognized compression injury characterized by normal radiographs and late physeal closure.[1,13,24,33,99,103,116,170,206]

Type I

Salter–Harris type I injuries are characterized by a transphyseal plane of injury, with no bony fracture line through either the metaphysis or the epiphysis. Radiographs of undisplaced type I physeal fractures, therefore, are normal except for associated soft tissue swelling, making careful patient examination particularly important in this injury. In the Olmstead County Survey of physeal fractures,[171] type I fractures occurred most frequently in the phalanges, metacarpals, distal tibia, and distal ulna. Epiphyseal separations

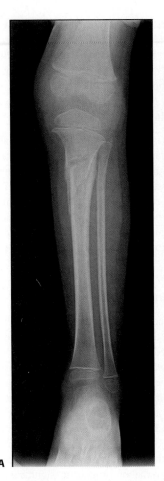
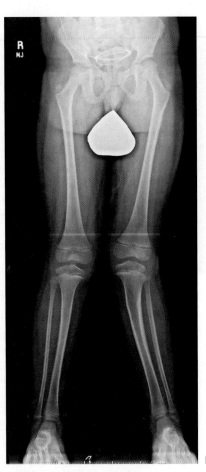

Figure 2-11. A: AP radiograph of the tibia of a 4 year old shows a proximal metaphyseal fracture with minimal displacement in the fibula intact. **B:** Two years later note the significant valgus deformity.

in infants occur most commonly in the proximal humerus, distal humerus, and proximal femur. If there is an urgency to make the diagnosis on patients suspected of having a type I injury, further imaging by ultrasound, magnetic resonance imaging (MRI),[46,60,108,172,196] or intraoperative arthrography

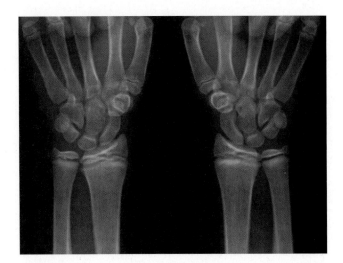

Figure 2-12. Stress injury of the distal radius and ulna in both wrists of a competitive gymnast. There was no history of specific injury. The wrists were tender to touch. Note distal radial and ulnar physeal widening and irregularity.

may be helpful.[6,89,139] Ultrasound is particularly helpful for assessing epiphyseal separations in infants (especially in the proximal femur and elbow regions) without the need for sedation, anesthetic, or invasive procedure.[37,66,67,98,188]

The fracture line of type I injuries is usually in the zone of hypertrophy of the physis, as the path of least resistance during the propagation of the injury (Fig. 2-15). As a consequence, in theory, the essential resting and proliferative zones are relatively spared, and, assuming that there is no vascular insult to these zones as a consequence of the injury, subsequent growth disturbance is relatively uncommon. As discussed above, however, studies have shown this to be a simplistic view of the fracture line through a physis, and that, because of uneven loading and macroscopic undulations in the physis, any zone of the physis can be affected by the fracture line.[35,109,148,183,189,197]

Because the articular surface and, at least in theory, the germinal and proliferative layers of the physis are not displaced, the general principles of fracture management are to secure a gentle and adequate reduction of the epiphysis on the metaphysis and stabilize the fragments as needed.

Type II

Type II injuries have physeal and metaphyseal components; the fracture line extends from the physeal margin peripherally across a variable portion of the physis and exits into the metaphysis at the opposite end of the fracture (Fig. 2-16). The epiphyseal fragment thus comprises all of the epiphysis and

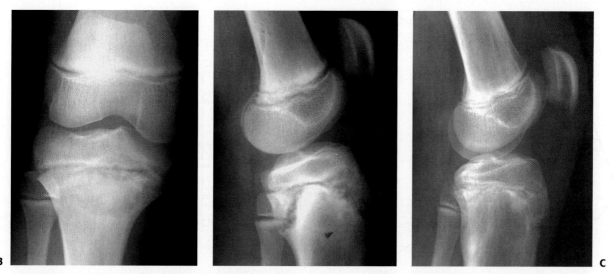

A, B   **C**

Figure 2-13. Stress injury of the proximal tibia in an elite soccer player. **A:** Anteroposterior radiograph film demonstrates subtle proximal tibial physeal widening. **B:** Lateral radiograph shows widening, a metaphyseal Thurston Holland fragment, and some posterior displacement of the proximal epiphysis. **C:** Significant radiograph improvement noted after discontinuing athletic activities for 3 months.

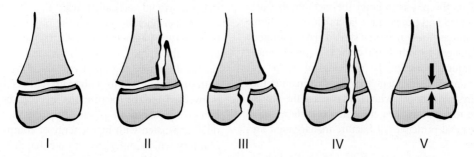

I   II   III   IV   V

Figure 2-14. Salter–Harris classification of physeal fractures. In Salter–Harris type I fractures, the fracture line is entirely within the physis, referred to by Poland as type I. In Salter–Harris type II fractures, the fracture line extends from the physis into the metaphysis; described by Poland as type II and Aitken as type I. In Salter–Harris type III fractures, the fracture enters the epiphysis from the physis and almost always exits the articular surface. Poland described this injury as type III and Aitken as type II. In Salter–Harris type IV, the fracture extends across the physis from the articular surface and epiphysis, to exit in the margin of the metaphysis. Aitken described this as a type III injury in his classification. Salter–Harris type V fractures were described by Salter and Harris as a crush injury to the physis with initially normal radiographs with late identification of premature physeal closure.

Figure 2-15. Scheme of theoretic fracture plane of Salter–Harris type I fractures. Because the hypertrophic zone is the weakest zone structurally, separation should occur at this level. Experimental and clinical studies have confirmed that the fracture plane is more complex than this concept and frequently involves other physeal zones as well.

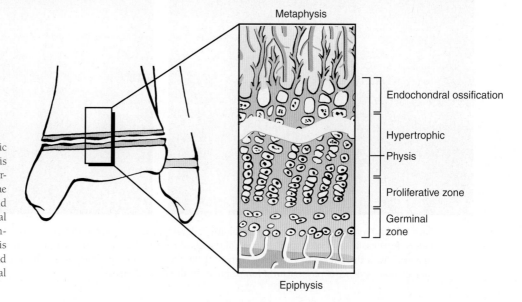

Metaphysis

Endochondral ossification

Hypertrophic
Physis

Proliferative zone

Germinal
zone

Epiphysis

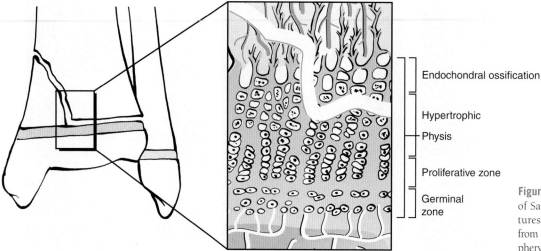

Endochondral ossification

Hypertrophic

Physis

Proliferative zone

Germinal zone

Figure 2-16. Fracture plane of Salter–Harris type II fractures. The fracture extends from the physis into the periphery of the metaphysis.

some portion of the peripheral metaphysis (the Thurston Holland fragment or sign). The physeal portion of this fracture has microscopic characteristics similar to those of type I injuries, but the fracture line exits the physis to enter the metaphysis (i.e., away from the germinal and proliferative layers) at one margin. Similar to type I injuries, these fractures should have a limited propensity to subsequent growth disturbance as a consequence of direct physeal injury. However, the metaphyseal "spike" of the diaphyseal/metaphyseal fragment may be driven into the physis of the epiphyseal fragment, which can damage the physis (Fig. 2-17). Similar to type I injuries, the articular surface is not affected and the general principles of fracture management are effectively the same.

Type III

Salter–Harris type III fractures begin in the epiphysis (with only rare exception) as a fracture through the articular surface and extend vertically toward the physis. The fracture then courses peripherally through the physis (Fig. 2-18). There are two fracture fragments: a small fragment consisting of a portion of the epiphysis and physis, and a large fragment consisting the remaining epiphysis and long bone. This fracture pattern is important for two main reasons: the articular surface is involved and the fracture line involves the germinal and proliferative layers of the physis. In addition, type III injuries are often associated with high-energy or compression mechanisms of injury, which imply greater potential disruption of the physis

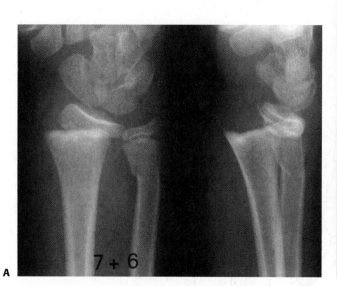
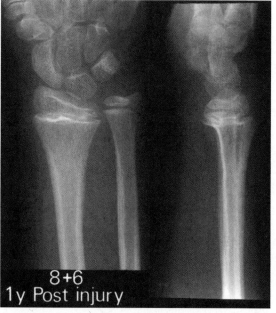

Figure 2-17. Potential mechanism of physeal arrest development after Salter–Harris type II fracture of the distal radius. **A:** Dorsally displaced type II fracture of the distal radius. Note the evidence of impaction of the epiphyseal fragment (with the physis) by the dorsal margin of the proximal fragment metaphysis. **B:** One year later, there is radiographic evidence of physeal arrest formation in the distal radial physis.

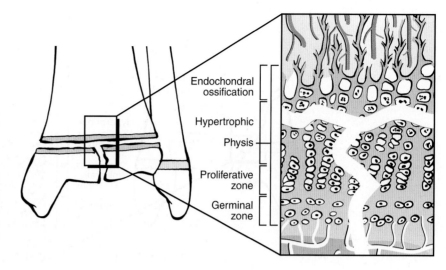

Figure 2-18. Scheme of fracture plane in Salter–Harris type III fractures. The fracture plane extends from the physis into the epiphysis and articular surface. "Extra-articular" type III fractures in which the articular surface is intact have been reported but are quite rare.

and higher risk of subsequent growth disturbance. Anatomic reduction (usually open) and stabilization are required to restore the articular surface and to minimize the potential for growth disturbance (Fig. 2-19).

Type IV

Type IV fractures are effectively vertical shear fractures, extending from the articular surface to the metaphysis (Fig. 2-20A). These fractures are important because they disrupt the articular surface, violate all the physeal layers in crossing from the epiphysis to the metaphysis, and, with displacement, may result in metaphyseal–epiphyseal cross union (Fig. 2-20B).[51,84] The latter occurrence almost invariably results in subsequent growth disturbance. This fracture pattern is frequent around the medial malleolus, but may occur in other epiphyses. Lateral condylar fractures of the distal humerus and intra-articular two-part triplane fractures of the distal tibia may be thought of as complex Salter–Harris type IV fractures.

General treatment principles include obtaining anatomic reduction and adequate stabilization to restore the articular surface and prevent metaphyseal–epiphyseal cross union.

Type V

The type V fracture described by Salter and Harris was not described by Poland or Aitken. Salter and Harris postulated that type V fractures represented unrecognized compression injuries with normal initial radiographs that later produced premature physeal closure. The existence of true type V injuries was questioned by Peterson and Burkhart[170] and subsequently became a subject of debate.[1,13,24,33,99,103,116,206] We believe that delayed physeal closure clearly occurs. The most common example of such an injury is closure of the tibial tubercle, often with the development of recurvatum deformity of the proximal tibia, after fractures of the femur or distal femoral epiphysis.[33,99,103] Although the mechanism of such injuries may be unclear (perhaps vascular rather than compression trauma), the traditionally held view that such injuries occurred as a result of inadvertent direct injury during the insertion of proximal tibial skeletal traction pins has been unequivocally discounted in some cases.[33,99,103] By definition, this pattern of injury is unrecognized on initial radiographs. Undoubtedly, more sophisticated imaging of injured extremities

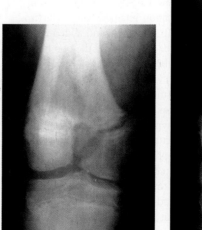
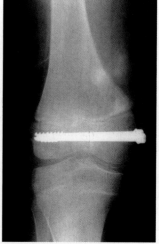

Figure 2-19. A: Salter–Harris type III fracture of the distal femur. **B:** Fixation with cannulated screws.

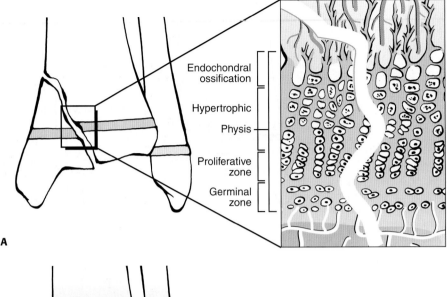

A

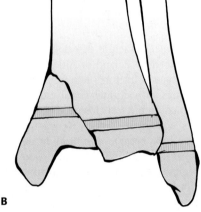

B

Figure 2-20. Scheme of the Salter–Harris type IV fracture. **A:** The fracture line extends across the physis from the epiphysis and articular surface into the peripheral metaphysis. **B:** Displacement of the fragments can lead to horizontal apposition (and cross union) of the epiphyseal and metaphyseal bones.

(such as with MRI) will identify physeal injuries in the presence of normal plain radiographs (Fig. 2-21). Although the mechanism of injury in type V injuries may be in dispute, in our opinion, the existence of such injuries is not.

Peterson Classification of Physeal Fractures

In an epidemiologic study of physeal injuries, Peterson et al.[170] identified several deficiencies of the Salter–Harris classification and subsequently developed a new classification of physeal fractures (Fig. 2-22). This classification retained Salter–Harris types I to IV as Peterson types II, III, IV, and V and added two new types.[168,169] It is important to be cognizant of the two new patterns that Peterson et al. described, because they are clinically relevant.

Peterson's type I is a transverse metaphyseal fracture with a longitudinal extension to the physis (Fig. 2-23). This pattern of injury is subclassified into four types, based on the extent of metaphyseal comminution and fracture pattern.

Peterson's type VI is a partial physeal loss. Unfortunately, this pattern of injury currently is common, largely as a consequence of lawn mower or "road-drag/abrasion" injuries. Soft tissue loss, neurovascular injury, and partial physeal loss (usually including the epiphysis so that articular impairment also results) further complicate this often devastating injury.

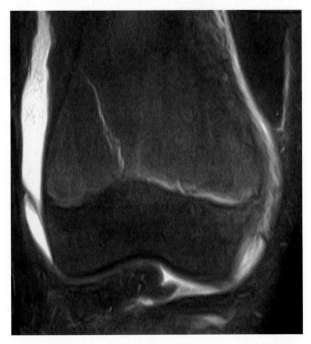

Figure 2-21. MRI of a patient after injury with normal radiographs. MRI clearly documents the presence of a Salter–Harris type II fracture of the distal femur.

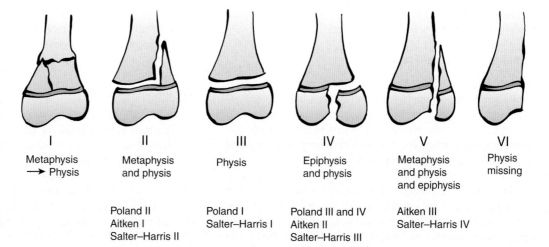

Figure 2-22. Peterson classification of physeal fractures. Type I is a fracture of the metaphysis extending to the physis. Peterson type VI is epiphyseal (and usually articular surface) loss. Lawn mower injuries are a frequent mechanism for type VI injuries.

I	II	III	IV	V	VI
Metaphysis → Physis	Metaphysis and physis	Physis	Epiphysis and physis	Metaphysis and physis and epiphysis	Physis missing
	Poland II Aitken I Salter–Harris II	Poland I Salter–Harris I	Poland III and IV Aitken II Salter–Harris III	Aitken III Salter–Harris IV	

Evaluation of Physeal Fractures

Modalities available for the evaluation of physeal injuries include plain radiographs, computed tomography (CT) scans, MRI scans,[46,60,81,108,109,172,196] arthrography,[6,65,89,139,211] and ultrasound.[37,66,67,98,188] Plain radiographs remain the preferred initial modality for the assessment of most physeal injuries. If a physeal injury is suspected, dedicated views centered over the suspected physis should be obtained to decrease parallax and increase detail. Oblique views may be of value in assessing minimally displaced injuries.

Although plain radiographs provide adequate detail for the assessment and treatment of most physeal injuries, occasionally greater anatomic detail is necessary. CT scans provide excellent definition of bony anatomy, particularly using reconstructed images. They may be helpful in assessing complex or highly comminuted fractures, as well as the articular congruency of minimally displaced fractures (Fig. 2-24). MRI scans are excellent for demonstrating soft tissue lesions and "bone bruises" which may not be seen using standard radiation techniques. MRI also has been shown to demonstrate entrapped periosteum in incomplete closed reduction of Salter–Harris type II fractures.[54,176] Arthrography, MRI, and ultrasound have been used to assess the congruency of articular surfaces. Arthrography and MRI may help define the anatomy in young patients with small or no secondary ossification centers in the epiphyses.[6,65,89,139,211]

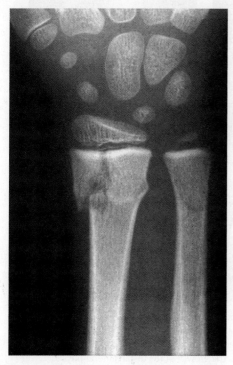

Figure 2-23. Peterson type I injury of the distal radius. These injuries typically have a benign course with respect to subsequent growth disturbance.

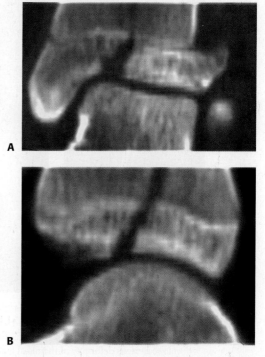

Figure 2-24. CT scans with or without reconstructed images can be helpful in the assessment of physeal fractures. Coronal (**A**) and sagittal (**B**) plane reconstructions of a triplane fracture of the distal tibia.

Ultrasonography is occasionally useful for diagnostic purposes to identify epiphyseal separation in infants.[37,65-67,98]

Treatment of Physeal Fractures

In general, fractures in children, including physeal injuries, heal more rapidly than in adults, and they are less likely to experience morbidity or mortality from prolonged immobilization. In addition, children are also often less compliant with postoperative activity restrictions, making cast immobilization a frequently necessary adjunct to therapy.

Physeal fractures, like all fractures, should be managed in a consistent methodical manner that includes a general assessment and stabilization of the polytraumatized patient, and evaluation of the neurovascular and soft tissue status of the traumatized limb; what constitutes an "acceptable" reduction is dictated in part by the fracture pattern and remodeling potential of the fracture. Intra-articular fractures (such as Salter–Harris types III and IV) require anatomic reduction to restore the articular surface and prevent epiphyseal–metaphyseal cross union. Salter–Harris type I and II fractures, particularly those that are the result of low-energy injuries, have minimal risk of growth disturbance (except injuries of the distal femur and proximal tibia) and excellent remodeling potential in most patients; in such patients, the surgeon must be cautious not to *create* physeal injury by excessive force or invasive reductions. When performing a closed reduction of physeal fractures the aphorism "90% traction, 10% translation" is useful to minimize iatrogenic injury to the physis which may occur as a physis grinds against a sharp bony metaphysis.

Complications of Physeal Fractures

Except for the possibility of subsequent growth disturbance, the potential complications of physeal injuries are no different than other traumatic musculoskeletal injuries. Neurovascular compromise and compartment syndrome represent the most serious potential complications.[36,160] Infection and soft tissue loss can complicate physeal fracture management, just as they can in other fractures. The one complication unique to physeal injuries is growth disturbance. Most commonly, this "disturbance" is the result of a tethering (physeal bar or arrest) that may produce angular deformity or shortening. However, growth disturbance may occur without an obvious tether or bar and growth acceleration also occurs (Fig. 2-25). Finally, growth disturbance may occur without recognized injury to the physis.

Physeal Growth Disturbance

An uncommon but important complication of physeal fracture is physeal growth disturbance.[141,150,178] The potential consequences

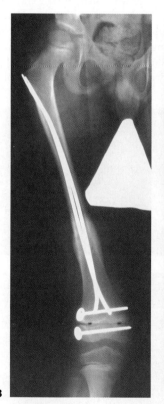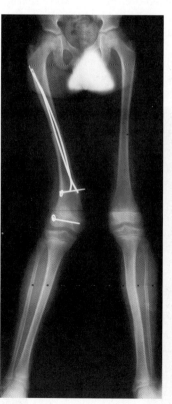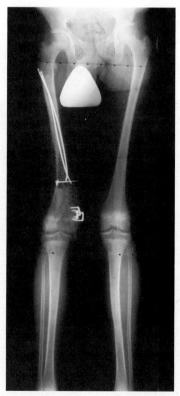

A, B   **C**

Figure 2-25. Growth deceleration in the absence of a true physeal arrest. This patient sustained concurrent ipsilateral femoral shaft and Salter–Harris type IV distal femoral epiphyseal fractures. **A:** Anteroposterior radiograph of the healed femur. Both fractures were treated with internal fixation. **B:** The patient developed valgus deformity of the distal femur because of asymmetric growth of the distal femoral physis. Note that the distance between the screws on either side of the physis has increased asymmetrically, confirming asymmetric growth rather than cessation of growth laterally. **C:** The angular deformity was treated with medial distal femoral epiphyseal stapling.

of physeal growth disturbance include the development of angular deformity, limb-length inequality, epiphyseal distortion, or various combinations of these. Development of these abnormalities, if any, depends on the physis affected, location within the affected physis, the duration of time present, and the skeletal maturity of the patient. Frequently, further surgery, often repeated and extensive, is required to correct or prevent deformity caused by an established growth disturbance.[35,38,91,113,124,128,186,210]

Etiology

Disturbance of normal physeal growth may result from physical loss of the physis (such as after Peterson type VI injuries), from disruption of normal physeal architecture and function without actual radiographic loss of the physis, or by the formation of a physeal arrest, also called bony bridges or physeal bars.[207]

Growth disturbance as a result of physeal injury may result from direct trauma (physeal fracture)[141,150,178] or associated vascular disruption.[167] Infection,[26,31] destruction by a space-occupying lesion such as unicameral bone cyst or enchondroma,[199] infantile Blount disease,[25] other vascular disturbances (such as purpura fulminans),[17,87,107,122] irradiation,[24,180] and other rare causes[27,39,48] also may result in physeal growth disturbance or physeal arrest.

Evaluation

Physeal growth disturbance may present as a radiographic abnormality noted on serial radiographs in a patient known to be at risk after fracture or infection, clinically with established limb deformity (angular deformity, shortening, or both), or occasionally incidentally on radiographs obtained for other reasons. The hallmark of plain radiographic features of physeal growth disturbance is the loss of normal physeal contour and the sharply defined radiolucency between epiphyseal and metaphyseal bones. Frank physeal arrests typically are characterized by sclerosis in the region of the arrest. If asymmetric growth has occurred, there may be tapering of a growth arrest line to the area of arrest,[90,154] angular deformity, epiphyseal distortion, or shortening (see Fig. 2-8). Physeal growth disturbance without frank arrest typically appears on plain radiographs as a thinner or thicker physeal area with an indistinct metaphyseal border because of alteration in normal endochondral ossification. There may be an asymmetric growth arrest line indicating angular deformity, but the arrest line will not taper to the physis itself.[154] This indicates altered physeal growth (either asymmetric acceleration or deceleration) but not a complete cessation of growth. This distinction is important, because the consequences and treatment are different from those caused by complete growth arrest.

If a growth arrest is suspected on plain radiographs in a skeletally immature child, further evaluation is often warranted. CT scanning with sagittal and coronal reconstructions (orthogonal to the area of interest) may demonstrate clearly an area of bone bridging the physis between the epiphysis and the metaphysis (Fig. 2-26). MRI is also a sensitive method of assessing physeal architecture.[46,69,81] Revealing images of the physis and the region of physeal growth disturbance can be obtained using three-dimensional (3D) spoiled recalled gradient-echo images with fat saturation or fast spin-echo proton density images with fat saturation (Fig. 2-27). MRI has the additional capability to

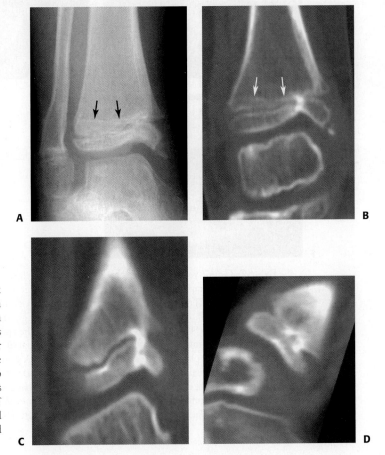

Figure 2-26. Harris growth arrest line tapering to the physis at the level of the growth arrest can serve as an excellent radiograph confirmation of the presence of the true growth arrest. Although most commonly noted on plain radiographs, these arrest lines can be seen on CT scans and MRIs as well. **A:** Anteroposterior radiograph of the distal tibia after Salter–Harris type IV fracture demonstrates a Harris growth arrest line (*arrows*) tapering to the medial distal tibial physis, where a partial physeal arrest has formed. **B:** Harris growth arrest line (*arrows*) as noted on CT. CT scans with coronal (**C**) and sagittal (**D**) reconstructions corrected for bone distortion provide excellent images of the location and size of the arrest.

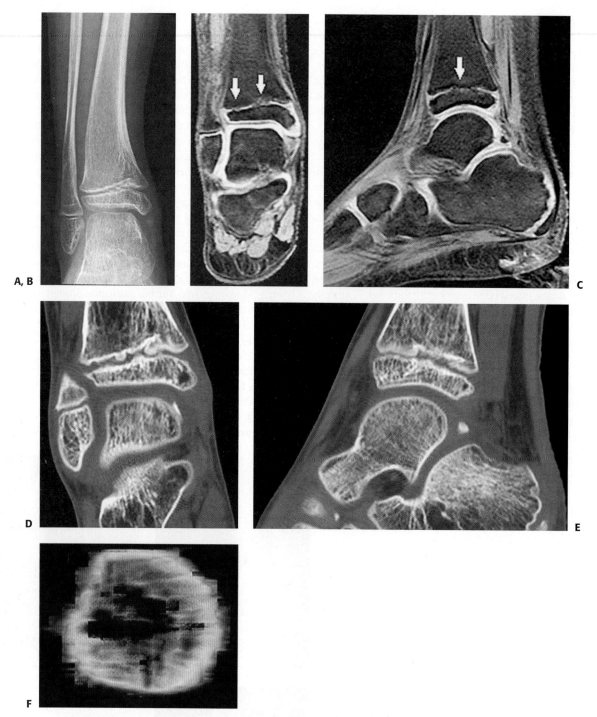

Figure 2-27. A 7-year-old girl presented with an ankle deformity after a trampoline injury 7 months prior. **A:** Frontal radiograph of the right ankle shows a varus deformity secondary to restriction of distal medial tibial growth. The growth plate, however, appears intact. Coronal and sagittal 3D SPGR MR images with fat suppression (**B, C**) of the ankle show two areas of bridging (*arrows*) across the growth plate on the coronal and sagittal views. These bridges are higher signal than the epiphyseal or metaphyseal bone and therefore may represent fibrous physeal bars. Corresponding coronal (**D**) and sagittal (**E**) CT reformations show narrowing of growth plate, but the actual bars are not seen. A volume-rendered model (**F**) of the growth plate is created by manually outlining the growth plate in the 3D SPGR sequence; a central U-shaped physeal bar with two free limbs is seen. Surface area occupied by the bar can then be calculated for treatment planning. (Reprinted by permission from Springer: Wang DC, Deeney V, Roach JW, et al. Imaging of physeal bars in children. *Pediatr Radiol.* 2015;45(9):1403–1412. Copyright © 2015 Springer-Verlag Berlin Heidelberg.)

assess the organization of the residual physis that may indicate its relative "health." This assessment may be helpful in cases of infection, irradiation, or tumor to determine if arrest resection is feasible based on the integrity of the remaining physis.

Although definitive assessment of physeal growth disturbance or arrest may require advanced imaging, further evaluation by plain radiographs is also beneficial. Radiographs of the entire affected limb should be obtained to document the magnitude of angular deformity. Existing limb-length inequality should be assessed by scanogram. Use of EOS low-dose biplanar radiographic imaging system is appealing for this purpose as it provides more accurate assessment of limb length than conventional radiographs and is associated with significantly lower dose of radiation.[71] An estimation of predicted growth remaining in the contralateral unaffected physis should be made based on a determination of the child's skeletal age and reference to an appropriate growth table.[14–16,86,94,95,138]

Growth Disturbance Without Arrest

Recognition

Growth disturbance may also occur without physeal arrest. Both growth deceleration and, less frequently, acceleration have been reported. Growth deceleration without arrest is characterized radiographically by the appearance of an injured physis (usually relative widening of the physis with indistinct metaphyseal boundaries). There may be associated clinical or radiographic deformity if the disturbance is severe and long standing. It is important to make a distinction between growth deceleration without complete cessation and true physeal arrest, because management and outcome are typically different in these two disorders. The concept of growth deceleration without arrest is most readily appreciated in patients with adolescent Blount disease and milder stages of infantile Blount disease. Recently, growth deceleration without physeal arrest has also been reported to produce distal femoral valgus deformity in obese adolescents.[195] Growth deceleration may also occur after infection and physeal fracture. In contrast to physeal arrests, there is no sclerotic area of arrest on plain radiographs (see Fig. 2-25). A growth arrest line, if present, may be asymmetric but will not taper to the physis, thereby suggesting growth asymmetry but not complete arrest. Furthermore, in some cases, deformity will not be relentlessly progressive and can actually improve over time.

Growth acceleration most classically occurs following proximal tibial fracture in young patients resulting in valgus deformity which usually spontaneously resolves.[104,111,156,194,195,214]

Management

Once a growth disturbance has been identified in a patient, its full impact should be assessed by determining the presence and extent of limb-length inequality and the calculated amount of potential growth remaining for the affected physis.

In some cases, the radiographic abnormality is stable and only longitudinal observation is required. This observation must be regular and careful, because progressive deformity will require treatment. If angular deformity is present or progressive, treatment options include hemiepiphysiodesis or physeal "tethering" with staples, screws, or tension plates[32,52,74,78,144,145,152,192,200,208] and corrective osteotomy, with or without completion of the epiphysiodesis. In the absence of frank arrest formation, hemiepiphysiodesis or "tethering" the affected physis with staples, screws, or tension plates on the convex side may result in gradual correction of the deformity. If correction occurs, options include completion of the epiphysiodesis (with contralateral epiphysiodesis if necessary to prevent the development of significant limb-length deformity) and removal of the tethering device with careful longitudinal observation for recurrence or overcorrection of deformity. Although there have been numerous publications regarding the various techniques and implants for physeal tethering, there is to date no solid evidence to support one technique. One pitfall to avoid is that a "tethering" technique (staples, plate, screw) opposite a known partial physeal arrest is unlikely to lead to correction of angular deformity, and is likely to lead to a complete growth arrest.

Corrective osteotomy is the other option for the management of growth disturbance with established angular deformity. The treating surgeon must decide whether to perform epiphysiodesis of the affected physis (with contralateral epiphysiodesis, if appropriate) to prevent recurrence or to ensure careful longitudinal observation of the growth performance of the affected physis until skeletal maturity.

PHYSEAL ARRESTS

Whenever a bridge of bone develops across a portion of the physis, tethering of the metaphyseal and epiphyseal bone together may result. Partial physeal arrests can result in angular deformity, joint distortion, limb-length inequality, or combinations of these, depending on the location of the arrest, the rate and extent of growth remaining in the physis involved, and the health of the residual affected physis.

Classification

Partial physeal arrests can be classified by etiology and anatomic pattern. Potential etiologies of physeal arrest include physeal fracture, Blount disease, infection, tumor, frostbite, and irradiation. Physeal arrests also can be classified based on the anatomic relationship of the arrest to the residual "healthy" physis. Three basic patterns are recognized (Fig. 2-28): central, peripheral, and linear. A *central* arrest is surrounded by a perimeter of normal

Figure 2-28. Anatomic classification of physeal arrests. Central arrests are surrounded by a perimeter of normal physis. Peripheral arrests are located at the perimeter of the physis. Linear arrests are "through-and-through" lesions with normal physis on either side of the arrest area.

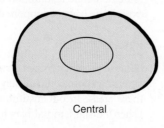

Central

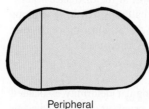

Peripheral

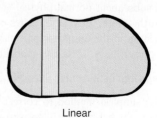

Linear

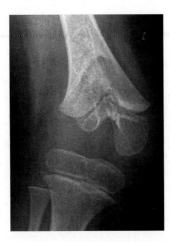

Figure 2-29. Central arrests are characterized by tenting of the articular surface. Variable shortening and angular deformity will develop, depending on the size and location of the arrest.

physis, like an island within the remaining physis. Central arrests are most likely to cause tenting of the articular surface, but also may result in angular deformity, if eccentrically located, and limb-length inequality (Fig. 2-29). A *peripheral* arrest is located at the perimeter of the affected physis. This type of arrest primarily causes progressive angular deformity and variable shortening. A *linear* arrest is a "through-and-through" lesion with anatomic characteristics of both central and peripheral arrests; specifically, the affected area starts at the perimeter of the physis and extends centrally with normal physis on either side of the affected area. Linear arrests most commonly develop after Salter–Harris type III or IV physeal fractures of the medial malleolus.

Management

Several management alternatives are available. It is important to be aware of these and to weigh carefully the appropriateness of each for the individual situation.

Prevention of Arrest Formation

Ideally, the surgeon should be proactive in the prevention of physeal arrest formation. Most commonly, this can be accomplished by adhering to the general treatment principles of physeal fractures: gentle, anatomic, and secure reduction of the fracture, especially Salter–Harris type III and IV injuries.

Physeal Distraction

Physeal arrests have been treated with the application of an external fixator spanning the arrest and gradual distraction until the arrest "separates."[44,61] Angular deformity correction and lengthening can be accomplished after separation as well. However, distraction injury usually results in complete cessation of subsequent normal physeal growth at the distracted level.[75] Furthermore, the fixation wires or half pins may have tenuous fixation in the epiphysis or violate the articular space, risking septic arthritis. Thus, this modality is rarely used.

Repeated Osteotomies During Growth

The simplest method to correct angular deformity associated with physeal arrests is corrective osteotomy in the adjacent

metaphysis. Of course, neither significant limb-length inequality nor epiphyseal distortion that may result from the arrest is corrected by this strategy. However, in young patients with a great deal of growth remaining in whom previous physeal arrest resection has been unsuccessful or is technically not possible, this treatment may be a reasonable interim alternative until more definitive completion of arrest and management of limb-length inequality is feasible.

Completion of Epiphysiodesis and Management of Resulting Limb-Length Discrepancy

An alternative strategy for the management of physeal arrests is to complete the epiphysiodesis to prevent recurrent angular deformity or epiphyseal distortion and manage the existing or potential limb-length discrepancy appropriately. Management of the latter may be by simultaneous or subsequent lengthening of the affected limb segment or contralateral epiphysiodesis if the existing discrepancy is tolerable and lengthening is not desired. We believe that this course of management is specifically indicated if arrest resection has failed to result in restoration of longitudinal growth and in patients in whom the amount of growth remaining does not warrant an attempt at arrest resection. In our opinion, this treatment should be considered carefully in all patients with a physeal arrest.

Partial Physeal Arrest Resection

Conceptually, surgical resection of a physeal arrest (sometimes referred to as *physiolysis* or *epiphysiolysis*) restoring normal growth of the affected physis is the ideal treatment for this condition.[35,38,51,79,113,125,127,128,141,158,209] The principle is to remove the bony tether between the metaphysis and the physis and fill the physeal defect with a bone reformation retardant, anticipating that the residual healthy physis will resume normal longitudinal growth.[35,79,124,127,128,158] However, this procedure can be technically demanding, and results in our practice are modest. To determine if this procedure is indicated, careful consideration must be given to the etiology, location, and extent of the arrest and the amount of longitudinal growth to be potentially salvaged.

Etiology of the Arrest

Arrests caused by trauma or infantile Blount disease have a better prognosis for resumption of normal growth, compared with those secondary to infection, tumor (or tumor-like conditions), or irradiation.

Anatomic Type of the Arrest

Central and linear arrests have been reported to be more likely to demonstrate resumption of growth after resection,[38] but our experience has not supported this observation.

Physis Affected

Because proximal humeral and proximal femoral lesions are difficult to expose, a technically adequate resection is less likely in these areas. In our institutional experience (currently unpublished), distal femoral bars have a poorer prognosis for growth after resection, whereas those of the distal tibia have a more favorable prognosis for the resumption of growth.

Extent of the Arrest

The potential for resumption of longitudinal growth after arrest resection is influenced by the amount of physeal surface area affected.[35,38,113] Arrests affecting more than 25% of the total surface area are unlikely to grow, and, except in patients in whom significant growth potential remains, alternative treatment strategies should be used.

Amount of Growth Remaining in the Physis Affected

Some authors[38,113,124,127,128,166] have stated that 2 years of growth remaining based on skeletal age determination is a prerequisite for arrest resection to be considered. Based on our results with this procedure, we find that 2 years of growth remaining is an inadequate indication for physeal arrest resection. We believe that the decision to perform arrest resection should be made based on a combination of the calculated amount of growth remaining in the affected physis and the likelihood of resumption of growth. A scanogram (Fig. 2-30) can be used to determine the existing discrepancy, determination of skeletal age and consultation with the growth remaining tables for the affected physis

(Table 2-1)[14–16,83,99,138] will allow calculation of the predicted discrepancy.

Preoperative Planning and Surgical Principles

If physeal arrest resection is considered appropriate, careful planning is required to maximize the opportunity for resumption of longitudinal growth. First, the extent and location of the arrest relative to the rest of the physis must be carefully documented. MRI is becoming the imaging study of choice. We currently prefer 3D spoiled recalled gradient-echo images with fat saturation or fast spin-echo proton density images with fat saturation to visualize the physis. CT images allow precise delineation of bony margins and, at the current time, are cheaper than MRI. An estimation of the affected surface area can be computed with the assistance of the radiologist using a modification of the method of Carlson and Wenger (Fig. 2-31).[47] The procedure should be planned with consideration of the following principles:

Minimize Trauma

The arrest must be resected in a manner that minimizes trauma to the residual physis. Central lesions should be approached either through a metaphyseal window (Fig. 2-32) or through

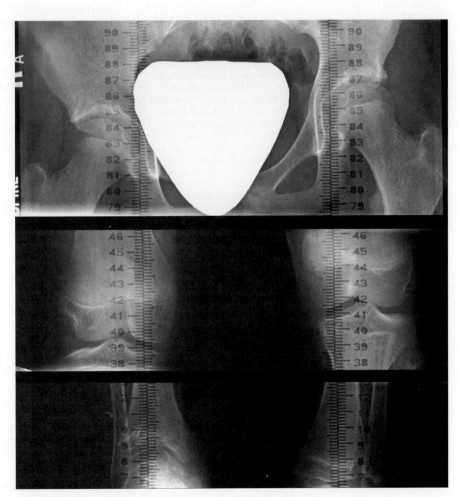

Figure 2-30. Scanogram indicates the existing limb-length inequality.

TABLE 2-1. Average Growth per Year (in mm) of Specific Physes of the Upper and Lower Extremities[a]

Location	Average Growth (mm/y)
Proximal humerus	7
Distal humerus	2
Proximal radius	1.75
Distal radius	5.25
Proximal ulna	5.5
Distal ulna	1.5
Proximal femur	3.5
Distal femur	9
Proximal tibia	6
Distal tibia	5
Proximal fibula	6.5
Distal fibula	4.5

[a]Estimations only. Gender, skeletal age, percentile height, and epiphyseal growth all influence magnitude of individual bone growth. Growth tables should be consulted when specific calculations are required. Adapted from growth studies.

Data from: Arriola F, Forriol F, Canadell J. Histomorphometric study of growth plate subjected to different mechanical conditions (compression, tension and neutralization): An experimental study in lambs. Mechanical growth plate behavior. *J Pediatr Orthop B.* 2001;10(4):334–338; Bright RW, Burstein AH, Elmore SM. Epiphyseal-plate cartilage. A biomechanical and histological analysis of failure modes. *J Bone Joint Surg Am.* 1974;56(4):688–703; Gomes LS, Volpon JB, Goncalves RP. Traumatic separation of epiphyses. An experimental study in rats. *Clin Orthop Relat Res.* 1988;236:286–295; Johnston RM, James WW. Fractures through human growth plates. *Orthop Trans.* 1980;4(295); Moen CT, Pelker RR. Biomechanical and histological correlations in growth plate failure. *J Pediatr Orthop.* 1984;4(2):180–184; Ogden JA. Skeletal growth mechanism injury patterns. *J Pediatr Orthop.* 1982;2(4):371–377; Rivas R, Shapiro F. Structural stages in the development of the long bones and epiphyses: A study in the New Zealand white rabbit. *J Bone Joint Surg Am.* 2002;84-A(1):85–100; Rudicel S, Pelker RR, Lee KE, et al. Shear fractures through the capital femoral physis of the skeletally immature rabbit. *J Pediatr Orthop.* 1985;5(1):27–31; Shapiro F. Epiphyseal growth plate fracture-separation: A pathophysiologic approach. *Orthopaedics.* 1982;5:720–736.

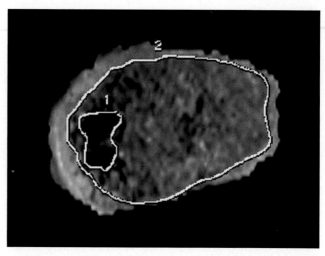

Figure 2-31. Reconstructed MRIs allow estimation of the percentage of surface area of the physis affected by a growth arrest. This workstation reconstruction delineates the perimeter of normal physis (border *2*) and that of the physeal arrest (border *1*). Surface area affected can be calculated from these reconstructions.

the intramedullary canal after a metaphyseal osteotomy. Peripheral lesions are approached directly, resecting the overlying periosteum to help prevent reformation of the arrest. Intraoperative imaging (fluoroscopy) is needed to keep the surgeon oriented properly to the arrest and the residual healthy physis. Care to provide adequate visualization of the surgical cavity is essential, because visualization is usually difficult even under "ideal" circumstances. A brilliant light source, magnification, and a dry surgical field are very helpful. An arthroscope can be inserted into a metaphyseal cavity to permit a circumferential view of the resection area. A high-speed burr worked in a gentle to-and-fro movement perpendicular to the physis is usually the most effective way to gradually remove the bony bridge and expose the residual healthy physis (Fig. 2-33). By the end of the resection, all of the bridging bone between the metaphysis and the epiphysis should be removed, leaving a void in the physis where the arrest had been, and the perimeter of the healthy residual physis should be visible circumferen-

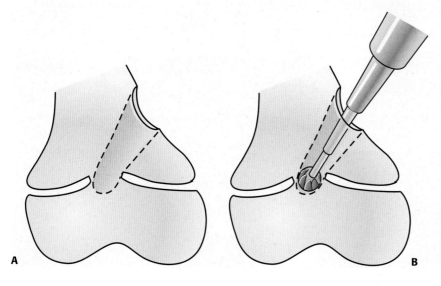

Figure 2-32. A: Central arrests are approached through a metaphyseal "window" or the medullary canal after metaphyseal osteotomy. **B:** The arrest is removed, leaving in its place a metaphyseal–epiphyseal cavity with intact physis surrounding the area of resection.

A   B

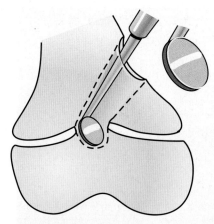

Figure 2-33. After complete resection, the healthy physis should be evident circumferentially within the cavity produced by the arrest resection.

tially at the margins of the surgically created cavity (Fig. 2-34). Recently, intraoperative CT has been reported to be an effective adjuvant to guide bar resection.[112]

Prevent Reforming of Bridge Between Metaphysis and Epiphysis

A bone-growth retardant or "spacer" material should be placed in the cavity created by the arrest resection to prevent reforming of the bony bridge between the metaphysis and the epiphysis. Four compounds have been used for this purpose either clinically or experimentally: autogenous fat,[38,113,124,127–130,210] methyl-methacrylate,[30,113,166] silicone rubber,[35] and autogenous cartilage.[23,25,76,88,114,133] Currently, only autogenous fat graft, harvested either locally or from the buttock, and methyl methacrylate are used clinically. Autogenous fat has at least a theoretic advantage of the ability to hypertrophy and migrate with longitudinal and interstitial growth (Fig. 2-35).[129,130] Methyl methacrylate is inert, but provides some immediate structural stability.[41] This feature may be important with large arrest resections in weight-bearing areas, as in the proximal tibia in association with infantile Blount disease. However, embedded methyl methacrylate, especially products without barium to clearly delineate its location on radiograph, can be extremely difficult to remove

and can jeopardize bone fixation if subsequent surgery is required. Pathologic fracture associated with methyl methacrylate migration from the metaphysis to diaphysis has also been reported.[191]

Marker Implantation

Metallic markers should be implanted in the epiphysis and metaphysis at the time of arrest resection to allow reasonably accurate estimation of the amount of longitudinal growth that occurs across the operated physis, as well as to identify the deceleration or cessation of that growth (see Fig. 2-35). We believe that precise monitoring of subsequent longitudinal growth is an important aspect of the management of patients after arrest resection. First, resumption of longitudinal growth may not occur despite technically adequate arrest resection in patients with good clinical indications. Perhaps more importantly, resumption of normal or even accelerated longitudinal growth may be followed by late deceleration or cessation of that growth.[91] It is imperative that the treating surgeon be alert to those developments, so that proper intervention can be instituted promptly. Embedded metallic markers serve those purposes admirably.

AUTHOR'S OBSERVATION

It has been our clinical observation that even patients who have significant resumption of growth following arrest resection will experience premature cessation of longitudinal growth of the affected physis relative to the contralateral uninvolved physis. We believe that even if growth resumes after bar resection, the previously injured physis will cease growing before the contralateral physis.

Our experience with physeal arrest resection prompted several conclusions and treatment recommendations.

* On average, approximately 60% of physeal arrests demonstrate clear radiograph evidence of resumption of longitudinal growth of the affected physis after physeal arrest resection.
* There is a correlation between the amount of surface area of the physis affected and the prognosis for subsequent longitudinal

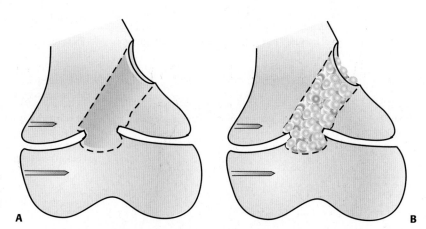

Figure 2-34. A: After the bar is resected, metallic markers are inserted in the epiphysis and metaphysis. **B:** Following marker placement fat graft is placed in the resection bed.

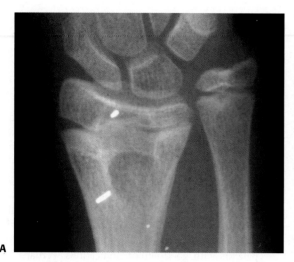 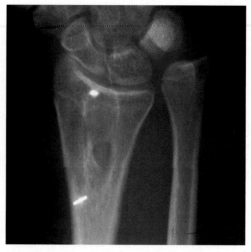

Figure 2-35. Fat used as an interposition material in partial physeal arrest resection can persist and hypertrophy during longitudinal growth. **A:** Radiograph appearance after traumatic distal radial physeal arrest resection. **B:** Appearance 5 years later. Longitudinal growth between the metallic markers is obvious. The fat-filled cavity created at physeal arrest resection has persisted and elongated with distal radial growth.

growth after arrest resection. Physeal arrests affecting less than 10% of the surface area of the physis have a better prognosis than larger arrests.

- Langenskiold stage VI infantile Blount disease has results comparable to posttraumatic physeal arrests.
- Etiologies other than posttraumatic and infantile Blount disease have poor prognoses for subsequent growth.
- Central and peripheral arrests have equivalent prognoses with respect to resumption of growth.
- Early growth resumption may be followed by cessation of longitudinal growth before skeletal maturity. As a consequence, patients must be evaluated regularly until skeletal maturity with some reliable method (such as metaphyseal

and epiphyseal radiograph markers) to detect such development as promptly as possible.

We believe that physeal bar resection has a role to play in patients with significant longitudinal growth remaining. However, the benefits of such surgery must be weighed against the actual amount of growth remaining, and the etiology, location, and extent of the physeal arrest must be considered. The appropriate time to add a corrective osteotomy to bony bar resection is controversial. Generally, when the angular deformity is more than 10 to 15 degrees from normal, corrective osteotomy should be considered.

Annotated References

Reference	Annotation
Langenskiold A. Surgical treatment of partial closure of the growth plate. *J Pediatr Orthop.* 1981;1(1):3–11.	This article reports the outcomes of 35 patients who had physeal bar resection and free fat interposition graft for partial physeal arrest. This case series includes patients treated from 1965 when this procedure was introduced by Langenskiold and is one of the first articles to discuss the factors that affect outcome.
Peterson HA. Physeal fractures: Part 2. Two previously unclassified types. *J Pediatr Orthop.* 1994;14(4):431–438.	This article describes two physeal fractures not classified in the Salter–Harris classification: a metaphyseal fracture with extension to the physis without extension of the fracture along the physis and an open fracture with a portion of the physis missing which almost always leads to premature physeal closure.
Salter R. Injuries involving the epiphyseal plate. *J Bone Joint Surg Am.* 1963;45:587–622.	Most commonly used classification for growth plate injuries. The classification includes type V compression injury which was not previously recognized. The classification is based on experimental and clinical observations and provides prognostic information.

REFERENCES

1. Abram LJ, Thompson GH. Deformity after premature closure of the distal radial physis following a torus fracture with a physeal compression injury. Report of a case. *J Bone Joint Surg Am.* 1987;69(9):1450–1453.
2. Aitken AP. The end results of the fractured distal tibial epiphysis. *J Bone Joint Surg Am.* 1936;18:685–691.
3. Aitken AP. Fractures of the epiphyses. *Clin Orthop Relat Res.* 1965;41:19–23.
4. Aitken AP. Fractures of the proximal tibial epiphysial cartilage. *Clin Orthop Relat Res.* 1965;41:92–97.
5. Aitken AP, Magill HK. Fractures involving the distal femoral epiphyseal cartilage. *J Bone Joint Surg Am.* 1952;34-A(1):96–108.
6. Akbarnia BA, Silberstein MJ, Rende RJ, et al. Arthrography in the diagnosis of fractures of the distal end of the humerus in infants. *J Bone Joint Surg Am.* 1986;68(4):599–602.
7. Akiyama H, Kim JE, Nakashima K, et al. Osteo-chondroprogenitor cells are derived from Sox9 expressing precursors. *Proc Natl Acad Sci U S A.* 2005;102(41):14665–14670.
8. Al Muderis M, Azzopardi T, Cundy P. Zebra lines of pamidronate therapy in children. *J Bone Joint Surg Am.* 2007;89(7):1511–1516.
9. Albanese SA, Palmer AK, Kerr DR, et al. Wrist pain and distal growth plate closure of the radius in gymnasts. *J Pediatr Orthop.* 1989;9(1):23–28.
10. Allen MR, Hock JM, Burr DB. Periosteum: biology, regulation, and response to osteoporosis therapies. *Bone.* 2004;35(5):1003–1012.
11. Amini S, Mortazavi F, Sun J, et al. Stress relaxation of swine growth plate in semi-confined compression: depth dependent tissue deformational behavior versus extracellular matrix composition and collagen fiber organization. *Biomech Model Mechanobiol.* 2013;12(1):67–78.
12. Amini S, Veilleux D, Villemure I. Tissue and cellular morphological changes in growth plate explants under compression. *J Biomech.* 2010;43(13):2582–2588.
13. Aminian A, Schoenecker PL. Premature closure of the distal radial physis after fracture of the distal radial metaphysis. *J Pediatr Orthop.* 1995;15(4):495–498.
14. Anderson M, Green WT. Lengths of the femur and the tibia; norms derived from orthoroentgenograms of children from 5 years of age until epiphysial closure. *Am J Dis Child.* 1948;75(3):279–290.
15. Anderson M, Green WT, Messner MB. Growth and predictions of growth in the lower extremities. *J Bone Joint Surg Am.* 1963;45-A:1–14.
16. Anderson M, Messner MB, Green WT. Distribution of lengths of the normal femur and tibia in children from one to eighteen years of age. *J Bone Joint Surg Am.* 1964;46:1197–1202.
17. Appel M, Pauleto AC, Cunha LA. Osteochondral sequelae of meningococcemia: radiographic aspects. *J Pediatr Orthop.* 2002;22(4):511–516.
18. Arikawa T, Omura K, Morita I. Regulation of bone morphogenetic protein-2 expression by endogenous prostaglandin E2 in human mesenchymal stem cells. *J Cell Physiol.* 2004;200(3):400–406.
19. Armulik A, Genove G, Betsholtz C. Pericytes: developmental, physiological, and pathological perspectives, problems, and promises. *Dev Cell.* 2011;21(2):193–215.
20. Augustin G, Antabak A, Davila S. The periosteum. Part 1: Anatomy, histology and molecular biology. *Injury.* 2007;38(10):1115–1130.
21. Bafico A, Liu G, Yaniv A, et al. Novel mechanism of Wnt signalling inhibition mediated by Dickkopf-1 interaction with LRP6/Arrow. *Nat Cell Biol.* 2001;3(7):683–686.
22. Ballock RT, O'Keefe RJ. Physiology and pathophysiology of the growth plate. *Birth Defects Res C Embryo Today.* 2003;69(2):123–143.
23. Barr SJ, Zaleske DJ. Physeal reconstruction with blocks of cartilage of varying developmental time. *J Pediatr Orthop.* 1992;12(6):766–773.
24. Beals RK. Premature closure of the physis following diaphyseal fractures. *J Pediatr Orthop.* 1990;10(6):717–720.
25. Beck CL, Burke SW, Roberts JM, et al. Physeal bridge resection in infantile Blount disease. *J Pediatr Orthop.* 1987;7(2):161–163.
26. Bergdahl S, Ekengren K, Eriksson M. Neonatal hematogenous osteomyelitis: risk factors for long-term sequelae. *J Pediatr Orthop.* 1985;5(5):564–568.
27. Bigelow D. The effects of frostbite in childhood. *J Bone Joint Surg Br.* 1963;45-B(1):122–131.
28. Bitgood MJ, McMahon AP. Hedgehog and Bmp genes are coexpressed at many diverse sites of cell-cell interaction in the mouse embryo. *Dev Biol.* 1995;172(1):126–138.
29. Blackwell KA, Raisz LG, Pilbeam CC. Prostaglandins in bone: bad cop, good cop? *Trends Endocrinol Metab.* 2010;21(5):294–301.
30. Bollini G, Tallet JM, Jacquemier M, et al. New procedure to remove a centrally located bone bar. *J Pediatr Orthop.* 1990;10(5):662–666.
31. Bos CF, Mol LJ, Obermann WR, et al. Late sequelae of neonatal septic arthritis of the shoulder. *J Bone Joint Surg Br.* 1998;80(4):645–650.
32. Bowen JR, Torres RR, Forlin E. Partial epiphysiodesis to address genu varum or genu valgum. *J Pediatr Orthop.* 1992;12(3):359–364.
33. Bowler JR, Mubarak SJ, Wenger DR. Tibial physeal closure and genu recurvatum after femoral fracture: occurrence without a tibial traction pin. *J Pediatr Orthop.* 1990;10(5):653–657.
34. Boyd KT, Batt ME. Stress fracture of the proximal humeral epiphysis in an elite junior badminton player. *Br J Sports Med.* 1997;31(3):252–253.
35. Bright RW. Operative correction of partial epiphyseal plate closure by osseous-bridge resection and silicone-rubber implant. An experimental study in dogs. *J Bone Joint Surg Am.* 1974;56(4):655–664.
36. Brogle PJ, Gaffney JT, Denton JR. Acute compartment syndrome complicating a distal tibial physeal fracture in a neonate. *Am J Orthop (Belle Mead NJ).* 1999;28(10):587–589.
37. Broker FH, Burbach T. Ultrasonic diagnosis of separation of the proximal humeral epiphysis in the newborn. *J Bone Joint Surg Am.* 1990;72(2):187–191.
38. Broughton NS, Dickens DR, Cole WG, Menelaus MB. Epiphyseolysis for partial growth plate arrest. Results after four years or at maturity. *J Bone Joint Surg Br.* 1989;71(1):13–16.
39. Brown FE, Spiegel PK, Boyle WE Jr. Digital deformity: an effect of frostbite in children. *Pediatrics.* 1983;71(6):955–959.
40. Buckwalter JA, Cooper RR. Bone structure and function. *Instr Course Lect.* 1987;36:27–48.
41. Bueche MJ, Phillips WA, Gordon J, et al. Effect of interposition material on mechanical behavior in partial physeal resection: a canine model. *J Pediatr Orthop.* 1990;10(4):459–462.
42. Burkus JK, Ogden JA. Development of the distal femoral epiphysis: a microscopic morphological investigation of the zone of Ranvier. *J Pediatr Orthop.* 1984;4(6):661–668.
43. Butler MS, Robertson WW Jr, Rate W, et al. Skeletal sequelae of radiation therapy for malignant childhood tumors. *Clin Orthop Relat Res.* 1990;(251):235–240.
44. Canadell J, de Pablos J. Breaking bony bridges by physeal distraction. A new approach. *Int Orthop.* 1985;9(4):223–229.
45. Caplan AI. Bone development and repair. *Bioessays.* 1987;6(4):171–175.
46. Carey J, Spence L, Blickman H, et al. MRI of pediatric growth plate injury: correlation with plain film radiographs and clinical outcome. *Skeletal Radiol.* 1998;27(5):250–255.
47. Carlson WO, Wenger DR. A mapping method to prepare for surgical excision of a partial physeal arrest. *J Pediatr Orthop.* 1984;4(2):232–238.
48. Carrera GF, Kozin F, Flaherty L, et al. Radiographic changes in the hands following childhood frostbite injury. *Skeletal Radiol.* 1981;6(1):33–37.
49. Carson WG Jr, Gasser SI. Little Leaguer's shoulder. A report of 23 cases. *Am J Sports Med.* 1998;26(4):575–580.
50. Carter SR, Aldridge MJ. Stress injury of the distal radial growth plate. *J Bone Joint Surg Br.* 1988;70(5):834–836.
51. Cass JR, Peterson HA. Salter-Harris Type-IV injuries of the distal tibial epiphyseal growth plate, with emphasis on those involving the medial malleolus. *J Bone Joint Surg Am.* 1983;65(8):1059–1070.
52. Castaneda P, Urquhart B, Sullivan E, et al. Hemiepiphysiodesis for the correction of angular deformity about the knee. *J Pediatr Orthop.* 2008;28(2):188–191.
53. Champagne CM, Takebe J, Offenbacher S, et al. Macrophage cell lines produce osteoinductive signals that include bone morphogenetic protein-2. *Bone.* 2002;30(1):26–31.
54. Chen J, Abel MF, Fox MG. Imaging appearance of entrapped periosteum within a distal femoral Salter-Harris II fracture. *Skeletal Radiol.* 2015;44(10):1547–1551.
55. Chen Y, Whetstone HC, Lin AC, et al. Beta-catenin signaling plays a disparate role in different phases of fracture repair: implications for therapy to improve bone healing. *PLoS Med.* 2007;4(7):e249.
56. Chen Y, Whetstone HC, Youn A, et al. Beta-catenin signaling pathway is crucial for bone morphogenetic protein 2 to induce new bone formation. *J Biol Chem.* 2007;282(1):526–533.
57. Cheon JE, Kim IO, Choi IH, et al. Magnetic resonance imaging of remaining physis in partial physeal resection with graft interposition in a rabbit model: a comparison with physeal resection alone. *Invest Radiol.* 2005;40(4):235–242.
58. Cheon SS, Wei Q, Gurung A, et al. Beta-catenin regulates wound size and mediates the effect of TGF-beta in cutaneous healing. *FASEB J.* 2006;20(6):692–701.
59. Cho TJ, Gerstenfeld LC, Einhorn TA. Differential temporal expression of members of the transforming growth factor beta superfamily during murine fracture healing. *J Bone Miner Res.* 2002;17(3):513–520.
60. Close BJ, Strouse PJ. MR of physeal fractures of the adolescent knee. *Pediatr Radiol.* 2000;30(11):756–762.
61. Connolly J. Physeal distraction treatment of fracture deformities. *Orthop Trans.* 1991;3(2):321–322.
62. Cooper C, Dennison EM, Leufkens HG, et al. Epidemiology of childhood fractures in Britain: a study using the general practice research database. *J Bone Miner Res.* 2004;19(12):1976–1981.
63. Dale GG, Harris WR. Prognosis of epiphysial separation: an experimental study. *J Bone Joint Surg Br.* 1958;40-B(1):116–122.
64. Dalton SE. Overuse injuries in adolescent athletes. *Sports Med.* 1992;13(1):58–70.
65. Davidson RS, Markowitz RI, Dormans J, et al. Ultrasonographic evaluation of the elbow in infants and young children after suspected trauma. *J Bone Joint Surg Am.* 1994;76(12):1804–1813.
66. Dias JJ, Lamont AC, Jones JM. Ultrasonic diagnosis of neonatal separation of the distal humeral epiphysis. *J Bone Joint Surg Br.* 1988;70(5):825–828.
67. Diaz MJ, Hedlund GL. Sonographic diagnosis of traumatic separation of the proximal femoral epiphysis in the neonate. *Pediatr Radiol.* 1991;21(3):238–240.
68. Dimitriou R, Tsiridis E, Giannoudis PV. Current concepts of molecular aspects of bone healing. *Injury.* 2005;36(12):1392–1404.
69. Ecklund K, Jaramillo D. Patterns of premature physeal arrest: MR imaging of 111 children. *AJR Am J Roentgenol.* 2002;178(4):967–972.
70. Einhorn TA. The cell and molecular biology of fracture healing. *Clin Orthop Relat Res.* 1998;(355 Suppl):S7–S21.
71. Escott BG, Ravi B, Weathermon AC, et al. EOS low-dose radiography: a reliable and accurate upright assessment of lower-limb lengths. *J Bone Joint Surg Am.* 2013;95(23):e1831–e1837.
72. Farnum CE, Lenox M, Zipfel W, et al. In vivo delivery of fluoresceinated dextrans to the murine growth plate: imaging of three vascular routes by multiphoton microscopy. *Anat Rec A Discov Mol Cell Evol Biol.* 2006;288(1):91–103.
73. Feldman DS, Jordan C, Fonseca L. Orthopaedic manifestations of neurofibromatosis type 1. *J Am Acad Orthop Surg.* 2010;18(6):346–357.
74. Ferrick MR, Birch JG, Albright M. Correction of non-Blount's angular knee deformity by permanent hemiepiphyseodesis. *J Pediatr Orthop.* 2004;24(4):397–402.
75. Fjeld TO, Steen H. Growth retardation after experimental limb lengthening by epiphyseal distraction. *J Pediatr Orthop.* 1990;10(4):463–466.
76. Foster BK, Hansen AL, Gibson GJ, et al. Reimplantation of growth plate chondrocytes into growth plate defects in sheep. *J Orthop Res.* 1990;8(4):555–564.

77. Foster BK, John B, Hasler C. Free fat interpositional graft in acute physeal injuries: the anticipatory Langenskiold procedure. *J Pediatr Orthop.* 2000;20(3):282–285.

78. Fraser RK, Dickens DR, Cole WG. Medial physeal stapling for primary and secondary genu valgum in late childhood and adolescence. *J Bone Joint Surg Br.* 1995; 77(5):733–735.

79. Freidenberg Z. Reaction of the epiphysis to partial surgical resection. *J Bone Joint Surg Am.* 1957;39-A(2):332–340.

80. Friberg KS. Remodelling after distal forearm fractures in children. I. The effect of residual angulation on the spatial orientation of the epiphyseal plates. *Acta Orthop Scand.* 1979;50(5):537–546.

81. Gabel GT, Peterson HA, Berquist TH. Premature partial physeal arrest. Diagnosis by magnetic resonance imaging in two cases. *Clin Orthop Relat Res.* 1991;(272):242–247.

82. Glorieux FH. Treatment of osteogenesis imperfecta: who, why, what? *Horm Res.* 2007;68 Suppl 5:8–11.

83. Goldfarb CA, Bassett GS, Sullivan S, et al. Retrosternal displacement after physeal fracture of the medial clavicle in children treatment by open reduction and internal fixation. *J Bone Joint Surg Br.* 2001;83(8):1168–1172.

84. Gomes LS, Volpon JB. Experimental physeal fracture-separations treated with rigid internal fixation. *J Bone Joint Surg Am.* 1993;75(12):1756–1764.

85. Govender S, Csimma C, Genant HK, et al. Recombinant human bone morphogenetic protein-2 for treatment of open tibial fractures: a prospective, controlled, randomized study of four hundred and fifty patients. *J Bone Joint Surg Am.* 2002;84-A(12):2123–2134.

86. Green WT, Anderson M. Skeletal age and the control of bone growth. *Instr Course Lect.* 1960;17:199–217.

87. Grogan DP, Love SM, Ogden JA, et al. Chondro-osseous growth abnormalities after meningococcemia. A clinical and histopathological study. *J Bone Joint Surg Am.* 1989; 71(6):920–928.

88. Hansen AL, Foster BK, Gibson GJ, et al. Growth-plate chondrocyte cultures for reimplantation into growth-plate defects in sheep. Characterization of cultures. *Clin Orthop Relat Res.* 1990;(256):286–298.

89. Hansen PE, Barnes DA, Tullos HS. Arthrographic diagnosis of an injury pattern in the distal humerus of an infant. *J Pediatr Orthop.* 1982;2(5):569–572.

90. Harris HA. Lines of arrested growth in the long bones of diabetic children. *Br Med J.* 1931;1(3668):700–714.3.

91. Hasler CC, Foster BK. Secondary tethers after physeal bar resection: a common source of failure? *Clin Orthop Relat Res.* 2002;(405):242–249.

92. Heck RK Jr, Sawyer JR, Warner WC, et al. Progressive valgus deformity after curettage of benign lesions of the proximal tibia. *J Pediatr Orthop.* 2008;28(7): 757–760.

93. Hedstrom EM, Svensson O, Bergstrom U, et al. Epidemiology of fractures in children and adolescents. *Acta Orthop.* 2010;81(1):148–153.

94. Hensinger R. Linear growth of long bones of the lower extremity from infancy to adolescence. In: Hensinger R, ed. *Standards in Pediatric Orthopaedics: Table, Charts, and Graphs Illustrating Growth.* New York: Raven Press Books; 1986: 232–233.

95. Hensinger R. *Standards in Pediatric Orthopaedics: Tables, Charts, and Graphs, Illustrating Growth.* New York: Raven Press Books; 1986.

96. Hill TP, Spater D, Taketo MM, et al. Canonical Wnt/beta-catenin signaling prevents osteoblasts from differentiating into chondrocytes. *Dev Cell.* 2005;8(5):727–738.

97. Houshian S, Holst AK, Larsen MS, et al. Remodeling of Salter-Harris type II epiphyseal plate injury of the distal radius. *J Pediatr Orthop.* 2004;24(5):472–476.

98. Howard CB, Shinwell E, Nyska M, et al. Ultrasound diagnosis of neonatal fracture separation of the upper humeral epiphysis. *J Bone Joint Surg Br.* 1992;74(3):471–472.

99. Hresko MT, Kasser JR. Physeal arrest about the knee associated with non-physeal fractures in the lower extremity. *J Bone Joint Surg Am.* 1989;71(5):698–703.

100. Hu H, Hilton MJ, Tu X, et al. Sequential roles of Hedgehog and Wnt signaling in osteoblast development. *Development.* 2005;132(1):49–60.

101. Huang W, Chung UI, Kronenberg HM, et al. The chondrogenic transcription factor Sox9 is a target of signaling by the parathyroid hormone-related peptide in the growth plate of endochondral bones. *Proc Natl Acad Sci U S A.* 2001;98(1):160–165.

102. Hui JH, Li L, Teo YH, et al. Comparative study of the ability of mesenchymal stem cells derived from bone marrow, periosteum, and adipose tissue in treatment of partial growth arrest in rabbit. *Tissue Eng.* 2005;11(5-6):904–912.

103. Hunter LY, Hensinger RN. Premature monomelic growth arrest following fracture of the femoral shaft. A case report. *J Bone Joint Surg Am.* 1978;60(6):850–852.

104. Ippolito E, Pentimalli G. Post-traumatic valgus deformity of the knee in proximal tibial metaphyseal fractures in children. *Ital J Orthop Traumatol.* 1984;10(1):103–108.

105. Jackson WF, Theologis TN, Gibbons CL, et al. Early management of pathological fractures in children. *Injury.* 2007;38(2):194–200.

106. Jacobsen FS. Periosteum: its relation to pediatric fractures. *J Pediatr Orthop B.* 1997;6(2):84–90.

107. Jacobsen ST, Crawford AH. Amputation following meningococcemia. A sequela to purpura fulminans. *Clin Orthop Relat Res.* 1984;(185):214–219.

108. Jain R, Bielski RJ. Fracture of lower femoral epiphysis in an infant at birth: a rare obstetrical injury. *J Perinatol.* 2001;21(8):550–552.

109. Jaramillo D, Kammen BF, Shapiro F. Cartilaginous path of physeal fracture-separations: evaluation with MR imaging–an experimental study with histologic correlation in rabbits. *Radiology.* 2000;215(2):504–511.

110. Jayakumar P, Barry M, Ramachandran M. Orthopaedic aspects of paediatric non-accidental injury. *J Bone Joint Surg Br.* 2010;92(2):189–195.

111. Jordan SE, Alonso JE, Cook FF. The etiology of valgus angulation after metaphyseal fractures of the tibia in children. *J Pediatr Orthop.* 1987;7(4):450–457.

112. Kang HG, Yoon SJ, Kim JR. Resection of a physeal bar under computer-assisted guidance. *J Bone Joint Surg Br.* 2010;92(10):1452–1455.

113. Kasser JR. Physeal bar resections after growth arrest about the knee. *Clin Orthop Relat Res.* 1990;(255):68–74.

114. Kawabe N, Ehrlich MG, Mankin HJ. Growth plate reconstruction using chondrocyte allograft transplants. *J Pediatr Orthop.* 1987;7(4):381–388.

115. Keaveny TM, Hayes WC. A 20-year perspective on the mechanical properties of trabecular bone. *J Biomech Eng.* 1993;115(4B):534–542.

116. Keret D, Mendez AA, Harcke HT, et al. Type V physeal injury: a case report. *J Pediatr Orthop.* 1990;10(4):545–548.

117. Kim HK, Stephenson N, Garces A, et al. Effects of disruption of epiphyseal vasculature on the proximal femoral growth plate. *J Bone Joint Surg Am.* 2009;91(5):1149–1158.

118. Kitase Y, Barragan L, Qing H, et al. Mechanical induction of PGE2 in osteocytes blocks glucocorticoid-induced apoptosis through both the beta-catenin and PKA pathways. *J Bone Miner Res.* 2010;25(12):2657–2668.

119. Kloen P, Doty SB, Gordon E, et al. Expression and activation of the BMP-signaling components in human fracture nonunions. *J Bone Joint Surg Am.* 2002;84-A(11):1909–1918.

120. Kolpakova E, Olsen BR. Wnt/beta-catenin–a canonical tale of cell-fate choice in the vertebrate skeleton. *Dev Cell.* 2005;8(5):626–627.

121. Kronenberg HM. Developmental regulation of the growth plate. *Nature.* 2003; 423(6937):332–336.

122. Kruse RW, Tassanawipas A, Bowen JR. Orthopedic sequelae of meningococcemia. *Orthopedics.* 1991;14(2):174–178.

123. Landin LA. Fracture patterns in children. Analysis of 8,682 fractures with special reference to incidence, etiology and secular changes in a Swedish urban population 1950–1979. *Acta Orthop Scand Suppl.* 1983;202:1–109.

124. Langenskiold A. The possibilities of eliminating premature partial closure of an epiphyseal plate caused by trauma or disease. *Acta Orthop Scand.* 1967;38:267–279.

125. Langenskiold A. Traumatic premature closure of the distal tibial epiphyseal plate. *Acta Orthop Scand.* 1967;38(4):520–531.

126. Langenskiold A. An operation for partial closure of an epiphysial plate in children, and its experimental basis. *J Bone Joint Surg Br.* 1975;57(3):325–330.

127. Langenskiold A. Surgical treatment of partial closure of the growth plate. *J Pediatr Orthop.* 1981;1(1):3–11.

128. Langenskiold A. Growth disturbance after osteomyelitis of femoral condyles in infants. *Acta Orthop Scand.* 1984;55(1):1–13.

129. Langenskiold A, Osterman K, Valle M. Growth of fat grafts after operation for partial bone growth arrest: demonstration by computed tomography scanning. *J Pediatr Orthop.* 1987;7(4):389–394.

130. Langenskiold A, Videman T, Nevalainen T. The fate of fat transplants in operations for partial closure of the growth plate. Clinical examples and an experimental study. *J Bone Joint Surg Br.* 1986;68(2):234–238.

131. Larsen E, Vittas D, Torp Pedersen S. Remodeling of angulated distal forearm fractures in children. *Clin Orthop Relat Res.* 1988;(237):190–195.

132. Lee EH, Chen F, Chan J, et al. Treatment of growth arrest by transfer of cultured chondrocytes into physeal defects. *J Pediatr Orthop.* 1998;18(2):155–160.

133. Lennox DW, Goldner RD, Sussman MD. Cartilage as an interposition material to prevent transphyseal bone bridge formation: an experimental model. *J Pediatr Orthop.* 1983;3(2):207–210.

134. Liebling MS, Berdon WE, Ruzal-Shapiro C, et al. Gymnast's wrist (pseudorickets growth plate abnormality) in adolescent athletes: findings on plain films and MR imaging. *AJR Am J Roentgenol.* 1995;164(1):157–159.

135. Lyons KM, Pelton RW, Hogan BL. Patterns of expression of murine Vgr-1 and BMP-2a RNA suggest that transforming growth factor-beta-like genes coordinately regulate aspects of embryonic development. *Genes Dev.* 1989;3(11): 1657–1668.

136. Mackie EJ, Tatarczuch L, Mirams M. The skeleton: a multi-functional complex organ: the growth plate chondrocyte and endochondral ossification. *J Endocrinol.* 2011;211(2):109–121.

137. Mann DC, Rajmaira S. Distribution of physeal and nonphyseal fractures in 2,650 long-bone fractures in children aged 0–16 years. *J Pediatr Orthop.* 1990;10(6):713–716.

138. Maresh MM. Linear growth of long bones of extremities from infancy through adolescence; continuing studies. *AMA Am J Dis Child.* 1955;89(6):725–742.

139. Marzo JM, d'Amato C, Strong M, et al. Usefulness and accuracy of arthrography in management of lateral humeral condyle fractures in children. *J Pediatr Orthop.* 1990;10(3):317–321.

140. Mayba II. Avulsion fracture of the tibial tubercle apophysis with avulsion of patellar ligament. *J Pediatr Orthop.* 1982;2(3):303–305.

141. Mayer V, Marchisello PJ. Traumatic partial arrest of tibial physis. *Clin Orthop Relat Res.* 1984;(183):99–104.

142. McKibbin B. The biology of fracture healing in long bones. *J Bone Joint Surg Br.* 1978;60-B(2):150–162.

143. Mendez AA, Bartal E, Grillot MB, et al. Compression (Salter-Harris Type V) physeal fracture: an experimental model in the rat. *J Pediatr Orthop.* 1992;12(1):29–37.

144. Metaizeau JP, Wong-Chung J, Bertrand H, et al. Percutaneous epiphysiodesis using transphyseal screws (PETS). *J Pediatr Orthop.* 1998;18(3):363–369.

145. Mielke CH, Stevens PM. Hemiepiphyseal stapling for knee deformities in children younger than 10 years: a preliminary report. *J Pediatr Orthop.* 1996;16(4):423–429.

146. Minina E, Wenzel HM, Kreschel C, et al. BMP and Ihh/PTHrP signaling interact to coordinate chondrocyte proliferation and differentiation. *Development.* 2001;128(22):4523–4534.

147. Mizuta T, Benson WM, Foster BK, et al. Statistical analysis of the incidence of physeal injuries. *J Pediatr Orthop.* 1987;7(5):518–523.

148. Moen CT, Pelker RR. Biomechanical and histological correlations in growth plate failure. *J Pediatr Orthop.* 1984;4(2):180–184.

149. Mudgal CS. Olecranon fractures in osteogenesis imperfecta. A case report. *Acta Orthop Belg.* 1992;58(4):453–456.

150. Navascues JA, Gonzalez-Lopez JL, Lopez-Valverde S, et al. Premature physeal closure after tibial diaphyseal fractures in adolescents. *J Pediatr Orthop.* 2000;20(2):193–196.

151. Ninomiya T, Hosoya A, Hiraga T, et al. Prostaglandin E(2) receptor EP(4)-selective agonist (ONO-4819) increases bone formation by modulating mesenchymal cell differentiation. *Eur J Pharmacol.* 2011;650(1):396–402.

152. Nouth F, Kuo LA. Percutaneous epiphysiodesis using transphyseal screws (PETS): prospective case study and review. *J Pediatr Orthop.* 2004;24(6):721–725.

153. Ogden JA. Skeletal growth mechanism injury patterns. *J Pediatr Orthop.* 1982;2(4):371–377.

154. Ogden JA. Growth slowdown and arrest lines. *J Pediatr Orthop.* 1984;4(4):409–415.

155. Ogden JA, Ganey T, Light TR, et al. The pathology of acute chondro-osseous injury in the child. *Yale J Biol Med.* 1993;66(3):219–233.

156. Ogden JA, Ogden DA, Pugh L, et al. Tibia valga after proximal metaphyseal fractures in childhood: a normal biologic response. *J Pediatr Orthop.* 1995;15(4):489–494.

157. Onishi T, Ishidou Y, Nagamine T, et al. Distinct and overlapping patterns of localization of bone morphogenetic protein (BMP) family members and a BMP type II receptor during fracture healing in rats. *Bone.* 1998;22(6):605–612.

158. Osterman K. Operative elimination of partial premature epiphyseal closure. An experimental study. *Acta Orthop Scand Suppl.* 1972:3–79.

159. Ozaki A, Tsunoda M, Kinoshita S, et al. Role of fracture hematoma and periosteum during fracture healing in rats: interaction of fracture hematoma and the periosteum in the initial step of the healing process. *J Orthop Sci.* 2000;5(1):64–70.

160. Pape JM, Goulet JA, Hensinger RN. Compartment syndrome complicating tibial tubercle avulsion. *Clin Orthop Relat Res.* 1993;(295):201–204.

161. Pathi S, Rutenberg JB, Johnson RL, et al. Interaction of Ihh and BMP/Noggin signaling during cartilage differentiation. *Dev Biol.* 1999;209(2):239–253.

162. Pearson OM, Lieberman DE. The aging of Wolff's "law": ontogeny and responses to mechanical loading in cortical bone. *Am J Phys Anthropol.* 2004;Suppl 39:63–99.

163. Peinado Cortes LM, Vanegas Acosta JC, Garzon Alvarado DA. A mechanobiological model of epiphysis structures formation. *J Theor Biol.* 2011;287:13–25.

164. Perren SM. Physical and biological aspects of fracture healing with special reference to internal fixation. *Clin Orthop Relat Res.* 1979;(138):175–196.

165. Peters W, Irving J, Letts M. Long-term effects of neonatal bone and joint infection on adjacent growth plates. *J Pediatr Orthop.* 1992;12(6):806–810.

166. Peterson HA. Partial growth plate arrest and its treatment. *J Pediatr Orthop.* 1984;4(2):246–258.

167. Peterson HA. Premature physeal arrest of the distal tibia associated with temporary arterial insufficiency. *J Pediatr Orthop.* 1993;13(5):672–675.

168. Peterson HA. Physeal fractures: Part 2. Two previously unclassified types. *J Pediatr Orthop.* 1994;14(4):431–438.

169. Peterson HA. Physeal fractures: Part 3. Classification. *J Pediatr Orthop.* 1994;14(4):439–448.

170. Peterson HA, Burkhart SS. Compression injury of the epiphyseal growth plate: fact or fiction? *J Pediatr Orthop.* 1981;1(4):377–384.

171. Peterson HA, Madhok R, Benson JT, et al. Physeal fractures: Part 1. Epidemiology in Olmsted County, Minnesota, 1979–1988. *J Pediatr Orthop.* 1994;14(4):423–430.

172. Petit P, Panuel M, Faure F, et al. Acute fracture of the distal tibial physis: role of gradient-echo MR imaging versus plain film examination. *AJR Am J Roentgenol.* 1996;166(5):1203–1206.

173. Planka L, Gal P, Kecova H, et al. Allogeneic and autogenous transplantations of MSCs in treatment of the physeal bone bridge in rabbits. *BMC Biotechnol.* 2008;8:70.

174. Poland Je. *Traumatic Separation of the Epiphysis.* London: E. Smith and Company; 1898.

175. Pontikoglou C, Deschaseaux F, Sensebe L, et al. Bone marrow mesenchymal stem cells: biological properties and their role in hematopoiesis and hematopoietic stem cell transplantation. *Stem Cell Rev.* 2011;7(3):569–589.

176. Raman S, Wallace EC. MRI diagnosis of trapped periosteum following incomplete closed reduction of distal tibial Salter-Harris II fracture. *Pediatr Radiol.* 2011;41(12):1591–1594.

177. Rapuano BE, Boursiquot R, Tomin E, et al. The effects of COX-1 and COX-2 inhibitors on prostaglandin synthesis and the formation of heterotopic bone in a rat model. *Arch Orthop Trauma Surg.* 2008;128(3):333–344.

178. Riseborough EJ, Barrett IR, Shapiro F. Growth disturbances following distal femoral physeal fracture-separations. *J Bone Joint Surg Am.* 1983;65(7):885–893.

179. Rivas R, Shapiro F. Structural stages in the development of the long bones and epiphyses: a study in the New Zealand white rabbit. *J Bone Joint Surg Am.* 2002;84-A(1):85–100.

180. Robertson WW Jr, Butler MS, D'Angio GJ, et al. Leg length discrepancy following irradiation for childhood tumors. *J Pediatr Orthop.* 1991;11(3):284–287.

181. Rogge EA, Romano RL. Avulsion of the ischial apophysis. *Clin Orthop.* 1957;9:239–243.

182. Roughley PJ, Rauch F, Glorieux FH. Osteogenesis imperfecta–clinical and molecular diversity. *Eur Cell Mater.* 2003;5:41–47; discussion 47.

183. Rudicel S, Pelker RR, Lee KE, et al. Shear fractures through the capital femoral physis of the skeletally immature rabbit. *J Pediatr Orthop.* 1985;5(1):27–31.

184. Sahm G, Witt E. Long-term results after childhood condylar fractures. A computer-tomographic study. *Eur J Orthod.* 1989;11(2):154–160.

185. Salter R. Injuries involving the epiphyseal plate. *J Bone Joint Surg Am.* 1963;45:587–622.

186. Scheffer MM, Peterson HA. Opening-wedge osteotomy for angular deformities of long bones in children. *J Bone Joint Surg Am.* 1994;76(3):325–334.

187. Schmitt JM, Hwang K, Winn SR, et al. Bone morphogenetic proteins: an update on basic biology and clinical relevance. *J Orthop Res.* 1999;17(2):269–278.

188. Sferopoulos NK. Fracture separation of the medial clavicular epiphysis: ultrasonography findings. *Arch Orthop Trauma Surg.* 2003;123(7):367–369.

189. Shapiro F. Epiphyseal growth plate fracture-separations: a pathophysiologic approach. *Orthopedics.* 1982;5(6):720–736.

190. Shapiro F, Holtrop ME, Glimcher MJ. Organization and cellular biology of the perichondrial ossification groove of ranvier: a morphological study in rabbits. *J Bone Joint Surg Am.* 1977;59(6):703–723.

191. Shea KG, Rab GT, Dufurrena M. Pathological fracture after migration of cement used to treat distal femur physeal arrest. *J Pediatr Orthop B.* 2009;18(4):185–187.

192. Shin SJ, Cho TJ, Park MS, et al. Angular deformity correction by asymmetrical physeal suppression in growing children: stapling versus percutaneous transphyseal screw. *J Pediatr Orthop.* 2010;30(6):588–593.

193. Siffert RS, Katz JF. Growth recovery zones. *J Pediatr Orthop.* 1983;3(2):196–201.

194. Skak SV. Valgus deformity following proximal tibial metaphyseal fracture in children. *Acta Orthop Scand.* 1982;53(1):141–147.

195. Skak SV, Jensen TT, Poulsen TD. Fracture of the proximal metaphysis of the tibia in children. *Injury.* 1987;18(3):149–156.

196. Smith BG, Rand F, Jaramillo D, et al. Early MR imaging of lower-extremity physeal fracture-separations: a preliminary report. *J Pediatr Orthop.* 1994;14(4):526–533.

197. Smith DG, Geist RW, Cooperman DR. Microscopic examination of a naturally occurring epiphyseal plate fracture. *J Pediatr Orthop.* 1985;5(3):306–308.

198. Stambolic V, Ruel L, Woodgett JR. Lithium inhibits glycogen synthase kinase-3 activity and mimics wingless signalling in intact cells. *Curr Biol.* 1996;6(12):1664–1668.

199. Stanton RP, Abdel-Mota'al MM. Growth arrest resulting from unicameral bone cyst. *J Pediatr Orthop.* 1998;18(2):198–201.

200. Stevens PM, Pease F. Hemiepiphysiodesis for posttraumatic tibial valgus. *J Pediatr Orthop.* 2006;26(3):385–392.

201. Stilli S, Magnani M, Lampasi M, et al. Remodelling and overgrowth after conservative treatment for femoral and tibial shaft fractures in children. *Chir Organi Mov.* 2008;91(1):13–19.

202. Sudmann E, Husby OS, Bang G. Inhibition of partial closure of epiphyseal plate in rabbits by indomethacin. *Acta Orthop Scand.* 1982;53(4):507–511.

203. Tobita M, Ochi M, Uchio Y, et al. Treatment of growth plate injury with autogenous chondrocytes: a study in rabbits. *Acta Orthop Scand.* 2002;73(3):352–358.

204. Trueta J, Morgan JD. The vascular contribution to osteogenesis. I. Studies by the injection method. *J Bone Joint Surg Br.* 1960;42-B:97–109.

205. Tschegg EK, Celarek A, Fischerauer SF, et al. Fracture properties of growth plate cartilage compared to cortical and trabecular bone in ovine femora. *J Mech Behav Biomed Mater.* 2012;14:119–129.

206. Valverde JA, Albinana J, Certucha JA. Early posttraumatic physeal arrest in distal radius after a compression injury. *J Pediatr Orthop B.* 1996;5(1):57–60.

207. Wattenbarger JM, Gruber HE, Phieffer LS. Physeal fractures, part I: histologic features of bone, cartilage, and bar formation in a small animal model. *J Pediatr Orthop.* 2002;22(6):703–709.

208. Wiemann JM 4th, Tryon C, Szalay EA. Physeal stapling versus 8-plate hemiepiphysiodesis for guided correction of angular deformity about the knee. *J Pediatr Orthop.* 2009;29(5):481–485.

209. Williams RM, Zipfel WR, Tinsley ML, et al. Solute transport in growth plate cartilage: in vitro and in vivo. *Biophys J.* 2007;93(3):1039–1050.

210. Williamson RV, Staheli LT. Partial physeal growth arrest: treatment by bridge resection and fat interposition. *J Pediatr Orthop.* 1990;10(6):769–776.

211. Yates C, Sullivan JA. Arthrographic diagnosis of elbow injuries in children. *J Pediatr Orthop.* 1987;7(1):54–60.

212. Yoo WJ, Choi IH, Chung CY, et al. Implantation of perichondrium-derived chondrocytes in physeal defects of rabbit tibiae. *Acta Orthop.* 2005;76(5):628–636.

213. Zhang AL, Exner GU, Wenger DR. Progressive genu valgum resulting from idiopathic lateral distal femoral physeal growth suppression in adolescents. *J Pediatr Orthop.* 2008;28(7):752–756.

214. Zionts LE, Harcke HT, Brooks KM, et al. Posttraumatic tibia valga: a case demonstrating asymmetric activity at the proximal growth plate on technetium bone scan. *J Pediatr Orthop.* 1987;7(4):458–462.

215. Zou H, Wieser R, Massague J, et al. Distinct roles of type I bone morphogenetic protein receptors in the formation and differentiation of cartilage. *Genes Dev.* 1997;11(17):2191–2203.

3

Cast and Splint Immobilization

Blaise A. Nemeth, Matthew A. Halanski, and Kenneth J. Noonan

INTRODUCTION

The past several decades have seen amazing enhancements in the management of adult orthopedic trauma; one of the most significant is the ability to operatively reduce fractures and to stabilize them safely with internal implants. These methods have resulted in less reliance on fracture manipulation and stabilization with external devices such as traction, splint, and cast immobilization. Gone are the days of extended skeletal traction and spica cast application for adult femur fractures; tibia shaft fractures in adults are rarely treated with time-honored methods of reduction in the emergency ward, long-leg cast application, followed by months of patellar tendon bearing a short-leg cast application. Although still used with some frequency in adult trauma, upper extremity cast and splint application is often considered temporary until definitive internal fixation.

Parallel to changes in fracture management, medicine has seen similar changes in medical education as well as who delivers certain health care. For instance, as a result of specialization, many adult orthopedists manage less trauma, rarely place casts, and even more rarely will they educate residents in the safe and effective use of these methods. As reimbursement for health care changes, orthopedic surgeons are called to do those things that only they can do—operate. Many other aspects of patients' care are assumed by advanced practitioners such as nurse practitioners or physician assistants (NPs or PAs) or other allied health specialists. In many emergency rooms and in most outpatient clinics, the patient who requires definitive cast immobilization will usually have these applied by cast technicians or nurses. As a result, large fracture clinics where orthopedic residents learn from senior residents or faculty to manage fractures with casting are replaced by cast technicians while residents learn who needs operations and how.

To a lesser degree and similar to adults, decades of advances in imaging and development of appropriate operative methods and implants have also benefited pediatric patients with orthopedic trauma. Despite wide changes in adult trauma, cast and splint methodology is still used with great frequency in the management of pediatric trauma. In children, requisite attention to perfect reduction and extensive immobilization is not needed because of the rapidity of fracture healing and the remodeling potential seen in children. Over 90% of adult forearm fractures are treated with surgery; in children, 90% of forearm fractures are treated with reduction and cast immobilization.

The purpose of this chapter is to review in detail the methods and pitfalls of nonoperative treatment that are common to all areas of pediatric trauma. In addition, we will review unique characteristics of children that are also of importance in all fracture locations and trauma. It is desired that this chapter, its figures, and video clips will serve as a primer of nonoperative pediatric orthopedic trauma management.

PAIN MANAGEMENT AND SEDATION FOR FRACTURE MANAGEMENT

In normally sensate children, reduction and immobilization of fractures is always associated with pain and anxiety. Advances in fracture management have been accompanied by improvements in methods to diminish anxiety, provide muscle relaxation, and to decrease pain during these noxious events. The most optimal location to perform these procedures is within the operating room where complete pain control, relaxation, and amnesia are provided by the anesthesia team.[54] This setting is ideal as it allows the orthopedist to focus completely on the fracture without worrying about the safety of the child, without the distractions of a suffering child, and with parents looming in the background. Unfortunately, this resource is not often available for our patients in a timely manner and the costs associated with general anesthesia and possible admission far outweigh the costs of fractures that are treated equally well in the emergency department.[33] In addition, the risks of general anesthesia are currently being evaluated and it is suspected that multiple long anesthetics may have some effect on child development. Yet one should consider reduction and cast application in the operating room for children with autistic spectrum disorders; children with medical comorbidities that preclude safe sedation in the emergency department; and in cases of fractures which could be very difficult to reduce (significant displacement and swelling) and will likely need operative stabilization anyway.

Procedural sedation methods include different routes of drug delivery (intranasal, IV, or inhalational) and can utilize differing combinations of agents. Although not an exhaustive list; a contemporary listing of systemic drugs used for these injuries include combinations of etomidate, ketamine, narcotics, midazolam, propofol, and nitrous oxide.[1,9,49,54,72] Some centers do not monitor these children who are sedated for procedures with nitrous oxide and oxygen.[9] Yet most centers recommend at least pulse oximetry and noninvasive blood pressure monitoring for all conscious sedation including nitrous oxide and oxygen.[65]

Ketamine appears to be a very popular agent for use in the ED with good sedative, amnestic, and analgesic effects; and reported doses include 0.75 to 2.0 mg/kg delivered IV or 2 to 4 mg/kg delivered IM. Its advantages include wide use and experience as a solitary agent, and can be administered IV or IM.[20] Side effects include nystagmus, lacrimation, salivation, vocalization, respiratory depression, and dissociative reactions that can occur at higher doses (2.5 mg/kg IV). Ketamine at lower doses may have decreased side effects but may require some redosing.[40] Some studies have augmented ketamine with small boluses of propofol (with its good antiemetic and anxiolytic properties); ketamine is helpful in mitigating the occasional hypotensive effects seen with propofol.[1,64]

Another popular agent for sedation is 50:50 nitrous oxide and oxygen (anxiolytic and analgesic); which is appealing because children don't need to be NPO and it is fast-acting, reversible, and doesn't require special staff to administer it. Nitrous oxide can be supplemented with hematoma block after a steady state of sedation has been achieved. Procedural sedation in combination with local block does have the advantage of not needing as much systemic sedation.

Some have suggested that regional anesthesia such as hematoma block could be the first line of pain management for upper extremity fractures as it is quicker and is well tolerated.[5,29] Conversion to sedation with ketamine of midazolam may be needed in a small proportion.[5] Regional Bier blocks have also been used in children with forearm and wrist fractures with good efficacy and has been shown to be safe, efficient, cost-effective and do not require patients to be fasting. When using a dose of 3.33 mg/kg of lidocaine, there are very few complications except for tourniquet pain. Despite the efficacy of regional blocks, recent research has suggested local hematoma block may not be as widely used today as many EDs are using ketamine or midazolam.[19]

GENERAL

Because of the growth and remodeling potential of pediatric bones, acceptable alignment rather than exact anatomic reduction is sufficient for many fractures, allowing the majority of pediatric fractures to be managed in a cast. Similarly, joint stiffness is not typically a long-term problem in children treated in a cast.[7] The goals of pediatric cast treatment are to protect and provide stability to the broken bone, maintain alignment, and protect from further injury until sufficient healing has occurred. In general, the alignment maintained in the cast should allow the child to eventually remodel to anatomic "normal" by the cessation of growth. The younger the child, the more malalignment may be acceptable. Likewise, deformity closer to the growth plate and in the plane of motion will typically remodel more than those elsewhere.

The duration of cast treatment is both age and site specific. Very young children, infants, and newborns will generally heal fractures quicker than adolescents. In general, fractures of the hands and feet require 4 weeks of immobilization; elbow fractures 3 to 6 weeks; tibial shaft fractures may take 12 to 16 weeks, whereas most other fractures require 6 weeks. Before discontinuing cast immobilization, fracture healing should be documented on radiographs and the child should be nontender at the fracture site.

In general, casts are utilized to *maintain* alignment. If a fracture is nondisplaced or has an acceptable alignment, the cast's purpose is to keep the child comfortable and maintain that alignment until the bone has healed. If a fracture has an unacceptable alignment, it should be reduced to an acceptable alignment and the cast placed to maintain that alignment. Fractures that should be treated operatively include injuries in which adequate alignment or length cannot be easily obtained or maintained, displaced intra-articular fractures, and many fractures involving the physis. Postoperatively, the limb may be protected with a splint or a cast if necessary. Problems may arise when a cast is used to *obtain* acceptable alignment. Pressure sores and soft tissue injuries have been documented when casts are used in this manner and should be done so with caution.[43,56,74]

To minimize motion at the fracture site, casts are placed to span the joint proximal, distal, or both. In general, the more proximal a fracture, the more likely joints at each end of the bone will be spanned. Increasing the length of the cast increases the resistance to rotation.[42] To maintain correct alignment, limbs may be casted in different positions to counteract specific displacing forces on the proximal or distal fragment of a given fracture. For example, in a subtrochanteric femur fracture, the proximal fragment is pulled into flexion, abduction, and external rotation by attached muscles, so the distal fragment must be positioned with this in mind. The distal fragment must be brought into a position of flexion to match the flexed proximal femur from pull of the psoas muscle.

CAST COMPLICATIONS

Although casting is often viewed as "conservative" treatment, the treating physician and family should recognize that this does not imply that this treatment is without complications. Although the true incidence of cast complications is unknown, a litigation history of a large multispecialty multilocation pediatric group showed that casts were the number one cause of litigation. Over 25% of children treated in a hip spica cast have been shown to have skin complications.[24] Over a 5-year period at one institution, 168 unplanned visits to the emergency room were because of cast issues. Twenty-nine percent of these visits were for a wet cast, 23% for a tight cast, and 13% for a loose cast.[63] Over a 10-year period, Physicians Insurers Association of America (PIAA) reported 1,023 claims on problems of immobilization and traction for which 16% of all claims had an associated issue including failure of consent. This implies that many physicians and patients may expect cast immobilization to be without risk. Thus, it is important to inform patients and their caregivers of the risks associated with cast treatment. For instance, a child with a tibia fracture can be told to expect pain in the pretibial area but they should also be aware that pain in other locations (such as over the point of the heal) is not fracture related and may imply an impending heel sore. When the expectations of cast immobilization are explained and risks of treatment are given, it is beneficial that these risks be written and delivered to the patient and their family.[39]

The Wet and Soiled Cast

Wet casts that are not made with synthetic material and waterproof liners (and thus can dry quickly) should be changed. Failure to do so may result in skin irritation, breakdown, and possible infection. Light moisture or spotting may be dried with

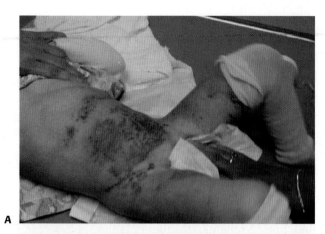

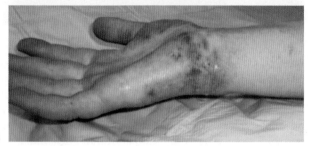

Figure 3-1. Examples of dermatitis related to wet casts. **A:** A soiled hip spica cast. **B:** Upper extremity cast that was wet. (*Property of UW Pediatric Orthopaedics.*)

a hair drier on cool or low heat, with instructions to check the temperature of the dryer with their hand to ensure that it is not too warm. A frankly wet cast or cast padding that cannot be dried as described above usually requires inspection of the skin and cast change (Fig. 3-1).[52] Although most limbs in these casts will only demonstrate skin maceration,[24] serious life-threatening complications such as toxic shock syndrome and necrotizing fasciitis have been reported.[22,57] Hip spica casts are often applied in the operating room and their removal and exchange at times require a general anesthetic. Parents should be well instructed on positioning to avoid soiling, frequent diaper changes, and inspecting the children for skin irritation. Anesthetic risks must be weighed with the perceived soft tissue and skin risk.

Thermal Injury

Plaster and fiberglass, the two most common casting materials, harden through exothermic chemical reactions. Plaster has a much higher setting temperature than fiberglass and therefore a higher risk for thermal injury when a cast is placed. Two factors strongly associated with thermal injuries are dip water temperature and the thickness of cast material. Several studies have shown that risk of thermal injury is significant if the dip water temperature is too hot (>50°C) or if the casts are too thick (>24 ply).[30,36,45] Each plaster manufacturer has recommended dip water temperatures that should not be exceeded. Using warmer temperatures to "speed up" the setting time beyond that recommended should be avoided. Casts in excess of 24 ply are rarely encountered; however, increased amounts of casting material are often placed in the concavities of extremities (antecubital fossa and dorsum of the ankle) because of material overlap.[36] Incorporating splints on the convexity, thus decreasing overlap in the concavity, can minimize this. Similarly, clinicians placing plaster splints of 10 to 15 ply on an extremity may breech safe thicknesses when the splint is too long and the edges are folded over thus creating a focal area of 20 to 30 ply, a thickness at which temperatures do become a risk.[36] Studies have shown that temperatures high enough to cause significant thermal injuries can also be reached when the clinician places a curing cast on a pillow.[30,36] The practice of reinforcing a curing plaster cast with fiberglass may place the limb at significant risk because the synthetic overlap prevents heat from effectively dissipating, as well as an increased risk of case burns at removal in our experience. The plaster must be allowed to cure before setting the casted limb on a support or applying fiberglass reinforcement. Failure to wait may place the insulated portion of the limb at significant risk.[36] Case reports demonstrating this potential complication do exist.[10] Those patients undergoing regional or general anesthesia may be at increased risk as they will not report burning pain that is associated with thermal injury.

Areas of Focal Pressure: Impending Pressure Sores

A key to preventing loss of fracture reduction is in the application of a well-molded cast. Cast padding should be applied between 3 and 5 layers thick over the limb being casted.[55,66] Bony prominences (heel, malleoli, patella, ASIS, and olecranon) and cast edges should be additionally padded to prevent irritation yet allow a cast to be molded to fit snugly without undue pressure. The use of foam padding in such areas may help decrease the incidence of pressure sores.[28]

Families and patients should be instructed to refrain from placing anything between a cast and the patients' skin, food, toys, writing utensils, money, and other items have been found down casts, and we have seen them erode through patients' skin.[12,71] Any patient with a suspected foreign body down their cast should have the cast removed and skin inspected (Fig. 3-2).

A loose cast (either too much padding from poor application or decreased swelling) may result in skin sores as a result of shear forces repeatedly applied to the limb or a loss of reduction.[38] Distal fingers or toes are often noted to "migrate" proximally (disappearing toes/fingers sign) when this occurs and should alert the parent and the clinician that there is a problem.[75] In a lower extremity cast, which migrates distally, the dorsum of the foot and ankle receives pressure from the anterior ankle crease of the cast, while the heel is pulled up and rests along the posterior calf portion of the cast. Prolonged positioning in such a manner may result in pressure sores.

Detecting Cast Complications

That "there are no hypochondriacs in casts" is an important aphorism to remember and every effort should be taken to resolve the source of complaint in an immobilized patient. A complication of casting should be considered whenever an immobilized patient has an unexplained increase in pain, irritability, or unexplained fevers.[22]

Some cast complications such as soiling and wetness can be detected on physical examination, whereas others may be more difficult to diagnose. A foul-smelling cast may be a sign of wound infection and the cast should be removed or windowed to inspect the source of the smell. Pressure sores may be diagnosed if the patient can localize an area of discomfort away from the fracture or operative site. Complaints of pain in high-risk areas such as the heel, dorsum of the foot, popliteal fossa, patella, and olecranon, must alert the clinician of an impending problem. However with pediatric patients, localization may not be possible. One must correlate history, the clinical examination findings, such as the "disappearing toes sign" with radiographs. These images can be used to critically evaluate not only the alignment of the fractured bone, but also the outline and contour of the cast padding and material, especially in the antecubital, the popliteal fossa, and over the dorsum of the foot. If there is a suspicion of a problem, the cast should be windowed or removed and the area inspected.

Certain pediatric patients may be at a higher risk for cast complications. These include the very young, developmentally delayed, or patients under anesthesia or sedation who may have difficulty responding to noxious stimuli such as heat or pressure during the cast application. Discerning problems in this group may be quite difficult and cast sores can occur despite appropriate and careful application.

Similarly, patients with impaired sensation are at increased risk for injuries related to excessive heat and pressure. In this group are those with spinal cord injuries,[60,67] myelomeningocele,[51] and systemic disorders such as diabetes mellitus.[34] Patients with CP are at increased risk for complications due to communication difficulties and poor nutrition, in addition to their spasticity.[47,68]

TREATING CAST COMPLICATIONS

Dermatitis

The majority of dermatitis under casts has to do with maceration of the skin and continued contact with wetness including fluids such as urine or feces. Often, removal of the cast, cleansing of the skin, and allowing the skin to "dry out" is all that is required. Some recommend applying over-the-counter skin moisturizers.[24] If fungal infection is suspected, half-strength nystatin cream and 1% hydrocortisone cream may be applied, followed by miconazole powder dusting twice daily.[24] If unstable, the fracture may be managed by a newly applied dry split cast or splint allowing time for the skin to recover. In rare cases, internal or external fixation may be chosen to manage the fracture and to allow treatment of the skin issues. Often, the skin will improve dramatically after a few days and a new cast may be applied. If significant concern for cellulitis exists, such as induration or fevers, laboratory tests should be ordered and empiric oral antibiotics prescribed.

Pressure Sores

Pressure sores are the result of a focal area of pressure, which exceeds perfusion pressure. Although there may be initial pain associated with this pressure, this can be difficult to separate

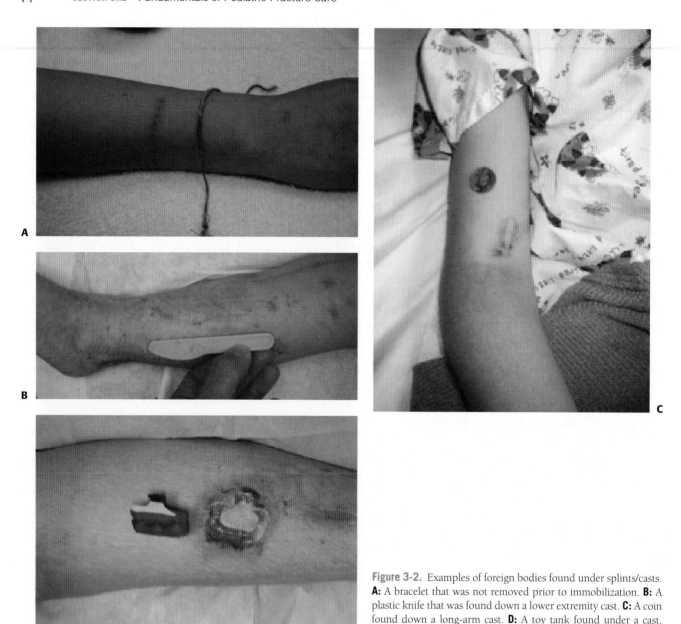

Figure 3-2. Examples of foreign bodies found under splints/casts. **A:** A bracelet that was not removed prior to immobilization. **B:** A plastic knife that was found down a lower extremity cast. **C:** A coin found down a long-arm cast. **D:** A toy tank found under a cast. (*Property of UW Pediatric Orthopaedics.*)

from the pain of the fracture or surgery. Any pain away from the injured area should be suspected to have a problem with focal pressure. The heel is the most common site. These sores may vary from areas of erythema, to black eschars, to full-thickness soft tissue loss and exposed bone (Fig. 3-3). In the benign cases, removal of the cast over the heel and either cessation or careful reapplication is all that is necessary. Typically, black eschars imply partial- to full-thickness injuries. If they are intact, non-fluctuant, nondraining, and mobile from the underlying bone, they may be treated as a biologic dressing with weekly wound checks. If any concern exists, a wound team and/or plastic surgery consult should be sought earlier rather than later. Often, dressing changes using topical enzymatic ointments and anti-biotic ointments can be used to treat these wounds (Fig. 3-4). Whenever exposed bone is present, osteomyelitis is a concern requiring aggressive intervention and possible intravenous

antibiotic therapy. In these severe cases, vacuum-assisted clo-sure (VAC) therapy, skin grafting, or flap coverage may be necessary.[46]

Joint Stiffness and Muscle Contractures

Determination of cast immobilization duration is often multi-factorial; however, the clinician must recognize that unwanted physiologic changes may occur. Although these changes are less pronounced in children than adults, excessive length of immobilization may lead to problems such as stiffness,[26] muscle atrophy, cartilage degradation, ligament weakening, and osteo-porosis.[7,14,15,35,69] This must be weighed against the bony healing gained in prolonged immobilizations. Alternatives such as Pav-lik harness bracing for infants with femur fractures,[58] patellar tendon bearing casts versus long-leg casts for tibial fractures,

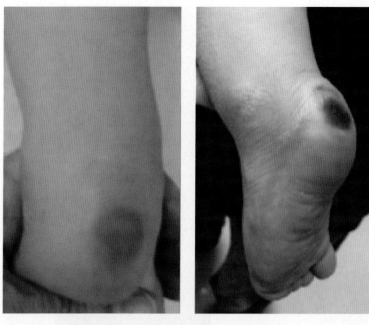
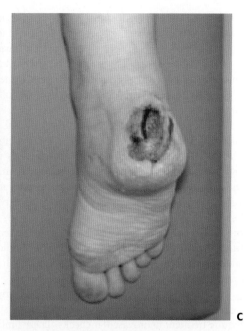

A, B   **C**

Figure 3-3. Examples of heel pressure sores. Mild erythema and superficial skin damage (**A**), intact eschar (**B**), and partial/full-thickness injury with exposed bone and fascia (**C**). (*Property of UW Pediatric Orthopaedics.*)

short-arm casts for distal forearm fractures, and other functional braces may minimize some of the risks of cast immobilization or at least decrease the duration of cast treatment.

The ankle, elbow, and fingers are often locations prone to stiffness. The duration of immobilization should be minimized if at all possible.

Compartment Syndrome

Most limbs with fresh fractures are more comfortable after immobilization. Therefore, increasing pain or neurovascular change should be fully evaluated to detect the above complications and possibly compartment syndrome. Fractures and surgery can result in progressive soft tissue swelling that might not have been present at the time of cast application and may lead to compartment syndrome. In this scenario,[63] the first intervention should be relieving the circumferential pressure by splitting the cast and all underlying padding, as leaving the padding intact has been shown to not fully relieve compartment pressure. Should splitting the cast fail to alleviate symptoms, cast removal should be considered. Fractures of the tibia,[27,32] forearm,[32] and elbow have increased risk of compartment

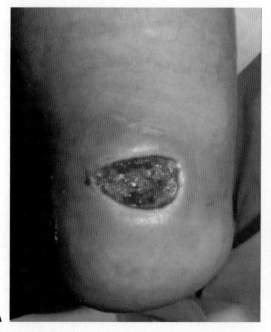
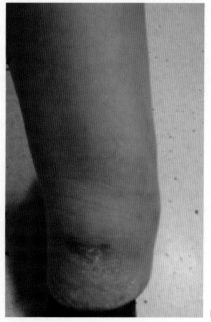

A   **B**

Figure 3-4. A: Picture of heel ulcer at clinical follow-up after operative debridement. **B:** After roughly 2 months of topical enzymatic and antibiotic treatment with dressing changes. (*Property of UW Pediatric Orthopaedics.*)

syndrome. High-energy fractures resulting from motor vehicle accidents, crush injuries, or two-level injuries such as a floating elbow should raise the treating physician's awareness to the possibility of an impending compartment syndrome. Any child unable to detect pain associated with compartment syndrome (a nerve injury or regional anesthesia) must be followed closely for the development of compartment syndrome.

Children do not usually exhibit the classical four Ps (pallor, paresthesias, pulseless, pain with passive stretch) associated with compartment syndrome until myonecrosis may be starting. Instead, the "three As" of increased agitation, anxiety, and analgesic requirements have been documented as the earliest signs of compartment syndrome in children. Any child exhibiting these symptoms that are not relieved with cast splitting should have the cast removed and limb inspected with a high suspicion of compartment syndrome. One should be ready to take the child to the operating room for formal compartment evaluation and decompression if needed.

Fractures with associated neurovascular injuries are at significant risk of developing a compartment syndrome and require frequent neurovascular checks. These limbs may be stabilized with a splint as opposed to circumferential cast application, which could worsen the risk of compartment syndrome. These limbs are most often treated with operative stabilization using internal or external fixation and/or splint immobilization. This allows continued neurovascular assessment, palpation of compartments, and inspection of the limb. For instance, the child with a floating elbow fracture and associated nerve palsy (at high risk for compartment syndrome) is usually best treated with internal fixation of the fractures, and either a splint, bivalved cast that is easily opened, or cast with thick foam to allow for swelling, with the volar forearm exposed to assess the compartments as well as the pulses.

Disuse Osteopenia and Pathologic Fractures Adjacent to Cast

Patients with paralytic conditions or cerebral palsy patients and those taking anticonvulsants may experience further disuse osteopenia with immobilization.[60,67] These patients are at significantly higher risk of pathologic fracture while casted or upon cast removal.[2,47] Strategies to prevent this includes minimizing immobilization (<4 weeks), weight-bearing casts, and the use of less rigid immobilization such as Soft Cast (3M Health Care Ltd., Loughborough, England) and splints and braces.

Delayed Diagnosis of Wound Infections

Many children are placed in postsurgical casts. The vast majority does well without incident. However, casts over wounds or pins may cause a delay in the diagnosis of a wound infection (Fig. 3-5). For instance, an estimated 1% to 4% of all pediatric supracondylar humerus fractures treated with pinning the elbow will develop a postoperative pin-tract inflammation or infection.[4,26] Therefore, unexplained fever beyond the perioperative period, increase in pain at pin sites, foul smell, or discharge from a cast should be evaluated by a member of the orthopedic team. The wound should be examined either with cast windowing or cast removal. Laboratory tests including

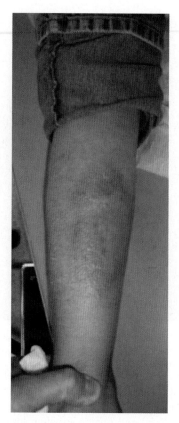

Figure 3-5. After getting a postoperative cast wet, dermatitis and possible cellulitis were found at the incision following a gastrocnemius recession. (*Property of UW Pediatric Orthopaedics.*)

CBC, ESR, and CRP may be advisable. In cases of early pin-site infection where the fracture is not yet healed, oral antibiotics may control the infection long enough to allow more fracture healing prior to pin removal. Infections of pins used for certain fractures may have a high chance of joint penetration (lateral condyle, supracondylar Humerus, distal femoral physeal, and proximal humerus) and thus superficial pin-tract infection could lead to a septic joint. This is much more serious than simple pin-site infections, and most often must be treated with surgical irrigation and debridement and pin removal should be considered despite the status of fracture healing.

TYPES OF CASTING MATERIALS

Before placing a cast, the limb must be inspected. Any dirt, operative skin prep, or jewelry should be removed before the cast is applied. Often, appropriate size stockinette or liner is applied against the skin, under the cast and cast padding. Although not essential, these liners minimize skin irritation; allow nice well-padded and polished edges to the cast to be applied. They also minimize the tendency of some children to "pick out" their cast padding. These liners are made of cotton, water-friendly synthetic materials such as polyester, sliver-impregnated cotton (to minimize bacterial growth), or Gore-Tex (W.L. Gore & Associates, Inc.; Newark, DE). Some in the care of children who require spica cast application favor water-permeable liners such as Gore-Tex. In addition to being more convenient for patients, these newer materials minimize skin irritation.

Cast Padding

Different materials are used to pad the extremity between the cast material and the patient's skin. A thin layer (3 to 5 layers) of padding is applied to the portion of the extremity that is not prone to pressure sores and it is applied without wrinkles.[55,66] Additional layers may be placed over bony prominences to minimize pressure in these areas. Cotton is the cheapest and is historically most commonly used. But casts with cotton padding cannot be made waterproof as the cotton padding retains water. Newer synthetic materials have variable water resistance and when paired with fiberglass, can allow patients to bathe and swim. However, these materials are considerably more expensive than their cotton counterparts. In addition, some synthetic padding is less resistant to a cast saw. If one applies Gore-Tex padding, the blue DE FLEX safety strip can be placed along the path that the cast saw will take to remove the cast.

Cast edges are often a source of skin irritation and abrasion. This is especially true for fiberglass casts. When making a cast, applying the stockinette and cast padding at least 1 cm beyond the edge of the fiberglass, and folding the stockinette and padding back over the first layer of fiberglass, will make a cast with well-padded edges. Closed-cell adhesive foam may also be applied to the edges of a cast and to pad bony prominences. It is important to recognize that some foam padding will accumulate moisture and will not be effectively wicked away from the liner and skin. Should difficulty be found in folding back the underlying stockinette or liner, the cast edges may be petaled with tape or moleskin adhesive. This involves placing a 1- to 2-in piece of tape on the inside of the liner and folding the taped liner over the opening of cast. Most commonly, petaling is performed on hip spica casts but may be performed on any cast.

Plaster of Paris

Plaster-impregnated cloth is the time-tested form of immobilization. It was first described in 1852 and has been the gold standard for cast immobilization for many years. This material is generally less expensive and is more moldable in comparison to the synthetic counterparts. Beyond more accurate molding, other major advantages of plaster over synthetic materials in the prevention of cast sores and limb compression are its increase in pliability and its effective spreading after univalving. Inconveniences associated with plaster include its poor resistance to water and its lower strength-to-weight ratio resulting in heavier (thicker) casts.

Plaster of Paris combines with water in a reaction that results in gypsum. In the process of setting up, the conversion to gypsum is an exothermic reaction with thermal energy as a by-product. In general, the amount of heat produced is variable between each of the manufactured plasters. However, within each product line, faster-setting plasters can be expected to produce more heat. As the speed of the reaction, amount of reactants, or

temperature of the system (dip water and/or ambient temperature) increase; the amount of heat given off can cause significant thermal injury.[30,36,45] The low strength-to-weight ratio may also increase risk of thermal injury as those unfamiliar with the amount (ply) of plaster to use may inadvertently use too much, resulting in a burn.

Fiberglass

More recently, synthetic fiberglass materials have been introduced. These materials have the benefit of being lightweight and strong. In addition, these materials can be combined with waterproof liners to allow patients to bathe and swim in their casts. These materials are often more radiolucent, allowing better imaging within the cast.

Risk of thermal injury is much lower and is a major advantage over plaster.[36] However, because of the increased stiffness, some feel these casts are more difficult to mold, whereas others prefer fiberglass as the strength of the molded portion is greater. To prevent increased areas of pressure and constriction of the limb, special precautions are recommended when applying fiberglass rolls.[21] In addition, fiberglass is more expensive than plaster (can be more than double). Finally, there may be a small long-term risk to those applying and removing these materials. The carcinogenic risks in the manufacturing and use of fiberglass materials are questioned.[70]

Other Casting Materials

In addition to the standard rigid casting materials of plaster and fiberglass, a less rigid class of nonfiberglass synthetic casting material is available. Although less rigid than standard casting materials, this Soft Cast (3M Health Care Ltd., Loughborough, UK) has several potential advantages. Experimental studies have shown that this material is more accommodating to increases in pressure than the other casting materials.[23] As this material is less rigid, it may be an ideal material to immobilize patients with severe osteopenia. Finally, this material can be removed without using a cast saw, which eliminates the risk of cast saw injury.[11]

Combination of Materials

Some combine plaster and fiberglass casting materials in hopes of obtaining the best features of both. One may reinforce a thin well-molded plaster cast by overwrapping it with fiberglass to increase its durability and minimize its weight. With this technique, one must ensure that the plaster has set before overwrapping with the fiberglass. Failure to do so may result in a thermal injury.[36] Shortcomings of this technique include the fact that the two layers of material may obscure fine radiographic detail. Finally, great care must be taken when removing such casts as it may be difficult to "feel" the depth of the cast saw blade and blade temperatures may be more elevated than usual. As a result of the increased risks of burns, it may be particularly advantageous to use plastic protection strips under the cast when using a standard vibrating cast saw for cast removal. Yet despite these shortcomings, fiberglass has become the most popular casting material in most centers;

this is because of the increased strength, decreased weight, improved radiographic quality, color choices, and ability to make water-friendly casts.

GENERAL CAST APPLICATION PRINCIPLES

While pain control and sedation are often required, techniques are needed for calming and distracting a child during cast application. Speak with a soft voice, sitting and placing oneself at a level at or below that of the child to present a less intimidating stature. Initial examination techniques should be soft and distant from the site of concern, progressing slowly to the area of concern.

Talking to the child and his parents helps identify the best approach for an individual child, and use of child life specialists proves extremely helpful in implementing the preferred approach.[17,62] For infants and toddlers, soft music, toys (especially those with lights or moving parts), and some interactive applications on handheld devices help with distraction and relaxation.[50] When using a cast saw for cutting the cast or cast removal, ear protection helps decrease anxiety.[13] For children with cognitive, behavioral, or autistic spectrum disorders, discussion of possible approaches with the parents reaps rewards as they have the best sense of what will be calming, as well as stimulatory, for their child.

Plaster of Paris depends on excellent handling techniques to maximize the benefits of mold ability and fit and also to maximize strength. Some like the plaster to be wet to mold better; others will like a drier roll to ease application (less slippery) and speed the curing process. It is optimal to keep the plaster roll in contact to the limb to avoid wrapping the material too tight (Fig. 3-6). The plaster should be unrolled with overlaps of one-half to one-third the width of the roll and tucks are taken to avoid the tendency of pulling and stretching the material (thus increasing tightness) to get a good distribution and fit of the plaster around the difficult concave areas of the ankle, knee, elbow, and thumb. The optimal cast technique requires frequent rubbing and incorporation of the plaster rolls as the cast is being applied (i.e., initial molding) and will improve the fit but will also flatten the tucks and incorporate the mineral portion of the plaster into the fiber mesh for optimal strength. Plaster splints should be dipped and vigorously molded together before applying to the convexity of the limb (back of elbow or ankle) or where additional strength is needed (anterior knee [long-leg cast] or posterior thigh [spica cast]).

Once the plaster cast is applied and the initial molding has been accomplished, the cast is supported by broad surfaces such as the palm of a hand; the thorax of the surgeon is an excellent broad surface to hold the plantar foot in neutral flexion and extension (Fig. 3-7). Statically holding a cast with the tips of fingers as it dries will leave indentations that can lead to pressure sores. If fingers are needed for molding, pressure should be applied and then withdrawn as the plaster reaches the final curing at which point, terminal molding of the cast can be done. Terminal molding is that point at which the plaster is fairly firm, somewhat pliable and warm; yet can be gently deformed without cracking the Plaster of Paris. This is

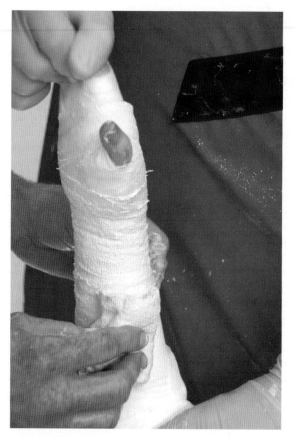

Figure 3-6. Plaster roll is not lifted off of the cast but kept in contact during application as it is "rolled" up the extremity with an overlap of 30% to 50%. (*Property of UW Pediatric Orthopaedics.*)

the appropriate time to do the final mold and hold of fracture fragments. As the cast goes through the final curing process, it can be supported on pillows, provided the cast is not too hot (the pillow prevents heat loss and will increase the temperature at the skin surface). A leg cast should be supported

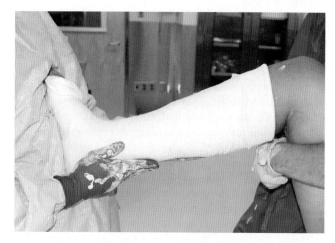

Figure 3-7. The foot is supported on the surgeon's thorax and this holds the foot at 90 degrees while the rest of the cast is molded. (*Property of UW Pediatric Orthopaedics.*)

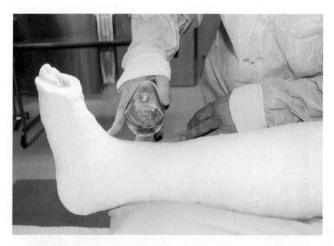

Figure 3-8. While the cooled cast is supported on the pillow, the heel is allowed to hang free and thus be at less risk for deformation and a heel sore. The cast is univalved with a cast saw that is supported by the surgeon's index finger. (*Property of UW Pediatric Orthopaedics.*)

under the calf and allowing the heel to hang free (Fig. 3-8) and thus prevent a gradual deformation of the heel into a point of internal skin pressure.

Fiberglass material is applied and molded in a slightly different manner and some believe its material properties make it harder to apply and mold in comparison to Plaster of Paris. Fiberglass material should be removed from its package and dipped in water just prior to application as it will cure and harden in the air. Fiberglass is often tacky in nature and therefore increased tension is needed to unroll the fiberglass, and can inadvertently result in a cast that is circumferentially too tight. To avoid this, fiberglass should be applied in a stretch relaxation manner[21]; the fiberglass roll is lifted off of the limb (in contradistinction to plaster which stays in contact); unrolled first then wrapped around the limb (Fig. 3-9). Difficulty exists when wrapping a wide roll into a concavity (anterior elbow or ankle) as the fiberglass can only lay flat if pulled too tight. Small

relaxing cuts in the fiberglass may be needed, as fiberglass does not tuck as easily as Plaster of Paris. Fiberglass is not as exothermic as Plaster of Paris and risk of burns is lower, yet the other principles of holding the cast as the fiberglass cures is the same as in Plaster of Paris.

CAST SPLITTING

Casts are cut and split to decrease the pressure the limb experiences after trauma or surgery. In general, the more trauma (either from the trauma or the surgery performed) a limb experiences, the more swelling that will ensue. Thus, minimally displaced fractures can often be managed without splitting a cast, while those requiring a closed or open reduction may initially need to be managed in a split cast or one padded with thick foam. Although splitting may be done prophylactically or as symptoms develop, the experienced clinician will often choose the former to avoid having to split the cast at a later time when the child is in pain, crying, anxious, and usually in the middle of the night. When splitting a cast, one must ensure that the plaster or fiberglass has set, that is hardened and cool, and that the blade temperature remains cool throughout the splitting process. Attempting to split a plaster cast before it is warm and hard (curing) or less than 10 minutes after application is more difficult and prone to result in inadvertent skin touches.

The effect of cast splitting depends on the material used, how it was applied, and whether or not the associated padding is split. Plaster cast cutting and spreading (univalve) can be expected to decrease 40% to 60% of the pressure and release of padding may increase this by 10% to 20%.[8,21,31,53] Fiberglass casts applied without stretch relaxation are known to be two times tighter than those applied with plaster[21] and in these cases, bivalving the fiberglass cast would be needed to see similar decreases in pressure. Casts that are applied with the stretch relaxation method are among the least constrictive of fiberglass casts and therefore univalving may be sufficient as long as the cast can be spread and held open with commercially available plastic cast wedges.

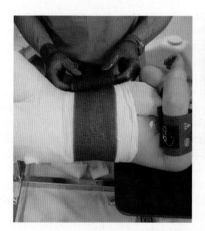
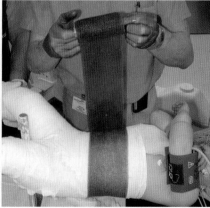
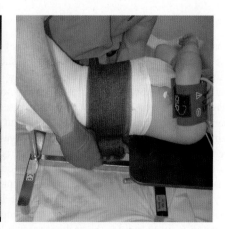

Figure 3-9. The fiberglass is applied with stretch relaxation method. The fiberglass is unrolled first then placed over the body. (*Property of UW Pediatric Orthopaedics.*)

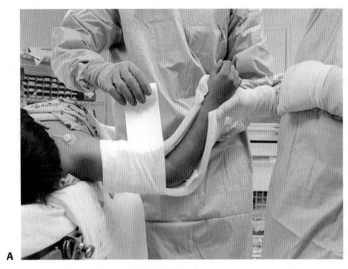
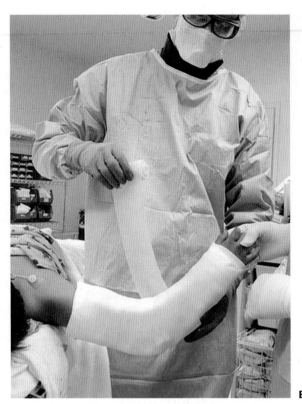

A **B**

Figure 3-10. A, B: Foam padding is placed on skin, followed by cast padding, then fiberglass casting material. This allows for welling and provides strength, but does not hold fracture reduction. Ideally, stockinette at the ends of the cast would make for better edges. (*Image property of Children's Hospital of Los Angeles.*)

Although splitting casts is the traditional means of relieving cast tightness and allowing for swelling, use of thick foam is gaining acceptance at many centers (Fig. 3-10). Half-inch sterile foam can be used on most postoperative casts when concern for swelling is present. The foam is placed directly on skin to ensure circumferential pressure is not caused by cast padding. Stockinette and cast padding are then applied, followed by fiberglass. This type of cast is not used to hold a closed reduction with cast molding, but works well for fractures made stable with internal fixation.

CAST REMOVAL

Casts are removed using an oscillating cast saw designed to cut the hard cast material and not soft material such as padding or skin. In one report, the incidence of cast saw burns occurring with the removal of casting material was found to be 0.72% (Fig. 3-11).[3] Studies have shown that increased cast thickness, decreased padding, and dull blade use result in higher blade temperatures.[41] The technician who removes the cast must be well trained in the use of the saws. One common pitfall is to slide the oscillating saw along the cast thus increasing the chance of a cut or burn. Proper technique dictates that the blade be used by alternating firm pressure with relaxation into the material and then withdrawn before replacing it at a different location.[66] Furthermore, the technician should intermittently feel the blade and pause during the removal process when necessary to allow the blade to cool.

Various safety shields are available; which, at the time of cast removal may be slid between the skin and the padding to prevent saw injury. Oftentimes, the safety shield cannot be slid up the entirety of the cast, so extreme care must be taken in these areas where the skin is not protected. Alternatively, safety strips may be incorporated into the cast at the time of cast application (Fig. 3-12). Finally, new advances in differing types of saws may improve the safety of cast removal.

CAST WEDGING

In a fresh fracture (usually less than 2 weeks old and prior to significant callus formation) in which initial reduction was obtained and subsequently is found to have an unacceptable loss of reduction, cast wedging of a well-fitting cast may be attempted. Many techniques for cast wedging have been described; however, the most recent description by Bebbington[6] appears to be easy to apply for simple angular deformities. The radiograph of the malaligned limb is used to trace the long axis of the bone onto a sheet of paper, which is then cut along this line. The cut edge of the paper is traced onto the cast, matching the position of the apex of the paper with the apex of the deformity. The cast is then cut, nearly circumferentially at this level, leaving a bridge of intact plaster only at the apex. Corks or cast wedges are applied opposite this bridge, until the line transferred on the cast is straight.

If this fails, the cast may need to be removed and the fracture either remanipulated or treated in some other fashion.

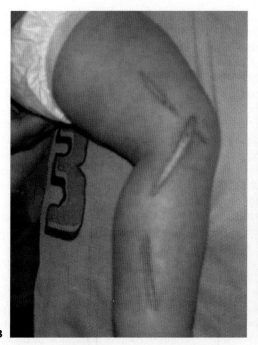
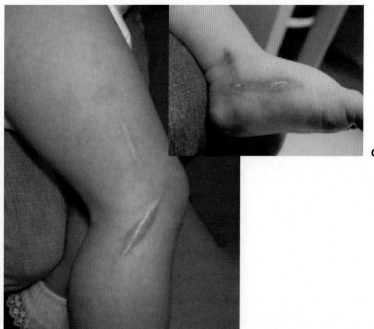

A, B   **C**

Figure 3-11. Examples of cast saw burns. Initial injury photo (**A**) and after healing (**B**). **C:** A separate injury.

Great care should be taken when performing cast wedging, especially in the tibia and in fractures where the patient may be already partially healed. The clinician needs to ensure that

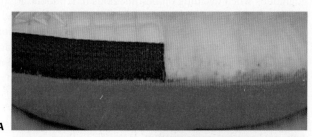

A

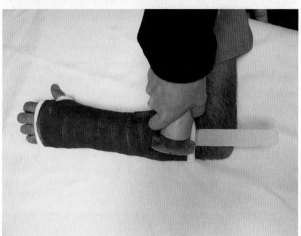

B

Figure 3-12. A: A cutaway picture showing the DE FLEX (W.L. Gore & Associates; Newark, Delaware) strip under the fiberglass casting tape. **B:** This strip will protect the skin from cast saw that has a propensity to cut easily through synthetic cast padding. (*Property of UW Pediatric Orthopaedics.*)

no excessive focal pressure is exerted at the bridge causing a pressure ulcer or nerve compression. Performing a "closing wedge" of a cast allows the bridge to be placed on the opposite side of the limb, which may be advantageous in certain circumstances, such as correcting a procurvatum or valgus deformity of the tibia. A disadvantage is that it may pinch soft tissue. After performing a cast wedging, it is wise to observe the patient in the clinic long enough to reasonably ensure that any pain associated with the correction has abated and no pain because of focal pressure exists. If any concern exists, a new cast should be applied or a different treatment course taken.

CASTING OVER SURGICAL WOUNDS AND IMPLANTS

Often, casts are applied over surgical wounds. While the majority of these heal uneventfully, special attention should be given to casts applied over traumatic or surgical wounds. When applying a stockinette over a surgical wound, care should be taken to ensure the dressing is not bunched up under the liner. It is vitally important that wounds should not be dressed with circumferential cotton gauze as they may become constrictive with dried blood over time and act as a tourniquet. We prefer to use sterile cast padding, which is able to stretch with swelling and we limit placement of the gauze to directly over the wound itself. Applying nonstick dressings directly to the wound aids in decreasing the anxiety of wound inspection during the cast removal process. Should unexplained pain, fevers, foul odors, drainage, or worsening pain occur; wounds should be inspected; however without these, routine inspection is not often necessary.

Bending the exposed ends of pins under a cast prevents excessive migration and allows for easy removal; however, migration of the bent end of the pin can occur. Sterile felt or antibiotic dressing may be placed at the pin site to help provide mechanical protection of soft tissue from migrating pins. Be aware that pin caps may become displaced and cause pressure sores. Cast padding should be placed over the pins to prevent them from sticking to the casting material as it hardens.

Although the technique of pins and plaster has largely disappeared from adult orthopedics, it can be used occasionally in pediatric orthopedics. In this technique, a fracture is reduced using pins that are placed percutaneously and incorporated into a cast to act essentially as an external fixator. The pin sites should be managed as any other exposed pin with an antibiotic dressing and/or sterile felt at the pin/skin interface. This technique allows the pins to be removed when callus formation is observed without removing the entire cast.

To inspect any area of concern under a cast, the cast can be removed, split, or windowed. The process of windowing involves localizing the area of concern and removing the overlying cast in this area without disrupting the alignment of the underlying bone. One may consider removing this window as a circular or oval piece to avoid creating any stress risers in the cast that may alter its structural integrity. However, attempting to cut "curves" with an oscillating saw places torque on the blade, increasing blade temperature. These factors should be remembered when windowing a cast. Once the cast and padding materials are removed, the wound can be inspected. Once satisfied, equal depth of padding should be replaced over the wound and the window replaced. It may be taped in place if serial examinations are required or it may be overwrapped with casting tape. Failure to replace the window can lead to swelling through the window aperture.

MEDICAL COMORBIDITIES THAT AFFECT CAST CARE

Even with application of a "perfect" cast, numerous medical issues may complicate tolerance of casting or lead to complications.[37] Children with myelomeningocele are susceptible to a number of casting complications. Pressure sores commonly occur in insensate children who do not experience or exhibit discomfort when irritation arises under the cast. Caution should be taken to avoid areas of increased pressure or overmolding when casting. In addition, the many fractures in children with myelomeningocele result from casting used for immobilization following elective surgery.[51] Iatrogenic fracture risk can be minimized by utilizing casting for as short a time frame as possible and/or use of a soft fiberglass casting material or a soft, bulky dressing that creates less of a stress riser on the bone.[51] Children with cerebral palsy are also at increased risk for pressure sores due to poor nutrition and an inability to articulate pain.[68] The contractures that likely contributed to the fracture may make casting or splinting difficult.[59] Similar approaches may be considered in children with malnutrition, renal osteodystrophy or other bone fragility disorders. An additional consideration in cases of malnutrition and diminished bone health includes increased duration of fracture healing that may require longer periods of protection to prevent refracture.[25]

Children with obesity present their own complications. Although there are no studies documenting the outcomes of casting in obese children, studies on surgical treatment have demonstrated complications of refracture, wound infection, and failure of surgical fixation,[48,73] issues that likely have non-operative correlates. Loss of alignment when adequate molding cannot occur because of increased soft tissues can occur. When casting an obese child, inclusion of an extra joint above and/or below the fracture may be required to maintain cast position. Diligent monitoring of alignment allows intervention with recasting, wedging, or transition to surgical intervention. Obese patients are more likely to undergo surgical treatment, as opposed to closed reduction, although it is unclear whether this is related to fracture severity or concerns regarding fracture stabilization.[61]

Alterations in casting materials or approaches may also be necessary in children with behavioral issues. Children with autistic spectrum disorder present additional complexity during cast application (see discussion on distraction techniques), but even prior to cast application considering their behavior guides decision making regarding the most appropriate immobilization. Children with violent tendencies pose even more risk once a cast is applied, not only to others but also to themselves. Administration of behavioral medications may improve tolerance of casting.[16] Soft splinting may be preferable, accepting some risk of malunion over likely secondary injury. Discussion and shared decision making with the parents result in the best management for an individual child and their family.

Children with dermatologic conditions require other considerations when deciding on best methods of immobilization. Children with atopic dermatitis may react to synthetic padding, so cotton may be more preferable. Splinting allows for better skin management, but when casting is required, minimizing duration or performing frequent cast changes allows for monitoring of skin conditions or early transition to splinting. Soft casting material contains diisocyanate which has been suspected, but not proven, as a skin irritant in isolated cases[44]; avoiding such material in children with significant skin sensitivity or disorders seems prudent. Windowing the cast over an area of skin breakdown or infection allows for monitoring of the area. Varicella presents an even more complex issue as widespread skin breakdown occurs, predisposing to superinfection and development of bacterial pyomyositis. Casting helps prevent skin breakdown by covering itchy lesions, but monitoring lesions is not possible. Again, splinting may be preferable to allow for monitoring if it does not compromise maintenance of fracture reduction; otherwise, windowing, or frequent cast changes may allow for skin monitoring. There should be a low threshold for removal of the cast if the child complains of pain to assess for not only compartment syndrome or infection, but also necrotizing fasciitis.[22,18]

LOCATION-SPECIFIC IMMOBILIZATION

SUGAR-TONG SPLINT IMMOBILIZATION

Sugar-tong splints provide effective temporary support to the wrist and forearm until definitive reduction and casting or

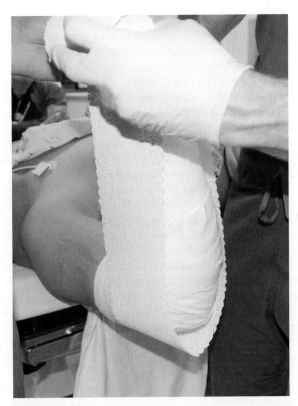

Figure 3-13. The plaster roll for the sugar-tong splint is measured and is chosen to be wider than the arm without allowing for overlapping once the plaster slab is dipped and applied. (*Property of UW Pediatric Orthopaedics.*)

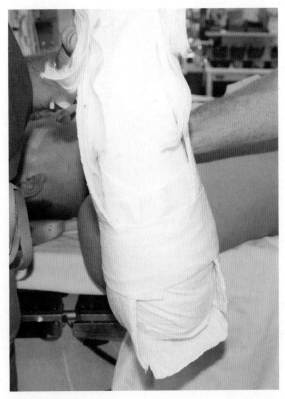

Figure 3-14. After being dipped and applied, the slab is held on by one layer of cotton while tucks are cut in the plaster at the elbow to allow for overlap and minimal bunching. (*Property of UW Pediatric Orthopaedics.*)

internal fixation, while allowing for swelling. Sugar-tong splints can be used for definitive treatment provided the splint is comfortable and is retightened after 3 to 5 days to accommodate the decrease in swelling. At that point, reapplication of an elastic bandage or overwrapping with fiberglass is appropriate.

Before treating, the contralateral uninjured limb may be used as a template to measure and prepare an appropriate slab of casting material which should be wide enough to fully support the volar and dorsal surfaces of the arm (without radial and ulnar overlap) and long enough to span the arm from the volar MP flexion crease in the hand, around the elbow (flexed at 90 degrees), and dorsally to the metacarpal heads (Fig. 3-13). It is important that plaster splints are no more than 10 layers thick and of appropriate length so that edges do not have to be folded over (increasing thickness and the heat from curing). The slab is further customized to cut out material around the thumb base and tuck cuts are made at the elbow to prevent bunching of the material during the application.

The injured arm is reduced and positioned as described above, it is wrapped with three to four layers of cotton padding from the hand and around the elbow (similar thickness as that used for long-arm casting). The slab is dipped in cool water, excess water is removed and the material is vigorously rubbed together so that the layers incorporate for strength. The ends of the slab have two to three layers of padding applied which will fold back and make the edges soft (Fig. 3-14). The splint is applied and held with one roll of cotton and then an

elastic bandage is tightly applied until the material is hardened (Fig. 3-15). After hardening, the tight Ace bandage is removed and replaced with a new elastic bandage applied without significant tension (Fig. 3-16). This method ensures an optimal fit without having the splint be too tight.

In the method described above, the arm is circumferentially wrapped with cotton and then a slab of plaster with padded ends is applied over it. This method is advantageous in ensuring a smooth interface of cotton without bunching under the

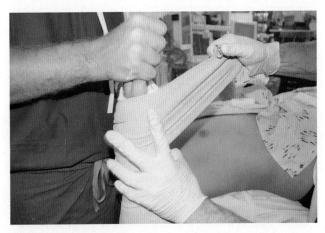

Figure 3-15. An elastic bandage is wrapped tightly to assist with terminal molding of the splint.

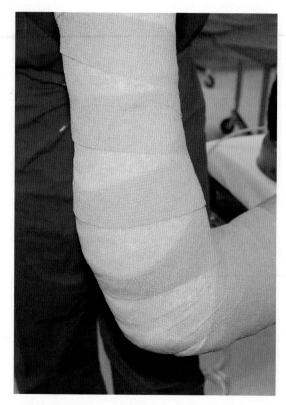

Figure 3-16. The elastic bandage has been removed and replaced with a self-adherent elastic tape that has been loosely applied. (*Property of UW Pediatric Orthopaedics.*)

plaster slab. If the clinician fears a lot of circumferential cotton padding could worsen swelling, an alternative method exists. In this instance, a long strip of padding is made by layering three to five layers of cotton and then the plaster slab is laid on top of it. The cotton is long and wide enough to ensure that there are no rough edges. The padded slab is then applied and wrapped as described above.

LONG-ARM 90-DEGREE CAST IMMOBILIZATION

Case study 1: A 7-year-old girl with a both-bone forearm fracture undergoes attempted closed reduction and long-arm cast application. She presents to clinic the following day, where radiographs reveal angulation of 18 degrees in the AP plane and 5 degrees in the lateral plane (Fig. 3-17). Critical review of this case demonstrates a cast applied with too much padding and thus a poor fit, is too short in the long-arm portion, has too much plaster applied throughout the cast and especially in the antecubital fossa (increased risk for burn), and has a curved ulnar border that allows the arm to settle into the angulation. She is indicated for cast removal and rereduction.

Fracture reduction and long-arm cast application are best done in a setting where the child is adequately sedated and where enough qualified personnel can apply the cast under fluoroscopic guidance, although this may not be possible in many locations. Fracture reduction technique may consist of longitudinal traction, manipulation recreating the deformity (Fig. 3-18), or reducing the fracture and placing the intact periosteum on tension.

Three-point molding can be used in completely displaced fractures at the same level in the forearm; hand rotation is the final position to account for, based on angulation. In both-bone forearm fractures in which the fractures are at differing levels, apex volar greenstick angulation is reduced with pronation and apex dorsal angulation is reduced with supination. It may be helpful to remember the (literal) "rule of thumb": rotating the thumb toward the apex of the deformity aids in reduction. Thus, an apex volar greenstick is reduced with pronation, an apex dorsal with supination. Optimal hand and wrist rotations can be ensured with fluoroscopy prior to cast application.

In this instance, longitudinal traction is used with an assistant while a thin layer of cotton padding is applied (Fig. 3-19). Alternatively, the fingers could be placed in finger traps with the elbow flexed just short of 90 degrees and with weights from the distal humerus. Individual strips of cotton are placed and torn with tension to fit intimately on the posterior elbow thus avoiding too much anterior padding (Fig. 3-20). Cotton is rolled high in the axilla to ensure enough padding for the proximal trimline (Fig. 3-21). After padding is applied to the entire arm, a small splint of five layers of Plaster of Paris is fashioned to fit into the first web space (Fig. 3-22) and then incorporated with sequential layers of plaster (Fig. 3-23); we find that this method allows for a better fit in the hand. Plaster is pushed and unrolled up the arm to the elbow (see Fig. 3-6) without lifting the plaster roll off the arm unless tucks are needed in the concavity. We prefer to apply Plaster of Paris or fiberglass to a limb in stages by focusing and immobilizing one joint at a time; for long-arm casts, we apply and mold the wrist and forearm and we extend the cast up over the elbow after the material has hardened. Once enough plaster is applied, the initial mold to incorporate the layers is started by rubbing the arm circumferentially (Fig. 3-24). As the plaster begins to harden, terminal molding of the arm is performed under fluoroscopy by flattening the plaster over the apex of the deformity (Fig. 3-25), molding the ulnar border with the flat of the hand (Fig. 3-26), and finally with some interosseus molding (Fig. 3-27) that will make the cast flatter and less cylindrical in cross section. Fluoroscopy images are obtained as the short-arm portion hardens before extending the cast up the humerus. If acceptable reduction is apparent, the antecubital fossa is inspected closely to detect and trim back cast material which may be too high and which could lead to neurovascular compromise. Decreased pressure in a limb can be obtained by using foam underneath the cast material or by cutting and spreading casts and after releasing the underlying padding. This method of applying the cast in two stages has the potential downside of edges of the short-arm cast digging into soft tissue proximally, so this must be avoided. As the cast is extended up the humerus, a small posterior splint can be applied to elbow convexity to decrease the tendency to fill the concavity of the elbow with thick exothermic plaster. The humerus portion is molded terminally by flattening the posterior humerus and molding along the supracondylar ridges. Plain radiographs are then obtained while the child is still sedated and if alignment is good, the forearm cast is univalved and spread. In general, the cast should be univalved and spread on the side of the arm which is opposite the direction of initial displacement; a fracture with a

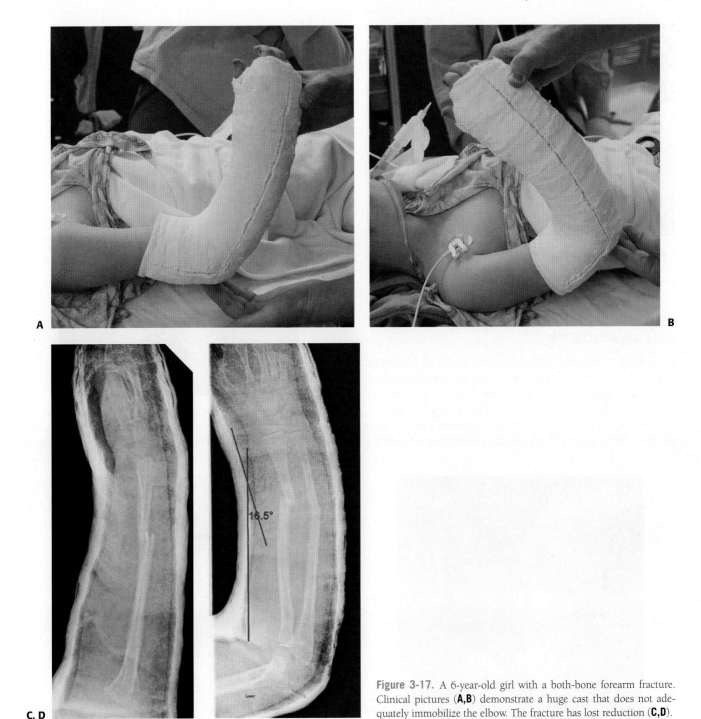

A **B** **C, D**

Figure 3-17. A 6-year-old girl with a both-bone forearm fracture. Clinical pictures (**A,B**) demonstrate a huge cast that does not adequately immobilize the elbow. The fracture has lost reduction (**C,D**).

propensity for dorsal displacement should be split volarly and a fracture with a propensity for volar displacement should be split and spread along the dorsal surface. After 2 weeks, the plain radiographs demonstrate improved reduction and a more improved fitting cast (Fig. 3-28).

SHORT-ARM CAST IMMOBILIZATION

It should be noted that the above description of a long-arm cast application utilizing plaster, staged casting, splints, and univalving is the traditional method of casting preferred in many centers for displaced both-bone diaphyseal fractures. Alternative methods include the use of fiber glass with the stretch relax technique, which generally does not require splints or univalving. As there are now good quality, randomized prospective studies showing that distal third both-bone fractures are treated equally well in short- or long-arm casts, short-arm cast immobilization is appropriate for most distal radius and ulnar fractures. The technique of application is similar to that presented above; however, it is important that the distal cast be oval in cross section (see Fig. 3-27) and the cast index (ratio of the AP cast width to lateral cast depth) to be near 0.7.

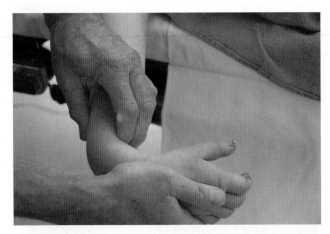

Figure 3-18. The deformity is accentuated and hyperflexion followed by reduction can allow the displaced ends to become opposed. (*Property of UW Pediatric Orthopaedics.*)

LONG ARM–THUMB SPICA EXTENSION CAST IMMOBILIZATION

Case study 2: A 6-year-old boy suffers a displaced both-bone forearm fracture that is treated with long-arm cast application. Proximal and middle third both-bone forearm fractures are harder to manage as there is less remodeling potential; further, when the radius is fractured proximal to the ulna, one can often see more difficulty in holding the fractures reduced when the

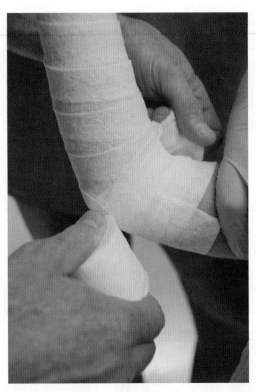

Figure 3-20. To pad the convexity of the elbow without excessively padding the concavity, cotton strips are placed and torn over the elbow to prevent cotton from bunching up in the antecubital fossa. (*Property of UW Pediatric Orthopaedics.*)

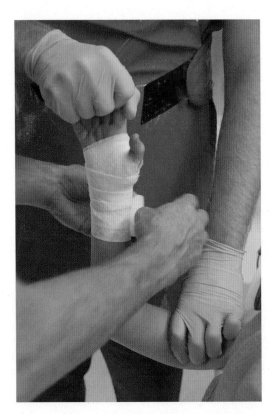

Figure 3-19. While the limb is held reduced with longitudinal traction applied by the assistant, cotton padding is applied and overlapped by 50%. (*Property of UW Pediatric Orthopaedics.*)

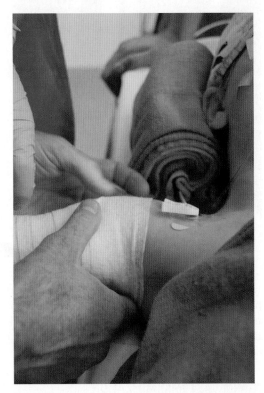

Figure 3-21. In this instance, stockinette was not used. Cotton is placed high in the axilla to have a soft edge at the proximal trimline of the plaster which will be applied more distal in the arm. (*Property of UW Pediatric Orthopaedics.*)

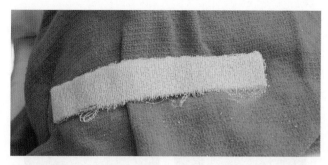

Figure 3-22. A small plaster splint fits nicely into the web space and will be incorporated in the plaster of the forearm portion. (*Property of UW Pediatric Orthopaedics.*)

elbow is flexed. At 1 week, radiographs demonstrate loss in reduction with 30 degrees of angulation at the radius and the need for rereduction (Fig. 3-29).

In this instance, we plan to reduce the arm with a combination of traction, pronation, and apex pressure with fluoroscopic guidance (Fig. 3-30). Once reduced, the arm is held with longitudinal traction, proximal and distal stockinette and cotton padding are applied for a long arm–thumb spica cast in extension (Fig. 3-31). Including the thumb in this cast will fully control forearm rotation while additionally maintaining the fracture out-to-length, which is obtained during the casting under traction. To prevent pressure sores over the thumb, extra padding is placed over the radial aspect of the anatomic snuffbox and thumb. The thumb spica portion of fiberglass is placed carefully out to the tip of the thumb while holding the thumb in neutral abduction and opposition (Fig. 3-32). The fiberglass is applied with 50% overlap and using the stretch relaxation technique, fluoroscopy is again utilized while terminal molding of the short-arm portion is performed in slight pronation and with broad pressure over the apex of the deformity (Fig. 3-33). The upper arm portion is next applied once the forearm portion is hardened and with the reduction confirmed under fluoroscopic imaging. As the upper fiberglass hardens, a supracondylar mold is applied with the arm in gentle traction as the butt of the surgeon's hand and thenar eminence terminally mold the

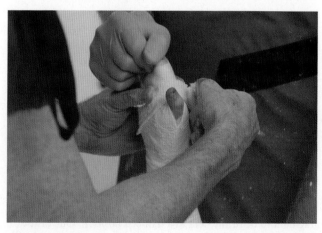

Figure 3-23. This splint is incorporated with rolls of plaster moving proximally. (*Property of UW Pediatric Orthopaedics.*)

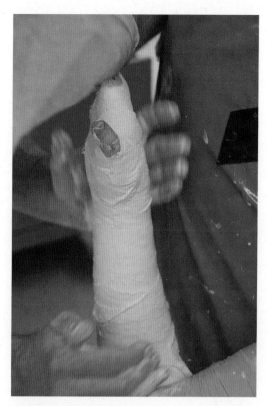

Figure 3-24. The cast is initially molded to incorporate the fiber and plaster to make it stronger and to improve the fit. (*Property of UW Pediatric Orthopaedics.*)

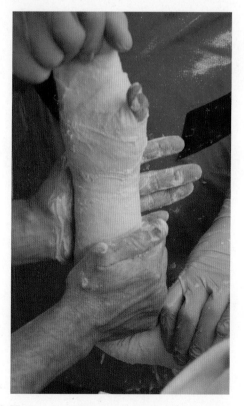

Figure 3-25. Initial molding is performed to flatten the cast with a flat surface applied over the apex of the deformity. (*Property of UW Pediatric Orthopaedics.*)

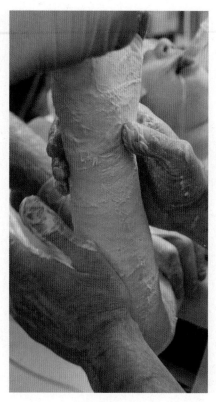

Figure 3-26. Initial and terminal molding of the ulnar border will allow the cast to be straight and will resist ulnar sag of fracture fragments when the swelling goes down. (*Property of UW Pediatric Orthopaedics.*)

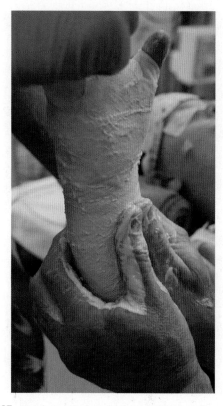

Figure 3-27. Gentle terminal interosseus mold keeps pressure on the apex, keeps the radius and ulna apart, and flattens the cast, maintaining optimal cast index. (*Property of UW Pediatric Orthopaedics.*)

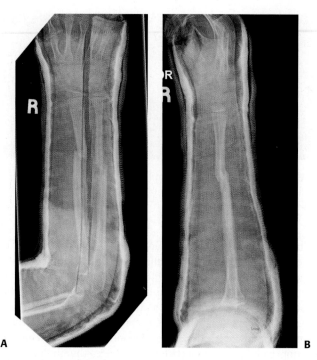

Figure 3-28. AP (**A**) and lateral (**B**) radiographs 2 weeks after the operative procedure demonstrate excellent maintenance of reduction and early healing. (*Property of UW Pediatric Orthopaedics.*)

fiberglass (Fig. 3-34); this mold in concert with the thumb spica mold should help to maintain rotation and length of the reduction. Final trimming and finishing the edges with the previously placed stockinette is done in the hand and the palmar trimline is cut back to allow MP finger flexion (Fig. 3-35). Finally, the dorsum of the cast can be univalved with a cast saw to allow for swelling; with fiberglass the cut edges of the cast need to be held open with commercially available spacers (Fig. 3-36) or other such material to keep the cast from springing closed; this is in contradistinction to plaster which can remain open once a terminally molded cast is spread. Plain radiographs after 3 weeks of immobilization confirm reduction of the fracture (Fig. 3-37).

THUMB SPICA CAST IMMOBILIZATION

Usual incorporation of the thumb is needed for the extension cast described above as well as carpal injuries. Some surgeons include the thumb in all short-arm casts too. Regardless, it's important to ensure the thumb is well padded and casted in a neutral position thumb abduction and opposition with well-padded distal trimline.

Shoulder Immobilization

Immobilization about the shoulder and the clavicle is somewhat limited when compared with other areas of the skeleton. Because of anatomic constraints about the shoulder, it is often very challenging to gain a reduction of a bone (proximal humerus, clavicle); and it is not practical to expect the fracture fragment to be firmly held in a reduced position. One historical exception may be the use of the shoulder spica cast for displaced proximal humerus fractures. Practically speaking, this

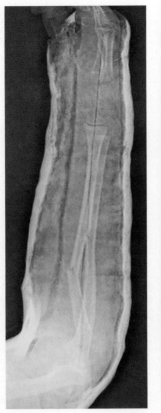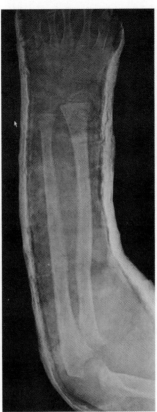

A   B

Figure 3-29. Radiographs of a 7-year-old boy with a proximal both-bone forearm fracture treated in a long-arm cast. The radius fracture is proximal to the ulna and this pattern is prone to loss of reduction in a long-arm flexed cast as seen in this case with unacceptable alignment. (*Property of UW Pediatric Orthopaedics.*)

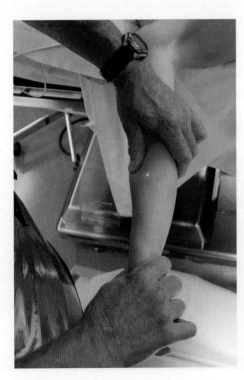

cast was challenging to apply and for the patient to wear; pediatric orthopedic trauma surgeons today would use internal fixation to maintain fracture reduction.

Despite the difficulty encountered when attempting reduction and firmly maintaining reduction with closed means, immobilization about the shoulder is used to provide comfort in the injured child. For clavicle fractures, a figure-of-eight collar or a shoulder sling can support the shoulder. Although the figure-of-eight collar was designed to retract the shoulder posteriorly and thus potentially reduce a shortened clavicle; practically

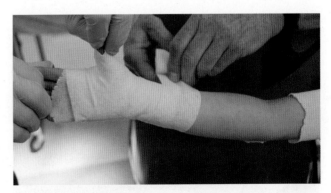

Figure 3-30. The arm is rotated under fluoroscopy to identify the rotation of the hand that best reduces the fracture. (*Property of UW Pediatric Orthopaedics.*)

Figure 3-31. The thumb spica cotton padding is applied. A moderate amount of padding is applied at the dorsal radial aspect of the thumb base. (*Property of UW Pediatric Orthopaedics.*)

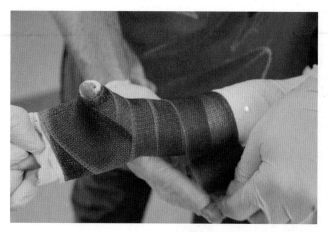

Figure 3-32. Fiberglass is applied with the stretch relaxation method. (*Property of UW Pediatric Orthopaedics.*)

the effect is minimal and the force needed to hold the shoulder back is often a challenge to the patient. Most patients find a personal preference between figure-of-eight collar and shoulder sling which is acceptable given equal clinical results between the two.

A proximal humerus fracture (whether treated nonoperatively or operatively) may be protected with immobilization with a sugar-tong splint. This splint is applied in stages. A slab of fiberglass or plaster is cut to a length that spans the proximal medial humerus (not too high in the axilla) and extends over the elbow and up the lateral aspect of the humerus up over the shoulder (Fig. 3-38). After dipping in water, the slab is placed on appropriate padding and then applied to the arm. We find it helpful to wrap sugar-tong splints very tightly with an elastic bandage as this improves the mold and fit. The elastic bandage is removed when the splint material is hard and is replaced loosely with a new one. The common pitfalls with this type of immobilization include the medial splint edge in the axilla that is too thick or too high. In addition, when the lateral splint edge is too low and ends close to a fracture level, it does not immobilize and actually increases the lever arm forces at the fracture. This is due to the fact that the adjacent joints which are immobilized, and that could normally move and decrease the length of the lever arm, cannot function as such.

Hanging arm casts can be used in proximal humerus surgical neck fractures and humeral shaft fractures. These synthetic

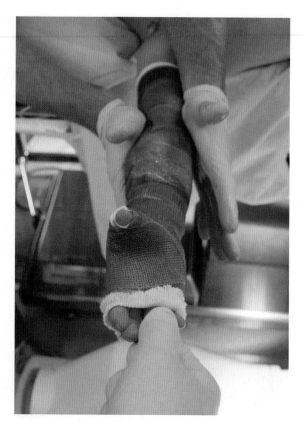

Figure 3-34. Supracondylar mold is applied above the elbow; this will prevent the cast from slipping down. (*Property of UW Pediatric Orthopaedics.*)

long-arm casts are applied with the concept that gravity will act upon the humerus fracture and can be effective in gradually improving alignment in children with fractures that are minimally angulated or bayonet opposed. The children will have to sleep in an upright position for several weeks until the fracture is healed enough to be converted to splint immobilization. These casts are simple long-arm casts that do not require intimate molding; the weight of the cast will provide gradual distraction that aligns the fracture. Common

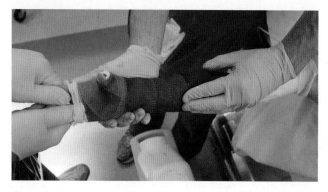

Figure 3-33. Initial molding of the fiberglass is performed over the apex of the deformity. (*Property of UW Pediatric Orthopaedics.*)

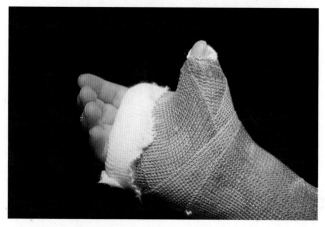

Figure 3-35. The hand portion is trimmed back to allow finger MP flexion and the spica portion of the cast is out to the tip of the thumb, which is neutrally placed. (*Property of UW Pediatric Orthopaedics.*)

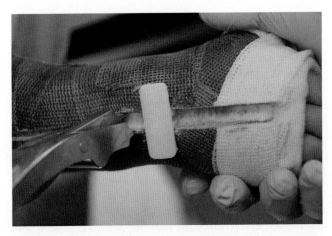

Figure 3-36. The fiberglass cast is held open with a plastic spacer, univalved fiberglass casts tend to spring back while plaster casts tend to stay open. (*Property of UW Pediatric Orthopaedics.*)

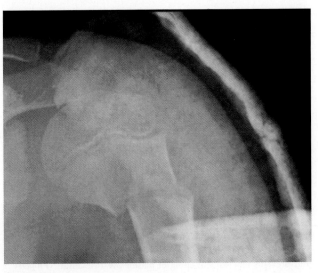

Figure 3-38. The plaster of a sugar-tong upper arm splint is folded over the shoulder and above the fractured proximal humerus fracture. (*Property of UW Pediatric Orthopaedics.*)

pitfalls include a patient who cannot sleep upright and placing the neck collar attachment on the forearm too close to the elbow, which could increase anterior angulation; or placing the attachment too close to the wrist, which could lead to posterior angulation.

SHORT-LEG CAST APPLICATION

Short-leg casts are applied with goals of fully immobilizing the lower leg and keeping the ankle at 90 degrees while avoiding complications such as pressure sores. After applying proximal

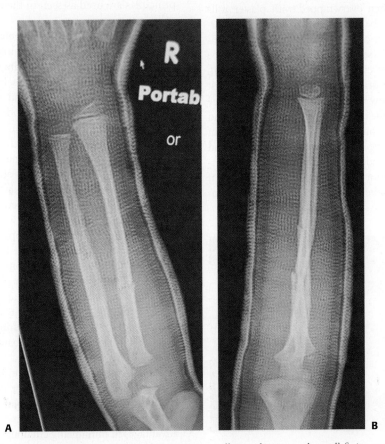

Figure 3-37. Radiographs obtained in the OR demonstrate excellent reduction and a well-fitting cast. (*Property of UW Pediatric Orthopaedics.*)

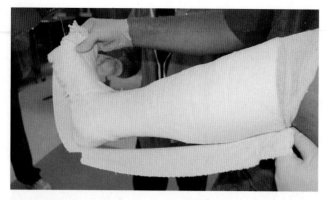

Figure 3-39. A 5 thickness posterior slab has been dipped and applied to the posterior foot and leg at the beginning of a short-leg cast. Cuts have been made at the ankle to allow good overlap without bunching. This posterior splint brings thickness and strength to the posterior part and prevents anterior bunching of plaster over the ankle. (*Property of UW Pediatric Orthopaedics.*)

and distal stockinette, the limb is wrapped with cotton padding and the ankle is held at 90 degrees. A potential pitfall is that as the casting material is placed, the ankle drifts into equinus; then as ankle flexion is restored to 90 degrees, casting material bunches up at the anterior ankle, which can cause soft tissue damage over time as well as neurovascular constriction. To avoid excessive Plaster of Paris cast material over the anterior ankle, a posterior splint of five layers thick is measured and applied (Fig. 3-39) and then overwrapped with plaster rolls (Fig. 3-40). The ankle can be held at 90 degrees by the surgeon's torso and the plaster is carefully molded around the malleoli and the pretibial crest (see Fig. 3-7). The cast should be hard and well cured before cutting; bivalving a wet cast will weaken it and the foot can drift into equinus. The cooled cast can be supported on a pillow with the ankle hanging free (see Fig. 3-8). Once hardened, the cast can be univalved and spread anteriorly, if needed, to accommodate swelling; if significant swelling is expected, then the cast can be bivalved and spread with release of the cotton padding. Using fiberglass for short-leg casts generally results in a lighter and stronger cast, but if fiberglass is improperly applied too tightly, it can cause compartment syndrome.

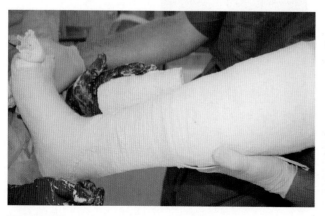

Figure 3-40. Plaster is overlapped by half and rolled up the leg over the splint. (*Property of UW Pediatric Orthopaedics.*)

LONG-LEG CAST APPLICATION

Long-leg cast application incorporates all of the techniques above; once the short-leg portion has hardened, the upper thigh is wrapped with padding and the knee (held in the chosen degree of flexion) and thigh are overwrapped with cast material. Care is needed to make sure the posterior trimline of the short-leg cast is not too high and which could be compressing in the popliteal fossa. The anterior knee portion can be reinforced with a splint and thus further decreasing the cast load in the popliteal fossa. Finally, a medial and lateral supracondylar mold (similar to that in long-arm cast) can be used to support the weight of the cast and prevent distal migration. Plaster long-leg casts can be heavy, as such we will use an all fiberglass cast or consider a composite cast whereby the short-leg portion is molded with Plaster of Paris and then when hardened, the proximal portion is placed with fiberglass.

SHORT-LEG SPLINT APPLICATION

Posterior short-leg splints are commonly used to immobilize the foot and ankle prior to definitive operative or nonoperative treatment and additionally to support the limb in the immediate postoperative period. These splints can accommodate significant swelling following trauma or surgery. Supplemental stirrup application may be needed in larger patients whose foot position cannot be controlled with a single posterior slab. In these cases, similar application methods and principles are used as seen in the upper extremity sugar-tong splint application.

Fundamental application includes holding the foot and ankle in 90 degrees of flexion while the limb is wrapped with four to six layers of cotton padding from the toes to the knee. A posterior slab of plaster is selected and should be wide enough to provide a medial and lateral trimline of an inch. It should be 10 layers thick and measured similarly to that seen in short-leg cast application described above. If needed, a U-stirrup of plaster five layers thick is measured and is usually 1 to 2 in narrower than the posterior plaster slab; this allows overlap of the two pieces of plaster without completely covering the anterior foot, ankle, and leg. Both the stirrup and the posterior slab are dipped in water and the proximal and distal trimlines are padded with three to four more layers of cast padding. The slab is applied posteriorly; any redundant material at the level of the heel can be cut away before the U-stirrup is applied with some overlap of the stirrup and the slab. The plaster is held in place with one layer of cast padding. An elastic bandage is applied tightly until the plaster is hard, and then removed to prevent constriction. This last layer of cast padding allows for easy removal of the final layer of loosely applied elastic bandage or self-adherent elastic tape.

Variances to this method are similar to sugar-tong splint application described above. For instance, some practitioners prefer to layer the wet plaster splint with 5 thicknesses of padding and apply the padded splint directly to the limb. This has advantages in minimizing circumferential wrapping of the limb with cotton; yet great care is needed to prevent inadvertent bunching or slipping of the padding.

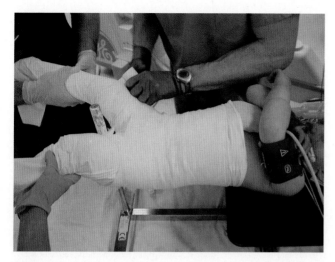

Figure 3-41. This 5-year-old child with a femur fracture is supported with four assistants as cotton padding is applied to the patient's body, which is covered with a waterproof liner over a stack of towels placed as a spacer for his belly. (*Property of UW Pediatric Orthopaedics.*)

SPICA CAST APPLICATION

Spica casts can be applied from infants to adolescents and the location of application can vary according to age and clinical problem. For instance, infants and most children with painful injuries will require sedation and application in the supine position on a spica table. In contrast, a single-leg spica cast can be used as an adjunct to internal fixation for femur fracture in large children or adolescents. These latter casts can be applied in a supine or even a standing position with a compliant and comfortable patient. Because of the size of the casts, most spica casts are constructed with synthetic cast material; Plaster of Paris still has utility in small infants where a more intimate mold is used and where it's hard to conform fiberglass rolls.

Spica cast application in children is performed on a well-padded spica table which should be firmly attached to the OR bed or cart; one person should be responsible for managing the torso and making sure the child does not fall off the table; one to two assistants will support the legs while the anesthesia team manages the head and airway—this leaves the last of a four- or five-person team to apply the cast.

Before placing the child on the spica table, a waterproof pantaloon or stockinette is applied to the torso and legs in some centers. Place a 2- to 4-in thick towel or other pad on the stomach and under the liner or stockinette that will be removed when the cast is dry, to have room for food and respiration. Note that if the patient starts to desaturate during spica cast application, pulling out the abdomen padding frequently resolves this. The child is lifted onto the table and 3 to 6 thicknesses of padding are applied, with more at bony prominences such as over the patella and heels. It is also wise to completely cover the perineum with padding and high over the thorax; it is extremely hard to add padding once the cast material is applied (Fig. 3-41). After padding is appropriately applied, the thorax is wrapped with synthetic cast material (see Fig. 3-9) and extended down over the uninjured thigh; care is needed to cover the "intern's triangle"; this is the posterior area of the cast at the junction of the thigh, buttock, and thorax. Once the uninjured leg portion is hardened, the injured leg is casted from proximal to distal. We recommend casting from the thorax, over the hip, and to the distal thigh then extending over the knee and onto the distal leg as soon as the hip and thigh portion is firm; once the knee and leg portion is hardened, then extend it down to include the foot and ankle. Care must be taken not to apply a short-leg cast first, and use it to apply traction across the femur as this is associated with soft tissue problems and compartment syndrome. In general, we include the foot in neuromuscular patients who are prone to develop an equinus contracture and whose distal tibia is osteoporotic and prone to fracture at the level of the distal trimline. The risk of including the foot in a spica cast is soft tissue problems over the dorsal ankle. Once the final cast is hardened, the perineal region is trimmed out and patient is removed from the spica table. The abdominal pad is removed and in some children, a hole can be cut for further room (Fig. 3-42). Next, appropriate radiographs are obtained and the trimlines are padded from rolling back

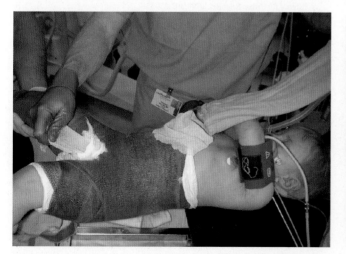
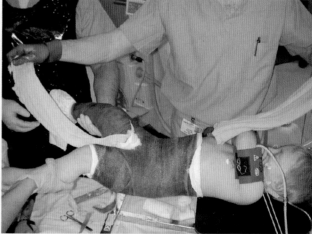

Figure 3-42. The abdominal pillow is removed after trimming away the perineal region.

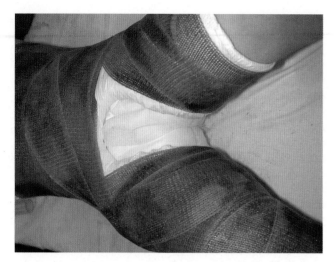

Figure 3-43. When finished, the spica edges are well padded and incorporated into the cast. A small diaper is placed into the perineal region and then another diaper will be placed over this to hold it in place. (*Property of UW Pediatric Orthopaedics.*)

the under padding and lining and incorporated with trim fiberglass. The decision to apply a bar from leg to leg is made based on the structural integrity of the cast. Usually, this is not needed in small children and infants. Should a bar be needed, then it is wise to wait until the cast is fully cured and the chance of a pressure sore is decreased. Non–toilet-trained infants and children need to have an absorbent pad (small diaper, ABD pad, or sanitary napkin) placed in the perineal region and then a diaper is placed over this (Fig. 3-43). Simply placing a diaper over the cast will not absorb the waste material, as the diaper will not be in contact before it tracks under the cast.

For length-stable diaphyseal femoral shaft fractures, many centers are now moving toward a single-leg spica cast, which does not include the contralateral thigh and positions the hip and knee in less flexion and gives the child the opportunity to ambulate with a walker or crutches.

CONCLUSION

In this chapter, we highlight the pearls and pitfalls of cast and splint application in children with pediatric orthopedic trauma. This orthopedic subspecialty is one of the few in which an injury is more likely treated with these methods than surgical treatment. A dearth of prospective studies means that much art and personal preferences remain in cast and splint application. As time moves along and there are more innovative methods to treat fractures with surgery, the role of casting will not be supplanted. There will always be a need for a technically well-done cast that helps speed recovery in pediatric trauma. In our minds, the many complications result from inappropriate use of the cast or splint to *obtain* correction; in contrast, the cast or splint should be used to *maintain* reduction achieved either open or closed. Tight casts and bandages are also commonly associated with compartment syndrome. Problems such as tight

casts, wet casts leading to infection, foreign objects in casts, and pressure ulcers are not uncommon. It is important to educate parents that small children may not adequately communicate problems occurring under a cast. It is good for us all to remember that in the words of Chad Price, MD, "there are no hypochondriacs in a cast."

REFERENCES

1. Aarons CE, Fernandez MD, Willsey M, et al. Bier block regional anesthesia and casting for forearm fractures: safety in the pediatric emergency department setting. *J Pediatr Orthop*. 2014;34:45–49.
2. Akbar M, Bresch B, Raiss P, et al. Fractures in myelomeningocele. *J Orthop Traumatol*. 2010;11:175–182.
3. Ansari MZ, Swarup S, Ghani R, et al. Oscillating saw injuries during removal of plaster. *Eur J Emerg Med*. 1998;5:37–39.
4. Bashyal RK, Chu JY, Schoenecker PL, et al. Complications after pinning of supracondylar distal humerus fractures. *J Pediatr Orthop*. 2009;29:704–708.
5. Bear DM, Friel NA, Lupo CL, et al. Hematoma block versus sedation for the reduction of distal radius fractures in children. *J Hand Surg Am*. 2015;40:57–61.
6. Bebbington A, Lewis P, Savage R. Cast wedging for orthopaedic surgeons! *Injury*. 2005;36:71–72.
7. Bernthal NM, Hoshino CM, Dichter D, et al. Recovery of elbow motion following pediatric lateral condylar fractures of the humerus. *J Bone Joint Surg Am*. 2011;93:871–877.
8. Bingold AC. On splitting plasters: a useful analogy. *J Bone Joint Surg Br*. 1979;61-B:294–295.
9. Borland M, Esson A, Babl F, et al. Procedural sedation in children in the emergency department: a PREDICT study. *Emerg Med Austral*. 2009;21:71–79.
10. Boyle PK, Badal JJ, Boeve JW. Severe cast burn after bunionectomy in a patient who received peripheral nerve blocks for postoperative analgesia. *Local Reg Anesth*. 2011;4:11–13.
11. Brewster MB, Gupta M, Pattison GT, et al. Ponseti casting: a new soft option. *J Bone Joint Surg Br*. 2008;90:1512–1515.
12. Carmichael KD, Goucher NR. Cast abscess: a case report. *Orthop Nurs*. 2006;25:137–139.
13. Carmichael KD, Westmoreland J. Effectiveness of ear protection in reducing anxiety during cast removal in children. *Am J Orthop (Belle Mead NJ)*. 2005;34:43–46.
14. Ceroni D, Martin X, Delhumeau C, et al. Effects of cast-mediated immobilization on bone mineral mass at various sites in adolescents with lower-extremity fracture. *J Bone Joint Surg Am*. 2012;94:208–216.
15. Ceroni D, Martin XE, Farpour-Lambert NJ, et al. Assessment of muscular performance in teenagers after a lower extremity fracture. *J Pediatr Orthop*. 2010;30:807–812.
16. Chambers H, Becker RE, Hoffman MT, et al. Managing behavior for a child with autism in a body cast. *J Dev Behav Pediatr*. 2012;33:506–508.
17. Chambers CT, Taddio A, Uman LS, et al. Psychological interventions for reducing pain and distress during routine childhood immunizations: a systematic review. *Clin Ther*. 2009;31(Suppl 2):S77–S103.
18. Clark P, Davidson D, Letts M, et al. Necrotizing fasciitis secondary to chickenpox infection in children. *Can J Surg*. 2003;46:9–14.
19. Constantine E, Steele DW, Eberson C, et al. The use of local anesthetic techniques for closed forearm fracture reduction in children. *Pediatr Emerg Care*. 2007;23:209–211.
20. Cudny ME, Wang NE, Bardas SL, et al. Adverse events associated with procedural sedation in pediatric patients in the emergency department. *Hosp Pharm*. 2013;48:134–142.
21. Davids JR. Rotational deformity and remodeling after fracture of the femur in children. *Clin Orthop Relat Res*. 1994;302:27–35.
22. Delasobera BE, Place R, Howell J, et al. Serious infectious complications related to extremity cast/splint placement in children. *J Emerg Med*. 2011;41:47–50.
23. Deshpande SV. An experimental study of pressure-volume dynamics of casting materials. *Injury*. 2005;36:1067–1074.
24. DiFazio R, Vessey J, Zurakowski D, et al. Incidence of skin complications and associated charges in children treated with hip spica casts for femur fractures. *J Pediatr Orthop*. 2011;31:17–22.
25. Dwyer AJ, John B, Mam MK, et al. Relation of nutritional status to healing of compound fractures of long bones of the lower limbs. *Orthopedics*. 2007;30:709–712.
26. Fletcher ND, Schiller JR, Garg S, et al. Increased severity of type III supracondylar humerus fractures in the preteen population. *J Pediatr Orthop*. 2012;32:567–572.
27. Flynn JM, Bashyal RK, Yeger-McKeever M, et al. Acute traumatic compartment syndrome of the leg in children: diagnosis and outcome. *J Bone Joint Surg Am*. 2011;93:937–941.
28. Forni C, Loro L, Tremosini M, et al. Use of polyurethane foam inside plaster casts to prevent the onset of heel sores in the population at risk. A controlled clinical study. *J Clin Nurs*. 2011;20(5–6):675–680.
29. Furia JP, Alioto RJ, Marquardt JD. The efficacy and safety of the hematoma block for fracture reduction in closed, isolated fracture. *Orthopedics*. 1997;20:423–426.
30. Gannaway JK, Hunter JR. Thermal effects of casting materials. *Clin Orthop Relat Res*. 1983;181:191–195.
31. Garfin SR, Mubarak SJ, Evans KL, et al. Quantification of intracompartmental pressure and volume under plaster casts. *J Bone Joint Surg Am*. 1981;63:449–453.
32. Grottkau BE, Epps HR, Di Scala C. Compartment syndrome in children and adolescents. *J Pediatr Surg*. 2005;40:678–682.

33. Gulati A, Dixit A, Taylor GJ. Pediatric fractures: temporal trends and cost implications of treatment under general anesthesia. *Eur J Trauma Emerg Surg.* 2012;38: 59–64.
34. Guyton GP. An analysis of iatrogenic complications from the total contact cast. *Foot Ankle Int.* 2005;26:903–907.
35. Haapala J, Arokoski J, Pirttimaki J, et al. Incomplete restoration of immobilization induced softening of young beagle knee articular cartilage after 50-week remobilization. *Int J Sports Med.* 2000;21:76–81.
36. Halanski MA, Halanski AD, Oza A, et al. Thermal injury with contemporary cast-application techniques and methods to circumvent morbidity. *J Bone Joint Surg Am.* 2007;89:2369–2377.
37. Halanski M, Noonan KJ. Cast and splint immobilization: complications. *J Am Acad Orthop Surg.* 2008;16:30–40.
38. Hang JR, Hutchinson AF, Hau RC. Risk factors associated with loss of position after closed reduction of distal radial fractures in children. *J Pediatr Orthop.* 2011; 31:501–506.
39. Hossieny P, Carey Smith R, Yates P, et al. Efficacy of patient information concerning casts applied post-fracture. *ANZ J Surg.* 2012;82:151–155.
40. Kannikeswaran N, Lieh-Lai M, Malian M, et al. Optimal dosing of intravenous ketamine for procedural sedation in children in the ED: a randomized controlled trial. *Am J Emerg Med.* 2016;34:1347–1353.
41. Killian JT, White S, Lenning L. Cast-saw burns: comparison of technique versus material versus saws. *J Pediatr Orthop.* 1999;19:683–687.
42. Kim JK, Kook SH, Kim YK. Comparison of forearm rotation allowed by different types of upper extremity immobilization. *J Bone Joint Surg Am.* 2012;94:455–460.
43. Large TM, Frick SL. Compartment syndrome of the leg after treatment of a femoral fracture with an early sitting spica cast. A report of two cases. *J Bone Joint Surg Am.* 2003;85-A:2207–2210.
44. Larsen TH, Gregersen P, Jemec GB. Skin irritation and exposure to diisocyanates in orthopedic nurses working with soft casts. *Am J Contact Dermat.* 2001;12: 211–214.
45. Lavalette R, Pope MH, Dickstein H. Setting temperatures of plaster casts. The influence of technical variables. *J Bone Joint Surg Am.* 1982;64:907–911.
46. Lee TG, Chung S, Chung YK. A retrospective review of iatrogenic skin and soft tissue injuries. *Arch Plast Surg.* 2012;39:412–416.
47. Leet AI, Mesfin A, Pichard C, et al. Fractures in children with cerebral palsy. *J Pediatr Orthop.* 2006;26:624–627.
48. Leet AI, Pichard CP, Ain MC. Surgical treatment of femoral fractures in obese children: does excessive body weight increase the rate of complications? *J Bone Joint Surg Am.* 2005;87:2609–2613.
49. Liddo LD, D'Angelo A, Nguyen B, et al. Etomidate versus midazolam for procedural sedation in pediatric outpatients: a randomized controlled trial. *Ann Emerg Med.* 2006;48:433–440.
50. Liu RW, Mehta P, Fortuna S, et al. A randomized prospective study of music therapy for reducing anxiety during cast room procedures. *J Pediatr Orthop.* 2007;27: 831–833.
51. Lock TR, Aronson DD. Fractures in patients who have myelomeningocele. *J Bone Joint Surg Am.* 1989;71:1153–1157.
52. Marks MI, Guruswamy A, Gross RH. Ringworm resulting from swimming with a polyurethane cast. *J Pediatr Orthop.* 1983;3:511–512.
53. Marson BM, Keenan MA. Skin surface pressures under short leg casts. *J Orthop Trauma.* 1993;7:275–278.
54. McKenna P, Leonard M, Connolly P, et al. A comparison of pediatric forearm fracture reduction between conscious sedation and general anesthesia. *J Orthop Trauma.* 2012;26:550–556.
55. Monument M, Fick G, Buckley R. Quantifying the amount of padding improves the comfort and function of a fibreglass below-elbow cast. *Injury.* 2009;40:257–261.
56. Mubarak SJ, Frick S, Sink E, et al. Volkmann contracture and compartment syndromes after femur fractures in children treated with 90/90 spica casts. *J Pediatr Orthop.* 2006;26:567–572.
57. Netzer G, Fuchs BD. Necrotizing fasciitis in a plaster-casted limb: case report. *Am J Crit Care.* 2009;18:288–287.
58. Podeszwa DA, Mooney JF 3rd, Cramer KE, et al. Comparison of Pavlik harness application and immediate spica casting for femur fractures in infants. *J Pediatr Orthop.* 2004;24:460–462.
59. Presedo A, Dabney KW, Miller F. Fractures in patients with cerebral palsy. *J Pediatr Orthop.* 2007;27:147–153.
60. Ragnarsson KT, Sell GH. Lower extremity fractures after spinal cord injury: a retrospective study. *Arch Phys Med Rehabil.* 1981;62:418–423.
61. Rana AR, Michalsky MP, Teich S, et al. Childhood obesity: a risk factor for injuries observed at a level-1 trauma center. *J Pediatr Surg.* 2009;44:1601–1605.
62. Rusy LM, Weisman SJ. Complementary therapies for acute pediatric pain management. *Pediatr Clin North Am.* 2000;47:589–599.
63. Sawyer JR, Ivie CB, Huff AL, et al. Emergency room visits by pediatric fracture patients treated with cast immobilization. *J Pediatr Orthop.* 2010;30:248–252.
64. Scheier E, Gadot C, Leiba R, et al. Sedation with the combination of ketamine and propofol in a pediatric ed: a retrospective case series analysis. *Am J Emerg Med.* 2015;33:815–817.
65. Schofield S, Schutz J, Babl F. Procedural sedation and analgesia for reduction of distal forearm fractures in the paediatric emergency department: a clinic survey. *Emerg Med Austral.* 2013;25:241–247.
66. Shuler FD, Grisafi FN. Cast-saw burns: evaluation of skin, cast, and blade temperatures generated during cast removal. *J Bone Joint Surg Am.* 2008;90:2626–2630.
67. Sobel M, Lyden JP. Long bone fracture in a spinal-cord-injured patient: complication of treatment—a case report and review of the literature. *J Trauma.* 1991;31:1440–1444.
68. Stasikelis PJ, Lee DD, Sullivan CM. Complications of osteotomies in severe cerebral palsy. *J Pediatr Orthop.* 1999;19:207–210.
69. Stevens JE, Walter GA, Okereke E, et al. Muscle adaptations with immobilization and rehabilitation after ankle fracture. *Med Sci Sports Exerc.* 2004;36:1695–1701.
70. Stone RA, Youk AO, Marsh GM, et al. Historical cohort study of U.S. man-made vitreous fiber production workers IX: summary of 1992 mortality follow up and analysis of respiratory system cancer among female workers. *J Occup Environ Med.* 2004;46:55–67.
71. Terzioglu A, Aslan G, Sarifakioglu N, et al. Pressure sore from a fruit seed under a hip spica cast. *Ann Plast Surg.* 2002;48:103–104.
72. Warrington SE, Kuhn RJ. Use of intranasal medications in pediatric patients. *Orthopedics.* 2011;34:456–459.
73. Weiss JM, Choi P, Ghatan C, et al. Complications with flexible nailing of femur fractures more than double with child obesity and weight >50 kg. *J Child Orthop.* 2009;3:53–58.
74. Weiss AP, Schenck RC Jr, Sponseller PD, et al. Peroneal nerve palsy after early cast application for femoral fractures in children. *J Pediatr Orthop.* 1992;12:25–28.
75. Wenger D, Pring ME, Rang M, eds. *Rang's Children's Fractures.* 3rd ed. Philadelphia, PA: Lippincott Williams & Wilkins; 2005.

4

Management of the Multiply Injured Child

Susan A. Scherl and Robert M. Kay

ROLE OF THE PEDIATRIC TRAUMA CENTER

✔ Role of the Pediatric Trauma Center: KEY CONCEPTS

- ❏ The American College of Surgeons has established specific criteria for pediatric trauma centers mirroring those in adult trauma centers, including the principles of rapid transport and rapid treatment by an in-house surgical team.
- ❏ Timely assessment and treatment during the "golden hour" decreases mortality.
- ❏ Pediatric trauma centers can provide improved outcomes for severely injured children, but there are relatively few such centers, and many children are stabilized or treated definitively at adult trauma centers.

Trauma centers have been established based on the premise that the first hour (the "golden hour") after injury is the most critical in influencing the rates of survival from the injuries.

The first trauma centers focused on adult patients, though pediatric trauma centers have recently been created due to differences between pediatric and adult polytrauma.[59] The American College of Surgeons has established comparable criteria for pediatric and adult trauma centers based on the principles of rapid transport and rapid treatment by an in-house surgical team. A pediatric general surgeon is in the hospital at all times and heads the pediatric trauma team. This surgeon evaluates the child first, and the other surgical specialists are immediately available. General radiographic services and computed tomography (CT) capability must be available at all times for patient evaluation, and an operating room must be immediately available.

There is increasing evidence that survival rates and outcomes for severely injured children are improved at trauma centers compared to community hospitals, with the best results often reported at pediatric trauma centers.[3,4,20,31,36,38,82,98,103,142]

Previous authors have reported better outcomes for children treated at pediatric trauma centers than at adult trauma centers[43] Data from adult trauma centers show significantly lower mortality rates in pediatric polytrauma patients treated at centers with added pediatric qualifications.[111,118,120] The authors of one of these studies further reported improved mortality rates in specific groups, including patients aged 3 to 12 years, those with injury severity scores above 25, and Glasgow Coma Scale (GCS) scores below 7.[111] Another recent study which queried the National Trauma Data Bank showed lower rates of complications, but no significant difference in mortality, in pediatric patients treated at hospitals verified as trauma centers by American College of Surgeons compared to those which were not.[55] Although adolescent trauma patients admitted to an adult surgical intensive care unit (SICU) have been reported to have similar outcomes to comparable patients admitted to a pediatric intensive care unit (PICU) in a single institution, those admitted to the SICU were more likely to be intubated and to have a Swan–Ganz catheter placed and had longer ICU stays and longer hospital stays.[129]

However, the costs associated with running a pediatric trauma center (particularly the costs of on-call personnel) have limited the number of such centers. As a result, pediatric trauma patients are often stabilized at other hospitals before either transfer to a pediatric trauma center or treatment at an adult trauma center. The use of a general trauma center for pediatric trauma care may be an acceptable alternative if it is not feasible to fund a separate pediatric trauma center.

INITIAL RESUSCITATION AND EVALUATION

✔ Initial Resuscitation and Evaluation: KEY CONCEPTS

❑ Following polytrauma, the initial medical management focuses on the life-threatening, nonorthopedic injuries.[77,99,141,151]
❑ Initial resuscitation follows the Advanced Trauma Life Support (ATLS) or Pediatric Advanced Life Support (PALS) protocols.
❑ The primary survey comprises the "ABCDEs": Airway, Breathing, Circulation, Disability (neurologic), and Exposure and screening radiographs (cervical spine, chest, and pelvis).
❑ Hypovolemia is the most common cause of shock in pediatric trauma patients so early and adequate fluid resuscitation is critical.

INITIAL EVALUATION

The initial steps in resuscitation of a child are essentially the same as those used for an adult.[77,88,99,141,151] The primary survey begins with assessment of the "ABCDEs"—airway, breathing, circulation, disability (neurologic), and exposure—followed by screening radiographs (cervical spine, chest, and pelvis). In severe injuries, the establishment of an adequate airway immediately at the accident site often means the difference between life and death. The cervical spine needs to be stabilized for transport if the child is unconscious, or in those with facial trauma and/or neck pain (Fig. 4-1). A special transport board with an occipital cutout is recommended for children younger than 6 years because head size is large, relative to body size, in young patients. If a young child is placed on a traditional transport board, the cervical spine is flexed, which may cause neurologic injury.[67]

FLUID REPLACEMENT

Once an adequate airway is established, the amount of hemorrhage from the injury, either internally or externally, is assessed. Because

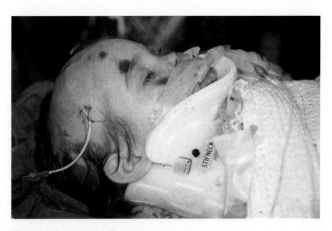

Figure 4-1. Temporary cervical spine stabilization is imperative in any child with multitrauma, especially those who are unconscious or complain of neck pain.

of the prevalence of blunt trauma in pediatric polytrauma patients, most of the blood loss is internal and is easily underestimated. The blood loss is replaced initially with intravenous (IV) crystalloid solution. In younger children, rapid IV access may be difficult. In this situation, a large-bore intraosseous needle can typically be inserted into the tibial metaphysis within 1 to 2 minutes and then used to deliver both fluids and drugs during resuscitation.[10,108] Bielski et al.,[13] in a rabbit tibia model, demonstrated no adverse effects on the histology of bone or the adjacent physis with intraosseous injection of various resuscitation drugs and fluids.

Because death is common if hypovolemic shock is not rapidly reversed, the child's blood pressure must be maintained at an adequate level for organ perfusion. A urinary catheter is used during the resuscitation to monitor urine output as a means of assessing organ perfusion. In some instances, a central venous catheter is used to more precisely monitor fluid resuscitation. In children with traumatic brain injuries, care is exercised during initial fluid resuscitation since overhydration can exacerbate cerebral edema. Excessive fluid resuscitation can also lead to fluid shifts and interstitial pulmonary edema, with potential drops in arterial oxygenation, particularly following thoracic trauma.

The "triad of death," consisting of acidosis, hypothermia, and coagulopathy, has been described in trauma patients as a result of hypovolemia and the systemic response to trauma.[167]

EVALUATION AND ASSESSMENT

✔ Evaluation and Assessment: KEY CONCEPTS

❑ Trauma rating systems have two functions: to aid in triage and to predict outcomes.
❑ Of the commonly used systems, the Injury Severity Score (ISS), Pediatric Trauma Score (PTS), and Glasgow Coma Scale (GCS) have prognostic value.
❑ The secondary survey is a systematic examination of the patient from head to toe. It includes a complete history, physical examination, focused radiographs, and adjunctive imaging studies such as CT and MRI scans.
❑ Because of many distracting injuries, serial examinations of the child may reveal initially undiagnosed injuries in the ensuing days to weeks.

TRAUMA RATING SYSTEMS

After initial resuscitation has stabilized the injured child's condition, it is essential to perform a quick but thorough check for other injuries. At this point in the evaluation, a trauma rating is often performed. The purpose of the trauma rating is twofold: To aid in triage and to predict outcomes. Several trauma rating systems have been validated for the pediatric population,[16,27,28,35,44,46,61,79,91,105,109] but the most commonly used are the GCS, the Injury Severity Score (ISS), and the Pediatric Trauma Score (PTS). Each of the scoring systems has strengths and weaknesses. The ISS is a valid, reproducible rating system that can be widely applied in the pediatric polytrauma setting (Table 4-1).[166] It is an ordinal, not a linear scale (i.e., a score of 40 is not twice as bad as a score of 20). It has been found to be a valid predictor of mortality, length of hospital stay, and cost of care.[18] Another injury-rating system for children that has been shown to be valid and reproducible is the PTS (Table 4-2).[166] It has good predictive value for injury severity, mortality, and the need for transport to a pediatric trauma center. However, it is a poor predictor of internal injury in children with blunt abdominal trauma.[128] The BIG score has been advocated by some centers for its prognostic value and ease of use.[16,35,46]

Trauma Quality Improvement Program (TQIP) is used by many trauma centers treating pediatric trauma patients.[63,64] It uses the National Trauma Data Bank and allows for stratification of risk. It is in its nascency and there are only limited data available.

Head injury is most often evaluated and rated by the GCS, which evaluates eye opening (1 to 4 points), motor function (1 to 6 points), and verbal function (1 to 5 points) on a total scale of 3 to 15 points (Table 4-3). GCS is of limited use in children

---

TABLE 4-1. Injury Severity Score

Abbreviated Injury Scale (AIS)

The AIS classifies injuries as moderate, severe, serious, critical, and fatal for each of the five major body systems. The criteria for each system into the various categories are listed in a series of charts for each level of severity. Each level of severity is given a numerical code (1–5). The criteria for severe level (Code 4) are listed below.

Severity Code	(AIS) Severity Category/ Injury Description	Policy Code
4	Severe (life-threatening, survival probable)	B

General

Severe lacerations and/or avulsions with dangerous hemorrhage; 30–50% surface second- or third-degree burns.

Head and Neck

Cerebral injury with or without skull fracture, with unconsciousness >15 min, with definite abnormal neurologic signs; posttraumatic amnesia 3–12 hrs; compound skull fracture.

Chest

Open-chest wounds; flail chest; pneumomediastinum; myocardial contusion without circulatory embarrassment; pericardial injuries.

Abdomen

Minor laceration of intra-abdominal contents (ruptured spleen, kidney, and injuries to tail of pancreas); intraperitoneal bladder rupture; avulsion of the genitals.

Thoracic and/or lumbar spine fractures with paraplegia.

Extremities

Multiple closed long-bone fractures; amputation of limbs.

Injury Severity Score (ISS)

The injury severity score (ISS) is a combination of values obtained from the AIS. The ISS is the sum of the squares of the highest AIS grade in each of the three most severely injured areas. For example, a person with a laceration of the aorta (AIS = 5), multiple closed long-bone fractures (AIS = 4), and retroperitoneal hemorrhage (AIS = 3) would have an injury severity score of 50 (25 + 16 + 9). The highest possible score for a person with trauma to a single area is 25. The use of the ISS has dramatically increased the correlation between the severity and mortality. The range of severity is from 0 to 75.

Adapted from Committee on Medical Aspects of Automotive Safety. Rating the severity of tissue damage. I. The abbreviated scale. *JAMA*. 1971;215(2):277–280; Baker SP, O'Neill B, Haddon W Jr, et al. The Injury Severity Score: a method for describing patients with multiple injuries and evaluating emergency care. *J Trauma*. 1974;4:187–196.

TABLE 4-2. Pediatric Trauma Score

Component	+2	+1	−1
		Category	
Size	≥20 kg	10–20 kg	<10 kg
Airway	Normal	Maintainable	Unmaintainable
Systolic blood pressure	≥90 mm Hg	90–50 mm Hg	<50 mm Hg
Central nervous system	Awake	Obtunded/LOC	Coma/decerebrate
Open wound	None	Minor	Major/penetrating
Skeletal	None	Closed fracture	Open/multiple fractures

This scoring system includes six common determinants of the clinical condition in the injured child. Each of the six determinants is assigned a grade: +2, minimal or no injury; +1, minor or potentially major injury; −1, major, or immediate life-threatening injury. The scoring system is arranged in a manner standard with advanced trauma life support protocol, and thereby provides a quick assessment scheme. The ranges are from −6 for a severely traumatized child to +12 for a least traumatized child. This system has been confirmed in its reliability as a predictor of injury severity.
Adapted from Tepas JJ III, Mollitt DL, Talbert JL, et al. The Pediatric Trauma Score as a predictor of injury severity in the injured child. *J Pediatr Surg.* 1987;22(1):14–18. Copyright © 1987 Elsevier. With permission.

who are preverbal or in the early stages of verbal development, but in other children, this rating system has been a useful guide for predicting early mortality and later disability.[15,27,28,61,169,172] Some authors have advocated a pediatric GCS for these younger children, though it has not yet proven to be as reliable as the GCS in older children.[15] Recent authors have reported predictive value in the motor component of the GCS, even without using other components of GCS, though it was not as predictive as was use of the entire GCS score.[28] A GCS score <8 points indicates a significantly worse chance of survival than does a

GCS >8. The GCS should be noted on arrival in the trauma center and repeated 1 hour later. Serial changes in the GCS correlate with improvement or worsening of the neurologic injury. Repeated GCS assessments over the initial 72 hours after injury may be of prognostic significance.

PHYSICAL ASSESSMENT

The secondary survey starts with a full history and physical examination. A careful abdominal examination allows early detection of injuries to the liver, spleen, pancreas, or kidneys. When present, ecchymosis on the abdominal wall must be noted, as it is often a sign of significant visceral or spinal injury.[23,40,78]

The extremities are checked for swelling, deformity, or crepitus. If extremity deformity is present, it is important to determine whether the fracture is open or closed. Sites of external bleeding are examined, and pressure dressings are applied if necessary to prevent further blood loss. Imaging studies facilitate surgical planning.

Pelvic fractures are high-energy injuries and often associated with significant morbidity and mortality.[33,37,112,133,140,144,161] A pelvic fracture combined with one or more other skeletal injuries has been suggested to be a marker for the presence of head and abdominal injuries.[160] Major arterial injuries associated with fractures of the extremity are usually diagnosed early by the lack of a peripheral pulse. In contrast, abdominal venous injuries caused by blunt trauma—half of which are fatal—are rare and often remain undiagnosed before exploratory laparotomy. Consequently, in children who continue to require substantial blood volume support after the initial resuscitation has been completed, abdominal venous injury should be considered.[51]

Initial splinting of suspected extremity fractures is routinely done in the field. However, once the injured child is in the hospital, the orthopedist should inspect the extremities to assess the injuries and determine the urgency of definitive treatment.

TABLE 4-3. Glasgow Coma Scale

Response	Action	Score
Best motor response	Obeys	M6
	Localizes	5
	Withdraws	4
	Abnormal flexion	3
	Extensor response	2
	Nil	1
Verbal response	Oriented	V5
	Confused conversation	4
	Inappropriate words	3
	Incomprehensible sounds	2
	Nil	1
Eye opening	Spontaneous	E4
	To speech	3
	To pain	2
	Nil	1

This scale is used to measure the level of consciousness using the eye-opening, best verbal, and best motor responses. The range of scores is from 3 for the most severe to 15 for the least severe. This is a measure of level and progression of changes in consciousness.
Adapted from Jennett B, Teasdale G, Galbraith S, et al. Severe head injuries in three countries. *J Neurol Neurosurg Psychiatry.* 1977;40(3):291–298, with permission from BMJ Publishing Group Ltd.

Any neurologic deficit is noted and extremity function is documented prior to treatment. The inability to obtain a reliable examination due to the child's age, mental status or pain from distracting injuries should be documented.

Head injuries and pain in other locations can result in injuries being missed initially. In a series of 149 pediatric polytrauma patients, 13 injuries were diagnosed an average of 15 days following the initial accident, including five fractures (one involving the spine), four abdominal injuries, two aneurysms, one head injury, and one facial fracture.[91] Given this 9% incidence of delayed diagnosis, polytrauma patients should be reexamined once they are more comfortable to reassess for potential sites of injury. Despite careful inpatient examinations, some pediatric injuries escape detection until follow-up visits. Children with head injuries need to be reassessed once they awaken enough to cooperate with reexamination. Families and patients should be informed of the frequency of delayed diagnosis of some injuries in polytrauma patients so they can help identify additional injuries, and are not surprised in the event of later diagnoses.

IMAGING STUDIES

Radiographs

Primary screening radiographs classically consist of a cross-table lateral cervical spine, anteroposterior chest, and anteroposterior pelvis. In some centers, a lateral cervical spine radiograph is obtained only if the child has a head injury or if neck pain is noted on physical examination.

The lateral cervical spine radiograph detects 80% of C-spine injuries.[88] If there is suspicion of a cervical spine injury on the neutral lateral view, a lateral flexion radiograph of the cervical spine taken in an awake patient will help detect any cervical instability safely.

The cervical spine of a young child is much more flexible than the cervical spine in an adult. Under the age of 12 years, the movement of C1 on C2 during flexion of the neck can normally be up to 5 mm, whereas in adults, this distance should be less than 3 mm. Likewise in this young age group, the distance between C2 and C3 is up to 3 mm. No forward movement of C2 on C3 should be present in a skeletally mature patient when the neck is flexed. Pseudosubluxation of C2 on C3 in a child should not be diagnosed as instability that requires treatment because this is a normal finding in young children.[26,42] Because it is difficult to detect a fracture of the thoracic or lumbar spine clinically, radiographs of this area, primarily a lateral view, should be carefully evaluated, particularly in a comatose child.

Imaging studies of any site of suspected musculoskeletal injury should be obtained as quickly as possible after the initial resuscitation and physical examination.

Computed Tomography

CT is essential in evaluating a child with multiple injuries and often provides useful information regarding injuries to the head, chest, abdomen, and pelvis.

CT of the pelvis is more sensitive for pelvic fractures than is a screening pelvic radiograph (Fig. 4-2). Pelvic CT is useful for

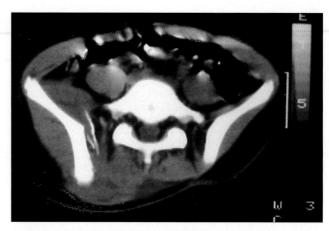

Figure 4-2. CT is more sensitive and specific for the identification and classification of pediatric pelvic fractures.

thoroughly evaluating fracture configuration and determining appropriate treatment options, both surgical and nonsurgical. In one study, a screening pelvic radiograph demonstrated only 54% of pelvic fractures identified on CT scan.[56] A more recent study showed that CT scan resulted in a change in diagnosis of the pelvic fracture (compared to plain radiograph findings) in 38% of cases, though treatment was not changed, as none of their 30 patients required surgery.[12] If abdominal CT is being done to evaluate visceral injury, the CT should be extended distally to include the pelvis.

CT of a fractured vertebra will provide the information needed to classify the fracture as stable or unstable and determine whether operative treatment is needed. Some centers evaluate the cervical spine with a CT scan in children with polytrauma who have neck pain, a traumatic brain injury (TBI), or who have been drinking alcohol.[130] Further workup with cervical spine magnetic resonance imaging (MRI) is necessary before cervical spine clearance in those who have persistent neck pain or tenderness despite normal plain films and CT, and should be considered in patients who remain obtunded.

Intravenous Pyelography

There is a strong correlation of urologic injury with anterior pelvic fractures, as well as with liver and spleen injury. Although CT and ultrasonography are used to evaluate renal injuries, the IV pyelogram still has a role in helping to diagnose bladder and urethral injuries (Fig. 4-3).[107]

Magnetic Resonance Imaging

MRI is used primarily for the detection of injury to the brain, spine, and spinal cord. In young children, the bony spine is more elastic than the spinal cord and spinal cord injury can occur without an obvious spinal fracture, particularly in automobile accidents.[6,17,42,45,49,170] In the spinal cord injury without radiographic abnormality (SCIWORA) syndrome, MRI is valuable in demonstrating the site and extent of spinal cord injury and in defining the level of injury to the disks or vertebral apophysis. A fracture through the vertebral apophysis is similar to a fracture through the physis of a long bone and may not be obvious on plain radiographs.

Ultrasonography

Ultrasound evaluation can detect hemopericardium and intraperitoneal fluid following injury.[21,68,123] The protocol most typically used is called "Focused Assessment with Sonography for Trauma" (FAST). FAST consists of a rapid ultrasound examination of four areas: the right upper abdominal quadrant, the left upper abdominal quadrant, the subxiphoid area, and the pelvis. Though FAST has been used as a rapid screening tool in pediatric polytrauma patients, it frequently misses intra-abdominal injuries following blunt trauma.[22,47,69,70,104,131] Typically, its sensitivity for visceral injuries is lower than its specificity. As a result, CT is more often used for assessment and monitoring of visceral injury in children sustaining multiple injuries. Despite these limitations, hemodynamically unstable children with a positive FAST are often taken for laparotomy rather than for CT scanning.

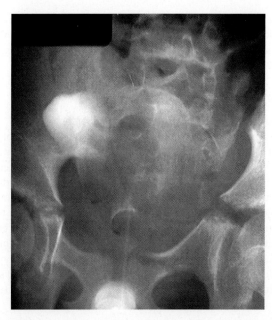

Figure 4-3. Genitourinary injuries typically involve the urethra and/or bladder, are more common in males than females, and are associated with anterior pelvic ring fractures.

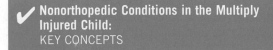

NONORTHOPEDIC CONDITIONS IN THE MULTIPLY INJURED CHILD

✔ **Nonorthopedic Conditions in the Multiply Injured Child:**
KEY CONCEPTS

- ❑ Head injury severity is the principle determinant of morbidity and mortality in a multiply injured child.
- ❑ Children often make substantial recovery from even severe head trauma.
- ❑ Management of orthopedic injuries in children with head trauma should be based on the presumption of full recovery from the head injury.
- ❑ Spasticity and contracture are common sequelae of brain injury, and should be addressed early.
- ❑ There is an association between pediatric pelvic fractures and both intra-abdominal and genitourinary injuries.
- ❑ Motion at the site of a long-bone fracture results in increased intracranial pressure (ICP). To control ICP, it is imperative that long-bone fractures are immobilized until definitive fracture care is provided.

HEAD INJURY

Prognosis for Recovery

Children recover more quickly and fully from significant head injuries than do adults, but head injuries remain the most common cause of ongoing disability in children following polytrauma.[32,43,93,169] Mild cognitive, problem-solving and/or learning deficits may persist, so educational testing needs to be considered for children who have had significant head injury.[162]

The severity of TBI is the single most important determinant of long-term outcome in polytraumatized children.[77] Better functional outcomes are reported at pediatric trauma centers

than at adult trauma centers following pediatric TBI, regardless of whether or not the adult trauma center has added qualification in pediatric trauma.[118] The resiliency of children in the face of TBI was evident in one recent series, with approximately 15% of children who presented with an initial GCS of 3 or 4 having a good outcome 10 years postinjury.[52]

Since children with brain injuries recover more fully than do adults, orthopedic care is based on the assumption of full neurologic recovery. Without optimal orthopedic care, the primary functional deficit may well result from ill-managed orthopedic injuries rather than from the initial neurologic injury.

Intracranial Pressure

After a head injury, ICP is commonly monitored. Elevated ICP may exacerbate the sequelae of TBI, leading to further permanent disability or death. ICP can be controlled by elevating the head of the bed, lowering the PCO_2 (via mechanical ventilation), and restricting IV fluids.

Since motion at the site of a long-bone fracture results in increased ICP, it is imperative that long-bone fractures are immobilized until definitive fracture is provided.[149]

Secondary Orthopedic Effects of Head Injuries

A head injury can have direct impact on the musculoskeletal system. Head injury can lead to spasticity, contractures, and heterotopic ossification (HO), and also accelerates fracture healing.

Spasticity

Spasticity may develop within a few days of head injury. An early effect of this spasticity is to cause shortening at the sites of long-bone fractures, despite traction or external immobilization.

Fracture displacement or shortening in a cast may cause skin breakdown and increase the risk of infection. Operative stabilization should be done as soon as possible because fracture healing is accelerated by a head injury.[149]

Contractures

Contractures commonly develop after polytrauma and TBI. The persistence of spasticity in the extremities often leads to contractures of the joints spanned by the spastic muscles, but attention to appropriate positioning and splinting in the trauma center can decrease contracture frequency and severity. If the child lies in bed with the hips and knees extended, this extensor positioning will usually result in plantarflexion of the ankles. Part-time positioning with the hips and knees flexed helps prevent early equinus contractures from developing. Stretching and splinting can often be effective in preventing contractures; casting may be needed if contractures develop. If these measures are not successful and are interfering with rehabilitation, the contractures may need to be released surgically.

Heterotopic Bone Formation

Heterotopic bone may form in the soft tissues within weeks after a significant head injury with persistent coma.[81,143] Although any joint can be affected, the most common sites are the hip and the elbow. There is some evidence that HO can be stimulated by surgical incisions and can form at the insertion site in head-injured children who undergo antegrade femoral intramedullary nailing.[80] HO should be considered in the differential diagnosis (along with a new fracture and deep vein thrombosis) if new swelling is noted in the extremity of a comatose child.[139] Technetium-99 bone scans show increased isotope uptake in the soft tissue where heterotopic bone forms.

The two primary approaches to managing HO are observation and excision.[81,143] Observation is the mainstay of treatment if the child remains comatose or if the child has recovered from the head injury but the HO does not interfere with rehabilitation. Excision is chosen if there is significant restriction of joint motion from the heterotopic bone which interferes with rehabilitation. The timing of the heterotopic bone excision is controversial, but resection should be considered whenever heterotopic bone significantly interferes with rehabilitation, rather than waiting 12 to 18 months for the bone to mature. After surgical excision, early postoperative prophylaxis with local low-dose radiation therapy or medications (salicylates or nonsteroidal anti-inflammatory drugs) decreases the risk of recurrence. Mital et al.[100] reported success in preventing recurrence of heterotopic bone after excision by use of salicylates at a dosage of 40 mg/kg/day in divided doses for 6 weeks postoperatively.

Fracture Healing Rates

Long-bone fractures heal more quickly in children and adults who have associated head injuries.[174] Delay in treatment of acute fractures can make reduction more difficult due to the often early, exuberant callus formation.

PERIPHERAL NERVE INJURIES

Although TBI most often accounts for persistent neurologic deficits in a child with multiple injuries, one clinical review of brain-injured children reported that 7% had evidence of an associated peripheral nerve injury documented by electrodiagnostic testing.[116] For closed injuries, the peripheral nerve injury is typically associated with an adjacent fracture or with a stretching injury of the extremity and observation is indicated in most cases because these injuries often recover spontaneously. However, if the nerve injury is at the level of an open fracture, then exploration of the nerve is indicated at the time of the initial surgery. If function does not return within 2 to 3 months following observation of a closed injury, then electrodiagnostic testing is indicated. If peripheral nerve injury is present, surgical repair with nerve grafts offers an excellent chance of functional recovery in children and adolescents.

THORACIC INJURIES AND PULMONARY CONTUSIONS

Thoracic injuries encompass a wide spectrum of injury.[114] Many are more limited with blunt trauma and associated pulmonary contusion, while others involve damage to the great vessels, with very high associated mortality. Isolated thoracic injuries in children typically have quite good outcomes. On the other end of the spectrum, children with combined thoracic and brain and/or abdominal injuries have reported mortality rates of 20% to 40%.[114]

Pulmonary contusions have much better outcomes in the pediatric population than in adults.[54,60] However, if the lungs have been severely contused, protein leaks into the alveolar spaces, making ventilation more difficult. This may be exacerbated by the systemic inflammatory response syndrome, which is commonly seen following severe trauma.[167] Surfactant dysfunction follows and is most abnormal in patients with the most severe respiratory failure. As the time from the injury increases, pulmonary function can deteriorate and general anesthesia becomes more risky. Orthopedic surgical treatment before such pulmonary deterioration limits the anesthetic risks in these patients. Bruises on the chest or rib fractures should alert the orthopedist to potential pulmonary contusions as a part of the injury complex. Initial chest radiographs may not clearly demonstrate the degree of pulmonary parenchymal injury, and oxygen saturation (and arterial blood gas measurements) is more useful in estimating the anesthetic risk of these patients during operative fracture care. Previous authors have reported that operative stabilization of fractures within the first 2 or 3 days after injury led to fewer complications, shorter hospital and intensive care unit stays, and a shorter time on ventilator assistance in children with multiple injuries.[96,97]

ABDOMINAL INJURIES

Abdominal injuries occur in approximately 10% to 30% of pediatric polytrauma patients.[22,39,91] Abdominal swelling, tenderness, and bruising are all signs of injury. Abdominal injury is common if a child in a motor vehicle accident (MVA) has been wearing a lap seat belt, regardless of whether a contusion is evident.[23,78,136,153] Sivit et al. noted that over half of their 61 patients with abdominal ecchymosis had spine fracture and/or abdominal viscus injury, including 21% with fracture, 23% with viscus injury, and 8% with both fracture and viscus injury.[136] Bond et al.[14] noted that the presence of multiple pelvic fractures strongly correlated (80%) with the presence of abdominal or genitourinary injury, whereas the child's age or mechanism of injury had no correlation with abdominal injury rates.

Most hepatic and splenic lacerations are treated nonoperatively, by monitoring the hematocrit, by performing serial abdominal examinations, and by serial CT.[24,29,30,36,76,103,119,147,156] Addition of a pediatric trauma center to a regional trauma system has been reported to decrease the rate of splenectomy following blunt abdominal trauma in children.[103] Once the child's overall condition has stabilized, the presence of nonoperative abdominal injuries should not delay fracture care.

GENITOURINARY INJURIES

Genitourinary system injuries are rare in the pediatric polytrauma population, though they have been reported in 9% to 24% of children with pelvic fractures.[33,107,134,146,150]

Injuries to the bladder and urethra are more common in males and are associated with fractures of the anterior pelvic ring (Fig. 4-4).[9] Although less common following pelvic fracture in girls, such injuries are often associated with injury to the vagina and rectum, with long-term concerns regarding continence, stricture formation, and childbearing.[41,117,125] If the iliac wings are displaced or the pelvic ring shape is changed, it may be necessary to reduce these fractures to reconstitute the birth canal in female patients. There are increased rates of cesarean section in young women who have had a pelvic fracture.[33] Adolescent females with displaced pelvic fractures should be informed of this potential problem with vaginal delivery. If the injury is severe, kidney injury may also occur, but most urologic injuries that occur with pelvic fractures are distal to the ureters.[1]

FAT EMBOLISM AND PULMONARY EMBOLISM

Fat embolism and acute respiratory distress syndrome are rare in children.[48,95,122,165] Though hypoxemia likely develops in some children after multiple fractures, the full clinical picture of fat embolism seldom develops. When fat embolism occurs, the signs and symptoms are the same as in adults: axillary petechiae,

hypoxemia, and radiograph changes of pulmonary infiltrates appearing within several hours of the fractures. If a child with multiple fractures without a head injury develops a change in sensorium and orientation, hypoxemia is the most likely cause. The other primary cause of mental status change after fracture is overmedication with narcotics.

If fat embolism is diagnosed, the treatment is the same as in adults, generally with endotracheal intubation, positive pressure ventilation, and hydration with IV fluid. The effect of early fracture stabilization, IV alcohol, or high-dose corticosteroids on fat embolism syndrome has not been studied well in children with multiple injuries.

Deep venous thrombosis and pulmonary thromboembolism are much rarer in pediatric trauma patients than in adults, with rates between 0.02% and 1.2%.[2,5,7,8,34,89,94,124,127,152,159,171] The risk of deep venous thrombosis and pulmonary embolism is increased in older children, those with higher ISS scores, and low GCS scores.[34,124,171] One recent study reported a 9% rate of DVT in pediatric trauma patients admitted to the ICU, with the greatest risk following TBI.[89] The role of prophylaxis for pediatric deep venous thrombosis and pulmonary thromboembolism is unclear and recommendations vary among surgeons and institutions.[2]

NUTRITIONAL REQUIREMENTS

Pediatric polytrauma patients have high caloric demands. If an injured child requires ventilator support for several days, caloric intake through enteral or parenteral supplementation may help avoid catabolism, improve healing, and minimize complications. Children on mechanical ventilation in a PICU have been reported to require 150% of the basal energy or caloric requirements for age and weight.[148] The institution of nutritional support guidelines in a pediatric ICU has been shown to improve energy and protein intake in critically ill patients.[83]

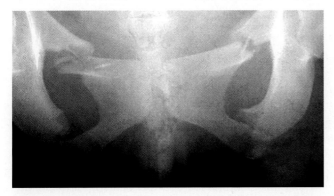

Figure 4-4. Bilateral superior and inferior pubic rami fractures. Genitourinary and abdominal injuries are common with severe pelvic fractures.

ORTHOPEDIC MANAGEMENT OF THE MULTIPLY INJURED CHILD

✔ **Orthopedic Management of the Multiply Injured Child:**
KEY CONCEPTS

☐ Most fractures in multiply injured children can be splinted initially and undergo definitive treatment urgently, not emergently.

☐ Pelvic fractures in children can typically be treated nonoperatively, but some may require urgent external fixation or placement of a pelvic binder if the child is hemodynamically unstable.

☐ Timely administration of IV antibiotics and appropriate irrigation and debridement are the most important steps in the treatment of open fractures.

☐ Tetanus status should be checked and updated in all patients with open fractures.

☐ Cultures should not routinely be performed for open fractures.

☐ Children will often heal open fractures that would necessitate amputation in an adult.

☐ If amputation is necessary, preserve as much stump length as possible.

TIMING

As noted, splinting is needed at the time of the initial resuscitation. In a child with multiple closed fractures, definitive treatment should proceed expeditiously once the child's condition has been stabilized. Loder[96] reported that operative stabilization of fractures within the first 2 or 3 days after injury led to fewer complications, shorter hospital and intensive care unit stays, and a shorter time on ventilator assistance in children with multiple injuries. A more recent study by Loder et al.[97] reported a trend toward a higher rate of complications in fractures treated after 72 hours. Although there appears to be other factors besides the timing of surgery that affect the eventual outcomes of polytrauma patients, the timing of surgery is a variable that can be controlled by the surgeon, and it seems prudent to complete fracture stabilization within 2 to 3 days of injury when possible.

PELVIC FRACTURES

Pelvic fractures occur in less than 1% of pediatric patients in the National Trauma Data bank, but have been reported in up to 7% of children referred to level I regional trauma centers.[37,138,144,161] More than half of pelvic fractures involve a pedestrian struck by a motor vehicle and over 90% result from three mechanisms: pedestrian struck by motor vehicle, MVA, or fall from height.[134,140,144] Most pediatric pelvic fractures do not require surgery, though the frequency is higher in adolescents.

In a series of 166 pelvic fracture patients, associated substantial head trauma was reported in 39%, chest trauma in 20%, and visceral/abdominal injuries in 19%.[134] Mortality in children following pelvic fractures has been reported to occur in 3.6% to 10.5% of cases in some series.[37,134,144] Other authors reported that 62% of children (8/13) with pelvic fractures had additional orthopedic injuries.[140]

Exsanguination may present an immediate threat to the life of a child following pelvic fracture, but death more frequently is due to other severe associated injuries in this patient population.[37,75,140,144,154] Survival after pelvic fracture is related to ISS and type of hospital.[161]

Most pelvic fractures in children are treated nonoperatively. However, in a child or preadolescent, an external fixator can be used to close a marked pubic diastasis or to control bleeding by stabilizing the pelvis for transport and other injury care. The external fixator will not reduce a displaced vertical shear fracture, but the stability provided is helpful to control the hemorrhage while the child's condition is stabilized. Another option for acute pelvic stabilization in the emergency department is a simple pelvic binder. Injury to the sciatic nerve or the lumbosacral nerve roots may result from hemipelvis displacement through a vertical shear fracture.

OPEN FRACTURES

Background

Most serious open fractures in children result from high-velocity blunt injury involving vehicles. However, even low-energy blunt injuries can cause puncture wounds in the skin adjacent to fractures, especially displaced radial, ulnar, and tibial fractures. In children with multiple injuries, approximately 10% of the fractures are open.[20,132] When open fractures are present, 25% to 50% of patients have additional injuries involving the head, chest, abdomen, and other extremities.[132]

Wound Classification

The classification used to describe the soft tissues adjacent to an open fracture is based on the system described by Gustilo and Anderson[57] and Gustilo et al.[58] Primary factors that are considered and ranked in this classification system are the size of the wound, the degree of soft tissue damage and wound contamination, and the presence or absence of an associated vascular injury (Table 4-4). Despite its widespread use, the Gustilo classification has only moderate interobserver reliability.[19,71,106]

Though type IIIC injuries are commonly associated with extensive soft tissue loss and contamination, a type IIIC injury may, in fact, be associated with even a small wound in some cases. Also, key distinguishing factors between types II and III fractures are the amount of periosteal stripping of the bone, and the severity of the damage to the surrounding soft tissues, not simply the size of the skin laceration (Fig. 4-5).

Some of the factors which determine the correct classification of the open fracture may not be known until the time of surgery; as such, the grade the orthopedic surgeon assigns to the open fracture may change at the time of surgery.

The final functional results of type III fractures in children appear to be superior to those in adults, likely because of their better peripheral vascular supply and the regenerative potential of pediatric periosteum.

TABLE 4-4. Gustilo Classification of Open Fractures	
Type	**Description**
I	An open fracture with a wound <1 cm long and clean
II	An open fracture with a laceration >1 cm long without extensive soft tissue damage, flaps, or avulsions
III	Massive soft tissue damage, compromised vascularity, severe wound contamination marked fracture instability
IIIA	Adequate soft tissue coverage of a fractured bone despite extensive soft tissue laceration or flaps, or high-energy trauma irrespective of the size of the wound
IIIB	Extensive soft tissue injury loss with periosteal stripping and bone exposure; usually associated with massive contamination
IIIC	Open fracture associated with arterial injury requiring repair

Adapted from Gustilo RB, Mendoza RM, Williams DN. Problems in the management of type III (severe) open fractures: a new classification of type III open fractures. *J Trauma*. 1984;24(8):742–746; Gustilo RB, Anderson JT. Prevention of infection in the treatment of one thousand and twenty-five open fractures of long bones: retrospective and prospective analyses. *J Bone Joint Surg Am*. 1976;58(4):453–458.

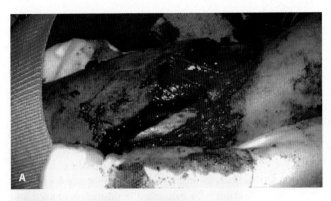
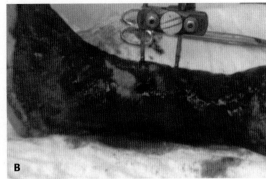
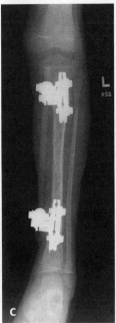
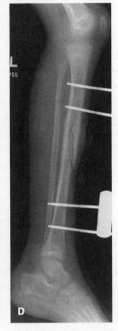

Figure 4-5. A: Grade IIIC open tibia fracture in a 9-year-old boy hit by a bus. **B:** Appearance of the wound after several debridements. **C, D:** AP and lateral radiographs showing external fixation of the fracture. Note the vascular clips distally, where an autologous vein graft from the popliteal trifurcation was anastomosed to the posterior tibial artery.

Author's Preferred Method

Three Stages

The treatment of open fractures in children is similar to that for open fractures in adults. The primary goals are to prevent infection of the wound and fracture site, while allowing soft tissue healing, fracture union, and return of optimal function. Initial emergency care includes the ABCDEs of resuscitation, application of a sterile povidone-iodine dressing, and preliminary alignment and splinting of the fracture. If significant bleeding is present, a compression dressing is applied to limit blood loss. Tetanus toxoid is given for patients whose immunization status is unknown, or if more than 5 years have passed since their last dose. The initial dose of IV antibiotics is given. All open fractures are treated with operative irrigation and debridement. The second stage of management is the primary surgical treatment, including initial and (if necessary) repeat debridement of the tissues in the area of the open fracture until the entire wound

appears viable. The fracture is reduced and stabilized at this time. If the bone ends are not covered with viable soft tissue, muscle or skin flap coverage is considered. Vacuum-assisted closure (VAC) therapy (Kinetic Concepts, Inc., San Antonio, TX) may be a useful adjunct to facilitate coverage and obviate the need for flaps in some patients.[66,90,102,106,163,164] VAC has been shown to shorten the time of healing of wounds associated with open fractures.[90] The third and final stage of management is bony reconstruction as needed if bone loss has occurred, followed by rehabilitation of the child.

Cultures

Previous studies have demonstrated poor correlation of growth on routine cultures with wound infections.[87,113,157] Lee[87] reported that neither pre- nor postdebridement cultures accurately predicted the risk of infection in open fractures, with only 20% (24/119) of predebridement wounds with positive cultures and only 28% (9/32) with positive postdebridement cultures becoming infected. Although postdebridement cultures were more predictive of infection, these cultures identified the causative organism in only 42% (8/19) of infected wounds. Valenziano et al.[157] found that cultures at the time of presentation to the trauma center also were of no value, with only 2 of 28 patients (7%) with positive cultures becoming infected, in comparison to 5 of 89 patients (6%) with negative initial cultures. Initial cultures were positive in only two of seven cases that became infected. A recent review of the literature found little data to support the routine use of pre- or postdebridement cultures in open fractures.[126] Open fractures do not need to be routinely cultured. Cultures should be obtained only at the time of reoperation in patients with clinical evidence of infection.

Antibiotic Therapy

Antibiotic therapy decreases the risk of infection in children with open fractures. Wilkins and Patzakis[168] reported a 13.9% infection rate in 79 patients who received no antibiotics after open fractures, and a 5.5% rate in 815 patients with similar injuries who had antibiotic prophylaxis. Bacterial contamination has been noted in 70% of open fractures in children, including both gram-positive and gram-negative organisms, depending on the degree of wound contamination and adjacent soft tissue injury. We limit antibiotic administration generally to 48 to 72 hours after each surgical treatment of the open fracture.

For all type I and some type II fractures, we use a first generation cephalosporin (cefazolin 100 mg/kg/day divided q8h, maximal daily dose 6 g). For more severe type II fractures and for type III fractures, we use a combination of a cephalosporin and aminoglycoside (gentamicin 5 to 7.5 mg/kg/day divided q8h).[86]

For farm injuries or grossly contaminated fractures, penicillin (150,000 units/kg/day divided q6h, maximal daily dose 24 million units) is added to the cephalosporin and aminoglycoside. All antibiotics are given intravenously for 24 to 72 hours. Although there is a trend toward a shorter duration (24 hours) of antibiotic prophylaxis, there is currently a lack of evidence-based medicine to support specific regimens of duration of antibiotic prophylaxis in children. Oral antibiotics are occasionally used if significant soft tissue erythema at the open fracture site remains after the IV antibiotics have been completed. Gentamicin levels should be checked after four or five doses (and doses adjusted as necessary) to minimize the risk of ototoxicity.

An additional 48-hour course is given around subsequent surgeries, such as those for repeat irrigation and debridement, delayed wound closure, open reduction and internal fixation of fractures, and secondary bone reconstruction procedures.

It should be noted, however, that the guidelines above were developed prior to the widespread prevalence of community-acquired methicillin-resistant *Staphylococcus aureus* (MRSA). If the patient is at risk for MRSA, consideration should be given to adding clindamycin or vancomycin to the regimen. Moreover, evidence-based guidelines published in 2006 found that the available data support the conclusion that a short course of a first-generation cephalosporin, combined with appropriate orthopedic management, does decrease risk of subsequent infection in open fractures. However, the data were inadequate to either support or refute additional practices such as adding an aminoglycoside for Gustilo type II fractures, or increasing the duration of antibiotic administration.[62]

Debridement and Irrigation

After the initial dose(s) of antibiotics are given, debridement and irrigation of the open fracture in the operating room is the next critical step in the primary management of open fractures in children. A multicenter study demonstrated an overall infection rate of 1% to 2% after open long-bone fractures, with no difference in infection rates between groups of patients treated with irrigation and debridement within 6 hours of injury and those treated between 6 and 24 hours following injury.[137] One likely reason for the low rates of infection in these two series is the early administration of IV antibiotics in both groups. Although up to a 24-hour delay does not appear to have adverse consequences regarding infection rates, it may be necessary to perform an earlier irrigation and debridement to minimize compromise of the soft tissue envelope. The debridement needs to be performed carefully and systematically to remove all foreign and nonviable materials from the wound. The order of debridement typically is (1) excision of the necrotic tissue from the wound edges, (2) extension of the wound to adequately explore the fracture ends, (3) debridement of the wound edges to bleeding tissue, (4) resection of necrotic skin, fat, muscle, and contaminated fascia, (5) fasciotomies as needed, and (6) thorough irrigation of the fracture ends and wound.

Two previous studies of pediatric type I open fractures reported a 2% to 2.5% infection rate with nonoperative treatment.[53,74] Both of these studies are significantly hampered by sample size. Given the potential for devastating complications in children with open fractures treated nonoperatively, we still advocate operative treatment of all such children.

For grade II and III fractures, since children generally heal better and have fewer comorbidities than adults, it is often possible to do a less aggressive debridement at the initial surgery, and wait until questionable tissue declares itself at a second look to determine the definitive necessary extent of debridement.

When debriding and irrigating an open diaphyseal fracture, we typically bring the proximal and distal bone ends into the wound to allow visual inspection and thorough irrigation and debridement. This often necessitates extension of the open wound, which is preferable to leaving the fracture site contaminated. We carefully remove devitalized bone fragments and contaminated cortical bone with curettes or a small rongeur. If there is a possible nonviable bone fragment, judgment is needed as to whether this bone fragment should be removed or left in place. Small fracture fragments without soft tissue attachments are removed, whereas very large ones may be retained if they are not significantly contaminated. Reconstruction of a large segmental bone loss has a better outcome in children than in adults because children have a better potential for bone regeneration and a better vascular supply to their extremities. Nearby major neurovascular structures in the area of the fracture are identified and protected. Debridement is complete when all contaminated, dead, and ischemic tissues have been excised; the bones' ends are clean with bleeding edges; and only viable tissue lines the wound bed.

Although a high-pressure lavage system can be used for irrigation, there have been reports of complications, including acute compartment syndrome, using these devices.[85,135] Therefore, gravity lavage using wide-bore cystoscopy tubing is a good alternative. Several recent studies, including the multicenter, randomized, blinded Fluid Lavage of Open Wound (FLOW) study have found that low-pressure lavage is safer and more effective than high-pressure lavage.[72,73,110,115] Based on the most recent data, it appears that using a soap solution to irrigate has a higher infection rate than irrigation with saline.[72] We routinely use 3 to 9 L of normal saline for the lower extremities and 2 to 6 L in the upper extremities because of the smaller compartment size.

After the debridement and irrigation are complete, local soft tissue is used to cover the neurovascular structures, tendons, and bone ends. If local soft tissue coverage is inadequate, consideration should be given to local muscle flaps or other coverage methods, including VAC. The area of the wound that has been incised to extend the wound for fracture inspection can be primarily closed. The traumatic wound should either be left open to drain or may be closed over one or more drains. Wounds that are left open can be dressed with a moistened povidone-iodine or saline dressing, but are probably better treated with a VAC. Types II and III fractures are routinely reoperated on every 48 to 72 hours for repeat irrigation and debridement until the wounds appear clean and the tissue viable. This cycle is repeated until the wound can be sutured closed or a split-thickness skin graft or local flap is used to cover it. If flap coverage is necessary, this is optimally accomplished within 1 week of injury.

Fracture Stabilization

Fracture stabilization in children with open fractures decreases pain, protects the soft tissue envelope from further injury, decreases the spread of bacteria, allows stability important for early soft tissue coverage, decreases cerebral pressure, and improves the fracture union rate.

Principles for stabilization of open fractures in children include allowing access to the soft tissue wound and the extremity for debridement and dressing changes, allowing weight bearing when appropriate, and preserving full motion of the adjacent joints to allow full functional recovery.

The concept of "damage-control" orthopedics, in which an external fixator is used to temporarily stabilize a long-bone fracture until the patient is systemically stable enough to undergo definitive fracture fixation, is well studied and accepted in the adults,[145,155] but we are aware of only one case series of three patients in the pediatric orthopedic literature.[101] External fixators can be put on quickly and safely in the ICU or at bedside without fluoroscopy for pelvic, femur, tibia, and other fractures for initial stabilization, with the understanding that definitive alignment can be achieved later.

Fracture management for specific anatomic locations is discussed throughout the other chapters of this book and will not be addressed here.

Wound Management

Serial irrigation and debridement are done every 2 to 3 days until the wounds are clean and all remaining tissue appears viable. Fracture fixation at the time of initial surgery (as described previously) facilitates wound management. We prefer to provide soft tissue coverage of the open fracture and adjacent soft tissue defect by 5 to 10 days after the injury to limit the risk of later infection. Most type I wounds heal with local dressing changes. For some type II and type IIIA fractures, we use delayed wound closure or a split-thickness skin graft over underlying muscle cover.

Large soft tissue loss is most often a problem with types IIIB and IIIC fractures. In the proximal tibia, plastic surgeons may be needed to provide a gastrocnemius rotational flap, followed by secondary coverage of the muscle with a skin graft. In the middle-third of the leg, a soleus flap is used with skin graft coverage, and a vascularized free muscle transfer is necessary if local coverage is inadequate. Free flaps may be required for coverage of the distal third of the tibia, especially in adolescents,[84,121] although there is a high complication rate. VAC sometimes can reduce the need for free tissue transfers. The VAC can convert wounds that need free tissue to ones that need split-thickness skin graft or can heal completely.[25,66,102,106]

The flaps and grafts used for reconstructing severe injuries are either muscle flaps or composite grafts. For a massive loss of soft tissue and bone, composite grafts of muscle and bone often are necessary. The younger the child, the better the likelihood that autogenous graft will fill in a bone defect if there is a well-vascularized bed from the muscle flap. Free flaps, especially from the latissimus

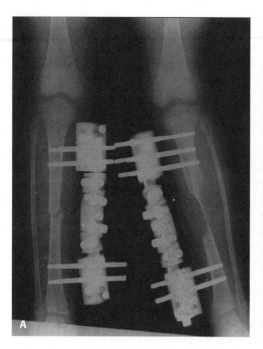
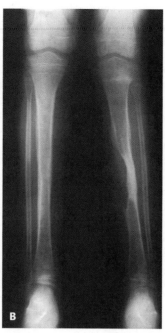

Figure 4-6. A: AP radiograph of a 6-year-old boy with bilateral open tibia fractures, fixed with external fixators. Despite the bone loss on the left, his periosteum was preserved. **B:** One year later, there is healing and hypertrophy of the cortical bone, without bone grafting.

dorsi, are useful in the mid-tibial and distal tibial regions to decrease infection rates and improve union rates. Vascularized fibular grafts rarely are used acutely to reconstruct bone defects, but may be useful after soft tissue healing.

For the rare case of significant bone defect in a child, we rely on the healing capacity of young periosteum and bone and the vascular supply of a child's extremity (Fig. 4-6). An external fixator is used to hold the bone shortened about 1 to 2 cm to decrease the size of the bone loss. In a growing child, 1 to 2 cm of overgrowth can be expected in the subsequent 2 years after these severe injuries, so the final leg length will be satisfactory. Autogenous bone graft can be used early, but if there is surviving periosteum at this site, spontaneous bone formation often is surprisingly robust and may preclude the need for bone grafting. In teenagers with bone loss, once the soft tissue has healed, bone transport using either a uniplanar lengthening device or a circular thin wire external fixator is our preferred method of reconstruction, although use of an allograft or vascularized fibular graft may be considered.

Amputation

In children, attempts should generally be made to preserve all extremities, even with type IIIC open fractures that are usually treated with primary amputation in adults. Wounds and fractures that do not heal in adults often heal satisfactorily in children, and preservation of limb length and physes are important in young children. Although the Mangled Extremity Severity Score (MESS) correlates well with the need for amputation in adults, the correlation is poor in children, and many limbs are salvageable despite a MESS of 7 or higher.[50] In one series,[50] the MESS predicted limb amputation or salvage correctly in 86% (31/36) of children, with 93% accuracy in salvaged limbs but only 63% in amputated limbs. Another study reported MESS of at least 6.5 had a sensitivity of only 73% and specificity of only 54% in children with open fractures due to polytrauma who underwent posttraumatic amputation.[11]

If amputation is absolutely necessary, as much length as possible should be preserved. For example, if the proximal tibial physis is preserved in a male with a below-knee amputation at age 7 years, 6 to 8 cm more growth of the tibial stump can be expected by skeletal maturity. Thus, even a very short tibial stump in a skeletally immature child may grow to an appropriate length by skeletal maturity. As a result, a short below-knee amputation at the time of injury would likely be superior to a knee disarticulation in final function.

Although amputations to treat congenital limb deficits usually are done through the joint to limit bone spike formation (overgrowth) at the end of the stump, we prefer to maintain maximal possible length if amputation becomes necessary as a result of a severe injury.

Management of Other Fractures

When a child with an open fracture is brought to the operating room for irrigation and debridement of the open fracture, the orthopedist may use this opportunity to treat the other fractures as well. In the setting of pediatric polytrauma, most long-bone fractures are treated surgically, to facilitate patient care and rehabilitation.

STABILIZATION OF FRACTURES

✔ Stabilization of Fractures:
KEY CONCEPTS

- ❑ Fracture stabilization aids in the overall care of the multiply injured child.
- ❑ Although many children who sustain polytrauma have some residual disability, optimal and timely treatment of their orthopedic injuries decreases their burden of musculoskeletal disability.

BENEFICIAL EFFECTS

Fracture stabilization provides a number of nonorthopedic benefits to a child with multiple injuries, including ease of patient mobilization and nursing care, decreased risks of pressure sores, and better wound access.

Operative Fixation

Operative stabilization of fractures is needed to facilitate and hasten patient mobilization and to decrease complications in the pediatric polytrauma patient. It appears that operative fracture fixation for multiply injured children within 3 days of injury leads to fewer complications, shorter stays in the hospital and ICU and less time on a ventilator, shorter hospital and ICU stays, and a shorter time on a ventilator, though such surgery does not appear to be requisite within the first 24 hours of injury.[65,96,97] The type of operative stabilization used in multiply injured children commonly depends on the training, experience, and personal preference of the orthopedist. The most common methods used are intramedullary rod fixation, external fixation, compression plating, and locking plating; Kirschner wires or Steinmann pins may be used in conjunction with casts. Optimal methods for various anatomic sites and fracture configurations are discussed in other chapters throughout this book.

OUTCOMES OF TREATMENT OF THE MULTIPLY INJURED CHILD

Though the vast majority of children survive following polytrauma, a large proportion remain disabled at follow-up. In one review of 74 children with multiple injuries, 59 (80%) survived, but after 1 year, 22% were disabled, mainly from a brain injury.[158] At 9 years after the injuries, 12% had significant physical disability, whereas 42% had cognitive impairment. In this group, however, the SF-36 or functional outcome survey did not differ from the control population. The best predictor of long-term disability was the GCS 6 weeks after injury and later.[158] Letts et al.[92] reported that 71.6% of multiply injured children made a full recovery, with a mean of 28 weeks until full recovery. Of the 53 residual deficits in their 48 patients, the common deficits were neurologic (38%), psychosocial (34%), and musculoskeletal (24%). Outcomes of children with pelvic fractures were near normal at 6 months.[133] Because of the obviously vital impact of central nervous system function on human performance, initial (including those made in the field by first responders) and follow-up measures of the GCS are excellent predictors of long-term disability in pediatric polytrauma patients.[15,27,28,44,105,173]

Whether operative or nonoperative fracture treatment is chosen for a child with multiple injuries, it is important that an orthopedist be involved in the care of the child from the start. Although recognizing the need to care for the other organ system injuries, it is important to advocate for expeditious treatment of the orthopedic injuries. Failure to do so will leave the multiply injured child with musculoskeletal disability once healing of the other injuries occurs.

ACKNOWLEDGMENTS

The authors gratefully acknowledge Vernon T. Tolo, MD and Frances Farley, MD, for their past contributions to this chapter.

Annotated References

Reference	Annotation
Bielski RJ, Bassett GS, Fideler B, et al. Intraosseous infusions: effects on the immature physis—an experimental model in rabbits. *J Pediatr Orthop.* 1993;13:511–515.	A rabbit study showing that intraosseous infusions did not result in physeal damage, thus supporting their potential use in young children requiring emergent fluid resuscitation in the setting of poor venous access.
Cattell HS, Filtzer DL. Pseudosubluxation and other normal variations in the cervical spine in children. A study of one hundred and sixty children. *J Bone Joint Surg Am.* 1965;47:1295–1309.	Classic work describing radiographic findings in the pediatric cervical spine, including pseudosubluxation.
Gustilo RB, Anderson JT. Prevention of infection in the treatment of one thousand and twenty-five open fractures of long bones: retrospective and prospective analyses. *J Bone Joint Surg Am.* 1976;58:453–458.	The first description of the Gustilo–Anderson classification system for open fractures.
Haller JA Jr, Shorter N, Miller D, et al. Organization and function of a regional pediatric trauma center: does a system of management improve outcome? *J Trauma.* 1983;23:691–696.	One of the earliest reports on the establishment, function, and outcomes at a dedicated pediatric trauma center.

Annotated References

Reference	Annotation
Herscovici D Jr, Sanders RW, Scaduto JM, et al. Vacuum-assisted wound closure (VAC therapy) for the management of patients with high-energy soft tissue injuries. *J Orthop Trauma*. 2003;17:683–688.	Consecutive, nonrandomized clinical series. Determined that VAC therapy does not obviate need for adequate debridement but can decrease need for free tissue transfer.
Herzenberg JE, Hensinger RN, Dedrick DK, et al. Emergency transport and positioning of young children who have an injury of the cervical spine. The standard backboard may be hazardous. *J Bone Joint Surg Am*. 1989;71:15–22.	Describes the anatomic characteristics that cause increased cervical spine flexion in young children on a standard backboard, along with recommendations for alternatives for safe transport.
Lee J. Efficacy of cultures in the management of open fractures. *Clin Orthop Relat Res*. 1997(339):71–75.	A study of 245 consecutive open fractures reported that pre- and postdebridement cultures were not useful in predicting later infection and infecting organisms.
Loder RT. Pediatric polytrauma: orthopaedic care and hospital course. *J Orthop Trauma*. 1987;1:48–54.	A study of 78 polytrauma patients showing decreased duration of stays in the ICU and hospital, along with less need for ventilator support in polytrauma patients undergoing orthopedic surgery within 72 hours of injury compared to those operated on more than 72 hours after injury.
Petrisor B, Sun X, Bhandari M, et al. Fluid lavage of open wounds (FLOW): a multicenter, blinded, factorial pilot trial comparing alternative irrigating solutions and pressures in patients with open fractures. *J Trauma*. 2011;71:596–606.	A randomized, blinded, multicenter trial that showed that low-pressure lavage with normal saline is the safest, most effective irrigation method.
Sivit CJ, Taylor GA, Newman KD, et al. Safety-belt injuries in children with lap-belt ecchymosis: CT findings in 61 patients. *AJR Am J Roentgenol*. 1991;157:111–114.	A study showing that more than 50% of children (32/61) with lap-belt bruising had spine fracture and/or abdominal viscus injury, including 21% with spine fracture, 23% with viscus injury, and 8% with both.
Skaggs DL, Friend L, Alman B, et al. The effect of surgical delay on acute infection following 554 open fractures in children. *J Bone Joint Surg Am*. 2005;87:8–12.	A multicenter, retrospective study of 554 children with open fractures reporting comparable infection rates for those undergoing surgery within 6 hours and those undergoing surgery 7 to 24 hours after injury.

REFERENCES

1. Abou-Jaoude WA, Sugarman JM, Fallat ME, et al. Indicators of genitourinary tract injury or anomaly in cases of pediatric blunt trauma. *J Pediatr Surg*. 1996;31(1):86–89.
2. Allen CJ, Murray CR, Meizoso JP, et al. Risk factors for venous thromboembolism after pediatric trauma. *J Pediatr Surg*. 2016;51(1):168–171.
3. Amini R, Lavoie A, Moore L, et al. Pediatric trauma mortality by type of designated hospital in a mature inclusive trauma system. *J Emerg Trauma Shock*. 2011;4(1):12–19.
4. Anders JF, Adelgais K, Hoyle JD Jr, et al. Comparison of outcomes for children with cervical spine injury based on destination hospital from scene of injury. *Acad Emerg Med*. 2014;21(1):55–64.
5. Askegard-Giesmann JR, O'Brien SH, Wang W, et al. Increased use of enoxaparin in pediatric trauma patients. *J Pediatr Surg*. 2012;47(5):980–983.
6. Aufdermaur M. Spinal injuries in juveniles. Necropsy findings in twelve cases. *J Bone Joint Surg Br*. 1974;56B(3):513–519.
7. Azu MC, McCormack JE, Scriven RJ, et al. Venous thromboembolic events in pediatric trauma patients: is prophylaxis necessary? *J Trauma*. 2005;59(6):1345–1349.
8. Babyn PS, Gahunia HK, Massicotte P. Pulmonary thromboembolism in children. *Pediatr Radiol*. 2005;35(3):258–274.
9. Batislam E, Ates Y, Germiyanoglu C, et al. Role of Tile classification in predicting urethral injuries in pediatric pelvic fractures. *J Trauma*. 1997;42(2):285–287.
10. Beaudin M, Daugherty M, Geis G, et al. Assessment of factors associated with the delayed transfer of pediatric trauma patients: an emergency physician survey. *Pediatr Emerg Care*. 2012;28(8):758–763.
11. Behdad S, Rafiei MH, Taheri H, et al. Evaluation of Mangled Extremity Severity Score (MESS) as a predictor of lower limb amputation in children with trauma. *Eur J Pediatr Surg*. 2012;22(6):465–469.
12. Bent MA, Hennrikus WL, Latorre JE, et al. Role of computed tomography in the classification of pediatric pelvic fractures-revisited. *J Orthop Trauma*. 2017;31(7):e200–e204.
13. Bielski RJ, Bassett GS, Fideler B, et al. Intraosseous infusions: effects on the immature physis—an experimental model in rabbits. *J Pediatr Orthop*. 1993;13(4):511–515.
14. Bond SJ, Gotschall CS, Eichelberger MR. Predictors of abdominal injury in children with pelvic fracture. *J Trauma*. 1991;31(8):1169–1173.
15. Borgialli DA, Mahajan P, Hoyle JD Jr, et al. Performance of the pediatric Glasgow Coma Scale in the evaluation of children with blunt head trauma. *Acad Emerg Med*. 2016;23(8):878–884.
16. Borgman MA, Maegele M, Wade CE, et al. Pediatric trauma BIG score: predicting mortality in children after military and civilian trauma. *Pediatrics*. 2011;127(4):e892–e897.
17. Bosch PP, Vogt MT, Ward WT. Pediatric spinal cord injury without radiographic abnormality (SCIWORA): the absence of occult instability and lack of indication for bracing. *Spine (Phila Pa 1976)*. 2002;27(24):2788–2800.
18. Brazelton T, Gosain A. *Classification of Trauma in Children*. 2017 ed. Waltham, MA: UpToDate; 2017.
19. Brumback RJ, Jones AL. Interobserver agreement in the classification of open fractures of the tibia: the results of a survey of two hundred and forty-five orthopaedic surgeons. *J Bone Joint Surg Am*. 1994;76(8):1162–1166.
20. Buckley SL, Gotschall C, Robertson W Jr, et al. The relationships of skeletal injuries with trauma score, injury severity score, length of hospital stay, hospital charges, and mortality in children admitted to a regional pediatric trauma center. *J Pediatr Orthop*. 1994;14(4):449–453.
21. Buess E, Illi OE, Soder C, et al. Ruptured spleen in children: 15-year evolution in therapeutic concepts. *Eur J Pediatr Surg*. 1992;2(3):157–161.
22. Calder BW, Vogel AM, Zhang J, et al. Focused Assessment with Sonography for Trauma (FAST) in children following blunt abdominal trauma: a multi-institutional analysis. *J Trauma Acute Care Surg*. 2017;83(2):218–224.
23. Campbell DJ, Sprouse LR II, Smith LA, et al. Injuries in pediatric patients with seatbelt contusions. *Am Surg*. 2003;69(12):1095–1099.
24. Canarelli JP, Boboyono JM, Ricard J, et al. Management of abdominal contusion in polytraumatized children. *Int Surg*. 1991;76(2):119–121.
25. Caniano DA, Ruth B, Teich S. Wound management with vacuum-assisted closure: experience in 51 pediatric patients. *J Pediatr Surg*. 2005;40(1):128–132.
26. Cattell HS, Filtzer DL. Pseudosubluxation and other normal variations in the cervical spine in children. A study of one hundred and sixty children. *J Bone Joint Surg Am*. 1965;47(7):1295–1309.
27. Chung CY, Chen CL, Cheng PT, et al. Critical score of Glasgow Coma Scale for pediatric traumatic brain injury. *Pediatr Neurol*. 2006;34(5):379–387.
28. Cicero MX, Cross KP. Predictive value of initial Glasgow Coma Scale score in pediatric trauma patients. *Pediatr Emerg Care*. 2013;29(1):43–48.
29. Cloutier DR, Baird TB, Gormley P, et al. Pediatric splenic injuries with a contrast blush: successful nonoperative management without angiography and embolization. *J Pediatr Surg*. 2004;39(6):969–971.
30. Coburn MC, Pfeifer J, DeLuca FG. Nonoperative management of splenic and hepatic trauma in the multiply injured pediatric and adolescent patient. *Arch Surg*. 1995;130(3):332–338.
31. Cochran A, Mann NC, Dean JM, et al. Resource utilization and its management in splenic trauma. *Am J Surg*. 2004;187(6):713–719.

32. Colombani PM, Buck JR, Dudgeon DL, et al. One-year experience in a regional pediatric trauma center. *J Pediatr Surg.* 1985;20(1):8–13.

33. Copeland CE, Bosse MJ, McCarthy ML, et al. Effect of trauma and pelvic fracture on female genitourinary, sexual, and reproductive function. *J Orthop Trauma.* 1997;11(2):73–81.

34. Cyr C, Michon B, Pettersen G, et al. Venous thromboembolism after severe injury in children. *Acta Haematol.* 2006;115(3–4):198–200.

35. Davis AL, Wales PW, Malik T, et al. The BIG Score and prediction of mortality in pediatric blunt trauma. *J Pediatr.* 2015;167(3):593–598.e1.

36. Davis DH, Localio AR, Stafford PW, et al. Trends in operative management of pediatric splenic injury in a regional trauma system. *Pediatrics.* 2005;115(1):89–94.

37. Demetriades D, Karaiskakis M, Velmahos GC, et al. Pelvic fractures in pediatric and adult trauma patients: are they different injuries? *J Trauma.* 2003;54(6):1146–1151.

38. Densmore JC, Lim HJ, Oldham KT, et al. Outcomes and delivery of care in pediatric injury. *J Pediatr Surg.* 2006;41(1):92–98.

39. Dereeper E, Ciardelli R, Vincent JL. Fatal outcome after polytrauma: multiple organ failure or cerebral damage? *Resuscitation.* 1998;36(1):15–18.

40. Deutsch RJ, Badawy MK. Pediatric cervical spine fracture caused by an adult 3-point seatbelt. *Pediatr Emerg Care.* 2008;24(2):105–108.

41. Dorairajan LN, Gupta H, Kumar S. Pelvic fracture-associated urethral injuries in girls: experience with primary repair. *BJU Int.* 2004;94(1):134–136.

42. Dormans JP. Evaluation of children with suspected cervical spine injury. *J Bone Joint Surg Am.* 2002;A(1):124–132.

43. Doud AN, Schoell SL, Weaver AA, et al. Disability risk in pediatric motor vehicle crash occupants. *J Trauma Acute Care Surg.* 2017;82(5):933–938.

44. Ehrlich PF, Brown JK, Sochor MR, et al. Factors influencing pediatric Injury Severity Score and Glasgow Coma Scale in pediatric automobile crashes: results from the Crash Injury Research Engineering Network. *J Pediatr Surg.* 2006;41(11):1854–1858.

45. Elgamal EA, Elwatidy S, Zakaria AM, et al. Spinal cord injury without radiological abnormality (SCIWORA). A diagnosis that is missed in unconscious children. *Neurosciences (Riyadh).* 2008;13(4):437–440.

46. El-Gamasy MA, Elezz AA, Basuni AS, et al. Pediatric trauma BIG score: predicting mortality in polytraumatized pediatric patients. *Indian J Crit Care Med.* 2016;20(11):640–646.

47. Eppich WJ, Zonfrillo MR. Emergency department evaluation and management of blunt abdominal trauma in children. *Curr Opin Pediatr.* 2007;19(3):265–269.

48. Eriksson EA, Rickey J, Leon SM, et al. Fat embolism in pediatric patients: an autopsy evaluation of incidence and etiology. *J Crit Care.* 2015;30(1):221.e1–e5.

49. Evans DL, Bethem D. Cervical spine injuries in children. *J Pediatr Orthop.* 1989;9(5):563–568.

50. Fagelman MF, Epps HR, Rang M. Mangled extremity severity score in children. *J Pediatr Orthop.* 2002;22(2):182–184.

51. Fayiga YJ, Valentine RJ, Myers SI, et al. Blunt pediatric vascular trauma: analysis of forty-one consecutive patients undergoing operative intervention. *J Vasc Surg.* 1994;20(3):419–424.

52. Fulkerson DH, White IK, Rees JM, et al. Analysis of long-term (median 10.5 years) outcomes in children presenting with traumatic brain injury and an initial Glasgow Coma Scale score of 3 or 4. *J Neurosurg Pediatr.* 2015;16(4):410–419.

53. Godfrey J, Choi PD, Shabtai L, et al. Management of pediatric type I open fractures in the emergency department or operating room: a multicenter perspective. *J Pediatr Orthop.* 2017.

54. Goedeke J, Boehm R, Dietz HG. Multiply trauma in children: pulmonary contusion does not necessarily lead to a worsening of the treatment success. *Eur J Pediatr Surg.* 2014;24(6):508–513.

55. Grossman MD, Yelon JA, Szydiak L. Effect of American College of Surgeons Trauma Center Designation on Outcomes: Measurable Benefit at the Extremes of Age and Injury. *J Am Coll Surg.* 2017;225(2):194–199.

56. Guillamondegui OD, Mahboubi S, Stafford PW, et al. The utility of the pelvic radiograph in the assessment of pediatric pelvic fractures. *J Trauma.* 2003;55(2):236–239.

57. Gustilo RB, Anderson JT. Prevention of infection in the treatment of one thousand and twenty-five open fractures of long bones: retrospective and prospective analyses. *J Bone Joint Surg Am.* 1976;58(4):453–458.

58. Gustilo RB, Mendoza RM, Williams DN. Problems in the management of type III (severe) open fractures: a new classification of type III open fractures. *J Trauma.* 1984;24(8):742–746.

59. Haller JA Jr, Shorter N, Miller D, et al. Organization and function of a regional pediatric trauma center: does a system of management improve outcome? *J Trauma.* 1983;23(8):691–696.

60. Hamrick MC, Duhn RD, Carney DE, et al. Pulmonary contusion in the pediatric population. *Am Surg.* 2010;76(7):721–724.

61. Hannan EL, Farrell LS, Meaker PS, et al. Predicting inpatient mortality for pediatric trauma patients with blunt injuries: a better alternative. *J Pediatr Surg.* 2000;35(2):155–159.

62. Hauser CJ, Adams CA Jr, Eachempati SR; Council of the Surgical Infection Society. Surgical Infection Society guideline: prophylactic antibiotic use in open fractures: an evidence-based guideline. *Surg Infect (Larchmt).* 2006;7(4):379–405.

63. Heaney JB, Guidry C, Simms E, et al. To TQIP or not to TQIP? That is the question. *Am Surg.* 2014;80(4):386–390.

64. Heaney JB, Schroll R, Turney J, et al. Implications of the TQIP inclusion of non-survivable injuries in performance benchmarking (TQIP Inclusion of non-survivable injuries). *J Trauma Acute Care Surg.* 2017;83(4):617–621.

65. Hedequist D, Starr AJ, Wilson P, et al. Early versus delayed stabilization of pediatric femur fractures: analysis of 387 patients. *J Orthop Trauma.* 1999;13(7):490–493.

66. Herscovici D Jr, Sanders RW, Scaduto JM, et al. Vacuum-assisted wound closure (VAC therapy) for the management of patients with high-energy soft tissue injuries. *J Orthop Trauma.* 2003;17(10):683–688.

67. Herzenberg JE, Hensinger RN, Dedrick DK, et al. Emergency transport and positioning of young children who have an injury of the cervical spine. The standard backboard may be hazardous. *J Bone Joint Surg Am.* 1989;71(1):15–22.

68. Hoffmann R, Nerlich M, Muggia-Sullam M, et al. Blunt abdominal trauma in cases of multiple trauma evaluated by ultrasonography: a prospective analysis of 291 patients. *J Trauma.* 1992;32(4):452–458.

69. Holmes JF, Brant WE, Bond WF, et al. Emergency department ultrasonography in the evaluation of hypotensive and normotensive children with blunt abdominal trauma. *J Pediatr Surg.* 2001;36(7):968–973.

70. Holmes JF, Gladman A, Chang CH. Performance of abdominal ultrasonography in pediatric blunt trauma patients: a meta-analysis. *J Pediatr Surg.* 2007;42(9):1588–1594.

71. Horn BD, Rettig ME. Interobserver reliability in the Gustilo and Anderson classification of open fractures. *J Orthop Trauma.* 1993;7(4):357–360.

72. Investigators F, Bhandari M, Jeray KJ, et al. A trial of wound irrigation in the initial management of open fracture wounds. *N Engl J Med.* 2015;373(27):2629–2641.

73. Investigators F, Petrisor B, Sun X, et al. Fluid lavage of open wounds (FLOW): a multicenter, blinded, factorial pilot trial comparing alternative irrigating solutions and pressures in patients with open fractures. *J Trauma.* 2011;71(3):596–606.

74. Iobst CA, Tidwell MA, King WF. Nonoperative management of pediatric type I open fractures. *J Pediatr Orthop.* 2005;25(4):513–517.

75. Ismail N, Bellemare JF, Mollitt DL, et al. Death from pelvic fracture: children are different. *J Pediatr Surg.* 1996;31(1):82–85.

76. Jacobs IA, Kelly K, Valenziano C, et al. Nonoperative management of blunt splenic and hepatic trauma in the pediatric population: significant differences between adult and pediatric surgeons? *Am Surg.* 2001;67(2):149–154.

77. Jakob H, Lustenberger T, Schneidmuller D, et al. Pediatric polytrauma management. *Eur J Trauma Emerg Surg.* 2010;36(4):325–338.

78. Jordan B. Lap belt complex: recognition and assessment of seatbelt injuries in pediatric trauma patients. *JEMS.* 2001;26(5):36–43.

79. Kaufmann CR, Maier RV, Rivara FP, et al. Evaluation of the Pediatric Trauma Score. *JAMA.* 1990;263(1):69–72.

80. Keret D, Harcke HT, Mendez AA, et al. Heterotopic ossification in central nervous system-injured patients following closed nailing of femoral fractures. *Clin Orthop Relat Res.* 1990(256):254–259.

81. Kluger G, Kochs A, Holthausen H. Heterotopic ossification in childhood and adolescence. *J Child Neurol.* 2000;15(6):406–413.

82. Knudson MM, Shagoury C, Lewis FR. Can adult trauma surgeons care for injured children? *J Trauma.* 1992;32(6):729–737.

83. Kyle UG, Lucas LA, Mackey G, et al. Implementation of nutrition support guidelines may affect energy and protein intake in the pediatric intensive care unit. *J Acad Nutr Diet.* 2016;116(5):844–851.e4.

84. Laine JC, Cherkashin A, Samchukov M, et al. The management of soft tissue and bone loss in type IIIB and IIIC pediatric open tibia fractures. *J Pediatr Orthop.* 2016;36(5):453–458.

85. Lauber S, Schulte TL, Gotze C, et al. Acute compartment syndrome following intramedullary pulse lavage and debridement for osteomyelitis of the tibia. *Arch Orthop Trauma Surg.* 2005;125(8):564–566.

86. Lavelle WF, Uhl R, Krieves M, et al. Management of open fractures in pediatric patients: current teaching in Accreditation Council for Graduate Medical Education (ACGME) accredited residency programs. *J Pediatr Orthop B.* 2008;17(1):1–6.

87. Lee J. Efficacy of cultures in the management of open fractures. *Clin Orthop Relat Res.* 1997(339):71–75.

88. Lee LK, Fleisher GR. *Trauma Management: Approach to the Unstable Child.* 2017 ed. Waltham, MA: *UpToDate*; 2017.

89. Leeper CM, Neal MD, McKenna C, et al. Abnormalities in fibrinolysis at the time of admission are associated with deep vein thrombosis, mortality, and disability in a pediatric trauma population. *J Trauma Acute Care Surg.* 2017;82(1):27–34.

90. Leininger BE, Rasmussen TE, Smith DL, et al. Experience with wound VAC and delayed primary closure of contaminated soft tissue injuries in Iraq. *J Trauma.* 2006;61(5):1207–1211.

91. Letts M, Davidson D, Lapner P. Multiple trauma in children: predicting outcome and long-term results. *Can J Surg.* 2002;45(2):126–131.

92. Letts M, Jarvis J, Lawton L, et al. Complications of rigid intramedullary rodding of femoral shaft fractures in children. *J Trauma.* 2002;52(3):504–516.

93. Levin HS, High WM Jr, Ewing-Cobbs L, et al. Memory functioning during the first year after closed head injury in children and adolescents. *Neurosurgery.* 1988;22(6 Pt 1):1043–1052.

94. Levy ML, Granville RC, Hart D, et al. Deep venous thrombosis in children and adolescents. *J Neurosurg.* 2004;101(1 Suppl):32–37.

95. Limbird TJ, Ruderman RJ. Fat embolism in children. *Clin Orthop Relat Res.* 1978(136):267–269.

96. Loder RT. Pediatric polytrauma: orthopaedic care and hospital course. *J Orthop Trauma.* 1987;1(1):48–54.

97. Loder RT, Gullahorn LJ, Yian EH, et al. Factors predictive of immobilization complications in pediatric polytrauma. *J Orthop Trauma.* 2001;15(5):338–341.

98. MacKenzie EJ, Rivara FP, Jurkovich GJ, et al. A national evaluation of the effect of trauma-center care on mortality. *N Engl J Med.* 2006;354(4):366–378.

99. Maksoud JG Jr, Moront ML, Eichelberger MR. Resuscitation of the injured child. *Semin Pediatr Surg.* 1995;4(2):93–99.

100. Mital MA, Garber JE, Stinson JT. Ectopic bone formation in children and adolescents with head injuries: its management. *J Pediatr Orthop.* 1987;7(1):83–90.

101. Mooney JF. The use of 'damage control orthopedics' techniques in children with segmental open femur fractures. *J Pediatr Orthop B.* 2012;21(5):400–403.

102. Mooney JF 3rd, Argenta LC, Marks MW, et al. Treatment of soft tissue defects in pediatric patients using the V.A.C. system. *Clin Orthop Relat Res.* 2000(376):26–31.

103. Murphy EE, Murphy SG, Cipolle MD, et al. The pediatric trauma center and the inclusive trauma system: impact on splenectomy rates. *J Trauma Acute Care Surg.* 2015;78(5):930–933.

104. Mutabagani KH, Coley BD, Zumberge N, et al. Preliminary experience with focused abdominal sonography for trauma (FAST) in children: is it useful? *J Pediatr Surg.* 1999;34(1):48–52.

105. Nesiama JA, Pirallo RG, Lerner EB, et al. Does a prehospital Glasgow Coma Scale score predict pediatric outcomes? *Pediatr Emerg Care.* 2012;28(10):1027–1032.

106. Okike K, Bhattacharyya T. Trends in the management of open fractures. A critical analysis. *J Bone Joint Surg Am.* 2006;88(12):2739–2748.

107. Onuora VC, Patil MG, al-Jasser AN. Missed urological injuries in children with polytrauma. *Injury.* 1993;24(9):619–621.

108. Orlowski JP, Porembka DT, Gallagher JM, et al. Comparison study of intraosseous, central intravenous, and peripheral intravenous infusions of emergency drugs. *Am J Dis Child.* 1990;144(1):112–117.

109. Ott R, Kramer R, Martus P, et al. Prognostic value of trauma scores in pediatric patients with multiple injuries. *J Trauma.* 2000;49(4):729–736.

110. Owens BD, White DW, Wenke JC. Comparison of irrigation solutions and devices in a contaminated musculoskeletal wound survival model. *J Bone Joint Surg Am.* 2009;91(1):92–98.

111. Oyetunji TA, Haider AH, Downing SR, et al. Treatment outcomes of injured children at adult level 1 trauma centers: are there benefits from added specialized care? *Am J Surg.* 2011;201(4):445–449.

112. Pascarella R, Bettuzzi C, Digennaro V. Surgical treatment for pelvic ring fractures in pediatric and adolescence age. *Musculoskelet Surg.* 2013;97(3):217–222.

113. Patzakis MJ, Bains RS, Lee J, et al. Prospective, randomized, double-blind study comparing single-agent antibiotic therapy, ciprofloxacin, to combination antibiotic therapy in open fracture wounds. *J Orthop Trauma.* 2000;14(8):529–533.

114. Peclet MH, Newman KD, Eichelberger MR, et al. Thoracic trauma in children: an indicator of increased mortality. *J Pediatr Surg.* 1990;25(9):961–965.

115. Petrisor B, Jeray K, Schemitsch E, et al. Fluid lavage in patients with open fracture wounds (FLOW): an international survey of 984 surgeons. *BMC Musculoskeletal Disord.* 2008;9:7.

116. Philip PA, Philip M. Peripheral nerve injuries in children with traumatic brain injury. *Brain Inj.* 1992;6(1):53–58.

117. Podesta ML, Jordan GH. Pelvic fracture urethral injuries in girls. *J Urol.* 2001;165(5):1660–1665.

118. Potoka DA, Schall LC, Ford HR. Improved functional outcome for severely injured children treated at pediatric trauma centers. *J Trauma.* 2001;51(5):824–832.

119. Potoka DA, Schall LC, Ford HR. Risk factors for splenectomy in children with blunt splenic trauma. *J Pediatr Surg.* 2002;37(3):294–299.

120. Potoka DA, Schall LC, Gardner MJ, et al. Impact of pediatric trauma centers on mortality in a statewide system. *J Trauma.* 2000;49(2):237–245.

121. Rinker B, Valerio IL, Stewart DH, et al. Microvascular free flap reconstruction in pediatric lower extremity trauma: a 10-year review. *Plast Reconstr Surg.* 2005;115(6):1618–1624.

122. Robinson CM. Current concepts of respiratory insufficiency syndromes after fracture. *J Bone Joint Surg Br.* 2001;83(6):781–791.

123. Roche BG, Bugmann P, Le Coultre C. Blunt injuries to liver, spleen, kidney and pancreas in pediatric patients. *Eur J Pediatr Surg.* 1992;2(3):154–156.

124. Rohrer MJ, Cutler BS, MacDougall E, et al. A prospective study of the incidence of deep venous thrombosis in hospitalized children. *J Vasc Surg.* 1996;24(1):46–49.

125. Rourke KF, McCammon KA, Sumfest JM, et al. Open reconstruction of pediatric and adolescent urethral strictures: long-term followup. *J Urol.* 2003;169(5):1818–1821.

126. Ryan SP, Pugliano V. Controversies in initial management of open fractures. *Scand J Surg.* 2014;103(2):132–137.

127. Ryan ML, Van Haren RM, Thorson CM, et al. Trauma induced hypercoagulablity in pediatric patients. *J Pediatr Surg.* 2014;49(8):1295–1299.

128. Saladino R, Lund D, Fleisher G. The spectrum of liver and spleen injuries in children: failure of the pediatric trauma score and clinical signs to predict isolated injuries. *Ann Emerg Med.* 1991;20(6):636–640.

129. Sanchez JL, Lucas J, Feustel PJ. Outcome of adolescent trauma admitted to an adult surgical intensive care unit versus a pediatric intensive care unit. *J Trauma.* 2001;51(3):478–480.

130. Sanchez B, Waxman K, Jones T, et al. Cervical spine clearance in blunt trauma: evaluation of a computed tomography-based protocol. *J Trauma.* 2005;59(1):179–183.

131. Scaife ER, Rollins MD, Barnhart DC, et al. The role of focused abdominal sonography for trauma (FAST) in pediatric trauma evaluation. *J Pediatr Surg.* 2013;48(6):1377–1383.

132. Schalamon J, Bismarck SV, Schober PH, et al. Multiple trauma in pediatric patients. *Pediatr Surg Int.* 2003;19(6):417–423.

133. Signorino PR, Densmore J, Werner M, et al. Pediatric pelvic injury: functional outcome at 6-month follow-up. *J Pediatr Surg.* 2005;40(1):107–112.

134. Silber JS, Flynn JM, Koffler KM, et al. Analysis of the cause, classification, and associated injuries of 166 consecutive pediatric pelvic fractures. *J Pediatr Orthop.* 2001;21(4):446–450.

135. Silva SR, Bosch P. Intramuscular air as a complication of pulse-lavage irrigation: a case report. *J Bone Joint Surg Am.* 2009;91(12):2937–2940.

136. Sivit CJ, Taylor GA, Newman KD, et al. Safety-belt injuries in children with lap-belt ecchymosis: CT findings in 61 patients. *AJR Am J Roentgenol.* 1991;157(1):111–114.

137. Skaggs DL, Friend L, Alman B, et al. The effect of surgical delay on acute infection following 554 open fractures in children. *J Bone Joint Surg Am.* 2005;87(1):8–12.

138. Smith WR, Oakley M, Morgan SJ. Pediatric pelvic fractures. *J Pediatr Orthop.* 2004;24(1):130–135.

139. Sobus KM, Sherman N, Alexander MA. Coexistence of deep venous thrombosis and heterotopic ossification in the pediatric patient. *Arch Phys Med Rehabil.* 1993;74(5):547–551.

140. Spiguel L, Glynn L, Liu D, et al. Pediatric pelvic fractures: a marker for injury severity. *Am Surg.* 2006;72(6):481–484.

141. Stafford PW, Blinman TA, Nance ML. Practical points in evaluation and resuscitation of the injured child. *Surg Clin North Am.* 2002;82(2):273–301.

142. Stylianos S, Egorova N, Guice KS, et al. Variation in treatment of pediatric spleen injury at trauma centers versus nontrauma centers: a call for dissemination of American Pediatric Surgical Association benchmarks and guidelines. *J Am Coll Surg.* 2006;202(2):247–251.

143. Sullivan MP, Torres SJ, Mehta S, et al. Heterotopic ossification after central nervous system trauma: a current review. *Bone Joint Res.* 2013;2(3):51–57.

144. Swaid F, Peleg K, Alfici R, et al. A comparison study of pelvic fractures and associated abdominal injuries between pediatric and adult blunt trauma patients. *J Pediatr Surg.* 2017;52(3):386–389.

145. Taeger G, Ruchholtz S, Waydhas C, et al. Damage control orthopedics in patients with multiple injuries is effective, time saving, and safe. *J Trauma.* 2005;59(2):409–416.

146. Tarman GJ, Kaplan GW, Lerman SL, et al. Lower genitourinary injury and pelvic fractures in pediatric patients. *Urology.* 2002;59(1):123–126.

147. Tataria M, Nance ML, Holmes JH 4th, et al. Pediatric blunt abdominal injury: age is irrelevant and delayed operation is not detrimental. *J Trauma.* 2007;63(3):608–614.

148. Tilden SJ, Watkins S, Tong TK, et al. Measured energy expenditure in pediatric intensive care patients. *Am J Dis Child.* 1989;143(4):490–492.

149. Tolo VT. Orthopaedic treatment of fractures of the long bones and pelvis in children who have multiple injuries. *Instr Course Lect.* 2000;49:415–423.

150. Torode I, Zieg D. Pelvic fractures in children. *J Pediatr Orthop.* 1985;5(1):76–84.

151. Tran A, Campbell BT. The art and science of pediatric damage control. *Semin Pediatr Surg.* 2017;26(1):21–26.

152. Truitt AK, Sorrells DL, Halvorson E, et al. Pulmonary embolism: which pediatric trauma patients are at risk? *J Pediatr Surg.* 2005;40(1):124–127.

153. Tso EL, Beaver BL, Haller JA Jr. Abdominal injuries in restrained pediatric passengers. *J Pediatr Surg.* 1993;28(7):915–919.

154. Tuovinen H, Soderlund T, Lindahl J, et al. Severe pelvic fracture-related bleeding in pediatric patients: does it occur? *Eur J Trauma Emerg Surg.* 2012;38(2):163–169.

155. Tuttle MS, Smith WR, Williams AE, et al. Safety and efficacy of damage control external fixation versus early definitive stabilization for femoral shaft fractures in the multiple-injured patient. *J Trauma.* 2009;67(3):602–605.

156. Uranus S, Pfeifer J. Nonoperative treatment of blunt splenic injury. *World J Surg.* 2001;25(11):1405–1407.

157. Valenziano CP, Chattar-Cora D, O'Neill A, et al. Efficacy of primary wound cultures in long bone open extremity fractures: are they of any value? *Arch Orthop Trauma Surg.* 2002;122(5):259–261.

158. van der Sluis CK, Kingma J, Eisma WH, et al. Pediatric polytrauma: short-term and long-term outcomes. *J Trauma.* 1997;43(3):501–506.

159. Van Haren RM, Valle EJ, Thorson CM, et al. Hypercoagulability and other risk factors in trauma intensive care unit patients with venous thromboembolism. *J Trauma Acute Care Surg.* 2014;76(2):443–449.

160. Vazquez WD, Garcia VF. Pediatric pelvic fractures combined with an additional skeletal injury is an indicator of significant injury. *Surg Gynecol Obstet.* 1993;177(5):468–472.

161. Vitale MG, Kessler MW, Choe JC, et al. Pelvic fractures in children: an exploration of practice patterns and patient outcomes. *J Pediatr Orthop.* 2005;25(5):581–587.

162. Wade SL, Cassedy AE, Fulks LE, et al. Problem-solving after traumatic brain injury in adolescence: associations with functional outcomes. *Arch Phys Med Rehabil.* 2017;98(8):1614–1621.

163. Webb LX. New techniques in wound management: vacuum-assisted wound closure. *J Am Acad Orthop Surg.* 2002;10(5):303–311.

164. Webb LX, Laver D, DeFranzo A. Negative pressure wound therapy in the management of orthopedic wounds. *Ostomy Wound Manage.* 2004;50(4A Suppl):26–27.

165. Weisz GM, Rang M, Salter RB. Posttraumatic fat embolism in children: review of the literature and of experience in the Hospital for Sick Children, Toronto. *J Trauma.* 1973;13(6):529–534.

166. Wesson DE, Spence LJ, Williams JI, et al. Injury scoring systems in children. *Can J Surg.* 1987;30(6):398–400.

167. Wetzel RC, Burns RC. Multiple trauma in children: critical care overview. *Crit Care Med.* 2002;30(11 Suppl):S468–S477.

168. Wilkins J, Patzakis M. Choice and duration of antibiotics in open fractures. *Orthop Clin North Am.* 1991;22(3):433–437.

169. Winogron HW, Knights RM, Bawden HN. Neuropsychological deficits following head injury in children. *J Clin Neuropsychol.* 1984;6(3):267–286.

170. Yalcin N, Dede O, Alanay A, et al. Surgical management of post-SCIWORA spinal deformities in children. *J Child Orthop.* 2011;5(1):27–33.

171. Yen J, Van Arendonk KJ, Streiff MB, et al. Risk factors for venous thromboembolism in pediatric trauma patients and validation of a novel scoring system: the risk of clots in kids with trauma score. *Pediatr Crit Care Med.* 2016;17(5):391–399.

172. Young B, Rapp RP, Norton JA, et al. Early prediction of outcome in head-injured patients. *J Neurosurg.* 1981;54(3):300–303.

173. Yousefzadeh-Chabok S, Kazemnejad-Leili E, Kouchakinejad-Eramsadati L, et al. Comparing Pediatric Trauma, Glasgow Coma Scale and Injury Severity scores for mortality prediction in traumatic children. *Ulus Travma Acil Cerrahi Derg.* 2016;22(4):328–332.

174. Zhao XG, Zhao GF, Ma YF, et al. Research progress in mechanism of traumatic brain injury affecting speed of fracture healing. *Chin J Traumatol.* 2007;10(6):376–380.

5

Compartment Syndrome in Children

Haleh Badkoobehi, John M. Flynn, and Milan V. Stevanovic

INTRODUCTION

Compartment syndrome (CS) in children is caused by sustained increased pressures within an fascial compartment resulting in circulatory compromise, ischemia, and ultimately tissue death. The importance of timely diagnosis and surgical intervention is critical to optimize clinical outcomes. Failure to address CS in an expeditious manner can lead to permanent disability in the affected limb.

DIAGNOSIS

A variety of injuries and medical conditions, including fractures, elective orthopedic procedures such as osteotomies, soft tissue injuries, burn eschar, animal and insect bites, external compression by tight dressings or casts, excessive flexion in a long-arm cast, intravenous infiltration, antishock garments, infection (Group B strep), and bleeding disorders can lead to CS and can involve the forearm, hand, thigh, leg and foot (Table 5-1). The most common cause of CS is trauma, secondary to motor vehicle accidents, falls, and sports.[15] Similar to adults, CS is up to four times more prevalent in boys than in girls.[2] The diagnosis of acute compartment syndrome (ACS) is challenging and can be more difficult in children, and particularly in infants. Additionally, a high index of suspicion must be maintained in obtunded or sedated patients.

The six Ps, including *pain, pressure, pallor, paresthesia, paralysis, and pulselessness* have been described as clinical markers of CS. The reliability of these clinical findings is questionable; however, as they may be difficult to obtain in the pediatric or obtunded patient or in a patient with delayed presentation in whom irreversible tissue damage has already occurred. Instead, in children, the *three As* may be more useful in making a diagnosis of CS in the pediatric population: *anxiety* (or restlessness), *agitation* (or crying), and an increasing *analgesia* requirement.[2]

TABLE 5-1. Causes of Compartment Syndrome

Intrinsic	Extrinsic
Fracture	Compressive casts, dressings
Soft tissue trauma without fracture	Pneumatic antishock garments
Vascular injury	
Penetrating trauma	
Burns	Burn eschar
Animal + insect bites	
Fluid infusion secondary to intravenous (or intraosseous) extravasation (also arthroscopy)	
Bleeding disorders	
Reperfusion injury following prolonged ischemia	
Elective orthopedic procedure—osteotomy	

Pain out of proportion to the injury, especially aggravated by passive motion of the ischemic compartment, is a sensitive and early physical finding of CS.[25] An increasing analgesia requirement, both in dose and frequency, is also a helpful early marker in children.[2]

A systematic review investigating if regional anesthesia (RA) or patient-controlled analgesia (PCA) masked the pain of CS in children reported mixed results, with 75% of studies after 2009 demonstrating that RA and PCA can safely be used in children without masking ACS. Authors postulate that modernized ultrasound-guided techniques for regional blocks allow for better targeting and thus lower volumes of injected anesthetic into a given compartment. Authors also argue that RA with complete motor and sensory blockade–masked nociceptive pain, *not* ischemic pain and therefore does not affect CS evaluation.[19] Despite this, there is currently not a strong recommendation for or against the use of RA or PCA in children when there is a concern for development of CS.[11]

In the case of "silent CS," there is an absence of pain.[1,25] Agitation and *anxiety* may be present instead. Pressure, swelling, and tenseness of the affected compartment may be objective but often unreliable findings of early CS.[25,34] Paralysis is a late and insensitive finding of CS.

In unclear clinical presentations, compartment pressure measurements are recommended. In the pediatric setting, compartment pressures are best measured under conscious sedation or anesthesia. Multiple measurements at different sites and depths within each compartment are recommended. Compartment pressure measurements close to the level of fracture may be most accurate. Historically, the threshold for lower leg fasciotomies in both adults and children were an absolute pressure greater than 30 mm Hg or pressures within 30 mm Hg of either the diastolic blood pressure or the mean arterial pressure. Application of this threshold to children may not be appropriate.

Baseline compartment pressures have been shown to be higher in children compared to adults: normal adult leg compartment pressures are between 5.2 and 9.7 mm Hg, whereas in children they are 13.3 to 16.6 mm Hg.[36] Also, children have been shown to tolerate compartment pressures above traditional thresholds for fasciotomies, and many do not develop ACS without surgical treatment. A prospective study identified 41 children with fractured forearms. Of these patients, 15 had needle manometry compartment pressure readings >30 mm Hg in the injured extremity. Only 1 in 15 went on to develop ACS. All the remaining children tolerated pressures greater than 30 mm Hg without developing ACS. Authors argue that traditional surgical cutoff pressure measurements may not apply to children, and that children may be closely observed and may ultimately avoid the need for fasciotomies.[40] We recommend serial evaluation of the at-risk extremity and decompressive fasciotomy when there are clinical signs of ACS development and elevated compartment pressure readings.

Risk factors that may delay diagnosis are altered level of consciousness, associated nerve injury, polytrauma, and altered pain perception. Delay in diagnosis may also be related to longer elapsed time between the initial injury and peak compartment pressures in the pediatric setting.[13] Extended close monitoring after injury is recommended when there is concern for development of CS in children. Near-infrared spectroscopy (NIRS) is a rarely used noninvasive method that measures oxygenation in at-risk tissues and has been shown to reliably estimate tissue intracompartmental pressure.[7,34]

CLASSIFICATION

Acute Compartment Syndrome: ACS occurs when tissue pressures rise high enough within an fascial compartment to cause tissue ischemia. The exact time of onset of ACS is difficult to determine and varies by patient.

Fracture ACS: The majority of cases of CS are associated with a fracture. Both high- and low-energy injuries can result in CS. Open fractures are associated with a higher incidence of CS than closed injuries.[15] Open fractures are generally associated with higher-energy injuries and the associated fascial disruption does not result in adequate decompression of all compartments.

Nonfracture ACS: Soft tissue injury without fracture can also lead to CS, especially in the setting of an underlying bleeding disorder or with the use of anticoagulants. CS in this setting has been associated with a high rate of disability.[17] A retrospective review over 16 years evaluating nonfracture CS identified 39 cases of which 29/39 (74%) involved the leg. In this series, CS was most commonly caused by vascular injury, followed by trauma and postoperative changes. Pain and swelling were the most common symptoms. Delay in diagnosis up to 48 hours was commonly seen and 21/39 (54%) had evidence of myonecrosis at time of surgery.[20] Muscle recovery is rare once myonecrosis has occurred.

Exercise-Induced or Exertional CS: Exercise-induced CS is a transient increased compartment pressure and reversible tissue ischemia caused by a noncompliant fascial compartment that does not accommodate muscle expansion occurring during a repetitive exercise such as running. It has been described in both the upper and lower extremities.[45] Exertional CS can be relieved with cessation of the offending activity or fasciotomies of affected compartments for refractory cases.

Neonatal: Neonatal CS has been reported. To our knowledge, it has only been reported in the upper extremity and is characterized by skin lesions that can be confused with other diagnoses. Due to this, diagnosis is usually delayed and patients develop Volkmann's contracture, as well as bone and nerve disturbances.[28] Early recognition and treatment can improve the functional outcome and growth; however, established neonatal Volkmann's contracture cannot be improved by emergent intervention.

TREATMENT

Potentially devastating complications of CS may be avoidable with early recognition and prompt intervention. The goal of treatment is to prevent tissue necrosis, neurovascular compromise, and permanent functional deficits.

The first step is to remove all possible extrinsic causes of pressure on the affected limb, including circumferential dressings, cast padding, and casts. A study simulating CS in the anterior leg compartment in healthy patients was performed using a pneumatic thigh cuff to elevate pressures in the studied leg, with the contralateral leg as control. Compartment pressures, microvascular blood flow, perfusion pressure, pH, and oxygenation were evaluated with the leg at heart level and 12 cm above heart level. Authors found that tissue oxygenation, blood flow, perfusion pressure, and pH all decrease as compartment pressure was increased, and leg elevation caused further decreases in all outcome variables.[8] Authors argue that in patients with ACS, the affected extremity should not be dependent, but also should not be elevated higher than the patient's heart to maximize perfusion while minimizing swelling. Optimizing overall medical management is also recommended, as shock and hypoxia may lower tissue pressure tolerance.[15]

If the diagnosis of CS is made, emergent fasciotomy, that is, release of the fascia overlying each affected compartment is necessary. At times, release of the epimysium is also necessary. Necrotic tissue should be excised. If in doubt as to the viability of soft tissue, questionable tissue should *not* be debrided at the index procedure because the potential for tissue recovery in a child is substantial.[12] The patient should return to the operating room for serial washouts and closure, at which time the tissue may have had time to declare itself. Late fibrosis of necrotic muscle can lead to compression of the adjacent nerves and result in disability of the extremity. Other procedures may be indicated based on the etiology of the CS, including vascular thrombectomy, repair, or grafting, nerve exploration, and fracture reduction and stabilization. Nerve repair or reconstruction should be performed at the time of definitive wound closure.

In the case of a delayed CS where there is no demonstrable muscle function in any segment of the involved limb, the limb can be splinted in a functional position. Fasciotomy is not indicated. For the upper extremity, if resources are available for immediate reconstruction with functional free muscle transfer, then early debridement and reconstruction can reduce the incidence of late contracture and can improve neurologic recovery.[32,37] Supportive care, usually in the form of vigorous intravenous hydration, should be given for the potential risk of myoglobinuria. Myoglobinuria, as well as metabolic acidosis and hyperkalemia, can also occur during reperfusion and requires medical management to prevent sequelae such as renal failure, shock, hypothermia, and cardiac arrhythmias and/or failure.

UPPER EXTREMITY

In the upper extremity, ACS most commonly involves the forearm and is typically associated with both bone fractures of the forearm and supracondylar fracture of the humerus.[5,13,15,18] The incidence of forearm CS following upper extremity injuries has been estimated at 1%.[15] High-risk fracture patterns include displaced SCH fractures with concomitant ipsilateral forearm fractures. In this case, the rate of CS is as high as 33%.[5] Additionally, SCH fractures with a median nerve injury are at high risk for CS, as the pain of CS is masked.[24] Other risk factors for developing CS after intramedullary nailing of forearm fractures include open fractures, longer intraoperative and fluoroscopic times, and younger age (mean age 6 compared to 10 years).[4,22,46]

The surgical incision for fasciotomy of the arm and forearm is extensile from the brachium to the carpal tunnel. The extent of the release performed is tailored to the clinical and intraoperative findings. Release of the dorsal forearm and compartments of the hand requires separate incisions when indicated (Table 5-2). Separate incisions for dermatomes of each finger may also be added to prevent skin necrosis and loss of fingers.

ARM

The anterior and posterior compartments of the arm can be decompressed through a single medial incision. This allows access to the neurovascular structures of the arm, the medial fascia of the biceps and brachialis in the anterior compartment, and the fascia of the triceps. Excision of the medial intermuscular septum will provide additional decompression of both compartments (Fig. 5-1). The incision can be extended to the elbow crease and incorporated with the incision for decompression of the forearm. This also allows release of the lacertus fibrosus and evaluation of the distal portion of the brachial artery. When there is no need to evaluate and decompress the neurovascular structures or extend the incision into the forearm, straight midline anterior and posterior fasciotomies may be performed to decompress the flexor and extensor compartments, respectively.

FOREARM

Several skin incisions have been described for the forearm. Since the surgical incisions are long and extensile, almost any

TABLE 5-2. Compartments of the Upper Extremity

Compartments			Contents
Arm	Anterior		Biceps and brachialis, brachial artery, and median nerve
	Posterior		Triceps, ulnar nerve, and radial nerve
Forearm	Volar	Superficial	FCR, PL, pronator teres, FCU, and FDS
		Deep	FDP, FPL, and pronator quadratus
			Anterior interosseous nerve and artery
	Dorsal	Mobile wad	Brachioradialis, ECRL, ECRB
		Extensor	EDC, ECU, EPL, APL, EPB, EIP, EDM, supinator,[a] posterior interosseous nerve
		Anconeus[b]	Anconeus
Hand	Thenar		Abductor pollicis brevis, opponens pollicis, and flexor pollicis brevis
	Hypothenar		Abductor digiti minimi, flexor digiti minimi, and opponens digiti minimi
	Adductor pollicis		Adductor pollicis (two heads)
	Dorsal interossei (4)		Each separate compartments
	Volar interossei (3)		Each separate compartments
Fingers			[c]

[a]Supinator is not typically a component of extensor compartment syndrome, but decompression can be done through the brachioradialis/ECRL interval.
[b]Not typically listed as a separate compartment, but should be assessed.
[c]Not technically a compartment, but compression of the neurovascular structures by rigid Cleland and Grayson's ligaments can lead to skin necrosis and/or loss of the finger.

incision can be used to decompress the forearm compartments (Fig. 5-2). Because the incisions are left open, we prefer the incision described in Figure 5-3C,D over the incision seen in Figure 5-3 A,B, as this minimizes exposure of neurovascular structures and can be extended proximally into the medial arm and distally into the carpal tunnel (see Fig. 5-3C,D).[33] After the skin incision is made, the antebrachial fascia is opened longitudinally from lacertus fibrosus to the wrist flexion crease. This decompresses the superficial flexor compartment. The deep flexor compartment is most easily and safely exposed through the ulnar side of the forearm.[29] Start at the mid to distal forearm and identify the interval between flexor carpi ulnaris and flexor digitorum superficialis. The flexor digitorum profundus and flexor pollicis longus fascia are exposed and released through this interval. This is the most important component of

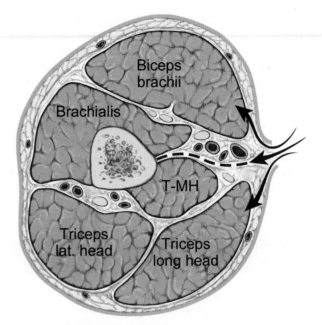

Figure 5-1. Cross-sectional anatomy of the arm is shown. The *dotted line* represents the plane of dissection for decompression of the anterior and posterior compartments through a medial incision. The intermuscular septum can be excised, which further decompresses both compartments. Alternatively, a straight anterior and posterior incision may be used to separately decompress the anterior and posterior compartments. (Courtesy of Dr. M. Stevanovic.)

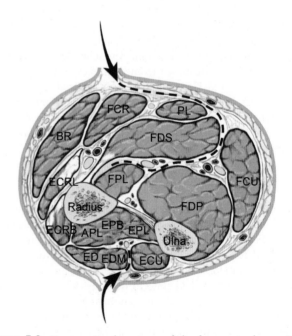

Figure 5-2. Cross-sectional anatomy of the forearm is shown. The *dotted lines* represent the plane of dissection for dorsal and volar compartments. The superficial flexor compartment can be released in the midline or any location, trying to avoid an incision over the radial or ulnar artery or median nerve. The deep flexor compartment is best released by opening the interval between flexor carpi ulnaris and the flexor digitorum superficialis. (Courtesy of Dr. M. Stevanovic.)

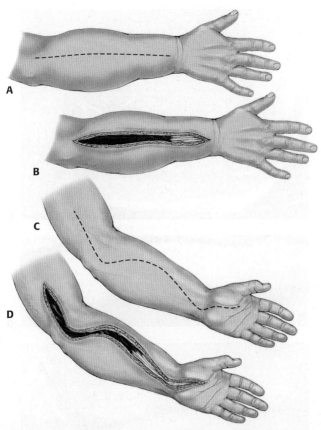

Figure 5-3. A: Dorsal (extensor) incision for forearm fasciotomy. **B:** Release of the extensor compartment. **C:** Volar (flexor) incision for forearm fasciotomy. This incision can be extended proximally into the medial arm and distally into the carpal tunnel as indicated by intra-operative findings. **D:** Release of the flexor compartment and carpal tunnel. (Courtesy of Dr. M. Stevanovic.)

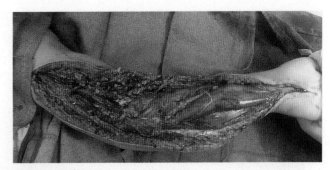

Figure 5-4. Intraoperative photograph of a patient with a SCH fracture and CS after forearm fasciotomy. (Courtesy of Dr. M. Stevanovic.)

this procedure, as the deep flexor compartment is usually the first and most affected by increased compartmental pressure. Through the same interval, the fascia overlying the pronator quadratus is also released.

During the dissection, if the muscles appear pale after release of the fascia, then additional release of the epimysium of the pale muscle should be performed. For these muscles, reperfusion injury will lead to more swelling in the muscle that will lead to further muscle injury if the epimysium is not released.

Clinical evaluation at this time of the remaining tension in the dorsal forearm compartment and/or hand should be done to determine whether additional release of the extensor compartments and hand should be added. The extensor compartments are released through a midline longitudinal dorsal incision extending from the lateral epicondyle to the distal radioulnar joint. This will allow release of the mobile wad and the extensor compartment (Fig. 5-3A). Figure 5-4 is an example of a patient with an SCH fracture and CS after the above-described fasciotomy. The following figure is another example of a patient with SCH and distal radius fractures and CS, including excellent functional clinical outcomes (Fig. 5-5).

HAND

The hand has 10 separate compartments. It is rarely necessary to release all the 10 compartments. Intraoperative assessment and/or measurement of compartment pressures should be used to determine the extent of release needed (Figs. 5-6 and 5-7).

Volar Release

Decompression should start with an extended carpal tunnel release. This will usually adequately release Guyon's canal without formally opening and decompressing the ulnar neurovascular structures. The carpal tunnel incision can be extended to the volar second web space. In the distal portion of the incision, the volar fascia of the adductor pollicis muscle can be released. Also, the fascia tracking to the long finger metacarpal (separating the deep radial and ulnar midpalmar space) can be decompressed. This will help decompress the volar interosseous muscles. The thenar and hypothenar muscles are decompressed through separate incisions as needed (Fig. 5-8A,C).

Dorsal Release

The dorsal interosseous muscles (and volar interosseous muscles) are decompressed through dorsal incisions between the second and third metacarpals and the fourth and fifth metacarpals. The first dorsal interosseous muscle is decompressed through an incision placed in the first dorsal web space. The dorsal fascia of the adductor pollicis can also be released through this incision (see Fig. 5-7B,D).

Fingers

Tense swollen fingers can result in skin and subcutaneous tissue necrosis. The tight fibers of Cleland and Grayson's ligaments can compress and obstruct the digital arteries and veins. Dermotomy of all involved fingers reduces the risk of necrosis of the skin and possible loss of the digit. Dermotomies should be done in the midaxial plane to prevent subsequent contracture. When possible, the dermotomy should be performed on the side that will cause the least amount of scar irritation. The preferred locations for finger and thumb dermotomies are shown in Figure 5-7A,B.

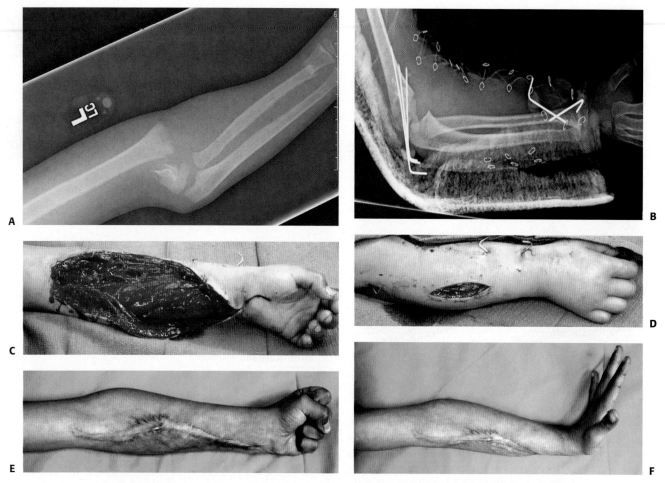

Figure 5-5. This 7-year-old patient fell while riding a bicycle, sustaining an ipsilateral displaced SCH fracture and distal radius fracture. He was seen about 4 hours after his initial injury. He was diagnosed with a compartment syndrome on presentation and taken emergently to the operating room for surgical stabilization and fasciotomy. **A:** Injury films showing displaced SCH fracture and distal radius fracture. **B:** Postoperative reduction and stabilization. **C:** Volar fasciotomy. **D:** Dorsal fasciotomy. **E:** Finger flexion at 1-year postinjury. **F:** Wrist and finger extension at 1-year postinjury. (Courtesy of Dr. M. Stevanovic.)

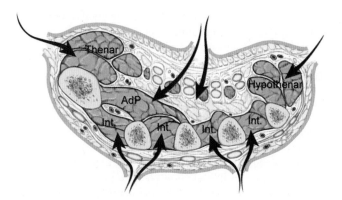

Figure 5-6. Cross-sectional anatomy of the hand. The *arrows* show the planes of dissection for decompression of the compartments of the hand. (Courtesy of Dr. M. Stevanovic.)

POSTOPERATIVE

All surgical incisions are left open. We do not like the use of retention sutures in children because even if there is minimal swelling of the muscle(s) during the primary release, muscle swelling will usually increase after perfusion has improved. If nerves and arteries are not exposed, a negative pressure wound vacuum can be used. If nerves or arteries are exposed, we prefer to use a moist gauze dressing. Dressing changes should be done in the operating room at 24 to 48 hours. Partial delayed primary wound closure can be performed at that time if swelling is decreased and/or to provide coverage over open neurovascular structures. Definitive wound closure should be performed only after swelling has considerably decreased. In the hand, only the incision for the carpal tunnel release should be considered for delayed primary wound closure. The other palmar and dorsal

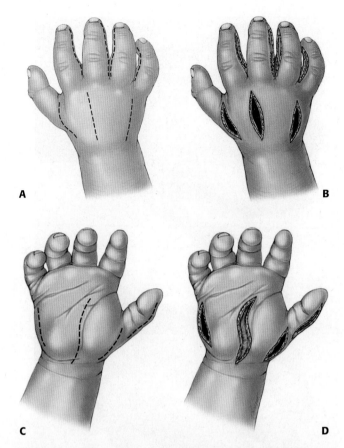

A

B

C

D

Figure 5-7. A, B: Dorsal incisions for fasciotomy of the hand and dermotomies of the fingers. **C, D:** Volar incisions for release of the thenar and hypothenar compartments, carpal tunnel release, and dermotomy of the thumb. (Courtesy of Dr. M. Stevanovic.)

TABLE 5-3. Compartments of the Thigh	
Compartment	Contents
Anterior	Quadriceps muscle Femoral artery, vein, and nerve
Medial	Adductor muscles Obturator nerve
Posterior	Hamstring muscles Sciatic nerve

with antishock trousers, and vascular injury with or without fracture of the femur. Children with femoral shaft fractures treated by skin or skeletal traction may also at risk for CS of the thigh.

Three compartments, anterior, medial, and posterior are described in the thigh (Table 5-3). A long single lateral incision on the thigh can adequately decompress the anterior and posterior compartments (Fig. 5-9). Occasionally, a medial adductor incision is required as well.[31]

LEG

The most common presentation of ACS in children involves the lower leg following a tibia and/or fibula fracture.[13,15] A retrospective review over 13 years identified 1,407 patients with tibial fractures. Of these patients, 160/1,407 (11%) developed CS. Youth was the strongest predictor of developing CS.[23] Treatment of tibial fractures with flexible nails has been shown to be associated with CS. Other risk factors include comminuted fractures, weight >50 kg or a neurologic deficit.[26] CS is also a well-known complication following tibial osteotomies for angular and/or rotational correction.

In the lower leg, a one- or two-incision technique can be employed for decompressive fasciotomy of all four compartments, including the anterior, lateral, superficial posterior, and deep posterior compartment (Table 5-4). In the two-incision technique (Fig. 5-10A), the anterolateral incision provides access to the anterior and lateral compartments. The posteromedial incision must be lengthy enough to allow for decompression of the superficial posterior compartment (more proximal) and deep posterior compartment (more distal). The soleus origin should be detached from the medial aspect of the tibia. All four compartments of the lower leg can also be adequately decompressed with a single-incision technique (Fig. 5-10B). The long lateral incision typically extends 3 to 5 cm within either end of the fibula. Identification of the septum between anterior and lateral compartments allows access to these compartments. Next, by elevating the lateral compartment musculature, the posterior intermuscular septum is visualized and access to the superficial and deep posterior compartments is possible.

FOOT

Foot CS in children is rare and usually caused by crush injuries, such as a car tire running over a foot. It is associated with Lisfranc

incisions as well as the dermotomy incisions will close quickly by secondary intention. If the skin cannot be closed without tension, then split-thickness skin grafting with or without dermal substitutes should be used.

Therapy should be started immediately postoperatively to maintain maximum active and passive range of motion of the fingers. Splinting should be done as long as needed for soft tissue stabilization or for treatment of other associated injuries. Therapy may need to be temporarily discontinued during healing of skin grafts, but should be resumed as soon as tissue healing allows. Once the soft tissues are adequately healed, we continue nighttime splinting to prevent contractures of the wrist and fingers. Splinting is continued until scars and soft tissues are mature and supple.

LOWER EXTREMITY

THIGH

CS involving the thigh is rare but has been reported in the pediatric population after blunt trauma, external compression

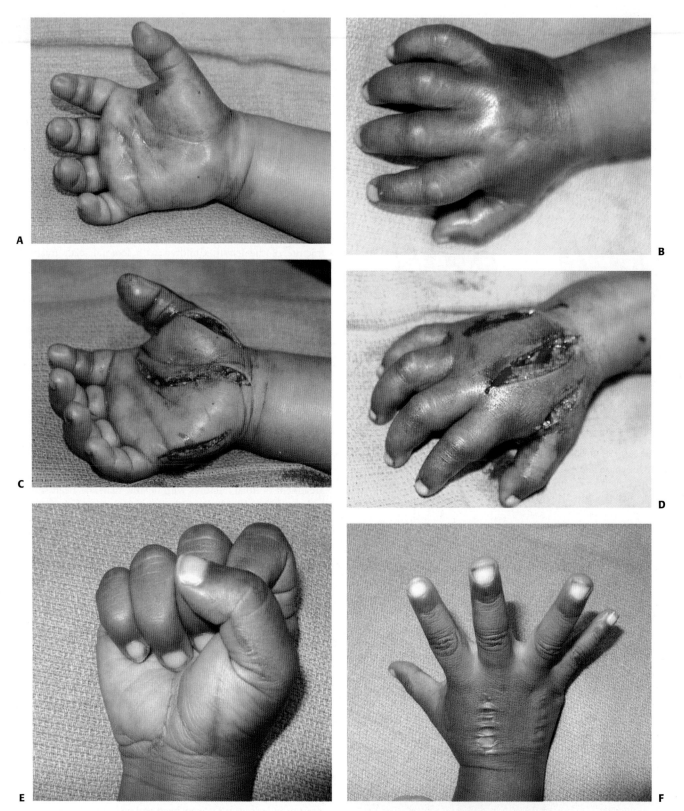

Figure 5-8. This 4-year-old girl placed a rubber band around her wrist before going to bed. She was brought to the emergency room the following morning because of swelling of her hand. She was taken immediately to the operating room for compartment release. **A:** Volar hand prior to fasciotomy. **B:** Dorsal hand prior to fasciotomy. **C:** Volar release. **D:** Dorsal release. **E:** Finger flexion at 6 months. **F:** Finger extension at 6 months. (Courtesy of Dr. M. Stevanovic.)

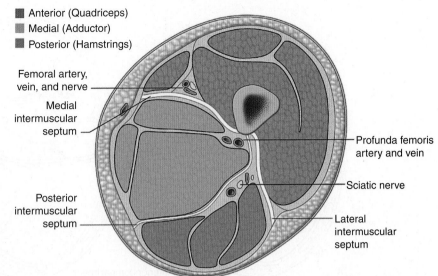

■ Anterior (Quadriceps)
■ Medial (Adductor)
■ Posterior (Hamstrings)

Femoral artery, vein, and nerve

Medial intermuscular septum

Posterior intermuscular septum

Profunda femoris artery and vein

Sciatic nerve

Lateral intermuscular septum

Figure 5-9. Cross-sectional anatomy of the thigh. Note the anterior (quadriceps), posterior (hamstrings), and medial (adductor) compartments. Entry sites for compartment pressure measurements should take into consideration the relationship between the intermuscular septa and the neurovascular structures of each compartment. (Modified with permission from Schwartz JT, Brumback RJ, Lakatos R, et al. Acute compartment syndrome of the thigh. A spectrum of injury. *J Bone Joint Surg Am.* 1989;71(3):392–400.)

fracture–dislocations and has been reported with fractures of the metatarsals and phalanges, but may occur in the absence of a fracture.[35] There are also reports of CS occurring following IV extravasation and with hemangioma of the foot.[10,16,39]

The foot has nine compartments, including the interosseous (4), adductor, central (2), medial, and lateral compartments. (Table 5-5). A dorsal approach through two longitudinal incisions centered over the second and fourth metatarsals may allow for adequate decompression of all nine compartments, though many authors recommend a third incision for the medial compartment (Fig. 5-11).

In a recent systematic review of pediatric foot CS spanning 12 years, 62 patients aged 7 months to 18 years with foot CS were reported on and all patients had fasciotomies.[44] There is a controversial trend toward not performing fasciotomies in adult foot CS because the main complication associated with untreated adult CS, that is, contractures leading to hammertoes, is viewed as less morbid than potential sequelae of performing fasciotomies. While this practice may apply to management of foot CS in skeletally mature adolescents, it may not be appropriate in children with significant growth remaining, as sustained compartment pressures may cause physeal arrest. Data toward this end are limited, although there are few reports of upper extremity CS causing growth arrest.[14] There are also case reports of fluid extravasation in the ankle causing growth arrest.[30,43] Authors speculate that this could be due to compression of the perichondrial vessels and damage to the perichondrium which leads to a bar formation, or from a physeal tether formed by scarring of soft tissue.[30] Premature physeal arrest has also been reported in the distal tibia in arterial insufficiency.[27] Given the limited data available, a low threshold for fasciotomies should be maintained especially in children with significant growth remaining, as long-term functional issues may develop if not treated.[44]

TABLE 5-4. Compartments of the Lower Leg

Compartment	Contents
Anterior	Tibialis anterior Extensor digitorum longus Extensor hallucis longus Peroneus tertius Deep peroneal (anterior tibial) vessels and nerve
Lateral	Peroneus longus Peroneus brevis Superficial peroneal nerve
Superficial posterior	Gastrocnemius Soleus Plantaris Sural nerve
Deep posterior	Tibialis posterior Flexor digitorum longus Flexor hallucis longus Posterior tibial nerve

TABLE 5-5. Compartments of the Foot

Compartments	Contents
Interosseous (4)	Interosseous muscles Digital nerves
Adductor	Adductor hallucis
Central (superficial)	Flexor digitorum brevis
Central (deep [or calcaneal])	Quadratus plantae
Medial	Abductor hallucis brevis Flexor hallucis brevis
Lateral	Flexor digiti minimi Abductor digiti minimi

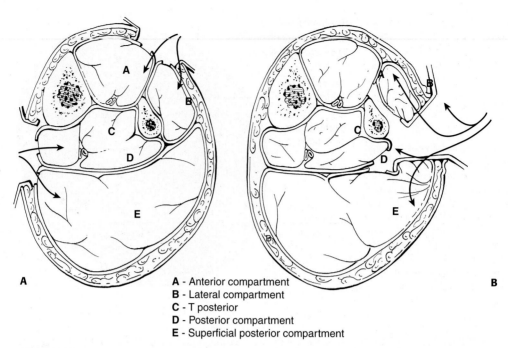

A - Anterior compartment
B - Lateral compartment
C - T posterior
D - Posterior compartment
E - Superficial posterior compartment

Figure 5-10. Decompressive fasciotomy of the lower leg. **A:** Two-incision approach. The anterolateral incision allows decompression of the anterior and lateral compartments. The medial incision allows decompression of the superficial posterior and the deep posterior compartments. The *arrows* are indicating the compartments that are released with each incision. **B:** One-incision approach. A single lateral incision allows decompression of all four compartments in the lower leg. (Courtesy of Paul Choi, MD.)

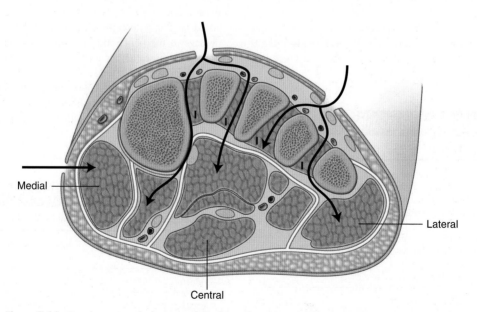

Figure 5-11. Decompressive fasciotomy of the foot. Through a dorsal approach, two longitudinal skin incisions over the second and fourth metatarsals can be utilized to decompress all nine compartments of the foot. The superficial fascia is divided over each interspace to decompress the interosseous (*I*) compartments (×4) (caution: Interosseous veins and the distal dorsalis pedis arterial branches in the first interspace). Next, the adductor, central (superficial and deep), medial, and lateral compartments are decompressed through each interspace. Many authors, however, recommend a third medial incision to decompress the medial/calcaneal compartment.

ESTABLISHED CONTRACTURE (VOLKMANN'S CONTRACTURE)

Volkmann's Ischemic Contracture: Volkmann's ischemic contracture is the end result of prolonged ischemia with irreversible tissue necrosis. The most commonly used classification system is that of Tsuge,[41] who classified Volkmann's contracture into mild, moderate, and severe types, according to the extent of the muscle involvement.

The *mild type,* also described as the localized type, involves the muscles of the deep flexor compartment of the forearm. It can involve all the flexor digitorum profundus and the flexor pollicis longus, although usually only involves the flexor digitorum profundus of the ring or middle fingers. Nerve involvement is absent or mild, typically involving sensory changes that resolve spontaneously. With wrist flexion, the fingers can be fully extended. The majority of the mild type resulted from direct trauma either from crush injury or forearm fractures, and was typically seen in young adults.

In the *moderate type,* muscle degeneration includes most or all of the flexor digitorum profundus and flexor pollicis longus with partial degeneration of the flexor superficialis muscles. Neurologic impairment is always present. Sensory impairment is generally more severe in the median than in the ulnar nerve, and the hand demonstrates an intrinsic minus posture. Moderate-type Volkmann's contracture was most commonly the result of SCH fractures in children between ages 5 and 10.

The *severe type* involves degeneration of all the flexor muscles of the fingers and of the wrist. There is central muscle necrosis, and varying involvement of the extensor compartment. Neurologic deficits are severe, including complete palsy of all the intrinsic muscles of the hand. Hallmarks of the severe type include fixed joint contractures, scarred soft tissue, or previously failed surgeries. As with the moderate cases, the severe cases were most commonly the result of SCH fractures in children.[41]

Treatment of established Volkmann's contracture depends on the severity of the contracture and neurologic deficits and the resultant functional losses.

Nonoperative management should be instituted early in most cases of established Volkmann's contracture. In children, there may be more recovery of nerve and muscle function over time than in adults, so we do not advocate immediate surgical intervention. A formal program of splinting and therapy can improve the outcome of later surgical intervention and may result in less extensive surgical corrections. Therapy should be directed toward maintenance of passive joint motion, preservation and strengthening of remaining muscle function, and correction of deformity through a program of splinting. We prefer the use of static progressive splinting or serial casting for fixed contractures of the wrist, fingers, and thumb web space. Mild contractures with minimal to no nerve involvement can often be treated only with a comprehensive program of hand therapy and rehabilitation. For moderate to severe involvement where surgery is anticipated, therapy is indicated only as long as necessary to achieve supple passive motion of the fingers. Preoperative therapy is also helpful in establishing a good patient and

parent rapport with the therapist and in gaining an understanding of the postsurgical therapy program.

A variety of surgical procedures have been used to treat Volkmann's ischemic contracture. These have included bony and soft tissue management. Surgical treatment should not be undertaken before soft tissue equilibrium is present. We do not recommend a shortening osteotomy of the radius and ulna and proximal row carpectomy to match the skeletal length to the shortened fibrotic muscle because the bones are already relatively shortened by the initial ischemic insult to the growth plates. Further, the principal contracture is usually on the flexor surface. Shortening the forearm indiscriminately lengthens the muscle resting length of both the flexor and extensor muscles, neglecting the predominant involvement of the contracture within the flexor compartment. Bony reconstructive procedures for long-standing contractures or for distal reconstruction required for neurologic injury include wrist fusion, trapeziometacarpal joint fusion, or thumb metacarpophalangeal joint fusion, which should be done after skeletal maturity. These may be considered in conjunction with some of the soft tissue procedures listed below.

Soft tissue procedures have included excision of the infarcted muscle, fractional or z-lengthening of the affected muscles, muscle sliding operations (flexor origin muscle slide), neurolysis, tendon transfers, and functional free tissue transfers, as well as combinations of the above procedures. Excision of scarred fibrotic nerves without distal function followed by nerve grafting has been described to try and establish some protective sensation in the hand. Fixed contractures of the joints can be addressed with soft tissue release including capsulectomy and collateral ligament recession or excision depending on the joints involved.

OUTCOMES

Full functional recovery within 6 months has been reported with timely management of CS in the pediatric population.[2] Late diagnosis of CS may increase the risk of severe complications, including infection, neurologic injury, need for amputation, and death. The duration of elevated tissue pressures before definitive surgical decompression may be the most important factor in determining outcome. In adults, prolonged ischemic insult to compartment musculature greater than 8 hours increases the risk of permanent sequelae.[13] Some studies have shown that after traumatic upper extremity injury in pediatric patients, delayed presentation and decompression of forearm CS after 48 hours results in significant morbidity, and can result in forearm muscle necrosis necessitating reconstructive surgery with a free gracilis muscle flap or long-term casting for long flexor tightness.[47] Despite this, many studies show good outcomes even with delayed diagnosis of CS, and authors postulate that the potential for recovery of muscle function may be greater in a child than in an adult. This is consistent with the increased potential for recovery observed from other types of injuries in children, such as fractures, traumatic brain injuries, and articular cartilage injuries.[9] Full recovery has been reported following CS of the lower leg in children even after delayed presentation.[9] Good results may be possible in children even when fasciotomy is performed as late as 72 hours after the injury.[13] A multicenter study spanning 15 years showed that CS in infants and toddlers is often delayed greater than 24 hours. Interestingly, even when fasciotomy is delayed by 48 to 72 hours, functional outcomes are excellent in most patients.[6]

Children may have a delayed *development* rather than delayed *diagnosis* of CS after the initial injury. Clinicians may diagnose and treat this late-developing CS acutely, which may result in good outcomes noted in studies. This is why it is imperative to continuously monitor children at risk for developing ACS. If muscle ischemia persists for longer than 6 to 8 hours, children are at risk for functional muscle loss, contracture, neurologic deficit (both motor and sensory distal to the level of injury), cosmetic deformity, growth arrest, and infection. Less commonly, loss of limb, rhabdomyolysis, multiorgan system failure, and death can be seen, especially in the setting of crush injury with severe large-volume muscle necrosis.

Delayed or missed diagnosis of CS is one of the most common causes of successful litigation against medical professionals in North America.[3] Of 66 closed cases involving CS, 48/66 (73%) were ruled in favor of the patient, with an average payment of $574,680.[21]

Patients who develop Volkmann's contracture of the upper extremity during childhood may have a permanently shortened extremity thereafter. After limb ischemia, muscles are generally more affected than bone, and thus muscles grow at a slower rate than the bone, which may lead to relative tightening of the muscles. Splinting the extremity in the functional position until age 18 may help combat contractures. Substantial improvements in hand function are noted in patients who undergo functional free muscle transfer. Tendon lengthening alone often results in recurrence of contracture. Finally, in patients who have sufficient remaining muscle, procedures which combine infarct excision, tenolysis, neurolysis, and tendon transfer when necessary produce good hand function.[42] Improvement in sensory function in conjunction with neurolysis has been noted.[38] In our experience, mild and moderate contractures can have significant functional improvement following flexor muscle slide and nerve reconstruction when indicated. Normal function is not anticipated, but a hand with protective sensation and functional grasp can often be achieved. Functional free muscle transfers can also restore gross grasp and have a much better outcome in patients with good intrinsic function.

Annotated References

Reference	Annotation
Bae DS, Kadiyala RK, Waters PM. Acute compartment syndrome in children: contemporary diagnosis, treatment, and outcome. *J Pediatr Orthop.* 2001;21(5):680–688.	This article examines 36 cases of compartment syndrome in children over 6 years at one institution. In this cohort, 75% of children who developed compartment syndrome had fractures. The authors demonstrated that previously used indicators of compartment syndrome such as pain, pallor, parasthesias, etc., were not reliable. Increasing analgesia requirement was a more reliable predictor of compartment syndrome in the children studied.
Broom A, Schur MD, Arkader A, et al. Compartment syndrome in infants and toddlers. *J Child Orthop.* 2016;10(5):453–460.	This article distinguishes the diagnosis of compartment syndrome in infants and toddlers from compartment syndrome in older children. Fifteen infants and toddlers who developed compartment syndrome were studied. In infants and toddlers, diagnosis was delayed compared to older children (>24 hours after injury), but regardless, outcomes were generally good even when fasciotomy was not performed for 48–72 hours after injury.
Flynn JM, Bashyal RK, Yeger-McKeever M, et al. Acute traumatic compartment syndrome of the leg in children: diagnosis and outcome. *J Bone Joint Surg Am.* 2011;93(10):937–941.	This article examines 43 cases of compartment syndrome of the leg in children. These children had an overall delay in the time between injury and fasciotomy. The authors raise awareness for late presentation and late development of compartment syndrome of the leg in children, and encourage monitoring of compartments in the days following injury.
Kalyani BS, Fisher BE, Roberts CS, et al. Compartment syndrome of the forearm: a systematic review. *J Hand Surg Am.* 2011;36(3):535–543.	This is a systematic review evaluating evidence on compartment syndrome of the forearm in children. This review provides information on the causes, diagnosis, treatment, and outcomes of compartment syndrome in the forearm of children.

REFERENCES

1. Badhe S, Baiju D, Elliot R, et al. The 'silent' compartment syndrome. *Injury.* 2009; 40(2):220–222.
2. Bae DS, Kadiyala RK, Waters PM. Acute compartment syndrome in children: contemporary diagnosis, treatment, and outcome. *J Pediatr Orthop.* 2001;21(5):680–688.
3. Bhattacharyya T, Vrahas MS. The medical-legal aspects of compartment syndrome. *J Bone Joint Surg Am.* 2004;86-A(4):864–868.
4. Blackman AJ, Wall LB, Keeler KA, et al. Acute compartment syndrome after intramedullary nailing of isolated radius and ulna fractures in children. *J Pediatr Orthop.* 2014;34(1):50–54.
5. Blakemore LC, Cooperman DR, Thompson GH, et al. Compartment syndrome in ipsilateral humerus and forearm fractures in children. *Clin Orthop Relat Res.* 2000;(376):32–38.
6. Broom A, Schur MD, Arkader A, et al. Compartment syndrome in infants and toddlers. *J Child Orthop.* 2016;10(5):453–460.
7. Cathcart CC, Shuler MS, Freedman BA, et al. Correlation of near-infrared spectroscopy and direct pressure monitoring in an acute porcine compartmental syndrome model. *J Orthop Trauma.* 2014;28(6):365–369.
8. Challa ST, Hargens AR, Uzosike A, et al. Muscle microvascular blood flow, oxygenation, ph, and perfusion pressure decrease in simulated acute compartment syndrome. *J Bone Joint Surg Am.* 2017;99(17):1453–1459.

9. Choi PD, Rose RK, Kay RM, et al. Compartment syndrome of the thigh in an infant: a case report. *J Orthop Trauma.* 2007;21(8):587–590.
10. Downey-Carmona FJ, Gonzalez-Herranz P, De La Fuente-Gonzalez C, et al. Acute compartment syndrome of the foot caused by a hemangioma. *J Foot Ankle Surg.* 2006;45(1):52–55.
11. Driscoll EB, Maleki AH, Jahromi L, et al. Regional anesthesia or patient-controlled analgesia and compartment syndrome in orthopedic surgical procedures: a systematic review. *Local Reg Anesth.* 2016;9:65–81.
12. Erdos J, Dlaska C, Szatmary P, et al. Acute compartment syndrome in children: a case series in 24 patients and review of the literature. *Int Orthop.* 2011;35(4):569–575.
13. Flynn JM, Bashyal RK, Yeger-McKeever M, et al. Acute traumatic compartment syndrome of the leg in children: diagnosis and outcome. *J Bone Joint Surg Am.* 2011;93(10):937–941.
14. Gauger EM, Casnovsky LL, Gauger EJ, et al. Acquired upper extremity growth arrest. *Orthopedics.* 2017;40(1):e95–e103.
15. Grottkau BE, Epps HR, Di Scala C. Compartment syndrome in children and adolescents. *J Pediatr Surg.* 2005;40(4):678–682.
16. Handler EG. Superficial compartment syndrome of the foot after infiltration of intravenous fluid. *Arch Phys Med Rehabil.* 1990;71(1):58–59.
17. Hope MJ, McQueen MM. Acute compartment syndrome in the absence of fracture. *J Orthop Trauma.* 2004;18(4):220–224.
18. Kalyani BS, Fisher BE, Roberts CS, et al. Compartment syndrome of the forearm: a systematic review. *J Hand Surg Am.* 2011;36(3):535–543.
19. Kucera TJ, Boezaart AP. Regional anesthesia does not consistently block ischemic pain: two further cases and a review of the literature. *Pain Med.* 2014;15(2):316–319.
20. Livingston K, Glotzbecker M, Miller PE, et al. Pediatric nonfracture acute compartment syndrome: a review of 39 cases. *J Pediatr Orthop.* 2016;36(7):685–690.
21. Marchesi M, Marchesi A, Calori GM, et al. A sneaky surgical emergency: acute compartment syndrome: retrospective analysis of 66 closed claims, medico-legal pitfalls and damages evaluation. *Injury.* 2014;45(Suppl 6):S16–S20.
22. Martus JE, Preston RK, Schoenecker JG, et al. Complications and outcomes of diaphyseal forearm fracture intramedullary nailing: a comparison of pediatric and adolescent age groups. *J Pediatr Orthop.* 2013;33(6):598–607.
23. McQueen MM, Duckworth AD, Aitken SA, et al. Predictors of compartment syndrome after tibial fracture. *J Orthop Trauma.* 2015;29(10):451–455.
24. Mubarak SJ, Carroll NC. Volkmann's contracture in children: aetiology and prevention. *J Bone Joint Surg Br.* 1979;61-B(3):285–293.
25. Olson SA, Glasgow RR. Acute compartment syndrome in lower extremity musculoskeletal trauma. *J Am Acad Orthop Surg.* 2005;13(7):436–444.
26. Pandya NK, Edmonds EW, Mubarak SJ. The incidence of compartment syndrome after flexible nailing of pediatric tibial shaft fractures. *J Child Orthop.* 2011;5(6):439–447.
27. Peterson HA. Premature physeal arrest of the distal tibia associated with temporary arterial insufficiency. *J Pediatr Orthop.* 1993;13(5):672–675.
28. Ragland R III, Moukoko D, Ezaki M, et al. Forearm compartment syndrome in the newborn: report of 24 cases. *J Hand Surg Am.* 2005;30(5):997–1003.
29. Ronel DN, Mtui E, Nolan WB III. Forearm compartment syndrome: anatomical analysis of surgical approaches to the deep space. *Plast Reconstr Surg.* 2004;114(3):697–705.
30. Sanpera I Jr, Fixsen JA, Hill RA. Injuries to the physis by extravasation: a rare cause of growth plate arrest. *J Bone Joint Surg Br.* 1994;76(2):278–280.
31. Schwartz JT Jr, Brumback RJ, Lakatos R, et al. Acute compartment syndrome of the thigh. A spectrum of injury. *J Bone Joint Surg Am.* 1989;71(3):392–400.
32. Seal A, Stevanovic M. Free functional muscle transfer for the upper extremity. *Clin Plast Surg.* 2011;38(4):561–575.
33. Sharpe MSaF. Compartment syndrome and Volkmann ischemic contracture. In: Wolfe S, Hotchkiss RN, Kozin SH, et al., eds. *Green's Operative Hand Surgery.* 7th ed. Philadelphia, PA: Elsevier Health; 2016:1708–1787.
34. Shuler MS, Reisman WM, Kinsey TL, et al. Correlation between muscle oxygenation and compartment pressures in acute compartment syndrome of the leg. *J Bone Joint Surg Am.* 2010;92(4):863–870.
35. Silas SI, Herzenberg JE, Myerson MS, et al. Compartment syndrome of the foot in children. *J Bone Joint Surg Am.* 1995;77(3):356–361.
36. Staudt JM, Smeulders MJ, van der Horst CM. Normal compartment pressures of the lower leg in children. *J Bone Joint Surg Br.* 2008;90(2):215–219.
37. Stevanovic M, Sharpe F. Management of established Volkmann's contracture of the forearm in children. *Hand Clin.* 2006;22(1):99–111.
38. Sundararaj GD, Mani K. Pattern of contracture and recovery following ischaemia of the upper limb. *J Hand Surg Br.* 1985;10(2):155–161.
39. Talbot SG, Rogers GF. Pediatric compartment syndrome caused by intravenous infiltration. *Ann Plast Surg.* 2011;67(5):531–533.
40. Tharakan SJ, Subotic U, Kalisch M, et al. Compartment pressures in children with normal and fractured forearms: a preliminary report. *J Pediatr Orthop.* 2016;36(4):410–415.
41. Tsuge K. Treatment of established Volkmann's contracture. *J Bone Joint Surg Am.* 1975;57(7):925–929.
42. Ultee J, Hovius SE. Functional results after treatment of Volkmann's ischemic contracture: a long-term followup study. *Clin Orthop Relat Res.* 2005;(431):42–49.
43. Wada A, Fujii T, Takamura K, et al. Physeal arrest of the ankle secondary to extravasation in a neonate and its treatment by the Gruca operation: a modern application of an old technique. *J Pediatr Orthop B.* 2003;12(2):129–132.
44. Wallin K, Nguyen H, Russell L, et al. Acute traumatic compartment syndrome in pediatric foot: a systematic review and case report. *J Foot Ankle Surg.* 2016;55(4):817–820.
45. Wilder RP, Magrum E. Exertional compartment syndrome. *Clin Sports Med.* 2010;29(3):429–435.
46. Yuan PS, Pring ME, Gaynor TP, et al. Compartment syndrome following intramedullary fixation of pediatric forearm fractures. *J Pediatr Orthop.* 2004;24(4):370–375.
47. Ziolkowski NI, Zive L, Ho ES, et al. Timing of presentation of pediatric compartment syndrome and its microsurgical implication: a retrospective review. *Plast Reconstr Surg.* 2017;139(3):663–670.

6

Pathologic Fractures and Nonaccidental Injuries

Alexandre Arkader and Richard M. Schwend

PATHOLOGIC FRACTURES

The definition of a pathologic fracture is one that occurs through abnormal bone. Pathologic fractures may result from a localized or generalized bone weakness, either from an intrinsic or extrinsic process, such as tumor or tumor-like lesions, osteopenia or osteoporosis of different etiologies.

The evaluation of a child with a pathologic fracture includes detailed history, physical examination, and imaging. The past medical history, use of medications, and prodromal symptoms, such as pain, may lead to the diagnosis. Radiographic evaluation helps in differentiating between a localized and a generalized process. If a bone lesion is identified, it is important to determine the nature of the lesion and level of aggressiveness.

An important concept is that the fracture is a result of the underlying cause for bone weakness; therefore, any attempt in "fixing" the fracture needs to be carried with adequate assessment and management of the underlying pathology. For that reason, at times the management of the fracture deviates from the classic principles of pediatric fractures treatment. The understanding of the natural history and prognosis related to the primary diagnosis will help guide treatment and anticipate outcomes, while preventing further complications. In the absence of an obvious diagnosis, temporizing methods, such as cast, brace, traction, are highly recommended to avoid burning bridges and complicating the management of the underlying condition. Below we will discuss the most common causes of pathologic fractures in children and highlight some of the issues associated with the treatment of this diagnosis.

TUMORS OR TUMOR-LIKE PROCESSES

UNICAMERAL BONE CYST

Unicameral bone cyst (UBC) is a benign, active, or latent solitary cystic lesion that involves the metaphysis or metadiaphysis of long bones.[20] The most common locations include the proximal humerus, proximal femur, and proximal tibia.[173] Although the etiology is unknown, it is thought that UBC is caused by an obstruction of the interstitial fluid drainage.[61]

Patients are usually in the first two decades, with male-to-female ratio of 2:1. UBCs are often asymptomatic and in approximately 80% of cases, the initial presentation is with a pathologic fracture.[47,72,242] The fractures are usually incomplete or minimally displaced, and tend to heal uneventfully, with an approximately 10% chance of cyst healing (partial or complete) (Fig. 6-1).[9] However, complications such as malunion, growth arrest, and avascular necrosis have been reported.[119,217]

On imaging, UBCs are a well-defined, centrally located, radiolucent/lytic cystic lesion. Cortical thinning and mild expansion are common. When a pathologic fracture occurs, there is periosteal reaction and the typical "fallen fragment" sign may be visualized (fragment of bone "floating" inside the fluid-filled cavity). Advanced imaging may be useful for lesions located in areas that are of difficult visualization (e.g., spine,

pelvis), to rule out minimally displaced fractures, evaluate adjacent physis, or differential diagnosis (e.g., aneurysmal bone cyst [ABC], fibrous dysplasia [FD], nonossifying fibroma [NOF], Fig. 6-2).

Most pathologic fractures through UBC, especially of upper extremities, should be treated conservatively. The main reasons are to allow possible spontaneous healing and because it is easier to treat a stable bone rather than two moving parts. While minimally or nondisplaced fractures of lower extremities can also be treated conservatively, displaced fractures or fractures around the hip often need surgical intervention and internal fixation. Large lesions involving more than 50% to 80% of the bone diameter, associated with cortical thinning, are at a high risk of fracture and may warrant prophylactic treatment (Figs. 6-3 and 6-4).[105] A CT model using a computerized regression system has been shown to predict the likelihood of fracture.[151]

There have been several described treatment strategies for UBCs (a detailed discussion of all available techniques is beyond the scope of this chapter). Our preferred approach when surgery is indicated is via a formal open curettage and bone grafting or utilizing a minimally invasive technique for decompression, curettage, and grafting (surgical technique below)[72,168]; complete cyst healing can be achieved in over 80% of the cases after one treatment.

SURGICAL TECHNIQUE

✔ Surgical Technique

- ☐ Under fluoroscopic guidance, a Jamshidi trocar needle (Cardinal Health, Dublin, OH) is percutaneously inserted into the cyst cavity, preferably in the middle of the cyst.
- ☐ The cyst is aspirated to confirm the presence of straw-colored fluid.
- ☐ Three to 10 mL of 50% diluted Renografin dye (E.R. Squibb, Princeton, NJ) is injected to perform a cystogram and confirm the single fluid-filled cavity.
- ☐ A 0.5-cm longitudinal incision is then made over the site of the aspiration and a 6-mm arthroscopy trocar is advanced into the cyst cavity through the same cortical hole. The cortical entry is then enlarged manually.
- ☐ Under fluoroscopic guidance, percutaneous removal of the cyst lining is done with curved curettes and a pituitary rongeur.
- ☐ An angled curette and/or flexible intramedullary nail is used to perform the intramedullary decompression in one direction (toward diaphysis) or in both directions (if the growth plate is far enough to avoid injury).
- ☐ Bone grafting is done with medical-grade calcium sulfate pellets (Osteoset, Wright Medical Technology, Arlington, TN) inserted through the same cortical hole and deployed to completely fill the cavity. The pellets do not offer structural support but act as scaffolding for new bone formation and cyst healing. Angled curettes can be used to advance pellets into the medullary canal, which also confirms adequate decompression. Tight packing of the cyst is preferred.
- ☐ The wound is closed in a layered fashion.

ANEURYSMAL BONE CYST

ABC is a benign but locally aggressive lesion, with an estimated incidence of approximately 1.4 cases per 100,000. The

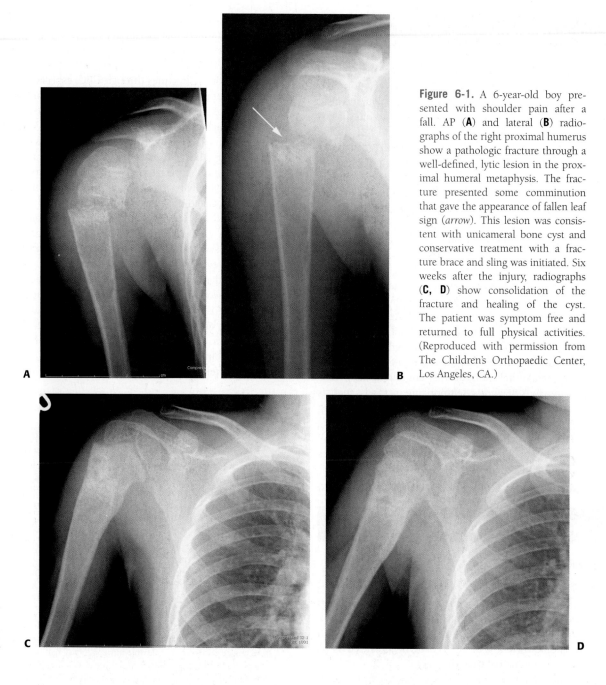

Figure 6-1. A 6-year-old boy presented with shoulder pain after a fall. AP (**A**) and lateral (**B**) radiographs of the right proximal humerus show a pathologic fracture through a well-defined, lytic lesion in the proximal humeral metaphysis. The fracture presented some comminution that gave the appearance of fallen leaf sign (*arrow*). This lesion was consistent with unicameral bone cyst and conservative treatment with a fracture brace and sling was initiated. Six weeks after the injury, radiographs (**C, D**) show consolidation of the fracture and healing of the cyst. The patient was symptom free and returned to full physical activities. (Reproduced with permission from The Children's Orthopaedic Center, Los Angeles, CA.)

neoplastic basis of primary ABCs has been in part demonstrated by the chromosomal translocation t(16;17)(q22; p13).[183]

These are well-defined, eccentric, expansile (often beyond adjacent growth plate), osteolytic, blood-filled lesions, most often seen in the metaphyseal region of long bones (~65%), especially the femur, tibia and humerus, and the spine (~25%), in particular in the posterior elements.[46,64] Approximately, a third of ABCs are associated with other benign and/or malignant tumors.

Pathologic fractures occur at a lower frequency than with UBC (11% to 35% of long-bone lesions; less than 20% of spinal lesions) and most lesions present with localized pain and/or swelling; spinal lesions may also present with radicular symptoms.[40,46,88,91,146] The humerus and femur are the most common

sites of pathologic fracture (Fig. 6-5).[88,145] MRI is helpful especially for axial lesions and demonstrates the characteristic double-density fluid level, septation, low signal on T1 images, and high intensity on T2 images.[224]

While conservative treatment of the fracture may be indicated, these lesions don't spontaneously heal and delayed surgical intervention is needed. Recurrence rates following intralesional curettage and bone grafting can be as high as 30%.[94] Several authors have shown that the recurrence is higher among younger children.[26,62,88] Serial embolization treatment utilizing n-butyl cyanoacrylate, concentrated bone marrow, doxyciclin, or others, has shown adequate results.[23,227] A four-step approach resection has been previously described with reported recurrence rate for appendicular lesions around

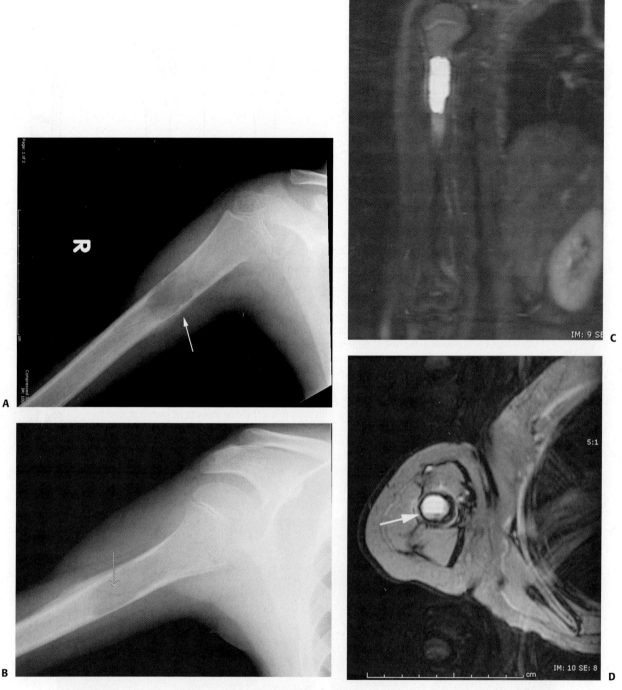

Figure 6-2. A 10-year-old boy presented with arm pain after low-energy trauma, 5 days prior. Antero-posterior (**A**) and lateral (**B**) radiographs of the right humerus show a nondisplaced pathologic fracture (*arrow* in **A**) through a lytic lesion in the proximal humerus. The lesion is difficult to visualize and the periosteal reaction is also of concern (*arrow* in **B**). T2-weighted coronal (**C**) and axial (**D**) MRI images show a well-defined, fluid-filled cystic lesion, with fluid–fluid levels (*arrow* in **D**) and no soft tissue mass or other worrisome signs cuts. The diagnosis was consistent with unicameral bone cyst and conservative treatment was recommended. (Reproduced with permission from The Children's Orthopaedic Center, Los Angeles, CA.)

Immature   **Mature**

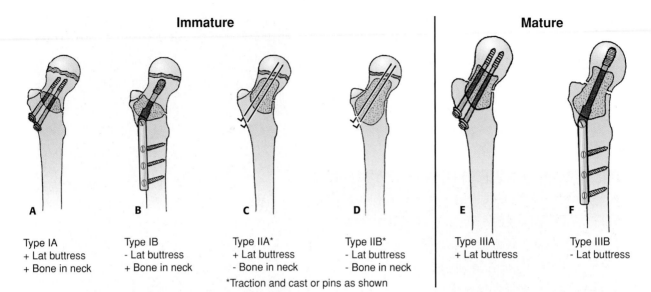

Type IA
+ Lat buttress
+ Bone in neck

Type IB
- Lat buttress
+ Bone in neck

Type IIA*
+ Lat buttress
- Bone in neck

Type IIB*
- Lat buttress
- Bone in neck

Type IIIA
+ Lat buttress

Type IIIB
- Lat buttress

*Traction and cast or pins as shown

For all: Curettage (with biopsy) and bone grafting with stabilization (as shown above) and spica cast

Figure 6-3. Classification system for the treatment of pathologic fractures of the proximal femur associated with bone cysts in children. **A:** In type IA, a moderately sized cyst is present in the middle of the femoral neck. There is enough bone in the femoral neck and lateral proximal femur (lateral buttress) to allow fixation with cannulated screws, avoiding the physis, after curettage and bone grafting. **B:** In type IB, a large cyst is present at the base of the femoral neck. There is enough bone proximally in the femoral neck but there is loss of lateral buttress, so a pediatric hip screw and a side plate should be considered rather than cannulated screws after curettage and bone grafting. **C, D:** In type IIA–B, a large lesion is present in the femoral neck, so there is not enough bone beneath the physis to accept screws. There are two options for treatment of these bone cysts: (1) after curettage and bone grafting, parallel smooth pins across the physis can be used in combination with spica cast; (2) the patient can be treated in traction until the fracture heals (with subsequent spica cast), followed by curettage and bone grafting. **E, F:** In type IIIA–B, the physis is closing or closed. The lateral buttress is present in type IIIA hips, so cannulated screws can be used to stabilize the fracture after curettage and bone grafting. In type IIIB hips, the loss of lateral buttress makes it necessary to use a pediatric hip screw and a side plate following curettage and bone grafting. In all types, we recommend spica cast immobilization after surgery.

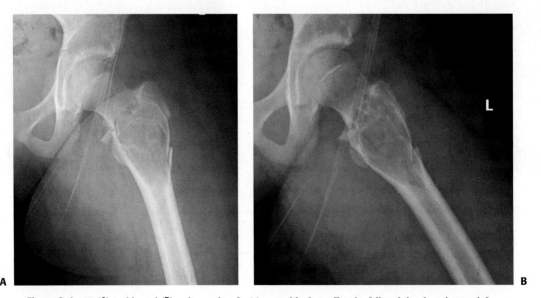

Figure 6-4. AP (**A**) and lateral (**B**) radiographs of a 12 year old who suffered a fall and developed acute left hip pain and inability to ambulate. There is a pathologic fracture through a well-defined, lytic, and loculated lesion in the proximal femur, with cortical thinning, no soft tissue mass or periosteal reaction. The patient underwent biopsy confirming the diagnosis of aneurysmal bone cyst, followed by curettage and allografting, supplemented by internal fixation with a variable hip screw and a cannulated antirotational screw (**C, D**).

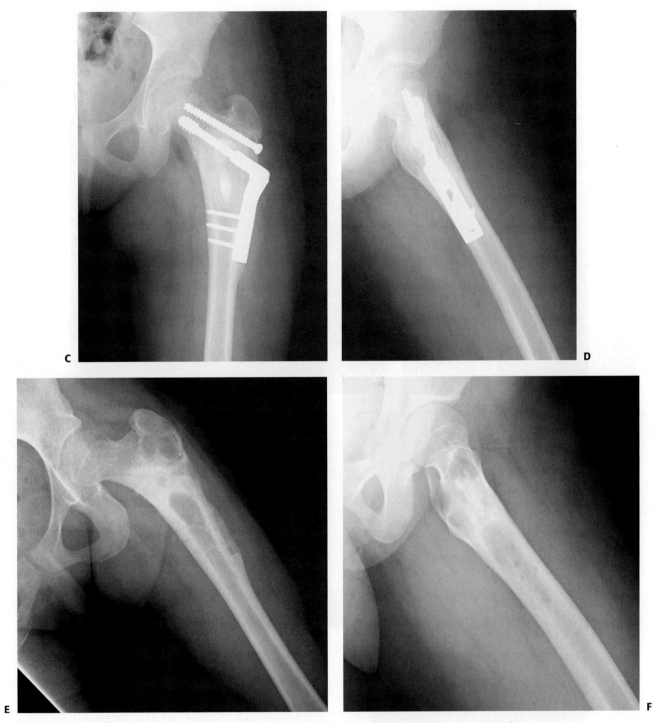

Figure 6-4. (*Continued*) The 4-year follow-up, short after hardware removal, shows no signs of recurrence or persistence of the lesion (**E, F**). AP and lateral views show no evidence of recurrence. (Figures reproduced with permission from The Children's Orthopaedic Center, Los Angeles, CA.)

8%. We recommend the use of headlamps for enhanced illumination and loupes for magnification. An image intensifier is available for intraoperative confirmation of complete tumor excision and appropriate bone grafting. Diagnostic tissue confirmation is an essential part of this technique. For large spinal tumors, preoperative embolization may be recommended (Fig. 6-6). If instrumentation is needed after spine tumor resection, we recommend titanium or cobalt chrome instrumentation that gives a much better visualization of the spine on future MRIs (less artifact) than stainless steel (Fig. 6-7).

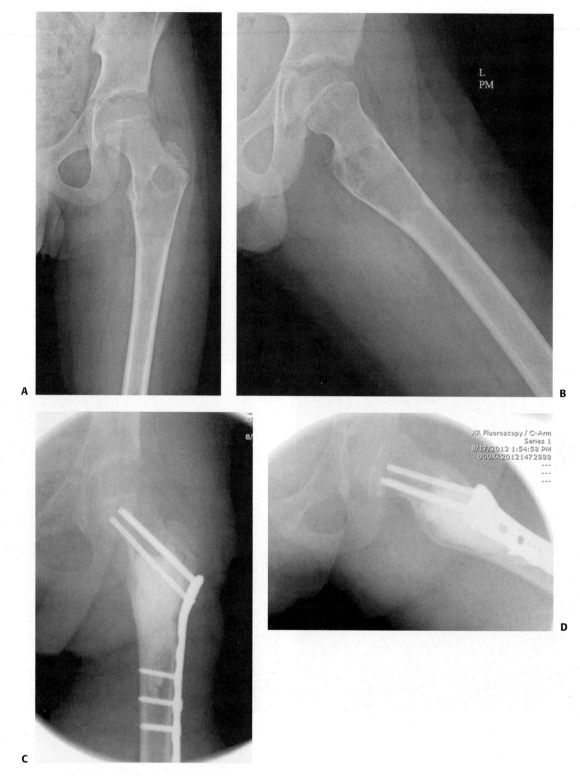

Figure 6-5. AP (**A**) and lateral (**B**) radiographs of a 10 year old who came in with chronic hip pain of several weeks duration. There is a well-defined, lytic lesion in the proximal femur, presenting with cortical thinning and some periosteal reaction, suggesting a healing stress pathologic fracture through a unicameral bone cyst. The patient underwent biopsy to confirm the diagnosis, followed by curettage and bone grafting, supplemented by internal fixation to improve the lateral buttress (**C, D**). (Reproduced with permission from The Children's Orthopaedic Center, Los Angeles, CA.)

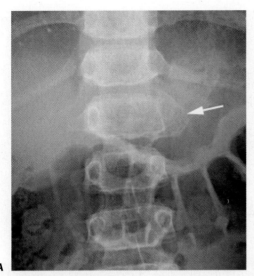

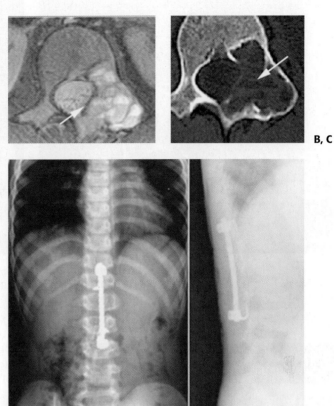

Figure 6-6. A 9-year-old boy presented with low back pain and abdominal discomfort. **A:** On plain radiographs of the abdomen, an expansile lesion (*arrow*) involving the left posterior elements of L1 was visualized. Axial T2-weighted MRI (**B**) and an axial CT scan (**C**) show the microfractures at the pedicle and lamina level (*arrow*) and the fluid–fluid levels. The patient underwent open biopsy that confirmed the diagnosis of aneurysmal bone cyst, followed by a four-step approach excision and bone grafting. **D:** Limited instrumentation of the spine was performed because of stability compromise. Nowadays, the author's preferred technique is pedicle screw fixation and fusion one level above and below the involved vertebra.

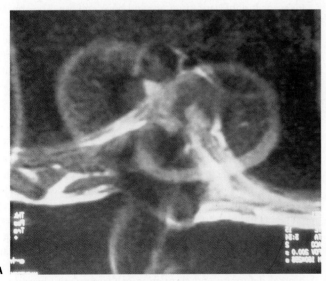

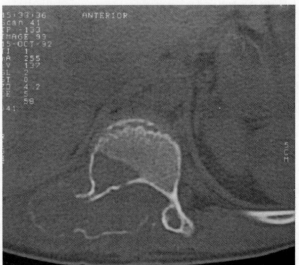

Figure 6-7. When dealing with pathologic fractures secondary to tumors or tumor-like processes of the spine, if instrumentation is needed, titanium instrumentation allows much better postoperative visualization with both CT and MRI for the detection of tumor recurrence as compared with standard stainless-steel instrumentation. **A:** Postoperative MRI of the spine with standard stainless-steel instrumentation showing a large degree of artifact that makes interpretation difficult. **B:** Preoperative CT scan of a patient with an ABC of the spine.

(continues)

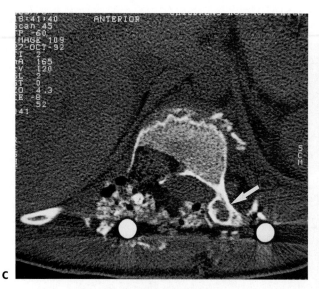
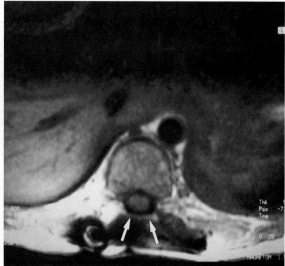

Figure 6-7. (*Continued*) **C:** Postoperative CT scan of the same patient showing an adequate view of the surgical area. **D:** Postoperative MRI of a patient with a previous spinal tumor again adequately showing the surgical site to monitor for recurrence or persistent tumor.

✔ Four-Step Approach Resection:
KEY SURGICAL STEPS

- ☐ Small incision over the cyst, respecting oncologic principles
- ☐ Lesional tissue is then retrieved and sent for frozen section for diagnostic confirmation; be prepared for possible excessive bleeding once cavity is opened
- ☐ A cortical window is enlarged to allow appropriate visualization and intralesional resection/curettage
- ☐ A high-speed burr is used, when possible, to extend the intralesional margins
- ☐ Electrocautery is used to help identify residual tumor pockets, to potentially kill residual tumor cells, and to coagulate the bleeding bone surface
- ☐ Adjuvants such as phenol solution 5%, or liquid nitrogen may be used
- ☐ Bone grafting is done with either a synthetic bone substitute or allograft
- ☐ Internal fixation is indicated on case-by-case basis; lesions of weight-bearing bones, particularly of the proximal femur, and some large vertebral lesions may warrant internal fixation/instrumentation

FIBROUS CORTICAL DEFECTS AND NONOSSIFYING FIBROMAS

Fibrous cortical defects (FCDs) and NOFs are the most common bone tumor or tumor-like condition seen in the growing child, with an estimated incidence of 20%. Most of these lesions are asymptomatic and incidentally found. Pathologic fractures may occur, especially through lesions involving more than 50% of the transverse cortical diameter, in boys between 6 and 14 years old, and with lower extremity lesions.[177]

These lesions present as a well-defined, cortical–based, lytic lesion in the metaphyseal region of long bones, surrounded by a sharp sclerotic border. FCDs are small, usually <2 cm, while NOFs are larger and can present as multiple lesions (1/3 of patients).[104]

The natural history of these lesions is of spontaneously healing over time. Pathologic fractures heal uneventfully but the lesion usually persists, and refracture may occur.[17,74,79,104]

Fractures are usually treated with immobilization until healing is obtained. If surgery is necessary due to high risk of further pathologic fractures, or chronic pain, it is best done after fracture healing. Although absolute size parameters may be useful in predicting pathologic fracture, they do not imply a requirement for prophylactic curettage and bone grafting. The appearance or stage of the lesion has been used as a predictor.[195] Most patients with large NOFs can be monitored without surgical intervention. Although we cannot readily identify an accurate denominator, we infer that many large NOFs remain unidentified and not problematic (Fig. 6-8).

ENCHONDROMA

Enchondromas are latent or active benign cartilaginous tumors. These lesions are often incidentally found, but can present with pain or pathologic fracture (more often with lesions in the phalanges of the hands or feet) (Fig. 6-9). The most common sites of involvement in decreasing order are the phalanges, metacarpals, metatarsals, humerus, and femur. Children may present with multiple enchondromas or enchondromatosis (Ollier's disease), which is usually diagnosed between 2 and 10 years of age. Although the lesion itself is similar to a solitary enchondroma, deformity and shortening of the extremity because of growth disturbance may occur (Fig. 6-10).[237]

On plain radiographs, enchondromas are central intramedullary lesions with stippled calcification. Larger lesions may cause cortical thinning and scalloping, predisposing to pathologic fractures. A typical radiographic finding of enchondromatosis is the presence of linear radiolucencies extending from the metaphysis down the shaft of the long bone, frequently seen in the hands.[194]

For asymptomatic patients with small lesions and classic radiographic findings, biopsy is not necessary. Younger patients with lesions in the fifth finger, especially in the distal phalanx, are at a higher risk for fractures. Curettage and bone grafting are necessary for those lesions with acute or impending pathologic fracture, or in cases of continued pain. Fixation is not necessary for lesions of the short tubular bones but may be

necessary for lesions of the proximal femur or long bone of the lower extremity. Standard fracture care is adequate to treat most pathologic fractures, but the bone quality may be compromised by the tumor, making fixation difficult.

OSTEOCHONDROMA

Osteochondromas are one of the most common bone tumors in children, and clinical symptoms are usually related to irritation

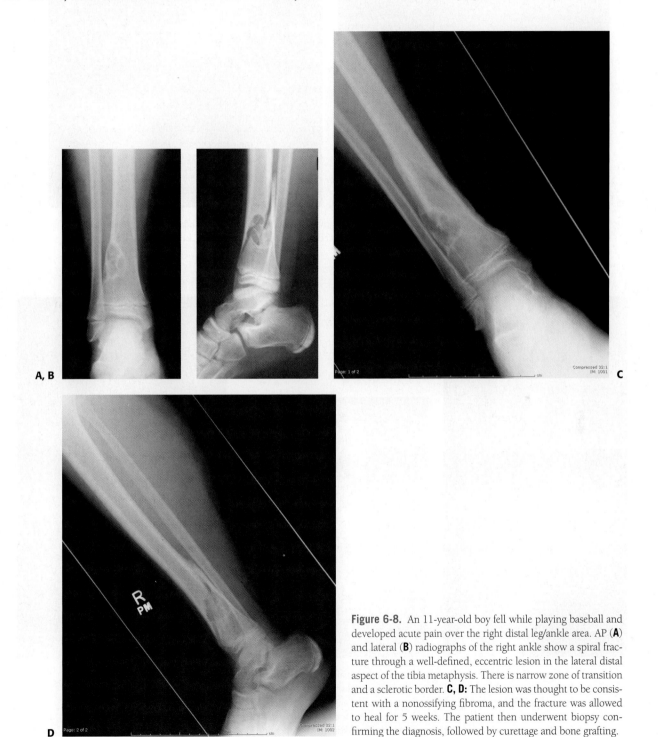

Figure 6-8. An 11-year-old boy fell while playing baseball and developed acute pain over the right distal leg/ankle area. AP (**A**) and lateral (**B**) radiographs of the right ankle show a spiral fracture through a well-defined, eccentric lesion in the lateral distal aspect of the tibia metaphysis. There is narrow zone of transition and a sclerotic border. **C, D:** The lesion was thought to be consistent with a nonossifying fibroma, and the fracture was allowed to heal for 5 weeks. The patient then underwent biopsy confirming the diagnosis, followed by curettage and bone grafting.

(*continues*)

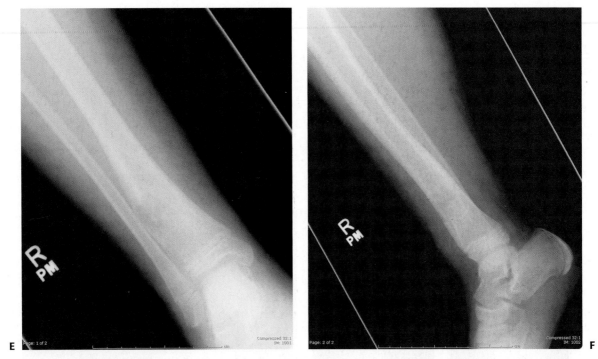

Figure 6-8. (*Continued*) **E, F:** Four months postoperatively, the lesion is completely healed and the patient resumed normal physical activities. (Figures reproduced with permission from The Children's Orthopaedic Center, Los Angeles, CA.)

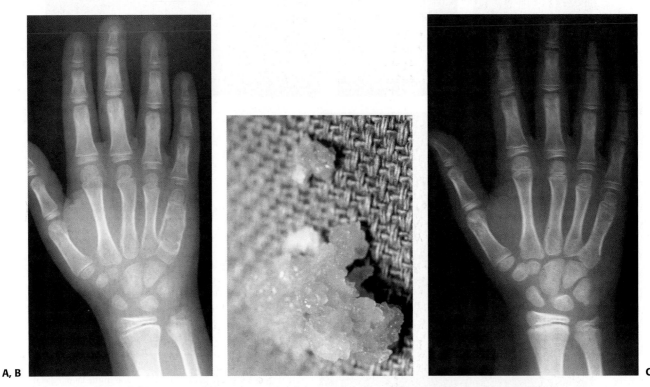

Figure 6-9. An 8-year-old boy presented with pain and swelling of the ulnar border of his right hand. **A:** Radiographic studies showed an expansile, lucent lesion of the diaphysis of the patient's right fifth metacarpal with microfractures. The patient had an open incisional biopsy with frozen section, which was consistent with enchondroma with subsequent curettage and bone grafting. **B:** Gross appearance of material removed at the time of surgery, which is consistent with enchondroma. **C:** At 6-month follow-up, the fracture is well healed, and there is no sign of recurrent tumor.

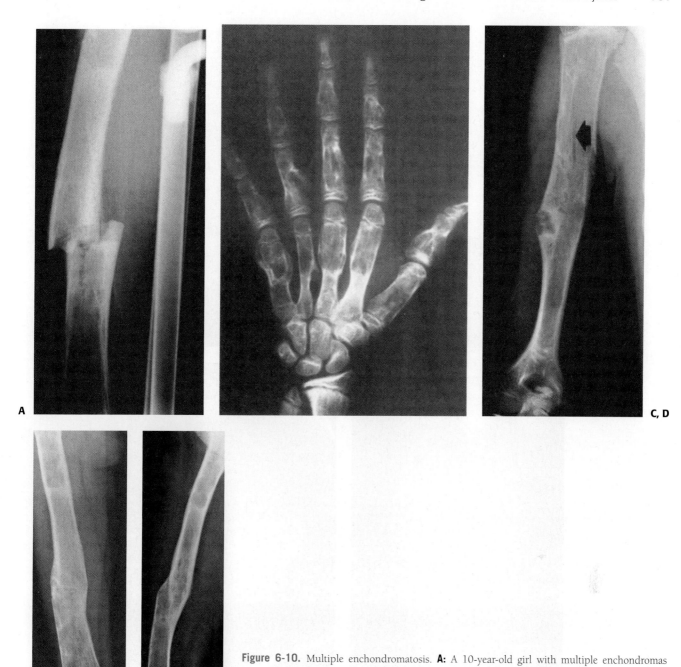

Figure 6-10. Multiple enchondromatosis. **A:** A 10-year-old girl with multiple enchondromas sustained a spontaneous pathologic fracture of the femur while running. The lateral radiograph shows overriding of the fracture. **B:** At 3-year follow-up, the fracture is well healed. **C:** The anteroposterior radiograph of the hand in this patient demonstrated multiple expansile enchondromas of the small bones. **D:** A radiograph of the humerus shows the streaked-mud appearance of the lateral humerus (*arrow*).

of the surrounding soft tissue structures. The radiographic appearance is pathognomonic, with a continuity of the host bone cortex with the outer cortex of the lesion and intramedullary cavities. Although fractures associated with osteochondromas are rare, they may occur through the base or stalk of a pedunculated tumor (Fig. 6-11).[49] Fractures through osteochondromas should be treated conservatively; however, excision in the acute phase may be considered because the fragment is "floating free" in the soft tissues.

FIBROUS DYSPLASIA

FD is a benign bone abnormality characterized by replacement of normal bone and marrow by fibrous–osseous tissue (woven bone formed by metaplasia with poorly oriented bone trabeculae) resulting in decrease of strength, deformity, and pathologic fracture. The disease may involve a single bone (monostotic FD) or several (polyostotic FD). When bone disease is associated with café-au-lait skin hyperpigmentation and endocrine dysfunction, it is referred as McCune–Albright syndrome.[182]

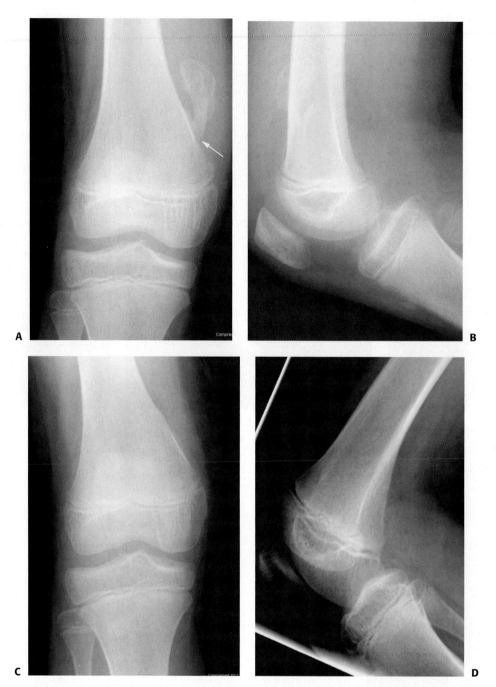

Figure 6-11. A 13-year-old girl presented with right knee pain following direct trauma to that area 10 days prior. On AP (**A**) and lateral (**B**) radiographs, there was a pathologic fracture through the base of a pedunculated osteochondroma (*arrow*). The patient was very tender around that area and elected surgical excision. **C, D:** Immediately after excision, there was improvement of the symptoms. Four weeks later, she returned to full activities. (Figures reproduced with permission from The Children's Orthopaedic Center, Los Angeles, CA.)

Most often, the lesions are asymptomatic and pathologic fracture may be the presenting symptom. Fractures of long bones can be minimally displaced or incomplete, many being microfractures presenting with pain and swelling.[148] The bones most commonly affected are the femur, tibia, and humerus. The age of first fracture, number of fractures, and fracture rate are related to the severity of the metabolic derangement and type of dysplasia (mono- vs. polyostotic). The endocrinopathy may lead to phosphaturia,

causing a rickets-type effect on the normal skeleton, leading to increased incidence of fractures.[148] The incidence of fractures in monostotic disease is around 5%.[97] Although the fractures heal rapidly, endosteal callus is poorly formed and periosteal callus is normal. With mild deformity, the cortex thickens on the concave side of the long bone, and a progressive deformity can issue.

On plain radiographs, FD is seen as a well-defined, mostly lytic and central lesion, located in the diaphysis of long bones.

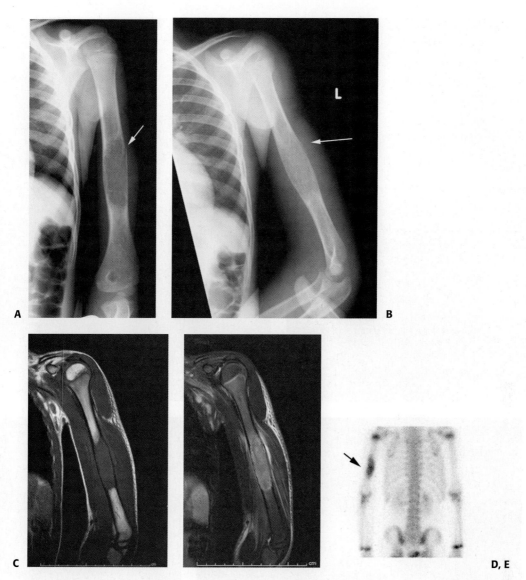

Figure 6-12. A 6-year-old girl presented with right arm acute pain after hitting the elbow in the bathtub. **A, B:** Radiographs of the humerus show a nondisplaced pathologic fracture through a humeral diaphyseal lesion (*arrows*). The lesion is well defined, mostly lytic but with definite matrix, cortical thinning, no periosteal reaction. MRI T1- (**C**) and T2-weighted (**D**) coronal images demonstrate absence of soft tissue mass or other aggressiveness signs. Bone scan shows increased activity at the lesion and fracture site (*arrow*). **E:** The patient underwent open incisional biopsy that confirmed the diagnosis of fibrous dysplasia. (Reproduced with permission from The Children's Orthopaedic Center, Los Angeles, CA.)

The metaplastic woven bone comprising the lesion creates the classic "ground-glass" appearance (Fig. 6-12). Bowing and/or angular deformity of tibia and femur are often seen. Differential diagnosis with UBC can be challenging.

Conservative treatment (at least at first) with immobilization is indicated for most, except for fractures through severely deformed long bones (especially in the lower extremities), and those through large cystic areas. Fractures in polyostotic disease often require more aggressive treatment. Proximal femoral pathologic fractures are especially troublesome because of the propensity for malunion or progressive deformity leading to coxa vara and *shepherd's crook* deformity.[71]

Curettage and grafting are usually not indicated since the bone graft is reabsorbed and replaced by FD bone; cortical allograft seems to be the most resistant graft. The use of bisphosphonates may prevent the occurrence and frequency of pathologic fractures in patients with severe/polyostotic FD. Pamidronate is a potent inhibitor of bone resorption and has a lasting effect on bone turnover. The major described effect however is decreased bone pain at the site of disease.[182] When pathologic fractures are managed surgically, internal fixation is key and intramedullary load-sharing fixation is preferred to decrease the metal–bone interface stress and preferably provide "total bone fixation" (Fig. 6-13).

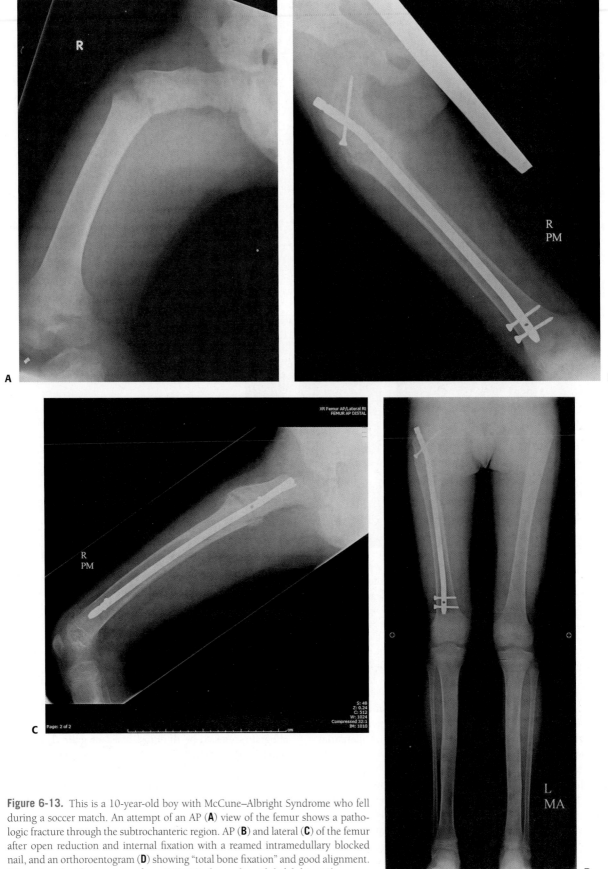

Figure 6-13. This is a 10-year-old boy with McCune–Albright Syndrome who fell during a soccer match. An attempt of an AP (**A**) view of the femur shows a pathologic fracture through the subtrochanteric region. AP (**B**) and lateral (**C**) of the femur after open reduction and internal fixation with a reamed intramedullary blocked nail, and an orthoroentogram (**D**) showing "total bone fixation" and good alignment. (Reproduced with permission from CHOP Orthopaedics, Philadelphia, PA).

MALIGNANT BONE TUMORS AND METASTASIS

Pathologic fractures can sometimes be the presenting symptom of a malignant bone tumor (Fig. 6-14). The two most common primary bone malignancies in children are osteosarcoma and Ewing sarcoma. Destructive bone lesions can also be caused by metastasis, being more common than primary tumors in certain age groups. Careful staging and biopsy are critical in the approach to children with bone tumors.[214] However, biopsy is not done without risks. One of the complications following

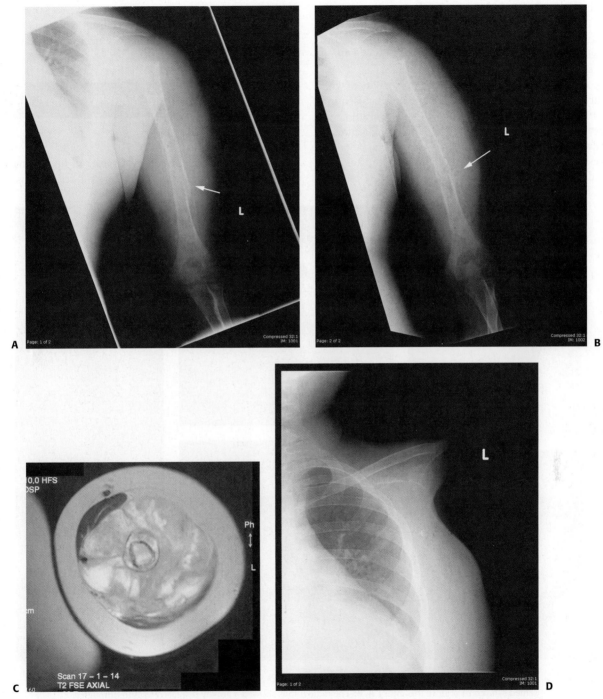

Figure 6-14. A 13-year-old boy presented with several months history of right arm pain and recent increase in pain following minor trauma. AP (**A**) and lateral (**B**) radiographs show a minimally displaced midshaft humeral pathologic fracture (*arrows*) through a poorly defined, permeative, aggressive-looking diaphyseal lesion. **C:** T2-weighted axial MRI shows a huge soft tissue mass associated with the bone lesion and involvement of the neurovascular bundle. The patient was diagnosed with Ewing sarcoma, received neoadjuvant chemotherapy, and had a shoulder disarticulation (**D**), followed by postoperative chemotherapy. (Reproduced with permission from The Children's Orthopaedic Center, Los Angeles, CA.)

open biopsies is pathologic fracture caused by a decrease in the torsional strength of the bone following cortical drilling. To prevent a pathologic fracture, an oval hole with smooth edges should be used, preferably in areas of less stress for weight-bearing bones. Sometimes, the biopsy hole can be filled with bone cement or other grafting material. Because most bone sarcomas are associated with a large soft tissue mass that can be sampled, drilling of the bone may be avoided. Nowadays, most biopsy can be safely done by percutaneous means with image guidance, with high accuracy and lower risk of secondary fracture.[239] Lytic lesions, especially larger ones, have the best accuracy rate.[239]

One of the major advances in the care of children with extremity sarcoma has been the development of limb-sparing surgical techniques for local control of the tumor. Pathologic fracture has previously been thought to be a contraindication to limb salvage because of concerns about tumor dissemination by fracture hematoma, leading to high local recurrence rate. Several studies, however, have shown that with adequate fracture care and modern neoadjuvant chemotherapy, free margin resection is achievable with no increased risk for local recurrence.[68] Some studies however show possible negative effect of pathologic fractures on survival rates (Fig. 6-15).[85] Pathologic fracture after limb-sparing surgery is another major complication, occurring most commonly after allograft reconstruction but also after limb salvage with endoprosthetic reconstruction.[35,236] Pathologic fractures in children as a result of metastatic disease tend to be mostly in the form of microfractures that can be successfully managed conservatively.

DISEASES OF THE BONE MARROW

GAUCHER DISEASE

Gaucher disease is a hereditary disorder of lipid metabolism. It is the most common lysosomal storage disease and is caused

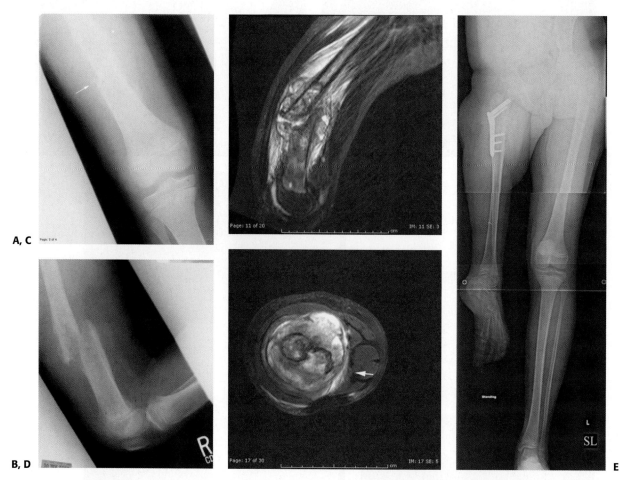

Figure 6-15. An 8-year-old girl sustained a pathologic fracture of the femur after falling off her bicycle. She denied symptoms prior to this injury. **A, B:** The radiographs showed a grossly displaced fracture through a poorly defined, mixed lesion in the midshaft of the femur (*arrow*); there is disorganized periosteal reaction with sunburst sign. T2-weighted coronal (**C**) and axial (**D**) MRIs showed extensive soft tissue mass; the neurovascular bundle (*arrow*) does not seem to be involved by the tumor mass. The patient underwent biopsy that confirmed osteogenic sarcoma and fracture stabilization with an external fixator at a referring institute. **E:** Note that the external fixator pins were inappropriately placed too far from the tumor and fracture site postoperative appearance following Van Ness rotationplasty. The patient is continuously free of disease, 5 years after surgery.

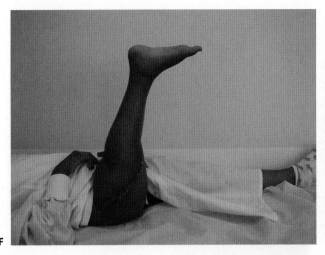
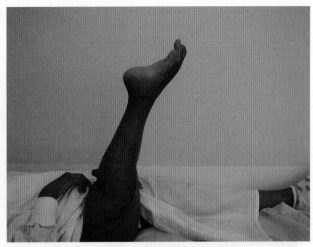

Figure 6-15. (*Continued*) **F, G:** Flexion and extension of the ankle, now used as a knee. (Figures reproduced with permission from The Children's Orthopaedic Center, Los Angeles, CA.)

by deficient production and activity of the lysosomal enzyme beta glucosidase (glucocerebrosidase), resulting in progressive accumulation of glucosylceramide (glucocerebroside) in macrophages of the reticuloendothelial system in the spleen, liver, and bone marrow. The most common sphingolipidosis is inherited as an autosomal recessive trait,[123] with most cases noted in Ashkenazi Jews of eastern European origin. There are three types of Gaucher disease: Type I represents more than 90% of all cases and is the most common type seen by orthopedic surgeons; it presents as a chronic nonneuropathic disease with visceral (spleen and liver) and osseous involvement, also known as the adult form, although patients present during childhood.[123] Type II is an acute, neuropathic disease with central nervous system (CNS) involvement and early infantile death. Type III is a subacute nonneuropathic type with chronic CNS involvement. Types II and III are both characterized as either infantile or juvenile, and are notable for severe progressive neurologic disease, usually being fatal.

Bone lesions are a result of marrow accumulation, and are most common in the femur, but they also occur in the pelvis, vertebra, humerus, and other locations. Infiltration of bone by Gaucher cells leads to vessel thrombosis, compromising the medullary vascular supply and leading to localized osteonecrosis of the long bones. Other radiographic findings include Erlenmeyer flask appearance of the metaphyseal bone, and pathologic fractures, especially of the spine and femoral neck.

Katz et al.[123] reported 23 pathologic fractures in nine children with Gaucher disease; seven had multiple fractures. In decreasing order of frequency, these involved the distal femur, femoral neck, spine, and proximal tibia. Fractures of the long bones were transverse and usually in the metaphysis. Fractures of the spine were either wedge shaped or centrally depressed at the endplate. The factors predisposing these children to fracture included significant medullary space infiltration, cortical bone erosion, osteonecrosis, and associated disuse osteoporosis. In another report of 53 patients with Gaucher disease aged 9 to 18 years,[124] 11 children had vertebral fractures, usually at two or three sites in

each patient, with either anterior wedging, central vertebral collapse, or total rectangular collapse.

Conservative treatment with immobilization and non-weight bearing is done for long-bone fractures when appropriate. Stable fractures of the femoral neck should be treated by immobilization with frequent follow-up radiographs, as varus malunion often occurs; internal fixation should be used in unstable femoral neck fractures. Preoperative planning is important, and the anesthesiologist must recognize that patients with Gaucher disease may be prone to upper airway obstruction because of infiltration of the upper airway with glycolipids and abnormal clotting function, even when clotting tests are normal.[231] Both delayed union and nonunion have been reported in older patients with Gaucher disease.

SICKLE CELL DISEASE

Sickle cell disease (SCD) is caused by the presence of sickle cell hemoglobin (HbS). The presence of the abnormal hemoglobin in red blood cells in SCD causes them to be mechanically fragile, and when they are deoxygenated, the cells assume a sickle shape, which makes them prone to clumping with blockage of the small vessels of the spleen, kidneys, and bones. The most common type of SCD, HbS-S, is a homozygous recessive condition in which individuals inherit the HbS globin gene from each parent. SCD affects approximately 1 in 400 African Americans. Chronic hemolytic anemia is present in most severely affected patients, and marrow hyperplasia is found in both the long bones and the short tubular bones. Sickle cell *trait* affects 8% to 10% of the African American population and other groups less frequently, but usually has no apparent clinical manifestations. These disorders are diagnosed by hemoglobin electrophoresis.

Fractures[32,80] may be one of the first symptoms of the disorder. Marrow hyperplasia may be a major contributing factor; not only does the hypercellular bone marrow expand the medullary canal with thinning of both trabecular and cortical bone, but it also extends into widened haversian and

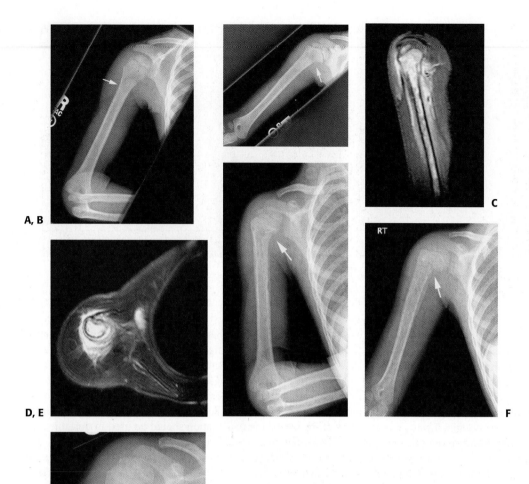

Figure 6-16. A 4-year-old boy with sickle cell disease presented with acute onset of right arm pain, swelling, increased warmth, and low grade fever. **A, B:** The initial radiographs show a poorly defined area of lucency in the proximal humeral metaphysis (*arrows*). T2-weighted sagittal (**C**) and axial (**D**) MRIs show intramedullary changes (enhancement) and periosteal reaction/abscess with no soft tissue mass. The clinical diagnosis of osteomyelitis was initially made and the patient was started on intravenous antibiotics. **E, F:** Three weeks later, there was little clinical improvement and new radiographs showed pathologic fracture/insufficiency fracture through the proximal humeral metaphysis (*arrows*). The patient underwent a biopsy that showed that this was an infarct with no superimposed infection. After clinical treatment, the patient's symptoms improved. **G:** At 6-month follow-up, he was completely asymptomatic and the radiographs showed remodeling and continued growth.

Volkmann canals. This process may weaken the bone, leading to fractures.[43] The prevalence of osteopenia and osteoporosis in young adults with SCD is extremely high and that can also predispose pathologic fractures (Fig. 6-16).[170] In a series of 81 patients with 198 long-bone infarcts with occasional concurrent osteomyelitis, Bohrer[38] found a 25% incidence of fractures associated with femoral lesions, and 20% with humeral lesions. The most common pattern was transverse diaphyseal fractures, especially the femur.[38]

Pathologic fractures in patients with SCD usually heal with conservative treatment. Furthermore, operative management may be hazardous. Extreme care must be taken to oxygenate the patient's tissues adequately during the procedure, and ideally, elective procedures should be preceded by transfusion regimen to raise hemoglobin levels to 10 g/dL and prevent perioperative complications. Intravenous hydration is very important, with one and a half to two times the daily fluid requirements needed in addition to routine replacement of fluid losses. The use of a tourniquet in surgery for patients with SCD is controversial due to the risk of thrombosis.

LEUKEMIA

Leukemia accounts for over 30% of cases of childhood cancer. Acute lymphocytic leukemia accounts for 80% of pediatric leukemias. There is an increased occurrence of lymphoid leukemias in patients with Down syndrome, immunodeficiencies, and ataxia telangiectasia. The peak incidence occurs at 4 years of age.

Approximately 50% to 75% of children with acute leukemia develop musculoskeletal signs and symptoms.[198,214] Skeletal lesions occur more frequently in leukemic children than in adults because leukemic cells can quickly replace the smaller marrow reserves in children. Diffuse osteopenia is the most frequent

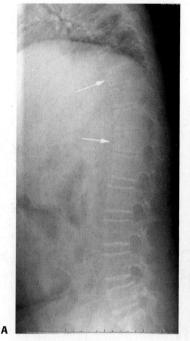
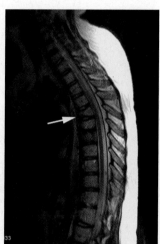

Figure 6-17. This 8-year-old girl presented with back pain, fever, malaise, and weight loss. **A:** Lateral radiographs of the spine showed diffuse osteopenia and compression/insufficiency fractures of the vertebral body (*arrows*). **B:** T1-weighted sagittal MRI confirms disease process within the vertebral body (*arrow*) and no soft tissue mass or intraspinal involvement. She was diagnosed with acute lymphoblastic leukemia. (Reproduced with permission from The Children's Orthopaedic Center, Los Angeles, CA.)

radiographic finding (Fig. 6-17).[123] Nonspecific juxtaepiphyseal lucent lines are often seen and are a result of generalized metabolic dysfunction[198,214]; these are usually bilateral and vary from 2 to 15 mm in width. Sclerotic bands of bone trabeculae are more typical in older children. Periosteal reaction is often present with osteolytic lesions and is most common in the posterior cortex of the distal femoral metaphysis, the medial neck of the femur, and the diaphysis of the tibia and fibula. Most bone lesions in leukemia improve after adequate response to treatment.

Pathologic fracture risk is around 20%.[14,143,198,214,225] The risk of pathologic fractures is higher for children with lower bone density at presentation, and tends to decrease with treatment. Fracture is most commonly associated with osteoporosis of the spine, particularly thoracic region, resulting in mild vertebral collapse (compression fracture).[165] A prompt diagnosis and initiation of chemotherapy is the main step in the treatment of pathologic fractures associated with leukemia. Most fractures are stable microfractures and can be treated with conservative treatment and symptomatic support, with emphasis on early ambulation to avoid further osteopenia. For vertebral fractures, a back brace or thoracolumbosacral orthosis may be used to alleviate symptoms.[14]

OSTEOMYELITIS

The pattern of pediatric osteomyelitis in North America has changed during the past several decades. Although the typical clinical picture of acute onset of pain, associated with fever and inability, or refusal to bear weight is still seen, subtle presentations and more aggressive ones have become frequent. Among the potential reasons for these changes are the increased use of empiric antibiotics, and the increased number of aggressive community-acquired pathogens such as methicillin-resistant *Staphylococcus aureus* (MRSA). Osteomyelitis can be classified according to the age of onset (neonatal, childhood, and adult

osteomyelitis); causative organism (pyogenic and granulomatous infections); onset (acute, subacute, and chronic); and routes of infection (hematogenous and direct inoculation). Although the acute form is still the most common, subacute osteomyelitis, or Brodie abscess, and chronic recurrent multifocal nonbacterial osteomyelitis are seen more frequently. Chronic osteomyelitis is defined as symptoms present for longer than 1 month (Fig. 6-18, Table 6-1).

At first, radiographs may be normal and the earliest finding is soft tissue swelling/loss of defined deep soft tissue planes. MRI has up to 98% sensitivity and 100% specificity for early detection of osteomyelitis.[145]

With early recognition and appropriate treatment, acute osteomyelitis rarely leads to a pathologic fracture. Pathologic fractures are more often associated with neglected or chronic osteomyelitis, neonatal osteomyelitis, or septic arthritis. During acute osteomyelitis, transitory osteopenia and surgical intervention can potentially predispose to fractures (Fig. 6-19). The presence of large subperiosteal abscess on MRI at the time of admission leads to greater incidence of fractures.[30]

These fractures may be difficult to treat and be associated with complications such as malunion and growth disturbance (Fig. 6-20).

The most important step in the treatment of fracture associated with osteomyelitis is to control the underlying infection. This requires biopsy for culture and sensitivities, drainage and debridement of the infection with appropriate immobilization and antibiotic therapy (Table 6-2). In advanced/chronic infections, sequestrectomy may be necessary. MRI is useful in identifying the sequestrum; an attempt should be made to leave as much supporting involucrum as possible at the time of sequestrectomy. Prolonged immobilization with either plaster casts or external fixation devices may be needed, and segmental bone loss can be treated with bone transport or grafting.

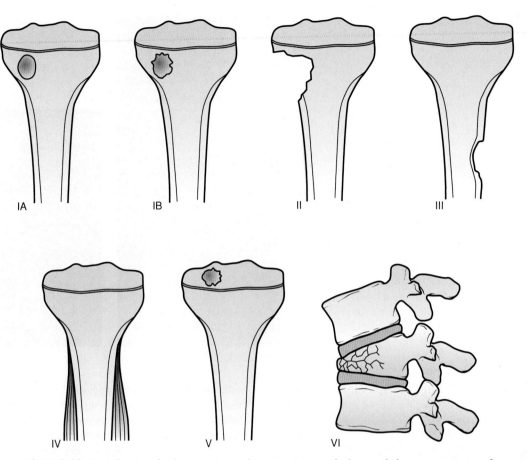

Figure 6-18. Classification of subacute osteomyelitis. Type IA, punched-out radiolucency suggestive of eosinophilic granuloma. Type IB, similar but with sclerotic margin; classic Brodie abscess. Type II, metaphyseal lesion with loss of cortical bone. Type III, diaphyseal lesion with excessive cortical reaction. Type IV, lesion with onionskin layering of subperiosteal bone. Type V, concentric epiphyseal radiolucency. Type VI, osteomyelitic lesion of vertebral body. (Adapted with permission from Dormans JP, Drummond DS. Pediatric hematogenous osteomyelitis: new trends in presentation, diagnosis, and treatment. *J Am Acad Orthop Surg.* 1994;2(6):333–341.)

TABLE 6-1. Comparison of Acute and Subacute Hematogenous Osteomyelitis		
Presentation	**Subacute**	**Acute**
Pain	Mild	Severe
Fever	Few patients	Majority
Loss of function	Minimal	Marked
Prior antibiotics	Often (30–40%)	Occasional
Elevated white blood cell count	Few	Majority
Elevated erythrocyte sedimentation rate	Majority	Majority
Blood cultures	Few positive	50% positive
Bone cultures	60% positive	85% positive
Initial x-ray study	Frequently abnormal	Often normal
Site	Any location (may cross physis)	Usually metaphysis

Reprinted with permission from Dormans JP, Drummond DS. Pediatric hematogenous osteomyelitis: new trends in presentation, diagnosis, and treatment. *J Am Acad Orthop Surg.* 1994;2(6):333–341.

PATHOLOGIC FRACTURES AFTER LIMB LENGTHENING

Limb lengthening has evolved dramatically; while the original Wagner method had rate of complications of over 90%, the use of gradual lengthening techniques, the combination of internal and external fixation techniques,[112,185] and the use of electromagnetic intramedullary devices have decreased the complication rates significantly.[109] Most lengthening is performed through the metaphysis, which has a larger bone diameter and better blood supply than the diaphysis, which decreases the incidence of fractures post device removal to around 3% to 10%.[44,212]

Pathologic fractures can occur during or after limb lengthening. The bone that is formed by distraction callotasis must be subjected to normal weight-bearing forces over a period of time before normal bony architecture is established. Fractures through the regenerate can occur either soon after removal of the fixator or years later (Fig. 6-21), but most often they occur in the first 4 weeks, especially following lengthening over 5 cm.[44] Some of the causes include disuse osteopenia, adjacent joint contracture, and pin tracks. Protective early weight

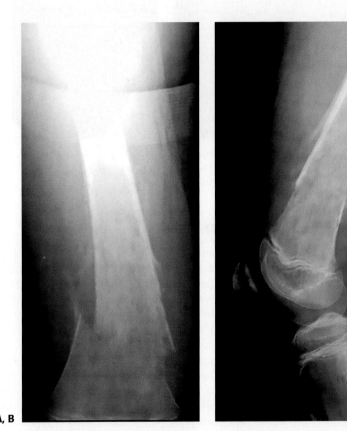

A, B

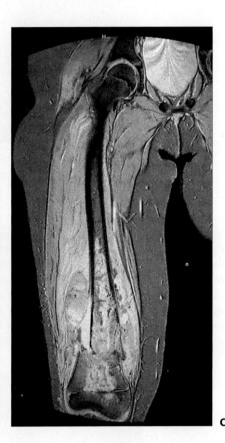

C

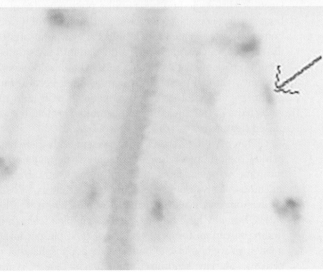

D

Figure 6-19. An 8-year-old girl sustained a fall from standing height and developed acute pain and deformity at the right knee. **A, B:** Radiographs at presentation demonstrated a pathologic fracture of the distal femur through a poorly defined, destructive lesion of the femur. **C:** MRI demonstrated soft tissue involvement abscess versus mass. **D:** A bone scan showed also increased uptake in the left proximal humerus. The patient underwent an open biopsy (**E**) of the lesion and was placed in a spanning external fixator until bone healing was evident (**F**).

(continues)

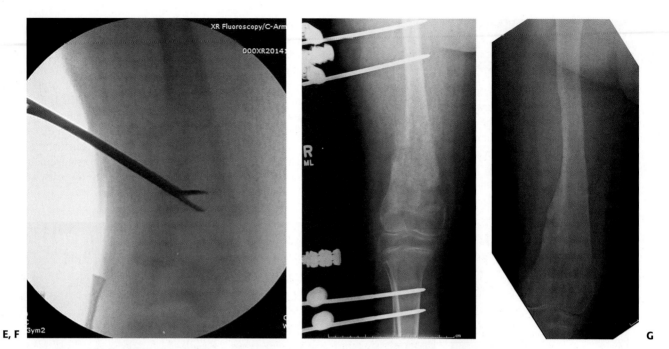

Figure 6-19. (*Continued*) The final diagnosis was consistent with a multifocal methicillin-sensitive *Staphylococcus aureus* infection and she responded to adequate antibiotics. **G:** The fracture healed in good alignment. (Reproduced with permission from The Children's Orthopaedic Center, Los Angeles, CA.)

bearing postoperatively, continued range of motion throughout the treatment, and using smaller screw diameter are some of the preventive measures.[212] These fractures often lead to loss of correction, inadequate alignment, and risk for further contracture; therefore, most need surgical treatment with internal or external fixation and early mobilization. The use of dual-energy x-ray absorptiometry to evaluate the quality of the regenerate prior to fixator removal has been suggested.[57]

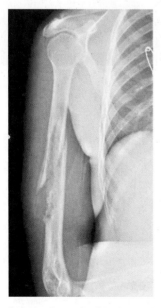

Figure 6-20. This lateral radiograph of the humeral shaft of a 17-year-old boy shows a pathologic fracture through chronic osteomyelitis of the humerus. (Courtesy of B. David Horn, MD.)

OSTEOGENESIS IMPERFECTA

Osteogenesis imperfecta (OI) is an inherited disorder in which the structure and function of type I collagen is altered or deficient. The fragile bone is susceptible to frequent fractures and progressive deformity. OI incidence is 1 in 20,000 total births, with an overall prevalence of approximately 16 per 1,000,000. The wide spectrum of clinical severity—from perinatal lethal forms to clinically silent forms—reflects the tremendous genotypic heterogeneity (more than 150 different mutations of the type I procollagen genes COL1A1 and COL1A2 have been described). Most forms (total of 13) of OI are the result of mutations in the genes that encode the pro alpha1 and pro alpha2 polypeptide chains of type I collagen.[180] Histologic findings reveal a predominance of woven bone, an absence of lamellar bone, and thinning of the cortical bone with osteopenia. From a practical viewpoint of orthopedic care, patients with OI can be divided into two groups: one group of patients with severe disease who develop long-bone deformity through repetitive fractures often needing surgical treatment, and another group of patients with mild disease with frequent fractures, but most injuries responding well to closed treatment.

Children with severe OI may present with a short trunk, marked deformity of lower extremities, prominence of the sternum, triangular faces, thin skin, muscle atrophy, and ligamentous laxity; some develop kyphoscoliosis,[98,171] basilar impression, and deafness (caused by otosclerosis).[99] Children with OI usually have normal intelligence. Blue sclera, a classic finding in certain forms of OI, can also be present in normal infants, as well as in children with hypophosphatasia, osteopetrosis, Marfan syndrome, and Ehlers–Danlos syndrome.

TABLE 6-2. Initial Antibiotic Therapy for Osteomyelitis

Patient Type	Probable Organism	Initial Antibiotic
Neonate	Group B Streptococcus, *Staphylococcus aureus,* gram-negative rods (*Haemophilus influenzae*)	Cefotaxime (100–120 mg/kg/24 hr) or oxacillin and gentamicin (5–7.5 mg/kg/24 hr)
Infants and children	*S. aureus* (90%) if allergic to penicillin[a]	Oxacillin (150 mg/kg/24 hr), Cefazolin (100 mg/kg/24 hr), Clindamycin (25–40 mg/kg/24 hr), or Vancomycin (40 mg/kg/24 hr)
Sickle cell disease	*S. aureus* or Salmonella	Oxacillin and ampicillin or chloramphenicol or cefotaxime (100–120 mg/kg/24 hr)

[a]Overall 80% because of *S. aureus.*

Children with OI also have a greater incidence of airway anomalies, thoracic anatomy abnormalities, coagulation dysfunction, hyperthyroidism, and an increased tendency to develop perioperative malignant hyperthermia.[220]

Pathologic fractures may present with swelling of the extremity, pain, low-grade fever, and a radiograph showing exuberant, hyperplastic, callus formation. The callus may occur without obvious fracture and can have a distinct butterfly shape, as opposed to the usual fusiform callus of most healing fractures. The femur is the most common site of pathologic fractures.[196]

The radiographic findings vary (Fig. 6-22). In severe OI, there is marked osteoporosis, thin cortical bone, and evidence of past fracture with angular malunion. Both anterior and lateral bowing

of the femur and anterior bowing of the tibia are common. Spinal radiographs may show compression of the vertebrae between the cartilaginous disc spaces (the so-called codfish vertebra).

When the diagnosis of OI is suspected, but cannot be made on classic clinical grounds, the diagnosis may be made by biochemical assay. Genetic testing of individuals with typical features of OI typically has disease-causing mutations in 98%.[24] The more severe the IO, the more genetic the variety beyond collagen type I encoding genes are involved. If IO is suspected but there are not the classic or typical signs, Pepin recommends DNA sequencing of COL1A1, COL1A2, and IFITM5, including duplication/deletion testing, but recommends no additional genetic testing if a variant is not identified.[186a] It is crucial, but

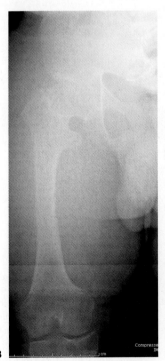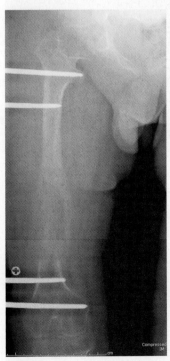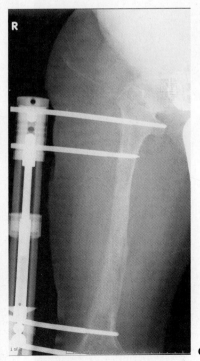

A, B   **C**

Figure 6-21. Radiograph of a 15-year-old boy with achondroplasia (**A**) who underwent femoral lengthening with a monolateral external fixator for limb-length discrepancy (**B**). **C, D:** The procedure and the lengthening were uneventful, and the device was removed after four cortices were visualized on radiographs.

(continues)

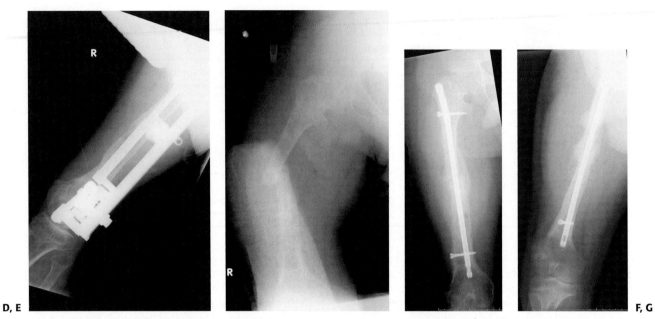

D, E

F, G

Figure 6-21. (*Continued*) **E:** Less than 2 months after external fixator removal, the patient fell and had a pathologic femoral fracture through the regenerated bone. **F, G:** He underwent ORIF with an intramedullary device and the fracture healed in approximately 3 months. (Figures reproduced with permission from The Children's Orthopaedic Center, Los Angeles, CA.)

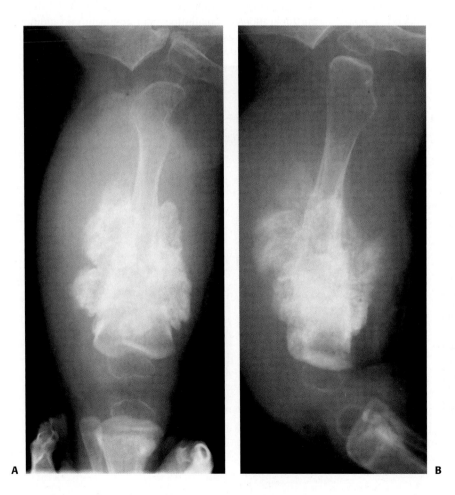

A

B

Figure 6-22. This 10-month-old boy with a history of osteogenesis imperfecta presented with a right thigh pain and swelling and refusal to bear weight. AP (**A**) and lateral (**B**) radiographs of the right femur show the extraordinarily abundant, hyperplastic callus—with the characteristic butterfly shape—that can occur in osteogenesis imperfecta. This appearance may be mistaken for an infection or a neoplastic process.

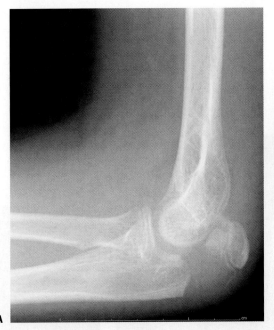
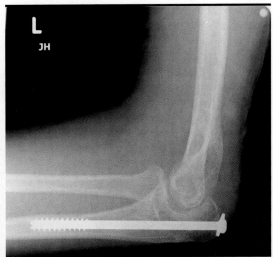

Figure 6-23. A 13-year-old boy with mild osteogenesis imperfecta presented after a fall on an outstretched arm, with inability to move his elbow, pain, and swelling. **A:** Radiographs showed a displaced olecranon fracture. This fracture pattern is commonly seen in children with osteogenesis imperfecta and is quite uncommon in healthy children. The patient underwent open reduction and internal fixation. **B:** The fracture healed after 6 weeks. (Figures reproduced with permission from The Children's Orthopaedic Center, Los Angeles, CA.)

often difficult, to distinguish OI from nonaccidental injury (NAI); before the diagnosis of OI is made, the parents may be presumed to be the cause of the fractures, with temporary removal of a child in 70% of cases.

Fractures tend to occur before skeletal maturity. Most pathologic fractures are transverse, diaphyseal, minimally displaced, and heal at a relatively normal rate.[209] Although nonunion may occur, they seem to be associated with inadequate fixation after osteotomies and fractures.[2] Recurrent fractures may result in angular deformities due to malunion, leading to coxa vara, genu valgum, and leg-length discrepancy. Olecranon sleeve (apophysis) avulsion fractures are essentially pathognomonic of OI (Fig. 6-23).[220]

The role of medical therapy in the prevention of fractures associated with OI has evolved. Bisphosphonates are a potent inhibitor of bone resorption and have been used for severe cases, with the goal to reduce chronic bone pain, decrease the rate of fractures, gain in muscle force, increase in bone density, thickening of bone cortex, and increase growth rate.[36,78,95,241] Some of the reported negative effects include decrease in bone remodeling rate, growth plate abnormalities, and delay in the healing of osteotomy.[78,95] New therapies with other antiresorptives as well as anabolic agents and transforming growth factor (TGF)-β antibodies are in development.

The orthopedist caring for children with OI must balance standard fracture care with the goal of minimizing immobilization to avoid a vicious circle: immobilization leading to weakness and osteopenia, leading to refracture.[13,171] Protected weight bearing is the goal for patients with severe OI. Close follow-up is necessary in the first few years of life, with protective splinting or soft cast for fractures. Orthoses are constructed for bracing of the lower extremities to aid in both standing and ambulation. Once ambulatory, the child is advanced to the use of a walker or independent ambulation. Severe bowing of the extremities, especially after recurrent fractures, is an indication for osteotomy and intramedullary rodding. Whenever possible, surgery is delayed until 6 or 7 years of age to allow for better fixation and decrease the chance of recurrence. Load-sharing devices (such as intramedullary rods) are used for internal fixation of long-bone fractures or osteotomies in children with OI (Fig. 6-24).[199,204] It is important to perform fixation without intent of hardware removal. Skeletally mature patients and patients with very small medullary canals are best treated with standard rods, whereas skeletally immature patients with adequate width of the medullary canal are best treated with extensible rods.[199] Complications after internal fixation of fractures or osteotomies and intramedullary fixation include fracture at the rod tip, migration of the fixation device, joint penetration, loosening of components of extensible rods, and fractures through the area of uncoupled rods.[204]

OSTEOPETROSIS

Osteopetrosis is a condition in which excessive density of bone occurs as a result of abnormal function of osteoclasts.[19,191,218,235] The resultant bone of these children is dense, brittle, and highly susceptible to pathologic fracture. The incidence of osteopetrosis is approximately 1 per 200,000 births. The inherent problem is a failure of bone resorption with continuing bone formation and persistent primary spongiosa. Osteopetrosis is classified into three main forms (malignant autosomal recessive, intermediate autosomal recessive, or benign autosomal dominant), leading to a severe infantile type or a milder form that presents later in life.[207,218]

Radiographically, the bones have a dense, chalk-like appearance. The spinal column may have a sandwich or "rugger-jersey" appearance because of dense, sclerotic bone at each end plate of the vertebrae and less involvement of the central portion. The

long bones tend to have a dense, marble-like appearance and may have an Erlenmeyer flask shape at their ends owing to deficient cutback remodeling. There may be bowing of the bones because of multiple fractures, spondylolysis, or coxa vara.[191] The small bones of the hands and feet may show a bone-within-bone appearance with increased density around the periphery.

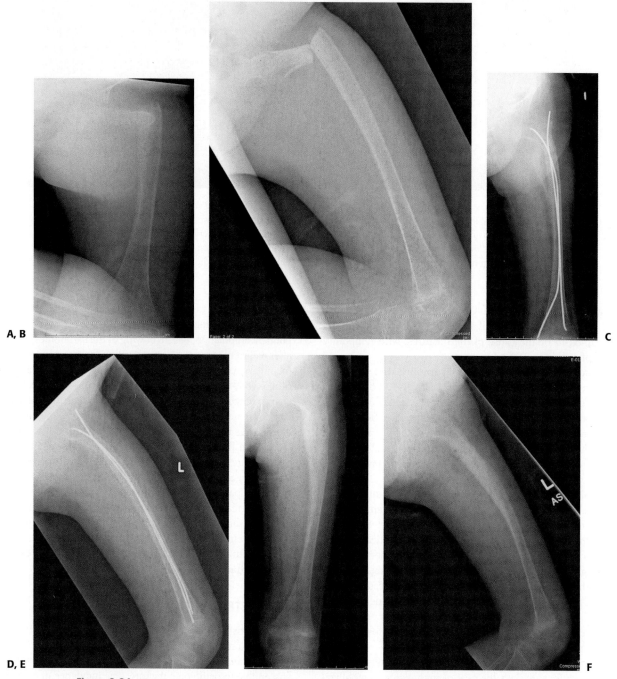

Figure 6-24. This 8-year-old girl presented with pain and deformity around the right hip after minor trauma. The patient had a known history of osteogenesis imperfecta. Initial radiographs (**A, B**) showed grossly displaced fracture of the proximal femur in the subtrochanteric area. The patient underwent closed reduction and internal fixation with titanium elastic nails, and the fracture healed after 5 weeks, with good alignment in both anteroposterior (**C**) and lateral (**D**) views. The nails were slightly prominent and the family elected removal of the hardware (**E, F**).

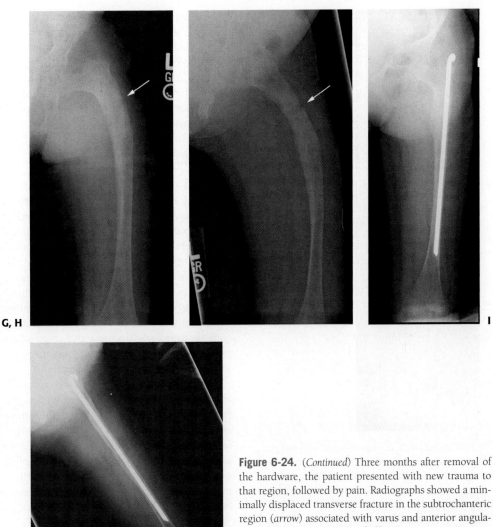

Figure 6-24. (*Continued*) Three months after removal of the hardware, the patient presented with new trauma to that region, followed by pain. Radiographs showed a minimally displaced transverse fracture in the subtrochanteric region (*arrow*) associated with varus and anterior angulation of the proximal femur (**G, H**). The patient underwent a Sofield procedure with Rush rods as the internal fixation. Ten weeks after the procedure, there was complete healing at the osteotomy/fracture site and adequate femoral alignment (**I, J**). (Figures reproduced with permission from The Children's Orthopaedic Center, Los Angeles, CA.)

The unusual radiographic appearance may initially obscure occult nondisplaced fractures (Fig. 6-25).[191,207,218] Patients with a severe form of the disease have more fractures than those with presentation later in childhood.

Patients with the severe, congenital disease have transverse or short oblique fractures of the diaphysis, particularly the femur. Distal physeal fractures with exuberant callus may be confused with osteomyelitis.[169] Common locations for fractures include the inferior neck of the femur, the proximal third of the femoral shaft, and the proximal tibia. Upper extremity fractures are also frequent.[19] The onset of callus formation after fracture in osteopetrosis is variable.

The orthopedist treating fractures in children with osteopetrosis should follow the principles of standard pediatric fracture care, with additional vigilance for possible delayed union (Fig. 6-26).[101,207] Armstrong et al.[19] surveyed the membership of the Pediatric Orthopaedic Society of North America and compiled the combined experience of 58 pediatric orthopedic surgeons with experience treating pathologic fractures in osteopetrosis. In this comprehensive review, they concluded that nonoperative treatment should be strongly considered for most diaphyseal fractures of the upper and lower limbs in children, but surgical management is recommended for femoral neck fractures and coxa vara. Open treatment of osteopetrotic fractures with fixation is technically difficult because of bone rigidity/density, and absence of intramedullary canal/sclerosis (leading to the use of multiple drill bits intraoperatively).

In addition to these technical difficulties, patients with osteopetrosis are at risk for excessive bleeding and infection, related to the hematopoietic dysfunction caused by obliteration of the marrow cavity.[207,218]

In the past, primary medical treatment for osteopetrosis included transfusions, splenectomy, and adrenal corticosteroids, but these techniques have proved ineffectual. Stimulation

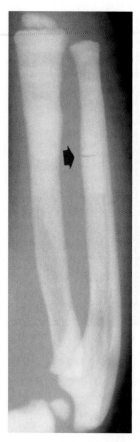

Figure 6-25. This 2-year-old with osteopetrosis presented with forearm pain. An anteroposterior radiograph shows the characteristic increased bone density and absence of a medullary canal, especially in the distal radius and ulna. There is a typical transverse, nondisplaced fracture (*arrow*) in the distal ulnar diaphysis.

of host osteoclasts has been attempted with calcium restriction, calcitriol, steroids, parathyroid hormone, and interferon. Bone marrow transplantation for severe infantile osteopetrosis has proved to be an effective means of treatment for some patients; however, it does not guarantee survival, and those due to deficiency of the pro-osteoclastogenic cytokine, RANKL, are not suitable for this.[55,59,93,218] There is still a need to identify other ways to treat this condition.

RICKETS

Rickets is a disease of the growing skeleton caused by either a deficiency of vitamin D or an abnormality of its metabolism. The osteoid of the bone is not mineralized, and broad unossified osteoid seams form on the trabeculae. With failure of physeal mineralization, the zone of provisional calcification widens and the ingrowth of blood vessels into the zone is disrupted. In the rickets of renal failure, the effects of secondary hyperparathyroidism (bone erosion and cyst formation) are also present. Regardless of the underlying cause, the various types of rickets share similar clinical and radiographic features (Fig. 6-27).

Both pathologic fractures and epiphyseal displacement can occur in rickets.[18,54,157] The treatment of rickets depends on identification of the underlying cause.

Recognition and treatment of the underlying metabolic abnormalities is the most important aspect in the care of pathologic fractures in rickets. In addition to nutritional rickets and lack of exposure to sunlight, many other diseases can affect vitamin D metabolism (Table 6-3). Most fractures of the long bones respond readily to cast or splint immobilization, with concurrent aggressive medical treatment of the underlying metabolic disease. Slipped capital femoral epiphysis may be the first presenting sign of renal osteodystrophy and renal

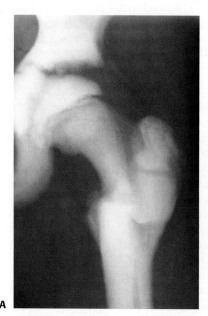
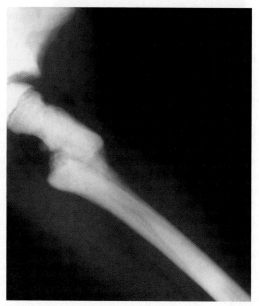

Figure 6-26. A: This 9 year old with osteopetrosis sustained similar bilateral subtrochanteric fractures of the femur over a 2-year period. Anteroposterior (**A**) and lateral (**B**) femoral radiographs show a healing transverse subtrochanteric fracture of the left femoral.

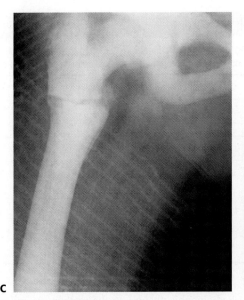

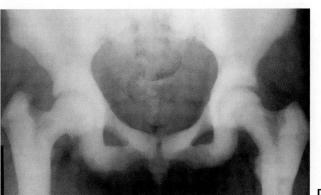

Figure 6-26. (*Continued*) **C:** One year later, at age 10, she sustained a similar right transverse minimally displaced subtrochanteric femur fracture, which was treated with reduction and a spica cast. **D:** This anteroposterior radiograph taken at age 14 years shows that both proximal and femoral fractures have healed and there is mild residual coxa vara, especially on the right side.

failure. The slip is bilateral in up to 95% of the patients and it is usually stable (Fig. 6-28).[157] The aggressive medical treatment of renal osteodystrophy, including administration of vitamin D, calcitriol, hemodialysis, renal transplantation, and parathyroidectomy, has improved the long-term survival and quality of life for these patients. A slipped capital femoral epiphysis should be stabilized with in situ screw fixation in older children, and multiple screws should be considered because the

underlying metaphyseal bone is quite soft, contralateral prophylactic fixation is recommended. Significant cysts should be treated with curettage and bone grafting. Angular deformities of the long bones should be corrected when the patient is close to maturity.

IDIOPATHIC OSTEOPOROSIS

Idiopathic osteoporosis is a rare cause of pathologic fractures in children. The etiology is likely multifactorial and incompletely understood; however, poor calcium intake during the adolescent growth spurt may play some role. Symptoms can persist for 1 to 4 years after diagnosis, with spontaneous resolution in most patients after the onset of puberty. The only consistent metabolic abnormality is a negative calcium balance with high rates of fecal excretion of calcium.

Idiopathic osteoporosis usually presents with bone pain, deformities, and fractures, most often of the spine.[21,56] Although many children present with back pain as the only complaint, the most severely affected present with generalized skeletal pain. Patients may have difficulty walking, and their symptoms may be initiated by mild trauma. Metaphyseal impaction/insufficiency fractures are a hallmark of this disorder.[56]

Serum calcium, phosphorus, and alkaline phosphatase levels are usually normal. Low plasma calcitriol, a vitamin D metabolite that aids calcium absorption in the gut, has been observed in juvenile osteoporosis.[56]

Lower extremity and vertebral fractures are the most common (Fig. 6-29). While there is no definitive treatment, many patients have been treated by both vitamin D and calcium supplements with equivocal benefit, and usually mineralization of the skeleton does not improve until puberty, when the disease spontaneously resolves. Low-dose pamidronate may be indicated.[90]

IATROGENIC OSTEOPOROSIS

Osteoporosis Associated With Cancer Treatment. Osteoporosis is commonly seen in children who are undergoing cancer

Figure 6-27. This 12-year-old girl with rickets associated with chronic kidney disease presented with complaints of knocked knees and wrist pain. Hip to ankle radiographs (**A**) showed typical rickets changes with valgus deformity at the knee level. Looser lines around the distal femur, and physeal widening. Wrist images (**B, C**) demonstrated marked physeal widening and metaphyseal flare of the distal radius and ulna. (Reproduced with permission from The Children's Orthopaedic Center, Los Angeles, CA.)

TABLE 6-3. Rickets: Metabolic Abnormalities

Disorder	Cause	1,25(OH)$_2$ Vitamin D	Parathyroid Hormone	Calcium	P	Alkaline Phosphate
Vitamin D deficiency rickets	Lack of vitamin D in the diet	↓	↑	↓ or →	↓	↑
Gastrointestinal rickets	Decreased gastrointestinal absorption of vitamin D or calcium	↓ or →	↑	↓	↓	↑
Vitamin D-dependent rickets	Reduced 1,25(OH)$_2$ vitamin D production	↓↓	↑	↓	↓	↑
Vitamin D-resistant rickets— end-organ insensitivity	Intestinal cell insensitivity to vitamin D causing decreased calcium absorption	↑ or →	↑	↓	↓	↑
Renal osteodystrophy	Renal failure causing decreased vitamin D synthesis, phosphate retention, hypocalcemia, and secondary hyperparathyroidism	↓↓	↑↑	↓	↑	↑

therapy. The cause of reduced bone mineral density is multifactorial. The disease itself may play a role (e.g., acute lymphoblastic leukemia, malignant bone tumors), but also the treatment including corticosteroids, chemotherapy (e.g., methotrexate, ifosfamide), and radiation (such as brain radiation that can reduce growth hormone secretion and cause hypogonadotropic hypogonadism), can contribute to the development of osteoporosis.[200] Methotrexate, for example, is believed to inhibit osteogenesis, causing both delayed union and nonunion of fractures. The incidence of pathologic fractures after methotrexate use ranges from 19% to 57%.[166]

Generalized demineralization of the skeleton is seen with marked radiolucency of the metaphyseal regions of the long bones. Radiographic changes in the metaphysis and epiphysis resemble those seen in scurvy. Minimally displaced transverse fractures or insufficiency type fractures occur in the long bones of both the upper and lower extremities and the small bones of the feet (Fig. 6-30).[166,191]

Prevention is the key and physical activity, adequate vitamin D intake, and sometimes bisphosphonates are some of the options.[200]

Immobilization Osteoporosis. Immobilization of an extremity for fracture treatment can result in loss of as much as a 44% of mineralization of trabecular bone. Immobilization leads to bone resorption, especially in unstressed areas.[219] Osteoporosis may persist for 6 months after an injury, but bone density returns

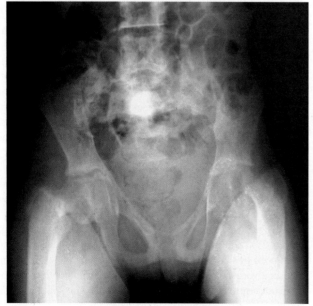
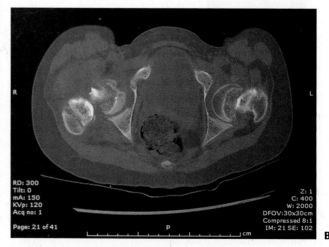

Figure 6-28. This 13-year-old boy with renal osteodystrophy presented with bilateral hip and thigh pain. **A:** Anteroposterior pelvic radiograph shows widening of the proximal femoral physes with sclerosis. Slipped capital femoral epiphyses were diagnosed. **B:** This anteroposterior pelvic radiograph taken 9 months after surgery shows narrowing of the physis and no evidence of further displacement of the capital femoral epiphyses. (Reproduced with permission from The Children's Orthopaedic Center, Los Angeles, CA.)

to normal in most by 1 year.[82] In an 11-year follow-up study of 30 patients, residual decrease in bone mineralization of the distal femur was present in 7%.[178] Persistent osteoporosis after cast immobilization for fracture can also contribute to refracture.[219]

CUSHING SYNDROME

Endogenous Cushing syndrome in children is a rare disorder that is most frequently caused by pituitary or adrenocortical tumors, resulting in excessive production of cortisol and its related compounds. If the hyperactivity of the adrenal cortex is caused by pituitary gland stimulation, the syndrome is known as Cushing disease. Exogenous Cushing occurs as a result of corticosteroid therapy. The elevated adrenal corticosteroids inhibit the formation of osteoblasts, resulting in increased resorption of the bone matrix and decreased bone formation.

Presenting symptoms include failure to thrive, short stature with excessive weight gain, moon facies, presence of a buffalo hump, hirsutism, weakness, and hypertension; mortality can be high.[150,161] In older children, the clinical picture is somewhat

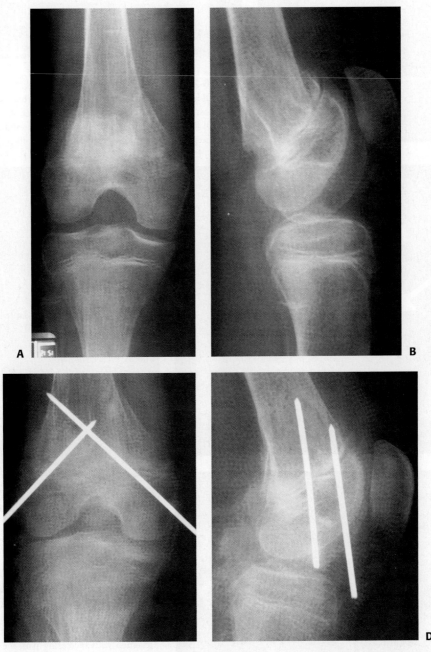

Figure 6-29. A: Multiple pathologic fractures in a previously healthy teenage boy who developed idiopathic osteoporosis. This anteroposterior radiograph of the right knee and this lateral radiograph (**B**) demonstrate a displaced distal femoral metaphyseal fracture with apex posterior angulation. **C:** This was treated with closed reduction and percutaneous pinning and application of a cast. **D:** This lateral radiograph shows satisfactory alignment with the pins in place.

(*continues*)

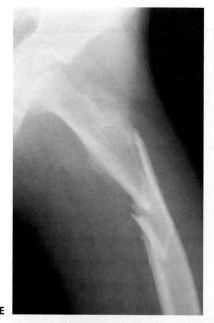

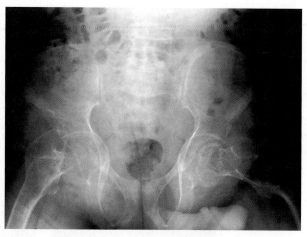

Figure 6-29. (*Continued*) **E:** A few months later, he sustained a left proximal femoral fracture, which was treated with a spica cast. **F:** This anteroposterior pelvic radiograph taken 3 years later shows healed proximal femoral fractures with varus angulation and severe osteopenia of the pelvis and femora with profusion of both acetabuli.

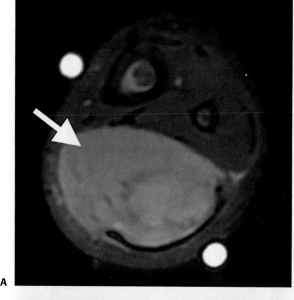

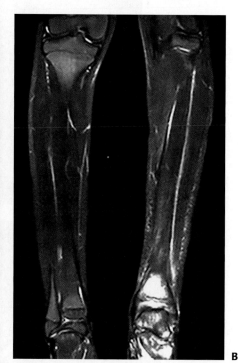

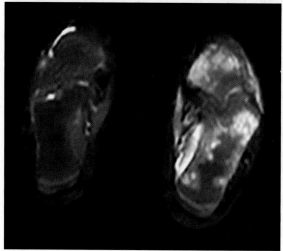

Figure 6-30. A: An 8-year-old boy who was diagnosed with a large alveolar rhabdomyosarcoma of the calf (*arrow*), as shown in the axial T1 MRI, was treated with chemotherapy, radiation, and surgical resection. **B, C:** At the end of treatment, he presented with increasing pain the affected ankle and foot area, and MRI showed increased signal changes and edema consistent with an insufficiency fracture of the distal tibia and calcaneus. (Reproduced with permission from CHOP Orthopaedics, Philadelphia, PA.)

different: truncal obesity, short stature, a lowered hairline, acne, weakness, emotional lability, hirsutism, cutaneous striae, hypertension, and ecchymosis.

Radiographic findings may include severe osteopenia and a delayed bone age. Fractures of the ribs, vertebrae, and long bones have been reported in children with Cushing syndrome.[161] Single cortisol value at midnight, followed by overnight high-dosage dexamethasone test leads to rapid and accurate confirmation and diagnostic differentiation, respectively, of hypercortisolemia caused by pituitary and adrenal tumors.[27]

The primary treatment of Cushing syndrome of childhood is total adrenalectomy.[161] The associated fractures usually can be treated with standard immobilization techniques, but care should be taken not to increase the extent of osteopenia through excessive immobilization. In patients taking steroids, dose modification is attempted when possible. Also, children and adolescents who have Cushing syndrome may have significant alterations in body composition that result in a small but significant decrease in bone mass and increase in visceral adiposity. Long-term monitoring of body fat and bone mass should be mandatory after treatment.[150]

SCURVY

Scurvy occurs in children who eat inadequate amounts of fresh fruit or vegetables leading to depletion in vitamin C. It takes up to 6 to 12 months before symptoms arise, and those may include asthenia, vascular purpura, bleeding, and gum abnormalities. In 80% of cases, the manifestations of scurvy include musculoskeletal symptoms consisting of arthralgia, myalgia, hemarthrosis, and muscular hematomas.[84] Because vitamin C

is essential for normal collagen formation, deficiency results in defective osteogenesis, vascular breakdown, delayed healing, and wound dehiscence. Children may experience severe lower limb pain related to subperiosteal bleeding. Although scurvy is often caused by a dietary deficiency of vitamin C,[174] both aspirin and phenytoin are associated with decreased plasma levels of ascorbic acid. Vitamin C deficiency may also be present in myelomeningocele, although its contribution to fracture in that population is unclear. Infants with scurvy may present with irritability, lower extremity tenderness, weakness, pseudoparalysis, and possibly bleeding gums (if teeth have erupted). Subperiosteal hemorrhages may exist as well as hemorrhage into the subcutaneous tissues, muscles, urinary system, and gastrointestinal tract.

Radiographs may show osteolysis, joint space loss, osteonecrosis, osteopenia, and/or periosteal proliferation. Trabecular and cortical osteoporosis is common. Profound demineralization is evident. In advanced disease, the long bones become almost transparent with a ground-glass appearance and extreme thinning of the cortex. Calcium accumulates in the zone of provisional calcification adjacent to the physis and becomes densely white (Fränkel line). Fractures generally occur in the scurvy line (Trummerfeld zone)—the radiolucent juxtaepiphyseal area above Fränkel line where the matrix is not converted to bone. Dense lateral spurs, known as the Pelken sign, may be seen. A characteristic finding of scurvy is the corner sign in which a peripheral metaphyseal defect exists where fibrous tissue replaces absorbed cortex and cartilage. The epiphysis becomes ringed with a thin, dense line (Wimberger sign). The periosteal elevation caused by hemorrhage calcifies within 10 days of treatment with vitamin C (Fig. 6-31).

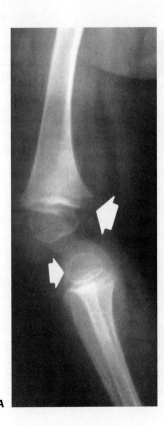
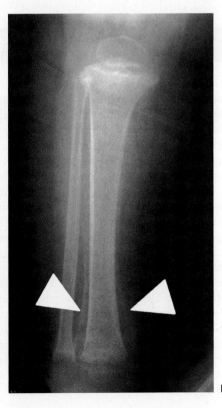

Figure 6-31. Scurvy. **A:** A 10-month-old boy presented with a 2-week history of refusal to walk with tenderness of the lower extremities. He had a history of milk and cereal intake only. There are signs of scurvy in the metaphysis (*large arrow*). The dense white line in the zone of the provisional calcification of the distal femur is known as the Fränkel line. The radiolucent juxtaepiphyseal line above the white line is known as the scurvy line. The peripheral metaphyseal defect, where fibrous tissue replaces absorbed cortex in cartilage, is known as the corner sign. Wimberger sign is a thin, dense line surrounding the epiphysis (*small arrow*). **B:** This is a child with healing scurvy. There is marked periosteal calcification around the distal tibia (*arrowheads*).

(continues)   **A**    **B**

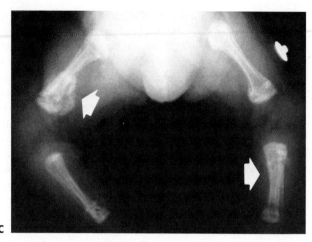

C

Figure 6-31. (*Continued*) **C:** A newborn with scurvy. Periosteal hemorrhage has become calcified in the bones of the lower extremity (*arrows*). (Courtesy of Bruce Mewborne, MD.)

The most common sites of fracture, in the order of frequency, are the distal femur, proximal humerus, costochondral junction of the ribs, and distal tibia. Fractures of the long bones generally are nondisplaced metaphyseal buckle fractures with mild angulation. In contrast, marked epiphyseal displacement occurs with a moderate amount of callus present even in untreated patients. Exuberant callus forms once vitamin C is administered. Standard immobilization, with administration of vitamin C, is adequate for most fractures. Remodeling potential is high in these patients. For infants who are older than 12 months of age and have begun weight bearing, spine films are recommended to rule out vertebral fractures.[158]

FRACTURES IN NEUROMUSCULAR DISEASE

Pathologic fractures occur with frequency in children with neuromuscular diseases. While different diagnosis may come with different predisposing factors, most neuromuscular diseases share a few characteristics that may lead to osteopenia and osteoporosis and pathologic fractures; among these are decreased ambulation, disease, joint contractures, comorbidities such as seizures, nutritional depletion, kidney disease, etc.

The main goal of treating pathologic fractures in this group of patients is to return them to their prefracture level of activity, minimize further osteopenia, and recover motion and ambulation (if applicable). The second goal is to prevent further fractures. After surgical intervention for deformities or contractures, minimizing cast immobilization is important. Foam abduction pillows and knee immobilizers and an intensive therapy program in the immediate postoperative period may avoid the deconditioning, osteopenia, and joint stiffness. For example, in ambulatory children who need hip osteotomies, use of rigid internal fixation allows standing and gait training, prevents not only osteopenia but also the risk that the child may never regain the full level of preoperative function after a prolonged period of cast immobilization.

CEREBRAL PALSY

The main causes of low bone density and osteoporosis in children and adolescents with cerebral palsy (CP) are lack of activity, nutritional (e.g., low vitamin D), and pharmacologic treatments (e.g., anticonvulsant drugs).[190,192,234] The diagnosis may be delayed because patients are often noncommunicative.

The literature points to several predisposing factors, namely GMFCS 5 and 4, presence of hip and knee contractures, and history of seizures and spasticity. The incidence of fractures varies from 4% to 14%.[192,234] Most fractures involve the lower extremities, especially the midshaft femur.[149,192]

While fractures in patients with cerebral palsy heal quickly with abundant callus, the challenges include a high rate of malunion (better tolerated in nonambulators) and around 20% risk of refracture. Closed treatment of these fractures is often preferred, but it can be complicated by the development of decubitus ulcers, or other skin issues. If a long-leg cast is used for a fracture of the lower extremity and the joint of the involved side is dislocated, the rigid cast may function as a lever arm, with the posterior fracture of the proximal femur beyond the cast.

If the patient is ambulatory, conventional forms of fracture treatment may be used (Fig. 6-32). When indicated, fixation with titanium elastic intramedullary nails can be a very effective way to treat femoral fractures (Fig. 6-33).

Fractures of the distal pole of the patella may occur in spastic ambulators with flexion contractures of the knees, patella alta, and a history of falls. If conservative treatment with extension casting is unsatisfactory, hamstring lengthening with correction of the knee flexion contracture can result in both healing of the fracture and relief of symptoms.

In a randomized controlled trial of standing program impact on bone mineral density in GMFCS 5 patients, participation in 50% longer periods of standing improved vertebral but not tibial bone density. The authors concluded that such intervention might reduce the risk of vertebral fractures but is unlikely to reduce the risk of lower limb fractures in children with CP.[51] The use of pamidronate has been shown to decrease the incidence of fractures in this population.

MYELOMENINGOCELE

Children with myelomeningocele are at a high risk of pathologic fractures of the lower extremities due to decreased bone mineral density from disuse, immobilization after reconstructive surgery, altered gait mechanics, decreased sensation (including protective sensation), and nephropathy (increased urinary calcium loss).[73,156,233] The incidence of fractures ranges from 12% to 31%. An important risk factor is the level of disease; myelomeningocele has a higher incidence (around 40%) than lower levels (10% for low lumbar/sacral levels).[156] The locations of these fractures, in the order of decreasing frequency, are midshaft of the femur, distal femur, midshaft of the tibia, proximal femur, femoral neck, distal femoral physis, and proximal tibia. Fractures tend to heal rapidly, except for physeal fractures, and nonunion is rare.[75,233]

Physeal fractures in patients with myelomeningocele may mimic infection, with elevated temperature and swelling, redness, and local warmth at the fracture site.[73,197,232] Both the white blood cell count and erythrocyte sedimentation rate are often elevated. Immobilization of these injuries usually results in a dramatic decrease in swelling and redness of the extremity within a few days. With healing, the radiographic picture can be alarming, with epiphyseal plate widening, metaphyseal fracture, and periosteal elevation. The radiographic differential diagnoses should include osteomyelitis, sarcoma, leukemia, and Charcot joint.[81] Recurrent trauma to the physis, from either

continued walking or passive joint motion after injury, results in an exuberant healing reaction (Fig. 6-34). Physeal fractures require lengthy immobilization with strict avoidance of weight bearing to avoid destructive repetitive trauma to the physis.[81]

Conservative treatment is best done with well-padded immobilization to avoid pressure sore and limited length to avoid further osteopenia.[156] In nonambulatory patients, mild malunion and shortening can be tolerated, and stable or minimally angulated fractures can be treated with either polyurethane splints

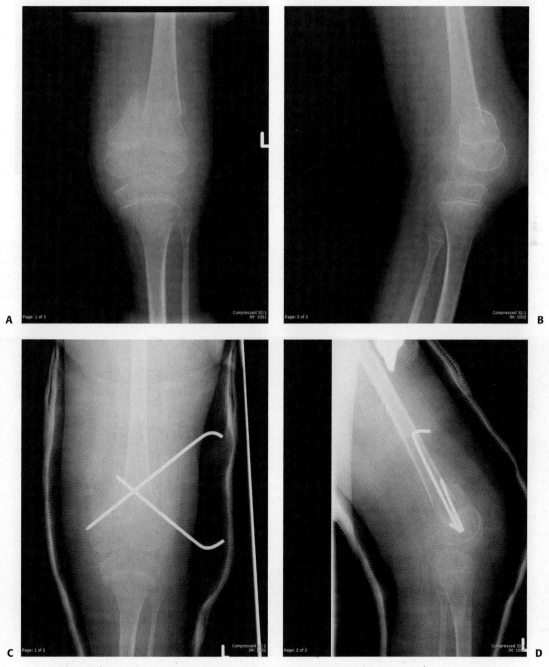

Figure 6-32. A, B: An 11-year-old boy with total body involvement cerebral palsy was receiving physical therapy when he developed pain and swelling around the left knee. Radiographs showed displaced femoral supracondylar fracture. **C, D:** To be able to fit to the brace adequately, closed reduction and percutaneous pinning were performed.

(continues)

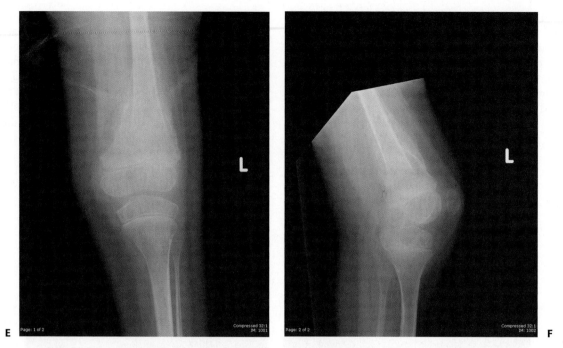

Figure 6-32. (*Continued*) **E, F:** The fracture healed in good alignment and the pins were removed after 6 weeks. (Reproduced with permission from The Children's Orthopaedic Center, Los Angeles, CA.)

or Webril dressings. In children who walk, fractures should be carefully aligned with heavily padded casts that allow continued protective weight bearing, if possible. Operative fixation may be associated with a high rate of infection, and it should also be noted that the incidence of latex allergy and malignant hyperthermia is higher in patients with myelomeningocele than in other children.[15,156] Between 18% and 40% of children with myelodysplasia are allergic to latex.[3] Any patient considered for operative intervention should be treated prophylactically with latex-free gloves and equipment.

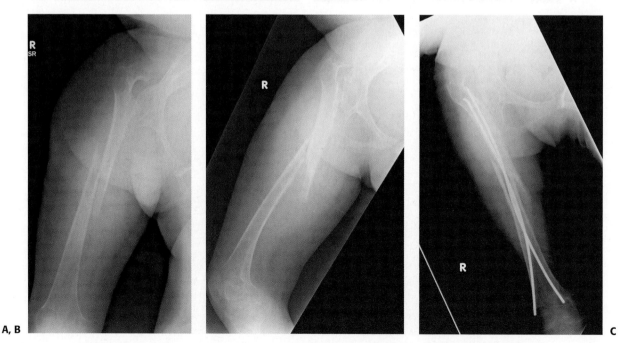

Figure 6-33. A 12-year-old girl with cerebral palsy and in-house-walking capabilities had an unwitnessed trauma to the right thigh, developing pain and deformity. **A, B:** Radiographs showed a displaced fracture of the femoral shaft. The patient underwent closed reduction, followed by titanium elastic nail fixation. **C, D:** At 6-week follow-up, there was abundant callus formation. (Reproduced with permission from The Children's Orthopaedic Center, Los Angeles, CA.)

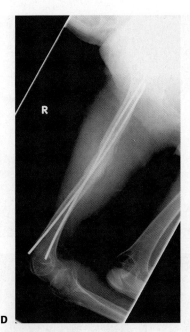

Figure 6-33. *(Continued)*

MUSCULAR DYSTROPHY

The main goal treating fractures of the lower extremity in children with Duchenne's muscular dystrophy is to avoid premature loss of the ability to walk or transfer.[113,163] In patients 9 to 10 years old, increasing muscle weakness and joint contractures contribute to falls, and a loss of normal muscle bulk and fat limit the cushioning on impact. Patients in lower extremity braces seem to sustain fewer fractures in falls, probably because the overlying orthoses provide some protection. Patients confined to a wheelchair can fall because they have poor sitting balance, and fractures are frequent because these patients are more osteoporotic than ambulatory individuals.

While corticosteroid therapy improves longevity, walking ability, and quality of life of children with Duchenne's, it also increases the rate of osteoporosis and risk of fracture.[29,129] Fractures tend to heal rapidly. The most commonly fractured bone is the femur, followed by the proximal humerus.

When ambulatory ability is tenuous, even minor bruises or ankle sprains may end walking ability. As little as 1 week in a wheelchair can prematurely end ambulation; patients at bed rest for more than 2 weeks will likely lose the ability to ambulate.[163] The patient should be mobilized as soon as possible in a lightweight cast or orthosis. Load-sharing devices, such as intramedullary nails, allow earlier weight bearing and are preferred over other methods of internal fixation (Fig. 6-35). Aggressive physical therapy should be used to maintain functional status.

ARTHROGRYPOSIS

Arthrogryposis is a group of rare and heterogeneous disorders affecting children in whom there are at least two or more joint contractures in multiple body areas, with an incidence of 3 in 10,000 live births.[238] Although the etiology is unknown and

likely multifactorial, there is a lack of fetal joint movement after initial normal development, leading to collagen proliferation, fibrotic replacement of muscle, a marked thickening of joint capsules, taut ligaments, and capsular tightness resulting in joint stiffness.[117] Dislocations can occur with severe shortening of the involved muscles.

Fractures may occur in 25% of infants with arthrogryposis.[70] Clinical symptoms included poor feeding, irritability, and fussiness when handled. The involved extremity was thickened, and there was often an increased white blood cell count. Short-term immobilization is adequate to treat nondisplaced fractures in these patients (Fig. 6-36). Postnatal fractures are most common in patients with either knee contracture or dislocation of the hip, and postnatal injury could possibly be reduced by avoidance of forceful manipulation of these extremities. Older patients with lower extremity contractures do not seem to have increased risk for pathologic fractures.

THE ORTHOPEDIC RECOGNITION OF CHILD MALTREATMENT

Child maltreatment is any act or failure to act on the part of a parent or caretaker which results in death, serious physical or emotional harm, sexual abuse or exploitation, or an act or failure to act which presents an imminent risk of serious harm.[5] Child maltreatment includes all types of abuse and neglect that occur among children under the age of 18 years.[193] The four common types of maltreatment include physical, sexual, and emotional abuse as well as child neglect.[115] Maltreatment can be acute or chronic over a number of years, with worse outcomes when inflicted over a number of years with multiple events.[118] Neglect is the most frequently encountered type of child maltreatment. Psychological maltreatment is increasingly recognized to be as harmful as other types of maltreatment.[106] Recent terminology for a battered child, physical abuse, or child abuse includes child maltreatment, NAI, inflicted injury, or nonaccidental trauma (NAT).[87]

Child abuse has been recognized as a legitimate medical and social issue for many decades. General public awareness of child abuse increased with the 1962 publication of a report by Kempe et al.[127] characterizing the problems as the battered-child syndrome. In 1974, Congress acknowledged the national importance of the prevention of child abuse by the passage of the Child Abuse Prevention and Treatment Act.[5] Because all health care professionals must be aware of reporting requirements for child maltreatment, there are recommendations for the establishment and management of hospital-based child multidiscipline collegial protection teams.[130]

EPIDEMIOLOGY

The National Child Abuse and Neglect Data System (NCANDS) was initiated in response to Public Law 93–247 to collect and analyze child abuse statistics.[5] NCANDS documents that the epidemic of child abuse continues to worsen in the United States, with approximately 3.4 million reports

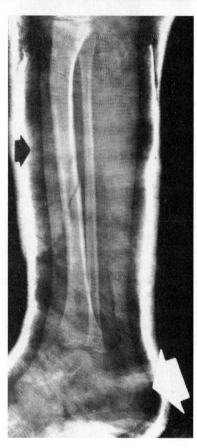

Figure 6-34. A 10-year-old boy with low-lumbar spina bifida and community ambulation (with braces) presented with chronic bilateral leg/ankle pain. Anteroposterior (**A, C**) and lateral (**B, D**) radiographs of both tibia and fibula show stress/insufficiency fracture of the distal tibial physis associated with extensive periosteal bone formation, characteristic of myelomeningocele.

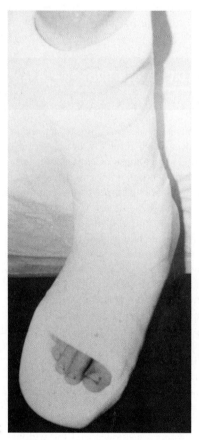

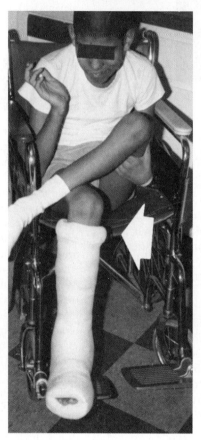

filed in federal fiscal year 2015 compared to 1.2 million in 1982.[6] Approximately, one-fifth (17.3%) of these children who received an investigation were confirmed to have been abused or neglected. This represents a victim rate of 9.2 per 1,000.[6] Approximately 60% of confirmed cases are neglect, 16% physical abuse, 10% sexual abuse, and 7% psychological abuse.[193] While children under the age of 4 years are at greatest risk for maltreatment, the victim rate is highest for infants, 24.2 per infant children. Abuse is second only to sudden infant death syndrome (SIDS) for mortality in infants 1 to 6 months of age and second only to accidental injury in children older than 1 year. Up to 11% of infants treated in

the emergency room for apparent life-threatening events are later confirmed to be victims of child abuse.[39] The incidence of abuse is three times that of developmental dysplasia of the hip or clubfoot.

The orthopedist becomes involved in the care of 30% to 50% of abused children.[12] Early recognition by the orthopedist is critical because children returned to their homes after an unrecognized episode of child abuse have a 25% risk of serious reinjury and a 5% risk of death.[201] However, orthopedic surgeons, especially those more experienced, do not always try to determine the underlying cause of the child's symptoms.[226] Jenny and Isaac have noted a threefold increased mortality rate

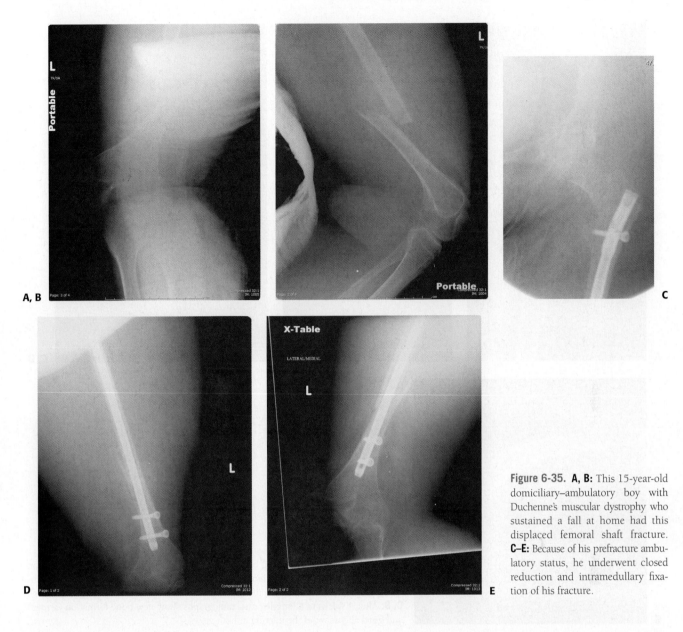

Figure 6-35. A, B: This 15-year-old domiciliary–ambulatory boy with Duchenne's muscular dystrophy who sustained a fall at home had this displaced femoral shaft fracture. **C–E:** Because of his prefracture ambulatory status, he underwent closed reduction and intramedullary fixation of his fracture.

of children who have been listed on state abuse registry for all types of abuse.[116] The mortality rate is highest for those who are physically abused, especially infants.[116]

THE RISK FACTORS FOR CHILD ABUSE

THE HOME AT RISK

In assessing where child abuse may occur, households in turmoil from marital separation, job loss, divorce, family death, housing difficulties, or financial difficulties are more likely to have abusive episodes.[76] Compared to single parent families, death caused by child abuse was noted to be 50 times higher in households that had unrelated adults; the perpetrator was the unrelated adult in 83.9% of these cases.[202] Parental substance abuse, whether alcohol or other drugs, makes child abuse more

likely.[102] Although the youngest, poorest, most socially isolated, and economically frustrated caretakers are the most likely to act violently toward their children, any adult from any social or economic level may abuse a child.[12] Day care may be an at-risk environment in situations where there is poor supervision of the child caregivers. Primary parental predictors of child abuse are listed in (Table 6-4).

THE CHILD AT RISK

Most reported cases of child abuse involve children younger than 3 years of age.[28,89] In one report of abused children,[28] 78% of all fractures reported were in children younger than 3 years of age and 50% of all fractures occurred in children younger than 1 year of age. Infants younger than 1 year are especially at risk for infant homicide, the most severe form of child abuse.[136] An infant may present to the emergency room dead or near-dead after an apparent "brief resolved

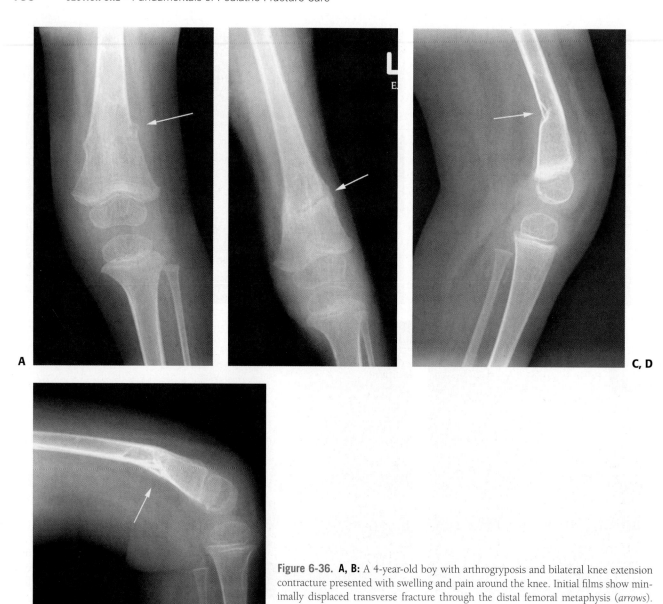

Figure 6-36. A, B: A 4-year-old boy with arthrogryposis and bilateral knee extension contracture presented with swelling and pain around the knee. Initial films show minimally displaced transverse fracture through the distal femoral metaphysis (*arrows*). **C, D:** After 4 weeks in a long-leg cast, radiographs show new bone formation (*arrows*) and good alignment of the fracture in both views.

unexplained event" which was previously termed "life-threatening event."[243] In these cases, it is important to be open to all diagnostic possibilities and use a multidisciplinary team approach to the evaluation.[176] Possible explanations for these events include SIDS, metabolic disease, cardiac disease, infection, as well as accidental or nonaccidental suffocation. Firstborn children, premature infants, stepchildren, and disabled children are at a greater risk for child abuse, as are twins and children of multiple births.[28] Up to 25% to 83% of children with a disability have been reported to be abused.[223] Physically abused children have a one in six chance of being sexually abused, whereas sexually abused children have a one in seven risk of being physically abused.[107]

Children who have experienced neglect or abuse or have been exposed to toxic stress, frequently have major health or behavior problems later in life, into adulthood.[206]

OBTAINING THE HISTORY

The history is critical in the diagnosis of child abuse, which is a team effort with the consulting pediatrician, social worker and other personnel from the hospital's child protective team, child protective services worker, law enforcement, and the appropriate consulting service. It is critical to inquire of the parent or caretaker if the information being provided is firsthand observation or secondhand recollection of another person. Physicians infrequently inquire about basic historic information such as the timing of the injury and who were the witnesses.[16]

When involved, the orthopedic surgeon performs a detailed musculoskeletal history and physical examination to characterize the features and mechanism of the obvious injury and to discover evidence of additional undocumented injuries. A delay

TABLE 6-4. Parental Predictors of Child Abuse

General

- Unrelated adult living in the home[a]
- Parent history of child abuse
- Divorce or separation of mother's parents
- Maternal history of being separated from mother, parental alcohol, or drug abuse
- Maternal history of depression
- Child attends a home day care

Mother

- Age less than 20 yrs
- Lower educational achievement
- History of sexual abuse
- Child guidance issues
- Absent father during childhood
- History of psychiatric illness

Father

- Age less than 20 yrs
- Lower educational achievement
- Child guidance issues
- History of psychiatric illness

[a]Fifty times the risk of death during infancy because of nonaccidental trauma.
Adapted from Sidebotham P, Golding J. The ALSPAC Study Team. Child maltreatment in the "Children of the Nineties"—a longitudinal study of parental risk factors. *Child Abuse Negl.* 2001;25(9):1177–1200. Copyright © 2001 Elsevier Science Inc. With permission.

in seeking medical care for an injured child is very suggestive of child abuse.[76] An infant who has sustained abusive head trauma (AHT) typically will develop immediate neurologic change and will invariably show symptoms within a few hours.

To make the diagnosis of child abuse, the orthopedic surgeon or child abuse team must determine if the history of trauma is adequate to explain the severity of injury.[53] This should be based on the experience in the care of fractures with knowledge of their mechanisms of injury and special insight into the types of trauma most likely to cause significant injury. We advise consultation with child abuse pediatricians for assistance matching the mechanism of the injury to the child's developmental abilities and family situation.

Details given as the reason for the injury should be carefully considered. Although it is not unusual for a young child to sustain an accidental fall, it is unusual to sustain a serious injury from that fall alone. Infants fall from a bed or a raised surface during a diaper change fairly frequently. A major injury or cluster of injuries in such falls is, however, extremely rare.[147] In another report, a much higher rate of fracture was seen in older children "falling" from furniture with 98% having fractures, mostly in the upper extremity, because of the child catapulting during play activity rather than sustaining a simple short-height fall.[103] More severe injuries occur with falls from greater heights. Stairway falls usually result in low-energy injuries, but there is increased risk of injury if the child is being carried by the caregiver. In a report of 363 stairway injuries,[127] 10 were infants who were dropped by their caretakers and four of those sustained skull fractures. In patients 6 months to 1 year of age, 60% were using walkers at the time of the stairway injury. Only 4% of patients had extremity fractures and 1% had

skull fractures. Reported short-height falls (<1.5 m) are rarely documented to cause death,[52] and fatally injured child from a reported short-height fall at home must receive expert postmortem investigation for child abuse.[8]

PHYSICAL EXAMINATION

After the initial musculoskeletal evaluation for acute fracture assessment, a detailed physical examination should follow, systematically evaluating from head to toes, to detect any signs of additional acute or chronic injury. Careful evaluation for signs of previous injury is useful because 50% of verified abuse cases show evidence of prior abuse. Acute and subacute fractures may cause local tenderness and swelling, whereas chronic fractures may produce swelling from the presence of callus and clinical deformity from malunion. Radiographs are obtained to confirm clinically suspected fractures. A skeletal survey must be performed in children under 2 years of age when there is reasonable suspicion of abuse,[1] and it should be considered an extension of the physical examination for this age group. A thorough examination should focus on the body areas commonly involved in child abuse including the skin, CNS, abdomen, and genitalia.[181]

SOFT TISSUE INJURIES

The child's entire body should be systematically evaluated to detect acute and chronic soft tissue trauma and is one of the most important physical findings to observe and to document. Sentinel injuries to observe and to document include the external ear for bruising, the eye for subconjunctival hemorrhage, and the tongue for tearing of the frenulum. Identification of sentinel injuries, such as rib fractures, abdominal trauma, or intracranial hemorrhage indicates abuse in more than 20%.[154] Soft tissue injuries are present in 81% to 92% of abused patients,[89,164] making them the most common abuse-related physical examination finding. The types of skin lesions commonly encountered include bruises, welts, abrasions, lacerations, scars, and burns.

Approximately 17% of mobile infants, 53% of toddlers, and most school children have bruises that aren't related to abuse.[160] Infants under 5 months of age have a much lower prevalence of accidental bruising (1.3%) compared to older infants (6.4%) or mobile toddlers.[160] Accidental bruises in babies are also typically noted over bony prominences.[48] The toddler may have multiple accidental bruises over bony prominences such as the chin, brow, knees, and shins.[201,222] Bruises on the back of the head, neck, arms, legs, buttocks, abdomen, cheeks, or genitalia may be suspicious for abuse.[12] Although any number of bruises may be present in any child, the location and configuration of the bruises and the mobility of the child, taken together with the rest of the medical and social history determine the suspicion for abuse (Fig. 6-37, Table 6-5). Photographs taken to document skin lesions must be done before cast placement, especially large spica casts.

BURNS

Burns are found in approximately 20% of abused patients[89] and are most likely to occur in patients younger than 3 years of

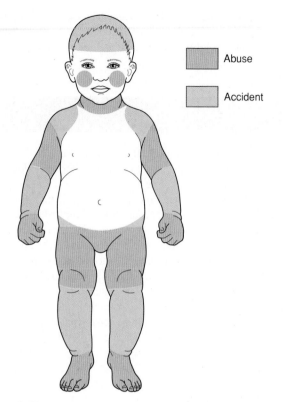

Figure 6-37. Schematic illustrates distribution of abusive versus accidental bruising. (Redrawn from original, courtesy of Samir Abedin, MD.)

age.[164] Scalds are the most frequent type of abusive burns and are caused either by a spill or an immersion.[144] Accidental spill burns are generally located on the trunk and proximal upper extremities (Fig. 6-38). Most accidental pour or spill burns occur on the front of the child, but accidental burns can also occur on the back as well. In accidental flowing liquid burns, the injury usually has an arrowhead configuration in which the burn becomes shallower and narrower as it moves downward, and there may be splash marks surrounding the lesion.[111] The pattern in accidental burns may also be indicative of flowing water.[208] Abuse should

---

TABLE 6-5. Evaluating Bruising in a Child—Implications for Practice

A bruise must never be interpreted in isolation and must always be assessed in the context of medical and social history, developmental stage, explanation given, full clinical examination, and relevant investigations.

Patterns of bruising that are suggestive of physical child abuse:
- Bruising in children who are not independently mobile
- Bruising in infants under 1 yr of age
- Bruises that are seen away from bony prominences
- Bruises to the face, back, abdomen, arms, buttocks, ears, hands
- Multiple bruises in clusters
- Multiple bruises of uniform shape
- Bruises that carry the imprint of implement used or a ligature

Adapted from Maguire S, Mann MK, Sibert J, et al. Are there patterns of bruising in childhood which are diagnostic or suggestive of abuse? A systematic review. *Arch Dis Child.* 2005;90(2):182–186, with permission from BMJ Publishing Group Ltd.

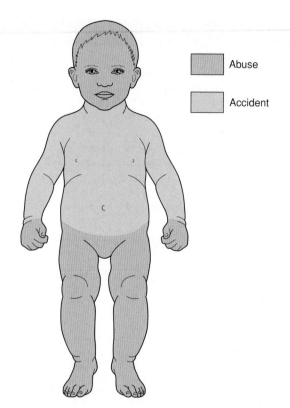

Figure 6-38. Schematic illustrates location of accidental versus abusive burns. Note the buttock and lower extremity distribution of nonaccidental immersion burns compared to thoracic distribution accidental burns. (Redrawn from original, courtesy of Samir Abedin, MD.)

be suspected when deep second- or third-degree burns are well demarcated with circumferential definition. Since burns are frequently intentional and are associated with evidence of previous abuse such as rib fractures, skeletal survey should be obtained on burned children less than 2 years of age.[83]

In accidental hot water immersion, an indistinct stocking or glove configuration may be seen with varying burn depths and indistinct margins. In deliberate immersion burns such as occurs when a child's buttocks are immersed in hot water, the burn demarcation has uniform depth and a well-demarcated water line.[111] The gluteal crease of the buttocks may be spared, giving a doughnut-like appearance to the burn. In accidental hot water immersion, the child is uniformly scalded about the lower extremities as the legs are quickly extended by the child to climb out of the water, but in deliberate, abusive immersion the child is lowered into the water and instinctively flexes the hips and knees, thus sparing the popliteal area.[89]

FRACTURES IN CHILD ABUSE

OVERVIEW

After skin lesions, fractures are the second most common physical presentation of abuse. The child abuse literature shows varying incidence of abuse-related fractures, depending on the age of the study population, institution, study entry criteria, selection bias, and time period when the study was published.[152] The younger the child with a fracture, especially under 18 months of age, the more likely abuse is the cause.[58,60,126] Particularly concerning is a bone that fractures under tension with torsion, rather than the physiologic loading of compression of normal childhood activity or falls. Pierce et al.[189] recommend that the clinician determines if the observed injury of a long bone and the stated mechanism are consistent (Table 6-6).

Kleinman ranked the specificity of skeletal fractures for abuse based on the location and type of fracture (Table 6-7).[131] He emphasized that both moderate and low specificity radiographic findings become more specific when there is an inadequate or inconsistent explanation for the injury. The location and the type of fracture can aid in distinguishing between an accident and child abuse, but is only one piece of information.

All types of fractures have been reported in the child abuse literature, and it is often the presence of multiple fractures that indicates NAT (Fig. 6-39, Table 6-8). King et al.[128] reported 429 fractures in 189 abused children. Fifty percent of these patients had a single fracture, and 17% had more than three fractures. Approximately 60% of fractures were found in roughly equal numbers in the humerus, femur, and tibia. Fractures also occurred in the radius, skull, spine, ribs, ulna, and fibula, in order of decreasing frequency. Another study found a similar incidence of fractures of the humerus, femur, and tibia in abused children, with skull fractures seen in 14%.[181] In contrast, Akbarnia et al.[10] found that rib fractures in abused patients were twice as prevalent as fractures of any one long bone; the next most frequently fractured bone was the humerus, followed by the femur and the tibia.

TABLE 6-6. Considerations When Evaluating a Child With a Long-Bone Fracture

1. What are the biodynamics of the injury event, the energies generated by the event, and how could certain factors of the injury environment contribute to the likelihood of injury?
2. What injuries are expected, and what is the likelihood that the event generated the specific load required to cause each and all of the injuries?
3. Did the energy of the event exceed the injury threshold, or was there a biologic abnormality such as decreased bone density that resulted in a lowering of the actual threshold for injury? Is there evidence of bone weakness or disease?
4. Is the fracture morphology consistent with the direction, magnitude, and rate of loading of the described mechanism?
5. Is the fracture pattern unusual, and one that requires an extremely unusual loading condition, as is the case with a classic metaphyseal lesion (also termed corner or bucket-handle fracture)?
6. What are the child's developmental capabilities, and could the child have generated the necessary energy independent of "outside" forces to cause the observed injury?
7. Does the fracture reflect a high-energy fracture? Did the event generate enough energy to cause a high-energy fracture? Or is the fracture a small cortical defect, or hairline crack, reflecting a smaller amount of energy required for propagation of the fracture type?
8. What regions of the bone have been injured and what are the structural components that affect the ultimate pattern of fracture that is being observed? Were there structural factors that contributed to the likelihood of fracture?

Adapted from Pierce MC, Bertocci GE, Vogeley E, et al. Evaluating long bone fractures in children: a biomechanical approach with illustrative cases. *Child Abuse Negl.* 2004;28(5):505–524.

TABLE 6-7. Specificity of Skeletal Trauma for Abuse[131]

High Specificity
- Classic metaphyseal lesions
- Posterior rib fracture
- Scapular fracture
- Spinous process fracture
- Sternal fracture

Moderate Specificity
- Multiple fractures, especially bilateral
- Fractures in various stages of healing
- Epiphyseal separation
- Vertebral body fracture or subluxation
- Digital fracture
- Complex skull fracture

Low Specificity
- Clavicular fracture
- Long-bone shaft fracture
- Linear skull fracture

Adapted from Pierce MC, Bertocci GE, Vogeley E, et al. Evaluating long bone fractures in children: A biomechanical approach with illustrative cases. *Child Abuse Negl.* 2004;28(5):505–524. Copyright © 2004 Elsevier Ltd. With permission.

Nearly a third of these patients had skull fractures. In a classic study of 31 postmortem infants, the fracture pattern was very different from clinical studies in living children.[137]

THE SKELETAL SURVEY

In addition to standard radiographic studies of the acute injury, a complete skeletal survey should be used to screen for additional fractures in all children younger than age 2 years when abuse is suspected.[1,125] Use of the skeletal survey in children suspected of abuse yielded positive findings in 10.8% of cases, most commonly in children with AHT, a life-threatening event, and in infants under 6 months of age in which the physical examination was less reliable.[77] Besides the index child, children under the age of 2 years in the same household of the injured abused child have an 11.9% risk of a positive skeletal survey, so are also recommended to have a skeletal survey.[155] A suspected metaphyseal lesion of the extremity is more likely to be detected when a lateral view is done in addition to the AP view.[122] Lateral views coned to the joints may help in diagnosing classic metaphyseal lesions (CMLs). Lateral views of the entire spine must always be included in the skeletal survey. Bilateral oblique views of the thorax are for the diagnosis of subtle rib fractures.[125] A "baby gram" has no place in diagnosing fractures of child abuse because the obliquity of the angle at which the radiographs transverse the skeleton may obscure many subtle fractures.[1] The standard views obtained on a skeletal survey recommended by the American College of Radiology[4] for imaging suspected child abuse in children less than 2 years of age with a low effective radiation dose of only 0.2 mSv[33,215] are listed in Table 6-9. Follow-up skeletal survey at 2 weeks increases the diagnosis of occult fractures, because some fractures, especially of the ribs, may not be seen until callus appears at 10 to 14 days. The second look skeletal survey better defines the fracture seen on the original survey and may help determine the age of the fracture.[125] Kleinman et al.[139] reported

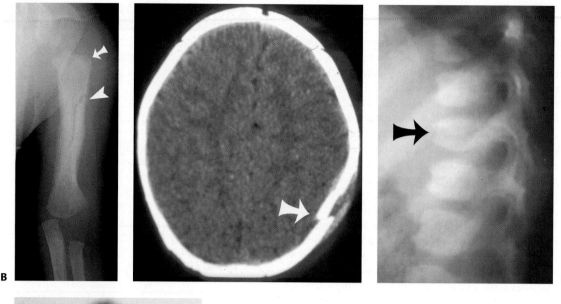

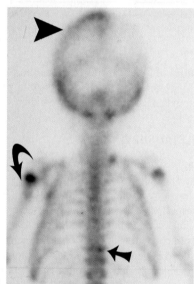

Figure 6-39. Multiple fractures in a 3-month-old female victim of inflicted injury. **A:** Frontal radiograph of the humerus shows proximal metaphyseal irregularity consistent with a corner fracture (*arrow*) and an oblique diaphyseal fracture with extensive periosteal reaction and healing (*arrowhead*). **B:** Axial CT image reveals a depressed left calvarial fracture (*arrow*). **C:** Lateral thoracolumbar radiograph suggests a T12 compression fracture (*arrow*), which is confirmed on nuclear bone scintigraphy (**D**) as a region of increased uptake (*arrow*). Bone scan also confirms left parietal (*arrowhead*) and humeral (*curved arrow*) fractures.

TABLE 6-8. Pearls and Pitfalls of Nonaccidental Trauma

- Be particularly cautious of a young infant with an injury.
- It is unusual for a young child to sustain a life-threatening injury from a fall alone, and he or she is highly unlikely to die from a short-height fall.
- Ask to describe in detail the mechanism of the injury and make sure that it is consistent with the observed injury. However, a parent may not have witnessed the injury or was distracted while it was occurring.
- Multiple rib fractures, fractures in various stages of healing, and classic metaphyseal fractures are highly specific.
- Injury mechanism stated by the parents should agree with the type and energy of the fracture.
- Failure to diagnose child abuse may result in 25% risk of repeat abuse and 5% chance of death.
- Concerning bruises and skin lesions are the most common presentation of abuse. However, the child with such bruises should receive a proper evaluation for bleeding disorder.
- Unexplained fractures are much more likely to represent abuse and not a rare disease such as osteogenesis imperfecta (OI). Always consider OI when multiple fractures are seen.
- Obtain skeletal survey in all children younger than 2 yr olds, and individualize for 2–5 yr olds when child abuse is suspected. Repeat in 2 wks.
- Involve the hospital child protective team early in the evaluation.
- Prepare records as though everything will be reviewed and read in court.

TABLE 6-9. Complete Skeletal Survey Table

Appendicular Skeleton
- Humeri (AP)
- Forearms (AP)
- Hands (PA)
- Femurs (AP)
- Lower legs (AP)
- Feet (AP)

Axial Skeleton
- Thorax (AP, lateral, right and left obliques), to include ribs, thoracic and upper lumbar spine
- Pelvis (AP), to include the mid lumbar spine
- Lumbosacral spine (lateral)
- Cervical spine (lateral)
- Skull (frontal and lateral)

Adapted from American Academy of Pediatrics. Section on Radiology. Diagnostic imaging of child abuse. *Pediatrics*. 2000;105(6):1345–1348.

that a follow-up skeletal survey 2 weeks after the initial series detected 27% more fractures and provided assistance in dating 20% of previously detected fractures. Fractures or questionable fractures diagnosed on the initial screening skeletal survey should be reimaged on the follow-up survey. Almost 10% of children who sustained suspected abuse have a normal initial skeletal survey, but have significant findings on a 2-week follow-up survey.[31,100] The sensitivity of skeletal surveys diminishes in patients older than 2 years of age. They have less value for children older than age 5 years because the older child can describe where the pain is located. For children between the ages of 2 and 5 years, the test should be individualized.[1]

DATING FRACTURES

Radiographic proof of unexplained fractures in various stages of healing is believed to be strong evidence of child abuse (Fig. 6-40).[10] The orthopedist often is asked to determine the age of fractures with some certainty to corroborate a history

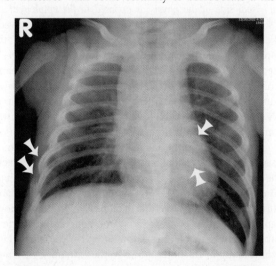

Figure 6-40. Rib fractures in multiple stages of healing in a 4-month-old female victim of nonaccidental injury. Frontal chest radiograph reveals acute (no periosteal reaction or healing) and subacute/healing (positive periosteal reaction) rib fractures (*arrows*).

of injury given by caretakers. Experienced orthopedists and radiologists can roughly estimate the age range of fractures by their radiographic appearance and their experience reading many radiographs of known dated injuries. There is limited evidence-based data for accurately predicting the age of healing fractures.[193] In a review of studies that met minimal evidence-based inclusion criteria, the following conclusions were reached: The science of fracture dating is inexact and periosteal reaction is seen as early as 4 days and is present in at least 50% of cases by 2 weeks with remodeling peaking at 8 weeks after the fracture. The most difficult fractures to date are those that are completely healed, with substantial remodeling, and often the only sign of a healed fracture is a thickened cortex.

EXTREMITY FRACTURES

There is no predominant pattern of diaphyseal fracture in child abuse. Traditionally, a midshaft spiral fracture such as in the femur was believed to be caused by a violent abusive twisting injury. However, this is not typically the case. However, others found that 71% of diaphyseal fractures were transverse in abused children, indicating a different plausible mechanism.[89] Transverse fractures are most commonly associated with either a violent bending force or a direct blow to the extremities, whereas spiral or oblique fractures of the long bones are caused by axial-loaded, twisting injuries, such as in a fall. Humeral shaft fractures in children under 3 years of age have an 18% risk of being due to probable abuse.[208] In delayed medical care, long-bone fractures may show exuberant callus because of lack of immobilization, and multiple fractures may be present in different stages of healing.[12]

Femur fractures in infants are especially suspicious for NAT; whereas children old enough to run can fall and accidentally fracture their femurs if there is a significant twisting motion at the time of injury.[230] Despite a high likelihood of NAT in an infant with a femoral fracture, an infant with a femur fracture may have accidental trauma as the cause, if the parent's reported mechanism is consistent with the injury. In a recent case series from Alberta, Canada, only 17% of femoral fractures in infants less than 1 year of age were from abuse, whereas the author's review of eight previous reports showed that NAT was the cause for 42% to 93% of cases.[110] As children get older and more active, a femur fracture is more likely to be from accidental injury than from abuse. Schwend et al.[203] reported that while 42% of femoral fractures in infants not walking were related to NAI, only 2.6% of femoral fractures in ambulatory toddlers were related to NAI. Blakemore et al.[37] noted that only 2% of femoral fractures from age 1 to 5 years were caused by abuse. Risk factors for abuse were age younger than 12 months, the child not yet walking, a questionable mechanism, and other associated injuries.

Humeral shaft fractures are frequently seen in NAT (Fig. 6-41). Fractures in unusual locations such as the distal clavicle, scapula, acromial tip, proximal humeral metaphysis, or distal humeral physis may result from violent blows or upper extremity traction injury and are suggestive of abuse in young children.[2] Infants may normally have a separate ossification center adjacent to the tip of the acromion, simulating a fracture[142] but a true fracture has sharp, demarcated edges, may be positive on bone scan, and will show callus or healing.

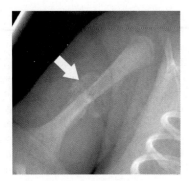

Figure 6-41. Humeral fracture in a 3-week-old boy after a difficult delivery. Radiograph shows a transverse mid diaphyseal fracture with extensive callus (*arrow*).

Fractures of the hands and feet are commonly due to accidental trauma in older children,[167] but are suspicious for abuse in infants. Nimkin et al.[179] reviewed 11 hand and foot fractures in abused children younger than 10 months of age and found mostly torus fractures either of the metacarpals or the proximal phalanges of the hand and similar fractures of the first metatarsals of the feet (Fig. 6-42). These injuries are best seen on the oblique views standard in the skeletal survey.

Metaphyseal and epiphyseal fractures of the long bones are classically associated with child abuse.[45,211] In infants and toddlers, these fractures can occur when the child is violently shaken by the extremities with direct violent traction or rotation of the extremity (see Fig. 6-41).[167] Buckle fractures may occur at multiple sites, seldom producing exuberant callus. Repeated injury may cause irregular metaphyseal deformities. Periosteal avulsion typically produces new bone formation within 2 to 3 weeks of injury and may be confused with osteomyelitis.[12] New bone formation may be delayed, particularly in children with malnutrition or rickets.

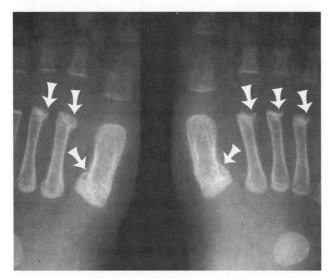

Figure 6-42. Metatarsal fractures in a 2-month-old female victim of nonaccidental trauma. Radiographic image from a skeletal survey shows multiple healing, bilateral, and symmetric proximal and distal metatarsal fractures (*arrows*).

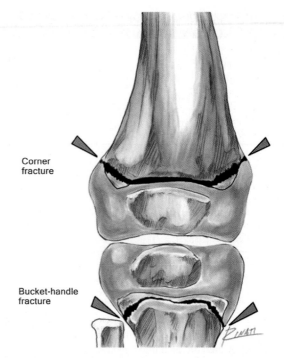

Figure 6-43. Schematic representation of classic metaphyseal lesions (CMLs). Illustration demonstrates the path of the CML. Depending on the angle at which the CML is viewed from, it may appear to extend across the width of the ossified physis (tibia illustrating a bucket-handle fracture) or only the margins of the physis (femur, illustrating a corner fracture). (Artwork courtesy of Gholamreza Zinati, MD.)

The almost pathognomonic fracture of child abuse is the CML, commonly termed the "corner" or "bucket-handle fracture."[12] These fractures are almost exclusively seen in NAI, but are not the most common fractures in abused children. The incidence of CML in large series ranges from 15% to 32%.[89,128] Radiographs show a corner fracture at the edge of the ossified portion of the zone of provisional calcification, *which is the metaphyseal side of the physis as opposed to the epiphyseal side*. If a significant portion of the metaphyseal rim is involved, a bucket-handle fracture pattern is produced. Based on their histopathologic autopsy study of metaphyseal fractures in abused infants, Kleinman et al.[135,136] found that bucket-handle or corner fractures are actually a full-thickness metaphyseal fracture extending through the primary spongiosa of bone just above the zone of provisional calcification (Fig. 6-43). Centrally, the amount of metaphysis remaining attached to the physis was thin, but peripherally the fracture line curved away from the physis so that a substantial metaphyseal rim remained attached to the physis (Fig. 6-44). On radiographic study, this metaphyseal rim formed the basis for both corner and bucket-handle fractures. In healing fractures, biopsy specimens showed metaphyseal extension of hypertrophied chondrocytes.[184] Metaphyseal corner fractures are most likely caused by either violent shaking or traction injuries to the extremity.[12] Even one CML noted on a skeletal survey is highly suspicious and specific for child abuse.[140,228] Subepiphyseal–metaphyseal lucency can also be caused by systematic disease such as rickets and leukemia, but there is evidence that CML is caused by rickets.[188]

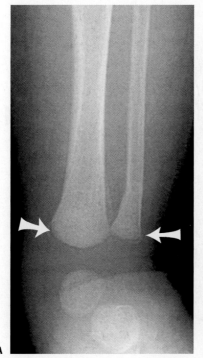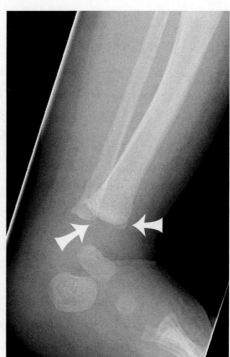

Figure 6-44. Classic metaphyseal fracture in a 2.5-month-old male victim of nonaccidental injury. **A:** Frontal radiograph of the tibia and fibula demonstrates transmetaphyseal lucencies or bucket-handle fractures (*arrows*). **B:** A lateral ankle radiograph reveals lucency at the tibial and fibular metaphyseal margins indicating corner fractures (*arrows*).

Lesions resembling corner fractures of the distal radius, ulna, tibia, and proximal humerus also have been reported with one variant of spondylometaphyseal dysplasia.[66] Because fracture callus does not reliably occur, dating the CML lesion is unreliable. The presence of callus suggests that the fracture is probably greater than 10 to 14 days.

RIB FRACTURES

Rib fractures are uncommon in childhood accidents, especially when located posterior and associated with other long-bone fractures. Although no single fracture is specific for abuse, rib fractures are highly suggestive of abuse if there is no plausible trauma or medical explanation.[125] Abusive rib fractures may be caused by squeezing of the chest by a caretaker,[45] hitting the child from behind, or stepping on the chest.[139,216] Kleinman et al.[138] postulated that severe shaking of an infant can cause front-to-back chest compression, which levers the posterior rib over the transverse process of the vertebral body, causing fractures of the posterior rib shaft at the transverse process and of the rib head adjacent to the vertebra (Fig. 6-45). One series showed that fractures of the first rib in children were only seen in abuse.[221] Barsness et al.[25] reported that rib fractures had a positive predictive value of NAI of 95% in children younger than 3 years of age. In this study, rib fracture(s) were the only skeletal manifestation of NAI in 29% of the children. Posterior rib fractures are difficult to diagnose acutely because they lack callus and are rarely displaced. Even with healing, the callus on radiography may be obscured by the overlying transverse process.[134] Oblique views of the chest are included in skeletal surveys because they better show these fractures. Posterior rib fractures are the most common location in child abuse, but fractures may occur anywhere along the arc of the rib, including disruption of the anterior costochondral junction (Fig. 6-46).

Posterior rib fractures tend to occur between T4 and T9. Rib fractures may be discovered in abused infants who have undergone resuscitation for cardiac arrest; in which case, there may be confusion about the etiology of the fractures. Older fractures of the ribs in NAT may form lytic, expansile lesions.[159]

In infant fatalities of suspicious origin, postmortem high-detailed preautopsy skeletal surveys and specimen radiographs are helpful in fully evaluating and diagnosing child abuse.[132] In a postmortem study of 31 infants who died of inflicted skeletal injury,[137] there were a total of 165 fractures (51% rib fractures, 39% metaphyseal long-bone fractures, 5% long-bone shaft fractures, 4% fractures of the hands and feet, 1% clavicular fractures, and less than 1% spinal fractures). Postmortem thoracic CT is more sensitive than radiography for pediatric anterior and posterior rib fractures.[108] If an abdominal CT is being performed for evaluation of NAT, inclusion of the chest may yield additional information about rib fractures, but with additional radiation of approximately 3 mSv.

SPINAL FRACTURES

Spinal fractures in abused children are infrequent but important to recognize. Based on autopsy findings, spinal fractures of fatally abused children generally involve 25% or less compression of the vertebrae.[133] In a report of 103 children with cervical spine injury, only three patients had injury because of abuse and all had spinal cord injury without radiographic abnormalities (SCIWORA).[42] Hangman's type fractures of the posterior elements have been described in infants as a result of child abuse.[141] CT is helpful in evaluating pediatric cervical trauma. Vertebral compression fractures can occur when a child's buttocks are forcibly slammed onto a flat surface with hyperflexion of the spine.[11] Carrion et al.[50] reported circumferential physeal fractures of the thoracolumbar spine associated with child abuse that required

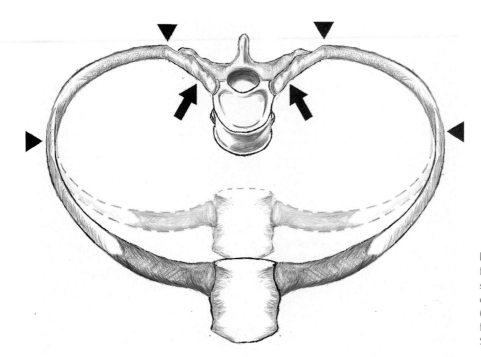

Figure 6-45. Schematic representation of rib fracture mechanism. Anterior chest compression causes the posterior ribs to be levered over the transverse processes of the vertebra (*arrows*) causing posterior and lateral rib fractures (*arrowheads*). (Artwork courtesy of Samir Abedin, MD.)

open reduction. Thoracolumbar fracture dislocations may occur in abused children with or without neurologic injury.[210] Flexion–distraction Chance fractures and synchondroses injuries (Fig. 6-47) may also be seen in NAT. Although neurologic injury in spinal fractures resulting from child abuse is uncommon,[65] any patient with abusive spinal injury should undergo thorough neurologic examination. Skeletal survey must include a lateral view of the cervical, thoracic, and lumbar spine. For children younger than 36 months, the cervical spine injury incidence is as high as 15%, so children suspected of AHT should also have cervical spine imaging.[22] Because of the potentially serious con-

sequences of a spinal injury in an infant or young child, clinical or radiographic suggestion of a spinal injury should be further evaluated with MRI. If a patient has evidence of AHT to require MRI, it should include the entire spine.[126]

LABORATORY STUDIES

An abused child should have a complete blood cell count with sedimentation rate, liver function studies, and urinalysis.

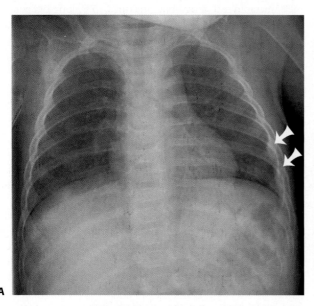
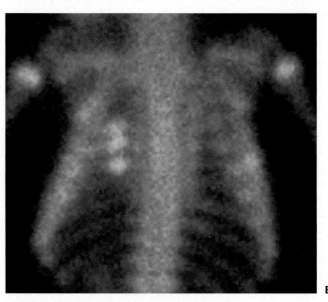

Figure 6-46. Rib fractures in a 9-month-old male victim of nonaccidental trauma. **A:** Chest radiograph reveals left lateral sixth and seventh rib fractures (*arrows*). **B:** Nuclear medicine bone scan confirms foci of increased uptake within the left lateral ribs as well as revealing additional hot foci in multiple right posterior lateral ribs.

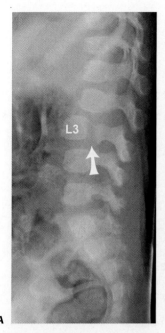 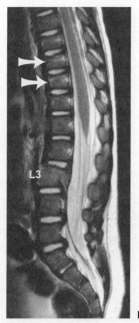

Figure 6-47. Lumbar spine fracture in a 16-month-old male victim of nonaccidental trauma. **A:** Lateral lumbar radiograph shows lucency through the L3 synchondrosis (*arrow*) with anterolisthesis of L3 body on L4. **B:** Sagittal T2-weighted MRI reveals hyperintense signal within the bone marrow of the fractured L3. Slight compression fractures of T10 and T11 are also noted (*arrows*).

Clotting studies, including prothrombin time and activated partial thromboplastin time, thrombin time, fibrinogen, factor VIII, factor IX, and von Willebrand factor antigen and activity should be performed in patients with bleeding or ecchymosis, to evaluate for bleeding diathesis. If bruising is the only finding of possible abuse, consultation with a hematologist may be necessary to fully evaluate for an unusual bleeding disorder.[229] Infants born prematurely are at risk for rickets and low bone density. Therefore, evaluation of calcium, phosphorous, alkaline phosphatase, and 25-OH vitamin D may be useful in such infants.

If there is suspicion of substance abuse by any family member, and the child has symptoms, a toxicology screen should also be performed on the patient.[89]

THE DIFFERENTIAL DIAGNOSIS

The most important consultation to request for a child with suspected inflicted injury is the child protective services team. In many major pediatric centers, a Child Abuse Pediatrician, who has received specialty training in this field, is the leader of this team. Any suspected abuse should initiate a minimum evaluation that includes an appropriate radiographic evaluation with a skeletal survey in the younger child and consultation by a child abuse specialist. Any significant nonorthopedic injury should prompt consultation by the appropriate subspecialty: neurosurgery, general surgery, plastic surgery, ophthalmology, or urology.[12]

Although it is extremely important not to miss the diagnosis of child abuse, it is equally important to maintain an objective, critical view and not to make the diagnosis in error.[114] Overdiagnosing child abuse can be harmful to the family, with the parents being placed at risk of losing custody of their children and also facing criminal charges.[121] Patients or family friends may make false statements about an abuse situation through misinterpretation, confabulation, fantasy, delusions, and other situations.[34]

Normal metaphyseal variations are seen occasionally and should not be confused with corner fractures of child abuse. These variants are seen most commonly in the proximal tibia, distal femur, proximal fibula, distal radius, and distal ulna. A bony beak may be seen medially in the proximal humerus or tibia, and is usually bilateral. Cortical irregularity in the medial proximal tibia may also be seen in 4% of normal infants and young toddlers and is bilateral in 25%.

The signs of child abuse found on radiographs can overlap with the findings of systemic diseases such as Caffey disease (infantile cortical hyperostosis), osteomyelitis, septic arthritis, insufficiency fracture, hypophosphatasia (Fig. 6-48), leukemia, metastatic neuroblastoma, OI, scurvy, vitamin D deficient and drug-induced rickets, congenital insensitivity to pain, osteopetrosis, kinky hair syndrome, prostaglandin therapy, osteoid osteoma, and other benign bone tumors.[12] Children with biliary atresia may present with osteopenia and fractures without history of significant injury, which should not be mistaken for child abuse.[69] There has been an increase in the incidence of syphilis in females of childbearing age, and, although extremely rare, congenital syphilis can mimic fractures of child abuse with diaphysitis, metaphysitis, and multiple pathologic fractures in different stages of healing.[153] Physiologic periostitis, in contrast to lesions from child abuse, is seen in young infants of about 6 months of age, is usually bilateral, symmetric, diaphyseal, located on the long bones—humerus, femur, and tibia—and has no periostitis of the metaphysis.[63] Insufficiency rib fractures may be seen in rickets of prematurity as well as rickets of low birth weight. The presence of metabolic disease and pathologic fractures does not exclude the possibility of child abuse.

Several diseases are commonly brought up in custodial hearings as alternative possibilities to nonaccidental traumatic injuries, and these diseases should be objectively considered in the differential diagnosis. Leukemia should always be considered in a child with diffuse osteopenia or metaphyseal lucencies. McClain et al.[162] reported a 2-year-old child who died of undiagnosed acute lymphoblastic leukemia, having been earlier reported as a possible victim of child abuse. Clinical signs of leukemia, including fever, pallor, petechia, purpura, adenopathy, hepatosplenomegaly, and bone pain, should be sought in children with bruising of unknown origin. Factor XIII deficiency may cause unexplained bleeding from minor trauma and be mistaken for child abuse because the standard coagulation profile may be negative and factor-specific tests may be negative if performed post transfusion.[175]

Undiagnosed OI should always be considered when a child presents with multiple fractures of unknown etiology, but may be a difficult diagnosis to make. Before the diagnosis of OI is

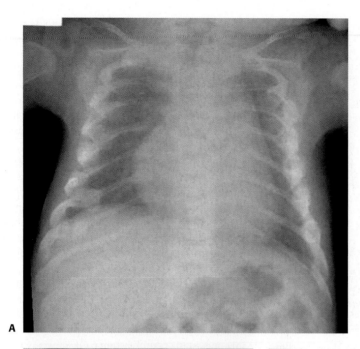

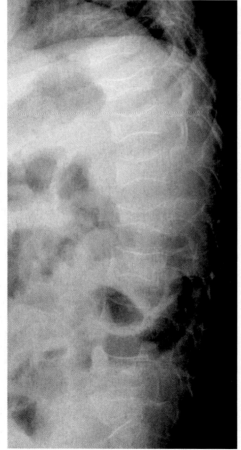

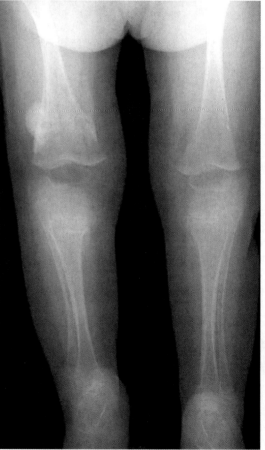

Figure 6-48. Hypophosphatasia in a 2-month-old female with multiple fractures. **A:** Chest radiograph shows severe osteopenia and multiple bilateral healing rib fractures. **B:** Lateral spine radiograph reveals multiple compressed vertebra. **C:** Lower extremity radiographs demonstrate multiple, bilateral healing femoral and lower leg fractures.

made, the parents may be presumed to be the cause of the fractures, with temporary removal of a child in 70% of cases.[213] Thoughtful review of the medical history and clinical evaluation identify most children with OI, without the need for genetic testing, which has low yield when there are no clinical findings.[240] However, when the diagnosis of OI is suspected, but cannot be made on classic clinical grounds, the diagnosis may be made by biochemical assay.[187] Genetic testing of individuals with typical features of OI typically has disease-causing mutations in 98%.[24] OI was further discussed earlier in this chapter; a more complete review of this topic is beyond the scope of this chapter.

POST-EMERGENCY ROOM TREATMENT AND LEGAL REPORTING REQUIREMENTS

Once NAT is recognized, the first step in treatment is hospital admission.[7] This is therapeutic in that it places the child in a safe, protected environment, provides the opportunity for additional diagnostic workup, and, more importantly, investigation of the family's social situation by appropriate personnel. In tertiary centers, multidisciplinary teams are available to evaluate and treat such children, but in other circumstances the orthopedist may be primarily responsible for coordinating both evaluation and treatment. Mandatory reporting functions as a screening test for suspected abuse. False positives are much preferred to a false negative, which could be fatal. Court custody may be required for children of uncooperative families who refuse admission, and hospitalization should be continued until a full investigation is completed by the appropriate child protective services and a safe disposition is established. In the United States, the physician is required by law to report all suspected abuse to appropriate child protective services or legal authorities. Although physicians have better reporting rates than most other professionals, 27% of injuries were considered likely to be caused by abuse and 76% of injuries that were considered possibly related to child abuse were not reported.[86] When the reporting is done in good faith, the physician has immunity against criminal or civil liability for these actions. The granting of absolute immunity, even for physicians, is not encouraged by the American legal system because in theory, it would protect individuals who make false reports of child abuse to harass families and would deprive the injured parties their legal right to seek damages for harmful actions. In contrast, physician immunity based on good faith reporting of suspected child abuse is contingent on the physician having a reasonable belief that abuse or neglect has occurred. Since the stakes for failure to report suspected child abuse are so high, physicians should always report suspicions of abuse.[12]

THE ORTHOPEDIC SURGEON'S LEGAL ROLE IN NONACCIDENTAL INJURY

The orthopedist may fill a dual role in the courtroom in child abuse proceedings. First, he or she serves as a material witness whose testimony is confined to the physician's personal involvement in the legal matter of the child's evaluation and treatment. The testimony may include clarification to the court of information contained in the medical record. As a material witness, the physician cannot render opinions about the facts as stated during his or her testimony. However, the physician may also be requested to be as an expert witness.[96,172,186] An expert witness is an individual considered by the court to have special knowledge and experience that qualifies him or her

to render opinions about certain facts presented in the courtroom. The limits of the physician's expertise usually are defined by the attorneys in court before the testimony of the expert witness.

Physicians may be reluctant to testify in court for many reasons. The courtroom is an unfamiliar setting for most physicians and the adversarial nature of the American legal system may be perceived as a hostile environment. In the courtroom, opposing attorneys are likely to search for inconsistencies in the testimony or unfamiliarity with the record to discredit the physician witness, which can be very uncomfortable for the physician not used to this behavior. When a physician is asked to be an expert witness or a material witness, consultation with the child's attorney is essential. Principles of testimony include a meticulous preparation of the case, an understanding of what to expect in a deposition, and thorough instruction by the attorney about what to expect in court. The key to deposition or court testimony is to understand and honestly answer the defense attorney questions as succinctly as possible. Testimony should be objective, honest, and thorough.[96] In child abuse cases, in particular, the testimony will lead to the fact that the abuse has occurred and that it has been appropriately diagnosed. In addition, the physician expert witness may be asked to give an opinion of the risk for subsequent abuse if the child returns to the home where the alleged abuse occurred. Questions regarding medical findings often will be prefaced in the courtroom by the words "reasonable medical certainty," a term that is poorly understood by most physicians. Chadwick[52] offered a definition of reasonable medical certainty as "certain as a physician should be in order to recommend and carry out treatment for a given medical condition."

During testimony, the orthopedist's words should be carefully chosen and understandable by a lay jury. Attorneys may frame questions in ways that are difficult to understand, and the orthopedist should not hesitate to ask the attorney to clarify a question.[52] Language should be straightforward, and visual aids may be used in providing clear testimony. The expert witness should use testimony as an educational process for the court, in which the common experience and knowledge of the jury are used to build understanding with common sense explanations of medical findings.[52] The material witness should provide answers that are brief, without volunteering extra information. The child's attorney should prepare the orthopedic surgeon for the rigors of cross-examination by the defense attorneys, which often works to question the physician's credibility. A strategy of aggressive cross-examination is to provoke the physician into arguments or unprofessional behavior that could discredit his or her testimony before the court. The physician witnesses are always expected to respond professionally, even under extreme duress.[67] Brent[41] assembled an excellent series of vignettes of expert medical witness case studies in court and provided detailed instructions with regard to the responsibilities of such experts.

ACKNOWLEDGMENTS

Thanks to Didja Hilmara for all her editing support.

Annotated References

Reference	Annotation
Belthur MV, Birchansky SB, Verdugo AA, et al. Pathologic fractures in children with acute *Staphylococcus aureus* osteomyelitis. *J Bone Joint Surg Am.* 2012;94(1):34–42.	The authors report on 17 children with acute osteomyelitis who developed pathologic fracture. MRI studies at the time of admission demonstrated a significantly greater prevalence and size of subperiosteal abscess in the pathologic fracture group.
Christian CW, Committee on Child Abuse and Neglect. The evaluation of suspected child physical abuse. *Pediatrics.* 2015;135(5):e1337–e1354. *Pediatrics.* 2015;136(3):583.	Comprehensive article describing the role of the physician in suspecting, reporting, and evaluating physical abuse.
Deng ZP, Ding Y, Puri A, et al. The surgical treatment and outcome of nonmetastatic extremity osteosarcoma with pathological fractures. *Chin Med J (Engl).* 2015;128(19):2605–2608.	In this retrospective review of a large Asian database, the authors demonstrate that patients with osteosarcoma and associated pathologic fracture can safely be treated with limb salvage, achieving comparable results to nonfracture group.
James KA, Cunniff C, Apkon SD, et al. Risk factors for first fractures among males with Duchenne or Becker muscular dystrophy. *J Pediatr Orthop.* 2015;35(6):640–644.	Retrospective review of 747 children with muscular dystrophy aiming to identify risk factors for first fracture. Incidence of fractures was 33% and full-time wheelchair use increased the risk of first fracture by 75%; corticosteroid use, bisphosphonate use, and calcium/vitamin D use did not significantly affect incidence of fractures.
Kocher MS, Kasser JR. Orthopaedic aspects of child abuse. *J Am Acad Orthop Surg.* 2000;8:10–20.	A concise review of the orthopedic detection of child abuse.
Laposata ME, Laposata M. Children with signs of abuse. When is it not child abuse? *Am J Clin Pathol.* 2005;123(Suppl 1):S1–S6.	Illustrates the need to keep an open mind regarding other diagnoses and the mimics of child abuse.
Leong NL, Anderson ME, Gebhardt MC, et al. Computed tomography-based structural analysis for predicting fracture risk in children with benign skeletal neoplasms: comparison of specificity with that of plain radiographs. *J Bone Joint Surg Am.* 2010;92(9):1827–1833.	The authors report on the use of quantitative computed tomography-based rigidity analysis for predicting the risk of fractures through UBCs.
Lindberg DM, Shapiro RA, Laskey AL, et al. Prevalence of abusive injuries in siblings and household contacts of physically abused children. *Pediatrics.* 2012;130(2):193–201.	Recommendation to obtain a skeletal survey in siblings and other contacts under age 2 years when a child is found to be abused.
Pierce MC, Bertocci GE, Vogeley E, et al. Evaluating long bone fractures in children: a biomechanical approach with illustrative cases. *Child Abuse Negl.* 2004;28(5):505–524.	Highly recommended for the orthopedic surgeon to develop a clearer understanding of underlying biomechanical plausible injury mechanisms.
Sees JP, Sitoula P, Dabney K, et al. Pamidronate treatment to prevent reoccurring fractures in children with cerebral palsy. *J Pediatr Orthop.* 2016;36(2):193–197.	This is a retrospective review of children with cerebral palsy GMFCS 3, 4, and 5 who underwent pamidronate treatment aiming to reduce the incidence of fractures. The posttreatment group showed 0.10 fracture/yr rate, compared to 2.4 fractures/yr in the pretreatment group.
Sheets LK, Leach ME, Koszewski IJ, et al. Sentinel injuries in infants evaluated for child physical abuse. *Pediatrics.* 2013;131(4):701–707.	27.5% of abused infants were noted to have a previous sentinel injury.
Sink EL, Hyman JE, Matheny T, et al. Child abuse: the role of the orthopaedic surgeon in nonaccidental trauma. *Clin Orthop Relat Res.* 2001;469:790–797.	Summary of the role for the orthopedic surgeon in child maltreatment.
Sugar NF, Taylor JA, Feldman KW. Bruises in infants and toddlers: those who don't cruise rarely bruise. Puget Sound Pediatric Research Network. *Arch Pediatr Adolesc Med.* 1999;153(4):399–403.	Bruising in infants under 9 months of age or atypical bruises in toddlers (trunk, hands, buttocks) are unusual and causes for concern.

REFERENCES

1. American Academy of Pediatrics. Section on Radiology: diagnostic imaging of child abuse. *Pediatrics.* 1991;87(2):262–264.
2. American Academy of Pediatrics. *A Guide to References and Resources in Child Abuse and Neglect.* Elk Grove Village, IL: American Academy of Pediatrics; 1994.
3. Allergic reactions to latex containing medical devices: FDA Medical Alert. *DHHS (NIOSH).* 1997;97–135.
4. American Academy of Radiology. *Imaging of the Child With Suspected Child Abuse.* Reston, VA: American College of Radiology; 1997.
5. Children's Bureau. *The Child Abuse Prevention and Treatment Act (CAPTA).* Washington, DC: US Dpt of Health and Human services; 2003.
6. *Child Maltreatment.* In: Services UDoHaH, ed. Washington, DC; 2006.
7. National Association of Children's Hospital and Related Institution. *Defining the Children's Hospital Role in Child Maltreatment.* Alexandria, VA: Author; 2006.
8. American Academy of Pediatrics. Policy statement—child fatality review. *Pediatrics.* 2010;126(3):592–596.
9. Ahn JI, Park JS. Pathological fractures secondary to unicameral bone cysts. *Int Orthop.* 1994;18(1):20–22.
10. Akbarnia B, Torg JS, Kirkpatrick J, et al. Manifestations of the battered-child syndrome. *J Bone Joint Surg Am.* 1974;56(6):1159–1166.

11. Akbarnia BA. Pediatric spine fractures. *Orthop Clin North Am*. 1999;30(3):521–536, x.
12. Akbarnia BA, Akbarnia NO. The role of orthopedist in child abuse and neglect. *Orthop Clin North Am*. 1976;7(3):733–742.
13. Alman B, Frasca P. Fracture failure mechanisms in patients with osteogenesis imperfecta. *J Orthop Res*. 1987;5(1):139–143.
14. Alos N, Grant RM, Ramsay T, et al. High incidence of vertebral fractures in children with acute lymphoblastic leukemia 12 months after the initiation of therapy. *J Clin Oncol*. 2012;30(22):2760–2767.
15. Anderson TE, Drummond DS, Breed AL, et al. Malignant hyperthermia in myelomeningocele: a previously unreported association. *J Pediatr Orthop*. 1981;1(4):401–403.
16. Anderst JD. Assessment of factors resulting in abuse evaluations in young children with minor head trauma. *Child Abuse Negl*. 2008;32(3):405–413.
17. Arata MA, Peterson HA, Dahlin DC. Pathological fractures through nonossifying fibromas. Review of the Mayo Clinic experience. *J Bone Joint Surg Am*. 1981;63(6):980–988.
18. Arkader A, Woon RP, Gilsanz V. Can subclinical rickets cause SCFE? A prospective, pilot study. *J Pediatr Orthop*. 2015;35(7):e72–e75.
19. Armstrong DG, Newfield JT, Gillespie R. Orthopedic management of osteopetrosis: results of a survey and review of the literature. *J Pediatr Orthop*. 1999;19(1):122–132.
20. Aycan OE, Camurcu IY, Ozer D, et al. Unusual localizations of unicameral bone cysts and aneurysmal bone cysts: a retrospective review of 451 cases. *Acta Orthop Belg*. 2015;81(2):209–212.
21. Bacchetta J, Wesseling-Perry K, Gilsanz V, et al. Idiopathic juvenile osteoporosis: a cross-sectional single-centre experience with bone histomorphometry and quantitative computed tomography. *Pediatr Rheumatol Online J*. 2013;11:6.
22. Baerg J, Thirumoorthi A, Vannix R, et al. Cervical spine imaging for young children with inflicted trauma: expanding the injury pattern. *J Pediatr Surg*. 2017;52(5):816–821.
23. Barbanti-Brodano G, Girolami M, Ghermandi R, et al. Aneurysmal bone cyst of the spine treated by concentrated bone marrow: clinical cases and review of the literature. *Eur Spine J*. 2017;26(Suppl 1):158–166.
24. Bardai G, Moffatt P, Glorieux FH, et al. DNA sequence analysis in 598 individuals with a clinical diagnosis of osteogenesis imperfecta: diagnostic yield and mutation spectrum. *Osteoporos Int*. 2016;27(12):3607–3613.
25. Barsness KA, Cha ES, Bensard DD, et al. The positive predictive value of rib fractures as an indicator of nonaccidental trauma in children. *J Trauma*. 2003;54(6):1107–1110.
26. Basarir K, Piskin A, Guclu B, et al. Aneurysmal bone cyst recurrence in children: a review of 56 patients. *J Pediatr Orthop*. 2007;27(8):938–943.
27. Batista DL, Riar J, Keil M, et al. Diagnostic tests for children who are referred for the investigation of Cushing syndrome. *Pediatrics*. 2007;120(3):e575–e586.
28. Beals RK, Tufts E. Fractured femur in infancy: the role of child abuse. *J Pediatr Orthop*. 1983;3(5):583–586.
29. Bell JM, Shields MD, Watters J, et al. Interventions to prevent and treat corticosteroid-induced osteoporosis and prevent osteoporotic fractures in Duchenne muscular dystrophy. *Cochrane Database Syst Rev*. 2017;1:CD010899.
30. Belthur MV, Birchansky SB, Verdugo AA, et al. Pathologic fractures in children with acute Staphylococcus aureus osteomyelitis. *J Bone Joint Surg Am*. 2012;94(1):34–42.
31. Bennett BL, Chua MS, Care M, et al. Retrospective review to determine the utility of follow-up skeletal surveys in child abuse evaluations when the initial skeletal survey is normal. *BMC Res Notes*. 2011;4:354.
32. Bennett OM, Namnyak SS. Bone and joint manifestations of sickle cell anaemia. *J Bone Joint Surg Br*. 1990;72(3):494–499.
33. Berger RP, Panigrahy A, Gottschalk S, et al. Effective radiation dose in a skeletal survey performed for suspected child abuse. *J Pediatr*. 2016;171:310–312.
34. Bernet W. False statements and the differential diagnosis of abuse allegations. *J Am Acad Child Adolesc Psychiatry*. 1993;32(5):903–910.
35. Berrey BH Jr, Lord CF, Gebhardt MC, et al. Fractures of allografts. Frequency, treatment, and end-results. *J Bone Joint Surg Am*. 1990;72(6):825–833.
36. Biggin A, Munns CF. Long-term bisphosphonate therapy in osteogenesis imperfecta. *Curr Osteoporos Rep*. 2017;15(5):412–418.
37. Blakemore LC, Loder RT, Hensinger RN. Role of intentional abuse in children 1 to 5 years old with isolated femoral shaft fractures. *J Pediatr Orthop*. 1996;16(5):585–588.
38. Bohrer SP. Acute long bone diaphyseal infarcts in sickle cell disease. *Br J Radiol*. 1970;43(514):685–697.
39. Bonkowsky JL, Guenther E, Filloux FM, et al. Death, child abuse, and adverse neurological outcome of infants after an apparent life-threatening event. *Pediatrics*. 2008;122(1):125–131.
40. Boriani S, De Iure F, Campanacci L, et al. Aneurysmal bone cyst of the mobile spine: report on 41 cases. *Spine (Phila Pa 1976)*. 2001;26(1):27–35.
41. Brent RL. The irresponsible expert witness: a failure of biomedical graduate education and professional accountability. *Pediatrics*. 1982;70(5):754–762.
42. Brown RL, Brunn MA, Garcia VF. Cervical spine injuries in children: a review of 103 patients treated consecutively at a level 1 pediatric trauma center. *J Pediatr Surg*. 2001;36(8):1107–1114.
43. Buison AM, Kawchak DA, Schall JI, et al. Bone area and bone mineral content deficits in children with sickle cell disease. *Pediatrics*. 2005;116(4):943–949.
44. Burke NG, Cassar-Gheiti AJ, Tan J, et al. Regenerate bone fracture rate following femoral lengthening in paediatric patients. *J Child Orthop*. 2017;11(3):210–215.
45. Caffey J. Multiple fractures in the long bones of infants suffering from chronic subdural hematoma. *Am J Roentgenol Radium Ther*. 1946;56(2):163–173.
46. Campanacci M, Capanna R, Picci P. Unicameral and aneurysmal bone cysts. *Clin Orthop Relat Res*. 1986;(204):25–36.
47. Capanna R, Dal Monte A, Gitelis S, et al. The natural history of unicameral bone cyst after steroid injection. *Clin Orthop Relat Res*. 1982;(166):204–211.
48. Carpenter RF. The prevalence and distribution of bruising in babies. *Arch Dis Child*. 1999;80(4):363–366.
49. Carpintero P, Leon F, Zafra M, et al. Fractures of osteochondroma during physical exercise. *Am J Sports Med*. 2003;31(6):1003–1006.
50. Carrion WV, Dormans JP, Drummond DS, et al. Circumferential growth plate fracture of the thoracolumbar spine from child abuse. *J Pediatr Orthop*. 1996;16(2):210–214.
51. Caulton JM, Ward KA, Alsop CW, et al. A randomised controlled trial of standing programme on bone mineral density in non-ambulant children with cerebral palsy. *Arch Dis Child*. 2004;89(2):131–135.
52. Chadwick DL. Preparation for court testimony in child abuse cases. *Pediatr Clin North Am*. 1990;37(4):955–970.
53. Chadwick DL, Bertocci G, Castillo E, et al. Annual risk of death resulting from short falls among young children: less than 1 in 1 million. *Pediatrics*. 2008;121(6):1213–1224.
54. Chapman T, Sugar N, Done S, et al. Fractures in infants and toddlers with rickets. *Pediatr Radiol*. 2010;40(7):1184–1189.
55. Chen CJ, Chao TY, Chu DM, et al. Osteoblast and osteoclast activity in a malignant infantile osteopetrosis patient following bone marrow transplantation. *J Pediatr Hematol Oncol*. 2004;26(1):5–8.
56. Chlebna-Sokol D, Loba-Jakubowska E, Sikora A. Clinical evaluation of patients with idiopathic juvenile osteoporosis. *J Pediatr Orthop B*. 2001;10(3):259–263.
57. Chotel F, Braillon P, Sailhan F, et al. Bone stiffness in children: part II. Objectives criteria for children to assess healing during leg lengthening. *J Pediatr Orthop*. 2008;28(5):538–543.
58. Clarke NM, Shelton FR, Taylor CC, et al. The incidence of fractures in children under the age of 24 months—in relation to non-accidental injury. *Injury*. 2012;43(6):762–765.
59. Coccia PF, Krivit W, Cervenka J, et al. Successful bone-marrow transplantation for infantile malignant osteopetrosis. *N Engl J Med*. 1980;302(13):701–708.
60. Coffey C, Haley K, Hayes J, et al. The risk of child abuse in infants and toddlers with lower extremity injuries. *J Pediatr Surg*. 2005;40(1):120–123.
61. Cohen J. Simple bone cysts. Studies of cyst fluid in six cases with a theory of pathogenesis. *J Bone Joint Surg Am*. 1960;42-A:609–616.
62. Cole WG. The Nicholas Andry Award—1996. The molecular pathology of osteogenesis imperfecta. *Clin Orthop Relat Res*. 1997;(343):235–248.
63. Conway JJ, Collins M, Tanz RR, et al. The role of bone scintigraphy in detecting child abuse. *Semin Nucl Med*. 1993;23(4):321–333.
64. Cottalorda J, Kohler R, Sales de Gauzy J, et al. Epidemiology of aneurysmal bone cyst in children: a multicenter study and literature review. *J Pediatr Orthop B*. 2004;13(6):389–394.
65. Cullen JC. Spinal lesions in battered babies. *J Bone Joint Surg Br*. 1975;57(3):364–366.
66. Currarino G, Birch JG, Herring JA. Developmental coxa vara associated with spondylometaphyseal dysplasia (DCV/SMD): "SMD-corner fracture type" (DCV/SMD-CF) demonstrated in most reported cases. *Pediatr Radiol*. 2000;30(1):14–24.
67. Dalton HJ, Slovis T, Helfer RE, et al. Undiagnosed abuse in children younger than 3 years with femoral fracture. *Am J Dis Child*. 1990;144(8):875–878.
68. Deng ZP, Ding Y, Puri A, et al. The surgical treatment and outcome of nonmetastatic extremity osteosarcoma with pathological fractures. *Chin Med J (Engl)*. 2015;128(19):2605–2608.
69. DeRusso PA, Spevak MR, Schwarz KB. Fractures in biliary atresia misinterpreted as child abuse. *Pediatrics*. 2003;112(1 Pt 1):185–188.
70. Diamond LS, Alegado R. Perinatal fractures in arthrogryposis multiplex congenita. *J Pediatr Orthop*. 1981;1(2):189–192.
71. DiCaprio MR, Enneking WF. Fibrous dysplasia. Pathophysiology, evaluation, and treatment. *J Bone Joint Surg Am*. 2005;87(8):1848–1864.
72. Dormans JP, Sankar WN, Moroz L, et al. Percutaneous intramedullary decompression, curettage, and grafting with medical-grade calcium sulfate pellets for unicameral bone cysts in children: a new minimally invasive technique. *J Pediatr Orthop*. 2005;25(6):804–811.
73. Dosa NP, Eckrich M, Katz DA, et al. Incidence, prevalence, and characteristics of fractures in children, adolescents, and adults with spina bifida. *J Spinal Cord Med*. 2007;30(Suppl 1):S5–S9.
74. Drennan DB, Maylahn DJ, Fahey JJ. Fractures through large non-ossifying fibromas. *Clin Orthop Relat Res*. 1974;(103):82–88.
75. Drummond DS, Moreau M, Cruess RL. Post-operative neuropathic fractures in patients with myelomeningocele. *Dev Med Child Neurol*. 1981;23(2):147–150.
76. Dubowitz H, Bross DC. The pediatrician's documentation of child maltreatment. *Am J Dis Child*. 1992;146(5):596–599.
77. Duffy SO, Squires J, Fromkin JB, et al. Use of skeletal surveys to evaluate for physical abuse: analysis of 703 consecutive skeletal surveys. *Pediatrics*. 2011;127(1):e47–e52.
78. Dwan K, Phillipi CA, Steiner RD, et al. Bisphosphonate therapy for osteogenesis imperfecta. *Cochrane Database Syst Rev*. 2016;10:CD005088.
79. Easley ME, Kneisl JS. Pathologic fractures through nonossifying fibromas: is prophylactic treatment warranted? *J Pediatr Orthop*. 1997;17(6):808–813.
80. Ebong WW. Pathological fracture complicating long bone osteomyelitis in patients with sickle cell disease. *J Pediatr Orthop*. 1986;6(2):177–181.
81. Edvardsen P. Physeo-epiphyseal injuries of lower extremities in myelomeningocele. *Acta Orthop Scand*. 1972;43(6):550–557.
82. Elsasser U, Ruegsegger P, Anliker M, et al. Loss and recovery of trabecular bone in the distal radius following fracture—immobilization of the upper limb in children. *Klin Wochenschr*. 1979;57(15):763–767.
83. Fagen KE, Shalaby-Rana E, Jackson AM. Frequency of skeletal injuries in children with inflicted burns. *Pediatr Radiol*. 2015;45(3):396–401.
84. Fain O. Musculoskeletal manifestations of scurvy. *Joint Bone Spine*. 2005;72(2):124–128.
85. Ferguson PC, McLaughlin CE, Griffin AM, et al. Clinical and functional outcomes of patients with a pathologic fracture in high-grade osteosarcoma. *J Surg Oncol*. 2010;102(2):120–124.
86. Flaherty EG, Sege RD, Griffith J, et al. From suspicion of physical child abuse to reporting: primary care clinician decision-making. *Pediatrics*. 2008;122(3):611–619.
87. Frasier L, Alexander R, Parrish R, et al. *Abusive Head Trauma in Infants and Children: A Medical, Legal and Forensic Reference*. St Louis, MO: GW Medical Publishing; 2006.
88. Freiberg AA, Loder RT, Heidelberger KP, et al. Aneurysmal bone cysts in young children. *J Pediatr Orthop*. 1994;14(1):86–91.

89. Galleno H, Oppenheim WL. The battered child syndrome revisited. *Clin Orthop Relat Res*. 1982;(162):11–19.
90. Gandrud LM, Cheung JC, Daniels MW, et al. Low-dose intravenous pamidronate reduces fractures in childhood osteoporosis. *J Pediatr Endocrinol Metab*. 2003;16(6):887–892.
91. Garg S, Mehta S, Dormans JP. Modern surgical treatment of primary aneurysmal bone cyst of the spine in children and adolescents. *J Pediatr Orthop*. 2005;25(3):387–392.
92. Gaulke R, Suppelna G. Solitary enchondroma at the hand. Long-term follow-up study after operative treatment. *J Hand Surg Br*. 2004;29(1):64–66.
93. Gerritsen EJ, Vossen JM, van Loo IH, et al. Autosomal recessive osteopetrosis: variability of findings at diagnosis and during the natural course. *Pediatrics*. 1994;93(2):247–253.
94. Gibbs CP Jr, Hefele MC, Peabody TD, et al. Aneurysmal bone cyst of the extremities. Factors related to local recurrence after curettage with a high-speed burr. *J Bone Joint Surg Am*. 1999;81(12):1671–1678.
95. Glorieux FH. Experience with bisphosphonates in osteogenesis imperfecta. *Pediatrics*. 2007;119(Suppl 2):S163–S165.
96. Halverson KC, Elliott BA, Rubin MS, et al. Legal considerations in cases of child abuse. *Prim Care*. 1993;20(2):407–416.
97. Han I, Choi ES, Kim HS. Monostotic fibrous dysplasia of the proximal femur: natural history and predisposing factors for disease progression. *Bone Joint J*. 2014;96-B(5):673–676.
98. Hanscom DA, Winter RB, Lutter L, et al. Osteogenesis imperfecta. Radiographic classification, natural history, and treatment of spinal deformities. *J Bone Joint Surg Am*. 1992;74(4):598–616.
99. Harkey HL, Crockard HA, Stevens JM, et al. The operative management of basilar impression in osteogenesis imperfecta. *Neurosurgery*. 1990;27(5):782–786; discussion 786.
100. Harper NS, Eddleman S, Lindberg DM. The utility of follow-up skeletal surveys in child abuse. *Pediatrics*. 2013;131(3):e672–e678.
101. Hasenhuttl K. Osteopetrosis: review of the literature and comparative studies on a case with a twenty-four-year follow-up. *J Bone Joint Surg Am*. 1962;44-A:359–370.
102. Helfer RE. The epidemiology of child abuse and neglect. *Pediatr Ann*. 1984; 13(10):745–751.
103. Hennrikus WL, Shaw BA, Gerardi JA. Injuries when children reportedly fall from a bed or couch. *Clin Orthop Relat Res*. 2003;(407):148–151.
104. Herget GW, Mauer D, Krauss T, et al. Non-ossifying fibroma: natural history with an emphasis on a stage-related growth, fracture risk and the need for follow-up. *BMC Musculoskelet Disord*. 2016;17:147.
105. Herring JA, Peterson HA. Simple bone cyst with growth arrest. *J Pediatr Orthop*. 1987;7(2):231–235.
106. Hibbard R, Barlow J, Macmillan H. Psychological maltreatment. *Pediatrics*. 2012;130(2):372–378.
107. Hobbs CJ, Wynne JM. The sexually abused battered child. *Arch Dis Child*. 1990;65(4):423–427.
108. Hong TS, Reyes JA, Moineddin R, et al. Value of postmortem thoracic CT over radiography in imaging of pediatric rib fractures. *Pediatr Radiol*. 2011;41(6):736–748.
109. Hood RW, Riseborough EJ. Lengthening of the lower extremity by the Wagner method: a review of the Boston Children's Hospital Experience. *J Bone Joint Surg Am*. 1981;63(7):1122–1131.
110. Hui C, Joughin E, Goldstein S, et al. Femoral fractures in children younger than three years: the role of nonaccidental injury. *J Pediatr Orthop*. 2008;28(3):297–302.
111. Hyden PW, Gallagher TA. Child abuse intervention in the emergency room. *Pediatr Clin North Am*. 1992;39(5):1053–1081.
112. Iobst CA, Dahl MT. Limb lengthening with submuscular plate stabilization: a case series and description of the technique. *J Pediatr Orthop*. 2007;27(5):504–509.
113. James KA, Cunniff C, Apkon SD, et al. Risk factors for first fractures among males with Duchenne or Becker muscular dystrophy. *J Pediatr Orthop*. 2015;35(6):640–644.
114. Jenny C. Evaluating infants and young children with multiple fractures. *Pediatrics*. 2006;118(3):1299–1303.
115. Jenny C. Recognizing and responding to medical neglect. *Pediatrics*. 2007; 120(6):1385–1389.
116. Jenny C, Isaac R. The relation between child death and child maltreatment. *Arch Dis Child*. 2006;91(3):265–269.
117. JG H. Arthrogryposis (multiple congential contractures): diagnostic approach to etiology, classification, genetics, and general principles. In: Rimoin D, Pyeritz R, Korf B, eds. *Emery and Rimion's Principles and Practice of Medical Genetics*. Vol. 168. 5th ed. Philadelphia, PA: Churchill Livingstone; 2007:3785–3856.
118. Jonson-Reid M, Kohl PL, Drake B. Child and adult outcomes of chronic child maltreatment. *Pediatrics*. 2012;129(5):839–845.
119. Kaelin AJ, MacEwen GD. Unicameral bone cysts: natural history and the risk of fracture. *Int Orthop*. 1989;13(4):275–282.
120. Kanagawa H, Masuyama R, Morita M, et al. Methotrexate inhibits osteoclastogenesis by decreasing RANKL-induced calcium influx into osteoclast progenitors. *J Bone Miner Metab*. 2016;34(5):526–531.
121. Kaplan JM. Pseudoabuse—the misdiagnosis of child abuse. *J Forensic Sci*. 1986; 31(4):1420–1428.
122. Karmazyn B, Duhn RD, Jennings SG, et al. Long bone fracture detection in suspected child abuse: contribution of lateral views. *Pediatr Radiol*. 2012;42(4):463–469.
123. Katz K, Cohen IJ, Ziv N, et al. Fractures in children who have Gaucher disease. *J Bone Joint Surg Am*. 1987;69(9):1361–1370.
124. Katz K, Sabato S, Horev G, et al. Spinal involvement in children and adolescents with Gaucher disease. *Spine (Phila Pa 1976)*. 1993;18(3):332–335.
125. Kemp AM, Butler A, Morris S, et al. Which radiological investigations should be performed to identify fractures in suspected child abuse? *Clin Radiol*. 2006;61(9):723–736.
126. Kemp AM, Joshi AH, Mann M, et al. What are the clinical and radiological characteristics of spinal injuries from physical abuse: a systematic review. *Arch Dis Child*. 2010;95(5):355–360.
127. Kempe CH, Silverman FN, Steele BF, et al. The battered-child syndrome. *JAMA*. 1962;181:17–24.
128. King J, Diefendorf D, Apthorp J, et al. Analysis of 429 fractures in 189 battered children. *J Pediatr Orthop*. 1988;8(5):585–589.
129. King WM, Ruttencutter R, Nagaraja HN, et al. Orthopedic outcomes of long-term daily corticosteroid treatment in Duchenne muscular dystrophy. *Neurology*. 2007;68(19):1607–1613.
130. Kistin CJ, Tien I, Bauchner H, et al. Factors that influence the effectiveness of child protection teams. *Pediatrics*. 2010;126(1):94–100.
131. Kleinman P. *Diagnostic Imaging of Child Abuse*. 2nd ed. St Louis, MO: Mosby; 1998.
132. Kleinman PK, Blackbourne BD, Marks SC, et al. Radiologic contributions to the investigation and prosecution of cases of fatal infant abuse. *N Engl J Med*. 1989;320(8):507–511.
133. Kleinman PK, Marks SC. Vertebral body fractures in child abuse. Radiologic-histopathologic correlates. *Invest Radiol*. 1992;27(9):715–722.
134. Kleinman PK, Marks SC, Adams VI, et al. Factors affecting visualization of posterior rib fractures in abused infants. *AJR Am J Roentgenol*. 1988;150(3):635–638.
135. Kleinman PK, Marks SC, Blackbourne B. The metaphyseal lesion in abused infants: a radiologic-histopathologic study. *AJR Am J Roentgenol*. 1986;146(5):895–905.
136. Kleinman PK, Marks SC Jr. Relationship of the subperiosteal bone collar to metaphyseal lesions in abused infants. *J Bone Joint Surg Am*. 1995;77(10):1471–1476.
137. Kleinman PK, Marks SC Jr, Richmond JM, et al. Inflicted skeletal injury: a postmortem radiologic-histopathologic study in 31 infants. *AJR Am J Roentgenol*. 1995;165(3):647–650.
138. Kleinman PK, Marks SC, Spevak MR, et al. Fractures of the rib head in abused infants. *Radiology*. 1992;185(1):119–123.
139. Kleinman PK, Nimkin K, Spevak MR, et al. Follow-up skeletal surveys in suspected child abuse. *AJR Am J Roentgenol*. 1996;167(4):893–896.
140. Kleinman PK, Perez-Rossello JM, Newton AW, et al. Prevalence of the classic metaphyseal lesion in infants at low versus high risk for abuse. *AJR Am J Roentgenol*. 2011;197(4):1005–1008.
141. Kleinman PK, Shelton YA. Hangman's fracture in an abused infant: imaging features. *Pediatr Radiol*. 1997;27(9):776–777.
142. Kleinman PK, Spevak MR. Variations in acromial ossification simulating infant abuse in victims of sudden infant death syndrome. *Radiology*. 1991;180(1):185–187.
143. Kobayashi D, Satsuma S, Kamegaya M, et al. Musculoskeletal conditions of acute leukemia and malignant lymphoma in children. *J Pediatr Orthop B*. 2005;14(3):156–161.
144. Kos L, Shwayder T. Cutaneous manifestations of child abuse. *Pediatr Dermatol*. 2006;23(4):311–320.
145. Kothari NA, Pelchovitz DJ, Meyer JS. Imaging of musculoskeletal infections. *Radiol Clin North Am*. 2001;39(4):653–671.
146. Kransdorf MJ, Sweet DE. Aneurysmal bone cyst: concept, controversy, clinical presentation, and imaging. *AJR Am J Roentgenol*. 1995;164(3):573–580.
147. Kravitz H, Driessen G, Gomberg R, et al. Accidental falls from elevated surfaces in infants from birth to one year of age. *Pediatrics*. 1969;44(Suppl 5):869–876.
148. Leet AI, Chebli C, Kushner H, et al. Fracture incidence in polyostotic fibrous dysplasia and the McCune-Albright syndrome. *J Bone Miner Res*. 2004;19(4):571–577.
149. Leet AI, Mesfin A, Pichard C, et al. Fractures in children with cerebral palsy. *J Pediatr Orthop*. 2006;26(5):624–627.
150. Leong GM, Abad V, Charmandari E, et al. Effects of child- and adolescent-onset endogenous Cushing syndrome on bone mass, body composition, and growth: a 7-year prospective study into young adulthood. *J Bone Miner Res*. 2007;22(1):110–118.
151. Leong NL, Anderson ME, Gebhardt MC, et al. Computed tomography-based structural analysis for predicting fracture risk in children with benign skeletal neoplasms: comparison of specificity with that of plain radiographs. *J Bone Joint Surg Am*. 2010;92(9):1827–1833.
152. Leventhal JM, Larson IA, Abdoo D, et al. Are abusive fractures in young children becoming less common? Changes over 24 years. *Child Abuse Negl*. 2007;31(3):311–322.
153. Lim HK, Smith WL, Sato Y, et al. Congenital syphilis mimicking child abuse. *Pediatr Radiol*. 1995;25(7):560–561.
154. Lindberg DM, Beaty B, Juarez-Colunga E, et al. Testing for abuse in children with sentinel injuries. *Pediatrics*. 2015;136(5):831–838.
155. Lindberg DM, Harper NS, Laskey AL, et al. Prevalence of abusive fractures of the hands, feet, spine, or pelvis on skeletal survey: perhaps "uncommon" is more common than suggested. *Pediatr Emerg Care*. 2013;29(1):26–29.
156. Lock TR, Aronson DD. Fractures in patients who have myelomeningocele. *J Bone Joint Surg Am*. 1989;71(8):1153–1157.
157. Loder RT, Hensinger RN. Slipped capital femoral epiphysis associated with renal failure osteodystrophy. *J Pediatr Orthop*. 1997;17(2):205–211.
158. Maclean AD. Spinal changes in a case of infantile scurvy. *Br J Radiol*. 1968; 41(485):385–387.
159. Magid N, Glass T. A "hole in a rib" as a sign of child abuse. *Pediatr Radiol*. 1990; 20(5):334–336.
160. Maguire S, Mann MK, Sibert J, et al. Are there patterns of bruising in childhood which are diagnostic or suggestive of abuse? A systematic review. *Arch Dis Child*. 2005;90(2):182–186.
161. McArthur RG, Cloutier MD, Hayles AB, et al. Cushing disease in children. Findings in 13 cases. *Mayo Clin Proc*. 1972;47(5):318–326.
162. McClain JL, Clark MA, Sandusky GE. Undiagnosed, untreated acute lymphoblastic leukemia presenting as suspected child abuse. *J Forensic Sci*. 1990;35(3):735–739.
163. McDonald DG, Kinali M, Gallagher AC, et al. Fracture prevalence in Duchenne muscular dystrophy. *Dev Med Child Neurol*. 2002;44(10):695–698.
164. McMahon P, Grossman W, Gaffney M, et al. Soft-tissue injury as an indication of child abuse. *J Bone Joint Surg Am*. 1995;77(8):1179–1183.
165. Meehan PL, Viroslav S, Schmitt EW Jr. Vertebral collapse in childhood leukemia. *J Pediatr Orthop*. 1995;15(5):592–595.
166. Meier L, van Tuyll van Sersooskerken AM, Liberton E, et al. Fractures of the proximal tibia associated with longterm use of methotrexate: 3 case reports and a review of literature. *J Rheumatol*. 2010;37(11):2434–2438.

167. Merten DF, Radkowski MA, Leonidas JC. The abused child: a radiological reappraisal. *Radiology.* 1983;146(2):377–381.

168. Mik G, Arkader A, Manteghi A, et al. Results of a minimally invasive technique for treatment of unicameral bone cysts. *Clin Orthop Relat Res.* 2009;467(11):2949–2954.

169. Milgram JW, Jasty M. Osteopetrosis: a morphological study of twenty-one cases. *J Bone Joint Surg Am.* 1982;64(6):912–929.

170. Miller RG, Segal JB, Ashar BH, et al. High prevalence and correlates of low bone mineral density in young adults with sickle cell disease. *Am J Hematol.* 2006;81(4):236–241.

171. Moorefield WG Jr, Miller GR. Aftermath of osteogenesis imperfecta: the disease in adulthood. *J Bone Joint Surg Am.* 1980;62(1):113–119.

172. Narang SK, Paul SR, Committee on Medical Liability and Risk Management. Expert witness participation in civil and criminal proceedings. *Pediatrics.* 2017;139(3): pii: e20164122.

173. Neer CS 2nd, Francis KC, Marcove RC, et al. Treatment of unicameral bone cyst. A follow-up study of one hundred seventy-five cases. *J Bone Joint Surg Am.* 1966;48(4):731–745.

174. Nerubay J, Pilderwasser D. Spontaneous bilateral distal femoral physiolysis due to scurvy. *Acta Orthop Scand.* 1984;55(1):18–20.

175. Newman RS, Jalili M, Kolls BJ, et al. Factor XIII deficiency mistaken for battered child syndrome: case of "correct" test ordering negated by a commonly accepted qualitative test with limited negative predictive value. *Am J Hematol.* 2002;71(4):328–330.

176. Newton AW, Vandeven AM. Unexplained infant and child death: a review of sudden infant death syndrome, sudden unexplained infant death, and child maltreatment fatalities including shaken baby syndrome. *Curr Opin Pediatr.* 2006;18(2):196–200.

177. Nielsen G, Kyriakos M. Fibrohistiocytic tumours. In: Fletcher C, Bridge J, Hogendom PCW, et al, eds. *WHO Classifications of Tumours of Bone and Soft Tissue.* Lyon: IARC Press; 2013:301–304.

178. Nilsson BE, Westlin NE. Restoration of bone mass after fracture of the lower limb in children. *Acta Orthop Scand.* 1971;42(1):78–81.

179. Nimkin K, Spevak MR, Kleinman PK. Fractures of the hands and feet in child abuse: imaging and pathologic features. *Radiology.* 1997;203(1):233–236.

180. Niyibizi C, Smith P, Mi Z, et al. Potential of gene therapy for treating osteogenesis imperfecta. *Clin Orthop Relat Res.* 2000;(379 Suppl):S126–S133.

181. O'Neill JA Jr, Meacham WF, Griffin JP, et al. Patterns of injury in the battered child syndrome. *J Trauma.* 1973;13(4):332–339.

182. O'Sullivan M, Zacharin M. Intramedullary rodding and bisphosphonate treatment of polyostotic fibrous dysplasia associated with the McCune-Albright syndrome. *J Pediatr Orthop.* 2002;22(2):255–260.

183. Oliveira AM, Hsi BL, Weremowicz S, et al. USP6 (Tre2) fusion oncogenes in aneurysmal bone cyst. *Cancer Res.* 2004;64(6):1920–1923.

184. Osier LK, Marks SC Jr, Kleinman PK. Metaphyseal extensions of hypertrophied chondrocytes in abused infants indicate healing fractures. *J Pediatr Orthop.* 1993;13(2):249–254.

185. Paley D, Herzenberg JE, Paremain G, et al. Femoral lengthening over an intramedullary nail: a matched-case comparison with Ilizarov femoral lengthening. *J Bone Joint Surg Am.* 1997;79(10):1464–1480.

186. Paul SR, Narang SK. Expert witness participation in civil and criminal proceedings. *Pediatrics.* 2017;139(3): pii: e20163862.

186a. Pepin MG, Byers PH. What every clinical geneticist should know about testing for osteogenesis imperfecta in suspected child abuse cases. *Am J Med Genet C Semin Med Genet.* 2015;169(4):307–313. doi: 10.1002/ajmg.c.31459. Epub 2015 Nov 14. Review.

187. Pereira EM. Clinical perspectives on osteogenesis imperfecta versus non-accidental injury. *Am J Med Genet C Semin Med Genet.* 2015;169(4):302–306.

188. Perez-Rossello JM, McDonald AG, Rosenberg AE, et al. Absence of rickets in infants with fatal abusive head trauma and classic metaphyseal lesions. *Radiology.* 2015;275(3):810–821.

189. Pierce MC, Bertocci GE, Vogeley E, et al. Evaluating long bone fractures in children: a biomechanical approach with illustrative cases. *Child Abuse Negl.* 2004;28(5):505–524.

190. Plotkin H, Sueiro R. Osteoporosis in children with neuromuscular diseases and inborn errors of metabolism. *Minerva Pediatr.* 2007;59(2):129–135.

191. Popoff SN, Marks SC Jr. The heterogeneity of the osteopetroses reflects the diversity of cellular influences during skeletal development. *Bone.* 1995;17(5):437–445.

192. Presedo A, Dabney KW, Miller F. Fractures in patients with cerebral palsy. *J Pediatr Orthop.* 2007;27(2):147–153.

193. Prosser I, Maguire S, Harrison SK, et al. How old is this fracture? Radiologic dating of fractures in children: a systematic review. *AJR Am J Roentgenol.* 2005;184(4):1282–1286.

194. Riester S, Ramaesch R, Wenger D, et al. Predicting fracture risk for enchondroma of the hand. *Hand (N Y).* 2016;11(2):206–210.

195. Ritschl P, Karnel F, Hajek P. Fibrous metaphyseal defects—determination of their origin and natural history using a radiomorphological study. *Skeletal Radiol.* 1988;17(1):8–15.

196. Roberts JB. Bilateral hyperplastic callus formation in osteogenesis imperfecta. *J Bone Joint Surg Am.* 1976;58(8):1164–1166.

197. Rodgers WB, Schwend RM, Jaramillo D, et al. Chronic physeal fractures in myelodysplasia: magnetic resonance analysis, histologic description, treatment, and outcome. *J Pediatr Orthop.* 1997;17(5):615–621.

198. Rogalsky RJ, Black GB, Reed MH. Orthopaedic manifestations of leukemia in children. *J Bone Joint Surg Am.* 1986;68(4):494–501.

199. Ruck J, Dahan-Oliel N, Montpetit K, et al. Fassier-Duval femoral rodding in children with osteogenesis imperfecta receiving bisphosphonates: functional outcomes at one year. *J Child Orthop.* 2011;5(3):217–224.

200. Sala A, Barr RD. Osteopenia and cancer in children and adolescents: the fragility of success. *Cancer.* 2007;109(7):1420–1431.

201. Schmitt B. *Child Abuse.* Philadelphia, PA: WB Saunders; 1984.

202. Schnitzer PG, Ewigman BG. Child deaths resulting from inflicted injuries: household risk factors and perpetrator characteristics. *Pediatrics.* 2005;116(5):e687–e693.

203. Schwend RM, Werth C, Johnston A. Femur shaft fractures in toddlers and young children: rarely from child abuse. *J Pediatr Orthop.* 2000;20(4):475–481.

204. Scollan JP, Jauregui JJ, Jacobsen CM, et al. The outcomes of nonelongating intramedullary fixation of the lower extremity for pediatric osteogenesis imperfecta patients: a meta-analysis. *J Pediatr Orthop.* 2017;37(5):e313–e316.

205. Sees JP, Sitoula P, Dabney K, et al. Pamidronate treatment to prevent reoccurring fractures in children with cerebral palsy. *J Pediatr Orthop.* 2016;36(2):193–197.

206. Sege RD, Amaya-Jackson L. Clinical considerations related to the behavioral manifestations of child maltreatment. *Pediatrics.* 2017;139(4): pii: e20170100.

207. Shapiro F, Glimcher MJ, Holtrop ME, et al. Human osteopetrosis: a histological, ultrastructural, and biochemical study. *J Bone Joint Surg Am.* 1980;62(3):384–399.

208. Shaw BA, Murphy KM, Shaw A, et al. Humerus shaft fractures in young children: accident or abuse? *J Pediatr Orthop.* 1997;17(3):293–297.

209. Shoenfeld Y. Osteogenesis imperfecta. Review of the literature with presentation of 29 cases. *Am J Dis Child.* 1975;129(6):679–687.

210. Sieradzki JP, Sarwark JF. Thoracolumbar fracture-dislocation in child abuse: case report, closed reduction technique and review of the literature. *Pediatr Neurosurg.* 2008;44(3):253–257.

211. Silverman FN. The roentgen manifestations of unrecognized skeletal trauma in infants. *Am J Roentgenol Radium Ther Nucl Med.* 1953;69(3):413–427.

212. Simpson AH, Kenwright J. Fracture after distraction osteogenesis. *J Bone Joint Surg Br.* 2000;82(5):659–665.

213. Singh Kocher M, Dichtel L. Osteogenesis imperfecta misdiagnosed as child abuse. *J Pediatr Orthop B.* 2011;20(6):440–443.

214. Sinigaglia R, Gigante C, Bisinella G, et al. Musculoskeletal manifestations in pediatric acute leukemia. *J Pediatr Orthop.* 2008;28(1):20–28.

215. Slovis TL, Strouse PJ, Strauss KJ. Radiation exposure in imaging of suspected child abuse: benefits versus risks. *J Pediatr.* 2015;167(5):963–968.

216. Smith FW, Gilday DL, Ash JM, et al. Unsuspected costo-vertebral fractures demonstrated by bone scanning in the child abuse syndrome. *Pediatr Radiol.* 1980;10(2):103–106.

217. Stanton RP, Abdel-Mota'al MM. Growth arrest resulting from unicameral bone cyst. *J Pediatr Orthop.* 1998;18(2):198–201.

218. Stark Z, Savarirayan R. Osteopetrosis. *Orphanet J Rare Dis.* 2009;4:5.

219. Stenevi Lundgren S, Rosengren BE, Dencker M, et al. Low physical activity is related to clustering of risk factors for fracture—a 2-year prospective study in children. *Osteoporos Int.* 2017;28(12):3373–3378.

220. Stott NS, Zionts LE. Displaced fractures of the apophysis of the olecranon in children who have osteogenesis imperfecta. *J Bone Joint Surg Am.* 1993;75(7):1026–1033.

221. Strouse PJ, Owings CL. Fractures of the first rib in child abuse. *Radiology.* 1995;197(3):763–765.

222. Sugar NF, Taylor JA, Feldman KW. Bruises in infants and toddlers: those who don't cruise rarely bruise. Puget Sound Pediatric Research Network. *Arch Pediatr Adolesc Med.* 1999;153(4):399–403.

223. Sullivan PM, Brookhouser PE, Scanlan JM, et al. Patterns of physical and sexual abuse of communicatively handicapped children. *Ann Otol Rhinol Laryngol.* 1991;100(3):188–194.

224. Sullivan RJ, Meyer JS, Dormans JP, et al. Diagnosing aneurysmal and unicameral bone cysts with magnetic resonance imaging. *Clin Orthop Relat Res.* 1999;(366):186–190.

225. te Winkel ML, Pieters R, Hop WC, et al. Bone mineral density at diagnosis determines fracture rate in children with acute lymphoblastic leukemia treated according to the DCOG-ALL9 protocol. *Bone.* 2014;59:223–228.

226. Tenenbaum S, Thein R, Herman A, et al. Pediatric nonaccidental injury: are orthopedic surgeons vigilant enough? *J Pediatr Orthop.* 2013;33(2):145–151.

227. Terzi S, Gasbarrini A, Fuiano M, et al. Efficacy and safety of selective arterial embolization in the treatment of aneurysmal bone cyst of the mobile spine: a retrospective observational study. *Spine (Phila Pa 1976).* 2017;42(15):1130–1138.

228. Thackeray JD, Wannemacher J, Adler BH, et al. The classic metaphyseal lesion and traumatic injury. *Pediatr Radiol.* 2016;46(8):1128–1133.

229. Thomas AE. The bleeding child; is it NAI? *Arch Dis Child.* 2004;89(12):1163–1167.

230. Thomas SA, Rosenfield NS, Leventhal JM, et al. Long-bone fractures in young children: distinguishing accidental injuries from child abuse. *Pediatrics.* 1991;88(3):471–476.

231. Tobias JD, Atwood R, Lowe S, et al. Anesthetic considerations in the child with Gaucher disease. *J Clin Anesth.* 1993;5(2):150–153.

232. Townsend PF, Cowell HR, Steg NL. Lower extremity fractures simulating infection in myelomeningocele. *Clin Orthop Relat Res.* 1979;(144):255–259.

233. Trinh A, Wong P, Brown J, et al. Fractures in spina bifida from childhood to young adulthood. *Osteoporos Int.* 2017;28(1):399–406.

234. Uddenfeldt Wort U, Nordmark E, Wagner P, et al. Fractures in children with cerebral palsy: a total population study. *Dev Med Child Neurol.* 2013;55(9):821–826.

235. Waguespack SG, Hui SL, Dimeglio LA, et al. Autosomal dominant osteopetrosis: clinical severity and natural history of 94 subjects with a chloride channel 7 gene mutation. *J Clin Endocrinol Metab.* 2007;92(3):771–778.

236. Wang J, Temple HT, Pitcher JD, et al. Salvage of failed massive allograft reconstruction with endoprosthesis. *Clin Orthop Relat Res.* 2006;443:296–301.

237. Watanabe K, Tsuchiya H, Sakurakichi K, et al. Treatment of lower limb deformities and limb-length discrepancies with the external fixator in Ollier's disease. *J Orthop Sci.* 2007;12(5):471–475.

238. Williams P. The management of arthrogryposis. *Orthop Clin North Am.* 1978;9(1):67–88.

239. Wu JS, Goldsmith JD, Horwich PJ, et al. Bone and soft-tissue lesions: what factors affect diagnostic yield of image-guided core-needle biopsy? *Radiology.* 2008;248(3):962–970.

240. Zarate YA, Clingenpeel R, Sellars EA, et al. COL1A1 and COL1A2 sequencing results in cohort of patients undergoing evaluation for potential child abuse. *Am J Med Genet A.* 2016;170(7):1858–1862.

241. Zeitlin L, Fassier F, Glorieux FH. Modern approach to children with osteogenesis imperfecta. *J Pediatr Orthop B.* 2003;12(2):77–87.

242. Zhao JG, Wang J, Huang WJ, et al. Interventions for treating simple bone cysts in the long bones of children. *Cochrane Database Syst Rev.* 2017;2:CD010847.

243. Zwemer E, Claudius I, Tieder J. Update on the evaluation and management of brief resolved unexplained events (previously apparent life-threatening events). *Rev Recent Clin Trials.* 2017;12(4):233–239.

Fractures and Dislocations of the Hand and Carpal Bones in Children

Nina Lightdale-Miric and Scott H. Kozin

Fractures of the Hand and Carpal Bones

INCIDENCE OF FRACTURES AND DISLOCATIONS OF THE HAND AND CARPAL BONES

The pediatric hand is exposed and vulnerable to injury during play as a curious child explores their surrounding world.[36,173,177] Hand injuries account for up to 25% of pediatric fractures (Table 7-1).[36,173] The reported annual incidence is approximately 26.4 fractures/10,000 children.[141]

Pediatric hand fractures occur primarily in a *biphasic* age distribution: toddler and adolescent. In toddlers, the injury occurs most often secondary to a crush[14,36,50]; for example, a closing door. In teenagers, however, the mechanism is more commonly from a torque, twist, or axial load sustained during contact activities and athletics.[85,114,149,153]

A higher incidence of pediatric upper extremity fractures is associated with certain youth sports, such as snow skiing, skateboarding, or ball sports.[64] Overweight adolescents can have poorer balance or increased body mass indices, which may explain their propensity for upper extremity fracture related to falls on an outstretched hand.[24] Hand fractures in children peak around age 13, coinciding with active participation in organized contact sports, random play, as well as punching.[148,184]

TABLE 7-1. Incidence of Pediatric Hand Injuries

Peak Age: 13 yrs

Annual incidence: 26.4/10,000 children

Percentage of all pediatric emergency patients: 1.7%

Right side incidence equals left

Male incidence is greater than female incidence

Most common fracture types

• Nonphyseal: Distal phalanx (crush)

• Physeal: Proximal phalanx

• Index and small fingers most commonly injured

The two most common pediatric hand fractures are distal phalanx crush injuries and Salter–Harris (S-H) II fractures of the proximal phalanx.[34,124,135,141,159,173] The border digits (thumb and small fingers) are the most vulnerable rays.[124,135,141,159,173,177] Dislocations are relatively uncommon in children. Forces are more often transmitted through the physis rather than the collateral ligaments in a child's hand because the growth plate is the path of least resistance.[97,135,141,149,173] Proximal phalanx S-H II fractures account for nearly 33% of all hand fractures in children. Although rare, the thumb metacarpophalangeal (MCP) joint is the most commonly dislocated joint in the skeletally immature hand.[55,125,155] The proximal interphalangeal (PIP) joint is the most commonly injured articular surface involving the volar plate or collateral ligament avulsion fractures.

Fractures and dislocations about the child's carpus are rare compared to injuries of the adjacent vulnerable physis of the distal radius.[70,141] The scaphoid is the most frequently injured carpal bone in children.[49,73,96] Pediatric scaphoid fractures have a peak incidence between the ages of 12 and 15 years.[138] Scaphoid fractures are extremely rare during the first decade of life.[27,32,73,97,132] Only a few reported cases involve children younger than 8 years of age, and the youngest patient reported is 4 years of age.[138]

Carpal ligament dissociation and tears of the triangular fibrocartilage complex (TFCC) do occur in children and adolescents, mostly common with athletic trauma or associated with skeletal trauma[105] such as distal radial fractures or as a consequence of radial growth arrest, positive ulnar variance, and ulnar carpal impaction.

APPLIED ANATOMY OF HAND AND CARPAL BONES

Children have distinct patterns of hand injury because of their underlying skeletal and soft tissue anatomy. Knowledge of the architecture of the physis, the soft tissue origins and insertions, and the surrounding periosteum is essential for the diagnosis and treatment of children's hand fractures.

OSSEOUS ANATOMY

Potential epiphyses exist at both the proximal and distal ends of all the tubular bones. Secondary ossification centers, however, develop only at the distal ends of the metacarpals of the index, long, ring, and small rays, and at the proximal end of the thumb. Conversely, the epiphyses are present only at the proximal ends of the phalanges in all digits.[149]

Secondary Ossification Centers

The pattern of carpal bone ossification and the appearance of secondary ossification sites in the metacarpals and phalanges are often used to predict the skeletal bone age and years of remaining growth (Fig. 7-1).[116] The fetal wrist begins as a single cartilaginous mass. By the 10th week of gestation, the carpus transforms into eight distinct entities with definable intercarpal separations. Although these precursors display minor differences in contour, the amatomic elements greatly resemble the individual carpal bones in their mature form.[62]

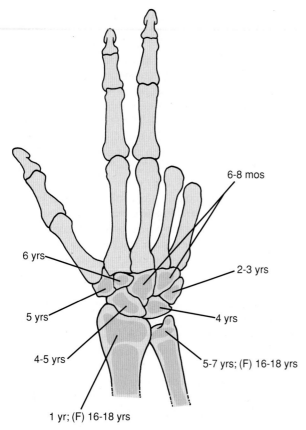

Figure 7-1. The age at the time of appearance of the ossific nucleus of the carpal bones and distal radius and ulna. The ossific nucleus of the pisiform (not shown) appears at about 6 to 8 years of age.

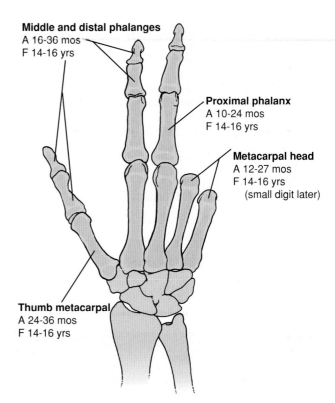

Figure 7-2. Appearance of secondary ossification centers (*A*). Fusion of secondary centers to the primary centers (*F*).

In boys, the secondary ossification centers within the proximal phalanges appear at 15 to 24 months and fuse by bone age of 16 years (Fig. 7-2).[116] In girls, the appearance and closure occur earlier, at 10 to 15 months and bone age of 14 years, respectively. The secondary ossification centers of the middle and distal phalanges appear later in both girls and boys, usually by 6 to 8 months. Fusion of the secondary ossification centers, however, occurs first distally then proximally with maturity. Within the metacarpal, the secondary ossification centers appear at 18 to 27 months in boys and at 12 to 17 months in girls. The proximal thumb metacarpal secondary ossification center appears 6 to 12 months after the fingers. The secondary centers within the metacarpals fuse between 14 and 16 years of age in girls and boys.

The capitate is the first carpal bone to ossify, usually within the first few months of life and certainly by 1 year of age. The hamate appears next, usually at about 4 months of age. The pattern of ossification proceeds stepwise from the distal row to the proximal row moving counterclockwise in a circular fashion when looking at the back of your left hand. The triquetrum appears during the second year, and the lunate begins ossification around the fourth year. The scaphoid begins to ossify in the fifth year, usually slightly predating the appearance of the trapezium.[32] Scaphoid ossification begins at the distal aspect and progresses in a proximal direction.[22] The trapezium and trapezoid ossify in the fifth year, with the trapezoid lagging slightly behind. The ossification pattern usually concludes with the pisiform in the ninth or tenth year. The scaphoid, trapezoid, lunate, trapezium, and pisiform may demonstrate multiple centers of ossification.[22,160] Although variations are well recognized, they may be confused with acute trauma or ligamentous rupture by the inexperienced observer. For example, since the scaphoid ossifies from proximal to distal, the distance between the scaphoid and lunate is greater in the immature wrist (pseudo-Terry Thomas sign). Contralateral x-rays or advanced imaging can clarify the anatomy and prevent misdiagnosis.

The ossific nucleus of each carpal bone is cloaked in a cartilaginous cover during development, which provides a unique shelter from injury.[34] This observation is supported by epidemiologic studies of scaphoid fractures that highlight the infrequent incidence in children younger than 7 years of age and the marked increase in teenagers.[32,73] The detection of injuries to the immature carpus is likely underappreciated because of difficulties in examining an injured child, and the limited ability of radiographs to reveal injury in ossifying carpal bones.[16,106]

PHYSEAL ANATOMY

The physis (growth plate) of the long bones of the hand provides longitudinal growth.[128] The physis is divided into four distinct zones: germinal, proliferative, hypertrophic, and provisional calcifications (zones I, II, III, and IV, respectively). The zone of chondrocyte hypertrophy (zone III) is the least resistant to mechanical stresses. This zone is devoid of the collagen that provides inherent stabilizing properties. Collagen is dominant in zones I and II while the calcium in zone IV provides the most structural strength.[20,34] Therefore, the fracture often propagates through zone III as the

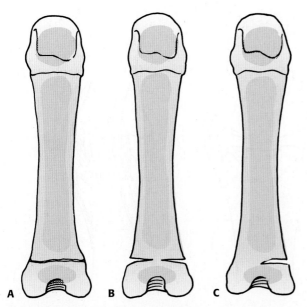

Figure 7-3. Abnormal epiphyseal appearance. **A:** Double epiphysis. **B:** Pseudoepiphysis. **C:** Notched epiphysis.

path of least resistance. High-energy injuries, however, may undulate through all four zones of the physis.[121,128]

The irregularity of the physeal zones in the phalanges and metacarpals increases near skeletal maturity.[19] Thus, a fracture line may be transmitted through several zones in adolescents. This variable path through irregular topography contributes to the increased risk of partial growth arrest following adolescent physeal fractures.[121] Physeal irregularity also explains the differing patterns of physeal injuries dependent on age: S-H I and II fractures tend to occur in younger patients compared to the S-H III or IV fractures that are more prevalent in children close to skeletal maturity.

Pseudoepiphyses, Double Epiphyses, and Periphyseal Notching

A persistent expression of the distal epiphysis of the thumb metacarpal is called a pseudoepiphysis.[143] The pseudoepiphysis appears earlier than the proximal epiphysis and fuses rapidly. By the sixth or seventh year, the pseudoepiphysis is incorporated within the metacarpal and is inconspicuous. Pseudoepiphyses also have been noted at the proximal ends of the finger metacarpals, usually of the index ray. The only clinical significance is radiologic differentiation from an acute fracture following an injury (Fig. 7-3).

Double epiphyses can be present in any bone of the hand, but these anomalies are more common in the metacarpals of the index finger and thumb. There are variable expressions of double epiphyses, but the true entity is considered only when a fully developed growth mechanism is present on both ends of a tubular bone. Double epiphyses are usually seen in children with other congenital anomalies, but their presence does not appear to influence overall bone growth.[117]

Periphyseal "notching" should not be confused with double epiphyses, pseudoepiphyses, or fracture.[117,143] The location of the notches can coincide with the physis or may be slightly more distant from the epiphysis. Notching is a benign condition

that does not influence the structural properties of the bone.[117] Clinical examination and x-rays of the contralateral noninjured hand are critical to clarify unique individual osseous anatomy from an acute injury.

SOFT TISSUE ANATOMY

The tensile strength of a younger child's soft tissues usually exceeds that of the adjacent physis and epiphysis.[98,128] For this reason, tendon or collateral ligament avulsions are less common compared to physeal or epiphyseal fractures in the skeletally immature hand.[98,145]

Tendons

The terminal tendon of the digital extensor mechanism and the extensor pollicis longus insert on the epiphyses of the distal phalanx. The central slip of the extensor mechanism inserts onto the epiphysis of the middle phalanx. The extensor pollicis brevis inserts onto the epiphysis of the proximal phalanx of the thumb. The abductor pollicis longus has a broad-based insertion onto both the radial epiphysis and metaphysis of the thumb metacarpal. These extensor tendinous insertions are broad to the thick periosteum, which predisposes bony avulsion injuries. The extensor digitorum communis for index through small finger connects into the sagittal band at the MCP joint, which in turn lifts the proximal phalanx into extension by its insertion along the volar plate.

The long digital flexor tendons (flexor digitorum profundus [FDP] and the flexor pollicis longus [FPL]) insert along the metadiaphyseal, not epiphyseal, region of their respective terminal phalanges of the fingers and thumb.[145] The flexor digitorum superficialis (FDS) inserts onto the central three-fifths of the middle phalanx.

Collateral Ligaments

The collateral ligaments at the interphalangeal joint originate from the collateral recesses of the phalangeal head, span the physis, and insert onto both the metaphysis and epiphysis of the middle and distal phalanges (Fig. 7-4). The collaterals also insert onto the volar plate to create a three-sided box that protects the physes and epiphyses of the interphalangeal joints from laterally directed forces.[55,145] This configuration explains the rarity of S-H III injuries at the interphalangeal joints.

In contrast, the collateral ligaments about the MCP joints originate from the metacarpal epiphysis and insert almost exclusively onto the epiphysis of the proximal phalanx (Fig. 7-5). This anatomic arrangement accounts for the frequency of S-H III injuries at the MCP joint level.

Volar Plate

The volar plate is a stout stabilizer of the interphalangeal joint and MCP joints and resists hyperextension forces. The volar plate originates from the metaphysis of the respective proximal digital segment and inserts onto the epiphysis of the distal segment (Fig. 7-4B). The plate receives insertional fibers from the accessory collateral ligaments to create a three-sided box that protects the joint. Hyperextension of the finger joints often results in avulsion injuries of the epiphysis or S-H III at the volar plate insertion site.

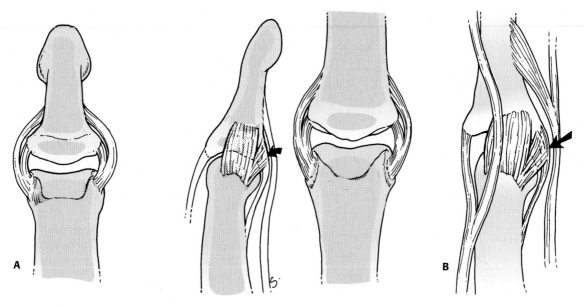

Figure 7-4. Anatomy of the collateral ligaments at the distal (**A**) and proximal (**B**) interphalangeal joints. The collateral ligaments at the interphalangeal joints originate in the collateral recesses and insert into both the metaphyses and epiphyses of their respective middle and distal phalanges. Additional insertion into the volar plane (*arrows*) is seen at the interphalangeal joints.

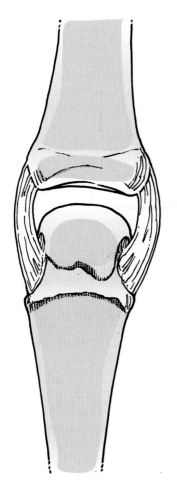

Figure 7-5. The collateral ligaments at the MCP joint originate and insert almost exclusively on the epiphyseal regions of the metacarpal and the proximal phalanges.

Periosteum

The periosteum is robust in a child's hand and can act as a considerable asset or liability in fracture management. On the positive side, the periosteal sleeve can minimize fracture displacement and aid in fracture reduction. On the negative side, the periosteum can shear off, become interposed between displaced fracture fragments, and prevent reduction.

Nail Matrix

The skin, nail elements, soft tissues, and bone of the distal digit are closely related (Fig. 7-6). The dorsal periosteum of the distal phalanx is the underlying nutritional and structural support for the sterile matrix and nail bed. The germinal matrix is responsible for generating the nail plate. The sterile matrix has a role in nail plate adherence as well as adding strength and thickness to the plate.

REMODELING OF HAND AND CARPAL BONES

A young child's ability to remodel displaced fractures in the hand and carpus must be incorporated into the treatment algorithm. Factors that influence remodeling potential include the patient's age, the proximity of the fracture to the physis, and the plane of motion of the adjacent joint. The remodeling capacity is greater in: (1) younger children, (2) fractures that are closer to the physis, and (3) deformity in the plane of motion.[34,75,140] Several clinicians have observed remodeling between 20 to 30 degrees in the sagittal plane in children under 10 years of age and 10 to 20 degrees in older children.[21,140] Remodeling potential in the coronal or adduction–abduction plane is rarely quantified but is likely greater than or equal to 50% of the remodeling potential in the sagittal plane. Rotational deformity remodeling never occurs unless there is rotatory joint motion (carpometacarpal [CMC] joint thumb) and is an indication for fracture management.

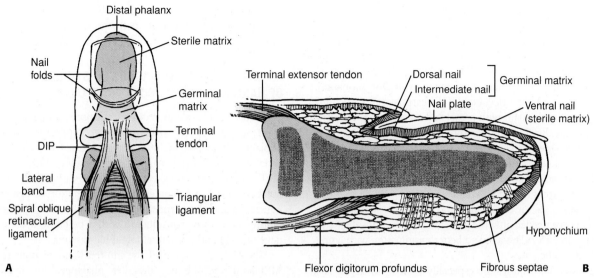

Figure 7-6. Anatomy about the distal phalanx. **A:** The skin, nail, and extensor apparatus share a close relationship with the bone of the distal phalanx. Specific anatomic structures at the terminal aspect of the digit are labeled. **B:** This lateral view of the nail demonstrates the tendon insertions and the anatomy of the specialized nail tissues.

The speed of healing in children is remarkable. In the skeletally immature hand, most fractures become clinically stable within 2 weeks. This rapid healing allows earlier motion and decreased stiffness; however, a delay in treatment of just 7 to 10 days may negate the possibility of closed reduction without osteoclasis.

ASSESSMENT OF HAND AND CARPAL BONE FRACTURES

MECHANISMS OF INJURY FOR HAND AND CARPAL BONE FRACTURES

Assessment of a child with a hand fracture should begin with a detailed description of the injury itself, timing of the injury, treatment prior to presentation, history of previous injuries to the same hand, and identification of potential penetrating or embedded materials such as glass, metal, or teeth.

Axial load injuries, such as punching, yield injury primarily to the metacarpals or CMC joints. Digital torsion or lateral bending forces most often propagate through the physis of the phalanx. Hyperextension injuries cause volar plate avulsion fractures.

INJURIES ASSOCIATED WITH CARPAL BONE FRACTURES

Pediatric carpal bone fractures and dislocations are relatively uncommon and associated with higher-velocity trauma. Motor vehicle accidents, contact sports, and falls from a height can cause carpal injury. Additional injuries to the head, cervical spine, wrist, elbow, or shoulder girdle may be present. In these polytrauma cases, treatment decision making may be driven by a need for earlier stabilization to allow mobilization of the child or to prevent fracture displacement during rehabilitation of concomitant injuries.

Children who have sustained carpal bone fractures and dislocations from crush injuries, penetrating trauma, mechanical equipment entrapment, or motor vehicle accidents may also have injuries to the soft tissue envelope of the fingers and hand. Nerve, artery, and tendon repair as well as flap or skin graft coverage may dictate the need for hand fracture stabilization.

SIGNS AND SYMPTOMS OF HAND AND CARPAL BONE FRACTURES

The evaluation of a child's hand, especially of traumatized infants and toddlers, can be more challenging than that of an adult. The child frequently is anxious, unable to understand instructions, and fearful of the physician. The examiner must be patient, engage the child, and often employ the parents to comfort the child. Patience with observation, bribery, and play are the tricks of the trade. The child's hand use, posture, and movements provide clues about the location and severity of the injury as the child interacts with toys, parents, and the environment in the examining area. A hurried examination or a frightened child can lead to an erroneous or missed diagnosis.

Fracture is diagnosed by swelling, ecchymosis, deformity, or limited movement of the fingers or hand. Fracture malrotation is noted by digital scissoring during active grasp or passive tenodesis. Tendon integrity is observed by digital posture at rest and during active grasp around objects of varying size. Passive wrist extension with finger flexion tenodesis is a critical part of the evaluation to accurately diagnose fracture malrotation.

The history, physical examination, and clinical suspicion are the essential elements to diagnosis of a scaphoid and carpus fracture.[99] The relative infrequency of this injury and the difficulty in interpreting radiographs of the immature wrist increase the likelihood of missing a pediatric scaphoid fracture. A distal pole fracture may present with swelling or tenderness over the scaphoid tuberosity. A scaphoid waist fracture typically presents with pain to palpation within the anatomic snuffbox and pain with ulnar deviation of the wrist.

For TFCC and carpal ligamentous injuries, pain is localized to the distal ulna, fovea, and ulnar carpal region. Forearm rotation may be limited and usually reproduces the pain, particularly at the extremes of supination and/or pronation. Compression and ulnar deviation of the carpus against the ulna may reproduce the pain with associated crepitus at times. The stability of the distal radioulnar joint should be compared to the contralateral side.[78,105]

In the relaxed child, the physician may palpate areas of tenderness and move injured joints to assess their integrity. Gentle comparative stress testing and joint stability should be recorded in the anteroposterior (AP) and lateral directions. Repeat examination may be needed after the pain and swelling subside. Reexamination in 5 to 7 days allows a better examination with ample time to intervene.

Neurovascular injuries are especially difficult to detect in a young child. The proper digital artery is dorsal to the proper digital nerve within the finger. Therefore, pulsatile bleeding is indicative of a digital artery injury and usually indicates a concomitant digital nerve laceration. Discriminatory sensibility testing is not reliable until 5 to 7 years of age. Therefore, meaningful objective data are difficult to obtain in the very young. A clinical clue to sensory impairment is that children often bypass a painful or anesthetic digit during grasp and pinch. A helpful examination maneuver is the wrinkle test. Immersion of an innervated digit in warm water for 5 minutes usually results in corrugation or wrinkling of the volar skin of the pulp. Wrinkling is absent in a digit without nerve innervation. If there is doubt about the integrity of the nerve, operative exploration is indicated.

IMAGING AND OTHER DIAGNOSTIC STUDIES OF HAND AND CARPAL BONE FRACTURES

A careful clinical evaluation directs a focused radiographic assessment. Several pediatric imaging factors complicate interpretation of plain radiographs, including unossified segments and normal variations. Lack of understanding of normal ossification pattern of the immature hand creates problems with the detection of fractures and also promotes false interpretation of ligamentous injuries. Accurate interpretation may require comparison to the uninjured hand or consultation with a pediatric atlas of child development and normal radiographic variants.[116]

Complete evaluation of the injured hand or digit requires AP, lateral, and oblique views. The phalangeal line test is useful in recognizing displaced fractures and joint malalignment. A line drawn from the center of the phalangeal neck through the center of the phalangeal metaphysis at the level of the physis, should pass through the exact center of the metacarpal or phalangeal head in a normal finger, regardless of joint flexion (Fig. 7-7).[181] Oblique views are particularly useful for assessing displacement and intra-articular extension. A common radiographic pitfall is failure to obtain a true lateral radiograph of the injured digit. Isolation of the affected digit on the film or splaying of the fingers (cascade lateral) projects a true lateral view.

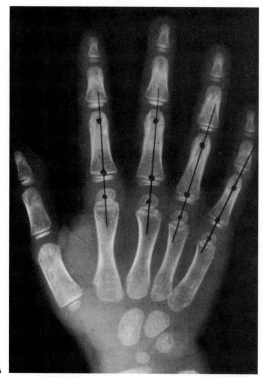
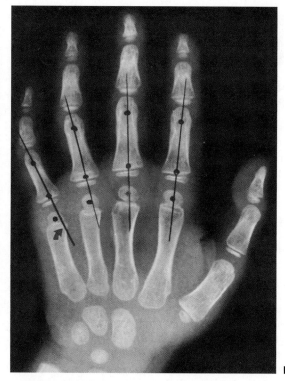

A **B**

Figure 7-7. The straight method of assessing alignment about the MCP joint. The long axes of the metacarpal and proximal phalanx should align, as they do in this normal hand (**A**). If there is a fracture in the proximal phalanges, as in this patient's opposite or injured hand (**B, C**), the axes will not be colinear (*arrows*). (Courtesy of Robert MC, MD and Campbell Jr, MD.)

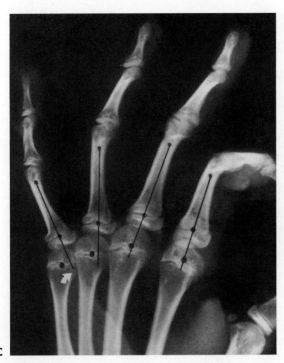

Figure 7-7. (*Continued*)

Stress views are rarely used for pediatric fracture evaluation. If the injury can be clinically isolated to a single digit, individual finger x-rays will demonstrate more detail than a zoomed out image of the entire hand.

Ultrasound, although operator dependent, is increasingly utilized in emergency rooms and clinical triage centers to diagnose a fracture of the upper extremity. Advanced imaging studies are rarely used for finger injuries, although they may provide additional detail in distal radius and carpal bone fractures.

Scaphoid fractures may or may not be evident on initial radiographs; however, sclerosis may appear after a few weeks. A scaphoid view places the scaphoid parallel to the film and reveals the scaphoid in its full size. If the clinical picture is consistent with a scaphoid fracture but the radiographs are negative, the patient should be immobilized. The child should either be instructed to return in 2 weeks for repeat examination and radiographs, or advanced imaging studies may be ordered. MRI can detect scaphoid fractures that are not visualized on the initial radiographs.[8,54,118,129,137] Johnson et al.[137] evaluated 56 children (57 injuries) with MRI within 10 days of injury. All children had a suspected scaphoid injury but negative radiographs. In 33 (58%) of the 57 injuries, the MRI was normal, and the patients were discharged from care. In 16 cases (28%), a fractured scaphoid was diagnosed, and treatment was initiated. Sedation is required for a young child having MRI, and the modality may be overly sensitive in identifying bone edema that never develops into a fracture.[54,175] CT images of the scaphoid can be useful to assess fracture displacement and fracture union. CT images must be made along the longitudinal axis of the scaphoid, which is different from CT imaging of the wrist.[35]

Portable mini-fluoroscopy units are invaluable and allow a real-time assessment. These units have considerable advantages in kids, allowing multiple imaging angles in real time and stress views. Mini-fluoroscopy emits a lower radiation exposure for both the physician and the patient.

DIFFERENTIAL DIAGNOSIS OF HAND AND CARPAL BONE FRACTURES

The differential diagnosis in a child who presents with hand trauma includes nontraumatic entities that may be interpreted as acute injuries. These diagnoses are uncommon but may cause swelling, deformity, or decreased motion.

Congenital or Acquired

A Kirner deformity is a palmar and radial curving of the terminal phalanx of the small digit. This deformity occurs spontaneously between the ages of 8 and 14 years and may be confused with an acute fracture or epiphyseal separation (Fig. 7-8). A trigger thumb or finger in a young child is sometimes mistaken for an interphalangeal joint dislocation. This misperception is caused by the fixed flexion posture, clinical feel of "joint reduction" with manipulative digital extension, and triggering of a nodule or tendon abnormality through the pulley system. The key diagnostic feature or sine qua non of a trigger thumb is the palpable nodule in the FPL (Notta's nodule). Familial camptodactyly or clinodactyly presents predominantly in adolescents. A traumatic event may lead to its recognition. X-rays will reveal an irregular trapezoidal or delta phalanges (aka longitudinal epiphyseal bracket). Thiemann disease is a rare disorder that is considered to be a form of avascular necrosis of the PIP joints. This osteochondrosis may cause epiphyseal narrowing and fragmentation. This hereditary entity (autosomal dominant) usually involves the middle and distal phalanges and presents with painless swelling. Over time, the swelling subsides although some permanent joint deformity may persist.[90,142]

Thermal Injury

Thermal injury to the growing hand (e.g., frostbite, burns from flame or radiation) causes unusual deformities from altered bone growth. Ischemic necrosis of the physes and epiphyses may occur (Fig. 7-9). The clinical result may yield altered bone width, length, or angulation secondary to the unpredictable thermal effect on the growing skeleton.[28]

Tumors

A tumor may be discovered after fracture of the weakened bone or confused with fracture secondary to swelling and pain. An enchondroma of the proximal phalanx is the classic benign tumor that fractures after minor trauma (Fig. 7-10). An isolated osteochondroma that grows into the joint (Trevor's Disease) or Nora's nodule (bizarre periosteal osteochondromatous proliferation) may cause angular alignment of the affected digit. Malignant bone, cartilage, or muscle tumors are rare. Radiographs reveal intrinsic destructive bony changes from a bony sarcoma or extrinsic compression from a malignant soft tissue tumor.

Inflammatory and Infectious Processes

Dactylitis from sickle cell anemia can masquerade as a traumatic injury. The affected digit presents with fusiform swelling

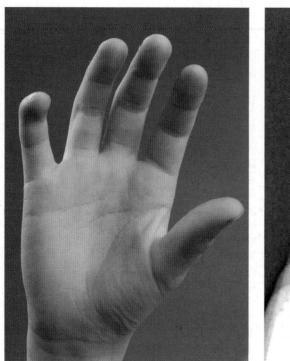

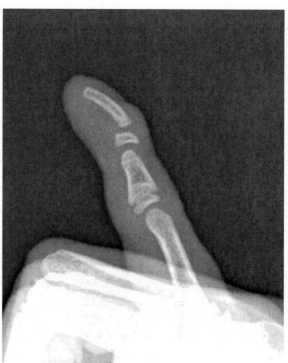

Figure 7-8. A, B: A 9-year-old girl with incurving of the tip of the right small finger. Similar findings are noted in family members. The AP and lateral radiographs show radial and palmar incurving of the distal phalanx characteristic of Kirner deformity.

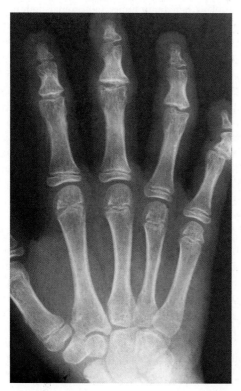

Figure 7-9. An 11-year-old girl sustained a frostbite injury to the right hand. Radiograph reveals premature fusion of the physis of the distal and proximal phalanges with irregularity of the bases of the shortened phalanges.

and decreased motion. The medical history usually is positive for sickle cell disease. The inflammatory arthropathies (e.g., juvenile rheumatoid arthritis, psoriatic arthritis, scleroderma, systemic lupus) may be confused with trauma (Fig. 7-11). A joint effusion and tenosynovitis are findings that require further diagnostic evaluation. An infectious process can be mistaken for injury, though local and systemic evaluation usually ascertains this diagnosis. Children with juvenile inflammatory arthritis often present with a history of trauma (Fig. 7-12). Stiffness and advanced skeletal maturity of the involved carpus are the diagnostic findings.

OUTCOMES OF HAND AND CARPAL BONE FRACTURES

Outcomes assessment following pediatric hand and carpal bone fractures include subjective and objective measures. Patient-reported outcomes are quickly replacing the legacy measures of motion and strength. Outcome instruments such as the Disabilities of the Arm, Shoulder and Hand (DASH), Pediatric Outcomes Data Collection Instrument (PODCI), and Michigan Hand Outcomes Questionnaire (MHQ) can be completed by parents or adolescent children to survey a broad spectrum of long- and short-term results. Newer outcome instruments try to include assessment of the child's ability to text, type on a computer, and play video games. Functional evaluations such as pinch and grip strength, pegboard test, dexterity, in-hand manipulation, and Jebsen–Taylor timed testing are examples of validated outcome instruments in the assessment of hand function in children.

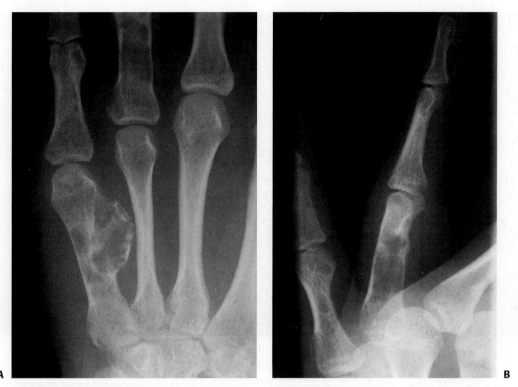

Figure 7-10. A, B: A 14-year-old girl with multiple enchondromas (Ollier disease), which weaken the bone and increase the susceptibility to fracture. (Courtesy of Shriners Hospitals for Children, Philadelphia, PA.)

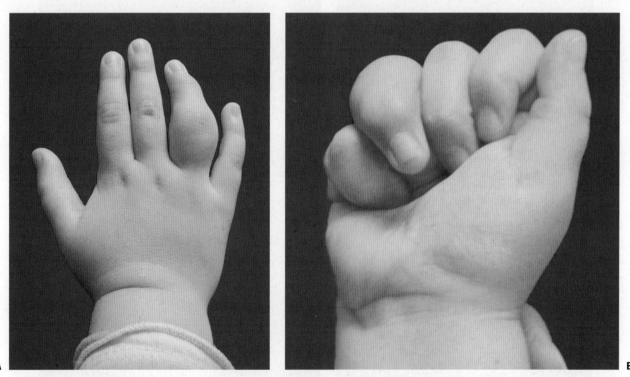

Figure 7-11. A: Images of a 3½-year-old girl with a history of 1 year of right ring finger swelling. Rheumatologic workup was negative. Repeat synovectomy was scheduled and the patient was seen for a second opinion. The surgery was cancelled and the patient was referred to pediatric rheumatologist and ultimately diagnosed with inflammatory arthritis. Photographs show right ring finger dactylitis (**A**) and decreased flexion (**B**).   (*continues*)

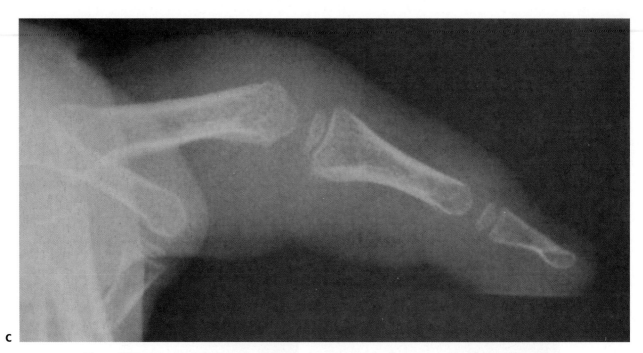

C

Figure 7-11. (*Continued*) **C:** Lateral radiograph shows fusiform soft tissue swelling and preservation of the joint structure. Workup revealed psoriatic arthritis. (Courtesy of Shriners Hospital for Children, Philadelphia, PA.)

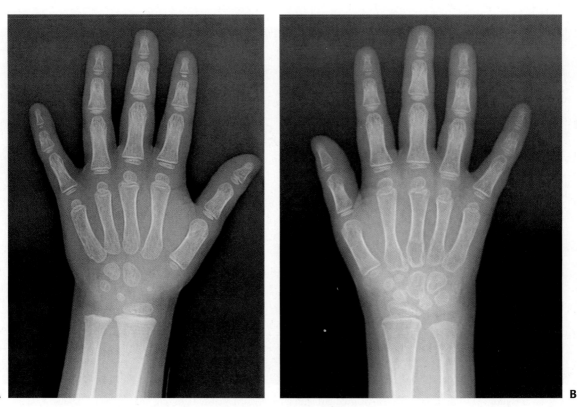

A   **B**

Figure 7-12. Posteroanterior radiographs of both wrists of a 4-year-old girl brought in for evaluation because of a 3-month history of stiffness in the right wrist that began when she fell from a swing. Rheumatology workup diagnosed juvenile inflammatory arthritis. (Courtesy of Shriners Hospital for Children, Philadelphia, PA.)

Fractures of the Distal Phalanx

Classification of Distal Phalangeal Fractures

- Extraphyseal
  - Transverse diaphysis
  - Longitudinal splitting
  - Comminuted separations
  - Avulsion of FDP tendon with bone (Jersey finger)

- Physeal
  - S-H I or II including Seymour fracture
  - S-H III with or without extensor tendon displacement "pediatric mallet finger"
  - S-H IV with articular extension

- Mechanism
  - Crush
  - Hyperflexion
  - Hyperextension

- Open versus closed

Fractures of the distal phalanx in children can be classified into extraphyseal and physeal injuries. Extraphyseal fractures range from a simple distal tuft fracture to an unstable diaphyseal fracture underlying a nail bed laceration. The extraphyseal fracture pattern can be divided into three types: transverse, longitudinal split, or comminuted (Fig. 7-13). A transverse fracture

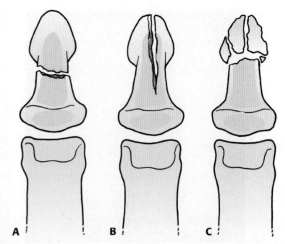

Figure 7-13. Three types of extraphyseal fractures of the distal phalanx. **A:** Transverse diaphyseal fracture. **B:** Cloven-hoof longitudinal splitting fracture. **C:** Comminuted distal tuft fracture with radial fracture lines.

(Fig. 7-12A) may occur either at the distal extent of the terminal phalanx or through the diaphysis. Displaced transverse fractures through the diaphysis are almost always associated with a considerable nail bed injury that requires repair. A longitudinal splitting-type fracture, much less common, is the result of excessive hoop stress within the tubular distal phalanx at the time of a crush injury (Fig. 7-13B). The "cloven-hoof" appearance of the fracture is characteristic (Fig. 7-14). This type of distal phalanx fracture may be contained within the shaft or can

Figure 7-14. A, B: Extraphyseal fracture of the distal phalanx: The cloven-hoof longitudinal splitting fracture. In this patient, the fracture line (*arrow*) does not appear to extend across the physis.

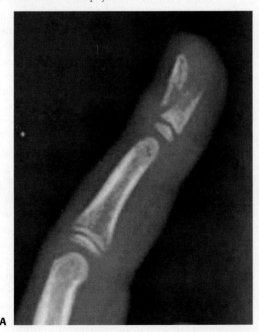

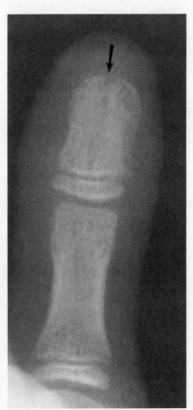

A

B

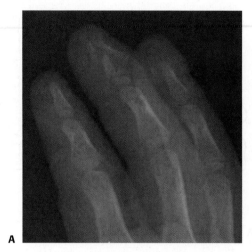
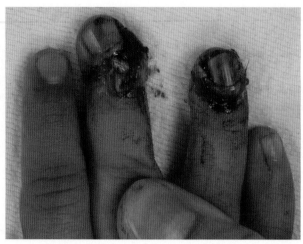

Figure 7-15. **A, B:** Stellate or comminuted extraphyseal fractures and clinical findings.

propagate through the physis and even into the joint. Comminuted or stellate fractures of the distal diaphysis also can occur and usually are often accompanied by extensive nail and soft tissue injury (Fig. 7-15).

Physeal fractures clinically often resemble a mallet finger. There are four basic fracture patterns, and most result in a flexed posture of the distal interphalangeal (DIP) joint (Fig. 7-16). An S-H I or II fracture with flexion of the distal fragment, known as

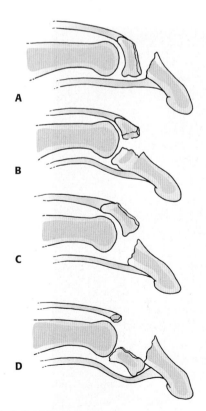

Figure 7-16. **A–D:** Mallet-equivalent fracture types.

a Seymour fracture,[107] occurs predominantly in young patients less than 12 years of age. The unopposed FDP flexes the distal fragment. The injury is often open and associated with a very proximal nail bed and plate injury. The proximal nail plate may lie on top of the dorsal nail fold, whereas the distal nail plate remains intact. This open fracture exposes the underlying bone to bacterial contamination and osteomyelitis. Closed reduction may also be blocked by interposition of the nail bed in the dorsal physis deep to the nail plate. Rarely, an S-H I or II fracture causes extrusion of the epiphyseal fragment.[44,171] This "epiphyseal dislocation" is challenging to diagnose with an "invisible" not yet ossified epiphysis. The remaining distal phalanx stays colinear with the axis of the digit, whereas the displaced unossified epiphysis is dorsally dislocated by the pull of the extensor tendon. A dorsal S-H III or IV fracture of the distal phalanx, "bony mallet finger," occurs in teenagers and results in an extension lag at the DIP joint and joint incongruity. Very rarely, the epiphysis may also separate from the terminal extensor tendon.[39]

Distal phalanx fractures can also be described by mechanism of injury including crush, hyperflexion, and hyperextension. A crush injury creates a spectrum of damage from minor tissue disruption with little need for intervention to severe tissue trauma that requires bony fixation, meticulous nail bed repair, and skin coverage (Fig. 7-17). A flexion force applied to the extended tip of the finger results in a mallet-like injury to the terminal tendon insertion or physeal separation with nail bed injury as described above. The DIP joint remains flexed whereas active extension is not possible in both types. A hyperextension force can produce a bony avulsion injury of the volar articular surface or rupture of the insertion of the FDP tendon (Jersey finger) (Fig. 7-18) although this is rarely reported in children.

Finally, fractures can be classified into open or closed injuries. A nail bed injury or a subungual hematoma greater than 50% creates a high index of suspicion for an open bony injury and displaced nail bed laceration (Fig. 7-19).[157]

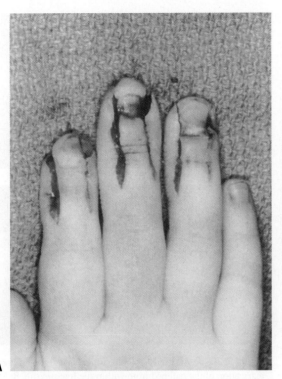
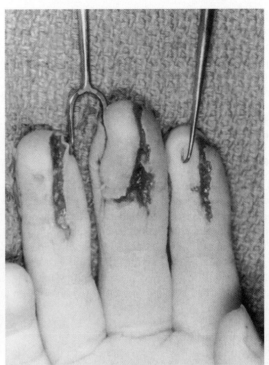

Figure 7-17. A, B: Crush injury to the fingers of a 4-year-old child with multiple fingernail bed lacerations requiring meticulous repair with absorbable suture.

DISTAL PHALANGEAL FRACTURE TREATMENT OPTIONS

INDICATIONS/CONTRAINDICATIONS

Nonoperative Treatment of Phalanx Fractures in Children:	
Indications	**Contraindications**
• Stable	• Unstable
• Closed	• Open
• Low risk of infection, nail deformity, joint instability, or growth plate arrest	• High risk of infection, nail deformity, joint instability, or growth plate arrest

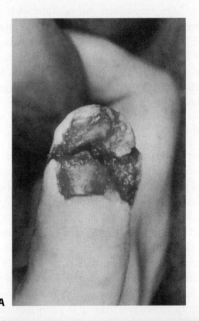

A

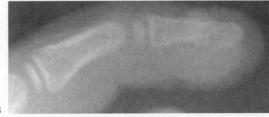

B

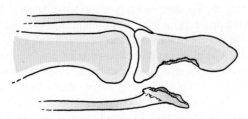

Figure 7-18. An FDP avulsion fracture of the distal phalanx (Jersey finger). This bony avulsion is apparent on radiographs, indicating the extent of proximal migration.

Figure 7-19. A: A crush injury to the thumb of a 4-year-old child with a stellate nail bed laceration and fracture of the tuft. **B:** Radiograph reveals a comminuted tuft fracture.

Distal phalanx fractures in children are frequently associated with nail bed lacerations. The soft tissue repair may be at the bed-side or in the operating room, depending on the emergency room facilities, operating room availability, and surgeon's preference. Any substantial nail bed laceration requires irrigation, debridement, and repair to prevent nail deformity and osteomyelitis.

NONOPERATIVE TREATMENT OF DISTAL PHALANGEAL FRACTURES

Immobilization

Most distal phalangeal fractures can be treated with nonoperative measures using a splint or cast. Mild and moderate displacement of extraphyseal fractures will heal in days to weeks. Clinical union precedes complete radiographic healing by about 1 month. Physeal injuries with mild displacement of the dorsal epiphyseal fragment and joint congruity, "bony mallet finger," have favorable results with hyperextension splinting. Extreme hyperextension is avoided because dorsal skin hypoperfusion and necrosis may result.[45]

Hematoma Evacuation

Indications for a hematoma evacuation, or trephination, have typically been described for subungual hematoma involving more than 50% of the nail plate or painful pressure under the nail in adults, although pediatric-specific indications are unknown.[14] Decompression can be done with a sterile hypodermic needle, heated paper clip, or electrocautery, but the heat can cause further nail bed injury if penetration is too deep. After 12 to 24 hours, the effectiveness of trephination decreases as the blood coagulates. The use of oral antibiotics in the setting of trephination, although theoretically protective against infection, has not been proven.[180]

Nail Bed Repair

A nail bed repair can be performed at bedside, in a clinical procedure room, in an emergency room under digital block and/or conscious sedation, and finally if needed, in the operating room. A digital tourniquet is often used but care has to be taken to remove the digital tourniquet at the end of the repair procedure. Nail bed repair is required for overt nail bed lacerations and potentially for subungual hematomas that involve more than 50% of the nail plate. After adequate anesthesia, a blunt Freer elevator is used to remove the nail plate, avoiding additional nail bed injury. Curved clamps should not be used as they can cause further nail matrix injury. Partial nail removal is rarely indicated for nail bed repair in children. Proximal exposure of the germinal matrix may require scalpel incisions along the eponychial folds and proximal retraction of the eponychial flap. The nail bed is repaired with interrupted 6-0 chromic or equivalent absorbable sutures under loupe magnification. Following repair, the nail bed is supported and the dorsal nail fold is kept open typically using the previously removed nail plate. Other substitutes are possible, such as the foil from the suture pack or a cut portion of a plastic culture tube.[157] Nail plate replacement surgeries are typically unnecessary in children and can lead to limited benefit and more complications.[93] Always remember to remove the digital tourniquet.

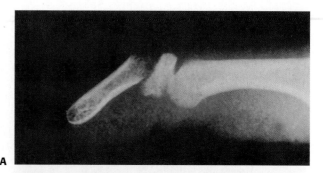

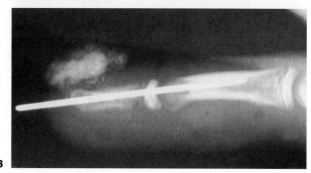

Figure 7-20. A: An irreducible distal phalangeal fracture that required extrication of the nail bed from within the fracture site. **B:** Stabilization of the fracture fragments with a longitudinal K-wire across the DIP joint.

OPERATIVE TREATMENT OF DISTAL PHALANGEAL FRACTURES

Unstable extraphyseal fractures with wide displacement require stabilization. Open injuries with severe displacement or irreducible fractures require reduction and stabilization (Fig. 7-20).[4,127,171] The Seymour fracture represents an open and potentially irreducible fracture that requires open reduction.[44,151,171] The sterile matrix must be extricated from the fracture site and repaired beneath the eponychium. Epiphyseal dislocations also require operative intervention to both restore growth potential and reestablish extensor tendon continuity. Physeal fractures with a dorsal fragment larger than 50% of the epiphysis or considerable DIP joint subluxation may require operative intervention.[55] Volar distal phalanx fractures associated with avulsion of the FDP require repair with tendon reinsertion. Surgery should be done as soon as possible to limit tendon ischemia and shortening. Delay in diagnosis may prohibit tendon reattachment.

Fingertip amputations often involve the distal phalanx. The injury may involve skin, nail tissue, and bone. Support for nail growth is a primary consideration. Minimal loss of tissue can be treated with local wound care and healing through secondary intention. A small amount of exposed bone does not preclude spontaneous healing in children. Debridement of minimally exposed bone will not negatively impact digital length and can expedite healing. The likelihood of nail deformity (hook nail or "parrot's beak") is high for amputations that involve more than 50% of the distal phalanx. Primary nail ablation may be indicated in children with loss of the majority of the distal phalanx to avoid a hook-nail deformity (Fig. 7-21).

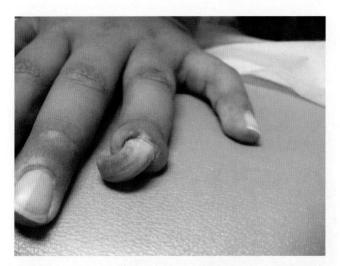

Figure 7-21. A hook nail can become symptomatic and require revision nail ablation. Adequate primary management can prevent this sequela.

Soft tissue coverage varies depending on the degree of tissue loss, direction of injury, and amount of bone exposed or at risk. Simple healing by primary closure is preferred for most volar oblique fingertip amputations. Dorsal oblique amputations are complicated by nail bed injury and are more difficult to cover. Composite grafts of skin and subcutaneous tissue from the amputated part have been used in young children under 3 years of age with variable results. Local flaps are another option for coverage of large volar or dorsal oblique amputations. Options include a variety of flaps, such as a V-Y volar advancement, a thenar flap, a cross-finger flap, a pedicled flap, or a neurovascular island flap (Figs. 7-22 and 7-23). Fortunately, coverage issues are rare in children as most heal with local wound care without flap reconstruction. An amputation of the distal thumb can also be covered with a bipedicle (Moberg) volar advancement flap or a unipedicle neurovascular flap. The choice of coverage depends on the degree and direction of soft tissue loss, age of the patient, amount of bone exposed, long-term outcome risks, and preference of the surgeon and family.

Preoperative Planning

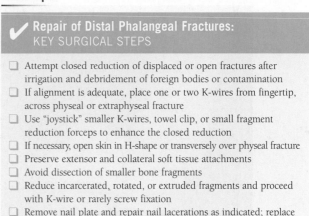

✔ Surgery of Distal Phalangeal Fractures: PREOPERATIVE PLANNING CHECKLIST	
OR table	❏ Hand table
Position	❏ Supine
Fluoroscopy	❏ Mini-fluoroscopy and perpendicular or opposite the surgeon
Equipment	❏ Hand tray instruments, wire driver
Tourniquet	❏ Nonsterile at approximately 200 mm Hg in small children or Esmark
Hardware	❏ 0.027, 0.035, or 0.045 K-wires, limited role for other fixation devices
Suture	❏ 6-0 chromic for nail bed in all patients ❏ 5-0 chromic skin closure in young children ❏ In older children, nonabsorbable monofilament can be used for soft tissue laceration or incision closure

Technique

✔ Repair of Distal Phalangeal Fractures: KEY SURGICAL STEPS
❏ Attempt closed reduction of displaced or open fractures after irrigation and debridement of foreign bodies or contamination
❏ If alignment is adequate, place one or two K-wires from fingertip, across physeal or extraphyseal fracture
❏ Use "joystick" smaller K-wires, towel clip, or small fragment reduction forceps to enhance the closed reduction
❏ If necessary, open skin in H-shape or transversely over physeal fracture
❏ Preserve extensor and collateral soft tissue attachments
❏ Avoid dissection of smaller bone fragments
❏ Reduce incarcerated, rotated, or extruded fragments and proceed with K-wire or rarely screw fixation
❏ Remove nail plate and repair nail lacerations as indicated; replace plate or substitute under dorsal nail fold

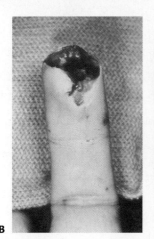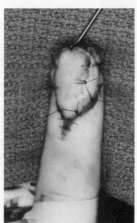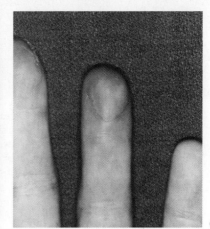

A, B   **C**

Figure 7-22. Volar V-Y advancement flap for coverage. **A:** A volar oblique tissue loss of the ring finger with intact nail bed. **B:** Flap designed with apex at the DIP joint and mobilized to cover the fingertip. The defect is closed proximal to the flap creating the Y. **C:** Satisfactory result with good durability and sensibility.

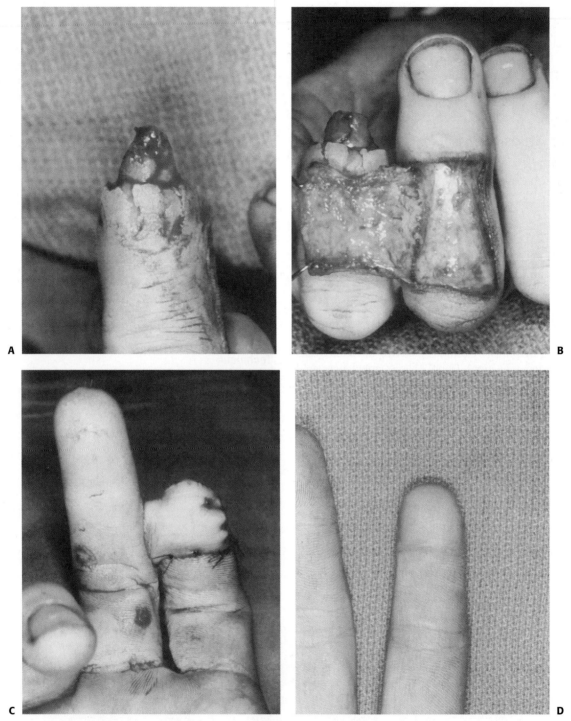

Figure 7-23. Cross-finger flap in a 17-year-old male with open distal phalangeal injury and tissue loss.
A: Extensive volar and distal soft tissue loss with preservation of the bone and nail bed. **B:** A cross-finger flap of skin and subcutaneous tissue is elevated from the dorsal aspect of the adjacent donor digit based on the side of the index finger. **C:** The vascular epitenon is preserved on the donor digit to support a skin graft. The flap is transferred to the volar aspect of the index finger to recreate the tuft. **D:** Satisfactory coverage and functional result.

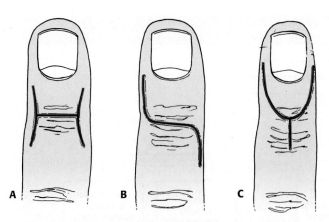

Figure 7-24. Exposures to the DIP joint. **A:** H-type flap with the transverse limb over the DIP joint. **B:** S-shaped exposure of the DIP joint. **C:** An extended exposure of the DIP joint. All exposures must avoid injury to the germinal matrix, which is located just proximal to the nail fold.

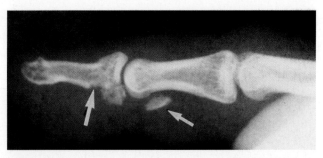

Figure 7-26. A 17-year-old athlete with an avulsion fracture from the FDP tendon. The fracture extends through the epiphysis and into the joint (*large arrow*). The FDP tendon with its attached bony fragment has retracted to the level of the A4 pulley (*small arrow*).

Closed manipulation with or without percutaneous K-wire fixation is usually effective treatment of displaced distal phalanx physeal fractures. One or two smooth 0.35 or 0.45 K-wires can be inserted retrograde through the tip of the finger and across the fracture for stabilization. A hypodermic needle can be used in an emergency as a substitute for smooth wires.[100] A DIP-immobilizing splint alone is often adequate in the older child; a cast is used in an older child. The assistance of joystick K-wires, towel clips, tenaculums, or forceps can be applied as external temporary fixation while final fixation is placed. After the fracture is stabilized, the nail may be repaired in the technique described previously.

In open injuries or fractures that will not reduce with closed technique, a dorsal or midlateral approach is used for most extraphyseal and physeal fractures (Fig. 7-24). The dorsal fragment is isolated and reduced (Fig. 7-25). A small portion of the collateral ligaments may be recessed to enhance exposure; however, soft tissue dissection should be limited to lessen risk of osteonecrosis of small bony fragments. Open fracture fixation can be accomplished with a smooth wire, pull-out wire, tension band, or heavy suture.[50,71,117,181] Fixation may be placed across the DIP joint to maintain joint and physeal congruity. A volar approach is used for FDP tendon avulsion injuries. In acute FDP avulsion injuries, the tendon is identified at the level of retraction and repaired to the distal phalanx with transosseous sutures or wires (Fig. 7-26). The transosseous sutures or wires ideally avoid the growth plate in young children.

Figure 7-25. A: Displaced mallet fracture with considerable articular involvement and dorsal prominence. **B:** Open reduction through a dorsal approach reveals the articular fragment attached to the terminal tendon.

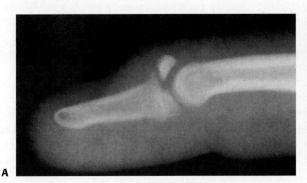

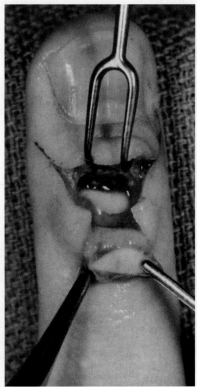

Authors' Preferred Treatment for Fractures of the Distal Phalanx (Algorithm 7-1)

Algorithm 7-1. Authors' preferred treatment for distal phalanx fractures.

Extraphyseal Fractures

Simple closed stable fractures are treated with immobilization in a splint or cast for 1 to 2 weeks, reevaluated and converted to early mobilization when healing is evident. Distal phalanx fractures with a substantial nail bed laceration or avulsion are treated with removal of the nail plate, fracture reduction, and nail bed repair. It takes several cycles of nail growth (3 to 6 months) before the final morphology of the nail is known. An unstable, displaced distal extraphyseal phalangeal fracture that penetrated through the nail bed or is irreducible requires open reduction and percutaneous pinning with a smooth K-wire across the DIP joint and physis (with or without nail bed repair). The pin is removed 3 to 4 weeks after injury, followed by early protected range of motion.

Physeal Fractures

Most closed pediatric S-H III physeal fractures, or bony mallet fingers, are treated with immobilization or by closed reduction and splinting of the DIP joint into neutral or mild hyperextension. Adequate healing requires full-time splinting for 4 to 6 weeks depending on the age of the child, size of the fracture fragment, and amount of bony apposition. Adolescent mallet fingers that are acute or chronic with soft tissue terminal tendon disruption are treated similarly to adults with 4 to 6 weeks of dorsal DIP joint splint immobilization. Operative repair of soft tissue or bony mallet fingers is rarely indicated, even for a delay in presentation. The loss of digital flexion associated with surgery can be more disabling than a minor extension lag.

Surgery is reserved for fractures that are open, grossly unstable, irreducible, or have unacceptable alignment (Fig. 7-25). Closed reduction and longitudinal percutaneous fixation is preferred. Entrapped soft tissue, osteochondral fragments, or epiphyseal dislocations require open reduction. Seymour fractures require irrigation, nail plate removal, fracture alignment, pinning, and nail bed repair (Fig. 7-27).

Jersey Finger

Avulsion injuries of the FDP require open repair (Fig. 7-26). Bone-to-bone fixation is preferred using pull-out wires or suture. Fragments that are too small for fixation require bone removal and repair of the tendon directly to the fracture bed. Repair of long-standing profundus avulsion is controversial and risky in patients with an intact FDS tendon.

Amputations

Mild to moderate loss of skin, subcutaneous tissue, and bone is best treated by wound cleansing, dressing changes, and healing by secondary intention. Acceptable functional and aesthetic results are uniform. Skin or composite grafts are rarely necessary for coverage in children. Extensive soft tissue loss with exposed bone requires more innovative coverage (Figs. 7-22 and 7-23).

Dorsal tissue loss is more difficult to reconstruct. The nail bed injury adds additional complexity. Mild loss can be treated by local wound care. Moderate to severe loss may require a reverse cross-finger flap or a more distant flap. Unfortunately, nail bed replacement techniques, such as partial-thickness grafting from the toe, often result in considerable nail deformity.

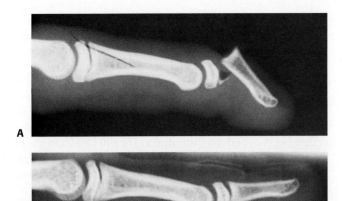

Figure 7-27. A: A 13-year-old boy sustained an open S-H type II fracture. **B:** The wound was cleansed, and acceptable alignment was obtained with closed reduction.

Postoperative Care and Rehabilitation

Children younger than 4 or 5 years of age are immobilized with long-arm mitten strapping, soft casts (3M, St. Paul, Minnesota), or rigid casts. As the child ages, the degree of immobilization is decreased. An adolescent with a simple distal phalangeal fracture or nail bed repair can usually be treated similar to an adult with only DIP joint immobilization. The use of adjunctive antibiotics and tetanus prophylaxis should be utilized in contaminated cases. Nonabsorbable suture should be removed after 2 weeks, but, whenever possible, absorbable suture is used in a child to avoid the trauma of suture removal. Percutaneous skeletal fixation (K-wire fixation) is removed in the office 3 to 4 weeks after surgery. Formal hand therapy is usually not required, though a home exercise program (HEP) with an emphasis on DIP joint motion is useful. Formal therapy is reserved for patients who fail to regain motion and strength after 3 to 4 weeks on a home program.

Potential Pitfalls and Preventive Measures

Distal Phalanx Fracture:
PITFALLS AND PREVENTIONS

Pitfall	Prevention
• Osteomyelitis	• Irrigation and debridement • Nail bed laceration repair • Monitor and treat infection signs early with repeat irrigations and antibiotic coverage
• Premature physeal closure	• Smooth wires • Minimize reduction attempts
• Hook nail	• Ablate nail matrix when majority distal phalanx amputated, avoid advancing nail matrix pulp during repair, use thenar flap closure to support nail
• Quadrigia	• Do not sew extensors or flexors to tip of amputated finger

• Extensor lag	• Neutral or 10-degree extension splint or pin fixation • Continue night, school, and sports splint use for additional 4 to 6 weeks after full-time day splint use discontinued to prevent recurrence
• Osteomyelitis	• Irrigation, debridement

Outcomes

There are few studies that assess outcomes following distal phalanx fractures. The cost-effectiveness of trephination and observation versus removal of the nail plate in nondisplaced nail lacerations over distal phalanx fractures has been studied in several case series.[13,126] These studies concluded that osteomyelitis and nail deformity were equivalent; however, trephination and observation were more cost-effective than nail bed repair. In a series of 200 children, S-H IV, bony mallet, and Seymour fracture patterns were shown to be associated with a higher risk of complications.[151] Identification of these high-risk injuries and early intervention can improve the outcome.[29,183] All studies emphasize the need for prospective randomized trials to better delineate the treatment paradigm.[93]

MANAGEMENT OF EXPECTED ADVERSE OUTCOMES AND UNEXPECTED COMPLICATIONS RELATED TO DISTAL PHALANX FRACTURES

Distal Phalanx Fractures:
COMMON ADVERSE OUTCOMES AND COMPLICATIONS

- Osseous: Nonunion, malunion, osteomyelitis
- Soft tissue: Scar, stiffness, extensor tendon insufficiency with extensor lag
- Nail: Split or hook-nail deformity, rides, ingrown lateral or dorsal nail fold

The overall results following distal phalangeal fractures are favorable. A small loss of motion has negligible functional impact. A small extensor lag or minor longitudinal nail ridge is well tolerated by most patients. Considerable nail irregularity or deformity is a source of dissatisfaction.

Bony complications from distal phalangeal fractures are uncommon. Potential problems include nonunion, malunion, and osteomyelitis. Nonunion and malunion are exceedingly rare, except in open injuries that result in avascular fracture fragments. Osteomyelitis can result from open fractures and requires application of the basic tenets for the treatment of infected bone. Debridement, removal of any sequestrum, and intravenous antibiotics are required to resolve the infection.

Soft tissue complications are more prevalent than bony problems. Difficulties may involve the skin, subcutaneous tissue, nail, and tendons. An inadequate soft tissue envelope can be reconstructed with replacement using a variety of local flaps.

Nail problems depend on the location and degree of nail bed injury. Damage to the germinal matrix produces deficient nail

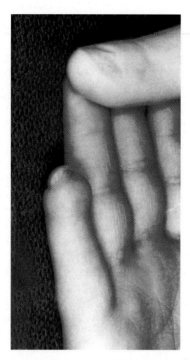

Figure 7-28. A hook-nail deformity of the small finger after a distal fingertip amputation.

growth and nail ridging. Injury to the sterile matrix causes poor nail adherence or nail ridging. Treatment options are limited and usually involve resection of the damaged segment and replacement with a full- or split-thickness skin or nail bed graft.[39,92,158] Adjacent digits or toes are potential sources of nail bed transfers. The results in children have been superior to those in adults, although not uniformly satisfying.[92,158,167,176] The hook nail or "parrot's beak" nail is a nail plate complication related to the underlying bony and soft tissue deficit. The nail plate curves over the abbreviated end of the distal phalanx (Fig. 7-28). Treatment requires restoring length to the shortened distal phalanx and creation of an adequate soft tissue envelope to support the nail plate (Fig. 7-29). In these situations, a thenar flap or composite graft is typically used to provide improved support for the nail bed.

A mild DIP joint or extensor tendon lag can occur after pediatric mallet fracture care. Often, this is an acceptable non-limiting deformity and no further treatment is warranted. Loss of extension is much less debilitating than loss of digital flexion. Chronic mallet fingers in children often still benefit from a course of hyperextension splinting. Severe DIP joint deformities are uncommon but may result in swan-neck positioning of the finger. Reconstruction options are similar to methods used in adults, such as a spiral oblique retinacular ligament reconstruction or central slip tenotomy.[3] In a young child, untreated

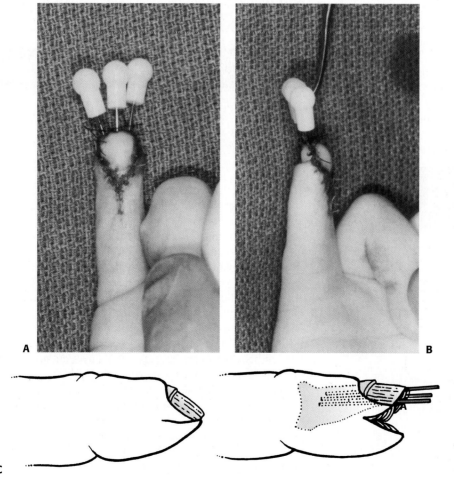

Figure 7-29. A, B: Postoperative photographs of the patient shown in Figure 7-28 after the antenna procedure. The procedure involved the optional technique of a volar V-Y advancement flap to cover the distal tip, elevation of the sterile matrix, and the nail supported using three K-wires. **C:** Line drawings demonstrating technique of elevation and support of the sterile matrix with wires. (**A, B:** Courtesy of William B. Kleinman, MD. **C:** Reprinted from Atasoy E, Godfrey A, Kalisman M. The "antenna" procedure for the "hook-nail" deformity. *J Hand Surg Am.* 1983;8(1):55–58. Copyright © 1983 American Society for Surgery of the Hand. With permission.)

lacerations proximal to the terminal tendon insertion may result in an extensor lag that can be repaired successfully with a teno-dermodesis repair.[146,170]

Middle and Proximal Phalangeal Fractures in Children

CLASSIFICATION OF MIDDLE AND PROXIMAL PHALANGEAL FRACTURES

Classification of Proximal and Middle Phalangeal Fractures

- Physeal
  - S-H I, II, III, IV

- Extraphyseal
  - Shaft
  - Phalangeal neck
  - Intra-articular (condylar)

Classification of middle and proximal phalangeal fractures in children is based primarily on anatomic location. There are four locations: physeal, shaft, neck, and condyles. The fracture pattern varies with the direction and amount of force incurred.

Most fractures of the proximal and middle phalanges result from a torsional or angular force combined with an axial load, such as catching a ball, falling on an outstretched hand, or colliding in sports. Crush injuries are less common in the proximal and middle phalanges than in the distal phalanx. The thumb proximal phalanx and MCP joint are subject to greater lateral bending forces.

Every fracture must be carefully examined for rotational deformity regardless of classification, mechanism of injury, or radiographic appearance. Active finger flexion will produce deviation of the plane of the nails or overt digital scissoring (Fig. 7-30). Passive wrist extension produces long-finger flexor tenodesis, and malrotation will manifest with an abnormal digital cascade or crossover.

Physeal Fractures

Physeal fractures of the proximal phalanx are reported in several series as the most common pediatric hand fracture.[20,50,173] Extra-articular S-H II fractures are more prevalent, and intra-articular S-H III and IV fractures are less common. A common fracture pattern is the S-H II fracture along the ulnar aspect of the proximal phalanx of the small digit. The small digit is angulated in an ulnar direction. This fracture has been termed the "extra-octave" fracture to denote its potential benefit to the span of a pianist's hand (Fig. 7-31).[75] Physeal fractures about the middle phalanx can involve the lateral, dorsal, or volar aspects of the physis. A lateral force across the PIP joint may cause an S-H III or IV fracture. Similarly, a flexion force may produce

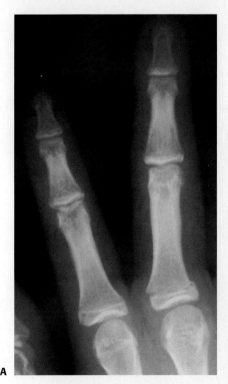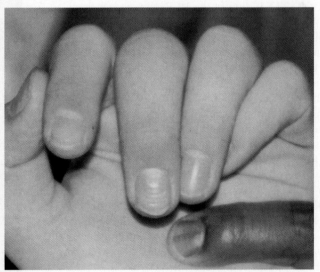

Figure 7-30. A: An AP radiograph of an S-H II fracture at the long-finger proximal phalanx. The radiograph reveals slight angulation and can appear benign. Clinical examination must be done to assess the digital cascade for malrotation. **B:** Tenodesis of the wrist with passive extension reveals unacceptable malrotation as evident by the degree of overlap of the middle finger on the ring finger.

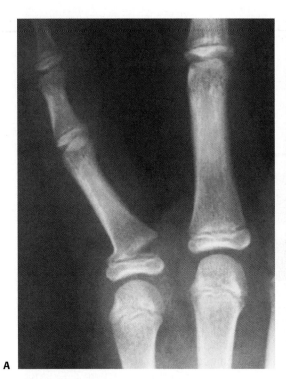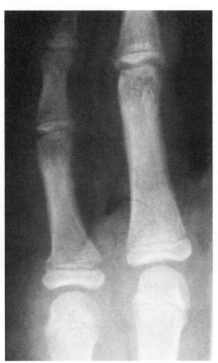

A   B

Figure 7-31. **A:** An extra-octave fracture in a 12-year-old girl. **B:** The fracture was reduced with the MCP joint in full flexion.

a dorsal S-H III fracture, indicative of a central slip avulsion fracture (pediatric boutonnière injury). A hyperextension injury produces small avulsion fragments from the middle phalangeal epiphysis associated with damage to the volar plate.

The thumb proximal phalanx is particularly susceptible to injury. An ulnar collateral ligament (UCL) avulsion injury at the base of the thumb proximal phalanx is similar to the adult gamekeeper's or skier's thumb. The mechanisms of injury, clinical findings of UCL laxity at the MCP joint, and physical symptoms of instability with grip and pinch will be similar to the adult soft tissue UCL injury. However, the fracture pattern is usually an S-H III injury, as the ligament typically remains attached to the epiphyseal fracture fragment (Fig. 7-32). Displaced injuries with articular incongruity or joint instability require open reduction and internal fixation (ORIF) to restore articular alignment and joint stability.[156–158] Similar to the adult counterpart, the epiphyseal fracture with the attached UCL can displace outside the adductor aponeurosis ("Stener's lesion").[156] This location prohibits healing and requires open reduction.

Children rarely sustain comminuted intra-articular fractures of the PIP joint, the so-called "pilon" fractures of the middle phalanx or fracture–dislocations. These injuries can occur in adolescent athletes and result from an axial load sustained while attempting to catch a ball or contacting an opponent. The fracture fragment from the volar side may have the volar plate attached, whereas the dorsal fragment is likely to have the central slip attached. The central aspect of the joint may be depressed and comminuted. The joint can be unstable and incongruent, requiring careful treatment.[121]

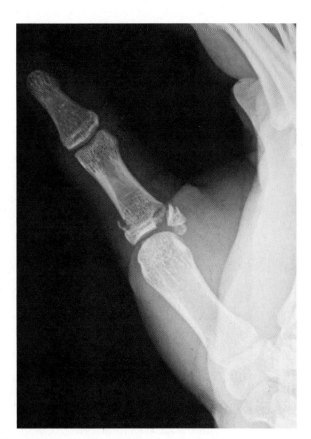

Figure 7-32. Bony gamekeeper's or skier's thumb is an S-H III fracture of the base of the thumb proximal phalanx attached to the UCL of the MCP joint.

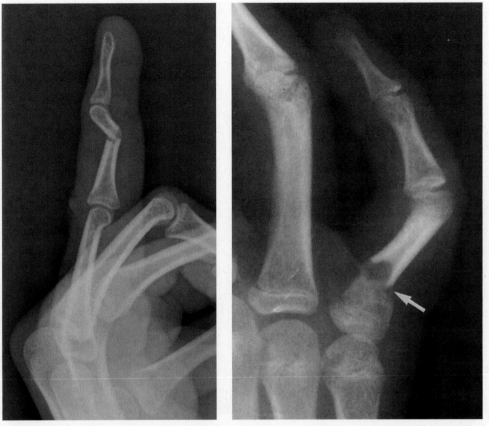

Figure 7-33. A, B: Radiographs of transverse middle and proximal phalangeal fractures respectively which demonstrate the characteristic apex volar deformity.

Shaft Fractures

Extraphyseal middle and proximal phalanx shaft fractures in children are less common. The fracture configuration may be transverse, spiral, or spiral oblique. The fracture may be comminuted. Proximal and middle phalangeal fractures are usually angulated in an apex volar pattern because the distal fragment is extended by the central slip and lateral band, and the proximal fragment is flexed by the FDS in the middle phalanx and by the intrinsic musculature in the proximal phalanx (Fig. 7-33). Oblique fractures often rotate and shorten. Careful clinical evaluation of rotational alignment is critical. Comminution is most often secondary to a high-energy injury or crush mechanism (Fig. 7-34).

Neck Fractures

Neck fractures of the phalanx are problematic with regard to treatment and functional outcome. Displaced neck fractures are also referred to as subcondylar fractures or "door jam fracture" as they often occur in young children as a result of finger entrapment (Fig. 7-35). The head fragment remains attached to the collateral ligaments and tends to rotate into extension.[162] This displacement disrupts the architecture of the subcondylar fossa, which normally accommodates the volar plate and base of the phalanx during interphalangeal joint flexion. Malunited neck fractures may result in a mechanical block to interphalangeal

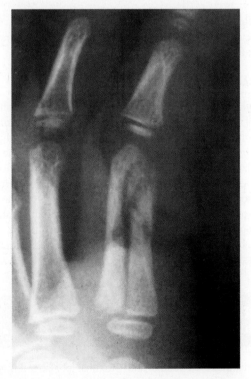

Figure 7-34. Comminuted fractures secondary to a crush injury with longitudinal splitting into the physis.

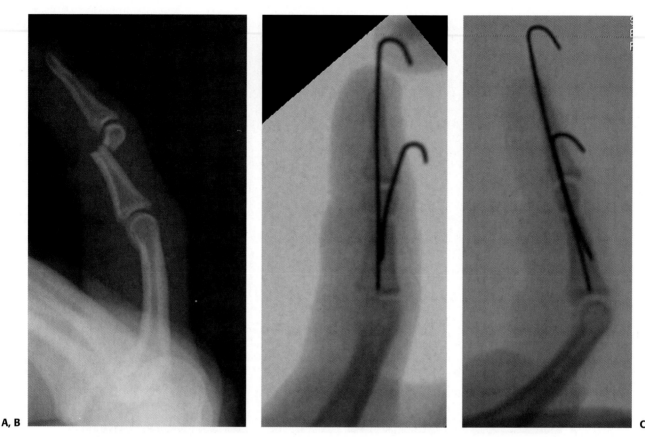

A, B   C

Figure 7-35. A: Phalangeal neck fractures are often unstable and rotated. These fractures are difficult to reduce and control by closed means because of the forces imparted by the volar plate and ligaments. **B, C:** Fixed with a closed reduction and hyperextension maneuver across the DIP joint as well as a derotational wire.

joint flexion. These fractures are inadequately imaged, under-appreciated, or misinterpreted as trivial when they are fractures at risk for poor outcome if left untreated.

Intra-Articular (Condylar) Fractures

Condylar fractures involve the joint and represent a constellation of fracture patterns, including small lateral avulsion fractures, unicondylar or intracondylar fractures, bicondylar or transcondylar fractures, and a rare shearing injury of the entire articular surface and its underlying subchondral bone from the distal aspect of the phalanx (Fig. 7-36). Condylar fractures can be associated with subluxations or dislocations of the joint. Many of these fractures are initially misdiagnosed as sprains[179] and too often present late with an articular malunion. Restoration of articular alignment and joint stability is critical to a successful outcome (Fig. 7-37).

TREATMENT OPTIONS FOR MIDDLE AND PROXIMAL PHALANX FRACTURES

The treatment of middle and proximal phalangeal fractures varies greatly with the type of injury. Nonoperative treatment

is overwhelmingly the most common management for most physeal and shaft nondisplaced fractures. Operative treatment is utilized most for neck and condylar fractures, especially fractures that are displaced or unstable.

NONOPERATIVE AND OPERATIVE TREATMENT OF MIDDLE AND PROXIMAL PHALANGEAL FRACTURES

Indications/Contraindications

Treatment of Middle and Proximal Phalangeal Fractures: INDICATIONS	
Nonoperative Indications	**Operative Indications**
• Stable initially or after closed reduction	• Unstable
• Closed, isolated	• Open, polytrauma
• Normal tenodesis (no malrotation)	• Malrotation (scissoring)
• Joint congruity and stability	• Joint incongruity (S-H III, neck, or condylar fractures)

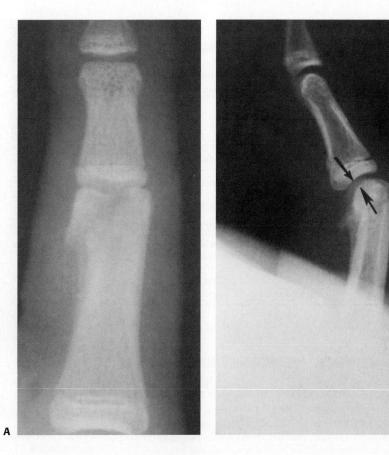

Figure 7-36. A: An AP radiograph reveals an intra-articular fracture of the small finger. **B:** Lateral view demonstrates the double-density sign indicative of displacement (*arrows*).

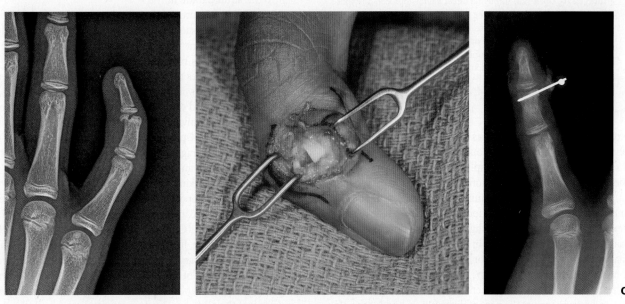

Figure 7-37. A 13-year-old male football player who injured right small finger during a game. **A:** Anteroposterior x-ray with displaced unicondylar fracture small finger distal interphalangeal joint. **B:** Dorsal exposure of distal interphalangeal joint with wide displacement of radial condyle. **C:** Postoperative x-ray with restoration of joint congruity after open reduction and internal fixation with K-wire. (Courtesy of Shriners Hospital for Children, Philadelphia, PA.)

Preoperative Planning

✔ **ORIF of Middle and Proximal Phalangeal Fractures:**
PREOPERATIVE PLANNING CHECKLIST

OR table	❑ Hand table
Position	❑ Supine
Fluoroscopy	❑ Perpendicular or opposite the surgeon
Equipment	❑ Hand tray instruments, wire driver
Tourniquet	❑ Nonsterile at approximately 200 mm Hg in small children or Esmark
Hardware	❑ 0.027, 0.035, or 0.045 K-wires; tension-band wires, modular screw set
Suture	❑ Nonabsorbable or absorbable suture for incision closure

Technique

✔ **ORIF of Middle and Proximal Phalangeal Fractures:**
KEY SURGICAL STEPS

❑ Attempt closed reduction of displaced or open fractures after irrigation and debridement of foreign bodies or contamination
❑ If alignment is adequate, place one or two K-wires parallel or crossed at fracture site, across physeal or extraphyseal fracture. Limit crossing of PIP joint
❑ Use "joystick" smaller K-wires, Freer elevator, dental pick, towel clip, or small fragment reduction forceps to enhance the closed reduction, osteoclasis for partially healed fractures
❑ If necessary, open skin through a direct lateral approach or expose the articular surface through the open fracture wound
   • Preserve extensor and collateral soft tissue attachments
   • Avoid dissection of smaller bone fragments
❑ Reduce incarcerated, rotated, or extruded fragments and proceed with K-wire or lag screw fixation.

Physeal Fractures

Nondisplaced physeal fractures of the proximal and middle phalanges are treated by nonoperative management. Minimal displacement is treated with splinting or functional casting in the intrinsic plus or safe position for 3 weeks.

Moderate displacement requires closed reduction with local anesthesia or conscious sedation. Placing the MCP joint into flexion tightens the collateral ligaments and facilitates fracture manipulation and reduction. In the "extra-octave" fifth proximal phalanx fracture, a pencil or digit in the fourth web space as a fulcrum may assist reduction.[111] Buddy tape and cast immobilization will maintain alignment until healing (Fig. 7-30). The age and compliance of the patient determine if buddy tape alone or combined with casting is necessary. Minimally displaced S-H III epiphyseal fractures at the base of the middle phalanx associated with volar plate avulsion are treated with early buddy tape or extension block splint. "Pediatric boutonnière" fractures or dorsal S-H III epiphyseal fractures can be treated with a PIP

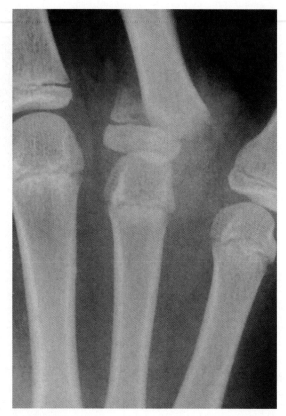

Figure 7-38. Displaced S-H II fracture of the proximal phalanx that was irreducible. The distal fragment was herniated through a rent in the periosteum and extensor mechanism that prohibited reduction.

extension splint and early DIP range-of-motion exercises similar to the adult paradigm.

Irreducible fractures of the physis may be caused by[5,50] any surrounding soft tissue structures, including periosteum and tendon. Open treatment with removal of the impeding tissue and fracture reduction is required for these rare injuries (Fig. 7-38). Some S-H II fractures may be reducible but unstable after reduction. These fractures require insertion of a smooth K-wire after reduction is required to maintain fracture alignment.[5,68] Another indication for operative management is a displaced S-H III fracture of the proximal phalangeal base with a sizable (more than 25%) epiphyseal fragment to restore articular congruity.[68,173] Operative exposure and fixation techniques are challenging with nonborder digit proximal phalangeal S-H III fractures.

A bony gamekeeper's or skier's thumb is an S-H III fracture of the proximal phalanx that requires closed reduction and percutaneous pinning (CRPP) or ORIF with K-wire or modular screw fixation if the fragment is large enough. Open visualization may be necessary for visualization of the articular reduction and reduction of the UCL. The approach is similar to the operative steps of an adult gamekeeper's thumb surgery with incision of the adductor aponeurosis for exposure, followed by later repair after fracture reduction (Fig. 7-39).

Beware of the "flipped physis" of the middle or proximal phalanx in younger children. The findings on x-ray may be subtle and only visible on the lateral view. Treatment most often requires open "flipping" of the physis, attempting to keep any

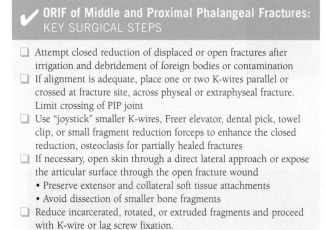

collateral ligaments or capsule intact. Surprisingly, appropriate management rarely results in growth arrest (Fig. 7-40).

Shaft Fractures

Nondisplaced shaft fractures are treated with simple immobilization. Safe position splinting for 3 to 4 weeks should be adequate for clinical union. Displaced or angulated fractures require closed reduction. The amount of acceptable angulation in the plane of motion is controversial.[97] In children less than 10 years of age, 20 to 30 degrees may be acceptable. In children older than 10 years, 10 to 20 degrees of angulation is acceptable. Less angulation is acceptable in the coronal plane. Malrotation is unacceptable.

Fractures that are unstable after reduction or irreducible by closed methods require operative intervention. A shaft

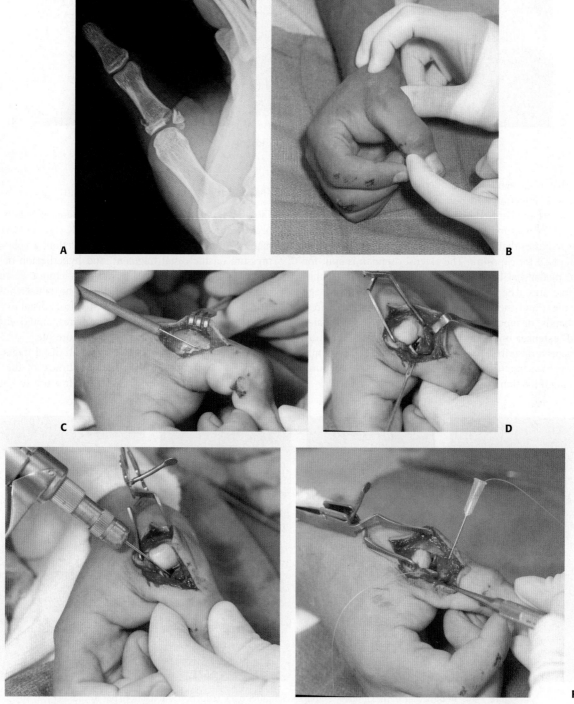

Figure 7-39. A–H: Open reduction and K-wire fixation of a bony gamekeeper's thumb, taking care to repair the UCL, articular surface, and adductor aponeurosis.   (*continues*)

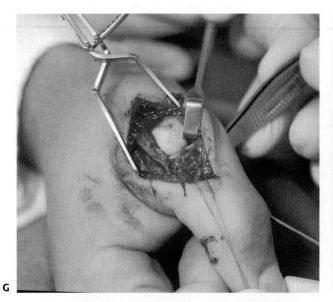

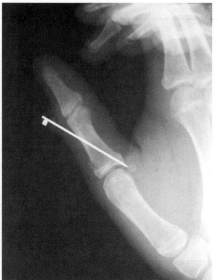

Figure 7-39. (*Continued*)

fracture that is unstable after reduction is managed primarily by closed reduction and percutaneous K-wire fixation in either a longitudinal or horizontal direction, depending on the obliquity of the fracture (Fig. 7-41).[127] Open reduction is indicated for fractures that cannot be reduced. A dorsal approach is usually used for exposure. The extensor tendon is split for proximal phalangeal fractures and elevated for middle phalangeal fractures. The choice of implant depends on the age of the patient and the fracture configuration. Smooth wires, tension bands, or modular set screws are preferable to plates to avoid extensor mechanism adherence.[83] Bone grafting alone has been described to provide rigid fixation to proximal phalangeal base fractures.[166] All malrotated fractures require reduction and fixation.

Phalangeal Neck Fractures

Closed treatment of fractures of the phalangeal neck is difficult because these fractures are often unstable (Fig. 7-35A). Closed manipulation is done with digital distraction, a volar-directed pressure on the distal fragment, and hyperflexion of the DIP or PIP joint depending on the phalanx fractured. Percutaneous pinning is usually necessary to maintain the reduced position.[162] Under fluoroscopy, K-wires are inserted from distal to proximal obliquely across the fracture. These wires should engage the contralateral cortex proximal to the fracture site.

An alternative technique with a small distal fragment is to insert the pins through the articular surface of the phalanx in a longitudinal fashion, crossing the fracture to engage the

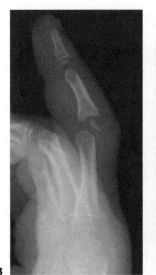
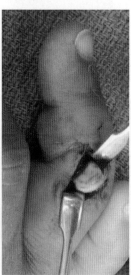
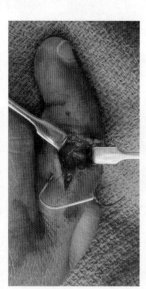
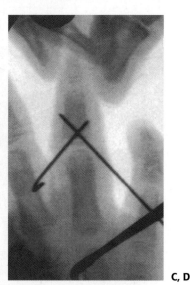

Figure 7-40. A–D: Beware of the "flipped" epiphysis. Requires open reduction and fixation, but in younger children may not even cause growth arrest. Higher risk of infection and growth arrest than other epiphyseal fractures. (Courtesy of Children's Hospital Los Angeles, CA.)

proximal fragment. For example, in the middle phalanx neck fracture, a longitudinal wire can be placed distal to proximal, across the physis of the distal phalanx with the DIP in hyperextension to engage the distal fragment and condyles of the middle phalanx. Then, the finger is flexed at the fracture site and the pin driven into the proximal middle phalanx with restoration of bony alignment (Fig. 7-35B,C). An easier percutaneous approach is to flex the injured joint, which reduces the phalangeal neck fracture. While the finger is held flexed, the K-wire is inserted into the articular surface of the reduced fragment and drilled retrograde to secure the reduction. The K-wire is then drilled out the skin and the wire driver placed over the proximal K-wire. Under fluoroscopic guidance, the K-wire is withdrawn until the distal end is just beneath the articular surface. The joint is then extended and the K-wire drilled antegrade and out the tip of the finger.[186] The wire driver is placed on the distal K-wire, which is then withdrawn until the proximal part is within the proximal phalanx. The distal K-wire is cut short and a pin cap applied (Video 7-1). (VIDEO Strauch Pinning)

Remodeling potential has been demonstrated in phalangeal neck fractures displaced in extension in children under the age of 2 years. Remarkable reforming of the anatomic condyles can occur despite being so far from the epiphysis. If very young children present late, allowing time for remodeling may obviate the need for any management (Fig. 7-42).[67]

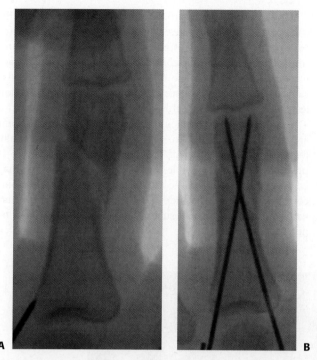

Figure 7-41. A, B: Closed reduction, percutaneous pinning of a proximal phalanx spiral oblique shaft fracture. (Courtesy of Children's Hospital Los Angeles, CA.)

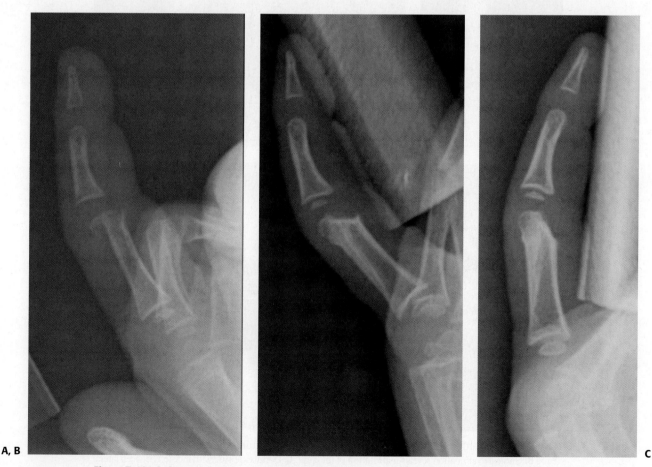

Figure 7-42. A–C: Remodeling potential of the subcondylar fracture in a very young child.

Intra-Articular Fractures

Nondisplaced fractures can be treated by immobilization. Weekly radiographs, often out of cast to gain acceptable visualization, are necessary to ensure maintenance of reduction. Displaced intra-articular fractures require closed or open reduction.[68] Closed or percutaneous reduction can be accomplished with traction and use of a percutaneous towel clip or reduction clamp to obtain provisional fracture reduction. Percutaneous fixation is used for definitive fracture fixation. Fractures not appropriate for closed manipulation require ORIF (Fig. 7-43). A dorsal, lateral, or rare volar incision is used for direct inspection of the fracture and articular surface. Care is taken to preserve the blood supply of the fracture fragments entering through the collateral ligaments. Fracture stabilization is either by K-wires (preferred) or mini-screws.

Certain unusual intra-articular fractures are especially difficult to treat. Shear fractures and osteochondral slice fractures are difficult to recognize. Treatment is by open reduction and smooth wire fixation. Osteonecrosis, especially of small fragments, is a concern. Some of these fractures require a volar surgical approach. Avoidance of extensive soft tissue dissection lessens the risk of osteonecrosis.

Comminuted pilon fracture–dislocations of the PIP joint are uncommon in children. Operative intervention is usually required to restore articular congruity. Anatomic reduction is preferred whenever possible (Fig. 7-44).[122] Bone grafting may be necessary to support the articular surface.[160] Extreme joint comminution may preclude anatomic reduction, and alternative treatment options, such as dynamic traction, may be necessary.[90]

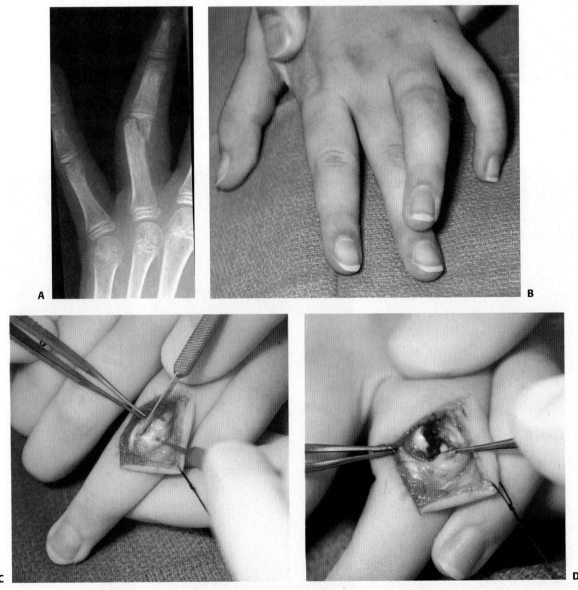

Figure 7-43. A: A 10-year-old girl with a displaced unicondylar fracture of the ring finger proximal phalanx. **B:** Clinical examination reveals malrotation of the digit. **C:** Dorsal exposure with incision between lateral band and central slip. **D:** Exposure of displaced fracture fragment.

Figure 7-43. (*Continued*) **E:** Fracture reduced with K-wire fixation. **F:** Postoperative radiograph shows restoration of articular surface. (Courtesy of Shriners Hospitals for Children, Philadelphia, PA.)

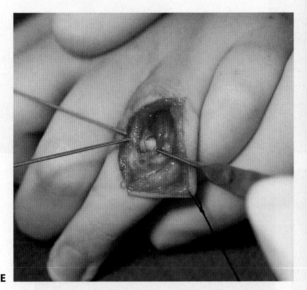

E

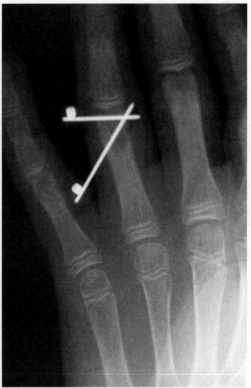

F

Complex Injuries

Combined injuries that affect several tissue systems are common in the digits. Skin, tendon, neurovascular structures, and bone may all be injured in the same digit (Fig. 7-45). Open fracture care is mandatory, followed by establishment of a stable bony foundation. Markedly comminuted fractures or injuries with bone loss may require external fixation followed by delayed bony reconstruction. Neurovascular and tendon reconstruction in children follows the same principles as for adults. Rehabilitation of complex injuries in children can be complicated by a lack of cooperation. Vascular injuries can affect subsequent growth.

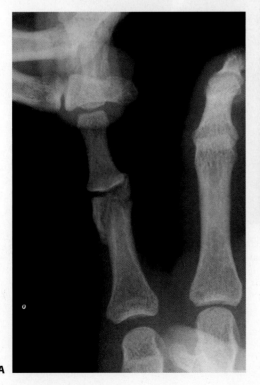

A

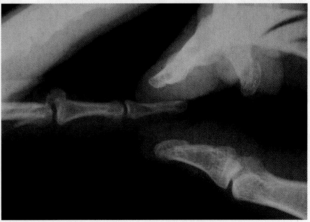

B

Figure 7-44. A: A 16-year-old girl with a severe intra-articular pilon fracture of the small finger PIP joint. **B:** Traction radiograph helps define fracture components.   (*continues*)

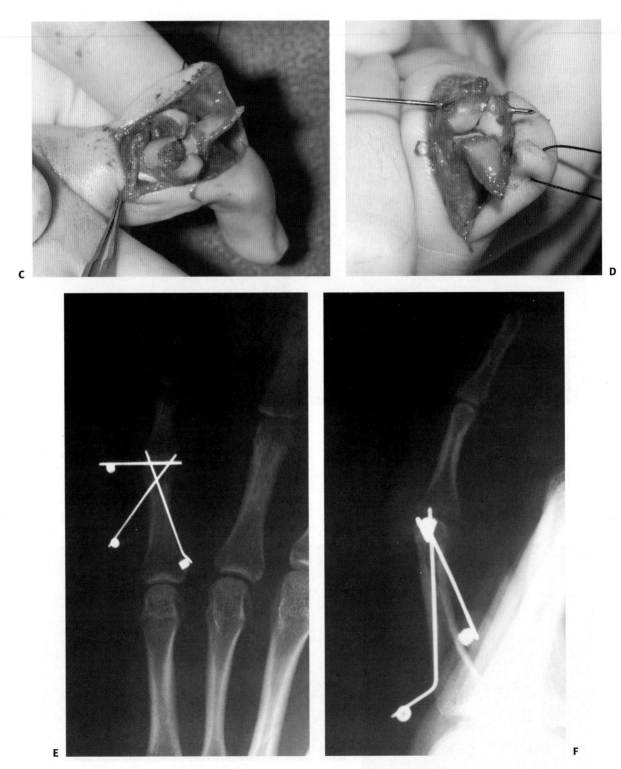

Figure 7-44. (*Continued*) **C:** Dorsal exposure reveals ulnar condyle outside of joint requiring incision of extensor tendon for reduction. **D:** Reduction of joint surface and K-wire fixation. **E:** Postoperative AP radiograph shows restoration of articular surface. **F:** Lateral radiograph shows sagittal alignment of condyles. (Courtesy of Shriners Hospitals for Children, Philadelphia, PA.)

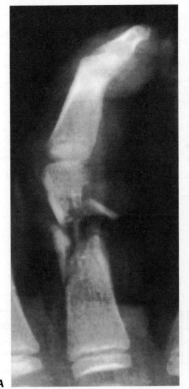
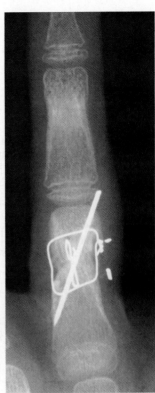

Figure 7-45. A: A 14-year-old boy sustained a near-amputation of his ring digit with severe soft tissue injury. **B:** Use of 90-90 intraosseous wiring was supplemented with K-wire fixation to provide a stable base for soft tissue repair.

Authors' Preferred Treatment for Middle and Proximal Phalangeal Fractures (Algorithm 7-2)

Physeal Fractures

Nondisplaced stable fractures are treated with early range of motion and buddy tape in the older child and immobilization in the younger or uncooperative child for 3 weeks. Displaced S-H I and II fractures are treated with closed reduction (Fig. 7-46). Alignment and rotation are verified by clinical examination and reduction is assessed with radiographs. Even subtle fractures can result in malrotation and digital scissoring, so all fractures need to be assessed with tenodesis out of cast before immobilization treatment is chosen or continued (Fig. 7-47). Physeal fractures that are open or unstable after closed reduction require smooth percutaneous pin fixation. Irreducible fractures require open reduction, removal of any interposed tissue, and fixation.

Dorsal S-H III or IV fractures that fail closed reduction of the middle phalangeal base often require open reduction and fixation to avoid the development of a boutonnière deformity (Fig. 7-48). Lateral S-H III fractures that are displaced more than 1.5 mm or involve more than 25% of the articular surface may also require ORIF.

Shaft Fractures

Nondisplaced fractures are treated with immobilization for 3 to 4 weeks. Displaced fractures are treated with CRPP fixation (Fig. 7-49). For a proximal phalangeal fracture, the MCP joint is flexed to relax the intrinsic muscle pull and to stabilize the proximal fragment. Open reduction is reserved for open or irreducible fractures.

Neck Fractures

Phalangeal neck fractures usually require CRPP. The pin(s) are placed through the collateral recesses to engage the proximal fragment in a crossed fashion or directly across the displaced fragment with the joint flexed as previously described. If closed reduction is unsuccessful, open reduction with preservation of the collateral ligament attachments to the bony fragment and pinning has been described. Late presentation of a neck fracture requires consideration of the time from injury, age of the patient, and fracture displacement. Considerable displacement requires treatment to regain joint flexion (Fig. 7-50). If the fracture line is still visible, a percutaneous pin osteoclasis is used.[65] The fracture is then stabilized with additional percutaneous pins (Video 7-2). A nascent or established malunion that cannot be reduced by osteoclasis can be treated by late open reduction or condylar advancement osteotomy (Fig. 7-51). Mild loss of the condylar recess can be treated with recession of the prominent volar bone rather than risk osteonecrosis associated with extensive fracture mobilization by osteotomy.[12,134] In addition, slow remodeling is feasible in very young children without rotational malalignment and with a family that is willing to wait up to 2 years for remodeling and restoration of normal motion.[21,172]

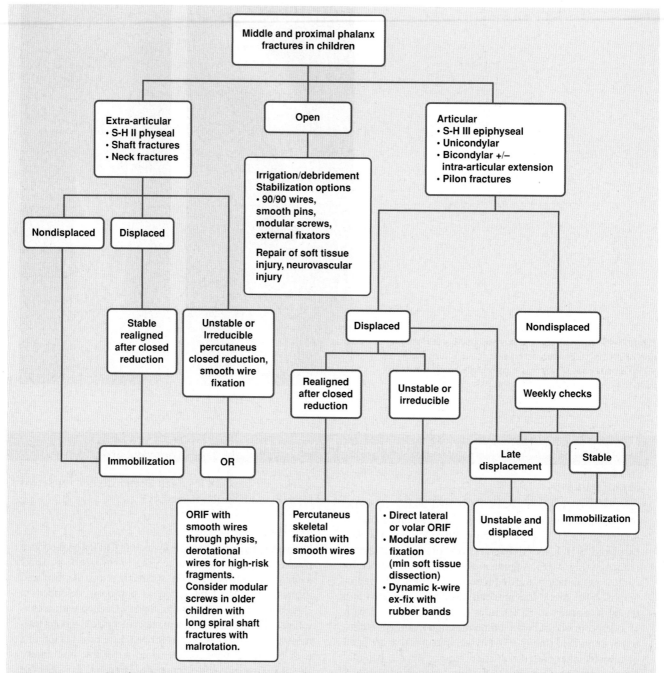

Algorithm 7-2. Authors' preferred treatment for middle and proximal phalangeal fractures in children.

Intra-Articular Fractures

Intra-articular fractures of the phalanges typically require percutaneous or open reduction. Unicondylar fractures that are mildly displaced can be treated with CRPP. Widely displaced unicondylar and bicondylar fractures require open reduction (Fig. 7-42).

Pilon fractures or intra-articular fracture–dislocations present a management dilemma.[122] Open reduction is worthwhile when the fragments are large and the joint surface can be reconstructed. Bone grafting may be necessary to support the reduction. Severe articular damage and comminution are best treated with dynamic traction.

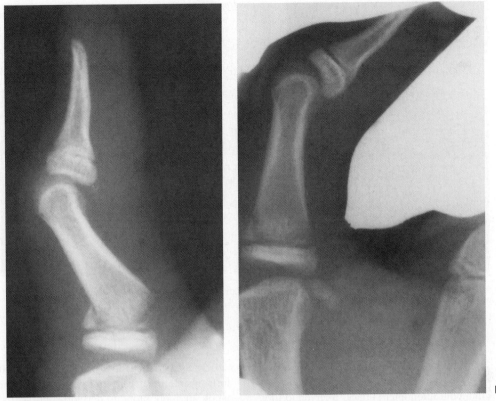

Figure 7-46. A: An S-H II fracture of the proximal phalanx of the thumb. **B:** Gentle closed reduction under fluoroscopic control obtained an anatomic reduction.

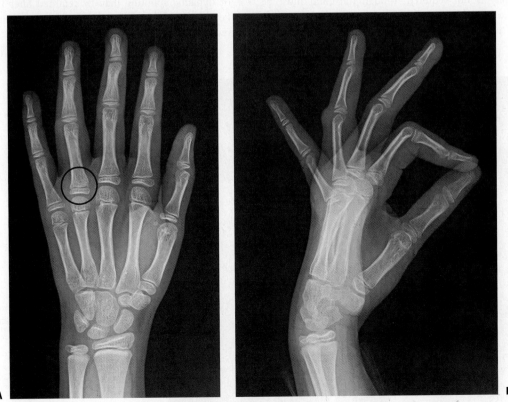

Figure 7-47. An 8 year old was in a bouncy ball doing cartwheels when she felt a crack in her left ring finger. **A:** Innocuous fracture of the left finger proximal phalanx. **B:** Lateral x-ray with fracture difficult to recognize. *(continues)*

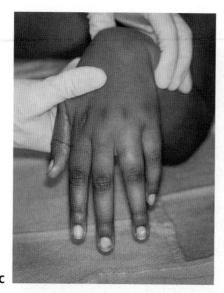
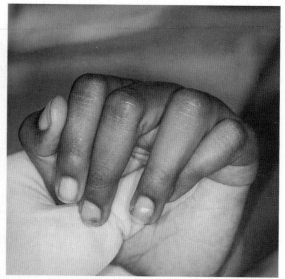

Figure 7-47. (*Continued*) **C:** Clinical examination benign with fingers in extension. **D:** Examination using wrist tenodesis for finger flexion demonstrated malrotation. (Courtesy of Shriners Hospital for Children, Philadelphia, PA.)

Postoperative Care

The duration of immobilization after surgical intervention for phalangeal fractures is usually 3 to 4 weeks. Percutaneous pins are removed at the time and motion instituted. Formal hand therapy usually is not required, though the child must be encouraged to reestablish a normal usage pattern to improve motion and flexibility. Periarticular fractures are monitored closely for persistent loss of motion that would benefit from formal hand therapy. Patients with complex fractures or replantation are more prone to develop stiffness. In these instances, therapy is routinely prescribed to regain motion. Therapy is directed at both flexion and extension of the injured digit. Static or dynamic splinting may be required after fracture healing. Persistent stiffness may require tenolysis and/or joint release to regain motion (Fig. 7-52).

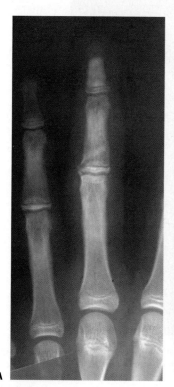
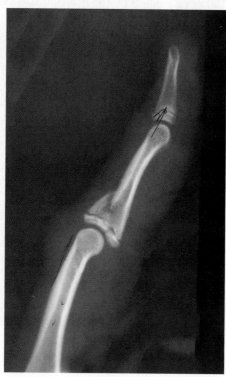

Figure 7-48. A, B: A 16-year-old male sustained a dorsal S-H IV fracture of the middle phalanx.

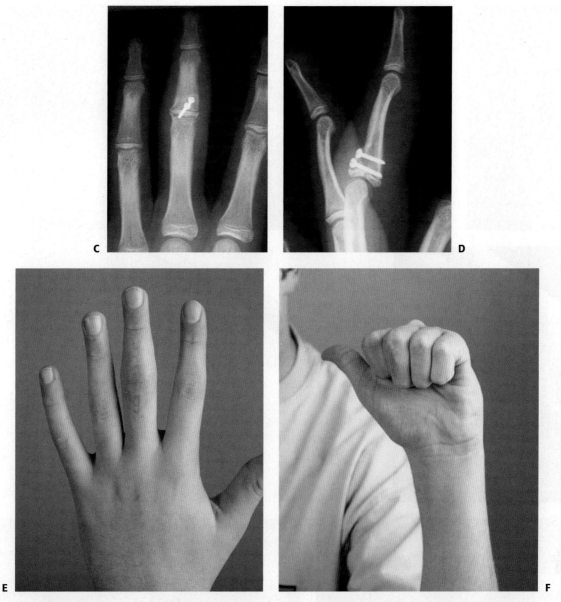

Figure 7-48. (*Continued*) **C:** Open reduction and internal screw fixation was accomplished through a dorsal approach. Radiographs show reduction of joint subluxation and fixation of fracture fragment. **D–F:** Postoperative extension and flexion with near-normal motion. (Courtesy of Shriners Hospitals for Children, Philadelphia, PA.)

Potential Pitfalls and Preventive Measures

Middle and Proximal Phalanx Fractures: SURGICAL PITFALLS AND PREVENTIONS	
Pitfall	**Prevention**
• Malrotation	• Check tenodesis intraoperatively • Use true lateral x-ray view to establish if radial and ulnar condyles of middle or proximal phalanx are overlapping
• Osteonecrosis	• Minimize open procedures and soft tissue stripping of fragile blood supply to condyles
• Pin-tract infection	• Bicortical fixation, relax any tension between the wire and skin
• Stiffness	• Allow early range of motion as soon as clinically stable; radiographic union will lag behind clinical union

Outcomes

The overall results following proximal and middle phalangeal fractures are positive. Considering the frequency of these fractures, the occurrence of complications and functional impairment is low. Despite appropriate treatment, however, some

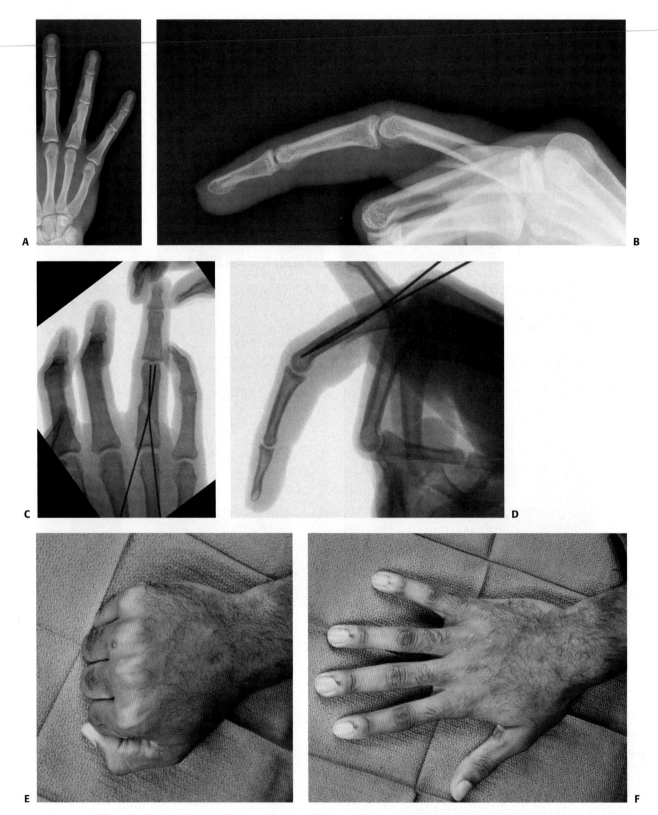

Figure 7-49. An 18-year-old male who injured his right finger 2 weeks earlier while tubing at camp. **A:** Anteroposterior x-ray with spiral fracture right ring finger proximal phalanx. **B:** Lateral x-ray with apex volar angulation. **C:** Anteroposterior fluoroscopic imaging demonstrating longitudinal traction and fracture reduction following intramedullary Kirschner-wire fixation. **D:** Fluoroscopic imaging demonstrating fracture reduction in the lateral plane. **E:** Clinical follow-up with full extension. **F:** Full flexion and fist formation. (Courtesy of Shriners Hospital for Children, Philadelphia, PA.)

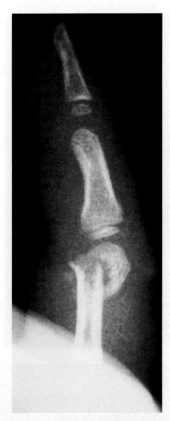

Figure 7-50. Displaced phalangeal neck fracture of the proximal phalanx revealing loss of subchondral fossa at the PIP joint. If this is not corrected to anatomic alignment, there will be a mechanical block to flexion.

children have permanent loss of motion, malunion, or growth disturbance. The major concern is to avoid rotational, articular, or periarticular malunion caused by the inappropriate diagnosis or treatment.

MANAGEMENT OF EXPECTED ADVERSE OUTCOMES AND UNEXPECTED COMPLICATIONS OF MIDDLE AND PROXIMAL PHALANGEAL FRACTURES

Middle and Proximal Phalangeal Fractures:
COMMON ADVERSE OUTCOMES AND COMPLICATIONS

- Malunion, malrotation, finger deformity
- Growth arrest
- Stiffness
- Osteonecrosis
- Degenerative joint changes
- Pin-tract infection, osteomyelitis

Complications associated with proximal and middle phalangeal fractures begin with failure to recognize the injury (Fig. 7-53). AP and true lateral x-ray views of the injured digit must be made orthogonal and scrutinized for subtle abnormalities. Questionable findings warrant additional views or advanced imaging

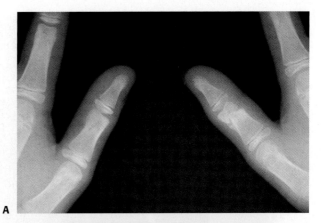

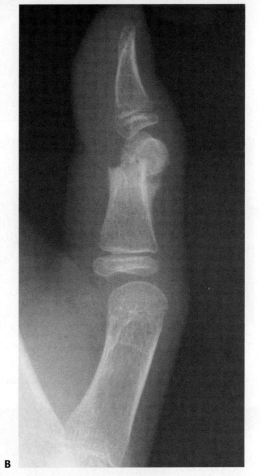

Figure 7-51. A: A 14-year-old girl with incipient malunion of right thumb proximal phalanx neck fractures that impede flexion. **B:** Lateral radiograph reveals loss of the subchondral fossa.   *(continues)*

studies. A common misdiagnosis is failure to recognize a displaced phalangeal neck fracture because of inadequate lateral radiographs of the finger.

Another early complication is false interpretation of a "nondisplaced" fracture that is malrotated. All children with phalangeal fractures require careful examination for rotational alignment. The clinical examination is the mainstay for

(text continues on page 196)

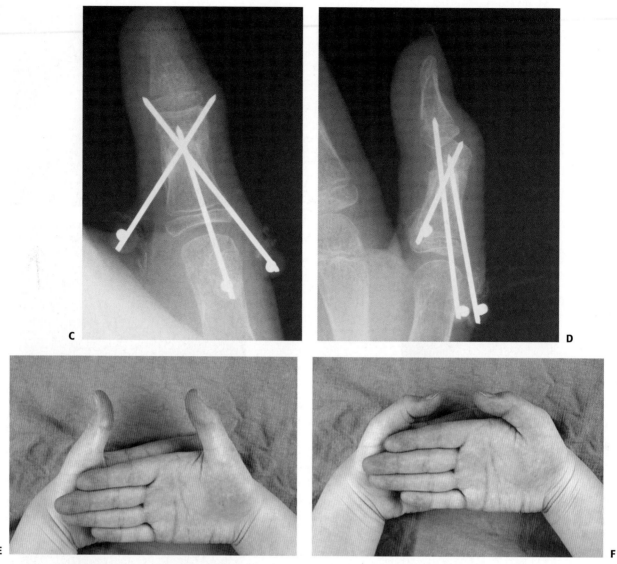

Figure 7-51. (*Continued*) **C:** An AP view after open reduction and K-wire fixation. **D:** Oblique view reveals restoration of subchondral fossa. **E, F:** Postoperative flexion and extension compared to the other side. (Courtesy of Shriners Hospitals for Children, Philadelphia, PA.)

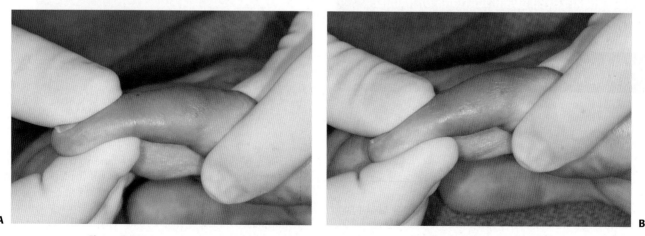

Figure 7-52. A 16-year-old girl with a severe intra-articular pilon fracture of the small finger PIP joint depicted in Figure 7-34 with healed fracture but limited motion after therapy. **A:** Passive extension. **B:** Passive flexion.

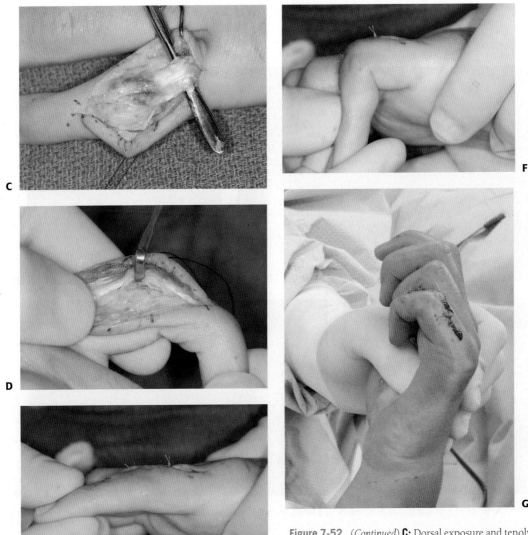

Figure 7-52. (*Continued*) **C:** Dorsal exposure and tenolysis under local anesthesia with sedation. **D:** Joint release. **E:** Passive extension. **F:** Passive flexion. **G:** Active flexion. (Courtesy of Shriners Hospitals for Children, Philadelphia, PA.)

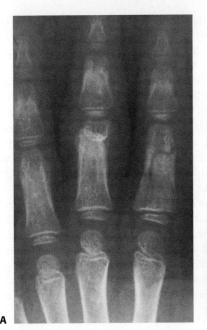

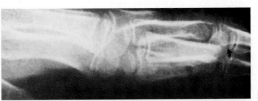

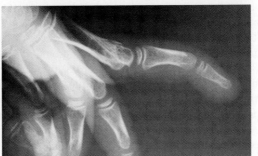

Figure 7-53. A: A 3-year-old girl sustained a fracture of the neck of the proximal phalanx of the index and middle fingers. The displaced fracture in the middle finger appears similar to an epiphysis at the distal end of the phalanx. **B:** No true lateral radiograph of the injured finger was obtained. Close scrutiny of this lateral view shows a dorsally displaced neck fracture, rotated almost 90 degrees (*arrow*). **C:** A lateral radiograph taken 18 months later reveals malunion with hyperextension of the PIP joint and loss of flexion.

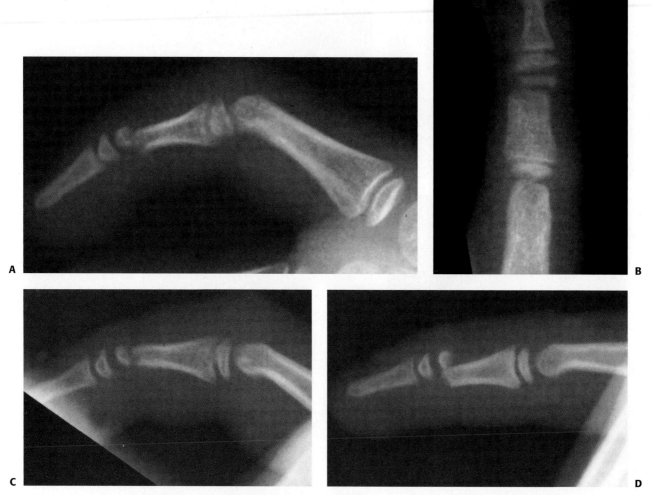

Figure 7-54. A, B: An 8-year-old girl with a mildly displaced fracture of the neck of the middle phalanx. **C:** Closed reduction was successful on the day of injury and a plaster splint was applied. **D:** Two weeks later, the fracture had markedly redisplaced.

determining fracture rotation. Digital scissoring is indicative of fracture malrotation and requires reduction. Regardless of radiographic appearance, rotational alignment should be evaluated by active finger flexion and passive finger tenodesis via wrist extension.

Most phalangeal fractures can be maintained in satisfactory alignment after closed reduction. Certain fractures, however, have a propensity for redisplacement (Fig. 7-54). Oblique shaft fractures, unicondylar articular fractures, and neck fractures are prime examples. Early follow-up to ensure maintenance of reduction is paramount. Displacement requires repeat manipulation and pin fixation. When in doubt, the digit should be examined out of cast carefully for malalignment and blocks to motion. Most of these unstable fractures are best treated with pin fixation after acceptable reduction.

Late complications include rare nonunion, malunion, osteonecrosis, growth disturbance, and arthritis. Nonunion is rare except in combined injuries with devascularization of the fracture fragments. Bone grafting is usually successful for union. Malunion can result in angulation or limited motion. Extra-articular

malunion can cause angulation or rotational abnormalities. The treatment depends on the child's age and ability to remodel according to fracture location, plane of malunion, and degree of deformity (Fig. 7-55). Considerable deformity may require osteotomy to realign the bone.[18] A subcondylar or intra-articular malunion is particularly difficult to treat. Early diagnosis within the first month offers the possibility of fracture realignment through the site of deformity. Treatment of a late diagnosis must include consideration of the risks and benefits associated with extensive surgery. Successful late osteotomies can restore normal digital alignment and functional recovery, but risk nonunion, stiffness, and pain (Fig. 7-56).

Osteonecrosis is usually related to extensive fracture comminution, soft tissue injury, or surgical dissection of an intra-articular fracture. In severe cases, reconstruction is limited to some form of joint transfer. Growth disturbance can result from any injury that involves the physis. A shortened or angulated digit may result. Fortunately, growth disturbance is rare because reconstruction options for children are limited. Angulation must be addressed by corrective osteotomy.

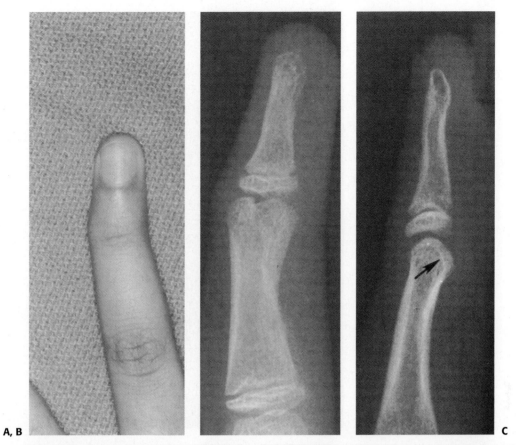

Figure 7-55. A: A 13-year-old boy with malunion of the ring finger middle phalanx articular surface. **B, C:** Radiographs reveal slight malunion of the radial condyle with mild intra-articular incongruity. The lateral view suggests a double-density shadow (*arrow*). The flexion and extension motion of the digit was normal, and reconstruction was not recommended.

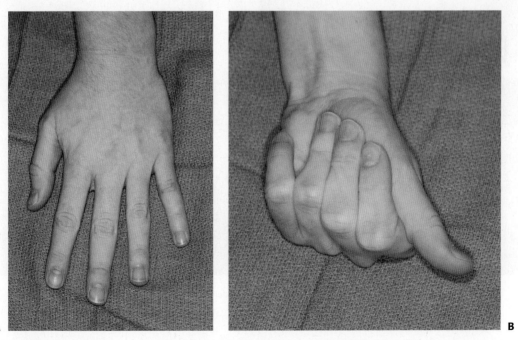

Figure 7-56. A–K: A 12-year-old girl with malunion of the small finger shaft proximal phalanx fracture. Operative steps for fixation and correction of tenodesis. (Courtesy of Shriners Hospitals for Children, Philadelphia, PA.)

(*continues*)

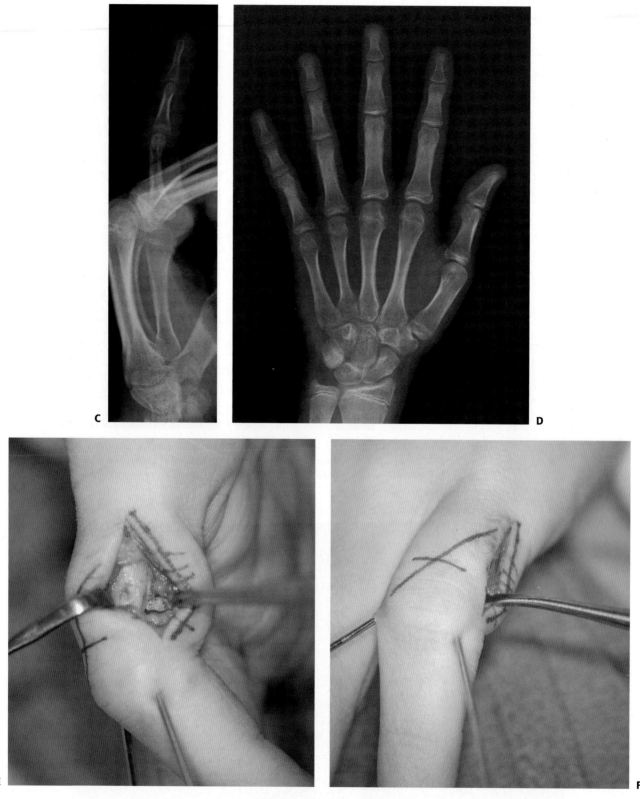

Figure 7-56. (*Continued*)

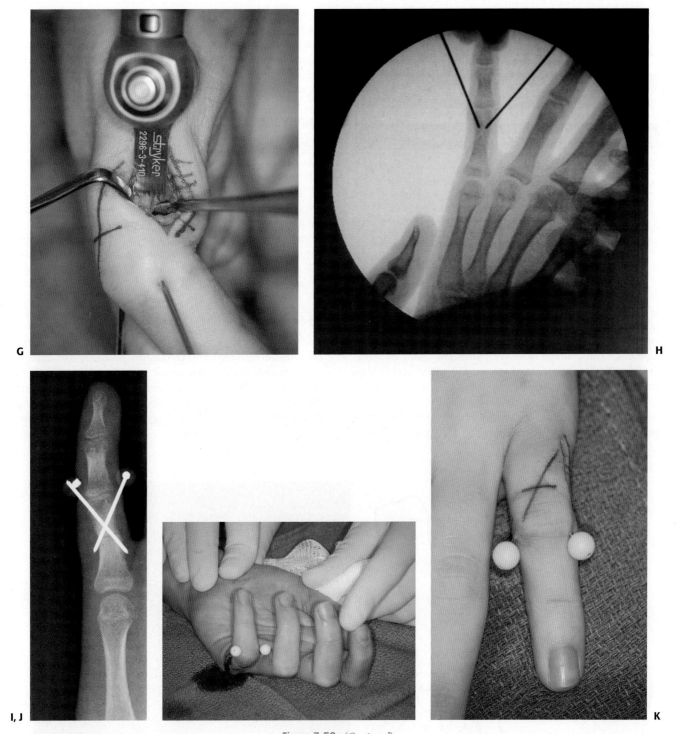

Figure 7-56. (*Continued*)

Posttraumatic degenerative joint disease is rare in children, but intra-articular injury and infection may result in arthrosis. Treatment is directed toward the child's symptoms and not the radiographic findings. Minimal pain and acceptable function often accompany arthritic changes on radiographs and warrant no treatment. Pain and functional limitations require treatment; options include a vascularized joint transfer, interposition or distraction arthroplasty, hemi-hamate osteochondral transfer, prosthetic joint replacement, and arthrodesis.[174] Arthrodesis in the most functional position is considered the most reliable procedure for children. Results are better for index and long than small and ring fingers.

Metacarpal Fractures in Children

CLASSIFICATION OF METACARPAL FRACTURES

Classification of Finger Metacarpal Fractures

- Physeal fractures

- Extraphyseal fractures
  - Neck fractures
  - Shaft fractures

- Metacarpal base fractures
  - Thumb
  - Fingers (other than thumb)

Metacarpal fractures in children are classified by location: head/epiphysis, physis, neck, shaft, or base. The metacarpals are surrounded by soft tissue and are relatively protected within the hand. Considerable variation exists in the relative mobility of the metacarpals through the CMC joints. The index and long rays have minimal CMC joint motion (10 to 20 degrees). In contrast, the ring and small rays possess more motion (30 to 40 degrees), and the thumb CMC joint has universal motion. Every metacarpal fracture must be examined for rotation. Malrotation will result in digital scissoring during active flexion or an abnormal digital cascade with passive tenodesis. Direct trauma, rotational forces, and axial loading all cause fractures of the metacarpal. Contact sports and punching are the most common mechanisms of injury. Pediatric thumb metacarpal fractures have unique anatomy and characteristic patterns and are discussed in a separate section.

EPIPHYSEAL AND PHYSEAL FRACTURES

Epiphyseal and physeal fractures of the metacarpal head are rare but occur most often in the small ray.[144,179,181] Physeal S-H II fractures of the small metacarpal occur among patients 12 to 16 years of age and are prone to partial closure of the physis.[22,144,150] Intra-articular, head-splitting fractures at the metacarpal epiphysis and physis consistent with S-H III and IV patterns seldom occur at the metacarpal level but are problematic when displaced (Fig. 7-57). There is a theoretical increased risk of head avascular necrosis after an epiphyseal fracture due to capsular hematoma.

METACARPAL NECK FRACTURES

The metacarpal neck is the most frequent site of metacarpal fractures in children. The metacarpal geometry and composition predispose the metacarpal neck to injury. The distal metacarpal neck angles as it approaches the MCP joint, and the cortical bone within the subcondylar fossa is relatively thin, making it vulnerable to injury. Neck fractures in children are analogous to boxer's fractures in adults (Fig. 7-58). Neck

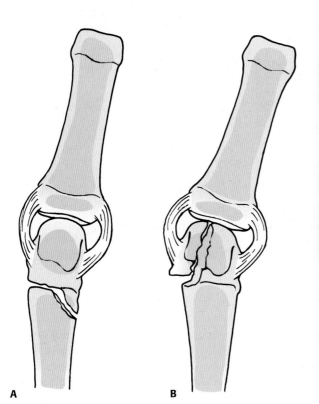
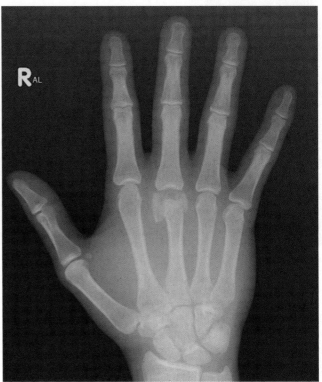

Figure 7-57. A: An S-H type II fracture of the metacarpal head. **B:** Head-splitting fracture of the metacarpal epiphysis. (Courtesy of Children's Hospital Los Angeles, CA.)

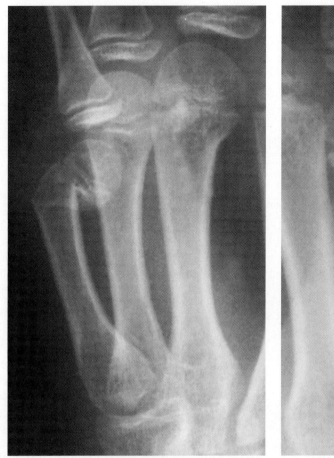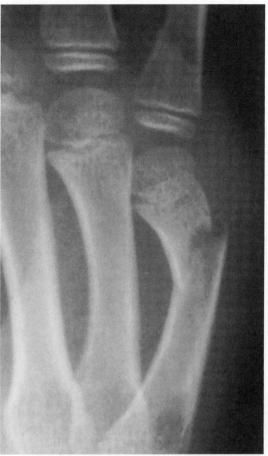

A   B

Figure 7-58. A: A true boxer's fracture of the metacarpal neck of the 5th ray. **B:** This fracture is more in the diaphysis and should not be considered a boxer's fracture.

fractures are more common in the small and ring fingers. Fortunately, these injuries are juxtaphyseal and have considerable remodeling potential.

METACARPAL SHAFT FRACTURES

Metacarpal shaft fractures are relatively common. Torsional forces combined with axial load cause long oblique and spiral fractures whereas direct trauma (being stepped on or a heavy object dropping onto the hand) produces short oblique or transverse fractures. An isolated shaft fracture of a central ray is suspended by the intermetacarpal ligaments, which limit displacement and shortening. In contrast, the border digits (index and small) displace more readily.

METACARPAL BASE FRACTURES

Metacarpal base fractures are less common in children. The base is protected from injury by its proximal location in the hand and the stability afforded by the bony congruence and soft tissue restraints. The small finger CMC joint is the most prone to injury. Fracture–dislocations of the small finger CMC joint are often unstable because of the proximal pull of the extensor carpi ulnaris (reverse Bennett fracture).

TREATMENT OPTIONS FOR METACARPAL FRACTURE

NONOPERATIVE AND OPERATIVE TREATMENT OF METACARPAL FRACTURES

Indications/Contraindications

Metacarpal Fractures:
INDICATIONS FOR NONOPERATIVE VERSUS OPERATIVE TREATMENT

Nonoperative	Operative
• Nondisplaced	• Multiple metacarpals
• Closed	• Open or extensive soft tissue injury
• Reducible	• Displaced articular
• Stable	• Unstable
	• Irreducible
	• Malrotation
	• Excessive shortening

The treatment of metacarpal fractures varies with the location, extent, and configuration of the fracture. Nonoperative or closed treatment is the primary mode of management for most fractures. Operative intervention is used for multiple metacarpal fractures, extensive soft tissue injury, intra-articular head-splitting fractures, malrotated fractures, and irreducible fractures.

Preoperative Planning

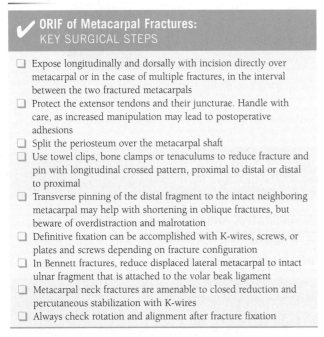

✔ ORIF of Metacarpal Fractures:
PREOPERATIVE PLANNING CHECKLIST

OR table	☐ Radiolucent hand table
Position	☐ Supine
Fluoroscopy	☐ Parallel or perpendicular to the patient's hands
Equipment	☐ Hand instrument set, small tenaculums, bone clamps, or towel clips, rare pediatric use of modular screw and plate tray
Tourniquet	☐ Nonsterile, upper arm, not elevated unless converted to open procedure

Technique

✔ ORIF of Metacarpal Fractures:
KEY SURGICAL STEPS

- ☐ Expose longitudinally and dorsally with incision directly over metacarpal or in the case of multiple fractures, in the interval between the two fractured metacarpals
- ☐ Protect the extensor tendons and their juncturae. Handle with care, as increased manipulation may lead to postoperative adhesions
- ☐ Split the periosteum over the metacarpal shaft
- ☐ Use towel clips, bone clamps or tenaculums to reduce fracture and pin with longitudinal crossed pattern, proximal to distal or distal to proximal
- ☐ Transverse pinning of the distal fragment to the intact neighboring metacarpal may help with shortening in oblique fractures, but beware of overdistraction and malrotation
- ☐ Definitive fixation can be accomplished with K-wires, screws, or plates and screws depending on fracture configuration
- ☐ In Bennett fractures, reduce displaced lateral metacarpal to intact ulnar fragment that is attached to the volar beak ligament
- ☐ Metacarpal neck fractures are amenable to closed reduction and percutaneous stabilization with K-wires
- ☐ Always check rotation and alignment after fracture fixation

Physeal Fractures

A metacarpal head-splitting fracture may be difficult to detect and requires special x-ray views. The Brewerton view is helpful and is performed with the dorsum of the hand against the cassette and the MCP joints flexed about 65 degrees. The central beam is angled 15 degrees to the ulnar side of the hand.[76] This projection focuses on the metacarpal heads and may highlight subtle bony abnormalities. An MRI or CT scan to assess articular alignment is diagnostic in complex injuries; however, advanced imaging is reserved for difficult cases.

Management is based on the amount of articular or fracture fragment displacement and stability detected on imaging studies. Many of these fractures can be treated by closed methods. Gentle reduction under metacarpal or wrist block anesthesia is followed by application of a splint in the safe position. If the fracture is reducible but unstable, percutaneous pin fixation is recommended. If the Thurston Holland fragment is large enough, the wire can secure the metaphyseal piece and avoid the physis. Otherwise, the wire must cross the physis to obtain stability. A small-diameter smooth K-wire is recommended, and multiple passes should be avoided.

Displaced intra-articular head-splitting fractures require ORIF to restore articular congruity. Many of these fractures have unrecognized comminution that complicates internal fixation. Wire or screw fixation is used depending on the age of the patient and size of the fragments. Transosseous suture repair may be necessary for small fragments.[153] Bone grafting may be necessary to support the articular reduction. The primary goal of surgical treatment is anatomic reduction of the joint. A secondary goal is stable fixation to allow early motion.

Metacarpal Neck Fractures

Metacarpal neck fractures are usually treated by closed methods. The amount of acceptable apex dorsal angulation in children as in adults is controversial. Greater angulation is allowable in the mobile ring and small rays compared to the index and long. Another consideration is the effect of remodeling over time, which is dependent on the age of the child. In general, 10 to 30 degrees of angulation greater than the corresponding CMC joint motion is acceptable. AP and lateral x-ray views may be supplemented by an oblique view to assess fracture configuration.

Considerable angulation can be treated with closed reduction with local anesthesia or conscious sedation and splint or cast application. The Jahss maneuver is commonly recommended and involves initial flexion of the MCP joint to 90 degrees to relax the deforming force of the intrinsic muscles and tighten the collateral ligaments.[31] Subsequently, upward pressure is applied along the proximal phalanx to push the metacarpal head in a dorsal direction whereas counter-pressure is applied along the dorsal aspect of the proximal metacarpal fracture. Jahss[175] suggested immobilization with the MCP and PIP joints flexed, but this type of immobilization is no longer advocated for fear of stiffness and skin breakdown. Immobilization in the intrinsic plus or safe position is the appropriate approach. A well-molded splint or ulnar gutter or outrigger cast is necessary. Three-point molding over the volar metacarpal head and proximal dorsal shaft is recommended. In addition, immobilization with the fingers more extended to maintain the fracture reduction is acceptable as MCP joint stiffness resolves over time in the young.[112] The PIP joints may or may not be included in the immobilization depending on the status of the reduction and reliability of the patient.

Uncommonly, a neck fracture may be extremely unstable and require percutaneous pinning. Pins can be inserted in a variety of configurations. Extramedullary techniques include crossed pinning or pinning to the adjacent stable metacarpal. Intramedullary techniques can also be used, similar to those used for metacarpal shaft and neck fractures in adults.[15,59] Intramedullary techniques are reserved for patients near physeal closure. Pre-bent K-wires or commercially available implants are inserted through the metacarpal base in an antegrade fashion. The wires can be used to assist in fracture reduction. Stability is obtained by stacking several wires within the canal and across the fracture site.

Open reduction of metacarpal neck fractures is seldom required in children and is reserved for irreducible fractures, unstable fractures in skeletally mature children, multiple metacarpal fractures, and combination injuries that require a stable bony platform.

Metacarpal Shaft Fractures

An isolated long or ring metacarpal fracture is often minimally displaced because the metacarpals are suspended by the intermetacarpal ligaments. Immobilization for 4 weeks is usually all that is necessary. In contrast, the index and small digits may require additional treatment, such as closed reduction and immobilization. Percutaneous pinning is reserved for unstable shaft fractures (Fig. 7-59). Pins can be inserted with extramedullary or intramedullary techniques. Diaphyseal fractures are slower to heal and more prone to malunion than neck fractures.

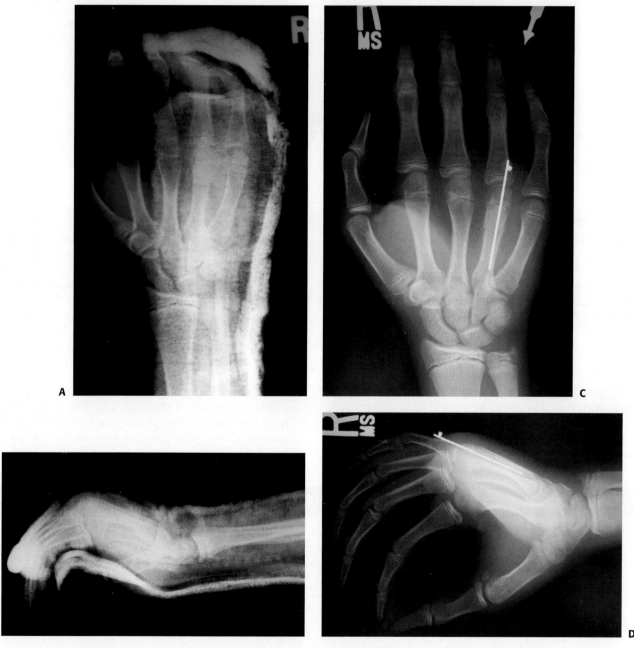

Figure 7-59. A 14-year-old boy with a reducible, but unstable, ring finger metacarpal shaft fracture. **A:** The injury on an AP radiograph appears reduced. **B:** Lateral radiograph shows persistent apex dorsal angulation. **C:** An AP radiograph after CRPP. **D:** Lateral radiograph reveals anatomic alignment.

(continues)

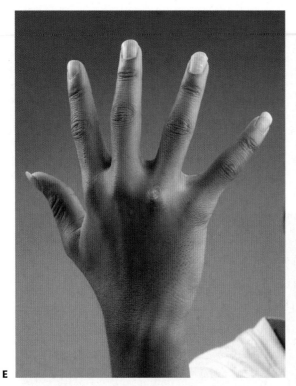
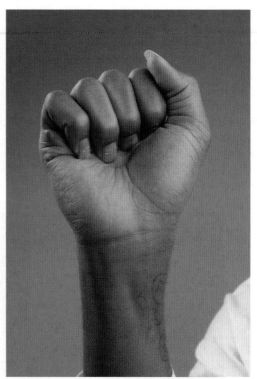

E   **F**

Figure 7-59. (*Continued*) **E:** Full extension after pin removal and home therapy. **F:** Full flexion with normal digital cascade. (Courtesy of Shriners Hospitals for Children, Philadelphia, PA.)

An ORIF approach to a metacarpal shaft fracture is rarely indicated in children unless there are multiple fractures or extensive soft tissue damage or the child is skeletally mature. However, a long spiral–oblique fracture with substantial malrotation and shortening may require mini-screw fixation to reestablish alignment.

Metacarpal Base Fractures

Fractures of the metacarpal base or fracture–dislocations at the CMC joint are usually high-energy injuries with substantial tissue disruption. Assessment for signs of hand compartment syndrome and careful neurovascular assessment are mandatory. Isolated fracture–dislocations of the small ray CMC joint are the most common metacarpal base fractures. A CT scan may better define articular congruity and comminution. A CRPP approach is usually sufficient to restore alignment and to resist the deforming force of the extensor carpi ulnaris.[104] The pins can be placed transversely between the small and ring metacarpals and/or across the CMC joint.

Open reduction may be necessary to achieve reduction and ensure stable fixation in high-energy injuries. A transverse or longitudinal incision can be used for exposure. Longitudinal incisions are recommended in patients with concomitant compartment syndrome to allow for simultaneous decompression. Fixation options are numerous, depending on the fracture configuration. Supplemental bone graft may be necessary for substantial comminution. Late presentation is especially difficult. Treatment often requires open reduction or CMC arthrodesis (Fig. 7-60).

Authors' Preferred Treatment for Metacarpal Fractures (Algorithm 7-3)

Epiphyseal and Physeal Fractures

Nondisplaced epiphyseal and S-H II metacarpal neck fractures with up to 30 to 35 degrees of sagittal angulation in adolescents are treated with immobilization as long as there is no rotation and sufficient growth remaining. A widely displaced, unstable fracture that is reducible requires percutaneous pinning to maintain the reduction. Displaced epiphyseal fractures with considerable intra-articular displacement require ORIF (Fig. 7-61).

Metacarpal Neck Fractures

Nonoperative and closed methods are the mainstays of treatment. Small and ring finger angulation greater than 30 to 45 or malrotation necessitates closed reduction. Index and ring finger angulations of more than 20 degrees are treated by closed reduction. Pin fixation is used for unstable fractures and open reduction is rarely necessary.

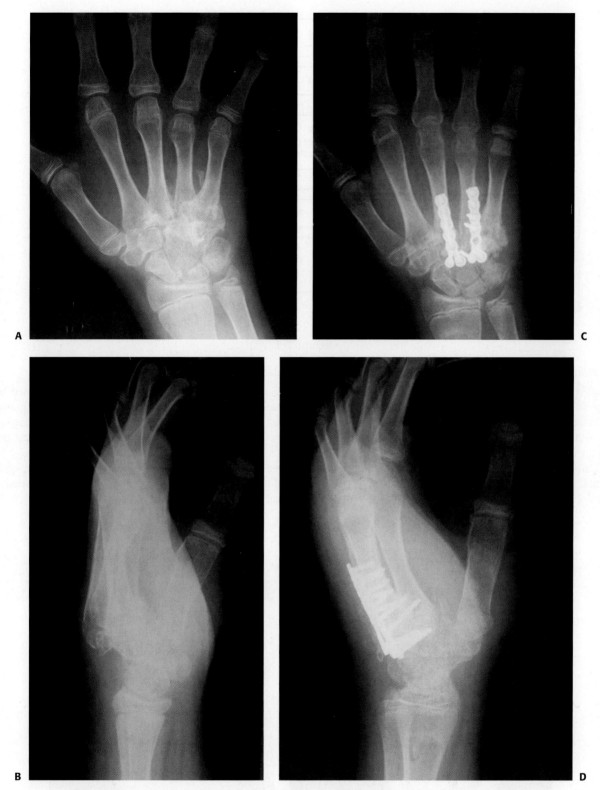

Figure 7-60. A 15-year-old boy with crush injury of the right hand requiring compartment release. He presented 6 weeks later with persistent pain and limited motion. **A:** An AP radiograph shows overlapping long, ring, and small CMC joints. **B:** Lateral radiographs reveal fracture–dislocations of long, ring, and small CMC joints. **C:** Postoperative AP radiograph after reduction and CMC fusion using miniplates. **D:** Lateral radiograph after reduction and CMC fusion. (Courtesy of Shriners Hospitals for Children, Philadelphia, PA.)

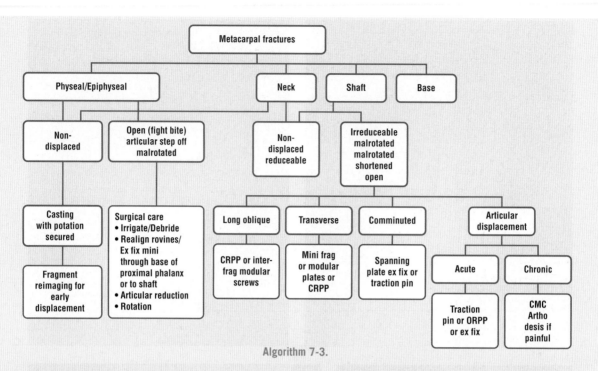

Algorithm 7-3.

Metacarpal Shaft Fractures

Isolated fractures that are minimally displaced require only immobilization. Isolated fractures that are displaced or malrotated require closed reduction and percutaneous fixation. An irreducible fracture or multiple fractures usually require open reduction (Fig. 7-59). The operative approach and internal fixation principles are similar in children and adults.

Metacarpal Base Fractures

Extra-articular metacarpal base fractures can be treated by closed reduction with or without percutaneous pinning. Intra-articular fracture–dislocations are more challenging. Percutaneous pinning is often required to stabilize the fracture and to reduce CMC joint subluxation (Fig. 7-62). Irreducible or multiple fracture–dislocations require open reduction. Late presentation with symptomatic degenerative changes requires CMC arthrodesis (Fig. 7-60).

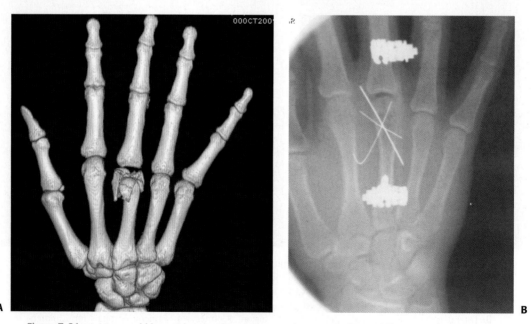

Figure 7-61. A 15-year-old boy with a punching injury causing an articular, multifragmented metacarpal head fracture (**A**). **B:** Fragments were pinned together with 0.035 and 0.028 K-wires. A mini-ex fix was utilized to provide distraction across the joint and alignment for collateral ligaments during healing.

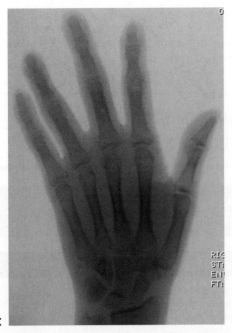

Figure 7-61. (*Continued*) **C:** Final results at ex fix removal. (Courtesy of Children's Hospital Los Angeles, CA.)

Postoperative Care

Most metacarpal fractures managed by closed treatment are immobilized for 4 weeks. Subsequently, a home program of range-of-motion exercises is started and formal therapy is not needed. In active children and young athletes, a light splint can be worn for protection and as a peer warning signal for an additional few weeks. If percutaneous pin fixation is used, the wires are removed in the office 4 weeks after surgery.

Rehabilitation of open fracture reduction depends on the stability of the fixation and the reliability of the patient to postoperative recommendations. Older and reliable patients with stable internal fixation are mobilized earlier, usually 5 to 7 days after surgery. A removable splint for protection between exercise sessions is used for 4 to 6 weeks.

Potential Pitfalls and Preventive Measures

Metacarpal Fractures: SURGICAL PITFALLS AND PREVENTIONS	
Pitfall	**Prevention**
• Malrotation	• Check tenodesis
	• After each K-wire or reduction maneuver, recheck tenodesis
• Malunion	• Stable fixation
	• Allow shaft metacarpals an extended healing time, as the diaphysis may be slower to consolidate than the neck
• Osteonecrosis of metacarpal head	• Consider joint aspiration; avoid dissection of fragments during open repair

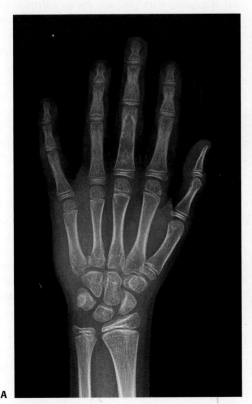
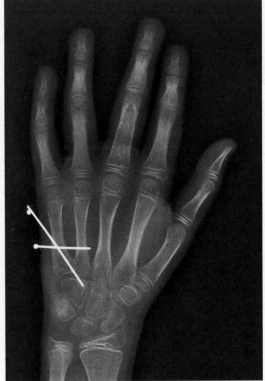

Figure 7-62. A 12-year-old boy fell off of the scooter, injuring his left hand. **A:** Anteroposterior x-ray with comminuted fracture at the base of the small metacarpal. **B:** Longitudinal traction resulted in anatomic reduction, followed by percutaneous pin fixation. (Courtesy of Shriners Hospital for Children, Philadelphia, PA.)

MANAGEMENT OF EXPECTED ADVERSE OUTCOMES AND UNEXPECTED COMPLICATIONS RELATED TO METACARPAL FRACTURES

Metacarpal Fractures:
COMMON ADVERSE OUTCOMES AND COMPLICATIONS

- Epiphyseal and physeal fractures: osteonecrosis, malreduction/malunion

- Neck fractures: excessive apex dorsal angulation, malrotation

- Shaft fractures:
  - Malrotation, soft tissue interposition, nonunion

- Metacarpal base fractures:
  - Loss of reduction, malreduction of articular fragments, late instability, arthritis

Most metacarpal fractures heal without sequelae. Mild deformity in the plane of motion is tolerated and may correct with remodeling. Considerable angulation or rotation creates a functional impairment that requires treatment.

Bony complications include malunion and osteonecrosis. Nonunion is rare.[22,102] Even a small amount (less than 10 degrees) of rotational malalignment may create overlap of the digits during flexion and a functional disturbance. Corrective osteotomy to realign the digit is often necessary. The osteotomy for rotational correction can be made at the site of fracture or anywhere along the metacarpal. The proximal shaft or base has certain advantages. This area provides ample bone for healing and offers the opportunity for internal fixation using wires or a plate. Diaphyseal malunions with symptomatic flexion deformity into the palm require a dorsal wedge osteotomy and internal fixation.

Osteonecrosis of the metacarpal head may occur after an intra-articular fracture. Factors include the degree of injury and the intracapsular pressure caused by the hemarthrosis.[48,150] Theoretically, early joint aspiration may diminish the intra-articular pressure. Fortunately, partial osteonecrosis in a growing child incites remarkable remodeling of the adjacent articular surface and often results in a functional joint. Part-time splint protection during the remodeling phase is recommended.

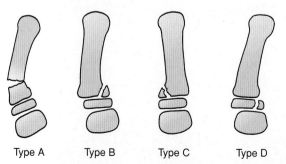

| Type A | Type B | Type C | Type D |

Figure 7-63. Classification of thumb metacarpal fractures. **Type A:** Metaphyseal fracture. **Types B and C:** S-H type II physeal fractures with lateral or medial angulation. **Type D:** An S-H type III fracture (pediatric Bennett fracture).

Considerable joint incongruity is rare and reconstruction options are limited.[174] However, recent experience with osteochondral autograft transplant surgery (OATS) transfer from the knee has been successful.[147]

Thumb Metacarpal Fractures in Children

CLASSIFICATION OF THUMB METACARPAL FRACTURES

Classification of Thumb Metacarpal Fractures

- Fractures of the head
- Fractures of the shaft
- Intra-articular S-H III or IV fractures of the thumb metacarpal base/epiphysis
- Physeal/epiphyseal S-H II fractures—Types A, B, C, D
- Thumb metacarpal shaft fractures
- Thumb metacarpal neck fractures
- Thumb metacarpal head fractures

Fractures of the thumb metacarpal can occur at the epiphysis, physis, neck, shaft, or base. Fractures of the neck and shaft and their treatment principles are similar to those of the fingers. Thumb metacarpal base fractures that involve the physis or epiphysis require unique considerations (Fig. 7-63).

The adductor pollicis, abductor pollicis longus, and thenar muscles play a role in fracture mechanics and can displace metacarpal fractures. The muscles' directions of pull dictate the direction of fracture displacement and deformity. The adductor pollicis inserts onto the proximal phalanx and into the extensor apparatus through the adductor aponeurosis. The abductor pollicis longus inserts onto the metacarpal base and is the primary deforming force in most fracture–dislocations about the thumb CMC joint (Bennett fractures[44] or pediatric equivalents).

Direct trauma, rotational forces, and axial loading may all cause thumb metacarpal fractures. Sporting endeavors are the prime events causing fractures. A valgus force to the MCP joint usually produces an epiphyseal fracture. Skiing, biking, and playing baseball catcher are specific activities that place the thumb MCP joint and metacarpal shaft in a vulnerable position. Adduction forces, such as direct trauma to a soccer goalie or basketball player during a fall or ball injury, place the thumb CMC joint and base of thumb metacarpal at risk.

THUMB METACARPAL BASE FRACTURES

Fractures of the base of the thumb metacarpal are subdivided according to their location. Type A fractures occur between the physis and the junction of the proximal and middle thirds of the bone. The fractures are often transverse or slightly oblique. There is often an element of medial impaction, and the fracture is angulated in an apex lateral direction (Fig. 7-64).

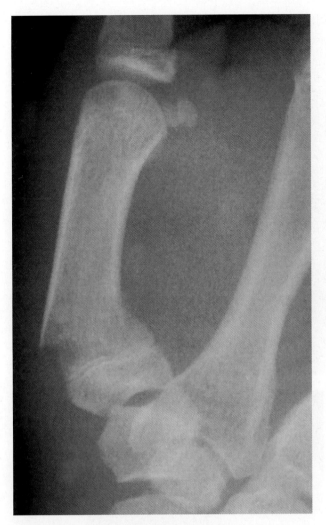

Figure 7-64. Metaphyseal thumb metacarpal fracture that does not involve the physis. Treatment consisted of closed reduction and cast immobilization.

Type B and C fractures are S-H II fractures at the thumb metacarpal base. Most patterns have the metaphyseal fragment on the medial side (type B) (Fig. 7-61). The shaft fragment is adducted by the pull of the adductor pollicis and shifted in a proximal direction by the pull of the abductor pollicis longus. Although this pattern resembles a Bennett fracture with respect to the deforming forces, there is no intra-articular extension. Type C fractures are the least common and have the reverse pattern, with the metaphyseal fragment on the lateral side and the proximal shaft displacement in a medial direction. This pattern often results from more substantial trauma and does not lend itself to closed treatment.

A type D fracture is an S-H III or IV fracture that most closely resembles the adult Bennett fracture.[34,68] The deforming forces are similar to a type B injury with resultant adduction and proximal migration of the base-shaft fragment.

Biplanar x-rays including a hyperpronated view of the thumb accentuate the view of the CMC joint. Examination under live fluoroscopy or CT scan may also be necessary for preoperative planning and classification of fracture severity.

TREATMENT OPTIONS FOR THUMB METACARPAL BASE FRACTURES

Thumb Metacarpal Fractures: INDICATIONS FOR NONOPERATIVE VERSUS OPERATIVE TREATMENT

Nonoperative	Operative
• Nondisplaced	• Displaced articular
• Closed	• Open or extensive soft tissue injury
• Reducible	• Irreducible
• Stable	• Unstable

TYPE A

Type A fractures can usually be treated by closed methods. Although swelling about the thenar eminence limits manipulation of the fracture and diminishes the effectiveness of immobilization, most fractures can still be treated successfully by closed reduction and immobilization. Because the CMC joint has near-universal motion and the physis is proximal in the metacarpal, remodeling is extensive in young patients. The multiplanar motion of the CMC joint combined with the potential for remodeling makes less than 20 to 30 degrees of angulation inconsequential. If reduction is attempted, pressure is applied to the apex of the fracture to effect reduction. Anatomic reduction is not required because remodeling is plentiful.[22] Unstable fractures with marked displacement require percutaneous pin fixation to maintain alignment (Fig. 7-65).

TYPES B AND C

Closed reduction is more difficult for type B and C fractures. The mobility of the metacarpal base and the swelling make closed reduction difficult. Comminution, soft tissue interposition, or transperiosteal "buttonholing" in type C fractures may further complicate reduction.[111] If closed reduction is accomplished and stable, then short-arm thumb spica splint or cast immobilization is possible. Repeat radiographic evaluation should be obtained 5 to 7 days later to ensure maintenance of reduction.

If closed reduction is possible but the reduction is unstable, percutaneous pinning is recommended (Fig. 7-66). There are multiple options for pin configuration including direct fixation across the fracture, pinning across the reduced CMC joint, and pinning between the first and second metacarpals. Open reduction is indicated for irreducible fractures. Type C fractures may require open reduction to remove any interposed periosteum that blocks reduction (Fig. 7-67).[111]

TYPE D

Type D fractures are unstable and require closed or open reduction to restore physeal and articular alignment.[95] An acceptable

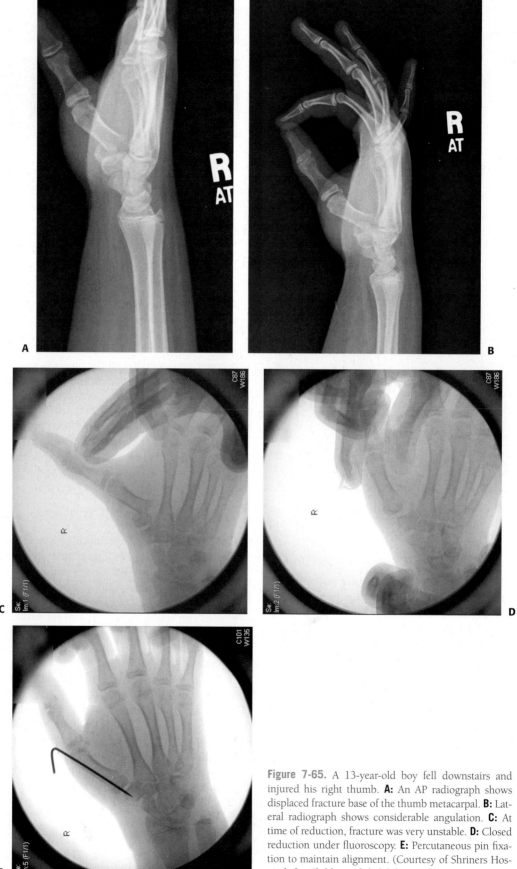

Figure 7-65. A 13-year-old boy fell downstairs and injured his right thumb. **A:** An AP radiograph shows displaced fracture base of the thumb metacarpal. **B:** Lateral radiograph shows considerable angulation. **C:** At time of reduction, fracture was very unstable. **D:** Closed reduction under fluoroscopy. **E:** Percutaneous pin fixation to maintain alignment. (Courtesy of Shriners Hospitals for Children, Philadelphia, PA.)

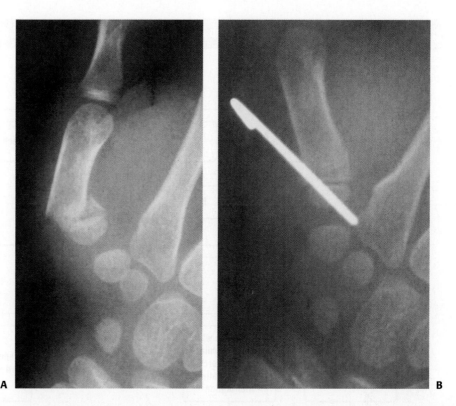

Figure 7-66. A: An 8-year-old boy with reducible, but unstable, fracture. **B:** A single percutaneous pin was placed to maintain alignment.

closed reduction is maintained by percutaneous pin fixation. An unacceptable closed reduction is rare but requires open reduction and fixation.[68] A hyperpronated view of the thumb accentuates the view of the CMC joint. The choice of implant must be individualized, though smooth wires are favored to minimize potential injury to the physis and articular cartilage.[34,68] Skeletal traction is an alternative treatment for complex injuries with severe bony or soft tissue damage.[94]

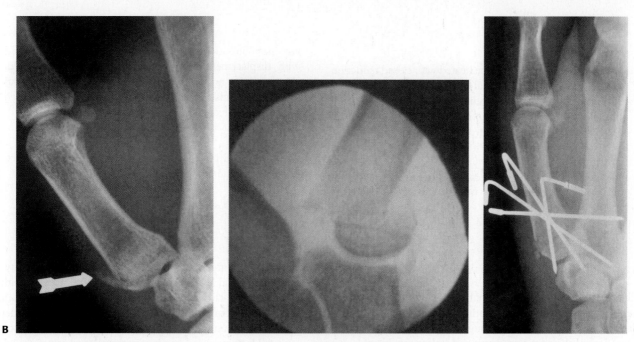

Figure 7-67. A: Fracture of the thumb metacarpal base with a small lateral metaphyseal flag that appears innocuous on radiograph (*arrow*). **B:** However, additional images revealed marked displacement of the distal fragment. **C:** Closed reduction was unsuccessful because of interposed tissue. After open reduction, K-wires were used to stabilize the fracture.

Authors' Preferred Treatment for Thumb Metacarpal Fractures (Algorithm 7-4)

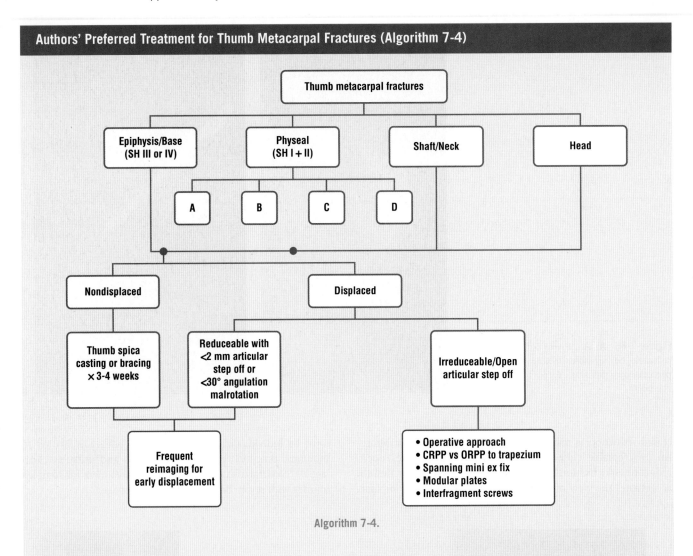

Algorithm 7-4.

Type A

Type A fractures can usually be treated with closed reduction and cast application. Residual angulation between 20 and 30 degrees is acceptable depending on the age of the child and clinical appearance of the thumb. Fractures that are reducible, but unstable, require percutaneous pinning (Fig. 7-65).

Types B and C

Mild angulation requires only cast application without reduction. Moderate angulation is treated with closed reduction and immobilization. Severe angulation is usually combined with displacement and requires reduction. A successful closed reduction is often augmented with percutaneous pin fixation. An unsuccessful closed reduction requires open reduction and fixation.

Type D

Displaced S-H III and IV fractures are rare and require closed or open reduction and internal fixation.

Postoperative Care

Closed treatment requires immobilization for 4 to 6 weeks depending on the fracture severity and degree of soft tissue damage. A home program for range of motion is started thereafter. Formal therapy is not instituted unless considerable soft tissue injury occurred. In active children and young athletes, a light splint may be worn for protection for an additional few weeks.

Open fracture management depends on the stability of the fixation and the reliability of the patient. Young children or marginal fracture fixations require 4 to 6 weeks of immobilization. Fracture union with mild stiffness takes precedence over fracture nonunion with excessive motion. Adolescents with stable fixation can be mobilized earlier, usually 5 to 7 days after surgery, provided they are trustworthy in terms of activity restrictions. A removable splint is used for protection between exercise sessions until union.

MANAGEMENT OF EXPECTED ADVERSE OUTCOMES AND UNEXPECTED COMPLICATIONS RELATED TO THUMB METACARPAL FRACTURES

Thumb metacarpal fractures usually heal without altering hand function. The remodeling capabilities of fractures near or involving the physis are extensive. The basilar thumb joint also allows multiplanar motion and can accommodate moderate fracture malunion. Residual deformity along the thumb metacarpal can be concealed through CMC joint motion, and the thumb tolerates malrotation better than the fingers (Fig. 7-68).

Complications are uncommon. Nonunion, malunion, and articular incongruity are potential problems.[80] Intra-articular incongruity may occur after incomplete reduction of an intra-articular fracture or inadequate fixation after an initial satisfactory reduction. Sequelae include pain, diminished motion, and arthrosis. Available treatment options include intra-articular osteotomy, fusion, or interposition arthroplasty.

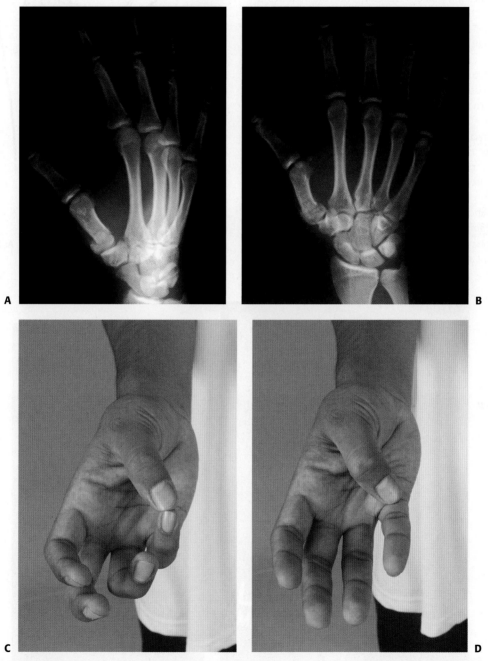

Figure 7-68. A 14-year-old boy presents 3 weeks after injury with mild pain and deformity at the base of right thumb. **A:** An AP radiograph shows a moderately displaced fracture at the base of the thumb metacarpal. **B:** Lateral radiograph shows mild angulation. **C:** Follow-up motion after splinting for an additional 2 weeks, and home therapy reveals excellent opposition. **D:** The thumb is able to touch the base of the small finger. (Courtesy of Shriners Hospitals for Children, Philadelphia, PA.)

Fractures of the Carpal Bones

SCAPHOID FRACTURES

The low incidence of scaphoid fractures in children is most likely related to the thick peripheral cartilage that covers and protects the ossification center. Therefore, fracture requires a considerable force to disrupt this cartilaginous shell and injure the underlying bone.[84] The pattern of pediatric scaphoid injury differs from that of adults because of the evolving ossification center.[138] During early stages of ossification, the scaphoid is more susceptible to avulsion fractures about the distal pole fracture.[27,119] As the ossification progresses from distal to proximal, the fracture pattern mirrors the adult forms by early adolescence (Fig. 7-69).

In children, fractures of the distal third of the scaphoid have traditionally been the most common injury pattern and often result from direct trauma.[27,84] However, scaphoid waist fractures are increasing in frequency in younger children as participation in contact athletics begins earlier.[131] Proximal pole fractures are rare in children and often represent an avulsion fracture of the scapholunate ligament. These fractures are at higher risk for nonunion and osteonecrosis. The scaphoid can also be fractured as a component of a greater arc perilunate injury (Fig. 7-70).[138]

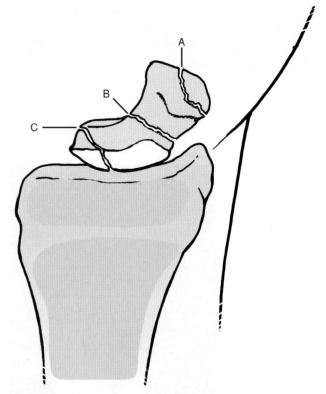

Figure 7-69. Three types of scaphoid fractures. **A:** Distal third. **B:** Middle third. **C:** Proximal pole.

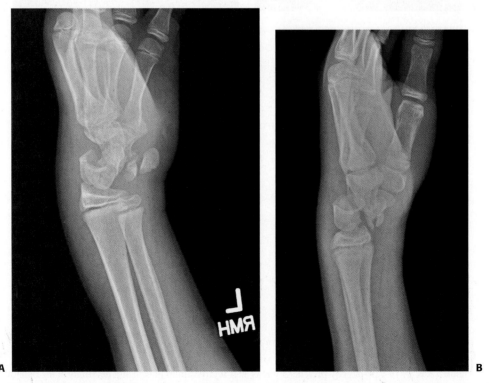

Figure 7-70. A 13-year-old boy who was playing tag at night when he jumped over a wall, falling 5 ft on his outstretched left wrist. A closed reduction and CT scan were performed at an outside institution. **A:** Lateral x-rays with volar perilunate and multiple carpal fractures. **B:** Semi-supinated lateral x-ray with markedly displaced carpal fractures.

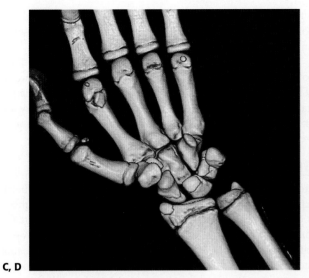
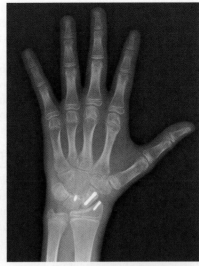
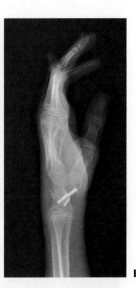

C, D   **E**

Figure 7-70. (*Continued*) **C:** 3D CT scan demonstrated fractures of the radial styloid, lunate, and triquetrum. **D:** Postoperative anteroposterior x-ray status post open reduction and internal fixation radial styloid, scaphoid fracture, and lunate fracture. **E:** Postoperative lateral x-ray after fixation of carpal fractures. (Courtesy of Shriners Hospital for Children, Philadelphia, PA.)

CLASSIFICATION OF SCAPHOID FRACTURES

Classification of Scaphoid Fractures		
A	•	Fractures of the distal pole
A1	•	Extra-articular distal pole fractures
A2	•	Intra-articular distal pole fractures
B	•	Fractures of the middle third (waist fractures)
C	•	Fractures of the proximal third

Type A: Fractures of the Distal Pole

Distal pole fractures are often secondary to direct trauma or avulsion with a dorsoradial or dorsovolar fragment.[27] The strong scaphotrapezial ligaments and capsular attachments produce mechanical failure through the bone (Fig. 7-71).[27,89] The fracture line and size of the avulsion fragment vary from an isolated chondral injury that is barely visible on radiographs to a large osteochondral fragment.

Type A1: Extra-articular distal pole fractures. The most important prognostic factor is the presence or absence of joint involvement. Extra-articular fractures may be either volar or dorsal avulsions (Fig. 7-72). A volar pattern is more common and is attributed to the stout scaphotrapezial ligaments. A dorsal fracture configuration is less common and is attributed to the dorsal intercarpal ligament. The fragments vary in size, and the radiographic appearance is age dependent.

Type A2: Intra-articular distal pole fractures. This type of fracture may be a variation of a type A1 fracture with an intra-articular extension (Fig. 7-73). Similar types (i.e., volar and dorsal) and mechanisms of injury are possible.

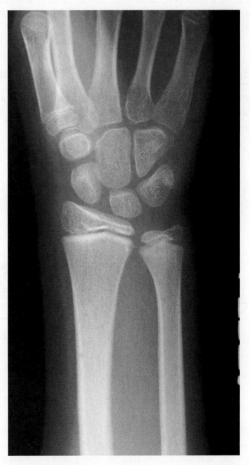

Figure 7-71. A 12-year-old boy fell on his right wrist and was tender over scaphoid tubercle. Radiograph reveals a small avulsion fracture of the distal scaphoid that might easily be overlooked. (Courtesy of Shriners Hospitals for Children, Philadelphia, PA.)

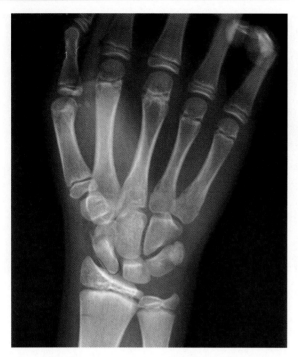

Figure 7-72. A 12-year-old boy fell playing ice hockey and complained of right wrist pain. Radiograph reveals an extra-articular distal pole scaphoid fracture with slight comminution. (Courtesy of Shriners Hospitals for Children, Philadelphia, PA.)

Type B: Fractures of the Middle Third (Waist Fractures)

Middle third fractures do occur in skeletally immature patients. The mechanism of injury is usually a fall onto the outstretched hand and pronated forearm, which exerts tensile forces acting across the volar portion of the scaphoid as the wrist extends.[138] Bony comminution may be present (Fig. 7-74). A careful scrutiny for other injuries about the carpus is mandatory.[49,63]

Dividing the bone into thirds or delineating the area bounded by the radioscaphocapitate ligament defines the waist of the scaphoid. Waist fractures occur in many forms. Pediatric fractures are incomplete, minimally displaced, or complete with or without displacement. Comminuted fractures are rare and are associated with higher-energy injuries.

Type C: Fractures of the Proximal Third

Proximal pole fractures are rare in children but have been reported in competitive adolescent athletes. The mechanism is often unclear and can be atypical, such as punching game machines or fighting.[4] A proximal pole fracture may propagate through the interface between newly ossified tissue and the cartilaginous anlage, or the injury may be strictly through the cartilage. Proximal fractures may cause destabilization of the scapholunate joint, as the scapholunate interosseous ligament remains attached to the avulsed fragment (Fig. 7-75).

Proximal third fractures present diagnostic and therapeutic dilemmas. The proximal pole is the last to ossify, which further complicates diagnosis. The tenuous blood supply of this region presents the same problems in children as adults in terms of nonunion and risks of osteonecrosis.

BIPARTITE SCAPHOID CONTROVERSY: TRAUMATIC VERSUS DEVELOPMENTAL

A bipartite scaphoid probably exists but is uncommon and may be associated with Down syndrome.[87,160] Criteria that must be met to diagnose a congenital bipartite scaphoid include the following: (a) similar bilateral appearance, (b) absence of historical

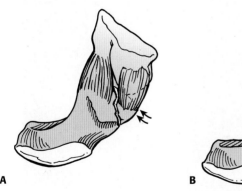
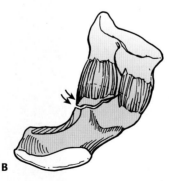

A   **B**

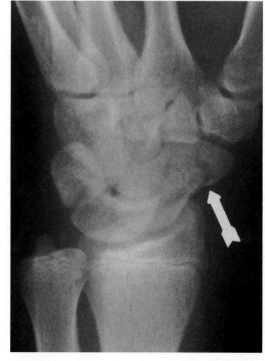

C

Figure 7-73. Two variations of an A2 intra-articular fracture of the scaphoid distal pole. **A:** The more prevalent type is on the radial aspect of the volar distal scaphoid. This fragment is attached to the radial portion of the scaphotrapezial ligament (*arrows*). **B:** The less common type is on the ulnar aspect of the volar distal scaphoid. This fragment is attached to the ulnar portion of the scaphotrapezial ligament (*arrows*). **C:** Radiograph of an intra-articular distal pole scaphoid fracture.

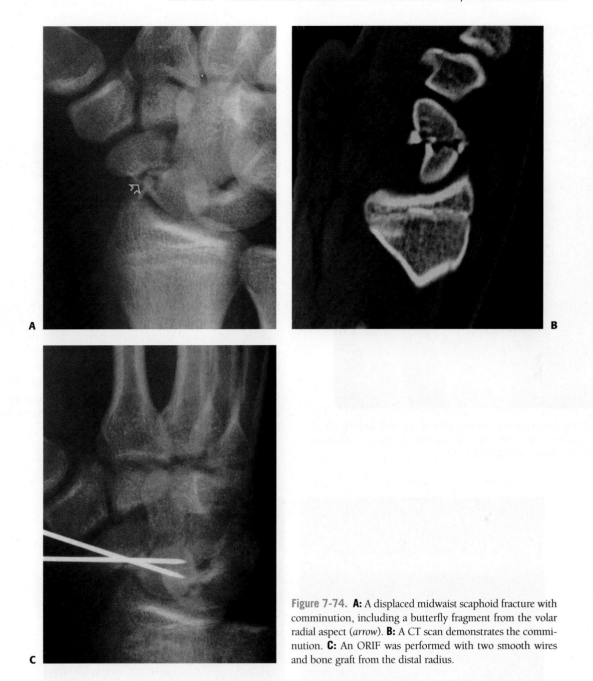

Figure 7-74. A: A displaced midwaist scaphoid fracture with comminution, including a butterfly fragment from the volar radial aspect (*arrow*). **B:** A CT scan demonstrates the comminution. **C:** An ORIF was performed with two smooth wires and bone graft from the distal radius.

or clinical evidence of antecedent trauma, (c) equal size and uniform density of each component, (d) absence of degenerative change between the scaphoid components or elsewhere in the carpus, and (e) smooth, rounded architecture of each scaphoid component. A unilateral "bipartite scaphoid" should be viewed as a posttraumatic scaphoid nonunion (Fig. 7-76).

CAPITATE FRACTURES

Isolated fractures of the capitate are rare and usually result from high-energy trauma.[96] Capitate fractures may represent a form of greater arc perilunar injury (Fig. 7-77). The force can prop-agate completely around the lunate and cause a perilunate or lunate dislocation.[49,109,123] The injury can also halt within the capitate and produce a scaphocapitate syndrome.[39,41]

Excessive dorsiflexion of the wrist is the most common mechanism. The waist of the capitate abuts the lunate or dorsal aspect of the radius. The fracture occurs through the waist with variable displacement. The wrist is usually markedly swollen and painful to palpation. The clinical presentation varies with the associated carpal injuries. Median nerve paresthesias may be present secondary to swelling within the carpal tunnel.

Standard AP and lateral views are usually adequate (Fig. 7-78). Careful scrutiny of the radiographs is necessary. The capitate fracture can be subtle, or the proximal capitate fragment can rotate 180 degrees. Either scenario can create a confusing

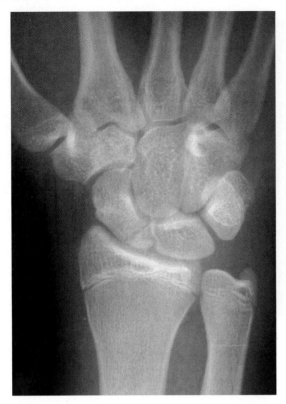

Figure 7-75. An AP radiograph of a 16-year-old male hockey player with a proximal one-third scaphoid fracture. (Courtesy of Shriners Hospitals for Children, Philadelphia, PA.)

image that often results in misinterpretation. Incomplete ossification further complicates radiographic diagnosis and degree of displacement. Small osteochondral fragments in the midcarpal region may indicate a greater arc injury or isolated capitate fracture. In these cases, advanced imaging studies, such as MRI or CT, may be useful (Fig. 7-79).

TRIQUETRUM FRACTURES

Dorsal avulsion fractures of the triquetrum are more common in adults than in children. The injury may occur in adolescents as carpal ossification nears completion. A fracture through the body of the triquetrum is rare and may occur with a perilunar injury as the path of the greater arc injury passes through the triquetrum (Fig. 7-70).[51] A fall on an outstretched wrist is the common event. The probable mechanism for a dorsal triquetrum fracture is a pulling force through the dorsal ligaments or abutment of the ulnar styloid. The wrist is mildly swollen and painful to palpation directly over the dorsal triquetrum. The clinical presentation is more severe with associated carpal injuries. Radiologic AP and lateral views may not show the avulsion fracture. A pronated oblique view highlights the dorsum of the triquetrum and can reveal the avulsed fragment. At times, CT scans are necessary for accurate diagnosis (Fig. 7-80).

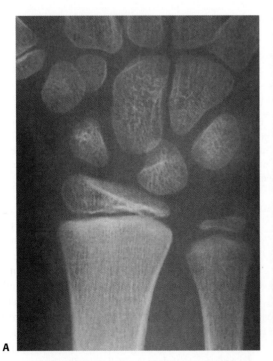
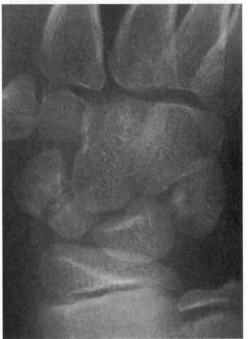

Figure 7-76. A: A 9-year-old boy who fell on an outstretched wrist and had radial-sided pain and tenderness; original radiographs failed to reveal any bony abnormalities. **B:** About 1.5 years later, he had persistent radial-sided wrist pain, and radiographs revealed a midwaist scaphoid nonunion. This would *not* be considered a bipartite scaphoid but instead an injury that was sustained when the cartilaginous anlage was present.

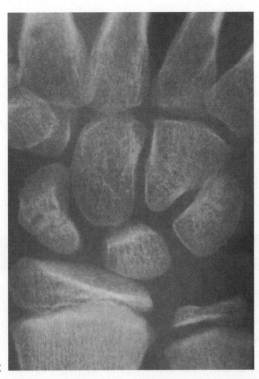

Figure 7-76. (*Continued*) **C:** After 2 months of casting, early fracture union is present.

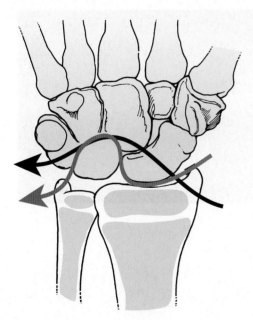

Figure 7-77. Progressive perilunar instability. The greater arc (*black arrow*) is associated with fractures of the carpal bones, which may include the scaphoid, lunate, capitate, hamate, and triquetrum. The *red arrow* depicts the lesser arc, in which forces are transmitted only through soft tissue structures. (Reprinted from Mayfield JK, Johnson RP, Kilcoyn RK. Carpal dislocations: Pathomechanics and progressive perilunar instability. *J Hand Surg Am.* 1980;5(3): 226–241. Copyright © 1980 American Society for Surgery of the Hand. With permission.)

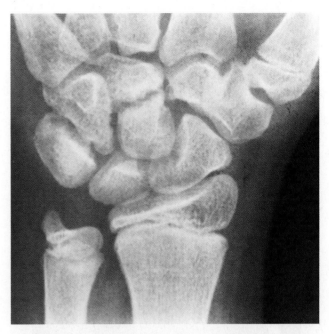

Figure 7-78. A 12-year-old boy sustained multiple carpal fractures attributed to a crushing injury. An established nonunion of the capitate is present 16 months later, which required bone grafting to obtain union. (Courtesy of James H. Dobyns, MD.)

HAMATE, PISIFORM, LUNATE, AND TRAPEZIUM FRACTURES

Pediatric fractures of the hamate, pisiform, lunate, and trapezium are rare. Hamate fractures are classified by their location in the hook, type I, or in the body, type II. Hook of the hamate fractures usually occur in adults but may occur in adolescents

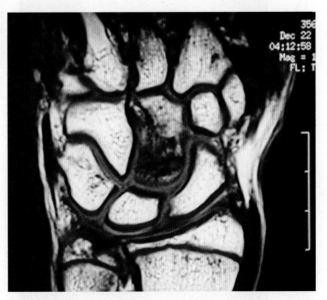

Figure 7-79. A 13-year-old boy with persistent midcarpal pain after a fall. An MRI scan shows a capitate fracture. (Courtesy of Shriners Hospitals for Children, Philadelphia, PA.)

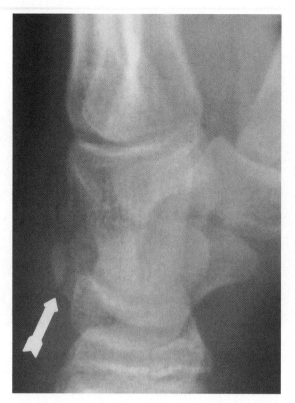

Figure 7-80. A minimally displaced dorsal triquetral avulsion fracture (*arrow*) that was treated with short-term immobilization.

who play baseball or golf or following a fall, usually bicycle related. If the fracture involved the distal third of the hook, it may have occurred from an avulsion injury secondary to pull from the transverse carpal ligament. A CT scan may be necessary for diagnosis if the fracture is not visible on the carpal tunnel view (Fig. 7-81). Dorsal or body hamate fractures can occur with axial load or punching injuries, as the bases of the fourth and fifth metacarpals act like pistons and shear off large or small pieces of the hamate.

Pisiform fractures are the result of direct trauma. Lunate fractures are associated with Kienbock disease,[17] which is relatively uncommon in children. Trapezium fractures can occur with CMC joint injuries about the thumb.

SOFT TISSUE INJURIES ABOUT THE CARPUS

Ligamentous injuries about the pediatric wrist are less common than osseous injuries.[25,108,123] The immature carpus and viscoelastic ligaments are relatively resistant to injury. Fracture–dislocations and isolated ligamentous injuries are usually caused by high-energy trauma (Fig. 7-82).[43] Motor vehicle accidents and sports-related injuries are potential causes of the rare fracture–dislocation. However, recurrent or chronic wrist pain is not uncommon in adolescents. Most recurrent ligamentous pain results from hypermobility and overuse during the adolescent growth spurt. This mechanism may result in joint

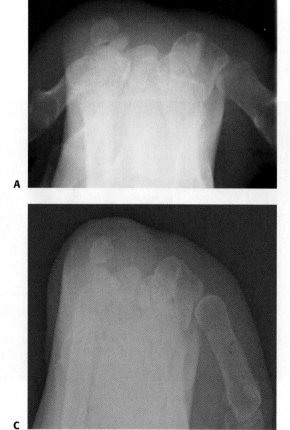

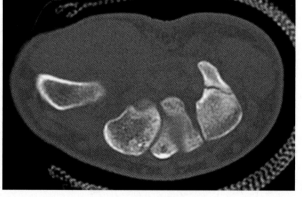

Figure 7-81. A: A 15-year-old baseball player with chronic pain over hypothenar eminence while batting. **B:** A CT scan coronal view demonstrated a base of the hook of the hamate fracture. **C:** After 3 months of immobilization and rest from baseball, the patient is elected for fragment removal. Returned to baseball wearing a silicone gel patch in his batting glove over the hypothenar area.

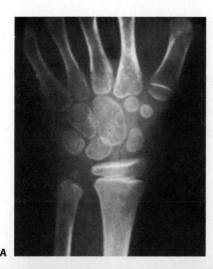

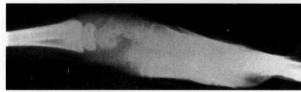

Figure 7-82. Radiographic AP (**A**) and lateral (**B**) views of a dorsal perilunate dislocation in a 6-year-old boy. (Courtesy of William F. Benson, MD.)

ASSESSMENT AND NONOPERATIVE AND OPERATIVE TREATMENT OF FRACTURES OF THE CARPAL BONES

Scaphoid Fractures

Nondisplaced Scaphoid Fractures

Normal radiographs do not preclude the presence of a scaphoid fracture. Clinical suspicion in the presence of normal radiographs warrants immobilization and reevaluation in 2 weeks.[49] The cast is removed, the wrist is examined, and repeat radiographs are obtained. Pain resolution and negative radiographs warrant discontinuation of immobilization and return to normal activities. Persistent pain with normal radiographs requires continued immobilization and advanced imaging studies. In this clinical setting, MRI scans have been shown to be diagnostically useful to avoid both misdiagnosis and overtreatment (Fig. 7-83).[8,54,118,129,137] However, MRI may be overly sensitive in identifying bone edema that fails to develop into a fracture.

If radiographs reveal a fracture, immediate treatment is required. Most pediatric scaphoid fractures can be treated with cast immobilization because children possess a great ability to heal. In addition, most scaphoid fractures in children are either incomplete (disrupting only a single cortex) or nondisplaced.

subluxation, chondral impingement, or ligamentous tears similar to patellofemoral injuries in adolescents.

A young child with an acute traumatic injury avoids use of the wrist and hand. The wrist is swollen and painful to palpation, making isolation of the injured segment difficult except in extremely cooperative children. Provocative maneuvers for carpal instability usually are not possible because of pain in the injured wrist.

Gross instability without pain on stress testing may indicate a hyperelasticity syndrome that is unrelated to trauma.[6] However, recurrent pain does occur in children with hypermobility, overuse, and relative muscular weakness. These children complain of diffuse pain, generalized tenderness, and limited strength on examination. Diagnosis is difficult particularly in patients with emotional overlay and somatization.

Radiologic AP and lateral views are routine. The incomplete ossification complicates radiographic interpretation, especially the assessment of carpal widening. Detection of slight widening or malalignment within the carpus is often difficult. Contralateral views are useful to compare ossification and carpal spacing.[136] Suspicion of a fracture warrants advanced imaging studies, such as arthrography, stress radiography, fluoroscopy, and MRI. Ligamentous injuries are best diagnosed with high-quality MRI scans.

As with the pediatric hand fractures, positive outcomes consist of healing, alignment, and painless return to function and sports. Because of the vascular anatomy of the carpus, avascular necrosis is rare but can occur after a proximal pole scaphoid fracture. Case series of children after carpal bone fractures and dislocations lack validated instrument scoring data.

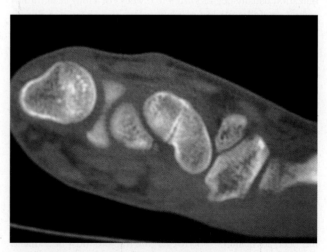

Figure 7-83. An MRI scan of a minimally displaced healing scaphoid fracture not seen on radiograph.

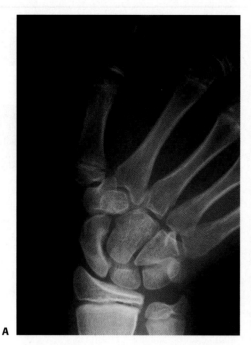 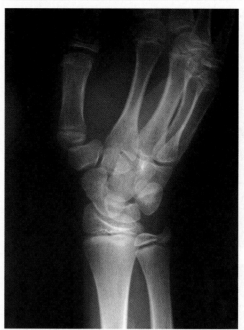

A   B

Figure 7-84. A 12-year-old boy depicted in Figure 7-83 after 8 weeks of casting. **A:** Scaphoid view demonstrates healing of the fracture. **B:** Pronated oblique radiograph further confirms fracture union. (Courtesy of Shriners Hospitals for Children, Philadelphia, PA.)

This principle is especially true for the distal pole, which is a frequent site of scaphoid fracture (Fig. 7-84).[138] Therefore, cast immobilization is the standard of treatment for most nondisplaced or minimally displaced (<2 mm) pediatric scaphoid fractures. For avulsion and incomplete fractures, a short-arm thumb spica cast for 4 to 6 weeks is recommended. In the young child, a long-arm cast is appropriate to prevent the cast from sliding off the arm. For complete, stable distal third and waist fractures, immobilization consisting of up to 6 to 8 weeks of casting is recommended until healing.

A longer period of immobilization (8 to 12 weeks) is recommended for nondisplaced proximal pole fractures, delayed diagnosis, or fractures with apparent bony resorption.[138] Immobilization usually begins with 4 to 6 weeks of a long-arm thumb spica cast, followed by up to 6 weeks of a short-arm thumb spica cast. The exact cast position and the joints immobilized are a matter of surgeon preference.[61,115,130] Most authors favor a long-arm thumb spica cast that permits thumb interphalangeal joint motion.[173]

Displaced Scaphoid Fractures

Closed Reduction and Casting

Historically, closed reduction of a displaced scaphoid fracture has been described.[65,66,115,130] Currently, ORIF is a more reliable method for restoring alignment and obtaining union.

Percutaneous Screw Fixation

In adults, percutaneous screw fixation for displaced fractures has been advocated.[9,142] However, the fracture must be reduced before placement of the screw fixation. Fracture reduction can be accomplished with manipulation, joysticks, or arthroscopic assistance. This technique can be applied to adolescent patients with displaced scaphoid fractures. Screws can be placed under fluoroscopic control either volarly (distal to proximal) or dorsally (proximal to distal) depending on fracture patterns and surgeon preference (Fig. 7-85).[10,156] This procedure is challenging in displaced scaphoid fractures (Video 7-3).

Open Reduction and Internal Fixation

Displacement of more than 1 mm or intrascaphoid angulation of more than 10 degrees on any image warrants ORIF. A volar or dorsal approach can be used depending on the fracture configuration and surgeon preference. The implant choice is individualized according to the fracture and patient. Scaphoid screws are the primary fixation techniques, though K-wires can be used (Fig. 7-86).[163] Smaller screws (mini and micro) may be necessary in the pediatric patient. Modern compression screws have been shown to speed up healing.[131]

Capitate Fractures

Treatment depends on the capitate fracture pattern, degree of displacement, and associated injuries. Distraction radiographs, MRI, or CT scans may be necessary to determine the exact pattern of injury. Nondisplaced fractures of the capitate and/or scaphoid can be treated with a long-arm cast for 6 to 8 weeks. Closed reduction of displaced fractures is not feasible.[109] Displaced fractures require open reduction to rotate the proximal capitate pole into anatomic position. Associated perilunar injuries also require internal fixation and ligamentous repair. The anatomic relationships within the carpus must be restored. Wire or osseous screw fixation can both be appropriate stabilization after open reduction.

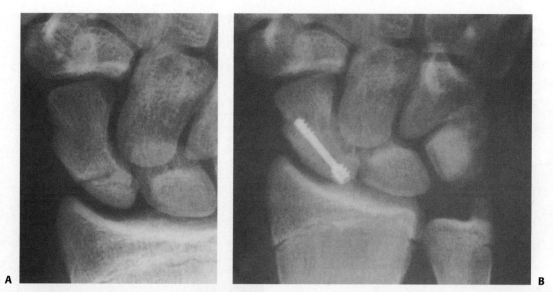

Figure 7-85. A: Nondisplaced proximal pole scaphoid fracture in a skeletally mature adolescent athlete. **B:** Treatment by percutaneous screw fixation led to healing.

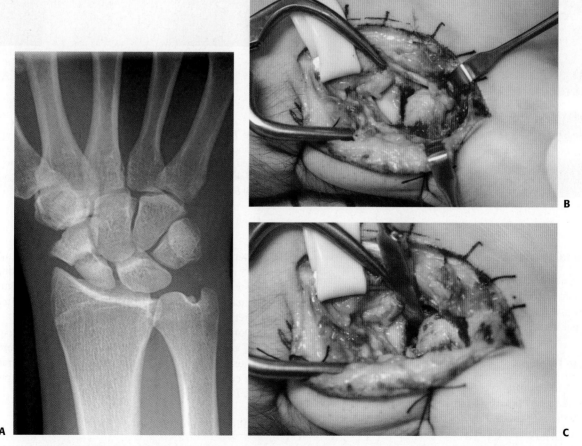

Figure 7-86. A: A 16-year-old male with a right scaphoid nonunion with resorption at the fracture site. **B:** Volar approach and exposure of the fracture site. **C:** The fracture site was debrided of fibrous material, and the humpback deformity was corrected.

(continues)

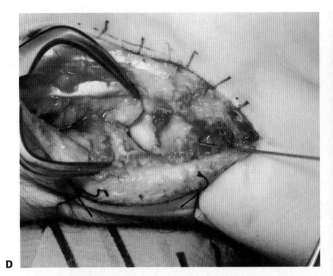

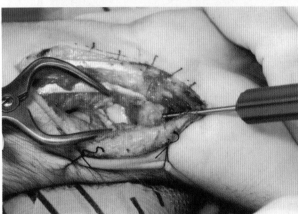

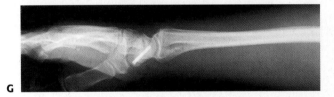

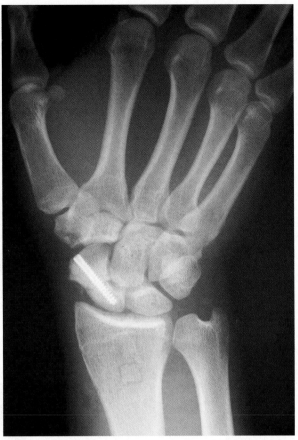

Figure 7-86. (*Continued*) **D:** The fracture site was packed with bone graft and a guidewire was placed for screw fixation. **E:** The screw was inserted over the guidewire. **F, G:** Radiographic AP and lateral views after fracture reduction, bone grafting, and screw placement. (Courtesy of Shriners Hospitals for Children, Philadelphia, PA.)

Triquetral Fractures

An avulsion fracture is treated with a short period of immobilization (3 to 6 weeks) followed by motion and return to activities. A fracture through the body of the triquetrum with a perilunar injury requires ORIF.

Hamate Fractures

Hook of the hamate, type I, fractures are often missed in the acute setting unless a carpal tunnel view is ordered or a CT scan of the wrist is obtained. Immobilization and avoidance of baseball batting, gymnastics, or golf may lead to complete union in children. After a period of casting, if imaging is consistent with a delayed union and the child is symptomatic, surgical fragment excision may be pursued (Fig. 7-81). Careful protection of the ulnar nerve motor branch and ulnar artery anatomy is required.

Subperiosteal dissection can minimize chances of neurovascular injury. Postoperative return to sports that requires direct pressure on the hypothenar eminence may be slow because of the hypersensitivity. Silicone patches or glove padding may facilitate return.

Dorsal body hamate, type II, fractures may be part of a CMC dislocation or isolated. Reduction of the hamate fracture usually reduces the CMC dislocation. If the fragment is large enough, ORIF with a headless screw may be performed (Fig. 7-87).

Carpal Ligamentous Injury

Treatment recommendations for traumatic dislocation injuries are lacking as the injury is rare. Decisive factors include the child's age, and extent of injury. Minor injuries are treated with immobilization for 3 to 6 weeks and reexamination. Resolution of symptoms and signs allows return to normal activities. Persistent pain warrants further clinical and radiographic evaluation. Overt ligamentous injuries with static instability and malalignment require accurate diagnosis and appropriate treatment. A complete ligament tear (e.g., an adolescent with a scapholunate injury) is treated according to principles similar to those for adults. Open reduction, anatomic reduction, and ligament repair are the basic tenets of treatment.

A child or adolescent with ligamentous laxity and persistent activity-related[177] pain is especially difficult to treat. Discriminating focal from nonfocal wrist pathology is imperative. Radiographs and MRI scans often are normal. Most of these children respond to therapeutic strengthening. Protective sports–specific wrist guards or taping may be appropriate (Fig. 7-88). A small subset of children has unresolved pain caused by chondral injuries or ligamentous tears that require arthroscopic treatment.[91]

ORIF of Fractures of the Scaphoid

Preoperative Planning

✔ ORIF of Fractures of the Scaphoid: PREOPERATIVE PLANNING CHECKLIST	
OR table	☐ Hand table, radiolucent preferable
Position	☐ Supine. A skilled wrist arthroscopic may perform an arthroscopic assisted reduction and fixation in which case a tower or wrist distraction system may be utilized
Fluoroscopy	☐ Mini-fluoroscopy in the small child or C-arm in adult-sized limbs
Equipment	☐ Headless conical or compression screw, K-wires
Tourniquet	☐ Nonsterile

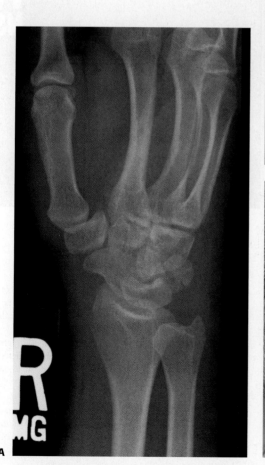

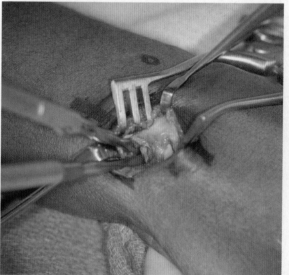

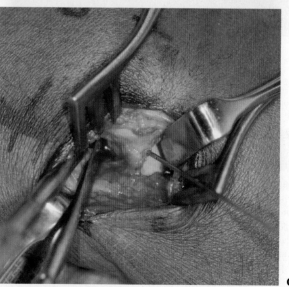

Figure 7-87. A: A 16-year-old male sustained a large dorsal hamate fracture from punching a wall. **B–E:** Dorsal exposure of fragment with cannulated headless screw fixation.

(continues)

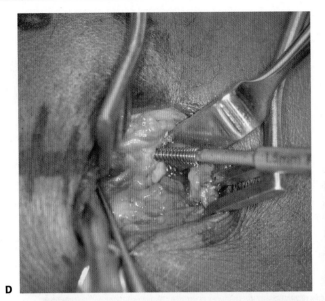

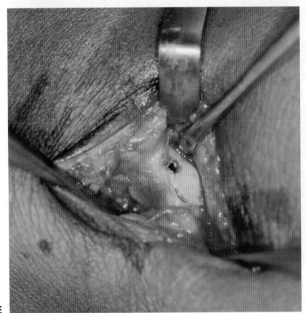

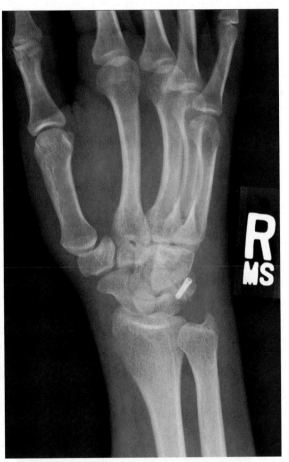

Figure 7-87. (*Continued*) **F:** Postoperative radiographs of healed fracture.

Technique

✔ ORIF of Fractures of the Scaphoid:
KEY SURGICAL STEPS

Dorsal Approach

❑ Small incision and spread soft tissue to avoid dorsal radial sensory nerve and extensor pollicis longus during pin or screw placement

❑ Flex the wrist to identify screw starting point on the scaphoid, adjacent to scapholunate ligament (need 90 degrees or greater for dorsal percutaneous screw placement)

❑ Aim guidewire down the thumb axis

❑ Verify guidewire placement in 1:1 position

❑ Follow standard sequence of steps to insert headless screw

Volar Approach

❑ Hockey stick incision over flexor carpi radialis and scaphoid tubercle

❑ Open sheath of flexor carpi radialis, protect radial artery, incision between the radiocapitate and radiotriquetral palmar radiocarpal ligaments

❑ Expose fracture and clear of fibrous debris or loose fragments

❑ Aim guidewire toward Lister's tubercle; use angiocatheter as guide

❑ Place pins or screws distal to proximal angled volar to dorsal

Joysticks

❑ In fractures with substantial dorsal intercalated segmental instability (DISI), consider reducing the lunate and the transradial lunate pinning with K-wire to hold the lunate and the proximal pole in neutral during fixation

❑ If fixation is stable, this K-wire can be removed

❑ If fixation is less than ideal, maintain K-wire for a few weeks

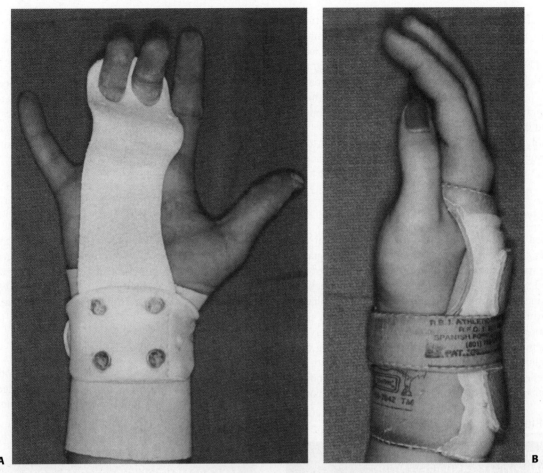

Figure 7-88. Wrist guards for gymnastics. **A:** The "lion's paw" protector used mainly for the vault. **B:** Hand and wrist protectors used primarily for the uneven parallel bars.

Authors' Preferred Treatment for Fractures of the Carpal Bones (Algorithm 7-5)

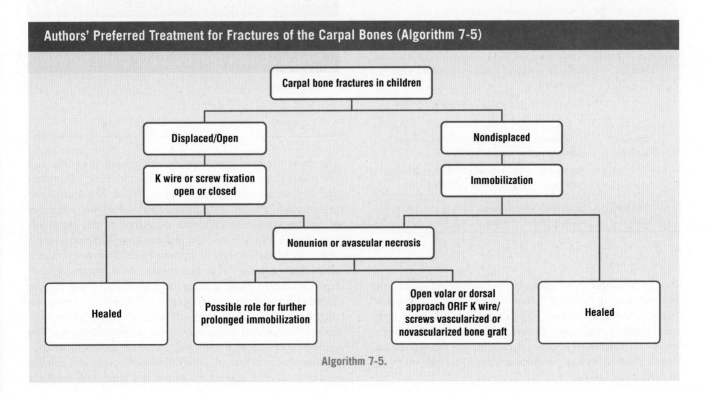

Algorithm 7-5.

Almost all nondisplaced scaphoid fractures are treated with cast immobilization. The preferred immobilization is a long-arm thumb spica cast for the initial 4 to 6 weeks, followed by a short-arm cast until clinical and radiographic union. Radiographs are obtained in the first 7 to 10 days to ensure alignment and then monthly until union. If there is doubt regarding anatomic alignment or subsequent union, a scaphoid CT scan is obtained.

Proximal pole fractures are at high risk for osteonecrosis and nonunion. Percutaneous or mini-open screw fixation is preferred to stabilize the fracture and promote union. Ideally, this is a dorsal proximal to distal screw placement to compress the fracture site and tighten the scapholunate ligament.

Indications for open reduction and fracture fixation are a waist fracture with more than 1 mm of displacement or an angular deformity of more than 10 degrees. Greater arc injuries, such as transscaphoid perilunate injuries, require operative management. Fractures of the middle and distal thirds are exposed through a volar approach. Proximal third fractures are exposed through a dorsal approach.[112]

Postoperative Care and Rehabilitation

Nondisplaced fractures are treated with immobilization until union. After the cast is removed, a home therapy program is started. Formal therapy usually is not necessary. Displaced fractures treated with ORIF require variable periods of immobilization. Fixation with K-wires necessitates prolonged immobilization and may involve formal therapy for the recovery of motion. Stable screw fixation allows early motion 10 to 14 days after surgery with a short-arm thumb spica splint worn for protection during vigorous activity until union. However, many adolescents will not wear the splint dependably and require longer periods of nonremovable immobilization to prevent loss of screw fixation and nonunion.

Potential Pitfalls and Preventive Measures

Fractures of the Carpal Bones:
POTENTIAL PITFALLS AND PREVENTIONS

Pitfall	Prevention
• Nonunion	• Early diagnosis and treatment
	• Long-arm thumb spica nonremovable immobilization
	• Identify displaced fractures
• Malunion	• Early recognition of lunate extension and DISI deformity
	• Three-dimensional advanced imaging, such as CT scan
• Avascular necrosis	• Early treatment of high-risk fractures, such as proximal pole of the scaphoid
	• Knowledge of the vascular supply to each carpal bone to avoid injury during dissection
• Intercarpal instability	• Static and dynamic examination of entire wrist to identify greater or lesser arc injuries

Scaphoid Fractures

Prompt treatment of a nondisplaced scaphoid fracture allows healing in most patients.[170] Nondisplaced pediatric scaphoid fractures have a better than 95% healing rate. A delay in treatment impedes healing and increases the possibility of displacement.[27,68,73] Displaced fractures require prompt recognition and open reduction because adequate reduction and fixation results in predictable union.[131]

Capitate Fractures

The rarity of this injury prevents broad generalizations. Early recognition and appropriate treatment lead to an acceptable outcome. Nonunion is rare and requires bone grafting (Fig. 7-77).[72] Despite the considerable rotation of the proximal pole in displaced fractures, osteonecrosis of the capitate is rare.

Triquetral Fractures

Avulsion fractures are relatively minor injuries. Treatment results in expedient and complete recovery. Body fractures associated with perilunate injuries have a guarded prognosis depending on the extent of concomitant injuries and treatment employed.

MANAGEMENT OF EXPECTED ADVERSE OUTCOMES AND UNEXPECTED COMPLICATIONS OF SCAPHOID FRACTURES

Scaphoid Fractures:
COMMON ADVERSE OUTCOMES AND COMPLICATIONS

- Nonunion
- Malunion
- Avascular necrosis
- Intercarpal instability

The most common complications are missed diagnosis and late presentation.[131] Scaphoid nonunions do occur in children and adolescents with the incidence as 20% to 25% due to late presentation.[49,69,152,165] Late presentation occurs for a number of reasons, including children's reluctance to tell their parents about a mechanism of injury, moderate symptoms seemingly not severe enough to warrant medical attention, and a child's fear of losing his or her position on a sporting team.[56] Open reduction, bone grafting, and internal fixation are the standard procedures for treatment of scaphoid nonunions (Fig. 7-89).[4,52,56,152] The approach varies according to the location of fracture and vascularity of the fracture fragments. The principles of operative scaphoid nonunion treatment in children are similar to those in adults. Persistent scaphoid nonunion results in altered kinematics within the wrist and produces

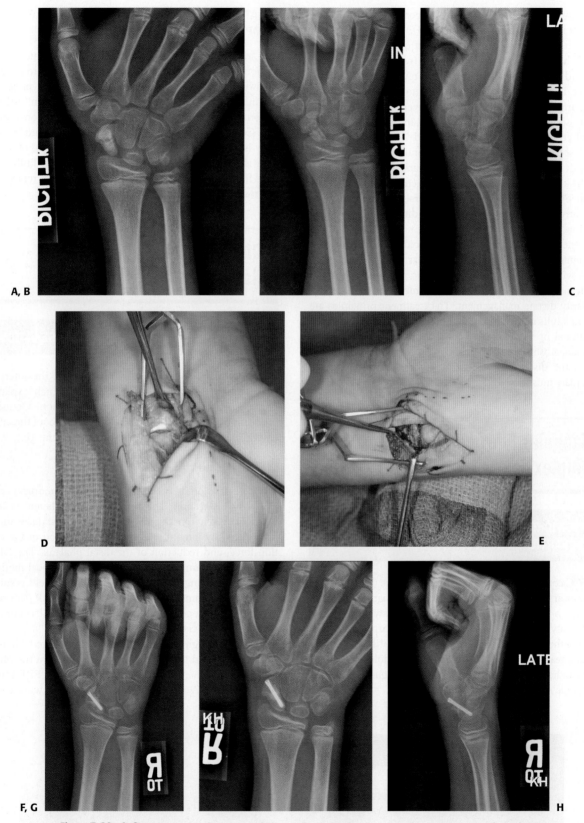

Figure 7-89. A–C: Radiographs of a 12-year-old boy with scaphoid nonunion and lunate extension through the fracture seen on the lateral view. **D:** Volar approach through the wrist to correct the mild humpback and flexion deformity. **E:** Iliac crest bone graft in place and headless screw fixation. **F–H:** Final radiographs after integration of graft, demonstrating correction of flexion deformity seen by lunate position on lateral. (Courtesy of Shriners Hospitals for Children, Philadelphia, PA.)

degenerative changes over time.[66,77] The goal is to obtain union to prevent long-term arthrosis (Video 7-4).

The long-term outcomes of treatment of nonunions of the scaphoid have been reported following treatment using both screws and K-wires. Masquijo and Willis reviewed 23 children, mean age 15.1 years old with scaphoid nonunions after bone grafting and fixation with a follow-up over 5 years. Scaphoid outcome scores were excellent in 66% and good in 33%.[164] Reigstad et al.[134] most recently reported 7-year outcomes in 11 adolescents with scaphoid waist nonunions treated with bone graft and K-wire fixation only. Range of motion, grip strength, key pinch strength, and subjective outcome scores were all excellent. No evidence of persistent nonunion or degenerative changes were evident on radiographs or from CT evaluation.

Osteonecrosis may result from a scaphoid fracture. The proximal fragment is more prone to avascular changes. Avascular changes within the proximal fragment do not preclude union after internal fixation. The size of the fragment and the extent of avascularity dictate management. The treatment principles are similar in adults and children. Options to obtain union include conventional or vascularized bone grafting.[58] With nonunion and osteonecrosis of the proximal pole, vascularized bone grafting from the distal radius has been successful, although the growth plate must be avoided.[58,161]

Triangular Fibrocartilage Complex Tears in Children

CLASSIFICATION OF TRIANGULAR FIBROCARTILAGE COMPLEX TEARS

The TFCC consists of the triangular fibrocartilage (TFC) and the volar ulnocarpal ligaments. The TFC spans the sigmoid notch of the radius to the fovea at the base of the ulnar styloid and provides stability to the distal radioulnar and ulnocarpal joints. The location of the tear determines the classification of TFCC tears.[105] Peripheral tears (type B) are most common in adolescents. Tears from the radial insertion (type D) are next in frequency, whereas central (type A) and volar (type C) tears are rare.[2,33]

TREATMENT OF TRIANGULAR FIBROCARTILAGE COMPLEX TEARS

The initial approach to adolescents with chronic wrist pain without instability incorporates rest until symptoms subside, followed by a strengthening program. If pain persists after regaining symmetric pinch and grip strength, then further evaluation is appropriate. If clinical examination is consistent with a TFCC tear or ulnar–carpal impaction, MRI and/or arthroscopy is appropriate. A partial TFCC tear or carpal chondromalacia is treated with arthroscopic debridement. Full-thickness tears from the fovea (type IB) require peripheral repair, usually arthroscopically or mini-open, to restore stability.

Dislocations of the Hand and Carpus

DISLOCATIONS OF THE INTERPHALANGEAL JOINTS

In children, the soft tissue stabilizers about the interphalangeal joints are stronger than the physis, which explains the propensity for fracture rather than dislocation. Occasionally, dislocations and fracture–dislocations occur about the interphalangeal and MCP joints, especially in adolescents (Fig. 7-90).

DISTAL INTERPHALANGEAL JOINT

A hyperextension or lateral force may result in dorsal or lateral DIP joint dislocation. The collateral ligaments and volar plate typically detach from the middle phalanx. Most dislocations can be reduced by longitudinal traction, recreation of the dislocation force, and reduction of the distal phalanx. The DIP joint reduction and congruity are confirmed by clinical motion and radiographs. Splinting of DIP joint for 2 to 3 weeks is sufficient, followed by a home program that focuses on DIP joint motion.

Irreducible or complex dislocations of the DIP occur primarily in adults but can occur in pediatric patients.[46,101,161,168] Open reduction through a dorsal approach is required for removal of the interposed tissue. The volar plate is often the offending agent, though the collateral ligaments and the FDP can block reduction.[46,168] A stable DIP joint is treated with DIP joint

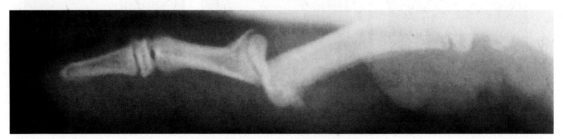

Figure 7-90. A dorsal dislocation of the PIP joint with an S-H type II fracture of the middle phalanx in a 15-year-old boy.

immobilization for 3 to 4 weeks. An unstable DIP joint requires pin fixation for 3 to 4 weeks.

PROXIMAL INTERPHALANGEAL JOINT

Dislocation of the PIP joint may occur in a variety of directions. Dorsal dislocations are the most common, though lateral and volar dislocations also occur. The differential diagnosis includes adjacent bony and tendon injuries.[110] Radiographs are required to assess the physis and to confirm joint alignment. The postreduction lateral radiograph must confirm concentric joint reduction. Persistent joint subluxation is unacceptable and detected by a slight offset between the proximal and middle phalanges along with a dorsal V-shaped space instead of smooth articular congruity.

Dorsal Proximal Interphalangeal Joint Dislocations

The middle phalanx is displaced dorsal to the proximal phalanx. The collateral ligaments and volar plate are disrupted. Many dorsal dislocations are probably joint subluxations that retain some of the collateral ligament or volar plate integrity. Some subluxations are reduced by the patient or trainer on the field and never receive medical evaluation.

Unreduced dorsal dislocations cause pain and obvious deformity. If necessary, anesthesia can usually be accomplished with a digital block. The dislocation is reduced with longitudinal traction, hyperextension, and palmar translation of the middle phalanx onto the proximal phalanx. The quality of the reduction and the stability of the joint must be assessed. Asking the patient to flex and extend the digit evaluates active motion. Most dislocations are stable throughout the normal range of motion, and radiographs confirm a concentric reduction. A stable joint requires a brief period (3 to 5 days) of splinting for comfort, followed by range of motion and buddy tape. Immediate motion may be started, though pain often prohibits movement and exacerbates swelling. Prolonged immobilization leads to PIP joint stiffness.

An unstable reduction tends to subluxate or dislocate during PIP joint extension. The radiographs must be scrutinized for subtle dorsal subluxation and concomitant fracture of the middle phalangeal base. Unstable PIP joint dislocations, with or without small fractures of the middle phalangeal base, have a stable arc of motion that must be defined. This stable arc is typically from full flexion to about 30 degrees of flexion. This arc is used to determine the confines of extension block splinting.[150] A short-arm cast is applied with an aluminum outrigger that positions the MCP joint in flexion and the PIP joint in 10 degrees less than the maximal extension that leads to joint

subluxation. Reduction is verified by lateral radiographs. The aluminum splint is modified every 7 to 10 days to increase PIP joint extension by 10 degrees. A lateral view or dynamic fluoroscopy is used to confirm concentric reduction. This process is continued over 4 to 5 weeks. The cast and splint are then discontinued and a home therapy program is instituted.

Extremely unstable injuries that dislocate in more than 30 degrees of flexion almost always involve considerable fracture of the middle phalanx. These injuries are regarded as pilon fractures or intra-articular fracture–dislocations. Treatment presents a management dilemma as discussed earlier.[122] Options range from open reduction to dynamic traction. Long-term subluxation, stiffness, and arthrosis are concerns. Aggressive surgical care has the best chance for, but does not guarantee, a good outcome.

Volar Proximal Interphalangeal Joint Dislocations

Volar PIP joint dislocations are uncommon in children,[23,81] and the diagnosis is often delayed.[23] Interposition of soft tissues or bony fragments can render the dislocation irreducible.[159] The proximal phalangeal head may herniate between the lateral band and the central tendon. Long-term results are often suboptimal if anatomic alignment is not restored. This outcome may be related to a delay in treatment or the degree of soft tissue involvement, especially the central slip.

Volar dislocations require closed or open reduction. Reducible dislocations are treated with 4 weeks of full-time PIP joint extension splinting to promote healing of the central slip.[166,178] Radiographs are necessary to confirm concentric reduction. An unstable reduction may require temporary pin fixation across the PIP joint. Irreducible dislocations require open reduction through a dorsal approach to extricate any interposed tissue. The central slip can be repaired to the middle phalanx. Postoperative immobilization consists of 4 weeks of full-time PIP joint extension splinting.

Lateral Proximal Interphalangeal Joint Dislocations

Pure lateral dislocations are uncommon, though dorsal dislocations may have a lateral component.[180] An isolated lateral dislocation represents severe disruption of the collateral ligament complex. The injury represents a spectrum of damage, beginning with the proper and accessory collateral ligaments and culminating in volar plate disruption.[80] Bony avulsion fragments may accompany the ligamentous failure. Closed reduction is uniformly successful. A brief period (5 to 7 days) of immobilization followed by buddy tape to protect the healing collateral ligament complex is the customary treatment.

Authors' Preferred Treatment of Proximal Interphalangeal Joint Dislocations (Algorithm 7-6)

The initial treatment of almost all PIP dislocations is an attempt at closed reduction followed by a stability assessment. If stable, a brief period of immobilization lessens pain and swelling. Subsequent mobilization prevents PIP joint stiffness.

Dorsal Dislocation

A stable reduction is treated with brief immobilization followed by early motion. An unstable reduction that can be held reduced in more than 30 to 40 degrees of flexion is

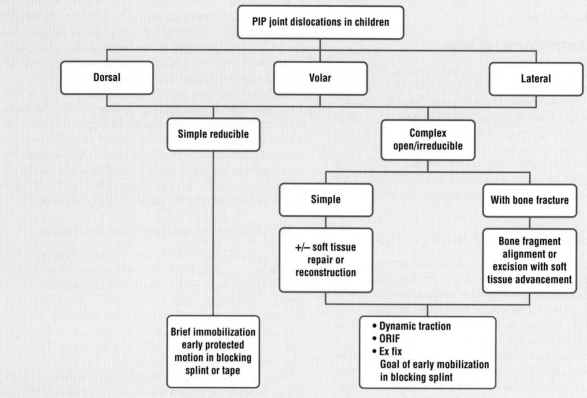

Algorithm 7-6.

treated with extension block splinting. Extremely unstable fracture–dislocations require open treatment, external fixation, or dynamic traction depending on the size of the fracture fragments.

Volar Dislocation

A stable congruent reduction is treated with immobilization for 4 weeks with the PIP joint in extension. Unstable reductions are treated with percutaneous pin fixation to maintain a concentric reduction. Irreducible dislocations require open reduction with repair of the central slip.

Lateral Dislocations

Closed reduction is usually obtainable, followed by a brief period of immobilization. Irreducible dislocations require open reduction with or without collateral ligament repair.

DISLOCATIONS OF THE METACARPOPHALANGEAL JOINT

The MCP joint is an uncommon site for dislocation in the child's hand.[125,155] The dislocation may involve a finger or thumb. The gamekeeper's or skier's thumb can be considered a subset of subluxation or dislocation.

DORSAL METACARPOPHALANGEAL JOINT

The most frequent dislocation of the MCP joint is dorsal dislocation of the index digit or thumb (Fig. 7-91), which results from a hyperextension force that ruptures the volar plate. The proximal phalanx is displaced dorsal to the metacarpal head. The diagnosis is readily apparent because the digit is shortened, supinated, and deviated in an ulnar direction. The interphalangeal joints are slightly flexed because of the digital flexor tendon tension. The volar skin is taut over the prominent metacarpal head.

Dislocations of the MCP joint are classified as simple or complex. Complex dislocations are irreducible because of volar plate interposition in the joint. The injury can be open with the metacarpal head penetrating the palmar skin (Fig. 7-92). Simple dislocations are in a position of hyperextension on radiographs. Irreducible dislocations have bayonet apposition of the proximal phalanx dorsal to the metacarpal head. The sesamoid bone(s) of the index finger or thumb may be seen within the joint. The position of the sesamoid bones is indicative of the site of the volar plate.[181] The most common irreducible dislocation is at the index MCP joint. Additional structures may impede reduction. There often is an impacted metacarpal head articular fracture. The metacarpal head becomes "picture-framed" by the flexor tendon on the ulnar side and the lumbrical on the radial side. The superficial transverse metacarpal ligament and the natatory ligaments can also entrap the metacarpal neck. The collar of the restraining tissue is tightened by longitudinal traction, and this reduction maneuver may convert a dislocation from reducible to irreducible.

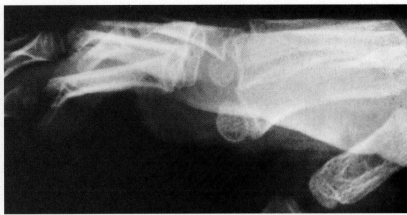

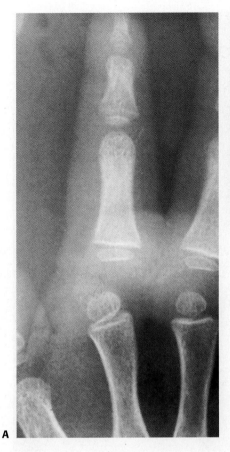

Figure 7-91. **A:** A 3-year-old boy with a complete complex dislocation of the index finger metacarpal joint. **B:** Note the parallelism in this lateral view. Open reduction was done through a volar approach.

Most simple dislocations can be reduced with distraction and volar manipulation of the proximal phalanx over the metacarpal head. Avoidance of hyperextension during reduction is important to prevent conversion of a simple to a complex dislocation. These reductions are usually stable. Reduction of a complex dislocation is problematic at best and usually not possible. The maneuver involves further hyperextension of the joint and palmar translation of the proximal phalanx. The goal

is to extricate the volar plate with the proximal phalanx during palmar translation. Intra-articular infiltration of anesthetic fluid may assist reduction through joint distention and "floating" of the volar plate from its displaced position. The success rate for conversion of an irreducible dislocation to a reducible dislocation is low; open reduction is necessary in almost all patients.

Open Reduction

> ✔ **Open Reduction of Dorsal Metacarpophalangeal Joint Dislocations:**
> KEY SURGICAL STEPS
>
> ❑ Volar or dorsal approach: Volar more at risk of NV injury; dorsal allows visualization of associated metacarpal head fracture if present. Both effective
> ❑ Protect neurovascular structures
> ❑ Remove interposed soft tissue, usually volar plate
> ❑ Pin fractures or ORIF if present
> ❑ Early motion after brief postoperative immobilization

Open reduction can be accomplished through a volar or dorsal approach. The volar approach provides excellent exposure of the metacarpal head and the incarcerated structures.[88,125,155] However, the digital nerves are draped over the articular surface of the metacarpal head and precariously close to the skin. A deep skin incision can cut these nerves. The skin is gently incised and soft tissue is dissected. The first annular pulley is incised. The metacarpal head is extricated from between the flexor tendon and the lumbrical.

Figure 7-92. A 17-year-old male after fall from height, with open index and middle finger dorsal dislocations. (Courtesy of Joshua Ratner, MD.)

The joint is evaluated for interposed structures, such as the volar plate, and then reduced under direct observation.

The dorsal approach offers a less extensive exposure but avoids the risk of digital nerve injury. Through a dorsal incision, the extensor tendon is longitudinally split over the MCP joint. A transverse or longitudinal capsulotomy is made if the injury has not torn the capsule. A Freer elevator is placed within the joint to clear it of any interposed tissue. Often, the interposed volar plate needs to be split longitudinally to reduce the joint. If the flexor tendon is wrapped around the metacarpal, the Freer is used to extricate the metacarpal head. If there is an impacted or displaced intra-articular metacarpal head fracture, it can be reduced and stabilized through this approach.

Regardless of the approach used, early motion as appropriate is best to optimize outcome.[88] The postoperative regimen is a 3- to 5-day immobilization period, followed by active motion. Rarely, a dorsal blocking splint is needed to prevent hyperextension that may foster repeat dislocation.

Dorsal dislocations of the other fingers are uncommon (Fig. 7-93).[154] Lateral fracture–dislocations are often S-H III fractures involving the base of the proximal phalanx (Fig. 7-94) and require ORIF of the displaced physeal fracture.

NEGLECTED METACARPOPHALANGEAL JOINT DISLOCATIONS

Early treatment is preferred for MCP joint dislocations, but delay of a few months may still result in an acceptable outcome. A delay of more than 6 months is associated with joint degeneration and a less predictable result. Late reduction may require a combined dorsal and volar approach for adequate exposure.[57] Collateral ligament release and temporary MCP joint pin fixation may be necessary.

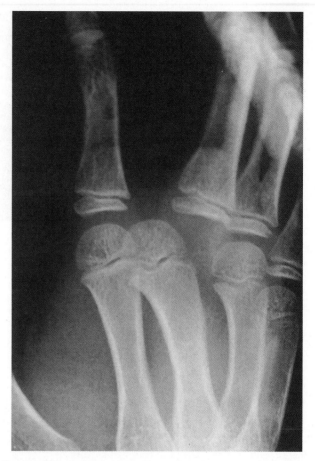

Figure 7-93. A rare dorsal dislocation of the long finger that was irreducible by closed means. A dorsal approach permitted inspection of the joint and extrication of the volar plate.

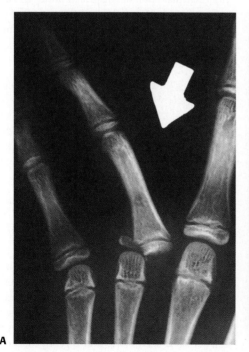
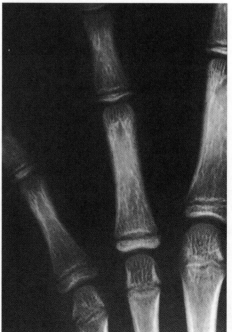

Figure 7-94. A: A 9-year-old girl sustained this radial fracture–dislocation of the middle fingers. **B:** Closed reduction restored joint and fracture alignment.

DORSAL DISLOCATION OF THE THUMB RAY

Thumb MCP joint dislocations are similar to those of the fingers, and hyperextension is the common mechanism. Thumb dislocations are classified according to the integrity and position of the volar plate, the status of the collateral ligaments, and the relative position of the metacarpal and proximal phalanx. The components of the classification are incomplete dislocation, simple complete dislocation, and complex complete dislocation (Fig. 7-95).

INCOMPLETE THUMB METACARPOPHALANGEAL JOINT DISLOCATION

An incomplete dislocation implies rupture of the volar plate with partial preservation of the collateral ligament integrity. The proximal phalanx perches on the dorsum of the metacarpal. Closed reduction is easily accomplished, and a 3-week course of immobilization is adequate. Return to sports requires protection for an additional 3 weeks.

SIMPLE COMPLETE THUMB METACARPOPHALANGEAL DISLOCATION

A simple complete dislocation implies volar plate and collateral ligament disruption. The proximal phalanx is displaced in a dorsal direction and is angulated 90 degrees to the long axis of the thumb metacarpal. Many of these dislocations can be reduced by closed means, though unnecessary longitudinal traction may convert a reducible condition into an irreducible situation (Fig. 7-96).[88] A successful reduction requires thumb spica immobilization for 3 to 4 weeks to allow healing of the volar plate and collateral ligaments.

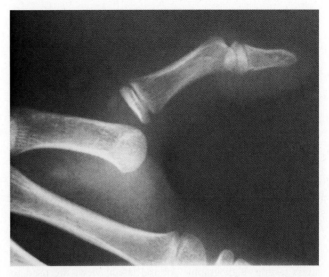

Figure 7-96. A 9-year-old boy with a complete simple dorsal dislocation of the thumb MCP joint.

COMPLEX COMPLETE THUMB METACARPOPHALANGEAL JOINT DISLOCATION

A complete or irreducible dislocation is the most severe form of this injury. The long axes of both the proximal phalanx and metacarpal are often parallel. Open reduction is usually required to extricate the volar plate from within the joint (Fig. 7-97).[53] A dorsal or volar approach is suitable and raises concerns similar to those for irreducible index MCP joint dislocations discussed above.[121]

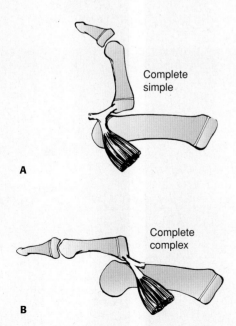

Figure 7-95. Simple and complex dorsal dislocations of the thumb MCP joint. Simple dislocations (**A**) are in extension and reducible. Complex dislocations (**B**) are in bayonet apposition and are irreducible because of the interposed volar plate.

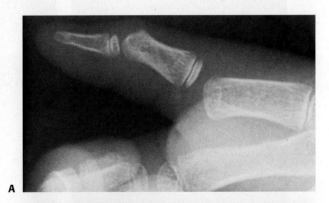

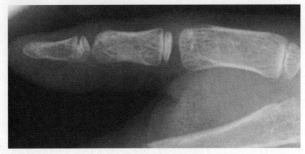

Figure 7-97. A: Irreducible dorsal MCP dislocation in a 7-year-old boy. **B:** After open reduction through a volar incision.

THUMB METACARPOPHALANGEAL ULNAR COLLATERAL LIGAMENT INJURY (GAMEKEEPER'S THUMB)

Injuries of the UCL are less prevalent in children than in adults. Forced abduction stress at a child's thumb MCP joint results in four types of injuries: (1) a simple sprain of the UCL, (2) a rupture or avulsion of the insertion or origin of the ligament, (3) an S-H I or II fracture of the proximal physis, or (4) an S-H III avulsion fracture that involves one-fourth to one-third of the epiphysis of the proximal phalanx (Figs. 7-98 and 7-99).[42,103]

The injury is most common in preadolescents and adolescents. A history of trauma is customary, especially involving sports. The thumb is swollen about the MCP joint with ecchymosis, and tenderness to palpation is well localized over the UCL. Pain is exacerbated by abduction stress. A complete rupture or displaced fracture lacks a discrete end point during stress testing. Radiographic AP and lateral views are used to diagnose and delineate fracture configuration. Stress views may be needed if the diagnosis is questionable. An MRI scan can be used to evaluate ligament disruption in complicated injuries, although rarely necessary.

Cast immobilization for 4 to 6 weeks is adequate for simple sprains, incomplete injuries, and nondisplaced fractures.

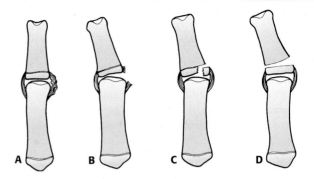

Figure 7-98. Ulnar instability of the thumb metacarpal joint. **A:** Simple sprain. **B:** Rupture of the ligament. **C:** Avulsion fracture (S-H type III). **D:** Pseudo-gamekeeper's injury resulting from an S-H type I or II fracture of the proximal phalanx.

A major concern is displacement of the ligament or fracture fragment outside the adductor aponeurosis known as a "Stener's lesion," which prohibits healing.[121,156] Complete ruptures, "Stener's lesion," or displaced fractures usually require operative intervention. Distal insertion avulsion without bony fracture will require suture anchor fixation for repair (Fig. 7-100).

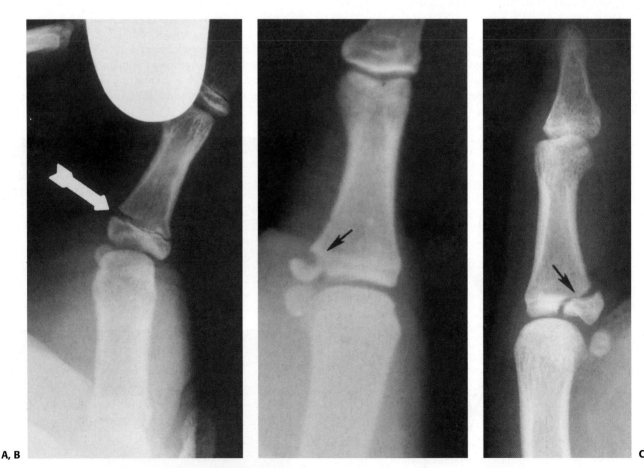

Figure 7-99. Spectrum of UCL injuries of the thumb. **A, B:** On stress examination, a widening of the physis is seen. Varying sizes of fragments (**B, C**) may be associated with UCL avulsion fractures (*arrows*). The size of the fragment is important with respect to the congruity of the MCP joint.

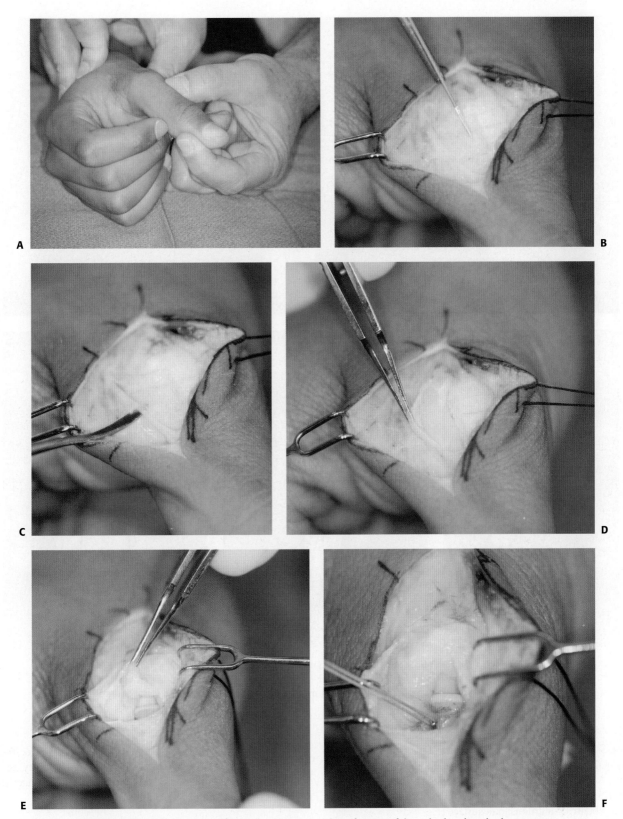

Figure 7-100. A: A 15-year-old boy with a UCL tear without fracture of the right thumb and valgus instability on stress testing. **B:** Exposure through an incision of the skin. **C:** Identification of the dorsal sensory nerve. **D, E:** Opening of the adductor aponeurosis and capsule; mobilization of the torn UCL. **F:** Placement of the bone anchor.

(*continues*)

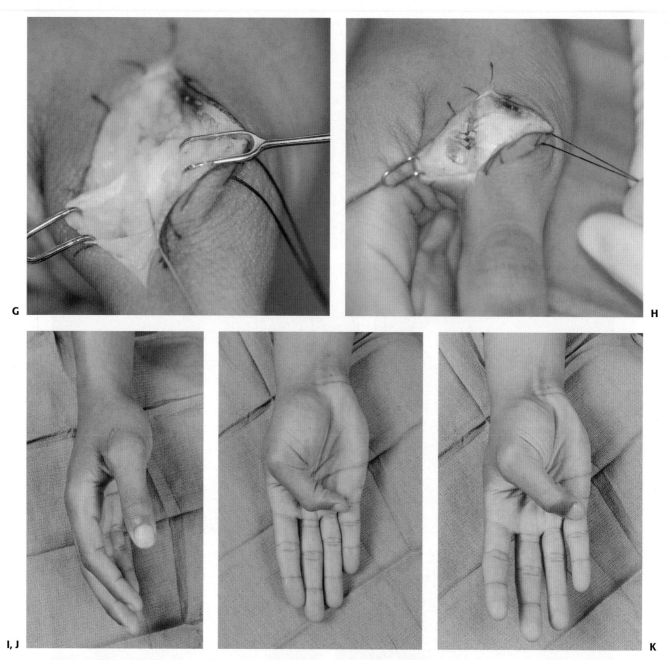

Figure 7-100. *(Continued)* **G:** Suture from the anchor passed through the ligament in a modified Kessler or similarly strong grasp technique. Tied in a figure-of-eight fashion. **H:** Knot buried under repair of the aponeurosis. **I–K:** Restoration of joint stability and maintenance of motion postoperatively. (Courtesy of Shriners Hospitals for Children, Philadelphia, PA.)

An S-H III fracture of the ulnar corner of the epiphysis of the proximal phalanx is the most common childhood gamekeeper's injury. A displaced fracture (fragment rotated or displaced more than 1.5 mm) requires ORIF to restore the integrity of the UCL and to obtain a congruous joint surface (Fig. 7-39).

Chronic UCL injuries are more difficult to manage. Treatment depends on the length of time since original injury, age of the patient, and current level of function. Options range from UCL reconstruction to MCP joint fusion.[174]

Authors' Preferred Treatment of Metacarpophalangeal Joint Dislocation (Algorithm 7-7)

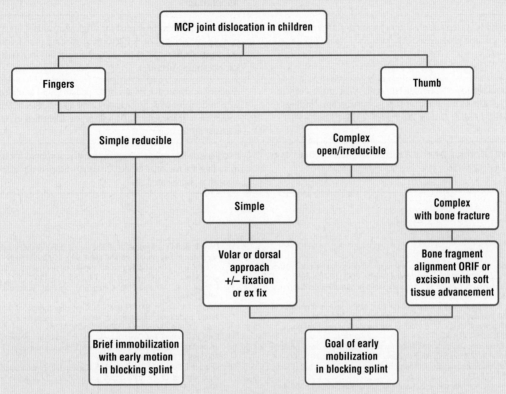

Algorithm 7-7.

The initial treatment for simple dislocations is closed reduction. Irreducible dislocations require open reduction. A dorsal or volar approach is used with removal of any interposed structure(s). The advantages and disadvantages of both approaches were discussed previously. Postoperative immobilization is used for 7 to 10 days, followed by active motion with splint protection.

Injuries of the UCL of the thumb are treated according to stability and displacement. Stable ligamentous injuries or minimally displaced fractures are treated with cast immobilization with reduced stress on fracture or ligament injury. Unstable complete ligamentous injuries or displaced fractures are treated with open reduction.

Annotated References

Reference	Annotation
Abzug JM, Dua K, Bauer AS, et al. Pediatric phalanx fractures. *J Am Acad Orthop Surg.* 2016;24(11):e174–e183.	Recent review articles that discuss pediatric phalanx fractures with an emphasis on diagnosis and treatment.
Gholson JJ, Bae DS, Zurakowski D, et al. Scaphoid fractures in children and adolescents: contemporary injury patterns and factors influencing time to union. *J Bone Joint Surg Am.* 2011;93(13):1210–1219.	Update on scaphoid fracture in children that notes changing trends in fracture patterns. Reconfirms that nonoperative treatment will heal nondisplaced fractures, although casting may be prolonged. Highlights the factors that directly affect treatment, healing, and outcome.
Godfrey J, Cornwall R. Pediatric metacarpal fractures. *Instr Course Lect.* 2017;66:437–445.	Review article of pediatric metacarpal fractures. Finger and thumb metacarpal fractures are discussed with an emphasis on clinical evaluation and management.

Annotated References

Reference	Annotation
Matzon JL, Cornwall R. A stepwise algorithm for surgical treatment of type II displaced pediatric phalangeal neck fractures. *J Hand Surg Am*. 2014;39(3):467–473.	Stepwise algorithm presented for surgical treatment of type II displaced pediatric phalangeal neck fractures. Algorithm produced 92% good to excellent results while minimizing the need for open reduction even in late-presenting fractures.
Ramavath AL, Unnikrishnan PN, George HL, et al. Wrist arthroscopy in children and adolescent with chronic wrist pain: arthroscopic findings compared with MRI. *J Pediatr Orthop*. 2017;37(5):e321–e325.	Authors' retrospective review of 32 pediatric and adolescent patients who underwent wrist arthroscopy after failing at least 4 months of conservative management. Pathology was identified in 32 of the 33 wrists at arthroscopy.
Ting B, Sesko Bauer A, Abzug JM, et al. Pediatric scaphoid fractures. *Instr Course Lect*. 2017;66:429–436.	Excellent review article covering pediatric scaphoid fractures. Diagnosis including the use of advanced imaging studies is discussed. Treatment algorithm is presented.

REFERENCES

1. Adolfsson L, Lindau T, Arner M. Acutrak screw fixation versus cast immobilization for undisplaced scaphoid waist fractures. *J Hand Surg Br*. 2001;26:192–195.
2. Aggarwal AK, Sangwan SS, Siwach RC. Transscaphoid perilunate dislocation in a child. *Contemp Orthop*. 1993;26:172–174.
3. Al-Qattan MM. Juxta-epiphyseal fractures of the base of the proximal phalanx of the fingers in children and adolescents. *J Hand Surg Br*. 2002;27:24–30.
4. Al-Qattan MM, Hashem F, Helmi A. Irreducible tuft fractures of the distal phalanx. *J Hand Surg Br*. 2003;28(1):18–20.
5. Al-Qattan MM. Extra-articular transverse fractures of the base of the distal phalanx (Seymour's fracture) in children and adults. *J Hand Surg Br*. 2001;26:201–206.
6. Anderson WJ. Simultaneous fracture of the scaphoid and capitate in a child. *J Hand Surg Am*. 1987;12:271–273.
7. Barton NJ. Fractures of the phalanges of the hand in children. *Hand*. 1979;11:134–143.
8. Beatty E, Light TR, Belsole RJ, et al. Wrist and hand skeletal injuries in children. *Hand Clin*. 1990;6(4):723–738.
9. Bhende MS, Dandrea LA, Davis HW. Hand injuries in children presenting to a pediatric emergency department. *Ann Emerg Med*. 1993;22:1519–1523.
10. Blitzer CM, Johnson RJ, Ettlinger CF, et al. Downhill skiing injuries in children. *Am J Sports Med*. 1984;12(2):142–147.
11. Bogumill GP. A morphologic study of the relationship of collateral ligaments to growth plates in the digits. *J Hand Surg Am*. 1983;8:74–79.
12. Bohart PG, Gelberman RH, Vandell RF, et al. Complex dislocations of the metacarpophalangeal joint. *Clin Orthop Relat Res*. 1982;(164):208–210.
13. Bond CD, Shin AY, McBride MT, et al. Percutaneous screw fixation or cast immobilization for nondisplaced scaphoid fractures. *J Bone Joint Surg Am*. 2001;83(4):483–488.
14. Brighton CT. Clinical problems in epiphyseal plate growth and development. *Instr Course Lect*. 1974;3:105–122.
15. Brydie A, Raby N. Early MRI in the management of clinical scaphoid fracture. *Br J Radiol*. 2003;76:296–300.
16. Buchler U, McCollam SM, Oppikofer C. Comminuted fractures of the basilar joint of the thumb: combined treatment by external fixation, limited internal fixation, and bone grafting. *J Hand Surg Am*. 1991;16(3):556–560.
17. Burge P. Closed cast treatment of scaphoid fractures. *Hand Clin*. 2001;17:541–552.
18. Campbell RM Jr. Operative treatment of fractures and dislocations of the hand and wrist region in children. *Orthop Clin North Am*. 1990;21:217–243.
19. Carr D, Johnson RJ, Pope MH. Upper extremity injuries in skiing. *Am J Sports Med*. 1981;12:142–147.
20. Cerezal L, del Pinal F, Abascal F, et al. Imaging findings in ulnar-sided wrist impaction syndromes. *Radiographics*. 2002;22(1):105–121.
21. Christodoulou AG, Colton CL. Scaphoid fractures in children. *J Pediatr Orthop*. 1986;6:37–39.
22. Cockshott WP. Distal avulsion fractures of the scaphoid. *Br J Radiol*. 1980;53:1037–1040.
23. Compson JP. Transcarpal injuries associated with distal radial fractures in children: a series of three cases. *J Hand Surg Br*. 1992;17:311–314.
24. Cook PA, Yu JS, Wiand W, et al. Suspected scaphoid fractures in skeletally immature patients: application of MRI. *J Comput Assist Tomogr*. 1997;21(4):511–515.
25. Cornwall R, Waters PM. Remodeling of phalangeal neck fracture malunions in children: case report. *J Hand Surg Am*. 2004;29:458–461.
26. Crick JC, Franco RS, Conners JJ. Fractures about the interphalangeal joints in children. *J Orthop Trauma*. 1987;1:318–325.
27. DaCruz DJ, Slade RJ, Malone W. Fractures of the distal phalanges. *J Hand Surg Am*. 1988;13:350–352.
28. D'Arienzo M. Scaphoid fractures in children. *J Hand Surg Br*. 2002;27(5):424–426.
29. De Boeck H, Jaeken R. Treatment of chronic mallet finger deformity in children by tenodermodesis. *J Pediatr Orthop*. 1992;12:351–354.
30. De Boeck H, Van Wellen P, Haentjens P. Nonunion of a carpal scaphoid fracture in a child. A case report. *J Orthop Trauma*. 1991;5:370–372.
31. Dean B, Becker G, Little C, et al. The management of the acute traumatic subungual haematoma: a systematic review. *Hand Surg*. 2012;17(1):151–154.
32. Dixon GL Jr., Moon NF. Rotational supracondylar fractures of the proximal phalanx in children. *Clin Orthop Relat Res*. 1972;83:151–156.
33. Doman AN, Marcus NW. Congenital bipartite scaphoid. *J Hand Surg Am*. 1990;15:869–873.
34. Dorsay TA, Major NM, Helms CA. Cost-effectiveness of immediate MR imaging versus traditional follow-up for revealing radiographically occult scaphoid fractures. *AJR Am J Roentgenol*. 2001;177:1257–1263.
35. Earp BE, Waters PM, Wyzykowski RJ. Arthroscopic treatment of partial scapholunate ligament tears in children with chronic wrist pain. *J Bone Joint Surg Am*. 2006;88(11):2448–2455.
36. Ebinger T, Roesch M, Wachter N, et al. Functional treatment of physeal and periphyseal injuries of the metacarpal and proximal phalangeal bones. *J Pediatr Surg*. 2001;36(4):611–615.
37. Elhassan BT, Shin AY, Kozin SH. Scaphoid fractures in children. In: Shin AY, ed. *Scaphoid Fractures*. Rosemont, IL: American Academy of Orthopaedic Surgeons Monograph Series; 2007:85–95.
38. Elson RA. Rupture of the central slip of the extensor hood of the finger. A test for early diagnosis. *J Bone Joint Surg Br*. 1986;68:229–231.
39. Ersek RA, Gadaria U, Denton DR. Nail bed avulsions treated with porcine xenografts. *J Hand Surg Am*. 1985;10:152–153.
40. Fabre O, De Boeck H, Haentjens P. Fractures and nonunions of the carpal scaphoid in children. *Acta Orthop Belg*. 2001;67(2):121–125.
41. Fischer MD, McElfresh EC. Physeal and periphyseal injuries of the hand. Patterns of injury and results of treatment. *Hand Clin*. 1994;10:287–301.
42. Foucher G. "Bouquet" osteosynthesis in metacarpal neck fractures: a series of 66 patients. *J Hand Surg Am*. 1995;20:S86–S90.
43. Garroway RY, Hurst LC, Leppard J, et al. Complex dislocations of the PIP joint. A pathoanatomic classification of the injury. *Orthop Rev*. 1984;13:21–28.
44. Gedda KO. Studies in Bennett fracture: anatomy, roentgenology, and therapy. *Acta Chir Scand Suppl*. 1954;193:1–114.
45. Gellman H, Caputo RJ, Carter V, et al. Comparison of short and long thumb-spica casts for nondisplaced fractures of the carpal scaphoid. *J Bone Joint Surg Am*. 1989;71(3):354–357.
46. Gerard FM. Posttraumatic carpal instability in a young child. A case report. *J Bone Joint Surg Am*. 1980;62(1):131–133.
47. Gholson JJ, Bae DS, Zurakowski D, et al. Scaphoid fractures in children and adolescents: contemporary injury patterns and factors influencing time to union. *J Bone Joint Surg Am*. 2011;93:1210–1219.
48. Giddins GE, Shaw DG. Lunate subluxation associated with a Salter-Harris type 2 fracture of the distal radius. *J Hand Surg Br*. 1994;19:193–194.
49. Gilbert A. Dislocation of the MCP joints in children. In: Tubiana R, ed. *The Hand*. Philadelphia, PA: W.B. Saunders; 1985:922–925.
50. Goldberg B, Rosenthal PP, Robertson LS, et al. Injuries in youth football. *Pediatrics*. 1988;81(2):255–261.
51. Gollamudi S, Jones WA. Corrective osteotomy of malunited fractures of phalanges and metacarpals. *J Hand Surg Br*. 2000;25:439–441.
52. Gonzalez MH, Igram CM, Hall RF Jr. Flexible intramedullary nailing for metacarpal fractures. *J Hand Surg Am*. 1995;20(3):382–387.
53. Goulding A, Jones IE, Taylor RW, et al. Dynamic and static tests of balance and postural sway in boys: effects of previous wrist bone fractures and high adiposity. *Gait Posture*. 2003;17(2):136–141.
54. Grad JB. Children's skeletal injuries. *Orthop Clin North Am*. 1986;17:437–449.
55. Green MH, Hadied AM, LaMont RL. Scaphoid fractures in children. *J Hand Surg Am*. 1984;9:536–541.
56. Greig A, Gardiner MD, Sierakowski A, et al. Randomized feasibility trial of replacing or discarding the nail plate after nail-bed repair in children. *Br J Surg*. 2017;104(12):1634–1639.
57. Griffiths JC. Bennett fracture in childhood. *Br J Clin Pract*. 1966;20:582–583.

58. Haims AH, Schweitzer ME, Morrison WB, et al. Limitations of MR imaging in the diagnosis of peripheral tears of the triangular fibrocartilage of the wrist. *AJR Am J Roentgenol.* 2002;178(2):419–422.

59. Haines RW. The pseudoepiphysis of the first metacarpal of man. *J Anat.* 1974; 117:145–158.

60. Hambidge JE, Desai VV, Schranz PJ, et al. Acute fractures of the scaphoid. Treatment by cast immobilisation with the wrist in flexion or extension? *J Bone Joint Surg Br.* 1999;81(1):91–92.

61. Hankin FM, Janda DH. Tendon and ligament attachments in relationship to growth plate in a child's hand. *J Hand Surg Br.* 1989;14:315–318.

62. Harryman DT II, Jordan TF III. Physeal phalangeal fracture with flexor tendon entrapment. A case report and review of the literature. *Clin Orthop Relat Res.* 1990;250:194–196.

63. Hastings H II, Simmons BP. Hand fractures in children. A statistical analysis. *Clin Orthop Relat Res.* 1984;188:120–130.

64. Hennrikus WL, Cohen MR. Complete remodeling of displaced fractures of the neck of the phalanx. *J Bone Joint Surg Br.* 2003;85:273–274.

65. Herbert TJ. Use of the Herbert bone screw in surgery of the wrist. *Clin Orthop Relat Res.* 1986;202:79–92.

66. Herbert TJ, Fisher WE. Management of the fractured scaphoid using a new bone screw. *J Bone Joint Surg Br.* 1984;66-B:114–123.

67. Hildebrand KA, Ross DC, Patterson SD, et al. Dorsal perilunate dislocations and fracture-dislocations: questionnaire, clinical, and radiographic evaluation. *J Hand Surg Am.* 2000;25(6):1069–1079.

68. Horii E, Nakamura R, Watanabe K. Scaphoid fracture as a "puncher's fracture." *J Orthop Trauma.* 1994;8:107–110.

69. Horton TC, Hatton M, Davis TR. A prospective, randomized controlled study of fixation of long oblique and spiral shaft fractures of the proximal phalanx: closed reduction and percutaneous Kirschner-wiring versus open reduction and lag screw fixation. *J Hand Surg Br.* 2003;28:5–9.

70. Ireland ML, Taleisnik J. Nonunion of metacarpal extraarticular fractures in children: report of two cases and review of the literature. *J Pediatr Orthop.* 1986;6(3): 352–355.

71. Jagodzinski N, Bavan L, McNab IS. Intraosseous suture fixation of a sagittal fracture of the distal phalanx. *J Hand Surg Eur.* 2016;41(4):458–459.

72. Jahss SA. Fractures of the metacarpals: a new method of reduction and immobilization. *J Bone Joint Surg.* 1938;20:178–186.

73. Johnson KJ, Haigh SF, Symonds KE. MRI in the management of scaphoid fractures in skeletally immature patients. *Pediatr Radiol.* 2000;30(10):685–688.

74. Jones NF, Jupiter JB. Irreducible palmar dislocation of the proximal interphalangeal joint associated with an epiphyseal fracture of the middle phalanx. *J Hand Surg Am.* 1985;10:261–264.

75. Kaawach W, Ecklund K, Di Canzio J, et al. Normal ranges of scapholunate distance in children 6 to 14 years old. *J Pediatr Orthop.* 2001;21(4):464–467.

76. Kardestuncer T, Bae DS, Waters PM. The results of tenodermodesis for severe chronic mallet finger deformity in children. *J Pediatr Orthop.* 2008;28(1):81–85.

77. Karl JW, White NJ, Strauch RJ. Percutaneous reduction and fixation of displaced phalangeal neck fractures in children. *J Pediatr Orthop.* 2012;32(2):156–161.

78. Kiefhaber TR, Stern PJ. Fracture dislocations of the proximal interphalangeal joint. *J Hand Surg Am.* 1989;23:368–380.

79. Kitay A, Waters PM, Bae DS. Osteochondral autograft transplantation surgery for metacarpal head defects. *J Hand Surg.* 2016;41:457–463.

80. Koshima I, Soeda S, Takase T, et al. Free vascularized nail grafts. *J Hand Surg Am.* 1988;13(1):29–32.

81. Krusche-Mandl I, Köttstorfer J, Thalhammer G, et al. Seymour fractures: retrospective analysis and therapeutic considerations. *J Hand Surg Am.* 2013;38(2):258–264.

82. Lane CS. Detecting occult fractures of the metacarpal head: the Brewerton view. *J Hand Surg Am.* 1977;2:131–133.

83. Lankachandra M, Wells CR, Cheng CJ, et al. Complications of distal phalanx fractures in children. *J Hand Surg Am.* 2017;42(7):574.

84. Larson B, Light TR, Ogden JA. Fracture and ischemic necrosis of the immature scaphoid. *J Hand Surg Am.* 1987;12:122–127.

85. Leddy JP, Packer JW. Avulsion of the profundus tendon insertion in athletes. *J Hand Surg Am.* 1977;2:66–69.

86. Leicht P, Mikkelsen JB, Larsen CF. Scapholunate distance in children. *Acta Radiol.* 1996;37(5):625–626.

87. Light TR. Injury to the immature carpus. *Hand Clin.* 1988;4(3):415–424.

88. Light TR, Ogden JA. Metacarpal epiphyseal fractures. *J Hand Surg Am.* 1987;12: 460–464.

89. Light TR, Ogden JA. Complex dislocation of the index metacarpophalangeal joint in children. *J Pediatr Orthop.* 1988;8:300–305.

90. Littlefield WG, Friedman RL, Urbaniak JR. Bilateral nonunion of the carpal scaphoid in a child: a case report. *J Bone Joint Surg Am.* 1995;77(1):124–126.

91. Louis DS, Calhoun TP, Gam SM, et al. Congenital bipartite scaphoid—fact or fiction? *J Bone Joint Surg Am.* 1976;58(8):1108–1112.

92. Mack GR, Bosse MJ, Gelberman RH, et al. The natural history of scaphoid nonunion. *J Bone Joint Surg Am.* 1984;66(4):504–509.

93. Mack MG, Keim S, Balzer JO, et al. Clinical impact of MRI in acute wrist fractures. *Eur Radiol.* 2003;13(3):612–617.

94. Mahabir RC, Kazemi AR, Cannon WG, et al. Pediatric hand fractures: a review. *Pediatr Emerg Care.* 2001;17(3):153–156.

95. Mallee W, Doornberg JN, Ring D, et al. Comparison of CT and MRI for diagnosis of suspected scaphoid fractures. *J Bone Joint Surg.* 2011;93:20–28.

96. Markiewitz AD, Andrish JT. Hand and wrist injuries in the preadolescent and adolescent athlete. *Clin Sports Med.* 1992;11:203–225.

97. Masquijo JJ, Willis BR. Scaphoid nonunions in children and adolescents: surgical treatment with bone grafting and internal fixation. *J Pediatr Orthop.* 2010; 30(2):119–124.

98. Matsumoto K, Sumi H, Sumi Y, et al. Wrist fractures from snowboarding: a prospective study for three seasons from. 1998 to 2001. *Clin J Sport Med.* 2004;14(2):64–71.

99. Mayfield JK, Johnson RP, Kilcoyne RK. Carpal dislocations: pathomechanics and progressive perilunar instability. *J Hand Surg Am.* 1980;5:226–241.

100. McElfresh EC, Dobyns JH. Intra-articular metacarpal head fractures. *J Hand Surg Am.* 1983;8:383–393.

101. McLaughlin HL. Complex "locked" dislocation of the metacarpophalangeal joints. *J Trauma.* 1965;5:683–688.

102. Melone CP Jr., Grad JB. Primary care of fingernail injuries. *Emerg Med Clin North Am.* 1985;3:255–261.

103. Michelinakis E, Vourexaki H. Displaced epiphyseal plate of the terminal phalanx in a child. *Hand.* 1980;12:51–53.

104. Minami M, Yamazaki J, Chisaka N, et al. Nonunion of the capitate. *J Hand Surg Am.* 1987;12(6):1089–1091.

105. Mintzer CM, Waters PM. Late presentation of a ligamentous ulnar collateral ligament injury in a child. *J Hand Surg Am.* 1994;19:1048–1049.

106. Mintzer CM, Waters PM. Acute open reduction of a displaced scaphoid fracture in a child. *J Hand Surg Am.* 1994;19:760–761.

107. Mintzer CM, Waters PM. Surgical treatment of pediatric scaphoid fracture nonunions. *J Pediatr Orthop.* 1999;19:236–239.

108. Mintzer CM, Waters PM, Brown DJ. Remodelling of a displaced phalangeal neck fracture. *J Hand Surg Br.* 1994;19:594–596.

109. Mizuta T, Benson WM, Foster BK, et al. Statistical analysis of the incidence of physeal injuries. *J Pediatr Orthop.* 1987;7(5):518–523.

110. Moen CT, Pelker RR. Biomechanical and histological correlations in growth plate failure. *J Pediatr Orthop.* 1984;4(2):180–184.

111. Muramatsu K, Doi K, Kuwata N, et al. Scaphoid fracture in the young athlete—therapeutic outcome of internal fixation using the Herbert screw. *Arch Orthop Trauma Surg.* 2002;122(9–10):510–513.

112. Murphy AF, Stark HH. Closed dislocation of the metacarpophalangeal joint of the index finger. *J Bone Joint Surg Am.* 1967;49(8):1579–1586.

113. Nafie SA. Fractures of the carpal bones in children. *Injury.* 1987;18:117–119.

114. Nakamura R. Diagnosis of ulnar wrist pain. *Nagoya J Med Sci.* 2001;64:81–91.

115. Nakazato T, Ogino T. Epiphyseal destruction of children's hands after frostbite: a report of two cases. *J Hand Surg Am.* 1986;11:289–292.

116. Nussbaum R, Sadler AH. An isolated, closed, complex dislocation of the metacarpophalangeal joint of the long finger: a unique case. *J Hand Surg Am.* 1986;11:558–561.

117. Obdeijn MC, van der Vlies CH, van Rijn RR. Capitate and hamate fracture in a child: the value of MRI imaging. *Emerg Radiol.* 2010;17(2):157–159.

118. Ogden JA. *Skeletal Injury in the Child.* Philadelphia, PA: W.B. Saunders; 1990.

119. Palmer AK, Linscheid RL. Irreducible dorsal dislocation of the distal interphalangeal joint of the finger. *J Hand Surg Am.* 1977;2:406–408.

120. Palmer AK, Werner FW. The triangular fibrocartilage complex of the wrist—anatomy and function. *J Hand Surg Am.* 1981;6(2):153–162.

121. Palmer AK. Triangular fibrocartilage complex lesions: a classification. *J Hand Surg Am.* 1989;14:594–606.

122. Peimer CA, Sullivan DJ, Wild DR. Palmar dislocation of the proximal interphalangeal joint. *J Hand Surg Am.* 1984;9:39–48.

123. Peiro A, Martos F, Mut T, et al. Transscaphoid perilunate dislocation in a child. A case report. *Acta Orthop Scand.* 1981;52(1):31–34.

124. Pennes DR, Braunstein EM, Shirazi KK. Carpal ligamentous laxity with bilateral perilunate dislocation in Marfan syndrome. *Skeletal Radiol.* 1985;13:62–64.

125. Perron AD, Brady WJ, Keats TE, et al. Orthopedic pitfalls in the ED: scaphoid fracture. *Am J Emerg Med.* 2001;19(4):310–316.

126. Pick RY, Segal D. Carpal scaphoid fracture and nonunion in an 8-year-old child. Report of a case. *J Bone Joint Surg Am.* 1983;65(8):1188–1189.

127. Pohl AL. Irreducible dislocation of a distal interphalangeal joint. *Br J Plast Surg.* 1976;29:227–229.

128. Prosser AJ, Irvine GB. Epiphyseal fracture of the metacarpal head. *Injury.* 1988;19:34–35.

129. Puckett BN, Gaston RG, Peljovich AE, et al. Remodeling potential of phalangeal distal condylar malunions in children. *J Hand Surg Am.* 2012;37(1):34–41.

130. Rajesh A, Basu AK, Vaidhyanath R, et al. Hand fractures: a study of their site and type in childhood. *Clin Radiol.* 2001;56(8):667–669.

131. Rang M. *Children's Fractures.* Philadelphia, PA: JB Lippincott; 1983.

132. Rasmussen F, Schantz K. Lunatomalacia in a child. *Acta Orthop Scand.* 1987;58:82–84.

133. Rayan GM, Mullins PT. Skin necrosis complicating mallet finger splinting and vascularity of the distal interphalangeal joint overlying skin. *J Hand Surg Am.* 1987; 12:548–552.

134. Reigstad O, Thorkildsen R, Grimsgaard C, et al. Excellent results after bone grafting and K-wire fixation for scaphoid non-union surgery in skeletally immature: a mid-term follow-up study of 11 adolescents after 6.9 years. *J Orthop Trauma.* 2012;27:285–289.

135. Rettig ME, Raskin KB. Retrograde compression screw fixation of acute proximal pole scaphoid fractures. *J Hand Surg Am.* 1999;24:1206–1210.

136. Reyes BA, Ho CA. The High risk of infection with delayed treatment of open Seymour fractures: Salter-Harris I/II or juxta-epiphyseal fractures of the distal phalanx with associated nailbed laceration. *J Pediatr Orthop.* 2017;37(4):247–253.

137. Roser SE, Gellman H. Comparison of nail bed repair versus nail trephination for subungual hematomas in children. *J Hand Surg Am.* 1999;24(6):1166–1170.

138. Roy S, Caine D, Singer KM. Stress changes of the distal radial epiphysis in young gymnasts: a report of 21 cases and a review of the literature. *Am J Sports Med.* 1985; 13:301–308.

139. Sanders WE. Evaluation of the humpback scaphoid by computed tomography in the longitudinal axial plane of the scaphoid. *J Hand Surg Am.* 1988;13:182–187.

140. Sandzen SC. Fracture of the fifth metacarpal resembling Bennett fracture. *Hand.* 1973;5:49–51.

141. Savage R. Complete detachment of the epiphysis of the distal phalanx. *J Hand Surg Br.* 1990;15:126–128.

142. Schantz K, Rasmussen F. Thiemann finger or toe disease. Follow-up of seven cases. *Acta Orthop Scand.* 1986;57:91–93.
143. Schenck RR. Dynamic traction and early passive movement for fractures of the proximal interphalangeal joint. *J Hand Surg Am.* 1986;11:850–858.
144. Segmuller G, Schonenberger F. Treatment of fractures in children and adolescents. In: Weber BG, Brunner C, Freuler F, eds. *Fracture of the Hand.* New York: Springer Verlag; 1980:218–225.
145. Seymour N. Juxta-epiphysial fracture of the terminal phalanx of the finger. *J Bone Joint Surg Br.* 1966;48:347–349.
146. Shepard GH. Nail grafts for reconstruction. *Hand Clin.* 1990;6:79–102.
147. Shibata M, Seki T, Yoshizu T, et al. Microsurgical toenail transfer to the hand. *Plast Reconstr Surg.* 1991;88(1):102–109.
148. Simmons BP, Lovallo JL. Hand and wrist injuries in children. *Clin Sports Med.* 1988;7:495–512.
149. Simmons BP, Peters TT. Subcondylar fossa reconstruction for malunion of fractures of the proximal phalanx in children. *J Hand Surg Am.* 1987;12(6):1079–1082.
150. Simmons BP, Stirrat CR. Treatment of traumatic arthritis in children. *Hand Clin.* 1987;3:611–627.
151. Slade JF III, Geissler WB, Gutow AP, et al. Percutaneous internal fixation of selected scaphoid nonunions with an arthroscopically assisted dorsal approach. *J Bone Joint Surg Am.* 2003;85-A(Suppl 4):20–32.
152. Smith DG, Geist RW, Cooperman DR. Microscopic examination of a naturally occurring epiphyseal plate fracture. *J Pediatr Orthop.* 1985;5(3):306–308.
153. Stahl S, Jupiter JB. Salter-Harris type II and IV epiphyseal fractures in the hand treated with tension-band wiring. *J Pediatr Orthop.* 1999;19:233–235.
154. Stanciu C, Dumont A. Changing patterns of scaphoid fractures in adolescents. *Can J Surg.* 1994;37(3):214–216.
155. Stein F. Skeletal injuries of the hand in children. *Clin Plast Surg.* 1981;8:65–81.
156. Steinmann SP, Bishop AT, Berger RA. Use of the 1,2 intercompartmental suprareti-nacular artery as a vascularized pedicle bone graft for difficult scaphoid nonunion. *J Hand Surg Am.* 2002;27:391–401.
157. Stener B. Displacement of the ruptured ulnar collateral ligament of the MCP joint of the thumb: a clinical and anatomical study. *J Bone Joint Surg Br.* 1962;44:869–879.
158. Stener B. Hyperextension injuries to the metacarpophalangeal joint of the thumb: rupture of ligaments, fracture of sesamoid bones, rupture of flexor pollicis brevis. An anatomical and clinical study. *Acta Chir Scand.* 1963;125:275–293.
159. Stern PJ, Roman RJ, Kiefhaber TR, et al. Pilon fractures of the proximal interphalangeal joint. *J Hand Surg Am.* 1991;16(5):844–850.
160. Strickler M, Nagy L, Buchler U. Rigid internal fixation of basilar fractures of the proximal phalanges by cancellous bone grafting only. *J Hand Surg Br.* 2001;26:455–458.
161. Stripling WD. Displaced intra-articular osteochondral fracture. Cause for irreducible dislocation of the distal interphalangeal joint. *J Hand Surg Am.* 1982,7.77–78.
162. Stuart HC, Pyle SI, Cornoni J, et al. Onsets, completions, and spans of ossification in the 29 bone growth centers of the hand and wrist. *Pediatrics.* 1962;29:237–249.
163. Tavassoli J, Ruland RT, Hogan CJ, et al. Three cast techniques for the treatment of extra-articular metacarpal fractures. Comparison of short-term outcomes and final fracture alignments. *J Bone Joint Surg.* 2005;87A:2196–2201.
164. Teoh LC, Yong FC, Chong KC. Condylar advancement osteotomy for correcting condylar malunion of the finger. *J Hand Surg Br.* 2002;27:31–35.
165. Terry CL, Waters PM. Triangular fibrocartilage injuries in pediatric and adolescent patients. *J Hand Surg Am.* 1998;23:626–634.
166. Thompson JS, Eaton RG. Volar dislocation of the PIP joint. *J Hand Surg Am.* 1977;2:232.
167. Thompson JS, Littler JW, Upton J. The spiral oblique retinacular ligament (SORL). *J Hand Surg Am.* 1978;3:482–487.
168. Toh S, Miura H, Arai K, et al. Scaphoid fractures in children: problems and treatment. *J Pediatr Orthop.* 2003;23(2):216–221.
169. Torre BA. Epiphyseal injuries in the small joints of the hand. *Hand Clin.* 1988;4:113–121.
170. Vahvanen V, Westerlund M. Fracture of the carpal scaphoid in children. A clinical and roentgenological study of 108 cases. *Acta Orthop Scand.* 1980;51(6):909–913.
171. Valencia J, Leyva F, Gomez-Bajo GJ. Pediatric hand trauma. *Clin Orthop Relat Res.* 2005;432:77–86.
172. Vance RM, Gelberman RH, Evans EF. Scaphocapitate fractures: patterns of dislocation, mechanisms of injury, and preliminary results of treatment. *J Bone Joint Surg Am.* 1980;62(2):271–276.
173. Waters PM, Benson LS. Dislocation of the distal phalanx epiphysis in toddlers. *J Hand Surg Am.* 1993;18(4):581–585.
174. Waters PM, Stewart SL. Surgical treatment of nonunion and avascular necrosis of the proximal part of the scaphoid in adolescents. *J Bone Joint Surg Am.* 2002;84(6):915–920.
175. Waters PM, Taylor BA, Kuo AY. Percutaneous reduction of incipient malunion of phalangeal neck fractures in children. *J Hand Surg Am.* 2004;29:707–711.
176. Watson HK, Ballet FL. The SLAC wrist: scapholunate advanced collapse pattern of degenerative arthritis. *J Hand Surg Am.* 1984;9:358–365.
177. Weiker GG. Hand and wrist problems in the gymnast. *Clin Sports Med.* 1992;11:189–202.
178. White GM. Ligamentous avulsion of the ulnar collateral ligament of the thumb of a child. *J Hand Surg Am.* 1986;11:669–672.
179. Wood VE. Fractures of the hand in children. *Orthop Clin North Am.* 1976;7:527–542.
180. Wood VE, Hannah JD, Stilson W. What happens to the double epiphysis in the hand? *J Hand Surg Am.* 1994;19:353–360.
181. Worlock PH, Stower MJ. Fracture patterns in Nottingham children. *J Pediatr Orthop.* 1986;6:656–660.
182. Worlock PH, Stower MJ. The incidence and pattern of hand fractures in children. *J Hand Surg Br.* 1986;11:198–200.
183. Yip HS, Wu WC, Chang RY, et al. Percutaneous cannulated screw fixation of acute scaphoid waist fracture. *J Hand Surg Br.* 2002;27(1):42–46.
184. Zaricznyj B, Shattuck LJ, Mast TA, et al. Sports-related injuries in school-aged children. *Am J Sports Med.* 1980;8(5):318–324.
185. Zook EG, Guy RJ, Russell RC. A study of nail bed injuries: causes, treatment, and prognosis. *J Hand Surg Am.* 1984;9:247–252.
186. Zook EG, Russell RC. Reconstruction of a functional and esthetic nail. *Hand Clin.* 1990;6:59–68.

8

Fractures of the Distal Radius and Ulna

William L. Hennrikus and Donald S. Bae

INTRODUCTION TO FRACTURES OF THE DISTAL RADIUS AND ULNA

Forearm fractures are the most common long-bone fractures in children, occurring with an annual incidence of approximately 1.5/100 children per year[33] and comprising up to 40% of all pediatric fractures.[13,30,33,107,122] Among all forearm fractures, the distal radius and ulna are most commonly affected.[30,122,214] Peak incidences of distal radius and ulna fractures occur during the preadolescent growth spurt.[13,30,122,214] The nondominant arm in males is most commonly affected. Several recent studies suggest that the frequency of pediatric distal radius fractures is rising, likely due to epidemiologic trends toward diminished bone density, increased body mass indices, higher-risk activities, and younger age at the time of initial sports participation.[82,83,116,181]

In children younger than 15 years of age, the frequency with which these fractures occur demonstrates considerable seasonal variation.[202] In a prior longitudinal study of 5,013 children over 1 year in Wales, the incidence of wrist and forearm fractures was roughly half (5.9/1,000 per year) in the three winter months compared with the rest of the year (10.7/1,000 per year). In addition, the non-winter fractures were more severe in terms of requiring reduction and hospitalization.

Because of the greater forces borne and imparted to the radius, as well as the increased porosity of the distal radial metaphysis, distal radial fractures are far more common than distal ulna fractures and so, isolated distal radius fractures do occur regularly. However, fractures of the distal ulna most often occur in association with fractures of the distal radius.[122,158] The metaphysis of the distal radius is the most common site of forearm fracture in children and adolescents.[13,116,122] The pediatric Galeazzi injury usually involves a distal radial metaphyseal fracture and a distal ulnar physeal fracture that result in a displaced distal radioulnar joint (DRUJ). Galeazzi fracture–dislocations are relatively rare injuries in children with a cited occurrence of 3% of pediatric distal radial fractures.[200]

Given the frequency with which these injuries occur, the evaluation and management of distal radius and ulna fractures in children remain a fundamental element of pediatric orthopedics. Despite established treatment principles, however, care of these injuries remains challenging due to the spectrum of injury patterns, issues of skeletal growth and remodeling, diversity of nonoperative and surgical techniques, evolving patient/family expectations, and increasing emphasis on cost-effective care.

MECHANISMS OF INJURY OF FRACTURES OF THE DISTAL RADIUS AND ULNA

Distal Radius and Ulna Fractures

The mechanism of injury is generally a fall on an outstretched hand. Typically, the extended position of the wrist at the time of loading leads to tensile failure on the volar side of the distal forearm (Fig. 8-1). Conversely, axial loading on the flexed wrist will produce a volarly displaced fracture with apex dorsal angulation (Fig. 8-2). Occasionally, a direct blow sustained to the distal forearm may result in fracture and displacement. In addition to the angular deformity caused by axial and bending loads applied to the distal forearm, rotational displacement may also occur, based on the position of the forearm and torsional forces sustained at the time of injury.

Fracture type and degree of displacement are also dependent on the height and velocity of the fall or injury mechanism.[214] Indeed, the spectrum of injury may range from nondisplaced torus (or "buckle") injuries (common in younger children with a minimal fall) or dorsally displaced fractures with apex volar angulation (more common in older children with higher-velocity injuries) (see Fig. 8-1). Displacement may be severe enough to cause foreshortening and bayonet apposition. Adult type injuries with intra-articular extension do occur. Rarely, a mechanism such as a fall from a height can cause a distal radial fracture associated with a more proximal fracture of the forearm or elbow (Fig. 8-3).[12,173] These "floating elbow" situations connote higher-energy trauma and as a result are associated with risks of neurovascular compromise and compartment syndrome.[12,173]

Fractures of the distal forearm in children typically occur when the radius and/or ulna are more susceptible to fracture secondary to biomechanical changes during skeletal development. Work based on load-to-strength ratio and other measures of bone quality has identified specific times during skeletal development where the biologic properties of the distal upper extremity produce relatively weaker bone, making a child more susceptible to fracture.[65,109,118,147] In these studies, prepubescent boys and girls were found to have lower estimates of bone strength compared to same-sex postpubertal peers. From these studies, it can be concluded that children are uniquely susceptible for fracture when longitudinal growth outpaces mineral accrual during rapid

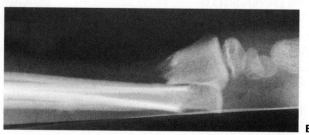

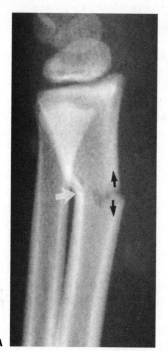

Figure 8-1. A: Tension failure greenstick fracture. The dorsal cortex is plastically deformed (*white arrow*), and the volar cortex is complete and separated (*black arrows*). **B:** Dorsal bayonet.

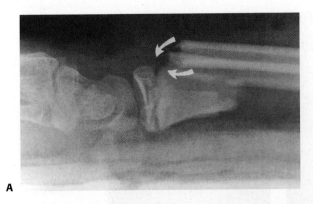

A

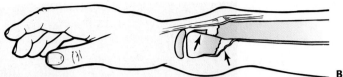

B

Figure 8-2. Reverse bayonet. **A:** Typical volar bayonet fracture. Often the distal end of the proximal fragment is buttonholed through the extensor tendons (*arrows*). (Reprinted from Wilkins KE, ed. *Operative Management of Upper Extremity Fractures in Children.* Rosemont, IL: American Academy of Orthopaedic Surgeons, 1994:27, with permission.) **B:** Intact volar periosteum and disrupted dorsal periosteum (*arrows*). The extensor tendons are displaced to either side of the proximal fragment.

growth.[13] As 90% of the radius growth is from the distal physis and accounts for 70% of the loading across the wrist, the radius is more prone to fracture than the ulna during rapid growth.[202] Fractures occur at the biomechanically weakest anatomic location of bone, which also varies over time. As the metaphyseal cortex of the radius is relatively thin and porous, fractures of the metaphysis are most common, followed by physeal.[140,191]

Usually, fractures occur during sports-related activities. Indeed, the trend toward increased sports participation in children has led to a substantial increase in the incidence of distal radius and/or ulna fractures.[102,213] Certain sports, such as skiing/snowboarding, basketball, soccer, football, rollerblading/skating, and hockey have been associated with an increased risk of distal radial fracture, though a fall or injury of sufficient severity may occur in any recreational activity.[190] Protective wrist guards have

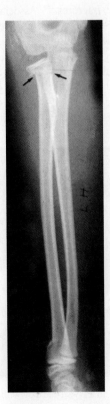

Figure 8-3. A 10-year-old girl with an innocuous-appearing distal radial fracture associated with an ipsilateral angulated radial neck fracture (*arrows.*)

been shown to decrease the injury rate in snowboarders, especially beginners and persons with rental equipment.[175]

As cited above, there is seasonal variation, with an increase in both incidence and severity of fractures in summer.[203] Children who are overweight, have poor postural balance, ligamentous laxity, or less bone mineralization are at increased risk for distal radial fractures.[83,117,123,167,182,214] Although bone quality measures predict that boys had lower risk of fracture than girls at every stage except during early puberty,[147] these fractures have been reported to be three times more common in boys. This may be due to relative risk-taking behaviors or participation in higher risk of injury activities. However, the increased participation in athletics by girls at a young age may change this ratio.

Radial Physeal Stress Fractures

Repetitive axial loading of the wrist may lead to physeal stress injuries, almost always involving the radius (Fig. 8-4). These physeal stress injuries are most commonly seen in competitive gymnasts.[29,47,52,193,194] Factors that predispose to this injury include excessive training, poor techniques, and attempts to advance too quickly in competitive level. Stress injuries have been also observed in other sports including wresting, break dancing, and cheerleading.[76]

Galeazzi Fracture

Axial loading of the wrist in combination with extremes of forearm rotation (Fig. 8-5) may result in distal radius fractures with associated disruption of the DRUJ, the so-called "pediatric Galeazzi fracture."[26,40,72,122,127,137,201] In adults, the mechanism of injury usually is an axially loading fall with hyperpronation. This results in a distal radial fracture with DRUJ ligament disruption and dorsal dislocation of the ulna. However, in children, both supination (apex volar) and pronation (apex dorsal) deforming forces have been described.[126,200] The mechanism of injury is most obvious when the radial fracture is incomplete. With an apex volar (supination) radial fracture, the distal ulna is displaced volarly; whereas with an apex dorsal (pronation) radial fracture, the distal ulna is displaced dorsally. This is evident both on clinical and radiographic examinations. In addition, the radius is foreshortened in a complete fracture, causing more radial deviation of the hand and wrist. In children, this injury may involve either disruption of the DRUJ ligaments or, more commonly, a distal ulnar physeal fracture (Fig. 8-6).[1,172]

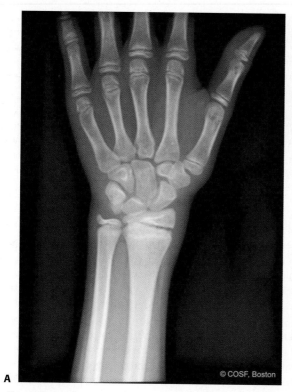
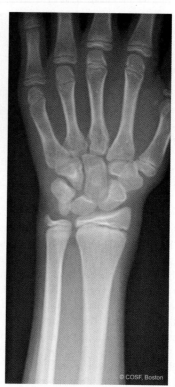

Figure 8-4. Radiographic images of the gymnast's wrist. **A:** AP radiograph of the left wrist in a 12-year-old female demonstrates physeal widening, cystic changes, and metaphyseal sclerosis. **B:** AP radiograph of the same wrist after 3 months of rest from gymnastics, demonstrating incomplete resolution of the physeal changes.

INJURIES ASSOCIATED WITH FRACTURES OF THE DISTAL RADIUS AND ULNA

The risk of associated injuries is significantly less in the skeletally immature as compared to skeletally mature patients.[58] The entire ipsilateral extremity should be carefully examined for fractures of the carpus, forearm, or elbow.[12,32,91,120,173,184,195] Indeed, 3% to 13% of distal radial fractures have associated ipsilateral extremity fractures.[184] Associated fractures of the hand and elbow regions need to be assessed because their presence implies more severe trauma. For example, the incidence of a compartment syndrome is higher with a "floating elbow" combination of radial, ulnar, and elbow fractures.[173]

With marked radial or ulnar fracture displacement, neurovascular compromise can occur.[15,44,205] Median neuropathy may be seen in severely displaced distal radius fractures, due to direct

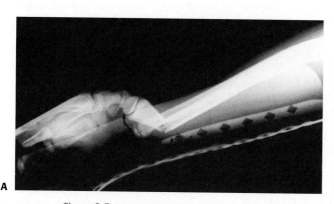
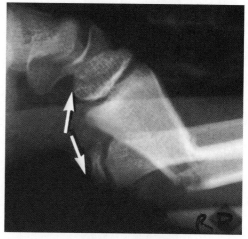

Figure 8-5. Supination-type Galeazzi fracture. **A:** View of the entire forearm of an 11-year-old boy with a Galeazzi fracture–dislocation. **B:** Close-up of the distal forearm shows that there has been disruption of the distal radioulnar joint (*arrows*). The distal radial fragment is dorsally displaced (apex volar), making this a supination type of mechanism. Note that the distal ulna is volar to the distal radius.

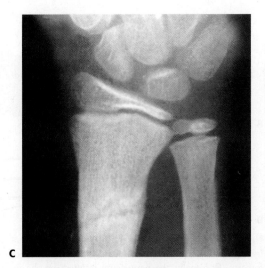
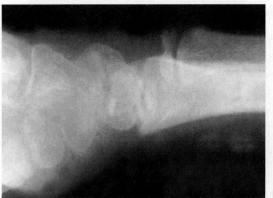

Figure 8-5. (*Continued*) **C, D:** The fracture was reduced by pronating the distal fragment. Because the distal radius was partially intact by its greenstick nature, the length was easily maintained, reestablishing the congruity of the distal radioulnar joint. The patient was immobilized in supination for 6 weeks, after which full forearm rotation and function returned.

nerve contusion sustained at the time of fracture displacement, persistent pressure or traction from an unreduced fracture, or an acute compartment syndrome (Fig. 8-7).[205] Ulnar neuropathy has been described with similar mechanisms, as well as entrapment or incarceration of the ulnar nerve within the fracture site.

Wrist ligamentous and articular cartilage injuries have been described in association with distal radial and ulna fractures in adults and less commonly in children.[12,55] Concomitant scaphoid fractures have occurred (Fig. 8-8).[32,41,196] Associated wrist injuries need to be treated both in the acute setting and in the patient with persistent pain after fracture healing. More

than 50% of distal radial physeal fractures have an associated ulnar fracture. This usually is an ulnar styloid fracture, but can be a distal ulnar plastic deformation, greenstick, or complete fracture.[33,107,123,191] Some patients with distal radial and ulna fractures are multitrauma victims. Care of the distal forearm fracture in these situations must be provided within the context of concomitant systemic injuries.

Isolated ulnar physeal fractures are rare injuries.[1,185] Most ulnar physeal fractures occur in association with radial metaphyseal or physeal fractures. Physeal separations are classified by the standard Salter–Harris criteria. The rare pediatric Galeazzi injury

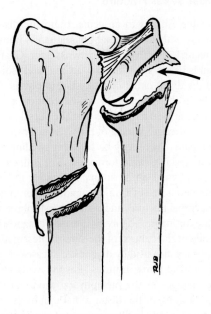

Figure 8-6. Galeazzi fracture–dislocation variant. Interposed periosteum can block reduction of the distal ulnar physis (*arrow*). This destabilizes the distal radial metaphyseal fracture. (Reprinted with permission from Lanfried MJ, Stenclik M, Susi JG. Variant of Galeazzi fracture–dislocation in children. *J Pediatr Orthop.* 1991;11(3):333–335.)

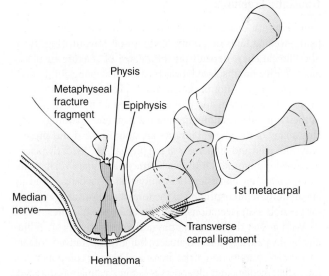

Figure 8-7. Volar forearm anatomy outlining the potential compression of the median nerve between the metaphysis of the radius and dorsally displaced physeal fracture. The taut volar transverse carpal ligament and fracture hematoma also are contributing factors. (Redrawn with permission from Waters PM, Kolettis GJ, Schwend R. Acute median neuropathy following physeal fractures of the distal radius. *J Pediatr Orthop.* 1994;14(2):173–177.)

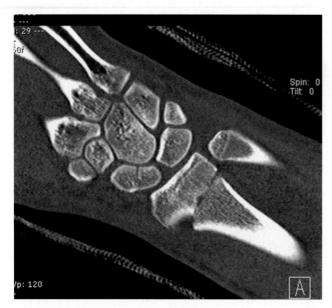

Figure 8-8. Coronal computed tomography (CT) image of an adolescent with ipsilateral distal radius and scaphoid fractures. (Courtesy of Children's Orthopaedic Surgery Foundation.)

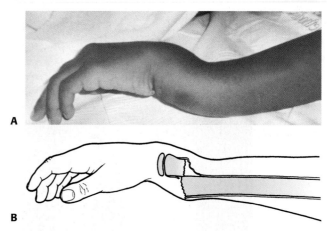

Figure 8-9. Dorsal bayonet deformity. **A:** Typical distal metaphyseal fracture with dorsal bayonet showing a dorsal angulation of the distal forearm. **B:** Usually, the periosteum is intact on the dorsal side and disrupted on the volar side.

usually involves an ulnar physeal fracture rather than a soft tissue disruption of the DRUJ. Another ulnar physeal fracture is an avulsion fracture off the distal aspect of the ulnar styloid.[1] Although an ulnar styloid injury is an epiphyseal avulsion, it can be associated with soft tissue injuries of the triangular fibrocartilage complex (TFCC) and ulnocarpal joint, though does not typically cause growth-related complications.

SIGNS AND SYMPTOMS OF FRACTURES OF THE DISTAL RADIUS AND ULNA

Traumatic Fractures

Children with distal radial and/or ulna fractures present with pain, swelling, and deformity of the distal forearm (Fig. 8-9). The clinical signs depend on the degree of fracture displacement. With a nondisplaced torus fracture in a young child, medical attention may not be sought until several days after injury; the intact periosteum and biomechanical stability are protective in these injuries, resulting in minimal pain and guarding. Similarly, many of the physeal injuries are nondisplaced and present only with pain and tenderness at the physis.[144,156] With displaced fractures, the typical dorsal displacement and apex volar angulation create an extension deformity that is usually clinically apparent. Careful inspection of the forearm is critical to evaluate for possible skin lacerations, wounds, and open fractures.

With greater displacement, physical examination is often limited by the patient's pain and anxiety, but it is imperative to obtain an accurate examination of the motor and sensory components of the radial, median, and ulnar nerves before treatment is initiated. Neurovascular compromise is uncommon but can occur.[205] A prior prospective study indicated an 8% incidence of nerve injury in children with distal radial fractures.[206] Median nerve irritability or dysfunction is most common, caused by direct trauma to the nerve at the time of injury or ongoing ischemic compression from the displaced fracture. Median nerve motor function is evaluated

by testing the abductor pollicis brevis (intrinsic) and flexor pollicis longus (extrinsic) muscles. Ulnar nerve motor evaluation includes testing the first dorsal interosseous (intrinsic), abductor digiti quinti (intrinsic), and flexor digitorum profundus to the small finger (extrinsic) muscles. Radial nerve evaluation involves testing the common digital extensors for metacarpophalangeal joint extension as well as thumb extensor pollicis longus. Sensibility to light touch and two-point discrimination should be tested. Normal two-point discrimination is less than 5 mm but may not be reliably tested in children younger than 5 to 7 years of age. Pinprick sensibility testing will only hurt and scare the already anxious child and should be avoided.

Radial Physeal Stress Fracture

In contrast to the child with an acute, traumatic distal radius fracture, patients with distal radial physeal stress injuries typically report recurring, activity-related wrist pain. Characteristically, this pain is described as diffuse "aching" and "soreness" in the region of the distal radial metaphysis and physis. Pain may be reproduced in the extremes of wrist extension and flexion, and usually there is local tenderness over the dorsal, distal radial physis. Resistive strength testing of the wrist extensors will also reproduce the pain. There may be fusiform swelling about the wrist if there is reactive bone formation. The differential diagnosis includes physeal stress injury, ganglion, inflammatory arthritis, ligamentous or TFCC injury, tendinosis or musculotendinous strain, carpal fracture, and osteonecrosis of the scaphoid (Preiser disease) or lunate (Kienbock disease). Diagnosis is made radiographically in the context of the clinical presentation.

Radiographs are also usually diagnostic in cases of suspected distal radial physeal stress injuries. Physeal widening, cystic and sclerotic changes in the metaphyseal aspect of the distal radial physis, beaking of the distal radial epiphysis, and reactive bone formation are highly suggestive of chronic physeal stress fracture. In advanced cases, premature physeal closure or physeal bar formation may be seen, indicating long-standing stress.[29,47,52,176,194,215] In these situations, continued ulnar growth leads to an ulnar positive variance with resulting pain from ulnocarpal impaction and/or TFCC tear.[12,176,215] Plain radiographs may not reveal early physeal stress fracture. If the diagnosis is suggested clinically, additional studies may be indicated. Technetium bone scanning is sensitive but nonspecific. Magnetic resonance imaging (MRI) is usually diagnostic, demonstrating the characteristic "double line" on coronal T1 and gradient echo sequences.[128]

Galeazzi Fracture

Children with Galeazzi injuries present with pain, limited forearm rotation, and limited wrist flexion and extension. Neurovascular impairment is rare. The radial deformity usually is clinically evident. Prominence of the ulnar head is seen with DRUJ disruption. Ligamentous disruption is often subtle and may be evident only by local tenderness and instability to testing of the DRUJ.

IMAGING AND OTHER DIAGNOSTIC STUDIES FRACTURES OF THE DISTAL RADIUS AND ULNA

Plain radiographs are diagnostic of the fracture type and degree of displacement. Standard anteroposterior (AP) and lateral radiographs usually are sufficient. Complete wrist, forearm, and elbow views are recommended in cases of high-energy injuries or when there is clinical suspicion for an ipsilateral fracture of the hand, wrist, or elbow. More extensive radiographic evaluation (e.g., computed tomography [CT], MRI) is typically reserved for evaluation of suspected or known intra-articular fractures or associated carpal injuries (e.g., scaphoid fractures, hook of hamate fractures, perilunate instability); these situations are most commonly encountered in older adolescents.

There has been increasing enthusiasm for the use of ultrasound in the diagnostic evaluation of distal radius and ulna fractures.[28,60,99,144,156,164] Two independent studies have demonstrated the feasibility and accuracy of bedside ultrasound for diagnosing nondisplaced fractures.[28,164] Ultrasonography is most useful in cases of suspected fractures in the absence of plain radiographic abnormalities, or in very young children in whom the skeletal structures are incompletely ossified. Since ultrasound machines are now commonplace in emergency departments and used by many nonradiology physicians, usage as a screening diagnostic tool is evolving.

Radiographic evaluation should be performed not only to confirm the diagnosis but also to quantify the degree of displacement, angulation, malrotation, and comminution (Fig. 8-10). Understanding of the normal radiographic parameters is essential in quantifying displacement. In adults, the normal distal radial inclination averages 22 degrees on the AP view and 11 degrees of volar tilt on the lateral projection.[73,139,150,183,222] Radial inclination is a goniometric measurement of the angle between the distal radial articular surface and a line perpendicular to the radial shaft on the AP radiograph. Volar tilt is measured by a line across the distal articular surface and a line perpendicular to the radial shaft on the lateral view. Pediatric values for radial inclination and volar tilt may vary from adult normative values, depending on the degree of skeletal maturity and the ossification of the epiphysis. Indeed, radial inclination is often less than 22 degrees in younger children, though volar tilt tends to be more consistent regardless of patient age.

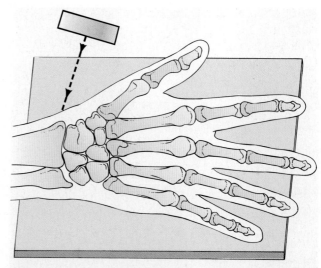

Figure 8-10. Angulation of the x-ray beam tangential to the articular surface, providing the optimal lateral view of the distal radius. The wrist is positioned as for the standard lateral radiograph, but the x-ray beam is directed 15 degrees cephalad. (Reprinted by permission from Springer: Johnson PG, Szabo RM. Angle measurements of the distal radius: A cadaver study. *Skel Radiol.* 1993;22(4):243–246. Copyright © 1993 International Skeletal Society.)

As noted above, advanced imaging may be helpful in cases of intra-articular extension to characterize fracture pattern and joint congruity. This may be done by AP and lateral tomograms, CT scans, or MRI. Dynamic motion studies with fluoroscopy can provide important information on fracture stability and the success of various treatment options. Dynamic fluoroscopy requires adequate pain relief and has been used more often in adult patients with distal radial fractures.

In Galeazzi fractures, the radial fracture is readily apparent on plain radiographs. Careful systematic evaluation of the radiographs will reveal concurrent injuries to the ulna and/or DRUJ (Fig. 8-11). A true lateral radiograph is essential to identify the direction of displacement and thus to determine the method of reduction. Rarely are advanced imaging studies, such as CT or MRI scan, necessary.

CLASSIFICATION OF FRACTURES OF THE DISTAL RADIUS AND ULNA

Distal Radius and Ulna Fractures

Distal Forearm Fractures: GENERAL CLASSIFICATION

Physeal fractures
    Distal radius
    Distal ulna

Distal metaphyseal (radius or ulna)
    Torus
    Greenstick
    Complete fractures

Galeazzi fracture–dislocations
    Dorsal displaced
    Volar displaced

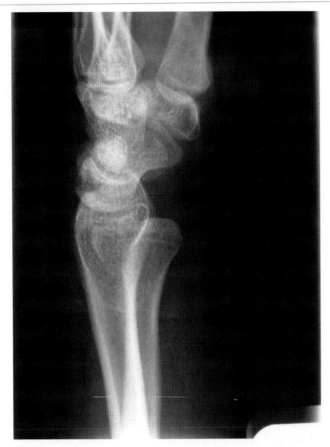

Figure 8-11. Lateral radiograph depicting volar subluxation of the distal ulna in relation to the distal radius, a pediatric Galeazzi equivalent. Careful inspection reveals a distal ulnar physeal fracture.

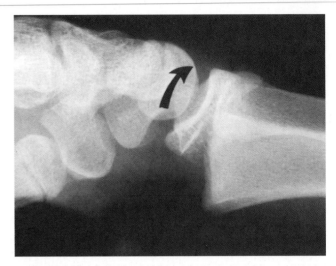

Figure 8-12. Dorsally displaced physeal fracture (type A). The distal epiphysis with a small metaphyseal fragment is displaced dorsally (*curved arrow*) in relation to the proximal metaphyseal fragment.

Distal radius and ulna fractures are classified according to fracture pattern, type of associated ulnar fracture, and direction of displacement, angulation, and rotation. Most distal radial metaphyseal fractures are displaced dorsally with apex volar angulation.[191] Volar displacement with apex dorsal angulation occurs less commonly with volar flexion mechanisms.

Distal radial and ulna fractures are then defined by their anatomic relationship to the physis. Physeal fractures are classified by the widely accepted Salter–Harris system (see below).[27,177] Metaphyseal injuries are often different from their adult equivalents, due to the thick periosteum surrounding the relatively thin metaphyseal cortex. Metaphyseal fractures are generally classified according to fracture pattern and may be torus fractures, greenstick or incomplete fractures, or complete bicortical injuries. Pediatric equivalents of adult Galeazzi fracture–dislocations involve a distal radial fracture and either a soft tissue disruption of the DRUJ or a physeal fracture of the distal ulna.

Physeal Injuries

The Salter–Harris system is the basis for classification of physeal fractures.[176] Most are Salter–Harris type II fractures.[27] In the more common apex volar injuries, dorsal displacement of the distal epiphysis and the dorsal Thurston–Holland metaphyseal fragment is evident on the lateral view (Fig. 8-12).

Salter–Harris type I fractures also usually displaced dorsally. Volar displacement of either a Salter–Harris type I or II fracture is less common (Fig. 8-13). Nondisplaced Salter–Harris type I fractures may be indicated only by a displaced pronator fat pad sign (Fig. 8-14),[177,220] ultrasound,[28,99,155] or tenderness over the involved physis.[143,155] A scaphoid fat pad sign may indicate a scaphoid fracture (Fig. 8-15).[94]

Salter–Harris type III fractures are rare and may be caused by a compression, shear, or avulsion of the radial origin of the volar radiocarpal ligaments (Fig. 8-16).[9,125] Triplane-equivalent fractures,[160] a combination of Salter–Harris type II and III fractures in different planes, have similarly been reported but are rare. CT scans may be necessary to define the fracture pattern and degree of intra-articular displacement in deciding best treatment options.

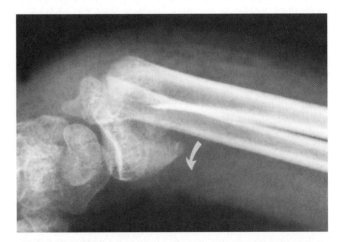

Figure 8-13. Volarly displaced physeal fracture (type B). Distal epiphysis with a large volar metaphyseal fragment is displaced in a volar direction (*curved arrow*). (Reprinted from Wilkins KE, ed. *Operative Management of Upper Extremity Fractures in Children.* Rosemont, IL: American Academy of Orthopaedic Surgeons; 1994:21, with permission.)

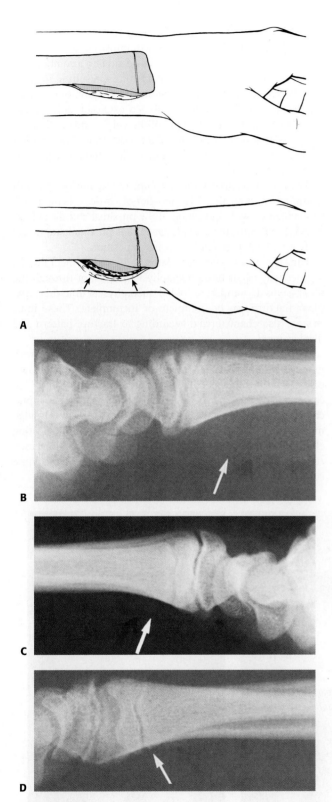

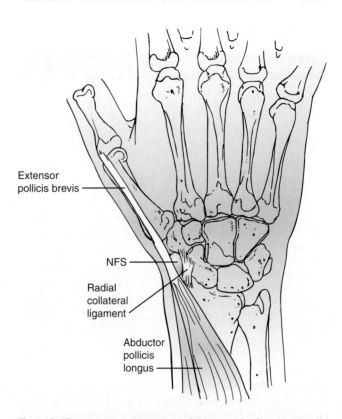

Figure 8-15. Anatomic relationships of the navicular fat stripe (NFS). The NFS, shaded black, is located between the combined tendons of the abductor pollicis longus and extensor pollicis brevis, and the lateral surface of the carpal navicular. (Adapted from Terry DW, Ramen JE. The navicular fat stripe. *Ham J Roent Rad Ther Nucl Med.* 1975;124:25, with permission.)

Figure 8-14. A: Subperiosteal hemorrhage from an occult fracture of the distal radius causes an anterior displacement of the normal pronator quadratus fat pad (*arrows*). **B:** A 13-year-old girl with tenderness over the distal radius after a fall. The only radiographic finding is an anterior displacement of the normal pronator quadratus fat pad (*arrow*). **C:** The opposite normal side (*arrow indicates normal fat pad*). **D:** Two weeks later, there is a small area of periosteal new bone formation (*arrow*) anteriorly, substantiating that bony injury has occurred.

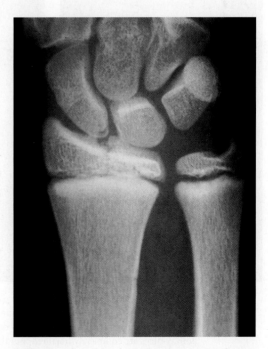

Figure 8-16. AP radiograph of Salter–Harris type III fracture of the distal radius.

Metaphyseal Injuries

Distal Metaphyseal Fractures: CLASSIFICATION

Directional displacement
 Dorsal
 Volar

Fracture combinations
 Isolated radius
 Radius with ulna
 Ulnar styloid
 Ulnar physis
 Ulnar metaphysis, incomplete
 Ulnar metaphysis, complete

Biomechanical patterns
 Torus
 Greenstick
 One cortex
 Two cortices
 Complete fracture
 Length maintained
 Bayonet apposition

Metaphyseal fracture patterns are classified as torus, incomplete or greenstick, and complete fractures (Fig. 8-17). This system of classification has been shown to have good agreement between experienced observers.[169] Torus fractures are axial compression injuries. The site of cortical failure is the transition from metaphysis to diaphysis.[128] As the mode of failure is compression, these injuries are inherently stable and are further stabilized by the intact surrounding periosteum. Rarely, they may extend into the physis, putting them at risk for growth impairment.[157–159]

Incomplete or greenstick fractures occur with a combination of compressive, tensile, and rotatory forces, resulting in complete failure of one cortex and plastic deformation of the other cortex. Most commonly, the combined extension and supination forces lead to tensile failure of the volar cortex and dorsal compression injury. The degree of force determines the amount of plastic deformation, dorsal comminution, and fracture angulation and rotation.

With greater applied loads, complete fracture occurs with disruption of both the volar and dorsal cortices. Length may be maintained with apposition of the proximal and distal fragments. Frequently, the distal fragment lies proximal and dorsal to the proximal fragment in bayonet apposition.

Ulna fractures often associated with radial metaphyseal injuries may occur in the metaphysis, physis, or through the ulnar styloid. Similar to radial metaphyseal fractures, the ulnar fracture can be complete or incomplete. These injuries are also characterized according to fracture pattern and displacement.

Distal radial fractures also can occur in conjunction with more proximal forearm fractures,[19,205] Monteggia fracture–dislocations,[18] supracondylar distal humeral fractures,[172,183] or carpal fractures.[32,41,91,119] The combination of a displaced supracondylar distal humeral fracture and a displaced distal radial metaphyseal fracture has been called the pediatric floating elbow. This injury combination is unstable and has an increased risk for malunion and neurovascular compromise including compartment syndrome.

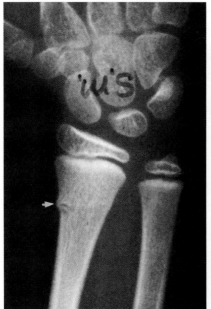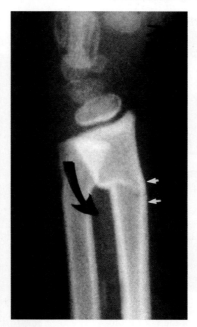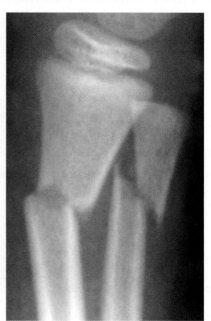

A, B   **C**

Figure 8-17. Metaphyseal biomechanical patterns. **A:** Torus fracture. Simple bulging of the thin cortex (*arrow*). **B:** Compression greenstick fracture. Angulation of the dorsal cortex (*large curved arrow*). The volar cortex is intact but slightly plastically deformed (*small white arrows*). **C:** Complete length maintained. Both cortices are completely fractured, but the length of the radius has been maintained. (Reprinted from Wilkins KE, ed. *Operative Management of Upper Extremity Fractures in Children.* Rosemont, IL: American Academy of Orthopaedic Surgeons; 1994:24, with permission.)

Distal Ulna Fractures

Isolated ulnar physeal fractures are rare, as most ulnar physeal injuries occur in association with radial metaphyseal or physeal fractures.[1,184] Physeal injuries are classified according to the Salter–Harris classification.[158] Ulnar physeal fractures may also be seen with the pediatric Galeazzi injuries,[171] which usually involve an ulnar physeal fracture rather than a soft tissue disruption of the DRUJ.

Avulsion fractures of the ulnar styloid also represent epiphyseal avulsion injuries. Most commonly associated with distal radial fractures,[1,184] these styloid fractures typically represent soft tissue avulsions of the ulnar insertion of the TFCC or ulnocarpal ligaments[12] and are rarely associated with growth-related complications.

Galeazzi Fracture

Galeazzi Fractures: CLASSIFICATION

Type I: Dorsal (apex volar) displacement of distal radius
  Radius fracture pattern
  Greenstick
  Complete
  Distal ulna physis
  Intact
  Disrupted (equivalent)

Type II: Volar (apex dorsal) displacement of distal radius
  Radius fracture pattern
  Greenstick
  Complete
  Distal ulna physis
  Intact
  Disrupted

Galeazzi fracture–dislocations are most commonly described by direction of displacement of either the distal ulnar dislocation or the radial fracture.[126] Letts preferred to describe the direction of the ulna: volar or dorsal.[77,200] Others classified pediatric Galeazzi injuries by the direction of displacement of the distal radial fracture. Dorsally displaced (apex volar) fractures were more common than volarly displaced (apex dorsal) injuries in their series. Wilkins and O'Brien[211] modified the Walsh and McLaren method by classifying radial fractures as incomplete and complete fractures and ulnar injuries as true dislocations versus physeal fractures. DRUJ dislocations are called true Galeazzi lesions and distal ulnar physeal fractures are called pediatric Galeazzi equivalents.[109,121,126]

PATHOANATOMY AND APPLIED ANATOMY RELATING TO FRACTURES OF THE DISTAL RADIUS AND ULNA

The distal radial epiphysis normally appears between 0.5 and 2.3 years in boys and 0.4 and 1.7 years in girls.[73,138,149] Initially transverse in appearance, it rapidly becomes more adult-like with its triangular shape. The contour of the radial styloid

progressively elongates with advancing skeletal maturity. The secondary center of ossification for the distal ulna appears at about age 7 years.[149] Similar to the radius, the ulnar styloid appears with the adolescent growth spurt. It also becomes more elongated and adult-like until physeal closure. On average, the ulnar physis closes at age 16 in girls and age 17 in boys, whereas the radial physis closes on average 6 months later than the ulnar physis.[174,222] The distal radial and ulnar physes contribute approximately 75% to 80% of the growth of the forearm and 40% of the growth of the upper extremity (Fig. 8-18).[150]

The distal radius articulates with the distal ulna at the DRUJ.[179] Both the radius and ulna articulate with the carpus, serving as the platform for the carpus and hand. The radial joint surface has three concavities for its articulations: the scaphoid and lunate fossa for the carpus and the sigmoid notch for the ulnar head. These joints are stabilized by a complex series of volar and dorsal radiocarpal, ulnocarpal, and radioulnar ligaments. The volar ligaments are the major stabilizers. Starting radially at the radial styloid, the radial collateral, radioscaphocapitate, radiolunotriquetral (long radiolunate), and radioscapholunate (short radiolunate) ligaments volarly stabilize the radiocarpal joint. The dorsal radioscaphoid and radial triquetral ligaments are less important stabilizers. The complex structure of ligaments stabilize the radius, ulna, and carpus through the normal wrist motion of 120 degrees of flexion and extension, 50 degrees of radial and ulnar deviation, and 150 degrees of forearm rotation.[152]

The TFCC is the primary stabilizer of the ulnocarpal and radioulnar articulations.[152] It extends from the sigmoid notch of the radius across the DRUJ and inserts into the base of the ulnar styloid. It also extends distally as the ulnolunate, ulnotriquetral, and ulnar collateral ligaments and inserts into the ulnar carpus and base of the fifth metacarpal.[152] The volar ulnocarpal ligaments (V ligament) from the ulna to the lunate and triquetrum are important ulnocarpal stabilizers.[22,180] The central portion of the TFCC is the articular disk (Fig. 8-19). The interaction between the bony articulation and the soft tissue attachments accounts for stability of the DRUJ during pronation and supination.[153] At the extremes of rotation, the joint is most stable. The compression loads between the radius and ulna are aided by the tensile loads of the TFCC to maintain stability throughout rotation.

The interosseous ligament of the forearm (Fig. 8-20) helps stabilize the radius and ulna more proximally in the diaphysis of the forearm. The ulna remains relatively immobile as the radius rotates around it. Throughout the mid-forearm, the interosseous ligament connects the radius to the ulna. It passes obliquely from the proximal radius to the distal ulna. However, the interosseous ligament is not present in the distal radius. Moore et al.[142] found that injuries to the TFCC and interosseous ligament were responsible for progressive shortening of the radius with fracture in a cadaveric study. The soft tissue component to the injury is a major factor in the deformity and instability in a Galeazzi fracture–dislocation.

The length relationship between the distal radius and ulna at the wrist is defined as ulnar variance. In adults, this is measured by the relationship of the radial corner of the distal ulnar articular surface to the ulnar corner of the radial articular

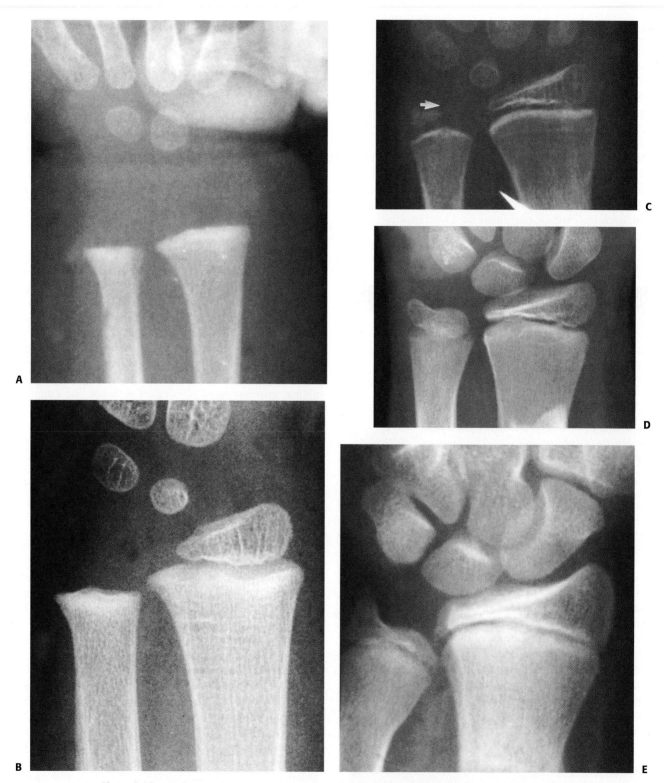

Figure 8-18. Ossification of the distal radius. **A:** Preossification distal radius with transverse ossification in a 15-month-old boy. **B:** The triangular secondary ossification center of the distal radius in a 2-year-old girl. **C:** The initial ossification center of the styloid in this 7-year-old girl progresses radially (*arrow*). **D:** Extension of the ulnar ossification center into the styloid process of an 11 year old. **E:** The styloid is fully ossified and the epiphyses have capped their relative metaphyses in this 13-year-old boy.

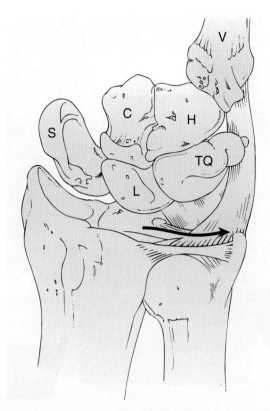

Figure 8-19. Diagrammatic drawing of the TFCC and the prestyloid recess. The meniscal reflection runs from the dorsoulnar radius to the ulnovolar carpus. The *arrow* denotes access under the reflection to the tip of the styloid, the so-called prestyloid recess. V, fifth metacarpal; S, scaphoid; C, capitate; H, hamate; L, lunate; TQ, triquetrum. (Redrawn from Bowers WH. *Green's Operative Hand Surgery*. New York: Churchill-Livingstone; 1993.)

and wrist placed on the cassette, with the shoulder abducted 90 degrees, elbow flexed 90 degrees, and forearm in neutral rotation (Fig. 8-22). The importance of ulnar variance relates to the force transmission across the wrist with axial loading. Normally, the radiocarpal joint bears approximately 80% of the axial load across the wrist, and the ulnocarpal joint bears 20%. Changes in the length relationship of the radius and ulna alter respective load bearing. Indeed, 2.5 mm of ulnar positive variance has been demonstrated to double the forces borne across the ulnocarpal articulation in adult biomechanical analyses.[105,153] Biomechanical and clinical studies have shown that this load distribution is important in fractures, TFCC tears (positive ulnar variance), and Kienbock disease (negative ulnar variance).[4,75]

The distal radius normally rotates around the relatively stationary ulna. The two bones of the forearm articulate at the proximal radioulnar joints and DRUJs. In addition, proximally the radius and ulna articulate with the distal humerus and distally with the carpus. These articulations are necessary for forearm pronation and supination. At the DRUJ, the concave sigmoid notch of the radius incompletely matches the convex, asymmetric, semicylindrical shape of the distal ulnar head.[22,153] This allows some translation at the DRUJ with rotatory movements. The ligamentous structures are critical in stabilizing the radius as it rotates about the ulna (Fig. 8-23).

TREATMENT OPTIONS FOR FRACTURES OF THE DISTAL RADIUS AND ULNA

NONOPERATIVE TREATMENT OF FRACTURES OF THE DISTAL RADIUS AND ULNA

The goal of pediatric distal radius fracture care is to achieve bony union within acceptable radiographic parameters to optimize long-term function and avoid late complications. Management is influenced tremendously by the remodeling potential of the distal radius in growing children (Fig. 8-24). In general, remodeling potential is dependent on the amount of skeletal growth remaining, proximity of the injury to the physis, and relationship of the deformity to plane of adjacent joint motion. Fractures in very young children, close to the distal radial physis, with predominantly sagittal plane angulation have the greatest remodeling capacity. Acceptable sagittal plane angulation of acute distal radial metaphyseal fractures has been reported to be from 10 to 35 degrees in patients under 5 years of age.[63,108,114,149,163,171,211] Similarly, in patients under 10 years of

surface.[100] However, measurement of ulnar variance in children requires modifications of this technique. Hafner et al.[89] described measuring from the ulnar metaphysis to the radial metaphysis to lessen the measurement inaccuracies related to epiphyseal size and shape, a technique recently validated by Goldfarb et al. (Fig. 8-21).[80] If the ulna and radius are of equal lengths, there is a neutral variance. If the ulna is longer, there is a positive variance. If the ulna is shorter, there is a negative variance. Variance measurement is made in millimeters.

Although not dependent on the length of the ulnar styloid,[22] the measurement of ulnar variance is dependent on forearm position and radiographic technique.[61] Radiographs of the wrist to determine ulnar variance should be standardized with the hand

Figure 8-20. The attachment and the fibers of the interosseous membrane are such that there is no attachment to the distal radius. (Redrawn from Kraus B, Horne G. Galeazzi fractures. *J Trauma*. 1985;25:1094.)

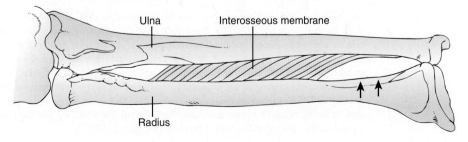

Ulna

Interosseous membrane

Radius

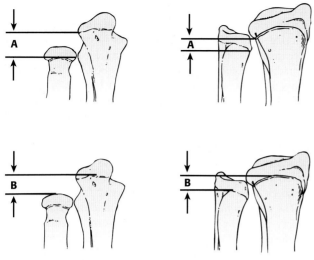

Figure 8-21. Hafner's technique to measure ulnar variance. **A:** The distance from the most proximal point of the ulnar metaphysis to the most proximal point of the radial metaphysis. **B:** The distance from the most distal point of the ulnar metaphysis to the most distal point of the radial metaphysis. (Adapted by permission from Springer: Hafner R, Poznanski AK, Donovan JM. Ulnar variance in children. Standard measurements for evaluation of ulnar shortening in juvenile rheumatoid arthritis, hereditary multiple exostosis and other bone or joint disorders in childhood. *Skel Radiol.* 1989;18(4):513–516. Copyright © 1989 International Skeletal Society.)

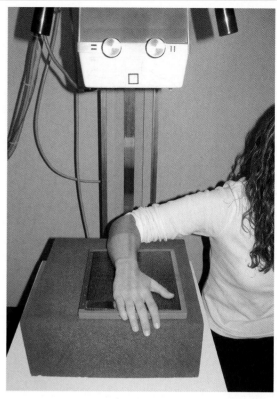

Figure 8-22. Technique for neutral rotation radiograph with wrist neutral, forearm pronated, elbow flexed 90 degrees, and shoulder abducted 90 degrees.

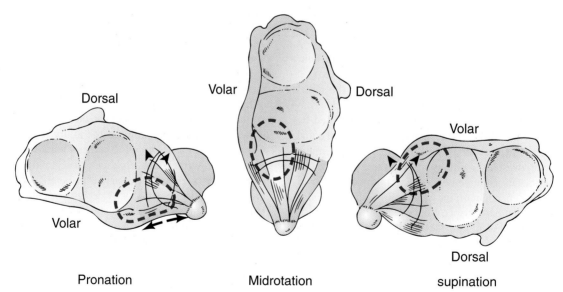

Pronation   Midrotation   supination

Figure 8-23. Distal radioulnar joint stability in pronation (**left**) is dependent on tension developed in the volar margin of the triangular fibrocartilage (TFCC, *small arrowheads*) and compression between the contact areas of the radius and ulna (volar surface of ulnar articular head and dorsal margin of the sigmoid notch, *large arrows*). Disruption of the volar TFCC would therefore allow dorsal displacement of the ulna in pronation. The reverse is true in supination, where disruption of the dorsal margin of the TFCC would allow volar displacement of the ulna relative to the radius as this rotational extreme is reached. The dark area of the TFCC emphasizes the portion of the TFCC that is not supported by the ulnar dome. The *dotted circle* is the arc of load transmission (lunate to TFCC) in that position. (Redrawn from Bowers WH. *Green's Operative Hand Surgery.* New York: Churchill-Livingstone; 1993.)

age, the degree of acceptable angulation has ranged from 10 to 25 degrees (Table 8-1).[63,108,114,149,163,171,211]

Criteria for what constitutes acceptable frontal plane deformity have been more uniform. The fracture tends to displace radially with an apex ulnar angulation. This deformity also has remodeling potential,[154,223] but less so than sagittal plane deformity. Most authorities agree that 10 degrees or less of acute malalignment in the frontal plane should be accepted. Greater magnitudes of coronal plane malalignment may not remodel and may result in limitations of forearm rotation.[42,44,54,62,210]

In general, 10 to 30 degrees maximum of sagittal plane angulation, 10 to 15 degrees maximum of radioulnar deviation, and even complete bayonet apposition will reliably remodel in younger children with at least 2 years of significant growth remaining.[50,70,97,223]

Indications/Contraindications

Nonoperative Treatment of Distal Radius Fractures:
INDICATIONS AND CONTRAINDICATIONS

Indications	Relative Contraindications
Torus fractures	Open fractures
Nondisplaced fractures	Neurovascular compromise or excessive swelling precluding circumferential cast immobilization
Displaced fractures within acceptable radiographic alignment	
Displaced fractures amenable to closed reduction and immobilization	Irreducible fracture in unacceptable alignment
Late-presenting physeal fractures	Unstable fractures failing initial reduction and cast immobilization
Distal radial physeal stress fractures	

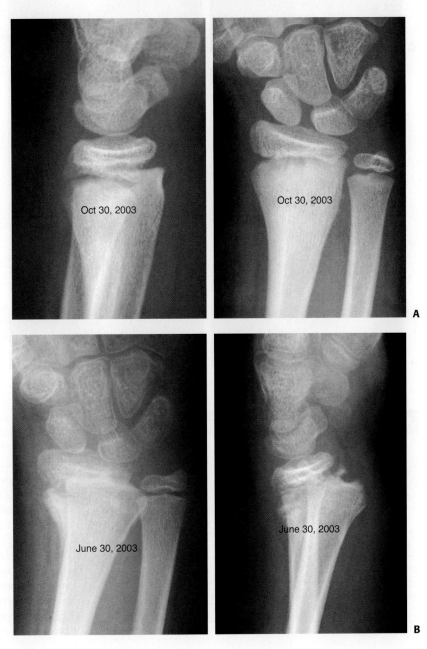

Oct 30, 2003

Oct 30, 2003

A

June 30, 2003

June 30, 2003

B

Figure 8-24. A: AP and lateral views of displaced radial physeal fracture. **B:** Healed malunion 1 month after radial physeal fracture.

(continues)

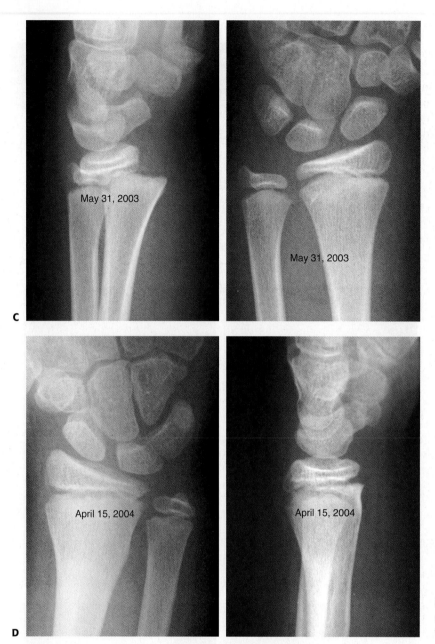

C

D

Figure 8-24. (*Continued*) **C:** Significant remodeling at 5 months after fracture. **D:** Anatomic remodeling with no physeal arrest.

TABLE 8-1. Angular Corrections in Degrees

| | Sagittal Plane | | |
Age (yrs)	Boys	Girls	Frontal Plane
4–9	20	15	15
9–11	15	10	5
11–13	10	10	0
>13	5	0	0

Acceptable residual angulation is that which will result in total radiographic and functional correction.

(Courtesy of B. De Courtivron, MD. Centre Hospitalie Universitaire de Tours. Tours, France.)

For the reasons cited above, most pediatric distal radius fractures can be successfully treated with nonoperative means (no reduction or closed reduction, cast immobilization). General indications for nonoperative treatment include torus fractures, displaced physeal or metaphyseal fractures within acceptable parameters of expected skeletal remodeling, displaced fractures with unacceptable alignment amenable to closed reduction and immobilization, and late-presenting displaced physeal injuries in which late closed reduction has high risk of growth arrest.

Contraindications to nonoperative care include open fractures, fractures with excessive soft tissue injury or neurovascular compromise precluding circumferential cast immobilization, irreducible fractures in unacceptable alignment, unstable fractures failing initial nonoperative care, and fractures with displacement that will not remodel sufficiently to be acceptable long term.

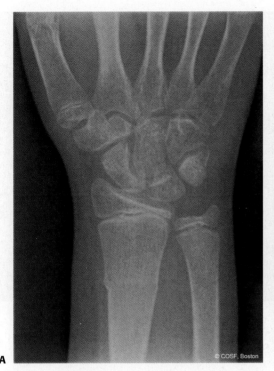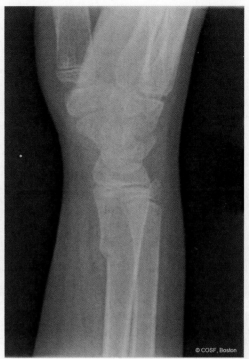

Figure 8-25. Anteroposterior (**A**) and lateral (**B**) radiographs of a distal radius torus fracture.

Splint Immobilization of Torus Fractures

By definition, torus fractures are compression fractures of the distal radial metaphysis and are therefore inherently stable (Fig. 8-25). There is typically minimal cortical disruption or displacement. As a result, treatment should consist of protected immobilization to prevent further injury and relieve pain. Multiple studies have compared the effectiveness and cost of casting, splinting, and simple soft bandage application in the treatment of torus fractures. As expected, there is little difference in outcome of the various immobilization techniques.[2,21,102,147,163,173,182,207]

Davidson et al.[43] randomized 201 children with torus fractures to plaster cast or removable wrist splint immobilization for 3 weeks. All patients went on to successful healing without complications or need for follow-up clinical visits or radiographs. Similarly, Plint et al.[161] reported the results of a prospective randomized clinical trial in which 87 children were treated with either short-arm casts or removable splints for 3 weeks. Not only were there no differences in healing or pain, but also early wrist function was considerably better in the splinted patients. West et al.[209] even challenged the need for splinting in their clinical study randomizing 39 patients to either plaster casts or soft bandages. Again, fracture healing was universal and uneventful, and patients treated with soft bandages had better early wrist motion.

Given the reliable healing seen with torus fracture healing, Symons et al.[186] performed a randomized trial of 87 patients treated with plaster splints to either hospital follow-up or home removal. No difference was seen in clinical results, and patient/families preferred home splint removal. A similar study by Khan et al.[115] confirmed these findings. No differences in outcomes were seen in 117 patients treated with either rigid cast removal in fracture clinic versus soft cast removal at home, and families preferred home removal of their immobilization.

A meta-analysis of torus and minimally displaced fractures treated by removable splints instead of circumferential casts was found to have improved secondary outcomes for the patient and family and with equal position at healing.[11] SCAMPs (Standardized Clinical Assessment and Management Plans) work from Boston Children's Hospital has indicated that reduction in casting and postinjury radiographs, coupled with phone call follow-up visits, have lessened direct and indirect costs, radiation and cast saw injury risk significantly, with no change or improved outcome for torus fractures.[130,131]

Therefore, simple splinting is sufficient, and once the patient is comfortable, range-of-motion exercises and nontraumatic activities may begin. Fracture healing usually occurs in 3 to 4 weeks.[2,10] Simple torus fractures heal without long-term sequelae or complications.

Cast Immobilization of Nondisplaced or Minimally Displaced Distal Radial Metaphyseal and Physeal Fractures

Nondisplaced fractures are treated with cast immobilization until appropriate bony healing and pain resolution have been achieved.[47,52,175] Although these fractures are radiographically well aligned at the time of presentation, fracture stability is difficult to assess and a risk of late displacement exists (Fig. 8-26). Serial radiographs are obtained in the first 2 to 3 weeks posttreduction to confirm maintenance of acceptable radiographic alignment. In general, most fractures will heal within 4 to 6 weeks.

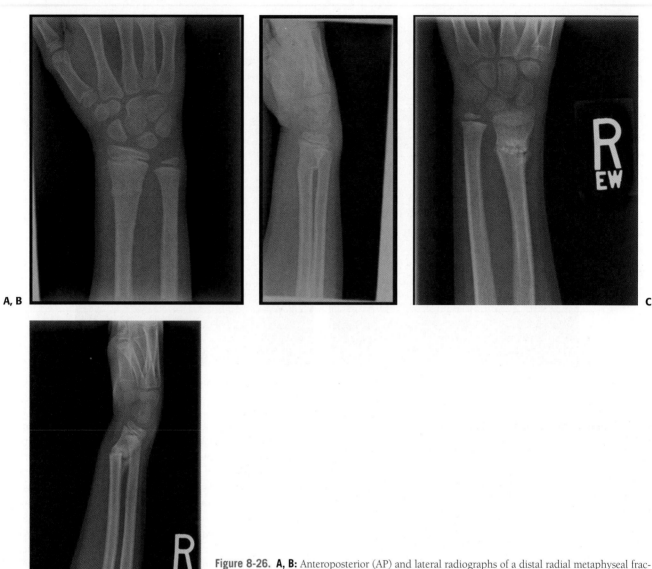

Figure 8-26. A, B: Anteroposterior (AP) and lateral radiographs of a distal radial metaphyseal fracture. This injury was initially assumed to be stable and was treated with cast immobilization with suboptimal mold. **C, D:** Subsequent radiographs taken 3 weeks after injury demonstrate loss of alignment and early bony healing. (Courtesy of Children's Orthopaedic Surgery Foundation.)

Simple immobilization without reduction may also be considered in minimally displaced fractures within acceptable alignment, based on patient age and remodeling potential. Hove and Brudvik[98] evaluated a cohort of 88 patients treated nonoperatively for distal radius fractures. Though eight patients had early loss of reduction with greater than 15 to 20 degrees angulation, all demonstrated complete remodeling and restoration of normal function later. Al-Ansari et al. similarly evaluated 124 patients with "minimally angulated" distal radius fractures. Even patients who healed with 30 to 35 degrees angulation went on to complete fracture remodeling and normal function.[5] Finally, in a prior randomized clinical trial, 96 patients between 5 and 12 years of age with distal radius fractures with less than 15 degrees of sagittal plane angulation were treated with either cast or splint immobilization.[21] No difference was seen in fracture alignment at 6 weeks in the two treatment groups, and functional outcomes did not differ, as measured by the Activity Scale for Kids. Though the risk of late displacement and issues of compliance and comfort exist, this investigation supports the concept that splint immobilization may be considered in younger patients (age <10 years) with minimal displacement. The high potential for remodeling of a distal radial metaphyseal malunion has led some clinicians to recommend immobilization alone.[50] Cast immobilization alone without fracture manipulation may even be effective in young patients with complete dorsal displacement and bayonet apposition with acceptable sagittal and coronal plane alignments. Crawford et al. prospectively evaluated 51 children under the age of 10 years treated with cast immobilization for shortened and bayoneted fractures of the distal radial metaphysis.[38,50] All patients went on to complete radiographic remodeling and full return of wrist motion.

Reduction and Immobilization of Incomplete Fractures of the Distal Radius and Ulna

Treatment of incomplete distal radial and ulna fractures is similarly dependent on patient age and remodeling potential, magnitude, and direction of fracture displacement and angulation, and the biases of the care provider and patient/family regarding fracture remodeling and deformity. In cases of incomplete or greenstick distal radius fractures—with or without ulnar involvement—with unacceptable deformity, closed reduction and cast immobilization are recommended.

The method of reduction for greenstick fractures depends on the pattern of displacement. With apex volar angulated fractures of the radius, the rotatory deformity is supination. Pronating the radius and applying a dorsal-to-volar reduction force is utilized to restore bony alignment. Conversely, fractures with apex dorsal angulation result from pronation mechanisms of injury. Supinating the distal forearm and applying a volar-to-dorsal force should reduce the incomplete fracture of the radius.[137] Though these fractures are incomplete and patients often present with minimal pain, adequate analgesia will facilitate bony reduction and quality of cast application. Typically, this is done with the assistance of conscious sedation.[64,79,114]

Following reduction, portable fluoroscopy may be used to evaluate fracture alignment. Once acceptable alignment is achieved, a cast is applied with appropriate rotation and three-point molds, based on the initial pattern of injury. Long-arm casting is typically used for the first 4 weeks, and bony healing is achieved in 6 weeks in the majority of patients. A short-arm cast with acceptable cast indices is equally effective.

As in the case of torus fractures,[197] there is a study indicating that soft bandages can be applied to treat incomplete greenstick forearm fractures[120]; however, as the greenstick fracture is substantially more unstable than the torus fracture,[168] the authors do not advocate soft bandage treatment of greenstick fractures.

Closed Reduction and Cast Immobilization of Displaced Distal Radial Metaphyseal Fractures

Closed reduction and cast immobilization remains the standard of care for children with displaced distal radial metaphyseal fractures presenting with unacceptable alignment. Again, fracture reduction maneuvers are dependent on injury mechanism and fracture pattern. In patients with typical dorsal displacement of the distal epiphyseal fracture fragment with apex volar angulation, closed reduction is performed with appropriate analgesia, typically conscious sedation or general anesthesia. Finger traps applied to the ipsilateral digits may facilitate limb positioning and stabilization during fracture reduction but application of weights may hinder reduction by increasing dorsal periosteal tension. Recently, the lower extremity-aided fracture reduction maneuver (LEAFR) has been proposed as a simple, effective, reproducible, and mechanically advantageous technique of effectuating closed reductions in children with bayoneted distal radius fractures.[59] Given the stout, intact dorsal periosteum in these injuries, pure longitudinal traction is often insufficient to restore bony alignment, particularly in cases of bayonet apposition. Fracture reduction is performed first by hyperextension and exaggeration of the deformity, which relaxes the dorsal periosteal sleeve (Fig. 8-27). Longitudinal traction is then applied to restore adequate length. Finally, the distal fracture fragment is flexed to correct the translational and angular displacement, with rotational correction imparted as well. If available, fluoroscopy may be utilized to confirm adequacy of reduction, and a well-molded cast is applied.

The optimal type of cast immobilization remains controversial. Both long- and short-arm casts have been proposed following distal radial fracture reduction.[31,88,93,207] Long-arm casts have the advantage of restricting forearm rotation and theoretically reducing the deforming forces imparted to the distal radius. However, above-elbow immobilization is more inconvenient

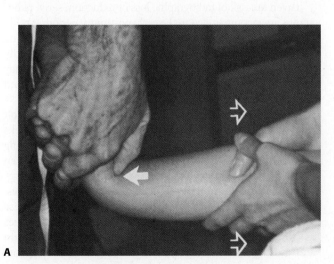

A

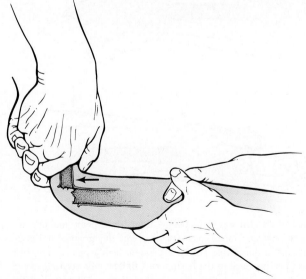

B

Figure 8-27. A, B: Use of the thumb to push the distal fragment hyperdorsiflexed 90 degrees (*solid arrow*) until length is reestablished. Countertraction is applied in the opposite direction (*open arrows*).

(continues)

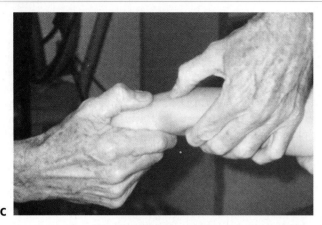

C

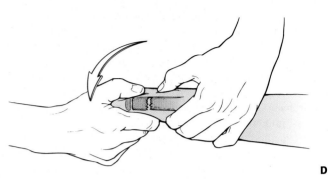

D

Figure 8-27. (*Continued*) **C, D:** Once length has been reestablished, the distal fragment is flexed into the correct position. Alignment is checked by determining the position of the fragments with the thumb and forefingers of each hand.

and has been associated with greater need for assistance with activities of daily living, as well as more days of school missed.[207] Prior randomized controlled trials have demonstrated that short-arm casts are as effective at maintaining reduction as long-arm casts, provided that acceptable alignment is achieved and an appropriate cast mold is applied.[20,207] A recent meta-analysis pooling the results of over 300 study subjects has further supported these findings.[93]

Perhaps more important than the length of the cast applied is the cast mold applied at the level of the fracture (Fig. 8-28). Appropriate use of three-point molds will assist in maintenance of alignment in bending injuries. Similarly, application of

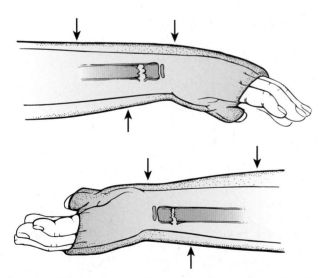

Figure 8-28. Three-point molding. **Top:** Three-point molding for dorsally angulated (apex volar) fractures, with the proximal and distal points on the dorsal aspect of the cast and the middle point on the volar aspect just proximal to the fracture site. **Bottom:** For volar angulated fractures, where the periosteum is intact volarly and disrupted on the dorsal surface, three-point molding is performed with the proximal and distal points on the volar surface of the cast and the middle point just proximal to the fracture site on the dorsal aspect of the cast.

interosseous mold will help to maintain interosseous space between the radius and ulna as well as coronal plane alignment. A host of radiographic indices have been proposed to quantify and characterize the quality of the cast mold, including the cast index, three-point index, gap index, padding index, Canterbury index, and second metacarpal/distal radius angle (Fig. 8-29).[10,57,90,164] Although the cast index is easily calculated and perhaps most widely utilized, some authorities tout the three-point index as the preferred index for this assessment and prediction of redisplacement.[48]

Complete fractures of the distal radius have a higher rate of loss of reduction after closed treatment than do incomplete fractures (Fig. 8-30). Indeed, prior investigations have demonstrated that 20% to 30% of patients will have radiographic loss of reduction following closed reduction and casting of displaced distal radius fractures. Risk factors for loss of reduction include greater initial fracture displacement and/or comminution, suboptimal reduction, suboptimal cast mold, and associated distal ulna fractures.[6,10,48,57,90,141,164]

Given the risk of radiographic loss of reduction, serial radiographs are recommended in the early postinjury period. Weekly radiographs are obtained in the first 2 to 3 weeks following reduction to confirm adequacy of alignment. Failure to identify and correct malalignment in the early postinjury period may lead to malunion and subsequent clinical loss of motion and upper limb function.

Malalignment of fractures during the development of soft tissue callus before bridging ossification (injury to 2 to 3 weeks after reduction) often can be realigned using cast wedging (Fig. 8-31).[14,17,36,85,101,191,208] Recently, this technique has been utilized less frequently given the advances in surgical management of fractures. Authors have advocated opening wedges, closing wedges, as well as a combination of each of these approaches. Most commonly we use open wedge techniques as closing wedges have the potential for pinching of the skin and causing accumulation of cast padding at the wedge site which may cause skin breakdown.[85,101] In addition, closing wedges also may shorten and reduce the volume of the cast thus decreasing fracture stability. There have been multiple

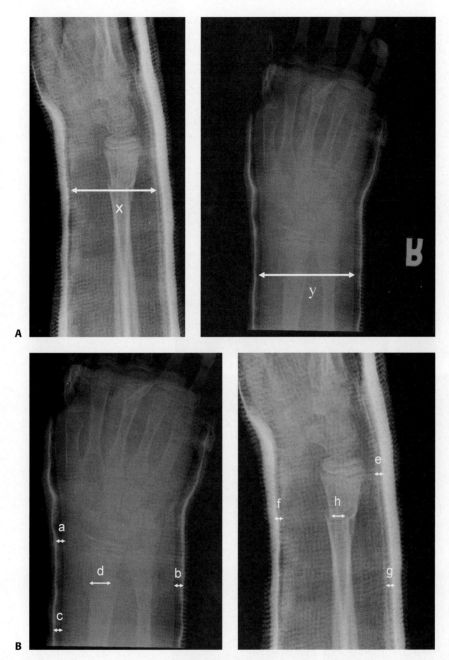

Figure 8-29. Radiographic evaluation of cast mold. **A:** Cast index (x/y) is the ratio of the inner cast diameter at the level of the fracture on the lateral projection (x) to the inner cast diameter at the level of the fracture as seen on the anteroposterior (AP) view (y). **B:** The three-point index is the sum of the three critical gaps divided by the contact area of the fracture fragments. The anteroposterior 3-point index is (a + b + c)/d. The lateral 3-point index is (e + f + g)/h. (Courtesy of Children's Orthopaedic Surgery Foundation.)

techniques proposed for predicting the size of a wedge. Bebbington et al.[14] suggested a technique that involves tracing the angle of displacement onto the cast itself thus representing the fracture fragments. Wedges are then inserted until the malalignment is reduced as the traced line becomes straight. Wells et al. recently described a technique in which the wedge position and opening angle are determined from the radiographic displacement and center of rotational alignment. Utilizing these methods on saw bones, they were able to reduce malalignment within 5 degrees with 90% success.[208] Regardless of the method, if utilized appropriately, cast wedging reduces the risk of additional anesthesia and potential surgery.

Displaced Distal Radial Physeal Fractures

Most displaced Salter–Harris I and II fractures are treated with closed reduction and cast stabilization. Closed manipulation of the displaced fracture is similarly performed with appropriate conscious sedation, analgesia, or, rarely, anesthesia to achieve pain relief and an atraumatic reduction.[64,79,114] Most of these

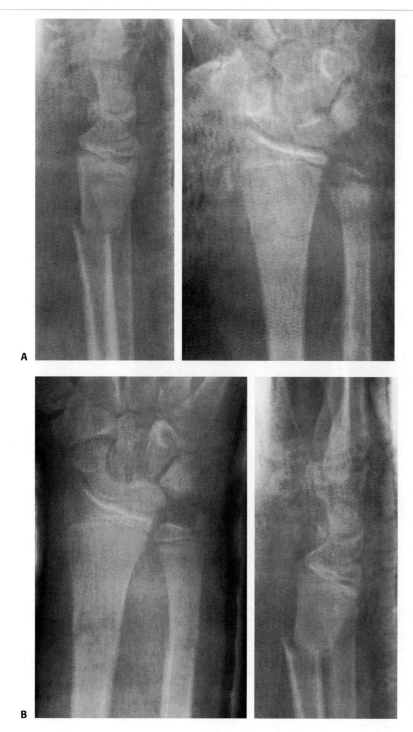

Figure 8-30. A: Serial radiographs at 3 days and 10 days (**B**) revealing slow loss of reduction that is common after closed reduction of distal radial metaphyseal fractures.

fractures involve dorsal and proximal displacement of the epiphysis with an apex volar extension deformity. Manipulative reduction is by gentle distraction and flexion of the distal epiphysis, carpus, and hand over the proximal metaphysis (Fig. 8-32). The intact dorsal periosteum is used as a tension band to aid in reduction and stabilization of the fracture. Unlike similar fractures in adults, finger trap distraction with pulley weights is often counterproductive. However, finger traps can help stabilize the hand, wrist, and arm for manipulative reduction and casting by applying a few pounds of weight for balance.

Otherwise, an assistant is helpful to support the extremity in the proper position for casting.

If portable fluoroscopy is available, immediate radiographic assessment of the reduction is obtained. Otherwise, a well-molded cast is applied and AP and lateral radiographs are obtained to assess the reduction. The cast should provide three-point molding over the distal radius to lessen the risk of fracture displacement and should follow the contour of the normal forearm. The distal dorsal mold should not impair venous outflow from the hand, which can occur if the mold is placed too

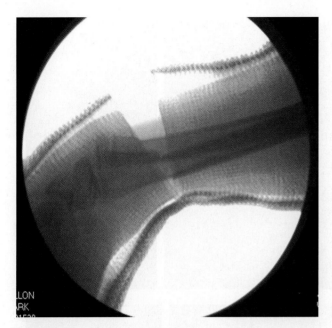

Figure 8-31. Lateral fluoroscopic projection of a distal radius fracture treated with dorsal cast wedging to correct loss of reduction. (Courtesy of Children's Orthopaedic Surgery Foundation.)

distal and too deep so as to obstruct the dorsal veins. Advocates of short-arm casting indicate at least equivalent results with proper casting techniques and more comfort during immobilization due to free elbow mobility. Instructions for elevation and close monitoring of swelling and the neurovascular status of the extremity are critical.

The fracture also should be monitored closely with serial radiographs to be certain that there is no loss of anatomic alignment (Fig. 8-33). Generally, these fractures are stable after closed reduction and cast immobilization. If there is loss of reduction after 7 days, the surgeon should be wary of repeat

reduction, as forceful remanipulation may increase the risk of iatrogenic physeal arrest.[27,125,176] Fortunately, remodeling of an extension deformity with growth is common if the patient has more than 2 years of growth remaining and the deformity is less than 20 degrees. Even marked deformity can remodel if there is sufficient growth remaining and the deformity is in the plane of motion of the wrist.

Galeazzi Fracture Repair

Nonoperative management remains the first-line treatment for pediatric Galeazzi fractures, distinguishing these injuries from their adult counterparts.[56,171,200] Indeed, the adult Galeazzi fracture has been often called a "fracture of necessity," given the near-universal need for surgical reduction and internal fixation to restore anatomic radial alignment and DRUJ congruity. In pediatric patients, however, the distal radial fracture often is a greenstick type that is stable after reduction; therefore, nonoperative treatment with closed reduction and cast immobilization is often sufficient.[109,171] Surgical treatment may be considered for adolescents with complete fractures and displacement, as their injury pattern, skeletal maturity, remodeling potential, and DRUJ instability concerns are more similar to the adult Galeazzi.

Incomplete fractures of the distal radius with either a true dislocation of the DRUJ or an ulnar physeal fracture are treated with closed reduction and long-arm cast immobilization. This can be done in the emergency room with conscious sedation or in the operating room with general anesthesia. Portable fluoroscopy is useful in these situations. If the radius fracture has apex volar angulation and dorsal displacement of the radius with associated volar dislocation of the ulnar head in relationship to the radius, pronation and volar-to-dorsal force on the radial fracture are used for reduction. Conversely, if the radius fracture is apex dorsal with volar displacement and dorsal dislocation of the distal ulna, supination and dorsal-to-volar force is utilized

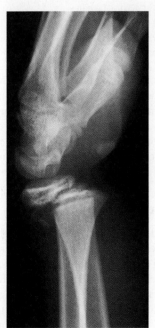
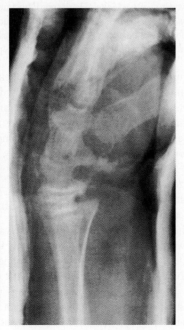

A, B

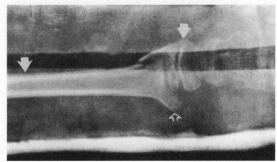

C

Figure 8-32. A: Lateral radiograph of dorsally displaced Salter–Harris type II fracture. **B:** Lateral radiograph after closed reduction and cast application. **C:** Reduction of the volar displaced fracture. The forearm was in supination with three-point molding anterior over the distal epiphysis and proximal shaft (*white arrows*). The third point is placed dorsally over the distal metaphysis (*open arrow*). (The dorsal surface of the cast is oriented toward the bottom of this figure.) (Reprinted from Wilkins KE, ed. *Operative Management of Upper Extremity Fractures in Children*. Rosemont, IL: American Academy of Orthopaedic Surgeons; 1994:17, with permission.)

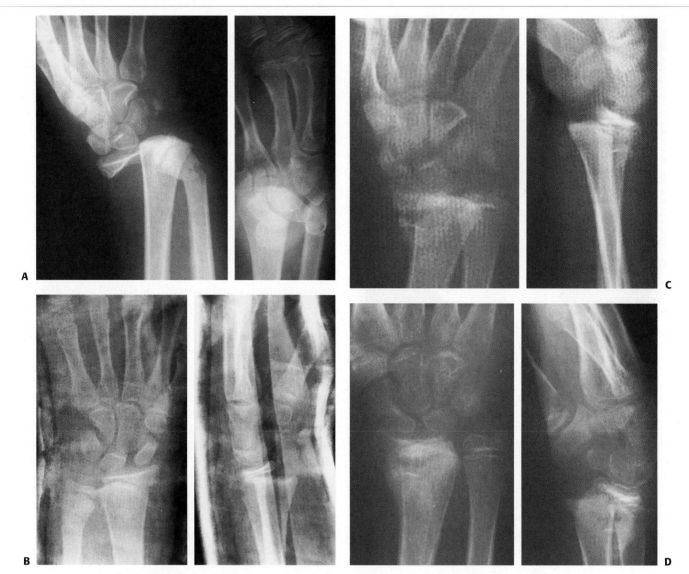

Figure 8-33 A: AP and lateral radiographs of severely displaced Salter–Harris type II fracture of the distal radius. **B:** Closed reduction shows marked improvement but not anatomic reduction. The case had to be bivalved due to excess swelling. **C:** Unfortunately, the patient lost reduction after a new fiberglass cast was applied. **D:** Out-of-cast radiographs show a healed malunion in a similar position to the prereduction radiographs.

during reduction. The reduction and stability of the fracture and DRUJ dislocation may then be checked on dynamic fluoroscopy; if both are anatomically reduced and stable, a long-arm cast with the forearm in the appropriate rotatory position of stability (i.e., pronation or supination) is applied. Six weeks of long-arm casting is recommended to allow for sufficient bony and soft tissue healing.

In patients with Galeazzi-equivalent injuries characterized by complete distal radius fractures associated with ulnar physeal fractures, both bones should be reduced. Usually, this can be accomplished with the same methods of reduction as when the radial fracture is incomplete. If there is sufficient growth remaining and the distal ulnar physis remains open, remodeling of a nonanatomic distal ulnar physeal reduction may occur. As long as the DRUJ is reduced, malalignment of less than 10 degrees can remodel in a young child. DRUJ congruity and stability, however, are dependent on distal ulnar alignment, and

great care should be taken in assessment of the DRUJ when accepting a nonanatomic distal ulnar reduction. Furthermore, the risk of ulnar growth arrest after a Galeazzi equivalent has been reported to be as high as 55%.[81] If the fracture is severely malaligned, the DRUJ cannot be reduced, or the patient is older and remodeling is unlikely, open reduction and smooth pin fixation are indicated.[211]

Distal Radial Physeal Stress Fracture Repair

Treatment of distal physeal stress injuries first and foremost involves rest. This activity restriction may be challenging in the pediatric athlete, depending on the level of the sports participation and the desires of the child, parents, and other stakeholders to continue athletic participation. Education regarding the long-term consequences of a growth arrest is important in these emotionally charged situations. Short-arm cast immobilization for several weeks may be the only way to restrict stress to the distal radial physis in some patients. Splint protection is appropriate in cooperative patients. Protection should continue until there is resolution of tenderness and pain with activity. The young athlete can maintain cardiovascular fitness, strength, and flexibility while protecting the injured wrist. Once the acute physeal injury has healed, return to weight-bearing and open-chain activities should be gradual. The process of return to sports should be protective, often 3 to 6 months, and adjustment of techniques and training methods is necessary to prevent recurrence. The major concern is development of a radial growth arrest in a skeletally immature patient, and consideration should be given to serial clinical and radiographic follow-up in high-risk patients to confirm maintenance of growth. A radial growth arrest will result in ulnar carpal impaction and risk of TFCC injury due to ulnar overgrowth.

Distal Ulna Physeal Fracture Repair

Treatment options are similar to those for radial physeal fractures: immobilization alone, closed reduction and cast immobilization, closed reduction and percutaneous pinning, and open reduction. Often, these fractures are minimally displaced or nondisplaced. Immobilization until fracture healing at 3 to 6 weeks is standard treatment. Closed reduction is indicated for displaced fractures with more than 50% translation or 20 degrees of angulation. Most ulnar physeal fractures reduce to a near-anatomic alignment with reduction of the concomitant radius fracture due to the attachments of the DRUJ ligaments and TFCC. Failure to obtain a reduction of the ulnar fracture may indicate that there is soft tissue interposed in the fracture site, necessitating open reduction and fixation.

Outcomes

Most of the published literature providing information on the short-term clinical and radiographic results of treatment for pediatric distal radius fractures indicates a positive outcome. With adherence to the principles and techniques described above, radiographic realignment, successful bony healing, and avoidance of complications are achieved in the majority of cases. Given the high healing capacity and remodeling potential of these injuries, there is less concern regarding long-term outcomes of nonoperative treatment compared with adult patients. In general, concerns regarding long-term outcomes have focused on patients who sustain distal radial physeal fractures and thus are at risk for subsequent growth disturbance and skeletal imbalance of the distal forearm.

The risk of growth disturbance following distal radial physeal fractures is approximately 4%. Cannata et al.[27] previously reported the long-term outcomes of 163 distal radial physeal fractures in 157 patients. Displaced fractures were treated with closed reduction and cast immobilization for 6 weeks. Mean follow-up was 25.5 years. Posttraumatic growth disturbance resulting in 1 cm or greater of length discrepancy was seen in 4.4% of distal radial and 50% of distal ulnar physeal fractures. In a similar prospective analysis of 290 children with distal radial physeal fractures, Bae and Waters[12] noted that 4% of patients went on to demonstrate clinical or radiographic distal

radial growth disturbance. Consideration should be given for follow-up radiographic evaluation following distal radial physeal fractures to assess for possible physeal arrest. In symptomatic patients with posttraumatic growth disturbance and growth remaining, surgical interventions including distal ulnar epiphysiodeses, corrective osteotomies of the radius, ulnar shortening osteotomies, and associated soft tissue reconstructions have been demonstrated to improve clinical function and radiographic alignment.[203]

OPERATIVE TREATMENT OF FRACTURES OF THE DISTAL RADIUS AND ULNA

Indications/Contraindications

Operative Treatment of Fractures of the Distal Radius and Ulna: INDICATIONS AND CONTRAINDICATIONS
Indications
Open fracture
Irreducible fracture
Floating elbow injury
Displaced, intra-articular fracture
Skeletally maturing adolescent patient with <2 years of growth remaining with an irreducible fracture or a fracture that lost initial acceptable reduction
Distal radius fractures with median neuropathy
Adolescent patients with a complete Galeazzi fracture
Contraindications
Young child with > 2 years of growth remaining, extra-articular fracture, displaced <20 degrees in the plane of motion
Physeal fracture >5 days after initial reduction that has lost reduction

Although surgical indications and techniques continue to evolve, in general surgical indications for pediatric distal radius and ulna fractures include open fractures, irreducible fractures, unstable fractures, floating elbow injuries, and fractures with soft tissue or neurovascular compromise precluding circumferential cast immobilization. Surgical reduction and fixation is also indicated in cases of joint incongruity associated with intra-articular Salter–Harris III, IV, or "triplane" fractures.

Distal radial fracture stability has been more clearly defined in adults[206] than in children. At present, an unstable fracture in a child is often defined as one in which closed reduction cannot be maintained. Pediatric classification systems have yet to more precisely define fracture stability, but this issue is critical in determining proper treatment management. As noted above, distal radial metaphyseal fractures have been shown to have a high degree of recurrent displacement and, therefore, inherent instability.[6,10,48,57,90,140,164,206] For these reasons, pediatric distal radial metaphyseal fractures are not classified in the same manner as adults in regard to stability. Instead, unstable fractures have been predominantly defined by the failure to maintain a successful closed reduction. Irreducible fractures usually are due to an entrapped periosteum or pronator quadratus.

Surgical treatment is similarly recommended in patients with neurovascular compromised and severely displaced injuries. Operative stabilization serves both to maintain adequate bony alignment and more importantly, minimize the risk of compartment syndrome due to excessive swelling and circumferential immobilization. Perhaps the best indication is a displaced radial physeal fracture with median neuropathy and significant volar soft tissue swelling (Fig. 8-34).[204] These patients are at risk for development of an acute carpal tunnel syndrome or forearm compartment syndrome with closed reduction and well-molded cast immobilization.[15,44,204] The torn periosteum volarly allows the fracture bleeding to dissect into the volar forearm compartments and carpal tunnel. If a tight cast is applied with a volar mold over that area, compartment pressures can increase dangerously. Percutaneous pin fixation allows the application of a loose dressing, splint, or cast without the risk of loss of fracture reduction.

Internal fixation usually is with smooth, small-diameter pins to lessen the risk of growth arrest. Plates and screws rarely are used unless the patient is near skeletal maturity because

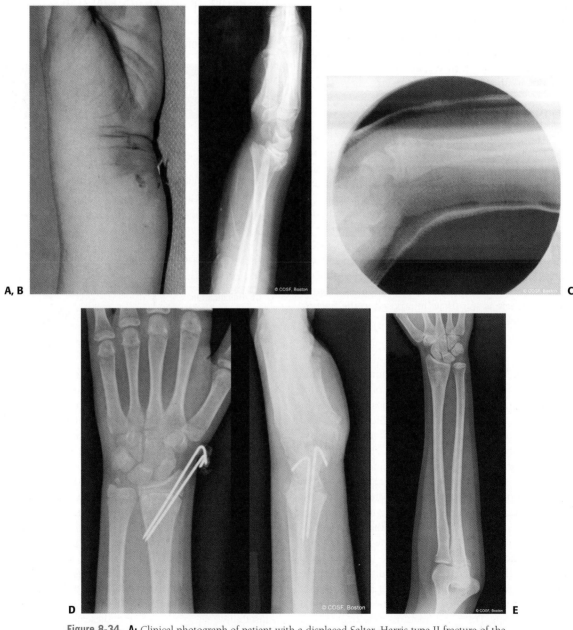

Figure 8-34. A: Clinical photograph of patient with a displaced Salter–Harris type II fracture of the distal radius. The patient has marked swelling volarly with hematoma and fracture displacement. The patient had a median neuropathy upon presentation. **B:** Lateral radiograph of the displaced fracture. **C:** Lateral radiograph following closed reduction and cast application. Excessive flexion has been utilized to maintain fracture reduction, resulting in persistent median neuropathy and increasing pain. **D:** Radiographs following urgent closed reduction and percutaneous pinning. **E:** Follow-up radiograph depicting distal radial physeal arrest and increased ulnar variance. (Courtesy of Children's Orthopaedic Surgery Foundation.)

of concerns about further physeal injury. In the rare displaced intra-articular Salter–Harris type III or IV fracture, internal fixation can be intraepiphyseal without violating the physis. If it is necessary to cross the physis, then smooth, small-diameter pins should be used to lessen the risk of iatrogenic physeal injury. Extra-articular external fixation also can be used to stabilize and align the fracture.

Closed Reduction and Pin Fixation of Displaced Distal Radial Fractures

Preoperative Planning

✔ Closed Reduction and Pin Fixation of Displaced Distal Radial Fractures: PREOPERATIVE PLANNING CHECKLIST	
OR table	☐ Standard; radiolucent hand table
Position/positioning aids	☐ Supine with affected limb supported by radiolucent hand table or image intensifier of fluoroscopy unit
Fluoroscopy location	☐ Variable, dependent on surgeon position
Equipment	☐ Smooth Kirschner (K)-wires, typically 0.045 or 0.062 in in diameter
Tourniquet	☐ Nonsterile

Preoperative planning begins with careful clinical and radiographic evaluation. Thorough neurovascular examination is performed to assess for signs and symptoms of nerve injury or impending compartment syndrome. Radiographs—both from the time of injury, after initial attempts at closed reduction, and any subsequent follow-up radiographs—are carefully evaluated to assess pattern of injury and direction of instability.

Given the relative simplicity of closed reduction and percutaneous fixation techniques, minimal equipment is required. Intraoperative fluoroscopy and surgical instrumentation for pin placement are typically sufficient.

Positioning

After adequate induction of general anesthesia, patients are positioned supine on a standard operating table, with the affected limb abducted and supported on a radiolucent hand table. While a nonsterile tourniquet may be applied to the proximal brachium, this is typically not utilized. Fluoroscopy may be brought in from the head, foot, or side of the patient, depending on surgeon position and preference. For example, as most pinning is performed from distal to proximal, the right-hand–dominant surgeon may wish to sit in the axilla and have the fluoroscopy unit come in from the head of the patients when pinning a left distal radius.

Surgical Approach

While percutaneous pinning may be performed without need for skin incision, placement of smooth C- or K-wires into the

region of the radial styloid carries the risk of iatrogenic radial sensory nerve or extensor tendon injury.[137] For this reason, a small longitudinal incision over the radial styloid at the site of pin insertion may be utilized to identify and retract adjacent soft tissues, facilitating safe pin passage. Alternatively, smooth pins may be inserted using an oscillating technique.

Technique

✔ Closed Reduction and Pin Fixation of Distal Radius Fractures: KEY SURGICAL STEPS
☐ Closed reduction of distal radius fracture
☐ Confirm bony alignment with intraoperative fluoroscopy
☐ Small incision over radial styloid
• Longitudinal spreading in subcutaneous tissues
• Retraction/protection of radial sensory nerve and extensor tendons
☐ Place smooth wire from distal fracture fragment, across fracture site, engaging the ulnar cortex of the proximal fracture fragment
• Fluoroscopic confirmation of pin trajectory and placement
☐ Assess fracture stability
☐ Place second wire if needed
• Cross-pinning may be performed from dorsoulnar corner of distal radial epiphysis proximally and radially into proximal fracture fragment
☐ Assess stability
☐ Bend and cut pins outside of skin
☐ Sterile dressing and cast application
☐ Pin removal after adequate bony healing, typically in 4 weeks

After appropriate anesthesia, closed reduction of the distal radius fracture into anatomic alignment is performed using the principles and techniques previously described. While maintaining fracture reduction, a skin incision is made over the radial styloid, long enough to ascertain there is no iatrogenic injury to the radial sensory nerve or extensor tendons (Fig. 8-35). Careful longitudinal spreading is performed in the subcutaneous tissues, and the radial sensory nerve and extensor tendons may be identified and carefully retracted. Pin fixation

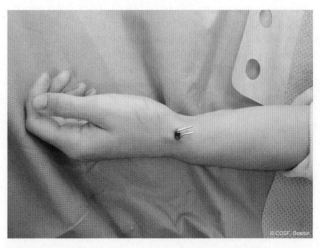

Figure 8-35. Small incision noted with pins left out of skin for removal at 4 weeks. (Courtesy of Children's Orthopaedic Surgery Foundation.)

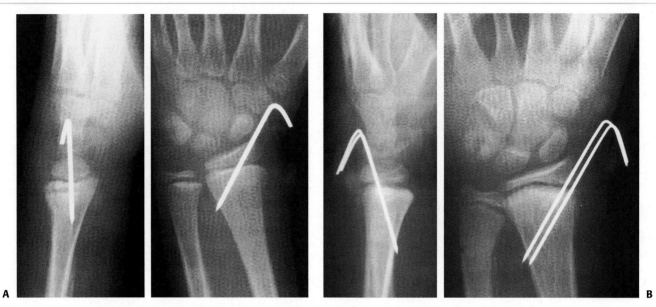

Figure 8-36. A: AP and lateral radiographs of displaced Salter–Harris type II fracture pinned with a single pin. **B:** After reduction and pinning with parallel pins.

can be either single or double, though often a single pin will suffice (Fig. 8-36). A smooth pin is then inserted into the distal fracture fragment and passed obliquely in a proximal and ulnar fashion, crossing the fracture site and engaging the far ulnar cortex proximal to the fracture line. Fluoroscopy is used to guide proper fracture reduction and pin placement.

Pin(s) may be placed within the distal radial epiphysis and passed across the physis before engaging the more proximal metaphyseal fracture fragment. Alternatively, smooth pins may be placed just proximal to the distal radial physis; while theoretically decreasing the risk of physeal disturbance, this has not been well demonstrated in the published literature.

Stability of the fracture should be evaluated with flexion and extension and rotatory stress under fluoroscopy. Often, in children and adolescents, a single pin and the reduced periosteum provide sufficient stability to prevent redisplacement of the fracture (Fig. 8-37). If fracture stability is questionable with a single pin, a second pin should be placed. The second pin can either parallel the first pin or, to create cross-pin stability, can be placed distally from the dorsal ulnar corner of the radial epiphysis between the fourth and fifth dorsal compartments and passed obliquely to the proximal radial portion of the metaphysis (Fig. 8-38). Again, the skin incisions for pin placement should be sufficient to avoid iatrogenic injury to the extensor tendons.

The pins are bent, left out of the skin, and covered with petroleum gauze and sterile dressing. Splint or cast immobilization is used but does not need to be tight, as fracture stability is conferred by the pins. The pins are left in until there is adequate fracture healing (usually 4 weeks). The pins can be removed in the office without sedation or anesthesia.

One of the arguments against pin fixation is the risk of additional injury to the physis by a pin.[23] The risk of physeal arrest is more from the displaced fracture than from a short-term, smooth pin. As a precaution, smooth, small-diameter pins should be used, insertion should be as atraumatic as possible,

and removal should be done as soon as there is sufficient fracture healing for fracture stability in a cast or splint alone.

Another pinning technique involves intrafocal placement of multiple pins into the fracture site to lever the distal fragment into anatomic reduction (Fig. 8-39). The pins are then passed through the opposing cortex for stability.[129,194] A supplemental, loose-fitting cast is applied.

Open Reduction and Fixation of Distal Radius Fractures

Preoperative Planning

✔	**Open Reduction and Fixation of Distal Radius Fractures:** PREOPERATIVE PLANNING CHECKLIST	
OR table	☐ Standard, radiolucent hand table
Position/positioning aids	☐ Supine
Fluoroscopy location	☐ Variable depending on surgeon preference
Equipment	☐ Smooth wires (0.0625-in diameter), small fragment 3.5-mm plates and screws, precontoured volar locking plates in older patients or intra-articular fractures
Tourniquet	☐ Nonsterile tourniquet placed on ipsilateral proximal brachium

Open reduction is indicated for open or irreducible fractures. Open fractures constitute approximately 1% of all distal radial metaphyseal fractures. Although treatment approaches to open fractures continue to evolve, at present the standard of care remains surgical irrigation and debridement, followed by

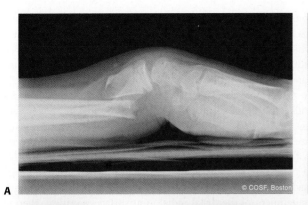

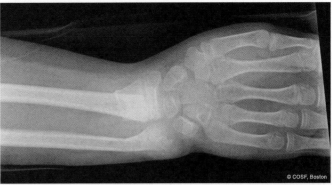

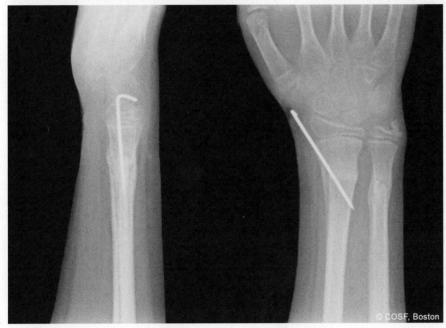

Figure 8-37. Severe swelling. **A, B:** Complete displacement and bayonet apposition of a distal radial fracture associated with severe swelling from a high-energy injury. **C:** Once reduced, the fragment is secured with an oblique percutaneous pin across the fracture site, sparing the distal radial physis.

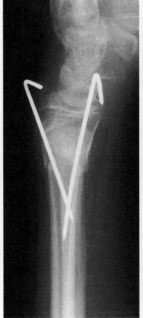

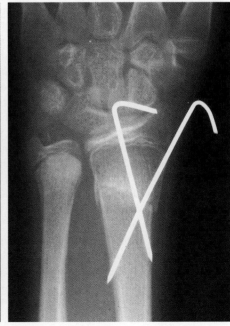

Figure 8-38. Crossed-pin technique for stabilization of distal radial metaphyseal fracture in a skeletally immature patient. (Courtesy of Children's Orthopaedic Surgery Foundation.)

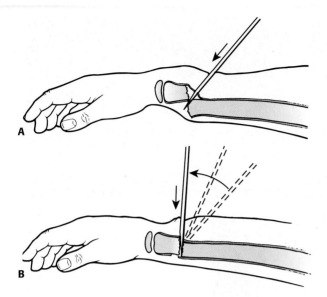

Figure 8-39. Pin leverage. **A:** If a bayonet is irreducible, after sterile preparation, a chisel-point Steinmann pin can be inserted between the fracture fragments from a dorsal approach. Care must be taken not to penetrate too deeply past the dorsal cortex of the proximal fragment. **B:** Once the chisel is across the fracture site, it is levered into position and supplementary pressure is placed on the dorsum of the distal fragment (*arrow*) to slide it down the skid into place. This procedure is usually performed with an image intensifier.

appropriate fracture care (also see Controversies) regarding nonoperative management of open fractures.

Irreducible metaphyseal or physeal fractures are rare and generally are secondary to interposed soft tissues. With dorsally displaced fractures, the interposed structure usually is the volar periosteum or pronator quadratus[95] and rarely the flexor tendons or neurovascular structures.[95,112,216] In volarly displaced fractures, the periosteum or extensor tendons may be interposed.

Closed reduction rarely fails if there is no interposed soft tissue. Occasionally, however, multiple attempts at reduction of a bayonet apposition fracture can lead to significant swelling that makes closed reduction impossible. If the patient is too old to remodel bayonet apposition, open reduction is appropriate.

Plate fixation can be used in more skeletally mature adolescents. Low-profile, fragment-specific fixation methods and locking plates also are now commonly used for internal fixation of distal radial fractures in adults. The utility of these anatomically contoured locking plates in children and skeletally immature adolescents is unknown, as is the deleterious effect, if any, on growth potential. Furthermore, the advantage of these more rigid constructs in younger patients in whom adequate stability may be achieved with pins is unclear, particularly given the reports of late tendon rupture and other soft tissue complications associated with fixed-angle volar plates.[167] Indications for skeletally mature adolescents are the same as for adults. Articular malalignment and comminution are assessed by CT preoperatively, and fracture-specific fixation is used as appropriate. These plates have proved to be quite useful in indicated cases.

Preoperative planning for open reduction and fixation is similar to the approach cited above, with a few additional considerations. Assessment of skeletal maturity and physeal status is important, particularly when considering use of implants which rigidly engage the distal radial epiphysis and when open reduction may potentially increase the risk of physeal disturbance. Secondly, children are not small adults, and care should be made to evaluate the width of the distal radial metaphysis and epiphysis. Use of precontoured volar locking plates typical of adult distal radius fractures may not be feasible, given size mismatch and/or presence of an open distal radial physis. With the numerous plate options available, it is quite feasible to match up sizes of plate and bone. Finally, care should be made to assess for articular extension of the fracture. Anatomic realignment of the distal radial joint surface is critical, even in the young child.

Positioning

Patients are positioned supine with the affected limb supported by a radiolucent hand table. Positioning of the fluoroscopic unit is similar to that in closed reduction and pinning techniques.

Surgical Approach

All open fractures, regardless of grade of soft tissue injury, should be irrigated and debrided in the operating room (Fig. 8-40). The open wound should be enlarged adequately to debride the contaminated and nonviable tissues and identify, protect, or if needed, repair the adjacent neurovascular structures. Judicious extension of the traumatic wound will allow for extensile exposure, facilitate fracture reduction, and allow for implant placement.

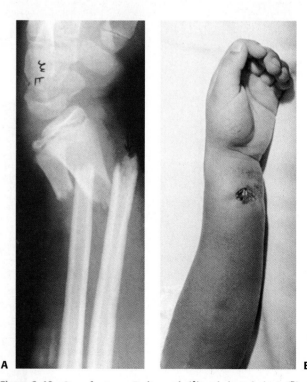

Figure 8-40. Open fractures. Radiograph (**A**) and clinical photo (**B**) of an open fracture of the distal radius. This patient needs formal irrigation and debridement in the operating room.

Open reduction for closed unstable or irreducible fractures is typically performed through a volar approach to the distal radius. A longitudinal incision overlying the flexor carpi radialis (FCR) tendon is created, centered on the fracture site with awareness of the location of the distal radial physis. Classically, superficial dissection is carried out in the interval between the radial artery and the FCR. In distal radius fractures, dissection may also be performed directly through the FCR sheath by incising the roof of the FCR sheath and retracting the tendon ulnarly; the intact radial FCR sheath, when retracted, will serve to protect the adjacent radial artery. Deep to the FCR, a fat plane will be encountered overlying the pronator quadratus. The pronator quadratus is incised along its radial border, leaving a small cuff of tissue for subsequent repair, and elevated in a subperiosteal fashion from radial to ulnar. Although this muscle can be interposed in the fracture site, the volar periosteum is more commonly interposed. This is evident only after elevation of the pronator quadratus. The periosteum is extracted from the physis with care to minimize further injury to the physis. Upon completion of pronator quadratus elevation, the fracture may be easily visualized.

Technique

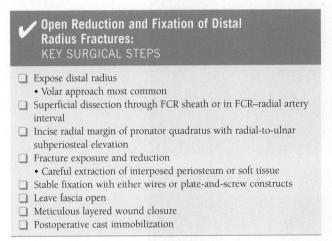

✔ **Open Reduction and Fixation of Distal Radius Fractures:**
KEY SURGICAL STEPS

☐ Expose distal radius
  • Volar approach most common
☐ Superficial dissection through FCR sheath or in FCR–radial artery interval
☐ Incise radial margin of pronator quadratus with radial-to-ulnar subperiosteal elevation
☐ Fracture exposure and reduction
  • Careful extraction of interposed periosteum or soft tissue
☐ Stable fixation with either wires or plate-and-screw constructs
☐ Leave fascia open
☐ Meticulous layered wound closure
☐ Postoperative cast immobilization

After adequate fracture exposure is obtained, bony reduction is performed easily using similar maneuvers as during closed manipulations. Once anatomic fracture alignment is achieved, percutaneous smooth K-wires may be used for stabilization of the reduction. The method of pin insertion is the same as after closed reduction; use of a small incision during wire insertion will minimize risk to the radial sensory nerve and extensor tendons.

Similarly for open fracture care, fracture reduction and fixation is performed, usually with two smooth wires, after thorough irrigation and debridement. In the uncommon open physeal fractures, care is taken with mechanical debridement to avoid injury to the physeal cartilage. If the soft tissue injury is severe, supplemental external fixation allows observation and treatment of the wound without jeopardizing the fracture reduction. The original open wound should not be closed primarily. Appropriate prophylactic antibiotics should be used depending on the severity of the open fracture.

Plate fixation may also be used for stabilization following open reduction. While the indications for plate fixation evolve and remain patient- and surgeon-dependent, plate fixation is more strongly considered in multitrauma patients, comminuted fractures, older patients nearing or at skeletal maturity, refractures, and fractures at the metaphyseal–diaphyseal junction in whom percutaneous pinning techniques are more challenging.

Following standard surgical exposure and fracture reduction, neutralization or dynamic compression plates are applied to the radius using techniques similar to adult fracture care, with a few caveats. Standard 3.5-mm implants may be too bulky for younger or smaller pediatric patients. In these situations, double-stacked one-third tubular plates, 2.7-mm plates, or 2.4-mm plates may be used. In addition, given the rapid bony healing, stout periosteum, and postoperative cast immobilization characteristic of pediatric fracture care, two cortices of fixation may be sufficient distal to the fracture site. Finally, in patients with skeletal growth remaining, implants should be placed sparing the distal physis.

In older adolescents at skeletal maturity or those with intra-articular injuries, volar locking plates may be used for internal fixation. Although a host of commercially available plates are available, the principles are constant: meticulous exposure, anatomic fracture reduction, and stable fixation proximal and distal to the fracture site. Care should be made in anatomically contoured volar locking plates to avoid penetration of obliquely angled distal locking screws into the radiocarpal joint, as well as excessive dorsal prominence of screws, which may lead to late extensor tendon irritation or rupture (Fig. 8-41).

Following fixation, the pronator quadratus, FCR sheath, and subcutaneous tissues are closed in layers, followed by skin closure. In cases of plate fixation, short-arm cast immobilization is sufficient postoperatively.

Fixation of Intra-Articular Fractures

Preoperative Planning

✔ **Open Reduction and Fixation of Intra-Articular Fractures:**
PREOPERATIVE PLANNING CHECKLIST

OR table	☐ Standard, radiolucent hand table
Position/positioning aids	☐ Supine
Fluoroscopy location	☐ Variable depending on surgeon preference
Equipment	☐ K-wires, small fragment plating systems, anatomically precontoured volar locking plates, small joint arthroscope
Tourniquet	☐ Nonsterile tourniquet placed on proximal brachium
Other	☐ Adequate preoperative imaging, including CT or MRI

The rare Salter–Harris type III or IV fracture or "triplane" fracture[157] may require open reduction if the joint or physis cannot be anatomically reduced via closed means. If anatomic

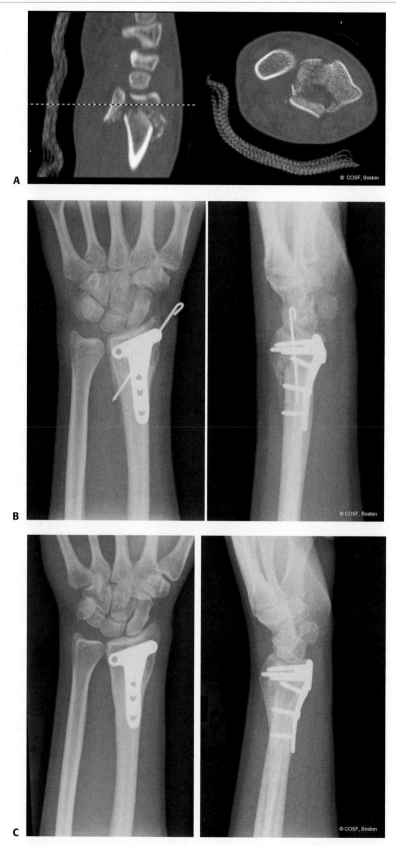

Figure 8-41. ORIF of distal radius with T plate and supplemental pin fixation. **A:** Injury CT scan revealing intra-articular displacement. **B:** ORIF with T buttress plate and supplemental styloid pin 1-month postoperative. **C:** One year after ORIF with anatomic alignment and asymptomatic hardware. (Courtesy of Children's Orthopaedic Surgery Foundation.)

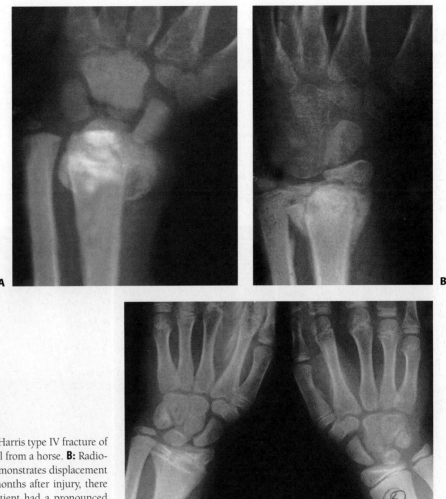

Figure 8-42. A: A markedly displaced Salter–Harris type IV fracture of the distal radius in an 11-year-old boy who fell from a horse. **B:** Radiograph taken 3 weeks after closed reduction demonstrates displacement of the comminuted fragments. **C:** Eighteen months after injury, there was 15 mm of radial shortening, and the patient had a pronounced radial deviation deformity of the wrist.

alignment of the physis and articular surface is not present, the risk of growth arrest, long-term deformity, or limited function is great (Fig. 8-42). Even minimal displacement (more than 2 mm) should not be accepted in this situation.

Preoperatively, CT or MRI scans are invaluable in defining fracture pattern, assessing articular congruity, and planning definitive treatment (Fig. 8-43). Based on these images, appropriate preoperative planning may be performed. There is great variation in fracture patterns, and treatment and fixation must be individualized to restore bony alignment and stability. In addition to traditional percutaneous and open techniques, arthroscopically assisted reduction may be helpful to align and stabilize these uncommon intra-articular fractures.[53] Although equipment-intensive, anatomic reduction and stabilization of the physis and articular surface can be achieved with arthroscopy, fluoroscopy, and combinations of external fixation or transphyseal fixation pins or screws (Fig. 8-44).

Positioning

Standard positioning is used, as described above. In cases where wrist arthroscopy is to be performed, use of a wrist traction tower with finger trap suspension applied to the index and long

fingers will stabilize the wrist and provide appropriate traction for arthroscopic visualization.

Surgical Approach

The volar surgical approach remains the standard workhorse exposure for distal radius fractures requiring open reduction. Often, more distal subperiosteal elevation is needed to visualize intra-articular fracture lines. This is more common in older, skeletally mature adolescents.

In many intra-articular fracture patterns, there are radial styloid and/or dorsal lunate facet fragments that necessitate exposure, reduction, and fixation. In these cases, supplemental dorsal approaches may need to be used. A longitudinal incision based over or ulnar to Lister's tubercle is most commonly used and provides a utilitarian approach. Superficial dissection is performed to the extensor retinaculum, with preservation of the dorsal veins if possible. In dorsal lunate facet fractures, incision of the retinaculum over the third or fourth extensor compartment and subsequent retraction of the extensor pollicis longus or extensor digitorum communis tendons, respectively, will provide access to the distal dorsal radius. Care is made to preserve the origins of the radiocarpal ligaments whenever possible.

Technique

✔ Fixation of Intra-Articular Fractures:
SURGICAL PRINCIPLES

- ❑ Careful preoperative evaluation of fracture pattern, comminution, and displacement
- ❑ Fracture-specific surgical approaches
- ❑ Articular realignment
  - • Use of traction, wrist arthroscopy, fluoroscopy, or arthrotomy to aid in visualization
- ❑ Stabilization of the articular surface to the proximal radius
- ❑ Fixation using K-wires, interfragmentary screws, or plate-and-screw constructs for maintenance of alignment

Given the spectrum of intra-articular distal radius fracture patterns, a sequential description of surgical steps is difficult; each patient must be treated in an individualized fashion according to fracture pattern, size of bony fragments, severity of displacement, and skeletal maturity. Universal surgical principles of adequate fracture reduction, anatomic realignment, and stable fixation will provide for optimal results. A few additional considerations are important.

Attempts should be made to achieve closed or minimally invasive reduction whenever possible. With adequate anesthesia, muscle relaxation, and traction, displaced articular fragments may often be anatomically realigned, facilitating percutaneous fixation or implant placement without violating

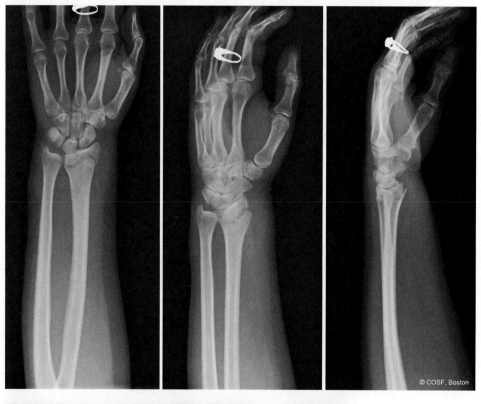

A

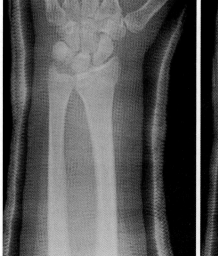 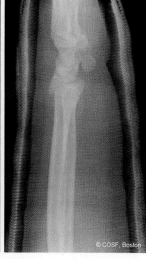

B

Figure 8-43. A: Displaced distal radius metaphyseal and intra-articular fracture. **B:** Emergency department postreduction radiographs in cast.

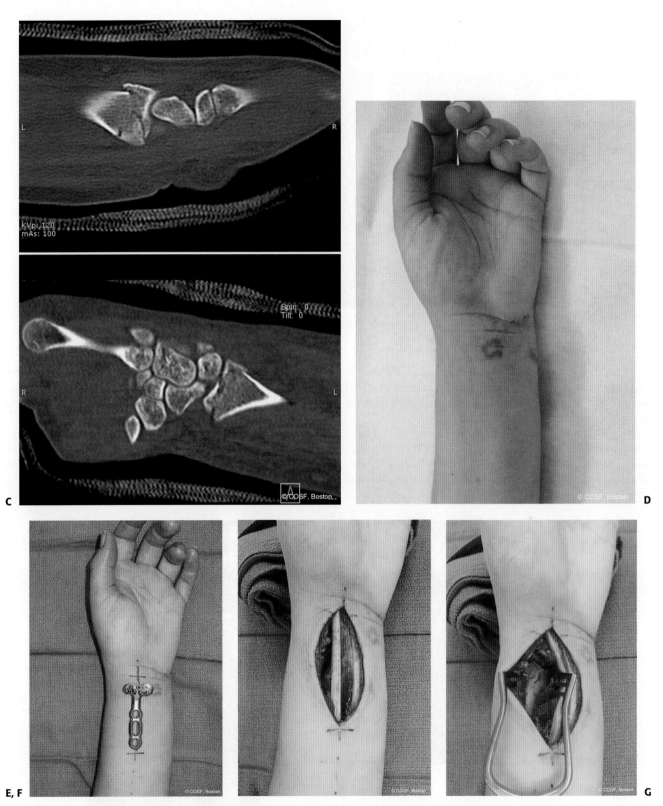

Figure 8-43. (*Continued*) **C:** Representative postreduction CT scan images revealing joint displacement. **D:** Clinical appearance after decreased swelling over 5 days preoperatively. **E:** Planned plate for fracture-fragment–specific volar fixation. **F:** Volar approach via FCR tendon sheath. **G:** Exposed fracture site with reduction.

(*continues*)

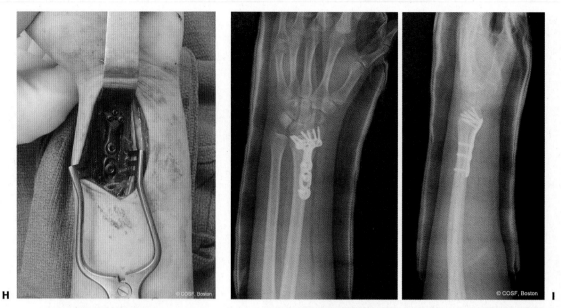

Figure 8-43. (*Continued*) **H:** Plate fixation of fracture anatomically. **I:** Radiographs of ORIF with volar plating system. (Courtesy of Children's Orthopaedic Surgery Foundation.)

the radiocarpal joint or physis. Furthermore, K-wires may be used to joystick-displaced fracture fragments or in an intrafocal fashion[194] to further assist in fracture reduction. Intraoperative fluoroscopy is invaluable in these cases.

Wrist arthroscopy may be a helpful adjunct for articular visualization.[35,53] With approximately 10 to 12 lb of distraction placed via finger traps to the index and long fingers, a small joint arthroscope (2.4 to 2.9 mm in diameter) may be inserted into the standard 3 to 4 wrist arthroscopy portal; this portal lies between the third and fourth extensor compartments and is typically 1 to 2 cm distal to Lister's tubercle. Care should be taken to avoid excessive extravasation of arthroscopy fluid into the zone of injury during arthroscopy; expeditious arthroscopy and use of low pressure and flow rates are helpful in these situations.

Finally, a wide spectrum of internal fixation options is available. Percutaneous K-wires are effective when properly positioned, particularly in younger patients with open physes in whom efforts are made to minimize the risk of iatrogenic growth

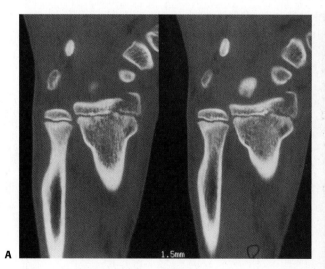

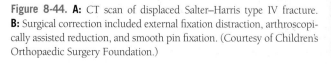

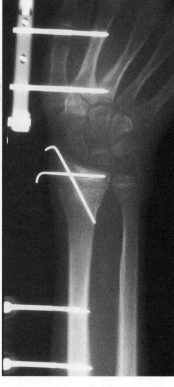

Figure 8-44. A: CT scan of displaced Salter–Harris type IV fracture. **B:** Surgical correction included external fixation distraction, arthroscopically assisted reduction, and smooth pin fixation. (Courtesy of Children's Orthopaedic Surgery Foundation.)

disturbance. Wires passed obliquely from distal to proximal are effective for radial styloid and dorsal lunate facet fracture fragments; similarly, transverse epiphyseal pins may impart stability to articular fracture fragments. In older patients nearing or at skeletal maturity, adult-like locking plate constructs may be used.

Reduction and Fixation of Distal Ulna Fractures

Open reduction is performed in cases where acceptable alignment is not achieved following radial reduction and attempted closed manipulation. This is an indication for open reduction.

Preoperative Planning

Preoperative planning and patient positioning are similar to that of displaced distal radius fractures.

Surgical Approach

Incisions for surgical exposure of the ulna are typically ulnar or dorsoulnar, though ideally, surgical exposure approaches the ulna from the side of periosteal disruption. In physeal fractures, the periosteum is typically torn opposite the Thurston–Holland fragment; in metaphyseal injuries, periosteal injury is opposite the direction of displacement. Deep dissection is most commonly made in the extensor carpi ulnaris—flexor carpi ulnaris interval ulnarly or the extensor digiti quinti—extensor carpi ulnaris intervals dorsally. Careful subperiosteal elevation may be performed in the zone of injury, which is typically already traumatized from the fracture. Interposed soft tissue (periosteum, extensor tendons, abductor digiti quinti, or flexor tendons) may then be identified and must be extracted from the fracture site.[1,81,184]

Technique

> ✔ **Fixation of Displaced Distal Ulna Fractures:**
> KEY SURGICAL STEPS
>
> ❑ Expose distal ulna
> • Preserve distal ulnar physis, capsular attachments of DRUJ and ulnocarpal joint, and ulnar wrist ligaments whenever possible
> ❑ Anatomic reduction of ulnar fracture
> ❑ Stable fixation based on fracture pattern and patient age
> • K-wire fixation
> • K-wire with tension-band construct
> • Plate-and-screw fixation
> ❑ Assess DRUJ alignment and stability intraoperatively
> ❑ Postoperative cast immobilization

Following exposure, soft tissue extraction, and bony reduction, if fracture instability persists, internal fixation is performed. Often, a single small-diameter smooth K-wire can be used to maintain alignment. This K-wire may be passed obliquely from distal to proximal, crossing the fracture site. In older patients with larger bones and greater instability, two parallel K-wires may be used, and this may be further supplemented by tension-band fixation (Fig. 8-45). A small drill hole made proximal to the fracture site is created, and a nonabsorbable braided suture or small-caliber stainless steel wire is passed through the drill hole and around the previously placed K-wires in a figure-of-eight fashion. Pins are typically removed after 4 weeks following radiographic confirmation of bony healing. Plate-and-screw fixation may also be performed in distal metaphyseal fractures and/or older, skeletally mature patients. Use of smaller implants, distal locking screws, or mini-fragment blade plates will assist in obtaining adequate

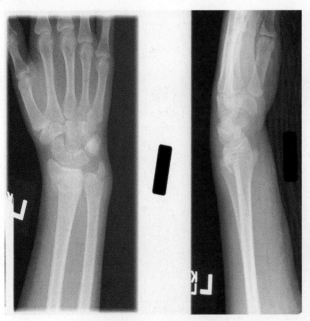
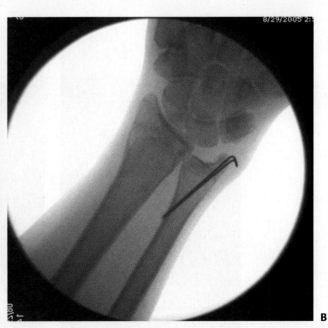

A   **B**

Figure 8-45. A: Plain radiographs depicting displaced distal radial metaphyseal and ulnar styloid fractures. Given the fracture and distal radioulnar joint instability, the injury was treated with closed reduction and percutaneous pinning of the distal radius as well as open reduction and tension-band fixation of the ulnar styloid. **B:** Follow-up radiograph following reduction and fixation demonstrates anatomic alignment. The prior radial pins have been removed, and the parallel smooth wires used for tension-band fixation of the ulnar styloid are seen. (Courtesy of Children's Orthopaedic Surgery Foundation.)

fixation in the often small distal ulnar fracture fragment. Further injury to the physis should be avoided during operative exposure and reduction because of the high risk of growth arrest.[81]

ORIF of Galeazzi Fractures

Open reduction of the radius is indicated in Galeazzi fractures or fracture equivalents in cases of failure to obtain or maintain fracture and DRUJ reduction. This most often occurs with unstable complete fractures in older adolescents.

Preoperative Planning

Preoperative planning and patient positioning are similar as described above. Unlike adult Galeazzi fracture dislocations, advanced imaging (e.g., CT or MRI) is rarely needed in pediatric patients.

Surgical Approach

Open reduction and internal fixation of complete radius fractures is performed through a standard volar approach, as described above. In the majority of acute injuries, with anatomic reduction of the radius, restoration of radial length and alignment will allow for spontaneous reduction of the DRUJ. Occasionally, however, the DRUJ dislocation cannot be reduced via closed means (Fig. 8-46). In these situations, the first intraoperative step is to reassess the quality of radial fracture reduction and fixation. Following this, open reduction of the DRUJ may be performed to remove any interposed soft tissues blocking reduction (periosteum, extensor carpi ulnaris tendon, extensor digiti quinti tendon, other ligamentous structures).[56,86,110,126,151,172,201]

The easiest approach for open reduction of the DRUJ is an extended ulnar approach. Care should be taken to avoid injury to the ulnar sensory nerve branches, which typically pass obliquely from proximal volar to distal dorsal in the region of the ulnar styloid. This approach allows exposure both volarly and dorsally to extract the interposed soft tissues and repair the torn structures. Alternatively, a Bowers' approach to the DRUJ may be used (Fig. 8-47). A curvilinear incision is made over the DRUJ. The fifth dorsal extensor compartment is incised and the extensor digiti quinti is retracted. The DRUJ lies immediately deep to this interval, and the joint may be opened and inspected, facilitating reduction.

Technique

> ✔ **ORIF of Galeazzi Fractures:**
> **SURGICAL STEPS**
>
> ❏ Expose distal radius fracture
> ❏ Anatomic reduction and stabilization of radius
>   • Plate fixation preferred
> ❏ Careful intraoperative assessment of forearm rotation and DRUJ stability
>   • Intraoperative fluoroscopy to confirm DRUJ alignment
> ❏ If DRUJ not reducible, open reduction via ulnar or Bowers' approach
> ❏ If DRUJ not reducible in setting of distal ulnar physeal fracture, open reduction and stabilization of ulnar fracture performed
> ❏ Radioulnar pinning in cases of reducible but unstable DRUJ reduction
> ❏ Long-arm cast immobilization for 6 weeks
>   • If utilized, radioulnar pin removal 4 to 6 weeks postoperatively

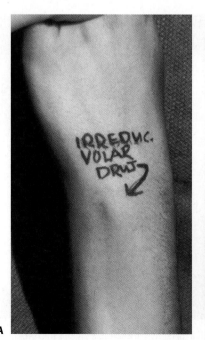 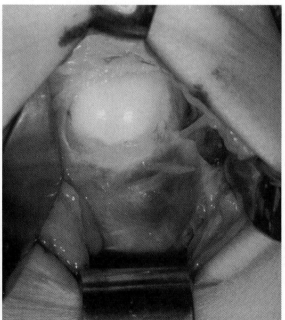

A **B**

Figure 8-46. An adolescent girl presented 4 weeks after injury with a painful, stiff wrist. **A:** By examination, she was noted to have a volar distal radioulnar dislocation that was irreducible even under general anesthesia. **B:** At the time of surgery, the distal ulna was found to have buttonholed out of the capsule, and there was entrapped triangular fibrocartilage and periosteum in the joint. (Courtesy of Children's Orthopaedic Surgery Foundation.)

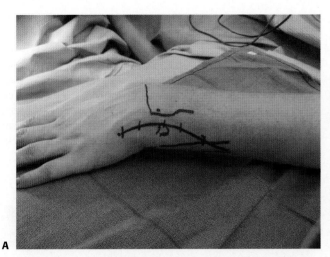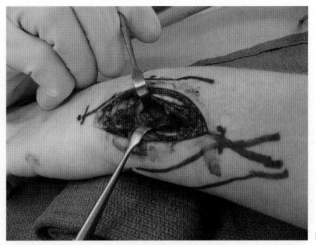

A   B

Figure 8-47. A: Clinical photograph depicting the dorsoulnar curvilinear incision used to approach the distal radioulnar joint in a patient with an irreducible Galeazzi fracture. **B:** Intraoperative photograph depicting the sigmoid notch of the distal radius. The ECU and EDQ tendons are seen retracted volarly and radially. The volarly displaced distal ulna remains dislocated. (Courtesy of Children's Orthopaedic Surgery Foundation.)

Open reduction and internal fixation of the radius is done through an anterior approach. Standard compression plating is preferred to intramedullary or cross-pinning techniques (Fig. 8-48). Stable, anatomic reduction of the radius almost always leads to stable reduction of the DRUJ dislocation. A long-arm cast is used for 6 weeks to allow fracture and soft tissue healing.

If the DRUJ dislocation cannot be reduced, it is exposed as described above. Typically after anatomic alignment of the radius and extraction of any soft tissues blocking DRUJ reduction, the joint is stable and no additional fixation is required. In cases of extreme instability and/or soft tissue compromise, smooth K-wire fixation of the DRUJ can be used to maintain reduction and allow application of a loose-fitting cast. The K-wire(s) are placed with the forearm in supination and passed transversely across from the reduced DRUJ from the ulna to the radius (usually all four cortices penetrated), and the pin(s) left

Figure 8-48. A: The patient with a pronation injury had a closed reduction and attempted fixation with pins placed percutaneously across the fracture site. However, this was inadequate in maintaining the alignment and length of the fracture of the distal radius. **B:** The length of the radius and the distal radioulnar relationship were best reestablished after internal fixation of the distal radius with a plate placed on the volar surface. The true amount of shortening present on the original injury film is not really appreciated until the fracture of the distal radius is fully reduced. (Reprinted from Wilkins KE, ed. *Operative Management of Upper Extremity Fractures in Children.* Rosemont, IL: American Academy of Orthopaedic Surgeons; 1994:34, with permission.)

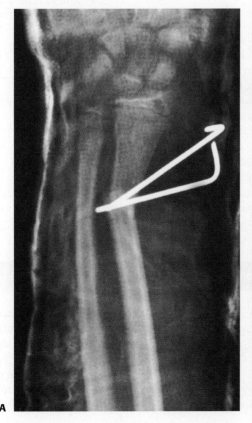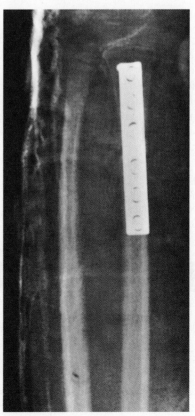

A   B

exposed out of the skin. Pin removal is in the office at 4 weeks with continuation of the cast for 6 weeks.

Ulnar physeal fractures may also be irreducible in Galeazzi-equivalent injuries. This also has been reported to be secondary to interposed periosteum, extensor tendons, or joint capsule.[56,86,122,127,151,172,201] Open reduction must be executed with care to avoid further violating the physis.

External Fixation

External fixation rarely is indicated for fractures in skeletally immature patients. Though a viable treatment option,[180] the success rates of both closed reduction and percutaneous pinning techniques make external fixation unnecessary for uncomplicated distal radial fractures in children. Presently, indications for external fixation include distal radius fractures with severe associated soft tissue injuries. Major crush injuries, open fractures, or replantations after amputation requiring additional soft tissue coverage are all indications for external fixation. Supplemental external fixation also may be necessary for severely comminuted fractures to maintain length and provide additional stability to pin or plate constructs. Standard application of the specific fixator chosen is done with care to avoid injury to the adjacent sensory nerves and extensor tendons.

Preoperative Planning

Preoperative planning and patient positioning are similar to as described above. A host of commercially available external fixators may be utilized, with selection of pin diameter based on fracture location and patient size.

Surgical Approach

In general, external fixation for distal radius fractures in children spans the radiocarpal articulation. Although nonbridging (or wrist joint sparing) constructs may be utilized, the small size of the distal radial epiphysis in young children often precludes the ability to obtain adequate purchase with external fixator pins. For this reason, typical constructs involve fixator pin placement through the index metacarpal and more proximal radial diaphysis.

Distally, a dorsoradial incision is made over the mid-diaphyseal region of the index metacarpal. Dissection is performed through the subcutaneous tissues. The periosteum may be incised via an open approach, and careful limited subperiosteal elevation will allow for the first dorsal interosseous and adductor pollicis muscles

to retract safely. Percutaneous techniques may also be utilized, with care taken to avoid inadvertent injury to the radial sensory nerve, extensor tendons, or intrinsic muscles.

Proximally, a dorsoradial approach in the region of the distal radial metadiaphysis is made. Again, identification and retraction of the radial sensory nerve are performed. Deep dissection will allow visualization of the characteristic "bare area" between the musculotendinous units of the first and second extensor compartments. A longitudinal periosteal incision is created, facilitating safe and direct placement of external fixator pins.

Technique

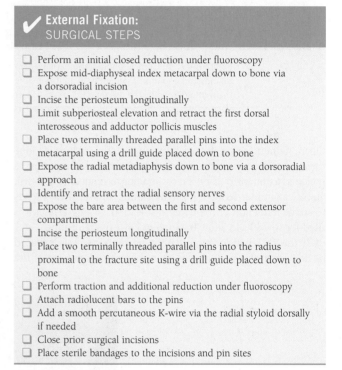

✔ **External Fixation:** SURGICAL STEPS

- ☐ Perform an initial closed reduction under fluoroscopy
- ☐ Expose mid-diaphyseal index metacarpal down to bone via a dorsoradial incision
- ☐ Incise the periosteum longitudinally
- ☐ Limit subperiosteal elevation and retract the first dorsal interosseous and adductor pollicis muscles
- ☐ Place two terminally threaded parallel pins into the index metacarpal using a drill guide placed down to bone
- ☐ Expose the radial metadiaphysis down to bone via a dorsoradial approach
- ☐ Identify and retract the radial sensory nerves
- ☐ Expose the bare area between the first and second extensor compartments
- ☐ Incise the periosteum longitudinally
- ☐ Place two terminally threaded parallel pins into the radius proximal to the fracture site using a drill guide placed down to bone
- ☐ Perform traction and additional reduction under fluoroscopy
- ☐ Attach radiolucent bars to the pins
- ☐ Add a smooth percutaneous K-wire via the radial styloid dorsally if needed
- ☐ Close prior surgical incisions
- ☐ Place sterile bandages to the incisions and pin sites

Exposure and pin placement are described as above. Following placement of two terminally threaded pins distal and proximal to the fracture, appropriate traction and reduction may be performed. Use of double-stacked radiolucent bars will increase construct rigidity and facilitate radiographic evaluation.

After fluoroscopic confirmation of pin placement and acceptable fracture alignment, prior surgical incisions may be closed primarily and sterile bandages and/or petroleum gauze may be applied to the pin sites.

Authors' Preferred Method of Treatment for Fractures of the Distal Radius and Ulna (Algorithm 8-1)

Torus Fractures

Torus fractures may be safely and effectively treated with removable splint immobilization for 3 weeks.

Incomplete Greenstick Fractures

Closed reduction and long-arm cast immobilization are performed for displaced greenstick fractures with greater than

10 degrees of angulation. With isolated distal radial fractures, it is imperative to reduce the DRUJ with appropriate forearm rotation. A long-arm cast with three-point molding is used for 3 to 4 weeks. Radiographs are obtained every 7 to 10 days until there is sufficient callus formation. A short-arm cast or volar wrist splint is then used until full healing, generally at 4 to 6 weeks after fracture reduction. Therapy rarely is required.

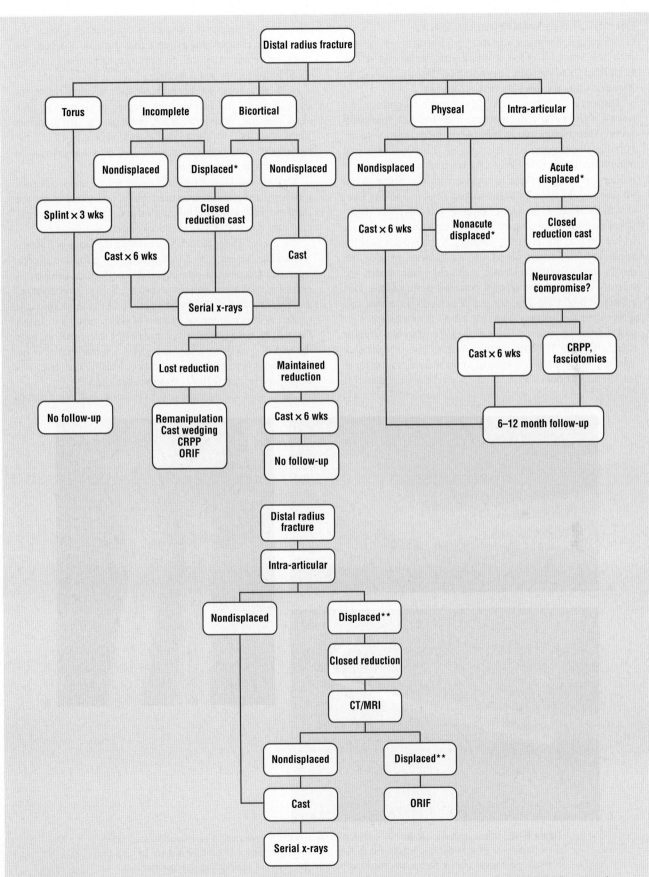

Algorithm 8-1. CRPP, closed reduction and percutaneous pinning; ORIF, open reduction and internal fixation; CT, computed tomography; MRI, magnetic resonance imaging.

Bicortical Complete Radial Metaphyseal Injuries

Nondisplaced bicortical metaphyseal fractures are treated with cast immobilization. A short-arm, well-molded cast is utilized. Radiographs are obtained for the first 2 to 3 weeks. Casts are discontinued at 6 weeks.

Displaced fractures with unacceptable alignment are treated with closed reduction and long-arm cast immobilization. This fracture can be reduced in the emergency room. Portable fluoroscopy is used. Loss of reduction with cast immobilization is more likely if the fracture is not completely reduced. A long-arm cast is applied with the elbow flexed 90 degrees, the wrist in slight palmar flexion, and the forearm in the desired rotation for stability and alignment. Rotational positioning and short- versus long-arm casting varies with each fracture and each surgeon. A three-point mold is applied at the fracture site as the cast hardens. In addition, molds are applied to maintain a straight ulnar border, the interosseous space, and straight posterior humeral line. This creates a "box" long-arm cast that lessens displacement risk rather than the "banana" cast that allows displacement. Portable fluoroscopy is used. The cast is split and spread anytime there are signs of neurovascular compromise or excessive swelling. The patient is instructed to maintain elevation for at least 48 to 72 hours after discharge and return immediately if excessive swelling or neurovascular compromise occurs. We inform our patients and parents that the risk of return for wedging, repeat reduction, or pinning under anesthesia is up to 30% during the first 3 weeks.

If there is loss of reduction, we individualize treatment depending on the patient's age, degree of deformity, time since fracture, and remodeling potential. A percutaneous pin is often used for the second reduction (Fig. 8-49). Occasionally, in pure bending injuries, loss of reduction can be corrected with cast wedging.

Cast immobilization usually is for 4 to 6 weeks. A protective volar splint is often used and activities are restricted until the patient regains full motion and strength for 2 weeks after cast removal. Physical therapy rarely is indicated.

In cases of loss of reduction exceeding the limits of fracture remodeling, repeat closed reduction and pin fixation is considered. Percutaneous pinning is also performed in cases of excessive swelling or signs of neurologic injury. Similarly, concurrent displaced supracondylar and distal radial fractures are treated with percutaneous fixation of both fractures to lessen the risk of neurovascular compromise. Older patients near the end of growth with bayonet apposition fractures also are treated with percutaneous pin fixation. Finally, open fractures usually are treated with pin fixation after I and D.

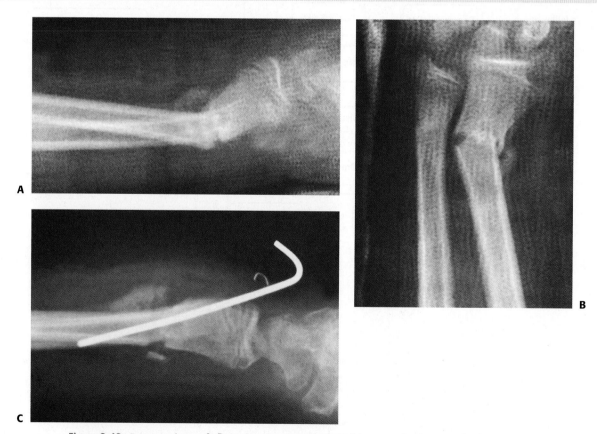

Figure 8-49. Remanipulation. **A, B:** Two weeks after what initially appeared to be a nondisplaced greenstick fracture, a 14-year-old boy was found to have developed late angulation of 30 degrees in both the coronal and sagittal planes. **C:** Because this was beyond the limits of remodeling, a remanipulation was performed. To prevent reangulation, the fracture was secured with a pin placed percutaneously obliquely through the dorsal cortex.

A small incision is made for the insertion of the pin to protect the radial sensory nerve and adjacent extensor tendons. Smooth pins are used and are removed in the office as soon as there is sufficient healing to make the fracture stable in a cast or splint (usually at 4 weeks).

Open reduction is typically reserved for open or irreducible fractures. Open fractures are irrigated and debrided in the operating room. The initial open wound is extended adequately to inspect and cleanse the open fracture site. After thorough irrigation and debridement, the fracture is reduced and stabilized. A cast rarely is applied in this situation because of concern about fracture stability, soft tissue care, and excessive swelling. Pin fixation often is used with Gustilo grade 1 or 2 open fractures. More severe soft tissue injuries may require external fixation. If flap coverage is necessary for the soft tissue wounds, the fixator pins should be placed in consultation with the microvascular surgeon planning the soft tissue coverage. In addition, open reduction internal fixation with volar plating is performed for unstable fractures in the skeletally mature adolescent.

Percutaneous pin fixation usually is used to stabilize the fracture in patients with open physes. If plate fixation is used, it should void violation of the physis (Fig. 8-50). Displaced intra-articular injuries in skeletally immature adolescents are adult-like and require open reduction and internal fixation.

Physeal Injuries

A patient with a displaced Salter–Harris type I or II physeal fracture associated with significant volar soft tissue swelling, median neuropathy, or ipsilateral elbow and radial fractures (floating elbow) is treated with closed reduction and percutaneous pinning[12,27] (Fig. 8-51). This avoids the increased risk of compartment syndrome in the carpal canal or volar forearm that is present if a well-molded, tight cast is applied. In addition, acute percutaneous pinning of the fracture prevents increased swelling, cast splitting, loss of reduction, and concerns about malunion or growth arrest with repeat reduction. The risk of growth arrest from a narrow-diameter, smooth pin left in place for 3 to 4 weeks is exceedingly small.[219]

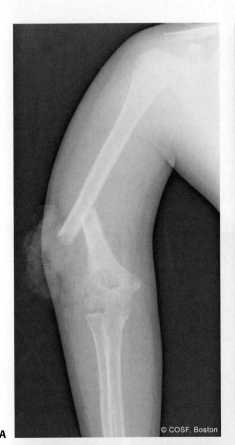
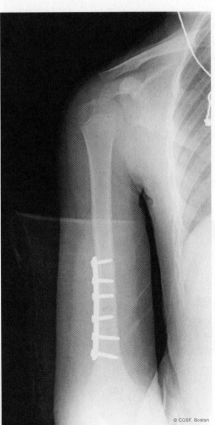
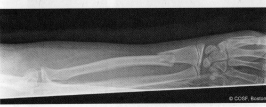

Figure 8-50. A: Radiograph of an open humeral diaphyseal fracture in the setting of a "floating elbow injury." **B:** Radiograph depicting a displaced distal radial metaphyseal fracture. **C:** Plate fixation following irrigation and debridement of the humerus fracture. *(continues)*

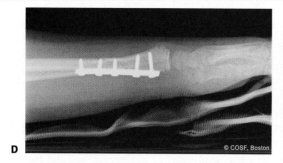

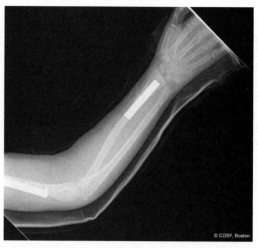

Figure 8-50. (*Continued*) **D, E:** Radiographs following open reduction and plate fixation of the radius fracture, sparing the distal radial physis. (Courtesy of Children's Orthopaedic Surgery Foundation.)

Open reduction is reserved for irreducible Salter–Harris type I and II fractures, open fractures, fractures with associated acute carpal tunnel or forearm compartment syndrome, displaced (more than 1 mm) Salter–Harris type III or IV fractures, or triplane-equivalent fractures. For an irreducible Salter–Harris type I or II fracture, exposure is from the side of the torn periosteum. Because these fractures usually are displaced dorsally, a volar exposure is used. Smooth pins are used for stabilization and are left in for 3 to 4 weeks. Open fractures are exposed through the open wound with proximal and distal extension for adequate debridement. All open debridements are performed in the operating room under general anesthesia. Acute compartment syndromes are treated with immediate release of the transverse carpal ligament or forearm fascia. The transverse carpal ligament is released in a Z-plasty fashion to lengthen the ligament and prevent volar bow-stringing and scarring of the median nerve against the palmar skin.

Intra-Articular Fractures

Displaced intra-articular fractures in the skeletally immature are best treated with arthroscopically assisted reduction and fixation. Distraction across the joint can be achieved with application of an external fixator or wrist arthroscopy traction devices and finger traps. Standard dorsal portals (3/4 and 4/5) are used for viewing the intra-articular aspect of the fracture and alignment of the reduction.[66,76] In addition, direct observation through the arthroscope can aid in safe placement of the intraepiphyseal pins.[53,87,92] Fluoroscopy is used to evaluate the extra-articular aspects of the fracture (triplane-equivalent and type IV fractures), the reduction, and placement of fixation pins.

In older patients near or at skeletal maturity with intra-articular comminution, volar locking plate fixation is performed, similar to adults.

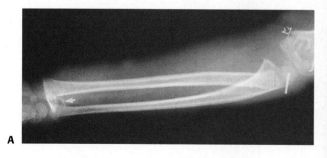

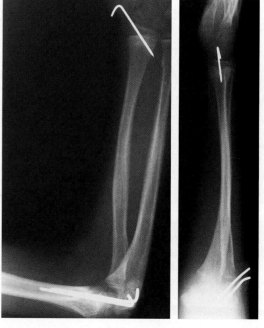

Figure 8-51. A: Ipsilateral distal radial physeal and supracondylar fractures. This 6 year old sustained both a dorsally displaced distal radial physeal fracture (closed arrow) and a type II displaced supracondylar fracture of the humerus (open arrow). **B:** Similar case treated with percutaneous pinning of radial physeal fracture and supracondylar humeral fracture.

Potential Pitfalls and Preventative Measures

Distal Radius Fractures:
POTENTIAL PITFALLS AND PREVENTIONS

Pitfall	Preventions
• Loss of reduction	• Correct diagnosis of bicortical disruption • Optimal fracture reduction • Well-molded cast application • Serial radiographic evaluation
• Posttraumatic growth arrest	• Avoidance of repeated forceful reduction maneuvers acutely • Avoidance of late manipulation for loss of reduction in children with considerable remaining growth
• Compartment syndrome	• Thorough neurovascular evaluation at time of initial presentation • Avoidance of excessive forceful manipulation during reduction maneuvers • Immediate pin fixation in patients with excessive soft tissue swelling or neurovascular compromise • Bivalve circumferential casts to avoid excessive external compression • Timely surgical stabilization with fasciotomies or carpal tunnel release in patients with impending compartment syndrome
• Radial sensory nerve injury	• Use of small incisions for nerve identification and retraction during pinning procedures • Pin placement using oscillating technique

MANAGEMENT OF EXPECTED ADVERSE OUTCOMES AND UNEXPECTED COMPLICATIONS IN FRACTURES OF THE DISTAL RADIUS AND ULNA

Distal Radial and Ulna Fractures:
COMMON ADVERSE OUTCOMES AND COMPLICATIONS

- Loss of reduction
- Malunion
- Nonunion
- Growth disturbance (radius or ulna)
- Ulnocarpal impaction
- TFCC tears
- Synostosis
- Neuropathy
- Infection

LOSS OF REDUCTION

Loss of reduction is a common occurrence after closed reduction and cast immobilization of displaced distal radius fractures (Fig. 8-52). Multiple studies demonstrate an incidence of loss of reduction of 20% to 30%.[6,7,10,48,57,90,103,133,136,141,165,166,200,207,218,221] From these studies, factors that have been identified as increasing the risk of loss of reduction with closed manipulation and

casting include poor casting, bayonet apposition, age greater than 10 years, translation of more than 50% the diameter of the radius, apex volar angulation of more than 30 degrees, isolated radial fractures, and radial and ulnar metaphyseal fractures at the same level. More specifically, Mani et al.[132] concluded that initial displacement of the radial shaft of over 50% was the single most reliable predictor of failure of reduction. Proctor et al.[165] found that complete initial displacement resulted in a 52% incidence of redisplacement of distal radial fractures in children and described remanipulation rates of 23%. Pretell et al.[164] found that postreduction translation of the radius greater than 10% in the sagittal plane resulted in 2.7 times more likely loss of reduction. Alemdaroğlu et al.[6,7] suggest that radial fractures with greater than 30 degrees of obliquity have 11.7 times more likelihood to redisplace than a straight transverse fracture.

In addition to the initial and postreduction angulation, a poor casting technique is often implicated as a cause of loss of reduction. It has become evident that casting alone is likely not sufficient to prevent loss of reduction for high-risk fractures. Miller et al.[138] reported that despite these optimal conditions, 30% of high-risk patients treated with cast immobilization alone sustained a loss of reduction that required remanipulation. These findings have generated enthusiasm for percutaneous pinning and casting as a preferable method to avoid loss of reduction.[78,219] Although the authors of these studies, and others,[219] conclude that pinning is a safe, effective means of treating distal radial metaphyseal fractures (see Controversies), the results of casting and pinning were equivalent after 2 years postfracture.[38,135]

In general, loss of reduction has been tolerated because of the remodeling potential of the distal radius.[70,155,223] However, given that remodeling can be incomplete leading to malunion (see Malunion section) with functional deficits, high rates of loss of reduction have led to considerable controversies regarding acceptable displacement, casting techniques, remanipulation, and need for initial percutaneous pinning. We prefer to reduce forearm fractures as near to perfect alignment as possible. No element of malrotation is accepted in the reduction. As indicated in the treatment sections, fractures at high risk of loss of reduction and malunion are treated with anatomic reduction and pin or, rarely, plate fixation. Fractures treated in a cast are followed closely and rereduced for any loss of alignment of more than 10 degrees. Although loss of forearm rotation can occur with anatomic healing,[146,191] it is less likely than with a malunion.

MALUNION

While complications from metaphyseal and physeal fractures of the radius are relatively rare, malunions do occur.[11,31,37–39,44,50,200] De Courtivron[45] reported that of 602 distal radial fractures, 14% had an initial malunion of more than 5 degrees. In addition, as noted above, the rate of loss of reduction for distal radius fractures ranges from 20% to 30%, and although many of these fractures will be rereduced, inevitably surgeons will encounter malunion of the distal radius, most often due to decisions to avoid injury to the physis from remanipulation beyond 7 days of injury or a patient may miss follow-up appointments before healing occurs. Fortunately, with significant growth remaining, many angular malunions of the distal radius will

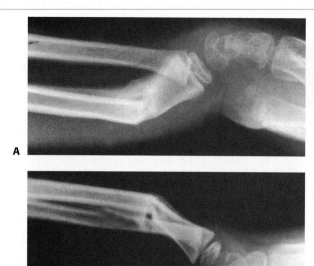

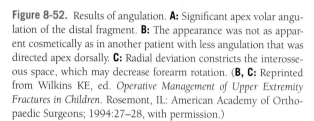

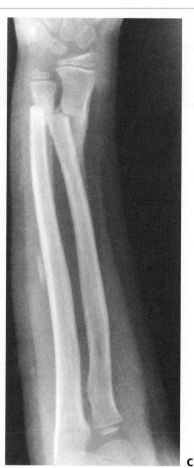

Figure 8-52. Results of angulation. **A:** Significant apex volar angulation of the distal fragment. **B:** The appearance was not as apparent cosmetically as in another patient with less angulation that was directed apex dorsally. **C:** Radial deviation constricts the interosseous space, which may decrease forearm rotation. (**B, C:** Reprinted from Wilkins KE, ed. *Operative Management of Upper Extremity Fractures in Children.* Rosemont, IL: American Academy of Orthopaedic Surgeons; 1994:27–28, with permission.)

remodel,[45,50,70,108,155,223] probably because of asymmetric physeal growth (see Fig. 8-24).[112,125] The younger the patient, the less the deformity, and the closer the fracture is to the physis, the greater the potential for remodeling. Distal radial fractures are most often juxtaphyseal, the malunion typically is in the plane of motion of the wrist joint (dorsal displacement with apex volar angulation), and the distal radius accounts for 60% to 80% of the growth of the radius. All these factors favor remodeling of a malunion.

The malunited fracture should be monitored over the next 6 to 12 months for remodeling. If the fracture does not remodel, persistent extension deformity of the distal radial articular surface puts the patient at risk for developing midcarpal instability[187,188] and degenerative arthritis of the wrist, though a recent report has raised the question of whether imperfect final radiographic alignment necessarily leads to symptomatic arthrosis.[69] For malunion correction, an opening-wedge (dorsal or volar) osteotomy is made, iliac crest bone of appropriate trapezoidal shape to correct the deformity is inserted, and either a plate or external fixator is used to maintain correction until healing.[68]

As there are controversies as to what degree of deformity is either less likely to remodel, or cause a functional loss (see Controversies), the degree and plane of loss of motion, as well as the individual affected, determine if this is functionally significant.[217] In cadaver studies, malangulation of more than 20 degrees of the radius or ulna caused loss of forearm rotation,[134,189] whereas less than 10 degrees of malangulation did

not alter forearm rotation significantly. Distal third malunion affected rotation less than middle or proximal third malunion. Radioulnar malunion affected forearm rotation more than volar–dorsal malunion. Excessive angulation may lead to a loss of rotation at a 1:2 degree ratio, whereas malrotation may lead to rotational loss at only a 1:1 degree loss.[171] The functional loss associated with rotational motion loss is difficult to predict. This has led some clinicians to recommend no treatment,[42,44] arguing that most of these fractures will remodel, and those that do not remodel will not cause a functional problem.[106] However, a significant functional problem is present if shoulder motion cannot compensate for loss of supination.

Intra-articular malunion is a potentially devastating complication, due to the risk of degenerative arthritis if the articular step-off is more than 2 mm.[119] MRI or CT scans can be useful in preoperative evaluations. Arthroscopy allows direct examination of the deformity and areas of impingement or potential degeneration. Intra-articular osteotomy with bone grafting in the metaphysis to support the reconstructed articular surface is controversial and risky; however, it has the potential to restore anatomic alignment to the joint and prevent serious long-term complications. This problem fortunately is uncommon in children because of the rarity of the injury and this type of malunion.

In Galeazzi fractures, malunion of the radius can lead to subluxation of the DRUJ, limited forearm rotation, and pain, usually secondary to persistent shortening and malrotation of the radial fracture. Most often, this occurs when complete fractures are treated with closed reduction and there is failure to either obtain or maintain reduction of the radial fracture. The ulna remains subluxed and heals with an incongruent joint. Treatment of this requires proper recognition and corrective osteotomy. If physical examination is not definitive for diagnosis, then a CT scan in pronation, neutral rotation, or supination may be helpful. MRI or wrist arthroscopy will aid in the diagnosis and management of associated ligamentous, chondral, or TFCC injuries that will benefit from debridement or repair. It is important to understand that if the DRUJ subluxation is caused by a radial malunion, a soft tissue reconstruction of the DRUJ alone will fail. In the true soft tissue disruption, repair of the TFCC will often stabilize the DRUJ. If there is no TFCC tear, soft tissue reconstruction of the DRUJ ligaments with extensor retinaculum or local tendon is appropriate.

NONUNION

Nonunion of a closed radial or ulnar fracture is rare. In children, nonunion has been universally related to a pathologic condition of the bone or vascularity.[27,84] Congenital pseudarthrosis or neurofibromatosis (Fig. 8-53) should be suspected in a young patient with a nonunion after a benign fracture.[111] This occurs most often after an isolated ulnar fracture.[81,185] The distal bone is often narrowed, sclerotic, and plastically deformed. These fractures rarely heal with immobilization. Vascularized fibular bone grafting usually is necessary for healing of a nonunion associated with neurofibromatosis or congenital pseudarthrosis.

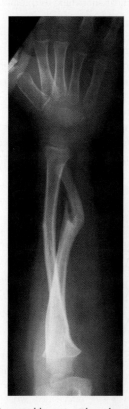

Figure 8-53. This 3 year old presented to the emergency room with pain after an acute fall on his arm. The ulna is clearly pathologic with thinning and deformity before this injury. This represents neurofibromatosis. (Courtesy of Children's Orthopaedic Surgery Foundation.)

If the patient is very young, this may include a vascularized epiphyseal transfer to restore distal growth.

Vascular impairment also can lead to nonunion. Distal radial nonunion has been reported in a child with an ipsilateral supracondylar fracture with brachial artery occlusion. Revascularization of the limb led to eventual union of the fracture. Nonunion also can occur with osteomyelitis and bone loss.[25] Debridement of the necrotic bone and either traditional bone grafting, osteoclasis lengthening, vascularized bone grafting, or creation of a single-bone forearm are surgical options. The choice depends on the individual patient.

CROSS-UNION

Cross-union, or posttraumatic radioulnar synostosis, is a rare complication of pediatric distal radial and ulna fractures. It has been described after high-energy trauma and internal fixation.[198,199] A single pin crossing both bones increases the risk of cross-union.[199] Synostosis take-down can be performed, but the results usually are less than full restoration of motion. It is important to determine if there is an element of rotational malunion with the cross-union because this will affect the surgical outcome.

Soft tissue contraction across both bones also has been described.[66] Contracture release resulted in restoration of forearm motion.

REFRACTURE

Fortunately, refractures after distal radial fractures are rare and much less common than after pediatric diaphyseal level radial and ulna fractures and fractures in adults. This is likely due to the unique biology in children where, as opposed to adults, remineralization after forearm fractures in children occurs rapidly with a transient elevation in bone mineral density.[71] Most commonly, refracture occurs with premature discontinuation of immobilization or early return to potentially traumatic activities. It is advisable to protectively immobilize the wrist until full radiograph and clinical healing (usually 6 weeks) and to restrict activities until full motion and strength are regained (usually an additional 1 to 6 weeks). Individuals involved in high-risk activities, such as downhill ski racing, snowboarding, or skateboarding, should be protected with a splint during those activities for much longer.

PHYSEAL ARREST OF THE DISTAL RADIUS

Distal radial physeal arrest can occur from either the trauma of the original injury (Fig. 8-54)[3,8,96] or late reduction of a displaced fracture. The incidence of radial growth arrest has been shown to be 4% to 5% of all displaced radial physeal fractures.[12,27,126] The trauma to the physeal cartilage from displacement and compression is a significant risk factor for growth arrest. However, a correlation between the risk of growth arrest and the degree of displacement, type of fracture, or type of reduction has yet to be defined. Similarly, the risk of further compromising the physis with late reduction at various time intervals is still unclear. The current recommendation is for an atraumatic reduction of a displaced physeal fracture less than 7 days after injury.

When a growth arrest develops, the consequences depend on the severity of the arrest and the amount of growth remaining.

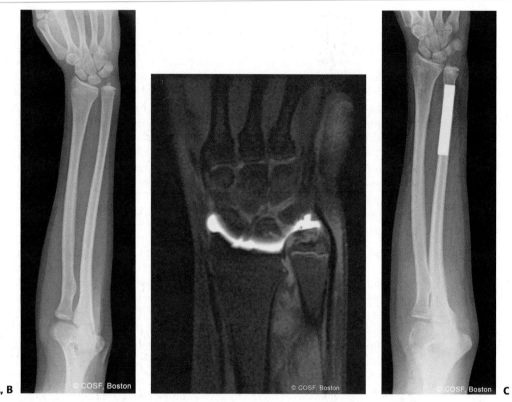

Figure 8-54. A: AP radiograph of growth arrest with open ulnar physis. **B:** MRI scan of large area of growth arrest that was not deemed respectable by mapping. Note is made of impaction of the distal ulna against the triquetrum and a secondary peripheral TFCC tear. **C:** Radiograph after ulnar shortening osteotomy, restoring neutral ulnar variance.

A complete arrest of the distal radial physis in a skeletally immature patient can be a serious problem. The continued growth of the ulna with cessation of radial growth can lead to incongruity of the DRUJ, ulnocarpal impaction, and development of a TFCC tear (Fig. 8-55).[12,204] The radial deviation deformity at the wrist can be severe enough to cause limitation of wrist and forearm motion. Pain and clicking can develop at the ulnocarpal or radioulnar joints, indicative of ulnocarpal impaction or a TFCC tear. The

deformity will progress until the end of growth. Pain and limited motion and function will be present until forearm length is rebalanced, until the radiocarpal, ulnocarpal, and radioulnar joints are restored, and until the TFCC tear and areas of chondromalacia are repaired or debrided.[12,152,192]

Ideally, physeal arrest of the distal radius will be discovered early before the consequences of unbalanced growth develop. Radiographic screening 6 to 12 months after injury can identify

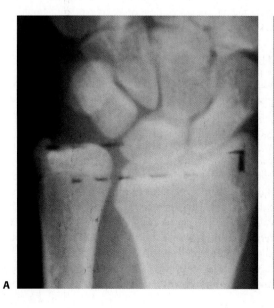

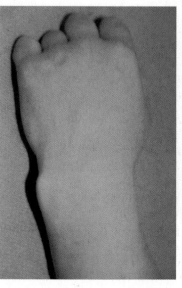

Figure 8-55. A: AP radiograph of radial growth arrest and ulnar overgrowth after physeal fracture. Patient complained of ulnar-sided wrist pain and clicking. **B:** Clinical photograph of ulnar overgrowth and radial deviation deformity. (Courtesy of Children's Orthopaedic Surgery Foundation.)

the early arrest. A small area of growth arrest in a patient near skeletal maturity may be clinically inconsequential. However, a large area of arrest in a patient with marked growth remaining can lead to ulnocarpal impaction and forearm deformity if intervention is delayed. MRI can map the area of arrest.[158] If it is less than 45% of the physis, a bar resection with fat interposition can be attempted.[124] This may restore radial growth and prevent future problems (Fig. 8-56). If the bar is larger than 45% of the physis, bar resection is unlikely to be successful. An early ulnar epiphysiodesis will prevent growth imbalance of the

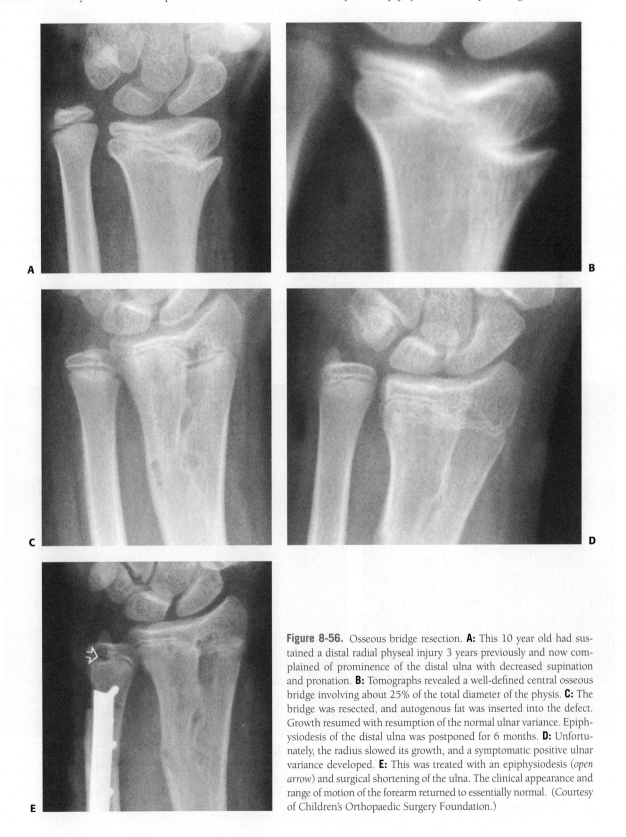

Figure 8-56. Osseous bridge resection. **A:** This 10 year old had sustained a distal radial physeal injury 3 years previously and now complained of prominence of the distal ulna with decreased supination and pronation. **B:** Tomographs revealed a well-defined central osseous bridge involving about 25% of the total diameter of the physis. **C:** The bridge was resected, and autogenous fat was inserted into the defect. Growth resumed with resumption of the normal ulnar variance. Epiphysiodesis of the distal ulna was postponed for 6 months. **D:** Unfortunately, the radius slowed its growth, and a symptomatic positive ulnar variance developed. **E:** This was treated with an epiphysiodesis (*open arrow*) and surgical shortening of the ulna. The clinical appearance and range of motion of the forearm returned to essentially normal. (Courtesy of Children's Orthopaedic Surgery Foundation.)

forearm.[204] The growth discrepancy between forearms in most patients is minor and does not require treatment. However, this is not the case for a patient with an arrest at a very young age, for whom complicated decisions regarding forearm lengthening need to occur.

If a radial growth arrest occurs associated with a radial physeal stress fracture, treatment depends on the degree of deformity and the patient's symptoms. Physeal bar resection often is not possible because the arrest is usually too diffuse in stress injuries. If there is no significant ulnar overgrowth, a distal ulnar epiphysiodesis will prevent the development of an ulnocarpal impaction syndrome. For ulnar overgrowth and ulnocarpal pain, an ulnar shortening osteotomy is indicated. Techniques include transverse, oblique, and Z-shortening osteotomies. Transverse osteotomy has a higher risk of nonunion than either oblique or Z-shortening and should be avoided. Even when oblique or Z-shortenings are used, making the osteotomy more distally in the metaphyseal region will lessen the risk of nonunion, owing to the more robust vascularity of the distal ulna. The status of the TFCC also should be evaluated by MRI or wrist arthroscopy. If there is an associated TFCC tear, it should be repaired as appropriate.

Growth arrest of the distal radius after metaphyseal fracture is extremely rare with only five cases reported in the literature. Wilkins and O'Brien[211] proposed that these arrests may be in fractures that extend from the metaphysis to the physis. This coincides with a Peterson type I fracture (Fig. 8-57)[159] and in

essence is a physeal fracture. These fractures should be monitored for growth arrest.

Both undergrowth and overgrowth of the distal radius after fracture were described by de Pablos.[46] The average difference in growth was 3 mm, with a range of −5 to +10 mm of growth disturbance compared with the contralateral radius. Maximal overgrowth occurred in the 9- to 12-year-old age group. As long as the patient is asymptomatic, under- or overgrowth is not a problem. If ulnocarpal impaction or DRUJ disruption occurs, then surgical rebalancing of the radius and ulna may be necessary.

Physeal Arrest Distal Ulna

Physeal growth arrest is frequent with distal ulnar physeal fractures (Fig. 8-58), occurring in 10% to 55% of patients.[81] It is unclear why the distal ulna has a higher incidence of growth arrest after fracture than does the radius. Ulnar growth arrest in a young child leads to relative radial overgrowth and bowing. The most common complication of distal ulnar physeal fractures is growth arrest. Golz et al.[81] described 18 such fractures, with growth arrest in 10%. If the patient is young enough, continued growth of the radius will lead to deformity and dysfunction. The distal ulnar aspect of the radial physis and epiphysis appears to be tethered by the foreshortened ulna (Fig. 8-59). The radial articular surface develops increased inclination toward the foreshortened ulna. This is similar to the deformity Peinado[154] created experimentally with arrest of the distal ulna

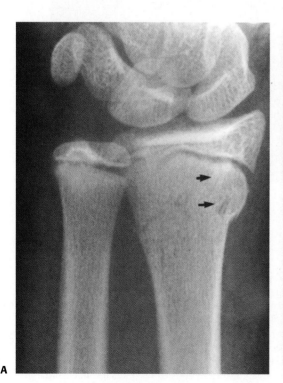
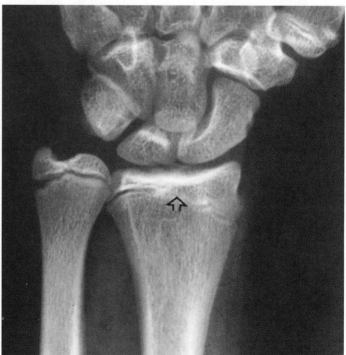

Figure 8-57. Physeal arrest in a Peterson type I fracture. **A:** Injury film showing what appears to be a benign metaphyseal fracture. Fracture line extends into the physis (*arrows*). **B:** Two years postinjury, a central arrest (*open arrow*) has developed, with resultant shortening of the radius. (Reprinted from Wilkins KE, ed. *Operative Management of Upper Extremity Fractures in Children.* Rosemont, IL: American Academy of Orthopaedic Surgeons; 1994:21, with permission.)

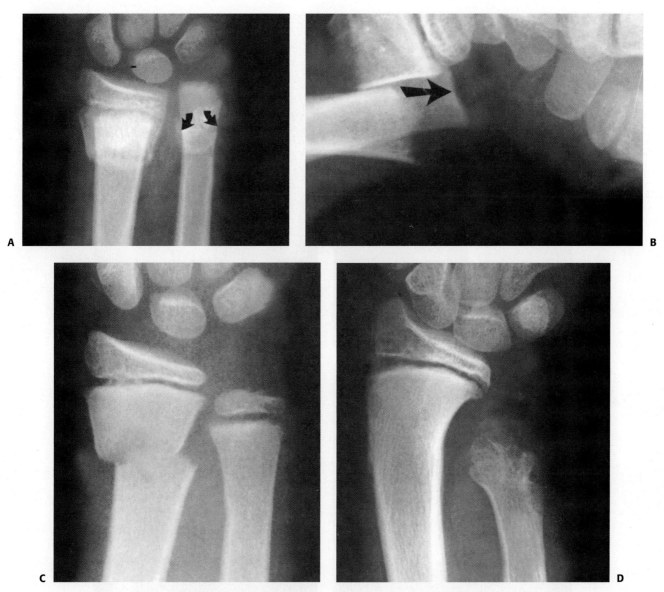

Figure 8-58. A, B: A 10-year-old boy sustained a closed Salter–Harris type I separation of the distal ulnar physis (*arrows*) combined with a fracture of the distal radial metaphysis. **C:** An excellent closed reduction was achieved atraumatically. **D:** Long-term growth arrest of the distal ulna occurred.

in rabbits' forelimbs. The distal ulna loses its normal articulation in the sigmoid notch of the distal radius. The metaphyseal–diaphyseal region of the radius often becomes notched from its articulation with the distal ulna during forearm rotation. Frequently, these patients have pain and limitation of motion with pronation and supination.[16]

Ideally, this problem is identified before the development of marked ulnar foreshortening and subsequent radial deformity. Because it is well known that distal ulnar physeal fractures have a high incidence of growth arrest, these patients should have serial radiographs at 6 to 12 months after fracture for early identification. Unfortunately, in the distal ulnar physis, physeal bar resection generally is unsuccessful. Surgical arrest of the radial physis can prevent radial deformity. Usually, this occurs toward

the end of growth so that the forearm length discrepancy is not a problem.

Rarely, patients present late with established deformity. Treatment involves rebalancing the length of the radius and ulna. The options include hemiphyseal arrest of the radius, corrective radial closing wedge osteotomy, and ulnar lengthening,[16,81,145] or a combination of these procedures. The painful impingement of the radius and ulna with forearm rotation can be corrected with reconstitution of the DRUJ. If the radial physis has significant growth remaining, a complete radial physeal arrest should be done at the same time as the surgical rebalancing of the radius and ulna. Treatment is individualized depending on the age of the patient, degree of deformity, and level of pain and dysfunction.

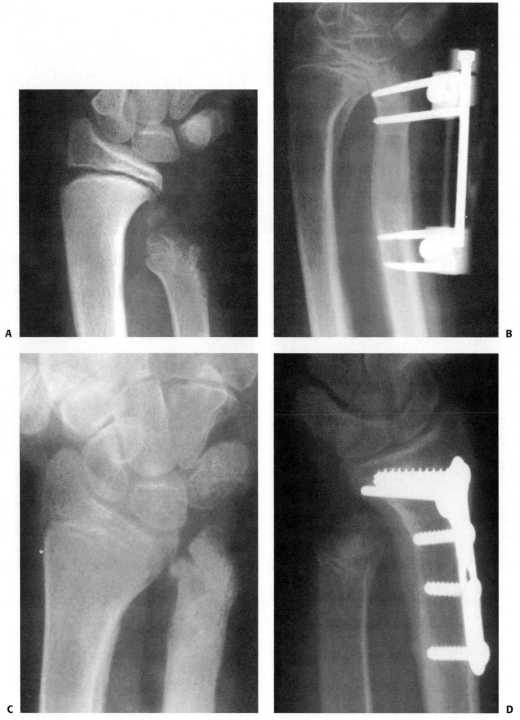

Figure 8-59. A: The appearance of the distal ulna in the patient seen in Figure 8-44, 3 years after injury, demonstrating premature fusion of the distal ulnar physis with 3.2 cm of shortening. The distal radius is secondarily deformed, with tilting and translocation toward the ulna. **B:** In the patient in Figure 8-44 with distal ulnar physeal arrest, a lengthening of the distal ulna was performed using a small unipolar distract- ing device. The ulna was slightly overlengthened to compensate for some subsequent growth of the distal radius. **C:** Six months after the lengthening osteotomy, there is some deformity of the distal ulna, but good restoration of length has been achieved. The distal radial epiphyseal tilt has corrected somewhat, and the patient has asymptomatic supination and pronation to 75 degrees. **D:** Similar case to **A–C,** but with more progressive distal radial deformity treated with corrective osteotomy and epiphysiodesis of the distal radius.

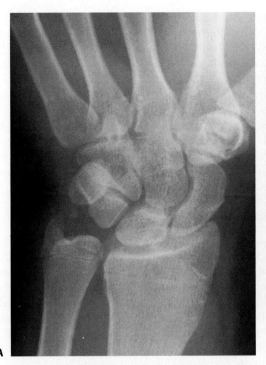
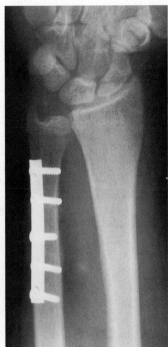
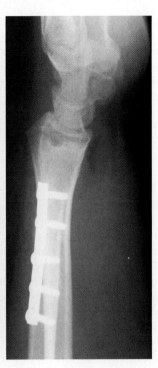

A

B

Figure 8-60. A: AP radiograph of distal radial growth arrest, ulnar overgrowth, and an ulnar styloid non-union. Wrist arthroscopy revealed an intact triangular fibrocartilage complex. **B:** AP and lateral radiographs after ulnar shortening osteotomy. (Courtesy of Children's Orthopaedic Surgery Foundation.)

Golz et al.[81] cited ulnar physeal arrest in 55% of Galeazzi-equivalent fractures. If the patient is young enough, this ulnar growth arrest in the presence of ongoing radial growth will lead to deformity. Initially, there will be ulnar shortening. Over time, the foreshortened ulna can act as a tether, causing asymmetric growth of the radius. There will be increased radial articular inclination on the AP radiograph and subluxation of the DRUJ. Operative choices include ulnar lengthening, radial closing wedge osteotomy, radial epiphysiodesis, and a combination of the above procedures that is appropriate for the individual patient's age, deformity, and disability.

Ulnocarpal Impaction Syndrome

The growth discrepancy between the radius and ulna can lead to relative radial shortening and ulnar overgrowth. The distal ulna can impinge on the lunate and triquetrum and cause pain with ulnar deviation, extension, and compression activities.[16] This is particularly true in repetitive wrist-loading sports such as field hockey, lacrosse, and gymnastics.[49] Physical examination loading the ulnocarpal joint in ulnar deviation and compression will recreate the pain. Radiographs show the radial arrest, ulnar overgrowth, and distal ulnocarpal impingement. The ulnocarpal impaction also may be caused by a hypertrophic ulnar styloid fracture union or an ulnar styloid nonunion.[25] MRI may reveal chondromalacia of the lunate or triquetrum, a tear of the TFCC, and the extent of the distal radial physeal arrest.

Treatment should correct all components of the problem. The ulnar overgrowth is corrected by either an ulnar shortening or radial lengthening osteotomy. Most often, a marked degree of positive ulnar variance requires ulnar shortening to neutral or

negative variance (Fig. 8-60). If the ulnar physis is still open, a simultaneous arrest should be done to prevent recurrent deformity. If the degree of radial deformity is marked, this should be corrected by a realignment or lengthening osteotomy. Criteria for radial correction are debatable, but we have used radial inclination of less than 11 degrees on the AP radiograph as an indication for correction.[204] In the rare case of complete arrest in a very young patient, radial lengthening is preferable to ulnar shortening to rebalance the forearm.

Triangular Fibrocartilage Complex Tears

Peripheral traumatic TFCC tears should be repaired. The presence of an ulnar styloid nonunion at the base often is indicative of an associated peripheral tear of the TFCC.[1,12,152,192] The symptomatic ulnar styloid nonunion is excised[25] and any TFCC tear is repaired. If physical examination or preoperative MRI indicates a TFCC tear in the absence of an ulnar styloid nonunion, an initial arthroscopic examination can define the lesion and appropriate treatment. Peripheral tears are the most common TFCC tears in children and adolescents and can be repaired arthroscopically by an outside-in suture technique. Tears off the sigmoid notch are the next most common in adolescents and can be repaired with arthroscopic-assisted, transradial sutures. Central tears are rare in children and, as opposed to adults with degenerative central tears, arthroscopic debridement usually does not result in pain relief in children. Distal volar tears also are rare and are repaired open, at times with ligament reconstruction.[192]

Some ulnar styloid fractures result in nonunion or hypertrophic union.[1,12,25,152,192] Nonunion may be associated with TFCC tears. Hypertrophic healing represents a pseudoulnar positive variance with resultant ulnocarpal impaction. Both cause ulnar-sided wrist pain. Compression of the lunate or triquetrum on the distal ulna reproduces the pain. Clicking with ulnocarpal compression or forearm rotation represents either a TFCC tear or chondromalacia of the lunate or triquetrum. Surgical excision of the nonunion or hypertrophic union with repair of the TFCC to the base of the styloid is the treatment of choice. Postoperative immobilization for 4 weeks in a long-arm cast followed by 2 weeks in a short-arm cast protects the TFCC repair.

Neuropathy

Median neuropathy can occur from direct trauma from the initial displacement of the fracture, traction ischemia from a persistently displaced fracture, or the development of a compartment syndrome in the carpal canal or volar forearm (see Fig. 8-7).[15,205] Median neuropathy and marked volar soft tissue swelling are indications for percutaneous pin stabilization of the fracture to lessen the risk of compartment syndrome in a cast. Median neuropathy caused by direct trauma or traction ischemia generally resolves after fracture reduction. The degree of neural injury determines the length of time to recovery. Recovery can be monitored with an advancing Tinel sign along the median nerve. Motor-sensory testing can define progressive return of neural function.

Median neuropathy caused by a carpal tunnel syndrome will not recover until the carpal tunnel is decompressed. After anatomic fracture reduction and pin stabilization, volar forearm and carpal tunnel pressures are measured. Gelberman[74] recommended waiting 20 minutes or more to allow for pressure–volume equilibration before measuring pressures. If the pressures are elevated beyond 40 mm Hg or the difference between the diastolic pressure and the compartment pressure is less than 30 mm Hg,[107] an immediate release of the affected compartments should be performed. The carpal tunnel is released through a palmar incision in line with the fourth ray, with care to avoid injuring the palmar vascular arch and the ulnar nerves exiting the Guyon canal. The transverse carpal ligament is released with a Z-plasty closure of the ligament to prevent late bow-stringing of the nerve against the palmar skin. The volar forearm fascia is released in the standard fashion.

Both the median and ulnar[34,197] nerves are less commonly injured in metaphyseal fractures than in physeal fractures. The mechanisms of neural injury in a metaphyseal fracture include direct contusion from the displaced fragment, traction ischemia from tenting of the nerve over the proximal fragment,[155] entrapment of the nerve in the fracture site,[212] rare laceration of the nerve, and the development of an acute compartment syndrome. If signs or symptoms of neuropathy are present, a prompt closed reduction should be performed. Extreme positions of immobilization should be avoided because this can lead to persistent traction or compression ischemia and increase the risk of compartment syndrome. If there is marked swelling, it is better to percutaneously pin the fracture than to apply a constrictive cast. If there is concern about compartment syndrome, the forearm and carpal canal pressures should be measured immediately. If pressures are markedly elevated, appropriate fasciotomies and compartment releases should be performed

immediately. Finally, if the nerve was intact before reduction and is out after reduction, neural entrapment should be considered, and surgical exploration and decompression may be required. Fortunately, most median and ulnar nerve injuries recover after anatomic reduction of the fracture.

Injuries to the ulnar nerve and anterior interosseous nerve have been described with Galeazzi fracture–dislocations.[56,137,172,201] These reported injuries have had spontaneous recovery. Moore et al.[143] described an 8% rate of injury to the radial nerve with operative exposure of the radius for internal fixation in their series. Careful surgical exposure, dissection, and retraction can decrease this risk.

Infection

Infection after distal radial fractures is rare and is associated with open fractures or surgical intervention (also see Controversies). Fee et al.[67] described the development of gas gangrene in four children after minor puncture wounds or lacerations associated with distal radial fractures. Treatment involved only local cleansing of the wound in all four and wound closure in one. All four developed life-threatening clostridial infections. Three of the four required upper limb amputations, and the fourth underwent multiple soft tissue and bony procedures for coverage and treatment of osteomyelitis.

Infections related to surgical intervention also are rare. Superficial pin-site infections can occur and should be treated with pin removal and antibiotics. Deep-space infection from percutaneous pinning of the radius has not been described.

CONTROVERSIES RELATED TO FRACTURES OF THE DISTAL RADIUS AND ULNA

ACCEPTABLE DEFORMITY

There is considerable controversy about what constitutes an acceptable reduction.[11,37–39,42,45,50,69] This is clearly age dependent; the younger the patient, the greater the potential for remodeling. Volar–dorsal malalignment has the greatest potential for remodeling because this is in the plane of predominant motion of the joint. A recent prospective study found excellent long-term clinical and radiographic results with reduced cost with nonsedated cast molding in patients with displaced fractures in preteen children.[38] Marked radioulnar malalignment is less likely to remodel. Malrotation will not remodel. The ranges for acceptable reduction according to age are given in the immobilization section on incomplete fractures and apply to complete fractures as well.

GREENSTICK FRACTURES

Controversy exists regarding completion of greenstick fractures.[44,170,178] Although some researchers advocate completion of the fracture to reduce the risk of subsequent loss of reduction from the intact periosteum and concave deformity acting as a tension band to redisplace the fracture, completing the fracture increases the risk of instability and malunion.[170,205,211]

IMMOBILIZATION

The position and type of immobilization after reduction also have been controversial. Recommendations for the position of postreduction immobilization include supination, neutral, and pronation. The rationale for immobilization in pronation is that reduction of the more common apex volar fractures requires correction of the supination deformity.[63] Following this rationale, apex dorsal fractures should be reduced and immobilized in supination. Pollen[162] believed that the brachioradialis was a deforming force in pronation and was relaxed in supination (Fig. 8-61) and advocated immobilization in supination for all displaced distal radial fractures. Kasser[113] recommended immobilization in slight supination to allow better molding of the volar distal radius. Some researchers advocate immobilization in a neutral position, believing this is best at maintaining the interosseous space and has the least risk of disabling loss of forearm rotation in the long term. Davis and Green[44] and Ogden[148] advocated that each fracture seek its own preferred position of stability. Gupta and Danielsson[88] randomized immobilization of distal radial metaphyseal greenstick fractures in neutral, supination, or pronation to try to determine the best position of immobilization. Their study showed a statistical improvement in final healing with immobilization in supination. More recently, Boyer et al.[24] prospectively randomized 109 distal third forearm fractures into long-arm casts with the forearm in neutral rotation, supination, or pronation following closed reduction. No significant differences in final radiographic position were noted among the differing positions of forearm rotation.

Another area of controversy is whether or not long- or short-arm cast immobilization is better. Historically, most publications on pediatric distal radial fracture treatment advocated long-arm cast treatment for the first 3 to 4 weeks of healing.[20,93,148,162] The rationale is that elbow flexion reduces the muscle forces acting to displace the fracture. In addition, a long-arm cast may further restrict the child's activity and therefore decrease the risk of

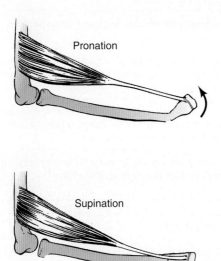

Figure 8-61. The brachioradialis is relaxed in supination but may become a deforming force in pronation. (Reprinted with permission from Pollen AG. *Fractures and Dislocations in Children.* 1st ed. Churchill Livingstone, MD: Williams & Wilkins; 1973.)

displacement. However, Chess et al.[31] reported redisplacement and reduction rates with well-molded short-arm casts similar to those with long-arm casts. They used a cast index (sagittal diameter divided by coronal diameter at the fracture site) of 0.7 or less to indicate a well-molded cast. In addition, two prospective studies have recapitulated these findings. The short-arm cast offers the advantage of elbow mobility and better patient acceptance of casting. Two recent randomized prospective clinical trials and a meta-analysis review compared the efficacy of short- and long-arm cast immobilization following closed reduction for pediatric distal radial fractures.[20,93] Bohm et al.[20] randomized 102 patients over the age of 4 years to either short- or long-arm casts following closed reduction of displaced distal radial metaphyseal fractures. No statistically significant difference was seen in loss of reduction rate between the two treatment groups. Webb et al.[207] similarly randomized 103 patients to short- or long-arm casts after reduction of distal radial fractures. No significant difference in rate of lost reduction was seen between the two cohorts. Patients in short-arm casts, however, missed fewer days of school and required less assistance with activities of daily living than those with long-arm casts. In both of these studies, quality of fracture reduction and cast mold were influential factors in loss of reduction rates. These studies have challenged the traditional teaching regarding the need for elbow immobilization to control distal radial fracture alignment.

IMMEDIATE PINNING OF DISPLACED DISTAL RADIUS FRACTURES

In the past decade or two, closed reduction and percutaneous pinning have become more common as the primary treatment of distal radial metaphyseal fractures in children and adolescents.[78,95,129,185,194,219] Despite this practice change, a meta-analysis review of the data comparing cast immobilization versus immediate pinning reveals equivalent long-term outcomes, despite more loss of reduction in the cast groups and more pin complications in the pin groups.[11] The indications cited include fracture instability and high risk of loss of reduction increasing the likelihood of the need for remanipulation,[7,48,57,90,103,132,135,140,164,165,221] excessive local swelling that increases the risk of neurovascular compromise,[15,44,204] and ipsilateral fractures of the distal radius and elbow region (floating elbow) that increase the risk of compartment syndrome.[19,172,183] In addition, surgeon's preference for pinning in a busy office practice has been considered an acceptable indication because of similar complication rates and long-term outcomes with pinning and casting[134,137] and the avoidance of remanipulation because alignment is secure.

OPEN FRACTURES

There have been multiple studies[51,104] demonstrating that the infection rate (2.5% to 4%) following nonoperative treatment of Gustilo grade 1 open fractures results in infection rates comparable to reported rates for operative[84] treatment (2.5%). However, these were retrospective studies and likely will not change the standard of care of these fractures until an appropriate prospective randomized study has been conducted. Even with prospective studies, it is unclear if the studies will be large enough to include the rare gas gangrene infection.

CONCLUSIONS

Fractures of the distal forearm are common in the pediatric population. Given their proximity to the distal physes of the radius and ulna, these fractures have tremendous remodeling capacity and as a result, the majority may be effectively treated with appropriate nonoperative means. The future direction for management of these fractures is primarily focused on prognosticating which fractures would be better served through surgical reduction and fixation, considering the relatively high rate of loss of reduction of these fractures.

Annotated References

Reference	Annotation
Chess DG, Hyman JC, Leahey JL, et al. Short arm plaster cast for distal pediatric forearm fracture. *J Pediatr Orthop*. 1994;14:211–213.	A forearm cast should be flat not round to maintain reduction. The "cast index"—the ratio of the cast diameter on the lateral compared to the AP radiograph—of less than or equal to 0.7 is a key cast-molding technique for successful maintenance of reduction of distal forearm fractures.
Crawford SN, Lee LS, Izuka BH. Closed reduction of overriding distal radius fractures without reduction in children. *J Bone Joint Surg*. 2012A;94:246–252.	A simple, effective, cost- and time-efficient method of treatment for displaced distal radius fractures in children which should eliminate the need to transfer 8 year olds with displaced distal radius fractures 3 hours in the middle of the night to children's hospitals from community hospitals.
Do TT, Strub WM, Foad SL, et al. Reduction versus remodeling in pediatric distal forearm fractures: a preliminary cost analysis. *J Pediatr Orthop B*. 2003;12:109–115.	A study ahead of its time that pre-dates the Michael Porter Value revolution—Porter ME. What is value in health care? *NEJM*. 2010;363:2477–2481.
Fee NF, Dobranski A, Bisia RS. Gas gangrene complicating open forearm fractures. Report of five cases. *J Bone Joint Surg*. 1977A;59:135–138.	An older study that tempers the enthusiasm for the Iobst et al. revolution for treating grade 1 open forearm fractures without a formal I and D in the operating room
Godambe SA, Elliot V, Matheny D, et al. Comparison of propofol/fentanyl versus ketamine/midazolam for brief orthopaedic procedural sedation in the emergency department. *Pediatrics*. 2003;112:116–123.	A prospective, controlled trial evaluating the advantages and disadvantages of two commonly used methods of conscious sedation in children for fracture reduction.
Hang JR, Hutchinson AF, Hau RC. Risk factors associated with loss of position after closed reduction of distal radial fractures in children. *J Pediatr Orthop*. 2011;31:501–506.	Completely displaced distal radius fractures and an ipsilateral ulna fracture that cannot be anatomically reduced is the best predictor for redisplacement.
Iobst CA, Spurdel C, Baitner AC, et al. A protocol for the management of pediatric type 1 open fractures. *J Child Orthop*. 2014;8:71–76.	Forty-five consecutive patients treated with wound cleansing in the ED, closed reduction under conscious sedation in the ED, IV antibiotics, and no formal I and D in the operating room resulted in uncomplicated fracture healing and no infections.
Khan S, Sawyer J, Pershad J. Closed reduction of distal forearm fractures by pediatric emergency room physicians. *Acad Emerg Med*. 2010;17:1169–1174.	The value revolution gone wild. Michael Porter would be proud.
Luther G, Miller PE, Mahan ST, et al. Decreasing utilization using standardized clinical assessment and management plans (SCAMPs). *J Pediatr Orthop*. 2016 Sept 15. [Epub ahead of print]	Using SCAMPs in the management of pediatric buckle fractures resulted in decreased practice variability, resource utilization, and cost of care with no change in outcomes.
McQuinn AG, Jaarsma RL. Risk factors for redisplacement of pediatric distal forearm and distal radius fractures. *J Pediatr Orthop*. 2012;32:687–692.	Initial displacement of >50% and inability to achieve an anatomic reduction are the major risk factors for redisplacement. The cast index is the most useful method to grade cast molding.
Plint AC, Perry JJ, Correll R, et al. A randomized, controlled trial of removable splinting versus casting for wrist buckle fractures in children. *Pediatrics*. 2006;117:691–697.	Removable splinting was superior to casting for function and bathing with equal outcomes noted for pain, healing, and reinjury.
Samora JB, Klingele KE, Beebe AC, et al. Is there still a place for cast wedging in pediatric forearm fractures? *J Pediatr Orthop*. 2014;34:246–252.	An update on the technique of cast wedging of the distal radius and ulna for the millennial generation.
Voto SJ, Weiner DS, Leighley B. Redisplacement after closed reduction of forearm fractures in children. *J Pediatr Orthop*. 1990;10:79–84.	Redisplacement occurs in about 7% of cases and can usually be successfully treated with a second closed reduction and casting.
Waters PM, Bae DS, Montgomery KD. Surgical management of post-traumatic distal radial growth arrest in adolescents. *J Pediatr Orthop*. 2002;22:717–724.	Growth arrest occurs in about 4% of fractures. Surgical options and outcomes are nicely outlined in this paper.

REFERENCES

1. Abid A, Accadbled F, Kany J, et al. Ulnar styloid fracture in children: a retrospective study of 46 cases. *J Pediatr Orthop B*. 2008;17(1):15–19.
2. Abraham A, Handoll HH, Khan T. Interventions for treating wrist fractures in children. *Cochrane Database Syst Rev*. 2008;(2):CD004576.
3. Abram LJ, Thompson GH. Deformity after premature closure of the distal radial physis following a torus fracture with a physeal compression injury. Report of a case. *J Bone Joint Surg Am*. 1987;69(9):1450–1453.
4. af Ekenstam F. Anatomy of the distal radioulnar joint. *Clin Orthop Relat Res*. 1992;(275):14–18.
5. Al-Ansari K, Howard A, Seeto B, et al. Minimally angulated pediatric wrist fractures: is immobilization without manipulation enough? *CJEM*. 2007;9(1):9–15.
6. Alemdaroğlu KB, Iltar S, Aydo˘gan NH. 3-point index in redisplacement of distal radial fractures in children: how should it be used? *J Hand Surg Am*. 2009;34(5):964; author reply 964–965.
7. Alemdaroğlu KB, Iltar S, Cimen O, et al. Risk factors in redisplacement of distal radial fractures in children. *J Bone Joint Surg Am*. 2008;90(6):1224–1230.
8. Aminian A, Schoenecker PL. Premature closure of the distal radial physis after fracture of the distal radial metaphysis. *J Pediatr Orthop*. 1995;15(4):495–498.
9. Arima J, Uchida Y, Miura H, et al. Osteochondral fracture in the distal end of the radius. *J Hand Surg Am*. 1993;18(3):489–491.
10. Bae DS. Pediatric distal radius and forearm fractures. *J Hand Surg Am*. 2008;33(10):1911–1923.
11. Bae DS, Howard AW. Distal radius fractures: what is the evidence? *J Pediatr Orthop*. 2012;32(Suppl 2):S128–S130.
12. Bae DS, Waters PM. Pediatric distal radius fractures and triangular fibrocartilage complex injuries. *Hand Clin*. 2006;22(1):43–53.
13. Bailey DA, Wedge JH, McCulloch RG, et al. Epidemiology of fractures of the distal end of the radius in children as associated with growth. *J Bone Joint Surg Am*. 1989;71(8):1225–1231.
14. Bebbington A, Lewis P, Savage R. Cast wedging for orthopaedic surgeons! *Injury*. 2005;36(1):71–72.
15. Bell CJ, Viswanathan S, Dass S, et al. The incidence of neurologic injury in paediatric forearm fractures requiring manipulation. *J Pediatr Orthop B*. 2010;19(4):294–297.
16. Bell MJ, Hill RJ, McMurtry RY. Ulnar impingement syndrome. *J Bone Joint Surg Br*. 1985;67(1):126–129.
17. Berberich T, Reimann P, Steinacher M, et al. Evaluation of cast wedging in a forearm fracture model. *Clin Biomech (Bristol A von)*. 2008;23(7):895–899.
18. Biyani A. Ipsilateral Monteggia equivalent injury and distal radial and ulnar fracture in a child. *J Orthop Trauma*. 1994;8(5):431–433.
19. Biyani A, Gupta SP, Sharma JC. Ipsilateral supracondylar fracture of humerus and forearm bones in children. *Injury*. 1989;20(4):203–207.
20. Bohm ER, Bubbar V, Yong Hing K, et al. Above and below-the-elbow plaster casts for distal forearm fractures in children. A randomized controlled trial. *J Bone Joint Surg Am*. 2006;88(1):1–8.
21. Boutis K, Willan A, Babyn P, et al. Cast versus splint in children with minimally angulated fractures of the distal radius: a randomized controlled trial. *CMAJ*. 2010;182(14):1507–1512.
22. Bowers W. *The Distal Radioulnar Joint*. New York: Churchill Livingstone; 1999.
23. Boyden EM, Peterson HA. Partial premature closure of the distal radial physis associated with Kirschner wire fixation. *Orthopedics*. 1991;14(5):585–588.
24. Boyer BA, Overton B, Schrader W, et al. Position of immobilization for pediatric forearm fractures. *J Pediatr Orthop*. 2002;22(2):185–187.
25. Burgess RC, Watson HK. Hypertrophic ulnar styloid nonunions. *Clin Orthop Relat Res*. 1988;(228):215–217.
26. Campbell RM Jr. Operative treatment of fractures and dislocations of the hand and wrist region in children. *Orthop Clin North Am*. 1990;21(2):217–243.
27. Cannata G, De Maio F, Mancini F, et al. Physeal fractures of the distal radius and ulna: long-term prognosis. *J Orthop Trauma*. 2003;17(3):172–179; discussion 179–180.
28. Chaar-Alvarez FM, Warkentine F, Cross K, et al. Bedside ultrasound diagnosis of nonangulated distal forearm fractures in the pediatric emergency department. *Pediatr Emerg Care*. 2011;27(11):1027–1032.
29. Chamay A. Mechanical and morphological aspects of experimental overload and fatigue in bone. *J Biomech*. 1970;3(3):263–270.
30. Cheng JC, Shen WY. Limb fracture pattern in different pediatric age groups: a study of 3,350 children. *J Orthop Trauma*. 1993;7(1):15–22.
31. Chess DG, Hyndman JC, Leahey JL, et al. Short arm plaster cast for distal pediatric forearm fractures. *J Pediatr Orthop*. 1994;14(2):211–213.
32. Christodoulou AG, Colton CL. Scaphoid fractures in children. *J Pediatr Orthop*. 1986;6(1):37–39.
33. Chung KC, Spilson SV. The frequency and epidemiology of hand and forearm fractures in the United States. *J Hand Surg Am*. 2001;26(5):908–915.
34. Clarke AC, Spencer RF. Ulnar nerve palsy following fractures of the distal radius: clinical and anatomical studies. *J Hand Surg Br*. 1991;16(4):438–440.
35. Cooney WP, Dobyns JH, Linscheid RL. Arthroscopy of the wrist: anatomy and classification of carpal instability. *Arthroscopy*. 1990;6(2):133–140.
36. Cozen L. Colles' fracture; a method of maintaining reduction. *Calif Med*. 1951;75(5):362–364.
37. Crawford AH. Pitfalls and complications of fractures of the distal radius and ulna in childhood. *Hand Clin*. 1988;4(3):403–413.
38. Crawford SN, Lee LS, Izuka BH. Closed treatment of overriding distal radial fractures without reduction in children. *J Bone Joint Surg Am*. 2012;94(3):246–252.
39. Creasman C, Zaleske DJ, Ehrlich MG. Analyzing forearm fractures in children. The more subtle signs of impending problems. *Clin Orthop Relat Res*. 1984;(188):40–53.
40. Dameron TB Jr. Traumatic dislocation of the distal radio-ulnar joint. *Clin Orthop Relat Res*. 1972;83:55–63.
41. D'Arienzo M. Scaphoid fractures in children. *J Hand Surg Br*. 2002;27(5):424–426.
42. Daruwalla JS. A study of radioulnar movements following fractures of the forearm in children. *Clin Orthop Relat Res*. 1979;(139):114–120.
43. Davidson JS, Brown DJ, Barnes SN, et al. Simple treatment for torus fractures of the distal radius. *J Bone Joint Surg Br*. 2001;83(8):1173–1175.
44. Davis DR, Green DP. Forearm fractures in children: pitfalls and complications. *Clin Orthop Relat Res*. 1976;(120):172–183.
45. De Courtivron B. *Spontaneous Correction of the Distal Forearm Fractures in Children. European Pediatric Orthopaedic Society Annual Meeting*. Brussels, Belgium; 1995.
46. de Pablos J, Franzreb M, Barrios C. Longitudinal growth pattern of the radius after forearm fractures conservatively treated in children. *J Pediatr Orthop*. 1994;14(4):492–495.
47. De Smet L, Claessens A, Lefevre J, et al. Gymnast wrist: an epidemiologic survey of ulnar variance and stress changes of the radial physis in elite female gymnasts. *Am J Sports Med*. 1994;22(6):846–850.
48. Devalia KL, Asaad SS, Kakkar R. Risk of redisplacement after first successful reduction in paediatric distal radius fractures: sensitivity assessment of casting indices. *J Pediatr Orthop B*. 2011;20(6):376–381.
49. DiFiori JP, Puffer JC, Aish B, et al. Wrist pain, distal radial physeal injury, and ulnar variance in young gymnasts: does a relationship exist? *Am J Sports Med*. 2002;30(6):879–885.
50. Do TT, Strub WM, Foad SL, et al. Reduction versus remodeling in pediatric distal forearm fractures: a preliminary cost analysis. *J Pediatr Orthop B*. 2003;12(2):109–115.
51. Doak J, Ferrick M. Nonoperative management of pediatric grade 1 open fractures with less than a 24-hour admission. *J Pediatr Orthop*. 2009;29(1):49–51.
52. Dobyns JH, Gabel GT. Gymnast's wrist. *Hand Clin*. 1990;6(3):493–505.
53. Doi K, Hattori Y, Otsuka K, et al. Intra-articular fractures of the distal aspect of the radius: arthroscopically assisted reduction compared with open reduction and internal fixation. *J Bone Joint Surg Am*. 1999;81(8):1093–1110.
54. Dumont CE, Thalmann R, Macy JC. The effect of rotational malunion of the radius and the ulna on supination and pronation. *J Bone Joint Surg Br*. 2002;84(7):1070–1074.
55. Earp BE, Waters PM, Wyzykowski RJ. Arthroscopic treatment of partial scapholunate ligament tears in children with chronic wrist pain. *J Bone Joint Surg Am*. 2006;88(11):2448–2455.
56. Eberl R, Singer G, Schalamon J, et al. Galeazzi lesions in children and adolescents: treatment and outcome. *Clin Orthop Relat Res*. 2008;466(7):1705–1709.
57. Edmonds EW, Capelo RM, Stearns P, et al. Predicting initial treatment failure of fiberglass casts in pediatric distal radius fractures: utility of the second metacarpal-radius angle. *J Child Orthop*. 2009;3(5):375–381.
58. Ehsan A, Stevanovic M. Skeletally mature patients with bilateral distal radius fractures have more associated injuries. *Clin Orthop Relat Res*. 2010;468(1):238–242.
59. Eichinger JK, Agochukwu U, Franklin J, et al. A new reduction technique for completely displaced forearm and wrist fractures in children: a biomechanical assessment and 4-year clinical evaluation. *J Pediatr Orthop*. 2011;31(7):e73–e79.
60. Eksioglu F, Altinok D, Uslu MM, et al. Ultrasonographic findings in pediatric fractures. *Turk J Pediatr*. 2003;45(2):136–140.
61. Epner RA, Bowers WH, Guilford WB. Ulnar variance—the effect of wrist positioning and roentgen filming technique. *J Hand Surg Am*. 1982;7(3):298–305.
62. Evans E. Rotational deformity in the treatment of fractures of both bones of the forearm. *J Bone Joint Surg Am*. 1945;27:373–379.
63. Evans EM. Fractures of the radius and ulna. *J Bone Joint Surg Br*. 1951;33-B(4):548–561.
64. Evans JK, Buckley SL, Alexander AH, et al. Analgesia for the reduction of fractures in children: a comparison of nitrous oxide with intramuscular sedation. *J Pediatr Orthop*. 1995;15(1):73–77.
65. Farr JN, Tomas R, Chen Z, et al. Lower trabecular volumetric BMD at metaphyseal regions of weight-bearing bones is associated with prior fracture in young girls. *J Bone Miner Res*. 2011;26(2):380–387.
66. Fatti JF, Mosher JF. An unusual complication of fracture of both bones of the forearm in a child. A case report. *J Bone Joint Surg Am*. 1986;68(3):451–453.
67. Fee NF, Dobranski A, Bisla RS. Gas gangrene complicating open forearm fractures. Report of five cases. *J Bone Joint Surg Am*. 1977;59(1):135–138.
68. Fernandez DL. Correction of post-traumatic wrist deformity in adults by osteotomy, bone-grafting, and internal fixation. *J Bone Joint Surg Am*. 1982;64(8):1164–1178.
69. Forward DP, Davis TR, Sithole JS. Do young patients with malunited fractures of the distal radius inevitably develop symptomatic post-traumatic osteoarthritis? *J Bone Joint Surg Br*. 2008;90(5):629–637.
70. Friberg KS. Remodelling after distal forearm fractures in children. III. Correction of residual angulation in fractures of the radius. *Acta Orthop Scand*. 1979;50(6 Pt 2):741–749.
71. Fung EB, Humphrey ML, Gildengorin G, et al. Rapid remineralization of the distal radius after forearm fracture in children. *J Pediatr Orthop*. 2011;31(2):138–143.
72. Galeazzi R. Di una particolare syndrome traumatica dello scheletro dell' avambraccio. *Atti Mem Soc Lomb Chir*. 1934;2:12.
73. Garn SM, Rohmann CG, Silverman FN. Radiographic standards for postnatal ossification and tooth calcification. *Med Radiogr Photogr*. 1967;43(2):45–66.
74. Gelberman RH. *Operative Nerve Repair and Reconstruction*. Philadelphia, PA: Lippincott; 1991.
75. Gelberman RH, Salamon PB, Jurist JM, et al. Ulnar variance in Kienbock's disease. *J Bone Joint Surg Am*. 1975;57(5):674–676.
76. Gerber SD, Griffin PP, Simmons BP. Break dancer's wrist. *J Pediatr Orthop*. 1986;6(1):98–99.
77. Giannoulis FS, Sotereanos DG. Galeazzi fractures and dislocations. *Hand Clin*. 2007;23(2):153–163, v.
78. Gibbons CL, Woods DA, Pailthorpe C, et al. The management of isolated distal radius fractures in children. *J Pediatr Orthop*. 1994;14(2):207–210.
79. Godambe SA, Elliot V, Matheny D, et al. Comparison of propofol/fentanyl versus ketamine/midazolam for brief orthopedic procedural sedation in a pediatric emergency department. *Pediatrics*. 2003;112(1 Pt 1):116–123.
80. Goldfarb CA, Strauss NL, Wall LB, et al. Defining ulnar variance in the adolescent wrist: measurement technique and interobserver reliability. *J Hand Surg Am*. 2011;36(2):272–277.

81. Golz RJ, Grogan DP, Greene TL, et al. Distal ulnar physeal injury. *J Pediatr Orthop*. 1991;11(3):318–326.
82. Goulding A, Jones IE, Taylor RW, et al. More broken bones: a 4-year double cohort study of young girls with and without distal forearm fractures. *J Bone Miner Res*. 2000;15(10):2011–2018.
83. Goulding A, Jones IE, Taylor RW, et al. Bone mineral density and body composition in boys with distal forearm fractures: a dual-energy x-ray absorptiometry study. *J Pediatr*. 2001;139(4):509–515.
84. Greenbaum B, Zionts LE, Ebramzadeh E. Open fractures of the forearm in children. *J Orthop Trauma*. 2001;15(2):111–118.
85. Guastavino TD. Technique of cast wedging in long bone fractures. *Orthop Rev*. 1987;16(9):691.
86. Gunes T, Erdem M, Sen C. Irreducible Galeazzi fracture-dislocation due to intra-articular fracture of the distal ulna. *J Hand Surg Eur Vol*. 2007;32(2):185–187.
87. Guofen C, Doi K, Hattori Y, et al. Arthroscopically assisted reduction and immobilization of intraarticular fracture of the distal end of the radius: several options of reduction and immobilization. *Tech Hand Up Extrem Surg*. 2005;9(2):84–90.
88. Gupta RP, Danielsson LG. Dorsally angulated solitary metaphyseal greenstick fractures in the distal radius: results after immobilization in pronated, neutral, and supinated position. *J Pediatr Orthop*. 1990;10(1):90–92.
89. Hafner R, Poznanski AK, Donovan JM. Ulnar variance in children—standard measurements for evaluation of ulnar shortening in juvenile rheumatoid arthritis, hereditary multiple exostosis and other bone or joint disorders in childhood. *Skeletal Radiol*. 1989;18(7):513–516.
90. Hang JR, Hutchinson AF, Hau RC. Risk factors associated with loss of position after closed reduction of distal radial fractures in children. *J Pediatr Orthop*. 2011;31(5):501–506.
91. Hastings H 2nd, Simmons BP. Hand fractures in children. A statistical analysis. *Clin Orthop Relat Res*. 1984;(188):120–130.
92. Hattori Y, Doi K, Estrella EP, et al. Arthroscopically assisted reduction with volar plating or external fixation for displaced intra-articular fractures of the distal radius in the elderly patients. *Hand Surg*. 2007;12(1):1–12.
93. Hendrickx RP, Campo MM, van Lieshout AP, et al. Above- or below-elbow casts for distal third forearm fractures in children? A meta-analysis of the literature. *Arch Orthop Trauma Surg*. 2011;131(12):1663–1671.
94. Hernandez JA, Swischuk LE, Bathurst GJ, et al. Scaphoid (navicular) fractures of the wrist in children: attention to the impacted buckle fracture. *Emerg Radiol*. 2002;9(6):305–308.
95. Holmes JR, Louis DS. Entrapment of pronator quadratus in pediatric distal-radius fractures: recognition and treatment. *J Pediatr Orthop*. 1994;14(4):498–500.
96. Horii E, Tamura Y, Nakamura R, et al. Premature closure of the distal radial physis. *J Hand Surg Br*. 1993;18(1):11–16.
97. Houshian S, Holst AK, Larsen MS, et al. Remodeling of Salter-Harris type II epiphyseal plate injury of the distal radius. *J Pediatr Orthop*. 2004;24(5):472–476.
98. Hove LM, Brudvik C. Displaced paediatric fractures of the distal radius. *Arch Orthop Trauma Surg*. 2008;128(1):55–60.
99. Hubner U, Schlicht W, Outzen S, et al. Ultrasound in the diagnosis of fractures in children. *J Bone Joint Surg Br*. 2000;82(8):1170–1173.
100. Hulten O. Uber anatomische variationen der hand-gelenkknochen. *Acta Radiol*. 1928;9:155–168.
101. Husted CM. Technique of cast wedging in long bone fractures. *Orthop Rev*. 1986;15(6):373–378.
102. Ibrahim T, Qureshi A, Sutton AJ, et al. Surgical versus nonsurgical treatment of acute minimally displaced and undisplaced scaphoid waist fractures: pairwise and network meta-analyses of randomized controlled trials. *J Hand Surg Am*. 2011;36(11):1759–1768.e1.
103. Iltar S, Alemdaroglu KB, Say F, et al. The value of the three-point index in predicting redisplacement of diaphyseal fractures of the forearm in children. *Bone Joint J*. 2013;95-B(4):563–567.
104. Iobst CA, Tidwell MA, King WF. Nonoperative management of pediatric type I open fractures. *J Pediatr Orthop*. 2005;25(4):513–517.
105. Ishii S, Palmer AK, Werner FW, et al. Pressure distribution in the distal radioulnar joint. *J Hand Surg Am*. 1998;23(5):909–913.
106. Johari AN, Sinha M. Remodeling of forearm fractures in children. *J Pediatr Orthop B*. 1999;8(2):84–87.
107. Jones IE, Cannan R, Goulding A. Distal forearm fractures in New Zealand children: annual rates in a geographically defined area. *N Z Med J*. 2000;113(1120):443–445.
108. Kalkwarf HJ, Laor T, Bean JA. Fracture risk in children with a forearm injury is associated with volumetric bone density and cortical area (by peripheral QCT) and areal bone density (by DXA). *Osteoporos Int*. 2011;22(2):607–616.
109. Kamano M, Honda Y. Galeazzi-equivalent lesions in adolescence. *J Orthop Trauma*. 2002;16(6):440–443.
110. Kameyama O, Ogawa R. Pseudarthrosis of the radius associated with neurofibromatosis: report of a case and review of the literature. *J Pediatr Orthop*. 1990;10(1):128–131.
111. Karaharju EO, Ryoppy SA, Mäkinen RJ. Remodelling by asymmetrical epiphyseal growth. An experimental study in dogs. *J Bone Joint Surg Br*. 1976;58(1):122–126.
112. Karlsson J, Appelqvist R. Irreducible fracture of the wrist in a child. Entrapment of the extensor tendons. *Acta Orthop Scand*. 1987;58(3):280–281.
113. Kasser JR. *Forearm Fractures*. Baltimore, MD: Lippincott Williams & Wilkins; 1993.
114. Kennedy RM, Porter FL, Miller JP, et al. Comparison of fentanyl/midazolam with ketamine/midazolam for pediatric orthopedic emergencies. *Pediatrics*. 1998;102(4 Pt 1):956–963.
115. Khan S, Sawyer J, Pershad J. Closed reduction of distal forearm fractures by pediatric emergency physicians. *Acad Emerg Med*. 2010;17(11):1169–1174.
116. Khosla S, Melton LJ 3rd, Dekutoski MB, et al. Incidence of childhood distal forearm fractures over 30 years: a population-based study. *JAMA*. 2003;290(11):1479–1485.
117. Kirmani S, Christen D, van Lenthe GH, et al. Bone structure at the distal radius during adolescent growth. *J Bone Miner Res*. 2009;24(6):1033–1042.
118. Knirk JL, Jupiter JB. Intra-articular fractures of the distal end of the radius in young adults. *J Bone Joint Surg Am*. 1986;68(5):647–659.
119. Kozin SH, Waters PM. Fractures and dislocations of the hand and carpus in children. In: Beaty JH, Kasser JR, eds. *Rockwood and Green's Fractures in Children*. Philadelphia, PA: Lippincott Williams & Wilkins; 2006:257–336.
120. Kropman RH, Bemelman M, Segers MJ, et al. Treatment of impacted greenstick forearm fractures in children using bandage or cast therapy: a prospective randomized trial. *J Trauma*. 2010;68(2):425–428.
121. Landfried MJ, Stenclik M, Susi JG. Variant of Galeazzi fracture-dislocation in children. *J Pediatr Orthop*. 1991;11(3):332–335.
122. Landin LA. Fracture patterns in children. Analysis of 8,682 fractures with special reference to incidence, etiology and secular changes in a Swedish urban population 1950–1979. *Acta Orthop Scand Suppl*. 1983;202:1–109.
123. Langenskiold A. Surgical treatment of partial closure of the growth plate. *J Pediatr Orthop*. 1981;1(1):3–11.
124. Larsen E, Vittas D, Torp-Pedersen S. Remodeling of angulated distal forearm fractures in children. *Clin Orthop Relat Res*. 1988;(237):190–195.
125. Lee BS, Esterhai JL Jr, Das M. Fracture of the distal radial epiphysis. Characteristics and surgical treatment of premature, post-traumatic epiphyseal closure. *Clin Orthop Relat Res*. 1984;(185):90–96.
126. Letts M, Rowhani N. Galeazzi-equivalent injuries of the wrist in children. *J Pediatr Orthop*. 1993;13(5):561–566.
127. Liebling MS, Berdon WE, Ruzal-Shapiro C, et al. Gymnast's wrist (pseudorickets growth plate abnormality) in adolescent athletes: findings on plain film and MR imaging. *AJR Am J Roentgenol*. 1995;164:157–159.
128. Light TR, Ogden DA, Ogden JA. The anatomy of metaphyseal torus fractures. *Clin Orthop Relat Res*. 1984;(188):103–111.
129. Low CK, Liau KH, Chew WY. Results of distal radial fractures treated by intra-focal pin fixation. *Ann Acad Med Singapore*. 2001;30(6):573–576.
130. Luther G1, Miller PE, Mahan ST, et al. Decreasing resource utilization using Standardized Clinical Assessment and Management Plans (SCAMPs). *J Pediatr Orthop*. 2016. [Epub ahead of print]
131. Luther G, Miller PE, Mahan ST, et al. Decreasing resource utilization using standardized clinical assessment and management plans (SCAMPs). [published online ahead of print September 15, 2016] *J Pediatr Orthop*. doi: 10.1097/BPO.0000000000000873.
132. Mani GV, Hui PW, Cheng JC. Translation of the radius as a predictor of outcome in distal radial fractures of children. *J Bone Joint Surg Br*. 1993;75(5):808–811.
133. Matthews LS, Kaufer H, Garver DF, et al. The effect on supination–pronation of angular malalignment of fractures of both bones of the forearm. *J Bone Joint Surg Am*. 1982;64(1):14–17.
134. McLauchlan GJ, Cowan B, Annan IH, et al. Management of completely displaced metaphyseal fractures of the distal radius in children. A prospective, randomised controlled trial. *J Bone Joint Surg Br*. 2002;84(3):413–417.
135. McQuinn AG, Jaarsma RL. Risk factors for redisplacement of pediatric distal forearm and distal radius fractures. *J Pediatr Orthop*. 2012;32(7):687–692.
136. Mikic ZD. Galeazzi fracture-dislocations. *J Bone Joint Surg Am*. 1975;57(8):1071–1080.
137. Miller BS, Taylor B, Widmann RF, et al. Cast immobilization versus percutaneous pin fixation of displaced distal radius fractures in children: a prospective, randomized study. *J Pediatr Orthop*. 2005;25(4):490–494.
138. Mino DE, Palmer AK, Levinsohn EM. Radiography and computerized tomography in the diagnosis of incongruity of the distal radio-ulnar joint. A prospective study. *J Bone Joint Surg Am*. 1985;67(2):247–252.
139. Mizuta T, Benson WM, Foster BK, et al. Statistical analysis of the incidence of physeal injuries. *J Pediatr Orthop*. 1987;7(5):518–523.
140. Monga P, Raghupathy A, Courtman NH. Factors affecting remanipulation in paediatric forearm fractures. *J Pediatr Orthop B*. 2010;19(2):181–187.
141. Moore DC, Hogan KA, Crisco JJ 3rd, et al. Three-dimensional in vivo kinematics of the distal radioulnar joint in malunited distal radius fractures. *J Hand Surg Am*. 2002;27(2):233–242.
142. Moore TM, Lester DK, Sarmiento A. The stabilizing effect of soft-tissue constraints in artificial Galeazzi fractures. *Clin Orthop Relat Res*. 1985;(194):189–194.
143. Musharafieh RS, Macari G. Salter-Harris I fractures of the distal radius misdiagnosed as wrist sprain. *J Emerg Med*. 2000;19(3):265–270.
144. Nelson OA, Buchanan JR, Harrison CS. Distal ulnar growth arrest. *J Hand Surg Am*. 1984;9(2):164–170.
145. Nilsson BE, Obrant K. The range of motion following fracture of the shaft of the forearm in children. *Acta Orthop Scand*. 1977;48(6):600–602.
146. Nishiyama KK, Macdonald HM, Moore SA, et al. Cortical porosity is higher in boys compared with girls at the distal radius and distal tibia during pubertal growth: an HR-pQCT study. *J Bone Miner Res*. 2012;27(2):273–282.
147. Oakley EA, Ooi KS, Barnett PL. A randomized controlled trial of 2 methods of immobilizing torus fractures of the distal forearm. *Pediatr Emerg Care*. 2008;24(2):65–70.
148. Ogden JA. *Skeletal Injury in the Child*. Philadelphia, PA: WB Saunders; 1990.
149. Ogden JA, Beall JK, Conlogue GJ, et al. Radiology of postnatal skeletal development. IV. Distal radius and ulna. *Skeletal Radiol*. 1981;6(4):255–266.
150. Ooi LH, Toh CL. Galeazzi-equivalent fracture in children associated with tendon entrapment—report of two cases. *Ann Acad Med Singapore*. 2001;30(1):51–54.
151. Palmer AK, Werner FW. The triangular fibrocartilage complex of the wrist—anatomy and function. *J Hand Surg Am*. 1981;6(2):153–162.
152. Palmer AK, Werner FW. Biomechanics of the distal radioulnar joint. *Clin Orthop Relat Res*. 1984;(187):26–35.
153. Peinado A. Distal radial epiphyseal displacement after impaired distal ulnar growth. *J Bone Joint Surg Am*. 1979;61(1):88–92.
154. Perona PG, Light TR. Remodeling of the skeletally immature distal radius. *J Orthop Trauma*. 1990;4(3):356–361.

155. Pershad J, Monroe K, King W, et al. Can clinical parameters predict fractures in acute pediatric wrist injuries? *Acad Emerg Med.* 2000;7(10):1152–1155.

156. Peterson HA. Partial growth plate arrest and its treatment. *J Pediatr Orthop.* 1984;4(2):246–258.

157. Peterson HA, Madhok R, Benson JT, et al. Physeal fractures: part 1. Epidemiology in Olmsted County Minnesota, 1979–1988. *J Pediatr Orthop.* 1994;14(4):423–430.

158. Peterson HA. Physeal fractures: part 2. Two previously unclassified types. *J Pediatr Orthop.* 1994;14(4):431–438.

159. Peterson HA. Physeal fractures: part 3. Classification. *J Pediatr Orthop.* 1994;14(4):439–448.

160. Peterson HA. Triplane fracture of the distal radius: case report. *J Pediatr Orthop.* 1996;16(2):192–194.

161. Plint AC, Perry JJ, Correll R, et al. A randomized, controlled trial of removable splinting versus casting for wrist buckle fractures in children. *Pediatrics.* 2006;117(3):691–697.

162. Pollen AG. *Fractures and Dislocations in Children.* Baltimore, MD: Lippincott Williams & Wilkins; 1973.

163. Pountos I, Clegg J, Siddiqui A. Diagnosis and treatment of greenstick and torus fractures of the distal radius in children: a prospective randomised single blind study. *J Child Orthop.* 2010;4(4):321–326.

164. Pretell Mazzini J, Rodriguez Martin J. Paediatric forearm and distal radius fractures: risk factors and re-displacement—role of casting indices. *Int Orthop.* 2010;34(3):407–412.

165. Proctor MT, Moore DJ, Paterson JM. Redisplacement after manipulation of distal radial fractures in children. *J Bone Joint Surg Br.* 1993;75(3):453–454.

166. Pullagura M, Gopisetti S, Bateman B, et al. Are extremity musculoskeletal injuries in children related to obesity and social status? A prospective observational study in a district general hospital. *J Child Orthop.* 2011;5(2):97–100.

167. Rampoldi M, Marsico S. Complications of volar plating of distal radius fractures. *Acta Orthop Belg.* 2007;73(6):714–719.

168. Randsborg PH, Sivertsen EA. Distal radius fractures in children: substantial difference in stability between buckle and greenstick fractures. *Acta Orthop.* 2009;80(5):585–589.

169. Randsborg PH, Sivertsen EA. Classification of distal radius fractures in children: good inter- and intraobserver reliability, which improves with clinical experience. *BMC Musculoskelet Disord.* 2012;13:6.

170. Rang M. *Children's Fractures.* Philadelphia, PA: Lippincott; 1983.

171. Rettig ME, Raskin KB. Galeazzi fracture-dislocation: a new treatment-oriented classification. *J Hand Surg Am.* 2001;26(2):228–235.

172. Ring D, Waters PM, Hotchkiss RN, et al. Pediatric floating elbow. *J Pediatr Orthop.* 2001;21(4):456–459.

173. Robert CE, Jiang JJ, Khoury JG. A prospective study on the effectiveness of cotton versus waterproof cast padding in the reduction of pediatric distal forearm fractures. *J Pediatr Orthop.* 2011;31(2):144–149.

174. Ronning R, Ronning I, Gerner T, et al. The efficacy of wrist protectors in preventing snowboarding injuries. *Am J Sports Med.* 2001;29(5):581–585.

175. Roy S, Caine D, Singer KM. Stress changes of the distal radial epiphysis in young gymnasts. A report of twenty-one cases and a review of the literature. *Am J Sports Med.* 1985;13(5):301–308.

176. Salter RHW. Injuries involving the epiphyseal plate. *J Bone Joint Surg Am.* 1963;45:587–622.

177. Sasaki Y, Sugioka Y. The pronator quadratus sign: its classification and diagnostic usefulness for injury and inflammation of the wrist. *J Hand Surg Br.* 1989;14(1):80–83.

178. Schranz PJ, Fagg PS. Undisplaced fractures of the distal third of the radius in children: an innocent fracture? *Injury.* 1992;23(3):165–167.

179. Schuind F, An KN, Berglund L, et al. The distal radioulnar ligaments: a biomechanical study. *J Hand Surg Am.* 1991;16(6):1106–1114.

180. Schuind F, Cooney WP 3rd, Burny F, et al. Small external fixation devices for the hand and wrist. *Clin Orthop Relat Res.* 1993;(293):77–82.

181. Skaggs DL, Loro ML, Pitukcheewanont P, et al. Increased body weight and decreased radial cross-sectional dimensions in girls with forearm fractures. *J Bone Miner Res.* 2001;16(7):1337–1342.

182. Solan MC, Rees R, Daly K. Current management of torus fractures of the distal radius. *Injury.* 2002;33(6):503–505.

183. Stanitski CL, Micheli LJ. Simultaneous ipsilateral fractures of the arm and forearm in children. *Clin Orthop Relat Res.* 1980;(153):218–222.

184. Stansberry SD, Swischuk LE, Swischuk JL, et al. Significance of ulnar styloid fractures in childhood. *Pediatr Emerg Care.* 1990;6(2):99–103.

185. Subramanian P, Kantharuban S, Shilston S, et al. Complications of Kirschner-wire fixation in distal radius fractures. *Tech Hand Up Extrem Surg.* 2012;16(3):120–123.

186. Symons S, Rowsell M, Bhowal B, et al. Hospital versus home management of children with buckle fractures of the distal radius. A prospective, randomised trial. *J Bone Joint Surg Br.* 2001;83(4):556–560.

187. Taleisnik J, Watson HK. Midcarpal instability caused by malunited fractures of the distal radius. *J Hand Surg Am.* 1984;9(3):350–357.

188. Tarr RR, Garfinkel AI, Sarmiento A, et al. The effects of angular and rotational deformities of both bones of the forearm. An in vitro study. *J Bone Joint Surg Am.* 1984;66(1):65–70.

189. Taylor BL, Attia MW. Sports-related injuries in children. *Acad Emerg Med.* 2000;7(12):1376–1382.

190. Terry CL, Waters PM. Triangular fibrocartilage injuries in pediatric and adolescent patients. *J Hand Surg Am.* 1998;23(4):626–634.

191. Thomas FB. Precise plaster wedging: fracture-angle/cast-diameter ratio. *Br Med J.* 1965;2(5467):921.

192. Thomas EM, Tuson KW, Browne PS. Fractures of the radius and ulna in children. *Injury.* 1975;7(2):120–124.

193. Tolat AR, Sanderson PL, De Smet L, et al. The gymnast's wrist: acquired positive ulnar variance following chronic epiphyseal injury. *J Hand Surg Br.* 1992;17(6):678–681.

194. Trumble TE, Wagner W, Hanel DP, et al. Intrafocal (Kapandji) pinning of distal radius fractures with and without external fixation. *J Hand Surg Am.* 1998;23(3):381–394.

195. Vahvanen V, Westerlund M. Fracture of the carpal scaphoid in children. A clinical and roentgenological study of 108 cases. *Acta Orthop Scand.* 1980;51(6):909–913.

196. Vance RM, Gelberman RH. Acute ulnar neuropathy with fractures at the wrist. *J Bone Joint Surg Am.* 1978;60(7):962–965.

197. Vernooij CM, Vreeburg ME, Segers MJ, et al. Treatment of torus fractures in the forearm in children using bandage therapy. *J Trauma Acute Care Surg.* 2012;72(4):1093–1097.

198. Vince KG, Miller JE. Cross-union complicating fracture of the forearm. Part II: Children. *J Bone Joint Surg Am.* 1987;69(5):654–661.

199. Voto SJ, Weiner DS, Leighley B. Redisplacement after closed reduction of forearm fractures in children. *J Pediatr Orthop.* 1990;10(1):79–84.

200. Walsh HP, McLaren CA, Owen R. Galeazzi fractures in children. *J Bone Joint Surg Br.* 1987;69(5):730–733.

201. Wang Q, Wang XF, Luliano-Burns S, et al. Rapid growth produces transient cortical weakness: a risk factor for metaphyseal fractures during puberty. *J Bone Miner Res.* 2010;25(7):1521–1526.

202. Wareham K, Johansen A, Stone MD, et al. Seasonal variation in the incidence of wrist and forearm fractures, and its consequences. *Injury.* 2003;34(3):219–222.

203. Waters PM, Bae DS, Montgomery KD. Surgical management of posttraumatic distal radial growth arrest in adolescents. *J Pediatr Orthop.* 2002;22(6):717–724.

204. Waters PM, Kolettis GJ, Schwend R. Acute median neuropathy following physeal fractures of the distal radius. *J Pediatr Orthop.* 1994;14(2):173–177.

205. Waters PM, Mih AD. Fractures of the distal radius and ulna. In: Beaty JH, Kasser JR, eds. *Rockwood and Green's Fractures in Children.* Philadelphia, PA: Lippincott Williams & Wilkins; 2006:337–398.

206. Waters PM, Mintzer CM, Hipp JA, et al. Noninvasive measurement of distal radius instability. *J Hand Surg Am.* 1997;22(4):572–579.

207. Webb GR, Galpin RD, Armstrong DG. Comparison of short and long arm plaster casts for displaced fractures in the distal third of the forearm in children. *J Bone Joint Surg Am.* 2006;88(1):9–17.

208. Wells L, Avery A, Hosalkar HH, et al. Cast wedging: a "forgotten" yet predictable method for correcting fracture deformity. *UPOJ.* 2010;20:113–116.

209. West S, Andrews J, Bebbington A, et al. Buckle fractures of the distal radius are safely treated in a soft bandage: a randomized prospective trial of bandage versus plaster cast. *J Pediatr Orthop.* 2005;25(3):322–325.

210. Wilkins KE. *Operative Management of Upper Extremity Fractures in Children.* Chicago, IL: AAOS; 1994.

211. Wilkins KE, O'Brien E. *Distal Radius and Ulnar Fractures.* Philadelphia, PA: Lippincott Williams & Wilkins; 2002.

212. Wolfe JS, Eyring EJ. Median-nerve entrapment within a greenstick fracture; a case report. *J Bone Joint Surg Am.* 1974;56(6):1270–1272.

213. Wood AM, Robertson GA, Rennie L, et al. The epidemiology of sports-related fractures in adolescents. *Injury.* 2010;41(8):834–838.

214. Worlock P, Stower M. Fracture patterns in Nottingham children. *J Pediatr Orthop.* 1986;6(6):656–660.

215. Yong-Hing K, Wedge JH, Bowen CV, et al. Chronic injury to the distal ulnar and radial growth plates in an adolescent gymnast. A case report. *J Bone Joint Surg Am.* 1988;70(7):1087–1089.

216. Young TB. Irreducible displacement of the distal radial epiphysis complicating a fracture of the lower radius and ulna. *Injury.* 1984;16(3):166–168.

217. Younger AS, Tredwell SJ, Mackenzie WG, et al. Accurate prediction of outcome after pediatric forearm fracture. *J Pediatr Orthop.* 1994;14(2):200–206.

218. Younger AS, Tredwell SJ, Mackenzie WG, et al. Factors affecting fracture position at cast removal after pediatric forearm fracture. *J Pediatr Orthop.* 1997;17(3):332–336.

219. Yung PS, Lam CY, Ng BK, et al. Percutaneous transphyseal intramedullary Kirschner wire pinning: a safe and effective procedure for treatment of displaced diaphyseal forearm fracture in children. *J Pediatr Orthop.* 2004;24(1):7–12.

220. Zammit-Maempel I, Bisset RA, Morris J, et al. The value of soft tissue signs in wrist trauma. *Clin Radiol.* 1988;39(6):664–668.

221. Zamzam MM, Khoshhal KI. Displaced fracture of the distal radius in children: factors responsible for redisplacement after closed reduction. *J Bone Joint Surg Br.* 2005;87(6):841–843.

222. Zerin JM, Hernandez RJ. Approach to skeletal maturation. *Hand Clin.* 1991;7(1):53–62.

223. Zimmermann R, Gschwentner M, Pechlaner S, et al. Remodeling capacity and functional outcome of palmarly versus dorsally displaced pediatric radius fractures in the distal one-third. *Arch Orthop Trauma Surg.* 2004;124(1):42–48.

9

Diaphyseal Radius and Ulna Fractures

Charles T. Mehlman and Eric J. Wall

INTRODUCTION TO DIAPHYSEAL RADIUS AND ULNA FRACTURES

Injuries to the shafts of the radius and ulna represent some of the most common reasons for children to receive orthopedic care[59,61,204] and are among the most challenging for the orthopedist because of their treatment complexity and risk of complications.[78,234,258] Because of numerous differences in both treatment and prognosis, shaft fractures are considered to be clinically distinct from fractures of the distal (metaphyseal fractures and physeal fractures) and proximal (radial neck fractures and physeal fractures) ends of the same bones.[70,145,283,323,328,329] Many shaft injuries in children are effectively treated with skillful closed fracture care,[162,257,355] but failures continue to occur despite good orthopedic intentions.[39] Care by reduction, splint/cast molding, remanipulation, and recasting, as well as treatment of delayed union, malunion, and refracture must be mastered.

Over the past 10 years, there has been a dramatic increase in surgical fixation of forearm shaft fractures,[139,300] primarily with elastic nails.[103] Shaft fractures of the forearm are also the most common reason for operative care of the forearm in children.[59,128] The evolving indications for surgical treatment of forearm shaft fractures and the resulting outcomes will be covered in detail in this chapter. Thus, it is very important for orthopedic surgeons who treat children to skillfully manage the cognitive and technical aspects of both nonoperative and operative treatment for injuries to the shafts of the radius and ulna.

Risk is a central concept in clinical epidemiology.[215] Landin[186] has shown that the overall risk of fracture in children slowly increases for both males and females until they are 11 or 12 years old and then drops for females and increases further for males (Fig. 9-1). This risk difference is starkly illustrated by the fact that males who are 13 years or older have approximately double the fracture rate of their female peers.[186]

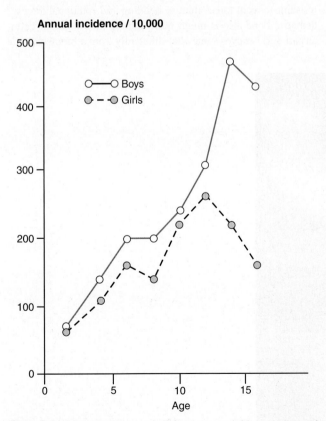

Annual incidence / 10,000

Figure 9-1. Annual incidence of all fractures in children. (Reprinted with permission from Landin LA. Epidemiology of children's fractures. *J Pediatr Orthop B.* 1997;6(2):79–83.)

Forearm fractures have been reported to be the most common pediatric fracture associated with backyard trampoline use[26] and the second most common one (supracondylar humeral fractures) was first associated with monkey bars.[341] Using a national database, Chung and Spilson[61] looked at the frequency of upper extremity fractures in the United States and found that the single largest demographic group was fractures of the radius and ulna in children aged 14 years or less, with a rate approaching 1 in 100. Two groups of researchers have recently evaluated the relationship between bone mineral density and forearm fractures in children. Using DXA scans, Andre Kaelin and his coauthors in Geneva, Switzerland prospectively studied 50 teenagers presenting with their first forearm fracture and 50 healthy controls and found no significant differences between the groups.[53] These same authors suggested that forearm fractures in such teenagers do not appear to be related to osteopenia.[53] However, Laura Tosi and her fellow researchers studied African American children (5 to 9 years of age) in Washington, DC and found that those who sustained forearm fractures did demonstrate lower bone mineral density and lower vitamin D levels.[277] Therefore, taking a calcium intake history on forearm fracture patients remains a prudent practice.

Large studies that distinguish distal radial fractures from forearm shaft fractures indicate that overall, radial shaft injuries rank as the third most common fracture of childhood (behind distal radial and supracondylar humeral fractures).[59] Open fractures in children are most often fractures of the shaft of the radius and ulna or tibial shaft fractures.[59] Among pediatric fractures, forearm shaft injuries are the most common site of refracture.[186] Forearm shaft fractures have been shown to occur most commonly in the 12- to 16-year-old age group, a challenging age group to treat.[59] The impact of increasing age on fracture incidence is further illustrated by Worlock and Stower,[353] who showed that the rate of forearm shaft fractures in school-age children (more than 5 years old) is more than double than that in toddlers (1.5 to 5 years old). Age also may have an effect on injury severity. Many experienced clinicians have pointed out the increasing level of treatment difficulty as the level of forearm fracture moves proximally,[70,145,244,328,329] and more proximal fractures tend to occur in older patients.[70]

MECHANISMS OF INJURY FOR DIAPHYSEAL RADIUS AND ULNA FRACTURES

The primary mechanism of injury associated with radial and ulnar shaft fractures is a fall on an outstretched hand that transmits indirect force to the bones of the forearm.[3,68,167] Biomechanical studies have suggested that the junction of the middle and distal thirds of the radius and a substantial portion of the shaft of the ulna have an increased vulnerability to fracture.[151] Often, a significant rotational component is associated with the fall, causing the radius and ulna to fracture at different levels (Fig. 9-2).[92,212] If the radial and ulna fractures are near the same

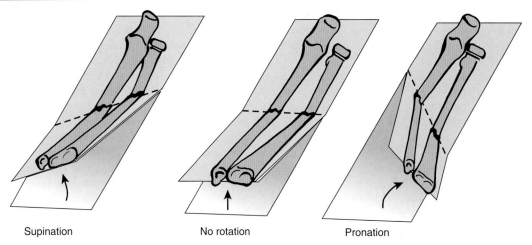

Figure 9-2. Radius and ulna shaft fractures occurring at different levels, implying rotational mechanism.

level, a minimal torsional component can be inferred (Fig. 9-3). If comminution is present, higher-energy trauma should be suspected.[83] Significant hyperpronation forces are associated with isolated shaft fractures of either the radius or the ulna and concomitant dislocation of either the distal (DRUJ) or the proximal radioulnar joint (PRUJ). Thus, in any single-bone forearm shaft fracture, these important joints need to be closely scrutinized. Galeazzi and Monteggia fracture–dislocations are discussed in Chapters 11 and 14, respectively.

A direct force to the arm (such as being hit by a baseball bat) can fracture a single bone (usually the ulna) without injury to the adjacent DRUJ or PRUJ.[32] Isolated ulnar shaft fractures have been referred to as "nightstick fractures." Alignment of

the radial head should be confirmed in any child with such a fracture to avoid a "missed Monteggia" injury.[149] Isolated radial shaft fractures are rare but notoriously difficult to reduce with closed methods.[64,93]

The mechanisms of injury of two particular forearm fracture patterns, traumatic bowing (also known as bow fractures or plastic deformation)[265] and greenstick fracture, also bear mentioning. The bone behaves differently based on the direction of the forces applied to it. This is the so-called anisotropic property of bone, and it can be simply explained as follows: Bone is more resistant to axial forces than to bending and rotational forces.[50] Pediatric bone also is much more porous than its adult counterpart and behaves somewhat differently from a biomechanical

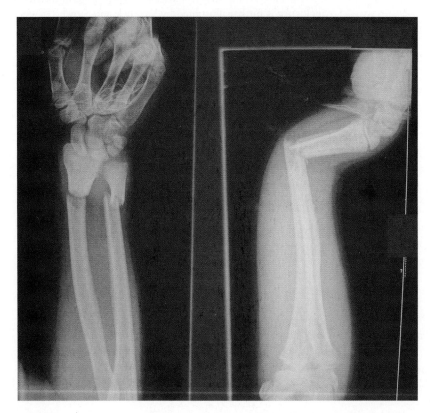

Figure 9-3. Radial and ulnar shaft fractures occurring at same level, implying no significant rotation.

standpoint.[54,236] Because of its porosity, pediatric bone absorbs significantly more energy prior to failure than the adult bone does.[73] When relatively slowly applied, longitudinal forces bend the immature bone beyond its elastic limits and into its plastic zone, resulting in traumatic bowing.[35,202] Thus, when a bending force is applied relatively slowly, many microfractures occur along the length of the bone, leading to macroscopic deformity without discernible radiographic fracture. This bending can usually be seen radiographically if suspected.

Greenstick fractures represent an intermediate step between plastic deformation and complete fractures.[51] On anteroposterior (AP) and lateral radiographs, greenstick fractures show cortical violation of one, two, or three of their radiographic cortices, and thus some bony continuity is preserved. Rotational deformity is considered to be intimately related to the clinical deformity seen with greenstick fractures of the forearm, and the analogy of a cardboard tube that tends to bend as it is twisted has been offered by Holdsworth.[145] Specifically, hyperpronation injuries usually are associated with apex-dorsal greenstick fractures of the forearm, and hypersupination injuries usually are associated with the opposite, apex-volar injuries.[93,224] The treatment of these greenstick fractures requires a derotation maneuver in addition to correction of any angulation.[51,133]

INJURIES ASSOCIATED WITH DIAPHYSEAL RADIUS AND ULNA FRACTURES

Most fractures of the shafts of the radius and ulna occur as isolated injuries, but wrist and elbow fractures may occur in conjunction with forearm fractures, and the elbow and wrist region needs to be included on standard forearm radiographs.[25,74,167,314,351,358] If clinical suspicion is high, then dedicated wrist and elbow films are necessary. The so-called floating elbow injury (fracture of the bones of the forearm along with ipsilateral supracondylar humeral fracture) is a well-described entity that must not be missed.[25,273,314,351] Surgical stabilization of both the supracondylar fracture and the forearm fractures has been recommended by multiple authors in recent years[29,138,272,273,319,322] to avoid the risk of a compartment syndrome. Galeazzi and Monteggia fracture–dislocations also must be ruled out. Compartment syndrome can also occur in conjunction with any forearm shaft fracture.[72,364] This rare but potentially devastating complication can lead to a Volkmann ischemic contracture, which has been shown to occur after forearm shaft fractures almost as often as it does after supracondylar humeral fractures in children.[225] Patients with severe pain unrelieved by immobilization and mild narcotic medication should be reassessed for excessive swelling and tight forearm compartments. If loosening of the splint, cast, and underlying cast materials fails to relieve pain, then measurement of compartment pressures and subsequent fasciotomy may be necessary.

Abrasions or seemingly small unimportant lacerations that occur in conjunction with forearm fractures must be carefully evaluated because they may be an indication of an open fracture. Clues to the presence of an open fracture include persistent slow bloody ooze from a small laceration near the fracture site and subcutaneous emphysema on injury films. Careful evaluation and, in some situations, sterile probing of suspicious

wounds will be necessary. Open forearm fractures are discussed later in this chapter.

Vascular or neurologic injuries are rarely associated with forearm shaft fractures, but the consequences of such injuries are far-reaching. Serial neurovascular examinations should be performed and documented. Radial and ulnar pulses along with distal digital capillary refill, in terms of number of seconds from blanching to return to full turgor, should be routinely evaluated. Davis and Green[78] reported nerve injuries in 1% (5/547) of their pediatric forearm fracture patients, with the most commonly injured nerve being the median nerve. Combined data from three large series of pediatric open forearm fractures reveal an overall nerve injury rate at presentation of 10% (17/173), with the median nerve once again being the one most commonly injured.[128,135,199] To screen for these rare but significant injuries, every child with a forearm fracture should routinely have evaluation of the radial, ulnar, and median nerves for both motor and sensory function.[64] Nerve injuries occurring at the time of injury must be differentiated from treatment-related or iatrogenic neurologic deficits.

Davidson[76] suggested using the game of "rock–paper–scissors" for testing the median, radial, and ulnar nerves (Fig. 9-4). The pronated fist is the rock and tests median nerve function (PT, FDP, FPL). The extended fingers and wrist depict paper and test radial nerve function (EDC, ECRB/L). Fully flexed small and ring fingers, an adducted thumb, and spreading the index and ring fingers mimic scissors and test ulnar nerve function (intrinsics). Further focused testing should also be done on two important nerve branches: the anterior interosseous nerve (branch of median nerve) and the posterior interosseous nerve (PIN) (branch of radial nerve). The anterior interosseous nerve provides motor function to the index flexor digitorum profundus, the flexor pollicis longus, and pronator quadratus and is best tested by having the patient make an "OK" sign. The PIN typically innervates the extensor carpi ulnaris, extensor digitorum communis, extensor digiti minimi, extensor indicis, and the three outcropping muscles of the thumb (abductor pollicis longus, extensor pollicis brevis, and extensor pollicis longus).[41] Its function is best documented by full extension of the phalangeal and metacarpophalangeal joints. This is especially difficult to test in a patient in a cast or splint that partially covers the fingers. Most injuries that occur in association with forearm fractures are true neurapraxias and typically resolve over the course of days to weeks.[72,78]

SIGNS AND SYMPTOMS OF DIAPHYSEAL RADIUS AND ULNA FRACTURES

The signs and symptoms indicating fracture of the shafts of the radius and ulna usually are not subtle. Deformity and pain are the classic findings. Patients typically experience exquisite pain emanating from the involved area. Decreased pronation and supination motion are also usually noted.[309] Neither practitioners nor parents are always reliable assessors of children's pain, and ideally patients should rate their own pain.[172,299] Significant anxiety and muscle spasm almost always amplify a child's painful experience.[45,116] It has been suggested that muscle spasm is a protective effort by the body to splint or otherwise protect the injured body part.[116] When such muscle

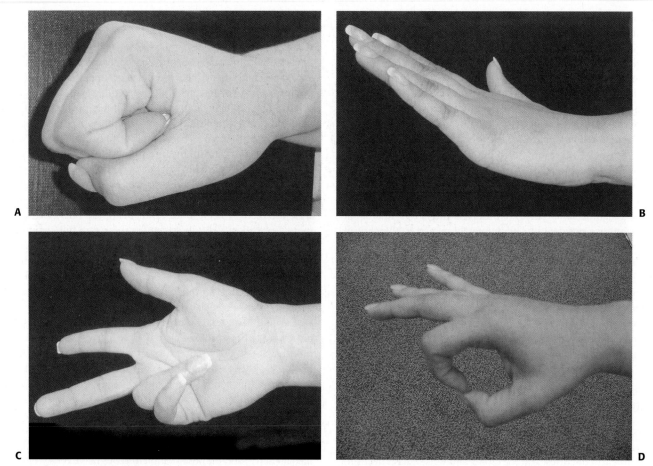

Figure 9-4. Upper extremity motor nerve physical examination. **A:** Rock position demonstrates median nerve motor function. **B:** Paper position demonstrates radial nerve motor function. **C:** Scissor position demonstrates ulnar nerve motor function. **D:** "OK" sign demonstrates function of anterior interosseous nerve.

spasm occurs in association with certain fracture patterns (e.g., a radial shaft fracture proximal to the pronator teres insertion), it produces predictable fracture displacement (e.g., a pronated distal radial fragment and a supinated proximal fragment).

More subtle fractures present special diagnostic challenges. Certain pathologic fractures of the forearm may occur in the absence of overt trauma.[157,181] Many minimally displaced fractures of the shafts of the radius and ulna can be mistaken for a "sprain" or "just a bruise" for several days to several weeks. This usually occurs in young children who continue to use the fractured arm during low-level play activities. As a general rule, a fracture should be suspected if the child has not resumed all normal arm function within 1 or 2 days of injury.

IMAGING AND OTHER DIAGNOSTIC STUDIES FOR DIAPHYSEAL RADIUS AND ULNA FRACTURES

Because important forearm fracture treatment decisions frequently are based on radiographic measurement of angular deformities, it must be remembered that these angles are projected shadows that are affected by rotation.[101] If angulation is present on both AP and lateral views (commonly called two orthogonal views), the true deformity is out of the plane of the

radiographs, and its true magnitude is greater than that measured on each individual view. Certain forearm shaft fracture deformities are clearly "two-plane deformities" whose maximal angular magnitude is in some plane other than the standard AP or lateral plane (Fig. 9-5).[15] Bär and Breitfuss[15] produced a table (based on the pythagorean theorem) that predicts the true maximal angulation. Accurate deformity measurement can be made when angulation is seen on only one view and there is no angulation on the other orthogonal view.

Evans pointed out the importance of tracking the rotational alignment of the free-moving radial fragment by ascertaining the relative location of the bicipital tuberosity. This was a major step forward in refining the orthopedic care of these forearm injuries. On a fully supinated AP radiograph of an unfractured forearm, the bicipital tuberosity points predominantly in a medial direction (nearly 180 degrees opposite of the radial tuberosity).[91] The radius and ulna are also nearly parallel to each other on such a view. On a fully pronated AP radiograph of an unfractured forearm, the bicipital tuberosity points in a lateral direction and the radial tuberosity is situated medially.[91] The radius also crosses over the ulna in a pronated AP view. Rang[264] noted that in an unfractured limb, the bicipital tuberosity tended to align with a point near the thenar eminence (Fig. 9-6), more

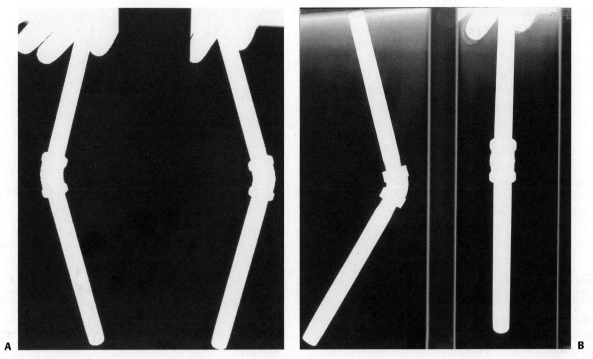

Figure 9-5. Underestimation of true angulation. **A:** "Out of the AP and lateral plane" underestimates angulation at 30 degrees. **B:** True AP and lateral demonstrates that true maximal angulation is 40 degrees.

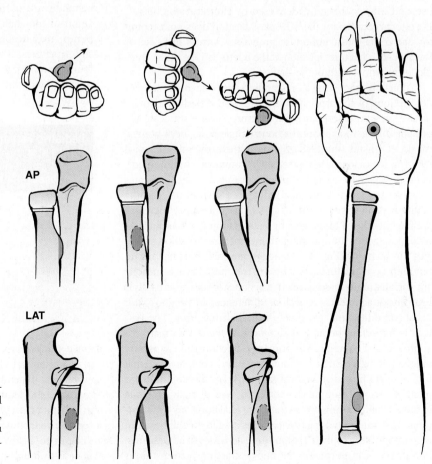

Figure 9-6. Rang's illustration depicting the position of the bicipital tuberosity on AP and lateral views with the forearm in pronation, supination, and neutral position. (Reprinted with permission from Rang M. *Children's Fractures.* 1st ed. Philadelphia, PA: JB Lippincott; 1974:96.)

nearly a 165-degree relationship than a true 180-degree one. These relationships are best assessed on standard radiographs that include the entire forearm on one film[74,258,329] rather than the specialized bicipital tuberosity view originally suggested by Evans.[91] A CT scan of both forearms with cuts through the bicipital tuberosity and the radial styloid is probably the best way to accurately identify a rotational malunion after a fracture that could be causing a loss of forearm rotation. The ulna can be similarly assessed by comparing the distal ulnar styloid to the proximal coronoid process on orthogonal views (similar to bicipital tuberosity and radial styloid, the coronoid process and ulnar styloid should be 180 degrees apart). CT scan cuts of the coronoid process and the ulnar styloid on the fractured and nonfractured sides are most reliable for measuring the rotational alignment of the ulna, but do carry the concern for irradiation to young children.

CLASSIFICATION OF DIAPHYSEAL RADIUS AND ULNA FRACTURES

Fractures of the shafts of the radius and ulna often are described in rather imprecise terms such as "both-bone forearm fracture" and "greenstick fracture." Radiographs confirm the diagnosis of forearm shaft fracture and are the basis for most classification systems. The most comprehensive classification of forearm fractures is the one adopted by the Orthopaedic Trauma Association (OTA).[10] Although this system is sound in concept, its 36 discrete subtypes[10] make it impractical for everyday clinical use, and it has not been widely used by clinical researchers.[270] Despite its complexity, the OTA classification does not account for one of the most important prognostic factors in pediatric forearm shaft fracture: location of the fracture in the distal, middle, or proximal third of the shaft.

Clinicians and clinical researchers have favored simpler descriptions of forearm shaft fractures. An orderly and practical approach to forearm shaft fracture classification should provide information about the bone (single bone, both bones), the level (distal, middle, or proximal third), and the pattern (plastic deformation, greenstick, complete, comminuted). Bone involvement is important because it not only indicates the severity of injury but also influences suspicion regarding additional soft tissue injury (e.g., single-bone injury increases the likelihood of a Monteggia or Galeazzi injury)[334] and affects reduction tactics (unique single-bone fracture reduction strategies can be used) (Fig. 9-7). Single-bone shaft fractures occur, but both-bone fractures are far more common. Level is important for anatomic reasons relative to muscle and interosseous ligament attachments, as well as differences in prognosis for distal-, middle-, and proximal-third shaft fractures. The pattern is important because it significantly alters the treatment approach. For example, the primary reduction strategy is very different for greenstick fractures (rotation) compared to that for complete fractures (vertical traction). Certain comminuted fractures (e.g., comminution of both bones) may preclude reduction and casting and require surgical fixation.[102,104] Fortunately, comminuted fracture patterns are rare in children, but increasingly seen in high-risk sporting activities of adolescents. For all practical purposes, the buckle fracture pattern that is

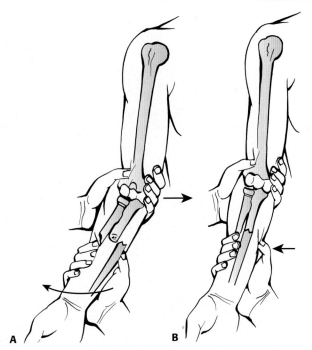

Figure 9-7. Isolated ulnar shaft reduction technique (Blount). Valgus force applied to fracture site and direct thumb pressure over distal ligament. **A:** Reductive force is applied as illustrated. **B:** The fracture is reduced.

common in the distal radial metaphysis never occurs in isolation in the shaft region. The typical buckle fracture "speed bump" may accompany either plastic deformation or greenstick fractures. Thus, there are two bones, three levels, and four common fracture patterns (Fig. 9-8). We believe this is a practical and clinically relevant way to describe forearm shaft fractures.[216]

Pediatric Forearm Shaft Fracture: PRACTICAL CLASSIFICATION		
Two Bones	**Three Levels**	**Four Patterns**
Radius	Distal one-third	Plastic deformation (Bow fracture)
Ulna	Middle one-third	Greenstick
	Proximal one-third	Complete
*beware of single-bone injuries due to risk to DRUJ and PRUJ	*completely displaced middle- and proximal-third fractures can be particularly troublesome	Comminuted

Once the forearm fracture has been described in the terms of this practical classification, fracture displacement must be evaluated. Fracture displacement can occur as angulation, rotation, shortening, or translation. Angulation is important in treatment decision making and can be measured with reasonable reliability.[190,320] Rotation is a simple concept, but it is difficult to assess clinically.[92,258] The best that usually can be done is to roughly estimate rotation within a 45-degree margin

Practical classification
Two bones

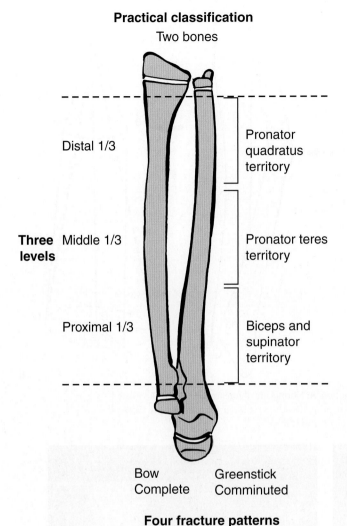

Distal 1/3

Pronator
quadrats
territory

Three Middle 1/3
levels

Pronator teres
territory

Proximal 1/3

Biceps and
supinator
territory

Bow   Greenstick
Complete   Comminuted

Four fracture patterns

Figure 9-8. Practical classification of forearm shaft fractures. (*Distal dotted line* defined by proximal extent of the Lister tubercle and *proximal dotted line* defined by proximal extent of bicipital tuberosity.)

of error.[70,258] Based on available clinical studies, it appears that less than 1 cm of shortening should be accepted in either single- or both-bone fracture patterns.[49,79,84,218,275] It has also been suggested that the shortening that accompanies displaced fractures may help preserve future motion through interosseous membrane relaxation.[258] Completely (100%) translated fractures of the middle third[70,258] and distal third[84,218,275] of the forearm have been shown to reliably remodel. Certain situations may raise concern regarding complete translation, such as isolated middle-third radial fractures with medial (ulnar) displacement that significantly narrows the interosseous space and translation in children who have less than 2 full years of growth remaining, because remodeling of the translated fracture site is less predictable in older than in younger children.[234,236]

OUTCOMES OF DIAPHYSEAL RADIUS AND ULNA FRACTURES

The fundamental reason for treating fractures of the shafts of the radius and ulna relates to the likelihood of bad results in the absence of adequate care. Data from certain developing countries may be as close as we come to natural history studies of untreated fractures. Archibong and Onuba[11] reported on 102 pediatric fracture patients treated in Southeastern Nigeria. Their patients most commonly had upper extremity fractures, and they frequently experienced significant delays in seeking medical treatment, which led to high rates of malunion requiring surgical treatment.[11] Other Nigerian authors have found that young age was not protective against fracture malunion (more than 50%) and nonunion (25%) following traditional bonesetter treatment.[239] It is unclear whether children treated in this fashion are better or worse off than if they had received no treatment at all. The rationale for treating pediatric forearm shaft fractures is thus based on the premise that the results of modern orthopedic treatment will exceed "pseudonatural histories" such as these.

The consequences of excessively crooked (and malrotated) forearm bones are both aesthetic and functional (Fig. 9-9).[27,30,145,211,233,329] Limited forearm supination following a forearm shaft malunion is illustrated in Figure 9-10. Despite their great concern to parents, aesthetic issues have not been formally studied, and as a result the practitioner must interpret forearm appearance issues on a case-by-case basis. Clinical experience has shown that the ulna appears to be less forgiving from an aesthetic standpoint because of its long subcutaneous border. Early and repeated involvement of the parents (or other legal guardians) in an informed and shared decision-making process is essential.

Bony malunion and soft tissue fibrosis have both been implicated as causes of limited forearm motion after forearm shaft fractures.[144,233] Limited forearm pronation and supination can have significant effects on upper extremity function.[25,246,258] Inability to properly pronate often can be compensated for with shoulder abduction (but can lead to fatigue with prolonged activities), and no easy compensatory mechanism exists for supination deficits.[64,145,246,258] Daruwalla[74] identified a nearly 53% rate of limited forearm rotation (subtle in some, dramatic in others) in his series of 53 children with forearm fractures and attributed it to angular deformity and rotational malalignment. Several patients in Price's[258] classic series of pediatric forearm malunions had severe forearm range-of-motion losses that significantly limited vocational and recreational activities. Trousdale and Linscheid[329] reported range-of-motion losses severe enough to prompt corrective osteotomies in many of their predominantly pediatric (less than 14 years old at time of injury) patients with forearm malunions. Meier[219] also reported significant range-of-motion deficits in association with pediatric forearm malunion.

Range-of-motion losses caused by deformity have been studied by numerous authors using adult cadaveric forearm specimens. Matthews et al.[211] studied 10- and 20-degree midshaft angular deformities of the radius and ulna in 10 forearm specimens. They found that 10-degree deformities of either bone individually resulted in little or no measurable motion loss (in the range of 3 degrees or less). When both bones were angulated 10 degrees dorsal, volar, or toward the interosseous membrane, larger motion losses were documented (approximately 10-degree pronation and 20-degree supination). Significantly

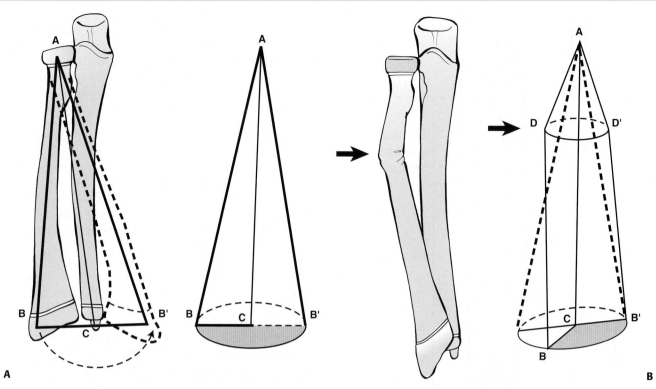

Figure 9-9. Effect of forearm malunion on forearm motion. **A:** Normal arc of forearm motion. **B:** Angulated radius leads to diminished arc of forearm motion. (Reprinted with permission from Ogden JA. *Skeletal Injury in the Child.* 1st ed. Philadelphia, PA: Lea & Febiger; 1982:56–57.)

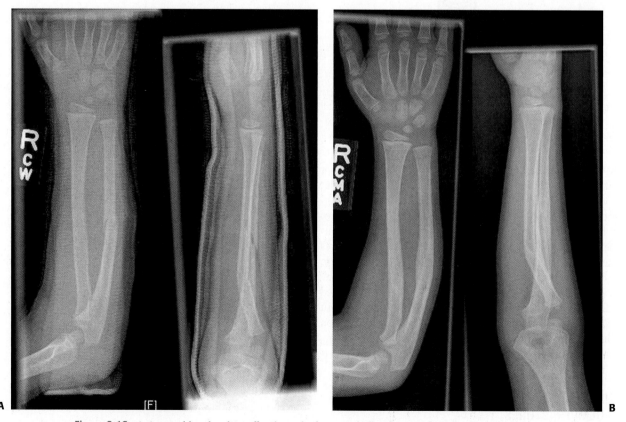

Figure 9-10. A 6-year-old male who suffered a right forearm shaft malunion. **A:** Radiograph one week after fracture showing complete midshaft ulnar and proximal third radial fractures. **B:** Healed fractures at 6-month follow-up.

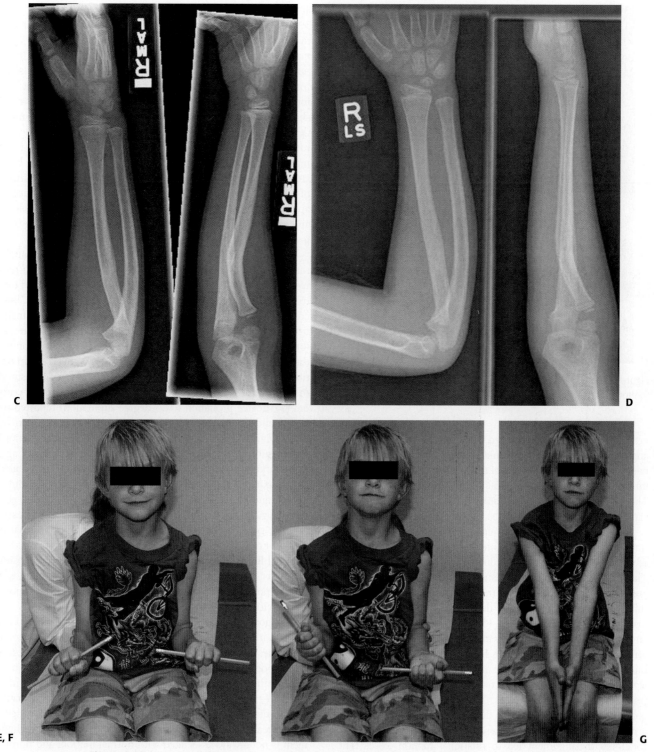

Figure 9-10. (*Continued*) **C:** Twenty-month follow-up. **D:** Twenty-six month follow-up. **E:** Symmetrical pronation. **F:** Limited supination on the right **G:** Axial alignment with palms together.

(*continues*)

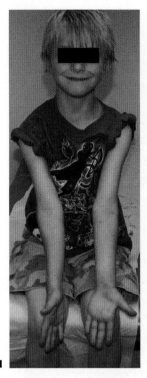
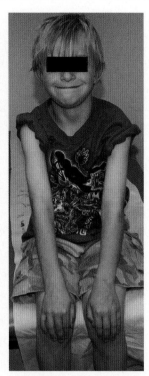

H   **I**

Figure 9-10. *(Continued)* **H:** An effort at supination. **I:** Axial alignment in pronation.

greater losses of motion occurred when one or both bones were angulated 20 degrees (approximately 40 degrees for both pronation and supination). Some of the 10-degree angulated specimens demonstrated "cosmetically unacceptable deformity."[211] These findings indicate that relatively small angular deformities can be clinically significant.

Additional important information about the influence of fracture level on forearm motion was provided by a series of adult cadaver experiments conducted by Sarmiento et al.[282,321] They found that fracture angulation of 15 to 30 degrees led to greater supination losses when the deformity was in the middle third of the forearm (40 to 90 degrees) and greater pronation losses when in the distal third (30 to 80 degrees).[321] Fracture angulation of 10 degrees or less in the proximal or middle forearm rarely resulted in more than 15 degrees of motion loss,[282,321] but the same angulation in the distal third of the forearm was at times (usually with isolated radius fracture) associated with pronation losses of 20 degrees.[282,321] These findings challenge commonly held beliefs that the distal-third fracture of the forearm is the most forgiving. These same authors asserted that rotational malalignment led to rotational motion losses that usually were equal in magnitude and opposite in direction to the deformity (e.g., a 10-degree pronation deformity led to a 10-degree loss of supination).[321]

Rotational malalignment of the forearm has been studied in greater detail in recent years, mostly in adults and in the laboratory.[87,169,330] In isolated midshaft radial fractures, more than 30 degrees of malrotation was a threshold for significant losses in motion (approximately 15 degrees).[169] Isolated midshaft ulna fracture malrotation did not alter the total

arc of forearm motion but did change the set point (e.g., a 30-degree pronation deformity took away 30 degrees of pronation and added 30 degrees of supination).[330] Larger ulnar axial malalignment of 45 degrees decreased overall forearm rotation by no more than 20 degrees.[330] Large residual ulnar shaft translation has similarly been found to have little impact on forearm rotation.[214] Simulated combined radial and ulnar midshaft rotational malunions resulted in the worst motion (more than 50% losses of pronation and supination when 60-degree rotational malunions were in opposite directions).[87] Rotational malunions that approximated recommended limits in the literature (45 degrees)[258] produced less extreme but real limitations of motion.[87] From these studies and our clinical experience, it appears that the radius is more sensitive to rotational problems and less sensitive regarding aesthetic issues, whereas the ulna is exactly the opposite.

Several generations of orthopedic surgeons have been taught that 50 degrees of pronation and 50 degrees of supination represent adequate forearm motion.[223] It must be remembered that this classic study performed by Morrey and his Mayo Clinic colleagues involving 33 normal subjects (18 female, 15 male) from 21 to 75 years of age is not the only study that addresses forearm motion. The average arc of normal forearm motion for the Mayo group (68-degree pronation to 74-degree supination)[223] was approximately 20 degrees less than that measured in 53 healthy male subjects who were not older than 19 years old (77-degree pronation to 83-degree supination) reported by Boone and Azen[34] and 35 degrees less than that reported by Rickert et al.[271] (75-degree pronation to 100-degree supination) in 141 subjects of both sexes between 20 and 30 years of age. Contemporary three-dimensional motion analysis has revealed that maximal pronation occurs when pouring liquid from a pitcher and maximal supination commonly occurs during personal hygiene activities.[263] Thus, it seems clear that the forearm motion "goals" reported by Morrey et al.[223] are not necessarily ideal or even optimal, but rather they may be considered as the minimal limits of forearm function. Stated another way, losing 20 degrees or 30 degrees of either pronation or supination carries the potential for significant functional impact upon important activities of daily living.

The goal of treatment is to achieve satisfactory healing of the forearm injury within the established anatomic and functional guidelines while also taking into account the reasonable degree of remodeling that can be expected in growing children.[155] Most of the time, these goals can be achieved with closed fracture care, and little or no radiographic or clinical abnormality can be detected following healing. A paradox exists in pediatric forearm fractures whereby anatomic radiographic alignment is not always associated with normal motion, and normal motion can be associated with nonanatomic radiographic healing.[144,229,233,321] Herein lies the inherent controversy between operative and nonoperative treatment approaches (Table 9-1). In patients with anatomic radiographs, range-of-motion problems usually have been attributed to scarring of the interosseous membrane.[170,246,258] With nonanatomic radiographs (incomplete remodeling), range-of-motion deficits usually are attributed to the radiographic abnormalities. Thus, treatment of forearm shaft fracture must balance the risk of allowing stiffness to occur

TABLE 9-1. Pros and Cons of Nonoperative Versus Operative Treatment

Treatment	Pros	Cons
Cast	Long track record	Stiffness may still occur
	Negligible infection risk	Frequent follow-up visits
	Fine-tuning possible	Anatomic reduction rare
Surgery	Anatomic reduction	Risk of infection
	Minimize immobilization	Need for implant removal
	Fewer follow-up visits	Stiffness from surgery

secondary to malunion against the risk of creating stiffness secondary to surgical procedures. Thus, the goal of surgical intervention is to provide sufficient stability to fracture(s) to allow for early motion to lessen risk of soft tissue stiffness and frature malunion.

The rationalization for the remodeling of pediatric forearm fractures has strong historical support,[21,32,46,242] but knowledge of the limits of remodeling must be taken into consideration. Established reduction criteria state that complete (100%) translation is acceptable,[218,258] as well as up to 15 degrees of angulation and up to 45 degrees of malrotation.[258] The fundamental reason for treating fractures of the shafts of the radius and ulna relates to the likelihood of bad results in the absence of adequate care or acceptable remodeling. As noted earlier, data from certain developing countries may be as close as we come to natural history studies of untreated fractures. Nigerian[11,239] studies indicate high rates of malunion with untreated or bonesetter treatment of diaphyseal fractures.

Published clinical studies have shown that pediatric forearm shaft fractures in children less than about 8 years of age have great remodeling potential that occurs through several mechanisms.[289] The distal radial epiphysis will redirect itself toward normal at about 10 degrees/yr. As long as the physis is open, this rate is relatively independent of age. Although the epiphysis will return to normal direction, it will have much less effect on correcting an angular deformity at the midshaft compared to fractures at the subphyseal level. Remodeling also occurs with lengthening of the bone through growth, which produces an apparent decrease in angulation, especially if measured as the difference between the proximal and distal ends of the bone. The bone also remodels by intramembranous apposition on the concave side and resorption on the convex side.[73,155,289] This occurs throughout life, but more rapidly when driven by the thick periosteum found in young children. Larsen[187] found that although the epiphyseal angle realigns quickly, children older than 11 years correct bone angulation less than the younger children. Thomas stated the following regarding pediatric forearm remodeling potential: "We should not fail to recall that the remodeling capabilities of the bones of children have not changed in the last million years and that open reduction and internal fixation must be undertaken only after due deliberation."[323] Others such as Johari[158] would state that if one critically evaluates the limits of forearm shaft remodeling capacity, you will find a much higher rate (approximately 50%) of incomplete remodeling in children over 10 years of age.

The perfect (or nearly perfect) pediatric diaphyseal forearm fracture outcome study has not yet been performed, therefore scientific answers regarding optimal treatment are lacking.[106] However, there is a growing consensus among pediatric orthopedic trauma surgeons that there are patient subsets (usually older patients with more proximal fractures) whose outcomes are clearly improved by flexible intramedullary nail surgical intervention.[347] A large retrospective cohort study focusing on radiographic outcomes has indicated that among pediatric forearm shaft fracture patients who underwent closed reduction treatment, most (51%) exceeded established radiographic criteria over the course of 2 to 4 weeks.[39] This is greatly concerning as a very clear relationship exists between radiographic and clinical outcomes for forearm shaft injuries in both adults and children.[36,86,166] For those patients deemed at higher risk, the risk–benefit ratio appears to be favorable as flexible nail surgical complications are mainly minor and in some respects, measurably lower than nonoperative forearm shaft fracture care.[280,301]

PATHOANATOMY AND APPLIED ANATOMY RELATING TO DIAPHYSEAL RADIUS AND ULNA FRACTURES

The forearm is a large nonsynovial joint with nearly a 180-degree arc of motion. Its bones, the radius and ulna, are not simple straight bony tubes. The shaft of the radius is a three-sided structure with two prominent curvatures. One major gradual convexity (approximately 10 degrees with its apex lateral-radial) is present along its midportion; a second, more acute curve of approximately 15 degrees with its apex medial occurs proximally near the bicipital tuberosity.[99,127,279] The deviation along the midportion is commonly referred to as the radial bow, and maintenance of this normal contour is a goal of forearm shaft fracture care (the radius is bowed so it can "radiate" around the ulna).[261,285,286] The most important bony landmarks of the radius are the radial styloid (lateral prominence) and the bicipital tuberosity (anteromedial prominence), which are oriented about 160 degrees away from each other (Fig. 9-11).[346] Maintenance of this styloid-tuberosity rotational relationship is another forearm shaft fracture principle. The nutrient artery of the radius enters the bone in its proximal half and courses anterior to ulnar (medial).[119] Such nutrient vessels typically are seen on only one orthogonal view and should not be confused with fracture lines. In cross section, most of the shaft of the ulna is also shaped like a classic three-sided prism, although its more distal and proximal portions are much more circular. The most important bony landmarks of the ulna are its styloid process (distally) and its coronoid process (proximally). These two landmarks are oriented nearly 180 degrees from one another, with the styloid aimed in a posterior (dorsal) direction and the coronoid in an anterior (volar) direction.[346] Tracking styloid–coronoid rotational alignment of the ulna is another part of forearm shaft fracture care. The ulnar shaft has mild curvatures in both its proximal (apex lateral/radial) and distal (apex medial/ulnar) portions but is otherwise relatively straight.[127,279] The nutrient artery to the ulna enters the bone in its proximal half and courses anterior to radial (lateral).[119]

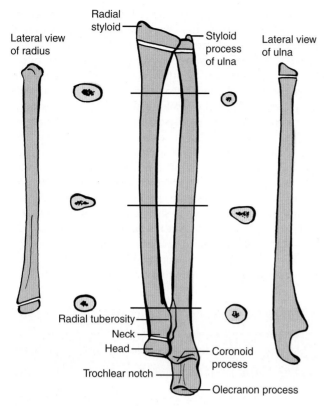

Figure 9-11. Radial and ulnar anatomy.

Lateral view of radius

Radial styloid

Styloid process of ulna

Lateral view of ulna

Radial tuberosity

Neck

Head

Trochlear notch

Coronoid process

Olecranon process

The classic works of Evans helped focus attention on rotational deformity associated with fractures of both bones of the forearm.[91,212,265] Evans stated, "The orthodox position in which to immobilize these fractures is that of full supination for the upper third, and the midposition for fractures of the middle and lower thirds, these positions being based on the anatomical arrangement of the pronators and supinators of the forearm. However, it

is unreasonable to suppose that all fractures at a given level will present the same degree of rotational deformity."[91] The radius and ulna are joined by three major passive restraints: the PRUJ, DRUJ, and the interosseous membrane complex, all of which have important stabilizing and load-transferring functions. These structures allow rotation of the radius about the ulna along an axis that runs approximately from the center of the radial head to the center of the distal ulna.[146,246] The PRUJ and DRUJ are discussed elsewhere in this book (Chapters 9 and 11). The structure and biomechanical function of the interosseous membrane have been studied extensively in recent years. Hotchkiss et al.[150] showed that the central band of the interosseous membrane (the interosseous ligament) courses from a point near the junction of the proximal and middle thirds of the radius to a point near the junction of the middle and distal thirds of the ulna. It is an important longitudinal stabilizer of the forearm in that 71% of forearm longitudinal stiffness is provided by the interosseous ligament after radial head excision.[150] Transverse vectors have also been identified[249] and reflect the stabilizing effect of the interosseous ligament during pronation and supination movements. The interosseous ligament demonstrates tensile properties comparable to the patellar tendon and the anterior cruciate ligament,[250] indicative of the magnitude of the arm forces to which this structure is subjected.

Although some difference of opinion still exists,[80,109,304] multiple studies have shown that the most strain in the central band of the interosseous membrane is generated when the forearm is in the neutral position.[207,208,304] These findings of maximal strain in neutral in cadaver studies also are consistent with radiographic measurement studies[70] and dynamic magnetic resonance imaging studies of the forearm showing that the interosseous space is maximal near a neutral position.[230] This may help explain certain pathologic situations such as the fixed supination deformity of neonatal brachial plexus palsy[213] as well as limitations of pronation and supination because of encroachment on the interosseous space from malangulated fractures (Fig. 9-12).[359] The interosseous membrane also serves

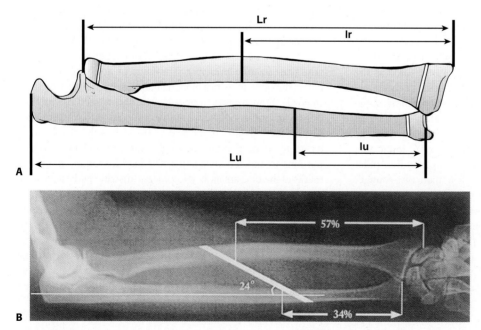

Figure 9-12. Anatomy of interosseous ligament. **A:** Central oblique orientation of interosseous ligament. **B:** Interosseous ligament attachment in terms of percentage forearm length. (Reprinted from Skahen JR III, Palmer AK, Werner FW, et al. Reconstruction of the interosseous membrane of the forearm in cadavers. *J Hand Surg Am.* 1997;22(6):986–994. Copyright © 1997 Elsevier Inc. With permission.)

as an important anchoring point for several forearm muscles: the flexor digitorum profundus, flexor pollicis longus, extensor indicis, and the outcropping muscles (extensor digitorum brevis, abductor pollicis longus).

The paired and seemingly balanced radial and ulnar bones have an unbalanced number of muscular connections. The ulna typically has 14 attached muscles and the radius 10 (Tables 9-2 and 9-3).[85,127] Powerful supinators attach to the proximal third of the forearm, whereas important pronators attach to its middle and distal thirds (Fig. 9-13). The accompanying vasculature of the forearm is complex: These muscles are supplied by more than 248 vascular pedicles arising from the brachial artery, its branches, or other collateral vessels.[269] The radial, ulnar, and median nerves (or their branches) along with the musculocutaneous nerve provide all of the key innervations to the motors that attach to the forearm bones. As mentioned earlier, the median nerve is the most commonly injured nerve with forearm fractures.[76,78,128,135]

The radial nerve proceeds from a posterior to anterior direction and enters the forearm after passing the lateral epicondyle between the brachialis and brachioradialis muscles (BRBr). Near this same level, it divides into superficial and deep terminal branches. The deep motor branch of the radial nerve is also known as the PIN. In addition to its routine innervation of the brachioradialis and extensor carpi radialis longus, most commonly (55% of the time), a motor branch arises from the radial nerve proper or its superficial terminal branch to innervate the extensor carpi radialis brevis, whereas the rest of the time (45%), this motor branch comes from the PIN.[2] The superficial branch travels along with and beneath the brachioradialis. The PIN enters the supinator muscle, passing the fibrous thickening called the arcade of Frohse shortly after branching from the radial nerve proper. It courses within the supinator past the proximal radius, later exiting this muscle dorsally (posteriorly) near the junction of the proximal and middle thirds of the radius. Following its

TABLE 9-2. Ten Muscles That Attach to the Radius and Their Innervation

Muscle	Innervation
Abductor pollicis longus	PIN
Biceps	Musculocutaneous nerve
Brachioradialis	Radial nerves
Extensor pollicis brevis	PIN
Extensor pollicis longus	PIN
Flexor digitorum superficialis	Median nerve
Flexor pollicis longus	AIN
Pronator quadratus	AIN
Pronator teres	Median nerve
Supinator	PIN

AIN, anterior interosseous innervation; PIN, posterior interosseous nerve.

TABLE 9-3. Fourteen Muscles That Attach to the Ulna and Their Innervation

Muscle	Innervation
Abductor pollicis longus	PIN
Anconeus	Radial nerve
Biceps	Musculocutaneous nerve
Brachialis	Musculocutaneous and small branches; median and radial nerves
Extensor carpi ulnaris	PIN
Extensor indicis proprius	PIN
Extensor pollicis longus	PIN[a]
Flexor carpi ulnaris	Ulnar nerve
Flexor digitorum profundus	AIN, index and long; ulnar nerve, ring and small
Flexor digitorum superficialis	Median nerve
Pronator teres	Median nerve
Pronator quadratus	AIN
Supinator	PIN
Triceps	Radial nerve

[a]Occasionally, the accessory head flexor pollicis longus (aka Gantzer muscle from coronoid region in 15% of specimens) is innervated by AIN.
AIN, anterior interosseous innervation; PIN, posterior interosseous nerve.

emergence from the supinator, the PIN branches repetitively to the superficial extensors and the deeper outcropping muscles. The ulnar nerve enters the forearm between the two heads of the flexor carpi ulnaris.[122] It traverses the forearm between the flexor carpi ulnaris and the flexor digitorum profundus. In the distal forearm, it lays just beneath the flexor carpi ulnaris. The median nerve enters the forearm as it passes between the two heads of the pronator teres.[56] It next passes beneath the archway created by the two heads of the flexor digitorum superficialis. The median nerve then continues down the course of the forearm nestled between the flexor digitorum superficialis and the flexor digitorum profundus. It becomes much more superficial as it nears the level of the carpal tunnel. The anterior interosseous branch arises from the median nerve at the level of the pronator and travels deep with the anterior interosseous vessels. Abundant muscles shield the radial, ulnar, and median nerves from the shafts of the radius and ulna through most of the forearm except for the PIN near the proximal radius.

COMMON SURGICAL APPROACHES TO DIAPHYSEAL RADIUS AND ULNA FRACTURES

The large exposure required for plate fixation of pediatric forearm fractures can be achieved with the Henry (anterior) or Thompson (posterior) approaches to the radial shaft and the direct (medial) approach to the ulnar shaft.[71,227] Compartment

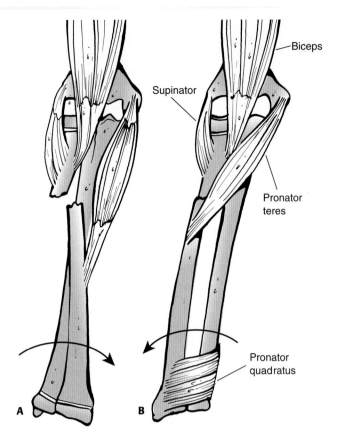

Figure 9-13. Muscle forces acting in proximal, middle, and distal thirds. **A:** Distal radial fragment significantly pronated by associated muscles while proximal fragment is flexed and supinated. **B:** The key involved muscles prior to significant displacement.

syndrome release usually requires the serpentine incision of McConnell's combined approach.[142] These approaches and their variations are well described and illustrated in detail elsewhere.[4,17,89,148,296] For open reduction of both the radius and the ulna, most authors favor separate incisions to minimize the possibility of communicating hematomas and the development of a radioulnar synostosis.[185,261,332] The Thompson approach to the radius is generally used for fractures of its proximal third[357] but requires special care to protect the PIN.[82,220,318] Other authors have emphasized the utility of the Henry approach for plating of the entire radius including the proximal aspect.[220] When open reduction is done in conjunction with other internal fixation

techniques (e.g., intramedullary fixation), limited versions of the same surgical approaches are used.

Indirect reduction and internal fixation of forearm fractures require knowledge of appropriate physeal-sparing entry portals about the distal and proximal forearm. Because of the relative inaccessibility of its proximal end, the radius usually is approached only distally through either a dorsal or radial entry point. The dorsal entry point is near the proximal base of the Lister tubercle or just lateral to it in a small bare area between the second and third dorsal compartments. This location is a short distance proximal to the physis of the distal radius. Another dorsal alternative is pin entry just medial to the Lister tubercle, between the third and fourth dorsal compartments,[276] but this may entail greater risk to the extensor tendons, especially the extensor pollicis longus. The most commonly used radial entry point is located in line with the styloid process just proximal to the physis.[355] Entry in this area passes adjacent to the first dorsal compartment, and thus the tendons of abductor pollicis longus and extensor pollicis brevis (as well as branches of the superficial radial nerve) must be protected (Fig. 9-14). Because of its extensive branching pattern, portions of the superficial branch of the radial nerve may also be at risk when dorsal or radial intramedullary entry points are used.[1,13]

Both distal and proximal intramedullary entry sites for the ulna have been described.[192,198,257,297,335] In the distal portion of the ulna, an entry site can be made proximal to the physis and in the interval between the extensor carpi ulnaris and flexor carpi ulnaris tendons. Care must be taken to avoid branches of the dorsal cutaneous sensory nerve. Ulnar entry is most easily accomplished in the proximal portion of the bone either along its lateral metaphyseal border just distal to the olecranon apophysis, piercing peripheral fibers of the anconeus (Fig. 9-15),[44,189,195] or directly through the olecranon apophysis. The metaphyseal anconeus entry site described by the Nancy group avoids the physis and avoids the painful bursa that tends to form over the "tip of the olecranon" pins.

Transphyseal approaches to both the distal radius[362,363,365] and the proximal ulna[7,198,318] have been suggested by some authors. Significant growth potential exists at the distal radius (approximately 10 mm/yr), whereas there is proportionately less from the olecranon apophysis (approximately 2 mm/yr). There is an unnecessary risk to the radial physis and few, if any, technical advantages to transphyseal entry of the radius in diaphyseal level fracture fixation. The ulna apophyseal entry site is used in many centers.

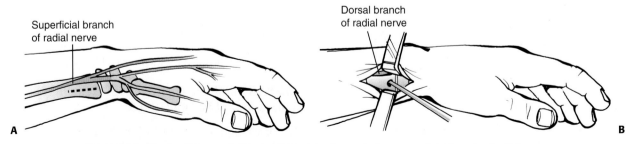

Figure 9-14. Distal radial entry. **A:** Distal radial incision in proximity to superficial branch of radial nerve. **B:** Distal radial entry position for intramedullary rod placement in relationship to superficial branch of radial nerve.

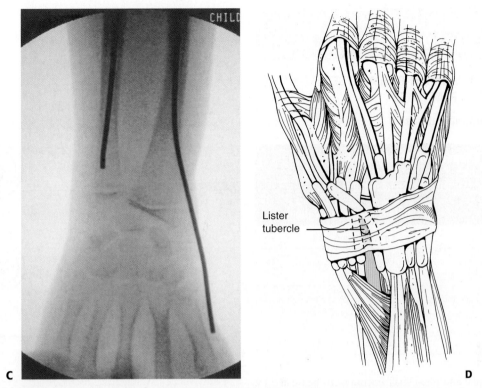

Figure 9-14. (*Continued*) **C:** Radiograph of lateral starting point for intramedullary nail. **D:** Alternate entry point just proximal to the Lister tubercle between second and third dorsal compartments.

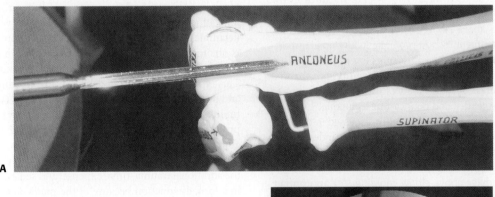

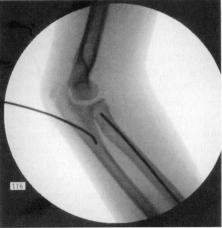

Figure 9-15. Proximal ulnar entry. **A:** Anconeus entry point. **B:** Radiograph of proximal ulnar entry point.

TREATMENT OPTIONS FOR DIAPHYSEAL RADIUS AND ULNA FRACTURES

NONOPERATIVE TREATMENT OF DIAPHYSEAL RADIUS AND ULNA FRACTURES

Indications/Contraindications

Nonoperative Treatment of Diaphyseal Radius and Ulna Fractures: INDICATIONS AND CONTRAINDICATIONS	
Indications	**Relative Contraindications**
• Closed fractures	• Open fractures
• Skeletally immature, displaced and nondisplaced	• Displaced and advanced skeletal maturity
• Reducible by closed means	• Unable to achieve reduction within accepted parameters
	• Tense swelling/impending compartment syndrome

Most pediatric radial and ulnar shaft fractures can be treated by nonoperative methods.[365] Low-energy, undisplaced, and minimally displaced forearm fractures can be immediately immobilized in a properly molded (three-point mold concept of Charnley) above-elbow cast.[7] If posttraumatic tissue swelling is a concern, noncircumferential splint immobilization (e.g., sugar-tong splint) can be used initially.[64,325,361] For fractures in the distal third of the forearm, below-elbow casting has been shown to be as effective as above-elbow casting in maintenance of satisfactory fracture alignment.[60,112] Appropriate follow-up is important for these minimally displaced fractures (an initial follow-up radiograph usually is taken 7 to 14 days after injury) because displacement may still occur for a variety of reasons: new trauma to the extremity, male gender, and poor casting technique.[64,113,290,361]

Good casting technique is infrequently discussed in contemporary orthopedic textbooks and sometimes is underemphasized during orthopedic residency training. The principles of good forearm casting technique include: (a) interosseous molding, (b) supracondylar above-elbow molding, (c) appropriate padding, (d) evenly distributed cast material, (e) straight ulnar border, and (f) three-point molding (Fig. 9-16). The risk of excessive cast tightness can be minimized through the use of the stretch–relax fiberglass casting technique described by Davids et al.[75] Chess et al.[60] described a cast index for distal radial fractures defined as the sagittal cast width divided by the coronal cast width at the level of the fracture site; a normal ratio is considered to be 0.70. The cast index has not been validated for forearm shaft fractures, but it embodies the sound concept of good interosseous molding. Techniques such as pins and plaster and cast wedging also have had a role in fracture care.[16,88] Cast wedging is almost always done with an opening wedge technique because this entails less risk of soft tissue impingement.[171]

Displaced fractures usually require reduction following appropriate analgesia.[84,333] Options include hematoma

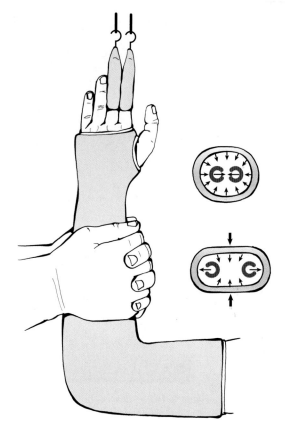

Figure 9-16. Interosseous mold technique.

block,[107,141,160] regional intravenous (IV) anesthesia[42,77,164] and inhalational methods,[94,129,141] and IV sedation with propofol or ketamine. After informed consent for sedation and reduction is obtained, monitored sedation can be used in the emergency department with a combination of narcotics and anxiolytics.[175] This typically requires a dedicated nurse to administer oxygen and perform appropriate monitoring functions (vital signs, continuous electrocardiogram, and pulse oximetry).[63,143] Ketamine protocols are also being used with increased frequency.[120,175] Young children with less than 5 or 10 degrees of angulation in the plane of wrist and elbow motion probably do not require the additional trauma, time, expense, and sedation risk involved in a formal reduction because of the predictable remodeling in this age group as long as immobilization brings stability to the fracture and prevents late displacement.[11] It has been shown that the more displaced the fracture, the more likely that formal monitored sedation techniques will be used for pediatric forearm fracture reduction as opposed to other techniques.[333]

More specific closed treatment options are discussed for pediatric forearm injuries in terms of their common fracture patterns: bow (plastic deformation), greenstick, complete, and comminuted.

Traumatic Bowing/Plastic Deformation

Although traumatic bowing was described by Rauber in 1876,[298] it was not widely recognized until Spencer Borden's classic paper was published in 1974.[35] This injury occurs almost exclusively

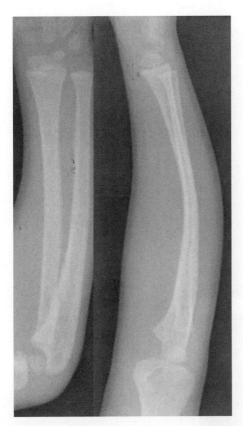

Figure 9-17. Bow fracture: approximately 15 degrees of apex-dorsal bowing of radius and ulna shaft.

with children's forearm fractures.[178] Bow fractures (Fig. 9-17) show no obvious macroscopic fracture line or cortical discontinuity, but they do demonstrate multiple microfractures (slip lines) along the length of the bow.[281] At times, a nearly classic buckle fracture (torus fracture) coexists with a bow fracture. The most common clinical scenario is a plastically deformed ulna along with a more typical fracture of the radius.[202]

Borden[35] and subsequent authors stressed the importance of natural remodeling potential in these injuries but voiced concern about this approach in older children (especially those over

10 years of age).[35,202,281] Vorlat and De Boeck[337] reported incomplete remodeling in 3 of 11 children at long-term follow-up (average 6.7 years) after traumatic bowing of the forearm. Because these three children were between the ages of 7 and 10 at the time of injury, the authors recommended more aggressive efforts at reduction in all patients with clinically significant deformity (more than 10 degrees) older than 6 years of age.[337] Traumatic bowing that causes aesthetically and/or functionally unacceptable angular deformity[278] should be manipulated under general anesthesia or deep sedation because strong (20 to 30 kg) gradual force applied over 2 to 3 minutes is required to obtain acceptable alignment (Fig. 9-18).[281] Application of this reductive pressure over a rolled towel, block, or surgeon's knee fulcrum followed by a three-point molded cast can substantially (although at times still incompletely) correct the deformity (Fig 9.19). Care must be taken to avoid direct pressure over adjacent epiphyses for fear of creating a physeal fracture.

Greenstick Fractures

Greenstick fractures present special issues in terms of diagnosis and treatment. Angulated greenstick fractures of the shafts of the radius and ulna at different levels indicate a significant rotational component to the injury (see Fig. 9-2). Evans, Rang, and others have stated that the apex-volar angulation pattern usually is associated with a supination-type injury mechanism, whereas most apex-dorsal greenstick fractures involve a pronation-type injury mechanism (Fig. 9-20),[91,93,234,264] although exceptions certainly occur.[93,132] Often, the apparent angular deformity can be corrected by simply reversing the forearm rotational forces (e.g., reducing an apex-dorsal pronation-type injury with supination). Noonan and Price[234] observed that it is difficult to remember whether to use pronation or supination reductive forces and suggested that most fractures can be reduced by rotating the palm toward the deformity. They also noted that most greenstick fractures are supination injuries with apex-volar angulation and thus can be reduced by a pronation movement.[234] Pediatric orthopedic researchers from the Arnold Palmer Hospital for Children have recently proposed the "radius crossover sign" as an indicator of significant angular and torsional deformity in greenstick fractures of the radial shaft.[354]

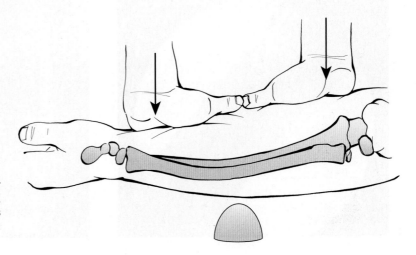

Figure 9-18. Reduction technique of bow fracture over fulcrum. (Reprinted with permission from Sanders WE, Heckman JD. Traumatic plastic deformation of the radius and ulna: a closed method of correction of deformity. *Clin Orthop Relat Res.* 1984;188:58–67.)

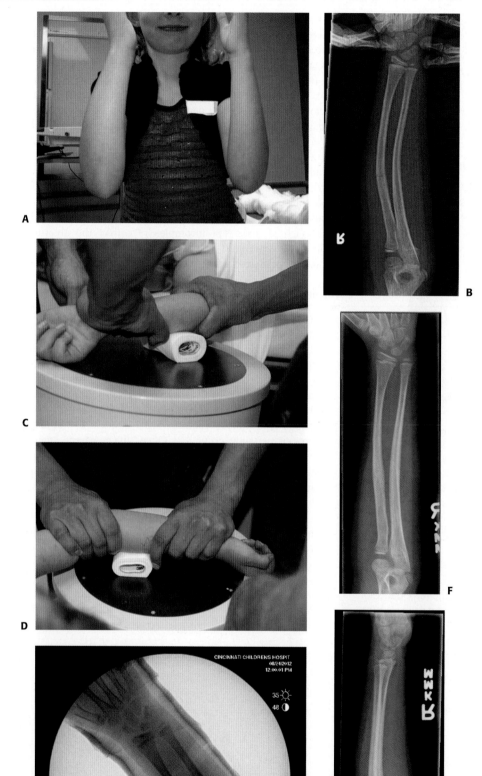

Figure 9-19. Reduction technique for plastic deformation. **A:** 7-year-3-month-old female demonstrating clinical deformity of her plastically deformed right forearm. **B:** Injury radiograph that pretty much looks exactly like her arm (some lucency in radius but cortices intact). **C:** Beginning of slow steady reduction maneuver over soft but firm bolster (roll of medical tape). **D:** End-of-reduction maneuver showing how force has corrected forearm and flattened tape. **E:** Intraoperative fluoroscopic image showing improved radiographic alignment. **F, G:** Anteroposterior and lateral radiographs at 2-month follow-up showing satisfactory healing and alignment.

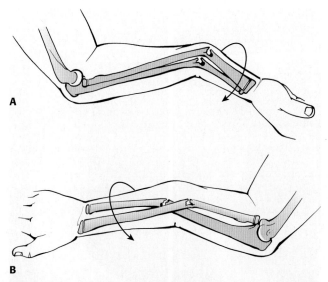

Figure 9-20. Shaft fractures at different levels imply rotational mechanism. **A:** Apex-volar angulation with supination deformity of the forearm. **B:** Apex-dorsal angulation with pronation deformity of the forearm.

Proper interpretation of this sign relies on full-length forearm films that include a good AP view of the distal humerus.

Greenstick fractures that occur near the same level probably have little to no rotational component and are best corrected by manipulative reduction and three-point molding techniques (see Fig. 9-3). Charnley believed that greenstick fractures of the forearm in children perfectly illustrated his dictum that "A curved plaster is necessary to make a straight limb."[58] He also stated that "The unsuspected recurrence of angular deformity in greenstick fractures of the forearm, while concealed in plaster, is an annoying event if it takes the surgeon by surprise and is not discovered until the plaster is removed. Parents, quite understandably, may be more annoyed about this happening to their children than if it had happened to themselves, and do not easily forgive the surgeon."[58] Despite these concerns, it is clear from large published reports that greenstick fractures can almost always be successfully treated with nonoperative manipulative reduction methods.[363]

Two philosophies are reflected in the literature regarding greenstick fracture reduction: one in which the greenstick fracture is purposely completed and another in which it is not. Those who favor completing the fracture (dating back at least to the 1859 work of Malgaigne) cite concerns about lost reduction and recurrent deformity that can be prevented only by converting the greenstick into a complete fracture.[22,32,102,153] Others prefer to maintain and perhaps exploit some of the inherent stability of the greenstick fracture.[5,60,78,93,323] In addition to the traditional view that loss of reduction is less likely if a greenstick fracture is completed, there also is the theoretical advantage of a lower refracture rate because of more exuberant callus formation.[60,234] To the best of our knowledge, these theories have not been validated in any controlled clinical studies. Davis and Green[78] advocated a derotational approach to greenstick fracture reduction and reported a 10% (16/151) reangulation rate in their series of patients with greenstick

fracture. They compared this to the 25% (12/47) reangulation rate in patients with complete fractures and questioned the wisdom of routinely completing greenstick fractures.[78] In a prospective study, Boyer et al.[40] showed statistically that greenstick fractures maintain their reduction better than complete forearm fractures.

Complete Fractures

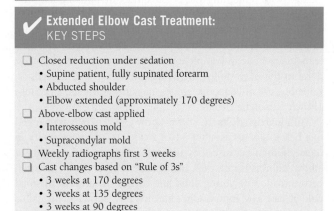

✔ Extended Elbow Cast Treatment:
KEY STEPS

☐ Closed reduction under sedation
  • Supine patient, fully supinated forearm
  • Abducted shoulder
  • Elbow extended (approximately 170 degrees)
☐ Above-elbow cast applied
  • Interosseous mold
  • Supracondylar mold
☐ Weekly radiographs first 3 weeks
☐ Cast changes based on "Rule of 3s"
  • 3 weeks at 170 degrees
  • 3 weeks at 135 degrees
  • 3 weeks at 90 degrees

Complete fractures in different regions of the shaft of the forearm behave differently from a clinical perspective and have classically been divided into distal-, middle-, and proximal-third fractures. Single-bone complete fractures usually are caused by direct trauma (nightstick fracture) and are difficult to reduce. Blount described a reduction technique that may be effective for reduction of a displaced single-bone shaft fracture. The intact bone is used as a lever to reestablish the length of the fractured bone, and then transverse forces are applied to realign the bone ends (see Fig. 9-7). Both-bone complete fractures (often with bayonet shortening) are common and are best treated with finger-trap or arm traction applied over 5 to 10 minutes. This stretches out the soft tissue envelope and aids in both reduction and cast or splint application. Traction allows complete fractures to "seek their own level of rotation" and allows correction of rotational malalignment.[78]

The position of immobilization for forearm fractures has been an area of debate since the days of Hippocrates.[32] Theoretically, the position of forearm rotation in an above-elbow cast or splint affects rotational alignment of complete fractures at all levels; however, a study of distal third forearm fractures found no significant effect of forearm rotation position on ultimate alignment.[40] We are aware of no similar studies analyzing the effects of forearm position on middle- or proximal-third shaft fractures, and treatment is influenced by certain anatomic considerations. Because of the strong supination pull of the biceps, aided by the supinator, complete proximal radial fractures may be best immobilized in supination so that the distal forearm rotation matches that of the proximal forearm (see Fig. 9-13). The position of immobilization of fractures in the middle third of the forearm commonly is dictated by whether the radial fracture occurs distal or proximal to the insertion of the pronator teres. Fractures proximal to its insertion are best treated by fully supinating the distal fragment, whereas those distal to its insertion are probably best treated in a neutral position. Fractures at different levels in the midshaft that require pronation or supination as part of the reduction maneuver should be immobilized in the position of reduction.

Manipulated fractures should be evaluated weekly for the first 2 to 3 weeks because most position loss can be recognized and corrected during this time.[182,338] Any significant shift in position between visits necessitates cast wedging or a cast change, with remolding and possible fracture remanipulation if unacceptable displacement is present. Voto et al.[338] found that, in general, 7% of forearm fractures redisplace; this can occur up to 24 days after the initial manipulation. Davis[78] reported a 25% reangulation rate in complete fractures. Remanipulation can be done in the office following administration of oral analgesics. Judicious use of benzodiazepines may also be valuable because of their anxiolytic effects.

Although in adults the above-elbow cast generally is changed to a below-elbow cast after 3 to 4 weeks, this is unnecessary in most children because they heal more quickly and permanent elbow stiffness is rare.[173] A cast change at week 3 or 4 also can be traumatic to a young child and carries the additional small risk of cast-saw injury. Once the fracture shows good callus formation, the cast can be removed. Because shaft fractures of the radius and ulna in children have a significant rate of refracture,[12,186,328] they should be splinted for an additional period of time.[66] Parents should be warned that forearm shaft fractures have the highest risk of the risk of refracture, which can occur even 6 to 12 months after the original injury.

Above-elbow casting with the elbow in extension has been suggested for some complete fractures of the middle and proximal thirds.[293,340,344] The supination moment exerted by the biceps has been shown to be diminished when the elbow is extended.[228] Walker and Rang[340] reported successful treatment of 13 middle- or proximal-third forearm shaft fractures with this method (some following failed flexed-elbow casting). They suggested that the "short fat forearms" of some young children prevented successful flexed-elbow casting.[340] Shaer et al.[293] also reported 20 children treated with this method and emphasized full supination of the forearm. Three of their patients required cast wedging, but at final follow-up 19 of the 20 patients had excellent results.[293] One patient who was lost to follow-up for 6 months (presumably removing his own cast) did suffer "mild residual deformity."[293] Walker and Rang[340] recommended that benzoin be applied to the skin, in addition to creation of an adequate supracondylar mold, to further secure the cast. Casting the thumb in abduction with extra padding may prevent the cast from sliding. Turco[293] suggested that reduction should be obtained with horizontal traction applied to the extended upper extremity, followed by additional steps outlined in the table above. Based on published clinical results, concerns related to cast slippage and elbow stiffness appear to have been overstated.[293,340] The main drawback of this technique is its awkwardness as compared to flexed-elbow casting (Fig. 9-21).[340]

Because radius and ulna shaft fractures have the highest rate of childhood refracture, casting is generally recommended for 6 to 8 weeks. This is followed with a forearm splint until all four cortices of each bone are healed and there

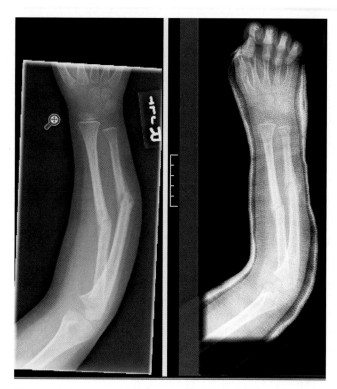

Figure 9-21. A forearm fracture lost of position while treated in an above-elbow cast with elbow at standard 90-degree elbow flexion. At 3 weeks postinjury, the arm was remanipulated and placed in an above-elbow cast with elbow extended down to only 45 degrees of flexion, with three- point mold placed. The fracture healed anatomically.

is no transverse lucency at the site of the original fracture (complete healing).

Comminuted Fractures

Although comminuted forearm fractures are less common in children than in adults,[323] they do occur.[23,102,104,153,185,357] Comminuted fractures tend to occur in conjunction with high-energy injuries, such as open fractures.[153,209] Comminuted forearm fractures deserve special attention because they often require specially tailored treatment approaches. If satisfactory reduction cannot be achieved or maintained by closed methods, then other treatment alternatives should be considered.

One option is to accept some shortening; according to Price,[258] this may help maintain motion through interosseous membrane slackening. Shortening of more than 1 cm is unacceptable in either single- or both-bone comminuted patterns. Standard closed fracture treatment generally is unsuccessful when both bones are comminuted, and surgical stabilization may be necessary.[102] Bellemans and Lamoureux[23] reported intramedullary nailing of all comminuted forearm fractures in their pediatric series. Other reported fixation methods for comminuted forearm fractures in children include plate-and-screw devices,[102,104] flexible intramedullary nailing for single-bone comminution,[270] and pins-and-plaster techniques.[339] Bone grafting is rarely if ever indicated in acute comminuted forearm features in children.

OPERATIVE TREATMENT OF DIAPHYSEAL RADIUS AND ULNA FRACTURES

Indications/Contraindications

Operative Treatment of Diaphyseal Radius and Ulna Fractures:
INDICATIONS AND CONTRAINDICATIONS

Indications	Contraindications
• High risk fracture patterns in older children	• Active infection
• Acceptable alignment not attained via casting (using age-adjusted criteria)	• Suspected malignancy requiring further work-up including biopsy
• Open fractures with significant instability	• No detectable clinical deformity in young child
• Status post compartment releases to facilitate wound care	
• Floating elbow injury pattern	

Duncan and Weiner[88] cited an "aggressive surgical mentality" as the reason for frequent operative treatment of pediatric forearm fractures, and Wilkins[350] expressed concern about "impetuous" surgeons who are too eager to operate. Cheng et al.[59] and Flynn et al.[103] documented a 10-fold and sevenfold increase in the rate of operative treatment of forearm shaft fractures in children, but it is unclear as to whether this increase in operative treatment has led to a commensurate improvement in clinical outcomes.

Operative treatment of radial and ulnar shaft fractures usually is reserved for open fractures, those associated with compartment syndrome, floating elbow injuries, and fractures that develop unacceptable displacement during nonoperative management. Residual angulation after closed treatment is much better tolerated by younger children than older adolescents and adults because of the increased remodeling potential in the younger age group.[112] As a consequence, adolescents are more likely to benefit from surgical treatment of their forearm fractures than are younger children. Although internal fixation is the standard of care for displaced forearm fractures in adults, the success of nonoperative methods and the complications associated with internal fixation have tempered enthusiasm for its routine application to pediatric forearm fractures. Compared to closed treatment methods, healing is slower after open reduction and internal fixation,[23] no matter what type of implant is used.[102] Crossed Kirschner wire (K-wire) fixation techniques that often are used successfully in the distal radius are technically difficult in the shaft region of the radius and ulna. In rare situations, external fixation has been used for pediatric forearm fixation, usually reserved for fractures with associated severe soft tissue injuries.[291]

Preoperative planning is essential regardless of which surgical technique is chosen. Assessment of the fracture, including rotation and the presence or absence of comminution, is important. Bone–plate mismatch (because of narrow bones and wide plates) and extensive soft tissue dissection are risks when adult-sized plates are applied to pediatric bones.[355] There

fortunately are many size options of plates available if sufficient advanced planning is performed. Before intramedullary nailing of fractures, the forearm intramedullary canal diameter should be measured, especially at the narrowest canal dimension; typically this is the central portion of the radius[305] and the distal portion of the ulna near the junction of its middle and distal thirds. Precise canal measurement can be difficult,[279,306] and the consequences of a nail or pin that is too large are probably worse than those of a nail or pin that is too small.[237,288] Modern digital radiography systems have made these measurements easier.[245]

Plate Fixation

Open reduction and internal fixation of pediatric forearm shaft fractures with plates and screws is a well-documented procedure in both pediatric series[243,310,324,332] and adult series that include patients as young as 13[57] and even 7[57] years of age. In one of the early series of pediatric forearm fractures fixed with plates,[81] dynamic compression plates and one-third tubular plates applied with standard AO (arbeitsgemeinschaft fuer osteosynthesefragen) technique (six cortices above and below the fracture site) obtained good results.[231] Four-cortex fixation on either side of the fracture site has been shown to be equally effective in pediatric forearm fractures.[357]

Plate fixation uses the standard adult approach and technique except that smaller plates (2.7-mm compression and stacked one-third tubular), fewer screws, and single-bone fixation often are acceptable.[357] Plate fixation may allow more anatomic and stable correction of rotational and angular abnormalities and restoration of the radial bow than with noncontoured intramedullary rods; however, the larger incisions and extensive surgical exposures required for plate fixation have raised concerns regarding unsightly scars[276,332,355] and muscle fibrosis with consequent motion loss.[357] Although the aesthetic concerns seem valid, ultimate forearm motion is similar with the two techniques, with only minor losses reported in the literature after both plating and intramedullary nailing.[72,170,297,331] Fernandez et al.[96] recently documented these precise issues very nicely in that they found no significant differences in functional outcome in their plate fixation versus intramedullary nailing patients, but they noted the longer operating room time and inferior appearance of the plated patients' scars.

Open reduction and internal fixation with plates and screws may be appropriate in the management of fractures with delayed presentation or fractures that angulate late in the course of cast care,[135,357] when significant fracture callus makes closed reduction and percutaneous passage of intramedullary nails difficult or impossible.[9] Other indications for plate fixation include shaft fractures with significant comminution[102] and impending or established malunion[329] or nonunion.[136,194,237] Several authors have reported good results with plate fixation of the radius only[47,105,243,264] or the ulna only (Fig. 9-22).[24] Bhaskar and Roberts[24] compared 20 children with both-bone plate fixation to 12 with ulna-only fixation and found significantly more complications in the dual plating group, although motion was equal at 1-year follow-up. Single-bone fixation requires satisfactory reduction of both bones. Stabilization of one bone, usually the ulna, allows rotation reduction of the other bone with intact

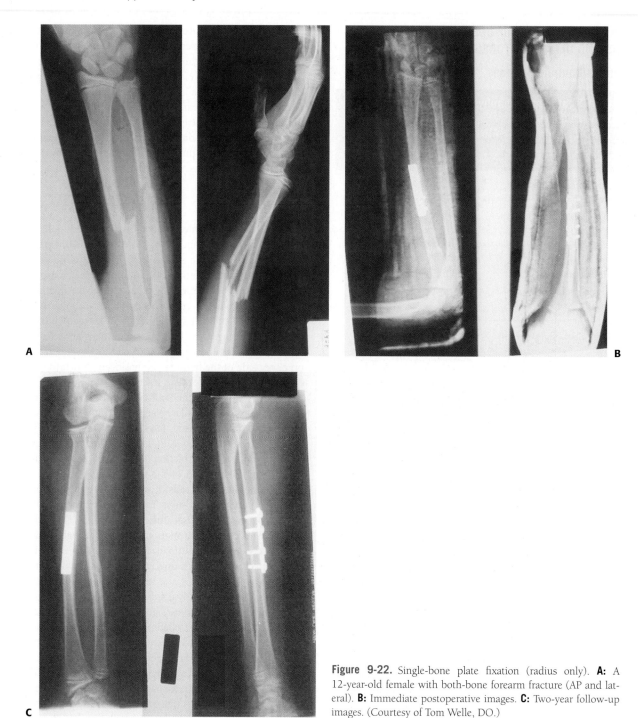

Figure 9-22. Single-bone plate fixation (radius only). **A:** A 12-year-old female with both-bone forearm fracture (AP and lateral). **B:** Immediate postoperative images. **C:** Two-year follow-up images. (Courtesy of Tom Welle, DO.)

periosteum acting as a tension band to maintain reduction. Flynn and Waters[105] stated that they usually performed intramedullary fixation of the ulna and manipulative reduction of the radius. However, when the radius is not reducible, it is usually due to interposed extensor muscle. In these less common cases, they preferentially plated the radius only when the fracture. Two patients in Bhaskar and Roberts'[24] study required open reduction and internal fixation of the radius when it was not adequately reduced after plate fixation of the ulna.

Kirschner Wire, Rush Rod, and Steinmann Pin Intramedullary Fixation

Currently, intramedullary fixation is the preferred method for internal fixation of forearm fractures in children.[7,44,185,192,198,261,262,335] Intramedullary fixation of children's forearm fractures dates back at least to Fleischer's 1975 report in the German literature in which he called it "marrow wiring."[100] Closed intramedullary nailing (also known as indirect reduction and internal fixation) of diaphyseal forearm fractures in adolescents was later reported in the English literature by Ligier et al.,[195] Amit et al.,[7] and others.[28,189,355] A variety of implants have been used for forearm intramedullary nailing, including K-wires, Rush rods, and Steinmann pins. Continued favorable reports from around the world (e.g., England, Germany, New Zealand, Turkey, and the United States) have established intramedullary fixation as the surgical treatment of choice.[52,115,163,192,268]

Intramedullary fixation has several advantages over plate fixation, including improved aesthetics because of smaller incisions and less deep tissue dissection, potentially leading to a lower risk of stiffness.[72,185,297,355] Contoured pins are used in the radius to preserve its natural anatomic bow[7,72,261,268,342]; contoured pins are not necessary for the ulna.[7] Although the rotational stability of pediatric forearm fractures treated with intramedullary fixation has been questioned, Blasier and Salamon[28] suggested that the strong periosteum in children resists torsional stresses. In a cadaver study of the rotational stability of fractures of the ulna and radius treated with Rush rods, Ono et al.[241] found that intramedullary fixation of both bones reduced fracture rotation to one-eighth of that in unfixed fractures.

Elastic Stable Intramedullary Nailing

In the early 1980s, Metaizeau et al.[221] described elastic stable intramedullary nailing (ESIN) of pediatric forearm fractures with small-diameter (1.5 to 2.5 mm) contoured implants.[195] No effort was made to fill the medullary canal as with other intramedullary nailing techniques,[270] and the "summit of the curve must be calculated preoperatively to lie at the level of the fracture."[189] The prebent flexible rods (known as Nancy nails) were reported to maintain satisfactory fracture alignment while encouraging development of normal physiologic fracture callus.[195,221,254] Biomechanically, these implants have been shown to act as internal splints provided the nails extend three or more diameters beyond the fracture site.[159] Good results with this technique have been reported by numerous authors (Figs. 9-23 and 9-24).[131,229,270,287,294,326,327,356]

Because the ESIN technique emphasizes the interdependence of the radius and ulna, if both bones are fractured, both bones are internally fixed.[189] It is also dependent on anchorage of the nails in the upper and lower metaphyseal portions of the

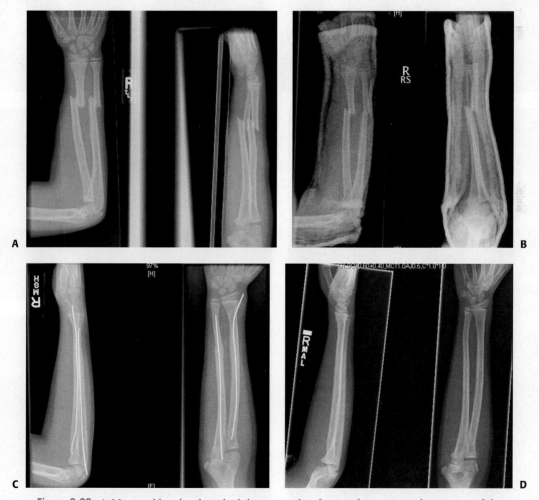

Figure 9-23. A 10-year-old male whose both-bone complete forearm fracture near the junction of the middle and distal thirds was treated with elastic stable intramedullary nailing (ESIN). **A:** Injury radiographs demonstrating completely displaced radial and ulnar shaft fractures. **B:** Postreduction radiographs reveal unsatisfactory angular alignment as well as significant loss of radial bow. **C:** Anatomic appearance following ESIN. **D:** One-and-a-half-year follow-up radiographs. Nails were removed 6 months postoperatively.

(continues)

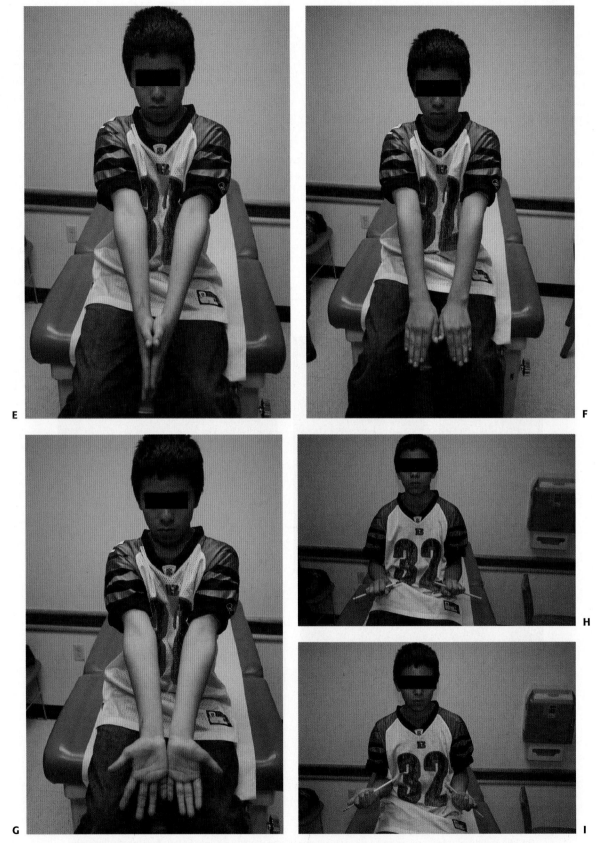

Figure 9-23. (*Continued*) **E:** Clinical appearance with extended elbows and forearm midposition. **F:** Clinical appearance with extended elbows and pronated forearms. **G:** Clinical appearance with extended elbows and supinated forearms. **H:** Symmetrical pronation. **I:** Symmetrical supination.

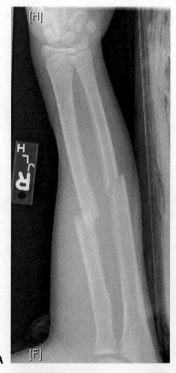

A

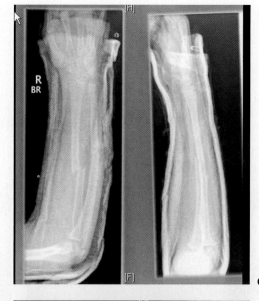

C

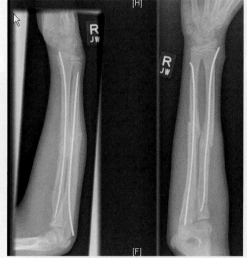

D

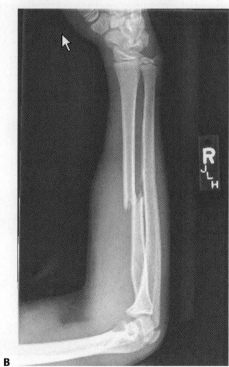

B

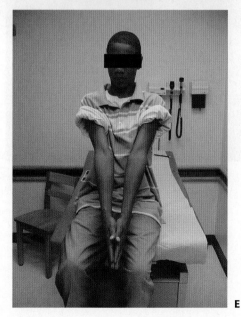

E

Figure 9-24. An 11-year-old male whose both-bone midshaft complete forearm shaft fracture was treated with ESIN. **A:** Injury AP radiograph. **B:** Injury lateral radiograph. **C:** Postreduction radiographs demonstrating unacceptable angular alignment. **D:** Improved alignment status after ESIN. **E:** Clinical appearance with extended elbows and forearm midposition.

(continues)

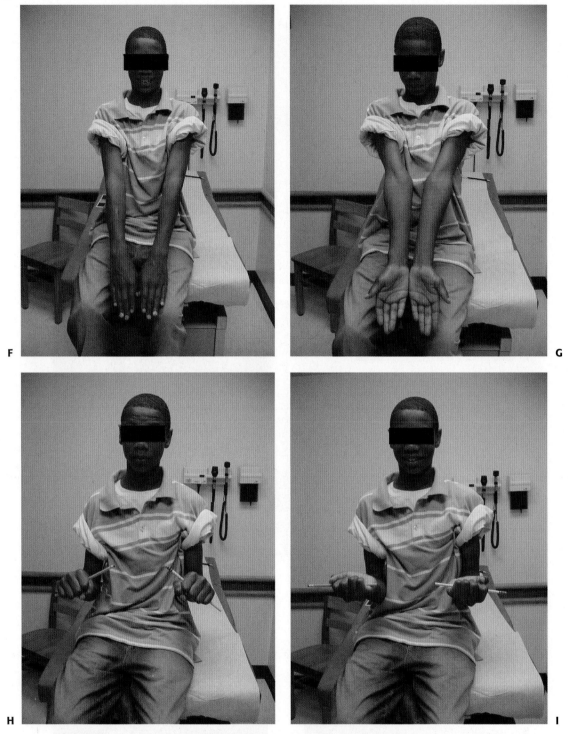

Figure 9-24. (*Continued*) **F:** Clinical appearance with extended elbows and pronated forearms. **G:** Clinical appearance with extended elbows and supinated forearms. **H:** Symmetrical pronation. **I:** Symmetrical supination.

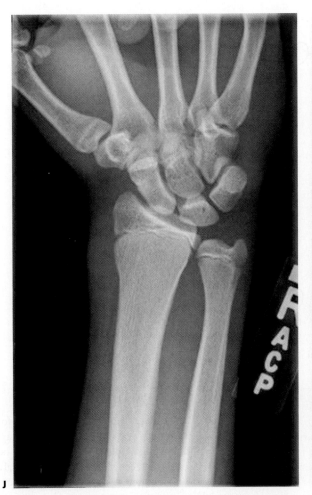
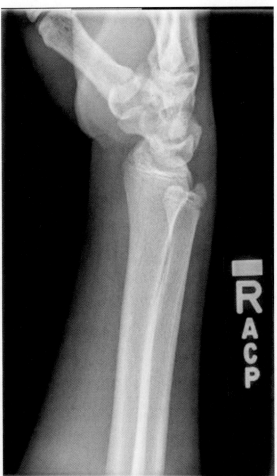

J

K

Figure 9-24. (*Continued*) **J:** Thirty-nine month follow-up AP wrist radiograph and lateral (**K**) wrist radiograph (taken because of new trauma) demonstrating normal bony anatomy. Nails were removed 6 months postoperatively.

bone to produce an internal three-point fixation construct.[189] Technique principles include fixing first the bone that is easiest to reduce, using physeal-sparing entry points, and using small nails varying in diameter from 1.5 to 2.5 mm.[189] A nail that is too large may lead to nail incarceration and distraction at the fracture site, especially in the ulna.[237] Large nails may also increase the fixation rigidity which may decrease the amount of callus formation, leading to delayed union and nonunion. Contouring of both nails is recommended, with particular attention to restoration of the appropriate radial bow (Fig. 9-25). Initially, nails were removed by about the fourth postoperative month, but several refractures led the originators of the technique to delay nail removal until one full year after surgery.[189] Pin ends should be cut short and buried to maintain prolonged fixation.

Immediate motion has been recommended by some authors after ESIN of pediatric forearm fractures,[23,131,189,335] whereas others have recommended immobilization for variable periods of time.[44] Early refracture with nails in place has been reported. Bellemans and Lamoureux[23] considered displaced oblique or comminuted midshaft forearm fractures in children older than 7 years of age to be an indication for ESIN. They considered bayonet apposition (overriding) to be unacceptable at any age because of concerns about rotational malalignment and frequent narrowing of the interosseous space.[23] Their fixation technique involved passage of the intramedullary nails, followed by rotation of each nail until the greatest distance between the two bones was achieved in full supination.[23]

The two largest contemporary published series of ESIN-treated pediatric forearm shaft fracture patients come from Bochum, Germany and Nashville, Tennessee.[184,210] Together these studies comprise over 400 cases and thus offer insight into the application of this technique as well as complications. The average age of the patients in each of these two studies was 9.7 years of age, with a range of a bit less than 2 years of age to 16 years of age. Fourteen percent of the forearm shaft fractures were open fractures. Refracture rate and infection rate were both 3% for the combined cohort. Malunion, EPL injury, significant stiffness, and nerve injury were all less than 1%.

MANAGEMENT OF OPEN FRACTURES OF DIAPHYSEAL RADIUS AND ULNA FRACTURES

In one large epidemiologic study, open fractures of the shafts of the radius and ulna and open tibial shaft fractures occurred with

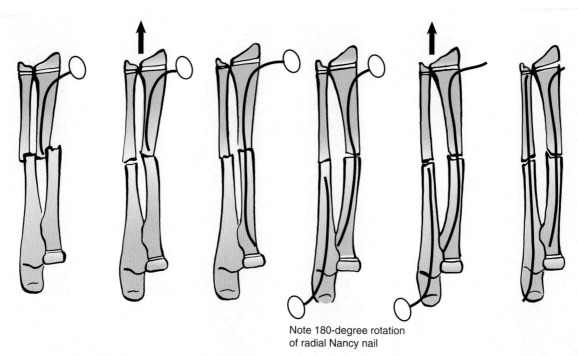

Note 180-degree rotation
of radial Nancy nail

Figure 9-25. Metaizeau ESIN technique. The radial rod is twisted 180 degrees in step 4 to reestablish the radial bow.

equal frequency, making them the most common open fractures in children.[59] Although the infection rate is extremely low for open fractures, even grade I open forearm fractures in children have been associated with serious complications such as gas gangrene.[95] Early irrigation and debridement[217,302] are indicated for open forearm fractures, and care should be taken to inspect and properly clean the bone ends.[167] Roy and Crawford[276] recommended routinely inspecting both of the bone ends for the presence of intramedullary foreign material (Fig. 9-26). Once debrided, open forearm fractures can be stabilized by any of the available internal fixation methods without undue risk of infection (Fig. 9-27).[128,135,199] Open fractures tend to be more unstable than closed fractures (because of soft tissue stripping and comminution) and more commonly require internal fixation. Internal fixation also may facilitate soft tissue management and healing.[357] Lim et al.[196] from the KK Children's Hospital in Singapore recently reminded us that internal fixation is not an absolute prerequisite and many children with such open fractures may still be successfully managed with casting alone.

The amount of periosteal stripping and possible foreign body reaction associated with open forearm fractures may produce an unusual radiographic appearance: the "ruffled border sign" (Fig. 9-28). Usually, this seems to represent a normal healing response in growing children, but occasionally it is an early sign of osteomyelitis. The infection rate ranges from 0% to 33% for open fractures in children.[72,128,135,182,199,234,243,258,357] Even grade I open forearm fractures in children can be complicated by gas gangrene or osteomyelitis, and therapeutic amputation has been reported.[78,95,153] Open fracture grade does not appear to correlate with the infection rate in childhood forearm fractures, with most of the serious forearm infections reported in the literature occurring after grade I fractures.

Some centers in the United States have evaluated emergency department based-treatment of grade I open fractures of the forearm, wrist, and tibia in children and concluded that there was no significant difference in infection rates.[121] We would strike a strong note of caution regarding this treatment approach for two main reasons. First, existing studies appear to

Intramedullary soil core
Benign skin laceration

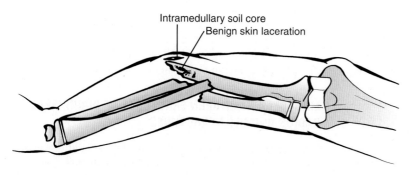

Figure 9-26. Intramedullary organic soil contamination from open forearm fracture with benign-appearing skin laceration.

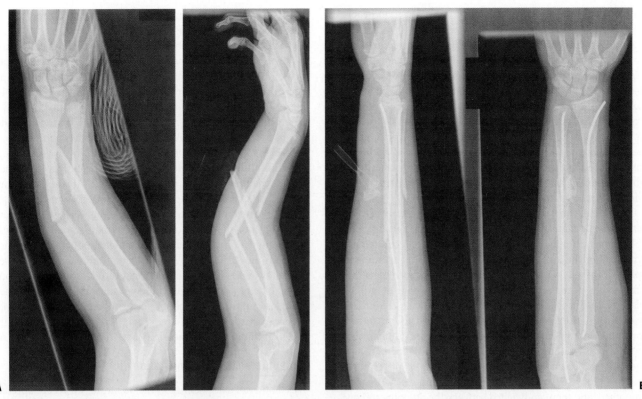

Figure 9-27. A 13-year-old female with open forearm fracture. **A:** AP and lateral radiographs; note extrusion of ulna on lateral view. **B:** After irrigation and debridement and flexible nail internal fixation. Note the Penrose drain in the ulnar wound.

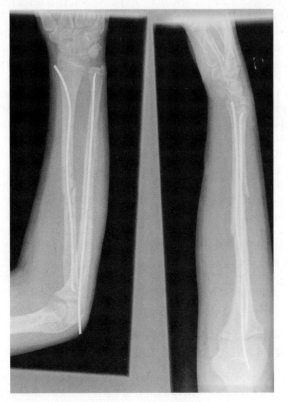

Figure 9-28. Ruffled border sign at the site of previous open fracture of ulna; same patient from Figure 9-24 at 1-month follow-up.

be at high risk of being underpowered (one infection occurred in the Godfrey et al. study and it was in the emergency department treatment group). Second, there is a dramatic difference in the nature of the two treatment approaches in that one involves formal surgical exposure and comprehensive visualization and cleansing of the bone ends, while the other might be characterized as rinsing the skin. The risk to the child of a limb- or life-threatening infection is juxtaposed to unnecessary resource utilization.

Fracture Reduction/Conscious Sedation Protocol

Significantly displaced forearm shaft fractures are usually manipulated in the emergency department using a conscious sedation (also known as deep sedation) protocol. After obtaining informed consent for conscious sedation and fracture manipulation, an IV line is started, and the child's blood pressure, pulse, respirations, electrocardiogram, and peripheral oxygen level are monitored during the procedure and for about 30 minutes after the procedure. We use ketamine/atropine or fentanyl/midazolam administered intravenously in divided doses. Although many children moan or cry briefly during the manipulation, very few recall pain. Two recent reports have drawn attention to ketamine-related concerns. Perez-Garcia et al. reported the disturbing complication of severe hypertension in a 12 year old who had undiagnosed coarctation of the aorta, and Kinder et al. found that children with a high body mass index were at greater risk for nausea and vomiting.[179,247] Reductions are done under mini-C-arm (fluoroscopy) control. The initial position of forearm rotation is based on the level of the fracture, and the final position is based on the best reduction under fluoroscopy. Small portable fluoroscopy units improve the quality of the reduction, decrease the radiation exposure to the patient, and decrease the need for repeat fracture reduction and save time.[10] The level of experience of the physician correlates to the level of radiation exposure risk to the patient and health professionals involved in reduction. Finger-trap traction with 10 to 15 lb of counterweight frequently is used for completely displaced both-bone forearm shaft fractures (especially those with shortening). We do not complete greenstick fractures because the partial bone continuity adds stability.

Because of concerns about soft tissue swelling, we place nonmanipulated and manipulated fractures into a plaster sugar-tong splint (incorporating the elbow). We avoid the circumferential wrapping of the arm with cast padding by using a "sandwich splint" technique. Before manipulation, the sugar-tong splint is prepared by laying out 7 to 10 layers of appropriate-length 3-in plaster casting material on top of a work surface. A four-layer matched length of cotton cast padding also is laid out and will form the inner padding (skin side) of the splint. A final single layer of cast padding is laid out and will form the outer layer of the splint to prevent elastic wrap adherence to the plaster. Once manipulation is completed, the plaster is dipped, wrung out, smoothed, and then sandwiched between the dry four- and one-ply cotton padding. This splint is then placed with the four-ply cotton side against the skin and secured with an elastic bandage (ace wrap). We prefer to avoid the circumferential application of cotton padding because it may limit splint expansion during follow-up swelling. If necessary, parents also can unwrap and loosen the elastic bandage at home to relieve pressure if swelling makes the splint too tight. Patients are given a prescription for mild narcotic analgesics, and discharge instructions to call back or return to the emergency room for pain not relieved by the pain medicine.

Patients usually return to the office within a week for repeat radiographs and clinical assessment. Provided that satisfactory alignment has been maintained, we remove the elastic wrap but leave the plaster sugar-tong splint in place. Nonmanipulated fractures can be converted to a conventional or waterproof cast on the first visit if it is more than 48 hours after the injury, but manipulated fractures that maintain good position are overwrapped with fiberglass for at least a week before converting to the definitive cast. The splint is "boxed in" by applying cotton cast padding over the splint and the exposed upper arm, and by wrapping with fiberglass to convert the splint into an above-elbow cast. Follow-up radiographs are taken of manipulated fractures at about 1-week intervals for the next 2 weeks. Fractures that are losing position but are still in acceptable alignment usually require removal and remolding of a new cast to prevent further position deterioration in the upcoming week. Fractures that show increasing displacement at the initial follow-up visits can continue to angulate up until 4 to 5 weeks postinjury. Minor remanipulations can be done in the office after appropriate administration of oral analgesics and anxiolytics. Major remanipulations are best done with general anesthesia. The decision regarding the need for remanipulation may be

tipped by viewing the arm position by the parents and physician after all splint and cast materials are removed.

We rarely convert an above-elbow cast to a below-elbow cast at 3 to 4 weeks postinjury as is common in adults. This step may be omitted in younger children because of their faster healing and their minimal inconvenience from temporary elbow immobilization.[173] Patients can return to sports after conversion to a below-elbow cast as long as the cast is padded during play and league rules allow casts. Patients usually are required to have a physician's note allowing sports participation with a cast. This decision is made with the patient's and parents' understanding of potential increase in refracture risk. Adequate fracture healing (4/4 cortices completely healed and no transverse shaft lucency) usually has occurred after several more weeks of cast treatment but should be confirmed by radiographic and physical examination before unlimited athletic participation. Older children are given home elastic band strengthening exercises and allowed to participate in normal activities while they continue to be protected in either a removable Velcro fracture brace or a customized thermoplastic forearm gauntlet brace. Formal physical therapy rarely is required. This fracture protocol is aimed at minimizing refracture risk.

Acceptable Limits of Angulation

Based on available evidence in the literature, we accept approximately 20 degrees of angulation in distal-third shaft fractures of the radius and ulna, 15 degrees at the midshaft level, and 10 degrees in the proximal third (for girls less than 8 years old and boys less than 10 years old).[360] We accept 100% translation if shortening is less than 1 cm. Although other authors recommend accepting up to 45 degrees of rotation, we find this extremely difficult to measure accurately using the bicipital tuberosity and radial styloid as landmarks because of the lack of anatomic distinction in younger children. Plastic deformation fractures seem to have less remodeling potential than other fractures, and radiographically or aesthetically unacceptable angulation may require gradual, forceful manipulation under sedation or general anesthesia. Children approaching skeletal maturity (less than 2 years of remaining growth) should be treated using adult criteria because of their reduced remodeling potential. Parents should be cautioned that even mild angulation of the ulna, especially posterior sag, will produce an obvious deformity after cast removal because of the subcutaneous location of the bone (Fig. 9-29). This aesthetic deformity is exacerbated by abundant callus formation, but it will ultimately remodel if it falls within acceptable angulation criteria. Ulnar sag may be countered by placing the child in an extended elbow cast or intramedullary fixation. Mild to moderate angulation of the radius usually produces much less aesthetic deformity but may limit motion more (Fig. 9-30).

SURGICAL REPAIR OF DIAPHYSEAL RADIUS AND ULNA FRACTURES

Most forearm shaft fractures continue to be successfully treated with closed methods at our institution. Our top two indications for surgical treatment of these injuries are open shaft fractures and shaft fractures that exceed our stated reduction limits. If surgical treatment

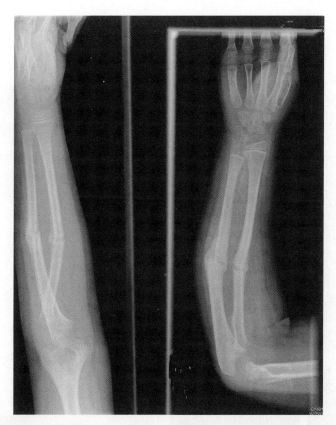

Figure 9-29. Ulnar sag on serial radiographs. Note the prominent ulna fracture callus.

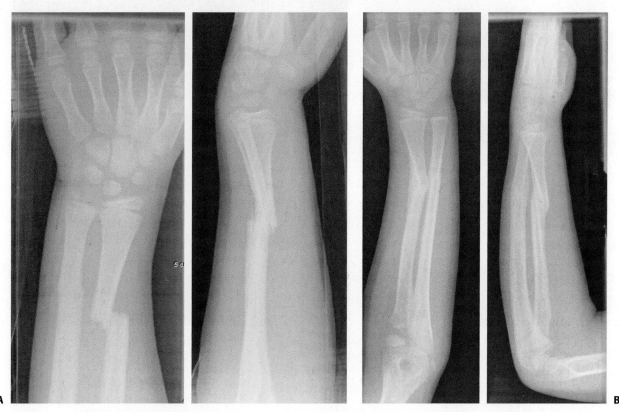

Figure 9-30. A 7-year-old female with left both–bone complete forearm fracture. **A:** AP and lateral injury radiographs. **B:** Two-month follow-up radiographs.

(*continues*)

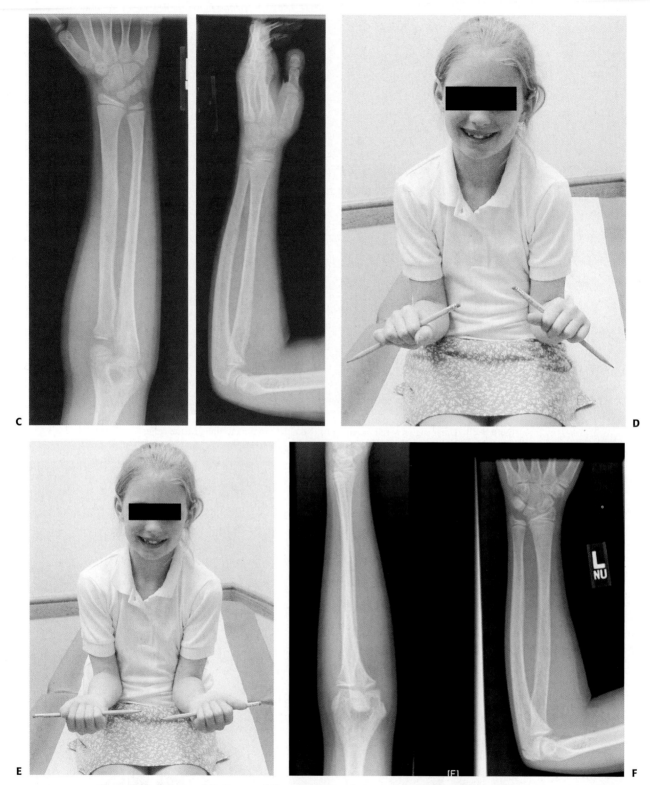

Figure 9-30. (*Continued*) **C:** Two-year follow-up radiograph shows mild residual deformity. **D:** Pronation.
E: Supination. **F:** Five-year follow-up radiographs of left forearm with mild loss of radial bow.

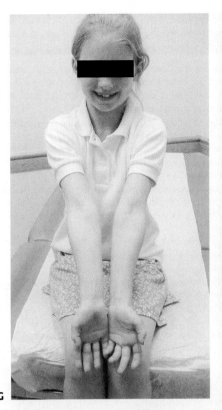

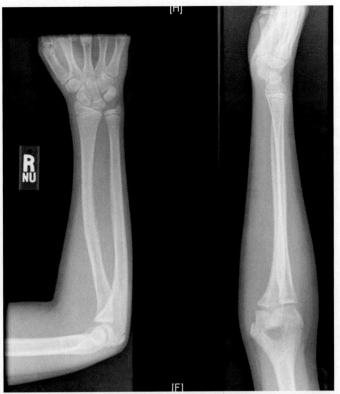

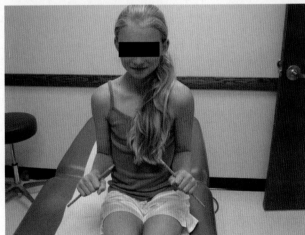

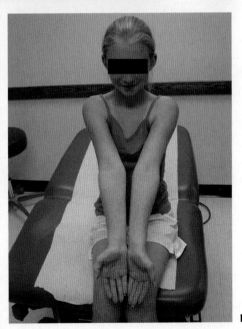

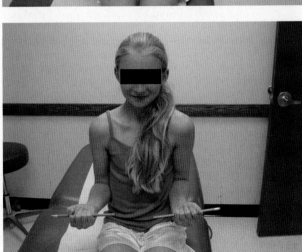

Figure 9-30. (*Continued*) **G**: Axial alignment at 2-year follow-up. **H**: Comparison radiographs of right forearm. **I**: Pronation. **J**: Supination. **K**: Axial alignment at 5-year follow-up.

is deemed necessary, intramedullary fixation is preferred over plate fixation because of reduced soft tissue disruption. We occasionally fix one bone when both bones are fractured if overall forearm alignment is acceptable and stable after single-bone fixation.

Intramedullary Nailing

Preoperative Planning

✓ Elastic Stable Intramedullary Nailing of Diaphyseal Radius and Ulna Fractures: PREOPERATIVE PLANNING CHECKLIST	
OR table	☐ Standard table with radiolucent hand table ☐ Rotate table 90 degrees to position arm opposite anesthesiologist
Position/positioning aids	☐ Supine with restraint strap across chest placed high in axilla ☐ Traction on arm must not pull patient's head off table
Fluoroscopy location	☐ Bring in parallel to the OR table on the foot (axilla) side ☐ One fluoro monitor should be on the opposite side of the table where anesthesiologist sits, and the other should be caudal to the arm
Equipment	☐ Elastic nail set, small bone wrench (small femoral wrench), vice grips, awl, nail grip device, mallet, ragnell retractors, small fragment set, bone reduction clamps, K-wire set
Tourniquet	☐ Placed high in axilla
Equipment	☐ To improve the torque needed to rotate the rod, a locking plier or extra heavy duty needle driver can be clamped to the rod near its insertion into the T-handle. The handle alone will frequently slip during rotation in the diaphysis ☐ Need a Kerlix gauze around distal humerus or a blunt mallet to apply countertraction against the hand with elbow flexed 90 degrees (see video)

Technique

Our preferred intramedullary ulnar entry site is just distal to the olecranon apophysis (anconeus starting point), just anterior to the subcutaneous border of the proximal ulna on its lateral side (Table 9-4). Care is taken not to enter the ulna more than 5 mm anterior to its subcutaneous crest to avoid encroachment into the region of the PRUJ. Pins placed directly through the tip of the olecranon apophysis have a strong tendency to cause bursitis and pain until removal. We prefer to open the cortex with an awl because it tends to wander less than motorized drills and it allows ulnar entry with little or no formal incision. The awl technique also simplifies operating room setup in that no pneumatic hose hookups or battery packs are necessary.

The patient is positioned supine with the arm abducted 90 degrees on a hand table. A wide sturdy strap is placed in the axilla to allow traction without pulling the patient off the table.

TABLE 9-4. Intramedullary Nailing of Diaphyseal Radius and Ulna Fractures: Key Surgical Steps

- Expose the radius first with a 1–2-cm incision, just proximal to the Lister tubercle between the second and third tendon compartments. Alternatively, perform a styloid approach through the first dorsal compartment just proximal to the physis.
- Avoid major branches of the superficial radial nerve and clearly identify the tendons to avoid damage.
- With the Lister approach, there is a "bare area" of bone between the EPL and ECRB tendons that is elevated clear of its periosteum (beware of branches of superficial radial nerve).
- Use an awl to create a start window in the "bare area" for the Lister approach, or between the APL/EPB and ECRL/B tendons for styloid approach (we feel this is superior to and safer than motorized drill techniques).
- Forcibly tighten the T-handle on the rod and insert the rod by hand with an oscillating twist motion.
- Pull traction on arm against the axillary strap.
- Use mallet to advance nail to fracture site if not possible by hand maneuvers. If rod fails to advance, the tip could be stuck in a rut. Tap the rod 5 mm backward; rotate the tip, then advance down the shaft again to the fracture.
- Pull heavy traction on the hand, manipulate the fracture, and use the small femoral wrench to align the bone ends. If you miss, pull the nail back, rotate the rod 90 degrees, reattempt to pass, and repeat.
- If the fracture ends remain 100% translated despite manipulation, try the "shoehorn" K-wire technique before opening.
- If you have to open, make a 3–4-cm incision, grip the bone ends with small reduction clamps, and hold reduced while assistant passes nail. Use the volar (Henry) approach to open, carefully avoiding the posterior interosseous nerve.
- Only advance the nail 1 cm past the fracture so it is just "perched." Full insertion will make it nearly impossible to manipulate the ulna next.
- Start the ulna about 3 cm distal to the olecranon tip about 4 mm lateral to the posterior crest. Palpate the radial head and stay clear of it. The starting incision can be 3–4 mm long and made percutaneously.
- Advance the nail with an oscillating twist technique to the fracture, past the rod similar to radial rod. With the radius rod just perched across the fracture by 1 cm, the ulna can be freely manipulated to ease nail passage across the ulna fracture.
- Insert nail about 1 cm short of the distal ulna physis to leave room for final impaction.
- Remove the T-handle, put about a 45-degree bend in the rod just as it enters the bone. Do not lever the rod against the bone because it will plough or fracture through the metaphyseal bone.
- Cut the nail as close to the bone as possible, then final impact the nail so only 3-mm stick is outside the bone for purchase during removal.
- Rotate the radial rod so that the bow in the nail follows the natural bow of the radius. Leave 1 cm short of the end of the bone to allow for final impaction after cutting the rod similar to the ulna.
- If using the Lister approach, make sure that the EPL tendon is not at risk for rubbing on the protruding nail end to avoid rupture.

Traction helps to gain length of overriding fracture ends and allows the bones to seek their normal rotation. If dual-bone fixation is elected, the radius is fixed first as it is usually more difficult to rod, and it is always more difficult to approach with an open reduction than the ulna. If the ulna is fixed first, it will limit forearm mobility and make it very difficult to manipulate the radius and pass the nail which forces a risky and complex open reduction on the radius. Optimizing the closed rodding of the radius by fixing it first makes the ulna reduction a little

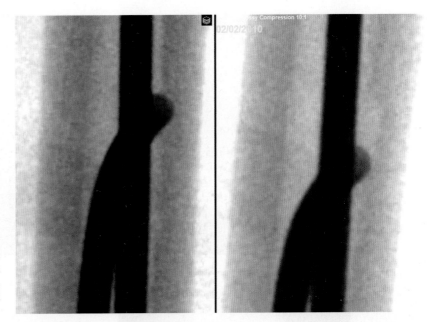

Figure 9-31. This illustrates the "rod rut" incurred during a femur Nancy nail insertion. In the **left** figure, the tip of the rod has dug a rut in the cortex and is stuck. It was backed up 5 mm, leaving behind a visible rut. The rod was twisted 90 degrees and then passed up the shaft freely.

more difficult, but open reduction of the ulna is vastly simpler than an open reduction of the radius fracture at any fracture level. The distal radial entry site can be either through a physeal-sparing direct lateral approach through the floor of the first dorsal compartment or dorsally near the proximal extent of the Lister tubercle between the second and third dorsal compartments. Both of these entry points are approximately 1 cm proximal to the physis of the distal radius. We insert the radial nail through a 1- to 2-cm incision, protecting the superficial radial nerve and the dorsal tendons with small blunt retractors. An awl is used to gain intramedullary access to the radius. We typically use small intramedullary nails (2 to 2.5 mm in diameter) to maintain some flexibility at the fracture site and stimulate appropriate callus formation. Larger nails may become incarcerated in either the narrow central canal of the radius or that of the distal third of the ulna. Care must be taken not to overbend the tip of the nail as this effectively increases the diameter of the implant and may impede its intramedullary

passage. If the rod gets stuck, the tip has often been pounded into a rut (Fig. 9-31).

Backing the rod up 5 mm and rotating it away from the rut will ease passage down the shaft isthmus. If the nail fails to engage the shaft on the other side of the fracture, tap it back to the fracture, rotate it 90 to 180 degrees and then retry. A "shoehorn" technique can be used to percutaneously align the fracture. A 2-mm K-wire is placed into the fracture between the two ends of the translated bone. It is then levered to allow the bone ends to translate into alignment. With the K-wire lever in place, pass the nail across the fracture (Fig. 9-32).

Failure to pass the intramedullary nail across the fracture site after several attempts may necessitate a limited open reduction with at least a 2-cm incision to directly pass the rod across the fracture site (Fig. 9-33). Because of the thick soft tissue envelope, an open approach to the radius needs to be twice this long. Placing a bone clamp on either side of the fracture allows bone alignment control. Persistence in attempting to achieve closed

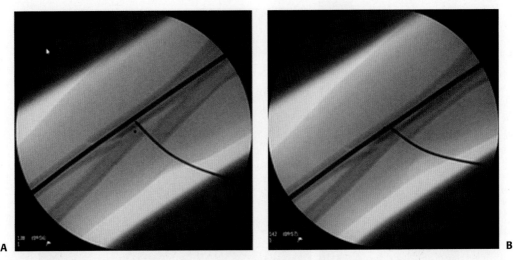

A   **B**

Figure 9-32. Shoehorn indirect reduction technique. **A:** Initial K-wire placement. **B:** Intrafocal location between fragments.

(continues)

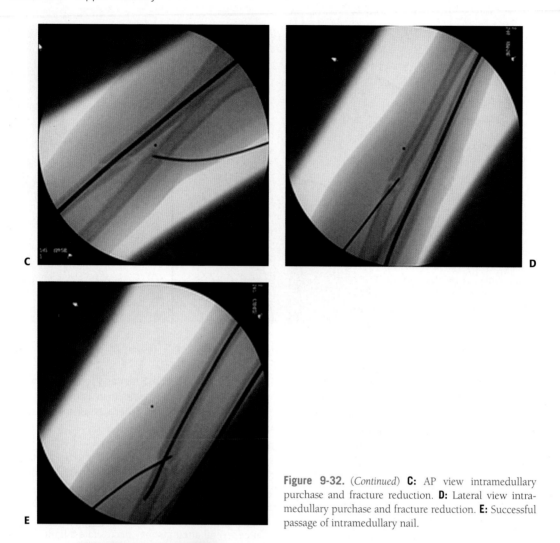

Figure 9-32. (*Continued*) **C:** AP view intramedullary purchase and fracture reduction. **D:** Lateral view intramedullary purchase and fracture reduction. **E:** Successful passage of intramedullary nail.

Figure 9-33. A 12-year-old female with midshaft both bone complete forearm fracture. **A:** AP and lateral injury radiographs.

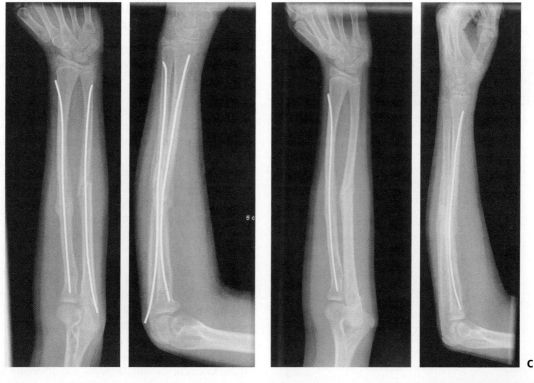

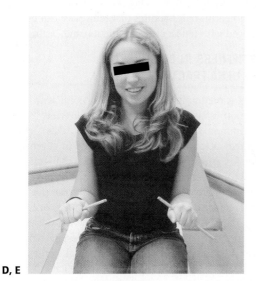

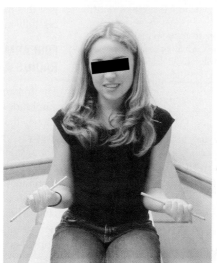

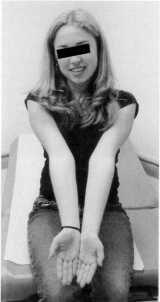

Figure 9-33. (*Continued*) **B:** Two-month follow-up radiographs. **C:** Six-month follow-up radiographs (ulnar nail removed). **D:** Pronation. **E:** Supination. **F:** Axial alignment.

reduction and rodding has been associated with compartment syndrome.[364] We are sensitive to both time and attempts during ESIN of forearm shaft fractures in our pediatric patients and recommend surgeons not to do prolonged attempts at reduction and fixation closed, and recommend relatively rapid conversion to a small open reduction if needed.

If single-bone fixation is done, the ulna usually is treated first because of its more benign entry site, subcutaneous location, and relatively straight canal compared to the radius. Plating is preferred to intramedullary nailing when early

malunion is present and callus formation is noted radiographically. Plating allows open osteoclasis and reduction. The plating technique is similar to that used in adults, except that smaller plates can be used and fewer cortices (often only four cortices above and below the fracture) are required for adequate fixation. In children with both-bone forearm fractures, plating of a single bone may be adequate and reduce the morbidity associated with dual-bone plating.[24] Significant comminution of both bones also may be an indication for plate fixation.

Potential Pitfalls and Preventive Measures

Intramedullary Nailing of Diaphyseal Radius and Ulna Fractures:
KEY SURGICAL STEPS

Pitfall	Prevention
• Refracture	• Keep elastic nails in place for nearly a year. Splint or cast for at least 6 to 8 weeks after elastic nailing
• Delayed union	• Use the smallest nail that will pass to allow callus formation (1.75 to 2.5 mm) • Use a plate instead of a nail after skeletal maturity
• Infection	• Wash out all open fractures, especially if they occur on organic surface (soccer field, fall from tree, dirt bike). Beware of the lawn biopsy in which a dirt clod gets stuck in the intramedullary canal
• Nail incarceration in canal	• Back up out of rut, rotate nail, then advance down canal
• Difficult nail passage across fracture	• Use a percutaneous K-wire to lever the ends of the fracture into alignment
• Muscle/tendon entrapment or rupture	• Make sure that elastic nail does not rub on or impale EPL tendon. Open fracture sites that are not reducible
• Neurapraxia	• Most will resolve spontaneously if noted prereduction. Fix radius first to minimize need to open which could injure PIN. Identify or avoid PIN during open reduction
• Compartment syndrome	• During elastic nailing, perform an open reduction if nail does not pass after multiple attempts (20 to 30 minutes). Perform fasciotomy in any patient who has increasing anxiety, analgesia requirements, and apprehension
• Complex regional pain syndrome	• Early recognition and referral to physical therapy or pain service for treatment

MANAGEMENT OF EXPECTED ADVERSE OUTCOMES AND UNEXPECTED COMPLICATIONS IN DIAPHYSEAL RADIUS AND ULNA FRACTURES

Diaphyseal Radius and Ulna Fractures:
COMMON ADVERSE OUTCOMES AND COMPLICATIONS

- Malunion
- Delayed union or nonunion
- Stiffness
- Refracture
- Nail prominence
- Compartment syndrome

REDISPLACEMENT/MALALIGNMENT IN DIAPHYSEAL RADIUS AND ULNA FRACTURES

The most common short-term complication of forearm shaft fracture treatment is loss of satisfactory reduction in a previously well-reduced and well-aligned fracture, a complication that occurs in 10%[55,62,78,162,339] to 25% of patients.[55,78] Initial follow-up radiographs are a screening test aimed at identifying redisplacement. Kramhøft and Solgaard[182] recommended that children with displaced diaphyseal forearm fractures have screening radiography at 1 and 2 weeks after reduction. Voto[338] also pointed out that most fractures that redisplace, do so within the first 2 weeks after injury. Inability to properly control fracture alignment with closed methods is the most commonly reported indication for operative intervention.[192,261,276,297,363]

The most common explanations for loss of fracture reduction are cast related (poor casting technique, no evidence of three-point molding).[60,339] The more experienced the surgeon, the greater the likelihood of successful reduction.[55] Other factors that have been found to be associated with forearm fracture redisplacement are quality of initial reduction,[361] missed follow-up appointments,[64] proximal third fractures,[70] and failure of the doctor to respond to early warning signs such as slight loss of reduction at 1-week follow-up.[113] Strategies for dealing with redisplacement include allowing the deformity to remodel,[144] cast wedging,[16,153,171] rereduction and recasting,[78,339] pins and plaster,[31,88,339] indirect reduction and internal fixation,[7] and open reduction and internal fixation.[357] Reports in the literature suggest that most forearm shaft fractures that redisplace can be successfully managed with repeat closed reduction and casting.[78,339]

FOREARM STIFFNESS IN DIAPHYSEAL RADIUS AND ULNA FRACTURES

The forearm is a predominantly nonsynovial joint with high-amplitude motion as its main function. Sardelli et al.[281a] have shown that common activities of daily living (ADLs) require nearly 75 degrees of pronation and 90 degrees of supination. The needs for forearm motion in ADLs may be changing with ever increasing computer and smartphone usage. The most common long-term complication of forearm shaft fracture treatment is significant forearm stiffness,[144] with pronation loss occurring almost twice as frequently as supination loss.[145] Loss of pronation or supination motion sometimes occurs despite perfectly normal-appearing radiographs.[170,233,258] Abnormal bony alignment of the forearm bones can lead to motion deficits.[168] However, stiffness can exceed that expected from bony malalignment alone[168] and stiffness can occur with normal radiographs and both situations may be indicative of fibrosis of the interosseous membrane and/or contracture of the interosseous ligament.[170,258]

With focused testing of forearm motion, between 18%[48] and 72%[145] of patients show at least some minor deficits after nonsurgical treatment. Most minor deficits are not even noticed by patients and rarely are associated with functional limitations.[48,74,233] More severe losses of forearm rotation have far greater impact.[223] In their series of malunited forearm fractures (thus strongly weighted to demonstrate forearm stiffness), Price et al.[258] reported a 15% (6/39) rate of mild stiffness (up to 25-degree loss) and an 8% (3/39) rate of severe forearm stiffness (loss of 45 degrees or more of either pronation or supination). Holdsworth's series of malunited pediatric forearm fractures had a similar rate (6%) of severe forearm stiffness. Holdsworth[145] told the classic story of a female whose inability to properly pronate caused her to elbow her neighbors when eating at the table. Patrick[246] pointed out that it is possible to compensate for pronation losses with shoulder abduction, but no similar compensation mechanism exists for supination losses. Such severe motion loss is a very undesirable outcome. For surgical treatment of these injuries to be a rational choice, the rates of stiffness after surgery must be lower than those after cast treatment.[130]

Bhaskar and Roberts[24] published one of the only studies of plated pediatric forearm fractures to report goniometric pronation and supination data. Both their single-bone (ulna) and both-bone plated patients showed mild forearm motion losses (maximal 18% loss of pronation).[24] Variable rates of mild forearm range-of-motion losses have been reported after intramedullary fixation. Amit et al.[7] reported a 40% rate of mild stiffness (5 to 10 degrees) in 20 pediatric patients after Rush rod fixation of forearm fractures. Combined data from five series of the flexible intramedullary nailing (K-wires, Steinmann pins, Nancy nails) revealed a 1.6% rate (2/128) of mild forearm stiffness (up to a 20-degree loss) and a 0% (0/128) rate of severe motion loss (40 degrees or more loss of either pronation or supination).[7,23,97,185,297,363] No published series of nonoperatively treated forearm shaft fracture patients has exceeded these results relative to preservation of forearm motion.

REFRACTURE IN DIAPHYSEAL RADIUS AND ULNA FRACTURES

Refracture occurs more often after forearm shaft fractures in children than after any other fracture.[186] Tredwell[328] found that forearm refractures occurred at an average of 6 months after original injury and were more common in males (3:1) and in older children (approximately 12 years old). Baitner and his San Diego colleagues suggested that middle- and proximal-third forearm shaft fractures created a higher risk of refracture for pediatric patients.[14] Refracture rates of 4%[97] to 8%[197] have been reported in pediatric diaphyseal forearm fractures. Bould and Bannister[38] reported that diaphyseal forearm fractures were eight times more likely to refracture than metaphyseal fractures. Schwarz et al.[292] found that 84% (21/28) of the forearm refractures in their series had initially presented as greenstick fractures. Based on the stage of bony healing, refractures may occur through the original

fracture site, through both the original site and partially through intact bone or completely through intact bone,[348] but most seem to occur through the original fracture site.

Several authors have suggested that internal fixation is necessary after refracture,[12,255,270] but Schwarz et al.[292] reported good results with repeat closed reduction and casting in 14 of 17 patients with refractures. Closed reduction of the fracture and the bent rods has been shown to be effective for forearm refractures that occur with flexible nails in place (Fig. 9-34).[226] The best treatment of refracture is prevention, and patients should be splint protected (removable forearm splint or thermoplastic gauntlet) for a period of 2 months depending on the activity after initial bone healing.[234,258] Refracture is rare during splint wear. Parents must be cautioned about the risk of refracture despite apparently adequate bone healing on radiographs.

Refracture after plate removal has been discussed frequently in the literature[102,231,257,331] and appears to be associated with decreased bone density beneath the plate.[176] This has led many authors to question the routine use of plate fixation for pediatric forearm fractures.[28,64,257,332] Refractures also have been reported after removal of intramedullary forearm fixation in children.[72,135,170,189,297,327,362] The main strategies aimed at decreasing the risk of refractures after implant removal are documentation of adequate bony healing before implant removal, and an additional period of splint protection after implant removal until the holes have filled in.

MALUNION IN DIAPHYSEAL RADIUS AND ULNA FRACTURES

Evaluation of pediatric forearm fracture malunion must take into account established malreduction limits and expected pediatric remodeling potential. Thus, a malunion of 30 degrees may become less than 10 degrees during the course of follow-up. The level of the malunited fracture also must be considered, because the consequences of malreduction vary according to level.[282,360] More deformity in the predominant plane of motion is acceptable in fractures near physes of long bones than in diaphyseal fractures. Normal motion can be preserved despite persistent radiographic abnormality (Fig. 9-35).

Malunion of radial and ulnar shaft fractures can lead to an aesthetic deformity and loss of motion; however, significant loss of function occurs in only a small percentage of patients.[48,74,233] Some authors have recommended more aggressive efforts at

(text continues on page 346)

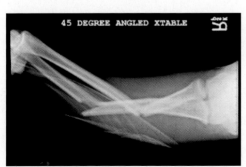
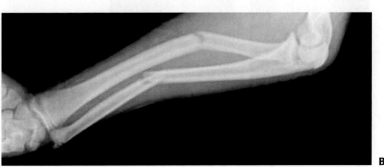

Figure 9-34. A 14-year-old ESIN patient who suffered refracture with the nails in place. **A:** Injury AP radiograph. **B:** Injury lateral radiograph. Skateboard mechanism.

(continues)

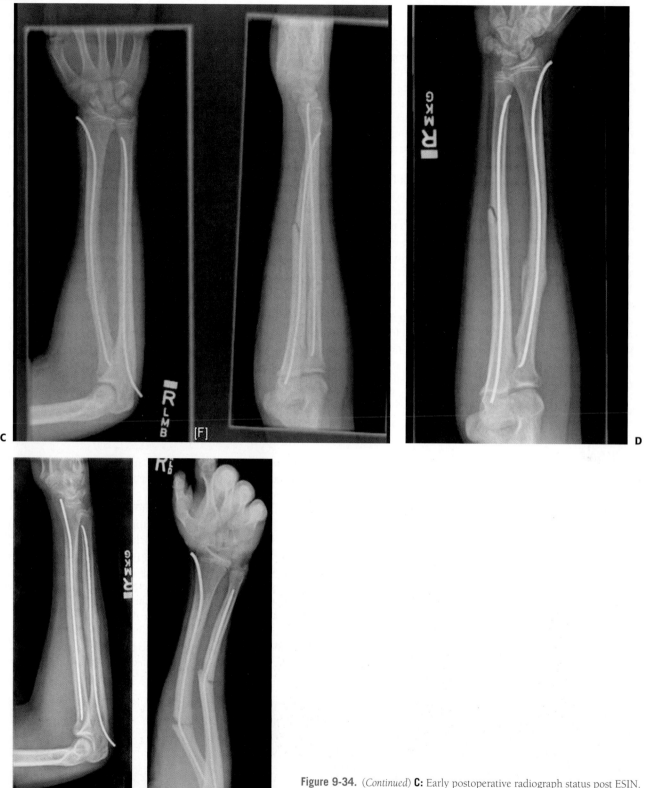

Figure 9-34. (*Continued*) **C:** Early postoperative radiograph status post ESIN. **D:** Two-month postoperative AP radiograph. **E:** Two-month postoperative lateral radiograph. **F:** Refracture at 2.5 months postoperative.

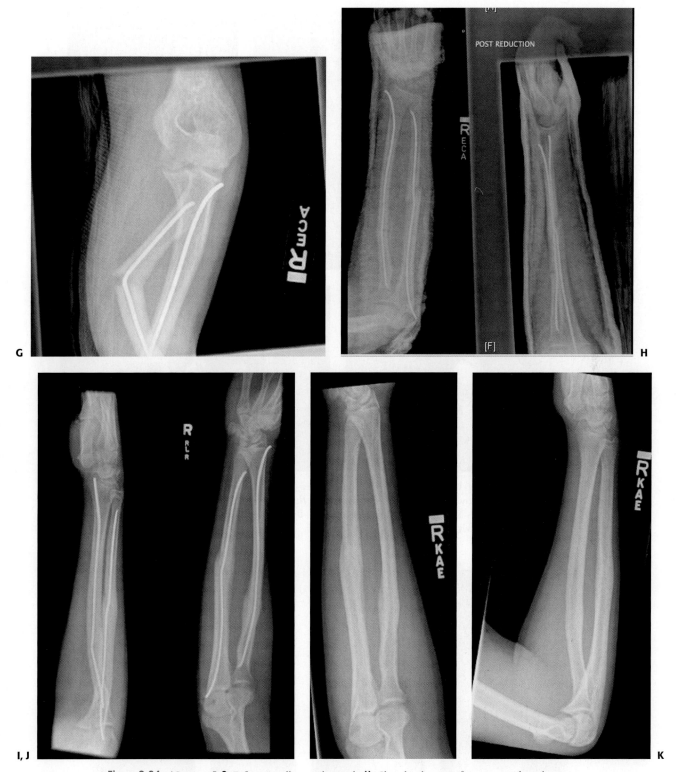

Figure 9-34. (*Continued*) **G:** Refracture elbow radiograph. **H:** Closed reduction of titanium nails and angulated radius and ulna fractures. **I:** Five months after refracture. **J:** AP radiograph 1 year after refracture. **K:** Lateral radiograph 1 year after refracture.

(*continues*)

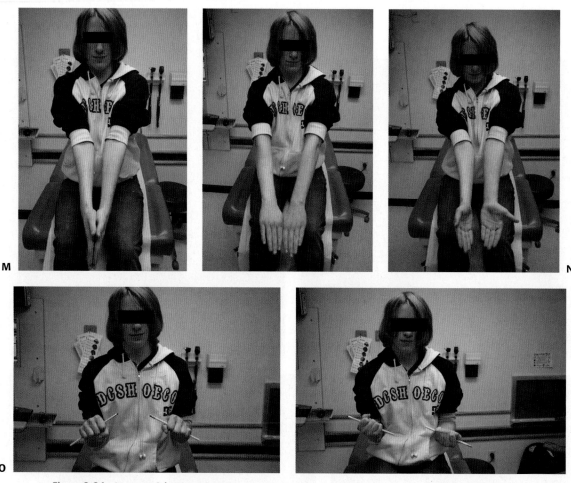

Figure 9-34. (*Continued*) **L:** Clinical appearance with extended elbows and forearm midposition. **M:** Clinical appearance with extended elbows and pronated forearms. **N:** Clinical appearance with extended elbows and supinated forearms. Note mild supination loss on right. **O:** Symmetrical pronation. **P:** Asymmetrical supination. Approximately 15-degree loss on right.

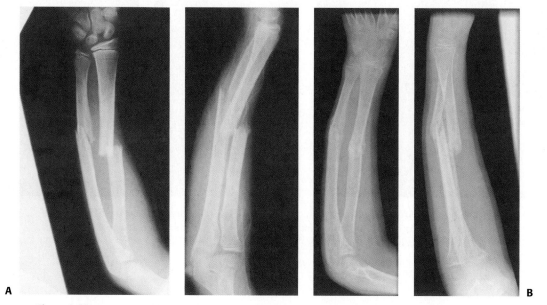

Figure 9-35 An 11-year old with midshaft both-bone complete forearm fracture. **A:** AP and lateral injury radiographs. **B:** One-month follow-up radiographs.

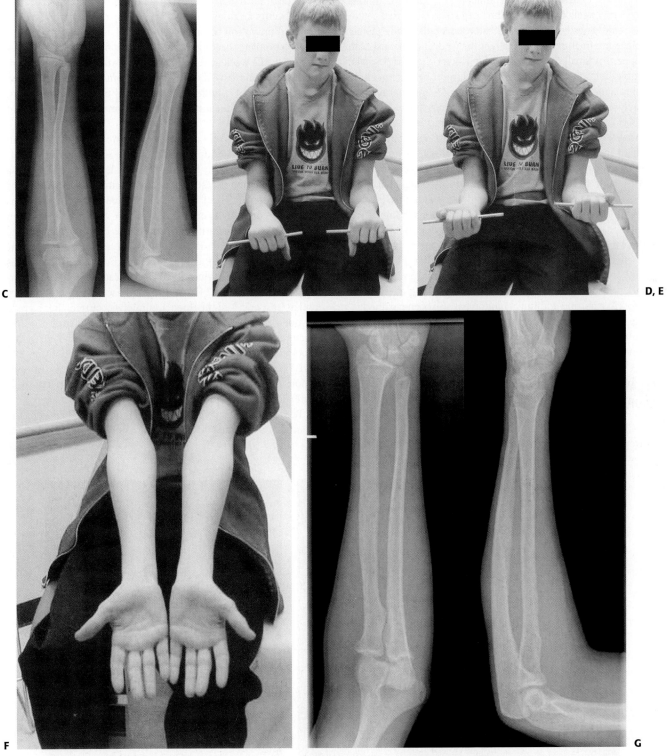

Figure 9-35. (*Continued*) **C:** Two-year follow-up radiographs. **D:** Pronation. **E:** Supination. **F:** Axial alignment. **G:** Six-year follow-up radiographs with substantial remodeling of radius and ulna fractures.

correction of forearm fracture malunions.[219,256] Early malunions (up to 4 or 5 weeks after injury) can be treated with closed osteoclasis under anesthesia. If closed osteoclasis fails to adequately mobilize the fracture, a minimally invasive drill osteoclasis can be done.[27] A small-diameter drill (or K-wire) is used to make multiple holes in the region of the malunion before forcefully manipulating the bone back into alignment.[27] Internal fixation is rarely needed if osteoclasis is performed in a timely fashion.

Once significant callus is present, indirect reduction and internal fixation with flexible intramedullary nails can be difficult or impossible because the intramedullary fracture site is now blocked with callus. Thus, established or impending malunions that cannot be adequately reduced closed and controlled with a cast may require formal open reduction and plate fixation (Figs. 9-36 and 9-37). Many fractures that heal with angulation or rotation of more than the established criteria regain full motion and have an excellent cosmetic outcome. Fractures may require corrective osteotomy if they fail to remodel after an adequate period of observation or if adequate motion fails to return.[219,329] Such corrective osteotomies have been done long after injury (up to 27 years) and additional motion has still been regained.[329] There is a minor subset of malunions that does not remodel, that has functional limits (especially when there is limited supination deformity), and is therefore a candidate for osteotomy.

DELAYED UNION/NONUNION IN DIAPHYSEAL RADIUS AND ULNA FRACTURES

The diagnosis of delayed union is based on documentation of slower-than-normal progression toward union.[194] Daruwalla[74]

stated that normal healing of closed pediatric forearm shaft fractures occurs at an average of 5.5 weeks (range 2 to 8 weeks). Delayed union can be practically defined as a failure to demonstrate complete healing (four cortices) on sequential radiographs by 12 weeks after injury, which exceeds the upper limit of normal healing by about 1 month. Nonunion can be defined as the absence of complete bony union by 6 months after injury, which exceeds the upper limit of normal healing by about 4 months.

Delayed unions and nonunions are rare after closed forearm shaft fractures in children.[98,194,308] In six large series of pediatric diaphyseal forearm fractures treated by closed methods, a less than 0.5% rate (1/263) of delayed union and no nonunions were reported.[48,74,145,170,182,258] Delayed unions and nonunions are more common after open reduction and internal fixation and open fractures. Particular concern has been raised about the potential of antegrade ulnar nailing (olecranon starting point) to distract the fracture site.[237] Combined data from four series of plated pediatric forearm fractures indicated a 3% (3/89) nonunion rate[24,231,332,357]; 24% (21/89) of these were open fractures and at least one[357] of the three nonunions occurred after a grade III open fracture.[231,332] Large series of open pediatric forearm fractures (treated by a variety of internal fixation methods) reported comparable numbers: 5% (8/173) delayed union rate and 1% (2/173) nonunion rate.[76,128,135] In a series of 30 nonunions in children, only 6 were in the forearm, and half of these were after open fractures.[194]

Because of the overall rarity of nonunions in children, the possibility of unusual diagnoses such as neurofibromatosis must

(text continues on page 353)

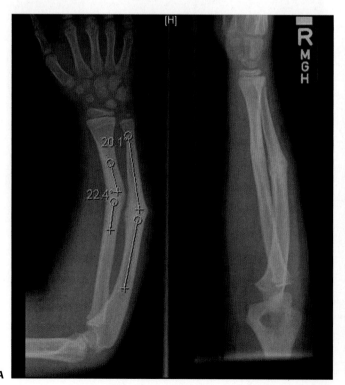 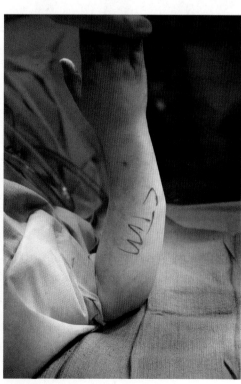

Figure 9-36. An 8-year-old male who underwent corrective osteotomy for forearm shaft malunion. **A:** Radiographs demonstrating significant angular malunion. **B:** Preoperative clinical appearance (dorsal view).

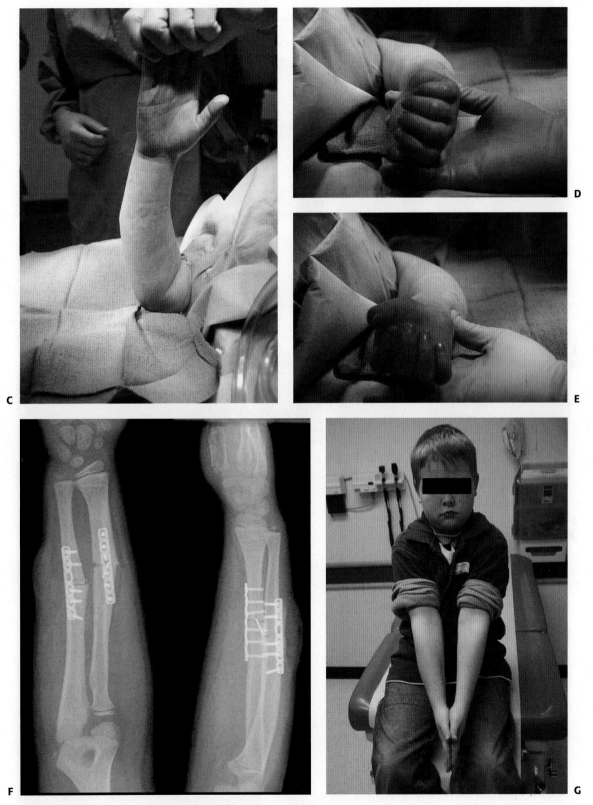

Figure 9-36. (*Continued*) **C:** Preoperative clinical appearance (volar view). **D:** Preoperative demonstration of full passive supination. **E:** Preoperative demonstration of marked limitation in passive pronation. **F:** Early postoperative radiographs following corrective osteotomies (note intraosseous Kirschner wire tip from provisional fixation). **G:** Clinical appearance with extended elbows and forearm midposition.

(continues)

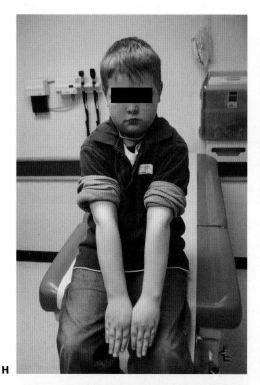

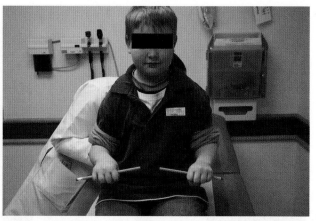

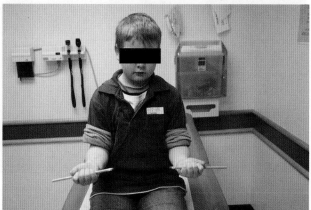

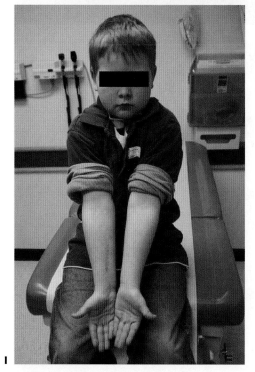

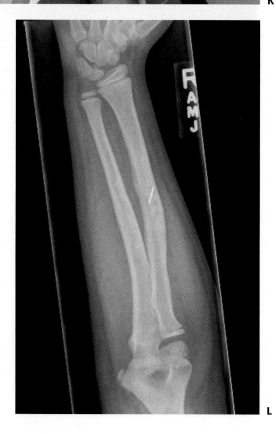

Figure 9-36. (*Continued*) **H:** Clinical appearance with extended elbows and pronated forearms. **I:** Clinical appearance with extended elbows and supinated forearms. **J:** Symmetrical pronation. **K:** Symmetrical supination. **L:** AP radiograph 18 months after osteotomies (plates and screws have been removed).

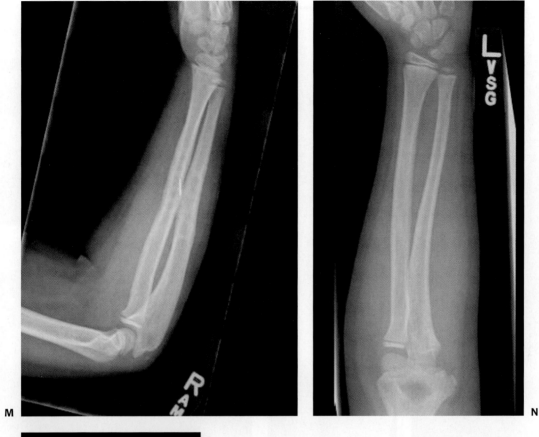

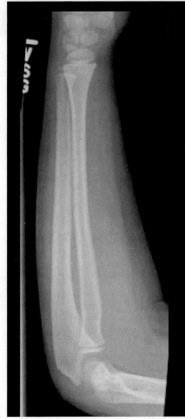

Figure 9-36. (*Continued*) **M:** Lateral radiograph at 18-month follow-up. **N:** AP radiograph uninjured left forearm. **O:** Lateral radiograph uninjured left forearm.

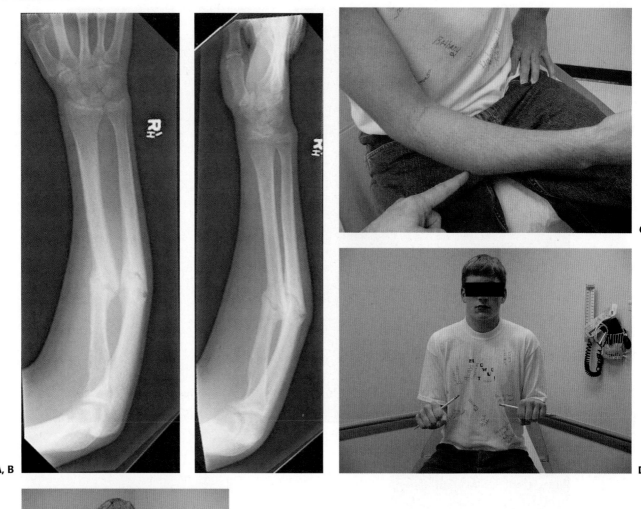

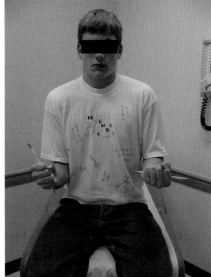

Figure 9-37. A 16-year-old boy who underwent corrective osteotomy for forearm shaft malunion. **A:** AP radiograph at time of presentation. **B:** Lateral radiograph at time of presentation. Note rotational malunion of radius in addition to angular abnormalities of both bones. **C:** Clinical deformity (bump). **D:** Relatively symmetrical pronation noted preoperatively. **E:** Dramatic lack of supination on the right noted preoperatively.

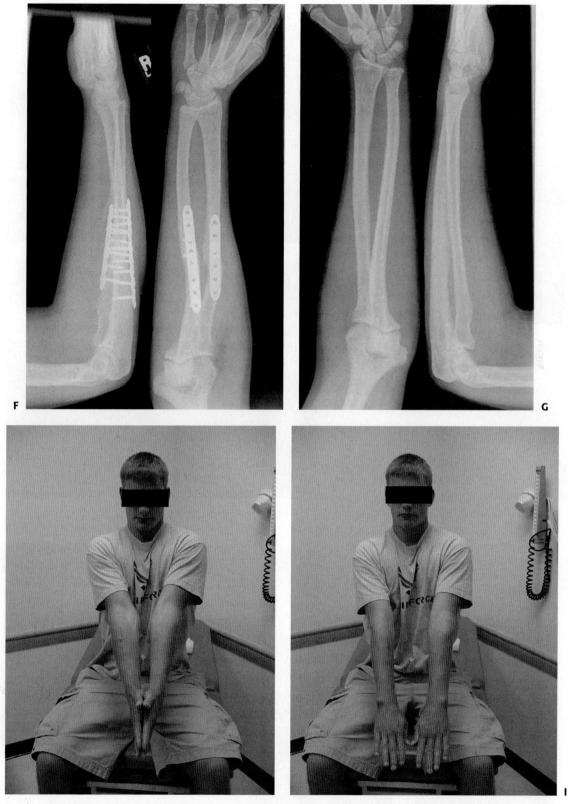

Figure 9-37. (*Continued*) **F:** One-year postoperative radiographs following osteotomies. Note improved rotational alignment of radius. **G:** Uninjured left forearm radiographs. **H:** Clinical appearance with extended elbows and forearm midposition. **I:** Clinical appearance with extended elbows and pronated forearms.

(continues)

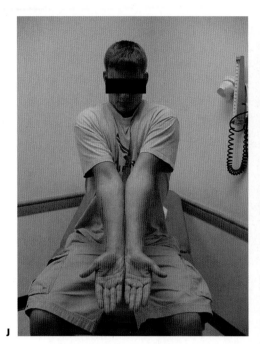

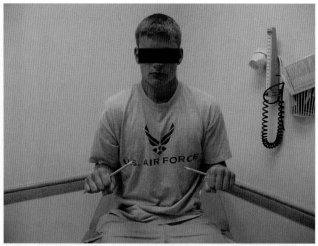

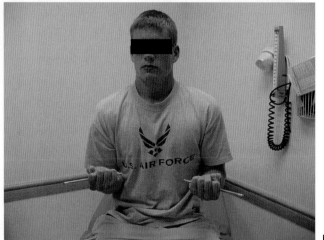

Figure 9-37. (*Continued*) **J:** Clinical appearance with extended elbows and supinated forearms. **K:** Symmetrical pronation. **L:** Symmetrical supination.

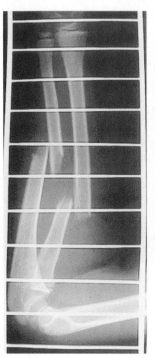

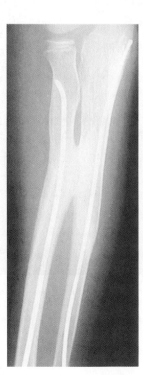

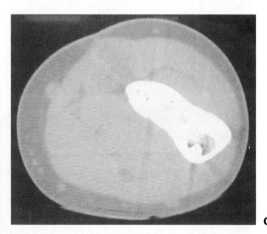

Figure 9-38. Radioulnar synostosis following closed injury. **A:** Injury radiographs. **B:** Plain radiographs showing synostosis. **C:** CT scan showing synostosis. (Courtesy of Alan Aner, MD.)

be considered.[67,69,156,206] After open injury or surgical intervention for other reasons, the possibility of septic nonunion must be ruled out. In the absence of such extraneous factors, nonunion of pediatric forearm fractures seems to be related to surgical treatment.[67,69,156,206,308] Weber and Cech[345] divided nonunions into atrophic and hypertrophic types. Atrophic nonunions probably are best treated with bone grafting and compression plating. Compression plating or other stable internal fixation without grafting usually is sufficient for hypertrophic nonunions.[191]

CROSS-UNION/SYNOSTOSIS IN DIAPHYSEAL RADIUS AND ULNA FRACTURES

Posttraumatic radioulnar synostosis results in complete loss of forearm rotation. Most cross-unions that form after pediatric forearm shaft fractures are type II lesions (diaphyseal cross-unions), as described by Vince and Miller (Fig. 9-39).[336] Although some series of adult forearm fractures have reported synostosis rates of 6% to 9%,[20,317] posttraumatic radioulnar synostosis is a rare complication of pediatric forearm shaft fractures.[336] In children, it is usually associated with high-energy injuries,[336] radial neck fractures,[274] and surgically treated forearm fractures.[72,238] Some have suggested a familial predisposition to this complication.[203] Postoperative synostosis after forearm fractures in children is almost exclusively associated with plate fixation.[352,357] The risk of cross-union is increased when open reduction and internal fixation of both-bone fractures are done through one incision.[20,64]

Both osseous and nonosseous cross-unions may form in the forearm,[8,62] but the more common type is osseous. After a synostosis matures (6 to 12 months), it can be excised along with any soft tissue interposition.[235,336] The results of synostosis resection may be better in adults than children,[336] perhaps because of the

more biologically active periosteum in children.[83,336] Complete synostoses have limited outcomes as compared to those with some lucency still present on CT scan between the two bones. Interposition of inert materials (such as Gore-Tex [W. L. Gore & Associates, Inc., Elkton, MD] or bone wax) and vascularized flaps has been used to decrease the chances of recurrent synostosis.[8,18,238,336] Nonsteroidal anti-inflammatory drugs and radiation treatment have been reported after synostosis excision in adults, but their use in children remains undefined. An alternative treatment is corrective osteotomy if the patient is synostosed in a position of either extreme pronation or supination. If the patient is stuck in a neutral position after posttraumatic synostosis, surgical intervention is usually not recommended.

INFECTION IN DIAPHYSEAL RADIUS AND ULNA FRACTURES

Infection occurs only in surgically treated forearm shaft fractures and open fractures. Appropriately timed preoperative antibiotic prophylaxis is believed to diminish the risk of infection. Children with open forearm fractures are considered to be at high risk for infection, and early (usually less than 24 hours)[302] irrigation and debridement in the operating room is indicated.[276] Whether in the backyard, the barnyard, the football field, or the hay field, open forearm fractures that occur in organic settings are best treated with early irrigation and debridement with inspection of the intramedullary canal of both bone ends, where soil contamination tends to occur during injury (see Fig. 9-26). Soil contamination has been reported to lead to gas gangrene and subsequent upper extremity amputation in children with grade I open forearm fractures.[95] Emergency room irrigation and debridement is not recommended and is considered inadequate with increased risk of serious infection.

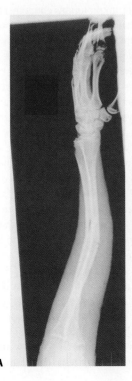

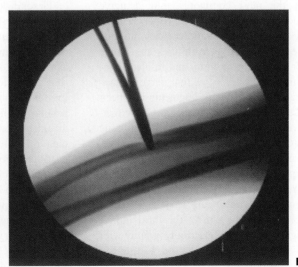

Figure 9-39. Muscle/tendon incarceration. **A:** Injury radiograph showing mild apex-volar fracture angulation. **B:** Flexor digitorum profundus entrapment in the ulna fracture site required surgical extirpation.

In four published series of plated pediatric forearm fractures (25% open fractures), deep infection (osteomyelitis) occurred in 5% (4/83).[223,231,332,357] Such deep infections usually require extensive additional surgical treatment to eradicate them. Combined data from 12 series of similar pediatric forearm fractures (15% open fractures) treated with intramedullary K-wires, Steinmann pins, or Rush rods revealed a deep infection rate of 0.46% (2/437)[7,44,72,185,198,261,262,297,342,363] and a superficial infection rate of 2.5% (11/437). Six studies of ESIN fixation reported a 0.2% (1/370) deep infection rate and a 3% (12/370) superficial infection rate.[44,131,189,205,270,335] Superficial infections may require oral antibiotics, pin removal, or both.

Open forearm fractures clearly are at increased risk for infection. Most (96%) open forearm fractures in children are Gustilo and Anderson[134] grade I or II.[128,135,199] It is often not possible to know if a fracture is grade I versus grade II open until more extensive exposure of deep tissues including the bone ends. Two studies specifically investigated the relationship between the time from injury until irrigation and debridement and the risk of later infection. Luhmann et al.[199] reported on 65 fractures (52 type I, 12 type II, 1 type III) that were irrigated and debrided an average of 5.6 hours (range 1.5 to 24 hours) after injury, and Greenbaum et al.[128] reported 62 fractures (58 type I, 4 type II) that were irrigated and debrided an average of 14.6 hours (range 1.7 to 37.8 hours) after injury. No statistically significant association was found in either of these studies; however, most (87%) of these fractures were grade I injuries. Pooled data revealed an overall 1.2% rate (2/173) of deep infection and a 0.6% rate (1/173) of superficial infection after current open fracture treatment protocols.[128,135,199]

NEURAPRAXIA IN DIAPHYSEAL RADIUS AND ULNA FRACTURES

The median nerve is the most commonly injured nerve with forearm shaft fractures (whether closed or open injuries),[78,128,135,199] but any peripheral nerve and at times multiple nerves may be involved.[72] Most of these injuries are simple neurapraxias that occur at the time of injury and resolve spontaneously over weeks to months.[78,134,232] Actual nerve entrapment within or perforation by the bony fragments has been reported,[6,111,117,118,152,259,260,313] most often with greenstick fractures.[118,152,259,260] Constricting fracture callus and fibrous tissue also have been known to cause nerve palsies.[260,313] In patients who fail to recover normal nerve function within a satisfactory time period,[6] nerve exploration, decompression, and possible nerve repair or reconstruction should be considered. If signs of progressive nerve recovery (e.g., advancing Tinel sign, return of function) are not present by the end of the third month after injury, further diagnostic workup (electromyography with nerve conduction studies) is indicated. Prolonged waiting can be harmful to long-term outcome.

Nerve injury after internal fixation is always a concern. Operative treatment of pediatric forearm fractures by either indirect reduction and internal fixation techniques or classic open reduction and internal fixation techniques requires fracture manipulation and soft tissue retraction, which have the potential to worsen existing subclinical nerve injury or to create a new injury. Such injuries are rare and may be underreported. Nerve injury after pediatric forearm plate fixation has been alluded to but not discussed extensively.[185] Luhmann et al.[198] reported an 8% (2/25) iatrogenic nerve injury rate after fixation with intramedullary K-wires or Rush rods: Both were ulnar nerve injuries that resolved in 2 to 3 weeks. Cullen et al.[72] reported one ulnar nerve injury that took 3 months to resolve in a group of 20 patients treated with K-wires or Rush rods.

Certain sensory nerves also are at risk for iatrogenic damage during surgical forearm fracture treatment, especially the superficial branch of the radial nerve.[44,198,315] Pooled data from six series that included 370 ESIN procedures revealed a 2% (7/370) rate of injury to the superficial branch of the radial nerve.[44,131,189,205,270,335] The branching pattern of this sensory nerve is complex, and efforts must be taken to protect it during insertion of intramedullary nails through distal radial entry points.[1,13]

MUSCLE OR TENDON ENTRAPMENT/TENDON RUPTURE IN DIAPHYSEAL RADIUS AND ULNA FRACTURES

Severely displaced forearm fractures may trap portions of muscle between the fracture fragments.[147,261] Often, interposed tissue can be effectively removed during standard fracture reduction, but the muscle may become an obstacle to successful closed reduction. Much of the volar aspects of the shafts of the radius and ulna are covered by the flexor pollicis longus and flexor digitorum profundus, respectively. Many displaced forearm shaft fractures also have apex-volar angulation.[234] As a result, portions of these muscles (or their tendons) are particularly prone to fracture site incarceration (Fig. 9-39). The pronator quadratus also is vulnerable to fracture site entrapment in the distal third of the radius and ulna, and it can block reduction of distal third forearm fractures.[147]

Flexor digitorum profundus entrapment within ulnar[140,180,267,295] and radial[343] shaft fractures has been reported. Entrapment of the flexor digitorum profundus typically causes an inability to fully extend the involved finger (usually index, long, or ring fingers alone or in combination).[140,295] Isolated ring finger flexor digitorum profundus entrapment has also recently been reported.[307] Even if identified early, this complication rarely responds to occupational or physical therapy. Surgical intervention is the preferred treatment and requires only a small incision (usually over the ulna) through which the adherent tissue is elevated with a blunt instrument from the bone at the site of the fracture. Excellent restoration of finger motion can be achieved, even when the release is done up to 2 years after the fracture.[267]

Extensor tendon injury has been reported after intramedullary nailing of pediatric forearm shaft fractures.[131,189,251,261] The extensor pollicis longus appears to be at particular risk for this injury if a dorsal entry point is utilized near the second and third dorsal compartments.[183,312] Primary tendon disruption may be caused by direct trauma during either nail insertion or extraction. Delayed tendon disruption is caused by slow erosion of the tendon as it glides past a sharp nail edge. The possibility of this complication can be minimized by using surgical incisions large enough to allow insertion of small blunt retractors to protect adjacent tendons during nail insertion and extraction. Avoidance of tendon erosion requires non-sharp ends and pin lengths that extend beyond the tendon level into either the subcutaneous tissues[72,297] or through the skin (external pins).[261] Conceivably, the pins could be buried completely within the bone, but this would require either accepting them as permanent implants (something not commonly practiced at this time) or significantly increasing the level of difficulty of nail removal. The extensor pollicis longus is more at risk near the Lister tubercle and may require a late tendon reconstruction with extensor indicis proprius transfer if ruptured.

COMPARTMENT SYNDROME IN DIAPHYSEAL RADIUS AND ULNA FRACTURES

Compartment syndrome is rare after closed forearm fractures in children, but its consequences can be devastating. Yuan et al.[364] found no compartment syndromes in 205 closed forearm injuries, and Jones and Weiner[162] reported no compartment syndromes in their series of 730 closed forearm injuries. A single compartment syndrome that developed during cast treatment of a 12-year-old female with a closed both-bone forearm fracture was reported by Cullen et al.[72] Because the diagnosis of compartment syndrome can be difficult in children,[266] the index of suspicion must be high.

Compartment syndrome should be suspected in any child who is not reasonably comfortable 3 to 4 hours after adequate reduction and immobilization of a forearm fracture.[65] The risk of compartment syndrome is higher with open fractures[135,364] and fractures that are difficult to reduce and require extended operative efforts.[364] Yuan et al.[364] voiced concern that the 10% (3/30) rate of compartment syndrome in their patients with closed fractures might be caused by multiple passes or "misses" with intramedullary devices during efforts at indirect reduction and internal fixation. Compartment syndrome was reported by Haasbeek and Cole[135] in 5 (11%) of 46 open forearm fractures in their series. The so-called floating elbow injury has been associated with a rate of compartment syndrome as high as 33%.[364] In children, the three As of increasing analgesia, anxiety, and agitation are the most reliable clinical signs of a pending compartment syndrome. Forearm compartment syndrome is best treated with fasciotomy, releasing both the superficial and deep volar compartments and the mobile wad. Both the lacertus fibrosus and the carpal tunnel should be released as part of the procedure.

COMPLEX REGIONAL PAIN SYNDROMES IN DIAPHYSEAL RADIUS AND ULNA FRACTURES

Complex regional pain syndromes such as reflex sympathetic dystrophy are uncommon complications after pediatric forearm shaft fractures.[332] Paradoxically, relatively minor injuries seem to place patients at greatest risk.[316,349] The most reliable sign in children is true allodynia: significant reproducible pain with light touch on the skin. Swelling and other vasomotor changes often are accompanying signs.[193] The diagnosis in children is made based almost exclusively on the history and physical examination, with little reliance on studies such as bone scans.[316] These pain syndromes are best treated initially with physical therapy aimed at range of motion and desensitization.[316,349] Failure to respond to physical therapy may warrant a referral to a qualified pediatric pain specialist.[174,193]

Authors' Preferred Treatment for Diaphyseal Radius and Ulna Fractures (Algorithm 9-1)

We agree with Jones and Weiner that "closed reduction still remains the gold standard for closed isolated pediatric forearm fractures."[162] Most nondisplaced and minimally displaced radial and ulnar shaft fractures can be splinted in the emergency department and referred for orthopedic follow-up within 1 week. Radiographs are repeated at the first orthopedic visit, and a cast is applied. During warmer weather, when fracture incidence peaks, we tend to use waterproof cast liners. We avoid flexing the elbow past 80 to 90 degrees in waterproof casts because the soft tissue crease that forms in the antecubital fossa tends to trap moisture. Because waterproof cast lining alone does not shield the skin from cast-saw cuts and burns as well as traditional padding does, specialized material may be added along the anticipated course of the cast saw to protect the skin during cast removal.

We prefer an above-elbow cast for all forearm fractures in children under the age of 4 years, because young children tend to lose or remove a below-elbow cast because of soft tissue differences (baby fat) common to the age group.[84] Most older children with forearm shaft fractures also are treated with above-elbow casting, except for those with distal third fractures. Good forearm casting technique should focus on the principles outlined earlier in this chapter. Patients with nondisplaced fractures usually are reevaluated radiographically in 1 to 2 weeks after initial immobilization to check for fracture displacement. Forearm shaft fractures heal more slowly than metaphyseal and physeal fractures of the distal radius and ulna.[12,78] The cast is removed in 6 to 8 weeks if adequate healing is present on radiographs. Because of the significant refracture rate after forearm shaft fractures, we splint these fractures for several weeks or even a few months until all transverse lucency of the original fracture disappears and all four cortices are healed. It is extremely helpful to warn patients and their parents about the high rate of refracture with forearm shaft fracture throughout their treatment. Fractures that heal in bayonet apposition (complete translation and some shortening) can take longer to heal than those with end-to-end apposition and may require prolonged splinting to prevent refracture.[84,275]

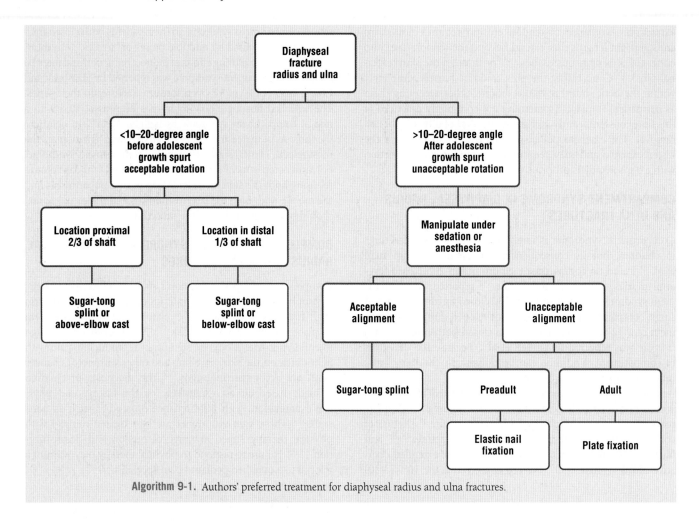

Algorithm 9-1. Authors' preferred treatment for diaphyseal radius and ulna fractures.

SUMMARY, CONTROVERSIES, AND FUTURE DIRECTIONS RELATED TO DIAPHYSEAL RADIUS AND ULNA FRACTURES

FRACTURE RISK/FRACTURE PREVENTION

Over the past three decades, the rate of forearm fractures has increased dramatically in the United States: 33% higher for males and 56% higher for females.[177] Certain risk-taking behaviors demonstrated by children, as well as increased use of roller blades, skateboards, scooters, trampolines, Heelys skate shoes, bicycle ramping, snowboarding, and motorized vehicles like all-terrain vehicles, may be at least partly to blame.[43,201] Increased general physical activity patterns and decreased calcium intake also have been suggested as explanations,[177] but gaps persist in our epidemiologic understanding. Preventing these injuries remains an admirable but elusive goal. Two main avenues of research have been explored: optimizing safety during activities known to be associated with forearm fractures and investigating biologic mechanisms related to fracture risk.

The relationship between in-line skating (rollerblading) and pediatric forearm fractures has been shown,[20,252] with 1 in 8 children sustaining a fracture on his or her first skating attempt.[222] Prevention efforts have focused largely on protective gear. Wrist guards have been shown to decrease distal forearm bone strain[311] and injury rates.[284] Similar protective effects of wrist guards in snowboarders have been shown.[240] Trampolines are another target of injury prevention efforts aimed at a specific play activity.[90] Dramatic increases in trampoline-related injuries were reported during the 1990s, with rates doubling[305] or even tripling.[108] Safety recommendations have ranged from constant adult supervision and one-child-at-a-time use[188] to outright bans on public trampoline use.[108,305]

A variety of biologic risk factors have been studied relative to forearm fractures. Children who avoid drinking milk have been shown to have increased fracture risk,[126] as well as those who prefer to drink fruit juice and soda.[248] Several studies have shown an increased risk of fractures in females aged 3 to 15 years with low bone density.[123,124] Diet, nutrition, and exercise are being explored as causative factors, but the precise reason for the low bone density has not been confirmed. Too little physical activity (as measured by television, computer, and video viewing) has been associated with increased fracture risk, presumably because of decreased bone mineral density.[200] Caution also must be exercised when obtaining dual-energy x-ray absorptiometry data in children, as up to 88% of scans may be misinterpreted.[110] Childhood obesity is a growing problem in our society.[114,154] Increased body weight and decreased cross-sectional dimensions of the forearm bones also have been found in females who fracture their forearms.[303] Other researchers have found an increased risk of forearm fracture in obese children.[125,161]

PARENTAL PRESENCE DURING FRACTURE REDUCTION IN DIAPHYSEAL RADIUS AND ULNA FRACTURES

Parental presence is becoming increasingly popular for pediatric emergency department procedures. Several studies on chest tubes, IV cannulation, lumbar puncture, and urethral catheterization have shown increased parental satisfaction when parents are allowed to stay for these procedures.[19,137,253] Parental presence during induction of anesthesia also has been shown to have favorable effects on children older than 4 years of age.[165] To the best of our knowledge, there are no published studies on parental presence during orthopedic procedures performed in the emergency department setting. There are also no parental presence studies on any emergency department procedures performed on children who are under sedation, when the child is probably not aware of the parent's presence.

Certain relationships between perceived procedural invasiveness and parental presence have been borne out in the literature. Four hundred parents from the Indiana area were surveyed, and with increasing invasiveness, the parents' desire to be present decreased.[33] A survey of academic emergency medicine attendings, residents, and nurses from across the country also showed that there is an inverse relationship between increasing invasiveness and support for parental presence.[21] Boudreaux et al. published their critical review of the parental presence literature and concluded that "randomized controlled trials are mixed regarding whether family presence actually helps the patient."[37]

Extrapolation of information from the previously mentioned studies to pediatric orthopedic settings should be done with caution. We typically allow parents to be present for the induction of sedation, and once the patient is sedated, the parents are asked to wait in a designated area. If parents are allowed to be present, we strongly recommend a dedicated employee to attend to the parent or parents (a "spotter"). Several parents (typically fathers) have fainted during such orthopedic procedures and injured themselves. Parents who stay for a reduction also should be counseled that the patient may moan or cry during reduction but will not remember it. Parents who are not present during reduction should be asked to wait far enough away from the procedure room so they cannot hear the child.

ACKNOWLEDGMENTS

The authors wish to acknowledge the priceless teaching and constructive feedback afforded us by our senior partner, Alvin H. Crawford, MD, FACS.

Annotated References

Reference	Annotation
Abrams RA, Brown RA, Botte MJ. The superficial branch of the radial nerve: an anatomic study with surgical implications. *J Hand Surg Am*. 1992;17:1037–1041.	These two adult cadaver dissection papers give us important anatomic information that relates to distal radial entry sites for flexible nailing of forearm shaft fractures. Multiple branches of the terminal superficial radial nerve must be respected. Abrams et al. showed that in addition to branches "in" the first dorsal compartment, there may be a branch as close as 5 mm to Lister tubercle.
Auerbach DM, Collins ED, Kunkle KL, et al. The radial sensory nerve: an anatomic study. *Clin Orthop Relat Res*. 1994;308:241–249.	Auerbach et al. showed an average of nearly six branches distally and 60% of specimens had branches overlying the so-called 3–4 wrist arthroscopy portal.
Bowman EN, Mehlman CT, Lindsell CJ, et al. Nonoperative treatment of both-bone forearm shaft fractures in children: predictors of early radiographic failure. *J Pediatr Orthop*. 2011;31:23–32.	This study retrospectively analyzed a cohort of 282 children with displaced complete both-bone forearm shaft fractures who underwent closed reduction. Over the course of up to 4 weeks of radiographic follow-up, age-dependent criteria were used to assess radiographic failure rates: 20/15/10 degrees (distal third, middle third, proximal third) for girls <8 years old and boys <10 years old, and >10 degrees for girls >8 years old and boys >10 years old. Overall, there was a 51% failure rate with age >10 for either sex having 3 times higher odds of failure and proximal-third fractures nearly 7 times higher.
Evans EM. Rotational deformity in the treatment of fractures of both bones of the forearm. *J Bone Joint Surg*. 1945;27:373–379.	These are two important and timeless contributions focusing on rotational forearm assessment. They include Evans' priceless and often reproduced figures of the different orientations of the bicipital tuberosity.
Evans EM. Fractures of the radius and ulna. *J Bone Joint Surg Br*. 1951;33:548–561.	Evans also emphasized important management differences between greenstick and complete fractures.

Annotated References

Reference	Annotation
Fee NF, Dobranski A, Bisla RS. Gas gangrene complicating open forearm fractures. Report of five cases. *J Bone Joint Surg Am.* 1977;59:135–138.	Four of the five patients presented in this paper were pediatric patients. All had outdoor injuries resulting in small grade 1 open forearm fractures. All had local wound care (rinsing the skin) and fracture reduction. Antibiotics were not routinely administered; an 8-year-old male, a 10-year-old female, and 11-year-old male all underwent upper extremity amputation while one 12-year-old male did not.
Lascombes P, Prevot J, Ligier JN, et al. Elastic stable intramedullary nailing in forearm shaft fractures in children: 85 cases. *J Pediatr Orthop.* 1990;10:167–171.	This is the classic paper produced by our French colleagues that effectively introduced this technique to the rest of the world. Eighty children with complete forearm shaft fractures (no greenstick fractures) were treated via their technique. 93% were middle-third fractures, 8% were open fractures, and 6% required open reduction. They used distal lateral radial and proximal ulnar "anconeus" entry points (both respectful of adjacent growth areas). Contoured stainless steel and titanium flexible nails (1.5 to 2.5 mm) were implanted. They recommended no postoperative casting and encouragement of immediate motion. Nail removal by 10 to 12 months was recommended. They reported 92% excellent results at an average of 3½-yr follow-up. There was an 8% rate of significant pronation/supination loss (>20 degrees) and a 16% rate of hypesthesia of superficial branch radial nerve.
Matthews LS, Kaufer H, Garver DF, et al. The effect on supination-pronation of angular malalignment of fractures of both bones of the forearm. *J Bone Joint Surg Am.* 1982;64:14–17.	Classic adult cadaver study where they created midshaft forearm malunions with steel fixation plates angulated 10 and 20 degrees. A 10-degree angulation of either single bone resulted in little measureable loss, while 10-degree angulation of both bones led to approximately 20 degrees of motion loss and 20-degree angulation of both bones created motion losses of 40 degrees or more for both pronation and supination.
Murphy HA, Jain VV, Parikh SN, et al. Extensor tendon injury associated with dorsal entry flexible nailing of radial shaft fractures in children: a report of 5 new cases and review of the literature. *J Pediatr Orthop* 2017; Epub ahead of print.	This paper summarizes 33 reported cases of EPL tendon injury and how every single one of them is associated with the so-called dorsal radial entry point.
Price CT, Knapp DR. Osteotomy for malunited forearm shaft fractures in children. *J Pediatr Orthop.* 2006;26:193–196.	This is a 9-patient forearm shaft malunion report that emphasizes a commonsense surgical technique for corrective osteotomy. Rotate the bones under fluoro to find the plane of maximum deformity and then do a closing wedge osteotomy with internal fixation to correct it. Rotation is also accounted for via anatomic landmarks.
Price CT, Scott DS, Kurzner ME, et al. Malunited forearm fractures in children. *J Pediatr Orthop.* 1990;10:705–712.	This is a study of 39 patients with forearm shaft malunions. 56% (22/39) had angular malunion exceeding 10 degrees (range 12 to 20 degrees) and/or rotational malunion (range 45 to 90 degrees). 23% (5/22) of this subgroup lost either pronation or supination ranging from 25 to 60 degrees.
Sardelli M, Tashjian RZ, MacWilliams BA. Functional elbow range of motion for contemporary tasks. *J Bone Joint Surg Am.* 2011;93-A:471–477.	This paper amounts to a sophisticated update (30 years later) to the classic Morrey & Askew paper from 1981 that produced numbers that any orthopedic resident worth their salt can recite: 30/130 and 50/50. It raises the stakes on what we should consider functional range of motion, pushing it as high as 20 to 155 degrees of elbow motion and nearly 75 degrees pronation and 90 degrees supination!!!
Trousdale RT, Linscheid RL. Operative treatment of malunited fractures of the forearm. *J Bone Joint Surg Am.* 1995;77:894–902.	Classic forearm shaft corrective osteotomy series (27 total patients) that is filled with patients whose injuries occurred while they were children)! Nearly 75% were less than 14 years old at the time of their initial injury and about 30% were actually less than 10 years old.
Younger AS, Tredwell SJ, Mackenzie WG, et al. Accurate prediction of outcome after pediatric forearm fracture. *J Pediatr Orthop.* 1994;14:200–206.	150 children (average age 8 years) with both-bone forearm shaft fractures were studied at an average of 4 years following injury. In conjunction with a concept they called axis deviation, they suggested cutoffs of 10 degrees in the midshaft, 12.5 degrees at the junction of middle and distal thirds, and 20 degrees in the distal third.

REFERENCES

1. Abrams RA, Brown RA, Botte MJ. The superficial branch of the radial nerve: an anatomic study with surgical implications. *J Hand Surg Am.* 1992;17:1037–1041.
2. Abrams RA, Ziets RJ, Lieber RL, et al. Anatomy of the radial nerve motor branches in the forearm. *J Hand Surg Am.* 1997;22:232–237.
3. Aktas S, Saridogan K, Moralar U, et al. Patterns of single segment nonphyseal extremity fractures in children. *Int Orthop.* 1999;23:345–347.
4. Allen PE, Vickery CW, Atkins RM. A modified approach to the flexor surface of the distal radius. *J Hand Surg Br.* 1996;21:303–304.
5. Alpar EK, Thompson K, Owen R, et al. Midshaft fractures of forearm bones in children. *Injury.* 1981;13:153–158.
6. al-Qattan MM, Clarke HM, Zimmer P. Radiological signs of entrapment of the median nerve in forearm shaft fractures. *J Hand Surg Br.* 1994;19:713–719.
7. Amit Y, Salai M, Chechik A, et al. Closing intramedullary nailing for the treatment of diaphyseal forearm fractures in adolescence: a preliminary report. *J Pediatr Orthop.* 1985;5:143–146.
8. Aner A, Singer M, Feldbrin Z, et al. Surgical treatment of posttraumatic radioulnar synostosis in children. *J Pediatr Orthop.* 2002;22:598–600.
9. Anonymous. The treatment of forearm fractures with pins. By Georg Schone, 1913. *Clin Orthop Relat Res.* 1988;234:2–4.
10. Anonymous. Fracture and dislocation compendium: Orthopaedic Trauma Association Committee for Coding and Classification. *J Orthop Trauma.* 1996;10:1–153.
11. Archibong AE, Onuba O. Fractures in children in south eastern Nigeria. *Cent Afr J Med.* 1996;42:340–343.
12. Arunachalam VS, Griffiths JC. Fracture recurrence in children. *Injury.* 1975;7:37–40.
13. Auerbach DM, Collins ED, Kunkle KL, et al. The radial sensory nerve: an anatomic study. *Clin Orthop Relat Res.* 1994;308:241–249.
14. Baitner AC, Perry A, LaLonde FD, et al. The healing forearm fracture: a matched comparison of forearm refractures. *J Pediatr Orthop.* 2007;27:743–747.
15. Bär HF, Breitfuss H. Analysis of angular deformities on radiographs. *J Bone Joint Surg Br.* 1989;71:710–711.
16. Bartl V, Gal P, Skotáková J, et al. Treatment of redislocated fragments of long bones using plaster cast wedging. *Rozhl Chir.* 2002;81:415–420.
17. Bass RL, Stern PJ. Elbow and forearm anatomy and surgical approaches. *Hand Clin.* 1994;10:343–356.
18. Bätz W, Hoffmann-v Kap-herr S, Pistor G. Posttraumatic radioulnar synostoses in childhood. *Aktuelle Traumatol.* 1986;16:13–16.
19. Bauchner H, Vinci R, Bak S, et al. Parents and procedures: a randomized controlled trial. *Pediatrics.* 1996;98:861–867.
20. Bauer G, Arand M, Mutschler W. Post-traumatic radioulnar synostosis after forearm fracture osteosynthesis. *Arch Orthop Trauma Surg.* 1991;110(3):142–145.
21. Beckman AW, Sloan BK, Moore GP, et al. Should parents be present during emergency department procedures on children and who should make the decision? A survey of emergency physician and nurse attitudes. *Acad Emerg Med.* 2002;9:154–158.
22. Beekman F, Sullivan JE. Some observations on fractures of long bones in children. *Am J Surg.* 1941;51:722–738.
23. Bellemans M, Lamoureux J. Indications for immediate percutaneous intramedullary nailing of complete diaphyseal forearm shaft fractures in children. *Acta Orthop Belg.* 1995;61(Suppl I):169–172.
24. Bhaskar AR, Roberts JA. Treatment of unstable fractures of the forearm in children: is plating of a single bone adequate? *J Bone Joint Surg Br.* 2001;83:253–258.
25. Biyani A, Gupta SP, Sharma JC. Ipsilateral supracondylar fractures of the humerus and forearm bone in children. *Injury.* 1989;20:203–207.
26. Black GB, Amadeo R. Orthopedic injuries associated with backyard trampoline use in children. *Can J Surg.* 2003;46:199–201.
27. Blackburn N, Ziv I, Rang M. Correction of the malunited forearm fracture. *Clin Orthop Relat Res.* 1984;188:54–57.
28. Blaisier RD, Salamon PB. Closed intramedullary rodding of pediatric adolescent forearm fractures. *Oper Tech Orthop.* 1993;3:128–133.
29. Blakemore LC, Cooperman DR, Thompson GH, et al. Compartment syndrome in ipsilateral humerus and forearm fractures in children. *Clin Orthop Relat Res.* 2000;376:32–38.
30. Blount WP. Osteoclasis for supination deformities in children. *J Bone Joint Surg.* 1940;22:300–314.
31. Blount WP. Forearm fractures in children. *Clin Orthop Relat Res.* 1967;51:93–107.
32. Blount WP, Schaefer AA, Johnson JH. Fractures of the forearm in children. *JAMA.* 1942;120:111–116.
33. Boie ET, Moore GP, Brummett C, et al. Do parents want to be present during invasive procedures performed on their children in the emergency department? A survey of 400 parents. *Ann Emerg Med.* 1999;34:70–74.
34. Boone DC, Azen SP. Normal range of motion of joints in male subjects. *J Bone Joint Surg Am.* 1979;61:756–759.
35. Borden S. Traumatic bowing of the forearm in children. *J Bone Joint Surg Am.* 1974;56:611–616.
36. Bot AG, Doornberg JN, Lindenhovius AL, et al. Long-term outcomes of fractures of both bones of the forearm. *J Bone Joint Surg Am.* 2011;93(6):527–532.
37. Boudreaux ED, Francis JL, Loyacano T. Family presence during invasive procedures and resuscitations in the emergency department: a critical review and suggestions for future research. *Ann Emerg Med.* 2002;40:193–205.
38. Bould M, Bannister GC. Refractures of the radius and ulna in children. *Injury.* 1999;30:583–586.
39. Bowman EN, Mehlman CT, Lindsell CJ, et al. Nonoperative treatment of both-bone forearm shaft fractures in children: Predictors of early radiographic failure. *J Pediatr Orthop.* 2011;31:23–32.
40. Boyer BA, Overton B, Schraeder W, et al. Position of immobilization for pediatric forearm fractures. *J Pediatr Orthop.* 2002;22:185–187.
41. Branovacki G, Hanson M, Cash R, et al. The innervation of the radial nerve at the elbow and in the forearm. *J Hand Surg Br.* 1998;23:167–169.
42. Bratt HD, Eyres RL, Cole WG. Randomized double-blind trial of low-and moderate-dose lidocaine regional anesthesia for forearm fractures in childhood. *J Pediatr Orthop.* 1996;16:660–663.
43. Brown RL, Koepplinger ME, Mehlman CT, et al. All-terrain vehicle and bicycle crashes in children: epidemiology and comparison of injury severity. *J Pediatr Surg.* 2002;37:375–380.
44. Calder PR, Achan P, Barry M. Diaphyseal forearm fractures in children treated with intramedullary fixation: outcome of K-wires versus elastic stable intramedullary nail. *Injury.* 2003;34:278–282.
45. Cameron ML, Sponseller PD, Rossberg MI. Pediatric analgesia and sedation for the management of orthopedic conditions. *Am J Orthop.* 2000;29:665–672.
46. Campbell WC. *Orthopedics of Childhood.* New York: Appleton and Company; 1930:154–156.
47. Campbell WC. *Campbell's Operative Orthopaedics.* 1st ed. St. Louis, MO: The CV Mosby Company; 1939.
48. Carey PJ, Alburger PD, Betz RR, et al. Both-bone forearm fractures in children. *Orthopedics.* 1992;15:1015–1019.
49. Carsi B, Abril JC, Epeldegui T. Longitudinal growth after nonphyseal forearm fractures. *J Pediatr Orthop.* 2003;23:203–207.
50. Carter DR, Spengler DM. Mechanical properties and composition of cortical bone. *Clin Orthop Relat Res.* 1978;135:192–217.
51. Casey PJ, Moed BR. Greenstick fractures of the radius in adults: a report of two cases. *J Orthop Trauma.* 1996;10:209–212.
52. Celebi L, Muratli HH, Dogan O, et al. The results of intramedullary nailing in children who developed redisplacement during cast treatment of both-bone forearm fractures. *Acta Orthop Traumatol Turc.* 2007;41:175–182.
53. Ceroni D, Martin X, Delhumeau-Cartier C, et al. Is bone mineral mass truly decreased in teenagers with a first episode of forearm fracture? A prospective longitudinal study. *J Pediatr Orthop.* 2012;32:579–586.
54. Chamay A. Mechanical and morphological aspects of experimental overload and fatigue in bone. *J Biomech.* 1970;3:263–270.
55. Chan CF, Meads BM, Nicol RO. Remanipulation of forearm fractures in children. *N Z Med J.* 1997;110:249–250.
56. Chantelot C, Feugas C, Guillem P, et al. Innervation of the medial epicondylar muscles: an anatomic study in 50 cases. *Surg Radiol Anat.* 1999;21:165–168.
57. Chapman MW, Gordon JE, Zissimos AG. Compression-plate fixation of acute fractures of the diaphysis of the radius and ulna. *J Bone Joint Surg Am.* 1989;71:159–169.
58. Charnley J. *The Closed Treatment of Common Fractures.* Edinburgh: Livingstone; 1957.
59. Cheng JC, Ng BK, Ying SY, et al. A 10-year study of the changes in the pattern and treatment of 6,493 fractures. *J Pediatr Orthop.* 1999;19:344–350.
60. Chess DG, Hyndman JC, Leahey JL, et al. Short arm plaster cast for distal pediatric forearm fractures. *J Pediatr Orthop.* 1994;14:211–213.
61. Chung KC, Spilson SV. The frequency and epidemiology of hand and forearm fractures in the United States. *J Hand Surg Am.* 2001;26:908–915.
62. Cleary JE, Omer GE Jr. Congenital proximal radio-ulnar synostosis: natural history and functional assessment. *J Bone Joint Surg Am.* 1985;67:539–545.
63. Committee on Drugs, American Academy of Pediatrics. Guidelines for monitoring and management of pediatric patients during and after sedation for diagnostic and therapeutic procedures. *Pediatrics.* 2002;110(4):836–838.
64. Crawford AH. Pitfalls and complications of fractures of the distal radius and ulna in childhood. *Hand Clin.* 1988;4:403–413.
65. Crawford AH. Orthopedic injury in children. In: Callaham ML, ed. *Current Practice of Emergency Medicine.* 2nd ed. Philadelphia, PA: BC Decker; 1991:1232–1233.
66. Crawford AH. Orthopedics. In: Rudolph CD, Rudolph AM, Hostetter MK, et al., eds. *Rudolph's Pediatrics.* 21st ed. New York: McGraw-Hill; 2002:2451.
67. Crawford AH Jr, Bagamery N. Osseous manifestations of neurofibromatosis in childhood. *J Pediatr Orthop.* 1986;6:672–688.
68. Crawford AH, Cionni AS. Management of pediatric orthopedic injuries by the emergency medicine specialist. In: *Pediatric Critical Illness and Injury: Assessment and Care.* Rockville, MD: Aspen System Publications; 1984:213–225.
69. Crawford AH, Schorry EK. Neurofibromatosis in children: the role of the orthopaedist. *J Am Acad Orthop Surg.* 1999;7:217–230.
70. Creasman C, Zaleske DJ, Ehrlich MG. Analyzing forearm fractures in children. The more subtle signs of impending problems. *Clin Orthop Relat Res.* 1984;188:40–53.
71. Crenshaw AH Jr. Surgical approaches. In: Canale ST, ed. *Campbell's Operative Orthopaedics.* 10th ed. St. Louis, MO: CV Mosby; 2003:107–109.
72. Cullen MC, Roy DR, Giza E, et al. Complications of intramedullary fixation of pediatric forearm fractures. *J Pediatr Orthop.* 1998;18:14–21.
73. Curry JD, Butler G. The mechanical properties of bone tissue in children. *J Bone Joint Surg Am.* 1975;57:810–814.
74. Daruwalla JS. A study of radioulnar movements following fractures of the forearm in children. *Clin Orthop Relat Res.* 1979;139:114–120.
75. Davids JR, Frick SL, Skewes E, et al. Skin surface pressure beneath an above-the-knee cast: plaster casts compared with fiberglass casts. *J Bone Joint Surg Am.* 1997;79:565–569.
76. Davidson AW. Rock, paper, scissors. *Injury.* 2003;34:61–63.
77. Davidson AJ, Eyres RL, Cole WG. A comparison of prilocaine and lidocaine for intravenous regional anaesthesia for forearm fracture reduction in children. *Paediatr Anaesth.* 2002;12:146–150.
78. Davis DR, Green DP. Forearm fractures in children: pitfalls and complications. *Clin Orthop Relat Res.* 1976;120:172–183.
79. de Pablos J, Franzreb M, Barrios C. Longitudinal growth pattern of the radius after forearm fractures conservatively treated in children. *J Pediatr Orthop.* 1994;14:492–495.
80. DeFrate LE, Li G, Zayontz SJ, et al. A minimally invasive method for the determination of force in the interosseous ligament. *Clin Biomech.* 2001;16:895–900.

81. Deluca PA, Lindsey RW, Ruwe PA. Refracture of bones of the forearm after the removal of compression plates. *J Bone Joint Surg Am*. 1988;70:1372–1376.
82. Dilberti T, Botte MJ, Abrams RA. Anatomical considerations regarding the posterior interosseous nerve during posterolateral approaches to the proximal part of the radius. *J Bone Joint Surg Am*. 2000;82:809–813.
83. Do T. Forearm. In: Cramer KE, Scherl SA, eds. *Orthopaedic Surgery Essentials*. Philadelphia, PA: Lippincott Williams & Wilkins; 2004:125–130.
84. Do TT, Strub WM, Foad SL, et al. Reduction versus remodeling in pediatric distal forearm fractures: a preliminary cost analysis. *J Pediatr Orthop B*. 2003;12:109–115.
85. Doyle JR, Botte MJ. *Surgical Anatomy of the Hand & Upper Extremity*. Philadelphia, PA: Lippincott Williams & Wilkins; 2003:34–40.
86. Droll KP, Perna P, Potter J, et al. Outcomes following plate fixation of fractures of both bones of the forearm in adults. *J Bone Joint Surg Am*. 2007;89(12):2619–2624.
87. Dumont CE, Thalmann R, Macy JC. The effect of rotational malunion of the radius and ulna on supination and pronation. *J Bone Joint Surg Br*. 2002;84:1070–1074.
88. Duncan J, Weiner D. Unstable pediatric forearm fractures: use of "pins and plaster." *Orthopedics*. 2004;27:267–269.
89. Elgafy H, Ebraheim NA, Yeasting RA. Extensile posterior approach to the radius. *Clin Orthop Relat Res*. 2000;373:252–258.
90. Esposito PW. Trampoline injuries. *Clin Orthop Relat Res*. 2003;409:43–52.
91. Evans EM. Rotational deformity in the treatment of fractures of both bones of the forearm. *J Bone Joint Surg*. 1945;27:373–379.
92. Evans EM. Pronation injuries of the forearm with special reference to the anterior Monteggia fracture. *J Bone Joint Surg Br*. 1949;31:578–588.
93. Evans EM. Fractures of the radius and ulna. *J Bone Joint Surg Br*. 1951;33:548–561.
94. Evans JK, Buckley SL, Alexander AH, et al. Analgesia for the reduction of fractures in children: a comparison of nitrous oxide with intramuscular sedation. *J Pediatr Orthop*. 1995;15:73–77.
95. Fee NF, Dobranski A, Bisla RS. Gas gangrene complicating open forearm fractures. Report of five cases. *J Bone Joint Surg Am*. 1977;59:135–138.
96. Fernandez FF, Egenolf M, Carsten C, et al. Unstable diaphyseal fractures of both bones of the forearm in children: plate versus intramedullary nailing. *Injury*. 2005;36:1210–1216.
97. Fiala M, Carey TP. Paediatric forearm fractures: an analysis of refracture rate. *Orthop Trans*. 1994–1995;18:1265–1266.
98. Fike EA, Bartal E. Delayed union of the distal ulna in a child after both-bone forearm fracture. *J South Orthop Assoc*. 1998;7:113–116.
99. Firl M, Wünsch L. Measurement of bowing of the radius. *J Bone Joint Surg Br*. 2004;86:1047–1049.
100. Fleischer H. Marrow wiring in lower-arm fractures of children. *Dtsch Med Wochenschr*. 1975;100:1278–1279.
101. Floyd AS. Is the measurement of angles on radiographs accurate? Brief report. *J Bone Joint Surg Br*. 1988;70:486–487.
102. Flynn JM. Pediatric forearm fractures: decision making, surgical techniques, and complications. *Instr Course Lect*. 2002;51:355–360.
103. Flynn JM, Jones KJ, Garner MR, et al. Eleven years experience in the operative management of pediatric forearm fractures. *J Pediatr Orthop*. 2010;30:313–319.
104. Flynn JM, Sarwark JF, Waters PM, et al. The surgical management of pediatric fractures of the upper extremity. *Instr Course Lect*. 2003;52:635–645.
105. Flynn JM, Waters PM. Single-bone fixation of both-bone forearm fractures. *J Pediatr Orthop*. 1996;16:655–659.
106. Franklin CC, Robinson J, Noonan K, et al. Evidence-based medicine: management of pediatric forearm fractures. *J Pediatr Orthop*. 2012;32(Suppl 2):S131–S134.
107. Furia JP, Alioto RJ, Marquardt JD. The efficacy and safety of the hematoma block for fracture reduction in closed isolated fractures. *Orthopedics*. 1997;20:423–426.
108. Furnival RA, Street KA, Schunk JE. Too many pediatric trampoline injuries. *Pediatrics*. 1999;103:e57.
109. Gabriel MT, Pfaeffle HJ, Stabile KJ, et al. Passive strain distribution in the interosseous ligament of the forearm: implications for injury reconstruction. *J Hand Surg Am*. 2004;29:293–298.
110. Gafni RI, Baron J. Overdiagnosis of osteoporosis in children due to misinterpretation of dual-energy x-ray absorptiometry (DEXA). *J Pediatr*. 2004;144:253–257.
111. Gainor BJ, Olson S. Combined entrapment of the median and anterior interosseous nerves in a pediatric both-bone forearm fracture. *J Orthop Trauma*. 1990;4:197–199.
112. Galpin RD, Webb GR, Armstrong DG, et al. A comparison of short and long-arm plaster casts for displaced distal-third pediatric forearm fractures: a prospective randomized trial. Paper presented at: Annual Meeting of the Pediatric Orthopaedic Society of North America; April 27–May 1, 2004; St. Louis, MO.
113. Gandhi RK, Wilson P, Mason Brown JJ, et al. Spontaneous correction of deformity following fractures of the forearm in children. *Br J Surg*. 1962;50:5–10.
114. Garcia VF, Langford L, Inge TI. Application of laparoscopy for bariatric surgery. *Curr Opin Pediatr*. 2003;15:248–255.
115. Garg NK, Ballal MS, Malek IA, et al. Use of elastic stable intramedullary nailing for treating unstable forearm fractures in children. *J Trauma*. 2008;65:109–115.
116. Gartland JJ. *Fundamentals of Orthopaedics*. 4th ed. Philadelphia, PA: WB Saunders; 1987:34.
117. Geissler WB, Fernandez DL, Graca R. Anterior interosseous nerve palsy complicating a forearm fracture in a child. *J Hand Surg Am*. 1990;15:44–47.
118. Genelin F, Karlbauer AF, Gasperschitz F. Greenstick fracture of the forearm with median nerve entrapment. *J Emerg Med*. 1988;6:381–385.
119. Giebel GD, Meyer C, Koebke J, et al. Arterial supply of forearm bones and its importance for the operative treatment of fractures. *Surg Radiol Anat*. 1997;19:149–153.
120. Godambe SA, Elliot V, Matheny D, et al. Comparison of propofol/fentanyl versus ketamine/midazolam for brief procedural sedation in a pediatric emergency department. *Pediatrics*. 2003;112:116–123.
121. Godfrey J, Choi PD, Shabtai L, et al. Management of pediatric type 1 open fractures in the emergency department or operating room: a multicenter perspective. *J Pediatr Orthop*. 2017. doi: 10.1097/BPO.0000000000000972
122. Gonzalez MH, Lotfi P, Bendre A, et al. The ulnar nerve at the elbow and its local branching: an anatomic study. *J Hand Surg Br*. 2001;26:142–144.
123. Goulding A, Cannan R, Williams SM, et al. Bone mineral density in girls with forearm fractures. *J Bone Miner Res*. 1998;13:143–148.
124. Goulding A, Jones IE, Taylor RW, et al. More broken bones: a 4-year double cohort study of young girls with and without distal forearm fractures. *J Bone Miner Res*. 2000;15:2011–2018.
125. Goulding A, Jones IE, Taylor RW, et al. Bone mineral density and body composition in boys with distal forearm fractures: a dual-energy x-ray absorptiometry study. *J Pediatr*. 2001;139:509–515.
126. Goulding A, Rockell JE, Black RE, et al. Children who avoid drinking cow's milk are at increased risk for prepubertal bone fractures. *J Am Diet Assoc*. 2004;104:250–253.
127. Gray H. *Gray's Anatomy: The Classic Collector's Edition*. New York: Bounty; 1977: 152–157.
128. Greenbaum B, Zionts LE, Ebramzadeh E. Open fractures of the forearm in children. *J Orthop Trauma*. 2001;15:111–118.
129. Gregory PR, Sullivan JA. Nitrous oxide compared with intravenous regional anesthesia in pediatric forearm fracture manipulation. *J Pediatr Orthop*. 1996;16:187–191.
130. Greiwe RM, Mehlman CT, Moon E, et al. Stiffness following displaced pediatric both-bone forearm fractures: a meta-analysis. Paper presented at: Annual Meeting of the Orthopaedic Trauma Association; October 5–7, 2006; Phoenix, AZ.
131. Griffet J, el Hayek T, Baby M. Intramedullary nailing of forearm fractures in children. *J Pediatr Orthop B*. 1999;8:88–89.
132. Griffin PP. Forearm fractures in children. *Clin Orthop Relat Res*. 1977;129:320–321.
133. Gupta RP, Danielsson LG. Dorsally angulated solitary metaphyseal greenstick fractures in the distal radius: results after immobilization in pronated, neutral, and supinated position. *J Pediatr Orthop*. 1990;10:90–92.
134. Gustilo RB, Anderson JT. Prevention of infection in the treatment of 1025 open fractures of long bones: retrospective and prospective analyses. *J Bone Joint Surg Am*. 1976;58:453–458.
135. Haasbeek JF, Cole WG. Open fractures of the arm in children. *J Bone Joint Surg Br*. 1995;77:576–581.
136. Hahn MP, Richter D, Muhr G, et al. Pediatric forearm fractures: diagnosis, therapy, and possible complications. *Unfallchirurg*. 1997;100:760–769.
137. Haimi-Cohen Y, Amir J, Harel L, et al. Parental presence during lumbar puncture: anxiety and attitude toward the procedure. *Clin Pediatr (Phila)*. 1996;35:2–4.
138. Harrington P, Sharif I, Fogarty EE, et al. Management of the floating elbow injury in children. *Arch Orthop Trauma Surg*. 2000;120:205–208.
139. Helenius I, Lamberg TS, Kääriäinen S, et al. Operative treatment of fractures in children is increasing: a population-based study from Finland. *J Bone Joint Surg Am*. 2009;91:2612–2616.
140. Hendel D, Aner A. Entrapment of the flexor digitorum profundus of the ring finger at the site of an ulnar fracture: a case report. *Ital J Orthop Traumatol*. 1992;18:417–419.
141. Hennrikus WL, Shin AY, Klingelberger CE. Self-administered nitrous oxide and a hematoma block for analgesia in the outpatient reduction of fractures in children. *J Bone Joint Surg Am*. 1995;77:335–339.
142. Henry AK. *Extensile Exposure*. 2nd ed. Edinburgh: Churchill Livingstone; 1966: 107–108.
143. Hoffman GM, Nowakowski R, Troshynski TJ, et al. Risk reduction in pediatric procedural sedation by application of an American Academy of Pediatrics/American Society of Anesthesiologists process model. *Pediatrics*. 2002;109:236–243.
144. Högström H, Nilsson BE, Willner S. Correction with growth following diaphyseal forearm fracture. *Acta Orthop Scand*. 1976;47:299–303.
145. Holdsworth BJ, Sloan JP. Proximal forearm fractures in children: residual disability. *Injury*. 1982;14:174–179.
146. Hollister AM, Gellman H, Waters RL. The relationship of the interosseous membrane to the axis of rotation of the forearm. *Clin Orthop Relat Res*. 1994;298:272–276.
147. Holmes JR, Louis DS. Entrapment of pronator quadratus in pediatric distal radius fractures: recognition and treatment. *J Pediatr Orthop*. 1994;14:498–500.
148. Hoppenfeld S, deBoer P. *Surgical Exposures in Orthopaedics*. 3rd ed. Philadelphia, PA: Lippincott Williams & Wilkins; 2003.
149. Hoppenfeld S, Zeide MS. *Orthopaedic Dictionary*. Philadelphia, PA: JB Lippincott; 1994:275.
150. Hotchkiss RN, An KN, Sowa DT, et al. An anatomic and mechanical study of the interosseous membrane of the forearm: pathomechanics of proximal migration of the radius. *J Hand Surg Am*. 1989;14:256–261.
151. Hsu ES, Patwardhan AG, Meade KP, et al. Cross-sectional geometrical properties and bone mineral content of the human radius and ulna. *J Biomech*. 1993;26:1307–1318.
152. Huang K, Pun WK, Coleman S. Entrapment and transection of the median nerve associated with greenstick fractures of the forearm: a case report and review of the literature. *J Trauma*. 1998;44:1101–1102.
153. Hughston JC. Fractures of the forearm in children. *J Bone Joint Surg Am*. 1962;44: 1678–1693.
154. Inge TH, Krebs NF, Garcia VF, et al. Bariatric surgery for severely overweight adolescents: concerns and recommendations. *Pediatrics*. 2004;114:217–223.
155. Jacobsen FS. Periosteum: its relation to pediatric fractures. *J Pediatr Orthop B*. 1997;6:84–90.
156. Jacobsen FS, Crawford AH. Complications in neurofibromatosis. In: Epps CH, Bowen JR, eds. *Complications in Pediatric Orthopaedic Surgery*. Philadelphia, PA: JB Lippincott; 1995:678–680.
157. Jacobsen ST, Hull CK, Crawford AH. Nutritional rickets. *J Pediatr Orthop*. 1986;6: 713–716.
158. Johari AN, Sinha M. Remodeling of forearm fractures in children. *J Pediatr Orthop B*. 1999;8:84–87.
159. Johnson CW, Carmichael KD, Morris RP, et al. Biomechanical study of flexible intramedullary nails. *J Pediatr Orthop*. 2009;29:44–48.
160. Johnson PQ, Noffsinger MA. Hematoma block of distal forearm fractures: is it safe? *Orthop Rev*. 1991;20:977–979.

161. Jones IE, Williams SM, Goulding A. Associations of birth weight and length, childhood size, and smoking with bone fractures during growth: evidence from a birth cohort study. *Am J Epidemiol*. 2004;159:343–350.
162. Jones K, Weiner DS. The management of forearm fractures in children: a plea for conservatism. *J Pediatr Orthop*. 1999;19:811–815.
163. Jubel A, Andermahr J, Isenberg J, et al. Outcomes and complications of elastic stable intramedullary nailing of forearm fractures in children. *J Pediatr Orthop B*. 2005;14:375–380.
164. Juliano PJ, Mazur JM, Cummings RJ, et al. Low-dose lidocaine intravenous regional anesthesia for forearm fractures in children. *J Pediatr Orthop*. 1992;12:633–635.
165. Kain ZN, Mayes LC, Caramico LA, et al. Parental presence during induction of anesthesia: a randomized controlled trial. *Anesthesiology*. 1996;84:1060–1067.
166. Kang SN, Mangwani J, Ramachandran M, et al. Elastic intramedullary nailing of paediatric fractures of the forearm: a decade of experience in a teaching hospital in the United Kingdom. *J Bone Joint Surg Br*. 2011;93(2):262–265.
167. Kasser JR. Forearm fractures. *Instr Course Lect*. 1992;41:391–396.
168. Kasten P, Krefft M, Hesselbach J, et al. Computer simulation of forearm rotation in angular deformities: a new therapeutic approach. *Injury*. 2002;33:807–813.
169. Kasten P, Krefft M, Hesselbach J, et al. How does torsional deformity of the radial shaft influence the rotation of the forearm? A biomechanical study. *J Orthop Trauma*. 2003;17:57–60.
170. Kay S, Smith C, Oppenheim WL. Both-bone midshaft forearm fractures in children. *J Pediatr Orthop*. 1986;6:306–310.
171. Keenan WNW, Clegg J. Intraoperative wedging of casts: correction of residual angulation after manipulation. *J Pediatr Orthop*. 1995;15:826–829.
172. Kelly AM, Powell CV, Williams A. Parent visual analogue scale ratings of children's pain do not reliably reflect pain reported by child. *Pediatr Emerg Care*. 2002;18: 159–162.
173. Kelly JP, Zionts LE. Economic considerations in the treatment of distal forearm fractures in children. Paper presented at: Annual Meeting of the American Academy of Orthopaedic Surgeons; February 28–March 4, 2001; San Francisco, CA.
174. Kemper KJ, Sarah R, Silver-Highfield E, et al. On pins and needles? Pediatric pain patients' experience with acupuncture. *Pediatrics*. 2000;105:941–947.
175. Kennedy RM, Porter FL, Miller JP, et al. Comparison of fentanyl/midazolam with ketamine/midazolam for pediatric orthopedic emergencies. *Pediatrics*. 1998;102: 956–963.
176. Kettunen J, Kroger H, Bowditch M, et al. Bone mineral density after removal of rigid plates from forearm fractures: preliminary report. *J Orthop Sci*. 2003;8: 772–776.
177. Khosla S, Melton LJ III, Dekutoski MB, et al. Incidence of childhood distal forearm fractures over 30 years: a population-based study. *JAMA*. 2003;290:1479–1485.
178. Kienitz R, Mandell R. Traumatic bowing of the forearm in children: report of a case. *J Am Osteopath Assoc*. 1985;85:565–568.
179. Kinder KL, Lehman-Huskamp KL, Gerard JM. Do children with high body mass indices have a higher incidence of emesis when undergoing ketamine sedation? *Pediatr Emerg Care*. 2012;28:1203–1205.
180. Kolkman KA, Von Niekerk JL, Rieu PN, et al. A complicated forearm greenstick fracture: case report. *J Trauma*. 1992;32:116–117.
181. Koo WW, Sherman R, Succop P, et al. Fractures and rickets in very low-birth-weight infants: conservative management and outcome. *J Pediatr Orthop*. 1989;9: 326–330.
182. Kramhøft M, Solgaard S. Displaced diaphyseal forearm fractures in children: classification and evaluation of the early radiographic prognosis. *J Pediatr Orthop*. 1989;9:586–589.
183. Kravel T, Sher-Lurie N, Ganel A. Extensor pollicis longus rupture after fixation of radius and ulna fracture with titanium elastic nail (TEN) in a child: a case report. *J Trauma*. 2007;63:1169–1170.
184. Kruppa C, Bunge P, Schildhauer TA, et al. Low complication rate of elastic stable intramedullary nailing (ESIN) of pediatric forearm fractures: a retrospective study of 202 cases. *Medicine*. 2017;96(16):e6669.
185. Kucukkaya M, Kabukcuoglu Y, Tezer M, et al. The application of open intramedullary fixation in the treatment of pediatric radial and ulnar shaft fractures. *J Orthop Trauma*. 2002;16:340–344.
186. Landin LA. Epidemiology of children's fractures. *J Pediatr Orthop B*. 1997;6:79–83.
187. Larsen E, Vittas D, Torp-Pedersen S. Remodeling of angulated distal forearm fractures in children. *Clin Orthop Relat Res*. 1988;237:190–195.
188. Larson BJ, Davis JW. Trampoline-related injuries. *J Bone Joint Surg Am*. 1995;77: 1174–1178.
189. Lascombes P, Prevot J, Ligier JN, et al. Elastic stable intramedullary nailing in forearm shaft fractures in children: 85 cases. *J Pediatr Orthop*. 1990;10:167–171.
190. Lautman S, Bergerault F, Saidani N, et al. Roentgenographic measurement of angle between shaft and distal epiphyseal growth plate of radius. *J Pediatr Orthop*. 2002;22:751–753.
191. Lavelle DG. Delayed union and nonunion of fractures. In: Canale ST, ed. *Campbell's Operative Orthopaedics*. 10th ed. St. Louis, MO: Mosby; 2003:3125–3127.
192. Lee S, Nicol RO, Stott NS. Intramedullary fixation for pediatric unstable forearm fractures. *Clin Orthop Relat Res*. 2002;402:245–250.
193. Lee BH, Scharff L, Sethna NF, et al. Physical therapy and cognitive-behavioral treatment for complex regional pain syndromes. *J Pediatr*. 2002;141:135–140.
194. Lewallen RP, Peterson HA. Nonunion of long bone fractures in children: a review of 30 cases. *J Pediatr Orthop*. 1985;5:135–142.
195. Ligier JN, Metaizeau JP, Prévot J, et al. Elastic stable intramedullary pinning of long bone shaft fractures in children. *Z Kinderchir*. 1985;40:209–212.
196. Lim YJ, Lam KS, Lee EH. Open Gustilo 1 and 2 midshaft fractures of the radius and ulna in children: is there a role for cast immobilization after wound debridement? *J Pediatr Orthop*. 2007;27:540–546.
197. Litton LO, Adler F. Refracture of the forearm in children: a frequent complication. *J Trauma*. 1963;3:41–51.
198. Luhmann SJ, Gordon JE, Schoenecker PL. Intramedullary fixation of unstable both-bone forearm fractures in children. *J Pediatr Orthop*. 1998;18:451–456.
199. Luhmann SJ, Schootman M, Schoenecker PL, et al. Complications and outcomes of open pediatric forearm fractures. *J Pediatr Orthop*. 2004;24:1–6.
200. Ma D, Jones G. Television, computer, and video viewing; physical activity; and upper limb fracture risk in children: a population-based case control study. *J Bone Miner Res*. 2003;18:1970–1977.
201. Ma D, Morley R, Jones G. Risk-taking coordination and upper limb fractures in children: population-based case-control study. *Osteoporos Int*. 2004;15:633–638.
202. Mabrey JD, Fitch RD. Plastic deformation in pediatric fractures: mechanism and treatment. *J Pediatr Orthop*. 1989;9:310–314.
203. Maempel FZ. Posttraumatic radioulnar synostosis. A report of two cases. *Clin Orthop Relat Res*. 1984;186:182–185.
204. Mann DC, Rajmaira S. Distribution of physeal and nonphyseal fractures in 2650 long-bone fractures in children aged 0 to 16 years. *J Pediatr Orthop*. 1990;10:713–716.
205. Mann DC, Schnabel M, Baacke M, et al. Results of elastic stable intramedullary nailing (ESIN) in forearm fractures in childhood. *Unfallchirurg*. 2003;106:102–109.
206. Manske PR. Forearm pseudarthrosis-neurofibromatosis: case report. *Clin Orthop Relat Res*. 1979;139:125–127.
207. Manson TT, Pfaeffle HJ, Herdon JH, et al. Forearm rotation alters interosseous ligament strain distribution. *J Hand Surg Am*. 2000;25:1058–1063.
208. Markolf KL, Lamey D, Yang S, et al. Radioulnar load-sharing in the forearm: a study in cadavers. *J Bone Joint Surg Am*. 1998;80:879–888.
209. Martin J, Marsh JL, Nepola JV, et al. Radiographic fracture assessments: which ones can we reliably make? *J Orthop Trauma*. 2000;14:379–385.
210. Martus JE, Preston RK, Schoenecker JG, et al. Complications and outcomes of diaphyseal forearm fracture intramedullary nailing: a comparison of pediatric and adolescent age groups. *J Pediatr Orthop*. 2013;33:598–607.
211. Matthews LS, Kaufer H, Garver DF, et al. The effect on supination-pronation of angular malalignment of fractures of both bones of the forearm. *J Bone Joint Surg Am*. 1982;64:14–17.
212. McGinley JC, Hopgood BC, Gaughan JP, et al. Forearm and elbow injury: the influence of rotational position. *J Bone Joint Surg Am*. 2003;85:2403–2409.
213. McGinley JC, Kozin SH. Interosseous membrane anatomy and functional mechanics. *Clin Orthop Relat Res*. 2001;383:108–122.
214. McHenry TP, Pierce WA, Lais RL, et al. Effect of displacement of ulna-shaft fractures on forearm rotation: a cadaveric model. *Am J Orthop*. 2002;31:420–424.
215. Mehlman CT. Clinical epidemiology. In: Koval KJ, ed. *Orthopaedic Knowledge Update*. 7th ed. Rosemont, IL: AAOS; 2002:82.
216. Mehlman CT. Forearm, wrist, and hand trauma: pediatrics. In: Fischgrund JS, ed. *Orthopaedic Knowledge Update 9*. Rosemont, IL: American Academy of Orthopaedic Surgeons; 2008:669–680.
217. Mehlman CT, Crawford AH, Roy DR, et al. Undisplaced fractures of the distal radius and ulna in children: risk factors for displacement. Paper presented at: Annual Meeting of the American Academy of Orthopaedic Surgeons; February 13–17, 2001; Dallas, TX.
218. Mehlman CT, O'Brien MS, Crawford AH, et al. Irreducible fractures of the distal radius in children. Paper presented at: Annual Meeting of Pediatric Orthopaedic Society of North America; May 1, 2001; Cancun.
219. Meier R, Prommersberger KJ, Lanz U. Surgical correction of malunited fractures of the forearm in children. *Z Orthop Ihre Grenzgeb*. 2003;141:328–335.
220. Mekhail AO, Ebraheim NA, Jackson WT, et al. Vulnerability of the posterior interosseous nerve during proximal radius exposures. *Clin Orthop Relat Res*. 1995;315:199–208.
221. Metaizeau JP, Ligier JN. Surgical treatment of fractures of the long bones in children. Interference between osteosynthesis and the physiological processes of consolidation. Therapeutic indications. *J Chir (Paris)*. 1984;121:527–537.
222. Mitts KG, Hennrikus WL. In-line skating fractures in children. *J Pediatr Orthop*. 1996;16:640–643.
223. Morrey BF, Askew LJ, Chao EY. A biomechanical study of normal functional elbow motion. *J Bone Joint Surg Am*. 1981;63:872–877.
224. Moseley CF. Obituary: Mercer Rang, FRCSC (1933–2003). *J Pediatr Orthop*. 2004;24:446–447.
225. Mubarak SJ, Carroll NC. Volkmann's contracture in children: aetiology and prevention. *J Bone Joint Surg Br*. 1979;61:285–293.
226. Muensterer OJ, Regauer MP. Closed reduction of forearm refractures with flexible intramedullary nails in situ. *J Bone Joint Surg Am*. 2003;85:2152–2155.
227. Müller ME, Allgöwer M, Schneider R, et al. *Manual of Internal Fixation: Techniques Recommended by the AO-ASIF Group*. 3rd ed. Berlin: Springer-Verlag; 1991:454–467.
228. Murray WM, Delp SL, Buchanan TS. Variation of muscle moment arms with elbow and forearm position. *J Biomech*. 1995;28:513–525.
229. Myers GJ, Gibbons PJ, Glithero PR. Nancy nailing of diaphyseal forearm fractures: single bone fixation for fractures of both bones. *J Bone Joint Surg Br*. 2004;86:581–584.
230. Nakamura T, Yabe Y, Horiuchi Y. In vivo MR studies of dynamic changes in the interosseous membrane of the forearm during rotation. *J Hand Surg Br*. 1999;24:245–248.
231. Nielson AB, Simonsen O. Displaced forearm fractures in children treated with AO plates. *Injury*. 1984;15:393–396.
232. Nieman R, Maiocco B, Deeney VF. Ulnar nerve injury after closed forearm fractures in children. *J Pediatr Orthop*. 1998;18:683–685.
233. Nilsson BE, Obrant K. The range of motion following fracture of the shaft of the forearm in children. *Acta Orthop Scand*. 1977;48:600–602.
234. Noonan KJ, Price CT. Forearm and distal radius fractures in children. *J Am Acad Orthop Surg*. 1998;6:146–156.
235. Ogden JA. *Skeletal Injury in the Child*. Philadelphia, PA: Lea & Febiger; 1982:56–57.
236. Ogden JA. Uniqueness of growing bones. In: Rockwood CA, Wilkins KE, King RE, eds. *Fractures in Children*. Philadelphia, PA: JB Lippincott; 1991:10–14.
237. Ogonda L, Wong-Chung J, Wray R, et al. Delayed union and nonunion of the ulna following intramedullary nailing in children. *J Pediatr Orthop B*. 2004;13:330–333.

238. Og˘ün TC, Sarlak A, Arazi M, et al. Posttraumatic distal radioulnar synostosis and distal radial epiphyseal arrest. *Ulus Travma Derg*. 2002;8:59–61.
239. OlaOlorun DA, Oladiran IO, Adeniran A. Complications of fracture treatment by traditional bonesetters in southwest Nigeria. *Fam Pract*. 2001;18:635–637.
240. O'Neil DF. Wrist injuries in guarded versus unguarded first-time snowboarders. *Clin Orthop Relat Res*. 2003;409:91–95.
241. Ono M, Bechtold JE, Merkow RL, et al. Rotational stability of diaphyseal fractures of the radius and ulna fixed with Rush pins and/or fracture bracing. *Clin Orthop Relat Res*. 1989;240:236–243.
242. Oönne L, Sandblom PH. Late results in fractures of the forearm in children. *Acta Chir Scand*. 1949;98:549–567.
243. Ortega R, Loder RT, Louis DS. Open reduction and internal fixation of forearm fractures in children. *J Pediatr Orthop*. 1996;16:651–654.
244. Ostermann PA, Richter D, Mecklenburg K, et al. Pediatric forearm fractures: Indications, technique, and limits of conservative management. *Unfallchirurg*. 1999; 102(10):784–790.
245. Parikh SN, Brody AS, Crawford AH. Use of a picture archiving and communication system (PACS) and computed plain radiography in preoperative planning. *Am J Orthop*. 2004;33:62–64.
246. Patrick J. A study of supination and pronation with special reference to the treatment of forearm fractures. *J Bone Joint Surg*. 1946;28:737–748.
247. Perez-Garcia MJ, Jimenez-Garcia R, Siles-Sanchez-Manjavacas A. Unexpected diagnosis of severe coarctation of the aorta after ketamine procedural sedation. *Pediatr Emerg Care*. 2012;28:1232–1233.
248. Petridou E, Karpathios T, Dessypris N, et al. The role of dairy products and non-alcoholic beverages in bone fractures among school-age children. *Scand J Soc Med*. 1997;25:119–125.
249. Pfaeffle HJ, Kischer KJ, Manson TT, et al. Role of the forearm interosseous ligament: is it more than just longitudinal load transfer? *J Hand Surg Am*. 2000;25:680–688.
250. Pfaeffle HJ, Tomaino MM, Grewal R, et al. Tensile properties of the interosseous membrane of the human forearm. *J Orthop Res*. 1996;14:842–845.
251. Ponet M, Jawish R. Stable flexible nailing of fractures of both bones of the forearm in children. *Chir Pediatr*. 1989;30:117–120.
252. Powell EC, Tanz RR. In-line skate and rollerskate injuries in childhood. *Pediatr Emerg Care*. 1996;12:259–262.
253. Powers KS, Rubenstein JS. Family presence during invasive procedures in the pediatric intensive care unit: a prospective study. *Arch Pediatr Adolesc Med*. 1999;153:955–958.
254. Prevot J, Guichet JM. Elastic stable intramedullary nailing for forearm fractures in children and adolescents. *J Bone Joint Surg*. 1996;20:305.
255. Prevot J, Lascombes P, Guichet JM. Elastic stable intramedullary nailing for forearm fractures in children and adolescents. *Orthop Trans*. 1996;20:305.
256. Price CT, Knapp DR. Osteotomy for malunited forearm shaft fractures in children. *J Pediatr Orthop*. 2006;26:193–196.
257. Price CT, Mencio GA. Injuries to the shafts of the radius and ulna. In: Beaty JH, Kasser JR, eds. *Rockwood & Wilkins Fractures in Children*. 5th ed. Philadelphia, PA: Lippincott Williams & Wilkins; 2001:452–460.
258. Price CT, Scott DS, Kurzner ME, et al. Malunited forearm fractures in children. *J Pediatr Orthop*. 1990;10:705–712.
259. Prosser AJ, Hooper G. Entrapment of the ulnar nerve in a greenstick fracture of the ulna. *J Hand Surg Br*. 1986;11:211–212.
260. Proubasta IR, De Sena L, Caceres EP. Entrapment of the median nerve in a greenstick forearm fracture: a case report and review of the literature. *Bull Hosp Jt Dis*. 1999;58:220–223.
261. Pugh DM, Galpin RD, Carey TP. Intramedullary Steinmann pin fixation of forearm fractures in children: long-term results. *Clin Orthop Relat Res*. 2000;376:39–48.
262. Qidwai SA. Treatment of diaphyseal forearm fractures in children by intramedullary Kirschner wires. *J Trauma*. 2001;50:303–307.
263. Raiss P, Rettig O, Wolf S, et al. Range of motion of shoulder and elbow in activities of daily life in 3D motion analysis. *Z Orthop Unfall*. 2007;145:493–498.
264. Rang M. *Children's Fractures*. Philadelphia, PA: JB Lippincott; 1974:126.
265. Rang M. *Children's Fractures*. 2nd ed. Philadelphia, PA: JB Lippincott; 1982:203.
266. Rang M, Armstrong P, Crawford AH, et al. Symposium: Management of fractures in children and adolescents, parts I & II. *Contemp Orthop*. 1991;23:517–548, 621–644.
267. Rayan GM, Hayes M. Entrapment of the flexor digitorum profundus in the ulna with fracture of both bones of the forearm: report of a case. *J Bone Joint Surg Am*. 1986;68:1102–1103.
268. Reinhardt KR, Feldman DS, Green DW, et al. Comparison of intramedullary nailing to plating for both-bone forearm fractures in older children. *J Pediatr Orthop*. 2008;28:403–409.
269. Revol MP, Lantieri L, Loy S, et al. Vascular anatomy of the forearm muscles: a study of 50 dissections. *Plast Reconstr Surg*. 1991;88:1026–1033.
270. Richter D, Ostermann PA, Ekkernkamp A, et al. Elastic intramedullary nailing: a minimally invasive concept in the treatment of unstable forearm fractures in children. *J Pediatr Orthop*. 1998;18:457–461.
271. Rickert M, Burger A, Gunther CM, et al. Forearm rotation in healthy adults of all ages and both sexes. *J Shoulder Elbow Surg*. 2008;17:271–275.
272. Ring D, Waters PM, Hotchkiss RN, et al. Pediatric floating elbow. *J Pediatr Orthop*. 2001;21:456–459.
273. Roposch A, Reis M, Molina M, et al. Supracondylar fractures of the humerus associated with ipsilateral fractures in children: a report of forty-seven cases. *J Pediatr Orthop*. 2001;21:307–312.
274. Roy DR. Radioulnar synostosis following proximal radial fracture in child. *Orthop Rev*. 1986;15:89–94.
275. Roy DR. Completely displaced distal radius fractures with intact ulnas in children. *Orthopedics*. 1989;12:1089–1092.
276. Roy DR, Crawford AH. Operative management of fractures of the shaft of the radius and ulna. *Orthop Clin North Am*. 1990;21:245–250.
277. Ryan LM, Teach SJ, Singer SA, et al. Bone mineral density and vitamin D status among African American children with forearm fractures. *Pediatrics*. 2012;130: e553–e560.
278. Rydholm U, Nilsson JE. Traumatic bowing of the forearm: a case report. *Clin Orthop Relat Res*. 1979;139:121–124.
279. Sage FP. Medullary fixation of fractures of the forearm: a study of the medullary canal of the radius and a report of 50 fractures of the radius treated with a prebent triangular nail. *J Bone Joint Surg Am*. 1959;41:1489–1516.
280. Salonen A, Salonen H, Pajulo O. A critical analysis of postoperative complications of antebrachium TEN-nailing in 35 children. *Scand J Surg*. 2012;101:216–221.
281. Sanders WE, Heckman JD. Traumatic plastic deformation of the radius and ulna: a closed method of correction of deformity. *Clin Orthop Relat Res*. 1984;188:58–67.
281a. Sardelli M, Tashjian RZ, MacWilliams BA. Functional elbow range of motion for contemporary tasks. *J Bone Joint Surg-Am*. 2011;93-A:471–477.
282. Sarmiento A, Ebramzadeh E, Brys D, et al. Angular deformities and forearm function. *J Orthop Res*. 1992;10:121–133.
283. Sauer HD, Mommsen U, Bethke K, et al. Fractures of the proximal and middle-third of the lower arm in childhood (author's transl). *Z Kinderchir Grenzgeb*. 1980;29:357–363.
284. Scheiber RA, Branche-Dorsey CM, Ryan GW, et al. Risk factors for injuries from inline skating and the effectiveness of safety gear. *N Engl J Med*. 1996;335: 1630–1635.
285. Schemitsch EH, Jones D, Henley MB, et al. A comparison of malreduction after plate and intramedullary nail fixation of forearm fractures. *J Orthop Trauma*. 1995;9:8–16.
286. Schemitsch EH, Richards RR. The effect of malunion on functional outcome after plate fixation of fractures of both bones of the forearm in adults. *J Bone Joint Surg Am*. 1992;74:1068–1078.
287. Schlickewei W, Salm R. Indications for intramedullary stabilization of shaft fractures in childhood: what is reliable and what is an assumption? *Kongressbd Dtsch Ges Chir Kongr*. 2001;118:431–434.
288. Schmittenbecker PP, Fitze G, Godeke J, et al. Delayed healing of forearm shaft fractures in children after intramedullary nailing. *J Pediatr Orthop*. 2008;28:303–306.
289. Schock CC. "The crooked straight": distal radial remodeling. *J Ark Med Soc*. 1987;84:97–100.
290. Schranz PJ, Fagg PS. Undisplaced fractures of the distal third of the radius in children: an innocent fracture? *Injury*. 1992;23:165–167.
291. Schranz PJ, Gultekin C, Colton CL. External fixation of fractures in children. *Injury*. 1982;23:80–82.
292. Schwarz N, Pienaar S, Schwarz AF, et al. Refracture of the forearm in children. *J Bone Joint Surg Br*. 1996;78:740–744.
293. Shaer JA, Smith B, Turco VJ. Midthird forearm fractures in children: an unorthodox treatment. *Am J Orthop*. 1999;28:60–63.
294. Shah MH, Heffernan G, McGuinness AJ. Early experiences with titanium elastic nails in a trauma unit. *Ir Med J*. 2003;96:213–214.
295. Shaw BA, Murphy KM. Flexor tendon entrapment in ulnar shaft fractures. *Clin Orthop Relat Res*. 1996;330:181–184.
296. Shenoy RM. Biplanar exposure of the radius and ulna through a single incision. *J Bone Joint Surg Br*. 1995;77:568–570.
297. Shoemaker SD, Comstock CP, Mubarak SJ, et al. Intramedullary Kirschner wire fixation of open or unstable forearm fractures in children. *J Pediatr Orthop*. 1999;19:329–337.
298. Simonian PT, Hanel DP. Traumatic plastic deformity of an adult forearm: case report and literature review. *J Orthop Trauma*. 1996;10:213–215.
299. Singer AJ, Gulla J, Thode HC Jr. Parents and practitioners are poor judges of young children's pain severity. *Acad Emerg Med*. 2002;9:609–612.
300. Sinikumpu JJ, Lautamo A, Pokka T, et al. The increasing incidence of paediatric diaphyseal both-bone forearm fractures and their internal fixation during the last decade. *Injury*. 2012;43:362–366.
301. Sinikumpu JJ, Lautamo A, Pokka T, et al. Complications and radiographic outcomes of children's both-bone diaphyseal forearm fractures after invasive and non-invasive treatment. *Injury*. 2013;44(4):431–436.
302. Skaggs DL, Kautz SM, Kay RM, et al. Effect of delay of surgical treatment on rate of infection in open fractures in children. *J Pediatr Orthop*. 2000;20:19–22.
303. Skaggs DL, Loro ML, Pitukcheewanont P, et al. Increased body weight and decreased radial cross-sectional dimensions in girls with forearm fractures. *J Bone Miner Res*. 2001;16:1337–1342.
304. Skahen JR III, Palmer AK, Werner FW, et al. Reconstruction of the interosseous membrane of the forearm in cadavers. *J Hand Surg Am*. 1997;22:986–994.
305. Smith GA. Injuries to children in the United States related to trampolines 1990–1995: a national epidemic. *Pediatrics*. 1998;101:406–412.
306. Soeur R. Intramedullary pinning of diaphyseal fractures. *J Bone Joint Surg*. 1946;28:309–331.
307. Song DJ, Kennebrew GJ Jr, Jex JW. Isolated ring finger flexor digitorum profundus entrapment after closed reduction and intramedullary fixation of both-bone forearm fracture. *Orthopedics*. 2012;35:e1283–e1285.
308. Song KS, Kim HK. Nonunion as a complication of an open reduction of a distal radial fracture in a healthy child: a case report. *J Orthop Trauma*. 2003;17:231–233.
309. Soong C, Rocke LG. Clinical predictors of forearm fracture in children. *Arch Emerg Med*. 1990;7:196–199.
310. Spiegel PG, Mast JW. Internal and external fixation of fractures in children. *Orthop Clin North Am*. 1980;11:405–421.
311. Staebler MP, Moore DC, Akelman E, et al. The effect of wrist guards on bone strain in the distal forearm. *Am J Sports Med*. 1999;27:500–506.
312. Stahl S, Calif E, Eidelman M. Delayed rupture of the extensor pollicis longus tendon following intramedullary nailing of a radial fracture in a child. *J Hand Surg Eur Vol*. 2007;32:67–68.
313. Stahl S, Rozen N, Michaelson M. Ulnar nerve injury following midshaft forearm fractures in children. *J Hand Surg Br*. 1997;22:788–789.

314. Stanitski CL, Micheli LJ. Simultaneous ipsilateral fractures of the arm and forearm in children. *Clin Orthop Relat Res.* 1980;153:218–222.
315. Stanley EA. Treatment of midshaft fractures of the radius and ulna utilizing percutaneous intramedullar pinning. *Orthop Trans.* 1996;20:305.
316. Stanton RP, Malcolm JR, Wesdock KA, et al. Reflex sympathetic dystrophy in children: an orthopaedic perspective. *Orthopedics.* 1993;16:773–780.
317. Stern PJ, Drury WJ. Complications of plate fixation of forearm fractures. *Clin Orthop Relat Res.* 1983;175:25–29.
318. Strauch RJ, Rosenwasser MP, Glazer PA. Surgical exposure of the dorsal proximal third of the radius: how vulnerable is the posterior interosseous nerve? *J Shoulder Elbow Surg.* 1996;5:342–346.
319. Tabak AY, Celebi L, Murath HH, et al. Closed reduction and percutaneous fixation of supracondylar fracture of the humerus and ipsilateral fracture of the forearm in children. *J Bone Joint Surg Br.* 2003;85:1169–1172.
320. Tachakra S, Doherty S. The accuracy of length and angle measurement in videoconferencing teleradiology. *J Telemed Telecare.* 2002;8(Suppl 2):85–87.
321. Tarr RR, Garfinkel AI, Sarmiento A. The effects of angular and rotational deformities of both bones of the forearm: an in vitro study. *J Bone Joint Surg Am.* 1984;66:65–70.
322. Templeton PA, Graham HK. The "floating elbow" in children: simultaneous supracondylar fractures of the humerus and of the forearm in the same upper limb. *J Bone Joint Surg Br.* 1995;77:791–796.
323. Thomas EM, Tuson KW, Browne PS. Fractures of the radius and ulna in children. *Injury.* 1975;7:120–124.
324. Thompson GH, Wilber JH, Marcus RE. Internal fixation of fractures in children and adolescents: a comparative analysis. *Clin Orthop Relat Res.* 1984;188:10–20.
325. Thorndike A Jr, Simmler CL Jr. Fractures of the forearm and elbow in children. *N Engl J Med.* 1941;225:475–480.
326. Till H, Huttl B, Knorr P, et al. Elastic stable intramedullary nailing (ESIN) provides good long-term results in pediatric long-bone fractures. *Eur J Pediatr Surg.* 2000;10:319–322.
327. Toussaint D, Vanderlinden C, Bremen J. Stable elastic nailing applied to diaphyseal fractures of the forearm in children. *Acta Orthop Belg.* 1991;57:147–153.
328. Tredwell SJ, Van Peteghem K, Clough M. Pattern of forearm fractures in children. *J Pediatr Orthop.* 1984;4:604–608.
329. Trousdale RT, Linscheid RL. Operative treatment of malunited fractures of the forearm. *J Bone Joint Surg Am.* 1995;77:894–902.
330. Tynan MC, Fornalski S, McMahon PJ, et al. The effects of ulnar axial malalignment on supination and pronation. *J Bone Joint Surg Am.* 2000;82:1726–1731.
331. Vainionpää S, Bostman O, Patiala H, et al. Internal fixation of forearm fractures in children. *Acta Orthop Scand.* 1987;58:121–123.
332. Van der Reis WL, Otsuka NY, Moroz P, et al. Intramedullary nailing versus plate fixation for unstable forearm fractures in children. *J Pediatr Orthop.* 1998;18:9–13.
333. Vanderbeek BL, Mehlman CT, Foad SL, et al. The use of conscious sedation for forearm fracture reduction in children: does race matter? *J Pediatr Orthop.* 2006;26:53–57.
334. Van Herpe LB. Fractures of the forearm and wrist. *Orthop Clin North Am.* 1976;7:543–556.
335. Verstreken L, Delronge G, Lamoureux J. Shaft forearm fractures in children: intramedullary nailing with immediate motion: a preliminary report. *J Pediatr Orthop.* 1988;8:450–453.
336. Vince KG, Miller JE. Cross-union complicating fracture of the forearm. Part II: children. *J Bone Joint Surg Am.* 1987;69:654–661.
337. Vorlat P, De Boeck H. Bowing fractures of the forearm in children: a long-term follow-up. *Clin Orthop Relat Res.* 2003;413:233–237.
338. Voto SJ, Weiner DS, Leighley B. Redisplacement after closed reduction of forearm fractures in children. *J Pediatr Orthop.* 1990;10:79–84.
339. Voto SJ, Weiner DS, Leighley B. Use of pins and plaster in the treatment of unstable pediatric forearm fractures. *J Pediatr Orthop.* 1990;10:85–89.
340. Walker JL, Rang M. Forearm fractures in children: cast treatment with the elbow extended. *J Bone Joint Surg Br.* 1991;73:299–301.
341. Waltzman ML, Shannon M, Bowen AP, et al. Monkeybar injuries: complications of play. *Pediatrics.* 1999;103:e58.
342. Waseem M, Paton RW. Percutaneous intramedullary elastic wiring of displaced diaphyseal forearm fractures in children. A modified technique. *Injury.* 1999;30:21–24.
343. Watson PA, Blair W. Entrapment of the index flexor digitorum profundus tendon after fracture of both forearm bones in a child. *Iowa Orthop J.* 1999;19:127–128.
344. Watson-Jones R. *Fractures and Other Bone and Joint Injuries.* 1st ed. Edinburgh: Livingstone; 1940:379–380.
345. Weber BG, Cech O. *Pseudarthrosis.* Bern, Switzerland: Hans Huber; 1976.
346. Weinberg DS, Park PJ, Boden KA, et al. Anatomic investigation of commonly used landmarks for evaluation rotation during forearm fracture reduction. *J Bone Joint Surg Am.* 2016;98-A:1103–1112.
347. Weiss JM, Mencio GA. Forearm shaft fractures: does fixation improve outcomes? *J Pediatr Orthop.* 2012;32(Suppl 1):S22–S24.
348. White AA, Panjabi MM, Southwick WO. The four biomechanical stages of fracture repair. *J Bone Joint Surg Am.* 1977;59:188–192.
349. Wilder RT, Berde CB, Wolohan M, et al. Reflex sympathetic dystrophy in children. *J Bone Joint Surg Am.* 1992;74:910–919.
350. Wilkins KE. Operative management of children's fractures: is it a sign of impetuousness or do the children really benefit? *J Pediatr Orthop.* 1998;18:1–3.
351. Williamson DM, Cole WG. Treatment of ipsilateral supracondylar and forearm fractures in children. *Injury.* 1992;23:159–161.
352. Wilson JC Jr, Krueger JC. Fractures of the proximal and middle thirds of the radius and ulna in children: study of the end results with analysis of treatment and complications. *Am J Surg.* 1966;112:326–332.
353. Worlock P, Stower M. Fracture patterns in Nottingham children. *J Pediatr Orthop.* 1986;6:656–660.
354. Wright PB, Crepeau AE, Herrera-Soto JA, et al. Radius crossover sign: an indication of malreduced radius shaft greenstick fractures. *J Pediatr Orthop.* 2012;32:e15–e19.
355. Wright J, Rang M. Internal fixation for forearm fractures in children. *Tech Orthop.* 1989;4:44–47.
356. Würfel AM, Voigt A, Linke F, et al. New aspects in the treatment of complete and isolated diaphyseal fractures of the forearm in children. *Unfallchirurgie.* 1995;21:70–76.
357. Wyrsch B, Mencio GA, Green NE. Open reduction and internal fixation of pediatric forearm fractures. *J Pediatr Orthop.* 1996;16:644–650.
358. Yasin MN, Talwalkar SC, Henderson JJ, et al. Segmental radius and ulna fractures with scaphocapitate fractures and bilateral multiple epiphyseal fractures. *Am J Orthop.* 2008;37:214–217.
359. Yasutomi T, Nakatsuchi Y, Koike H, et al. Mechanism of limitation of pronation/supination of the forearm in geometric models of deformities of the forearm bones. *Clin Biomech (Bristol, Avon).* 2002;17:456–463.
360. Younger AS, Tredwell SJ, Mackenzie WG, et al. Accurate prediction of outcome after pediatric forearm fracture. *J Pediatr Orthop.* 1994;14:200–206.
361. Younger AS, Tredwell SJ, Mackenzie WG. Factors affecting fracture position at cast removal after pediatric forearm fracture. *J Pediatr Orthop.* 1997;17:332–336.
362. Yung SH, Lam CY, Choi KY, et al. Percutaneous intramedullary Kirschner wiring for displaced diaphyseal forearm fractures in children. *J Bone Joint Surg Br.* 1998;80:91–94.
363. Yung PS, Lam CY, Ng BK, et al. Percutaneous transphyseal intramedullary Kirschner wire pinning: A safe and effective procedure for treatment of displaced forearm fracture in children. *J Pediatr Orthop.* 2004;24:7–12.
364. Yuan PS, Pring ME, Gaynor TP, et al. Compartment syndrome following intramedullary fixation of pediatric forearm fractures. *J Pediatr Orthop.* 2004;24:370–375.
365. Zionts LE, Zalavras CG, Gerhardt MB. Closed treatment of displaced both-bone forearm fractures in older children and adolescents. *J Pediatr Orthop.* 2005;25:507–512.

10

Radial Neck and Olecranon Fractures

Mark A. Erickson and Sumeet Garg

INTRODUCTION TO FRACTURES OF THE PROXIMAL RADIUS AND ULNA

Fractures of the proximal radius in skeletally immature patients usually involve the metaphysis or physis. True isolated radial head fractures are rare. In the proximal ulna, the olecranon, which biomechanically is a metaphysis, often fails with a greenstick pattern. Fractures in this area also may involve the physis. Fractures of the olecranon associated with proximal radioulnar joint (PRUJ) disruption are considered part of the Monteggia fracture pattern and are discussed in Chapter 11.

Fractures of the radial neck account for 1% to 3% of all children's fractures.[21] Radial neck fractures make up approximately 5% to 10% of elbow fractures in children.[10,21,34,48,51,60,79] Radial head fractures are uncommon but concerning if there is articular displacement, and when they occur usually are Salter–Harris type IV injuries. The median age at injury is 9 to 10 years in the pediatric population.[26,48,58,78,97,114,123,128] There is little difference in the occurrence rates between males and females[26,48,78]; however, this injury seems to occur on an average approximately 2 years earlier in girls than in boys.[114]

Fractures of the proximal ulna in skeletally immature children present in three different patterns: fractures involving the proximal apophysis, metaphyseal fractures of the olecranon, and fractures of the coronoid process.

Few fractures of the ulnar apophysis are described in the English literature, most recently by Carney.[15,43,89,103,108] In addition to acute injuries in children, some have been described in young adults with open physes.[57,86,107,124] Most reports of apophyseal olecranon fractures describe patients with osteogenesis imperfecta, who seem predisposed to this injury, and are often treated using tension-band wiring.[87]

Isolated metaphyseal fractures of the olecranon are relatively rare but beware of associated Monteggia lesions (Table 10-1). They are often associated with other fractures about the elbow. In the combined series of 4,684 elbow fractures reviewed, 230 were olecranon fractures, for an incidence of 4.9%. This agrees with the incidence of 4% to 6% in the major series reported.[32,65,82] Only 10% to 20% of the total fractures reported in these series required an operation. Six reports totaling 302 patients with fractures of the olecranon in children are in the English literature.[39,43,65,78] Considering all age groups, 25% of olecranon fractures in these reports occurred in the first decade and another 25% in the second decade.[58] During the first decade, the peak age for olecranon fracture was between age 5 and 10 years.[44,79] Approximately 20% of patients had an associated fracture or dislocation of the elbow, most involving the proximal radius. Only 10% to 20% required an operation.

The incidence of fracture of the coronoid varies from less than 1% to 2% of elbow fractures.[65]

Fractures of the Proximal Radius

ASSESSMENT OF FRACTURES OF THE PROXIMAL RADIUS

MECHANISMS OF INJURY FOR FRACTURES OF THE PROXIMAL RADIUS

Most fractures of the proximal radius occur at the neck. Fractures of the proximal radius most commonly occur after a fall on an outstretched arm with elbow extended and valgus stress at the elbow.[41,48,51,78,79,132] The immature radial head is primarily cartilaginous and intra-articular radial head fractures in children and adolescents are rare. The radial head is entirely articular cartilage and the primary blood supply comes from the metaphysis. This may predispose the radial head to avascular necrosis and nonunion with significant displacement. The cartilaginous head absorbs the force and transmits it to the weaker physis or metaphysis of the neck.[132] These fractures characteristically produce an angular

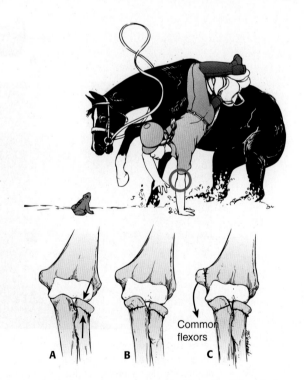

Figure 10-1. The most common mechanism of radial neck fractures involves a fall on the outstretched arm. This produces an angular deformity of the neck (**A**). Further valgus forces can produce a greenstick fracture of the olecranon (**B**) or an avulsion of the medial epicondylar apophysis (**C**). (Redrawn with permission from Jeffery CC. Fractures of the head of the radius in children. *J Bone Joint Surg Br.* 1950;32:314–324.)

TABLE 10-1. Incidence of Metaphyseal Fractures of the Olecranon
Age distribution: first decade, 25%; second decade, 25%; third decade, 50%
Peak age: 5–10 yrs
Extremity predominance: left (55%)
Sex predominance: male (65%)
Associated elbow injuries: 20%
Requiring surgical intervention: 19%

deformity of the head with the neck (Fig. 10-1A). The direction of angulation depends on whether the forearm is in a supinated, neutral, or pronated position at the time of the fall. Vostal showed that in neutral, the pressure is concentrated on the lateral portion of the head and neck. In supination, the pressure is concentrated anteriorly, and in pronation it is concentrated posteriorly.[132]

Proximal radial fractures also may occur in association with elbow dislocation. The fracture will usually occur during the dislocation event, typically displaced anterior. Alternatively, the fracture may occur during spontaneous reduction of the distal humerus, driving the displacement of the proximal radius posteriorly (Fig. 10-2).

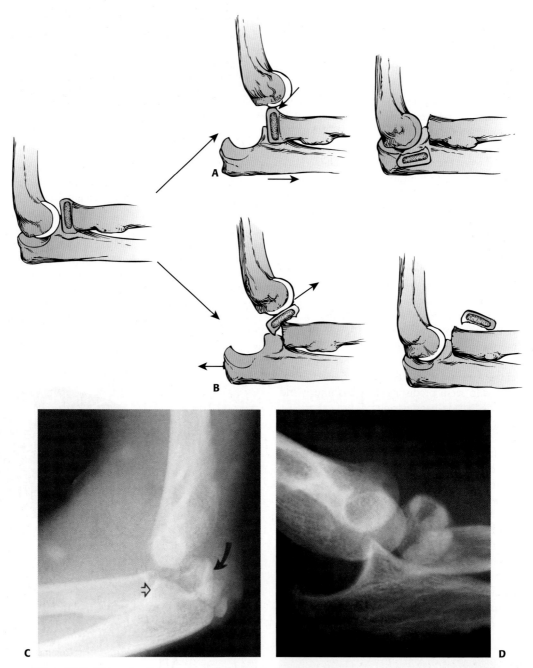

Figure 10-2. Dislocation fracture patterns. **A:** Type D: The radial neck is fractured during the process of reduction by the capitellum pressing against the distal lip of the radial head.[140] **B:** Type E: The radial neck is fractured during the process of dislocation by the capitellum pressing against the proximal lip of the radial head.[105] (Reprinted with permission from Sessa S, Lascombes P, Prevot J, et al. Fractures of the radial head and associated elbow injuries in children. *J Pediatr Orthop B.* 1996;5(3):200–209.) **C:** Radiographs of a radial head that was fractured during the reduction of the dislocation (type D). The radial head (*solid arrow*) lies posterior to the distal humerus, and the distal portion of the neck (*open arrow*) is anterior. (Courtesy of Richard E. King, MD.) **D:** Radiograph of the dislocated elbow in which the fracture of the radial neck occurred during the process of dislocation (type E).

INJURIES ASSOCIATED WITH FRACTURES OF THE PROXIMAL RADIUS

Proximal radius fractures can occur concomitantly with distal humerus, ulna, radial shaft, or distal radius fractures.[41,51,52,79,114] Fractures in combination with ulnar fractures often are part of the Monteggia fracture pattern detailed in Chapter 11. Presence of associated fractures portends a poor prognosis for patients with proximal radius fractures with higher rates of persistent stiffness and pain compared to those with isolated proximal radius fractures.[117] As detailed further in Chapter 15, proximal radius fractures can also occur during traumatic elbow dislocations. The posterior interosseous nerve (PIN) wraps around the proximal radius and occasionally can be injured in association with proximal radius fractures. More typically, however, the nerve is at risk during percutaneous manipulation or open reduction of proximal radius fractures.

SIGNS AND SYMPTOMS OF FRACTURES OF THE PROXIMAL RADIUS

Following a fracture, palpation over the radial head or neck is painful. The pain is usually increased with forearm rotation more so than with elbow flexion and extension. Displaced fractures frequently result in visible bruising on the lateral aspect of the elbow with soft tissue swelling. Neurologic examination should in particular evaluate the PIN (test for wrist, digital and thumb extension). Occasionally in a young child, the primary complaint may be wrist pain, and pressure over the proximal radius may accentuate this referred wrist pain.[3] The wrist pain may be secondary to radial shortening and subsequent distal radioulnar joint dysfunction. This reinforces the principle of obtaining radiographs of both ends of a fractured long bone and complete examination of the entire affected extremity.

IMAGING AND OTHER DIAGNOSTIC STUDIES FOR FRACTURES OF THE PROXIMAL RADIUS

Displaced proximal radius fractures are usually easy to identify on standard anteroposterior (AP) and lateral radiographs. Some variants in the ossification process can resemble a fracture. Most of these involve the radial head, although a step-off can also develop as a normal variant of the metaphysis. There may be a persistence of the secondary ossification centers of the epiphysis. Comparison views of the contralateral elbow are useful for evaluation of unusual ossification centers after an acute elbow injury.

If the elbow cannot be extended because of pain, special views are necessary to see the AP alignment of the proximal forearm and distal humerus. A regular AP view with the elbow flexed may not show the fracture because of obliquity of the beam and overlap of proximal forearm and distal humerus bones. One view is taken with the beam perpendicular to the distal humerus, and the other with the beam perpendicular to the proximal radius. The perpendicular views show the proximal radial physis in clear profile.

With a minimally displaced fracture, the fracture line may be difficult to see because it is superimposed on the proximal ulna, and oblique views of the proximal radius may be helpful.[12,132] One oblique view that is especially helpful is the radiocapitellar view suggested by Greenspan et al.[45,46] and Hall-Craggs et al.[47] This view projects the radial head anterior to the coronoid process (Fig. 10-3), and is especially helpful if full supination and

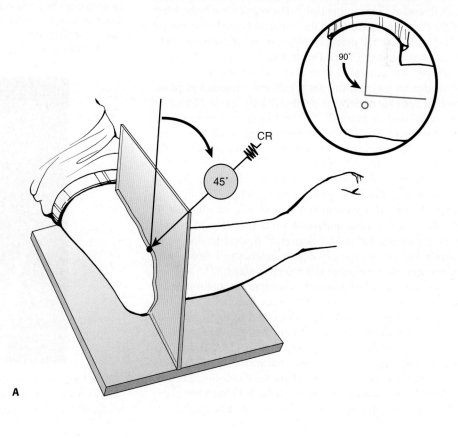

Figure 10-3. A: Radiocapitellar view.   **A**
(*continues*)

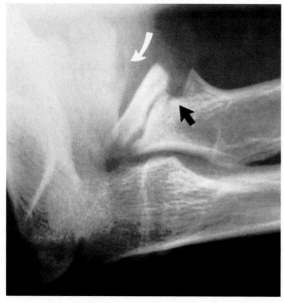

Figure 10-3. (*Continued*) **B:** Angular stress deformity: Anterior angulation of the radial head and neck in a 12-year-old baseball pitcher. There is evidence of some disruption of the normal growth of the anterior portion of the physis (*black arrow*). The capitellum also shows radiographic signs of osteochondritis dissecans (*white arrow*). (Courtesy of Kenneth P. Butters, MD.)

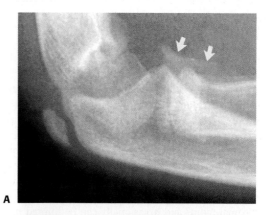

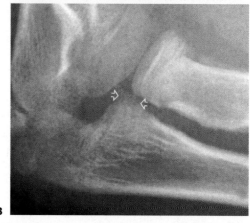

Figure 10-4. The radiocapitellar view. **A:** Radiographs of a 10-year-old female who sustained a radial neck fracture associated with an elbow dislocation. There is ectopic bone formation (*arrows*). In this view, it is difficult to tell the exact location of the ectopic bone. **B:** The radiocapitellar view separates the radial head from the coronoid process and shows that the ectopic bone is from the coronoid process (*arrows*) and not the radial neck.

pronation views are difficult to obtain because of acute injury (Fig. 10-4).

The diagnosis of a partially or completely displaced fracture of the radial neck may be difficult in children whose radial head remains unossified.[99] The only clue may be irregularity in the smoothness of the proximal metaphyseal margin (Fig. 10-5). The full extent of the injury is seen with magnetic resonance imaging (MRI). Displacement of the supinator fat pad may also indicate fracture of the proximal radius[101]; however, this fat pad and the distal humeral anterior and posterior fat pads are not always displaced with occult fractures of the radial neck or physis.[49,104,106] Arthrogram, ultrasound, and MRI are helpful to assess the extent of the displacement and the accuracy of reduction in children with an unossified radial epiphysis (Fig. 10-6).[20,50,59]

In the preossification stage, on the AP radiograph, the edge of the metaphysis of the proximal radius slopes distally on its lateral border. This angulation is normal and not a fracture. In the AP view, the lateral angulation varies from 0 to 15 degrees, with the average being 12.5 degrees.[128] In the lateral view, the angulation can vary from 10 degrees anterior to 5 degrees posterior, with the average being 3.5 degrees anterior.[12]

Recently described posterior radiocapitellar subluxation following what appeared to be fairly innocuous radial head fractures has been attributed to undiagnosed ligamentous injury associated with the fracture. Waters and Kasser include this among lesions described by the acronym TRASH for "The Radiographic Appearance Seemed Harmless."[135] MRI provides excellent anatomic detail of the elbow joint and should be considered when evaluating displaced radial head fractures, particularly if change in position is noted on serial radiographs.

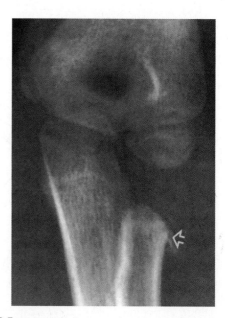

Figure 10-5. Preosseous fracture. The only clue to the presence of a fracture of the radial neck with displacement of the radial head was loss of smoothness of the metaphyseal margin (*arrow*).

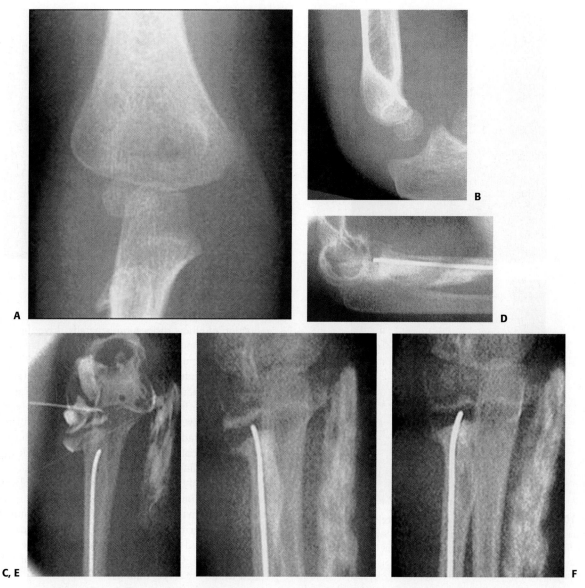

Figure 10-6. A, B: AP and lateral radiographs demonstrating a radial neck fracture in a patient with a non-ossified proximal radial epiphysis. **C:** Arthrogram prior to reduction demonstrating location/displacement of nonossified proximal radial epiphysis. **D–F:** Arthrogram/radiographs after reduction with intramedullary technique. (From Javed A, Guichet JM. Arthrography for reduction of a fracture of the radial neck in a child with a nonossified radial epiphysis. *J Bone Joint Surg Br*. 2001;83-B:542–543, with permission.)

CLASSIFICATION OF FRACTURES OF THE PROXIMAL RADIUS

Chambers' Classification of Proximal Radial Fractures

Chambers' Classification of Fractures Involving the Proximal Radius[17]

Group I: Primary displacement of the radial head (most common)

Valgus fractures
Type A—Salter–Harris type I and II injuries of the proximal radial physis
Type B—Salter–Harris type IV injuries of the proximal radial physis
Type C—Fractures involving only the proximal radial metaphysis

Fractures associated with elbow dislocation
Type D—Reduction injuries
Type E—Dislocation injuries

Group II: Primary displacement of the radial neck
A. Angular injuries (Monteggia type III variant)
B. Torsional injuries

Group III: Stress injuries
A. Osteochondritis dissecans or osteochondrosis of the radial head
B. Physeal injuries with neck angulation

Head-Displaced Fractures (Group I)

With valgus elbow injuries, the fracture pattern can be one of three types (A, B, or C) (Fig. 10-7). In the first two types,

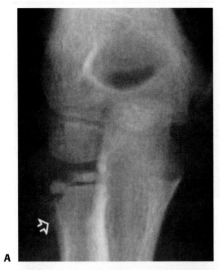

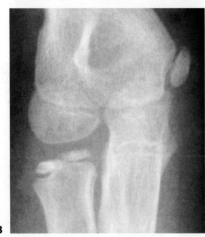

Figure 10-7. Valgus (type B) injury. **A:** Three weeks after the initial injury, there was evidence of distal migration of this Salter–Harris type IV fracture fragment. Periosteal new bone formation has already developed along the distal metaphyseal fragment (*arrow*). **B:** Six months after the initial injury, there was evidence of an osseous bridge formation between the metaphysis and the epiphysis. Subsequently, the patient had secondary degenerative arthritis with loss of elbow motion and forearm rotation.

the fracture line involves the physis. Type A represents either a Salter–Harris type I or II physeal injury. In a Salter–Harris type II injury, the metaphyseal fragment is triangular and lies on the compression side. In type B fractures, the fracture line courses vertically through the metaphysis, physis, and epiphysis to produce a Salter–Harris type IV fracture pattern (see Fig. 10-7). This is the only fracture type that involves the articular surface of the radial head. In type C fractures, the fracture line lies completely within the metaphysis (Fig. 10-8), and the fracture can be transverse or oblique. Type B fractures, intra-articular radial head fractures, are rare. These can have poor long-term results if posterior radiocapitellar subluxation develops (Fig. 10-9).[129,135] The incidences of types A and C fractures are approximately equal.[114]

In two rare types of fractures of the radial neck associated with elbow dislocation, the head fragment is totally displaced from the neck.[6,14,35,51,78,134] Fractures occurring during spontaneous

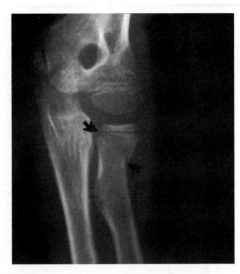

Figure 10-8. Valgus type C injury. The fracture line is totally metaphyseal and oblique (*arrows*).

reduction of elbow dislocation generally drive the radial head dorsal as the capitellum applies a dorsally directed force to the radial neck during reduction (type D) (Fig. 10-2A).[51,134] Fractures occurring during the dislocation event generally drive the radial head anteriorly as the capitellum applies an anteriorly direct force during the process of dislocating (type E) (Fig. 10-2B).[6,78,128] Even with spontaneous or manipulative elbow reduction, the radial head fragment will usually remain anterior to the radial shaft with the fractured radial neck articulating with the capitellum.

Regardless of the type of fracture pattern, displacement can vary from minimal angulation to complete separation of the radial head from the neck (see Fig. 10-10). With minimal angulation, the congruity of the PRUJ is usually retained. If the radial head is displaced in relation to the radial neck, the congruity of the PRUJ is lost. Completely displaced fractures are often associated with more severe injuries.

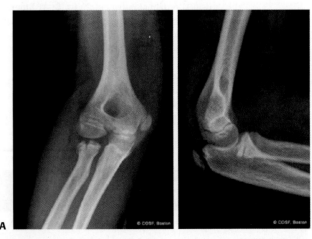

Figure 10-9. A: Acute injury films revealing small displacement of radial head fracture on the flexed elbow anteroposterior (AP) view and subtle posterior subluxation not originally appreciated on the lateral view.

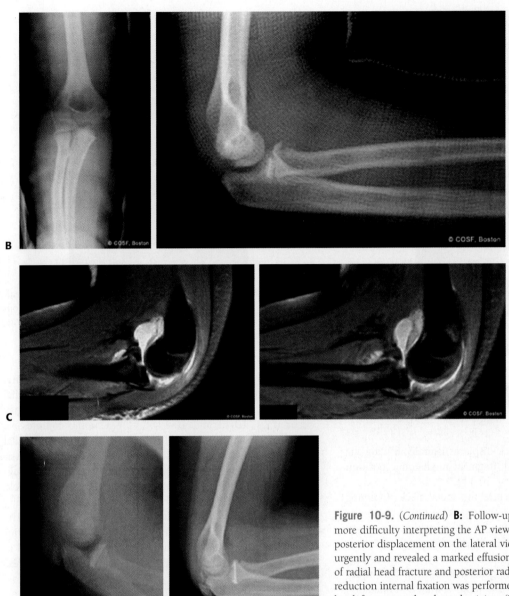

Figure 10-9. (*Continued*) **B:** Follow-up radiographs at 1 week noted more difficulty interpreting the AP view in cast, and more radiocapitellar posterior displacement on the lateral view. An MRI scan (**C**) was ordered urgently and revealed a marked effusion and intra-articular displacement of radial head fracture and posterior radiocapitellar subluxation. **D:** Open reduction internal fixation was performed to anatomically align the radial head fracture and reduce the joint. (Reprinted with permission from Waters PM, Beaty J, Kasser J. Elbow "TRASH" (The Radiographic Appearance Seemed Harmless) Lesions. *J Pediatr Orthop.* 2010;30:S77–S81.)

Neck-Displaced Fractures (Group II)

Rarely, angular or torsional forces cause a primary disruption or deformity of the neck while the head remains congruous within the PRUJ. Treatment of these fractures is manipulation of the distal neck fragment to align it with the head. For the neck-displaced fractures, there are two subgroups: angular and torsional.

An angular fracture of the radial neck may be associated with a proximal ulnar fracture. This association is recognized as a Monteggia variant. A Monteggia type III fracture pattern is created when a varus force is applied across the extended elbow, resulting in a greenstick fracture of the olecranon or proximal ulna and a lateral dislocation of the radial head.[140] Occasionally, however, the failure occurs at the radial neck (Monteggia III

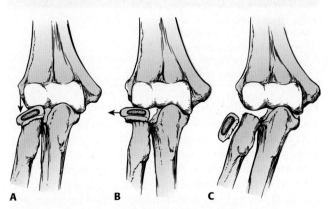

Figure 10-10. Displacement patterns. The radial head can be angulated (**A**), translated (**B**), or completely displaced (**C**).

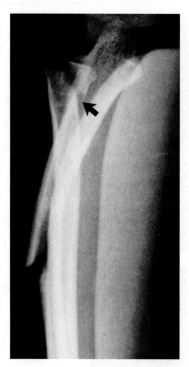

Figure 10-11. Angular forces. This 8-year-old sustained a type III Monteggia equivalent in which the radial neck fractured (*arrow*), leaving the radial head reduced proximally. (*Courtesy of Ruben D. Pechero, MD.*)

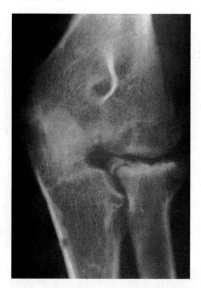

Figure 10-12. Osteochondritis dissecans. Radiograph of this 11-year-old Little League pitcher's elbow shows fragmentation of the subchondral surfaces of the radial head. These changes and the accelerated bone age are evidence of overuse.

equivalent) and the radial neck displaces laterally, leaving the radial head and proximal neck fragment in anatomic position under the annular ligament (Fig. 10-11).[80]

Rotational forces may fracture the radial neck in young children before ossification of the proximal radial epiphysis. This has been described only in case reports with a supination force.[40,48] Reduction was achieved by pronation of the forearm. Diagnosis of these injuries is difficult and may require arthrography or an examination under general anesthesia. This injury should be differentiated from the more common subluxation of the radial head ("nursemaid's elbow"), in which the forearm usually is held in pronation with resistance to supination.

Stress Injuries (Group III)

A final mechanism of injury is chronic repetitive stress, both longitudinal and rotational, on either the head or the proximal radial physis. These injuries are usually the result of athletic activity in which the upper extremity is required to perform repetitive motions. Repetitive stresses disrupt growth of either the neck or the head with eventual deformity. A true stress fracture is not present.

In the United States, the popularity of organized sports has produced a number of unique injuries in children related to repetitive stress applied to growth centers. Most elbow stress injuries are related to throwing sports such as baseball. Most of this "Little League" pathology involves tension injuries on the medial epicondyle. In some athletes, however, the lateral side is involved as well because of the repetitive compressive forces applied to the capitellum and radial head and neck. Athletes

involved in sports requiring upper extremity weight bearing, such as gymnastics or wrestling, are also at risk. In the radial head, lytic lesions similar to osteochondritis dissecans may occur (Figs. 10-12 and 10-13).[28,125,139] Chronic compressive loading may cause an osteochondrosis of the proximal radial epiphysis, with radiographic signs of decreased size of the ossified epiphysis, increased radiographic opacity, and later fragmentation. If the stress forces are transmitted to the radial neck, the anterior portion of the physis may be injured, producing an angular deformity of the radial neck (see Fig. 10-3).[29] The more complex aspect of this injury spectrum is loss of anterior radial head height, joint instability and malalignment, and at times, nonunion and avascular necrosis of the radial head stress fracture.

Judet and O'Brien Classification of Radial Neck Fractures

Judet Classification of Radial Neck Fractures[53]
Type I: Nondisplaced
Type II: <30 degrees of angulation
Type III: 30 to 60 degrees of angulation
Type IVA: 60 to 80 degrees of angulation
Type IVB: >80 degrees of angulation

Radial neck fractures, the most common type of proximal radius fracture (Groups IA and IC), have also been classified based on angulation by Judet.[53] Increasing grade has generally been associated with poorer outcomes with both nonoperative and operative care as discussed in the section on treatment outcomes. O'Brien described a similar classification of radial neck fractures specifically for pediatric patients with slightly different grading: type I: <30 degrees angulation, type II: 30 to 60 degrees angulation, type III: >60 degrees angulation.[79]

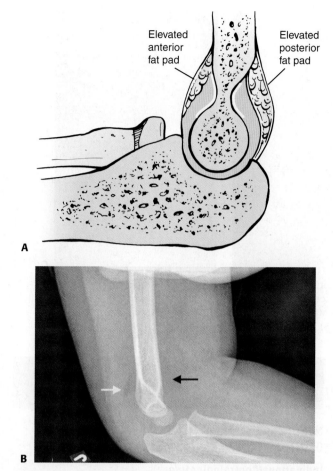

Elevated anterior fat pad   Elevated posterior fat pad

A

B

Figure 10-13. Elevated anterior and posterior fat pads. **A:** Illustration. (Adapted with permission from Skaggs DL, Mirzayan R. The posterior fat pad sign in association with occult fracture of the elbow in children. *J Bone Joint Surg Am.* 1999;81(10):1429–1433.) **B:** *White arrow:* Posterior fat pad sign. *Black arrow:* Anterior fat pad sign.

TABLE 10-2. The Mayo Clinic Performance Index for the Elbow[a]	
Function	**Point Score**
Pain (45 points)	
None	45
Mild	30
Moderate	15
Severe	0
Motion (20 points)	
Arc 100 degrees	20
Arc 50–100 degrees	15
Arc 2 degrees	5
Stability[b] (10 points)	
Stable	10
Moderate instability	
Gross instability	0
Daily Function (25 points)	
Combing hair	5
Feeding oneself	5
Hygiene	5
Putting on shirt	5
Putting on shoes	5
Maximum Possible Total	**100**

[a]90 points or more, excellent; 75–89 points, good; 60–74 points, fair; and less than 60 points, poor.
[b]Stable, no apparent varus-valgus laxity clinically; moderate instability, less than 10 degrees of varus-valgus laxity; and gross instability, 10 degrees or more of varus-valgus laxity.
Reprinted with permission from Mayo Elbow Performance Score. *J Orthop Trauma.* 2006;20(8):S127.

OUTCOME MEASURES FOR FRACTURES OF THE PROXIMAL RADIUS

Most previously published literature on the outcomes of pediatric proximal radius fractures has used nonvalidated functional outcome measures. Various iterations of "excellent," "good," "fair," and "poor" with individualized descriptions have been utilized. The growing emphasis in orthopedics on critical functional assessments following injury or surgery should improve the quality of future evidence on this topic. It is hoped that validated functional measures for upper extremity function and global pediatric and adolescent function be utilized in future research efforts in this area. Several recent papers reporting on radial head and neck fractures have used the Mayo Elbow Performance Score as a more objective functional measure (Table 10-2).[18,36,38,66,119,133]

Range of motion following treatment of proximal radius fractures is a critical component of outcome. Usually, assessments have been done manually using a goniometer but have poor reliability within and between observers. The wider availability of digital motion capture technology will hopefully provide more accurate measures of range of motion following extremity trauma in future studies.

PATHOANATOMY AND APPLIED ANATOMY RELATING TO FRACTURES OF THE PROXIMAL RADIUS

In the embryo, the proximal radius is well defined by 9 weeks of gestation. By 4 years of age, the radial head and neck have the same contours as in an adult.[79] Ossification of the proximal radius epiphysis begins at approximately 5 years of age as a small, flat nucleus (Fig. 10-14). This ossific nucleus can originate as a small sphere or it can be bipartite, which is a normal variation and should not be misinterpreted as a fracture.[12,67,106]

No ligaments attach directly to the radial neck or head. The radial collateral ligaments attach to the annular ligament, which originates from the radial side of the ulna. The articular capsule attaches to the proximal third of the neck. Distally, the capsule protrudes from under the annular ligament to form a pouch (recessus sacciformis). Thus, only a small portion of the neck lies within the articular capsule.[132] Because much of the neck is extracapsular, fractures involving only the neck may not produce an intra-articular effusion, and the fat pad sign may be negative with fracture of the radial neck.[12,49,106]

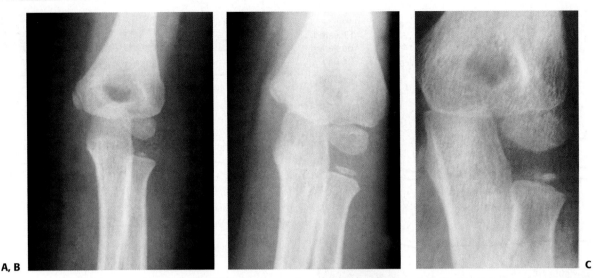

A, B   **C**

Figure 10-14. Ossification pattern. **A:** At 5 years, ossification begins as a small oval nucleus. **B:** As the head matures, the center widens but remains flat. **C:** Double ossification centers in developing proximal radial epiphysis. (Reprinted with permission from Silberstein MJ, Brodeur AE, Graviss ER. Some vagaries of the radial head and neck. *J Bone Joint Surgery Am.* 1982;64(8):1153–1157.)

The PRUJ has a precise congruence. The axis of rotation of the proximal radius is a line through the center of the radial head and neck. When a displaced fracture disrupts the alignment of the radial head on the center of the radial neck, the arc of rotation changes. Instead of rotating smoothly in a pure circle, the radial head rotates with a "cam" effect. This disruption of the congruity of the PRUJ (as occurs with displaced fractures of the proximal radius) may result in a loss of the range of motion in supination and pronation (Fig. 10-15).[137]

Table 10-3 lists the proposed mechanisms for fractures of the radial head and neck in children.

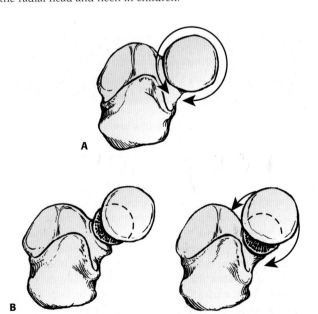

A

B

Figure 10-15. A: Normal rotation of the forearm causes the radial head to circumscribe an exact circle within the proximal radioulnar joint. **B:** Any translocation of the radial head limits rotation because of the "cam" effect described by Wedge and Robertson.[137]

TREATMENT OPTIONS FOR FRACTURES OF THE PROXIMAL RADIUS

NONOPERATIVE TREATMENT OF FRACTURES OF THE PROXIMAL RADIUS

Indications/Contraindications

Nonoperative Treatment of Proximal Radius Fractures: INDICATIONS AND CONTRAINDICATIONS

Indications	Relative Contraindications
<2-mm displacement of the radial head or neck	Open fracture
<30 to 45-degree angulation of the radial neck (<30 degrees if age >10, <45 degrees if age <10) (relative indication depending on motion)	Incongruent elbow joint
Full forearm pronation and supination	

TABLE 10-3. Proposed Mechanisms of Fractures of the Radial Head and Neck in Children

Primary Displacement of the Head (incongruous)
Valgus injuries
Associated with dislocation of the elbow
  • During reduction
  • During dislocation

Primary Displacement of the Neck
Angular forces
Rotational forces
Chronic stress forces

Nonoperative treatment is indicated for the majority of proximal radius fractures. Remodeling of the proximal radius can be expected in skeletally immature children. Based on multiple retrospective case series, radial neck angulation of 30 to 45 degrees can remodel if the radial head is not dislocated and conservative treatment will lead to good results.[21,26,31,76,78,114,128,144] It is critical to assess forearm rotation, and if a block to full rotation is appreciated, an attempt at reduction should be considered. Intra-articular aspiration of hematoma and injection of local anesthetic can assist with pain relief and assessment of range of motion.

In the case of nondisplaced radial head fractures (Salter–Harris IV, Group IB in the Chambers' classification), close follow-up with serial radiographs is warranted to monitor radiocapitellar alignment. If subluxation is suspected, advanced imaging with ultrasound or MRI along with consideration of operative treatment should be considered.

Closed reduction techniques should be attempted if there is displacement or unacceptable angulation at the fracture site, especially with a malaligned joint. The goal should be to restore the alignment to accepted indications below with full forearm rotation. Internal fixation is usually not necessary if successful closed reduction can be accomplished.

Patients not requiring closed reduction should be immobilized for a short period of time to allow for comfort and soft tissue healing. This is generally 1 to 3 weeks based on extent of injury and age. After fracture pain has subsided, patients should work on progressively increasing range of motion and resumption of activities as symptoms allow. Short-term immobilization can be accomplished with a sling, posterior arm splint, elbow-hinged brace, or long-arm cast based on surgeon and patient preference.

Closed Reduction Techniques

Several closed reduction techniques for proximal radius fractures have been described in the literature, all of which have reported generally good results. The surgeon should be familiar with multiple techniques and apply them as needed because closed treatment of proximal radius fractures has generally been shown to have improved results compared to open treatment. No technique has yet been demonstrated to have superiority over another. Techniques are variations on either manipulating the proximal fragment to the fixed radial shaft or manipulating the radial shaft to the fixed proximal fragment; and on rare occasions both.

Patterson[85] described a reduction technique for the radial neck in 1934. Conscious sedation or general anesthesia is recommended in children to allow for adequate relaxation during the procedure. The annular ligament should be intact to stabilize the proximal radial head fragment.[67] An assistant grasps the arm proximal to the elbow joint with one hand (Fig. 10-16) and places the other hand medially over the distal humerus to provide a medial fulcrum for the varus stress applied across the elbow. The surgeon applies distal traction with the forearm supinated to relax the supinators and biceps. A varus force is then placed on the elbow with added direct lateral pressure on the radial head in an attempt to reduce the fracture. Kaufman et al.[54] proposed another technique in which the elbow is manipulated in the flexed position. The surgeon presses his or her thumb against the anterior surface of the radial head with the forearm in pronation.

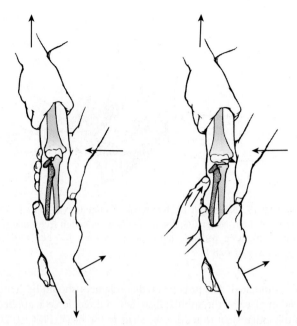

Figure 10-16. The Patterson manipulation technique. **Left:** An assistant grabs the arm proximally with one hand placed medially against the distal humerus. The surgeon applies distal traction with the forearm supinated and pulls the forearm into varus. **Right:** Digital pressure applied directly over the tilted radial head completes the reduction. Arrows indicate direction of force applied by the manipulating hands. (Redrawn with permission from Patterson RF. Treatment of displaced transverse fractures of the neck of the radius in children. *J Bone Joint Surg.* 1934;16(3):695–698.)

Although forearm supination relaxes the supinator muscle, supination may not be the best position for manipulation of the head fragment. Jeffrey[51] pointed out that the tilt of the radial head depends on the position of the forearm at the time of injury. The direction of maximal tilt can be confirmed by radiograph and is also when fracture deformity will be most palpable clinically. The best position for reduction is the degree of rotation that places the radial head most prominent laterally. If the x-ray beam is perpendicular to the head in maximal tilt, it casts an oblong or rectangular shadow; if not, the shadow is oval or almost circular.[51] With a varus force applied across the extended elbow, the maximal tilt directed laterally and the elbow in varus, the radial head can be reduced with the pressure of a finger (Fig. 10-16, right). An alternative technique with the elbow in extension was described by Neher and Torch.[75] An assistant uses both thumbs to place a laterally directed force on the proximal radial shaft while the surgeon applies a varus stress to the elbow. Simultaneously, the surgeon uses his other thumb to apply a reduction force directly to the radial head (Fig. 10-17).[75]

The Israeli technique involves stabilization of the proximal fragment with the thumb anteriorly while rotating the forearm into full pronation to reduce the shaft to the proximal fragment.[54] The elbow should be flexed to 90 degrees for the manipulation (Figs. 10-18 and 10-19). Another technique emphasizing reduction of the shaft to the proximal fragment was recently described by Monson.[71] After adequate sedation or anesthesia, the elbow is flexed to 90 degrees and forearm

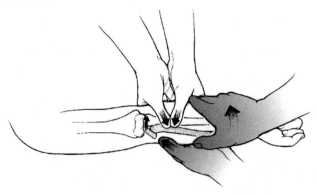

Figure 10-17. Neher and Torch reduction technique. (Reprinted with permission from Neher CG, Torch MA. New reduction technique for severely displaced pediatric radial neck fractures. *J Pediatr Orthop.* 2003;23(5):626–628.)

fully supinated. The proximal radial fragment should be stabilized in place by the annular ligament. A direct force is applied to the radial shaft to reduce the shaft to the head (Figs. 10-20 and 10-21). Initial experience with this technique in six children has been reported with excellent results and no further need for additional procedures.[71]

Lastly, use of an Esmarch bandage wrap, as is done for limb exsanguination prior to tourniquet use in extremity surgery, has been described to serendipitously promote fracture reduction (Fig. 10-22).[17] This can be used as an easy adjunct in nearly all of the described closed reduction techniques.

Regardless of the technique chosen, alignment should be assessed by fluoroscopy. Radial neck angulation should be

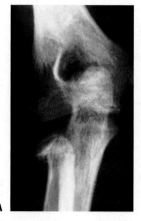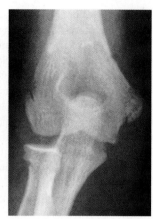

Figure 10-18. Flexion–pronation (Israeli) reduction technique. **A:** Radiograph of the best reduction obtained by the Patterson[85] method. (Reprinted with permission from Klitscher D, Richter S, Bodenschatz K, et al. Evaluation of severely displaced radial neck fractures in children treated with elastic stable intramedullary nailing. *J Pediatr Orthop.* 2009;29(7):698–703.) **B:** Position of the radial head after the flexion–pronation method. (Reprinted with permission from Patterson RF. Treatment of displaced transverse fractures of the neck of the radius in children. *J Bone Joint Surg.* 1934;16(3):695–698.)

reduced to less than 45 degrees in children under 10 years of age, and less than 30 degrees in children greater than 10 years of age. The radiocapitellar joint needs to be congruent. The elbow joint must be stable to stress. Immobilization for a short duration is recommended for pain control and soft tissue healing. Early range of motion should be encouraged once the acute pain has resolved, generally within 1 to 3 weeks.

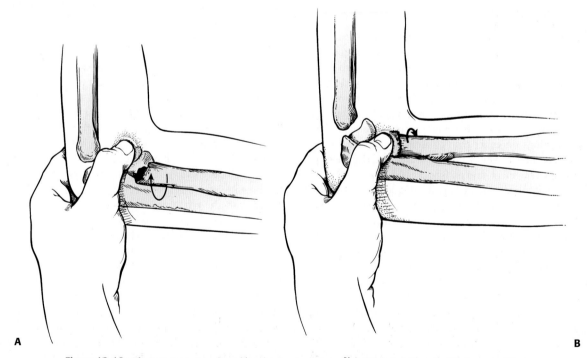

Figure 10-19. Flexion–pronation (Israeli) reduction technique.[54] **A:** With the elbow in 90 degrees of flexion, the thumb stabilizes the displaced radial head. Usually the distal radius is in a position of supination. The forearm is pronated to swing the shaft up into alignment with the neck (*arrow*). **B:** Movement is continued to full pronation for reduction (*arrow*).

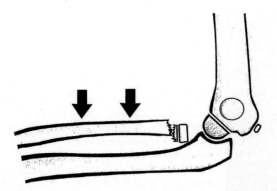

Figure 10-20. As the fracture is usually displaced laterally, placing the forearm in supination results in the apex being anterior. The radial head is relatively stable and locked by the annular ligament. Pressure on the proximal radial shaft (*solid arrows*) with the arm in supination reduces the shaft to the radial head. (Reprinted with permission from Monson R, Black B, Reed M. A new closed reduction technique for the treatment of radial neck fractures in children. *J Pediatr Orthop.* 2009;29(3):243–247.)

OPERATIVE TREATMENT OF FRACTURES OF THE PROXIMAL RADIUS

Indications/Contraindications

Operative Treatment of Fractures of the Proximal Radius:
INDICATIONS AND CONTRAINDICATIONS

Indications
- Displacement remains over 2 mm following closed alignment
- Angulation is greater than 45 degrees (age <10)
- Angulation is greater than 30 degrees (age >10)

Contraindications
- Acceptable alignment can be achieved with closed means
- No persistent elbow instability
- Unrestricted range of motion after closed treatment

Surgical treatment is indicated when acceptable alignment cannot be achieved with closed means, or if there is persistent elbow instability or restricted range of motion after closed treatment. Most fractures of the proximal radius present to the surgeon with minimal deformity and do not require treatment other

than a short period of immobilization. Operative treatment is considered when displacement remains over 2 mm, angulation is greater than 45 degrees (age <10) or greater than 30 degrees (age <10)—most importantly joint incongruity, and for open injuries. Nerve palsy is generally not an indication for surgery because most will recover function over time.

Instrument-Assisted Closed Reduction

Preoperative Planning

✔ Instrument-Assisted Closed Reduction of Proximal Radius Fractures: PREOPERATIVE PLANNING CHECKLIST	
OR table	☐ Standard with radiolucent hand table
Position/positioning aids	☐ Turn table 90 degrees, bring patient to edge of table toward hand table. Secure head with blanket/towel and tape. Safety strap over torso
Fluoroscopy location	☐ In line with affected extremity, perpendicular to OR table
Equipment	☐ Smooth K-wires
Tourniquet	☐ Nonsterile
Other	☐ Esmarch bandage

Positioning

The patient should be positioned supine on the operating table with a radiolucent hand table attached to the operating bed. The affected extremity should be placed directly in the middle of the hand table. The entire operating table should be rotated 90 degrees from standard position to place the injured extremity opposite the anesthesiologist. Fluoroscopy will be brought in directly in line with the injured extremity with surgeon and assistant on either side of the hand table (Fig. 10-23). The patient should be brought to the lateral edge of the bed and head secured to the operating room table. We suggest a towel or blanket draped over the head, surrounded by strong tape from one edge of the table to the other (Fig. 10-24). This is especially important for small patients, to allow for the fluoroscopy unit to be able to image the area of interest and not be blocked by the table. The torso should be secured to the table

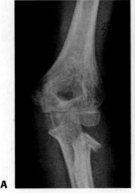
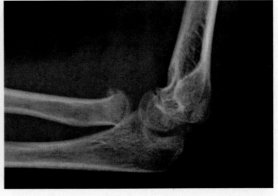

Figure 10-21. A: Preoperative anteroposterior and lateral radiographs of left elbow of a 9-year-old girl showing 34 degrees of angulation and 50% displacement.

(continues)   **A**

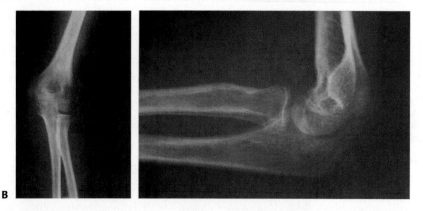

B

Figure 10-21. (*Continued*) **B:** Anteroposterior and lateral radiographs of the fracture 5 months postreduction showing maintenance of reduction with good callus formation. (Reprinted with permission from Monson R, Black B, Reed M. A new closed reduction technique for the treatment of radial neck fractures in children. *J Pediatr Orthop.* 2009;29(3):243–247.)

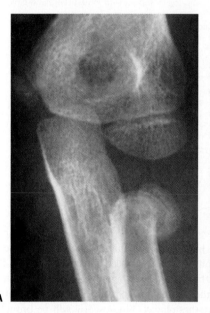

A

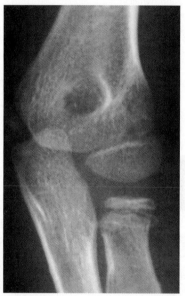

B

Figure 10-22. Elastic bandage wrap reduction. **A:** The final position achieved after manipulation by the Patterson[85] method. (Reprinted with permission from Patterson RF. Treatment of displaced transverse fractures of the neck of the radius in children. *J Bone Joint Surg.* 1934;16(3):695–698.) **B:** Position of the radial head after applying an elastic bandage to exsanguinate the extremity.

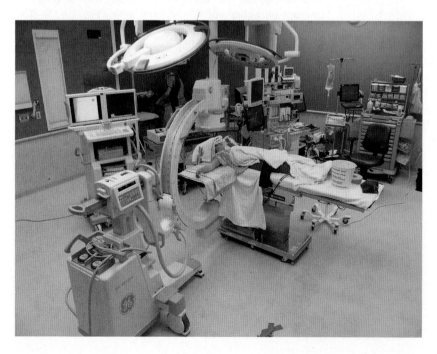

Figure 10-23. Preferred positioning and operative room setup for operative treatment of proximal radius and ulna fractures.

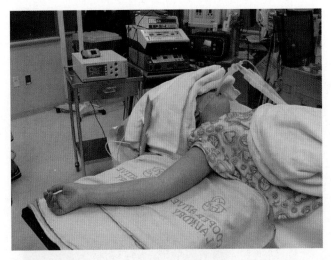

Figure 10-24. Detailed view of showing recommended method of securing head safely to the operative table while allowing for appropriate elbow positioning on the hand table for intraoperative fluoroscopy.

with a safety strap. A nonsterile tourniquet should be applied to the humerus. Surgeons may be standing or seated per their preference.

Surgical Approach

Percutaneous direct lateral approach is utilized as described in the technique below to minimize risk of injury to the PIN.

Technique

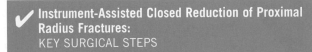

> **✓ Instrument-Assisted Closed Reduction of Proximal Radius Fractures:**
> **KEY SURGICAL STEPS**
>
> ❑ Attempt closed reduction
> ❑ Percutaneous insertion of blunt end K-wire lateral forearm
> ❑ Reduce fracture by pushing on proximal fragment
> ❑ Assess stability and range of motion
>   • If stable: Immobilize in long-arm cast
>   • If unstable: Antegrade K-wire fixation
> ❑ Alternatively—use leverage technique described in text

Simple steel smooth Kirschner wires (K-wires) generally are appropriate to assist with closed reduction. Size will range from 2 to 2.7 mm based on the size of the child. Other instruments utilized include Steinmann pins, periosteal elevators, or a double-pointed bident.[4,38,98] Fluoroscopy is used to localize the fracture site and intended entry site of the wire. This should be along the direct lateral cortex of the radial shaft to decrease risk of injury to the PIN. Pronating the forearm further moves the PIN away from the surgical field. Skin is incised with a small stab wound and a small curved clamp is utilized to bluntly dissect through the muscle to the radial cortex. The sharp end of the wire is cut for surgeon safety and the blunt end is inserted down to the radial cortex. Fluoroscopic guidance is used to localize the fracture site, and the blunt end of the wire can be used to push the distal fracture fragment back into an appropriate position (Fig. 10-25). Arthrography can be helpful to assess congruency

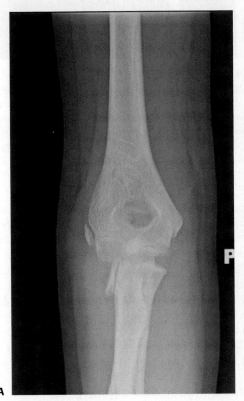
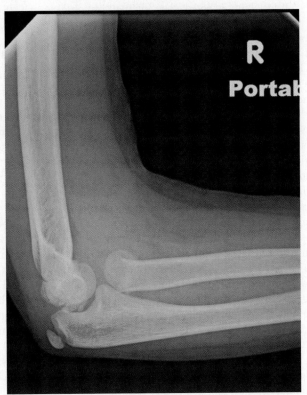

Figure 10-25. Instrument-assisted closed reduction of the proximal radius. **A:** AP radiograph of an angulated radial neck fracture in a 10-year-old female. **B:** Lateral radiograph of the same patient.

(continues)

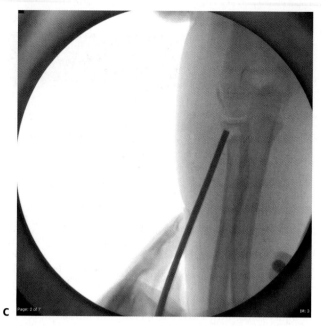

Figure 10-25. (*Continued*) **C:** Intraoperative fluoroscopy showing blunt end of a K-wire assisting with reduction of the fracture by direct manipulation of the proximal fragment.

of the elbow joint in the young.[23] Once the fracture is reduced to within appropriate guidelines, the pin is removed and stability and range of motion are assessed. If the fracture remains stable through a normal arc of motion, no internal fixation is needed.[9,78,137] If instability is noted, then internal fixation can be placed. Small antegrade K-wires can be placed percutaneously to transfix the fracture[24,34,52] (Fig. 10-26). Pins should stay lateral to minimize injury to the PIN. Pins traversing the capitellum into the proximal radius should be avoided because they have a high rate of migration and/or pin breakage.[34,78,104,137] Various iterations of this technique have been described in the literature.[4,8,24,88,113]

Alternatively, the sharp end of the wire can be retained and introduced to the fracture site and the wire used as a lever to correct angulation.[16,18,111,142] Similarly, if stable after pin removal, then further fixation is not necessary. However, if unstable, then once corrected, the pin can be driven from proximal to distal across the radial cortex and serve as a buttress against recurrent angulation of the distal fragment. In this instance, the wire is introduced through the skin closer to the fracture site than in the prior described technique, to prevent soft tissue from blocking appropriate leverage of the distal fracture fragment. The pin is cut short but left out of the skin and underneath postoperative immobilization. It may be removed in 1 to 3 weeks when the surgeon is comfortable allowing range of motion at the elbow (Fig. 10-27). A slight variation of this technique was recently described in which the pin was temporarily inserted into the proximal fracture fragment instead of the fracture site. Similar leverage technique is used to reduce the fracture followed by intramedullary fixation with a separate wire as described in the next section, followed by removal of the temporary wire in the proximal fragment.[133]

A modification described by Wallace utilizes an instrument to provide counterforce on the radial shaft. Fluoroscopy in an

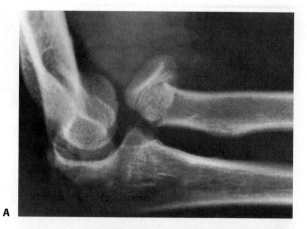

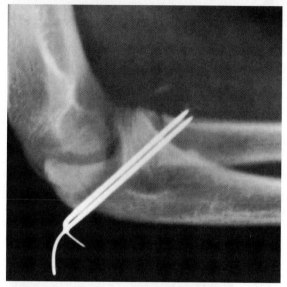

Figure 10-26. Oblique pin. **A:** Displaced fracture of the radial neck in a 10 year old. **B:** A closed reduction was performed, and to stabilize the head fragment, two pins were placed percutaneously and obliquely across the fracture site from proximal to distal. If open reduction and pinning are done, the preferred alignment is obliquely across the fracture site from distal to proximal. (From Wilkins KE, ed. *Operative Management of Upper Extremity Fractures in Children.* Rosemont, IL: American Academy of Orthopaedic Surgeons; 1994:57, with permission.)

AP projection is used to determine the forearm rotation that exposes the maximum amount of deformity of the fracture, and the level of the bicipital tuberosity of the proximal radius is marked. A 1-cm dorsal skin incision is made at that level just lateral to the subcutaneous border of the ulna. A periosteal elevator is gently inserted between the ulna and the radius, with care not to disrupt the periosteum of the radius or the ulna. The radial shaft is usually much more ulnarly displaced than expected, and the radial nerve is lateral to the radius at this level. While counter pressure is applied against the radial head, the distal fragment of the radius is levered away from the ulna. An assistant can aid in this maneuver by gently applying traction and rotating the forearm back and forth to disengage the fracture fragments. The proximal radial fragment can be reduced either manually with thumb pressure or assisted by a percutaneous instrument as described (Figs. 10-28 and 10-29).

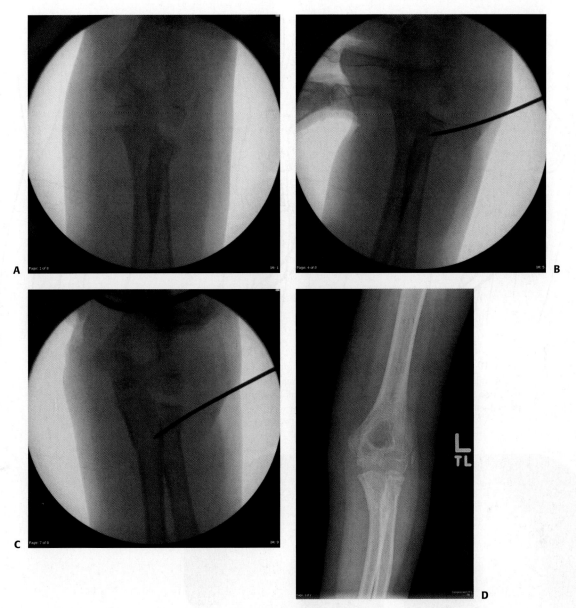

Figure 10-27. Leverage technique of instrument-assisted closed reduction of the proximal radius (**A**). Intraoperative AP fluoroscopy image demonstrating angulated radial neck fracture (**B**). K-wire inserted at fracture site and levering proximal fragment into a reduced position (**C**). AP view of elbow following pin removal in clinic showing anatomic alignment of proximal radius fracture (**D**). Same wire driven through the opposite cortex to hold reduced position of the proximal fragment.

Intramedullary Nail Reduction/Fixation

Preoperative Planning

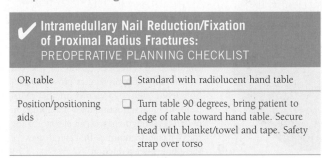

✔ Intramedullary Nail Reduction/Fixation of Proximal Radius Fractures: PREOPERATIVE PLANNING CHECKLIST	
OR table	☐ Standard with radiolucent hand table
Position/positioning aids	☐ Turn table 90 degrees, bring patient to edge of table toward hand table. Secure head with blanket/towel and tape. Safety strap over torso

Fluoroscopy location	☐ In line with affected extremity, perpendicular to OR table
Equipment	☐ Smooth K-wires
Tourniquet	☐ Nonsterile
Other	☐ Esmarch bandage

Implant size should be estimated prior to surgery. The technique was initially described using K-wires, which are readily available and inexpensive. Some prefer using titanium flexible nails that also work well but are more costly. The isthmus of

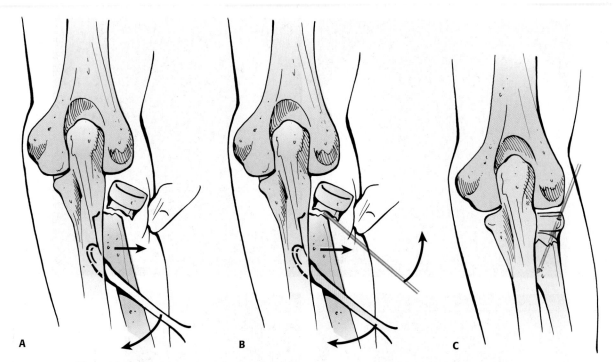

Figure 10-28. Wallace radial head reduction technique. **A:** A periosteal elevator is used to lever the distal fragment laterally while the thumb pushes the proximal fragment medially. **B:** K-wires are used to assist the reduction if necessary. Arrows indicate direction of movement of bone and instruments. **C:** The position of the reduction can be fixed with an oblique Kirschner wire.

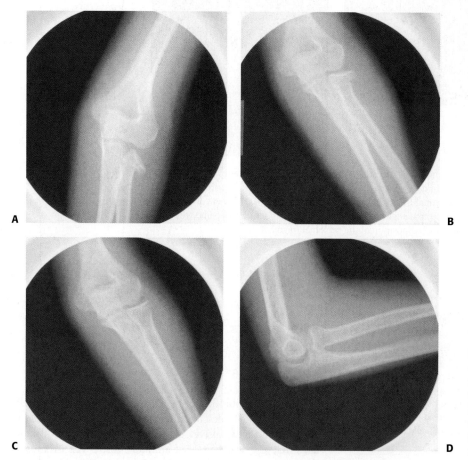

Figure 10-29. A: Radial neck fracture angulated 45 degrees in a 14-year-old female. **B:** Radiograph after closed reduction using thumb pressure on the radial head. **C:** Final reduction after manipulation of the distal fragment with an elevator using the Wallace technique. **D:** Lateral view of the elbow after reduction.

the radius should be measured on both AP and lateral views and implant size should be chosen to easily pass. Generally, an implant 60% to 70% of the width of the isthmus will pass without too much difficulty. In adolescents, this will usually be 2- or 2.4-mm K-wires. It is advised to have one size larger and smaller than planned available if needed.

Positioning

Same as for instrument-assisted closed reduction.

Surgical Approach(es)

The implant is inserted at the distal radius via a radial entry. The distal radial physis should be localized with fluoroscopy. A direct lateral incision of 1 to 2 cm is made just proximal to the physis of the distal radius. Careful scissor dissection to the lateral radial cortex is made with care taken not to injure the superficial radial nerve. It is not required to search for the nerve; however, if encountered, it should be gently retracted. Extensor tendons from the first dorsal compartment may also be encountered and should be retracted.

Alternatively, the implant may be inserted via a direct dorsal approach over the dorsal tubercle of the radius. Either longitudinal or transverse incisions may be utilized. Extensor tendons, especially extensor pollicis longus, will be encountered and should be protected during opening of the radial cortex at the dorsal tubercle.

Technique

> ✔ **Intramedullary Nail Reduction/Fixation of Proximal Radius Fractures:**
> KEY SURGICAL STEPS
>
> ❑ Pre-bend implant at distal end
> ❑ Open distal radial cortex via radial or dorsal approach
> ❑ Advance implant to the fracture site
> ❑ Closed manipulation of fracture to allow implant to enter distal fragment
> ❑ Advance implant into distal fragment
> ❑ Rotate implant as needed to reduce fracture
> ❑ Assess stability and range of motion
> ❑ Cut implant distally under the skin
> ❑ Close surgical wound
> ❑ Immobilize to allow for soft tissue healing

Intramedullary reduction and fixation of proximal radius fractures was described by Metaizeau in 1980.[70] After selection of an appropriate-sized implant (K-wire or titanium flexible nail), the distal 3 to 4 mm of the implant should be bent sharply about 40 degrees. Either a dorsal or radial approach can be utilized at the entry site of the distal radius. The wire is advanced through the radial canal to the fracture site. If necessary, closed maneuvers should be used to improve alignment at the fracture site to allow for successful passage of the distal tip of the implant into the proximal fragment. The implant should be impacted into the epiphysis to achieve maximal fixation prior to reduction attempts with the implant. Once advanced appropriately, the nail should be rotated 90 to 180 degrees as needed

to reduce the proximal fragment. The forearm should be held by the assistant to prevent the radial shaft from rotating with the implant (Fig. 10-30). Stability at the elbow joint and range of motion are assessed. The implant should be cut distally, balancing need for ease of recovery during implant removal with soft tissue irritation from implant prominence at the distal radius. Rigid immobilization is not necessary with use of an intramedullary implant; however, most surgeons will immobilize the extremity in a long-arm splint or cast for 7 to 10 days for pain relief and to allow for soft tissue healing. Early range of motion is encouraged to minimize postoperative stiffness.

Open Reduction Internal Fixation

Preoperative Planning

> ✔ **ORIF of Proximal Radius Fractures:**
> PREOPERATIVE PLANNING CHECKLIST

OR table	❑ Standard with radiolucent hand table
Position/positioning aids	❑ Turn table 90 degrees, bring patient to edge of table toward hand table. Secure head with blanket/towel and tape. Safety strap over torso
Fluoroscopy location	❑ In line with affected extremity, perpendicular to OR table
Equipment	❑ 2- to 2.7-mm screws; mini-fragment plates versus fracture-specific plates (radial neck, radial head)
Tourniquet	❑ Nonsterile
Other	❑ Esmarch bandage

Appropriate implants should be available if rigid internal fixation is planned. These may include mini-fragment screws, mini- or modular-fragment plates, or specialty proximal radius plates. Small fragment screws and plates are often too large for fixation of the proximal radius. Specialty plates are produced by numerous manufacturers, but are designed for adult patients. Many will be too large for children and young adolescents; however, they may fit appropriately in the older adolescent. Recently, bioabsorbable rods and pins (poly-L-lactic acid) have been reported in small case series for fixation of radial head and neck fractures in children.[36,115]

Positioning

Same as for instrument-assisted closed reduction.

Surgical Approach(es)

A lateral approach to the proximal radius should be used for open reduction of proximal radius fractures. Either the lateral Kocher or Kaplan approach provides appropriate exposure. In the Kocher, dissection is between the anconeus and extensor carpi ulnaris. Usually, the interval is easier to identify distally and can be traced back proximally. The muscle fibers will be seen to run in divergent directions distally, which assist with location

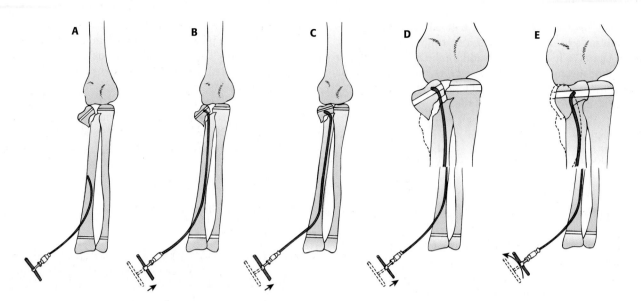

Figure 10-30. Intramedullary pin reduction. **A:** The insertion point for the curved flexible pin is in the metaphysis. **B:** The curved end of the rod passes in the shaft and engages the proximal fragment. **C:** Manipulation of the rod disimpacts the fracture. **D, E:** Once disimpacted, the head fragment is rotated into position with the intramedullary rod. (Reprinted with permission from Metaizeau JP, Lascombes P, Lemelle JL, et al. Reduction and fixation of displaced radial neck fractures by closed intramedullary pinning. *J Pediatr Orthop.* 1993;13(3):355–360.)

of the interval. The Kaplan approach is more anterior and is ligament sparing. Often the annular ligament will be traumatically disrupted and also the joint capsule will be disrupted. Care should be taken to stay superior to the lateral collateral ligament of the elbow to prevent adding iatrogenic instability. The supinator may be released distally, if needed, for plate application.

When exposing the proximal radius, the forearm should be kept in a pronated position to move the PIN further away from the surgical field. Vigorous retraction should be avoided anteriorly to limit traction on the PIN.

Technique

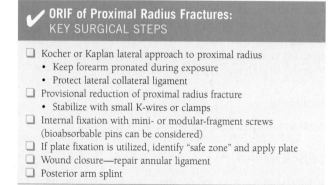

✔ **ORIF of Proximal Radius Fractures:**
  KEY SURGICAL STEPS

❏ Kocher or Kaplan lateral approach to proximal radius
  • Keep forearm pronated during exposure
  • Protect lateral collateral ligament
❏ Provisional reduction of proximal radius fracture
  • Stabilize with small K-wires or clamps
❏ Internal fixation with mini- or modular-fragment screws
  (bioabsorbable pins can be considered)
❏ If plate fixation is utilized, identify "safe zone" and apply plate
❏ Wound closure—repair annular ligament
❏ Posterior arm splint

After adequate exposure of the fracture site, the anatomy of the fracture should be evaluated. Radial neck fractures are more common and can be reduced using manual pressure or instrumented manipulation. Often, a dental pick is useful to hold a reduced position after manual reduction. The fracture can be either definitively or provisionally fixed at this point with small K-wires. Radial head fractures are usually more complex and may have multiple fragments. Attempts should be made to reduce the radial head in children and adolescents with use of small pins or bone clamps to hold provisional reduction. Radial head excision is a salvage operation and should be considered as a primary treatment only if there is extensive comminution prohibiting reconstruction. Results have been uniformly poor after excision with high incidence of cubitus valgus and radial deviation at the wrist.[25,48,52] Radial head replacement has not been described for children or adolescents but is increasingly utilized for adults.

When proceeding with open reduction, most surgeons elect to place more rigid fixation to allow for early range of motion. Screw fixation with mini-fragment screws or small headless screws provides stable fixation of radial head and neck fractures (Figs. 10-31 and 10-32).[109] Plates have been utilized for fixation of radial neck fractures requiring open reduction (Fig. 10-33). They should be placed in the "safe zone" of the proximal radius. This is an area of about 100 to 110 degrees of the circumference of the proximal radius that does not articulate with the proximal ulna during forearm rotation. With the forearm in 10 degrees of supination, the "safe zone" is directly lateral.[110,112] It is also found in the interval between the radial styloid and Lister's tubercle. Screws should be kept unicortical to prevent perforation into the PRUJ. Plate application requires more extensive dissection than isolated screw fixation and has led some authors to strongly advocate for multiple screw fixation alone for radial head and neck fractures. There is no good quality evidence supporting one form of internal fixation over another in the treatment of fractures of the proximal radius.

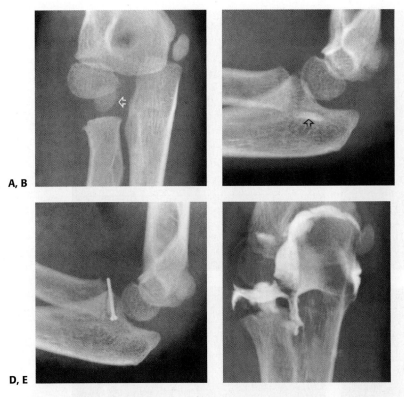

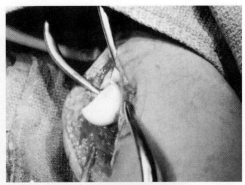

A, B

C

D, E

Figure 10-31. Miniscrew fixation. **A, B:** Anteroposterior and lateral views of the elbow of a 6-year-old male in whom the head fragment lies posterior to the capitellum (*arrows*). **C:** At the time of open reduction, a Salter–Harris type III fracture through the epiphysis and proximal physis was apparent. The fragment involved 60% of the head diameter and had soft tissue attached. **D:** A screw placed through the epiphysis fixed the reduction. **E:** Six months after surgery, an arthrogram showed maintenance of the architectural structure of the medial head after screw removal. The patient had 60 degrees of supination and pronation. (From Wilkins KE, ed. *Operative Management of Upper Extremity Fractures in Children.* Rosemont, IL: American Academy of Orthopaedic Surgeons; 1994:58, with permission.)

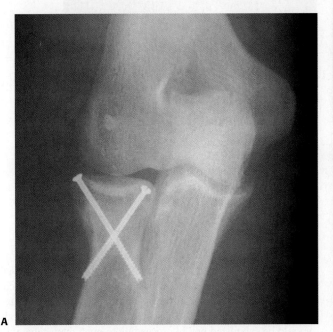

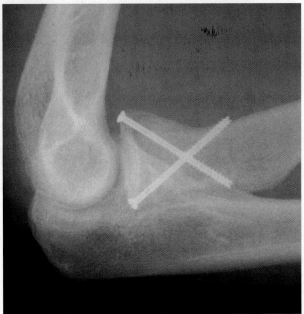

A

B

Figure 10-32. Patient underwent operative intervention using low-profile fixation with 3-mm cannulated screws and repair of a torn lateral ulnar collateral ligament complex. Gentle range of motion was started on postoperative day 1 and progressed as tolerated. Anteroposterior (**A**) and lateral (**B**) radiographs of the elbow at 3-month follow-up demonstrated healing of the fracture, and clinical assessment demonstrated full function and range of motion. (Reprinted with permission from Smith AM, Morrey BF, Steinmann SP. Low profile fixation of radial head and neck fractures: Surgical technique and clinical experience. *J Orthop Trauma.* 2007;21(10):718–724.)

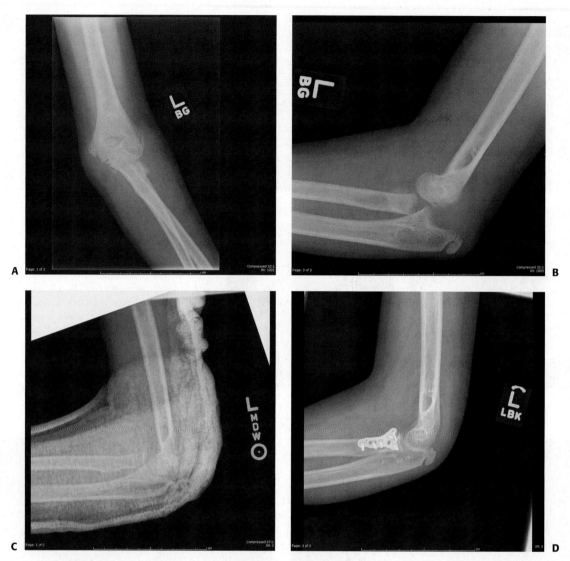

Figure 10-33. Open reduction internal fixation of a proximal radius fracture. **A:** AP radiograph of an 11-year-old female with elbow dislocation and radial neck fracture. **B:** Lateral radiograph of the same patient. **C:** Lateral radiograph in splint after closed reduction showing persistent radiocapitellar subluxation. Examination under anesthesia demonstrated very unstable elbow joint and therefore decision made to proceed with open reduction internal fixation. **D:** Lateral radiograph after open reduction internal fixation with a fracture-specific plate.

During closure, the annular ligament and joint capsule should be repaired if injured during the trauma or surgical dissection. The arm should be immobilized in a posterior splint for 1 to 2 weeks to allow for soft tissue healing before initiating range of motion. A regional anesthetic block prior to surgery or after surgery can provide improved patient comfort postoperatively. A detailed neurologic examination should be conducted preoperatively prior to regional nerve block and postoperatively after surgical exposure.

Outcomes

Severities of initial displacement and angulation are the best predictors of results after treatment. A higher incidence of good outcomes is found in patients who do not require fracture manipulation (closed or open) and present with fractures with minimal angulation and displacement.[78,123] For patients having operative treatment, closed methods generally lead to improved results compared to open treatments when the joint is aligned. This is again largely because of increased severity of fractures requiring open reduction. All closed and percutaneous methods should be exhausted before proceeding to open management of proximal radius fractures.

The overall incidence of poor results in large series varies from 15% to 33%.[7,21,31,34,48,52,114,128,144] Considering only severely displaced fractures, the incidence of poor results was as high as 50%.[114] A multivariable model developed in Boston identified degree of displacement at presentation as the only predictor of outcome with a 25% rate of unsuccessful outcomes with 35% displacement and 50% rate of unsuccessful outcomes with 76% displacement.[144] It is wise to counsel the parents before beginning treatment if poor prognostic factors are present. These include higher amounts of displacement or angulation, age >10 years, high-energy mechanism, associated injuries such as elbow dislocation, olecranon fracture, or other fractures of the elbow.[34,60,101,114]

Various tolerances for residual angulation have been described, and most authors believe that good results and remodeling can be achieved when there are less than 30 to 45 degrees of angulation.[9,26,60,67,78,79,92,128,131] D'Souza evaluated the results in 100 children from 1972 to 1990 and described better results with closed compared to open treatment. Overall, 86 patients had results described as "good" or "excellent." More recently, Tan and Mahadev[117] reported on 108 children with radial neck fractures. The majority were treated nonsurgically with only eight requiring a closed reduction, seven requiring instrument-assisted closed reduction, and seven requiring open reduction. Results were "excellent" in 93 children. Adverse outcomes were more likely in older patients and those with associated fractures about the elbow. Most believe that ability to achieve less than 30 to 45 degrees of angulation with closed treatment provides superior outcomes compared to patients having open reduction even with anatomic alignment.

As opposed to substantial angulation, displacement is not well tolerated because of the "cam effect" described. More recently, there has been increased attention paid to intra-articular radial head fractures in children.[1] These are problematic injuries and must be monitored closely. Progressive posterior radiocapitellar subluxation has been described, leading to severe cartilage deterioration (Fig. 10-34). Most patients with progressive subluxation presenting in a delayed manner end up requiring radial head excision.[129] Functional outcomes are very poor when this is identified and treated in a delayed manner.

An increasing number of reports with good results after intramedullary wire technique for angulated and displaced proximal radius fractures have been published recently.[133] Self-determined "excellent" results are described in 80% to 90% patients in these reported series.[27,44,56,69,88,127,133]

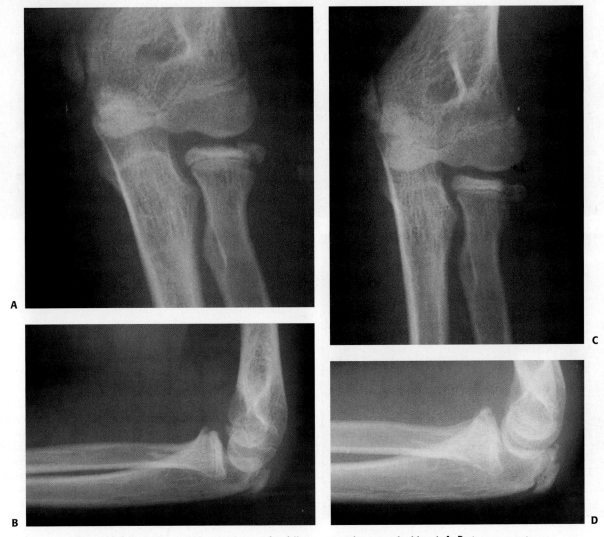

Figure 10-34. A 10-year-old male patient after fall on pronated outstretched hand. **A, B:** Anteroposterior and lateral radiographs of the injured elbow. Salter–Harris III fracture of radial epiphysis without evidence of subluxation. **C, D:** Anteroposterior and lateral radiographs 6 weeks after the injury. No evidence of osseous union with posterolateral subluxation.

(continues)

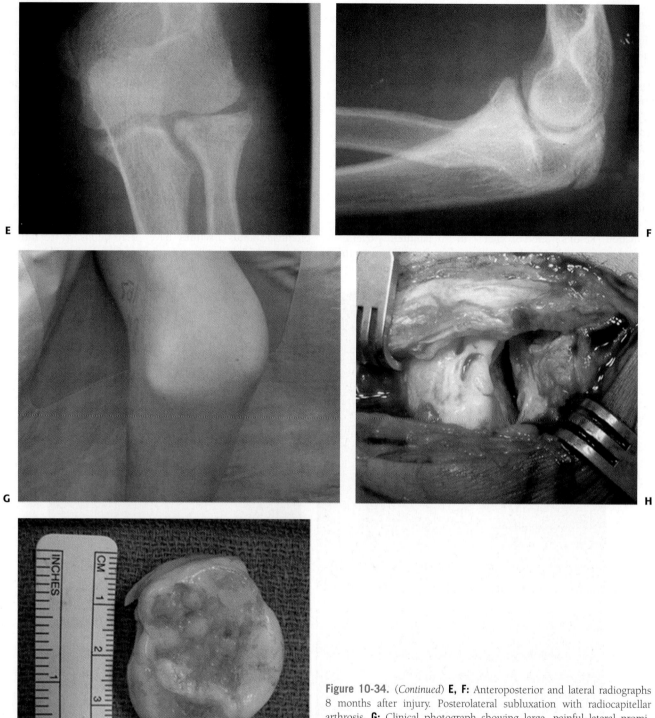

Figure 10-34. (*Continued*) **E, F:** Anteroposterior and lateral radiographs 8 months after injury. Posterolateral subluxation with radiocapitellar arthrosis. **G:** Clinical photograph showing large, painful lateral prominence. **H:** Intraoperative photograph showing severe radiocapitellar arthrosis. **I:** Gross, pathologic photograph of excised radial heal. (Reprinted with permission from Van Zeeland NL, Bae DS, Goldfarb CA. Intra-articular radial head fracture in the skeletally immature patient: Progressive radial head subluxation and rapid radiocapitellar degeneration. *J Pediatr Orthop.* 2011;31(2):124–129.)

Authors' Preferred Treatment for Fractures of the Proximal Radius (Algorithm 10-1)

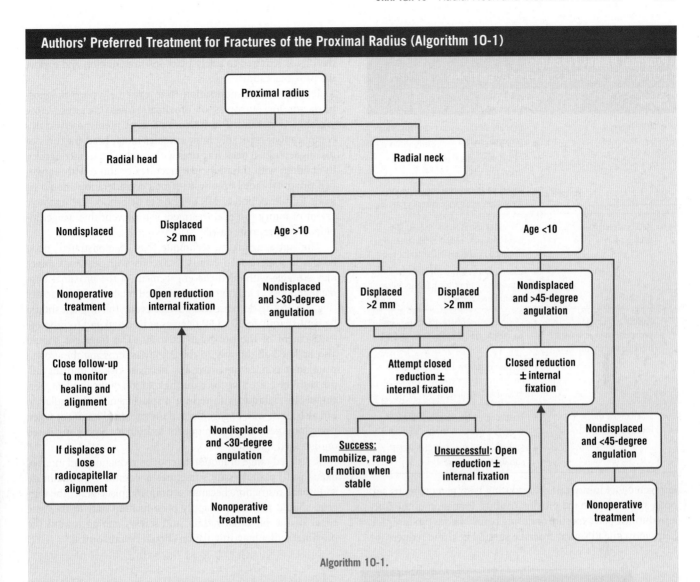

Algorithm 10-1.

Nonoperative management is our preferred treatment for most proximal radius fractures. Operative treatment should aim to reduce displacement of the radial head/neck to less than 2 mm, restore angulation of radial neck fractures to less than 30 to 45 degrees (based on child's age), and reduce the joint while also confirming normal arc of forearm rotation. Open approaches are avoided if these goals can be achieved closed. Necessity for internal fixation should be evaluated on an individual basis and avoided if possible. We have become more aggressive with operative treatment of radial head fractures because of the increased reports of adverse outcomes with progressive posterior radiocapitellar subluxation, articular incongruity, and joint malalignment. Low-profile internal fixation with mini-fragment screws and if needed, a mini-fragment plate and/or headless screw(s) is utilized for stable fixation to allow for early range of motion. MRI is utilized more frequently in the evaluation of radial head fractures because of its improved ability to assess for associated soft tissue injuries and evaluation of the radiocapitellar joint in skeletally immature patients.

Postoperative Care

Immobilization should only be for symptomatic relief from surgical trauma and soft tissue healing. Generally, 1 to 2 weeks is sufficient in patients with open reduction internal fixation or intramedullary fixation. Longer immobilization times of 2 to 3 weeks may be required for some patients treated without open reduction and internal fixation to achieve enough symptom relief before mobilization. Collar and cuff, posterior splint, and long-arm cast are all appropriate methods of immobilization. Range of motion should be allowed and encouraged when acute fracture pain has resolved and surgical scar has healed to lessen risk of permanent stiffness.

Potential Pitfalls and Preventative Measures

Proximal Radius Fractures:
POTENTIAL PITFALLS AND PREVENTIONS

Pitfall	Prevention
• PIN injury	• Pronate forearm when approaching proximal radius in open approaches
	• Avoid vigorous retraction during open reduction
	• Insert percutaneous implants for reduction assistance directly lateral
• Radiocapitellar subluxation	• Consider ultrasound or MRI for intra-articular radial head fractures, displaced extra-articular fractures
	• Close radiographic surveillance out of cast/splint for patients with radial head fracture
• Failure to engage proximal fragment with intramedullary implant	• Choose appropriate-sized implant based on preoperative templating
	• Ensure distal end of implant has an appropriate bend to capture proximal fragment
• Mechanical block to forearm rotation	• Ensure any plate fixation of the proximal radius is in the "safe zone"
	• Screws aiming toward the PRUJ should be unicortical

Iatrogenic PIN injury can occur during both percutaneous and open approaches to the proximal radius. Pronation of the forearm during open exposure or during percutaneous pin insertion helps move the PIN away from the surgical field and reduces the risk of nerve injury. Vigorous anterior retraction during open exposure should also be avoided. Knowledge of the anatomy of the PIN is required to safely place instrumentation and expose the proximal radius.

Radiocapitellar subluxation is an extremely poor prognostic factor for outcomes of proximal radius fractures. Close vigilance is warranted in fracture patterns predisposed to this complication, especially intra-articular radial head fractures or malaligned radial neck fractures with residual joint incongruity. In children with intra-articular fractures or those with unossified proximal radial epiphysis, strong consideration should be made for ultrasound or MR imaging to determine the anatomic extent of injury. Surgical treatment can prevent this dangerous pitfall in appropriate cases.

The intramedullary technique has demonstrated good results in experienced hands. Surgeons with less experience may struggle with adequate engagement of the proximal fragment and loss of fixation with attempted rotation of the implant (Fig. 10-35). To decrease this adverse event, the implant should be bent sharply to 30 to 40 degrees at its distal end to promote engagement of the proximal fragment. The fragment should also be fixed all the way to the epiphysis, crossing the growth plate, to maximize purchase, and decrease risk of implant failure with the corrective force during rotation of the implant. Percutaneous techniques to reduce displacement and angulation can also assist with engagement of the proximal fragment when using intramedullary technique for fixation for highly angulated or displaced fractures.

Restricted range of motion after open reduction and internal fixation of proximal radius fractures is common. To minimize additional restriction because of implant placement, the surgeon should take care to apply plate fixation only to the "safe zone" of the proximal radius, and screws aiming toward the proximal radioulnar articulation should be unicortical.

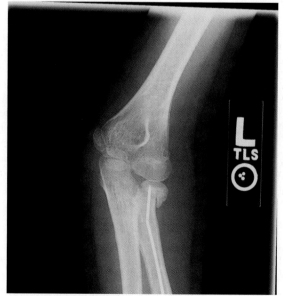 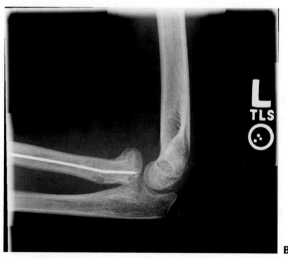

Figure 10-35. Failure of fixation with intramedullary technique for proximal radius fracture. **A:** AP view showing loss of fixation of the proximal fragment. **B:** Lateral view showing loss of fixation of the proximal fragment.

MANAGEMENT OF EXPECTED ADVERSE OUTCOMES AND UNEXPECTED COMPLICATIONS IN FRACTURES OF THE PROXIMAL RADIUS

Proximal Radius Fractures:
COMMON ADVERSE OUTCOMES AND COMPLICATIONS

- Loss of range of motion
- Radial head overgrowth
- Avascular necrosis of the radial head
- Nonunion
- Malunion
- Proximal radioulnar synostosis
- Cubitus valgus
- PIN injury

Loss of Range of Motion

Loss of motion is secondary to a combination of loss of joint congruity and posttraumatic or postoperative soft tissue scarring. Loss of pronation is more common than loss of supination. Flexion and extension are rarely significantly limited. Very little improvement in motion occurs after 6 months. Steinberg et al.[114] found that range of motion in their patients at 6 months was almost equal to that when the patients were examined years later. Patients should be encouraged to start range of motion early with both nonoperative and operative treatment to minimize loss of motion from posttraumatic stiffness. Both static and dynamic splinting can be useful along with aggressive therapy in the treatment of posttraumatic or postoperative elbow sand forearm stiffness.

Radial Head Overgrowth

Next to loss of range of motion of the elbow and forearm, radial head overgrowth is probably the most common sequela (20% to 40%).[26,128] The increased vascularity following the injury may stimulate epiphyseal growth, but the mechanisms of overgrowth following fractures are poorly understood. Radial head overgrowth usually does not compromise functional results,[24,52] but it may produce some crepitus or clicking with forearm rotation.[26]

Premature Physeal Closure

Many series report premature physeal closure[34,40,78,79,114,137] after fractures of the radial head and neck. This complication did not appear to affect the overall results significantly, except in one patient described by Fowles and Kassab,[34] who had a severe cubitus valgus. Newman[78] found that shortening of the radius was never more than 5 mm compared with the opposite uninjured side.

Osteonecrosis

The incidence of osteonecrosis is probably higher than recognized. D'Souza et al.[26] reported the frequency to be 10% to 20% in their patients, 70% of whom had open reductions. In patients with open reduction, the overall rate of osteonecrosis was 25%. Jones and Esah[52] and Newman[78] found that patients

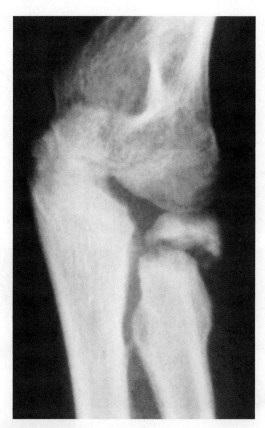

Figure 10-36. Osteonecrosis with nonunion in a radial head 1 year after open reduction. Both nonunion and osteonecrosis of the radial neck and head are present. Severe degenerative arthritis developed subsequently. (Courtesy of Richard E. King, MD.)

with osteonecrosis had poor functional results. It has been our experience, however, that revascularization can occur without any significant functional loss. Only in those in whom a residual functional deficit occurs is osteonecrosis considered a problem (Fig. 10-36).

Malunion

Failure to reduce a displaced and angulated proximal radial fracture in a young child often results in an angulated radial neck with subsequent incongruity of both the PRUJ and the radiocapitellar joint (Fig. 10-37). Partial physeal arrest can also create this angulation (see Fig. 10-3). In our experience, this malunion, because of the incongruity of the radiocapitellar joint, often results in erosion of the articular surface of the capitellum, with subsequent degenerative joint disease.

Nonunion

Nonunion of the radial neck is rare; union may occur[104] even after prolonged treatment (Fig. 10-38). Waters and Stewart[136] reported nine patients with radial neck nonunions, all of whom were treated with open reduction after failed attempts at closed reduction. These authors recommended observation of patients with radial neck nonunions who have limited symptoms and a functional range of motion. They suggested open reduction for displaced nonunions, patients with limited range of motion,

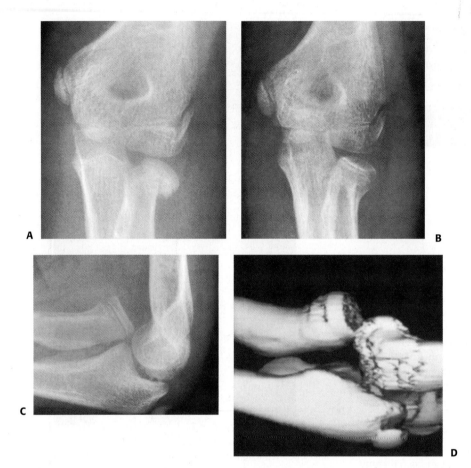

Figure 10-37. Angulation. **A:** Injury film showing 30 degrees of angulation and 30% lateral translocation of a radial neck fracture in a 10 year old. **B:** Radiograph appearance of the proximal radius taken about 5 months later, showing lateral angulation of the neck. **C:** Lateral view showing the anterior relationship of the radial neck with proximal migration. At this point, the patient had full supination and pronation but a clicking sensation with forearm rotation in the area of the radial head. **D:** Three-dimensional reconstruction showing the incongruity of the proximal radiocapitellar joint. (Courtesy of Vince Mosca, MD.)

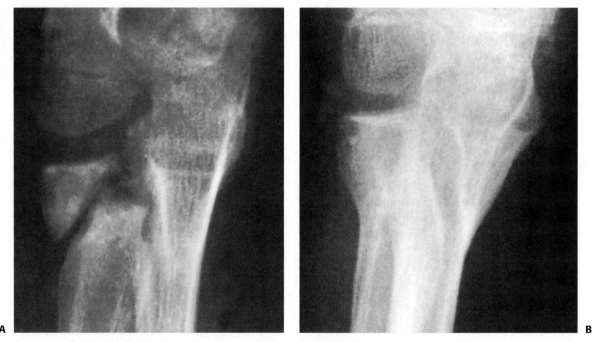

Figure 10-38. Nonunion. **A:** Eight months after radial neck fracture in an 8.5-year-old female. Patient had mild aching pain, but no loss of motion. There was some suggestion of proximal subluxation of the distal radioulnar joint. **B:** Three months later, the fracture is united after long-arm cast immobilization and external electromagnetic stimulation. (Courtesy of Charles T. Price, MD.)

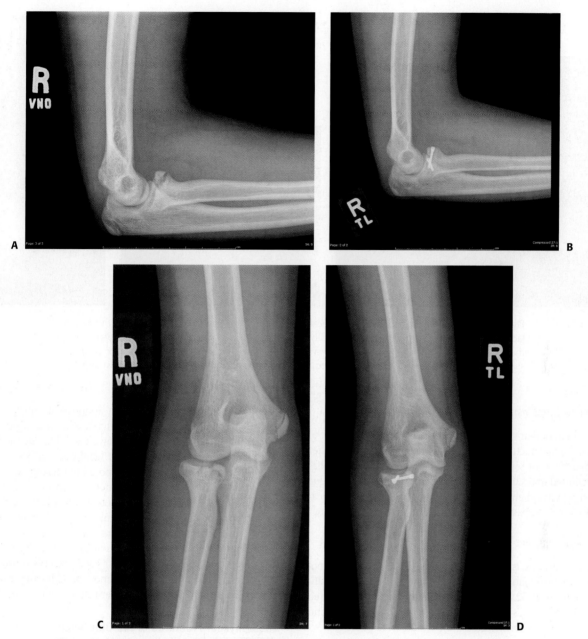

Figure 10-39. Nonunion of intra-articular radial head fracture. This 15-year-old female presented 1 year after elbow injury because of persistent pain. **A:** AP radiograph demonstrating nonunion of the radial head fracture. **B:** Lateral radiograph after open reduction and internal fixation. **C:** AP radiograph after open reduction and internal fixation. **D:** Lateral radiograph of the same patient.

and patients with restricting pain. Nonunion of intra-articular radial head fractures can also occur and should be treated with open reduction internal fixation if symptomatic and radiocapitellar joint has remained congruent (Fig. 10-39). In many cases, nonunion of these fractures leads to progressive radiocapitellar subluxation and cartilage destruction as previously described.

Changes in Carrying Angle (Cubitus Valgus)

In patients who have fractures of the radial neck, the carrying angle often is 10 degrees more (increased cubitus valgus) than on the uninjured side.[26,52] The increase in the carrying angle

appears to produce no functional deficit and no significant deformity.

Nerve Injuries

Partial ulnar nerve injury[48] and PIN injury may occur as a direct result of the fracture, but most injuries to the PINs are caused by surgical exploration[26] or percutaneous pin reduction.[6] These PIN injuries usually are transient and exploration is not generally warranted. However, if there is failure of recovery in a timely manner, then electrodiagnostics and surgical exposure are indicated.

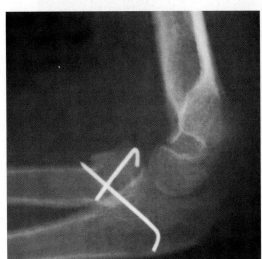
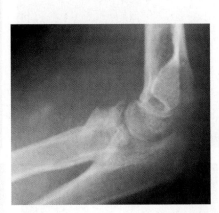
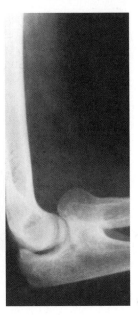

A, B   C

Figure 10-40. Radioulnar synostosis. **A:** Surgical intervention with wire fixation was necessary for a satis-factory reduction in this patient who had a totally displaced radial neck fracture. **B:** Six weeks after surgery, there was evidence of a proximal radioulnar synostosis. **C:** Radiograph taken 6 months after reduction shows a solid synostosis with anterior displacement of the proximal radius. (Courtesy of R.E. King, MD.)

Radioulnar Synostosis

Proximal radioulnar synostosis can occur following treatment of proximal radius fractures (Fig. 10-40). It occurs most often after open reduction of severely displaced fractures,[41,48,78,113] but has been reported to occur after closed reduction. Case reports argue that delayed treatment increases the likelihood of this complication. Treatment is based on functional limitation and disability.

Myositis Ossificans

Myositis ossificans is relatively common but usually does not impair function. Vahvanen[128] noted that some myositis ossificans occurred in 32% of his patients. In most, it was limited to the supinator muscle. If ossification was more extensive and was associated with a synostosis, the results were poor.

Fractures of the Proximal Ulna

ASSESSMENT OF FRACTURES OF THE PROXIMAL ULNA

MECHANISMS OF INJURY FOR FRACTURES OF THE PROXIMAL ULNA

Fractures Involving the Proximal Apophysis

The location of the triceps expansive insertion on the ulnar metaphysis, distal to the apophysis, probably accounts for the rarity of fracture along the apophyseal line. Only a few reports

mention the mechanism of these apophyseal injuries. In our experience, this fracture is usually caused by avulsion forces across the apophysis with the elbow flexed, like the more common flexion metaphyseal injuries. Children with osteogenesis imperfecta seem especially predisposed to this injury.[22,72]

Stress fractures of the olecranon apophysis can occur in athletes (especially throwing athletes) who place considerable recurrent tension forces on the olecranon.[37,83] Stress injuries also have been reported in surfers, elite gymnasts,[62] and tennis players.[96] If the recurring activity persists, a symptomatic nonunion can develop.[86,96,124,126,138] Paci[81] described use of cannulated screw fixation of an olecranon stress fracture leading to union and return to play in an overhead throwing athlete.

Metaphyseal Fractures of the Olecranon

Three main mechanisms produce metaphyseal olecranon fractures. First, in injuries occurring with the elbow flexed, posterior tension forces play an important role. Second, in injuries where the fracture occurs with the elbow extended, the varus or valgus bending stress across the olecranon is responsible for the typical fracture pattern. Third, a less common mechanism involves a direct blow to the elbow that produces an anterior bending or shear force across the olecranon. In this type, the tension forces are concentrated on the anterior portion of the olecranon.

Flexion Injuries

A fall with the elbow in flexion places considerable tension forces across the posterior aspect of the olecranon process. Proximally, the triceps applies a force to the tip of the olecranon process. Distally, there is some proximal pull by the insertion of the brachialis muscle. Thus, the posterior cortex is placed

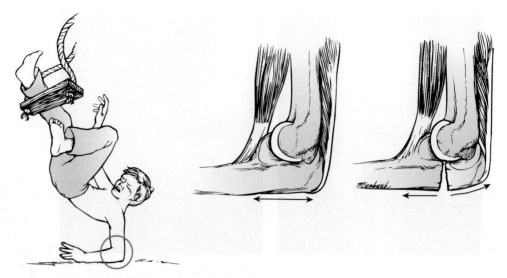

Figure 10-41. Mechanism of flexion injuries. **Center:** In the flexed elbow, a tension force develops on the posterior aspect of the olecranon (*small double arrow*). **Right:** Failure occurs on the tension side, which is posterior as a result of the muscle pull or a direct blow to the prestressed posterior olecranon. Arrows represent pull of brachialis (*left arrow*) and triceps (*right arrow*).

in tension. This tension force alone, if applied rapidly enough and with sufficient force, may cause the olecranon to fail at its midportion (Fig. 10-41). A direct blow applied to the posterior aspect of the stressed olecranon makes it more vulnerable to failure. With this type of mechanism, the fracture line is usually transverse and perpendicular to the long axis of the olecranon (Fig. 10-42). Because the fracture extends into the articular surface of the semilunar notch, it is classified as intra-articular.

The degree of separation of the fracture fragments depends on the magnitude of the forces applied and the integrity of the soft tissues. The low incidence of displaced olecranon fractures indicates that the soft tissues are quite resistant to these avulsion forces. In flexion injuries, there are relatively few associated soft tissue injuries or other fractures.[77]

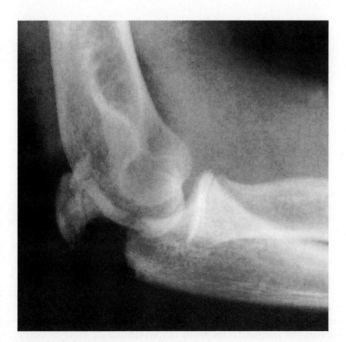

Figure 10-42. Radiograph of flexion injury showing greater displacement on the posterior surface.

Extension Injuries

Because children tend to have more ligamentous laxity, the elbow tends to hyperextend when a child breaks a fall with the outstretched upper extremity. In this situation, the olecranon may become locked into the olecranon fossa. If the elbow goes into extreme hyperextension, usually the supracondylar region of the distal humerus fails. If, however, the major direction of the force across the elbow is varus or valgus, a bending moment stresses the olecranon. Most of this force concentrates in the distal portion of the olecranon. Because the olecranon is metaphyseal bone, the force produces greenstick-type longitudinal fracture lines (Fig. 10-43). Most of these fracture lines are linear and remain extra-articular. In addition, because the fulcrum of the bending force is more distal, many of the fracture lines may extend distal to the coronoid process and into the proximal ulnar shaft regions. The major deformity of the olecranon with this type of fracture is usually an angulated greenstick type of pattern.

Many of these fractures are associated with other injuries in the elbow region, which depend on whether the bending force is directed toward varus or valgus. If a child falls with the forearm in supination, the carrying angle tends to place a valgus stress across the elbow. The result may be a greenstick fracture of the ulna with an associated fracture of the radial neck or avulsion of the medial epicondylar apophysis (Fig. 10-44). If the fracture involves the radial neck, Bado[5] classified it as an equivalent of the type I Monteggia lesion.

Shear Injuries

Anterior tension failure is a rare injury that can occur when a direct blow to the proximal ulna causes it to fail with an anterior tension force; the PRUJ maintains its integrity. The most common type of shear injury is caused by a force applied directly to the posterior aspect of the olecranon, with the distal fragment displacing anteriorly (Figs. 10-45 and 10-46). The intact PRUJ displaces with the distal fragment. In this type of injury, the elbow may be either flexed or extended when the direct shear force impacts the posterior aspect of the olecranon.

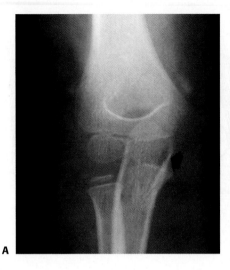
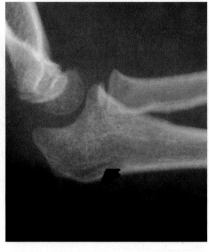

Figure 10-43. A: Anteroposterior view of a linear greenstick fracture line (*arrow*) in the medial aspect of the olecranon. **B:** Lateral view showing the posterior location of the fracture line (*arrow*).

These fractures are caused by a failure in tension, with the force concentrated along the anterior cortex. This is opposite to the tension failure occurring on the posterior aspect of the cortex in the more common flexion injuries. In the shear-type injury, the fracture line may be transverse or oblique. The differentiating feature from the more common flexion injury is that the thick posterior periosteum usually remains intact. The distal fragment is displaced anteriorly by the pull of the brachialis and biceps muscles. Newman[78] described one patient in whom a shear force was directed medially; the radial neck was fractured, and the radial head remained with the proximal fragment.

Fractures of the Coronoid Process

Isolated coronoid fractures are theoretically caused by avulsion stress from the brachialis or secondary to an elbow dislocation that reduced spontaneously. When associated with elbow

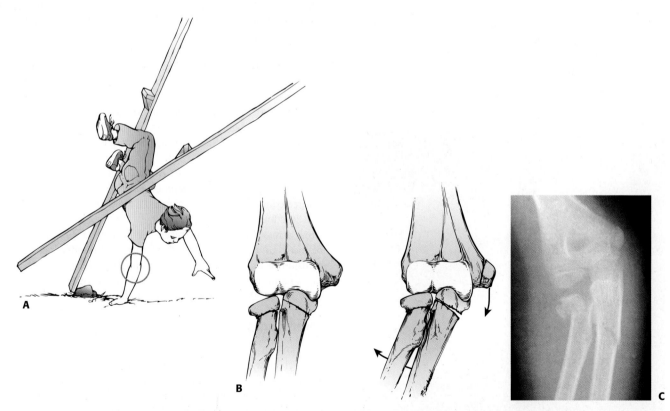

Figure 10-44. Valgus pattern of an extension fracture. **A:** A fall with the elbow extended places a valgus stress on the forearm. **B:** With increased valgus, a greenstick fracture of the olecranon can occur with or without a fracture of the radial neck or avulsion of the medial epicondylar apophysis (arrows denote direction of fracture displacement). **C:** Radiograph of a valgus extension fracture of the olecranon with an associated fracture of the radial neck.

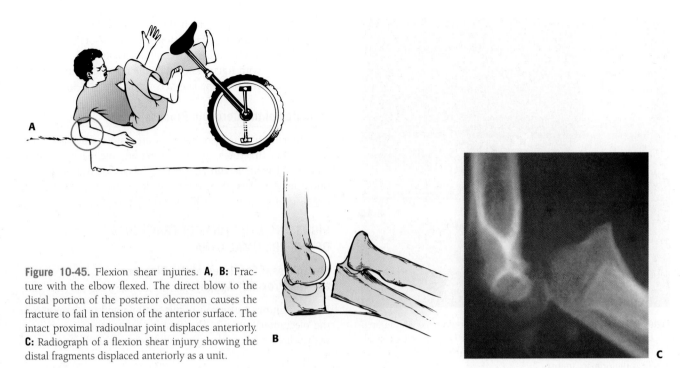

Figure 10-45. Flexion shear injuries. **A, B:** Fracture with the elbow flexed. The direct blow to the distal portion of the posterior olecranon causes the fracture to fail in tension of the anterior surface. The intact proximal radioulnar joint displaces anteriorly. **C:** Radiograph of a flexion shear injury showing the distal fragments displaced anteriorly as a unit.

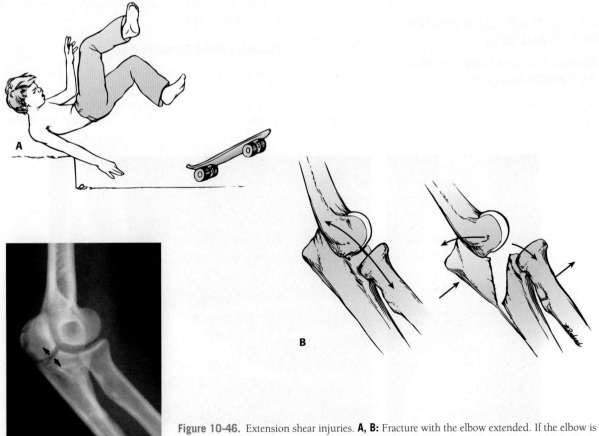

Figure 10-46. Extension shear injuries. **A, B:** Fracture with the elbow extended. If the elbow is extended when the direct blow to the posterior aspect of the elbow occurs, the olecranon fails in tension but with an oblique or transverse fracture line (*arrows*). **C:** With the elbow extended, the initial failure is in the anterior articular surface (*arrows*).

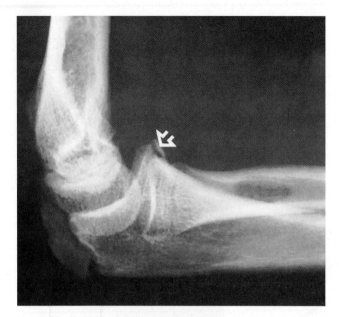

Figure 10-47. Lateral radiograph of an 11-year-old male who injured his left elbow. Displaced anterior and posterior fat pads, plus a small fracture of the coronoid (*arrow*), indicate a probable partially dislocated elbow as the primary injury.

dislocations, there is typically a hemarthrosis and a small avulsion of the tip of the olecranon process (Fig. 10-47).

INJURIES ASSOCIATED WITH FRACTURES OF THE PROXIMAL ULNA

Metaphyseal Fractures of the Olecranon and the Proximal Apophysis

Associated injuries occur in 48% to 77% of patients with olecranon fractures,[13,44,82,121] especially varus and valgus greenstick

extension fractures, in which the radial head and neck most commonly fracture (see Fig. 10-43). Other associated injuries include fractures of the ipsilateral radial shaft,[116] Monteggia type I lesions with fractures of both the ulnar shaft and olecranon,[80] and fractures of the lateral condyle (Fig. 10-48).[11]

Fractures of the Coronoid Process

Although most coronoid fractures are associated with elbow dislocations, fractures of the olecranon, medial epicondyle, and lateral condyle can also occur.[78] The fracture of the coronoid may be part of a greenstick olecranon fracture (i.e., the extension-type metaphyseal fracture; Fig. 10-49).

SIGNS AND SYMPTOMS OF FRACTURES OF THE PROXIMAL ULNA

Metaphyseal Fractures of the Olecranon and the Proximal Apophysis

Flexion injuries cause soft tissue swelling and tenderness over the olecranon fracture. The abrasion or contusion associated with a direct blow to the posterior aspect of the elbow provides a clue as to the mechanism of injury. If there is wide separation, a defect can be palpated between the fragments. In addition, there may be weakness or even lack of active extension of the elbow, which is difficult to evaluate in an anxious young child with a swollen elbow. Associated proximal radius fractures may be noted clinically by swelling and tenderness laterally with palpation in this region.

Fractures of the Coronoid Process

Because of the common association of these fractures with elbow dislocations, a high index of suspicion is necessary when evaluating these injuries. Significant soft tissue swelling about the elbow is a consistent finding. The patient may also recall the

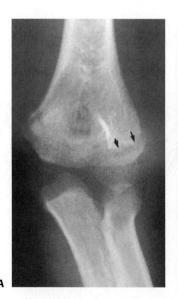

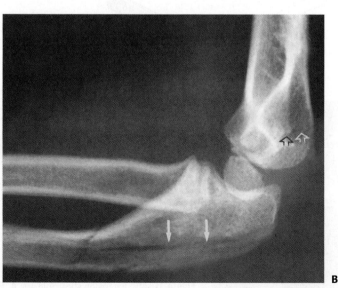

Figure 10-48. A: Undisplaced fracture of the lateral condyle (*arrows*) associated with a varus greenstick fracture of the olecranon. **B:** Lateral view showing greenstick fractures in the olecranon (*solid arrows*) and a nondisplaced fracture of the lateral condyle (*open arrows*).

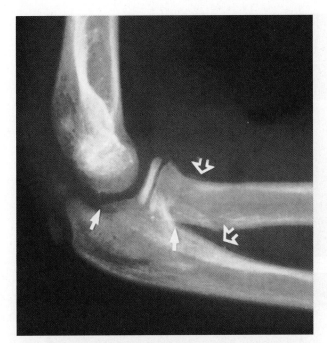

Figure 10-49. Fracture of the coronoid (*solid arrows*) as part of an extension valgus olecranon fracture pattern. There was an associated fracture of the radial neck. Both the neck fracture and the distal portion of the coronoid process show periosteal new bone formation (*open arrows*).

"clunking" sensation of dislocation and spontaneous relocation with specific inquiry.

IMAGING AND OTHER DIAGNOSTIC STUDIES FOR FRACTURES OF THE PROXIMAL ULNA

Metaphyseal Fractures of the Olecranon and the Proximal Apophysis

The radiographic diagnosis may be difficult before ossification of the olecranon apophysis. The only clue may be

a displacement of the small ossified metaphyseal fragment (Fig. 10-50), and the diagnosis may be based only on the clinical sign of tenderness over the epiphyseal fragment. If there is any doubt about the degree of displacement, injection of radiopaque material into the joint (arthrogram) may delineate the true nature of the fracture. Alternatively, an MRI may be useful if uncertainty remains.

Fractures of the Coronoid Process

The radiographic diagnosis of this fracture is often difficult because on the lateral view, the radial head is superimposed over the coronoid process. Evaluation of a minimally displaced fracture may require oblique views (Fig. 10-51).[114] The radiocapitellar view (see Fig. 10-4) shows the profile of the coronoid process.

CLASSIFICATION OF FRACTURES OF THE PROXIMAL ULNA

Fractures Involving the Proximal Apophysis

Apophyseal Injuries of the Olecranon: CLASSIFICATION
Type I: Apophysitis
Type II: Incomplete stress fracture
Type III: Complete fractures
A. Pure apophyseal avulsions
B. Apophyseal–metaphyseal combinations

Injuries to the apophysis of the olecranon can be classified as one of three types. Type I is a simple apophysitis in which there is irregularity in the secondary ossification center (Fig. 10-52A).[19,62] The apophyseal line may widen. Type II is an incomplete stress fracture that involves primarily the apophyseal line, with widening and irregularity (Fig. 10-52B). A small adjacent cyst may form, but usually the architecture of the

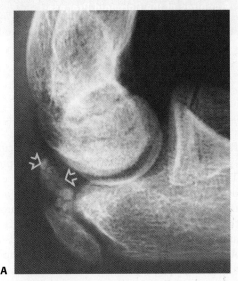

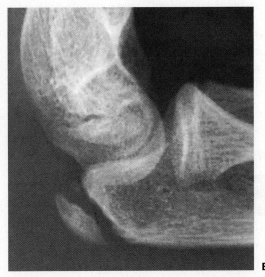

Figure 10-50. Apophysitis. **A:** Chronic stimulation with irregular ossification of the articular apophyseal center (*arrows*) in a basketball player who practiced dribbling 3 hours per day. **B:** Normal side for comparison.

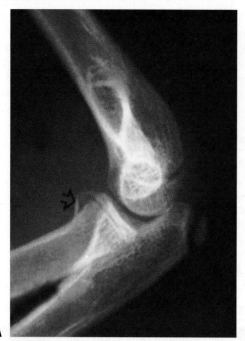
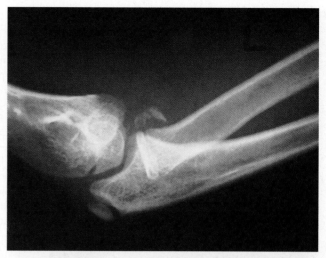
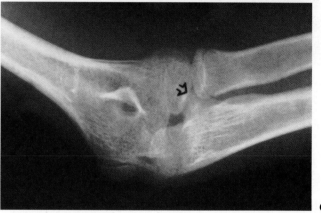
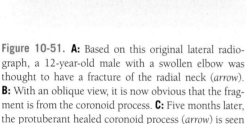
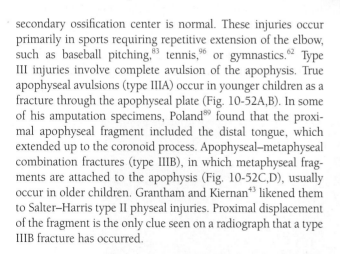

Figure 10-51. A: Based on this original lateral radiograph, a 12-year-old male with a swollen elbow was thought to have a fracture of the radial neck (*arrow*). **B:** With an oblique view, it is now obvious that the fragment is from the coronoid process. **C:** Five months later, the protuberant healed coronoid process (*arrow*) is seen on this radiocapitellar view.

secondary ossification center is normal. These injuries occur primarily in sports requiring repetitive extension of the elbow, such as baseball pitching,[83] tennis,[96] or gymnastics.[62] Type III injuries involve complete avulsion of the apophysis. True apophyseal avulsions (type IIIA) occur in younger children as a fracture through the apophyseal plate (Fig. 10-52A,B). In some of his amputation specimens, Poland[89] found that the proximal apophyseal fragment included the distal tongue, which extended up to the coronoid process. Apophyseal–metaphyseal combination fractures (type IIIB), in which metaphyseal fragments are attached to the apophysis (Fig. 10-52C,D), usually occur in older children. Grantham and Kiernan[43] likened them to Salter–Harris type II physeal injuries. Proximal displacement of the fragment is the only clue seen on a radiograph that a type IIIB fracture has occurred.

Metaphyseal Fractures of the Olecranon

Metaphyseal Fractures of the Olecranon: **CLASSIFICATION**
Group A: Flexion injuries
Group B: Extension injuries 　1. Valgus pattern 　2. Varus pattern
Group C: Shear injuries

The classification is based on the mechanism of injury, flexion/extension/shear. This classification system is useful in guiding treatment options.

Fractures of the Coronoid Process

Fractures of the Coronoid Process: **CLASSIFICATION**[95]
Type I: Involves only tip of coronoid
Type II: A single or comminuted fragment involving <50% of the coronoid process
Type III: A single or comminuted fragment involving >50% of the coronoid process

Regan and Morrey[95] classified coronoid fractures into three types based on the amount of the coronoid process involved. This classification is useful in predicting the outcome and in determining the treatment. Type I fractures involve only the tip of the process (Fig. 10-47), type II fractures involve more than just the tip but less than 50% of the process (Fig. 10-51), and type III fractures involve more than 50% of the process. Additionally, Mellema[68] identified several relationships between specific injury patterns and their ability to predict the type of fracture as well as the distribution of subsequent fracture lines, which are also helpful for diagnosis and treatment planning.

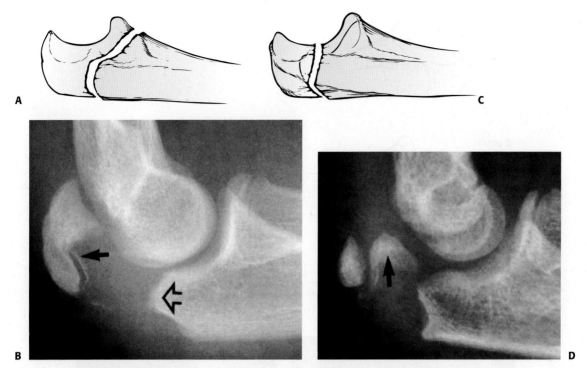

Figure 10-52. Apophyseal avulsions. Pure apophyseal avulsions. **A:** The fracture follows the contour of the apophyseal line. **B:** The distal fracture line is in the shape of the apophyseal line (*open arrow*) with a small metaphyseal flake attached to the apophysis (*solid arrow*). Apophyseal–metaphyseal combination. **C:** The fracture line follows the line of tension stress. **D:** A large portion of the metaphysis (*arrow*) is often with the proximal metaphyseal fragment.

OUTCOME MEASURES FOR FRACTURES OF THE PROXIMAL ULNA

The current literature is deficient in functional outcome instruments for fractures of the proximal ulna. The previously published studies on the outcomes of these fractures have used descriptive assessments that are currently nonvalidated techniques. Elbow range of motion after these injuries continues to be a driver of functional outcomes. As such, there is a definite need for both accurate methods of measuring range of motion as well as validated techniques for reporting the results.

PATHOANATOMY AND APPLIED ANATOMY RELATING TO FRACTURES OF THE PROXIMAL ULNA

At birth, the ossification of the metaphysis of the proximal ulna extends only to the midportion of the semilunar notch. At this age, the leading edge of the metaphysis is usually perpendicular to the long axis of the olecranon (Fig. 10-53A,B). As ossification progresses, the proximal border of the metaphysis becomes more oblique. The anterior margin extends proximally and to three-fourths of the width of the semilunar notch by 6 years of age. At this age, the physis extends distally to include the coronoid process (Fig. 10-52C). A secondary center of ossification occurs in the coronoid process. Just before the development of the secondary center of ossification in

the olecranon, the leading edge of the metaphysis develops a well-defined sclerotic margin.[103] Ossification of the olecranon occurs in the area of the triceps insertion at approximately 9 years of age (Fig. 10-53D).[103] Ossification of the coronoid process is completed about the time that the olecranon ossification center appears.[89]

The secondary ossification center of the olecranon may be bipartite (Fig. 10-53E).[90] The major center within the tip of the olecranon is enveloped by the triceps insertion. This was referred to by Porteous[90] as a traction center. The second and smaller center, an articular center, lies under the proximal fourth of the articular surface of the semilunar notch.

Fusion of the olecranon epiphysis with the metaphysis, which progresses from anterior to posterior, occurs at approximately 14 years of age. The sclerotic margin that defines the edge of the metaphysis may be mistaken for a fracture (Fig. 10-53F).[103] Rarely, the physeal line persists into adulthood.[57,86,124] If this does occur, it is usually in athletes who have used the extremity in repetitive throwing activities.[19,96,107,126,138] The chronic tension forces applied across the apophysis theoretically prevent its normal closure.

Occasionally, a separate ossification center called a patella cubiti develops in the triceps tendon at its insertion on the tip of the olecranon.[122] This ossicle is separate and can articulate with the trochlea. It is usually unilateral, unlike other persistent secondary ossification centers, which are more likely to be bilateral and familial. Zeitlin[141] believed that the patella cubiti was a traumatic ossicle rather than a developmental variation.

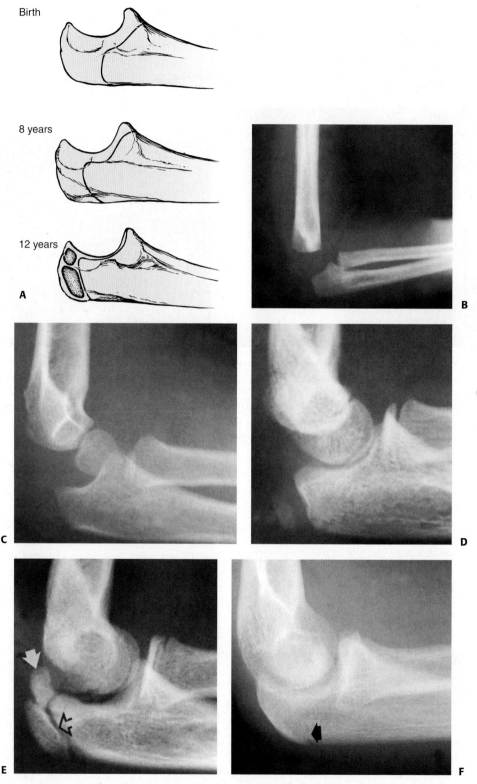

Figure 10-53. Olecranon ossification. **A:** Limits of the border of ossification at birth, 8 years, and 12 years. **B:** Lateral view of olecranon at 6 months of age. The proximal margin is perpendicular to the long axis of the ulna. **C:** Lateral view of the olecranon at 6 years of age. The proximal margin is oblique. **D:** Secondary ossification center developing in the olecranon in a 10 year old. A sclerotic border has developed on the proximal metaphyseal margin. **E:** Bipartite secondary ossification center. The larger center is the traction center (*open arrow*). The smaller, more proximal center is the articular center (*white arrow*). **F:** Before complete fusion, a partial line remains (*arrow*), bordered by a sclerotic margin.

Metaphyseal Fractures of the Olecranon

Because the olecranon is a metaphyseal area, the cortex is relatively thin, allowing for the development of greenstick-type fracture deformities. The periosteum in children is immature and thick, which may prevent the degree of separation seen in adults. Likewise, the larger amount of epiphyseal cartilage in children may serve as a cushion to lessen the effects of a direct blow to the olecranon. In the production of supracondylar fractures, ligamentous laxity in this age group tends to force the elbow into hyperextension when the child falls on the outstretched upper extremity. This puts a compressive force across the olecranon and locks it into the fossa in the distal humerus, where it is protected. An older person, whose elbow does not go into hyperextension, is more likely to fall with the elbow partially flexed. This unique biomechanical characteristic of the child's olecranon predisposes it to different fracture patterns than those in adults.

Fractures of the Coronoid Process

Up to age 6 years, the coronoid process consists of epiphyseal cartilage and physeal cartilage at the distal end of a tongue extending from the apophysis of the olecranon. The coronoid process does not develop a secondary center of ossification, but instead ossifies along with the advancing edge of the metaphysis (Fig. 10-53).

TREATMENT OPTIONS FOR FRACTURES OF THE PROXIMAL ULNA

NONOPERATIVE TREATMENT OF FRACTURES INVOLVING THE PROXIMAL APOPHYSIS OF THE ULNA

Indications/Contraindications

Nonoperative Treatment of Fractures Involving the Proximal Apophysis of the Ulna: INDICATIONS AND CONTRAINDICATIONS	
Indications	**Relative Contraindications**
• Nondisplaced fractures	• Displaced fractures
• Apophysitis	• Open fractures

For apophysitis and nondisplaced stress fractures, we ask the patient to cease the offending activity. During this period of rest, the patient should maintain upper extremity strength with a selective muscle exercise program as well as maintain cardiovascular conditioning.

In a recently published series by Rath,[93] isolated epiphyseal fractures of the olecranon were met with good long-term outcomes after nonoperative management with up to 2 mm of displacement.

Techniques

With minimal displacement of the fracture, satisfactory closed reduction can be obtained with the elbow extended. The elbow can then be immobilized in extension with a long-arm cast.

Outcomes

In general, these injuries recover well and the patients return to full activities quickly. The highest-risk group for failure of nonoperative management are the stress injuries.

NONOPERATIVE TREATMENT OF METAPHYSEAL FRACTURES OF THE OLECRANON OF THE PROXIMAL ULNA

Indications/Contraindications

Nonoperative Treatment of Metaphyseal Fractures of the Olecranon of the Proximal Ulna: INDICATIONS AND CONTRAINDICATIONS	
Indications	**Relative Contraindications**
• Nondisplaced fractures	• Nonreducible fractures
• Fractures reducible to anatomic alignment by closed methods	• Open fractures

Flexion injuries are the most common type of olecranon fractures. In those with minimal displacement, nonoperative treatment is the preferred option. Nonoperative management is contraindicated in displaced olecranon fractures.

Treatment of extension injuries requires both adequate realignment of the angulation of the olecranon and treatment of the secondary injuries. Indications for nonoperative treatment in these injuries include the ability to restore anatomic alignment.

Zimmerman[143] reported that the original angulation tends to redevelop in some fractures. If a varus force produced the fracture, the proximal ulna or olecranon may drift back into varus, which can cause a painful subluxation of the radial head. A secondary osteotomy of the proximal ulna or olecranon may be necessary if the angulation is significant.

For anterior shear fractures, the key to management is recognition that the distal fragment is displaced anteriorly and the posterior periosteum remains intact. The intact posterior periosteum can serve as an internal tension band to facilitate reduction.

Techniques

Flexion Injuries

Most displace minimally and require immobilization with the elbow in no more than 75 to 80 degrees of flexion (Fig. 10-54). Even if the fracture displaces significantly, immobilization in full or partial extension usually affords satisfactory healing and alignment.[32,108,143]

Extension Injuries

Often in varus injuries, correction of the alignment of the olecranon also reduces the radial head. The olecranon angulation corrects with the elbow in extension. This locks the proximal olecranon into the olecranon fossa of the humerus so that the distal angulation can be corrected at the fracture site with a valgus force applied to the forearm. Occasionally, in extension

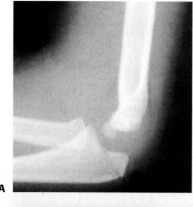

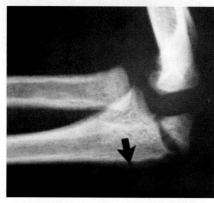

Figure 10-54. Simple immobilization of a flexion injury. **A:** Injury film, lateral view, showing minimal displacement. **B:** Three weeks later, the fracture has displaced further. Periosteal new bone is along the posterior border of the olecranon (*arrow*). Healing was complete with a normal range of motion. (Courtesy of Jesse C. DeLee, MD.)

fractures, complete separation of the fragments requires open reduction and internal fixation (Fig. 10-55).

Shear Injuries

Some of these fractures are reduced better in flexion, and the posterior periosteum serves as a compressive force to maintain the reduction. Smith[108] reported treatment of this fracture using an overhead sling placed to apply a posteriorly directed force against the proximal portion of the distal fragment. The weight

of the arm and forearm helps supplement the tension-band effect of the posterior periosteum.

Outcomes

Most nondisplaced proximal ulna fractures can be treated successfully with nonoperative methods. However, these injuries need to be followed closely to ensure maintenance of alignment. Any loss of reduction/alignment should be recognized and lead to surgical management.

NONOPERATIVE TREATMENT OF FRACTURES OF THE CORONOID PROCESS OF THE PROXIMAL ULNA

Indications/Contraindications

Nonoperative Treatment of Fractures of the Coronoid Process of the Proximal Ulna: INDICATIONS AND CONTRAINDICATIONS	
Indications	**Relative Contraindications**
• Elbow stability	• Elbow instability
• Mild displacement (Types I and II)	• Type III fractures

The degree of displacement or the presence of elbow instability guides the treatment. The associated injuries are also a factor in treatment. Regan and Morrey[94,95] treated type I and II fractures with early motion if there were no contradicting associated injuries.

Techniques

For initial immobilization, if the fracture is associated with an elbow dislocation, the elbow is placed in approximately 100 degrees of flexion, with the forearm in full supination.[78] Occasionally, in partial avulsion fractures, the fracture reduces more easily with the elbow in extension. In these rare cases, the brachialis muscle may be an aid in reducing the fragment in extension.[77]

Outcomes

Regan and Morrey[95] found that the elbow often was unstable in type III fractures, and they secured these fractures with internal fixation. They had satisfactory results with type I and II

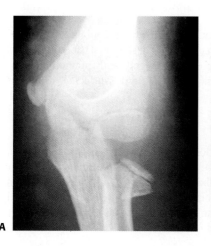

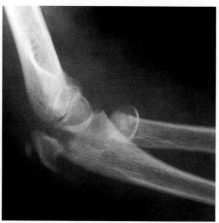

Figure 10-55. Open reduction of a valgus extension injury. **A:** Anteroposterior injury film shows complete displacement of the radial head. **B:** Lateral view also shows the degree of displacement of the olecranon fracture. This patient required surgical intervention with internal fixation to achieve a satisfactory reduction.

fractures, but in only 20% of type III fractures were the results satisfactory with nonoperative treatment.

OPERATIVE TREATMENT OF FRACTURES INVOLVING THE PROXIMAL APOPHYSIS AND OLECRANON METAPHYSIS OF THE ULNA

Indications/Contraindications

Operative Treatment of Fractures Involving the Proximal Apophysis and Olecranon Metaphysis of the Ulna: INDICATIONS AND CONTRAINDICATIONS
Indications • Significant displacement • Acceptable alignment cannot be achieved with closed methods • Fractures with >4-mm displacement • Fractures with incongruent intra-articular surface
Contraindications • Acceptable alignment achieved with closed methods • Fractures with ≤4-mm displacement • Fractures with congruent intra-articular surface • Percutaneous pinning allows stabilization of closed reduction

Apophyseal Fractures

There is no standard method of treatment of fractures of the apophysis, because few such fractures have been described. Surgical treatment is indicated in situations where acceptable alignment cannot be achieved with closed methods. A recently published manuscript determined that fractures with more than 4 mm of displacement or with a noncongruent intra-articular surface should be treated surgically to achieve a better reduction and surgical outcome.[93] With mild to moderately displaced fractures, if a satisfactory closed reduction can be obtained, percutaneous pinning will stabilize the reduction. This can allow for casting in flexion, which is often better tolerated. For fractures with significant displacement, treatment is usually open reduction with internal fixation using a combination of axial pins and tension-band wiring (Fig. 10-56).[43,89,108] Gortzak et al.[42] and Kim et al.[55] described techniques of open reduction using percutaneously placed K-wires and absorbable sutures instead of wires for the tension band. The percutaneously placed wires are subsequently removed 4 to 5 weeks postoperatively, eliminating the need for implant removal. Most stress injuries respond to simple rest from the offending activity. However, a chronic stress fracture can result in a symptomatic nonunion. Use of a compressive screw alone across the nonunion often is sufficient,[62] but supplemental bone grafting may be necessary to achieve union.[57,86]

Metaphyseal Olecranon Fractures

Flexion Injuries

If the fracture is significantly displaced or comminuted, open reduction with internal fixation is usually required. Recommended fixation devices vary from absorbable or nonabsorbable suture[64] to an axial screw,[63] tension-band wiring with axial pins,[30,43,64,100,102,108] or a plate.[118,120] Internal fixation allows early motion.

Extension Injuries

Treatment of extension injuries requires both adequate realignment of the angulation of the olecranon and treatment of the secondary injuries. Occasionally, in extension fractures, complete separation of the fragments requires open reduction and internal fixation (Fig. 10-55).

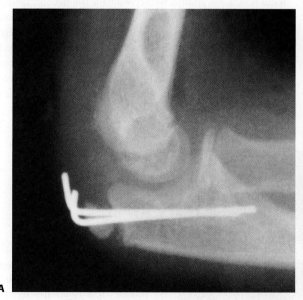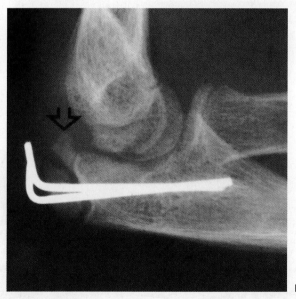

Figure 10-56. Operative treatment of an apophyseal fracture. **A:** Postoperative radiograph of apophyseal fracture, which was stabilized with small Steinmann pins alone. **B:** Five months later, growth has continued in the traction center and the articular center is ossified (*arrow*).

(continues)

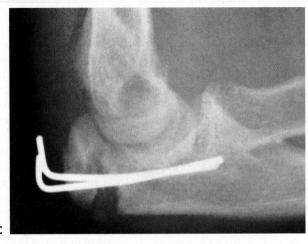

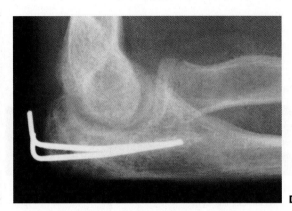

C   D

Figure 10-56. (*Continued*) **C:** One year after injury, the apophysis was partially avulsed a second time. The two secondary ossification centers are now fused. **D:** Three months after the second fracture, the fracture gap has filled in, producing a normal olecranon.

Shear Injuries

For anterior shear fractures, the key to management is recognition that the distal fragment is displaced anteriorly and the posterior periosteum remains intact. The intact posterior periosteum can serve as an internal tension band to facilitate reduction. If the periosteum is torn or early motion is desirable, Zimmerman[143] advocated internal fixation of the two fragments with an oblique screw perpendicular to the fracture line (Fig. 10-57).

Closed Reduction and Percutaneous Pinning

Preoperative Planning

✔ Closed Reduction and Percutaneous Pinning of Fractures Involving the Proximal Apophysis and Olecranon Metaphysis of the Ulna: PREOPERATIVE PLANNING CHECKLIST	
OR table	❑ Standard with radiolucent hand table
Position/positioning aids	❑ Turn table 90 degrees, bring patient to edge of table toward hand table. Secure head with blanket/towel and tape. Safety strap over torso

Fluoroscopy location	❑ In line with affected extremity, perpendicular to OR table
Equipment	❑ Smooth K-wires; power drill; tension-band equipment available
Tourniquet	❑ Nonsterile

To adequately prepare for this technique, we must carefully assess the fracture pattern and determine that an attempt at closed reduction is feasible. It is good practice to also prepare for the possibility that this technique may need to be abandoned and transitioned to an open procedure if an adequate closed reduction is not attainable. Accordingly, the patient, family, and operating room team should all be informed of these possibilities. The OR table, positioning of the patient, and equipment necessary for both closed and open procedures should be identified and available before beginning the surgery. Equipment needed for a potential open procedure can be left unopened in the sterile packaging, but should be visually accounted for and immediately available.

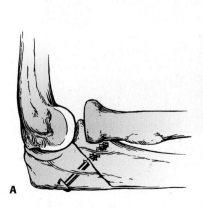

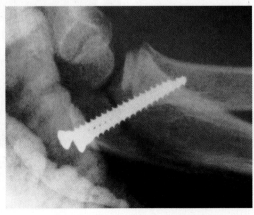

A   B

Figure 10-57. Operative treatment of extension shear fractures. **A:** If the periosteum is insufficient to hold the fragments apposed, an interfragmentary screw can be used. **B:** An extension shear type of fracture secured with two oblique interfragmentary screws.

Positioning

Same as for instrument-assisted closed reduction of proximal radius fractures.

Surgical Approach(es)

A percutaneous approach is used, starting at the subcutaneous border of the tip of the olecranon.

Technique

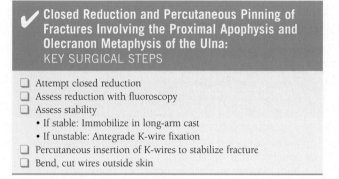

✔ **Closed Reduction and Percutaneous Pinning of Fractures Involving the Proximal Apophysis and Olecranon Metaphysis of the Ulna:** KEY SURGICAL STEPS

- ❑ Attempt closed reduction
- ❑ Assess reduction with fluoroscopy
- ❑ Assess stability
  - • If stable: Immobilize in long-arm cast
  - • If unstable: Antegrade K-wire fixation
- ❑ Percutaneous insertion of K-wires to stabilize fracture
- ❑ Bend, cut wires outside skin

Simple steel K-wires are appropriate to use for this technique. Size will range from 2 to 2.7 mm based on the size of the child. Fluoroscopy is used to localize the fracture site and intended entry site of the wire. The fracture is then reduced with simultaneous elbow extension and thumb pressure over the olecranon. Once the fracture reduction is achieved, percutaneous K-wires are driven from the tip of the olecranon across the fracture site, and exit the far cortex. Fracture stability and pin configuration are then assessed with fluoroscopy. The pins are then cut and bent outside of the skin. We prefer placing a sterile felt pad between the cut pins and the skin, followed by a long-arm cast for immobilization. The pins are then removed in the office after the fracture has healed, typically 3 to 4 weeks.

Open Reduction and Tension-Band Fixation

Preoperative Planning

✔ **Open Reduction and Tension-Band Fixation of Fractures Involving the Proximal Apophysis and Olecranon Metaphysis of the Ulna:** PREOPERATIVE PLANNING CHECKLIST

OR table	❑ Standard with radiolucent hand table
Position/positioning aids	❑ Turn table 90 degrees, bring patient to edge of table toward hand table. Secure head with blanket/towel and tape. Safety strap over torso
Fluoroscopy location	❑ In line with affected extremity, perpendicular to OR table
Equipment	❑ Smooth K-wires; tension-band equipment available
Tourniquet	❑ Nonsterile

Once it has been determined that satisfactory reduction is not achievable by closed methods, an open reduction is indicated. The preparation for this procedure includes ensuring proper OR table, fluoroscopy, patient positioning, and necessary equipment.

Positioning

The positioning for this procedure is the same as for the closed reduction and percutaneous pinning technique described above.

Surgical Approach(es)

A standard posterior approach to the proximal ulna is used, with the incision spanning from 1 to 2 fingerbreadths proximal to the tip of the olecranon to 2 to 3 cm distal to the fracture site. The subcutaneous location of the ulna in this location allows for quick access to the fracture site. However, particularly close attention needs to be paid to delicate handling of the soft tissue envelope as there is commonly a fair amount of soft tissue trauma locally from the injury. It is recommended to shape the incision in a curvilinear fashion proximally to avoid placing the scar directly over the bony prominence of the olecranon.

Technique

✔ **Open Reduction and Tension-Band Fixation of Fractures Involving the Proximal Apophysis of the Ulna:** KEY SURGICAL STEPS

- ❑ Expose proximal ulna
- ❑ Reduce fracture and provisionally stabilize with reduction clamp
- ❑ Assess reduction with fluoroscopy
- ❑ Insert two parallel antegrade K-wires in preparation for tension band
- ❑ Bend the proximal tip for later impaction
- ❑ Prepare bone tunnel in distal fragment for tension band
- ❑ Pass tension-band material through bone tunnel and around K-wires
- ❑ Stabilize fracture by securing the tension band
- ❑ Impact the proximal K-wires into the olecranon

Once the fracture is exposed, a reduction can be performed with a bone reduction forceps. The reduction maneuver can be facilitated by first placing a small unicortical drill hole distal to the fracture site along the diaphysis of the ulna. Then with one tine of the forceps in the drill hole and the other tine at the tip of the olecranon, applying gentle compression with the forceps will help reduce and stabilize the fracture.

With the fracture now reduced, two K-wires are driven in an antegrade fashion, parallel to each other, starting near the tip of the olecranon and coursing obliquely to cross the fracture site and exit the cortex of the anterior ulna. The fracture reduction and K-wire position are then assessed with fluoroscopy. The K-wires are then bent and cut in preparation for capture of the tension band. The wires are pulled back 3 to 4 mm at this point so that when fully impacted later, they will not protrude too far beyond the anterior ulnar cortex.

In preparation for tension-band application, a transverse tunnel is created in the ulnar diaphysis 1- to 2-cm distal to the fracture site. It is critical to leave an intact cortical bridge of bone along the posterior aspect of the ulna superficial to the tunnel. A drill is used to perforate the medial and lateral cortex of the ulna at the desired level of tunnel creation. A towel clip can then be inserted into these two pilot drill holes to finish creating the ulnar bone tunnel.

The tension-band material is then selected, either 18- to 20-gauge wire or large absorbable or nonabsorbable suture. We frequently utilize no. 2 polyethylene core braided polyester suture (Fiber Wire, Arthrex, Naples, FL) or no. 1 polydioxanone suture (PDS) instead of wire. The tension band is then passed through the ulnar bone tunnel and around the previously placed K-wires. Twisting the wires or tying the sutures tightens the tension band. At this point, the reduction clamp is removed and fracture stability assessed with elbow flexion/extension and fluoroscopy. The previously cut and bent K-wires are then impacted into the olecranon, finalizing the capture of the tension band.

Open Reduction and Compression Screw Fixation

Preoperative Planning

> ✔ **Open Reduction and Compression Screw Fixation of Fractures Involving the Proximal Apophysis and Olecranon Metaphysis of the Ulna:**
> PREOPERATIVE PLANNING CHECKLIST

OR table	☐ Standard with radiolucent hand table
Position/positioning aids	☐ Turn table 90 degrees, bring patient to edge of table toward hand table. Secure head with blanket/towel and tape. Safety strap over torso
Fluoroscopy location	☐ In line with affected extremity, perpendicular to OR table
Equipment	☐ Large fragment set (4.5- and 6.5-mm screws); smooth K-wires; tension-band equipment
Tourniquet	☐ Nonsterile

The preparation for this procedure is the same as for the above tension-band technique except for equipment/implant differences.

Positioning

The positioning for this procedure is the same as for the closed reduction and percutaneous pinning technique described above.

Surgical Approach

The approach for this procedure is the same as for the tension-band technique described above.

Technique

> ✔ **Open Reduction and Compression Screw Fixation of Fractures Involving the Proximal Apophysis of the Ulna:**
> KEY SURGICAL STEPS

- ☐ Expose proximal ulna
- ☐ Reduce fracture and provisionally stabilize with reduction clamp
- ☐ Assess reduction with fluoroscopy
- ☐ Insert antegrade guidewire for appropriate-sized screw
- ☐ Starting point at tip of olecranon
- ☐ Drill/tap over guidewire
- ☐ Place appropriate-sized screw over guidewire

Once the fracture is exposed, a reduction can be performed with a bone reduction forceps. The reduction maneuver can be facilitated by first placing a small unicortical drill hole distal to the fracture site along the diaphysis of the ulna. Then with one tine of the forceps in the drill hole and the other tine at the tip of the olecranon, applying gentle compression with the forceps will help reduce and stabilize the fracture.

With the fracture now reduced, the guide pin from the cannulated screw system can be placed in an antegrade fashion starting near the tip of the olecranon, across the fracture site, and into the intramedullary canal of the ulna. Most commonly a 6.5-mm cancellous bone screw is selected. The screw tract is then drilled and tapped over the guidewire, followed by placement of the appropriate-sized screw. The alignment and stability are then assessed with elbow flexion/extension and fluoroscopy.

Authors' Preferred Treatment for Fractures of the Proximal Ulna (Algorithm 10-2)

Apophyseal Fractures and Nondisplaced Fractures

For apophysitis and nondisplaced stress fractures, we ask the patient to cease the offending activity. During this period of rest, the patient should maintain upper extremity strength with a selective muscle exercise program as well as maintain cardiovascular conditioning. When a persistent nonunion of the olecranon in an adolescent does not demonstrate healing after a reasonable period of simple rest, we place a cannulated compression screw across the apophysis to stimulate healing.

Displaced Fractures

With minimal displacement of the fracture, satisfactory closed reduction can be obtained with the elbow extended. We usually immobilize the elbow in a long-arm cast in extension. Percutaneous pinning will stabilize the reduction if there is any concern about loss of reduction. Completely displaced fractures are treated operatively using a tension-band technique. In young children, we use small Steinmann or Kirschner pins. Patients with large ossification

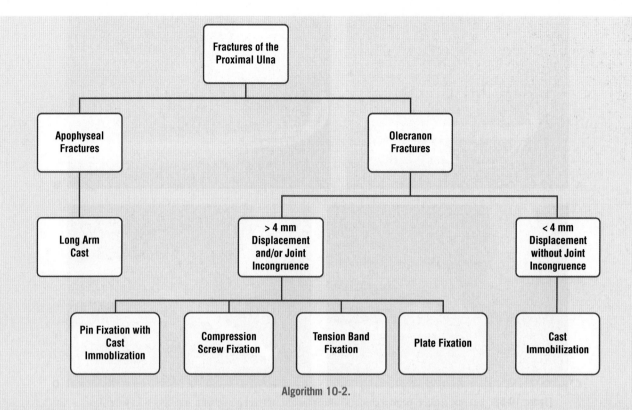

Algorithm 10-2.

centers are treated with a compression screw like those with metaphyseal fractures.[33]

Metaphyseal Olecranon Fractures

We use a classification based on the mechanism of injury in choosing the method of treatment.

Flexion Injuries

We immobilize most nondisplaced flexion injuries with the elbow in 5 to 10 degrees of flexion for approximately 3 weeks. It is important to obtain radiographs of these fractures after approximately 5 to 7 days in the cast to ensure that there has not been any significant displacement of the fragment.

To determine which injuries need internal fixation, we palpate the fracture for a defect and flex the elbow to determine the integrity of the posterior periosteum. If the fragments separate with either of these maneuvers, they are unstable and are fixed internally so that active motion can be started as soon as possible.

We prefer a modification of the tension-band technique. Originally, we used the standard AO technique with axial K-wires or Steinmann pins and figure-of-eight stainless steel as the tension band (Fig. 10-58A). Because removal of the wire often required reopening the entire incision, we now often use an absorbable suture for the figure-of-eight tension band. No. 1 PDS suture, which is slowly absorbed over a few months, is ideal (Fig. 10-58B). When rigid internal fixation is applied, rapid healing at the fracture site produces internal stability before the PDS absorbs.

We prefer K-wires in patients who are very young and have very little ossification of the olecranon apophysis (see Fig. 10-56). If the axial wires become a problem, we remove them through a small incision. Most recently, we have used a combination of an oblique cortical screw with PDS as the tension band (Fig. 10-58C,D), and are pleased with the results. In the past, we had to remove almost all the axial wires; very few of the screws cause enough symptoms to require removal. Occasionally, we use the tension-band wire technique with 16- or 18-gauge wire in a heavier patient.

Extension Injuries

For extension injuries, we anesthetize the patient to allow a forceful manipulation of the olecranon while it is locked in its fossa in extension. Because this is a greenstick fracture, we slightly overcorrect to prevent the recurrence of angular deformity. These fractures may require further manipulation in 1 to 2 weeks if the original angulation recurs. Associated fractures are treated simultaneously.

Shear Injuries

Most shear fractures can be treated nonoperatively. We usually immobilize them in enough flexion to hold the fragments together, if the posterior periosteum is intact (Fig. 10-59). If the periosteum is torn, an oblique screw is an excellent way to secure the fracture (Fig. 10-57). If considerable swelling prevents the elbow from being hyperflexed enough to use the posterior periosteum as a tension band, an oblique screw is a good choice.

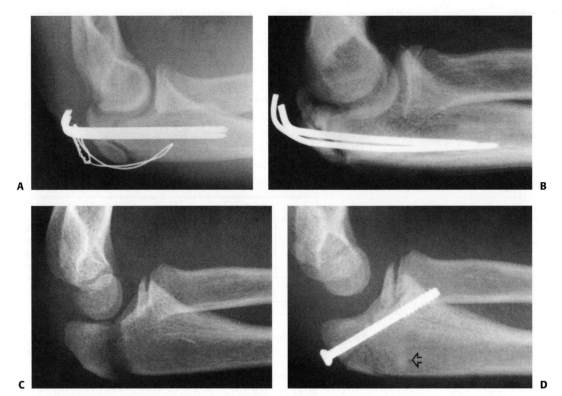

Figure 10-58. Internal tension-band techniques. **A:** Standard AO technique with stainless steel wire. The wire can be prominent in the subcutaneous tissues. **B:** Axial wires plus polydioxanone sutures (PDSs) 6 weeks after surgery. **C:** A displaced flexion-type injury in an 11-year-old male. There is complete separation of the fracture fragments. **D:** A cancellous lag screw plus PDS. The screw engages the anterior cortex of the coronoid process. The PDS passes through a separate drill hole in the olecranon (*open arrow*) and crosses in a figure-of-eight manner over the fracture site and around the neck of the screw.

Postoperative Care

A critical advantage of surgical management is the ability to allow and encourage early motion. Accordingly, with stable fixation, a brief period of immobilization postoperatively is in order. Typically, this would entail 10 to 14 days of immobilization to allow for wound healing, followed by active measures geared toward resumption of elbow/forearm range of motion.

Potential Pitfalls and Preventive Measures

Proximal Ulna Apophyseal and Metaphyseal Olecranon Fractures: POTENTIAL PITFALLS AND PREVENTIONS	
Pitfall	**Prevention**
Prominent implants	Attention to detail
	Plan for implant impaction
	Incision planning
	Consider use of suture instead of wire for tension band
Nonunion	Consider bone grafting
	Compression techniques
Loss of reduction in extension type	Reduce in extension, "over" reduce
	Pin if stability questionable

Murphy et al.[73] compared the failure of various fixation devices under rapid loading: (a) figure-of-eight wire alone, (b) cancellous screw alone, (c) AO tension band, and (d) cancellous screw with a figure-of-eight wire combination. The cancellous screw alone and figure-of-eight wire alone were by far the weakest. The greatest resistance to failure was found in the combination of a screw plus figure-of-eight wire, followed closely by the AO tension-band fixation. In their clinical evaluation of patients, comparing the AO tension band and combination of screw and figure-of-eight wire, they found more clinical problems associated with the AO technique.[74] The main problem with the AO technique is the subcutaneous prominence of the axial wires.[61,84] To prevent proximal migration of these wires, Montgomery[72] devised a method of making eyelets in the proximal end of the wires through which he passed the figure-of-eight fixation wire.

Zimmerman[143] reported that the original angulation tends to redevelop in some extension type olecranon fractures. If a varus force produced the fracture, the proximal ulna or olecranon may drift back into varus, which can cause a painful subluxation of the radial head. A secondary osteotomy of the proximal ulna or olecranon may be necessary if the angulation is significant.

Outcomes

There are no validated outcome measures on this population in the current literature. In general, the limited studies available

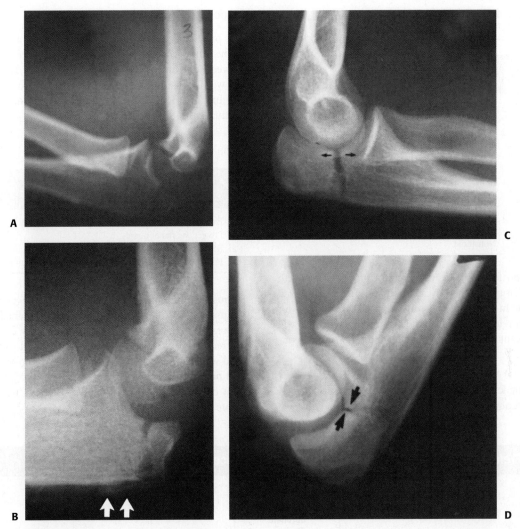

Figure 10-59. Shear injuries. **A:** Flexion pattern: Radiograph of the patient seen in Figure 11.45A after the elbow was flexed. The intact posterior periosteum acted as a tension band and held the fracture reduced. **B:** Radiograph taken 4 weeks after surgery shows new bone formation under the intact periosteum (*arrows*) on the dorsal surface of the olecranon. **C:** Extension pattern: Radiograph of patient with an extension shear injury showing an increase in the fracture gap (*arrows*). **D:** Because the dorsal periosteum and cortex were intact, the fracture gap (*arrows*) closed with flexion of the elbow.

report good-to-excellent outcomes with the techniques described above.

OPERATIVE TREATMENT OF FRACTURES OF THE CORONOID PROCESS OF THE PROXIMAL ULNA

Indications/Contraindications

Operative Treatment of Fractures of the Coronoid Process of the Proximal Ulna:
INDICATIONS AND CONTRAINDICATIONS

Indications
- Type III fractures
- Unstable fracture with external fixation
- Large fragment
- Marked displacement

Contraindications
- Type I or II fractures
- Stability achieved with external fixation

Regan and Morrey[95] found that the elbow often was unstable in type III fractures, and they secured these fractures with internal fixation. They had satisfactory results with type I and II fractures, but in only 20% of type III fractures were the results satisfactory that were treated nonoperatively. These indications were further supported by Aksu et al.,[2] who recommend surgical management for all type III injuries.

The presence of a coronoid fracture alerts us to be especially thorough in looking for other injuries. In children, surgery is rarely necessary. If there is a large fragment and marked displacement, open reduction is indicated.

ORIF of Coronoid Fractures

Preoperative Planning

✔ ORIF of Coronoid Fractures: PREOPERATIVE PLANNING CHECKLIST	
OR table	☐ Standard with radiolucent hand table
Position/positioning aids	☐ Turn table 90 degrees, bring patient to edge of table toward hand table. Secure head with blanket/towel and tape. Safety strap over torso
Fluoroscopy location	☐ In line with affected extremity, perpendicular to OR table
Equipment	☐ Mini-fragment set (2- to 2.75-mm screws); dental picks
Tourniquet	☐ Nonsterile

The preparation for ORIF of the coronoid process starts with ensuring familiarity with the local anatomy and anterior approach to this region. In addition, the surgeon needs to prepare for dealing with a relatively small-sized fracture fragment that will require significant precision for reduction and screw placement.

Positioning

The positioning for this technique is the same as described previously in the apophyseal and metaphyseal fracture section.

Surgical Approach

This procedure is performed through a Henry anterior approach to the elbow. The anatomic plane of the deep dissection lies between the brachioradialis and brachialis. The radial nerve lies within this interval, and needs to be protected. The fracture fragment will likely have at least partial attachment of the brachialis.

Technique

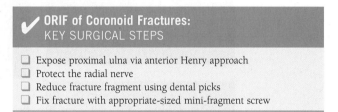

✔ ORIF of Coronoid Fractures: KEY SURGICAL STEPS
☐ Expose proximal ulna via anterior Henry approach
☐ Protect the radial nerve
☐ Reduce fracture fragment using dental picks
☐ Fix fracture with appropriate-sized mini-fragment screw

Because of the confined space anatomically in this location, the use of fracture reduction forceps will be challenging if not impossible. Accordingly, dental picks are very useful in obtaining reduction of this fracture. Once reduced, the fragment is fixed with a mini-fragment screw or sewn in place through two drill holes in the posterior aspect of the ulna. If there is significant comminution or the fragment is small, the pull through suture technique is superior.

Authors' Preferred Treatment for Fractures of the Coronoid Process (Algorithm 10-3)

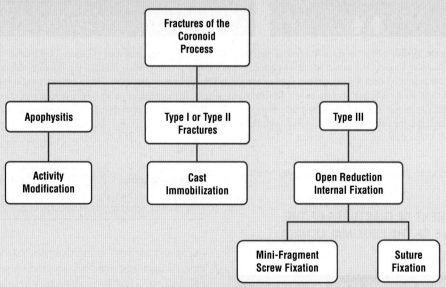

Algorithm 10-3.

We usually treat coronoid fractures with early motion, much as we do elbow dislocations. The presence of a coronoid fracture alerts us to be especially thorough in looking for other injuries. In children, surgery is rarely necessary. If there is a large fragment and marked displacement, open reduction is done through a Henry anterior approach to the elbow. The fragment is fixed with a mini-fragment screw or sewn in place through two drill holes in the posterior aspect of the ulna.

Postoperative Care

A short period of immobilization, 10 to 14 days, followed by active range of motion is preferred. However, tenuous fixation may be encountered when treating these injuries. Intraoperative assessment of fixation and stability is warranted, and depending on the assessment, the postoperative care may need to be adjusted accordingly.

POTENTIAL PITFALLS AND PREVENTIVE MEASURES

Coronoid Fractures: POTENTIAL PITFALLS AND PREVENTIONS	
Pitfall	**Prevention**
• Loss of fixation	• Assess intraoperatively • Cast longer if fixation tenuous
• Elbow instability	• Treat type III injuries operatively
• Fragment comminution	• Be prepared for pull through suture technique

Outcomes

As noted previously, Regan and Morrey[95] found that the elbow often was unstable in type III fractures, and they secured these fractures with internal fixation. They had satisfactory results with type I and II fractures, but in only 20% of type III fractures were the results satisfactory that were treated non-operatively.

MANAGEMENT OF EXPECTED ADVERSE OUTCOMES AND UNEXPECTED COMPLICATIONS IN FRACTURES OF THE PROXIMAL ULNA

Fractures of the Proximal Ulna: COMMON ADVERSE OUTCOMES AND COMPLICATIONS
Fractures of the Proximal Apophysis and Olecranon Metaphysis of the Ulna • Spur formation • Nonunion • Apophyseal arrest • Loss of reduction • Olecranon elongation • Prominent implants
Coronoid Fractures • Elbow stiffness • Recurrent elbow instability

Fractures of the Proximal Apophysis and Olecranon Metaphysis of the Ulna

Spur Formation

Overgrowth of the epiphysis proximally may produce a bony spur. Symptomatic spurs can be treated with surgical excision.

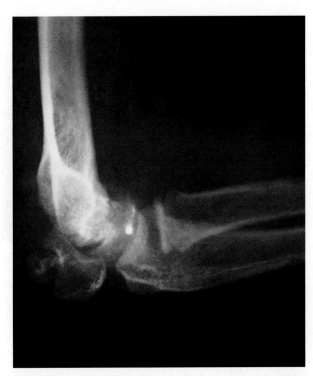

Figure 10-60. Congenital pseudarthrosis of the olecranon in a 9-year-old female who had limited elbow extension and no antecedent trauma. The edges of the bone were separated by thick fibrous tissue. (Courtesy of Michael J. Rogal, MD.)

Nonunion

Nonunion is a rare event in these fractures, most likely occurring in apophysitis/overuse injuries. Bone grafting the nonunion and ensuring stable fixation with compression is the most efficacious method of treatment. Nonunion is unusual and should not be confused with congenital pseudarthrosis of the ulna, which is rare (Fig. 10-60). In the latter condition, there is no antecedent trauma.

Apophyseal Arrest

Apophyseal arrest appears to have no significant effect on elbow function (Fig. 10-61). There has been concern that applying compressive forces across the apophysis might cause premature growth arrest. In our experience, fusion of the apophysis to the metaphysis is accelerated. Apophyseal fractures usually occur when the physis is near natural closure. The growth proximally is appositional rather than longitudinal across the apophyseal plate. Thus, we have not found any functional shortening of the olecranon because of the early fusion of the apophysis to the metaphysis (Fig. 10-56D). In practice, the use of a compression screw across an ossified olecranon fracture causes no loss of ulnar length. Children who sustain injuries before the development of the secondary ossification center may develop a deformity that is visible on radiographs (Fig. 10-61). Although there may be shortening of the olecranon, it does not appear to produce functional problems. There are no reports of the effects of this injury in very young children or infants.

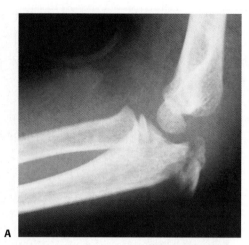 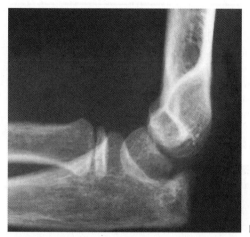

Figure 10-61. Preosseous apophyseal arrest. **A:** Comminuted fracture of the proximal olecranon from a direct blow to the elbow in an 8-year-old male. This fracture was treated nonoperatively. **B:** Radiograph 18 months later shows cessation of the proximal migration of the metaphyseal margin and a lack of development of a secondary ossification center. Despite this arrest of the apophysis, the patient had a full range of elbow motion.

Irreducibility

An and Loder[3] reported inability to reduce the fracture in one of their patients because the proximal fragment was entrapped in the joint.

Delayed Union

Delayed radiographic union usually is asymptomatic.[64] In Mathews' series,[64] one fracture treated with suture fixation ultimately progressed to a nonunion. Despite this, the patient had only a 10-degree extension lag and grade 4 triceps strength. An accessory ossicle, such as a patella cubiti, is not a nonunion.

Compartment Syndrome

Mathews[64] described one patient with Volkmann ischemic contracture after a nondisplaced linear fracture in the olecranon.

Nerve Injuries

Zimmerman[143] reported ulnar nerve neurapraxia from the development of a pseudarthrosis of the olecranon where inadequate fixation was used.

Elongation

Elongation of the tip of the olecranon may complicate healing of a fracture. Figure 10-62 illustrates a delayed union in which the

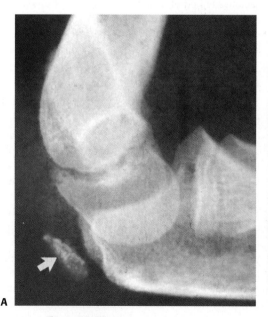 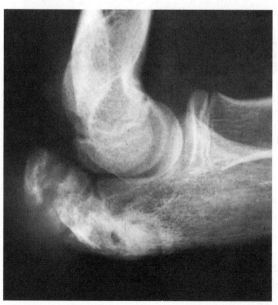

Figure 10-62. A: Injury film showing partial avulsion of the tip of the olecranon apophysis (*arrow*). **B:** Radiograph taken 4 years later shows a marked elongation and irregular ossification of the apophysis. (Courtesy of Joel Goldman, MD.)

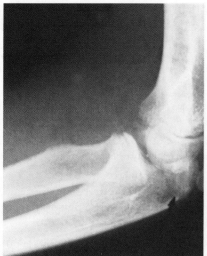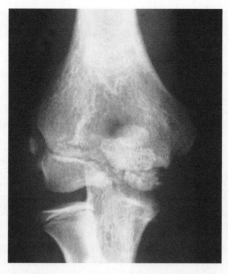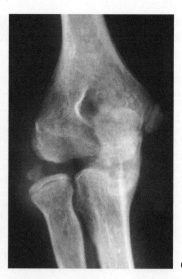

A, B   C

Figure 10-63. Loss of reduction. **A:** Lateral radiograph of what appeared to be a simple undisplaced fracture (*arrow*) of the olecranon in a 10-year-old female. **B:** On the anteroposterior film, the fracture also appears undisplaced. The mild lateral subluxation of the radial head was not recognized. **C:** Radiographs taken 5 months later showed further lateral subluxation with resultant incongruity of the elbow joint. (Courtesy of Richard W. Williamson, MD.)

apophysis became elongated to the point that it limited extension. This proximal overgrowth of the tip of the apophysis has occurred in olecranon fractures after routine open reduction and internal fixation.[82]

Loss of Reduction

Apparently stable fractures treated with external immobilization may lose reduction, which results in a significant loss of elbow function (Fig. 10-63).

Fractures of the Coronoid Process

Because of the high association of these coronoid fractures with elbow dislocations, postinjury stiffness is a concern. Accordingly, treatment modalities are selected to allow for early range of motion when possible. Complications are rare. In fractures with a large fragment (type III), the elbow may be unstable and prone to recurrent dislocations. Nonunion with the production of a free fragment in the joint occurs rarely in children.[83]

SUMMARY, CONTROVERSIES, AND FUTURE DIRECTIONS RELATED TO FRACTURES OF THE PROXIMAL RADIUS AND ULNA

A large portion of proximal radius and ulna fractures in children can be treated successfully by nonoperative methods. The surgical techniques described in this chapter are effective in achieving fracture union and good clinical results. However, the current literature is deficient in functional outcome instruments for fractures of the proximal ulna and radius in children. The previously published studies on the outcomes of these fractures have used descriptive assessments that are currently nonvalidated techniques. Elbow range of motion after these injuries continues to be a driver of functional outcomes. As such, there is a definite need for both accurate methods of measuring range of motion as well as validated techniques for reporting the results.

Annotated References

Reference	Annotation
Furushima K, Itoh Y, Iwabu S, et al. Classification of olecranon stress fractures in baseball players. *Am J Sports Med.* 2014;42(6):1343–1351.	Classification system for olecranon stress fractures to help guide treatment
Gortzak Y, Mercado E, Atar D, et al. Pediatric olecranon fractures: open reduction and internal fixation with removable K-wires and absorbable sutures. *J Pediatr Orthop.* 2006;26:39–42.	Surgical technique for tension-band fixation utilizing suture instead of wire to minimize need for secondary implant removal following surgical fixation
Greenspan A, Norman A. The radial head-capitellum view: useful technique in elbow trauma. *AJR Am J Roentgenol.* 1982;138:1186–1188.	Radiographic technique to assist in evaluation of radial head fractures
Metaizeau JP, Lascombes P, Lemelle JL, et al. Reduction and fixation of displaced radial neck fractures by closed intramedullary pinning. *J Pediatr Orthop.* 1993;13:355–360.	Surgical technique and results for closed intramedullary fixation of displaced radial neck fractures

Annotated References

Reference	Annotation
Regan W, Morrey BF. Classification and treatment of coronoid process fractures. *Orthopedics*. 1992;15:845–848.	Classification system for coronoid process fractures to help guide treatment
Smith GR, Hotchkiss RN. Radial head and neck fractures: Anatomic guidelines for proper placement of internal fixation. *J Shoulder Elbow Surg*. 1996;5(2 Pt 1):113–117.	Anatomic study describing safe surgical exposure and implant placement for radial head and neck fractures
Van Zeeland NL, Bae DS, Goldfarb CA. Intra-articular radial head fracture in the skeletally immature patient: progressive radial head subluxation and rapid radiocapitellar degeneration. *J Pediatric Orthop*. 2011;31:124–129.	Case series describing high morbidity of untreated intra-articular radial head fractures in children
Waters PM, Beaty J, Kasser J. TRASH (The Radiographic Appearance Seemed Harmless). *J Pediatr Orthop*. 2010;30:S77–S81.	Overview of fracture patterns with high morbidity that appear harmless on initial review of radiographs
Zimmerman RM, Kalish LA, Hresko MT, et al. Surgical management of pediatric radial neck fractures. *J Bone Joint Surg Am*. 2013;95(20):1825–1832.	Large case series describing treatment of radial neck fractures in 151 children. 31% overall poor results. Risk of poor result higher with age >10 years, higher initial displacement, and need for open surgical procedures.

REFERENCES

1. Ackerson R, Nguyen A, Carry PM, et al. Intra-articular radial head fractures in the skeletally immature patient: complications and management. *J Pediatr Orthop*. 2015;35(5):443–448.
2. Aksu N, Korkmaz MF, Gogus A, et al. [Surgical treatment of elbow dislocations accompanied by coronoid fractures]. *Acta Orthop Traumatol Turc*. 2008;42(4):258–264.
2a. An HS, Loder RT. Intraarticular entrapment of a displaced olecranon fracture: a case report. *Orthopedics*. 1989;12(2):289–291.
3. Anderson TE, Breed AL. A proximal radial metaphyseal fracture presenting as wrist pain. *Orthopedics*. 1982;5:425–428.
4. Angelov AA. New method for treatment of the dislocated radial neck fracture in children. In: Chapchal G, ed. *Fractures in Children*. New York: Georg Thieme; 1981:192–194.
5. Bado JL. The Monteggia lesion. *Clin Orthop Relat Res*. 1967;50:71–86.
6. Baehr FH. Reduction of separated upper epiphysis of the radius. *N Engl J Med*. 1932;24:1263–1266.
7. Basmajian HG, Choi PD, Huh K, et al. Radial neck fractures in children: experience from two level-1 trauma centers. *J Pediatr Orthop B*. 2014;23(4):369–374.
8. Bernstein SM, McKeever P, Bernstein L. Percutaneous pinning for radial neck fractures. *J Pediatr Orthop*. 1993;13:84–88.
9. Blount WP. Fractures in children. *AAOS Instr Course Lect*. 1950;7:194–202.
10. Boyd HB, Altenberg AR. Fractures about the elbow in children. *Arch Surg*. 1944;49:213–224.
11. Bracq H. Fractures de l'olecrane. *Rev Chir Orthop*. 1987;73:469–471.
12. Brodeur AE, Silberstein JJ, Graviss ER. *Radiology of the Pediatric Elbow*. Boston, MA: GK Hall; 1981.
13. Burge P, Benson M. Bilateral congenital pseudarthrosis of the olecranon. *J Bone Joint Surg Br*. 1987;69:460–462.
14. Carl AL, Ain MC. Complex fracture of the radial neck in a child: an unusual case. *J Orthop Trauma*. 1994;8:255–257.
15. Carney JR, Fox D, Mazurek MT. Displaced apophyseal olecranon fracture in a healthy child. *Mil Med*. 2007;172(12):1225–1227.
16. Cha SM, Shin HD, Kim KC, et al. Percutaneous reduction and leverage fixation using K-wires in paediatric angulated radial neck fractures. *Int Orthop*. 2012;36(4):803–809.
17. Chambers HG. Fractures of the proximal radius and ulna. In: Kasser JR, Beaty JH, eds. *Rockwood and Wilkins' Fractures in Children*. 5th ed. Philadelphia, PA: Lippincott Williams & Wilkins; 2001:483–528.
18. Cossio A, Cazzaniga C, Gridavilla G, et al. Paediatric radial neck fractures: one-step percutaneous reduction and fixation. *Injury*. 2014;45(Suppl 6):S80–S84.
19. Danielson LG, Hedlund ST, Henricson AS. Apophysitis of the olecranon: a report of four cases. *Acta Orthop Scand*. 1983;54:777–778.
20. Davidson RS, Markowitz RI, Dormans J, et al. Ultrasonographic evaluation of the elbow in infants and young children after suspected trauma. *J Bone Joint Surg Am*. 1994;76(12):1804–1813.
21. De Mattos CB, Ramski DE, Kushare IV, et al. Radial neck fractures in children and adolescents: an examination of operative and nonoperative treatment and outcomes. *J Pediatr Orthop*. 2016;36(1):6–12.
22. Di Cesare PE, Sew-Hoy A, Krom W. Bilateral isolated olecranon fractures in an infant as presentation of osteogenesis imperfecta. *Orthopedics*. 1992;15:741–743.
23. Dormans JP. Arthrographically assisted percutaneous manipulation of displaced and angulated radial neck fractures in children: description of a technique for reduction and a new radiographic sign. *J Orthop Tech*. 1994;2:77–81.
24. Dormans JP, Rang M. Fractures of the olecranon and radial neck in children. *Orthop Clin North Am*. 1990;21:257–268.
25. Dougall AJ. Severe fracture of the neck of the radius in children. *J R Coll Surg Edinb*. 1969;14:220–225.
26. D'Souza S, Vaishya R, Klenerman L. Management of radial neck fractures in children. A retrospective analysis of 100 patients. *J Pediatr Orthop*. 1993;13:232–238.
27. Eberl R, Singer J, Fruhmann A, et al. Intramedullary nailing for the treatment of dislocated pediatric radial neck fractures. *European J Pediatr Surg*. 2010;4:250–252.
28. Ellman H. Osteochondrosis of the radial head. *J Bone Joint Surg Am*. 1972;54:1560.
29. Ellman H. Anterior angulation deformity of the radial head. *J Bone Joint Surg Am*. 1975;57:776–778.
30. Fahey JJ. Fractures of the elbow in children. *AAOS Instr Course Lect*. 1980;17:13–46.
31. Falciglia F, Giordano M, Aulisa AG, et al. Radial neck fractures in children: results when open reduction is indicated. *J Pediatr Orthop*. 2014;34(8):756–762.
32. Fogarty EE, Blake NS, Regan BF. Fracture of the radial neck with medial displacement of the shaft of the radius. *Br J Radiol*. 1983;56:486–487.
33. Foruria AM, Augustin S, Morrey BF, et al. Heterotopic ossification after surgery for fractures and fracture-dislocations involving the proximal aspect of the radius or ulna. *J Bone Joint Surg Am*. 2013;95(10):e66.
34. Fowles JV, Kassab MT. Observations concerning radial neck fractures in children. *J Pediatr Orthop*. 1986;6:51–57.
35. Fraser KE. Displaced fracture of the proximal end of the radius in a child. A case report of the deceptive appearance of a fragment that had rotated 180 degrees. *J Bone Joint Surg Am*. 1995;77:782–783.
36. Fuller CB, Guillen PT, Wongworawat MD, et al. Bioabsorbable pin fixation in late presenting pediatric radial neck fractures. *J Pediatr Orthop*. 2016;36(8):793–796.
37. Furushima K, Itoh Y, Iwabu S, et al. Classification of olecranon stress fractures in baseball players. *Am J Sports Med*. 2014;42(6):1343–1351.
38. Futami T, Tsukamoto Y, Itoman M. Percutaneous reduction of displaced radial neck fractures. *J Shoulder Elbow Surg*. 1995;4:162–167.
39. Gaddy BC, Strecker WB, Schoenecker PL. Surgical treatment of displaced olecranon fractures in children. *J Pediatr Orthop*. 1997;17:321–324.
40. Gaston SR, Smith FM, Boab OD. Epiphyseal injuries of the radial head and neck. *Am J Surg*. 1953;85:266–276.
41. Gille P, Mourot M, Aubert F, et al. Fracture par torsion du col du radius chez l'enfant. *Rev Chir Orthop*. 1978;64:247–248.
42. Gortzak Y, Mercado E, Atar D, et al. Pediatric olecranon fractures: open reduction and internal fixation with removable Kirschner wires and absorbable sutures. *J Pediatr Orthop*. 2006;26:39–42.
43. Grantham SA, Kiernan HA. Displaced olecranon fractures in children. *J Trauma*. 1975;15:197–204.
44. Graves SC, Canale ST. Fractures of the olecranon in children: long-term follow-up. *J Pediatr Orthop*. 1993;13:239–241.
45. Greenspan A, Norman A. The radial head-capitellum view: useful technique in elbow trauma. *AJR Am J Roentgenol*. 1982;138:1186–1188.
46. Greenspan A, Norman A, Rosen H. Radial head-capitellum view in elbow trauma: clinical application and radiographic-anatomic correlation. *AJR Am J Roentgenol*. 1984;143:355–359.
47. Hall-Craggs MA, Shorvon PJ, Chapman M. Assessment of the radial head-capitellum view and the dorsal fat-pad sign in acute elbow trauma. *AJR Am J Roentgenol*. 1985;145:607–609.
48. Henrikson B. Isolated fracture of the proximal end of the radius in children. *Acta Orthop Scand*. 1969;40:246–260.
49. Irshad F, Shaw NJ, Gregory RJ. Reliability of fat-pad sign in radial head/neck fractures of the elbow. *Injury*. 1997;28:433–435.
50. Javed A, Guichet JM. Arthrography for reduction of a fracture of the radial neck in a child with a nonossified radial epiphysis. *J Bone Joint Surg Br*. 2001;83(4):542–543.
51. Jeffery CC. Fractures of the head of the radius in children. *J Bone Joint Surg Br*. 1950;32:314–324.

52. Jones ER, Esah M. Displaced fracture of the neck of the radius in children. *J Bone Joint Surg Br.* 1971;53:429–439.

53. Judet H, Judet J. *Fractures et orthopédie de l'enfant. Indications et Techniques.* Ed. Maloine SA, Paris; 1974.

54. Kaufman B, Rinott MG, Tanzman M. Closed reduction of fractures of the proximal radius in children. *J Bone Joint Surg Br.* 1989;71:66–67.

55. Kim JY, Lee YH, Gong HS, et al. Use of Kirschner wires with eyelets for tension band wiring of olecranon fractures. *J Hand Surg Am.* 2013;38(9):1762–1767.

56. Klitscher D, Richter S, Bodenschatz K, et al. Evaluation of severely displaced radial neck fractures in children treated with elastic stable intramedullary nailing. *J Pediatr Orthop.* 2009;29(7):698–703.

57. Kovach JI, Baker BE, Mosher JF. Fracture-separation of the olecranon ossification center in adults. *Am J Sports Med.* 1985;13:105–111.

58. Landin LA, Danielsson LG. Elbow fractures in children: an epidemiological analysis of 589 cases. *Acta Orthop Scand.* 1986;57:309.

59. Lazar RD, Waters PM, Jaramillo D. The use of ultrasonography in the diagnosis of occult fracture of the radial neck: a case report. *J Bone Joint Surg Am.* 1998;80:1361–1364.

60. Lindham S, Hugasson C. Significance of associated lesions including dislocation of fracture of the neck of the radius in children. *Acta Orthop Scand.* 1979;50:79–83.

61. Macko D, Azabo RM. Complications of tension band wiring of olecranon fractures. *J Bone Joint Surg Am.* 1985;67:1396–1401.

62. MacLennan A. Common fractures about the elbow joint in children. *Surg Gynecol Obstet.* 1937;64:447–453.

63. Maffulli N, Chan D, Aldridge MJ. Overuse injuries of the olecranon in young gymnasts. *J Bone Joint Surg Br.* 1992;74:305–308.

64. Mathews JG. Fractures of the olecranon in children. *Injury.* 1981;12:207–212.

65. Maylahn DJ, Fahey JJ. Fractures of the elbow in children. *JAMA.* 1958;166:220–228.

66. Mayo elbow performance score. *JOT.* 2006;20(8):S127.

67. McCarthy SM, Ogden JA. Radiology of postnatal skeletal development. *Skeletal Radiol.* 1982;9:17–26.

68. Mellema JJ, Doornberg JN, Dyer GS, et al. Distribution of coronoid fracture lines by specific patterns of traumatic elbow instability. *J Hand Surg Am.* 2014;39(10):2041–2046.

69. Metaizeau JP, Lascombes P, Lemelle JL, et al. Reduction and fixation of displaced radial neck fractures by closed intramedullary pinning. *J Pediatr Orthop.* 1993; 13:355–360.

70. Metaizeau JP, Prevot J, Schmitt M. Reduction et fixation des fractures et decollements epiphysaires de la tete radiale par broche centromedullaire. *Rev Chir Orthop.* 1980;66:47–49.

71. Monson R, Black B, Reed M. A new closed reduction technique for the treatment of radial neck fractures in children. *J Pediatr Orthop.* 2009;29:243–247.

71a. Montgomery RJ. A secure method of olecranon fixation: a modification of tension band wiring technique. *J R Coll Surg Edinb.* 1986;31:179–182.

72. Mudgal CS. Olecranon fractures in osteogenesis imperfecta: a case report. *Acta Orthop Belg.* 1992;58:453–456.

73. Murphy DF, Greene WB, Dameron TB. Displaced olecranon fractures in adults. *Clin Orthop Relat Res.* 1987;224:215–223.

74. Murphy DF, Greene WB, Gilbert JA, et al. Displaced olecranon fractures in adults. Biomedical analysis of fixation methods. *Clin Orthop Relat Res.* 1987;224:210–214.

75. Neher CG, Torch MA. New reduction technique for severely displaced pediatric radial neck fractures. *J Pediatr Orthop.* 2003;23:626–628.

76. Nenopoulos SP, Beslikas TA, Gigis JP. Long-term follow-up of combined fractures of proximal radius and ulna in childhood. *J Pediatr Orthop B.* 2009;18:252–260.

77. Newell RLM. Olecranon fractures in children. *Injury.* 1975;7:33–36.

78. Newman JH. Displaced radial neck fractures in children. *Injury.* 1977;9:114–121.

79. O'Brien PI. Injuries involving the proximal radial epiphysis. *Clin Orthop Relat Res.* 1965;41:51–58.

80. Olney BW, Menelaus MB. Monteggia and equivalent lesions in childhood. *J Pediatr Orthop.* 1989;9:219–223.

81. Paci JM, Dugas JR, Guy JA, et al. Cannulated screw fixation of refractory olecranon stress fractures with and without associated injuries allows a return to baseball. *Am J Sports Med.* 2013;41(2):306–312.

82. Papavasiliou VA, Beslikas TA, Nenopoulos S. Isolated fractures of the olecranon in children. *Injury.* 1987;18:100–102.

83. Pappas AM. Elbow problems associated with baseball during childhood. *Clin Orthop Relat Res.* 1982;164:30–41.

84. Parent S, Wedemeyer M, Mahar AT, et al. Displaced olecranon fractures in children: a biomechanical analysis of fixation methods. *J Pediatr Orthop.* 2008;28(2):147–151.

85. Patterson RF. Treatment of displaced transverse fractures of the neck of the radius in children. *J Bone Joint Surg.* 1934;16:695–698.

86. Pavlov H, Torg JS, Jacobs B, et al. Nonunion of olecranon epiphysis: two cases in adolescent baseball pitchers. *AJR Am J Roentgenol.* 1981;136:819–820.

87. Persiani P, Ranaldi FM, Graci J, et al. Isolated olecranon fractures in children affected by osteogenesis imperfecta type I treated with single screw or tension band wiring system: outcomes and pitfalls in relation to bone mineral density. *Medicine (Baltimore).* 2017;96(20):e6766.

88. Pesudo JV, Aracil J, Barcelo M. Leverage method in displaced fractures of the radial neck in children. *Clin Orthop.* 1982;169:215–218.

89. Poland J. *A Practical Treatise on Traumatic Separation of the Epiphyses.* London: Smith, Elder & Co; 1898.

90. Porteous CJ. The olecranon epiphyses. *Proc J Anat.* 1960;94:286.

91. Prathapkumar KR, Garg NK, Bruce CE. Elastic stable intramedullary nail fixation for severely displaced fractures of the neck of the radius in children. *J Bone Joint Surg Br.* 2006;88(3):358–361.

92. Radomisli TE, Rosen AL. Controversies regarding radial neck fractures in children. *Clin Orthop Relat Res.* 1998;353:30–39.

93. Rath NK, Carpenter EC, Thomas DP. Traumatic pediatric olecranon injury: a report of suture fixation and review of the literature. *Pediatr Emerg Care.* 2011;27(12):1167–1169.

94. Regan W, Morrey BF. Fractures of the coronoid process of the ulna. *J Bone Joint Surg Am.* 1989;71:1348–1354.

95. Regan W, Morrey BF. Classification and treatment of coronoid process fractures. *Orthopedics.* 1992;15:845–848.

96. Retrum RK, Wepfer JF, Olen DW, et al. Case report 355: delayed closure of the right olecranon epiphysis in a right-handed tournament-class tennis player. *Skeletal Radiol.* 1986;15:185–187.

97. Robert M, Moulies D, Longis B, et al. Les fractures de l'extremite superieure du radius chez l'enfant. *Chir Pediatr.* 1986;27:318–321.

98. Rodriguez-Merchan EC. Displaced fractures of the head and neck of the radius in children: open reduction and temporary transarticular internal fixation. *Orthopedics.* 1991;14:697–700.

99. Rodriguez-Merchan EC. Percutaneous reduction of displaced radial neck fractures in children. *J Trauma.* 1994;37:812–814.

100. Roe SC. Tension band wiring of olecranon fractures: a modification of the AO technique. *Clin Orthop Relat Res.* 1994;308:284–286.

101. Rogers SL, Mac Ewan DW. Changes due to trauma in the fat plane overlying the supinator muscle: a radiologic sign. *Radiology.* 1969;92:954–958.

102. Rowland SA, Burkhart SS. Tension band wiring of olecranon fractures. A modification of the AO technique. *Clin Orthop Relat Res.* 1992;277:238–242.

103. Saberstein MJ, Brodeur AE, Graviss ER, et al. Some vagaries of the olecranon. *J Bone Joint Surg Am.* 1981;63:722–725.

104. Scullion JE, Miller JH. Fracture of the neck of the radius in children: prognostic factors and recommendations for management. *J Bone Joint Surg Br.* 1985;67:491.

105. Sessa S, Lascombes P, Prevot J, et al. Fractures of the radial head and associated elbow injuries in children. *J Pediatr Orthop B.* 1996;5:200–209.

106. Silberstein MJ, Brodeur AE, Graviss ER. Some vagaries of the radial head and neck. *J Bone Joint Surg Am.* 1982;64:1153–1157.

107. Skak SV. Fracture of the olecranon through a persistent physis in an adult: a case report. *J Bone Joint Surg Am.* 1993;75:272–275.

108. Smith FM. *Surgery of the Elbow.* Philadelphia, PA: WB Saunders; 1972.

109. Smith AM, Morrey BF, Steinmann SP, et al. Low profile fixation of radial head and neck fractures: surgical technique and clinical experience. *J Orthop Trauma.* 2007;21(10):718–724.

110. Smith GR, Hotchkiss RN. Radial head and neck fractures: anatomic guidelines for proper placement of internal fixation. *J Shoulder Elbow Surg.* 1996;5(2 Pt 1):113–117.

111. Song KS, Kim BS, Lee SW. Percutaneous leverage reduction for severely displaced radial neck fractures in children. *J Pediatr Orthop.* 2015;35(4):e26–e30.

112. Soyer AD, Nowotarski PJ, Kelso TB, et al. Optimal position for plate fixation of complex fractures of the proximal radius: a cadaver study. *J Orthop Trauma.* 1998; 12(4):291–293.

113. Steele JA, Graham HK. Angulated radial neck fractures in children: a prospective study of percutaneous reduction. *J Bone Joint Surg Br.* 1992;74:760–764.

114. Steinberg EL, Golomb D, Salama R, et al. Radial head and neck fractures in children. *J Pediatr Orthop.* 1988;8:35–40.

115. Su Y, Xie Y, Qin J, et al. Internal fixation with absorbable rods for the treatment of displaced radial neck fractures in children. *J Pediatr Orthop.* 2016;36(8):797–802.

116. Suprock MD, Lubahn JD. Olecranon fracture with unilateral closed radial shaft fracture in a child with open epiphysis. *Orthopedics.* 1990;13:463–465.

117. Tan BH, Mahadev A. Radial neck fractures in children. *J Orthop Surg (Hong Kong).* 2011;19:209–212.

118. Tarallo L, Mugnai R, Adani R, et al. Simple and comminuted displaced olecranon fractures: a clinical comparison between tension band wiring and plate fixation techniques. *Arch Orthop Trauma Surg.* 2014;134(8):1107–1114.

119. Tarallo L, Mugnai R, Fiacchi F, et al. Management of displaced radial neck fractures in children: percutaneous pinning vs. elastic stable intramedullary nailing. *J Orthop Traumatol.* 2013;14(4):291–297.

120. Teasdall R, Savoie FH, Hughes JL. Comminuted fractures of the proximal radius and ulna. *Clin Orthop Relat Res.* 1993;292:37–47.

121. Theodorou SD, Ierodiaconou MN, Roussis N. Fracture of the upper end of the ulna associated with dislocation of the head of the radius in children. *Clin Orthop Relat Res.* 1988;228:240–249.

122. Thijn CJP, van Ouwerkerk WP, Scheele PM, et al. Unilateral patella cubiti: A probable posttraumatic disorder. *Eur J Radiol.* 1992;14:60–62.

123. Tibone JE, Stoltz M. Fracture of the radial head and neck in children. *J Bone Joint Surg Am.* 1981;63:100–106.

124. Torg JS, Moyer R. Nonunion of a stress fracture through the olecranon epiphyseal plate observed in an adolescent baseball pitcher. *J Bone Joint Surg Am.* 1977;59:264–265.

125. Tullos HS, King JW. Lesions of the pitching arm in adolescents. *JAMA.* 1972; 220:264–271.

126. Turtel AH, Andrews JR, Schob CJ, et al. Fractures of unfused olecranon physis: a reevaluation of this injury in three athletes. *Orthopedics.* 1995;18:390–394.

127. Ugutmen E, Ozkan K, Ozkan FU, et al. Reduction and fixation of radius neck fractures in children with intramedullary pin. *J Pediatr Orthop B.* 2010;19(4):289–293.

128. Vahvanen V. Fracture of the radial neck in children. *Acta Orthop Scand.* 1978;49: 32–38.

129. Van Zeeland NL, Bae DS, Goldfarb CA. Intra-articular radial head fracture in the skeletally immature patient: progressive radial head subluxation and rapid radiocapitellar degeneration. *J Pediatric Orthop.* 2011;31:124–129.

130. Veranis N, Laliotis N, Vlachos E. Acute osteomyelitis complicating a closed radial fracture in a child: a case report. *Acta Orthop Scand.* 1992;63:341–342.

131. Vocke AK, Von Laer L. Displaced fractures of the radial neck in children: long-term results and prognosis of conservative treatment. *J Pediatr Orthop B.* 1998;7:217–222.

132. Vostal O. Fracture of the neck of the radius in children. *Acta Chir Orthop Traumatol Cech.* 1970;37:294–301.

133. Wang J, Chen W, Guo M, et al. Percutaneous reduction and intramedullary fixation technique for displaced pediatric radial neck fractures. *J Pediatr Orthop B.* 2013;22(2):127–132.

134. Ward WT, Williams JJ. Radial neck fracture complicating closed reduction of a posterior elbow dislocation in a child: case report. *J Trauma*. 1991;31:1686–1688.

135. Waters PM, Beaty J, Kasser J. TRASH (The Radiographic Appearance Seemed Harmless). *J Pediatr Orthop*. 2010;30:S77–S81.

136. Waters PM, Stewart SL. Radial neck fracture nonunion in children. *J Pediatr Orthop*. 2001;21:570–576.

137. Wedge JH, Robertson DE. Displaced fractures of the neck of the radius. *J Bone Joint Surg Br*. 1982;64:256.

138. Wilkerson RD, Johns JC. Nonunion of an olecranon stress fracture in an adolescent gymnast: a case report. *Am J Sports Med*. 1990;18:432–434.

139. Wood SK. Reversal of the radial head during reduction of fractures of the neck of the radius in children. *J Bone Joint Surg Br*. 1969;51:707–710.

140. Wright PR. Greenstick fracture of the upper end of the ulna with dislocation of the radio-humeral joint or displacement of the superior radial epiphysis. *J Bone Joint Surg Br*. 1963;45:727–731.

141. Zeitlin A. The traumatic origin of accessory bones at the elbow. *J Bone Joint Surg*. 1935;17:933–938.

142. Zhang FY, Wang XD, Zhen YF, et al. Treatment of severely displaced radial neck fractures in children with percutaneous K-wire leverage and closed intramedullary pinning. *Medicine (Baltimore)*. 2016;95(1):e2346.

143. Zimmerman H. Fractures of the elbow. In: Weber BG, Brunner C, Freuler F, eds. *Treatment of Fractures in Children and Adolescents*. New York: Springer-Verlag; 1980.

144. Zimmerman RM, Kalish LA, Hresko MT, et al. Surgical management of pediatric radial neck fractures. *J Bone Joint Surg Am*. 2013;95(20):1825–1832.

11

Monteggia Fracture–Dislocation in Children

Apurva S. Shah and Julie Balch Samora

INTRODUCTION TO MONTEGGIA FRACTURE–DISLOCATIONS

Monteggia fracture–dislocations are a rare but complex injury usually involving a fracture of the ulna associated with proximal radioulnar joint dissociation and radiocapitellar dislocation. These injuries comprise less than 1% of all pediatric forearm fractures and typically affect patients between 4 and 10 years of age.[78,161] Unfortunately, this rare injury can have very serious consequences if not treated appropriately acutely. The annual incidence of Monteggia fracture–dislocations in children is less than 1 in 100,000.[78] In 1814, Giovanni Battista Monteggia, a surgical pathologist and public health official in Milan, Italy, first described a variation of the injury that now bears his name as "a traumatic lesion distinguished by a fracture of the proximal third of the ulna and an anterior dislocation of the proximal epiphysis of the radius."[94,110,118] In 1967, José Luis Bado, while director of National Institute of Orthopaedics and Traumatology in Montevideo, Uruguay, published his classic monograph on the classification of Monteggia lesions.[8,10] He described a

Monteggia lesion as a radial head fracture or dislocation in association with a fracture of the middle or proximal ulna. Over the last century, numerous authors have made significant contributions on pathoanatomy, classification, diagnosis, treatment, and complications.[7,21,32,34,37,38,49,53,56,66,71,82,84,91,92,102,109,120,123,131,135,165]

Despite the increased understanding of Monteggia lesions, the injury continues to represent a challenge for the orthopedic surgeon. In 1943, Sir Watson-Jones wrote that "no fracture presents so many problems; no injury is beset with greater difficulty; no treatment is characterized by more general failure."[163] Unfortunately, despite the increased awareness and understanding of Monteggia lesions, the initial diagnosis is still missed by qualified radiologists, emergency room physicians, and orthopedic surgeons among others.[18,42,43,49,51,61,82,85,111,123,125,131,135,155,165,168] In addition, less than optimal treatment of recognized but unstable injuries has also resulted in chronic Monteggia lesions.[34,38,49,58,63,71,75,120,122,123,166] A chronic Monteggia lesion can result in substantial morbidity, and is far more complex in terms of surgical decision making and management than an acute injury.[18,29,33,43,51,61,67,85,125,129]

ASSESSMENT OF MONTEGGIA FRACTURE–DISLOCATIONS

CLASSIFICATION OF MONTEGGIA FRACTURE–DISLOCATIONS

Bado Classification

Bado's original classification[8,10] has stood the test of time with minimal modifications except for the addition of various equivalent lesions (Fig. 11-1). The classification system is based on the direction of the radial head dislocation and the apex of the associated ulna fracture. Bado's[8,10] four true Monteggia types are as follows:

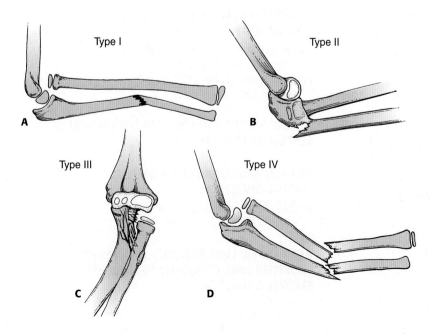

Figure 11-1. Bado classification. **A:** Type I (anterior dislocation): The radial head is dislocated anteriorly and the ulna has a short oblique or greenstick fracture in the diaphyseal or proximal metaphyseal area. **B:** Type II (posterior dislocation): The radial head is posteriorly or posterolaterally dislocated; the ulna is usually fractured in the metaphysis in children. **C:** Type III (lateral dislocation): There is lateral dislocation of the radial head with a greenstick metaphyseal fracture of the ulna. **D:** Type IV (anterior dislocation with radial shaft fracture): The pattern of injury is the same as with a type I injury, with the inclusion of a radial shaft fracture distal to the level of the ulnar fracture.

Bado Type I

A Bado type I lesion is an anterior dislocation of the radial head associated with an apex anterior ulnar diaphyseal fracture at any level. This is the most common Monteggia lesion in children and represents approximately 70% to 75% of all injuries.[38,54,82,123,161]

Bado Type II

A Bado type II lesion is a posterior or posterolateral dislocation of the radial head associated with an apex posterior ulnar diaphyseal or metaphyseal fracture. This pattern is the most common Monteggia lesion in adults, but is relatively rare in children.[108,109,123] Type II lesions account for 6% of Monteggia lesions in children,[78] and are usually found in older patients[108] who have sustained significant trauma.[41,120,121]

Bado Type III

A Bado type III lesion is a lateral dislocation of the radial head associated with a varus (apex lateral) fracture of the proximal ulna. This is the second most common pediatric Monteggia lesion.[13,49,101,106,165] When an injury is characterized by an olecranon fracture and a lateral or anterolateral radiocapitellar dislocation but no radioulnar dissociation, the injury is not a true Monteggia lesion.[64,122,150]

Bado Type IV

A Bado type IV lesion is an anterior dislocation of the radial head associated with fractures of both the ulna and the radius. The original description was of a radial fracture at the same level or distal to the ulna fracture. Type IV lesions are relatively rare in children.

EXPANSION OF THE BADO CLASSIFICATION: MONTEGGIA-EQUIVALENT LESIONS

Bado[8,10] classified certain injuries as equivalents to true Monteggia lesions because of their similar mechanisms of injury, radiographic appearance, or treatment methods. Since his original publication, the list of equivalent lesions has expanded case report by case report.

Type I Equivalent Fractures

Bado type I equivalents (Fig. 11-2) include isolated anterior dislocations of the radial head without ulnar fracture. This subclassification includes a "pulled elbow" or "nursemaid's elbow" because the mechanism of longitudinal traction, pronation, and hyperextension is similar to a true type I lesion. In nursemaid's elbow cases, the radiographs are normal. It is debatable if a "nursemaid's elbow" is really a part of the Monteggia spectrum but we will include it in this chapter for completeness. In type I equivalent lesions, the radial head is malaligned in its relationship to the capitellum and proximal ulna. However, the ulnar bow sign (Fig. 11-3) is normal as opposed to subtle plastic deformation of the ulna which will have a concave ulnar bow and can be misdiagnosed as a type I equivalent when the injury is really a Bado I lesion. This distinction can be critical in terms of operative decision making in that the type I equivalent lesion requires an

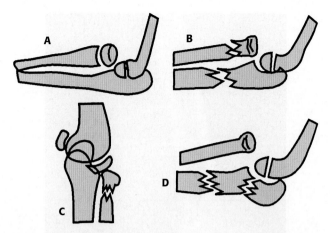

Figure 11-2. Type I equivalents. **A:** Isolated anterior radial head dislocation. **B:** Ulnar fracture with fracture of the radial neck. **C:** Isolated radial neck fractures. **D:** Elbow (ulnohumeral) dislocation with or without fracture of the proximal radius.

open repair of the displaced ligament while the Bado type I lesion with plastic deformation requires correction of the ulnar deformity. Other type I equivalents (Fig. 11-2) include anterior dislocation of the radial head with ulnar metaphyseal or diaphyseal fracture and radial neck fracture; anterior dislocation of the radial head with radial diaphyseal fracture more proximal to ulnar diaphyseal fracture; anterior radial head dislocation with ulnotrochlear dislocation (Fig. 11-4)[123]; and anterior dislocation of the radial head with segmental ulna fracture.[2,54,64,113,127,150] More case reports will probably expand this subclassification over time. The type I equivalents have been shown to have poorer outcomes and require more frequent operative intervention than true Monteggia lesions.[54,101] Poor outcomes may relate to intra-articular injury, coronoid fracture, comminution of the ulna fracture, and comminution of the radial head fracture.[130]

Type II Equivalents

Bado[8,10] described type II equivalents to include posterior radial head dislocations associated with fractures of the proximal radial epiphysis or radial neck.

Type III and Type IV Equivalents

Bado[8,10] did not have equivalent lesions for the true type III and type IV lesions. Because mechanism of injury allows for this subclassification, case reports have emerged over time to include fractures of the distal humerus (supracondylar,

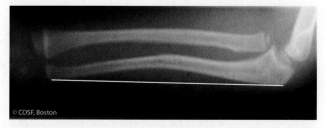

Figure 11-3. The ulnar bow line. This line, drawn between the distal ulna and the olecranon, defines the ulnar bow. The ulnar bow sign is a deviation of the ulnar border from the reference line by more than 1 mm.

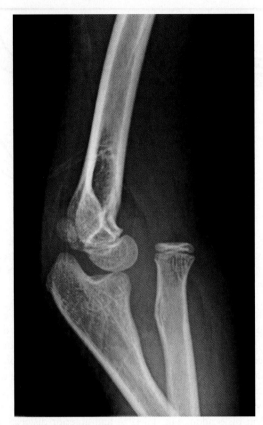

Figure 11-4. Type I equivalent that includes elbow subluxation in addition to the radioulnar dislocation.

Monteggia equivalents

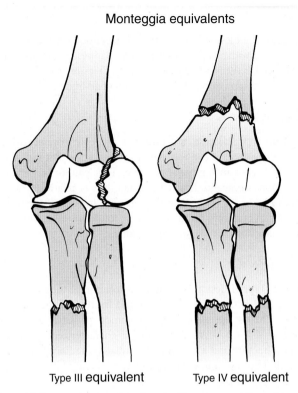

Type III **equivalent**   Type IV **equivalent**

Figure 11-5. Type III equivalent described by Ravessoud.[72] An oblique fracture of the ulna with varus alignment and a displaced lateral condylar fracture. Type IV equivalent described by Arazi[63]: fractures of the distal humerus, ulnar diaphysis, and radial neck.

lateral condylar) in association with proximal forearm fractures (Fig. 11-5).[5,16,17,36,46,52,54,55,89,98,113,119,124,127,133]

Letts Classification

Letts et al.[82] have described an alternate classification schedule for pediatric Monteggia fracture–dislocations based both

on direction of radial head dislocation and the type of ulnar fracture (Fig. 11-6). Letts types A, B, and C are analogous to Bado type I lesions and are characterized by anterior dislocation of the radial head with an associated ulnar fracture. In a type A lesion, there is plastic deformation of the ulna; in a type B lesion, there is an incomplete or greenstick ulnar fracture; and in a type C lesion, there is a complete ulnar

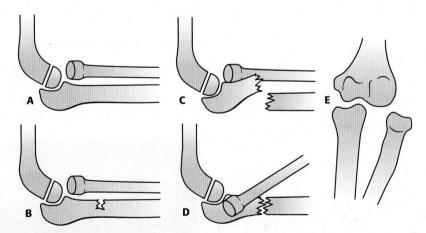

Figure 11-6. Pediatric Monteggia fracture–dislocation classification by Letts et al.[19] **A:** Anterior dislocation of the radial head with plastic deformation of the ulna. **B:** Anterior dislocation of the radial head with greenstick fracture of the ulna. **C:** Anterior dislocation of the radial head with complete fracture of the ulna. **D:** Posterior dislocation of the radial head with fracture of the ulnar metaphysis. **E:** Lateral dislocation of the radial head and metaphyseal greenstick fracture of the ulna.

fracture. The A, B, and C aspects of the Letts classification are useful for aiding in treatment decisions (see Ring, Jupiter, and Waters classification). Letts type D lesions are equivalent to Bado type II injuries and are characterized by posterior radial head dislocation. Letts type E lesions are equivalent to Bado type III injuries and are characterized by lateral radial head dislocation.

Authors' Preferred Classification

Monteggia Fracture–Dislocations: AUTHORS' PREFERRED CLASSIFICATION		
Type	**Dislocation**	**Fracture**
True Lesions		
I	Anterior	Metaphysis–diaphysis
II	Posterior	Metaphysis–diaphysis
III	Lateral	Metaphysis
IV	Anterior	Radial diaphysis, ulnar diaphysis
Hybrid lesion	Anterior, posterior, or lateral	Metaphysis or olecranon
Type	**Description**	
Equivalent Lesions		
I	Isolated dislocation of radial head	
	Radial neck fracture (isolated)	
	Radial neck fracture in combination with a fracture of the ulnar diaphysis	
	Radial and ulnar fractures with the radial fracture above the junction of the middle and proximal thirds	
	Fracture of ulnar diaphysis with anterior dislocation of radial head and an olecranon fracture	
II	Posterior dislocation of the elbow	
III	Ulnar fracture with displaced fracture of the lateral condyle	
IV	None described	

Ring, Jupiter, and Waters[122,123] defined a Monteggia lesion as a proximal radioulnar joint dislocation in association with a forearm fracture. In this classification system, it is the character of the ulnar fracture, more so than the direction of the radial head dislocation, that is most useful in determining the optimal treatment of Monteggia fracture–dislocations in both adults and children. Stable anatomic reduction of the ulnar fracture almost always results in anatomic, stable reduction of the radial head, proximal radioulnar joint, and radiocapitellar joint in the acute setting. The ulnar fracture is defined similarly to all pediatric forearm fractures: plastic deformation, incomplete or greenstick fractures, and complete fractures. Complete fractures are further subdivided into transverse, short oblique, long oblique, and comminuted fractures. Treatment directly relates to the fracture type: closed reduction for plastic deformation and greenstick fractures; intramedullary fixation for transverse and short

oblique fractures; and open reduction and internal fixation with plate and screws for long oblique and comminuted fractures.

MECHANISMS OF INJURY FOR MONTEGGIA FRACTURE–DISLOCATIONS

Type I Mechanism of Injury

Three separate mechanisms of type I lesions have been described: direct trauma,[10,22,27,42,99,116,120,135,155] hyperpronation,[22,120] and hyperextension.

Direct Blow Theory

The first theory proposed in English literature was the direct blow mechanism described by Speed and Boyd[135] and endorsed by Smith (Fig. 11-7).[131] This theory was actually proposed by Monteggia,[94] who noted that the fracture occurs when a direct blow on the posterior aspect of the forearm first produces a fracture through the ulna. Then, either by continued deformation or direct pressure, the radial head is forced anteriorly with respect to the capitellum, causing the radial head to dislocate. Monteggia[94] explained that these injuries sometimes resulted from a blow by a staff or cudgel on the forearm raised to protect the head.

The parry fracture, another term for the Monteggia fracture–dislocation, has been mentioned in the literature. During the American Civil War, Monteggia fractures were frequent because of direct blows on the forearm received while attempting to parry the butt of a rifle during hand-to-hand combat. The major argument against this theory as the mechanism is that in the usual clinical situation, there rarely is evidence of a direct blow to the posterior aspect of the forearm, such as a contusion or laceration.[42,155]

Hyperpronation Theory

In 1949, Evans[42] published his observations regarding anterior Monteggia fracture–dislocations. Previous investigators had based their direct blow theory on hypothesis and clinical observation, but Evans used cadaveric investigation to support

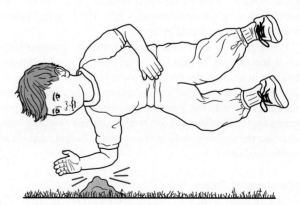

Figure 11-7. Mechanism of injury for type I Monteggia lesions: direct blow theory. The fracture–dislocation is sustained by direct contact on the posterior aspect of the forearm, either by falling onto an object or by an object striking the forearm. The continued motion of the object forward dislocates the radial head after fracturing the ulna.

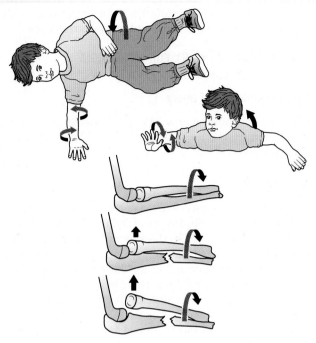

Figure 11-8. Mechanism of injury for type I Monteggia lesions: hyperpronation theory (Evans).[32] Rotation of the body externally forces the forearm into pronation. The ulnar shaft fractures with further rotation, forcibly dislocating the radial head.

his hyperpronation theory. He demonstrated that hyperpronation of the forearm produced a fracture of the ulna with a subsequent dislocation of the radial head. He postulated that during a fall, the outstretched hand, initially in pronation, is forced into further pronation as the body twists above the planted hand and forearm (Fig. 11-8). This hyperpronation forcibly rotates the radius over the middle of the ulna, resulting in either anterior dislocation of the radial head or fracture of the proximal third of the radius, along with fracture of the ulna. In actual patients reported on by Evans, the ulnar fractures demonstrated a pattern consistent with anterior tension and shear or longitudinal compression. His cadaveric investigation, however, showed the ulnar fracture pattern to be consistent with a spiral or rotational force. The hyperpronation theory was also supported by Bado.[9]

Two arguments have been used to dispute the hyperpronation mechanism.[155] First, the ulnar fracture rarely presents clinically in a spiral pattern; it is often oblique, indicating an initial force in tension with propagation in shear rather than rotational. Second, the Evans experiments, which were performed on totally dissected forearms,[42] did not take into consideration the dynamic muscle forces at play during a fall on an outstretched hand.

Hyperextension Theory

In 1971, Tompkins[155] analyzed both theories and presented good clinical evidence that type I Monteggia fracture–dislocations were caused by a combination of dynamic and static forces. His study postulated three steps in the fracture mechanism: hyperextension, radial head dislocation, and ulnar fracture

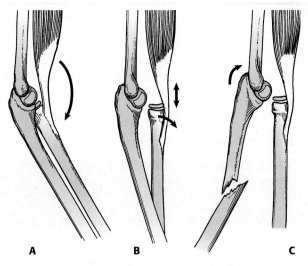

Figure 11-9. Mechanism of injury for type I Monteggia lesions: hyperextension theory (Tompkins).[39] **A:** Forward momentum caused by a fall on an outstretched hand forces the elbow into hyperextension. **B:** The biceps contracts, forcibly dislocating the radial head. **C:** Continued forward momentum causes the ulna to fracture because of tension on the anterior surface.

(Fig. 11-9). The patient falls on an outstretched arm with forward momentum, forcing the elbow joint into hyperextension. The radius is first dislocated anteriorly by the violent reflexive contracture of the biceps, forcing the radius away from the capitellum. Once the proximal radius dislocates, the weight of the body is transferred to the ulna. Because the radius is usually the main load-bearing bone in the forearm, the ulna cannot handle the transmitted longitudinal force and, subsequently, fails in tension. This tension force produces an oblique fracture line or a greenstick fracture in the ulnar diaphysis or at the diaphyseal–metaphyseal junction. In addition to the momentum of the injury, the anterior angulation of the ulna results from the pull of the intact interosseous membrane on the distal fragment, causing it to follow the radius. The brachialis muscle causes the proximal ulnar fragment to flex.

Summary of Type I Mechanism of Injury

The type I lesion can probably be caused by any of the three proposed mechanisms, but the most common mechanism is a fall on an outstretched hand that forces the elbow into complete extension, locking the olecranon into the humerus. The forearm is in a rotational position of neutral to midpronation. As the proximal ulna locks into the distal humerus, the bending force stresses the proximal radioulnar joint. Because of the relatively pronated position of the joint, the ligamentous restraints are lax, providing only tenuous stability for the radial head. The anterior bending force, combined with a reflexive contraction of the biceps, violently dislocates the radial head anteriorly. The radioulnar joint and its ligamentous complex are at risk because of the ligamentous laxity and the decreased contact area between the proximal radius and ulna created by the rotation of the forearm. At midrotation, the short axis of the elliptical radial head is perpendicular to the ulna, causing the annular ligament and the dense anterior portion of the quadrate ligament to be relaxed. The contact area of the proximal radioulnar joint, because of the shape of the radial head, is also decreased, further reducing the stability of the joint. The ulna, now the main weight-bearing structure of the forearm, is loaded by a continued bending moment, causing tension on the anterior cortex and producing failure. The force at the site of failure is propagated in shear at approximately 45 degrees to the long axis of the ulna. This mechanism may produce plastic deformation with an anterior bow, a greenstick fracture, or an oblique fracture pattern, all of which are observed clinically. As the anterior bending movement continues, the vector of the biceps changes and acts as a tether and resists any further advance of the proximal radius. The distal fragment of the ulna continues to advance, acting as a fulcrum against the radial shaft. The anteriorly directed force of the distal ulnar fragment, combined with the retrograde resistance of the biceps, may create a fracture of the radius, or a type IV lesion.

Type II Mechanism of Injury

The cause of the type II Monteggia lesion is subject to debate. Bado[10] thought the lesion was caused by direct force and sudden supination. Penrose[111] analyzed seven fractures in adults and noted that a proximal ulnar fracture was the typical pattern. He postulated that the injury occurred by longitudinal loading rather than by direct trauma.[135] Olney and Menelaus[101] reported four type II lesions in their series of pediatric Monteggia fractures. Three of these patients had proximal ulnar fractures and one had an oblique midshaft fracture, suggesting two different mechanisms of injury.

The mechanism proposed and experimentally demonstrated by Penrose[111] was that type II lesions occur when the forearm is suddenly loaded in a longitudinal direction with the elbow in approximately 60 degrees of flexion. This investigation demonstrated that a type II lesion occurred consistently if the ulna fractured; otherwise, a posterior elbow dislocation was produced (Fig. 11-10). The difference in bone strength of the ulna may explain the reason for the high incidence of type II Monteggia lesions in older adults and their rarity in children. Penrose[111] further noted that the rotational position of the forearm did not seem to affect the type of fracture produced.

Haddad et al.[59] described type II injuries caused by low-velocity injuries in six adults, five of whom were on long-term corticosteroid therapy. They suggested that this supports the theory that the type II Monteggia injury is a variant of posterior elbow dislocation, in that it occurs when the ulna is weaker than the ligaments surrounding the elbow joint, resulting in an ulnar fracture before the ligament disruption required for dislocation.

Type III Mechanism of Injury

Wright[168] studied fractures of the proximal ulna with lateral and anterolateral dislocations of the radial head and concluded that the mechanism of injury was varus stress at the level of the elbow, in combination with an outstretched hand planted firmly against a fixed surface (Fig. 11-11). This usually produces a greenstick ulnar fracture with tension failure

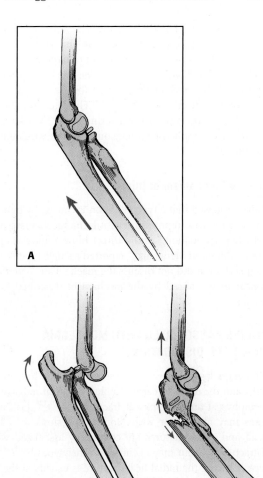

Figure 11-10. Mechanism of injury for type II Monteggia lesions. **A:** With the elbow flexed approximately 60 degrees, a longitudinal force is applied parallel to the long axis of the forearm. **B:** This force may result in a posterior elbow dislocation. **C:** If the integrity of the anterior cortex of the ulna is compromised, a type II fracture–dislocation occurs.

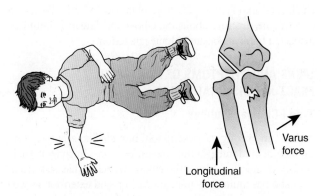

Figure 11-11. Mechanism of injury for type III Monteggia lesions. A forced varus stress causes a greenstick fracture of the proximal ulna and a true lateral or anterolateral radial head dislocation.

radially and compression medially. The radial head dislocates laterally, rupturing the annular ligament. Hume[64] suggested that type III lesions may be the result of hyperextension of the elbow combined with pronation of the forearm. Other authors confirmed the mechanism of varus force at the elbow as the cause of type III injuries.[10,38,96,109,150] The direction of the radial head dislocation is probably determined by the rotational and angular force applied simultaneously to the varus moment at the elbow.[96]

Type IV Mechanism of Injury

Bado[8] proposed that a type IV lesion is caused by hyperpronation. Of the case reports discussing the mechanism of injury, both hyperpronation[49] and a direct blow[124] have been postulated. Olney and Menelaus[101] reported a single type IV lesion in their series but did not discuss the mechanism. Type IV lesions appear to be caused by the mechanism described for type I lesions.

INJURIES ASSOCIATED WITH MONTEGGIA FRACTURE–DISLOCATIONS

Monteggia lesions have been associated with fractures of the wrist and the distal forearm,[10] including distal radial and ulnar metaphyseal and diaphyseal fractures.[10,65,67,124] Galeazzi fractures may also occur with Monteggia lesions.[10,27,28,81] Radial head and neck fractures are commonly associated with type II fractures[10,78] but may occur with other types.[1,45,50,145] With a type II lesion, the radial head fracture is usually at the anterior rim.[41,108] Strong et al.[144] reported two type I equivalent lesions consisting of a fractured radial neck and midshaft ulnar fracture. This injury pattern is notable because of significant medial displacement of the distal radial fragment. Obtaining and maintaining reduction of the radius proved difficult with a closed technique.

Fractures of the distal humerus lateral condyle have also been associated with Monteggia fractures.[31,109] Ravessoud[119] reported an ipsilateral ulnar shaft lesion and a lateral condylar fracture without loss of the radiocapitellar relation, suggesting a type II equivalent (Fig. 11-5). Kloen et al.[73] reported a bilateral Monteggia fracture–dislocation and described the operative technique for its treatment. Despite surgical and rehabilitative challenges, excellent results were obtained in both elbows. In essence, any fracture about the elbow and forearm should be inspected for an associated Monteggia lesion.

SIGNS AND SYMPTOMS OF MONTEGGIA FRACTURE–DISLOCATIONS

Type I Clinical Findings

Bado,[8,10] in his original description, provided an accurate clinical picture of Monteggia fracture–dislocations. In general, there is fusiform swelling about the elbow. The child has significant pain and has limitations in elbow flexion and extension as well as forearm pronation and supination. Usually, an angular change in the forearm itself is evident, with the apex shifted anteriorly and mild valgus apparent. There may be tenting of the skin

or an area of ecchymosis on the volar aspect of the forearm. It is imperative to check for an open fracture wound. With displaced fracture dislocations, the child may not be able to extend the fingers at the metacarpophalangeal joints or retropulse the thumb secondary to a posterior interosseous nerve (PIN) palsy. Later, as the swelling subsides, anterior fullness may remain in the cubital fossa for the typical type I lesion. However, this finding may be subtle because children will usually have an elbow flexion posture following injury. If the injury is seen late, there will be a loss of full flexion at the elbow and a palpable anterior dislocation of the radial head. The radial head–distal humerus impingement that occurs may be a source of pain with activities. There is usually loss of forearm rotation with late presentation. Progressive valgus may occur if the anterior radial head dislocation worsens. With plastic deformation injuries, the clinical findings may be subtle, leading to late presentation or difficult radiographic diagnosis.

Type II Clinical Findings

Similar to type I lesions, the elbow region is swollen but exhibits posterior angulation of the proximal forearm and a marked prominence in the area posterolateral to the normal location of the radial head. The entire upper extremity should be examined because of the frequency of associated injuries.[75,108]

Type III Clinical Findings

Lateral swelling, varus deformity of the elbow, and significant limitation of motion (especially supination) are the hallmarks of type III Monteggia fracture–dislocations. Again, these signs can be subtle and missed by harried clinicians. Injuries to the radial nerve, particularly the posterior interosseous branch, occur more frequently with type III lesions than other Monteggia fracture–dislocations.[13,123,138]

Type IV Clinical Findings

The appearance of the limb with a type IV lesion is similar to that of a type I lesion. However, more swelling and pain can be present because of the magnitude of force required to create this complex injury. Particular attention should be given to the neurovascular status of the limb, anticipating the possible increased risk for a compartment syndrome.

Clinical Findings in Monteggia Equivalents and Associated Injuries

In a Monteggia-equivalent injury, clinical findings are similar to those for the corresponding Bado lesion, with the common triad of pain, swelling, and deformity. Given the frequency of associated skeletal injuries, a careful examination of the entire upper extremity should be performed. This involves careful inspection of the skin and palpation of the distal humerus lateral condyle, the distal radius, and the distal radioulnar joint. Given the high frequency of radial nerve injuries with Monteggia fracture–dislocations,[13,14,64,99,123,131,138] a careful examination of neurologic examination should be performed. Because the posterior interosseous branch is most commonly injured, the clinician should routinely examine motor function of the extensor digitorum communis and the extensor pollicis longus. Failure to extend the fingers at the metacarpophalangeal joints or retropulse the thumb are concerning for a PIN palsy.

IMAGING AND OTHER DIAGNOSTIC STUDIES FOR MONTEGGIA FRACTURE–DISLOCATIONS

The standard evaluation of a Monteggia fracture–dislocation includes anteroposterior (AP) and lateral radiographs of the forearm and elbow. Any disruption of the ulna, including subtle changes in ulnar bowing, should alert the clinician to look for disruption of the proximal radioulnar joint.[30,32,69,71,84] Unfortunately, the dislocated radial head is all too often missed in the acute setting. It must be stressed that every forearm and elbow injury requires close scrutiny of the radial head–capitellar relationship. In cases where plain radiographs are concerning but equivocal, fluoroscopic imaging or cross-sectional imaging such as magnetic resonance imaging (MRI) or ultrasound scan should be strongly considered. The goal for every radiologist, orthopedist, and emergency department physician should be to never miss a Monteggia lesion in the acute setting.

Type I Radiographic Evaluation

The radiographic alignment of the radial head and capitellum is particularly important and is best defined by a true lateral view of the elbow (Fig. 11-12). In a type I Monteggia fracture–dislocation, the radiocapitellar relationship may appear normal on an AP radiograph despite obvious disruption on the lateral view. If there is any doubt regarding the radiocapitellar alignment, further radiographic evaluation must be obtained. Smith[131] and later Storen[142] noted that a line drawn through the center of the radial neck and head should extend directly through the center of the capitellum. This alignment should remain intact regardless of the degree of flexion or extension of the elbow (Fig. 11-13). In some instances, there is disruption of the radiocapitellar line in a normal elbow. Miles and Finlay[93] pointed out that the radiocapitellar line passes through the center of the capitellum only on a true lateral projection. They reported five patients in whom the elbow was clinically normal but the radiocapitellar line appeared disrupted. In analyzing the radiographs, they found that the radiographic projection of the elbow was usually an oblique view or that the forearm was pronated in the radiograph. If this disruption appears on radiographs in a child with an acute injury, however, it is the treating surgeon's responsibility to ensure that it is an insignificant finding.

It is still too frequent an occurrence that a highly qualified, distraught, orthopedic surgeon will call for referral of a chronic Monteggia lesion that was missed acutely (Fig. 11-14). With late presentation of a chronic Monteggia injury, an MRI scan may be useful to determine the congruency of the radial head and capitellum. If the radial head is

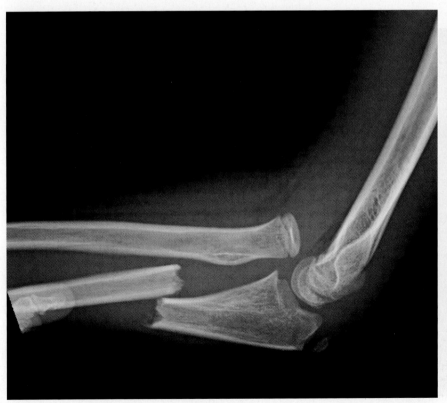
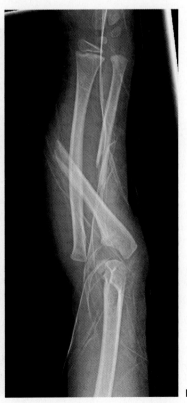

A   **B**

Figure 11-12. Two examples of a Bado type I Monteggia fracture with anterior dislocation of the radial head. **A:** Proximal ulna fracture in the metadiaphyseal region. **B:** Midshaft diaphyseal ulna fracture. Note the disruption of the radiocapitellar line in both.

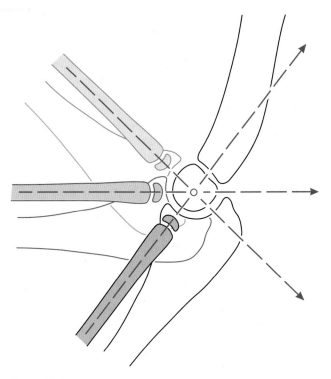

Figure 11-13. Radiocapitellar line. A composite drawing with the elbow in various degrees of flexion. A line drawn down the long axis of the radius bisects the capitellum of the humerus regardless of the degree of flexion or extension of the elbow.

no longer centrally concave or the capitellum is no longer symmetrically convex, surgical reduction may fail to improve pain or restore motion.

Type II Radiographic Evaluation

Standard AP and lateral radiographs of the forearm demonstrate the pertinent features for classifying type II Monteggia fracture–dislocations. The typical findings include a proximal metaphyseal fracture of the ulna, with possible extension into the olecranon (Fig. 11-15).[41,101,151] Oblique diaphyseal ulnar fractures can also result in a type II Monteggia lesion.[8,41,101] The radial head is dislocated posteriorly or posterolaterally[10] and should be carefully examined for other injuries. Accompanying fractures of the anterior margin of the radial head have been noted.[41,108] Initially, these rim fractures are subtle in children but can lead to progressive subluxation and make late reconstruction difficult. Cross-sectional imaging, such as an MRI or ultrasound scan, should be obtained if further characterization of the injury pattern is deemed warranted.

Type III Radiographic Evaluation

In type III lesions, the radial head is displaced laterally or antero-laterally,[107,109] which is best visualized on the AP radiograph (Fig. 11-16). The ulnar fracture often is in the metaphyseal region,[10,13,64,70,95,123,168] but it can also occur more distally.[10,11,47,167] Varus deformity is common to all ulna fractures, regardless of the level. Radiographs of the entire forearm should be obtained

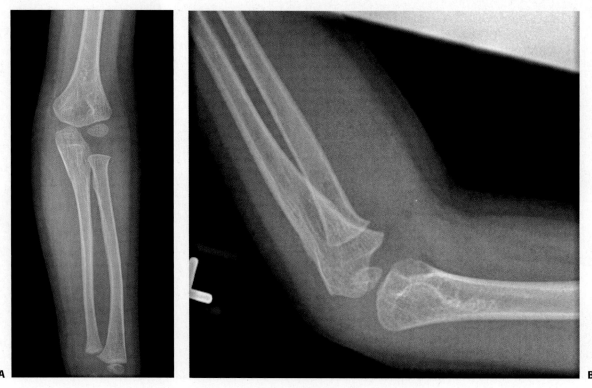

A   B

Figure 11-14. A 3-year-old boy fell from a fence and presented with acute compartment syndrome of the forearm. **A, B:** His initial x-rays did not demonstrate adequate views of the elbow. He underwent fasciotomies, but no bony injuries were addressed. He presented at age 15 with a "clunk" in his elbow.

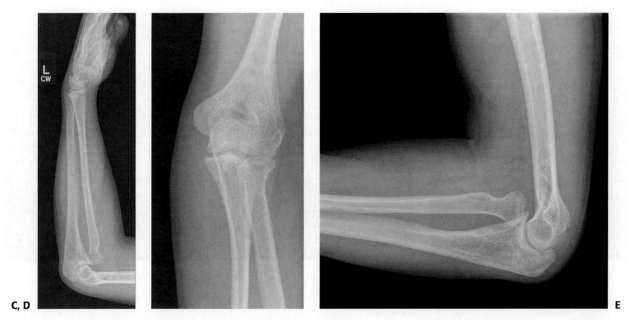

Figure 11-14. (*Continued*) **C–E:** Radiographs demonstrate a chronic anterior dislocation with a convex, misshapen radial head.

because of the association of distal radial and ulnar fractures with this complex elbow injury.[151] As with all Monteggia injuries, the acute lesion can be missed if proper radiographs are not obtained and careful evaluation of the studies is not performed.

Type IV Radiographic Evaluation

In a type IV Monteggia fracture–dislocation, the anterior radial head dislocation is similar to that in a type I lesion (Fig. 11-17).

The radial and ulnar fractures generally are in the middle third of the shaft,[39] with the radial fracture typically distal to the ulnar fracture. The fractures may be incomplete or complete. Although this injury pattern is uncommon in adults and rare in children, the radiocapitellar joint should be examined in all mid-shaft forearm fractures to avoid missing the proximal radioulnar joint disruption (Fig. 11-18). Failure to recognize the radial head dislocation is the major complication of this fracture.[12]

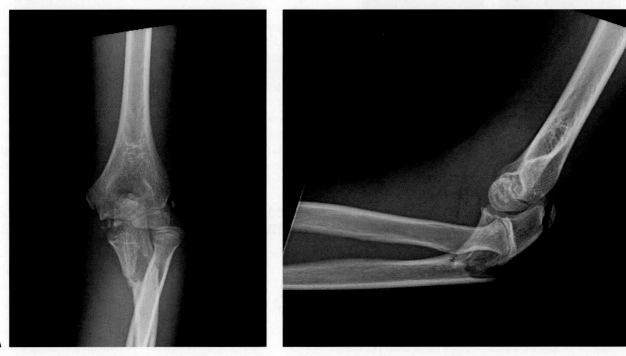

Figure 11-15. Bado type II lesion, with posterolateral dislocation of the radial head (**A**) with apex posterior ulna fracture (**B**).

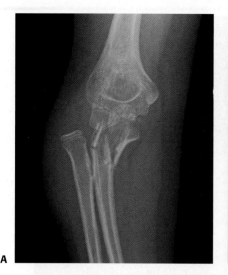
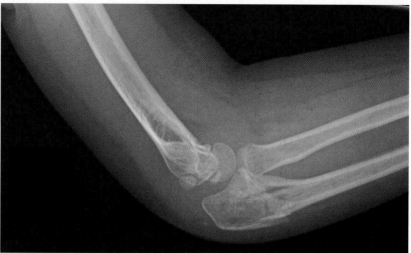

Figure 11-16. AP (**A**) and lateral (**B**) radiographs of a Bado type III fracture pattern, with lateral dislocation of the radius and apex lateral fracture of the proximal ulna.

Radiographic Evaluation of Monteggia Equivalents

As with the true Bado types, careful radiographic study should be made with at least two orthogonal views of the elbow in addition to standard views of the forearm. Special views such as

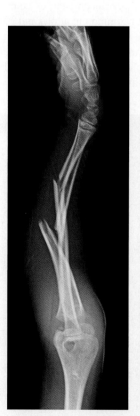
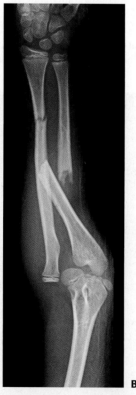

Figure 11-17. Bado type IV lesion with anterior dislocation of the radial head associated with a both bone forearm fracture. Type IV lesion. There is an anterior dislocation of the radial head. The radial and ulnar fractures are usually in the middle third of the shaft, with the radial fracture distal to the ulnar fracture.

obliques should be obtained to clearly delineate the associated injuries (e.g., radial head or neck fracture, distal humerus lateral condyle fracture) and allow adequate pretreatment planning. Cross-sectional imaging, such as an MRI or ultrasound scan, should be obtained as needed if further characterization of the injury is required.

Radiographic Determination of *Traumatic* Versus *Congenital* Dislocation

Distinguishing between chronic traumatic (Fig. 11-14) and congenital radial head dislocations (Fig. 11-19) can be challenging. When radiocapitellar alignment is disrupted radiographically, evaluation of the shape of the radial head and capitellum can help determine the cause of the disruption, especially if there is no history of trauma or the significance of the trauma is questioned. The presence of a hypoplastic capitellum and a convex deformed radial head suggests a congenital etiology (Fig. 11-19).[90] True congenital radial head dislocations are usually (but not always) posterior, may be bilateral, and can be associated with various syndromes such as Ehlers–Danlos and nail–patella.[3,84] To avoid missing the diagnosis of an acute Monteggia fracture–dislocation, all anterior radial head dislocations should be at least suspected of having a traumatic origin.[3,26,85]

OUTCOME MEASURES FOR MONTEGGIA FRACTURE–DISLOCATIONS

To assess recovery and patient outcome following closed or open treatment of Monteggia lesions, the clinician should carefully measure union rate, time to union, pain, patient satisfaction, elbow flexion and extension, and forearm rotation. Common treatment complications must be accurately recorded, especially because acute Monteggia injuries continue to be missed or inadequately treated, resulting in the development of chronic Monteggia lesions. An improved understanding of return to sports and functional outcomes is critical.

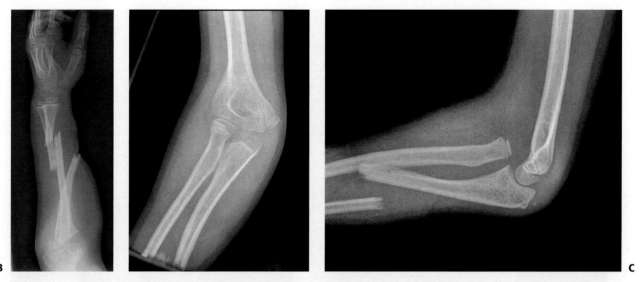

A, B   **C**

Figure 11-18. A: Forearm radiograph of a both bone fracture, which does not adequately visualize the elbow. AP (**B**) and lateral (**C**) radiographs of the elbow clearly demonstrate the disrupted radiocapitellar line.

The disabilities of the arm, shoulder, and hand (DASH) score can be used to measure the disability following Monteggia fracture–dislocations, but has not been validated in children. Joint-specific outcome measures have been developed for the elbow, but many of these measures would benefit from further research into their validity, reliability, and applicability in children.[132] For pediatric patients, the pediatric outcomes data collection instrument (PODCI) offers a validated tool, but its upper limb disability measurement is broad and not joint or disease specific. The development and validation of pediatric upper limb outcome measures are needed and recent work with PROMIS is encouraging.

PATHOANATOMY AND APPLIED ANATOMY RELATING TO MONTEGGIA FRACTURE–DISLOCATIONS

Understanding the anatomy of the proximal radioulnar joint, radiocapitellar joint, and proximal forearm is critical to understanding the treatment of acute and chronic Monteggia lesions. The bony architecture, joint contour, and periarticular ligaments provide stability to the proximal forearm and elbow. The muscle insertions and origins affect stability and determine surgical exposure along with the neighboring neurovascular structures.

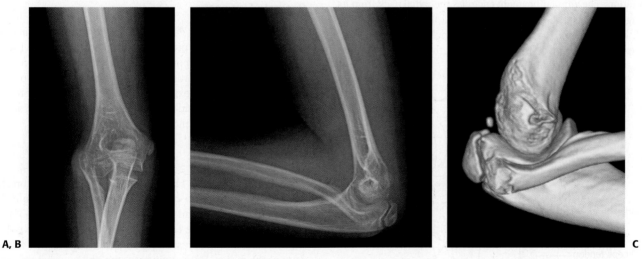

A, B   **C**

Figure 11-19. Congenital dislocation versus synostosis. AP (**A**) and lateral (**B**) elbow radiographs and 3D CT scan (**C**) demonstrating a dysplastic radial head, posterior dislocation, and hypoplastic capitellum. All of these findings are consistent with congenital radial head dislocation.

(continues)

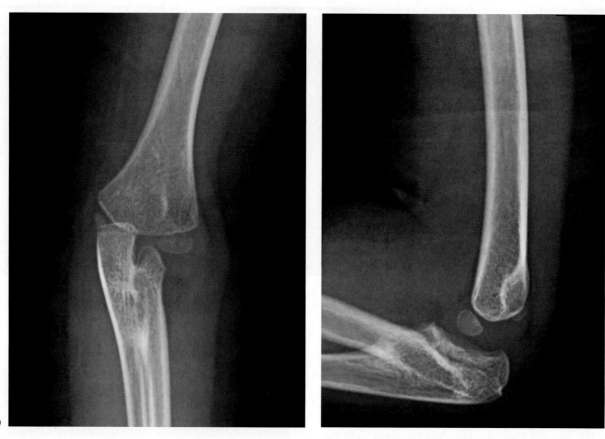

D   **E**

Figure 11-19. (*Continued*) AP (**D**) and lateral (**E**) elbow radiographs of a child with congenital radioulnar synostosis and posterior radial head dislocation. This is a case of congenital radioulnar synostosis.

LIGAMENTS

Annular Ligament

The annular (or orbicular) ligament (Fig. 11-20) is one of the prime stabilizers of the proximal radioulnar joint during forearm rotation. The annular ligament encircles the radial neck from its origin and insertion on the proximal ulna. Because of the shape of the radial head, the annular ligament tightens in supination. The annular ligament is confluent with the remainder of the lateral collateral ligamentous complex which provides stability to the radiocapitellar and proximal radioulnar joints and resists varus stress. Displacement of the annular ligament occurs in a Monteggia lesion.[148]

Quadrate Ligament

The quadrate ligament[35,68,157] is just distal to the annular ligament and connects the proximal radius and ulna (Fig. 11-20). It has a dense anterior portion, thinner posterior portion, and even thinner central portion. The quadrate ligament also provides stability to the proximal radioulnar joint during forearm rotation. The anterior and posterior borders become taut at the extremes of supination and pronation, respectively.

Oblique Cord

The oblique cord (Fig. 11-21), also known as the Weitbrecht ligament, extends at a 45-degree angle from the ulna proximally to the radius distally and is present in approximately 53% of forearms.[156] The oblique cord originates just distal to the radial notch of the ulna and inserts just distal to the bicipital tuberosity of the radius. With supination, the oblique cord tightens and may provide a marginal increase in stability to the proximal radioulnar joint. The clinical relevance of this structure is uncertain.

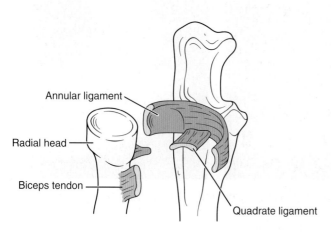

Annular ligament

Radial head

Biceps tendon

Quadrate ligament

Figure 11-20. Ligamentous anatomy of the proximal radioulnar joint.

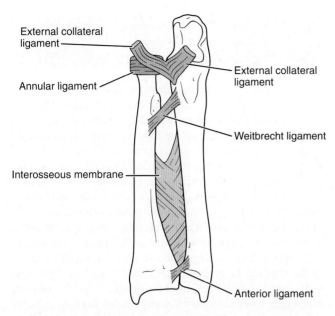

Figure 11-21. Ligaments of the forearm. In supination, the annular ligament, quadrate ligament, Weitbrecht ligament (oblique cord), and interosseous membrane are taut, providing increased stability to the proximal radioulnar joint.

Interosseous Ligament

The interosseous ligament (Fig. 11-21) is distal to the oblique ligament with its primary fibers running in the opposite direction (from radius proximally to ulna distally) to the oblique cord. However, similar to the oblique cord, it tightens in supination and provides further stability to the proximal radioulnar joint. The central band of the interosseous ligament is the stiffest stabilizing structure of the forearm.[164]

BONY ARCHITECTURE

The bony architecture of the elbow creates a relatively constrained hinge. The concave surface of the radial head matches the convex surface of the capitellum and provides stability to the radiocapitellar joint. In contrast, the bony geometry of the proximal radioulnar joint provides minimal inherent stability.

Radius

The shape of the radial head is generally elliptical in cross section (Fig. 11-22).[25] In supination, the long axis of the ellipse is perpendicular to the proximal ulna, causing the annular ligament and the anterior portion of the quadrate ligament to tighten and stabilize the proximal radioulnar joint. In addition, the contact area between the radius and the radial notch of the ulna increases in supination because of the broadened surface of the elliptical radial head proximal to distal in that position. This may provide some additional stability.

The radius "radiates" around the ulna. For this reason, the radius must have an anatomic bow to achieve full forearm rotation while maintaining stability at the proximal and distal radioulnar joints (Fig. 11-22). With the radius in supination,

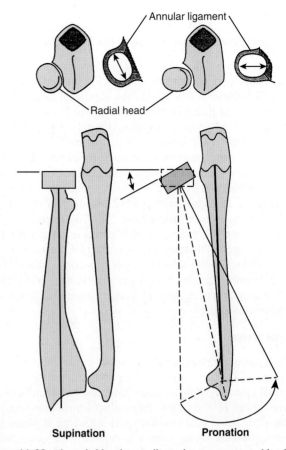

Supination **Pronation**

Figure 11-22. The radial head is an elliptical structure secured by the annular ligament, which allows movement while providing stability. Because of the shape of the radial head, the stability provided by the annular ligament is maximized in supination.

the bow tightens the oblique cord and interosseous ligament, thereby increasing stability of the proximal radioulnar joint.

MUSCULATURE

Biceps Brachii

The biceps brachii inserts into the bicipital tuberosity of the radius and acts as both flexor of the elbow and supinator of the forearm. The biceps acts as a deforming force in anterior Monteggia fracture–dislocations, pulling the radius anteriorly as the elbow is forcibly extended (Fig. 11-9).[155] During treatment of type I and IV lesions, care is taken to maintain the elbow in flexion to prevent recurrent anterior subluxation of the radial head while the soft tissues heal.

Anconeus

The anconeus may act as a dynamic stabilizer of the elbow joint by providing a valgus moment at the joint during extension and pronation.[11,155] It may also act as a deforming force, along with the forearm flexors, on complete fractures of the ulna in a Monteggia lesion. Surgical exposure of the proximal radioulnar and radiocapitellar joints is usually performed through the anconeus–extensor carpi ulnaris interval.

NERVES

Posterior Interosseous Branch of the Radial Nerve

The radial nerve (Fig. 11-23) passes the distal humerus in the brachialis–brachioradialis interval. As the nerve descends into the forearm, it divides into the superficial radial sensory branch and the posterior interosseous motor branch. The PIN passes under the Arcade of Frohse (Fig. 11-23) and between the two heads of the supinator, when present, or beneath the supinator when there is only one head. The nerve's close proximity to the radial head and neck makes it susceptible to injury with Monteggia fracture–dislocations.[71] Injuries to the PIN occur more frequently with type III lesions than other types of Monteggia fracture–dislocations.[13,123,138] Walton et al.[160] propose radiographic parameters that can possibly predict PIN palsy. In chronic Monteggia lesions, the PIN can be adherent to the dislocated radial head or, less commonly, entrapped in the radiocapitellar joint.[125] Care must be taken to avoid injury to the radial nerve in surgical reconstructions of the chronic anterior dislocation.

Ulnar Nerve

The ulnar nerve passes posterior to the medial intermuscular septum of the arm, through the cubital tunnel behind the medial epicondyle of the distal humerus, and then between both heads of the flexor carpi ulnaris into the forearm. The ulnar nerve is at risk for injury with type II Monteggia lesions because of the stretch associated with varus deformity and also with ulnar lengthening in chronic Monteggia reconstructions.

GENERAL TREATMENT PRINCIPLES FOR MONTEGGIA FRACTURE–DISLOCATIONS

Although most treatment algorithms for Monteggia fracture–dislocations are based on the Bado classification, Ring and Waters[123] recommended that treatment choices be based on the type of ulnar fracture rather than on the Bado type. They recommended plastic deformation of the ulna be treated with closed reduction of the ulnar bow to obtain stable reduction of the radiocapitellar joint. Incomplete (greenstick or buckle) fractures of the ulna are similarly treated with closed reduction and casting. In children, most type I Monteggia injuries with plastic deformation of the ulna or incomplete ulnar fractures are stable when immobilized in 100 to 110 degrees of elbow flexion and full forearm supination.

However, any Monteggia lesion with a complete fracture of the ulna can be unstable after closed reduction. Therefore, with complete transverse or short oblique ulnar fractures or Monteggia lesions associated with a radial fracture (type IV lesions), intramedullary fixation is recommended. Long oblique or comminuted ulnar fractures, which can develop shortening and malalignment even with intramedullary fixation, are best stabilized with plate and screw fixation. Using this treatment protocol, Ring and Waters[123] reported excellent results in all 28 patients treated within 24 hours of injury.

As noted, successful treatment is dependent on three goals: anatomical correction of the ulnar deformity, achieving a stable congruent reduction of the radiocapitellar joint, and maintenance of ulnar length and fracture stability (see Algorithm 11-1). For plastic deformation and incomplete

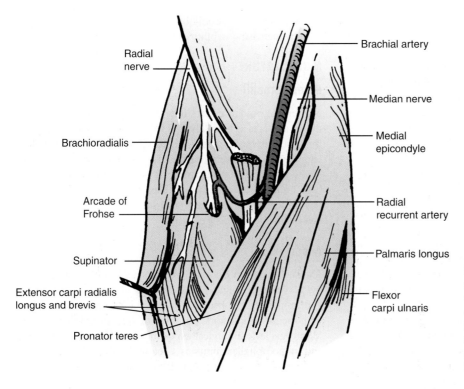

Figure 11-23. Dissection of the anterior elbow. Note the course of the radial nerve which emerges from the biceps–brachioradialis interval and then divides into the superficial radial sensory branch and the posterior interosseous branch. The posterior interosseous nerve then passes under the Arcade of Frohse.

fractures, these goals can usually be achieved with closed reduction and cast immobilization. For complete fractures, fracture instability after closed reduction may lead to loss of anatomic ulnar length and redislocation of the radial head. These injuries are generally treated with internal fixation. This ulnar-based strategy treatment algorithm was verified as reliable in a multicenter study of 112 pediatric Monteggia fracture–dislocations.[117]

TREATMENT OPTIONS FOR TYPE I MONTEGGIA FRACTURE–DISLOCATIONS

NONOPERATIVE TREATMENT OF TYPE I MONTEGGIA FRACTURE–DISLOCATIONS

Indications/Contraindications

Nonoperative Treatment of Type I Monteggia Fracture–Dislocations: INDICATIONS AND CONTRAINDICATIONS	
Indications	**Relative Contraindications**
• Plastic deformation of the ulna • Incomplete (greenstick or buckle) ulnar fracture	• Open fracture • Unstable ulnar fracture pattern • Transverse or short oblique ulnar fracture • Long oblique or comminuted ulnar fracture • Residual or recurrent loss of congruency at radiocapitellar joint

Closed reduction and cast immobilization is recommended as an initial treatment strategy for all type I Monteggia fracture–dislocations in which the ulna is plastically deformed or there is an incomplete fracture (greenstick or buckle). Operative intervention is recommended if there is a failure to obtain and maintain ulnar fracture reduction or a failure to obtain and maintain a congruent reduction of the proximal radioulnar and radiocapitellar joints. In patients with complete transverse or oblique fractures of the ulna, closed reduction alone risks loss of reduction in a cast and development of a chronic Monteggia lesion. In these fractures, operative intervention is recommended to facilitate maintenance of ulnar alignment and the radiocapitellar reduction.

Closed Reduction and Immobilization

Reduction of the Ulnar Fracture

The first step of the closed reduction is to reestablish the length of the ulna by longitudinal traction and manual correction of any angular deformity. The forearm is held in relaxed supination as longitudinal traction is applied with manual pressure directed over the apex of the deformity until the angulation is corrected clinically and radiographically (Figs. 11-24 and 11-25). With plastic deformation fractures, this may necessitate significant force that usually requires general anesthesia.

Type I

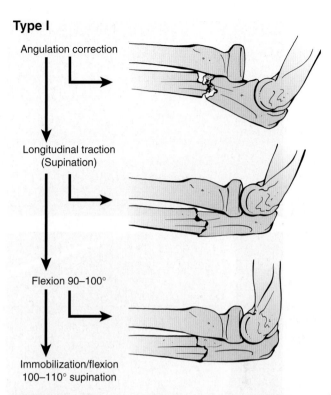

Angulation correction

↓

Longitudinal traction (Supination)

↓

Flexion 90–100°

↓

Immobilization/flexion 100–110° supination

Figure 11-24. Reduction technique for a type I Monteggia fracture–dislocation.

With incomplete fractures, the correction of the ulnar deformity and radial head reduction can often be achieved with conscious sedation in the emergency room. Some papers have cited successful treatment of acute Monteggia lesions (defined as maintenance of the radiocapitellar reduction) with nonanatomic alignment of the ulnar fracture (Fig. 11-26).[49,114,116] However, anatomic reduction and healing of the ulna fracture are strongly advocated.

Reduction of the Radial Head

Once ulnar length and alignment have been reestablished, the radial head can be relocated. This is often accomplished by simply flexing the elbow to 90 degrees or more, thus producing spontaneous reduction (Fig. 11-27). Occasionally, posteriorly directed pressure over the anterior aspect of the radial head is necessary for reduction of the radial head. Flexion of the elbow to 110 to 120 degrees stabilizes the reduction. Once the radial head position is established, it should be scrutinized radiographically in numerous views to ensure a concentric reduction. With a type I lesion, the optimal radiographic view is a true lateral of the elbow with the forearm held in supination. The longitudinal axis of the radius should pass directly through the center of the capitellum (Fig. 11-27).

Radiographic Evaluation and Immobilization

Once the concentric reduction of the radial head is confirmed, the elbow should be placed in approximately 110 to 120 degrees

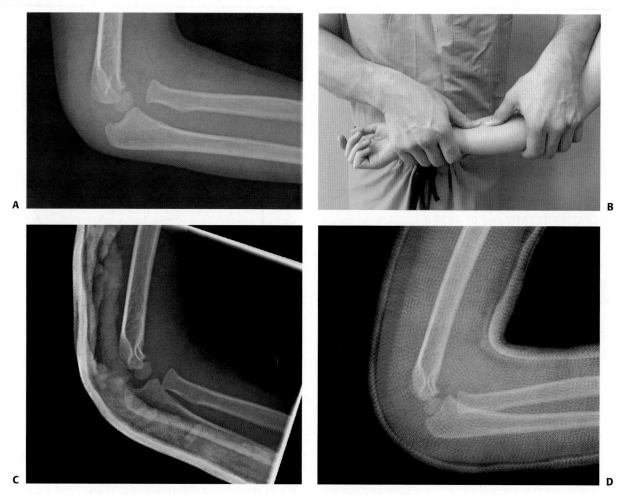

Figure 11-25. Closed reduction for type I lesion. **A:** Typical type I lesion in a 6 year old. Plastic deformation of the ulna must be corrected to prevent recurrence of the angular deformity, which allows reduction of the radial head and prevents its late subluxation. The deformity of the ulna is corrected first (**B**), but the radial head is still anteriorly subluxed because the ulna still has some anterior plastic deformation (**C**). **D:** By hyperflexing the elbow, the radiocapitellar line is restored.

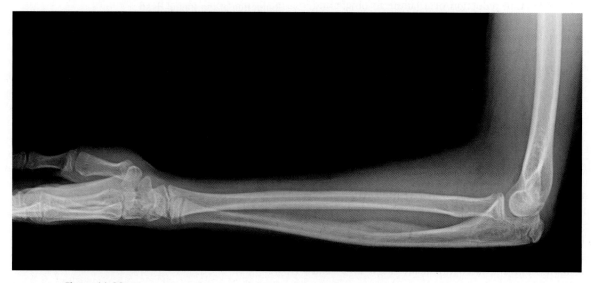

Figure 11-26. Nonanatomic alignment of the ulna fracture, with a residual posterior bow, but anatomic reduction of the radiocapitellar joint.

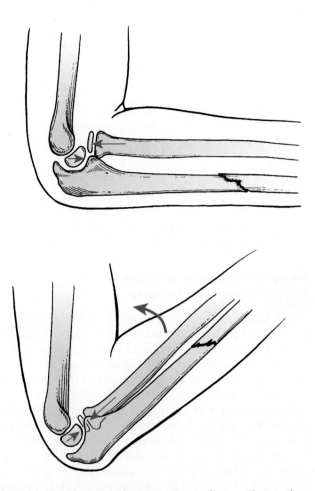

Figure 11-27. Schematic reduction maneuvers for type I lesion. Flexing the elbow spontaneously reduces the radial head. Occasionally, manual pressure is required in combination with flexion.

of flexion to alleviate the force of the biceps, which could redislocate the radial head. The forearm is placed in a position of midsupination to neutral rotation to alleviate the forces of the biceps, supinator muscle and the anconeus, as well as the forearm flexors, which tend to produce radial angulation of the ulna. After the fracture is reduced and the position of stability is established, a molded long-arm splint or cast is applied to hold the elbow joint in the appropriate amount of flexion, usually 110 to 120 degrees. Once the casting is completed, careful radiographic assessment should establish the concentric reduction of the radial head with respect to the capitellum, as well as satisfactory alignment of the ulna (Fig. 11-28).

Postreduction Care

The patient is followed at 1- to 2-week intervals to confirm continued satisfactory reduction by radiography. At 4 to 6 weeks after the initial reduction, if there is radiographic evidence of consolidation of the ulnar fracture and stability of the radial head, the long-arm cast can be removed with progressive guarded return to full activity. A final set of radiographs should be obtained when the patient has achieved full motion to be certain the radiocapitellar and proximal radioulnar joints remain anatomically aligned.

Outcomes

In all series,[4,10,21,22,38,49,82,101,120,123,131,165] type I Monteggia lesions in children have uniformly good results when treated by manipulative closed reduction, if the radial head is properly aligned and the ulnar fracture is reduced with length preserved. These results most clearly apply to plastic deformation and incomplete fractures, which make up the majority of type I

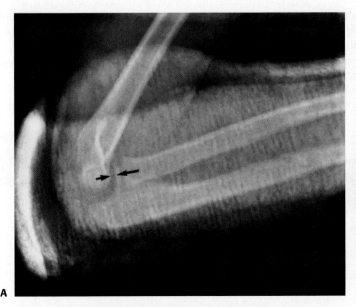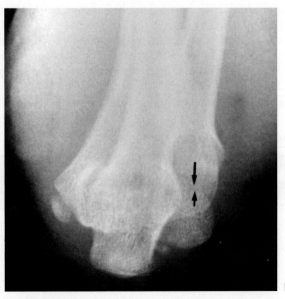

Figure 11-28. Once the closed reduction is complete, radiographs should be analyzed for reestablishment of the radiocapitellar line (*arrows*) and ulnar alignment on both the lateral (**A**) and Jones (**B**) views.

Monteggia lesions. No deterioration of results appears to occur at long term.[80,104]

OPERATIVE TREATMENT OF TYPE I MONTEGGIA FRACTURE–DISLOCATIONS

Indications/Contraindications

Operative Treatment of Type I Monteggia Fracture–Dislocations: INDICATIONS AND CONTRAINDICATIONS	
Indications	**Relative Contraindications**
• Open fracture • Unstable ulnar fracture pattern • Inability to obtain (or maintain) good alignment of the ulna and radiocapitellar joint • Transverse or short oblique ulnar fracture • Long oblique or comminuted ulnar fracture	• Plastic deformation of the ulna • Incomplete (greenstick or buckle) ulnar fracture • Good alignment with closed reduction and casting

There are two principal indications for operative treatment of type I fracture–dislocations: failure to obtain and maintain ulnar fracture reduction and a failure to obtain and maintain a congruent reduction of the radiocapitellar joint. The fractures most at risk for loss of reduction with nonoperative management are complete ulnar fractures. In these fractures, operative fixation of the ulna is recommended to facilitate maintenance of ulnar alignment and radiocapitellar reduction. In some cases, closed reduction of the radiocapitellar joint cannot be achieved, even after restoration of ulnar length and stabilization by intramedullary or plate fixation of the ulna. It is important not to accept a nonanatomic reduction as an imperfect reduction, which can result in further joint malalignment and the development of a chronic Monteggia lesion. In these cases, the annular ligament is almost always avulsed or entrapped.[148] There is a high likelihood that annular ligament and/or periosteal interposition is preventing congruent reduction of the radiocapitellar joint. In these situations, an open reduction of the radiocapitellar joint should be performed with restoration of the annular ligament to its normal position.[148,155]

Preoperative Planning

✔ **Operative Treatment of Monteggia Fracture–Dislocations:** PREOPERATIVE PLANNING CHECKLIST	
OR table	❑ Standard OR table with radiolucent arm board, table turned 90 degrees with operative limb pointing toward operating room
Position/positioning aids	❑ Patient supine with adequate padding of heels and other bony prominences
Fluoroscopy location	❑ Generally from below arm (medial to lateral)
Equipment	❑ Standard operating instruments, drill, Kirschner (K) wire or flexible titanium nail set, small fragment set, nonabsorbable 2-0 and 3-0 suture, splinting or casting supplies
Tourniquet	❑ Nonsterile tourniquet generally sufficient
[Other]	

Routine preoperative planning is required before embarking on any of the operative treatment pathways described below.

Intramedullary Fixation of Transverse or Short Oblique Ulnar Fractures

In patients with complete transverse or short oblique fractures, closed reduction alone can result in loss of reduction in a cast. In these cases, closed reduction and intramedullary fixation of the ulna is recommended to facilitate maintenance of ulnar alignment and length along with reduction of the radiocapitellar joint. The quality of the ulnar reduction affects the ability to reduce the radial head, which is of primary importance. If an ulnar fracture can be reduced but not maintained because of the obliquity of the fracture, internal fixation is also indicated.[49,101] Intramedullary fixation is standard in most series of Monteggia fracture–dislocations in children (Fig. 11-29).[8,10,38,47,49,77,79,88,101,115,123,126,142,165] Percutaneous intramedullary fixation reliably maintains alignment and preserves length without the additional concerns of open surgery or implant retention. This method of fixation can be accomplished using image intensification and with Steinmann pins, K-wires, or flexible titanium nails (Synthes, West Chester, PA). Steinmann pins and K-wires have the advantage of being universally available and inexpensive. Their stainless steel composition and smooth tip also permit easy removal in the office without need for additional anesthesia. Note that K-wires may not be of sufficient length for use in older children with longer, stronger forearms.

Technique

✔ **Intramedullary Fixation of Transverse or Short Oblique Ulnar Fractures:** KEY SURGICAL STEPS
❑ Cortical entry through the apophysis or proximal metaphysis of the ulna
❑ Introduce appropriately sized intramedullary device (K-wire, Steinmann pin, or flexible titanium nail)
❑ Perform closed reduction based on mechanism of injury • Intramedullary device can be used in the proximal fragment to joystick the reduction
❑ Stabilize fracture with the intramedullary device, utilize fluoroscopy to confirm appropriate ulnar and radiocapitellar reduction, as well as proper placement of the intramedullary device

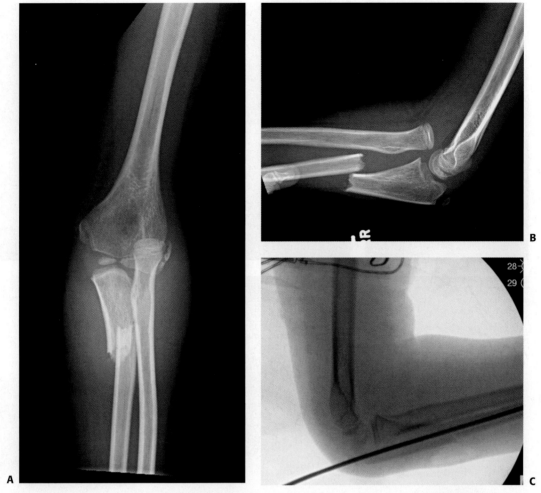

Figure 11-29. AP (**A**) and lateral (**B**) type I fracture pattern. Entry site is via the olecranon apophysis. A smooth Steinmann pin (**C**) or a titanium elastic nail can be utilized.

❑ Bend and cut intramedullary K-wire outside of skin to facilitate subsequent removal in the office; titanium nails or buried wires need to be removed in day surgery unit
❑ Apply long-arm splint, cast, or bivalved cast in a position of elbow flexion and supination appropriate for the specific Bado type

Entry can be through the apophysis or proximal metaphysis of the ulna depending on the level of the fracture and surgeon's preference. For type I lesions, a closed reduction maneuver is performed as described above. At times, an intramedullary device in the proximal fragment can be used to joystick the reduction. Intraoperative fluoroscopy is utilized to confirm appropriate ulnar and radiocapitellar reduction, as well as proper interosseous placement of the intramedullary device. Because ulnar fractures heal rapidly in children, the intramedullary device can generally be bent and cut outside of the skin to facilitate subsequent office removal. Some surgeons prefer to leave the intramedullary rod in a long time and therefore bury it beneath the skin. A long-arm splint, cast (if minimal manipulation needed), or bivalved cast is then applied with the elbow in 90 to 110 degrees of flexion and

forearm supination, which provides additional stability to the radiocapitellar joint.

Open Reduction and Plate Fixation of Long Oblique or Comminuted Ulnar Fractures

Although intramedullary fixation is preferred for transverse and short oblique fractures, long oblique and comminuted fractures may redisplace even with intramedullary fixation.[123] Plate and screw fixation (Fig. 11-30) is preferred with these rarer fractures.[79,107,112,123,153,158,167]

Technique

✔ **Open Reduction and Plate Fixation of Long Oblique or Comminuted Ulnar Fractures:** KEY SURGICAL STEPS

❑ Longitudinal incision over subcutaneous border of the ulna
❑ Develop interval between extensor carpi ulnaris and flexor carpi ulnaris
❑ Carefully incise periosteum and preserve for subsequent repair
❑ Perform open reduction

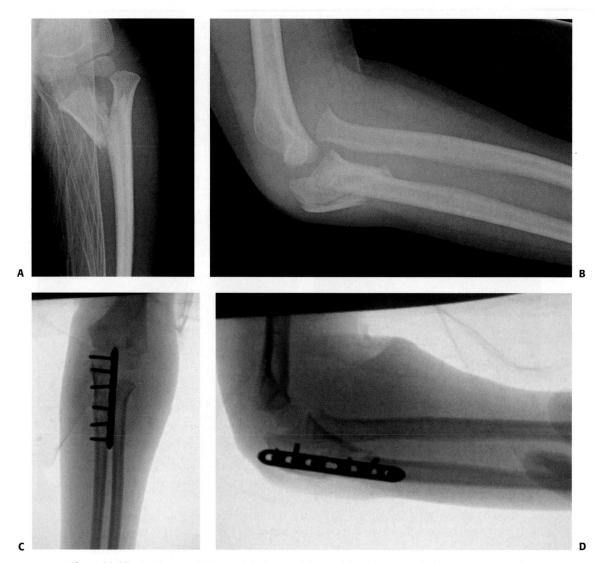

Figure 11-30. ORIF of type I Monteggia lesion in a 10-year-old male associated with a comminuted ulna fracture. Injury AP (**A**) and lateral (**B**) radiographs demonstrating the dislocated radial head and ulnar fracture pattern. Intraoperative AP (**C**) and lateral (**D**) images demonstrating plate and screw fixation.

❏ Apply double-stacked one-third tubular plate or 3.5-mm dynamic compression plate
 • Four to six cortices of fixation both proximal and distal to the fracture
❏ Utilize fluoroscopy to confirm appropriate ulnar and radiocapitellar reduction, as well as proper placement of the plate and screws
❏ Repair periosteum over the fracture site and implant
❏ Layered wound closure
❏ Apply long-arm splint, cast, or bivalved cast in a position of elbow flexion and supination appropriate for the specific Bado type

A longitudinal incision, centered at the apex of the fracture, is made along the subcutaneous border of the ulna, at the extensor carpi ulnaris–flexor carpi ulnaris interval. An open reduction is performed, and a double-stacked one-third tubular

plate or 3.5-mm dynamic compression plate (Synthes, West Chester, PA) is applied utilizing standard AO techniques. Four to six cortices of fixation are generally required both proximal and distal to the fracture. Intraoperative fluoroscopy is used to confirm appropriate ulnar and radiocapitellar reduction. The periosteum is repaired over the fracture site and implant. Again, a long-arm splint, cast, or bivalved cast is then applied with the elbow in 90 to 110 degrees of flexion and forearm supination, which provides additional stability to the radiocapitellar joint.

Open Reduction of the Annular Ligament

On occasion, a congruent closed reduction of the radiocapitellar joint cannot be achieved, even after intramedullary fixation or plate fixation of the ulna. In these situations, the position of the radial head may be improved, but the reduction remains imperfect. The surgeon may not feel a definitive clunk associated with an anatomic reduction, but instead may feel a soft or rubbery resistance during manipulation. This suggests soft tissue interposition of either the annular ligament and/or periosteum.[155,167] An open reduction of the radiocapitellar joint with restoration of the annular ligament to its normal position is recommended. Soft tissue interposition more commonly occurs in type III lesions, but can also occur in type I lesions. Interposed cartilaginous or osteochondral fractures in the radiocapitellar joint or proximal radioulnar joint may also prevent complete reduction of the radial head.[155] Morris[95] described a patient in whom reduction of the radial head was obstructed by radial nerve entrapment between the radial head and ulna.

Technique

✔ **Open Reduction of the Annular Ligament:**
KEY SURGICAL STEPS

❑ Posterolateral (Kocher) approach to the elbow under tourniquet control
❑ Develop interval between extensor carpi ulnaris and anconeus, maintain forearm in pronation to protect radial nerve from iatrogenic injury
❑ Perform elbow capsulotomy
❑ Identify annular ligament
  • Ligament typically in continuity, usually torn off the ulna with a periosteal sleeve (generally not torn mid-substance)
❑ Reduce annular ligament over the radius, repair as needed with 2-0 and/or 3-0 nonabsorbable suture
❑ Layered wound closure
❑ Apply long-arm splint, cast, or bivalved cast in a position of elbow flexion and supination appropriate for the specific Bado type

The most direct approach to the radiocapitellar joint is from the posterolateral aspect of the elbow. The interval between the anconeus and the extensor carpi ulnaris, using the distal portion of a Kocher incision, provides sufficient exposure of the radial head and the interposed structures.[57,143] This approach protects the PIN when the forearm is pronated. A more extensile approach was described by Boyd (Fig. 11-31).[20] This exposure is begun by making an incision following the lateral border of the triceps posteriorly to the lateral condyle and extending it along the radial side of the ulna. The incision is carried under the anconeus and extensor carpi ulnaris in an extraperiosteal manner, elevating the fibers of the supinator from the ulna. This carries the approach down to the interosseous membrane, allowing exposure of the radiocapitellar joint, excellent visualization of the annular ligament, access to the proximal fourth of the entire radius, and approach to the ulnar fracture all through the same incision.[20,21,135] In addition, elevation of the extensor–supinator mass from the lateral epicondyle allows more proximal exposure of the dislocated radial head if entrapped behind the displaced capsule and annular ligament.

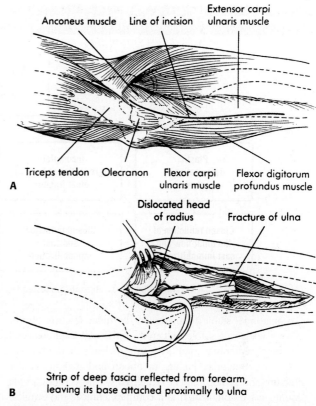

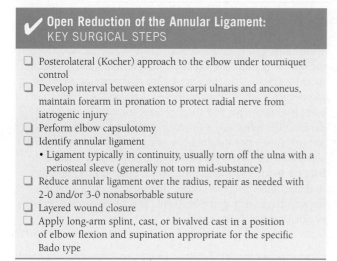

Figure 11-31. Boyd approach. **A:** The incision is carried under the anconeus and extensor carpi ulnaris to expose the radial head and annular ligament. **B:** The incision can be extended distally to allow exposure of the ulnar fracture and proximally to facilitate harvesting of a fascial strip for annular ligament reconstruction, if necessary.

After obtaining adequate surgical exposure through either approach, a capsulotomy is performed and the elbow joint is inspected. Careful exploration is required to identify the annular ligament. The ligament is not typically torn in its mid-substance, but rather remains in continuity and tears of the ulna with a periosteal sleeve. The displaced in continuity ligament usually slips off the radial neck over the radial head into the joint. Once the opening in the annular ligament is identified, a Freer elevator, forceps, soft tissue probe, or a small curette is used to reduce the annular ligament over the radial head. If a repair is required, 2-0 or 3-0 nonabsorbable sutures can be utilized. The congruency of the radiocapitellar and proximal radioulnar joint reductions should be confirmed under direct visualization. Stability can then be confirmed by rotating the forearm under careful fluoroscopic imaging. If the radial head is still unstable, look for missed plastic deformation of the ulna. If present, closed reduction of the ulna, or at times opening wedge osteotomy of the ulna, is required to anatomically and stably reduce the radial head. A layered wound closure is performed, followed by application of a long-arm splint or bivalved cast with the forearm in supination (see Algorithm 11-1).

Authors' Preferred Treatment for Type I Monteggia Fracture–Dislocations (Algorithm 11-1)

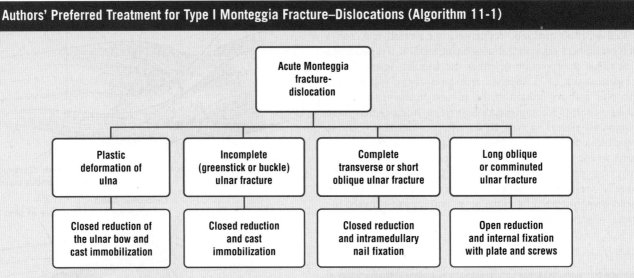

Algorithm 11-1. Authors' preferred treatment of all Monteggia fracture–dislocations.

An anatomic, stable reduction of the ulnar fracture almost always leads to a stable reduction of the radiocapitellar and proximal radioulnar joint. This in turn leads to an excellent long-term outcome. Failure to obtain and maintain ulnar fracture and radiocapitellar reduction will lead to a chronic Monteggia lesion, which is a complex clinical and surgical problem with risk of a suboptimum outcome. If a closed reduction can be achieved with a cast, close follow-up is warranted. If the reduction is lost at any point in the weekly follow-up evaluations, operative treatment is indicated. Although some authors have advocated conservative treatment,[48] it is not wrong to be very aggressive in treatment of

acute Monteggia fracture–dislocations and proceed directly to the operating room for stabilization. Overtreatment has been more successful than undertreatment in preventing a chronic Monteggia lesion.[117] Percutaneous intramedullary fixation of complete transverse and short oblique ulna fractures is standard. Open reduction and internal fixation with plate and screws of the rarer long oblique and comminuted fracture is also standard.[117] Any irreducible or unstable radial head after fracture reduction and stabilization is approached surgically to define and correct the cause. This usually involves reducing an interposed annular ligament. This aggressive approach avoids late complications.[123]

POSTOPERATIVE CARE

After closed or open reduction of the ulna fracture and closed or open reduction of the radial head, a long-arm cast is used for 4 to 6 weeks with the forearm in slight supination and the elbow flexed 90 to 110 degrees depending on the degree of swelling. Radiographs are obtained every 1 to 2 weeks until fracture healing. Intramedullary hardware is removed with fracture healing. Plate and screw fixation may be removed after 6 to 12 months if there is any discomfort. Home rehabilitation is begun at 6 weeks and return to sports is dependent on restoration of motion and strength.

POTENTIAL PITFALLS AND PREVENTIVE MEASURES

Monteggia Fracture–Dislocations:
POTENTIAL PITFALLS AND PREVENTIONS

Pitfall	Prevention
• Failure to identify radial head dislocation leading to chronic Monteggia lesion	• Always obtain dedicated elbow radiographs with forearm fractures to evaluate congruency of radiocapitellar reduction
• Loss of radiocapitellar reduction leading to chronic Monteggia lesion	• Intramedullary fixation or plate fixation for unstable ulnar fractures • Regular postoperative radiographs every 1 to 2 weeks until fracture healing
• Inadequate reduction of radial head leading to chronic Monteggia lesion	• Never accept an imperfect reduction of the radial head; always perform an open reduction of radiocapitellar joint with restoration of the annular ligament to its normal position
• Radial nerve palsy	• During posterolateral approach to the elbow, pronate forearm to protect radial nerve from iatrogenic injury • During chronic Monteggia reconstructions, identify and protect radial nerve
• Compartment syndrome	• Monitor high-energy injuries in hospital with frequent neurovascular monitoring • Perform prophylactic volar and dorsal forearm fasciotomies during chronic Monteggia reconstructions • Consider bivalving postoperative casts

TREATMENT OPTIONS FOR TYPE II MONTEGGIA FRACTURE–DISLOCATIONS

The indications for nonoperative and operative treatment of type II lesions are similar to type I lesions as the ulnar fracture pattern dictates initial decision making. Following ulnar fracture reduction, any residual lack of congruency at the radiocapitellar joint should be treated surgically.

NONOPERATIVE TREATMENT OF TYPE II MONTEGGIA FRACTURE–DISLOCATIONS

As with type I injuries, incomplete type II fractures usually have a satisfactory result after closed reduction.[82,101,109,116,165] The ulnar fracture is reduced by longitudinal traction in line with the long axis of the forearm while the elbow is held at 60 degrees of flexion (Fig. 11-32). The radial head may reduce spontaneously or may require gentle, anteriorly directed pressure applied to its posterior aspect. The elbow is extended once the radial head is reduced and immobilized in that position to stabilize the radial head and allow molding posteriorly to maintain the ulnar reduction.[38,109,159] If the ulnar alignment cannot be maintained, an intramedullary Steinmann pin or K-wire should be used.

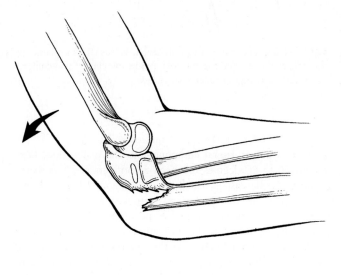

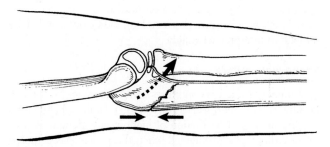

Figure 11-32. Schematic reduction maneuvers for type II lesion. Longitudinal traction and pronation of the forearm and immobilization in 60-degree flexion or complete extension.

OPERATIVE TREATMENT OF TYPE II MONTEGGIA FRACTURE–DISLOCATIONS

Treatment goals are stable concentric reduction of the radial head and alignment of the ulnar fracture. When there is an unstable, complete ulnar fracture, percutaneous intramedullary fixation, or open reduction and internal fixation with plate and screws are used similar to type I Monteggia fracture–dislocations.[107,112] The radial head should be reduced by open technique if there is interposed soft tissue or the Monteggia lesion is accompanied by a fractured capitellum or radial head.

With incomplete fractures, ulnar length is reestablished by applying longitudinal traction and straightening the angular deformity (Fig. 11-32). The radial head may reduce spontaneously or with gentle, anteriorly directed force over the radial head. Once reduced, the position of the head can be stabilized by holding the elbow in extension. If the ulnar fracture is stable, it can be maintained by cast immobilization with the elbow in extension. However, if there is any doubt, percutaneous intramedullary fixation is preferred. Comminuted or very proximal fractures may require open reduction and internal fixation with plate and screws or tension band fixation. Postoperative radiographs are obtained approximately every 7 to 14 days to confirm continued reduction of the radial head.

The Boyd approach (Fig. 11-31) can be used to obtain reduction of the radial head if it cannot be obtained through closed manipulation. Management of the annular ligament is the same as described for type I Monteggia lesions. Associated compression fractures of the radial head require early detection to avoid late loss of alignment. Open reduction and internal fixation may be required to maintain radiocapitellar joint stability. Osteonecrosis and nonunion are complications of this rare injury pattern. Cast immobilization is continued until fracture and soft tissue healing, usually 6 weeks. Home rehabilitation is performed until restoration of motion and strength.[109]

TREATMENT OPTIONS FOR TYPE III MONTEGGIA FRACTURE–DISLOCATIONS

Like type I lesions, there are two principal indications for operative treatment of type III fracture–dislocations: failure to obtain and maintain ulnar fracture reduction or a failure to obtain and maintain a congruent reduction of the radiocapitellar joint. Soft tissue interposition more commonly occurs in type III lesions, and open reduction of the radial head may be required more frequently as a consequence.[13,64,123,149,167,168] Nonoperative treatment by manipulative closed reduction is usually effective in pediatric patients with metaphyseal, incomplete, or plastic deformation fractures.[10,38,51,64,82,96,101,109,150,165,168] However, the rate of operative treatment has been reported to be as high as 12%.[101]

NONOPERATIVE TREATMENT OF TYPE III MONTEGGIA FRACTURE–DISLOCATIONS

Closed Reduction

A closed reduction is carried out by reversing the mechanism of injury.[38,96,109,151] The elbow is held in extension with longitudinal traction. Valgus stress is placed on the ulna at the fracture site, restoring anatomic realignment (Fig. 11-33). The radial head may spontaneously reduce or may need assistance with gentle pressure applied laterally (Fig. 11-34). Reduction of the radial head sometimes produces a palpable click.[151] Ulnar length and alignment must be nearly anatomic to ensure stability of the radial head.[49] Fluoroscopic radiographs are obtained to confirm radial head reduction (Fig. 11-35).[93] Stability of the ulnar fracture is tested. Any malalignment of the radiocapitellar joint in any view implies the possibility of interposed tissue or persistent malalignment of the ulna fracture.

Radiographic Evaluation and Immobilization

Radiographs are taken in the AP and lateral planes to confirm the reduction of the radial head and assess the ulnar alignment. Up to 10 degrees of ulnar angulation is acceptable in younger children, provided the radial head reduction is concentric and stable. Range-of-motion testing of stability is appropriate and necessary with plastic deformation fractures because radiocapitellar alignment can be difficult to assess AP radiographs in the cast.

Reduction is maintained by the application of a long-arm splint, cast, or bivalved cast with a valgus mold and with the elbow in relative flexion. The degree of flexion varies depending on the direction of the radial head dislocation. When the radial head is dislocated in a straight lateral or anterolateral position,

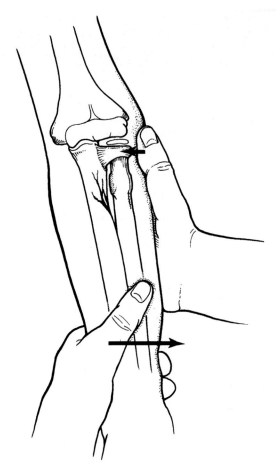

Figure 11-34. Reduction of type III lesion. Valgus stress is placed on the ulna at the fracture site (*arrows*), producing clinical realignment. The radial head may spontaneously reduce.

flexion to 100 to 110 degrees improves stability.[41,96,116,165] If there is a posterolateral component to the dislocation, flexion to 70 to 80 degrees has been recommended.[151] Forearm rotation in the cast is usually in supination, which tightens the interosseous membrane and further stabilizes the reduction.[10,38,96,165] Some have suggested positions of immobilization from pronation[150] to slight supination.[151] Ramsey and Pedersen[116] recommended neutral as the best position of rotation to avoid loss of motion; their patients showed no loss of reduction using this position. It must be emphasized that the ulnar fracture and radial head reduction need to be truly stable for closed treatment because postreduction radiographs in cast are difficult to interpret accurately.

Postreduction Care

Cast immobilization is continued until fracture and soft tissue healing, usually by 6 weeks (Fig. 11-35). Home rehabilitation is performed until restoration of motion and strength. A final set of radiographs is obtained when the patient has achieved full motion and strength to be certain that there is continued anatomic reduction of the proximal radioulnar and radiocapitellar joints.

Type III

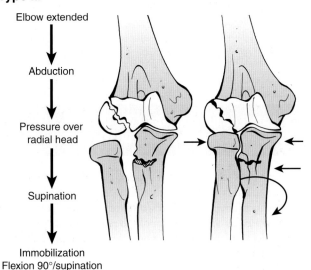

Elbow extended
↓
Abduction
↓
Pressure over radial head
↓
Supination
↓
Immobilization
Flexion 90°/supination

Figure 11-33. Schematic reduction maneuvers for type III lesion.

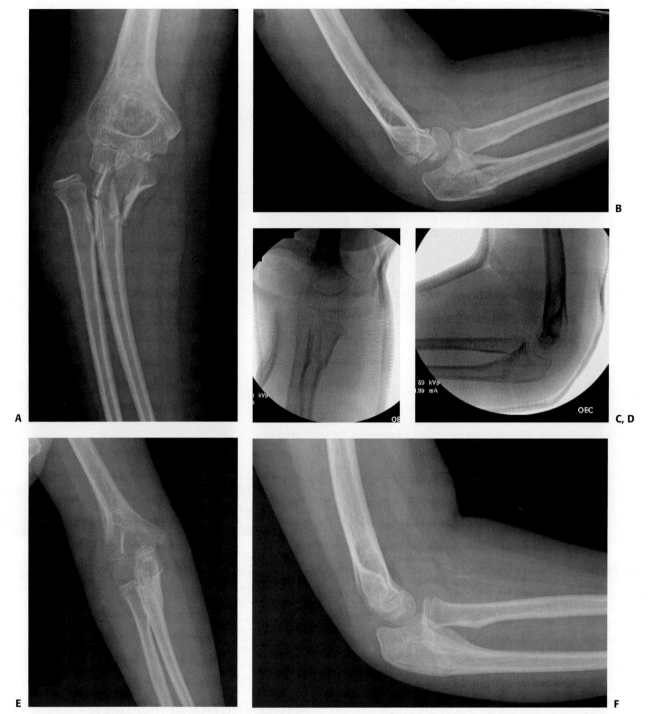

Figure 11-35. AP (**A**) and lateral (**B**) type III fracture pattern. AP (**C**) and lateral (**D**) intraoperative images demonstrating adequate reduction and an aggressive lateral mold/valgus stress. Final AP (**E**) and lateral (**F**) images demonstrating good healing. The patient had full return of motion.

OPERATIVE TREATMENT OF TYPE III MONTEGGIA FRACTURE–DISLOCATIONS

As noted earlier, the goals of surgical intervention are reduction and stabilization of both the ulnar fracture and the radial head. If there is an inability to obtain and maintain anatomic alignment of the ulnar fracture, proximal radioulnar joint, or radiocapitellar joint, then operative treatment is clearly indicated.

Ulnar Stabilization

Ulnar malalignment may prevent anatomic relocation of the radial head. The ulnar fracture can usually be reduced closed, but internal fixation may be necessary if the ulnar fracture is unstable to prevent recurrent lateral dislocation of the radial head. Persistent varus alignment, particularly with oblique ulnar fractures, can lead to recurrent subluxation of the radial

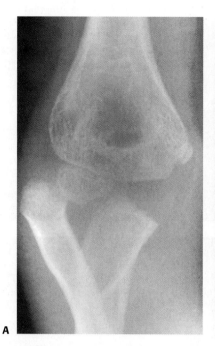 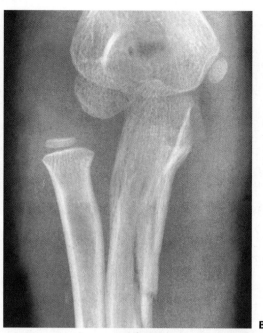

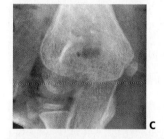

Figure 11-36. Irreducible type III lesion. **A:** Injury films showing typical greenstick olecranon fracture and lateral dislocation of a type III lesion. **B:** After manipulation and correction of the ulnar deformity, the radial head still remained dislocated. **C:** An open reduction was performed to extract the interposed torn annular ligament.

head, radiocapitellar incongruence, and risk of a poor outcome (Fig. 14-15).[49,101] Anatomic reduction of the ulna and fixation with plates and screws[49] or intramedullary wires[8] will yield excellent results.[117]

Open Reduction of the Annular Ligament

Failed closed reduction of the radial head with anatomic alignment of the ulna fracture implies interposition of soft tissue, which is repaired through a Boyd approach (Fig. 11-31).[20,167] This allows removal of the interposed tissues[155,167] and repair or reconstruction of the annular ligament and the periosteum of the ulna as necessary (Fig. 14-36).[14,23,49,51,135,149] The surgical technique is essentially the same as previously described for a type I Monteggia fracture–dislocation.

Authors' Preferred Treatment for Type III Monteggia Fracture–Dislocations

As with any Monteggia lesion, treatment is primarily aimed at obtaining and maintaining reduction of the radial head, either by an open or closed technique. This is usually performed by anatomic, stable closed reduction of the ulnar fracture, which in turn leads to a stable reduction of the proximal radioulnar and radiocapitellar joints.

TREATMENT OPTIONS FOR TYPE IV MONTEGGIA FRACTURE–DISLOCATIONS

This complex lesion has been treated by both closed[101] and open[10] techniques. Percutaneous intramedullary fixation of the radial and ulnar fractures with flexible rods and closed reduction of the radial has also been described.[52,124] The goals of treatment for a type IV Monteggia lesion are similar to those of other Bado types. The presence of the free-floating proximal radial fragment hampers the ability to reduce the radial head. Stabilization of the radial fracture converts a type IV lesion to a type I lesion, making treatment simpler.

NONOPERATIVE TREATMENT OF TYPE IV MONTEGGIA FRACTURE–DISLOCATIONS

Closed reduction should be attempted initially, with the aim of transforming the type IV lesion to a type I lesion (Fig. 11-36), especially if the radial and ulnar fractures have greenstick patterns. Use of the image intensifier allows immediate confirmation of reduction, especially of the radial head (Fig. 11-37). Closed treatment can occasionally be successful for type IV lesions (Fig. 11-38), but closed treatment of unstable ulnar lesions should not be attempted. If the initial fracture reduction cannot be obtained, an anatomic stable reduction with either intramedullary or plate fixation is performed.

Type IV

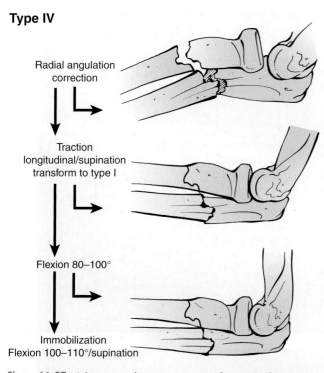

Radial angulation
correction

↓ →

Traction
longitudinal/supination
transform to type I

↓ →

Flexion 80–100°

↓ →

Immobilization
Flexion 100–110°/supination

Figure 11-37. Schematic reduction maneuvers for type IV lesion.

OPERATIVE TREATMENT OF TYPE IV MONTEGGIA FRACTURE–DISLOCATIONS

Type IV fractures are usually unstable and the reduction of the radial head is easier to obtain and maintain after stable fixation of the radius. In young patients, this may be achieved by intramedullary fixation. In children older than 12 years, plating of the radius through a volar Henry extensile approach[60] provides more rigid stabilization. Once stability is achieved, a closed reduction of the radial head is attempted. This is usually successful, but any intra-articular obstruction can be removed through a Boyd approach (Fig. 11-31).

Authors' Preferred Treatment for Type IV Monteggia Fracture–Dislocations

As with any Monteggia lesion, treatment is primarily aimed at obtaining and maintaining reduction of the radial head, either by an open or closed technique. Percutaneous intramedullary fixation is frequently necessary because of inherent fracture instability (Fig. 11-39). At times, there can be both a proximal and distal radius fracture, which requires special consideration (Fig. 11-40).

(text continues on page 451)

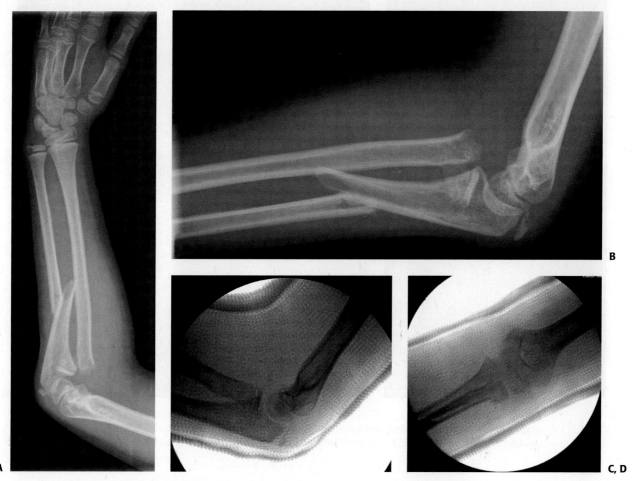

Figure 11-38. A, B: Type IV Monteggia fracture with radial neck fracture.

(continues)

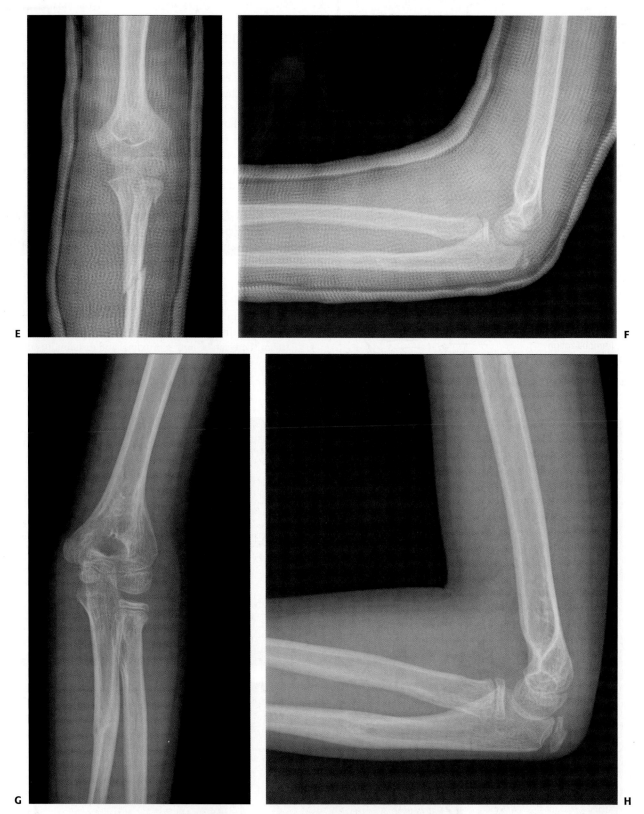

Figure 11-38. (*Continued*) **C, D:** Closed reduction and casting in the emergency department under conscious sedation. One-week follow-up AP (**E**) and lateral (**F**) radiographs demonstrating maintained alignment of the ulna fracture, radial neck fracture, and radiocapitellar line. Final follow-up AP (**G**) and lateral (**H**) images.

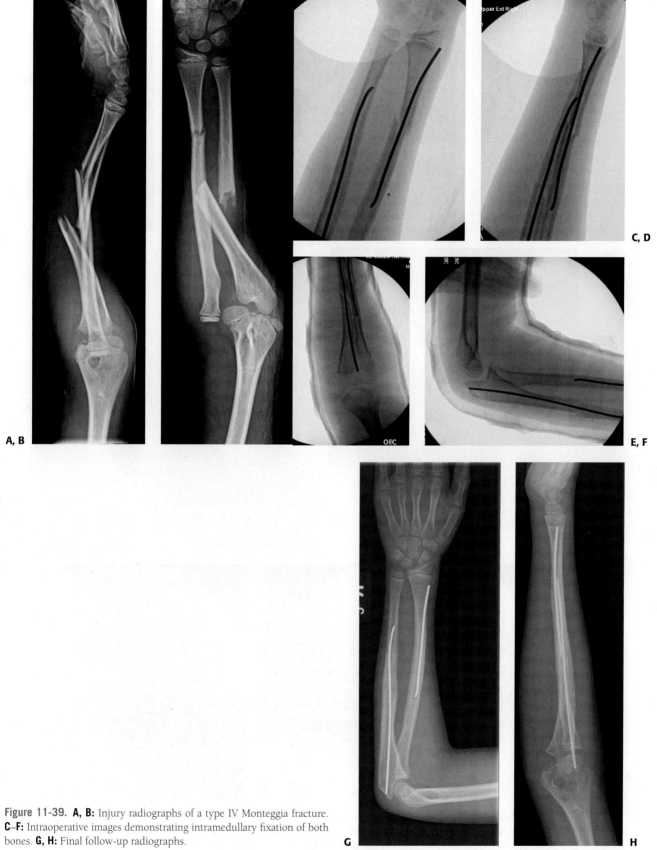

Figure 11-39. A, B: Injury radiographs of a type IV Monteggia fracture. **C–F:** Intraoperative images demonstrating intramedullary fixation of both bones. **G, H:** Final follow-up radiographs.

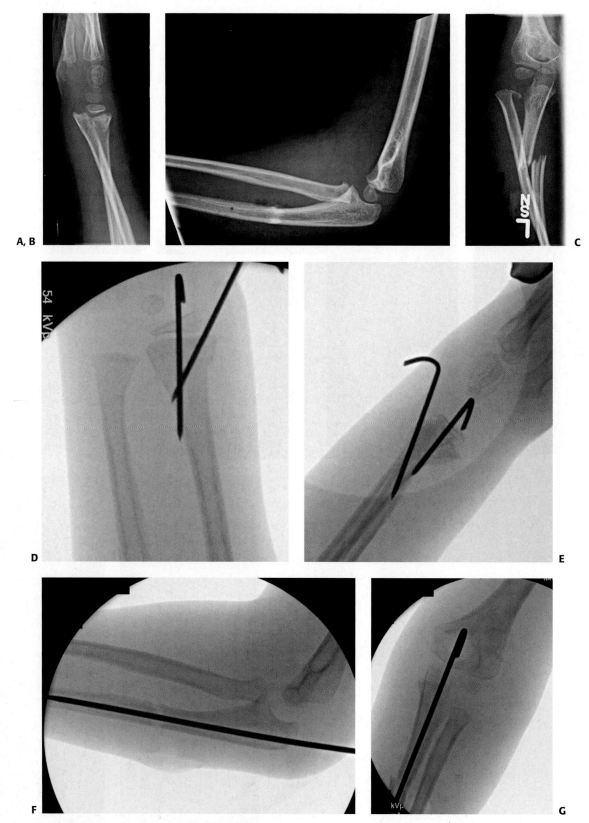

Figure 11-40. A, B: Distal radius and radial neck fractures, in addition to disruption of the radiocapitellar alignment. **C, D:** Start with percutaneous pinning of the Salter–Harris 2 distal radius fracture with smooth pins. **E, F:** Then proceed to reduce the ulna, radial neck, and radiocapitellar joint. In this case, the ulna was opened to achieve appropriate reduction, but the radial neck fracture was close reduced. Intramedullary fixation of the ulna fracture maintained the alignment of the radiocapitellar joint.

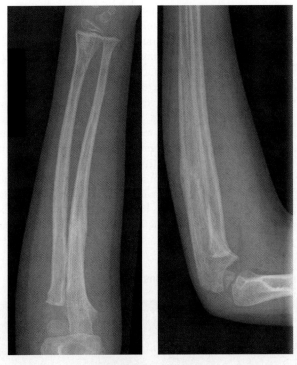

Figure 11-40. (*Continued*)

Following open treatment, the elbow is immobilized in a long-arm cast for 4 to 6 weeks in 110 to 120 degrees of flexion with the forearm in neutral rotation. A short-arm cast can be used thereafter if additional fracture protection is necessary. Home rehabilitation is performed until restoration of motion and strength. Final radiographs are obtained with full restoration of motion and strength to be certain there is anatomic reduction of the proximal radioulnar and radiocapitellar joints.

TREATMENT OPTIONS FOR CHRONIC MONTEGGIA FRACTURE–DISLOCATIONS

A late-presenting, previously undetected dislocation of the radial head is not as uncommon as orthopedic surgeons would prefer.[32,34,38,43,51,52,74,103,105,131,146] The diagnosis of an acute Monteggia fracture–dislocation is often missed by skilled radiologists, emergency room physicians, pediatricians, and orthopedic surgeons, particularly when the ulnar injury is subtle or in the form of plastic deformation. The shape of the ulna in patients with a seemingly isolated dislocation of the radial head usually indicates persistent plastic deformation or malunion of the ulna and a traumatic etiology to the radial head dislocation (Figs. 11-3 and 11-41).[84,93,131,142] Isolated radial head dislocations with remote trauma have also been mistaken for congenital radial head dislocations.[90] Elbow radiographs or MRI can help distinguish a chronic Monteggia lesion from congenital dislocation of the radial head. As noted previously, the shape of the radial head is concave in most chronic Monteggia lesions but is convex in congenital radial head dislocation. In congenital radial head dislocation, the capitellum is often hypoplastic which can serve as another distinguishing radiographic feature.

Chronic Monteggia lesions have been diagnosed as early as several weeks after injury follow-up for a misdiagnosed, isolated ulnar fracture, or years later because of pain, restriction of motion, or extremity malalignment. Even a few weeks after injury, treatment becomes much more complicated than acute recognition and intervention. Proper recognition and appropriate treatment of a dislocated radial head at the time of injury can prevent the difficult problem of a chronic Monteggia lesion. When a previously undetected proximal radioulnar and radiocapitellar dislocation is encountered (Fig. 11-42), there is controversy regarding subsequent care. At present, there are limited levels of evidence and conflicting retrospective literature on this problem. Some reports indicate that the natural history of the untreated lesion is not problematic.[99,128,140] Fahey[44] suggested that although persistent dislocations can do well in the short

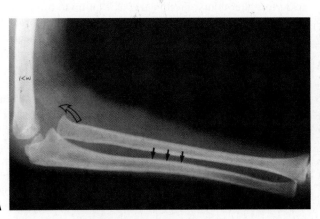

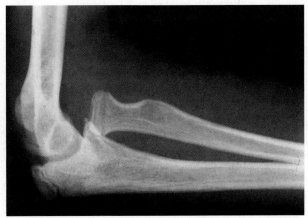

Figure 11-41. Chronic Monteggia lesion with ulnar bow line. **A:** The injury radiograph of an 8-year-old girl who fell, spraining her arm. Note the anterior bow of the ulna (*black arrows*) and loss of the radiocapitellar relation (*open arrow*). The diagnosis of a Monteggia lesion was not established. **B:** Radiograph at time of late diagnosis. Note the persistent ulnar bow and overgrowth of radius.

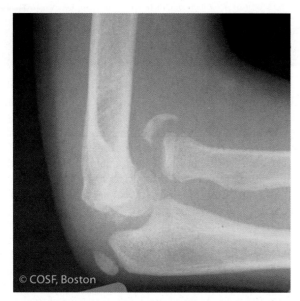

Figure 11-42. Chronic Monteggia lesion with a persistent anterior radial head dislocation and ossification of the displaced annular ligament.

term, problems arise over time, resulting in substantial patient morbidity. In fact, the majority of reports support the view that the natural history of persistent dislocation is not benign and is associated with restricted motion, deformity, functional impairment, pain, potential degenerative arthritis, and late neuropathy.[1,6,15,18,26,51,54,64,65,67,68,84] Kalamchi[67] reported pain, progressive valgus deformity, and restricted motion, especially loss of forearm rotation and elbow flexion. Tardy ulnar, median, and PIN palsy have been reported secondary to cubitus valgus and radial head dislocation in the setting of chronic Monteggia lesions.[1,6,62,85] Unless there is concern regarding the morphology of the radial head or capitellum (convex radial head, flattening of capitellum) that will prevent congruency of reduction, we believe that symptomatic patients with chronic Monteggia lesions are candidates for surgical reconstruction. In more chronic lesions, MRI can be obtained to further delineate cartilage quality and potential radiocapitellar and proximal radioulnar joint congruity. Patients with radial head enlargement or deformity, flattening of the capitellum, or joint arthrosis are not candidates for reconstruction (Fig. 11–14). In these patients, surgical decompression by radial head excision or ulnar lengthening can be considered if pain does not resolve with nonoperative treatment, but may place the patient at risk of developing wrist pain or progressive cubitus valgus.

OPERATIVE TREATMENT OF CHRONIC MONTEGGIA FRACTURE–DISLOCATIONS

Descriptions of surgical reconstruction for pediatric chronic Monteggia lesions have been variable and include (i) annular ligament repair or reconstruction alone,[58] (ii) ulnar osteotomy alone,[66,76] combined ulnar osteotomy with annular ligament repair or reconstruction,[34,63,97] and (iii) radial osteotomy.[33] The relative merit of each surgical technique has not been well defined and is likely to vary by patient and lesion. However, almost every expert advocates for an ulnar realignment

osteotomy when reconstructing a chronic Monteggia lesion. The principal controversy revolves around whether an annular ligament reconstruction should be performed in addition to the ulnar osteotomy. The original technique for delayed open reduction of the radial head and annular ligament reconstruction for chronic Monteggia fracture–dislocations is attributed to Bell Tawse,[14] who used the surgical approach described by Boyd (Fig. 11-31).[20] Other surgical approaches have been developed.[57,143] Nakamura et al.[97] reported long-term clinical and radiographic outcomes in patients undergoing ulnar osteotomy with annular ligament reconstruction. At a mean follow-up of 7 years, they reported excellent results in 19 out of 22 patients. Of concern, the radial head remained subluxated in five patients at the time of latest follow-up. Radiographic results did deteriorate when surgical reconstruction was performed more than 3 years after injury or in patients above 12 years of age.

Indications/Contraindications

Operative Treatment of Chronic Monteggia Fracture–Dislocations: INDICATIONS/CONTRAINDICATIONS	
Indications	**Contraindications**
• Symptomatic patients with a chronic Monteggia lesion (indication) • Asymptomatic patients with a chronic Monteggia lesion (relative indication)	• Radial head enlargement or deformity • Flattening of the capitellum joint arthrosis

Treatment indications have ranged from offering all patients with chronic Monteggia lesions surgical correction to limiting intervention to patients with pain, restricted motion, and functional disability. That wide spectrum of expert opinions makes individual case decisions difficult for patients, parents, and clinicians. Fowles et al.[49] suggested that reconstruction provides the best results in patients who have had a dislocation for 3 to 6 months or less. They also reported successful relocations up to 3 years after injury; Freedman et al.[51] for up to 6 years after injury. Throughout the literature, the appropriate age for radial head reduction seems to be younger than 10 to 12 years.[141] Hirayama et al.[61] suggested that the reduction of a chronically dislocated radial head should be avoided if there is significant deformation of the radiocapitellar joint architecture including permanent irregularity of the radial head or flattening of the capitellum (Fig. 11–14). Seel and Peterson[129] suggested that the age of the patient and the duration of the dislocation are unimportant. Their criteria for surgical repair were (1) normal concave radial head articular surface and (2) normal shape and contour of the ulna and radius (deformity of either, correctable by osteotomy). They treated seven patients ranging in age from 5 to 13 years for chronic dislocations that had been present from 3 months to 7 years. All seven were fully active with no elbow pain or instability at an average of 4 years after surgery.

Although they recommended surgical treatment of chronic Monteggia lesions in children because of the long-term sequelae,

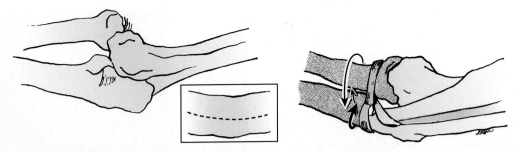

Figure 11-43. Bell Tawse reconstruction. The central slip of the triceps is used to reconstruct an annular ligament in Bell Tawse reconstruction. The direction of stability is posterior (*large arrow*).

Rodgers et al.[125] cautioned that the results of reconstructive procedures could be unpredictable and associated with a number of complications including malunion of the ulnar shaft, recurrent radiocapitellar subluxation, and radial and ulnar neuropathy.

At present, most authors advocate surgical reconstruction of a chronic Monteggia when (i) the diagnosis is made early, (ii) there is preservation of the normal concave radial head and convex capitellum, (iii) especially when there is progressive deformity (i.e., valgus), loss of motion and pain, and (iv) the patient and family are well aware of the concerns with operative reconstruction.

Annular Ligament Repair or Reconstruction

Most but not all authors advocate surgical repair or reconstruction of the annular ligament in conjunction with an ulnar osteotomy for a pediatric chronic Monteggia lesion.[34,63,97,125] Annular ligament repair or reconstruction without an osteotomy is very rarely indicated.[24] Kalamchi[67] restored stability after open reduction and osteotomy by utilizing the native annular ligament. The native ligament is generally present, even years later. The central opening can be dilated with a probe and/or surgical hemostat or by radial incisions. The annular ligament is then brought back over the radial head and down to its anatomic location on the neck before repair to the proximal ulna periosteum. Bell Tawse[14] used a strip of triceps tendon to reconstruct the annular ligament, as did Lloyd-Roberts[85] and Hurst.[65] Bell Tawse[14] used the central portion of the triceps tendon passed through a drill hole in the ulna and around the radial neck to stabilize the reduction and immobilized the elbow in a long-arm cast in extension (Fig. 11-43). Bucknill[23] and Lloyd-Roberts[85] modified the Bell Tawse procedure by using the lateral portion of the triceps tendon, with a transcapitellar pin for stability. The elbow was immobilized in flexion. Hurst and Dubrow[65] used the central portion of the triceps tendon but carried the dissection of the periosteum distally along the ulna to the level of the radial neck, which provided more stable fixation rather than stopping dissection at the olecranon as described by Bell Tawse.[14] They also used a periosteal tunnel rather than a drill hole for fixation of the tendinous strip to the ulna. Other authors have used other soft tissues for reconstruction, including the lacertus fibrosus,[29] a strip of the forearm fascia (Fig. 11-31),[134] palmaris longus free tendon graft,[162] and free fascia lata graft.[154]

Seel and Peterson[129] described the use of two holes drilled in the proximal ulna. The holes are placed at the original attachments of the annular ligament and allow repair of the annular ligament (frequently avulsed from one attachment and trapped within the joint) or reconstruction of the annular ligament with triceps tendon. This technique secures the radial head in its normal position from any dislocated position and allows osteotomy for correction of any accompanying deformity of the ulna or radius. Seel and Peterson[129] noted that the Bell Tawse procedure tends to pull the radius posterolaterally (Fig. 11-44A). A tight annular ligament reconstruction may constrict the neck of the radius, potentially limiting the growth of the radial neck ("notching") and reducing forearm rotation. Seel and Peterson[129] placed a single drill hole obliquely across the ulna to exit medially at the site of the medial attachment of the annular ligament on the coronoid process of the ulna (Fig. 11-44B). The tendon was routed through the tunnel, brought around the neck, and sutured to the lateral side of the ulna. With this construct, the direction of stability was posteromedial. The use of two drill holes to secure the annular ligament or other reconstructive tendon at both normal attachments of the annular ligament on the ulna achieved a more normal posteromedial holding force on the neck of the radius. Alternatives to holes drilled in the bone are small-bone staples or bone-anchoring devices.

Ulnar Osteotomy

The majority of surgeons advocate an ulnar osteotomy, with or without ligament repair or reconstruction, for a chronic

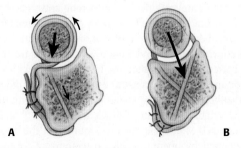

Figure 11-44. Schematic representation of annular ligament reconstruction techniques. **A:** The Bell Tawse reconstruction which results in a posteriorly directed force. **B:** The technique suggested by Seel and Peterson. In this technique, crossing drill holes are created at the anterior and posterior rim of the lesser sigmoid notch. The resulting reconstruction may improve stability of the radial head.

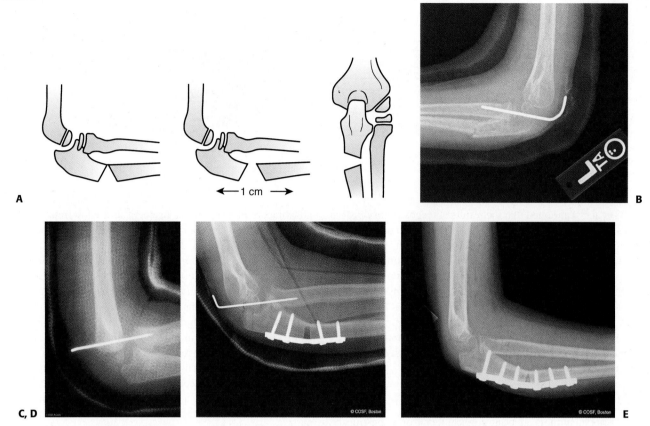

Figure 11-45. **A:** Diagram of floating open ulnar osteotomy without fixation or bone graft. **B:** Similar ulnar osteotomy with radiocapitellar pin fixation. **C:** Unfortunately in this case, the radial head was never reduced and the pin was placed without anatomic alignment. **D:** In this situation, the osteotomy was plated without bone graft, the radiocapitellar joint pinned anatomically for 4 weeks. **E:** Long-term follow-up with anatomic healing.

pediatric Monteggia lesion. Various types of osteotomies have been used to facilitate reduction of the radial head and prevent recurrent subluxation (Fig. 11-45). Kalamchi[67] reported using a "drill hole" ulnar osteotomy to obtain reduction of the radial head in two patients. Minimal periosteal stripping with this technique allowed the osteotomy to heal rapidly. Hirayama et al.[61] used a 1-cm distraction ulnar osteotomy approximately 5 cm distal to the tip of the olecranon with plate and screw fixation, but complications with loosening and plate breakage occurred. Mehta[91,92] used an osteotomy of the proximal ulna stabilized with bone graft. In neither series was annular ligament repair performed. Inoue and Shionoya[66] compared the results of simple corrective ulnar osteotomy in six patients with those of posterior angular (overcorrected) osteotomy in six others, and found that better clinical outcomes were obtained with the overcorrected, angular osteotomy. Tajima and Yoshizu,[147] in a series of 23 neglected Monteggia fractures, found that the best results were obtained by opening wedge osteotomy of the proximal ulna without ligament reconstruction. Exner[43] reported that in patients with chronic dislocation of the radial head after missed type I Monteggia lesions, reduction was successfully obtained with ulnar corticotomy and gradual lengthening and angulation of the ulna using an external fixator. Another option for chronic

type IV Monteggia lesion is a shortening osteotomy of the radius, usually indicated for angulation of the radius without angulation of the ulna. More recently, surgeons have advocated performing osteotomies and then external fixation.[19,86]

Ulnar Osteotomy and Open Reduction of the Radial Capitellar and Radioulnar Joints With Annular Ligament Reconstruction

In patients younger than 10 to 12 years of age with delayed diagnosis of a Monteggia lesion, reduction and stabilization of the radial head to its anatomic relationship with the capitellum is indicated if the radial head remains concave. Even though the child may do well in the short term without reduction of the radial head, problems usually develop in adolescence or adulthood when progressive instability, pain, weakness of the forearm, and restriction of motion are likely. Appropriate discussion with the patient and family regarding the risks and complications of surgery is performed. This is not an operation for the inexperienced surgeon or uninformed patient and family. We perform an ulnar osteotomy and open reduction of the radiocapitellar and proximal radioulnar joints with annular ligament repair or reconstruction.

Technique

> ✔ **Ulnar Osteotomy and Open Reduction of the Radial Capitellar and Radioulnar Joints With Annular Ligament Reconstruction:**
> KEY SURGICAL STEPS

❏ An extensile curvilinear posterolateral incision is planned

❏ The midportion of the incision allows access to the radiocapitellar joint at the Kocher interval (between the anconeus and extensor carpi ulnaris)

❏ Incision extended proximally for identification of the radial nerve between the brachialis and brachioradialis, and harvesting of the triceps fascia if required for annular ligament reconstruction

❏ Incision extended distally to allow access to the ulna for osteotomy between the extensor carpi ulnaris and the flexor carpi ulnaris

❏ Interval between the anconeus and extensor carpi ulnaris developed, the extensor–supinator mass can be elevated off of the anterior lateral epicondyle and lateral supracondylar if needed for visualization, elbow capsule incised anterior to the lateral ulnar collateral ligament in order to preserve the integrity of lateral ligamentous complex and ulnohumeral stability

❏ Pulvinar and synovitis are carefully debrided from the radiocapitellar joint to permit visualization of the radial head, annular ligament, and capitellum

❏ The lesser sigmoid notch should also be thoroughly debrided in order to permit reduction of the proximal radioulnar joint

❏ The annular ligament can generally be identified, careful dissection and dilation of its aperture allows reconstitution of its typical ring shape, dilation performed by making small radial incisions extending from the center toward the periphery

❏ At this stage, the surgeon must decide whether the native annular ligament can be salvaged (the native ligament is generally usable)

❏ If the annular ligament can be salvaged, attempt should be made to reduce it over the radial head

❏ If the ligament cannot be reduced over the radial head, the ligament may be incised along its posterior insertion (at or adjacent to the posterior rim of the lesser sigmoid notch) and repaired following reduction of the radial head

❏ If the annular ligament can be salvaged, the reduction of the radial head is evaluated with fluoroscopy

❏ If there is anatomic restoration of radiocapitellar alignment, annular ligament repair alone may be sufficient (this is very unusual, typically ulnar osteotomy is required)

❏ If the annular ligament cannot be salvaged, its remnant is sharply excised in preparation for subsequent annular ligament reconstruction

❏ Annular ligament repair or reconstruction alone does not usually result in a congruent, stable radiocapitellar reduction due to the deforming force created by concomitant ulnar malunion

❏ Opening wedge osteotomy of the ulna is normally required

❏ Opening wedge osteotomy of the ulna is usually performed at the apex of the malunion

❏ When the ulnar injury is characterized by plastic deformation, the osteotomy should be made proximal to the apex (closer to the elbow) in order to more effectively correct of radiocapitellar malalignment

❏ Temporary pinning of the radiocapitellar joint can help determine the size of the opening wedge osteotomy

❏ The radiocapitellar and proximal radioulnar joints are anatomically reduced and a K-wire is temporarily inserted across the radiocapitellar joint to stabilize the reduction

❏ Anatomic reduction of the radial head allows the ulnar osteotomy to open the necessary amount to maintain the reduction

❏ The osteotomy is then stabilized with appropriately contoured plate and screw fixation

❏ We prefer double-stacked one-third tubular plates in younger patients or a 3.5-mm dynamic compression plate in larger patients (Synthes, West Chester, PA)

❏ The radiocapitellar wire is then removed and fluoroscopy should be used to confirm stable reduction of the radial head

❏ If the annular ligament was not salvageable, a reconstruction should be performed with triceps fascia

❏ The extensor–supinator fascia may be used as an alternative

❏ Limited prophylactic fasciotomies of the volar and dorsal forearm compartments are performed to minimize risk of postoperative compartment syndrome

❏ Final orthogonal fluoroscopy imaging should be obtained to confirm stable reduction of the radiocapitellar and proximal radioulnar joints

The surgical approach is extensile (Fig. 11-46B). The posterolateral skin incision is curvilinear to allow for proximal triceps tendon harvesting, if necessary, and distally for an ulnar opening wedge osteotomy. Initially, only the proximal portion is opened. The radial nerve is identified between the brachialis and brachioradialis (Fig. 11-46C). Dissection of the nerve is performed distally to its motor (PIN) and sensory branches (Fig. 11-23). Generally, the PIN is adherent to the dislocated radial head. The nerves are mobilized and protected throughout the remainder of the reconstruction.

Next, the Kocher interval (between the anconeus and extensor carpi ulnaris) interval is utilized to expose the radiocapitellar joint. The joint exposure is carried proximal with elevation of the extensor–supinator mass and capsule as a single tissue plane off the anterior aspect of the lateral epicondyle and the lateral supracondylar ridge. This improves visualization of the elbow joint. The radial head is usually dislocated anteriorly and superiorly with a wall of interposed capsule and ligament blocking reduction. Pulvinar and synovitis are thoroughly debrided from the elbow joint. Particular attention is paid to a thorough debridement of the proximal radioulnar joint to allow the radial head to fit anatomically into place once reduced. At this stage, a decision needs to be made if the native annular ligament can be salvaged (Fig. 11-46D). There is usually a central perforation in the capsular wall that separates the dislocated radial head from the joint. This perforation indicates the site of the opening of the original ligament. Dilation and radial incisions extending from the center outward are made to enlarge this opening. This usually enables the native annular ligament to be reduced over the radial neck. Capsular adhesions are removed from the radial head to assist in reduction of the radial head and neck back into the joint. The native ligament usually detaches from the ulna with a large periosteal sleeve (the site of ossification on the radiographs of a chronic Monteggia lesion (Fig. 11-42), and this can be the site for suture reattachment to the ulna of the native ligament. If the native ligament cannot be used, and most of the time it can, then it is thoroughly debrided in preparation for harvesting of triceps fascia for ligament reconstruction.

A radial head reduction is then attempted. The reduction is scrutinized for congruity between the radial head and the

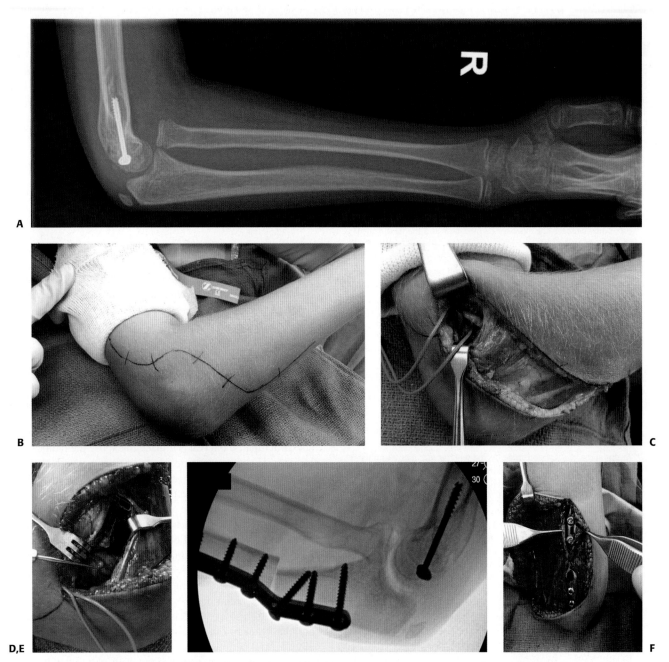

Figure 11-46. Authors' preferred technique for chronic Monteggia reconstruction. **A:** Lateral forearm radiograph in an 8-year-old female with a chronic Bado type I Monteggia lesion, a prior history of ipsilateral medial epicondyle fracture that underwent open reduction and internal fixation. Note the positive ulnar bow sign with associated anterior dislocation of the radial head. **B:** Extensile incision for annular ligament reconstruction and ulnar osteotomy. **C:** Radial nerve identified and tagged in the interval between the brachialis and the brachioradialis. **D:** The annular ligament was identified and was dilated to allow delivery of the radial head through the aperture of the ligament. A nerve hook was used to reduce the annular ligament into its native position. Ulnar opening wedge osteotomy is performed proximal to the apex of the deformity which is recommended in cases of plastic deformation to best facilitate reduction of the radial head. **E:** Fixation is achieved with contoured double-stacked one-third tubular plates. **F:** Limited prophylactic forearm fasciotomies are performed to minimize potential for compartment syndrome and to facilitate closure of the periosteum and fascia over the hardware.

capitellum. If this is satisfactory, ligamentous repair or reconstruction alone can be done. This is exceedingly unusual. If the radius cannot be reduced, an ulnar osteotomy is made at the site of maximal deformity. If the ulnar injury is characterized by plastic deformation, the osteotomy can be made proximal to the apex and closer to the elbow in order to more effectively correct of radiocapitellar malalignment. Subperiosteal dissection of the ulna is performed at the planned osteotomy site. An opening wedge osteotomy is made with a laminar spreader to allow the radial head to align itself with the capitellum without pressure (Fig. 11-45). Partial overcorrection of the ulnar alignment is the goal. A clever way to do this is to anatomically pin the radiocapitellar joint and allow the ulnar osteotomy to open the necessary amount for this reduction (Fig. 11-47). When reduced anatomically, the ulnar osteotomy is then fixed partially proximally and distally with contoured plate(s) and screws. Further testing of a complete stable arc of rotation of the radial head is performed in order to be certain that the correct level and degree of osteotomy were obtained to maintain radiocapitellar and radioulnar alignment. If a temporary radiocapitellar pin was used, it is removed for this testing. If correct, the fixation is completed. No bone graft is used, and the periosteum is repaired. We prefer fixation with double-stacked one-third tubular plates in small children and 3.5 dynamic compression plates in larger children (Synthes, West Chester, PA).

At this stage, the annular ligament repair or reconstruction is completed. Some authors have demonstrated repositioning of the annular ligament as an option.[87] If the native ligament is used, and it usually is in situations that are a year or less out from injury, then nonabsorbable braided sutures are placed in the annular ligament and the ligament is repaired through ulnar periosteal tunnels. None of the radial sutures are tightened until all are placed. If reconstruction is necessary, an 8- to 10-cm strip of triceps fascia is developed from proximal to distal,

carefully elevating the periosteum from the proximal ulna down to the level of the radial neck. Over the olecranon apophysis, this dissection will be delicate so as not to inadvertently amputate the fascia. The strip of tendon is then passed through the periosteum, around the radial neck, and then brought back and sutured to itself and the ulnar periosteum. The passage and securing in the periosteum are similar in design to the drill holes advocated by Seel and Peterson.[129] At this stage, the radial head and capitellum alignment should be anatomic throughout full rotation. Final closure involves repair of the capsule and extensor–supinator origin back to the lateral epicondylar region of the humerus. Final radiographs and fluoroscopic testing of a stable arc of motion in both flexion–extension and pronation–supination planes are gently tested before completion of closure. Prophylactic volar and dorsal forearm fasciotomies are carefully performed through the original incision with elevation of the skin and subcutaneous tissues and a long tenotomy scissors. Final inspection of the radial nerve is performed before skin closure.

Radiocapitellar or radioulnar pin fixation is rarely needed if the osteotomy and soft tissue repair tension are correct. As mentioned, at times, pin fixation is used intraoperatively for temporary stability to get the corrective ulnar osteotomy correct; it is then removed to test the range of motion. If there is radial head deformity in very chronic reconstructions, pinning the joint is sometimes useful for 3 to 4 weeks postoperatively. In our experience, this has been occasionally necessary in repeat surgery for a chronic Monteggia lesion in which options are limited and the patient has pain and marked limitation of motion. Then, the radiocapitellar joint is secured by passing a smooth, transcapitellar pin through the posterior aspect of the capitellum into the radial head and neck with the elbow at 90 degrees and the forearm in supination. A pin of sufficient size is mandatory to avoid pin failure[72]; a small pin may fatigue and break. An alternative

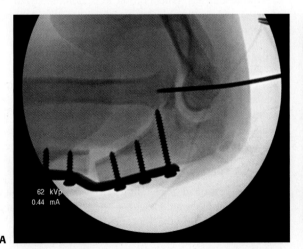
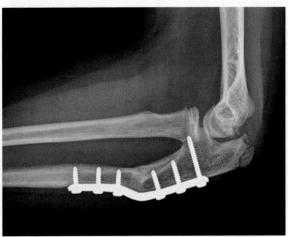

Figure 11-47. A: After completion of the ulnar osteotomy, the radial head can be anatomically reduced with the respect to the capitellum and the lesser sigmoid notch. As seen in this radiograph, the radiocapitellar joint can be temporarily pinned, which allows the ulnar osteotomy to open to the necessary amount to maintain the reduction. The ulnar osteotomy should then be stabilized with contoured plates and screws. The temporary wire is then removed so that fluoroscopy can be used to confirm stability of the reduction. **B:** Radiographs of the elbow 6 months after ulnar osteotomy and annular ligament repair demonstrate a healed osteotomy and anatomic reduction of the radiocapitellar joint.

technique to secure the reduction of the radius is transversely pinning the radius to the ulna.[82]

After wound closure, a bivalved long-arm cast is applied with the forearm in 60 to 90 degrees of supination and the elbow is flexed 80 to 90 degrees. The cast is maintained for 4 to 6 weeks and is then changed to a removable bivalved cast to allow active motion, especially pronation and supination. Elbow flexion and extension return more rapidly than rotary motion of the forearm which may take up to 6 months to improve, with pronation possibly limited, though minimally, permanently.[124] The final desired result is not determined until radiographs are anatomic with full restoration of motion.

MANAGEMENT OF EXPECTED ADVERSE OUTCOMES AND UNEXPECTED COMPLICATIONS RELATED TO MONTEGGIA FRACTURE–DISLOCATIONS

Monteggia Fracture–Dislocations:
COMMON ADVERSE OUTCOMES AND COMPLICATIONS

- Chronic Monteggia lesion
- Acute radial nerve palsy or PIN palsy
- Tardy radial nerve palsy
- Acute ulnar nerve palsy
- Acute anterior interosseous nerve palsy
- Myositis ossificans
- Compartment syndrome

NERVE INJURIES

Radial Nerve Injury

The literature reflects a 10% to 20% incidence of radial nerve injury, making it the most common complication associated with Monteggia fractures.[64] It is most commonly associated with type I and III injuries.[14,99,131] The PIN is most commonly injured because of its proximity to the radial head and its intimate relation to the Arcade of Frohse (Fig. 11-23). The arcade may be thinner and therefore more pliable in children than in adults.[136] In addition, the periosteum is much thicker in pediatric patients. This may account in part for the rapid resolution of the nerve injury in children. A radial nerve injury in a child is treated expectantly. Nerve function usually returns by 12 weeks after reduction, if not sooner.[137,139] A review of a series of pediatric Monteggia lesions[101] recommends waiting 6 months before intervention for a PIN injury. Most series report 100% resolution in both fractures treated promptly and those treated late.[1,6,83]

Two reports[95,134] of irreducible Monteggia fractures caused by interposition of the radial nerve posterior to the radial head documented return of function approximately 4 months after the nerve was replaced to its normal anatomic position and the radial head was reduced. Morris,[95] in cadaver studies, showed that significant anterior dislocation of the radial head and varus angulation of the elbow allowed the radial nerve to slide posterior to the radial head and, with subsequent reduction of the radial head, become entrapped. If a chronic reconstruction is

undertaken in the presence of a persistent radial nerve lesion, it is highly recommended that radial nerve exploration and decompression be performed before joint debridement. Rodgers et al.[125] cited a partial nerve injury during similar circumstances that was then microscopically repaired with full recovery. Rang[118] acknowledged the same experience in an open educational forum.

Ulnar Nerve Injury

Bryan[22] reported one adult with an ulnar nerve lesion associated with a type II Monteggia lesion with spontaneous resolution. Stein et al.[139] reported three combined radial and ulnar nerve injuries, two of which underwent exploration and decompression for functional return of the nerve.

Median Nerve Injury

Median nerve injuries are uncommon with Monteggia fractures, but injury to the anterior interosseous nerve has been reported.[162,165] Stein et al.,[139] in their report specifically examining nerve injuries in Monteggia lesions, reported no median nerve deficits. Watson and Singer[162] reported entrapment of the main trunk of the median nerve in a greenstick ulnar fracture in a 6-year-old girl. Completion of the fracture was necessary for release of the nerve. At 6 months after surgery, there was full motor recovery but the sensation was slightly reduced in the tips of the index finger and thumb.

Tardy Radial Nerve Palsy

Tardy radial nerve palsy associated with radial head dislocation has been infrequently reported.[1,6,62,83,169] Although reported treatment has varied, excision of the radial head with exploration and neurolysis of the nerve generally produced good results,[1,6] whereas exploration of the nerve alone produced variable results.[62,83] Yamamoto et al.[169] combined radial head resection and nerve exploration with tendon transfers, producing good results in two patients.

PERIARTICULAR OSSIFICATION

Two patterns of ossification after Monteggia fracture–dislocations have been noted radiographically: ossification around the radial head and myositis ossificans. Ossification around the radial head and neck[14,64,83,85,140,142] appears as a thin ridge of bone in a cap-like distribution and may be accompanied by other areas resembling sesamoid bones. This typically resorbs with time. Ossification may also occur in the area of the annular ligament,[40] including in a chronic Monteggia with a displaced annular ligament (Fig. 11-42). Elbow function generally is not affected by the formation of these lesions[14,64,85,140,142] as long as the radial head and neck are anatomically reduced.

The other form of ossification is true myositis ossificans, reported to occur in approximately 3% of elbow injuries and 7% of Monteggia lesions in adults and children.[100,152] Myositis ossificans has a good prognosis in patients younger than 15 years of age, appearing at 3 to 4 weeks after injury and resolving in 6 to 8 months. Its occurrence is related to the severity of the initial injury, association with a fractured radial head, the number of remanipulations during treatment, and passive motion of the elbow during the postoperative period.[100,152]

SUMMARY, CONTROVERSIES, AND FUTURE DIRECTIONS RELATED TO MONTEGGIA FRACTURE–DISLOCATIONS

Adherence to several fundamental principles helps ensure a good outcome after Monteggia fracture–dislocations in children:

1. With a high index of suspicion and careful radiographic evaluation, acute Monteggia injuries can be accurately diagnosed. Evaluation of radiocapitellar alignment requires AP and true lateral views of the elbow. All forearm fractures require careful inspection of the proximal radioulnar joint and the radiocapitellar joint before treatment.
2. The radiocapitellar line must be anatomic in all views.
3. If the radial head is dislocated, always look for ulnar fracture or plastic deformation. Conversely, if the ulna is fractured or plastically deformed, always look for a radial head subluxation or dislocation.
4. Stability of the ulnar reduction is required to maintain reduction of the radial head. Stability may be inherent to the fracture pattern (plastic deformation or incomplete fractures) or achieved by internal fixation (intramedullary fixation for short oblique and transverse fractures; plate and screw fixation for long oblique and comminuted fractures).

5. Radial head reduction confirmed by an intact radiocapitellar line must be achieved by open or closed means.
6. If the radial head is irreducible or unstable, removal of interposed soft tissue is required. An annular ligament repair or reconstruction may be required.
7. Treatment of an acute Monteggia lesion is more straightforward and much more successful than reconstruction of a chronic Monteggia lesion.
8. Reconstruction of a chronic Monteggia lesion is not an operation for the uninitiated. There is a high risk of recurrent or residual radial head subluxation and iatrogenic nerve injury.

Refining treatment recommendations for acute and chronic Monteggia lesions in the future will require prospective multicenter, scientific inquiry. To date, there are no prospective investigations with a large number of pediatric patients and sufficient duration of follow-up. The vast majority of published studies report limited outcomes data. Studies that report functional outcomes in addition to union rates, motion, and pain scores will permit surgeons to accurately counsel and monitor patient recovery and progress.

ACKNOWLEDGMENT

The authors wish to recognize contributions of the authors of previous editions of this chapter, Drs. Earl Stanley, Jose de la Garza, and Peter M. Waters.

Annotated References

Reference	Annotation
Bado JL. *The Monteggia Lesion*. Springfield, IL: Charles C Thomas; 1962.	The original classification system that has stood the test of time.
Bell Tawse AJ. The treatment of malunited anterior Monteggia fractures in children. *J Bone Joint Surg Br*. 1965;47:718–723.	
Boyd HB, Boals JC. The Monteggia lesion: a review of 159 cases. *Clin Orthop Relat Res*. 1969;66:94–100.	Large early case series of this fracture pattern.
Foran I, Upasani VV, Walace CD, et al. Acute pediatric Monteggia fractures: a conservative approach to stabilization. *J Pediatr Orthop*. 2017;37(6):e335–e341.	Multicenter study demonstrating safety of a trial of conservative treatment for Monteggia fractures.
Inoue G, Shionoya K. Corrective ulnar osteotomy for malunited anterior Monteggia lesions in children. 12 patients followed for 1 to 12 years. *Acta Orthop Scand*. 1998;69:73–76.	Comparison of simple corrective ulna osteotomy with posterior angular osteotomy for chronic Monteggia lesions; finding the patients with angular osteotomies had better outcomes.
Leonidou A, Pagkalos J, Lepetsos P, et al. Pediatric Monteggia fractures: a single-center study of the management of 40 patients. *J Pediatr Orthop*. 2012;32(4):352–356.	Large single-center retrospective study with outcomes reported using Bruce–Harvey–Wilson scoring system demonstrating excellent outcomes with a conservative approach.
Letts M, Locht R, Wiens J. Monteggia fracture-dislocations in children. *J Bone Joint Surg Br*. 1985;67:724–727.	Alternate classification system for Monteggia fractures based both on direction of radial head dislocation and the type of ulnar fracture.
Nakamura K, Hirachi K, Uchiyama S, et al. Long-term clinical and radiographic outcomes after open reduction for missed Monteggia fracture-dislocations in children. *J Bone Joint Surg Am*. 2009;91(6):1394–1404.	Single-center retrospective study demonstrating outcomes after open reduction for chronic Monteggia fractures using objective outcomes criteria (postoperative Mayo Elbow Performance Index).

Annotated References

Reference	Annotation
Ramski DE, Hennrikus WP, Bae DS, et al. Pediatric Monteggia fractures: a multicenter examination of treatment strategy and early clinical and radiographic results. *J Pediatr Orthop.* 2015;35(2):115–120.	Retrospective study at two large institutions analyzing the following treatment protocol: closed reduction for greenstick fractures, intramedullary fixation for transverse/short oblique fractures, and ORIF for long oblique/comminuted fractures.
Ring D, Waters PM. Operative fixation of Monteggia fractures in children. *J Bone Joint Surg Br.* 1996;78:734–739.	Large case series describing the importance of the characteristics of the ulna fracture influencing the treatment choice.
Rodgers WB, Waters PM, Hall JE. Chronic Monteggia lesions in children: complications and results of reconstruction. *J Bone Joint Surg Am.* 1996;78:1322–1329.	This is an important study demonstrating the vast complications that could occur with surgical intervention of chronic Monteggia fractures.
Seel MJ, Peterson HA. Management of chronic posttraumatic radial head dislocation in children. *J Pediatr Orthop.* 1999;19:306–312.	

REFERENCES

1. Adams JR, Rizzoli HV. Tardy radial and ulnar nerve palsy: a case report. *J Neurosurg.* 1959;16:342–344.
2. Agarwal A. Type IV Monteggia fracture in a child. *Can J Surg.* 2008;51(2):E44–E45.
3. Almquist EE, Gordon LH, Blue AI. Congenital dislocation of the head of the radius. *J Bone Joint Surg Am.* 1969;51:1118–1127.
4. Anderson HJ. Monteggia fractures. *Adv Orthop Surg.* 1989;4:201–204.
5. Arazi M, Ogun TC, Kapicioglu MI. The Monteggia lesion and ipsilateral supracondylar humerus and distal radius fractures. *J Orthop Trauma.* 1999;13(1):60–63.
6. Austin R. Tardy palsy of the radial nerve from a Monteggia fracture. *Injury.* 1976;7(3):202–204.
7. Babb A, Carlson WO. Monteggia fractures: beware! *S D J Med.* 2005;58(7):283–285.
8. Bado JL. La lesion de Monteggia. *Intermedica Sarandi.* 1958;328.
9. Bado JL. *The Monteggia Lesion.* Springfield, IL: Charles C Thomas; 1962.
10. Bado JL. The Monteggia lesion. *Clin Orthop Relat Res.* 1967;50:71–86.
11. Basmajian JV, Griffen WR Jr. Function of anconeus muscle: an electromyographic study. *J Bone Joint Surg Am.* 1972;54:1712–1714.
12. Beaty JH. Fractures and dislocations about the elbow in children: section on Monteggia fractures. *AAOS Instr Course Lect.* 1991;40:373–384.
13. Beddow FH, Corkery PH. Lateral dislocation of the radio-humeral joint with greenstick fracture of the upper end of the ulna. *J Bone Joint Surg Br.* 1960;42B:782–784.
14. Bell Tawse AJ. The treatment of malunited anterior Monteggia fractures in children. *J Bone Joint Surg Br.* 1965;47:718–723.
15. Best TN. Management of old unreduced Monteggia fracture dislocations of the elbow in children. *J Pediatr Orthop.* 1994;14:193–199.
16. Bhandari N, Jindal P. Monteggia lesion in a child: variant of a Bado type-IV lesion. A case report. *J Bone Joint Surg Am.* 1996;78(8):1252–1255.
17. Biyani A. Ipsilateral Monteggia equivalent injury and distal radial and ulnar fracture in a child. *J Orthop Trauma.* 1994;8(5):431–433.
18. Blasier D, Trussell A. Ipsilateral radial head dislocation and distal fractures of both forearm bones in a child. *Am J Orthop (Belle Mead NJ).* 1995;24:498–500.
19. Bor N, Rubin G, Rozen N, et al. Chronic anterior Monteggia lesions in children: report of 4 cases treated with closed reduction by ulnar osteotomy and external fixation. *J Pediatr Orthop.* 2015;35:7–10.
20. Boyd HB. Surgical exposure of the ulna and proximal one third of the radius through one incision. *Surg Gynecol Obstet.* 1940;71:86–88.
21. Boyd HB, Boals JC. The Monteggia lesion: a review of 159 cases. *Clin Orthop Relat Res.* 1969;66:94–100.
22. Bryan RS. Monteggia fracture of the forearm. *J Trauma.* 1971;11:992–998.
23. Bucknill TM. Anterior dislocation of the radial head in children. *Proc R Soc Med.* 1977;70(9):620–624.
24. Cappellino A, Wolfe SW, Marsh JS. Use of a modified Bell Tawse procedure for chronic acquired dislocation of the radial head. *J Pediatr Orthop.* 1998;18(3):410–414.
25. Captier G, Canovas F, Mercier N, et al. Biometry of the radial head: biomechanical implications in pronation and supination. *Surg Radiol Anat.* 2002;24(5):295–301.
26. Caravias DE. Some observations on congenital dislocation of the head of the radius. *J Bone Joint Surg Br.* 1957;39-B:86–90.
27. Castillo Odena I [Milch H, transl]. Bipolar fracture-dislocation of the forearm. *J Bone Joint Surg Am.* 1952;34:968–976.
28. Cheung EV, Yao J. Monteggia fracture-dislocation associated with proximal and distal radioulnar joint instability: a case report. *J Bone Joint Surg Am.* 2009;91(4):950–954.
29. Corbett CH. Anterior dislocation of the radius and its recurrence. *Br J Surg.* 1931;19:155.
30. Curry GJ. Monteggia fracture. *Am J Surg.* 1947;73:613–617.
31. Dattani R, Patnaik S, Kantak A, et al. Distal humerus lateral condyle fracture and Monteggia lesions in a 3-year old child: a case report. *Acta Orthop Belg.* 2008;74(4):542–545.

32. David-West KS, Wilson NI, Sherlock DA, et al. Missed Monteggia injuries. *Injury.* 2005;36(10):1206–1209.
33. De Boeck H. Radial neck osteolysis after annular ligament reconstruction. A case report. *Clin Orthop Relat Res.* 1997;342:94–98.
34. Degreef I, De Smet L. Missed radial head dislocations in children associated with ulnar deformation: treatment by open reduction and ulnar osteotomy. *J Orthop Trauma.* 2004;18(6):375–378.
35. Denucé P. *Memoire sun les luxations du coude.* Paris: These de Paris; 1854.
36. Deshpande S, O'Doherty D. Type I Monteggia fracture dislocation associated with ipsilateral distal radial epiphyseal injury. *J Orthop Trauma.* 2001;15(5):373–375.
37. Devnani AS. Missed Monteggia fracture dislocation in children. *Injury.* 1997;28(2):131–133.
38. Dormans JP, Rang M. The problem of Monteggia fracture-dislocations in children. *Orthop Clin North Am.* 1990;21:251–256.
39. Eady JL. Acute Monteggia lesions in children. *JSC Med Assoc.* 1975;71:107–112.
40. Earwaker J. Posttraumatic calcification of the annular ligament of the radius. *Skeletal Radiol.* 1992;21:149–154.
41. Edwards EG. The posterior Monteggia fracture. *Am Surg.* 1952;18:323–337.
42. Evans EM. Pronation injuries of the forearm, with special reference to the anterior Monteggia fracture. *J Bone Joint Surg Br.* 1949;31B(4):578–588.
43. Exner GU. Missed chronic anterior Monteggia lesion. Closed reduction by gradual lengthening and angulation of the ulna. *J Bone Joint Surg Br.* 2001;83(4):547–550.
44. Fahey JJ. Fractures of the elbow in children: Monteggia's fracture-dislocation. *AAOS Instr Course Lect.* 1960;17:39.
45. Fahmy NRM. Unusual Monteggia lesions in kids. *Injury.* 1980;12:399–404.
46. Faundez AA, Ceroni D, Kaelin A. An unusual Monteggia type-I equivalent fracture in a child. *J Bone Joint Surg Br.* 2003;85(4):584–586.
47. Fernandez FF, Egenolf M, Carsten C, et al. Unstable diaphyseal fractures of both bones of the forearm in children: plate fixation versus intramedullary nailing. *Injury.* 2005;36(10):1210–1216.
48. Foran I, Upasani VV, Walace CD, et al. Acute pediatric Monteggia fractures: a conservative approach to stabilization. *J Pediatr Orthop.* 2017;37(6):e335–e341.
49. Fowles JV, Sliman N, Kassah MT. The Monteggia lesion in children. Fracture of the ulna and dislocation of the radial head. *J Bone Joint Surg Am.* 1983;65:1276–1282.
50. Frazier JL, Buschmann WR, Insler HP. Monteggia type I equivalent lesion: diaphyseal ulna and proximal radius fracture with a posterior elbow dislocation in a child. *J Orthop Trauma.* 1991;5:373–375.
51. Freedman L, Luk K, Leong JC. Radial head reduction after a missed Monteggia fracture: brief report. *J Bone Joint Surg Br.* 1988;70:846–847.
52. Gibson WK, Timperlake RW. Orthopedic treatment of a type IV Monteggia fracture-dislocations in a child. *J Bone Joint Surg Br.* 1992;74:780–781.
53. Giustra PE, Killoran PJ, Furman RS, et al. The missed Monteggia fracture. *Radiology.* 1974;110(1):45–47.
54. Givon U, Pritsch M, Levy O, et al. Monteggia and equivalent lesions: a study of 41 cases. *Clin Orthop Relat Res.* 1997;(337):208–215.
55. Givon U, Pritsch M, Yosepovich A. Monteggia lesion in a child: variant of a Bado type-IV lesion. A case report. *J Bone Joint Surg Am.* 1997;79(11):1753–1754.
56. Gleeson AP, Beattie TF. Monteggia fracture-dislocation in children. *J Accid Emerg Med.* 1994;11(3):192–194.
57. Gorden ML. Monteggia fracture: a combined surgical approach employing a single lateral incision. *Clin Orthop Relat Res.* 1967;50:87–93.
58. Gyr BM, Stevens PM, Smith JT. Chronic Monteggia fractures in children: outcome after treatment with the Bell-Tawse procedure. *J Pediatr Orthop B.* 2004;13(6):402–406.
59. Haddad ES, Manktelow AR, Sarkar JS. The posterior Monteggia: a pathological lesion? *Injury.* 1996;27:101–102.
60. Henry AK. *Extensile Exposure.* Baltimore, MD: Lippincott Williams & Wilkins; 1970.
61. Hirayama T, Takemitsu Y, Yagihara K, et al. Operation for chronic dislocation of the radial head in children. *J Bone Joint Surg Br.* 1987;69:639–642.

62. Holst-Nielson F, Jensen V. Tardy posterior interosseus nerve palsy as a result of an unreduced radial head dislocation in Monteggia fractures: a report of two cases. *J Hand Surg Am.* 1984;9:572–575.
63. Hui JH, Sulaiman AR, Lee HC, et al. Open reduction and annular ligament reconstruction with fascia of the forearm in chronic Monteggia lesions in children. *J Pediatr Orthop.* 2005;25(4):501–506.
64. Hume AC. Anterior dislocation of the head of the radius associated with undisplaced fracture of olecranon in children. *J Bone Joint Surg Br.* 1957;39-B:508–512.
65. Hurst LC, Dubrow EN. Surgical treatment of symptomatic chronic radial head dislocation: a neglected Monteggia fracture. *J Pediatr Orthop.* 1983;3:227–230.
66. Inoue G, Shionoya K. Corrective ulnar osteotomy for malunited anterior Monteggia lesions in children. 12 patients followed for 1 to 12 years. *Acta Orthop Scand.* 1998;69:73–76.
67. Kalamchi A. Monteggia fracture-dislocation in children. Late treatment in two cases. *J Bone Joint Surg Am.* 1986;68:615–619.
68. Kaplan EB. The quadrate ligament of the radio-ulnar joint in the elbow. *Bull Hosp Joint Dis.* 1964;25:126–130.
69. Karachalios T, Smith EJ, Pearse MF. Monteggia equivalent injury in a very young patient. *Injury.* 1992;23:419–420.
70. Kay RM, Skaggs DL. The pediatric Monteggia fracture. *Am J Orthop (Belle Mead NJ).* 1998;27(9):606–609.
71. Kemnitz S, De Schrijver F, De Smet L. Radial head dislocation with plastic deformation of the ulna in children. A rare and frequently missed condition. *Acta Orthop Belg.* 2000;66(4):359–362.
72. King RE. Treating the persistent symptomatic anterior radial head dislocation. *J Pediatr Orthop.* 1983;3:623–624.
73. Kloen P, Rubel IF, Farley TD, et al. Bilateral Monteggia fractures. *Am J Orthop (Belle Mead NJ).* 2003;32(2):98–100.
74. Koslowsky TC, Mader K, Wulke AP, et al. Operative treatment of chronic Monteggia lesion in younger children: a report of three cases. *J Shoulder Elbow Surg.* 2006;15(1):119–121.
75. Kristiansen B, Eriksen AF. Simultaneous type II Monteggia lesion and fracture separation of the lower radial epiphysis. *Injury.* 1986;17:51–52.
76. Ladermann A, Ceroni D, Lefevre Y, et al. Surgical treatment of missed Monteggia lesions in children. *J Child Orthop.* 2007;1(4):237–242.
77. Lambrinudi C. Intramedullary Kirschner wires in the treatment of fractures: (Section of Orthopaedics). *Proc R Soc Med.* 1940;33:153–157.
78. Landin LA. Fracture patterns in children. *Acta Paediatr Scand Suppl.* 1983;54:192.
79. Lascombes P, Prevot J, Ligen JN, et al. Elastic stable intramedullary nailing in forearm shaft fractures in children: 85 cases. *J Pediatr Orthop.* 1990;10:167–171.
80. Leonidou A, Pagkalos J, Lepetsos P, et al. Pediatric Monteggia fractures: a single-center study of the management of 40 patients. *J Pediatr Orthop.* 2012;32(4):352–356.
81. Letta C, Schmied M, Haller A, et al. Combined Monteggia and Galeazzi lesions of the forearm: a rare injury. *Unfallchirurg.* 2012;115(11):1034–1037.
82. Letts M, Locht R, Wiens J. Monteggia fracture-dislocations in children. *J Bone Joint Surg Br.* 1985;67:724–727.
83. Lichter RL, Jacobsen T. Tardy palsy of posterior interosseous nerve with Monteggia fracture. *J Bone Joint Surg Am.* 1975;57:124–125.
84. Lincoln TL, Mubarak SJ. "Isolated" traumatic radial-head dislocation. *J Pediatr Orthop.* 1994;14:454–457.
85. Lloyd-Roberts GC, Bucknill TM. Anterior dislocation of the radial head in children: aetiology, natural history, and management. *J Bone Joint Surg Br.* 1977;59-B:402–407.
86. Lu X, Kun Wang Y, Zhang J, et al. Management of missed Monteggia fractures with ulnar osteotomy, open reduction, and dual-socket external fixation. *J Pediatr Orthop.* 2013;33(4):398–402.
87. Lu X, Yan G, Wang Y, et al. Repositioning of the annular ligament in the management of missed Monteggia fracture. *J Pediatr Orthop.* 2017;37(1):20–22.
88. Luhmann SJ, Gordon JE, Schoenecker PL. Intramedullary fixation of unstable both-bone forearm fractures in children. *J Pediatr Orthop.* 1998;18(4):451–456.
89. Maeda H, Yoshida K, Doi R, et al. Combined Monteggia and Galeazzi fractures in a child: a case report and review of the literature. *J Orthop Trauma.* 2003;17(2):128–131.
90. McFarland B. Congenital dislocation of the head of the radius. *Br J Surg.* 1936;24:41–49.
91. Mehta SD. Flexion osteotomy of ulna for untreated Monteggia fracture in children. *Indian J Surg.* 1985;47:15–19.
92. Mehta SD. Missed Monteggia fracture. *J Bone Joint Surg Br.* 1993;75:337.
93. Miles KA, Finlay DB. Disruption of the radiocapitellar line in the normal elbow. *Injury.* 1989;20:365–367.
94. Monteggia GB. *Instituzioni Chirurgiche.* Milan: Maspero; 1814.
95. Morris AH. Irreducible Monteggia lesion with radial nerve entrapment. A case report. *J Bone Joint Surg Am.* 1974;56:1744–1746.
96. Mullick S. The lateral Monteggia fracture. *J Bone Joint Surg Am.* 1977;59:543–545.
97. Nakamura K, Hirachi K, Uchiyama S, et al. Long-term clinical and radiographic outcomes after open reduction for missed Monteggia fracture-dislocations in children. *J Bone Joint Surg Am.* 2009;91(6):1394–1404.
98. Nakashima H, Kondo K, Saka K. Type II Monteggia lesion with fracture-separation of the distal physis of the radius. *Am J Orthop (Belle Mead NJ).* 2000;29(9):717–719.
99. Naylor A. Monteggia fractures. *Br J Surg.* 1942;29:323.
100. Neviaser RJ, LeFevre GW. Irreducible isolated dislocation of the radial head: a case report. *Clin Orthop Relat Res.* 1971;80:72–74.
101. Olney BW, Menelaus MB. Monteggia and equivalent lesions in childhood. *J Pediatr Orthop.* 1989;9:219–223.
102. Oner FC, Diepstraten AF. Treatment of chronic posttraumatic dislocation of the radial head in children. *J Bone Joint Surg Br.* 1993;75:577–581.
103. Osamura N, Ikeda K, Hagiwara N, et al. Posterior interosseous nerve injury complicating ulnar osteotomy for a missed Monteggia fracture. *Scand J Plast Reconstr Surg Hand Surg.* 2004;38(6):376–378.
104. Ovesen O, Brok KE, Arreskov J, et al. Monteggia lesions in children and adults: an analysis of etiology and long-term results of treatment. *Orthopedics.* 1990;13(5):529–534.
105. Papandrea R, Waters PM. Posttraumatic reconstruction of the elbow in the pediatric patient. *Clin Orthop Relat Res.* 2000;(370):115–126.
106. Papavasilou VA, Nenopoulos SP. Monteggia-type elbow fracture in childhood. *Clin Orthop Relat Res.* 1988;(233):230–233.
107. Parsch KD. Die Morote-Drahtung bei proximalen und mittleren Unterarm Schaft Frakturen des Kindes. *Operat Orthop Traumatol.* 1990;2:245–255.
108. Pavel A, Pitman JM, Lance EM, et al. The posterior Monteggia fracture: a clinical study. *J Trauma.* 1965;5:185–199.
109. Peiró A, Andres F, Fernandez-Esteve F. Acute Monteggia lesions in children. *J Bone Joint Surg Am.* 1977;59:92–97.
110. Peltier LF. Eponymic fractures: Giovanni Battista Monteggia and Monteggia's fracture. *Surgery.* 1957;42:585–591.
111. Penrose JH. The Monteggia fracture with posterior dislocation of the radial head. *J Bone Joint Surg Br.* 1951;33-B:65–73.
112. Pérez Sicialia JE, Morote Jurado JI, Corbach Girones JM, et al. Osteosintesis percutanea en fracturas diafisaris de ante brazo en ninos y adolescentes. *Rev Esp Cir Ost.* 1977;12:321–334.
113. Powell RS, Bowe JA. Ipsilateral supracondylar humerus fracture and Monteggia lesion: a case report. *J Orthop Trauma.* 2002;16(10):737–740.
114. Price CT, Scott DS, Kurener ME, et al. Malunited forearm fracture in children. *J Pediatr Orthop.* 1990;10:705–712.
115. Pugh DM, Galpin RD, Carey TP. Intramedullary Steinmann pin fixation of forearm fractures in children. Long-term results. *Clin Orthop Relat Res.* 2000;(376):39–48.
116. Ramsey RH, Pedersen HE. The Monteggia fracture-dislocation in children. Study of 15 cases of ulnar-shaft fracture with radial-head involvement. *JAMA.* 1962;82:1091–1093.
117. Ramski DE, Hennrikus WP, Bae DS, et al. Pediatric Monteggia fractures: a multicenter examination of treatment strategy and early clinical and radiographic results. *J Pediatr Orthop.* 2015;35(2):115–120.
118. Rang M. *The Story of Orthopaedics.* Philadelphia, PA: Saunders; 2000.
119. Ravessoud FA. Lateral condyle fracture and ipsilateral ulnar shaft fracture: Monteggia equivalent lesions? *J Pediatr Orthop.* 1985;5:364–366.
120. Reckling F. Unstable fracture-dislocations of the forearm (Monteggia and Galeazzi lesions). *J Bone Joint Surg Am.* 1982;64:857–863.
121. Reckling FW, Cordell LD. Unstable fracture-dislocations of the forearm. The Monteggia and Galeazzi lesions. *Arch Surg.* 1968;96:999–1007.
122. Ring D, Jupiter JB, Waters PM. Monteggia fractures in children and adults. *J Am Acad Orthop Surg.* 1998;6(4):215–224.
123. Ring D, Waters PM. Operative fixation of Monteggia fractures in children. *J Bone Joint Surg Br.* 1996;78:734–739.
124. Rodgers WB, Smith BG. A type IV Monteggia injury with a distal diaphyseal radius fracture in a child. *J Orthop Trauma.* 1993;7:84–86.
125. Rodgers WB, Waters PM, Hall JE. Chronic Monteggia lesions in children: complications and results of reconstruction. *J Bone Joint Surg Am.* 1996;78:1322–1329.
126. Rodríguez-Merchán EC. Pediatric fractures of the forearm. *Clin Orthop Relat Res.* 2005;(432):65–72.
127. Ruchelsman DE, Klugman JA, Madan SS, et al. Anterior dislocation of the radial head with fractures of the olecranon and radial neck in a young child: a Monteggia equivalent fracture-dislocation variant. *J Orthop Trauma.* 2005;19(6):425–428.
128. Salter RB, Zaltz C. Anatomic investigations of the mechanism of injury and pathologic anatomy of "pulled elbow" in young children. *Clin Orthop Relat Res.* 1971;77:134–143.
129. Seel MJ, Peterson HA. Management of chronic posttraumatic radial head dislocation in children. *J Pediatr Orthop.* 1999;19:306–312.
130. Singh AP, Dhammi IK, Jain AK, et al. Monteggia fracture dislocation equivalents: analysis of eighteen cases treated by open reduction and internal fixation. *Chin J Traumatol.* 2011;14(4):221–226.
131. Smith FM. Monteggia fractures: an analysis of 25 consecutive fresh injuries. *Surg Gynecol Obstet.* 1947;85:630–640.
132. Smith MV, Calfee RP, Baumgarten KM, et al. Upper extremity-specific measures of disability and outcomes in orthopaedic surgery. *J Bone Joint Surg Am.* 2012;94(3):277–285.
133. Sood A, Khan O, Bagga T. Simultaneous Monteggia type I fracture equivalent with ipsilateral fracture of the distal radius and ulna in a child: a case report. *J Med Case Reports.* 2008;2:190.
134. Spar I. A neurologic complication following Monteggia fracture. *Clin Orthop Relat Res.* 1977;(122):207–209.
135. Speed JS, Boyd HB. Treatment of fractures of ulna with dislocation of head of radius: Monteggia fracture. *JAMA.* 1940;125:1699.
136. Spinner M. The arcade of Frohse and its relationship to posterior interosseous nerve paralysis. *J Bone Joint Surg Br.* 1968;50:809–812.
137. Spinner M, Freundlich BD, Teicher J. Posterior interosseous nerve palsy as a complication of Monteggia fracture in children. *Clin Orthop Relat Res.* 1968;58:141–145.
138. Spinner M, Kaplan EB. The quadrate ligament of the elbow—its relationship to the stability of the proximal radioulnar joint. *Acta Orthop Scand.* 1970;41:632–647.
139. Stein F, Grabias SL, Deffer PA. Nerve injuries complicating Monteggia lesions. *J Bone Joint Surg Am.* 1971;53:1432–1436.
140. Stelling FH, Cote RH. Traumatic dislocation of head of radius in children. *JAMA.* 1956;160:732–736.
141. Stoll TM, Willis RB, Paterson DC. Treatment of the missed Monteggia fracture in the child. *J Bone Joint Surg Br.* 1992;74:436–440.
142. Storen G. Traumatic dislocation of radial head as an isolated lesion in children; report of one case with special regard to roentgen diagnosis. *Acta Chir Scand.* 1959;116:144–147.
143. Strachen JCH, Ellis BW. Vulnerability of the posterior interosseous nerve during radial head reduction. *J Bone Joint Surg Br.* 1971;53:320–332.

144. Strong ML, Kopp M, Gillespie R. Fracture of the radial neck and proximal ulna with medial displacement of the radial shaft. *Orthopedics*. 1989;12:1577–1579.
145. Sur YJ, Park JB, Song SW. Pediatric posterior Monteggia lesion: a greenstick fracture of the proximal ulnar metaphysis with radial neck fracture: a case report. *J Orthop Trauma*. 2010;24(2):e12–e16.
146. Tait G, Sulaiman SK. Isolated dislocation of the radial head: a report of two cases. *Injury*. 1988;19:125–126.
147. Tajima T, Yoshizu T. Treatment of long-standing dislocation of the radial head in neglected Monteggia fractures. *J Hand Surg Am*. 1995;20:S91–S94.
148. Tan JW, Mu MZ, Liao GJ, et al. Pathology of the annular ligament in paediatric Monteggia fractures. *Injury*. 2008;39(4):451–455.
149. Thakore HK. Lateral Monteggia fracture in children (case report). *Ital J Orthop Traumatol*. 1983;9(1):55–56.
150. Theodorou SD. Dislocation of the head of the radius associated with fracture of the upper end of ulna in children. *J Bone Joint Surg Br*. 1969;51:700–706.
151. Theodorou SD, Ierodiaconou MD, Rousis N. Fracture of the upper end of the ulna associated with dislocation of the head of the radius in children. *Clin Orthop Relat Res*. 1988;(228):240–249.
152. Thompson HC 3rd, Garcia A. Myositis ossificans: aftermath of elbow injuries. *Clin Orthop Relat Res*. 1967;50:129–134.
153. Thompson GH, Wilber JH, Marcus RE. Internal fixation of fractures in children and adolescents. A comparative analysis. *Clin Orthop Relat Res*. 1984;(188):10–20.
154. Thompson JD, Lipscomb AB. Recurrent radial head subluxation treated with annular ligament reconstruction. A case report and follow-up study. *Clin Orthop Relat Res*. 1989;(246):131–135.
155. Tompkins DG. The anterior Monteggia fracture: observations on etiology and treatment. *J Bone Joint Surg Am*. 1971;53:1109–1114.
156. Tubbs RS, O'Neil JT Jr, Key CD, et al. The oblique cord of the forearm in man. *Clin Anat*. 2007;20(4):411–415.
157. Tubbs RS, Shoja MM, Khaki AA, et al. The morphology and function of the quadrate ligament. *Folia Morphol (Warsz)*. 2006;65(3):225–227.
158. Verstreken L, Delronge G, Lamoureux J. Shaft forearm fractures in children: intramedullary nailing with immediate motion: a preliminary report. *J Pediatr Orthop*. 1988;8:450–453.
159. Walker JL, Rang M. Forearm fractures in children: cast treatment with the elbow extended. *J Bone Joint Surg Br*. 1991;73:299–301.
160. Walton RD, Ormsby NM, Brookes-Fazakerley SD, et al. Stability-based assessment of Monteggia-type injuries predicts failure of treatment. *J Pediatr Orthop B*. 2017;26(1):27–31.
161. Waters PM, Bae DS. *Pediatric Hand and Upper Limb Surgery: A Practical Guide*. Philadelphia, PA: Lippincott Williams & Wilkins; 2012:351–365.
162. Watson JA, Singer GC. Irreducible Monteggia fracture: beware nerve entrapment. *Injury*. 1994;25:325–327.
163. Watson-Jones R. *Fractures and Joint Injuries*. 3rd ed. Baltimore, MD: Lippincott Williams & Wilkins; 1943.
164. Werner FW, Taormina JL, Sutton LG, et al. Structural properties of 6 forearm ligaments. *J Hand Surg Am*. 2011;36(12):1981–1987.
165. Wiley JJ, Galey JP. Monteggia injuries in children. *J Bone Joint Surg Br*. 1985;67:728–731.
166. Wilkins KE. Changes in the management of Monteggia fractures. *J Pediatr Orthop*. 2002;22(4):548–554.
167. Wise RA. Lateral dislocation of the head of radius with fracture of the ulna. *J Bone Joint Surg*. 1941;23:379.
168. Wright PR. Greenstick fracture of the upper end of the ulna with dislocation of the radio-humeral joint or displacement of the superior radial epiphysis. *J Bone Joint Surg Br*. 1963;45:727–731.
169. Yamamoto K, Yoshiaki Y, Tomihara M. Posterior interosseous nerve palsy as a complication of Monteggia fractures. *Nippon Geka Hokan*. 1977;46:46–56.

12

Evaluation of the Injured Pediatric Elbow

Peter M. Waters

INTRODUCTION

To the uninitiated, pediatric elbow fractures can be difficult to properly diagnose. The absence of ossification in the young, the vagaries of secondary centers of ossification, and the limits of plain radiographs in the skeletally immature all contribute to risk of misdiagnosis, improper management, and poor outcome in some patients. Since most of these children present with their injuries initially to urgent care and emergency care units that may not have experienced pediatric orthopedic surgeons and radiologists on site, the risk magnifies. Even for experienced caregivers, a select group of injuries, the correct diagnosis, and thus management can be elusive. At the end of the 19th century, Sir Robert Jones[30] echoed the opinion of that era about elbow injuries: "The difficulties experienced by surgeons in making an accurate diagnosis; the facility with which serious blunders can be made in prognosis and treatment; and the fear shared by so many of the subsequent limitations of function, serve to render injuries in the neighborhood of the elbow less attractive than they might otherwise have proved." These concerns are applicable even today. The importance of correct diagnosis was emphasized in a study of litigation against the National Health Service in England: Over half of the cases involved missed or incorrectly diagnosed injuries, most of which were fractures about the elbow.[4] The difficulty in correctly diagnosing elbow injuries in children was shown by Shrader et al., who found that emergency room physicians accurately diagnosed elbow fractures in children only 53% of the time.[57] On the other hand, diagnostic errors with overcalls (1.1%) and miss rate (1.6%) of 1,235 abnormal cases and 2,630 normal cases were reported by Bisset and Crowe when senior certificate of added qualification pediatric radiologists read the films.[9]

In other bones and joints, good results can often be obtained with minimal treatment, but in the elbow, more aggressive diagnostic testing and surgical treatment are often required to avoid complications. This was emphasized in paper and text by Waters et al., on TRASH (**T**he **R**adiographic **A**ppearance **S**eemed **H**armless) lesions of the pediatric elbow.[68,69] An understanding of the basic anatomy and radiographic landmarks of the elbow is essential in choosing appropriate treatment.

EPIDEMIOLOGY

Because children tend to protect themselves with their outstretched arms when they fall, upper extremity fractures account for 65% to 75% of all fractures in children. The most common area of the upper extremity injured is the distal forearm[5,36] Ten to twelve percent of all pediatric fractures involve the elbow but the highest complication rate of upper extremity fractures involve the elbow.

The distal humerus accounts for approximately 86% of fractures about the elbow region. Supracondylar fractures are the most frequent elbow injuries in children, reported to occur in 55% to 75% of patients with elbow fractures. Lateral condylar and radial neck are the second most common fractures,[26] followed by medial epicondylar fractures. Fractures of the radial head, medial condyle, and T-condylar fractures are much less common. Olecranon fractures can be occult initially and seen more commonly on follow-up than original x-rays.[26]

Elbow injuries are much more common in children and adolescents than in adults.[11] Voth et al.[67] reported on 15,300 patients presenting to a level 1 trauma center for care of major and minor injuries. Of the 3,953 patients with a major injury, 76% were fractures and 3% were dislocations. The majority were in the upper limb (73%), with the most common (16%) being fractures about the elbow. The peak age for fractures of the distal humerus is between 5 and 10 years old.[28] Houshian et al.[37] reported that the average age of 355 children with elbow fractures was 7.9 years (7.2 years in boys and 8.5 years in girls). Contrary to most reports, these investigators found elbow fractures more frequent in girls (54%) than in boys. In a study of 450 supracondylar humeral fractures, Cheng et al.[18] found a median age of 6 years (6.6 years in boys and 5 years in girls) and a predominance of injuries (63%) in boys. In a series of 1,297 consecutive supracondylar humeral fractures, including 873 type III fractures, Fletcher et al. found that 18% occurred in children older than 8 years; these children had more open fractures from high-energy mechanisms than younger children.[27] Stoneback et al. reported that elbow dislocations were most frequent in those aged 10 to 19 years; 44% were sustained in sports.[63]

Physeal injuries in most parts of the body occur in older children between the ages of 10 and 13; however, the peak age for injuries to the distal humeral physes is 4 to 5 years in girls and 5 to 8 years in boys. In most physeal injuries, the increased incidence with advanced age is believed to be due to weakening of the perichondrial ring as it matures (see Chapter 2). Thus, some different biomechanic forces and conditions must exist about the elbow to make the physis more vulnerable to injuries at an earlier age. (For more data on the relationship of fractures about the elbow to all types of fractures, see Chapter 1.)

Finally, patient-specific carrying angle can predispose to fracture type with injury. Elbow alignment may influence the transmission of traumatic force with a fall on an outstretched arm with varus alignment more commonly resulting in lateral condyle fractures and valgus alignment more commonly with radial neck fractures.

ANATOMY

The elbow is a complex joint composed of three individual joints contained within a common articular cavity. Several anatomic concepts are unique to the growing elbow.

THE OSSIFICATION PROCESS

The process of differentiation and maturation begins at the center of the long bones and progresses distally. The ossification process begins in the diaphyses of the humerus, radius, and ulna at the same time. By term, ossification of the humerus has extended distally to the condyles. In the ulna, it extends to more than half the distance between the coronoid process and the tip of the olecranon. The radius is ossified proximally to the level of the neck. The bicipital tuberosity remains largely unossified (Table 12-1).[21] Brodeur et al.[14] compiled a complete atlas of ossification of the structures about the elbow, and their work is an excellent reference source for finer details of the ossification process about the elbow.

Distal Humerus

Ossification of the distal humerus proceeds at a predictable rate. In general, the rate of ossification in girls exceeds that of boys.[20,21,24] In some areas, such as the olecranon and lateral epicondyle, the difference between boys and girls in ossification age may be as great as 2 years.[20] During the first 6 months, the ossification border of the distal humerus is symmetric (Fig. 12-1).

Lateral Condyle

On average, the ossification center of the lateral condyle appears just before 1 year of age but may be delayed as late as 18 to 24 months.[11] When the nucleus of the lateral condyle first appears, the distal humeral metaphyseal border becomes asymmetric. The lateral border slants and becomes straight to conform with the ossification center of the lateral condyle (Fig. 12-2). By the end of the second year, this border becomes well defined, possibly even slightly concave. The capitellar

TABLE 12-1. Sequence and Timing of Ossification in the Elbow

	Girls (yr)	Boys (yr)
Capitellum	1.0	1.0
Radial head	5.0	6.0
Medial epicondyle	5.0	7.5
Olecranon	8.7	10.5
Trochlea	9.0	10.7
Lateral epicondyle	10.0	12.0

Data from Cheng JC, Wing-Man K, Shen WY, et al. A new look at the sequential development of elbow-ossification centers in children. *J Pediatr Orthop.* 1998;18:161–167.

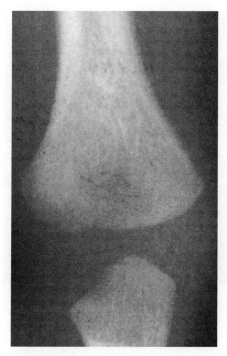

Figure 12-1. During the first 6 months, the advancing ossifying border of the distal humerus is fairly symmetric. Later, the lateral column becomes more vertical compared to the relatively more horizontal medial column on AP views.

ossification center is usually spherical when it first appears. It becomes more hemispherical as the distal humerus matures,[10] and the ossific nucleus extends into the lateral ridge of the trochlea (Fig. 12-3). On the lateral view, the physis of the capitellum is wider posteriorly. This is a normal variation and should not be confused with a fracture.[10]

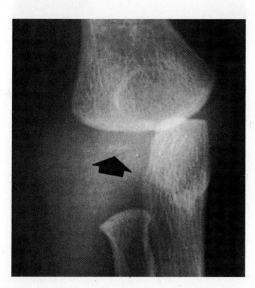

Figure 12-2. Ossification at 12 months. As the ossification center of the lateral condyle develops (*arrow*), the lateral border of the metaphysis becomes straighter. The initial ossification is usually elliptical and often appears fragmented, not to be confused with fracture.

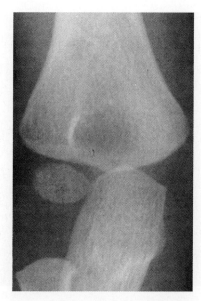

Figure 12-3. At 24 months, the oval-shaped secondary ossification center of the lateral condyle extends into the lateral crista of the trochlea. The lateral border of the neck (metaphysis) of the radius is normally angulated both anteriorly and laterally. The secondary center of ossification of the radial head is usually not yet present.

Medial Epicondyle

At about 5 to 6 years of age, a small concavity develops on the medial aspect of the metaphyseal ossification border. In this area, a medial epicondyle begins to ossify (Fig. 12-4).

Trochlea

At about 9 to 10 years of age, the trochlea begins to ossify. Initially, it may be irregular with multiple centers (Fig. 12-5).

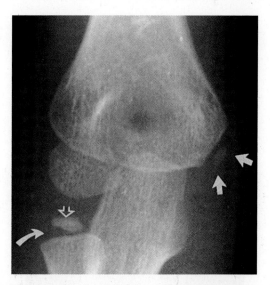

Figure 12-4. At about 5 or 6 years of age, a secondary center develops in the medial epicondylar apophysis (*white arrows*). At this same time, the ossification center of the radial head also develops (*open arrow*). Note that the physis of the proximal radius is widened laterally (*curved arrow*). Again, none of these findings should be viewed as fracture related.

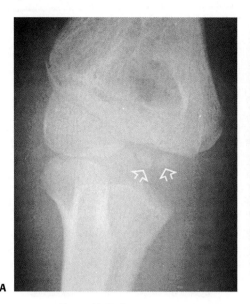
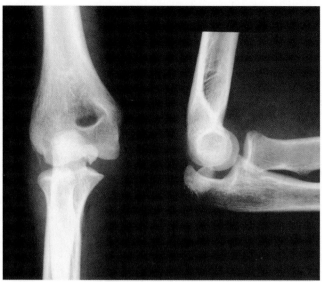

Figure 12-5. A: At about 9 years of age, the ossification of the medial crista of the trochlea may begin as two well-defined centers (*arrows*). These multiple centers can give the trochlea a fragmented appearance. This is not to be confused with avascular necrosis of the trochlea. Also, remember what the trochlea ossification center normally looks like so an entrapped medial epicondyle (**B**) will not be mistaken for normal ossification. Anteroposterior radiographs after a closed reduction. Note the entrapment of the medial epicondyle in the joint.

Lateral Epicondyle

The lateral epicondyle is last to ossify and is not always visible (Fig. 12-6). At about 10 years of age, it may begin as a small, separate oblong center, rapidly fusing with the lateral condyle.[10]

THE FUSION PROCESS

Just before completion of growth, the capitellum, lateral epicondyle, and trochlea fuse to form one epiphyseal center.

Metaphyseal bone separates the extra-articular medial epicondyle from this common humeral epiphyseal center (Fig. 12-7). The common epiphyseal center ultimately fuses with the distal humeral metaphysis. The medial epicondyle may not fuse with the metaphysis until the late teens.

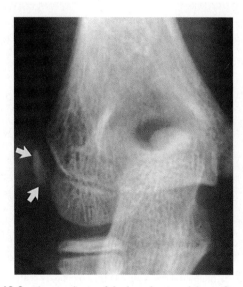

Figure 12-6. The apophysis of the lateral epicondyle ossifies as either an oblong or a triangular center (*arrows*). The wide separation of this center from the metaphyseal and epiphyseal borders of the lateral condyle is normal. Fractures in this region are exceedingly rare.

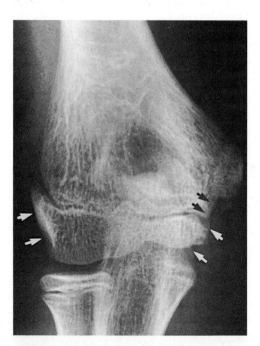

Figure 12-7. The secondary ossification centers of the lateral condyle, trochlea, and lateral epicondylar apophysis fuse to form one center (*white arrows*). This common distal humerus epiphyseal ossification center is separated from the medial epicondylar apophysis by advancing metaphyseal bone (*black arrows*).

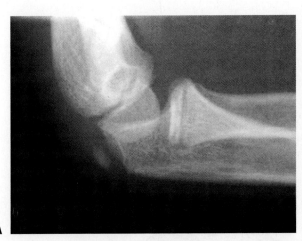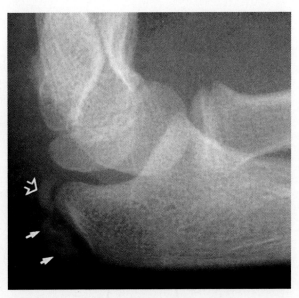

Figure 12-8. Ossification of the olecranon. **A:** Secondary ossification begins as an oblique oblong center at about 6 to 8 years of age. **B:** It may progress as two separate ossification centers: articular (*open arrow*) and traction (*closed arrows*).

Proximal Radius

The head of the radius begins to ossify at about the same time as the medial epicondyle (Fig. 12-4). The ossification center is present in at least 50% of girls by 3.8 years of age but may not be present in the same proportion of boys until around 4.5 years.[19] Initially, the ossification center is elliptical, and the physis is widened laterally due to the obliquity of the proximal metaphysis. The ossification center flattens as it matures. At about age 12, it develops a concavity opposite the capitellum.[10]

Ossification of the radial head may be bipartite or may produce an irregularity of the second center. These secondary or irregular ossification centers should not be interpreted as fracture fragments.

Olecranon

There is a gradual proximal progression of the proximal ulnar metaphysis. At birth, the ossification margin lies halfway between the coronoid process and the tip of the olecranon. By about 6 or 7 years of age, it appears to envelop about 66% to 75% of the capitellar surface. The final portion of the olecranon ossifies from a secondary ossification center that appears around 6.8 years of age in girls and 8.8 years in boys (Fig. 12-8A).[53] Peterson[51] described two separate centers: one articular and the other a traction type (Fig. 12-8B). This secondary ossification center of the olecranon may persist late into adult life.[40]

Fusion of the Ossification Centers

The epiphyseal ossification centers of the distal humerus fuse as one unit and then fuse later to the metaphysis. The medial epicondyle is the last to fuse to the metaphysis. The ranges of onset of the ossification of various centers and their fusion to other centers or the metaphysis are summarized in Figure 12-9.

Each center contributes to the overall architecture of the distal humerus (Fig. 12-9C).

Fusion of the proximal radial and olecranon epiphyseal centers with their respective metaphyses occurs at around the same time that the common distal humeral epiphysis fuses with its metaphysis (i.e., between 14 and 16 years of age).[6,8,46]

Noting that the pattern and ossification sequence of the six secondary ossification centers around the elbow were mainly derived from studies conducted more than 30 years ago, Cheng et al.[18] evaluated elbow radiographs of 1,577 Chinese children. They found that the sequence of ossification was the same in boys and girls—capitellum, radial head, medial epicondyle, olecranon, trochlea, and lateral epicondyle—but ossification was delayed by about 2 years in boys in all ossification centers except the capitellum (see Table 12-1).

BLOOD SUPPLY

Extraosseous

There is a rich arterial network around the elbow (Fig. 12-10).[49] The major arterial trunk, the brachial artery, lies anteriorly in the antecubital fossa. Most of the intraosseous blood supply of the distal humerus comes from the anastomotic vessels that course posteriorly.

Three structural components govern the location of the entrance of the vessels into the developing epiphysis. First, there is no communication between the intraosseous metaphyseal vasculature and the ossification centers.[73] Second, vessels do not penetrate the articular surfaces. The lateral condyle is nonarticular only at the origin of the muscles and collateral ligaments. Third, the vessels do not penetrate the articular capsule except at the interface with the surface of the bone. Thus, only a small portion of the lateral condyle posteriorly is both nonarticular and extracapsular (Fig. 12-11).[25]

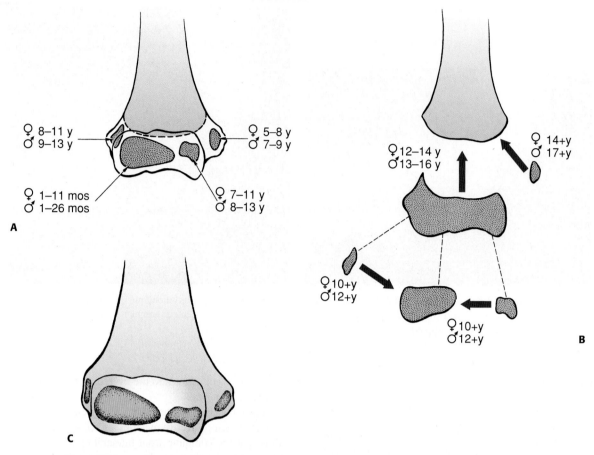

Figure 12-9. Ossification and fusion of the secondary centers of the distal humerus. **A:** The average ages for the onset of ossification of the various ossification centers are shown for both boys and girls. **B:** The ages at which these centers fuse with each other are shown for both boys and girls. (Modified and reprinted with permission from Haraldsson S. On osteochondrosis deformans juvenilis capituli humeri including investigation of intraosseous vasculature in distal humerus. *Acta Orthop Scand.* 1959;Suppl 38:1–232.) **C:** The contribution of each secondary center to the overall architecture of the distal humerus is represented by the stippled areas.

Intraosseous

The most extensive study of the intraosseous blood supply of the developing distal humerus was conducted by Haraldsson (Fig. 12-12),[32,33] who demonstrated that there are two types of vessels in the developing lateral condyle. These vessels enter the posterior portion of the condyle just lateral to the origin of the capsule and proximal to the articular cartilage near the origin of the anconeus muscle. They penetrate the nonossified cartilage and traverse it to the developing ossific nucleus. In a young child, this is a relatively long course (Fig. 12-12A). These vessels communicate with one another within the ossific nucleus but do not communicate with vessels in either the metaphysis or nonossified chondroepiphysis. Thus, for practical purposes, they are end vessels.

The ossification center of the lateral condyle extends into the lateral portion of the trochlea. Thus, the lateral crista or ridge of the trochlea derives its blood supply from these condylar vessels. The medial ridge or crista remains unossified for a longer period of time. The trochlea is covered entirely by articular cartilage and lies totally within the confines of the articular capsule. The vessels that supply the nucleus of the ossific centers of the trochlea must therefore traverse the periphery of the physis to enter the epiphysis.

Haraldsson's[32,33] studies have shown two sources of blood supply to the ossific nucleus of the medial portion of the trochlea (Fig. 12-12B). The lateral vessel, on the posterior surface of the distal humeral metaphysis, penetrates the periphery of the physis and terminates in the trochlear nucleus. Because this vessel supplying the trochlea is an end vessel, it is especially vulnerable to injury by a fracture that courses through either the physis or the very distal portion of the humeral metaphysis. Injury to this vessel can markedly decrease the nourishment to the developing lateral ossific nucleus of the trochlea. The medial vessel penetrates the nonarticulating portion of the medial crista of the trochlea. This multiple vascular source may account for the development of multiple ossification centers in the maturing trochlea, giving it a fragmented appearance (see Fig. 12-5). When growth is complete, metaphyseal and epiphyseal vessels anastomose freely. The blood supply from the central nutrient vessel of the shaft reaches the epicondylar regions in the skeletally mature distal humerus.[33]

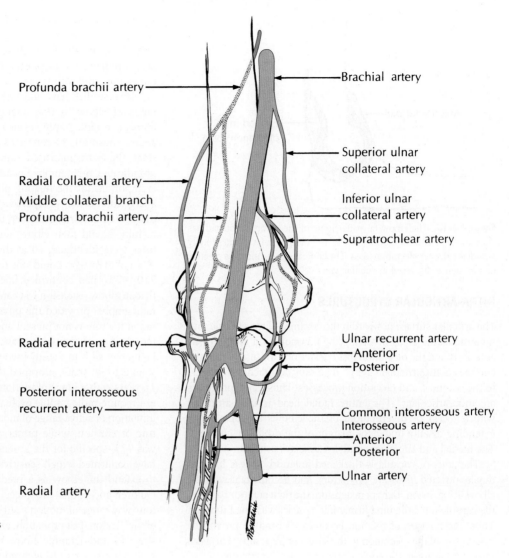

Profunda brachii artery

Brachial artery

Radial collateral artery

Middle collateral branch
Profunda brachii artery

Superior ulnar
collateral artery

Inferior ulnar
collateral artery

Supratrochlear artery

Radial recurrent artery

Ulnar recurrent artery
Anterior
Posterior

Posterior interosseous
recurrent artery

Common interosseous artery
Interosseous artery
Anterior
Posterior

Ulnar artery

Radial artery

Figure 12-10. The major arteries about the anterior elbow.

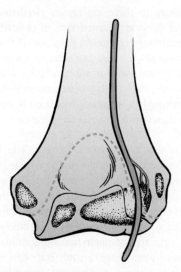

Figure 12-11. The vessels supplying the lateral condylar epiphysis enter the posterior aspect of the condyle, which is extra-articular. (Modified and reprinted with permission from Haraldsson S. On osteochondrosis deformans juvenilis capituli humeri including investigation of intraosseous vasculature in distal humerus. *Acta Orthop Scand Suppl.* 1959;38:1–232.)

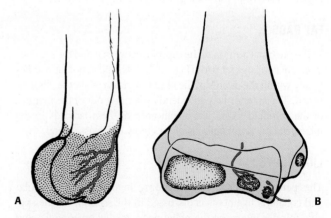

Figure 12-12. Intraosseous blood supply of the distal humerus. **A:** The vessels supplying the lateral condylar epiphysis enter on the posterior aspect and course for a considerable distance before reaching the ossific nucleus. **B:** Two definite vessels supply the ossification center of the medial crista of the trochlea. The lateral vessel enters by crossing the physis. The medial one enters by way of the nonarticular edge of the medial crista. (Modified and reprinted with permission from Haraldsson S. On osteochondrosis deformans juvenilis capituli humeri including investigation of intraosseous vasculature in distal humerus. *Acta Orthop Scand Suppl.* 1959;38:1–232.)

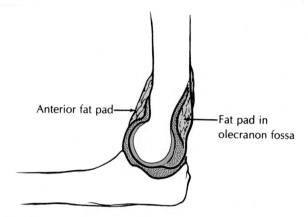

Figure 12-13. The elbow fat pads. Some of the coronoid fat pad lies anterior to the shallow coronoid fossa. The olecranon fat pad lies totally within the deeper olecranon fossa. The clinical significance of a positive fat pad sign is discussed in detail in text.

INTRA-ARTICULAR STRUCTURES

The articular surface lies within the confines of the capsule, but nonarticulating areas involving the coronoid and radial fossae anteriorly and the olecranon fossa posteriorly are also within the confines of the articular cavity.[48] The capsule attaches just distal to the coronoid and olecranon processes. Thus, these processes are intra-articular.[29] The entire radial head is intra-articular, with a recess or diverticulum of the elbow's articular cavity extending distally under the margin of the orbicular ligament. The medial and lateral epicondyles are extra-articular.

The anterior capsule is thickened anteriorly. These longitudinally directed fibers are very strong and become taut with the elbow in extension. In hyperextension, the tight anterior bands of the capsule force the ulna firmly into contact with the humerus. Thus, the fulcrum of rotation becomes transmitted proximally into the tip of the olecranon in the supracondylar area. This is an important factor in the etiology of supracondylar fractures.

FAT PADS

At the proximal portion of the capsule, between it and the synovial layer, are two large fat pads (Fig. 12-13). The posterior fat pad lies totally within the depths of the olecranon fossa when the elbow is flexed. The anterior fat pad extends anteriorly out of the margins of the coronoid fossa. The significance of these fat pads in the interpretation of radiographs of the elbow is discussed later.

LIGAMENTS

The pertinent ligamentous anatomy involving the orbicular and collateral ligaments is discussed in the sections on the specific injuries involving the radial neck, medial epicondyle, and elbow dislocations (see Chapters 13 and 18).[71]

RADIOGRAPHIC FINDINGS

Because of the ever-changing ossification pattern, identification and delineation of fractures about the elbow in the immature skeleton may be subject to misinterpretation. The variables of ossification of the epiphyses should be well known to the orthopedic surgeon who treats these injuries. Even with that expertise, supplemental diagnostic use of contralateral radiographs, ultrasound, and MRI scans may be appropriate and necessary.

Many studies have indicated that children with a normal range of elbow motion after elbow trauma do not require immediate radiographic evaluation.[34,55] Since cumulative radiation exposure is of concern in the pediatric population, and since there are increased unnecessary costs associated with unindicated radiographs, awareness of this body of literature is important for the treating physician in the acute setting. In a large multicenter prospective study, Appelboam et al.[3] found that of 780 children evaluated for elbow trauma, 289 were able to fully extend their elbow; among these, only 12 (4%) fractures were identified, all at their first evaluation. Among the 491 children who could not fully extend their injured elbow, 210 (43%) had confirmed fractures. These authors suggested that an elbow extension test can be used to rule out the need for radiographs, provided the physician is confident that an olecranon fracture is not present and that the patient can return for reevaluation if symptoms have not resolved in 7 to 10 days. Lennon et al.,[46] in a study involving 407 patients ranging in age from 2 to 96 years, proposed that patients aged no more than 16 years with a range of motion equal to the unaffected side do not require radiographic evaluation. Darracq et al.[20] found that limitation of active range of motion was 100% sensitive for fracture or effusion, while preservation of active range of motion was 97% specific for the absence of fracture. Other studies[17,35] have confirmed a high sensitivity (91% to 97%) of an inability to extend the elbow as a predictor of elbow fracture in both children and adults. Most recently, Vinson et al. noted that the four-way range of motion test (full elbow extension, 90 degrees elbow flexion, full pronation, and full supination) was 99% sensitive for radiographic elbow injuries and 100% sensitive for elbow injuries requiring surgical intervention in 251 patients seen prospectively in three emergency departments.[66] However, Baker and Borland[5] warned that in children with blunt trauma, a normal range of motion does not rule out significant injury and should not be used as a screening tool. In their 177 patients, an abnormal range of motion had a negative predictive value of only 77%.[5] In these circumstances, ultrasound is becoming increasingly a screening tool used in emergency care to assess for indications for formal radiographs.[23,54]

Waters et al.[68,69] described a subset of serious injuries to the pediatric elbow that they termed TRASH (**T**he **R**adiographic **A**ppearance **S**eemed **H**armless) lesions (Table 12-2). These lesions represent predominantly intra-articular osteochondral injuries in children younger than 10 years of age who have sustained high-energy trauma; the lesions are often associated with unrecognized, spontaneously reduced elbow dislocations (Fig. 12-14). Similarly, transphyseal separations in the very young (less than 2 years of age) are rare but often misdiagnosed. Usually, the elbow is quite swollen and the range of motion is limited. Any elbow dislocation in a child younger than 10 years of age should raise concern about a displaced, intra-articular osteochondral fracture, especially with a high-energy mechanism of injury and more swelling than the seemingly benign

TABLE 12-2. Elbow "TRASH" Lesions

- Unossified medial condylar humeral fractures
- Unossified transphyseal distal humeral fractures
- Entrapped medial epicondylar fractures
- Complex osteochondral elbow fracture–dislocation in a child younger than 10 years of age
- Osteochondral fractures with joint incongruity
- Radial head anterior compression fractures with progressive radiocapitellar subluxation
- Monteggia fracture–dislocations
- Lateral condylar avulsion shear fractures

Modified with permission from Waters PM, Beaty J, Kasser J. Elbow "TRASH" (the radiographic appearance seemed harmless) lesions. *J Pediatr Orthop.* 2010; 30 (2 Suppl):S77–S81.

radiograph demonstrates. In the children less than 2 years of age with a radiograph revealing posteromedial displacement of the radius and ulna relative to the distal humeral metaphysis and unossified epiphysis, a transphyseal injury should be suspected.[64] Ultrasound or magnetic resonance imaging (MRI) is diagnostic.[31,64] Since these young children are often victims of nonaccidental trauma and at risk not only for malunion, but importantly more serious body harm in the future, accurate diagnosis, treatment of the fracture, and evaluation of the human and social factors leading to injury are critical (see Chapter 6 for full details). Thus, a high index of suspicion and early additional imaging (ultrasound, arthrogram, or MRI) usually contribute to a more accurate diagnosis and best treatment of these injuries.[68,69]

When radiographs are indicated, a number of anatomic landmarks and angles should be evaluated and measured, including any displacement of the fat pads about the elbow. It is important to be familiar with these landmarks and angles and to be aware of the significance of any deviation from normal.

STANDARD VIEWS

The standard radiographs of the elbow include an anteroposterior (AP) view with the elbow fully extended and a lateral view with the elbow flexed to 90 degrees and the forearm neutral.

AP OF THE DISTAL HUMERUS (JONES VIEW)

It is often difficult for a child to fully extend the injured elbow, and an axial view of the elbow, the Jones view, may be helpful (Fig. 12-15). The injured distal humerus is often difficult to interpret due to the superimposed proximal radius and ulna when the elbow is flexed. In addition to AP and lateral views of the distal humerus, if there is a high index of suspicion for a fracture, but none is visible on routine AP and lateral radiographs, then internal and external oblique views may be helpful. This

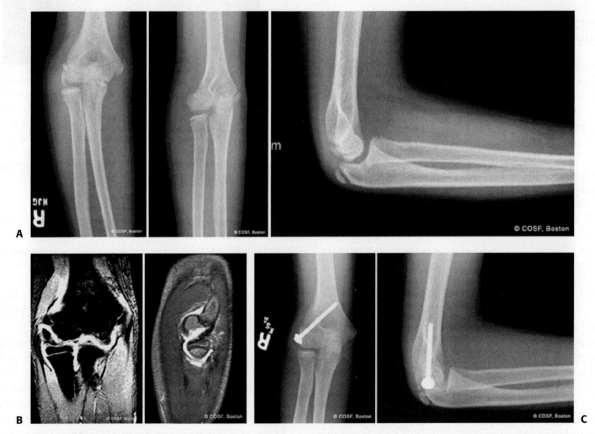

Figure 12-14. A: Anteroposterior, lateral, and oblique views of an osteochondral fracture of the lateral condyle. If unrecognized, this can lead to painful nonunion and intra-articular incongruity. **B:** Magnetic resonance imaging scan documenting displacement and operative indications. **C:** Percutaneous reduction and screw fixation were done based on MRI findings. (Reprinted with permission from Waters PM, Beaty J, Kasser J. Elbow "TRASH" (the radiographic appearance seemed harmless) lesions. *J Pediatr Orthop.* 2010;30(2 suppl):S77–S81.)

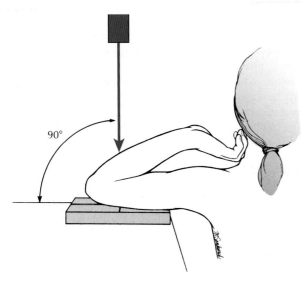

Figure 12-15. AP of the distal humerus (Jones axial radiographic view) that is important in acute trauma and follow-up care as an AP of the elbow will have overlapping radius and ulna and obscure injuries.

is especially true in identifying fractures of the radial head and coronoid process and judging displacement in lateral condylar and supracondylar humerus fractures.

MEASUREMENT OF DISPLACEMENT: MEDIAL EPICONDYLAR FRACTURES

The determination of the amount of fracture displacement is critical to the choice of treatment of medial epicondylar fractures.[70,72] The general consensus among pediatric orthopedic surgeons seems to be that fractures with less than 2 mm of displacement can be treated nonoperatively, while those with more than 5 mm of displacement should be treated operatively. A difference of 1 or 2 mm in the measurement of displacement can change the management of these fractures. To determine the reliability of displacement measurements, Pappas et al.[50] had radiographs of 38 children with fractures of the medial humeral epicondyle evaluated by five reviewers with different levels of orthopedic training. Pappas et al. found that the reviewers disagreed an average of 87% of the time about measurements on the lateral view, 64% of the time about measurements on the oblique view, and 54% about measurements on the AP view. The findings cast doubt on whether the amount of perceived displacement should be used as a criterion for choosing operative or nonoperative treatment of fractures of the medial epicondyle. Proposed methods for improving displacement measurement were (1) measuring displacement on AP views and (2) measuring displacement as the maximal distance between the fragment and the bone location from which it came (Fig. 12-16). In contrast, Edmonds[24] suggested that internal oblique views appear to best approximate the true anterior displacement. In addition, Edmonds et al. found that comparison of measurements of displacement on radiographs to those on three-dimensional computed tomography (CT) scans demonstrated that fractures that appear to be minimally displaced or nondisplaced on radiographs, especially

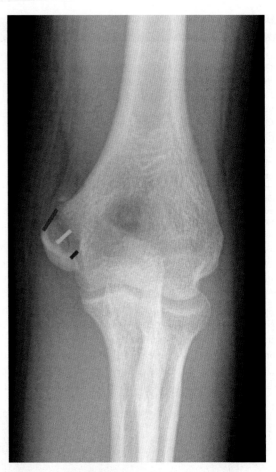

Figure 12-16. On anteroposterior radiograph of a left elbow with a medial epicondylar fracture, there are three different places where displacement could be measured. The *red line* represents 2 mm of displacement; the *green line*, 3 mm; and the *blue line*, 5 mm. (Reprinted with permission from Pappas N, Lawrence JT, Donegan D, et al. Intraobserver and interobserver agreement in the measurement of displaced humeral medial epicondyle fractures in children. *J Bone Joint Surg Am.* 2010;92(2):322–327.)

AP and lateral views, may have more than 1 cm of anterior displacement by CT scan. However, CT scans of all medial epicondylar fractures to assess accurate displacement would bring increased radiation exposure and risk to children. Klatt and Aoki[41] revealed that the center of the medial epicondyle throughout skeletal maturation consistently rests 0.5 mm (SD 2 mm) inferior to the olecranon line and 1.2 mm (SD 1.2 mm) anterior to the posterior humeral line.

Mini C-arm is increasingly used in the emergency setting for diagnosis and to assist and assess reduction of pediatric fractures. While extremely convenient and accurate, caregivers need to be aware of the risks of radiation exposure to the injured children, hospital employees, and themselves if overutilized. Sumko et al. reported on increased exposure averaging 53 mrem with mini C-arm use in ED compared with 20 mrem with standard AP, lateral radiographs of the elbow in their institution.[65] For these reasons, in emergency department, ultrasound screening is increasingly used for children with suspected fractures.

ANTEROPOSTERIOR LANDMARKS

Baumann Angle

In the standard AP view, the major landmark is the angulation of the physeal line between the lateral condyle and the distal humeral metaphysis. The ossification center of the lateral condyle extends into the radial or lateral crista of the trochlea (see Fig. 12-9C). This physeal line forms an angle with the long axis of the humerus. The angle formed by this physeal line and the long axis of the humerus is the Baumann angle (Fig. 12-17A).[6] The Baumann angle is not equal to the carrying angle of the elbow in older children.[9] This is a consistent angle when both sides are compared, and the x-ray beam is directed perpendicular to the long axis of the humerus. Acton and McNally[1] reviewed the descriptions of the Baumann angle in a number of commonly used textbooks and discovered three variations of measurement technique. They recommended that the angle should always be measured between the long axis of the humerus and the inclination of the capitellar physis, as Baumann described, and that it should be called the "shaft-physeal" angle to avoid confusion.

Caudad–cephalad angulation of the x-ray tube, or right or left angulation of the tube by as much as 30 degrees, changes the Baumann angle by less than 5 degrees. If, however, the tube becomes angulated in a cephalad–caudad direction by more than 20 degrees, the angle is changed significantly and the measurement is inaccurate. In their cadaver studies, Camp et al.[16] found that rotation of the distal fragment or the entire reduced humerus could also alter the projection of the Baumann angle. They found that to be accurate, the humerus must be parallel to the x-ray plate, with the beam directed perpendicular to the film as well. Thus, in the routine AP radiographs of the distal humerus, including the Jones view, the Baumann angle is a good measurement of any deviation of the angulation of the distal humerus.[15,59,62]

Other Angles

Two other angles measured on AP radiographs are commonly used to determine the proper alignment of the distal humerus or carrying angle. The *humeral–ulnar angle* is determined by lines longitudinally bisecting the shaft of the humerus with the shaft of the ulna on an AP view (Fig. 12-17B).[4,40] The *metaphyseal–diaphyseal angle* is determined by a line that longitudinally bisects the shaft of the humerus with a line that connects the widest points of the metaphysis of the distal humerus (Fig. 12-17C).[39] The humeral–ulnar angle is the most accurate in determining the true carrying angle of the elbow. The Baumann angle also has a good correlation with the clinical carrying angle, but it may be difficult to measure in adolescents in whom the ossification center of the lateral condyle is beginning to fuse with other centers. The metaphyseal–diaphyseal angle is the least accurate of the three.

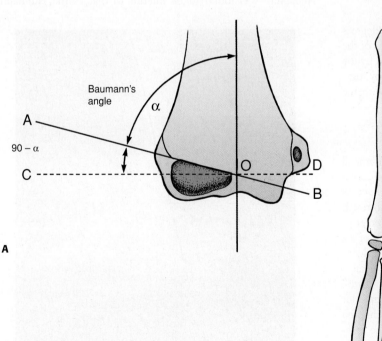

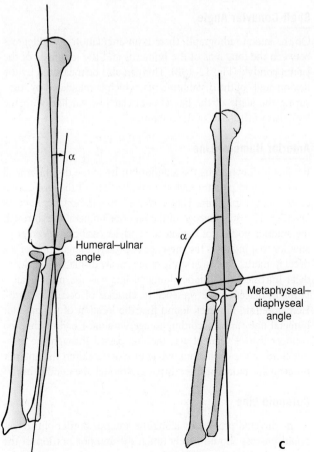

Figure 12-17. AP radiographic angles of the elbow. **A:** Baumann angle. **B:** The humeral–ulnar angle. **C:** The metaphyseal–diaphyseal angle. (Reprinted with permission from O'Brien WR, Eilert RE, Chang FM, et al. *The Metaphyseal–Diaphyseal Angle as a Guide to Treating Supracondylar Fractures of the Humerus in Children. Presented at 54th Annual Meeting of AAOS*, San Francisco, CA; 1987.)

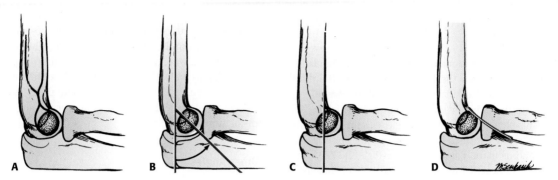

Figure 12-18. Lateral radiograph lines of the distal humerus. **A:** The teardrop of the distal humerus. **B:** The angulation of the lateral condyle with the shaft of the humerus. **C:** The anterior humeral line. **D:** The coronoid line. (Reprinted with permission from Shank CF, Wiater BP, Pace JL, et al. The lateral capitellohumeral angle in normal children: mean, variation, and reliability in comparison to Baumann's angle. *J Pediatr Orthop.* 2011;31(3):266–271.)

LATERAL LANDMARKS

Teardrop

The lateral projection of the distal humerus presents a teardrop-like shadow above the capitellum.[46] The anterior dense line making up the teardrop represents the posterior margin of the coronoid fossa. The posterior dense line represents the anterior margin of the olecranon fossa. The inferior portion of the teardrop is the ossification center of the capitellum. On a true lateral projection, this teardrop should be well defined (Fig. 12-18A).

Shaft-Condylar Angle

On the lateral radiograph, there is an angulation of 40 degrees between the long axis of the humerus and the long axis of the lateral condyle (Fig. 12-18B). This can also be measured by the flexion angle of the distal humerus, which is calculated by measuring the angle of the lateral condylar physeal line with the long axis of the shaft of the humerus.[44]

Anterior Humeral Line

If a line is drawn along the anterior border of the distal humeral shaft, it should pass through the middle third of the ossification center of the capitellum. This is referred to as the *anterior humeral line* (Fig. 12-18C). Passage of the anterior humeral line through the anterior portion of the lateral condylar ossification center or anterior to it indicates the presence of posterior angulation of the distal humerus. In a large study of minimally displaced supracondylar fractures, the anterior humeral line was the most reliable factor in detecting the presence or absence of occult fractures. Herman et al., however, found that the location of the anterior humeral line varied according to age: in almost half of children younger than 4 years of age, the line passed through the anterior third of the capitellum, while in older children the anterior humeral line more consistently passed through the middle third.[36]

Coronoid Line

A line directed proximally along the anterior border of the coronoid process should barely touch the anterior portion of the lateral condyle (Fig. 12-18D). Posterior displacement of the lateral condyle projects the ossification center posterior to this coronoid line.[46]

Lateral Humerocapitellar Angle

Shank et al.[58] described measurement of the *lateral humerocapitellar angle (LHCA)* using digital measurement tools and digital radiographs (Fig. 12-19). This angle measures the angular relationship between the humeral shaft and the capitellum as seen on the lateral view. In normal elbows, the LHCA averaged 51 degrees and was not affected by age, sex, or side. Its reliability was found to be inferior to that of the Baumann

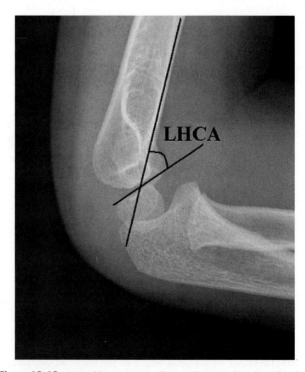

Figure 12-19. Lateral humerocapitellar angle (LHCA) on lateral radiograph of normal elbow. (From Shank CF, Wiater BP, Pace JL, et al. The lateral capitellohumeral angle in normal children: mean, variation, and reliability in comparison to Baumann's angle. *J Pediatr Orthop.* 2011;31:266–271.)

angle but improved with increasing patient age. The correlation between the LHCA and clinical outcome is unclear, with some studies finding no correlation and others reporting a strong correlation between the LHCA and loss of flexion at skeletal maturity.[60] Although the exact relationship between the LHCA and clinical outcome is unclear, the authors suggested that a LHCA of more than three standard deviations from normal (more than 69 degrees) should be accepted with reservation, especially in older patients, because some studies have suggested unpredictable remodeling of angular deformity.[60]

Pseudofracture

Some vagaries of the ossification process about the elbow may be interpreted as a fracture.[46] For example, the ossification of the trochlea may be irregular, producing a fragmented appearance (Fig. 12-5). This fragmentation can be misinterpreted, especially if the distal humerus is slightly oblique or tilted. These secondary ossification centers may be mistaken for fracture fragments lying between the semilunar notch and lateral condyle (Fig. 12-20).

On the lateral view, the physeal line between the lateral condyle and the distal humeral metaphysis is wider posteriorly. This appearance may give a misinterpretation that the lateral condyle is fractured and tilted.[10]

On the AP view before the radial head ossifies, there is normally some lateral angulation to the radial border of the neck of the radius that may give the appearance of subluxation (see Fig. 12-3). The true position of the radial head can be confirmed by noting the relationship of the proximal radius to the ossification center of the lateral condyle on the lateral projection.[45]

Fat Pad Signs of the Elbow

There are three areas in which fat pads overlie the major structures of the elbow. Displacement of any of the fat pads can indicate an occult fracture.[12] The first two areas are the fat pads that overlie the capsule in the coronoid fossa anteriorly and the olecranon fossa posteriorly. Displacement of either or both of these

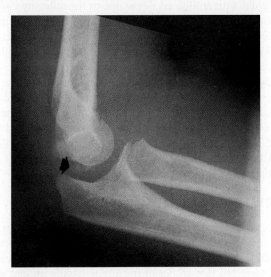

Figure 12-20. Pseudofracture of the elbow. The trochlea with its multiple ossification centers may be misinterpreted as fracture fragments lying between the joint surfaces (*arrow*).

fat pads is usually referred to as the *classic elbow fat pad sign*. A third accumulation of fat overlies the supinator muscle as it wraps around the proximal radius.

Olecranon (Posterior) Fat Pad

Because the olecranon fossa is deep, the fat pad here is totally contained within the fossa. It is not visible on a normal lateral radiograph of the elbow flexed to 90 degrees (Fig. 12-21A).

Distention of the capsule with an effusion, as occurs with an occult intra-articular fracture, a spontaneously reduced dislocation, or even an infection, can cause the dorsal or olecranon fat pad to be visible.[50]

Coronoid (Anterior) Fat Pad

Likewise, the ventral or coronoid fat pad may be displaced anteriorly (Fig. 12-21B).[7] Because the coronoid fossa is shallow, the fat pad in this area projects anterior to the bony margins and can be seen normally as a triangular radiolucency anterior to the distal humerus. Although displacement of the classic elbow fat pads is a reliable indication of an intra-articular effusion, there may be instances in which only one of the fat pads is displaced. Brodeur et al.[13] and Kohn[43] have shown that the coronoid fat pad is more sensitive to small effusions than the olecranon fat pad. The coronoid fat pad can be displaced without a coexistent displacement of the olecranon fat pad (Fig. 12-21C). Blumberg et al. analyzed the radiographs of 197 consecutive patients with elbow trauma and found that 113 (57%) had normal anterior fat pads; of these, only two had fractures, giving a 98% negative predictive value to the presence of a normal anterior fat pad.[11]

Supinator Fat Pad

A layer of fat on the anterior aspect of the supinator muscle wraps around the proximal radius. This layer of fat or fat pad may normally bow anteriorly to some degree. Brodeur et al.[14] stated that displacement may indicate the presence of an occult fracture of the radial neck. Displacement of the fat line or pad is often difficult to interpret; in a review of fractures involving the proximal radius, Schunk et al.[56] found it to be positive only 50% of the time.

Fat Pad Variations

For the fat pads to be displaced, the capsule must be intact. This can explain why there may be no displacement of the fat pads with an elbow dislocation that has spontaneously reduced due to capsule rupture. Murphy and Siegel[48] described other variations of classic fat pad displacement. If the elbow is extended, the fat pad is normally displaced from the olecranon fossa by the olecranon (Fig. 12-21D). Distal humeral fractures may cause subperiosteal bleeding and may lift the proximal portion of the olecranon fat pad without the presence of an effusion (Fig. 12-21E). These false-negative and false-positive determinations must be kept in mind when interpreting the presence or absence of a fat pad finding with an elbow injury.

To date, fat pad studies draw disparate conclusions. Corbett's[19] review of elbow injuries indicated that if a displacement

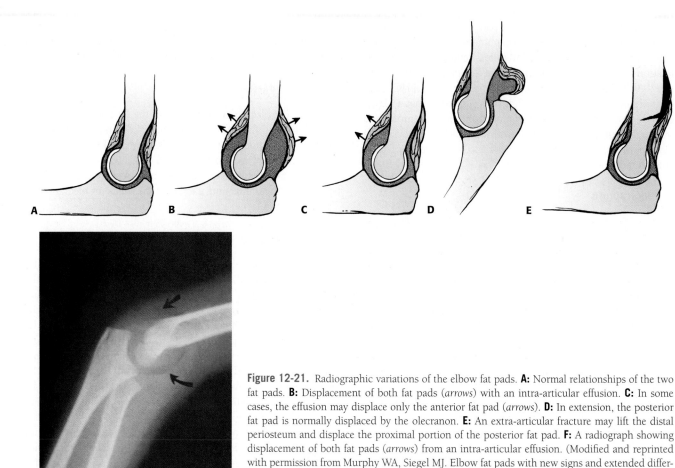

Figure 12-21. Radiographic variations of the elbow fat pads. **A:** Normal relationships of the two fat pads. **B:** Displacement of both fat pads (*arrows*) with an intra-articular effusion. **C:** In some cases, the effusion may displace only the anterior fat pad (*arrows*). **D:** In extension, the posterior fat pad is normally displaced by the olecranon. **E:** An extra-articular fracture may lift the distal periosteum and displace the proximal portion of the posterior fat pad. **F:** A radiograph showing displacement of both fat pads (*arrows*) from an intra-articular effusion. (Modified and reprinted with permission from Murphy WA, Siegel MJ. Elbow fat pads with new signs and extended differential diagnosis. *Radiology*. 1977;124:656–659.)

of the posterior fat pad existed, a fracture was almost always present. Displacement of the anterior fat pad alone, however, could occur without a fracture. Corbett[19] also determined that the degree of displacement bore no relation to the extent of the fracture. Skaggs and Mirzayan[61] reported that 34 of 45 children (76%) with a history of elbow trauma and an elevated posterior fat pad had radiographic evidence of elbow fractures at an average of 3 weeks after injury, though AP, lateral, and oblique radiographs at the time of injury showed no other evidence of fracture. They recommended that a child with a history of elbow trauma and an elevated fat pad should be treated as if a nondisplaced elbow fracture were present. Donnelly et al.,[22] however, found evidence of fracture in only 9 of 54 children (17%) who had a history of trauma and elbow joint effusion but no identifiable fracture on initial radiographs. Donnelly et al. concluded that joint effusion without a visible fracture on initial radiographs does not correlate with the presence of occult fracture in most patients (83%). Persistent effusion did correlate with occult fracture: 78% of those with occult fractures had persistent effusions, whereas effusions were noted in only 16% of those without fractures. More recently, in a prospective MRI study of 26 children with positive fat pad signs, Al-Aubaidi and Torfing[2] concluded that the presence of a positive fat pad sign is not synonymous with an occult fracture. All 26 children had a positive fat pad sign on lateral radiographs, but MRI scans obtained an average of 7 days later found occult fractures in

only six patients, none of whom had a change in fracture treatment. Most (73%) had bone bruise by MRI.

COMPARISON RADIOGRAPHS

Although it is often tempting to order comparison radiographs in a child with an injured elbow due to the difficulty evaluating the irregularity of the ossification process, the indications for ordering comparison radiographs are rare. Kissoon et al.[42] found that using routine comparison radiographs in children with injured elbows did not significantly increase the accuracy of diagnosis, regardless of the interpreter's training. Petit et al.[52] reviewed 3,128 radiographs of 2,470 children admitted to a pediatric emergency department for osteoarticular trauma and found that only 22% of the radiographs revealed abnormal findings; 33% of elbow radiographs revealed abnormalities. Fewer than half of clinically suspected fractures were confirmed by radiograph.

MAGNETIC RESONANCE IMAGING

Major and Crawford[47] used MRI to evaluate seven children who had radiographs that showed effusion but no fractures; four of the children had fractures identified by MRI. These investigators suggested that an occult fracture is usually present when effusion occurs, even if a fracture is not visible on radiograph. Griffith et al.[30] reviewed the radiographs and MRI scans of

50 children with elbow trauma. Radiographs identified effusions in 34% of the children and fractures in 52%; MRI identified effusions in 96% and fractures in 74%. Although MRI revealed a broad spectrum of bone and soft tissue injury beyond that shown on radiographs (bone bruising, muscle and ligament injuries, physeal injury, fracture), the additional information provided by MRI had little influence on patient treatment and no value in predicting clinical outcome. We have found MRI to be helpful in evaluating articular and osteochondral fractures to identify fracture pattern and extent, fragment position, and any interposed structure.

OTHER IMAGING MODALITIES

Sonography and arthrography can be useful in examining children with posttraumatic elbow effusions, but these can be painful (ultrasound with direct pressure) and invasive (arthrograms usually in operating rooms). The use of CT in the young can be limited by the need for sedation. In adolescent T condylar humerus fractures, CT is extremely helpful for planning operative intervention. The development of multidetector CT (MDCT) technology allows examinations to be completed in seconds, eliminating the need for sedation in most cases. Studies using MDCT can also be reformatted and evaluated in multiple planes, reducing the manipulation necessary for a series of radiographs. Chapman et al.[17] reported that, in a series of 31 children with posttraumatic elbow effusion and normal radiographs, MDCT depicted occult injuries in 52%. Besides the minimal manipulation required, making it relatively easy and pain-free, and the speed with which the image is obtained, they cited as additional advantages of MDCT the lower radiation dose than conventional radiographs, its sensitivity (92%), specificity (79%), and high negative predictive value (92%). A limitation of this method may be its high cost compared to standard radiographic examination.

REFERENCES

1. Acton JD, McNally MA. Baumann's confusing legacy. *Injury.* 2001;32(1):41–43.
2. Al-Aubaidi Z, Torfing T. The role of the fat pad sign in diagnosing occult elbow fractures in the pediatric patient: a prospective magnetic resonance imaging study. *J Pediatr Orthop B.* 2012;21:514–519.
3. Appelboam A, Reuben AD, Benger JR, et al. Elbow extension test to rule out elbow fracture: multicentre, prospective validation, and observational study of diagnostic accuracy in adults and children. *BMJ.* 2008;337:a2428.
4. Atrey A, Nicolaou N, Katchburian M, et al. A review of reported litigation against English health trusts for the treatment of children in orthopaedics: present trends and suggestions to reduce mistakes. *J Child Orthop.* 2010;4:471–476.
5. Baker M, Borland M. Range of elbow movement as a predictor of bony injury in children. *Emerg Med J.* 2011;28:666–669.
6. Baumann E. Beitrage zur Kenntnis dur Frackturen am Ellbogengelenk. *Bruns Beitr F Klin Chir.* 1929;146:1–50.
7. Beals RK. The normal carrying angle of the elbow. A radiographic study of 422 patients. *Clin Orthop Relat Res.* 1976;(119):194–196.
8. Beekman F, Sullivan JE. Some observations on fractures of long bones in children. *Am J Surg.* 1941;51:722–738.
9. Bisset GS 3rd, Crowe J. Diagnostic errors in interpretation of pediatric musculoskeletal radiographs at common injury sties. *Pediatr Radiol.* 2014;44:552–557.
10. Blount WP, Schulz I, Cassidy RH. Fractures of the elbow in children. *J Am Med Assoc.* 1951;146:699–704.
11. Blumberg SM, Kunkov S, Crain EF, et al. The predictive value of a normal radiographic fat pad sign following elbow trauma in children. *Pediatr Emerg Care.* 2011;27:596–600.
12. Bohrer SP. The fat pad sign following elbow trauma: its usefulness and reliability in suspecting "invisible" fractures. *Clin Radiol.* 1970;21:90–94.
13. Brodeur AE, Silberstein JJ, Graviss ER. *Radiology of the Pediatric Elbow.* Boston: GK Hall; 1981.
14. Brodeur AE, Silberstein JJ, Graviss ER, et al. The basic tenets for appropriate evaluation of the elbow in pediatrics. *Curr Prob Diagn Radiol.* 1983;12(5):1–29.
15. Buhr AJ, Cooke AM. Fracture patterns. *Lancet.* 1959;1:531–536.
16. Camp J, Ishizue K, Gomez M, et al. Alteration of Baumann's angle by humeral position: implications for treatment of supracondylar humerus fractures. *J Pediatr Orthop.* 1993;13:521–555.
17. Chapman V, Grottkau B, Albright M, et al. MDCT of the elbow in pediatric patients with posttraumatic elbow effusions. *AJR Am J Roentgenol.* 2006;187:812–817.
18. Cheng JC, Wing-Man K, Shen WY, et al. A new look at the sequential development of elbow-ossification centers in children. *J Pediatr Orthop.* 1998;18:161–167.
19. Corbett RH. Displaced fat pads in trauma to the elbow. *Injury.* 1978;9:297–298.
20. Darracq MA, Vinson DR, Panacek EA. Preservation of active range of motion after acute elbow trauma predicts absence of elbow fracture. *Am J Emerg Med.* 2008;26:779–782.
21. Docherty MA, Schwab RA, Ma OJ. Can elbow extension be used a test of clinically significant injury? *South Med J.* 2002;95:539–541.
22. Donnelly LF, Klostermeier TT, Klosterman LA. Traumatic elbow effusions in pediatric patients: are occult fractures a risk factor? *AJR Am J Roentgenol.* 1998;171:243–245.
23. Eckert K, Janssen N, Ackermann O, et al. Ultrasound diagnosis of supracondylar fractures in children. *Eur J Trauma Emerg Surg.* 2014;40:159–168.
24. Edmonds EW. How displaced are "nondisplaced" fractures of the medial humeral epicondyle in children? Results of a three-dimensional computed tomography analysis. *J Bone Joint Surg Am.* 2010;92:2785–2791.
25. Elgenmark O. The normal development of the ossific centers during infancy and childhood. *Acta Paediatr Scand.* 1946;33(Suppl 1):1–79.
26. Emery KH, Zingula SN, Anton CG, et al. Pediatric elbow injuries: a new angle on an old topic. *Pediatr Radiol.* 2016;46:61–66.
27. Fletcher ND, Schiller JR, Garg S, et al. Increased severity of type III supracondylar humerus fractures in the preteen population. *J Pediatr Orthop.* 2012;32:567–572.
28. Francis CC. The appearance of centers of ossification from 6 to 15 years. *Am J Phys Anthro.* 1940;27:127–138.
29. Gray DJ, Gardner E. Prenatal development of the human elbow joint. *Am J Anat.* 1951;88:429–469.
30. Griffith JF, Roebuck DJ, Cheng JC, et al. Acute elbow trauma in children: spectrum of injury revealed by MR imaging not apparent on radiographs. *AJR Am J Roentgenol.* 2001;176(1):53–60.
31. Guffler H, Schulze CG, Wagner S, et al. MRI for occult physeal fracture detection in children and adolescents. *Acta Radiol.* 2013;54:467–472.
32. Haraldsson S. The intra-osseous vasculature of the distal end of the humerus with special reference to capitulum; preliminary communication. *Acta Orthop Scand.* 1957;27:81–93.
33. Haraldsson S. On osteochondrosis deformans juvenilis capituli humeri including investigation of intraosseous vasculature in distal humerus. *Acta Orthop Scand Suppl.* 1959;38:1–232.
34. Hawksworth CR, Freeland P. Inability to fully extend the injured elbow: an indicator of significant injury. *Arch Emerg Med.* 1991;8:253–256.
35. Henrikson B. Supracondylar fracture of the humerus in children. A late review of end-results with special reference to the cause of deformity, disability and complications. *Acta Chir Scand Suppl.* 1966;369:1–72.
36. Herman MJ, Boardman MJ, Hoover JR, et al. Relationship of the anterior humeral line to the capitellar ossific nucleus: variability with age. *J Bone Joint Surg Am.* 2009;91:2188–2193.
37. Houshian S, Mehdi B, Larsen MS. The epidemiology of elbow fracture in children: analysis of 355 fractures, with special reference to supracondylar humerus fractures. *J Orthop Sci.* 2001;6(4):312–315.
38. Ippolito E, Caterini R, Scola E. Supracondylar fractures of the humerus in children. Analysis at maturity of 53 patients treated conservatively. *J Bone Joint Surg Am.* 1986;68:333–344.
39. Jenkins FA Jr. The functional anatomy and evolution of the mammalian humeroulnar articulation. *Am J Anat.* 1973;137:281–298.
40. Johansson O. Capsular and ligament injuries of the elbow joint. A clinical and arthrographic study. *Acta Chir Scand Suppl.* 1962;287:1–159.
41. Klatt JB, Aoki SK. The location of the medial humeral epicondyle in children: position based on common radiographic landmarks. *J Pediatr Orthop.* 2012;32:477–482.
42. Kissoon N, Galpin R, Gayle M, et al. Evaluation of the role of comparison radiographs in the diagnosis of traumatic elbow injuries. *J Pediatr Orthop.* 1995;15:449–453.
43. Kohn AM. Soft tissue alterations in elbow trauma. *Am J Roentgenol Radium Ther Nucl Med.* 1959;82:867–874.
44. Lamprakis A, Vlasis K, Siuampou E, et al. Can elbow-extension test be used as an alternative to radiographs in primary care? *Eur J Gen Pract.* 2007;13:221–224.
45. Landin LA, Danielsson LG. Elbow fractures in children: an epidemiological analysis of 589 cases. *Acta Orthop Scand.* 1986;57:309–312.
46. Lennon RI, Riayt MS, Hilliam R, et al. Can a normal range of elbow movement predict a normal elbow x-ray? *Emerg Med J.* 2007;24:86–88.
47. Major NM, Crawford ST. Elbow effusions in trauma in adults and children: is there an occult fracture? *AJR Am J Roentgenol.* 2002;178(2):413–418.
48. Murphy WA, Siegel MJ. Elbow fat pad with new signs and extended differential diagnosis. *Radiology.* 1977;124:659–665.
49. O'Brien WR, Eilert RE, Chang FM, et al. *The Metaphyseal Diaphyseal Angle as a Guide to Treating Supracondylar Fractures of the Humerus in Children.* Presented at and published in proceedings of 54th Annual Meeting of AAOS, San Francisco, CA: 1987.
50. Pappas N, Lawrence JT, Donegan D, et al. Intraobserver and interobserver agreement in the measurement of displaced humeral medial epicondyle fractures in children. *J Bone Joint Surg Am.* 2010;92:322–327.
51. Peterson CA, Peterson HA. Analysis of the incidence of injuries to the epiphyseal growth plate. *J Trauma.* 1972;12:275–281.
52. Petit P, Sapin C, Henry G, et al. Rate of abnormal osteoarticular radiographic findings in pediatric patients. *AJR Am J Roentgenol.* 2001;176(4):987–990.
53. Porteous CJ. The olecranon epiphyses. *J Anat.* 1960;94:286.
54. Rabiner JE, Khine H, Avner JR, et al. Accuracy of point of care ultrasonography for diagnosis of elbow fractures in children. *Ann Emerg Med.* 2013;61:9–17.

55. Sandegrad E. Fracture of the lower end of the humerus in children: treatment and end of the elbow in children. *J Bone Joint Surg Am.* 1999;81:1429–1433.

56. Schunk VK, Grossholz M, Schild H. Der Supinatorfettkorper bei Frakturen des Ellbogengelenkes. *ROFO.* 1989;150:294–296.

57. Shrader MW, Campbell MD, Jacofsky DJ. Accuracy of emergency room physicians' interpretation of elbow fractures in children. *Orthopedics.* 2008;31(12):1117–1119.

58. Shank CF, Wiater BP, Pace JL, et al. The lateral capitellohumeral angle in normal children: mean, variation, and reliability in comparison to Baumann's angle. *J Pediatr Orthop.* 2011;31:266–271.

59. Silva M, Pandarinath R, Farng E, et al. Inter- and intra-observer reliability of the Baumann angle of the humerus in children with supracondylar humeral fractures. *Int Orthop.* 2010;34:553–557.

60. Simanovsky N, Lamdan R, Hiller N, et al. The measurements and standardization of humerocondylar angle in children. *J Pediatr Orthop.* 2008;28:463–465.

61. Skaggs DL, Mirzayan R. The posterior fat pad sign in association with occult fracture of the elbow in children. *J Bone Joint Surg Am.* 1999;81:1429–1433.

62. Smith L. Deformity following supracondylar fractures of the humerus. *J Bone Joint Surg Am.* 1960;42-A:235–252.

63. Stoneback JW, Owens BD, Sykes J, et al. Incidence of elbow dislocations in the United States population. *J Bone Joint Surg Am.* 2012;94:240–245.

64. Sukakul N, Hicks RA, Caltoum CB, et al. Distal humeral epiphyseal separation in young children: an often-missed fracture-radiographic signs and ultrasound confirmatory diagnosis. *AJR Am J Roentgenol.* 2015;204:W192–W198.

65. Sumko MJ, Hennrikus W, Slough J, et al. Measurement of radiation exposure when using mini C-arm to reduce pediatric upper extremity fractures. *J Pediatr Orthop.* 2016;36:122–125.

66. Vinson DR, Kann GS, Gaona SD, et al. Performance of the 4-way range of motion test for radiographic injuries after blunt elbow trauma. *Am J Emerg Med.* 2016;34:235–239.

67. Voth M, Lustenberger T, Auner B, et al. What injuries should we expect in the emergence room? *Injury.* 2017;48:2119–2124.

68. Waters PM, Bae DS. *Elbow TRASH Lesions in Pediatric Hand and Upper Extremity Surgery: A Practical Guide.* Philadelphia, PA: Wolters Kluwer/Lippincott Williams & Wilkins; 2012:379–390.

69. Waters PM, Beaty J, Kasser J. Elbow "TRASH" (the radiographic appearance seemed harmless) lesions. *J Pediatr Orthop.* 2010;30(2 Suppl):S77–S81.

70. Wilkins KE. Fractures and dislocations of the elbow region. In: Rockwood CA Jr, Wilkins KE, Beaty JH, eds. *Fractures in Children.* 4th ed. Philadelphia, PA: Lippincott-Raven; 1996:653–904.

71. William PL, Warwick R. *Gray's Anatomy.* Philadelphia, PA: WB Saunders; 1980.

72. Wilson PD. Fractures and dislocations in the region of the elbow. *Surg Gynecol Obstet.* 1933;56:335–359.

73. Yang Z, Wang Y, Gilula LA, et al. Microcirculation of the distal humeral epiphyseal cartilage: implications for posttraumatic growth deformities. *J Hand Surg Am.* 1998;23:165–172.

13

Supracondylar Fractures of the Distal Humerus

David L. Skaggs and John M. Flynn

Supracondylar Fractures of the Distal Humerus

INTRODUCTION TO SUPRACONDYLAR FRACTURES OF THE DISTAL HUMERUS

Current evidence and consensus suggest that displaced supracondylar fractures are best treated operatively with fixation.[3,72,115,121] Modern techniques for the treatment of supracondylar humerus (SCH) fractures in children have dramatically decreased the rates of malunion and compartment syndrome.[3,15,82,95,99,115,148] Although there have been more than 500 peer-reviewed articles on supracondylar fractures over the last decade, there remains poor consensus on many areas of treatment. An 88-question survey of 35 pediatric orthopedic surgeons on the treatment of SCH fractures found consensus on only 27% of the questions.[73]

A database search showed that over 10,000 pediatric supracondylar fractures are seen in emergency rooms each year in the United States.[71] Of the 24% of these treated surgically, 87% are closed reduced, and this proportion is growing over time (Fig. 13-1). Transfer rates for these fractures increased from 5.6% in 2006 to 9.1% in 2011, generally transferring from general or rural hospitals to academic or urban centers. One study comparing the treatment of supracondylar fractures by pediatric orthopedic fellowship–trained surgeons to general orthopedic surgeons found no statistical difference in the complication rate, though patients treated by non–fellowship-trained surgeons were about four times more likely to have inadequate fixation and 10 times more likely to have an open reduction.[43] There appears to be a trend toward pediatric orthopedic specialists treating a higher proportion of these injuries,[79] with one center reporting over a 100% increase in less than a decade.[159]

SCH fractures are the most common elbow fractures seen in children,[42] and the most common fracture requiring surgery in children. The peak age range at which most supracondylar fractures occur is 5 to 6 years.[28]

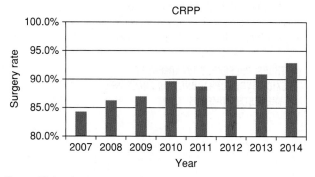

Figure 13-1. The percentage of patients who underwent CRPP for the treatment of a supracondylar humeral fracture. A significant increase in the rate of CRPP ($p < 0.0001$) was demonstrated.

ASSESSMENT OF SUPRACONDYLAR FRACTURES OF THE DISTAL HUMERUS

An elbow or forearm fracture should be suspected in a child with elbow pain or failure to use the upper extremity after a fall. A careful examination of the entire arm should be performed, and any area with tenderness or swelling should have radiographs as multiple fractures (such as a supracondylar fracture and a radius/ulna fracture) are not uncommon (Fig. 13-2). In children with acute elbow pain and failure to use the upper extremity, the differential diagnosis should include fracture, nursemaid's elbow, inflammatory arthritis, and infection.

With a type I supracondylar fracture, there is tenderness about the distal humerus and restriction of motion, particularly lack of full elbow extension. X-rays may be negative except for a posterior fat pad sign. In type III fractures, gross displacement of the elbow is evident (Fig. 13-3).

An anterior pucker sign may be present if the proximal fragment has penetrated the brachialis and the anterior fascia of the elbow (Fig. 13-4). Skin puckering results from the proximal segment piercing the brachialis muscle and engaging the deep dermis. This is a sign of considerable soft tissue damage. If any bleeding from a punctate wound is present, this should be considered an open fracture.

Careful motor, sensory, and vascular examinations should be performed in all patients, this may be difficult in a young child but should be attempted and recorded accurately. Sensation should be tested in discrete sensory areas of the radial nerve (dorsal first web space), median nerve (palmar index fingertip), and ulnar nerve (ulnar side little fingertip). If a child is not cooperative or has altered mental status, a wet cloth may be wrapped around the hand and checked for wrinkling of the skin, though in practice this is rarely done. In this test, a lack of sensation is demonstrated in areas where the skin does not wrinkle. Motor examination should include finger, wrist, and thumb extension (radial nerve), index finger distal interphalangeal flexion and thumb interphalangeal flexion (anterior interosseous nerve, or AIN), finger flexion strength (median), and interossei (ulnar nerve) muscle function. In young children, the interosseous nerve may be tested by asking the child to pinch something with their thumb and first finger, while palpating the first dorsal interosseous for muscle contracture. If you cannot determine sensory and/or motor function accurately preoperatively, it should be documented in the medical record and communicated to appropriate caregivers. Misinformation preoperatively makes decision making postoperatively difficult when a nerve or vascular deficit is discovered.

The vascular examination should include determining the presence of pulse, as well as warmth, capillary refill, and color of the hand. Assessment of the vascular status is essential, as series report up to 20% of displaced fractures present with vascular compromise.[31,124,140] The vascular status may be classified into one of three categories:

- Hand well perfused (warm and red), radial pulse present
- Hand well perfused (warm and red), radial pulse absent
- Hand poorly perfused (cool and blue or blanched), radial pulse absent

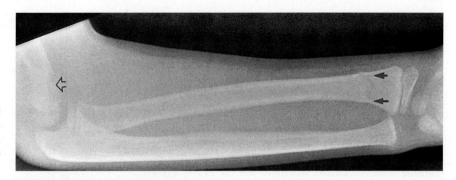

Figure 13-2. Occult ipsilateral fracture. Type II supracondylar fracture (*open arrow*) with an occult distal radial fracture (*solid arrows*). (Reproduced with permission of Children's Orthopaedic Center, Los Angeles, CA.)

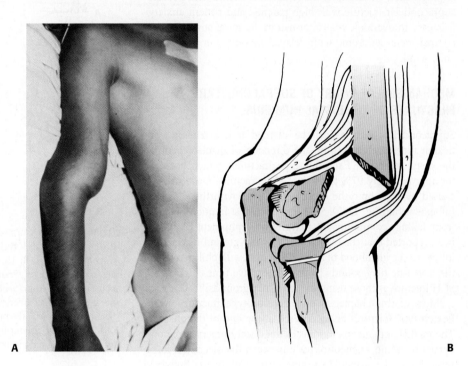

Figure 13-3. A: Clinical appearance. **B:** The S-shaped configuration is created by the anterior prominence of the proximal fragment's spike and extension of the distal fragment.

A

B

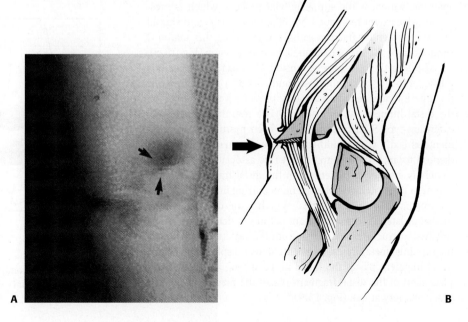

Figure 13-4. The pucker sign. This patient had penetration of the proximal fragment's spike into the subcutaneous tissue. **A:** In the AP view, there is a large puckering or defect in the skin where the distal fragment has pulled the skin inward (*arrow*). **B:** Laterally, there is puckering of the skin (*arrow*) in the area where the spike has penetrated into the subcutaneous tissue.

A

B

During the physical examination, a very high index of suspicion is needed in order not to miss a developing compartment syndrome in fractures with considerable swelling and/or ecchymosis, anterior skin puckering, and/or absent pulse. Possible firmness of the volar compartment should be evaluated, and excessive swelling about the elbow should be noted. Pain with passive finger extension and flexion should be noted. Recent studies show that increasing anxiety and need for pain medicine may be the earliest warnings of compartment syndrome. Pediatric patients with compartment syndromes often present with the three As: anxiety, agitation, and increasing analgesic requirement.[12] In the initial examination of a child with a severe supracondylar fracture with high parental and patient anxiety, it is easy to overlook vital information. Be more suspicious of compartment syndrome with delayed presentation or dysvascular hand.

MECHANISMS OF INJURY OF SUPRACONDYLAR FRACTURES OF THE DISTAL HUMERUS

Supracondylar fractures can be divided into extension and flexion types, depending on the direction of displacement of the distal fragment. Extension-type fractures, which account for approximately 97% to 99% of SCH fractures[100] are usually caused by a fall onto the outstretched hand with the elbow in full extension (Fig. 13-5). SCH fractures most frequently result from falling, commonly off playground equipment.[147] It has been reported that the overall safety of playground design can influence the likelihood of an SCH fracture, with children using the least safe playgrounds having almost five times the rate of SCH fracture as those using the safest playgrounds.[120]

Most of this chapter is on extension-type fractures, with flexion-type fractures being covered at the end of the chapter. The medial and lateral columns of the distal humerus are connected by a thin segment of bone between the olecranon fossa posteriorly and coronoid fossa anteriorly, resulting in a high risk of fracture to this area (Fig. 13-6). In a normal anatomic variant, the olecranon fossa may be absent (Fig. 13-7). Another normal anatomic variant is the supracondylar process, which is present to some extent in about 1.5% of adult cadavers and should not be mistaken for fracture pathology. However, this anatomic variant can be the site of median nerve compression (Fig. 13-8).

With forced elbow hyperextension, the olecranon forcefully pushes into the olecranon fossa and acts as a fulcrum, while the anterior capsule simultaneously provides a tensile force on the distal humerus at its insertion. The resulting injury is an extension-type SCH fracture. It has been postulated that ligamentous laxity with resulting elbow hyperextension may predispose to an SCH fracture,[112] but this association is unclear. Generally, medial displacement of the distal fragment is more common than lateral displacement, occurring in approximately 75% of patients in most series. Whether the displacement is medial or lateral is also important because it determines which soft tissue structures are at risk from the penetrating injury of the proximal metaphyseal fragment. Medial displacement of the distal fragment places the radial nerve at risk, and lateral displacement of the distal fragment places the median nerve and brachial artery at risk (Fig. 13-9).[98]

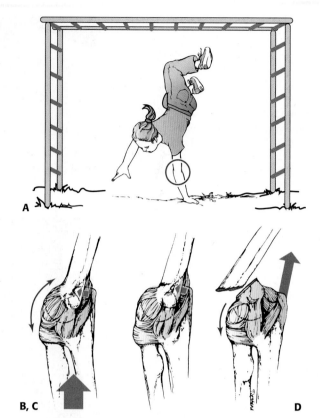

Figure 13-5. Mechanism of injury—elbow hyperextension. **A:** Most children attempt to break their falls with the arm extended, and the elbow then hyperextends. **B:** The linear applied force (*large arrow*) leads to an anterior tension force. Posteriorly, the olecranon is forced into the depths of the olecranon fossa (*small arrow*). **C:** As the bending force continues, the distal humerus fails anteriorly in the thin supracondylar area. **D:** When the fracture is complete, the proximal fragment can continue moving anteriorly and distally, potentially harming adjacent soft tissue structures such as the brachialis muscle, brachial artery, and median nerve.

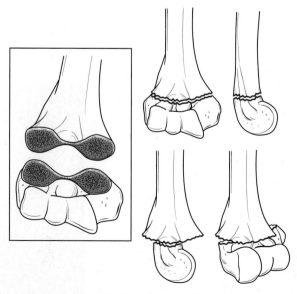

Figure 13-6. Supracondylar fractures occur through the thinnest portion of the distal humerus in the AP plane. The thin bone makes the fracture unstable.

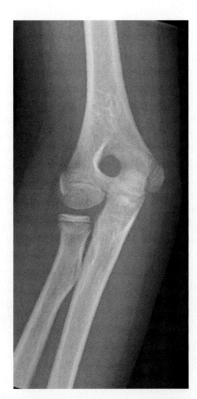

Figure 13-7. Normal anatomic variant in which there is no bone in the olecranon fossa. Note the minimally displaced radial neck fracture. (Reproduced with permission of Children's Orthopaedic Center, Los Angeles, CA.)

IMAGING AND OTHER DIAGNOSTIC STUDIES OF SUPRACONDYLAR FRACTURES OF THE DISTAL HUMERUS

All patients with a history of a fall onto an outstretched hand as well as pain and inability to use the extremity should undergo a thorough radiologic evaluation. If physical examination does not localize the trauma to the elbow alone, this may include obtaining anteroposterior (AP) and lateral views of the entire

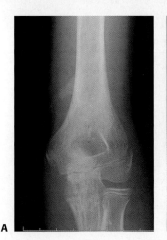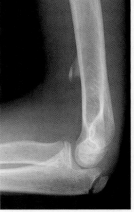

Figure 13-8. A: AP radiograph of the distal humerus demonstrating a supracondylar process, a normal anatomic variant. **B:** Lateral radiograph demonstrating a supracondylar process. (Reproduced with permission of Children's Orthopaedic Center, Los Angeles, CA.)

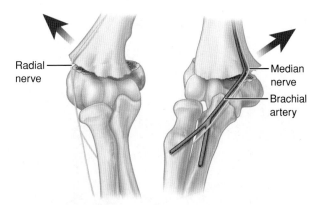

Figure 13-9. Relationship to neurovascular structures. The proximal metaphyseal spike penetrates laterally with posteromedially displaced fractures and places the radial nerve at risk; with posterolaterally displaced fractures, the spike penetrates medially and places the median nerve and brachial artery at risk. (Reprinted with permission from Choi PD, Skaggs DL. Closed reduction and percutaneous pinning of supracondylar fractures of the humerus. In: Wiesel S, ed. *Operative Techniques in Orthopaedic Surgery.* 2nd ed. Philadelphia, PA: Lippincott William & Wilkins; 2010.)

upper extremity. Comparison views are rarely required by an experienced orthopedist, but occasionally may be useful to evaluate an ossifying epiphysis. Beware that the emergency room physician's interpretation of elbow fractures in children has been reported to have an overall accuracy of only 53%.[142]

Radiographic examination begins with a true AP view of the distal humerus. (In contrast, an AP of an elbow in 90 degrees of flexion will give a roughly 45-degree angulated view of the distal humerus and proximal radius and ulna.) A true AP view of the distal humerus allows a more accurate evaluation of the distal humerus and decreases the error in determining Baumann's angle. The lateral film should be taken as a true lateral with the humerus held in the anatomic position and not externally rotated (Fig. 13-10). Oblique views of the distal humerus occasionally may be helpful when a supracondylar fracture or occult condylar fracture is suspected but not seen on standard AP and lateral views, but should not be routinely ordered to evaluate for a supracondylar fracture.

Initial radiographs may be negative except for a posterior fat pad sign (Fig. 13-11). A series of patients with traumatic elbow pain and a posterior fat pad sign but no visible fracture found that 53% (18/34) had an SCH fracture, 26% (9/34) a fracture of the proximal ulna, 12% (4/34) a fracture of the lateral condyle, and 9% (3/34) a fracture of the radial neck.[151]

Two main radiographic parameters are used to evaluate the presence of a supracondylar fracture. The anterior humeral line (AHL) should cross the capitellum on a true lateral of the elbow. Previous editions of this text and others have stated that in a normal elbow, the AHL should pass through the middle third of the capitellum. However, it has been demonstrated by Herman that in a normal elbow, the AHL passes through the middle third of the capitellum only 52% of the time in children under 10 years of age, and in children younger than 4 years of age, the AHL is equally likely to pass through the anterior third of the capitellum as the middle third (Fig. 13-12).[68] Ryan et al.[134] found that the AHL should pass through the center of the

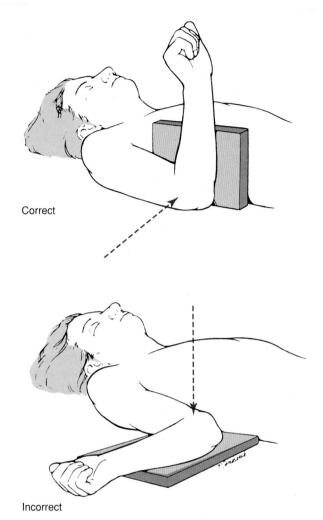

Correct

Incorrect

Figure 13-10. X-ray positioning. The correct method of taking a lateral view is with the upper extremity directed anteriorly rather than externally rotated.

capitellum in all children 5 years and older, and if it does not, pathology should be suspected. In an extension-type supracondylar fracture, the capitellum is posterior to this line. Note that the "hourglass" should be tilted slightly forward in a true lateral view of a normal elbow (see Fig. 13-11A) and can help aid in the diagnosis of a type II SCH fracture.

Baumann's angle, also referred to as the humeral capitellar angle, is the angle between the long axis of the humeral shaft and the physeal line of the lateral condyle (normal range, about 9 to 26 degrees) (Fig. 13-13). Interpretation of Baumann's angle is open to variability. One study reports one of five observers measure Baumann's angle from the same radiograph greater than 7 degrees different from the other four observers.[145] A rule of thumb is that a Baumann's angle of at least 10 degrees is okay. A decrease in Baumann's angle compared to the other side is a sign that a fracture is in varus angulation.

If the AP and lateral views show a displaced type II or III supracondylar fracture but do not show full detail of the distal humeral fragment, we usually obtain further x-ray evaluation to define the fracture anatomy with particular emphasis on impaction of the medial column, supracondylar comminution, and vertical split

of the epiphyseal fragment. T-condylar fractures (Fig. 13-14) can initially appear to be supracondylar fractures, but these generally occur in children over 10 years of age, in whom supracondylar fractures are less likely (see Chapter 17).

In a young child, an epiphyseal separation can mimic an elbow dislocation.[174] In an epiphyseal separation, the fracture propagates through the physis without a metaphyseal fragment. This fracture occurs in very young children with primarily chondral epiphyses. On physical examination, the patient appears to have a supracondylar fracture with gross swelling about the elbow and marked discomfort. The key to making the diagnosis and differentiating this injury from an elbow dislocation radiographically is seeing that the capitellum remains aligned with the radial head. A thin metaphyseal fragment, which may make one think of a lateral condyle fracture, usually can be seen, which technically makes this a Salter type II fracture (Fig. 13-15). In such cases, more data is required to make the diagnosis and initiate treatment. An arthrogram may be helpful (Fig. 13-16). In selected patients, magnetic resonance imaging or ultrasonography[174] may also aid in evaluating the injury to the unossified epiphysis.

CLASSIFICATION OF SUPRACONDYLAR FRACTURES OF THE DISTAL HUMERUS

Gartland Classification

A modified Gartland classification of SCH fractures is the most commonly accepted and used system.[3,56,115] The modified Gartland classification had less intra- and interobserver variability than did any fracture classification systems previously studied according to a study by Barton et al.[14] A recent study of functional outcomes following operative treatment of 652 patients using PODCI and QuickDASH did not find a relationship of outcomes and Gartland type, or direction of displacement.[45] As outcomes were generally excellent, this may be due to a basement effect of the outcome instruments.

Supracondylar Fractures of the Distal Humerus: MODIFIED GARTLAND CLASSIFICATION		
Type	**Description**	**Comments**
Type I	<2-mm displacement	Fat pad present acutely
Type II	Hinged posteriorly	Only sagittal plane displacement, AHL anterior to capitellum with greater displacement
Type III	Displaced	Sagittal and coronal plane displacement, variable amount of cortical continuity
Type IV	Displaces into extension and flexion	Usually diagnosed with manipulation under fluoroscopic imaging
Medial comminution (not truly a separate type)	Collapse of medial column	Loss of Baumann's angle, requires reduction

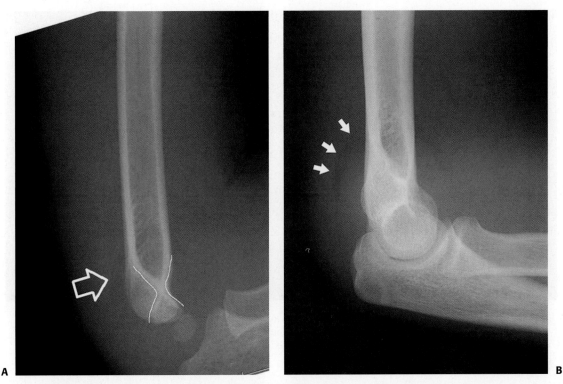

Figure 13-11. A: Lateral radiograph demonstrating an elevated posterior fat pad (*white open arrow*) and a normal hourglass which is anteriorly tilted if there is not a displaced fracture. **B:** Another example of an elevated fat pad (*solid white arrows*). (Reproduced with permission of Children's Orthopaedic Center, Los Angeles, CA.)

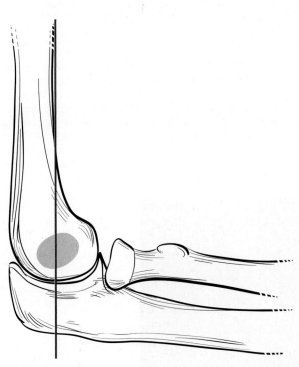

Figure 13-12. Anterior humeral line should cross the capitellum on a true lateral of the elbow, though not necessarily through the middle third of the capitellum as was previously believed. (From Tolo VT, Skaggs DL, eds. *Master Techniques in Orthopaedic Surgery: Pediatrics.* Philadelphia, PA: Lippincott Williams & Wilkins; 2007:1–15.)

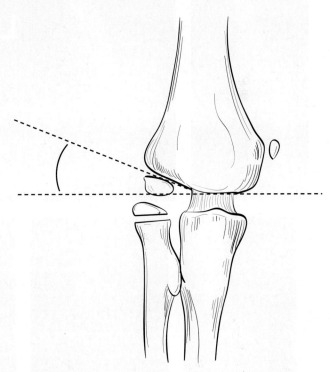

Figure 13-13. Baumann's angle is between the line perpendicular to the long axis of the humeral shaft and the physeal line of the lateral condyle. A decrease in Baumann's angle may indicate medial comminution. (From Tolo VT, Skaggs DL, eds. *Master Techniques in Orthopaedic Surgery: Pediatrics.* Philadelphia, PA: Lippincott Williams & Wilkins; 2007:1–15.)

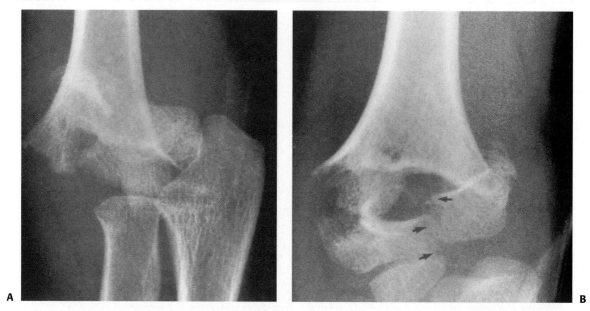

Figure 13-14. Occult T-condylar fracture. **A:** Original x-rays appear to show a type III posteromedial supracondylar fracture. **B:** After manipulation, the vertical intercondylar fracture line (*arrows*) was visualized.

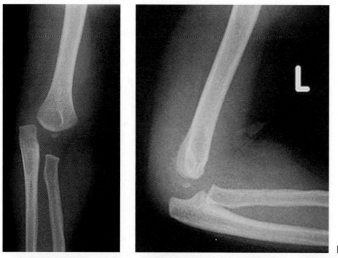

Figure 13-15. Twelve month old, Salter II fracture resulting from child abuse. **A:** Note the radius points to the capitellum in all views, so this is not a dislocation. **B:** Lateral view. **C:** Oblique view shows the thin metaphyseal fragment, which defines this as a Salter II fracture. **D:** This fracture was not recognized at presentation to the emergency department. This AP view is 1 month old. **E:** Lateral view 1 month after injury. (Reproduced with permission of Children's Orthopaedic Center, Los Angeles, CA.)

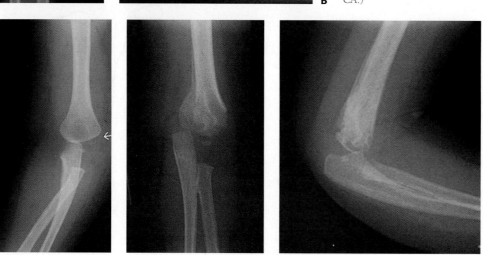

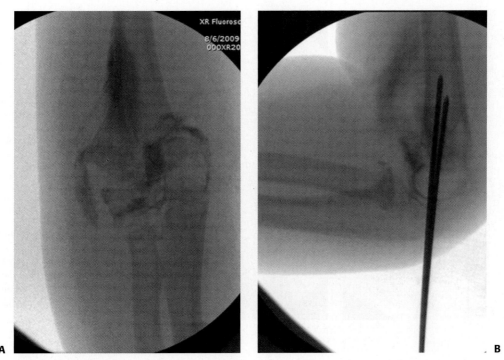

Figure 13-16. A: Salter II fracture in a 20 month old is a bit easier to appreciate on arthrogram. **B:** Lateral view after reduction and pinning. (Reproduced with permission of Children's Orthopaedic Center, Los Angeles, CA.)

Type I

A Gartland type I fracture is a nondisplaced or minimally displaced (<2 mm) supracondylar fracture with an intact AHL. There may or may not be any evidence of osseous injury: The posterior fat pad sign may be the only evidence of fracture. There should be an intact olecranon fossa, no medial or lateral displacement, no medial column collapse, and a normal Baumann's angle. These fractures are stable.

Type II

A Gartland type II fracture is a pure sagittal plane deformity. It is displaced (>2 mm) with a presumably intact, yet hinged, posterior cortex. The AHL is usually anterior to the capitellum on a true lateral of the elbow (Fig. 13-17), though in mildly displaced fractures, the AHL may touch the capitellum (Fig. 13-18). If there is significant rotation in the coronal or transverse plane, it is a type III fracture. There is little benefit in dividing type II

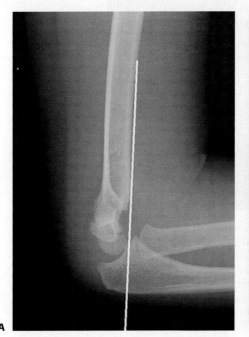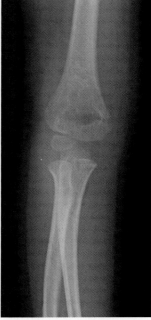

Figure 13-17. A: Type II SCH fracture with anterior humeral line anterior to the capitellum. **B:** AP radiograph of a type II SCH fracture in a 6-year-old girl. Note that Baumann's angle is intact.

(continues)

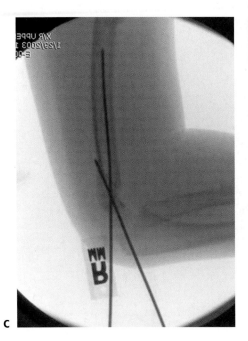

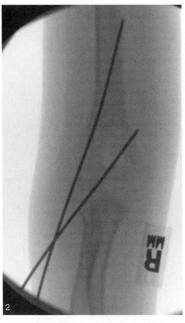

Figure 13-17. (*Continued*) **C:** In the reduced position, the anterior humeral line crosses the capitellum. **D:** AP radiograph following reduction and pinning. Note the good position of the pins demonstrating wide separation of the pins at the fracture site. (Reproduced with permission of Children's Orthopaedic Center, Los Angeles, CA.)

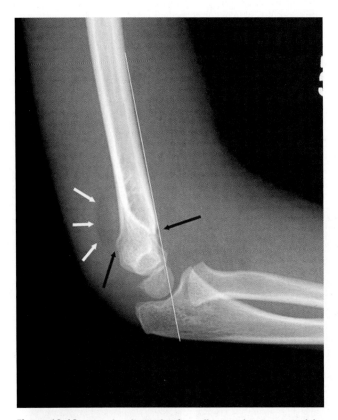

Figure 13-18. Lateral radiograph of an elbow with a supracondylar humerus fracture (*black arrows*) and an elevated posterior fat pad (*white arrows*). The anterior humeral line (*thin white line*) passes through the capitellum, but not through the middle third, so some posterior angulation is present. This fracture may be considered borderline between a type II fracture (since there is some posterior angulation) and a type I fracture, as the anterior humeral line touches the capitellum. (Reproduced with permission of Children's Orthopaedic Center, Los Angeles, CA.)

fractures into subtypes, although clearly this is a clinical continuum with some injuries more severe and unstable than others.

Type III

A Gartland type III fracture is a displaced supracondylar fracture with a range of cortical contact (Figs. 13-19 and 13-20).

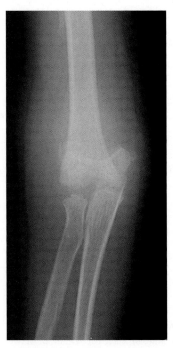

Figure 13-19. Type III supracondylar fracture. AP view shows overlap of distal and proximal fragments. (Reproduced with permission of Children's Orthopaedic Center, Los Angeles, CA.)

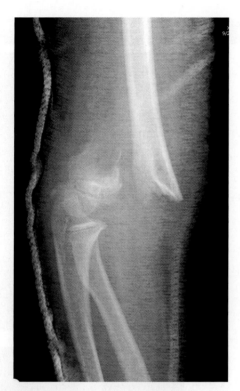

Figure 13-20. Lateral view of fracture demonstrating no meaningful cortical continuity. (Reproduced with permission of Children's Orthopaedic Center, Los Angeles, CA.)

There is usually extension in the sagittal plane and rotation in the frontal and/or transverse planes. The periosteum is extensively torn, and soft tissue and neurovascular injuries often accompany this fracture.

Type IV

Leitch et al. retrospectively reviewed 297 displaced extension-type supracondylar fractures and described 9 of 297 (3%) with multidirectional instability. These fractures are characterized by an incompetent periosteal hinge circumferentially and defined by being unstable in both flexion and extension.[97] This multidirectional instability is usually determined under anesthesia at the time of operation when on a lateral view the capitellum is anterior to the AHL with elbow flexion, and posterior to the AHL with elbow extension (Figs. 13-21 and 13-22). This pattern of instability may result from the initial injury or may occur iatrogenically during a forceful attempted reduction. Classifying this as a separate type of fracture is warranted as it has treatment implications, as discussed later in this chapter, and has gained wide acceptance.[3] As a type I fracture is treated nonoperatively, and type II fractures are treated operatively, the lateral radiograph, which distinguishes these two fractures, deserves special consideration. Assume the AP radiographs have a normal Baumann's angle (Table 13-1).

Pediatric Comprehensive Classification

An alternative classification system was described in 2006 that could cause confusion as it unfortunately uses similar terms

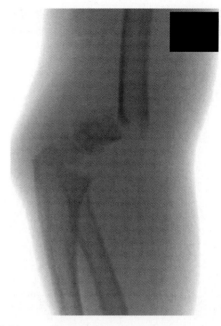

Figure 13-21. Intraoperative imaging demonstrates distal fragment falls into extension. (Reprinted with permission from Leitch KK, Kay RM, Femino JD, et al. Treatment of multidirectionally unstable supracondylar humeral fractures in children: a modified Gartland type-IV fracture. *J Bone Joint Surg Am.* 2006;88(5):980–985.)

(types I to IV) as the established Gartland classification, but with different definitions.[154] According to the Arbeitsgemeinschaft für Osteosynthesefragen (AO) Pediatric Comprehensive Classification, these fractures are classified with regard to the

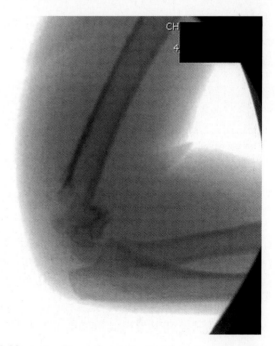

Figure 13-22. As the elbow is flexed, the distal fragment falls into flexion, thus defining a Gartland type IV fracture. (Reprinted with permission from Leitch KK, Kay RM, Femino JD, et al. Treatment of multidirectionally unstable supracondylar humeral fractures in children: a modified Gartland type IV fracture. *J Bone Joint Surg Am.* 2006;88(5):980–985.)

TABLE 13-1. Decision Making Using Lateral X-Rays

This is a typical type I fracture. The anterior humeral line (AHL) clearly goes through the capitellum. Cast with no more than 90 degrees of elbow flexion.

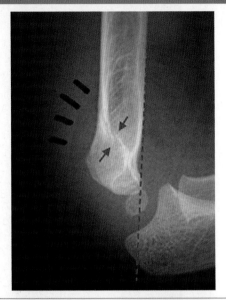

This technically is a type I fracture by definition as the AHL touches the capitellum. However, this fracture is at risk for displacement as the hourglass is not tilting forward, and the posterior cortex is broken as well. Initial treatment is casting at no more than 90 degrees of elbow flexion with the need for close follow-up stressed.

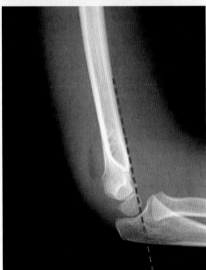

This is a typical type II fracture, with the AHL missing the capitellum and the distal fragment hinged posteriorly. This is treated with closed reduction and pinning.

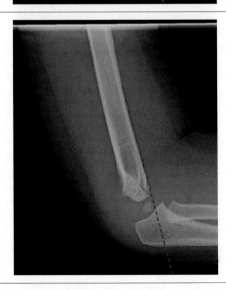

As there is a hint of translation at the posterior cortex, this may be considered a type III fracture and should be reduced and pinned.

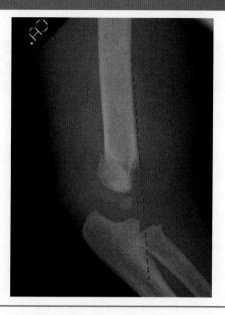

degree of displacement at four levels (I to IV): no displacement (type I), displacement in one plane (type II), rotation of the distal fragment with displacement in two planes (type III), and rotation with displacement in three planes (or no contact between bone fragments) (type IV).[154]

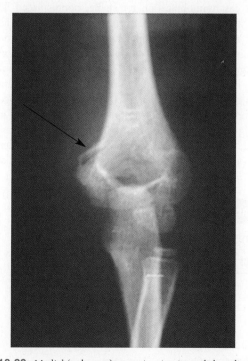

Figure 13-23. Medial (*red arrow*) comminution is a subtle radiographic finding and indicates a more unstable variant which may collapse into the varus if not treated appropriately. (From Tolo VT, Skaggs DL, eds. *Master Techniques in Orthopaedic Surgery: Pediatrics.* Philadelphia, PA: Lippincott; 2007:1–15.)

The Special Case of Medial Comminution in Supracondylar Fractures of the Distal Humerus

A potential pitfall is to underappreciate the extent of loss of normal alignment in fractures with comminution and collapse of the medial column (Fig. 13-23). Medial collapse signifies malrotation in the frontal plane (which defines the injury as at least a type II fracture) and is associated with a loss of Baumann's angle and varus malalignment. The lateral view (Fig. 13-24) may show reasonable alignment, which may lull the inexperienced into not appreciating the seriousness of this fracture, which requires reduction and usually pin fixation to prevent late malunion.

Bahk et al.[13] reported that fractures with greater than 10 degrees of obliquity in the coronal plane or 20 degrees in the

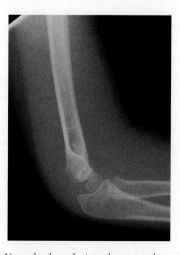

Figure 13-24. Note the lateral view does not show significant displacement. This view alone would suggest nonoperative treatment may be sufficient. (Reproduced with permission of Children's Orthopaedic Center, Los Angeles, CA.)

sagittal plane were more likely than fractures with less obliquity to result in malunion.

TREATMENT OPTIONS FOR SUPRACONDYLAR FRACTURES OF THE DISTAL HUMERUS

See Table 13-2 for treatment options for subcondylar fractures of the distal humerus based on fracture type.

INITIAL MANAGEMENT OF SUPRACONDYLAR FRACTURES OF THE DISTAL HUMERUS

Displaced supracondylar fractures requiring a reduction should be initially splinted with the elbow in a comfortable position of approximately 20 to 40 degrees of flexion, while avoiding tight bandaging. If the arm is pulseless, gentle traction and elbow flexion alone frequently restore a pulse. Excessive flexion or extension may compromise the limb's vascularity and increase compartment pressure.[16,103] The elbow and hand should then be gently elevated above the heart.

Urgency of Treatment

Several studies have concluded that delay of surgery of even over 24 hours did not have any deleterious effects on the outcomes of children with supracondylar fractures.[55,63,143] These studies were all retrospective and may have reported good results in large part because of the selection bias of experienced pediatric orthopedic surgeons selecting which fractures required urgent treatment, such as those with neurovascular injuries.[55] A recent survey of 309 members of the Pediatric Orthopaedic Society of North America found that 81% of the respondents would treat a type III supracondylar humerous fracture (SCHF) presenting after normal work hours by splinting overnight and fixing the following morning, if there were no issues necessitating emergent fixation.[27] Type II fractures may be a special case in this regard. Larson et al. reported on 399 consecutive cases in which it appears that timing for the operative treatment of type II fractures did not affect outcome, with 52% of the fractures having surgery more than 24 hours after injury.[93] There were no compartment syndromes or vascular injury in this group. Although there is little published data to support our opinion, we and others believe that if conditions such as poor perfusion, pulselessness, an associated displaced forearm fracture, firm compartments, skin puckering, antecubital ecchymosis, or very considerable swelling are present, operative treatment should not be unduly delayed.[3,110,121,129]

How Late Can Fractures Be Reduced?

Little has been written about how long after injury a fracture can still be closed reduced. Silva et al.[146] reported on 42 type II SCH fractures treated 7 to 15 days after injury. They found that closed anatomic reduction was achieved in all fractures, with equal outcomes to fractures treated within 7 days of injury. We would caution that in very young children, reliable fracture reduction 2 weeks after injury with early callus formation is less likely. Two children closed reduced 8 days after injury developed avascular necrosis of the trochlea.[146] Although these numbers are small, this phenomenon seems worthy of further study. Lal and Bhan[90] reported that delayed open reduction (11 to 17 days after injury) did not increase the frequency of myositis ossificans. If a supracondylar fracture is unreduced or poorly reduced, delayed open reduction and pin fixation appear to be justified.

NONOPERATIVE MANAGEMENT OF SUPRACONDYLAR FRACTURES OF THE DISTAL HUMERUS

Closed Reduction and Casting

Closed reduction and casting of SCH fractures is not practiced in most modern centers. Most pediatric orthopedic surgeons reserve cast immobilization for stable, nondisplaced fractures (type I) that do not require reduction. Mildly displaced fractures can be reduced closed, using the intact posterior periosteum as a stabilizing force and then holding reduction by flexing the elbow greater than 120 degrees. Less flexion increases the risk of loss of reduction. The concern with closed reduction and flexion greater than 120 degrees is the risk of vascular compromise and/or compartment syndrome in the presence of anterior swelling and compression. If closed reduction and casting is performed, the patients need to be monitored closely for neurovascular compromise and loss of reduction. Follow-up radiographs

TABLE 13-2. Treatment Options for Subcondylar Fractures of the Distal Humerus

Treatment	Fracture Type			
	I	II	III	IV
Casting without reduction	Almost always			
Closed reduction and casting		Rarely indicated, do *not* flex elbow >90 degrees		
Closed reduction and pinning		Great majority of cases	Great majority of cases	Most cases
Open reduction and fixation		Uncommonly necessary	If closed reduction inadequate	If closed reduction inadequate

require AP views of the distal humerus to interpret with elbow flexion beyond 120 degrees. If necessary, rereduction or conversion to pinning needs to occur before full healing occurs, so, close radiographic follow-up is necessary in the first 3 weeks.

Traction

Traction as definitive treatment for supracondylar fractures in children is largely of historic interest now. Indications for traction may include lack of anesthesia, medical conditions prohibiting anesthesia, lack of an experienced surgeon, or severe open wounds. Devnani[40] reported using traction in the gradual reduction of eight fractures with late presentation (mean of 5.6 days), though 18% of these children went on to a corrective osteotomy for malunion. Rates of cubitus varus from 9% to 33% have been reported in some series,[70,127] whereas others have reported excellent results.[54,170] Traction is difficult to justify economically due to prolonged hospitalization necessary, given the excellent results with closed reduction and pinning, which usually requires no more than one-night hospitalization and is associated with a low rate of intraoperative complications.

OPERATIVE MANAGEMENT OF SUPRACONDYLAR FRACTURES OF THE DISTAL HUMERUS

Closed Reduction and Pinning

Closed reduction and pinning is the most common operative treatment of supracondylar fractures. An initial attempt at closed reduction is indicated in almost all displaced supracondylar fractures that are not open fractures. Under general anesthesia, the fracture is first reduced in the frontal plane with fluoroscopic verification. The elbow is then flexed while pushing the olecranon anteriorly to correct the sagittal deformity and reduce the fracture. Criteria for an acceptable reduction include restoration of Baumann's angle (generally >10 degrees) on the AP view, intact medial and lateral columns on oblique views, and the AHL passing through the middle third of the capitellum on the lateral view. As there is considerable rotation present at the shoulder, minor rotational malalignment in the axial plane can be tolerated at the fracture site. However, any rotational malalignment is detrimental to fracture stability, so if present, be extra careful in assessing stability of reduction.

The fracture reduction is generally held with two to three Kirschner wires (K-wires) by lateral entry with divergence of pins. The elbow is immobilized in 40 to 60 degrees of flexion depending on the amount of swelling and vascular status. If there is a considerable gap in the fracture site or the fracture is irreducible with a "rubbery" feeling on attempted reduction, the median nerve and/or brachial artery may be trapped in the fracture site and an open reduction should be performed (Fig. 13-25).

Crossed Pins Versus Lateral Entry Pins

Recent papers suggest that lateral entry pins are being used more commonly than cross-pins for most supracondylar fractures.[1,5,17,27,86,101] A recent survey of 309 members of the Pediatric Orthopaedic Society of North America found that 70% of respondents prefer lateral pins.[27] Some series report that

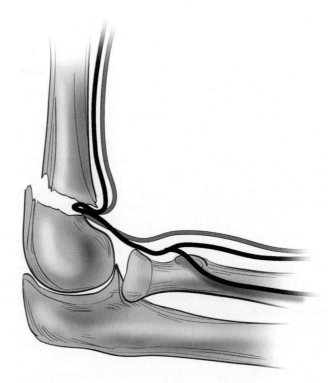

Figure 13-25. Brachial artery and median nerve may be trapped at the fracture site. If a reduction feels rubbery, and a gap at the fracture site is seen on imaging, entrapment is possible, especially in the setting of vascular compromise or median nerve or anterior interosseous nerve injury. (From Tolo VT, Skaggs DL, eds. *Master Techniques in Orthopaedic Surgery: Pediatrics*. Philadelphia, PA: Lippincott; 2007:1–15.)

when a medial pin is used, there are more complications[168] or longer surgical time,[86] and other series find no difference.[55,169]

The two main issues with crossed pin versus lateral entry pinning of SCH fractures are risk of ulnar nerve injury and risk of loss of reduction. Iatrogenic injury to the ulnar nerve with use of crossed pins has been reported to be as low as 0% but three large series of supracondylar fractures at major pediatric centers have shown the prevalence to be 5% (17 of 345), 5% (14/297), and 6% (19 of 331).[1,24,38,99,130,150,171] Others have reported that these injuries occur more commonly.[166] A meta-analysis of 1,158 patients in seven randomized controlled trials (RCTs) and six prospective comparative cohorts found iatrogenic ulnar nerve injury was over 10 times more likely when a medial pin was used, compared to lateral entry pins (4.1% [20/493] vs. 0.3% [2/666]) but no difference in loss of fixation between the two techniques.[38] Smaller series reported a 13% (5/39) risk of iatrogenic ulnar nerve injury when pediatric orthopedic fellowship–trained surgeons used a medial pin,[43] and one series even reported 21% (10/48) rate of iatrogenic ulnar nerve injury with a medial pin.[17]

Three recent meta-analyses have examined the issue of pin configuration and iatrogenic nerve injury. In 2010, Slobogean et al.[153] reported on 32 trials with 2,639 patients and found there was an iatrogenic ulnar nerve injury for every 28 patients treated with crossed pins compared to lateral-pinning. In the same year, Babal et al.[10] reported on a systematic review of 35 articles discussing medial and lateral-pinning versus lateral entry pinning and found that iatrogenic ulnar nerve injury occurred in 40 of 1,171 (3.4%) of cross-pins and 5 of 738 (0.7%) of lateral entry pins. The 2012 report by Woratanarat et al.[168] included 18 studies and 1,615 SCH fractures. They reported the risk of iatrogenic ulnar nerve injury to be 4.3 times higher in cross-pinning compared to lateral-pinning. They found no difference in loss of fixation, late deformity, or Flynn criteria between the two types of pinning.

A prospective, surgeon-randomized study was performed on 104 children with type III SCH fractures, with surgeons using their preferred techniques of cross-pins or lateral entry pins. The authors found no statistical difference in the radiographic outcomes between lateral entry and cross-pin techniques, but two cases of iatrogenic injury to the ulnar nerve occurred with medially placed pins.[57]

Zaltz et al.[171] reported that in children less than 5 years of age, when the elbow is flexed more than 90 degrees, the ulnar nerve migrated over, or even anterior to, the medial epicondyle in 61% (32/52) of children. Wind et al.[166] showed that the location of the ulnar nerve cannot be adequately determined by palpation to allow blind medial pinning. Unfortunately, even making an incision over the medial epicondyle to make certain the ulnar nerve is not directly injured by a pin does not ensure protection of the nerve.[150]

In a series of six cases of iatrogenic ulnar nerve injuries with early exploration, the nerve was directly penetrated by the pin in two of six cases (33.3%), with constriction of the cubital tunnel occurring in three of six cases (50%), and the nerve being fixed anterior to the medial epicondyle in one of six (16.7%) cases.[130] Thus, even if direct penetration of the ulnar nerve is avoided, simply placing a medial epicondyle entry pin adjacent to the nerve can cause injury, presumably by constriction of the cubital tunnel or kinking of the nerve. Iatrogenic ulnar nerve injuries usually resolve, but there have been several reports of permanent iatrogenic ulnar nerve injuries.[128,130,150]

A series of 345 SCH fractures[150] treated by percutaneous pinning showed that the use of a medial pin was associated with a 4% (6/149) risk of ulnar nerve injury when the medial pin was placed without hyperflexion and 15% (11/71) if the medial pin was placed with hyperflexion. None of the 125 fractures treated with lateral entry pins alone resulted in iatrogenic injury. This is consistent with the findings of Zaltz et al.[171] of anterior subluxation of the ulnar nerve with elbow flexion beyond 90 degrees. Thus, one apparently undeniable conclusion is that if a medial pin is used, the lateral pins should be placed first, then the elbow extended and the medial pin placed without hyperflexion of the elbow.

The second issue with pin configuration is stability of pin configuration. Biomechanical studies of stability of various pin configurations have been somewhat misleading. Two studies evaluated the torsional strength of pin configurations and found crossed pins to be stronger than two lateral pins.[116,172] Unfortunately, in these studies, the two lateral pins were placed immediately adjacent to each other and not separated at the fracture site as is recommended clinically for lateral entry pins.[67,122,137,148] In synthetic humeri study, Srikumaran et al.[155] found cross-pins to be stronger than two lateral entry pins, but did not test three lateral entry pins. Lee et al.[96] found that two divergent lateral pins separated at the fracture site were superior to crossed pins in extension loading and varus but were equivalent in valgus (Fig. 13-26). The greater strength seen with divergence of the pins was attributed to the location of the intersection of the two pins and greater divergence between the two pins, which would allow for some purchase in the medial column as well as the lateral column.

Bloom et al.[19] reported that three lateral entry divergent pins were equivalent to cross-pinning and both were stronger than two lateral divergent pins. Another study with simulated medial comminution showed that three lateral divergent pins had equivalent torsional stability to standard medial and lateral crossed pinning.[94] Feng et al.[48] reported that two and three lateral entry pins had comparable construct stiffness to each other, and both were greater than crossed pins to all types of stress, except in valgus, in which cross-pins had greater stiffness. Thus, contemporary biomechanical studies mostly support clinical recommendations of lateral entry pins.[3,115,137,148]

Multiple biomechanical studies have reported that larger pins provide more stability.[61,126,155]

A series of 124 consecutive fractures treated with lateral entry pins reported no malunions or loss of fixation.[148] From this successful series, combined with a failure analysis of eight fractures performed outside of this series, the authors concluded the important technical points for fixation with lateral entry pins as follows[148]:

- Maximize separation of the pins at the fracture site.[122]
- Engage the medial and lateral columns proximal to the fracture.
- Engage sufficient bone in both the proximal segment and the distal fragment.
- Maintain a low threshold for use of a third lateral entry pin if there is concern about fracture stability or the location of the first two pins.
- Use three pins for type III fractures.

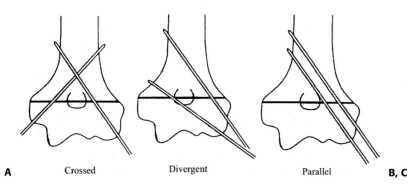

A   Crossed   Divergent   Parallel   **B, C**

Figure 13-26. Three pinning techniques in study by Lee et al.[96] **A:** Crossed: one medial and one lateral pin. **B:** Divergent: two divergent lateral pins. **C:** Parallel: two parallel lateral pins. (Reprinted with permission from Lee YH, Lee SK, Kim BS, et al. Three lateral divergent or parallel pin fixations for the treatment of displaced supracondylar humerus fractures in children. *J Pediatr Orthop.* 2008;28(4):417–422.)

In a study of eight other cases of SCH fractures, which lost reduction, Sankar et al. reported that loss of fixation in all cases was because of technical errors that were identifiable on the intraoperative fluoroscopic images and that could have been prevented with proper technique. They identified three types of pin-fixation errors[137]: failure to engage both fragments with two or more pins, failure to achieve bicortical fixation with two pins or more, and failure to achieve adequate pin separation (>2 mm) at the fracture site. A systematic review of 35 articles reported loss of reduction in 0 of 849 of crossed pins and 4 of 606 (0.7%) of lateral entry pins.[22] Based on this study and the previous series by Skaggs et al.,[148] we recommend a minimum of two pins for a type II fracture and three pins for a type III fracture.

A recent study of 192 patients concluded that pin spread is an important factor associated with preventing loss of reduction, with the goal of pin spacing at least 13 mm or one-third the width of the humerus at the level of the fracture.[122]

Two prospective randomized clinical trials comparing lateral- and cross-pinning techniques in the treatment of displaced SCH fractures showed no statistically significant difference between the two treatment groups in any radiographic or clinical outcome measures,[82,158] including nerve injury. It is interesting that following the randomized clinical trial,[82] the same eight surgeons who used cross-pins in 59% of SCH fractures pretrial changed their practice to use cross-pins in only 15% of cases posttrial.[101]

An alternative technique using antegrade insertion of elastic intramedullary nailing has been described.[41] This technique seems needlessly invasive to the uninvolved upper humerus when pinning of the fracture site reliably results in excellent results in most cases.

Open Reduction

Open reduction is indicated in cases of failed closed reduction, a loss of pulse, poor perfusion, or nerve injury following reduction, and open fractures. Over time, the rate of open reductions in the United States has been steadily decreasing over time, with about 6% in the most recent year reported (Fig. 13-27).[71] Specialized pediatric trauma centers report even lower numbers, such as 0.7% (9/1,296) at Denver Children's Hospital,[55] and 2% (8/339) at Children's Hospital Los Angeles.[150] In the past, open reductions led to concerns of elbow stiffness, myositis ossificans, scarring, and iatrogenic neurovascular injury. However, several reports have shown the low rate of complications associated with open reduction, and this is in the setting of more severe soft tissue and bony injuries. Ay et al.[9] found no loss of motion or clinical deformity in 61 patients treated with open reduction. In a prospective, randomized controlled study of 28 children, Kaewpornsawan[75] compared closed reduction and percutaneous pin fixation with open reduction (through a lateral approach); the patients treated with percutaneous pin fixation showed no differences with regard to cubitus varus, neurovascular injury, the range of motion (ROM), the infection rate, the union rate, or the criteria of Flynn et al.[53] In older children with SCH fractures (8 to 14 years of age), Mollon et al.[107] reported a mean loss of 30 degrees of elbow flexion at final follow-up in those patients treated with open reduction internal fixation

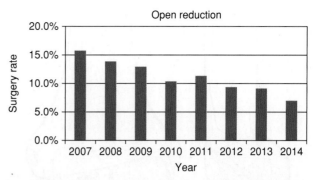

Figure 13-27. The percentage of patients who underwent open reduction for the treatment of a supracondylar humeral fracture. A significant decrease in the rate of open reduction ($p < 0.0001$) over time was demonstrated.

compared with those treated with closed reduction percutaneous pinning. Twenty-two-year follow-up of 49 patients in Turkey showed 84% good functional outcome, with a mean of 4 degrees varus/valgus difference from the contralateral side, and a mean of 5 degrees flexion deficit and 4 degrees extension deficit.[65]

Surgical Approach

The direct anterior approach to the elbow is extremely useful for open reduction, particularly in cases of neurovascular compromise. The anterior approach has the advantages of allowing direct visualization of the brachial artery and median nerve as well as the fracture fragments. The exposure is through the torn periosteum and disrupted brachialis and therefore does not further destabilize the fracture. When performed through a relatively small (5 to 8 cm) transverse incision above the cubital fossa at the fracture site, the resulting scar is much more aesthetic than that of the lateral approach, and scar contraction limiting elbow extension is not an issue. A series of 26 patients treated with the anterior approach showed equivalent results to the traditional lateral or combined lateral with medial approach in terms of malunion, Flynn criteria,[53] and ROM.

The posterior approach for an extended supracondylar fracture risks a higher rate of loss of motion, further fracture instability with exposure through intact periosteum, and, most importantly, the risk of avascular necrosis secondary to disruption of the posterior end arterial supply to the trochlea of the humerus[5,87,106,167] (Fig. 13-28). This approach is not recommended.

OPERATIVE TREATMENT BY FRACTURE TYPE

Type I (Nondisplaced)

Simple immobilization at 60 to 90 degrees of elbow flexion, with the forearm in neutral rotation is all that is necessary.[164] If there is unequivocally no significant swelling about the elbow, a circumferential cast may be used; with significant swelling, initial splinting may be best. Caregivers are educated on elevation and the signs and symptoms of compartment syndrome. The elbow should not be flexed greater than 90 degrees. Using Doppler examination of the brachial artery after supracondylar fractures, Mapes and Hennrikus[103] found that flow was decreased in the brachial artery in positions of pronation and increased

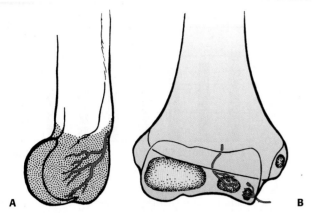

Figure 13-28. Intraosseous blood supply of the distal humerus. **A:** The vessels supplying the lateral condylar epiphysis enter on the posterior aspect and course for a considerable distance before reaching the ossific nucleus. **B:** Two definite vessels supply the ossification center of the medial crista of the trochlea. The lateral vessel enters by crossing the physis. The medial one enters by way of the nonarticular edge of the medial crista. (Redrawn after Haraldsson S. On osteochondrosis deformans juvenilis capituli humeri including investigation of the intraosseous vasculature in the distal humerus. *Acta Orthop Scand.* 1959;38(Suppl):1–232.)

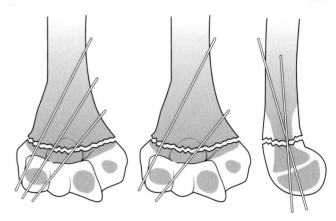

Figure 13-29. Properly placed divergent lateral entry pins. On the AP view, there should be maximal pin separation at the fracture site, the pins should engage both medial and lateral columns just proximal to the fracture site, and they should engage an adequate amount of bone proximal and distal to the fragments. On the lateral view, pins should incline slightly in the anterior to posterior direction in accordance with normal anatomy. (Reprinted with permission from Skaggs DL, Cluck MW, Mostofi A, et al. Lateral-entry pin fixation in the management of supracondylar fractures in children. *J Bone Joint Surg Am.* 2004;86(4):702–707.)

flexion. Before the splint is applied, it should be confirmed that the pulse is intact and that there is good capillary refill with the amount of elbow flexion intended during immobilization.

X-rays are obtained 3 to 7 days after fracture to document lack of displacement. If there is evidence of significant distal fragment extension, as judged by lack of intersection of the AHL with the capitellum, the fracture should be treated with closed reduction and percutaneous pinning to secure the reduction.

An acceptable position is determined by the AHL transecting the capitellum on the lateral x-ray, a Baumann's angle of greater than 10 degrees or equal to the other side, and an intact olecranon fossa. The duration of immobilization for supracondylar fractures is 3 weeks, whether type I, II, or III. In general, no physical therapy is required after this injury. Patients may be seen 4 to 6 weeks after immobilization is removed to ensure that ROM and strength are returning normally. As the outcome in type I fractures is predictably excellent if alignment is maintained at the time of early healing, follow-up visits are optional depending on family and medical circumstances.

Remember that the initial x-ray is a static representation of the actual injury that may involve soft tissue disruption much greater than one might expect from the minimal bony abnormality. Excessive swelling, nerve or vascular disruption, or excessive pain are indicative of a more significant injury that a type I fracture, in which case periosteal disruption, may render this fracture inherently unstable. Also, beware of any medial comminution that could allow the fracture to collapse into varus during immobilization.

Type II Fracture (Hinged Posteriorly, With Posterior Cortex in Continuity)

The optimal treatment of type II fractures has evolved to the current trend of operative intervention with closed reduction and percutaneous pinning rather than cast immobilization.

The fracture is reduced with flexion, the reduction is confirmed with AP, lateral and oblique fluoroscopy, and two lateral pins are placed[137,148,150] through the distal humeral fragment, engaging the opposite cortex of the proximal fragment (Fig. 13-29, see Figs. 13-4 and 13-17C,D) (see Closed Reduction and Pinning). This is generally sufficient fixation, though in many series three pins are often used.[148] The posterior cortex and intact periosteum provide some degree of inherent stability. Cross-pinning of a type II fracture is generally not needed. The pins are left protruding through the skin and are removed at 3 weeks after fixation, generally without the need for sedation or anesthesia.

Casting Versus CRPP of Type II Supracondylar Fractures of the Distal Humerus

The distal humerus provides 20% of the growth of the humerus and thus has little remodeling potential. The upper limb grows approximately 10 cm during the first year, 6 cm during the second year, 5 cm during the third year, 3.5 cm during the fourth year, and 3 cm during the fifth year of life.[42] In toddlers (<3 years), some remodeling potential is present, so the surgeon may accept nonoperative treatment of a type II fracture in which the capitellum abuts the AHL but does not cross it. In a child who is 8 to 10 years old, however, there is only 10% of growth of the distal humerus remaining, so adequate reduction and stabilization is essential to prevent malunion.

Three studies support the initial treatment of type II fractures with closed reduction and casting. Hadlow et al.[66] make the point that pinning all type II fractures in their series of initial closed reduction and casting meant that 77% (37 of 48) of patients would have undergone an unnecessary operative procedure. However, 23% (11 of 48) of the patients in that series lost reduction following closed reduction and underwent delayed operative fixation. Fourteen percent (2 of 14) that were followed had a poor outcome by Flynn criteria.[53]

A retrospective review of 25 elbows treated with closed reduction and casting by Parikh et al.[119] showed a 28% (7 of 25) loss of reduction, 20% (5 of 25) need for delayed surgery, and 2% (2 of 25) unsatisfactory outcome according to Flynn criteria.

Similarly, Fitzgibbons et al.[49] reported 20% lost reduction in the closed treatment of 61 type II fractures. They noted that failure was more likely to occur in more displaced fractures in which the AHL did not touch the capitellum, and in those children with wider upper arms. They concluded that "a reasonable protocol" would involve urgent pinning of fractures in which the capitellum extends beyond the AHL, whereas fractures that are less displaced could undergo reduction and casting and then be followed at 1-week intervals.[49] In a series of 155 type II SCH fractures treated nonoperatively, Camus et al.[26] reported that fractures were found to have radiographic evidence of sagittal plane (80% with abnormal AHL, decreased humerocapitellar angle), coronal plane (47% with abnormal Baumann's angle), and rotational (44%) deformities. An additional consideration when treating SCH fractures nonsurgically is the likelihood of the child following up with an orthopedic surgeon soon enough for a loss of reduction to be rereduced. Fletcher et al.[51] reported that children with supracondylar fractures seen at a large urban hospital in the United States were almost three times less likely to be seen back in clinic if they had public insurance or no insurance.

In contrast to the frequent loss of fixation from casting and reduction of type II fractures, closed reduction and percutaneous pinning has predictably good results. A consecutive series of 69 children with type II fractures treated with closed reduction and pinning reported no radiographic or clinical loss of reduction, no cubitus varus, no hyperextension, and no loss of motion. There were no iatrogenic nerve palsies, and no patient required additional surgery.[148] In another study of type II fractures, 189 consecutive cases of closed reduction and percutaneous pinning were reviewed. There were 2% (4/189) pin-tract infections, of which three were treated successfully with oral antibiotics and pin removal 1.5% (3/191) and one (0.5%) underwent operative irrigation and debridement for a wound infection not involving the joint. There were no nerve or vascular injuries, and no loss of reduction, delayed unions, or malunions. The authors conclude that pinning type II supracondylar fractures leads to a high probability of satisfactory outcome compared with previous studies of closed reduction without pinning.[152]

Another reason for advocating operative treatment of these injuries is that the amount of hyperflexion needed to maintain reduction in unpinned type II fractures would predispose these patients to increased compartment pressures.[16] A study by Mapes and Hennrikus[103] showed that a pulse was lost to Doppler when type II fractures are flexed more than 110 degrees and type III fractures are flexed more than 70 degrees. Pronation also decreased flow in the brachial artery. Pinning these fractures obviates the need for immobilization with considerable elbow flexion. To truly stabilize an extension fracture treated closed, greater than 120 degrees of flexion is required.[85] The basic concept is that any fracture that would require elbow flexion greater than 90 degrees to hold reduction increases the risk of neurovascular compromise and therefore, should instead have the reduction held by pins, and immobilized with the elbow in less flexion (usually about 45 to 70 degrees).

Type III Fractures

The standard of care in most modern centers for the treatment of type III fractures is operative reduction and pinning. In most series,[3,85,124] the results of type III fractures treated with closed reduction and cast immobilization are not as good as those treated with pinning. Hadlow et al.,[66] reported only 61% of type III and 77% of type II fractures were successfully treated without pinning. It must be emphasized that flexion of the elbow with a type III supracondylar fracture up to 90 degrees or greater significantly increases the risk of compartment syndrome and should rarely, if ever, be done if modern operative facilities and an experienced surgeon are available. Type III fractures are more likely than type to lose reduction and require return to surgery by one report.[114]

Posteromedial Versus Posterolateral Displacement of Extension-Type Supracondylar Fractures of the Distal Humerus

The periosteum plays a key role with regard to treatment. With extension-type injuries, the anterior periosteum is likely torn. The intact posterior periosteal hinge provides stability to the fracture and facilitates reduction with a flexion reduction maneuver. Many authors have described adding forearm pronation to assist in reduction, but this should not be automatic. The direction of fracture displacement often indicates whether the medial or lateral periosteum remains intact. With a posteromedially displaced fracture, the medial periosteum is usually intact. Elbow flexion and forearm pronation places the medial and posterior periosteum on tension, which corrects varus and extension malalignment and adds to stability of fracture reduction (Fig. 13-30). The medial periosteum, however, is often torn in a posterolaterally displaced fracture, in which case pronation may be counterproductive. Instead, in a posterolaterally displaced supracondylar fracture, forearm supination in addition to flexion may be better because the lateral periosteum is usually intact (Table 13-3). If the posterior periosteal hinge is also disrupted, the fracture becomes unstable in both flexion and extension and this has been described as a multidirectionally unstable, modified Gartland type IV fracture.[97]

The Special Case of Medial Column Comminution

Fractures with medial comminution may not have the dramatic displacement of most type III fractures, but must be treated with operative reduction because collapse of the medial column will lead to varus deformity in an otherwise minimally displaced supracondylar fracture (see Fig. 13-23). De Boeck et al.[37] recommended closed reduction with percutaneous pinning when a fracture had medial comminution even in otherwise minimally displaced fractures, to prevent cubitus varus. In this retrospective review, none of the six patients with medial comminution who underwent operative fixation had cubitus varus whereas four of seven (57%) patients who were treated nonoperatively developed cubitus varus.

The technique for reduction of a medial comminuted fracture is significant valgus force applied across a straight elbow. Often, so much force is required that one is fearful of creating a new fracture. Well-placed lateral entry pins are sufficient to hold the reduction.

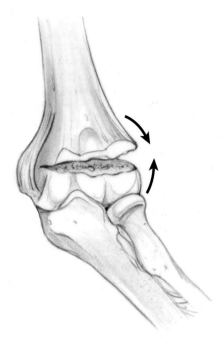

Figure 13-30. Laterally torn periosteum in a posteromedially displaced supracondylar humerus fracture. (From Skaggs DL. Closed reduction and pinning of supracondylar humerus fractures. In: Tolo VT, Skaggs DL, eds. *Master Techniques in Orthopaedic Surgery: Pediatrics.* Philadelphia, PA: Lippincott Williams & Wilkins; 2007.)

Open Fractures

Open supracondylar fractures generally have an anterior puncture wound where the metaphyseal spike penetrates the skin (Fig. 13-31). Even if the open wound is only a small puncture in the center of an anterior pucker, open irrigation and debridement are indicated. The anterior approach, using a transverse incision based on the open wound with medial or lateral extension as needed, is recommended. The neurovascular bundle (NVB) is usually directly under the skin and tented over the metaphyseal fragment, so care should be taken in approaching this fracture surgically. The skin incision can be extended medially proximally (to follow the brachial artery and median nerve) and laterally distally if needed. However, usually only the transverse portion of the incision is required, which gives a better aesthetic result. The brachialis muscle is usually transected because it is a muscle belly to its insertion on the coronoid attachment and is highly vulnerable to trauma from the proximal metaphyseal fragment. The fracture surfaces are examined and washed, and a curette is used to remove any dirt or entrapped soft tissue. Once the debridement and washing are

TABLE 13-3. Forearm Rotation to Aid in Reduction as a Function of Direction of Fracture Displacement

Displacement	Periosteum Is Torn	Forearm Rotation to Aid in Reduction
Posterior medial	Lateral	Pronation
Posterior lateral	Medial	Supination

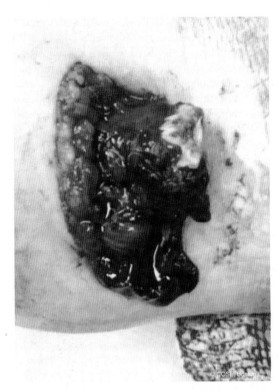

Figure 13-31. Open supracondylar humerus fracture. The distal humerus metaphysis is completely protruding through the transverse open wound. Fortunately, the pulse was intact, and the hand was viable. (Reprinted with permission from Waters PM, Bae DS, eds. *Pediatric Hand and Upper Limb Surgery: A Practical Guide.* 1st ed. Philadelphia, PA: Wolters Kluwer Health/Lippincott Williams & Wilkins; 2012.)

complete, the fracture is reduced by mobilizing the periosteum out of the way and flexing the distal humerus. Stabilization is with K-wires. All patients with open fractures are also treated with antibiotics: generally, cefazolin for Gustilo type I, II, and IIIA injuries, with the addition of appropriate antibiotics to cover gram-negative organisms for type IIIB and C fractures.

OPERATIVE TECHNIQUES

Closed Reduction and Percutaneous Pinning

Preoperative Planning

✔ Closed Reduction and Percutaneous Pinning: PREOPERATIVE PLANNING CHECKLIST	
OR table	❑ Radiolucent arm board
Position	❑ Supine, with the fractured elbow on a short radiolucent arm board
Fluoroscopy location	❑ X-ray unit from foot of bed, monitor opposite the surgeon
Equipment	❑ K-wires (most commonly, 0.062-in smooth K-wires are used, but smaller or larger sizes may be considered if the child is particularly small or large), sterile coban, sterile felt, sterile foam

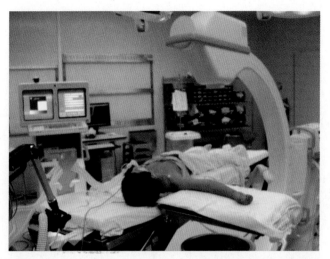

Figure 13-32. Positioning the fluoroscopy monitor on the opposite side of the bed allows the surgeon to easily see the images while operating. (From Tolo VT, Skaggs DL, eds. *Master Techniques in Orthopaedic Surgery: Pediatrics*. Philadelphia, PA: Lippincott Williams & Wilkins; 2007:1–15.)

Positioning

In the operating room, the patient receives a general anesthetic and prophylactic antibiotics. We prefer to have the fluoroscopy monitor opposite to the surgeon for ease of viewing (Fig. 13-32).

The patient is positioned supine on the operating table, with the fractured elbow on a short radiolucent arm board.[148] Some surgeons use the wide end of the fluoroscopy unit as the table, which is probably fine for type II fractures, but this setup will not allow for rotation of the fluoroscopy unit to obtain lateral images of the elbow which is useful in very unstable fractures, such as type IV. It is essential that the child's arm is far enough onto the arm board that the elbow can be well visualized with fluoroscopy. In very small children, this may mean having the child's shoulder and head on the arm board (Fig. 13-33).

Technique

Prep and drape the injured arm with an extremity drape. Apply traction with the elbow flexed at about 20 degrees to avoid the possibility of tethering neurovascular structures over an anteriorly displaced proximal fragment. For badly displaced fractures, hold significant traction for 60 seconds to allow soft tissue

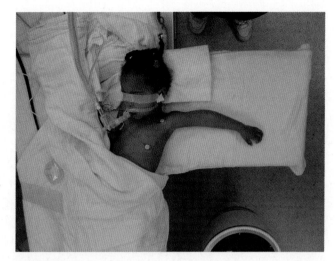

Figure 13-33. In small children, imaging of the elbow may be difficult if the arm is not long enough to reach the center of the fluoroscopy unit. By placing the child's head in the crack between the operating room table and the arm board, the elbow is more easily imaged, and the child's head is unlikely to be inadvertently pulled off the side of the bed during the procedure. (From Tolo VT, Skaggs DL, eds. *Master Techniques in Orthopaedic Surgery: Pediatrics*. Philadelphia, PA: Lippincott Williams & Wilkins; 2007:1–15.)

realignment, with the surgeon grasping the forearm with both hands, and the assistant providing countertraction in the axilla (Fig. 13-34). With the elbow almost straight, varus and valgus angular alignment is corrected by movement of the forearm. Medial and lateral fracture translation is realigned with direct movement of the distal fragment by the surgeon with image confirmation. The elbow is then slowly flexed while applying anterior pressure to the olecranon with the surgeon's thumb (Fig. 13-35). Pronate the forearm for posterior medially displaced fractures, and supinate for posterior laterally displaced fractures.

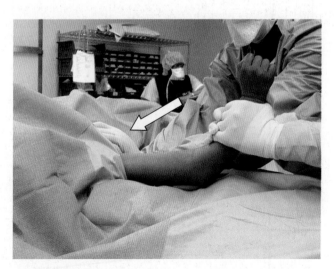

Figure 13-34. Reduction maneuver: Traction with elbow flexed 20 to 30 degrees. Assistant provides countertraction against patient's axilla (*white arrow*) to allow for significant traction to be applied. (From Tolo VT, Skaggs DL, eds. *Master Techniques in Orthopaedic Surgery: Pediatrics*. Philadelphia, PA: Lippincott Williams & Wilkins; 2007:1–15.)

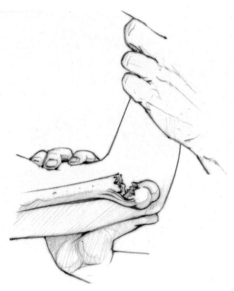

Figure 13-35. Reduction maneuver: Flex elbow while pushing anteriorly on olecranon with the thumb(s). (From Tolo VT, Skaggs DL, eds. *Master Techniques in Orthopaedic Surgery: Pediatrics*. Philadelphia, PA: Lippincott; 2007:1–15.)

The reduction is then checked by fluoroscopic images in AP, lateral, and oblique planes. Verify four points to check for a good reduction: (1) the AHL intersects the capitellum (Fig. 13-36), (2) Baumann's angle is greater than 10 degrees (Fig. 13-37), and (3 and 4) the medial *and* lateral columns are intact on oblique views (Fig. 13-38). We will accept some translation of the distal

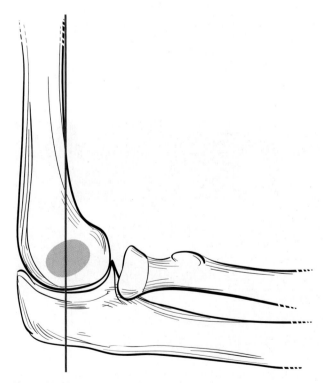

Figure 13-36. Anterior humeral line should cross the capitellum on a true lateral of the elbow. (From Tolo VT, Skaggs DL, eds. *Master Techniques in Orthopaedic Surgery: Pediatrics*. Philadelphia, PA: Lippincott Williams & Wilkins; 2007:1–15.)

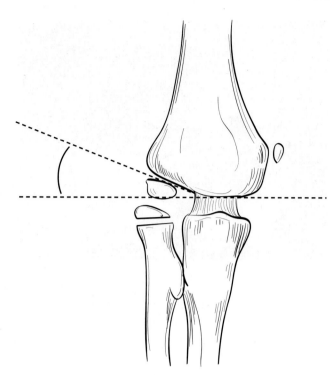

Figure 13-37. The Baumann's angle is between the line perpendicular to the long axis of the humeral shaft and the physeal line of the lateral condyle. A decrease in the Baumann's angle may indicate medial comminution. (From Tolo VT, Skaggs DL, eds. *Master Techniques in Orthopaedic Surgery: Pediatrics*. Philadelphia, PA: Lippincott Williams & Wilkins; 2007:1–15.)

fragment (up to perhaps 5 mm), as long as the above criteria are met. Once reduction is satisfactory, tape the elbow in the reduced position of elbow hyperflexion with elastic tape to prevent loss of reduction while pinning (Fig. 13-39).

Position elbow on a folded towel. Palpate the lateral humeral condyle. The K-wire is placed against the lateral condyle without piercing skin and checked under AP fluoroscopic guidance to assess the starting point. The K-wire is held free in the surgeon's hand at this point, not in the drill, to allow maximum control. If the starting point and trajectory are correct, the wire may be pushed through the skin and into the cartilage, using the cartilage of the distal lateral condyle as a pincushion (Fig. 13-40) that will hold the K-wire in place while the surgeon carefully examines the AP and lateral images. Place pins to maximally separate the pins at the fracture site to engage both the medial and lateral columns (see Fig. 13-29). In the sagittal plane, to engage the most bone with the K-wire in the distal fragment, the reduced capitellum lies slightly anterior to the plane of the fracture, thus the pin may start a bit anterior to the plane of the fracture and angulate about 10 to 15 degrees posteriorly to maximize osseous purchase. If imaging verifies correct pin placement, then advance the pin with a drill. After pin placement, the elbow is extended and the reduction is again checked under fluoroscopy with lateral, oblique, and AP views (Fig. 13-41). Stress is applied in varus and valgus under fluoroscopy to ensure stable reduction. If there is any instability, you want to know about it now, rather than a week later. If there is instability, we will add a third lateral entry pin (Fig. 13-42).

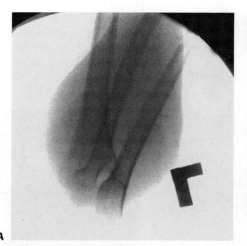 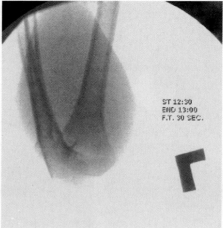

Figure 13-38. A: Oblique fluoroscopic view of the elbow demonstrating continuity of the medial column following adequate fracture reduction. **B:** Demonstration of lateral column continuity. (From Tolo VT, Skaggs DL, eds. *Master Techniques in Orthopaedic Surgery: Pediatrics.* Philadelphia, PA: Lippincott Williams & Wilkins; 2007:1–15.)

Vascular status is assessed. The wires are bent and cut. Take care to leave the wires at least 1 to 2 cm off the skin after, to prevent migration of the wires under the skin. A sterile felt square with a slit cut into it is then placed around the wires to protect the skin (Fig. 13-43). Foam is applied to the arm on the anterior and posterior aspects of the elbow to allow for swelling[139] (Fig. 13-44). The cast is then applied in 45 to 70 degrees of elbow flexion, as flexion to 90 degrees may needlessly increase the risk of compartment syndrome (Fig. 13-45).

Medial Pin

In the exceptionally rare instance when three lateral pins do not stabilize the fracture, or there is an oblique fracture pattern preventing multiple lateral entry pins, a medial pin may be considered. After placing lateral entry pins, the elbow is fully extended to relax tension on the ulnar nerve and surrounding tissue, and the surgeon can palpate the medial epicondyle which is posterior to the center plane of the distal humerus. The entry site for medial pin placement is anterior on the medial epicondyle. A small incision is made to expose and protect the ulnar nerve. A drill guide is used to prevent binding of the perineural soft tissues that could kink the nerve. After desired pin placement is confirmed on fluoroscopy, the medial epicondyle and nerve are inspected to be certain there is no injury, impingement, or kinking of the nerve throughout flexion–extension arc of motion.

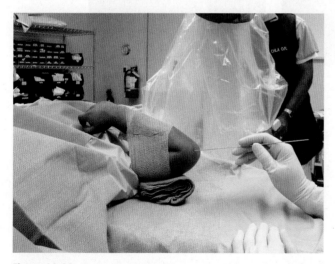

Figure 13-39. Fracture reduction is maintained by taping elbow in hyperflexed position. The wire may be pushed through the skin and into the cartilage using the cartilage of the distal lateral condyle as a pincushion that will hold the K-wire in place while carefully examining the AP and lateral images. (Reproduced with permission of Children's Orthopaedic Center, Los Angeles, CA.)

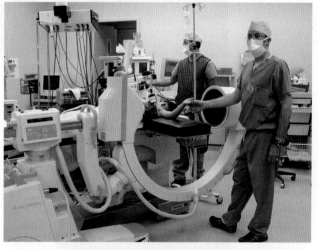

Figure 13-40. In very unstable fractures, rotation of the shoulder into external rotation to obtain a lateral image of the elbow may lead to a loss of reduction. In these rare instances, rotation of the C-arm, rather than the elbow, is a useful trick. (From Tolo VT, Skaggs DL, eds. *Master Techniques in Orthopaedic Surgery: Pediatrics.* Philadelphia, PA: Lippincott Williams & Wilkins; 2007:1–15.)

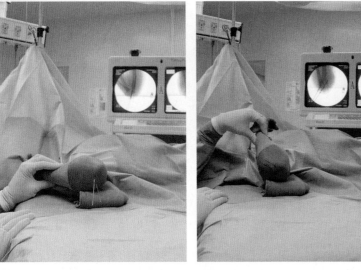
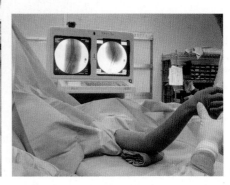

A, B   **C**

Figure 13-41. A: Assessment of sagittal alignment with lateral view. **B:** Both oblique views are checked to assess reduction of medial and lateral columns. **C:** If the lateral and oblique views show good reduction, the tape is removed and reduction and pin placement are checked in the AP view with elbow in relative elbow extension. (From Tolo VT, Skaggs DL, eds. *Master Techniques in Orthopaedic Surgery: Pediatrics.* Philadelphia, PA: Lippincott Williams & Wilkins; 2007:1–15.)

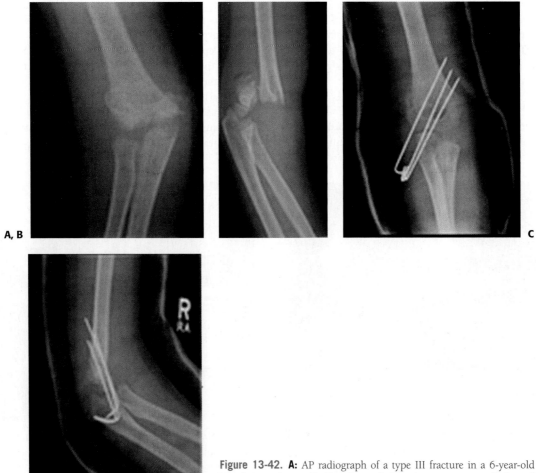

A, B   **C**

D

Figure 13-42. A: AP radiograph of a type III fracture in a 6-year-old boy. **B:** Lateral view. **C:** AP radiograph 3 weeks postoperative. **D:** Lateral view. (Reproduced with permission of Children's Orthopaedic Center, Los Angeles, CA.)

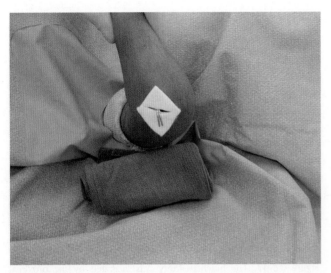

Figure 13-43. Skin is protected from pins with felt squares. (From Tolo VT, Skaggs DL, eds. *Master Techniques in Orthopaedic Surgery: Pediatrics.* Philadelphia, PA: Lippincott Williams & Wilkins; 2007:1–15.)

Postreduction Perfusion

If there is any question of perfusion following fracture reduction in the operating room, the surgical prep (Betadine) is removed to evaluate the skin color. In addition, a Doppler is used to assess for a triphasic pulse. In the case of a poorly perfused hand following reduction, open exploration and decompression or repair of the artery is required. In a case where the hand was well perfused prior to reduction and then poorly or not perfused after reduction and pinning, one must assume the artery, or adjacent tissue that kinks the vessel, is entrapped in the fracture site. The pins should be immediately removed and the fracture allowed to return to its unreduced position. If the hand is still avascular or dysvascular, open exploration of the artery is required. Either decompression or reconstruction will

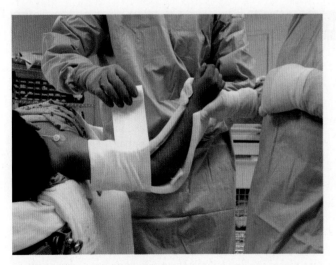

Figure 13-44. Sterile foam is placed directly on skin. If there is any circumferential dressing placed under the foam, it may be restricting. (From Tolo VT, Skaggs DL, eds. *Master Techniques in Orthopaedic Surgery: Pediatrics.* Philadelphia, PA: Lippincott Williams & Wilkins; 2007:1–15.)

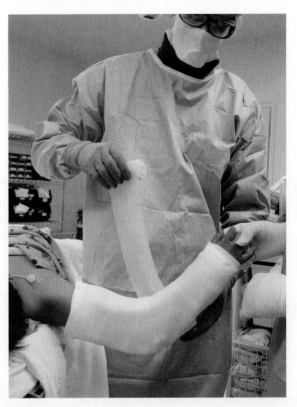

Figure 13-45. Cast with elbow flexion no more than 70 degrees and less flexion for very swollen elbows. (From Tolo VT, Skaggs DL, eds. *Master Techniques in Orthopaedic Surgery: Pediatrics.* Philadelphia, PA: Lippincott Williams & Wilkins; 2007:1–15.)

be necessary, followed by open reduction and repinning of fracture. If there is no pulse postoperatively in an arm that had no pulse preoperatively, but the hand is warm and well perfused, our preference is prolonged observation of the child in hospital for 48 hours with the arm mildly elevated (Fig. 13-46). This is especially true if there is associated median neuropathy preoperatively as the patient will not have the expected level of pain with a pending compartment syndrome. The rich collateral circulation about the elbow is generally sufficient to keep the hand viable but any alteration in vascularity requires prompt operative intervention.

Open Reduction and Pinning

Technique

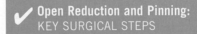
Open Reduction and Pinning:
KEY SURGICAL STEPS

- ☐ Exposure through a 4- to 5-cm transverse anterior incision above and parallel to the antecubital fossa at the fracture site
- ☐ Retract brachialis muscle and identify neurovascular bundle; untether or extract if constrained by fracture
- ☐ Remove periosteum
- ☐ Reduce and stabilize fracture, placing K-wires in the same manner as in closed reduction with percutaneous pinning
- ☐ Repair artery or reconstruct with vein graft if required
- ☐ Release forearm compartments

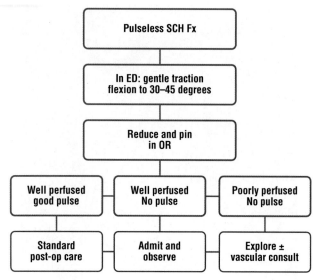

Figure 13-46. Algorithm for management of the pulseless supracondylar humerus fracture.

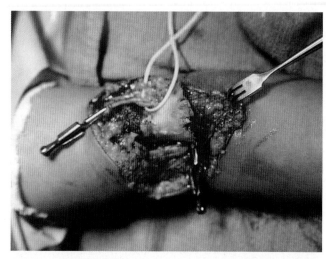

Figure 13-47. The brachial artery was lacerated by the proximal fragment. Bulldog clips have been placed on each end of the artery to control bleeding, and the median nerve is within the vessel loop. (Reproduced with permission from Children's Orthopaedic Center, Los Angeles, CA.)

Make a transverse anterior incision above and parallel to the antecubital fossa at the fracture site about 4 to 5 cm long, which allows access to the neurovascular structures and is aesthetic (see Fig. 13-42C). Retract the disrupted brachialis muscle and identify NVB proximal and distal to fracture site. Follow NVB to and across fracture site. If not unconstrained, untether or extract NVB from fracture site. If more visualization is needed, this incision can be extended medially or laterally based on displacement. Remove periosteum, which is often entrapped in the fracture site. Open

reduce and stabilize fracture. Place K-wires in the same manner as in closed reduction with percutaneous pinning. Just medial to the biceps tendon the brachial artery is noted, with the median nerve just medial to the artery. If the artery cannot be located in a patient presenting with a pulseless, poorly perfused hand search for the lacerated ends of a torn artery, which may have retracted proximally and distally (Fig. 13-47). Repair artery or reconstruct with vein graft if required. Release forearm compartments to prevent reperfusion compartment syndrome with arterial reconstruction.

Authors' Preferred Treatment for Supracondylar Fractures of the Distal Humerus

Type I to III Fractures (Algorithm 13-1)

Type I fractures are managed in a long-arm cast with approximately 60 to 90 degrees of elbow flexion for approximately 3 weeks. Follow-up x-rays at 1 week are recommended for assessment of fracture position.

We prefer closed reduction and pinning of most type II supracondylar fractures. Two lateral pins are chosen as the initial postreduction fixation method in nearly all cases (see Fig. 13-17). If two lateral pins fail to provide acceptable fixation, we do not hesitate to place a third lateral pin. We believe it is safer to hold a type II fracture reduced with pins, rather than flex the elbow greater than 90 degrees.

For type III fractures, CRPP is attempted first. If closed reduction cannot be obtained, open reduction with pinning is performed. A well-padded cast with sterile foam is applied, with x-rays at postoperative weeks 1 and 3, and pin removal at week 3.

Type IV Fractures (Algorithm 13-2)

Although this extremely unstable fracture could be treated with open reduction, we follow the protocol recommended by Leitch et al.[97] First, place two K-wires into the distal fragment. Next, the fracture is reduced in the AP plane and verified by imaging. At this point, rather than rotating the arm for a lateral image as is commonly done in more stable fracture patterns, the fluoroscopy unit is rotated into the lateral view (see Fig. 13-38B). The fracture is then reduced in the sagittal plane and the K-wires are driven across the fracture site. The reduction often is in midposition of flexion and extension (~60 degrees) and requires holding the reduction with distraction by the surgeon while the assistant places the first lateral entry stabilizing pin. Subsequent studies have also reported that over 80% of type IV fractures can be closed reduced and pin stabilized with good results.[144]

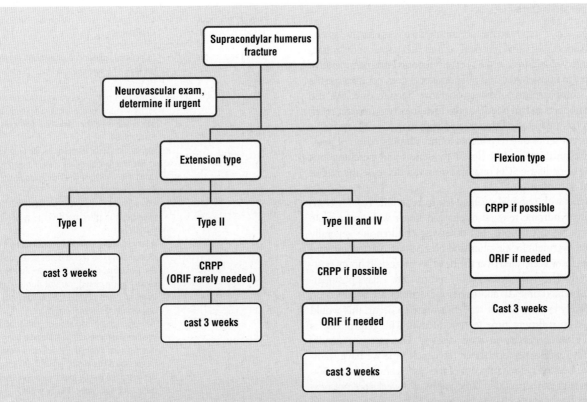

Algorithm 13-1. Authors' preferred treatment for type I to III supracondylar fractures of the distal humerus.

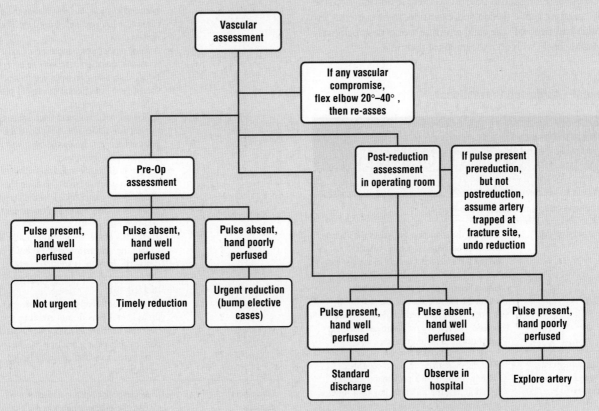

Algorithm 13-2. Authors' preferred treatment for type IV supracondylar fractures of the distal humerus.

Postoperative Care

Swanson et al.[156] reported that acetaminophen is as effective as narcotic analgesics for providing pain control after supracondylar fracture surgery in children, and Kay et al.[80] reported that perioperative ketorolac (a nonsteroidal anti-inflammatory) does not increase the risk of complications following operative fracture care. We use acetaminophen and an NSAID as the first-line drugs for pain relief, as narcotics are historically associated with more side effects.

A recent series of 618 patients found administration of postoperative antibiotics after closed reduction and percutaneous pinning of pediatric SCH fractures does not decrease the rate of surgical-site infection.[138]

Patients with minimal swelling felt to be at little risk for compartment syndrome may be discharged home with appropriate postoperative instructions, but otherwise children are generally admitted overnight for elevation and observation. We recommend that the elbow is elevated over the heart for at least 48 hours postoperatively. The patient customarily returns 5 to 7 days postoperatively at which time AP and lateral radiographs are obtained. In the unlikely event a loss of reduction were to occur, this would be noted in sufficient time for rereduction. This return visit is probably not necessary in most cases.[125] The cast is generally removed 3 weeks postoperatively, at which time we have traditionally obtained radiographs out of the cast. A study of over 500 patients suggest that routine radiographs at 3 weeks are not necessary as they did not change treatment.[78] The authors suggested only taking radiographs at 3 weeks if clinically indicated by pain, deformity, or a severe fracture pattern. The pins are removed in the outpatient setting at this time. ROM exercises are taught to the family, targeting gentle flexion and extension, to be started a few days after cast removal. The child returns 6 weeks postoperatively for a ROM check, with no radiographs at that time.

Potential Pitfalls and Preventions

Operative Treatment of Supracondylar Fractures of the Distal Humerus:
POTENTIAL PITFALLS AND PREVENTIONS

Pitfall	Prevention
Closed Reduction and Percutaneous Pinning	
Nerve entrapment	• If during the reduction maneuver the fracture does not stay reduced, and a "rubbery" feeling is encountered instead of the desired "bone-on-bone" feeling, the median nerve and/or brachial artery may be trapped within the fracture site (see Fig. 13-25). If this occurs, an open reduction is generally necessary to remove the neurovascular structures from the fracture site.
Proximal fragment has pierced the brachialis	• "Milking maneuver"[126]: the biceps are forcibly "milked" in a proximal to distal direction past the proximal fragment, often culminating in a palpable release of the humerus posteriorly through the brachialis (Fig. 13-48).
Inability to obtain closed reduction	• Milking maneuver; try pronation and/or supination
Loss of reduction	• In general, plan on a minimum of two pins for type II fractures and three pins for type III fractures. • If the first pin is in between where you really wanted two pins, just leave it and place one on either side of it for a total of three pins. • Aim to separate the pins as far as possible at the fracture site—at least 13 mm or one-third the width of the humerus at the level of the fracture. • Pin separation is more important than whether the pins are divergent or parallel. • A key element to ensure a correctly placed pin is to feel the pin go through the proximal cortex. If this feeling is not clearly appreciated, careful fluoroscopic imaging often reveals the pin did not engage the proximal fragment. • To optimize pin placement, think of the cartilaginous distal humerus as a pincushion. With the K-wires in your fingers (not the drill), push them into the cartilage in the exact location and trajectory you want. Verify with imaging, then advance the pin with a drill. • It is acceptable to cross the olecranon fossa, which adds two more cortices to improve fixation, but this means the elbow cannot be fully extended until the pins are removed. • A small amount of translation or axial rotational malalignment may be accepted rather than doing an open reduction, but accept very little frontal or sagittal plane angular malalignment. • Following reduction and fixation, stress the fracture under live imaging to the point where you are confident it will not fall apart postoperatively. • If there is difficulty maintaining fracture reduction when eternally rotating the shoulder for a lateral view of the elbow, move the C-arm instead of the patient's arm (see Fig. 13-40). • The child's elbow should sufficiently flex so that the fingers touch the shoulder. If not, the fracture is still likely not reduced and is in too much extension (Fig. 13-49). • In the exceptionally rare instance when three lateral pins do not stabilize the fracture, or there is an oblique fracture pattern preventing multiple lateral entry pins, a medial pin may be considered.
Ulnar nerve damage	• If you choose to place a medial pin, extend the elbow when placing the pin to keep the ulnar nerve posteriorly out of harm's way.

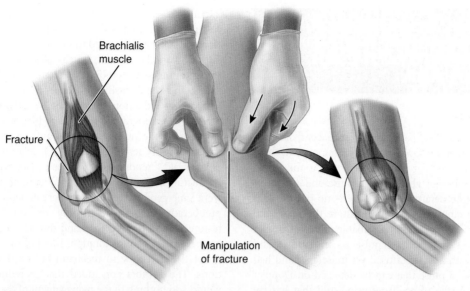

Figure 13-48. Brachialis muscle interposition is indicated on the left. The "milking maneuver" frees the brachialis muscle from its location in the fracture, allowing a closed reduction.

Decreased elbow flexion	• We save the images in which the reduction looks the "worst," particularly if some translational or rotational malreduction is accepted, to have them for comparison during postoperative visits to determine if movement of the fracture occurred. It has been noted that if the AHL is anterior to the capitellum following fracture healing, the child will go on to have less elbow flexion than if the AHL touches the capitellum, and even the AHL crossing the anterior third of the capitellum is associated with less elbow flexion than crossing the middle or posterior third.[76]

Compartment syndrome	• Cast the elbow in significantly less than 90 degrees of flexion; the pins are holding the reduction, not the cast. • Be attentive to the three As postoperatively: analgesia requirements increasing, anxiety, agitation
Postreduction perfusion	• If any question of perfusion, remove Betadine to evaluate the skin color; undertake Doppler assessment for a triphasic pulse. • Open exploration and decompression or repair of the artery may be required.

Open Reduction and Pinning

Damage to NVB	• Care must be taken in dissection as the NVB may be immediately superficial as it is pushed against the skin by the proximal fragment. • With an avascular or dysvascular hand, the NVB is usually tethered by soft tissues in fracture site and needs to be gently teased out of fracture without harm. Sometimes, the artery is in fracture site and requires atraumatic extraction. Rarely, it is completely lacerated and retracted away from fracture site proximally and distally.
Reduction difficulty	• A Freer can be used as a lever to elevate the periosteum out of entrapped position in the fracture site to assist the reduction. • Be certain to obtain anatomic alignment before pinning. • Reconstruct the artery if needed once the fracture is anatomic and stable.
Compartment syndrome	• Release the forearm compartments if revascularization is required to lessen risk of reperfusion compartment syndrome.

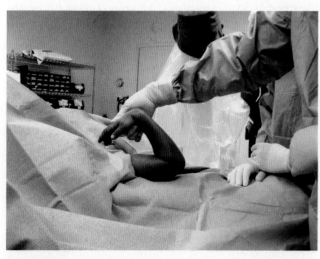

Figure 13-49. If fingers cannot touch shoulder, flexion deformity may not be reduced.

MANAGEMENT OF EXPECTED ADVERSE OUTCOMES AND UNEXPECTED COMPLICATIONS RELATED TO SUPRACONDYLAR FRACTURES OF THE DISTAL HUMERUS

VASCULAR INJURIES

Approximately 1% to 15% of patients with supracondylar fractures present with an absent pulse but only a minority of these patients will require vascular repair.[11,31,55,62,140] At the initial evaluation, the presence or absence of a pulse and perfusion of the hand should be determined. If there is no pulse, slight traction and gentle elbow flexion often restore the pulse and improve perfusion.[108] If there is not a palpable pulse, a Doppler may be used to assess for a triphasic pulse. As one study found that every patient with a well-perfused yet pulseless hand had a Dopplerable pulse, a pulse that can be detected on Doppler may be an objective sign of good perfusion, but that has yet to be proven clinically.[55] Perfusion of the hand is estimated by color, warmth, pulp turgor, and arterial capillary refill, but there is no study yet with clear evidence of the degree of reliability and validity of these standards. Capillary refill by itself can be deceiving. For example, after wrapping a rubber band around a finger, there is instant venous capillary refill but no artery inflow or venous outflow, so this must be differentiated from normal arterial capillary refill. Generally accepted normal perfusion criteria (viable hand) are capillary refill equivalent to the opposite side and less than 3 to 5 seconds, normal pulp turgor, and pink color. The clinician must distinguish between the nonviable and viable hand upon presentation and throughout care.

Hand perfusion, not presence or absence of a pulse, appears to be predictive of the need for arterial repair and risk of compartment syndrome. Choi et al.[31] reported on 25 pulseless patients whose hands were well perfused at presentation, and none (0%) required vascular repair or developed a compartment syndrome. In contrast, of eight patients who presented with poor distal perfusion, compartment syndrome developed in 25% and 38% underwent vascular repair. Garg et al.[55] reported on 54 pulseless supracondylar fractures. Twenty-six of the patients (48%) had a return of palpable pulse following reduction. Twenty of these patients observed postreduction had a well-perfused hand with a pulse that could not be palpated but that could be detected on Doppler, one of which required vascular repair after loss of hand perfusion 9 hours after the operative reduction. All of the other observed 19 patients had restoration of a palpable pulse by their first postoperative visit.

An absent radial pulse is not in itself an emergency, as collateral circulation may keep the limb well perfused in the short term and potentially even long term. In the case of a pulseless, well-perfused hand, urgent, but nonemergent, reduction with pinning in the operating room is indicated.[115,135,140] However, in the presence of an associated median nerve injury, there is higher risk of a compartment syndrome and more cautious close observation until surgery is indicated.[109] If the arm is pulseless and also has signs of poor perfusion (white color, decreased turgor, and/or slow capillary refill), this is an emergency.[3] When a patient with a severely displaced supracondylar fracture presents to the emergency room and has compromised vascularity to the limb, the arm should be repositioned with the elbow in approximately 20 to 40 degrees of flexion which may improve vascular flow.[108,115] Regardless of return of pulse after repositioning of the elbow, the fracture should be reduced and pinned in a timely fashion.[108]

Fracture reduction should not be delayed by any waiting time for an angiographic study, as reduction of the fracture usually restores the pulse.[3,30] Several authors state angiography is an unnecessary test that should not delay treatment.[33,108,124,140] Shaw et al.[140] reported on a series of 143 type III supracondylar fractures, 17 of which had vascular compromise. All underwent emergent reduction and percutaneous pinning without preoperative angiogram. In only 3 of the 17 (18%) patients, restored blood flow to the hand did not occur after reduction and required open exploration. In 14 of the 17 (82%) patients, restored blood flow to the hand occurred without complications. The authors concluded that prereduction angiography would add nothing to the management of these injuries. Copley et al.[33] used angiography in 4 of 17 (24%) dysvascular SCH fractures and found that the angiogram did not alter the course of management in any of the cases. Choi et al.[30] reported that of 25 patients presenting with a pulseless but well-perfused hand, 100% did well clinically without arterial repair—52% (11) had a palpable pulse following surgery, and 48% (10) remained pulseless but well perfused. Cheng et al.[28] in a series of 623 supracondylar fractures reported nine cases presenting with an absent radial pulse (1.4%), of which only one required exploration. Garg et al.[55] reported on 54 pulseless fractures, of which 9% (5/54) required vascular intervention.

Pulseless Hand

Prereduction White, Pulseless Hand

Standard treatment for a pulseless hand is closed reduction and percutaneous pinning. After closed reduction and stabilization, the pulse and perfusion of the hand should be evaluated. Usually, hand perfusion is restored. Most extension-type supracondylar fractures are reduced and pinned with the elbow in hyperflexion. With more than 120 degrees of elbow flexion, the radial pulse generally is lost, and the hand becomes pale, even in patients with an initially intact pulse and a viable hand. Following pinning when the arm is extended, the pulse frequently does not return immediately. This is presumably secondary to arterial spasm, aggravated by swelling about the artery and decreased peripheral perfusion in the anesthetized, somewhat cool intraoperative patient.

Because of this phenomenon, up to 10 to 15 minutes should be allowed for recovery of perfusion in the operating room before any decision is made regarding the need for exploring the brachial artery and restoring flow to the distal portion of the extremity. Because most patients without a palpable pulse regain and maintain adequate distal perfusion, the absence of a pulse alone is not an indication for exploring a brachial artery. However, hand viability is imperative and all poorly perfused hands require exploration.

If there is a prolonged poor or absent pulse, and/or poor perfusion, there is a high risk of compartment syndrome and a low threshold for intraoperative compartment pressure measurements and documentation. In cases of poor limb perfusion for over 6 hours, prophylactic forearm compartment release should be considered.

Postreduction White (Poorly Perfused), Pulseless Hand

Following reduction and pinning, a poorly perfused pulseless hand requires urgent treatment.[3,115] If there was a pulse before fracture reduction, but not after reduction, one must assume the artery or surrounding tissue is trapped at the fracture site, and pins should be pulled, and artery explored if the pulse does not return quickly. If there was not adequate perfusion before fracture reduction, and the hand remains poorly perfused after reduction, arterial exploration should be performed emergently.

Exploration through an anterior approach allows evaluation of arterial kinking by entrapped adjacent soft tissues or incarceration of the artery between the fracture fragments.[8,50] Once the artery is freed from the fracture, associated arterial spasm may be relieved by application of lidocaine, warming, and 10 to 15 minutes of observation. Following anatomic fracture reduction and decompression of the NVB of a pulseless limb, if the hand remains poorly perfused, vascular reconstruction is indicated by an appropriate specialist.

Postreduction Pink (Perfused), Pulseless Hand

If the pulse does not return, but the hand is well perfused following reduction, treatment is controversial.[108,133] Our practice is to admit the child to the hospital with gentle arm elevation and careful observation for at least 48 hours.[11] We have found the presence of a triphasic pulse by Doppler reassuring, but it does not necessarily change treatment. One study found that every patient (20/20) with a well-perfused yet pulseless hand had a pulse that was detectable on Doppler, suggesting this may be an objective sign of good perfusion.[55] A vascular consult may be called, particularly if there is no pulse by Doppler. The patient should be observed for increasing narcotic requirements, increasing pain, and decreased passive finger motion (i.e., the three As of a pending pediatric compartment syndrome: increasing anxiety, agitation, and analgesic requirement). Multiple authors report good results with observation of the postreduction pink pulseless hand.[3,30,62] However, a very low threshold for returning to the operating room for vascular exploration, decompression, and/or reconstruction along with forearm fasciotomies must be maintained rather than assuming that perfusion from collaterals is sufficient. There are known disastrous cases of permanent impairment in this setting.

Alternatively, vascular reconstruction may be performed in the pink pulseless hand. There has been some variance of results of reconstruction long term. Sabharwal et al.[135] have shown that early repair of the brachial artery has a high rate of symptomatic reocclusion or residual stenosis and recommended a period of close observation with frequent neurovascular checks before more invasive correction of this problem is contemplated. Many other studies report good results following vascular repair,[84,140] including an analysis of 19 studies with a patency rate of 91% in 54 patients with surgically repaired arteries.[163] Repair by microscopic techniques appears to have better long-term results.

Alves et al.[6] reported on 20 patients with brachial artery reconstruction with interposition vein grafting studied by duplex sonography, 19 of which had patent grafts with normal flow patterns and one had increased collateralization with reconstitution of normal flow distal to the elbow.

Lally et al.[92] reported on the long-term follow-up of 27 patients who had brachial artery ligation as a child for renal transplant. Decreased mean systolic pressure was noted in the affected limb in about 25% of patients and 67% had mildly decreased exercise tolerance. There was no significant difference in limb circumference or length.

VASCULAR STUDIES

There is currently no generally accepted evidence that further vascular studies beyond pulse and perfusion lead to improved outcomes, though this is an area of active research.[11] A review of articles subsequent to 1980 in the vascular surgical literature concludes, "Both angiography and color duplex ultrasound provide little benefit in the management of these patients. A child with a pink pulseless hand postfracture reduction can be managed expectantly unless additional signs of vascular compromise develop, in which exploration should be undertaken."[62] Similarly, some surgeons in the past have recommended pulse oximetry[131] for evaluating postreduction circulation, though this has not been shown to discriminate the nonviable from the viable hand.

PULSELESS ARM WITH MEDIAN NERVE INJURY

If the arm is pulseless and has a median nerve deficit, special attention is warranted.[133] With injury to both the brachial artery and a nerve, we can assume that significant soft tissue damage has occurred, which places the child at higher risk for a compartment syndrome. The pain of a compartment syndrome may be masked by the nerve injury, so, very careful assessment and monitoring for a compartment syndrome are needed throughout the perioperative period, with a low threshold for vascular exploration and/or compartment release.[109] Mangat et al.[102] reported on seven patients who were pulseless with a median nerve injury, and all seven patients were found to have the brachial artery trapped or tethered at the fracture site. They recommend early exploration of the brachial artery in a Gartland type III supracondylar fracture in patients who present with an absent pulse and a coexisting anterior interosseous or median nerve palsy, as these appear to be strongly predictive of nerve and vessel entrapment. In contrast, they found only 20% of pulseless extremities without a nerve deficit had the artery trapped or tethered.

EXPLORATION OF THE BRACHIAL ARTERY

Often, during the open reduction of the fracture, release of a fascial band or an adventitial tether resolves the problem of obstructed flow. In some patients, however, a formal vascular repair and/or vein grafting is required, at which time many orthopedic surgeons will consult colleagues with vascular expertise. The brachial artery is approached through an anteromedial transverse incision at the level of the fracture above the antecubital fossa. Often, this provides excellent exposure of the fracture site and NVB. Distal and proximal extension can be performed with Z-limbs if necessary, as described in the authors' preferred method for open reduction (see Fig. 13-42C).

If the hand is still nonviable after reduction and pinning the fracture, care must be taken because the NVB may be difficult to identify when it is surrounded by hematoma or lies in a very superficial position. At the level of the fracture, the artery may seem to disappear into the fracture site, covered with shredded brachialis muscle. The artery is likely tethered by a fascial band or arterial adventitia attached to the proximal metaphyseal spike pulling the artery in the fracture site. Dissection is often best accomplished proximally to distally, along the brachial artery, identifying both the artery and the median nerve. Arterial injury is generally at the level of the supratrochlear artery (Fig. 13-50), which provides a tether, making the artery vulnerable at this location. Arterial transection or direct arterial injury can be identified at this level.

If arterial spasm is the cause of inadequate flow, and collateral flow is not sufficient to maintain the hand, attempts to relieve the spasm may be tried. Once the artery is no longer kinked or tethered, direct application of papaverine or local anesthetic to the artery has been found to be beneficial. Sympathetic block with a stellate ganglion block may prolong the vasodilatory effect. If these techniques do not relieve the spasm, and if collateral flow is insufficient to maintain a viable hand, there most likely is an intimal injury and occlusion. In these rare situations, the injured portion of the vessel is excised and a reverse vein graft of appropriate size is inserted, usually from the same extremity. Prophylactic release of forearm fascia is indicated in cases of prolonged ischemia to prevent a reperfusion compartment syndrome. When flow is restored, the wound is closed, the patient is placed in a splint or foam and cast with the elbow in approximately 60 degrees of flexion, and the forearm is in neutral pronation and supination. Postoperative monitoring should include frequent examinations of perfusion and for signs of compartment syndrome or ischemia. Although injecting urokinase has been suggested to increase flow,[25] we no longer advocate that technique because of systemic risks.

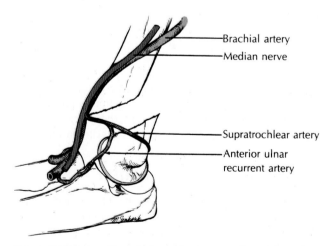

Figure 13-50. Arterial pathology. The supratrochlear branch that arises from the anterior ulnar recurrent artery may bind the main trunk of the brachial artery against the sharp end of the proximal fragment. (Reprinted from Rowell PJW. Arterial occlusion in juvenile humeral supracondylar fracture. *Injury.* 1974;6(3):254–256. Copyright © 1975 Elsevier Ltd. With permission.)

Compartment Syndrome

The prevalence of compartment syndrome in the setting of a supracondylar fracture is estimated to be 0.1% to 0.5%.[15,16] The classic five Ps for the diagnosis of compartment syndrome—pain, pallor, pulselessness, paresthesias, and paralysis—are poor indicators of a compartment syndrome in children. Bae et al.[12] reported increasing analgesia requirement in combination with other clinical signs is a more sensitive and earlier indicator of compartment syndrome in children. They found that 10 children with access to patient-controlled or nurse-administered analgesia had increasing requirement for pain medication. Resistance to passive finger movement and dramatically increasing pain after fracture are clinical signs of compartment syndrome of the forearm. Special attention must be paid to supracondylar fractures with median nerve injuries, as the patient will not feel pain in the volar compartment.[109] A compartment syndrome of the forearm may occur with or without brachial artery injury and in the presence or absence of a radial pulse.

If the supracondylar fracture's mechanism of injury is high energy as evidenced by crushing or associated fractures, there is an increased risk for compartment syndrome. A small series of patients suggested that an associated forearm fracture is associated with compartment syndrome, but Muchow reported a larger series of 1,288 patients that did not find an associated increased risk of compartment syndrome.[110] Such retrospective studies are difficult to interpret, because those patients with forearm fractures may have been treated differently (more urgently, elevation, etc.). Ring et al.[132] found 6 of 10 pediatric floating elbows with pending or true compartment syndromes and recommend pinning of both forearm and SCH fractures. An arterial injury in association with multiple injuries or crush injury further diminishes blood flow to the forearm musculature and increases the probability of a compartment syndrome.

In a multicenter review, Ramachandran et al.[129] identified 11 cases in which children with supracondylar fracture developed compartment syndrome despite presenting with closed, low-energy injuries and no associated fractures or vascular compromise. This series is disturbing as it demonstrates that compartment syndrome still occurs with modern treatment, even in children who may be thought to be at low risk. They found that in 10 of 11 patients' charts, excessive swelling was noted at time of presentation. The 10 cases with severe elbow swelling documented at presentation had a mean delay until surgery of 22 hours. This study suggests excessive swelling combined with delay in treatment is a risk factor for development of compartment syndrome. The authors also noted that even if distal pulse is found by palpation or Doppler examination, an evolving compartment syndrome may be present.

If one is concerned that a compartment syndrome may be evolving, initial management includes removing all circumferential dressings. Battaglia et al.[16] documented the relationship between increasing elbow flexion above 90 degrees and increasing volar compartment pressure, so the elbow should be extended to a position well below 90 degrees. The volar compartment should be palpated, and the elbow should be extended. We believe that the fracture should be immediately stabilized with K-wires to allow proper management of the soft tissues.

Another factor that contributes to the development of compartment syndrome is warm ischemic time after injury. When blood flow is compromised and the hand is pale with no arterial flow, muscle ischemia is possible, depending on the time of oxygen deprivation. After fracture reduction and flow restoration, the warm ischemic time should be noted. If this time is more than 6 hours, compartment syndrome secondary to ischemic muscle injury is likely. Prophylactic volar compartment fasciotomy can be performed at the time of arterial reconstruction. The exact indication for prophylactic fasciotomy in the absence of an operative revascularization is uncertain. Even when the diagnosis is delayed or if the compartment syndrome is chronic, fasciotomy has been shown to be of some value.

Blakey et al.[18] reported on the experience of their specialized center over a 21-year period. At a mean of 3 months after sustaining an SCH fracture, 23 children with ischemic contractures of the forearm were referred. The authors recommend that urgent exploration of the vessels and nerves in a child with a "pink pulseless hand" following fracture reduction with persistent and increasing pain suggests critical ischemia. No further conclusions regarding acute care of patients with a pink pulseless hand that does not have increasing pain suggestive of ischemia can be drawn from this retrospective study of established ischemic contractures.

Neurologic Deficit

A meta-analysis of 3,457 extension-type SCH fractures found an overall neurapraxia rate of 13%, with the AIN (5%) being the most common, followed by the radial nerve (4%).[10] The largest single-center study of type III fractures reported 12% nerve injuries at presentation, with a rate of 19% of nerve injuries if there was an associated forearm fracture that required reduction.[55] A prospective study limited to examinations of operatively treated SCHFs performed by pediatric fellowship–trained surgeons on patients the surgeons felt could give a reliable examination, found a rate of 16% nerve injury: median 12% (12/100) (including 8 AIN injuries), radial 8% (8/100), ulnar 3% (3/100). A trend was seen between fracture severity and rate of a preoperative nerve injury: type II 7% (2/28), type III 19% (9/58), and type IV 36% (5/14) (P = 0.058).[74] A recent single-center study[141] of 244 nerve injuries associated with SCH fractures revealed 11% of extension fractures have a nerve injury: 86% were single nerve involvement (14% multiple nerves injured) and 29% had concurrent vascular injury. The most common nerve injured was also median nerve (62%).

AIN palsy presents as paralysis of the long flexors of the thumb (FPLY) and index finger (FDP II) without sensory changes. Complete median nerve injury occurs from a more severe contusion, entrapment, or even rare transection of the nerve at the level of the fracture and presents with sensory loss in the median nerve distribution as well as motor loss of all muscles innervated by the median nerve (extrinsic and intrinsic). Nerve transections are rare and almost exclusively involve the radial nerve.[104,105]

The direction of the fracture's displacement determines the nerve most likely to be injured. If the distal fragment is displaced posteromedially, the radial nerve is more likely to be injured. Conversely, if the displacement of the distal fragment is posterolateral, the NVB is stretched over the proximal fragment, injuring the complete median nerve or isolated AIN. In a flexion-type supracondylar fracture, which is rare, the ulnar nerve is the most likely nerve to be injured (see Fig. 13-9).

Open reduction and exploration of the injured nerve are not necessarily indicated in cases of nerve injury in a closed fracture. Neural recovery, regardless of which nerve is injured, generally occurs with observation, but may take 6 months or more.[24,141] In the large series of 244 displaced extension SCH fractures with nerve injuries out of Boston Children's Hospital, 60% of median nerve injuries had recovery at 3 months and 92% had complete recovery at follow-up, with median time to recovery of 2.3 months. Isolated median nerve injuries recovered faster (70% by 3 months) than median nerve injuries associated with multiple nerve injuries, which took 54% longer to recovery. Radial nerve injuries took 30% longer to recover, with only 42% having recovered by 3 months.[141]

Culp et al.[35] reported identification of eight injured nerves in five patients in which spontaneous recovery did not occur by 5 months after injury. Neurolysis was successful in restoring nerve function in all but one patient. Shore et al.[141] noted five cases with poor recovery requiring surgery, none of which had decompression as part of open reduction internal fixation of fracture. None of the patients who had nerve decompression as part of operative treatment of the fracture and/or vascular injury had a long-term nerve deficit. Nerve grafting may be indicated for nerves not in continuity at the time of exploration. Release of tethering and entrapment with neurolysis for perineural fibrosis are generally successful in restoring nerve function. There is no indication for early electromyographic analysis or treatment other than observation for nerve deficit until 3 to 6 months after fracture. Failure to observe an advancing Tinel's sign and expected neural recovery as outlined above leads to exploration and treatment.

In their series of radial nerve injuries with humeral fractures, Amillo et al.[7] reported that of 12 injuries that did not spontaneously recover within 6 months of injury, only one was associated with a supracondylar fracture. Perineural fibrosis was present in four patients, three nerves were entrapped in callus, and five were either partially or totally transected.

In the supracondylar area, nerve compression and perineural fibrosis appears to be the most common cause of prolonged nerve deficit. Although nerve injury is related to fracture displacement, a neural deficit can exist with even minimally displaced fractures. Sairyo et al.[136] reported one patient in whom radial nerve palsy occurred with a slightly angulated fracture that appeared to be a purely extension-type fracture on initial x-rays. Even in patients with mild injuries, a complete neurologic examination should be performed before treatment. An irreducible fracture with nerve deficit is an indication for open reduction of the fracture to ensure that there is no nerve entrapment. Chronic nerve entrapment in healed callus can give the appearance of a hole in the bone, Metev's sign.

Iatrogenic injury to the ulnar nerve has been reported to occur in 1% to 15% of patients with supracondylar fractures.[24,44,130,150] In a large series of type III supracondylar fractures, the rate of iatrogenic injury to the radial nerve was less than 1%. The course of the ulnar nerve through the cubital tunnel, between the medial epicondyle and the olecranon, makes it vulnerable when a medial pin is placed. Rasool[130] demonstrated with operative exploration that the pin usually did not impale the ulnar nerve, but more commonly constricted the nerve within the cubital tunnel by tethering adjacent soft tissue. These findings were later confirmed by an ultrasonographic study by Karakurt et al.[77] Zaltz et al.[171] reported that in children less than 5 years of age, when the elbow is flexed more than 90 degrees, the ulnar nerve migrated over, or even anterior to, the medial epicondyle in 61% (32/52) of children. It has been suggested that placement of lateral entry pins first, followed by elbow extension to relax tension on the ulnar nerve and subsequent placement of a medial pin, could decrease the risk of iatrogenic nerve injury. Using this technique, Edmonds et al. reported a 1.1% (2/187) rate of iatrogenic ulnar nerve injury with medial pins.[44]

If an iatrogenic ulnar nerve injury occurs following placement of a medial pin, there is a lack of literature on which to base treatment. Lyons et al.[99] reported on 17 patients with iatrogenic ulnar nerve injuries presumably due to a medial pin. All 17 patients had complete return of function, though many not until 4 months. Only 4 of the 17 (24%) had the medial pins removed. This study demonstrates that ulnar nerve function may eventually return without pin removal. Brown and Zinar[24] reported four ulnar nerve injuries associated with pinning of supracondylar fractures, all of which resolved spontaneously 2 to 4 months after pinning. Rasool[130] reported six patients with ulnar nerve injuries in whom early exploration was performed. In two patients, the nerve was penetrated, and in three, it was constricted by a retinaculum over the cubital tunnel, aggravated by the pin. In one patient, the nerve was subluxed and was fixed anterior to the cubital tunnel by the pin. Full recovery occurred in three patients, partial recovery in two, and no recovery in two. Spontaneous recovery of ulnar nerve function was reported in three patients. One nerve that was explored had direct penetration, and the pin was replaced in the proper position. Two patients had late-onset ulnar nerve palsies discovered during healing, and the medial pin was removed.

If an immediate postoperative neural injury is documented, we prefer to explore the ulnar nerve and to replace the pin in the proper position or convert to a lateral pin construct. Common sense suggests that removal of the causative factor (the medial pin) earlier rather than later may lead to a quicker recovery of the nerve.[24,130,171]

Preventing ulnar nerve injury is obviously more desirable than treating ulnar neuropathy. Because of the frequency of ulnar nerve injury with crossed pinning, most surgeons prefer to use two or three lateral pins if possible and no medial pin. Successful maintenance of alignment of type III supracondylar fractures with lateral pins has been reported in many series.[82,148,150] In our opinion, the only technique for avoiding iatrogenic ulnar nerve injury across is to use lateral entry pins, and avoid the use of cross-pins if not needed for fracture fixation. However, one meta-analysis of 3,457 extension-type fractures reported an iatrogenic neurapraxia rate of 1.9% for laterally placed pins.[10] Remember, any nerve can be injured by any aberrant pin placement.

Elbow Stiffness

Clinically significant loss of motion after extension-type supracondylar fractures is rare in children. In a study of 45 children with SCH fractures who did not undergo physical therapy, 90% ROM returned at 30 days for extension and 39 days for flexion.[161] In another report of 63 patients with closed reduction percutaneous pinning of supracondylar fractures of the humerus stabilized with either two or three lateral entry pins, elbow ROM returned to 72% of contralateral elbow motion by 6 weeks after pinning and progressively increased to 86% by 12 weeks, 94% by 26 weeks, and 98% by 52 weeks.[173] Pins were removed by 3 to 4 weeks. No patient participated in formal physical therapy.

Although most children do not require formal physical therapy, we generally teach the parents ROM exercises to be performed at home following pin and cast removal at about 3 to 4 weeks. A follow-up appointment to assess ROM is scheduled about 4 to 8 weeks later, and if motion is not nearly normal at that time, a physical therapy to improve elbow motion is begun.

Significant loss of flexion can be caused by a lack of anatomic fracture reduction: either posterior distal fragment angulation, posterior translation of the distal fragment with anterior impingement, or medial rotation of the distal fragment with a protruding medial metaphyseal spike proximally (Fig. 13-51). In young children with significant growth potential, there may be significant remodeling of anterior impingement, and any corrective surgery should be delayed for at least 1 year. Although anterior impingement can significantly remodel, there is risk of limited remodeling of persistent posterior angulation or hyperextension.

Pin-Tract Infections

The reported prevalence of pin-tract infections in SCH fractures ranges from less than 1% to 2.5% with closed reduction and standard pinning techniques[16,55,148] in most series, though one series reports a rate of 4.3% (21/490), noting that about half of the patients with infections did not receive preoperative antibiotics.[118] In a retrospective review of 622 operative treated patients, one patient developed a deep infection with septic arthritis and osteomyelitis (0.2%). Five additional patients had superficial skin infections and were treated with oral antibiotics for a total infection rate of 6 of 622 patients (1%).[15] Lateral entry pins can enter the risk of carry risk of deep-spaced infection, so expedient care of superficial infections is appropriate.

Pin-tract infections generally resolve with pin removal and antibiotics. Fortunately, by the time a pin-tract infection develops, the fracture is usually stable enough to remove the pin without loss of reduction. However, an untreated pin-tract infection can result in a septic joint and should thus be treated as soon as is recognized or suspected. Interviews of patients 18 years after infected pin tracts show no long-term sequelae.[118]

Pin Migration

In one retrospective series of 622 patients,[15] the most common complication was pin migration, necessitating unexpected

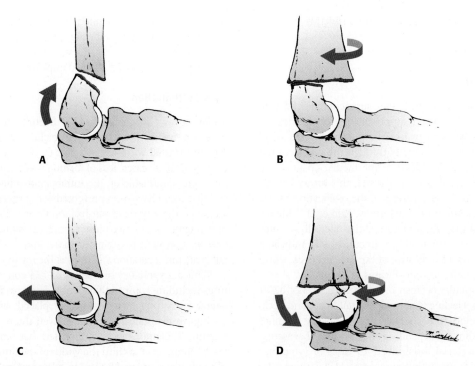

Figure 13-51. Distal fragment rotation. **A:** Posterior angulation only of the distal fragment. **B:** Pure horizontal rotation without angulation. **C:** Pure posterior translocation without rotation or angulation. **D:** Horizontal rotation with coronal tilting, producing a cubitus varus deformity. There is a positive crescent sign. **C, D:** (Redrawn after Marion J, LaGrange J, Faysse R, et al. Les fractures de l'extremite inferieure de l'humerus chez l'enfant. *Rev Chir Orthop*. 1962;48:337–413.)

return to the operating room for pin removal in 11 patients (1.8%). This complication can be minimized by both bending at least 1 cm of pin at a 90-degree angle, at least 1 cm from the skin, and protecting the skin with thick felt over the pin (see Fig. 13-42A) or using commercially available pin covers.

Myositis Ossificans

Myositis ossificans is a remarkably rare complication of supracondylar fractures, but it can occur (Fig. 13-52). This complication has been described after closed and open reductions due to disruption of the brachialis with injury, but vigorous postoperative manipulation or physical therapy is believed to be an associated factor.[124]

In a report of two patients with myositis ossificans after closed reduction of supracondylar fractures, Aitken et al.[4] noted that limitation of motion and calcification disappeared after 2 years. Postoperative myositis ossificans can be observed with the expectation of spontaneous resolution of both restricted motion and the myositis ossificans. There is no indication for early excision. O'Driscoll et al.[113] reported a single case of myositis ossificans associated with sudden onset of pain posttrauma in which a 1-year-old lesion of myositis ossificans was fractured. With excision, the pain was relieved and full ROM returned.

Nonunion

The distal humeral metaphysis is a well-vascularized area with remarkably rapid healing, and nonunion of a supracondylar

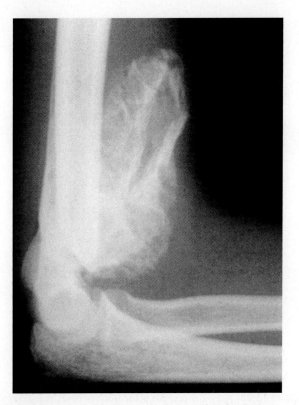

Figure 13-52. Myositis ossificans. Ossification of the brachialis muscle developed in this 8 year old who had undergone multiple attempts at reduction. (Courtesy of John Schaeffer, MD.)

fracture is rare. We have not seen nonunion of this fracture. With infection, devascularization, and soft tissue loss, the risk of nonunion would presumably increase.

Avascular Necrosis

Avascular necrosis of the trochlea after supracondylar fracture has been reported.[46] The blood supply of the trochlea's ossification center is fragile, with two separate sources. One small artery is lateral and courses directly through the physis of the medial condyle. It provides blood to the medial crista of the trochlea. If the fracture line is very distal, this artery can be injured, producing avascular necrosis of the ossification center and resulting in a classic fishtail deformity. Kim et al.[81] identified 18 children with trochlear abnormalities after elbow injuries, five of which were supracondylar fractures. MRI indicated low-signal intensity on T2 indicative of cartilage necrosis. Cubitus varus deformity developed in all cases.

Symptoms of avascular necrosis of the trochlea do not occur for months or years. Healing is normal, but mild pain and occasional locking develop with characteristic radiologic findings and motion may be limited depending on the extent of avascular necrosis. Glotzbecker et al.[58] described 15 cases of symptomatic fishtail deformity presenting an average of 4.7 years after fracture, 80% of whom had mechanical symptoms of locking, catching, and painful limited motion. An important risk for AVN of the trochlea is following an open reduction of a supracondylar fracture through a posterior approach, which presumably disrupts the blood supply of the trochlea (Fig. 13-53). Treatment

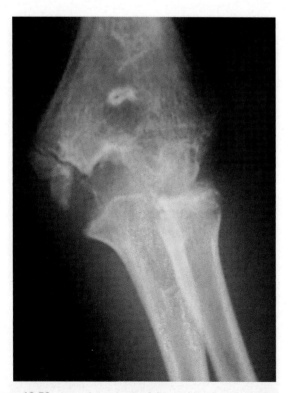

Figure 13-53. Avascular necrosis of the trochlea developed following open reduction through a posterior approach. The child had limited motion and symptoms of occasional catching. (Reproduced with permission from Children's Orthopaedic Center, Los Angeles, CA.)

options at present are limited but medial and lateral column growth arrests to stop deformity progression; and arthroscopic debridement and removal of osteochondral loose bodies have been reported to provide clinical improvement.

Loss of Reduction

Sankar et al.[137] in a series of 322 fractures reported 2.9% had postoperative loss of fixation. All eight were Gartland type III fractures treated with just two pins (seven lateral entry and one cross-pin). In all cases, loss of fixation was due to technical errors that were identifiable on the intraoperative fluoroscopic images and that could have been prevented with proper technique. They identified three types of pin-fixation errors: (1) failure to engage both fragments with two pins or more, (2) failure to achieve bicortical fixation with two pins or more, and (3) failure to achieve adequate pin separation (>2 mm) at the fracture site (Fig. 13-54).

Clinical experience of a series of 124 consecutive SCH fractures including completely unstable fractures has taught us that lateral entry pins, when properly placed, are usually strong enough to maintain reduction of even the most unstable SCH fracture.[148] Pennock et al.[122] reported that pins separated by at least 13 mm, or one-third the width of the humerus, at the level of the fracture on an AP view is an important factor in helping to prevent loss of reduction.

When loss of reduction is noted within the first 1 to 2 weeks, revision closed reduction is usually effective. A report of 21 supracondylar fractures that lost reduction underwent revision surgery at a mean of 7.6 days (range, 3 to 18 days). Seventeen were treated with closed reduction and four required open reduction. Two cases resulted in cubitus varus, and three patients lacked 10 degrees of motion at final follow-up.[117]

Cubitus Varus

Cubitus varus, also known as a "gunstock deformity," has a characteristic appearance in the frontal plane (Fig. 13-55). The malunion also includes hyperextension, which leads to increased elbow extension and decreased elbow flexion (Fig. 13-56). The appearance of cubitus varus deformity is distinctive upon x-ray. On the AP view, the angle of the physis of the lateral condyle (Baumann's angle) is more horizontal than normal (Fig. 13-57). On the lateral view, hyperextension of the distal fragment posterior to the AHL goes along with the clinical findings of increased extension and decreased flexion of the elbow (Fig. 13-58).

It has been proposed that unequal growth in the distal humerus causes cubitus varus deformity, but this seems unlikely, as there is not enough growth in this area to cause cubitus varus within the time it is recognized. The most common reason for cubitus varus in patients with supracondylar fractures is likely malunion rather than growth arrest. Cubitus varus can be prevented by making certain Baumann's angle is intact at the time of reduction and remains so during healing by achieving stable fixation. Pirone et al.[124] reported cubitus varus deformities in 8 of 101 (7.9%) patients treated with cast immobilization compared to 2 of 105 (1.9%) patients with pin fixation, with ages ranging from 1.5 to 14 years (mean of 6.4 years). A decrease in frequency of cubitus varus deformity after the use of percutaneous pin fixation has been reflected in other series.[53,124]

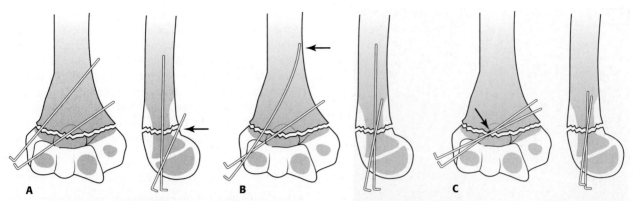

Figure 13-54. Illustrations depicting errors in pin-fixation technique. **A:** The *black arrow* demonstrates the anterior pin failing to transfix the proximal bone. **B:** The *black arrow* demonstrates one pin without bicortical purchase. **C:** The *black arrow* demonstrates pins too close together at the fracture site.

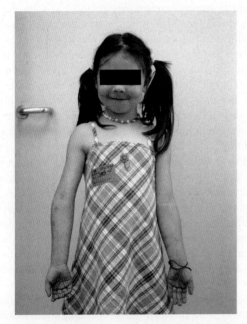

Figure 13-55. Five-year-old girl with cubitus varus of right elbow following a malunion of a supracondylar humerus fracture. (Reproduced with permission of Children's Orthopaedic Center, Los Angeles, CA.)

The distal humerus growth is 20% of that of its overall length. In a 5 year old then, the amount of distal humeral growth in 1 year is approximately 2 mm, making it unlikely that growth asymmetry is a significant cause of varus deformity that occurs within the first 6 to 12 months after fracture. Avascular necrosis of the trochlea or medial portion of the distal humeral fragment can result in progressive varus deformity. However, in a series of 36 varus deformities reported by Voss et al.,[160] only four patients had medial growth disturbance and distal humeral avascular necrosis as a cause of progressive varus deformity.

Treatment for cubitus varus has in the past been considered for aesthetic reasons only. However, there are several consequences of cubitus varus such as an increased risk of lateral condyle fractures, pain, and tardy posterolateral rotatory instability, which may be indications for an operative reconstruction with a supracondylar humeral osteotomy.[2,113] Our experience suggested many patients have elbow discomfort with significant cubitus varus. Takahara et al.[157] reported nine patients with distal humeral fractures complicating varus deformity. Supracondylar fractures as well as epiphyseal separations were included in these nine fractures. Further problems complicating varus deformity involved the shoulder. Tardy ulnar nerve palsy has also been associated with varus and internal rotational malalignment.[64]

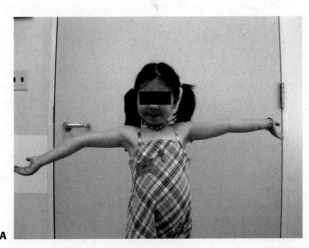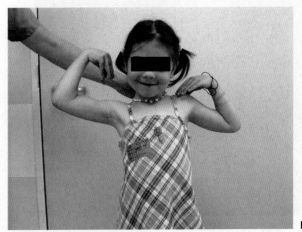

Figure 13-56. A: Hyperextension of right elbow. **B:** Decreased flexion of right elbow. (Reproduced with permission of Children's Orthopaedic Center, Los Angeles, CA.)

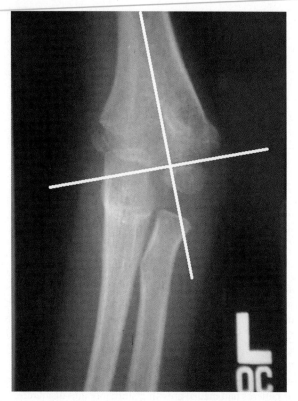

Figure 13-57. AP radiograph of the girl in preceding clinical photos. (Reproduced with permission of Children's Orthopaedic Center, Los Angeles, CA.)

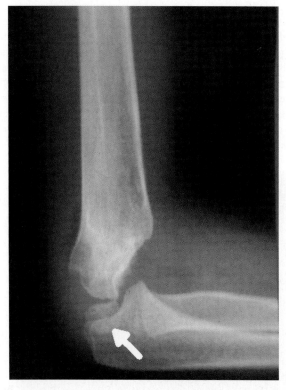

Figure 13-58. Lateral radiograph shows overlapping of the distal humerus with the olecranon (*arrow*) producing the typical crescent sign. Note the anterior humeral line is anterior to the capitellum.

Cubitus varus deformity is also associated with a significant increase in late ulnar nerve palsies, as reported in the Japanese literature.[2] With a cubitus varus deformity, the olecranon fossa moves to the ulnar side of the distal humerus, and the triceps shifts a bit ulnarward. Investigators theorized that this ulnar shift might compress the ulnar nerve against the medial epicondyle, narrowing the cubital tunnel and resulting in chronic neuropathy. A fibrous band running between the heads of the flexor carpi ulnaris was thought to cause ulnar nerve compression.[2]

Treatment

As for the treatment of any posttraumatic malalignment, options include observation with expected remodeling, hemiepiphysiodesis and growth alteration, and corrective osteotomy. Observation is generally not successful in achieving anatomic alignment as hyperextension may remodel to some degree in a young child (Fig. 13-59), but in an older child, insufficient remodeling occurs even in the joint's plane of motion.

Hemiepiphysiodesis of the distal humerus is rarely of value in restoring anatomic alignment, only to prevent cubitus varus deformity from developing in a patient with clear medial growth arrest or trochlear avascular necrosis. If untreated, medial growth disturbance will lead to lateral overgrowth and progressive deformity. Lateral epiphysiodesis will not correct the deformity, but will prevent it from increasing. Because of the slow growth rate in the distal humerus, we do not believe there is any role for lateral epiphysiodesis in correcting a varus deformity in a child with otherwise normal physis.

Osteotomy is the only way to correct a cubitus varus deformity with a high probability of success. High complication rates in historic series have led to some controversy about the value of a distal humeral corrective osteotomy for cubitus varus deformity. In a review of 41 patients undergoing distal humeral osteotomies for malunions following SCH fractures at two major pediatric centers, Weiss et al.[162] reported a complication rate of 53% with a 32% return to the operating room in surgeries performed between 1987 and 1997. However, in surgeries performed from 1998 to 2002, the complication rate was 14% with a 0% reoperation rate. This group found that when lateral entry pins were used to fix the osteotomy, there were significantly less complications.[162]

Because malunion is the cause of most cubitus varus deformities, the angular deformity usually occurs at the level of the fracture. Rotation and hypertension may contribute to the deformity, but varus is the most significant factor.[29] Hyperextension can produce a severe deformity in some patients. An oblique configuration (Fig. 13-60) places the corrective osteotomy's center of rotation as close to the actual level of the deformity as possible. On an AP x-ray of the humerus with the forearm in full supination, the size of the wedge and the angular correction needed are determined. An "incomplete" lateral closing wedge osteotomy may be performed, leaving a small medial hinge of bone intact. This protects the ulnar nerve and provides rotational stability to the osteotomy. The osteotomy usually is fixed with two K-wires placed laterally (two or three with spread and divergence). In the absence of an intact medial hinge, two lateral wires probably are not sufficient to secure

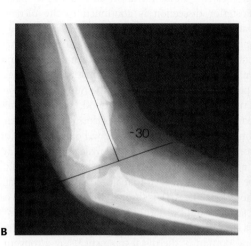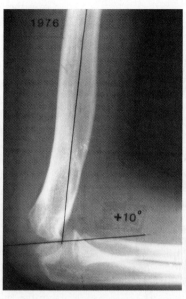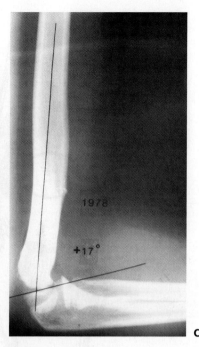

Figure 13-59. A hyperextension deformity in the distal humerus may remodel somewhat, whereas varus and valgus deformities do not. **A:** Hyperextension deformity in the distal humerus after fracture. **B:** Four years later, a more normal distal humeral anatomy is seen with remodeling of the hyperextension deformity. **C:** Two years after that, a normal distal humeral anatomy has been reinstated.

this osteotomy.[160] Crossed wires may be useful in this situation. In general, an oblique lateral closing wedge osteotomy with a medial hinge will correct the varus deformity, with minor correction of hyperextension unless one of the two osteotomy cuts has slightly more anterior wedge removed at the time of lateral wedge excision.[160] A transverse lateral closing wedge has more risk of a lateral bump with poor aesthetics. Residual rotational

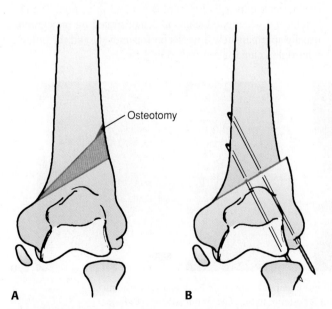

Figure 13-60. A: By moving the apex of the closing wedge distally, the osteotomy's center of rotation is moved closer to the deformity. **B:** Upon closing a distally based wedge osteotomy, there is less translational effect than in a more proximally based osteotomy.

deformity was not found to be a significant problem in studies by Voss et al.,[160] which is logical given the amount of rotation available from the shoulder.

Higaki and Ikuta[69] described a dome osteotomy in which a curved osteotomy is made in the supracondylar area. Proponents of this osteotomy suggest that multiplane correction is possible without inducing translation in the distal fragment and that rotation can be corrected. DeRosa and Graziano[39] described a step-cut osteotomy in which the distal fragment is slotted into the proximal fragment and the osteotomy is secured with a single screw. Functional outcomes are generally good, but the preoperative functional deficit is nearly always minor in patients with cubitus varus deformities.

Hyperextension deformity may remodel over time (see Fig. 13-57), but correction is slow and inconsistent. In one series,[160] hyperextension deformities remodeled as much as 30 degrees in very young children, but in older children, there was no significant remodeling in the flexion/extension plane. If hyperextension appears to be a major problem, osteotomy should also be directed at this deformity rather than simple correction of the varus deformity; this situation requires a multiplane osteotomy.

We prefer to use a Wiltse-type osteotomy, similar to that described by DeRosa and Graziano but with the complete transverse cut distal as possible, just superior to the olecranon fossa, to have the axis of rotation of the osteotomy as close as possible to the deformity (Fig. 13-61).[149] This technique is adopted from the osteotomy described on the distal tibia by Wiltse.[165] Preoperative templating is performed to determine the angle of correction required for correction of the varus and, if necessary, for correction of any extension deformity. Templating is based

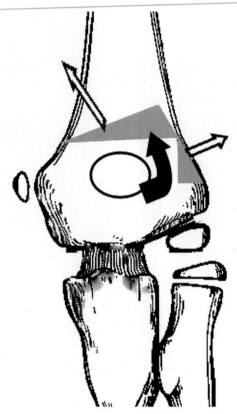

Figure 13-61. This osteotomy can address frontal and sagittal plane malalignment, and offer some inherent bony stability, while not producing a lateral bump which occurs with simple closing wedge osteotomies. *Hollow arrows* show triangles of bone that are removed, *solid arrow* shows rotation of fragment.

on AP of bilateral upper extremities centered on the elbow combined with clinical examination comparing one arm to the other in terms of frontal plane appearance and arc of motion. For example, if the affected arm has 20 degrees more extension and 20 degrees less flexion than the contralateral arm, a 20-degree wedge is planned in the sagittal plane.

Technique

A longitudinal incision measuring approximately 6 cm is made over the lateral distal humerus. Dissection is carried out in the interval between the brachioradialis and triceps. Subperiosteal dissection is performed to expose the distal humerus. There is sometimes scarring from fracture healing about the area of fracture. Posterior dissection is continued to the olecranon fossa as a landmark, but not distal to it to prevent harming the blood supply to the trochlea. Chandler retractors are used for circumferential protection with special care medially near the ulnar nerve. An osteotomy is performed just above the olecranon fossa perpendicular to the shaft of the humerus. The proximal humerus is delivered out of the wound, to allow the more complex part of the osteotomy to be performed with maximal visualization and protection. At this second cut, the osteotomy is angled correctly to account for sagittal malalignment. On average, about a 20-degree anterior closing wedge is performed, but this may be adjusted as needed to make certain the postfixation image demonstrates the AHL is through the midthird of the capitellum. A small lateral portion of the proximal fragment is left intact and a similarly shaped area with a 90-degree angle is made in the lateral portion of the distal fragment using a rongeur to allow the pieces to fit together for added stability. This prevents excessive lateral translation of the distal fragment, keeps the axis of rotation near the site of deformity, and has some inherent stability if done correctly. Once correction is achieved, bony contact is maximized by further cuts if needed. Three 0.062-in or 2-mm K-wires are then placed across the osteotomy site from lateral to medial with spread, divergence, and bicortical fixation. Stability is tested with stress under fluoroscopy. The wound is irrigated, a small amount of local bone graft from the excised wedge is packed around the osteotomy site but making certain bone graft is not in the olecranon fossa. The periosteum is reapproximated. A long-arm cast is applied in 60 to 80 degrees of flexion with the arm at neutral in regard to supination and pronation. The cast is removed when good callus is demonstrated on radiographs, usually approximately 4 weeks postoperatively, and the pins are removed in clinic at that time (Fig. 13-62).

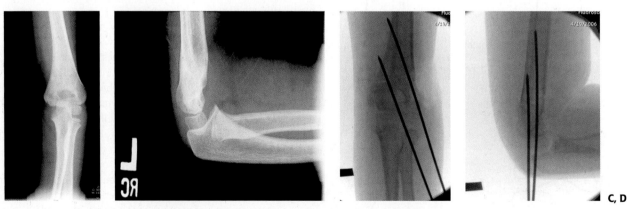

A, B   C, D

Figure 13-62. A: AP radiograph of elbow of 5-year-old girl in cubitus varus with Baumann's angle about 0 degrees. **B:** Lateral radiograph demonstrates capitellum is posterior to the anterior humeral line. **C:** Intraoperative AP image demonstrates restoration of Baumann's angle after Wiltse-type osteotomy. **D:** Lateral intraoperative image demonstrates the anterior humeral line now intersects the capitellum. Postoperatively, a normal arc of elbow flexion and extension was restored. (Reproduced with permission from Children's Orthopaedic Center, Los Angeles, CA.)

Flexion-Type Supracondylar Fractures of the Distal Humerus

INTRODUCTION TO FLEXION-TYPE SUPRACONDYLAR FRACTURES OF THE DISTAL HUMERUS

Flexion-type supracondylar humeral fractures account for about 2% of humeral fractures.[100] A flexion pattern of injury may not be recognized until reduction is attempted because initial radiographs are inadequate. A flexion-type supracondylar fracture is unstable in flexion, whereas extension-type fractures generally are stable in hyperflexion. A laterally displaced supracondylar fracture may actually be a flexion-type injury.

ASSESSMENT OF FLEXION-TYPE SUPRACONDYLAR FRACTURES OF THE DISTAL

A meta-analysis of 146 flexion-type SCH fractures found an overall neurapraxia rate of 15%, with the ulnar nerve injury as the most common nerve injured (91%),[10] as the flexed displaced fracture fragment places the nerve under tension. Mahan et al.[100] and Flynn et al.[52] together noted a higher rate of open

reduction for flexion-type supracondylar humeral fractures with an associated ulnar nerve injury.

MECHANISMS OF INJURY FOR FLEXION-TYPE SUPRACONDYLAR FRACTURES OF THE DISTAL HUMERUS

The mechanism of injury is generally believed to be a fall directly onto the elbow rather than a fall onto the outstretched hand with hyperextension of the elbow (Fig. 13-63). The distal fragment is displaced anteriorly and may migrate proximally in a totally displaced fracture. The ulnar nerve is vulnerable in this fracture pattern.[100] Rarely, it may be entrapped in the fracture or later in the healing callus.[91]

IMAGING AND OTHER DIAGNOSTIC STUDIES FOR FLEXION-TYPE SUPRACONDYLAR FRACTURES OF THE DISTAL HUMERUS

Anterior displacement may be accompanied by medial or lateral translation. Associated fractures of the proximal humerus and radius can occur and any tenderness in these areas mandates full x-ray evaluation of the upper extremity. Fracture classification is similar to extension-type supracondylar fractures[56]: type I, nondisplaced fracture; type II, flexion angulations only with anterior cortical contact; and type III, totally unstable displaced distal fracture fragment.

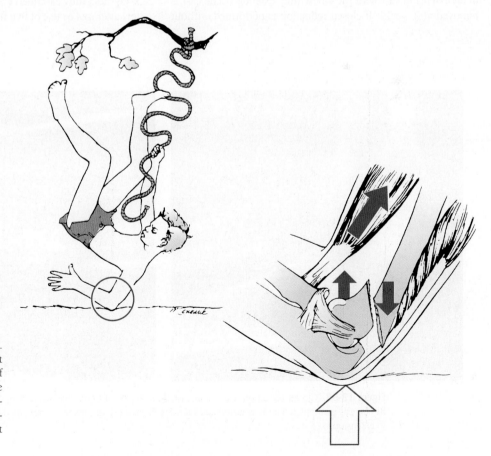

Figure 13-63. Flexion mechanism. Flexion-type fractures usually result from a blow to the posterior aspect of the elbow. The obliquity of the fracture line may be opposite that of an extension type. The large *white arrow* demonstrates the usual direction of fragment displacement.

TREATMENT OPTIONS FOR FLEXION-TYPE SUPRACONDYLAR FRACTURES OF THE DISTAL HUMERUS

NONOPERATIVE TREATMENT OF FLEXION-TYPE SUPRACONDYLAR FRACTURES OF THE DISTAL HUMERUS

In general, type I flexion-type supracondylar fractures are stable nondisplaced fractures that can simply be protected in a long-arm cast. If mild angulation, as in a type II fracture, requires some reduction in extension, the arm can be immobilized with the elbow fully extended. X-ray evaluation with the elbow extended is easily obtained and accurate in determining the adequacy of reduction. Reduction is assessed by evaluating Baumann's angle, the AHL intersecting the lateral condyle, and the integrity of the medial and lateral columns at the olecranon fossa. If reduction cannot be obtained, as is often the case, or if rotation persists, soft tissue interposition, possibly the ulnar nerve, should be suspected. De Boeck[36] studied 22 flexion-type supracondylar fractures. He found cast treatment to be satisfactory in nondisplaced cases. In the other 15 cases, closed reduction and percutaneous pinning was successful in most patients.

Type I and II fractures (Figs. 13-64 and 13-65) are generally reduced if any angular displacement is seen on fluoroscopic intraoperative evaluation. Type II fractures can be immobilized in an extension cast with the elbow fully extended. The cast is removed at 3 weeks. If closed reduction is performed without

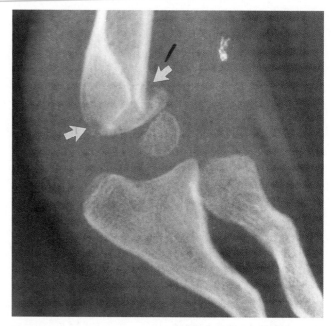

Figure 13-64. Type I flexion injury. A type I flexion supracondylar fracture pattern (*arrows*) in a 6-year-old below-the-elbow amputee. There is only about a 10-degree increase in the shaft condylar angle. The patient was treated with a simple posterior splint.

skeletal stabilization, follow-up x-rays usually are taken at 1 week and when the cast is removed at 3 weeks. True lateral x-rays in a fully extended cast are important, and may require a few attempts or use of live fluoroscopy.

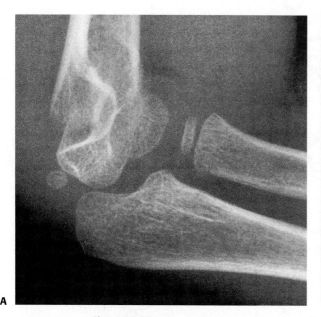

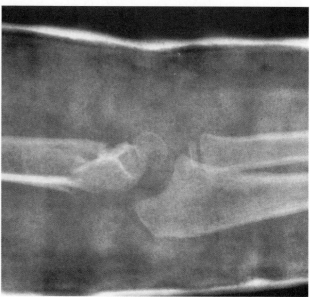

A

B

Figure 13-65. Closed reduction, extension cast. **A:** A 5-year-old girl sustained a type II flexion pattern. **B:** She was manipulated into extension and found to be stable, and thus was maintained in a long-arm cast in extension.

OPERATIVE TREATMENT OF FLEXION-TYPE SUPRACONDYLAR FRACTURES OF THE DISTAL HUMERUS

Pinning of Unstable Flexion-Type Supracondylar Fractures

Pinning is generally required for unstable type II and III flexion supracondylar fractures. The pinning technique described for extension-type supracondylar fractures is not appropriate for these fractures, because its instability in flexion precludes pinning with the elbow hyperflexed. In a flexion-type supracondylar fracture, the posterior periosteum is torn, so reduction can be obtained in extension which places tension across the intact anterior periosteum. In general, a slightly less than anatomic reduction can be accepted as long as three conditions are met: there is no soft tissue interposition of tissue, Baumann's angle is acceptable to the other side, and neither flexion nor extension is seen on the lateral view. Although rotating the arm is often possible for a lateral view of extension supracondylar fracture, the C-arm must be moved to obtain satisfactory x-ray results when pinning a flexion-type supracondylar fracture, because they are often rotationally unstable even when reduced (see Fig. 13-40).

Technique

> **✔ Pinning of Flexion-Type Supracondylar Fractures: KEY SURGICAL STEPS**
>
> ❑ Place pin in distal fragment
> ❑ Check pin placement in both AP and lateral planes
> ❑ Place second parallel or divergent pin
> ❑ Reduce fracture in both planes
> ❑ Drive pins across fracture site
> ❑ Assess reduction and stability of reduction
> ❑ Cut and bend pins
> ❑ Apply cast

Place a lateral entry pin in the distal fragment. Check pin placement in the AP plane then the lateral plane by rotating the C-arm, not the elbow. Adjust pin placement as needed, then place a second parallel or divergent pin. Reduce fracture in the AP plane. Rotate the C-arm and reduce fracture in the lateral plane, either by extension and flexion of the elbow, or using the "push–pull" technique[32] (Fig. 13-66). Drive the pins across the fracture site and through the cortex of the proximal bone. Assess reduction with AP and lateral images; Baumann's angle should be at least 10 degrees, and the AHL should go through the capitellum (Fig. 13-67). Assess stability of reduction with stress under live imaging. Cut and bend pins, protect skin with sterile felt or other barrier, and cast to allow for swelling, with less than 90 degrees of elbow flexion.

Open Reduction of Flexion-Type Supracondylar Fractures

Open reduction is required for flexion-type supracondylar fractures in up to 23% of cases; and if the ulnar nerve is injured, the open reduction rate is 60% (6/10) in one series.[52] In an earlier series, the open reduction rate of displaced flexion type SCH fractures was 31% and ulnar nerve injury rate was 19%.[100] Open reduction through a medial or posterior approach is used if an anatomic closed reduction cannot be obtained. If a posterior approach is used, care is taken to avoid posterior soft tissue dissection of distal fragment to avoid injuring the blood supply to the trochlea. The ulnar nerve is identified and protected throughout the exposure and fracture stabilization.

> **Authors' Preferred Treatment for Flexion-Type Supracondylar Fractures of the Distal Humerus (Algorithm 13-3)**
>
> In general, we treat type I flexion supracondylar fractures with a splint or cast with the elbow flexed for comfort. Minimally displaced type II fractures that reduce in extension are treated in an extension cast. Unstable type II and III fractures are pinned, open if needed.

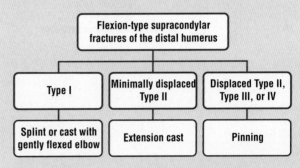

Algorithm 13-3. Authors' preferred treatment for flexion-type supracondylar fractures of the distal humerus.

> **Operative Treatment of Flexion-Type Supracondylar Humerus Fractures: POTENTIAL PITFALLS AND PREVENTIONS**

Pitfall	Prevention
Loss of fracture reduction	• Pins spaced at least 13 mm or one-third the width of the humerus at the level of the fracture • Use three pins in type III and IV fractures
Iatrogenic compartment syndrome	• Do not flex humerus >70 degrees if elbow very swollen
Not recognizing compartment syndrome	• Three As: analgesia requirements increasing, anxiety, agitation
Inability to reduce closed	• Milking maneuver, try pronation and/or supination

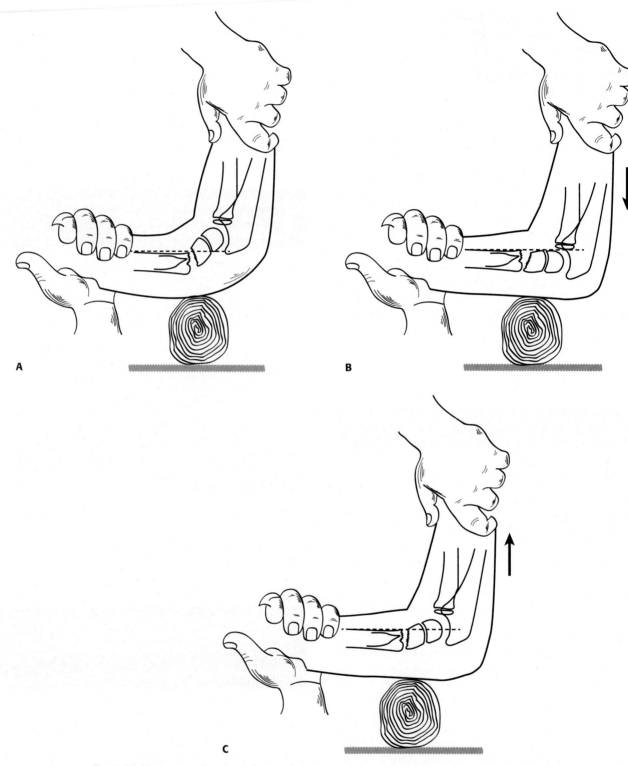

Figure 13-66. The "push–pull" method. **A:** Prereduction with a rolled towel used as a fulcrum. **B:** Push with overreduction into extension. **C:** Pull back to align the anterior humeral line with the middle third of the capitellum. (Reprinted with permission from Chukwunyerenwa C, Orlik B, El-Hawary R, et al. Treatment of flexion-type supracondylar fractures in children: the 'push–pull' method for closed reduction and percutaneous K-wire fixation. *J Pediatr Orthop B*. 2016;25(5):412–416.)

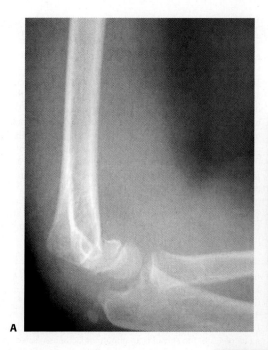
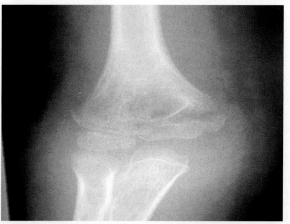
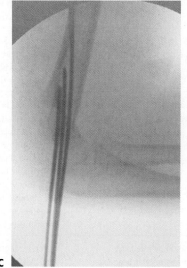
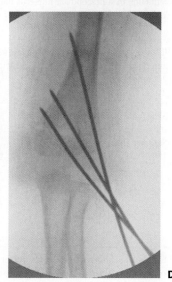

Figure 13-67. Lateral view of a flexion-type supracondylar fracture. **A:** The capitellum in front of the anterior humeral line. **B:** AP view of fracture often underestimates the amount of displacement if an AP is taken of a bent elbow rather than a true AP of the distal humerus. **C:** Intraoperative view shows anatomy has been restored, with the anterior humeral line crossing the middle third of the capitellum. **D:** AP view demonstrates three well-placed lateral pins with maximal separation at fracture site, with all pins engaging solid bone.

Annotated References

Reference	Annotation
Bae DS, Kadiyala RK, Waters PM. Acute compartment syndrome in children: contemporary diagnosis, treatment, and outcome. *J Pediatr Orthop.* 2001;21(5):680–688.	Pain, pallor, paresthesia, paralysis, and pulselessness were relatively unreliable signs and symptoms of compartment syndrome in children. An increasing analgesia requirement in combination with other clinical signs such as anxiety and agitation was a more sensitive indicator of compartment syndrome: All 10 patients with access to patient-controlled or nurse-administered analgesia demonstrated an increasing requirement for pain medication.
De Boeck H, De Smet P, Penders W, et al. Supracondylar elbow fractures with impaction of the medial condyle in children. *J Pediatr Orthop.* 1995;15(4):444–448.	In this retrospective review, none of six patients with medial comminution who underwent operative fixation had cubitus varus whereas four of seven (57%) patients who were treated nonoperatively developed cubitus varus. De Boeck et al. recommended closed reduction with percutaneous pinning when a fracture had medial comminution even in otherwise minimally displaced fractures, to prevent cubitus varus.

Annotated References

Reference	Annotation
Leitch KK, Kay RM, Femino JD, et al. Treatment of multidirectionally unstable supracondylar humeral fractures in children: a modified Gartland type-IV fracture. *J Bone Joint Surg Am*. 2006;88(5):980–985.	Type IV fractures with multidirectional instability are described. These fractures are characterized by an incompetent periosteal hinge circumferentially and defined by being unstable in both flexion and extension. This multidirectional instability is usually determined under anesthesia at the time of operation when on a lateral view the capitellum is anterior to the AHL with elbow flexion, and posterior to the AHL with elbow extension. This pattern of instability may result from the initial injury or may occur iatrogenically during a forceful attempted reduction. A specialized approach to closed reduction of this type of fracture is described in this chapter.
Mapes RC, Hennrikus WL. The effect of elbow position on the radial pulse measured by Doppler ultrasonography after surgical treatment of supracondylar elbow fractures in children. *J Pediatr Orthop*. 1998;18(4):441–444.	Doppler is not able to detect pulse when type II fractures are flexed >110 degrees, and type III fractures are flexed >70 degrees. Supination also decreased flow in the brachial artery.
Parikh SN, Wall EJ, Foad S, et al. Displaced type II extension supracondylar humerus fractures: do they all need pinning? *J Pediatr Orthop*. 2004;24(4):380–384.	In type II fractures treated initially with casting, there was a 28% (7 of 25) loss of reduction, 20% (5 of 25) need for delayed surgery, and 2% (2 of 25) unsatisfactory outcome according to Flynn criteria.
Pennock AT, Charles M, Moor M, et al. Potential causes of loss of reduction in supracondylar humerus fractures. *J Pediatr Orthop*. 2014;34(7):691–697.	Loss of reduction after percutaneous fixation of supracondylar fractures occurs at a rate of 4.2%. Pin spread is an important factor associated with preventing loss of reduction with a goal of pin spacing at least 13 mm or 1/3 the width of the humerus at the level of the fracture.
Ryan DD, Lightdale-Miric NR, Joiner ERA, et al. Variability of the anterior humeral line in normal pediatric elbows. *J Pediatr Orthop*. 2016;36(2):e14–e16.	In children 5 years and older, the AHL goes through the middle third of the capitellum in all patients, so if it does not, it is appropriate to look for pathology. However, with decreasing age, variability increases, with the AHL going through the anterior third of the capitellum in almost 1/3 of children under age 2 years.
Skaggs DL, Cluck MW, Mostofi A, et al. Lateral-entry pin fixation in the management of supracondylar fractures in children. *J Bone Joint Surg Am*. 2004;86(4):702–707.	A series of 345 SCH fractures treated by percutaneous pinning showed that the use of a medial pin was associated with a 4% (6/149) risk of ulnar nerve injury when the medial pin was placed without hyperflexion and 15% (11/71) if the medial pin was placed with hyperflexion. None of the 125 fractures treated with lateral entry pins alone resulted in iatrogenic injury. Thus one apparently undeniable conclusion is that if a medial pin is used, place the lateral pin(s) first, then extend the elbow and place the medial pin without hyperflexion of the elbow. Unfortunately, even making an incision over the medial epicondyle to make certain the ulnar nerve is not directly injured by a pin does not ensure protection of the nerve.
Skaggs DL, Sankar WN, Albrektson J, et al. How safe is the operative treatment of Gartland type 2 supracondylar humerus fractures in children? *J Pediatr Orthop*. 2008;28(2):139–141.	189 consecutive cases of type II fractures treated with closed reduction and percutaneous pinning were reviewed. There were 2% (4/189) pin-tract infections, of which three were treated successfully with oral antibiotics and pin removal 1.5% (3/191) and one (0.5%: 1/191) had operative irrigation and debridement for a wound infection not involving the joint. There were no nerve or vascular injuries, and no loss of reduction, delayed unions, or malunions. Pinning type II supracondylar fractures leads to a high probability of satisfactory outcome compared with previous studies of closed reduction without pinning.
Woratanarat P, Angsanuntsukh C, Rattanasiri S, et al. Meta-analysis of pinning in supracondylar fracture of the humerus in children. *J Orthop Trauma*. 2012;26(1):48–53.	Eighteen of 1,829 studies were included with 1,615 supracondylar fractures (837 and 778 children with cross and lateral-pinning, respectively). The average age was 6.1 ± 0.9 years. The risk of iatrogenic ulnar nerve injury was 4.3 (95% confidence interval, 2.1–9.1) times higher in cross-pinning compared with lateral-pinning. There was no significant difference for loss of fixation, late deformity, or Flynn criteria between the two types of pinning. Conclusions: Lateral-pinning is preferable to cross-pinning for fixation of pediatric supracondylar humerus fractures as a result of decreased risk of ulnar nerve injury.
Zaltz I, Waters PM, Kasser JR. Ulnar nerve instability in children. *J Pediatr Orthop*. 1996;16(5):567–569.	In children less than 5 years of age, when the elbow is flexed more than 90 degrees, the ulnar nerve migrated over, or even anterior to, the medial epicondyle in 61% (32/52) of children.

REFERENCES

1. Abbott MD, Buchler L, Loder RT, et al. Gartland type III supracondylar humerus fractures: outcome and complications as related to operative timing and pin configuration. *J Child Orthop*. 2014;8(6):473–477.
2. Abe M, Ishizu T, Shirai H, et al. Tardy ulnar nerve palsy caused by cubitus varus deformity. *J Hand Surg Am*. 1995;20(1):5–9.
3. Abzug JM, Herman MJ. Management of supracondylar humerus fractures in children: current concepts. *J Am Acad Orthop Surg*. 2012;20(2):69–77.
4. Aitken AP, Smith L, Blackette CW. Supracondylar fractures in children. *Am J Surg*. 1943;59:161–171.
5. Aktekin CN, Toprak A, Ozturk AM, et al. Open reduction via posterior triceps sparing approach in comparison with closed treatment of posteromedial displaced Gartland type III supracondylar humerus fractures. *J Pediatr Orthop B*. 2018;17(4):171–178.
6. Alves K, Spencer H, Barnewolt CE, et al. Early outcomes of vein grafting for reconstruction of brachial artery injuries in children. *J Hand Surg Am*. 2017;43(3):287–e1.
7. Amillo S, Barrios RH, Martínez-Peric R, et al. Surgical treatment of the radial nerve lesions associated with fractures of the humerus. *J Orthop Trauma*. 1993;7(3):211–215.
8. Aronson DC, van Vollenhoven E, Meeuwis JD. K-wire fixation of supracondylar humeral fractures in children: results of open reduction via a ventral approach in comparison with closed treatment. *Injury*. 1993;24(3):179–181.
9. Ay S, Akinci M, Kamiloglu S, et al. Open reduction of displaced pediatric supracondylar humeral fractures through the anterior cubital approach. *J Pediatr Orthop*. 2005;25(2):149–153.
10. Babal JC, Mehlman CT, Klein G. Nerve injuries associated with pediatric supracondylar humeral fractures: a meta-analysis. *J Pediatr Orthop*. 2010;30(3):253–263.
11. Badkoobehi H, Choi PD, Bae DS, et al. Management of the pulseless pediatric supracondylar humeral fracture. *J Bone Joint Surg*. 2015;97(11):937–943.
12. Bae DS, Kadiyala RK, Waters PM. Acute compartment syndrome in children: contemporary diagnosis, treatment, and outcome. *J Pediatr Orthop*. 2001;21(5):680–688.
13. Bahk MS, Srikumaran U, Ain MC, et al. Patterns of pediatric supracondylar humerus fractures. *J Pediatr Orthop*. 2008;28(5):493–499.
14. Barton KL, Kaminsky CK, Green DW, et al. Reliability of a modified Gartland classification of supracondylar humerus fractures. *J Pediatr Orthop*. 2001;21(1):27–30.
15. Bashyal RK, Chu JY, Schoenecker PL, et al. Complications after pinning of supracondylar distal humerus fractures. *J Pediatr Orthop*. 2009;29(7):704–708.
16. Battaglia TC, Armstrong DG, Schwend RM. Factors affecting forearm compartment pressures in children with supracondylar fractures of the humerus. *J Pediatr Orthop*. 2002;22(4):431–439.
17. Begovic N, Paunovic Z, Djuraskovic Z, et al. Lateral pinning versus others procedures in the treatment of supracondylar humerus fractures in children. *Acta Orthop Belg*. 2016;82(4):866–871.
18. Blakey CM, Biant LC, Birch R. Ischaemia and the pink, pulseless hand complicating supracondylar fractures of the humerus in childhood. *J Bone Joint Surg Br*. 2009;91-B(11):1487–1492.
19. Bloom T, Robertson C, Mahar A, et al. Biomechanical analysis of supracondylar humerus fracture pinning for slightly malreduced fractures. *J Pediatr Orthop*. 2008;28(7):766–772.
20. Böstman O, Mäkelä EA, Södergård J, et al. Absorbable polyglycolide pins in internal fixation of fractures in children. *J Pediatr Orthop*. 1993;13(2):242–245.
21. Boyd DW, Aronson DD. Supracondylar fractures of the humerus: a prospective study of percutaneous pinning. *J Pediatr Orthop*. 1992;12(6):789–794.
22. Brauer CA, Lee BM, Bae DS, et al. A systematic review of medial and lateral entry pinning versus lateral entry pinning for supracondylar fractures of the humerus. *J Pediatr Orthop*. 2007;27(2):181–186.
23. Bronfen CE, Geffard B, Mallet JF. Dissolution of the trochlea after supracondylar fracture of the humerus in childhood: an analysis of six cases. *J Pediatr Orthop*. 2007;27(5):547–550.
24. Brown IC, Zinar DM. Traumatic and iatrogenic neurological complications after supracondylar humerus fractures in children. *J Pediatr Orthop*. 1995;15(4):440–443.
25. Cairns RA, MacKenzie WG, Culham JA. Urokinase treatment of forearm ischemia complicating supracondylar fracture of the humerus in three children. *Pediatr Radiol*. 1993;23(5):391–394.
26. Camus T, MacLellan B, Cook PC, et al. Extension type II pediatric supracondylar humerus fractures: a radiographic outcomes study of closed reduction and cast immobilization. *J Pediatr Orthop*. 2011;31(4):366–371.
27. Carter CT, Bertrand SL, Cearley DM. Management of pediatric type III Supracondylar humerus fractures in the United States: results of a national survey of pediatric orthopaedic surgeons. *J Pediatr Orthopaed*. 2013;33(7):750–754.
28. Cheng JC, Lam TP, Maffulli N. Epidemiological features of supracondylar fractures of the humerus in Chinese children. *J Pediatr Orthop B*. 2001;10(1):63–67.
29. Chess DG, Leahey JL, Hyndman JC. Cubitus varus: significant factors. *J Pediatr Orthop*. 1994;14(2):190–192.
30. Choi PD, Melikian R, Skaggs DL. *Management of Vascular Injuries in Pediatric Supracondylar Humeral Fractures*. San Francisco, CA: Presented at the Annual Meeting of American Academy of Pediatrics, Section of Orthopaedics; 2008.
31. Choi PD, Melikian R, Skaggs DL. Risk factors for vascular repair and compartment syndrome in the pulseless supracondylar humerus fracture in children. *J Pediatr Orthop*. 2010;30(1):50–56.
32. Chukwunyerenwa C, Orlik B, El-Hawary R, et al. Treatment of flexion-type supracondylar fractures in children: the 'push–pull' method for closed reduction and percutaneous K-wire fixation. *J Pediatr Orthop B*. 2016;25(5):412–416.
33. Copley LA, Dormans JP, Davidson RS. Vascular injuries and their sequelae in pediatric supracondylar humeral fractures: toward a goal of prevention. *J Pediatr Orthop*. 1996;16(1):99–103.
34. Cotton FJ. Elbow fractures in children. *Ann Surg*. 1902;35:252–269.
35. Culp RW, Osterman AL, Davidson RS, et al. Neural injuries associated with supracondylar fractures of the humerus in children. *J Bone Joint Surg Am*. 1990;72(8):1211–1215.
36. De Boeck H. Flexion-type supracondylar elbow fractures in children. *J Pediatr Orthop*. 2001;21(4):460–463.
37. De Boeck H, De Smet P, Penders W, et al. Supracondylar elbow fractures with impaction of the medial condyle in children. *J Pediatr Orthop*. 1995;15(4):444–448.
38. Dekker A, Krijnen P, Schipper I. Results of crossed versus lateral entry K-wire fixation of displaced pediatric supracondylar humeral fractures: a systematic review and meta-analysis. *Injury*. 2016;47(11):2391–2398.
39. DeRosa GP, Graziano GP. A new osteotomy for cubitus varus. *Clin Orthop Relat Res*. 1988;236:160–165.
40. Devnani AS. Late presentation of supracondylar fracture of the humerus in children. *Clin Orthop Relat Res*. 2005;(431):36–41.
41. Dietz HS, Schmittenbecher PP, Slongo T, et al. *AO Manual of Fracture Management: Elastic Stable Intramedullary Nailing in Children*. Stuttgart: Thieme Medical Publishers; 2006.
42. Dimeglio A. Growth in pediatric orthopaedics. In: Morrissy RT, Weinstein SL, eds. *Lovell and Winters's Pediatric Orthopaedics*. 6th ed. Philadelphia, PA: Lippincott Williams & Wilkins; 2006:35–65.
43. Dodds SD, Grey MA, Bohl DD, et al. Clinical and radiographic outcomes of supracondylar humerus fractures treated surgically by pediatric and non-pediatric orthopedic surgeons. *J Child Orthop*. 2015;9(1):45–53.
44. Edmonds EW, Roocroft JH, Mubarak SJ. Treatment of displaced pediatric supracondylar humerus fracture patterns requiring medial fixation: a reliable and safer cross-pinning technique. *J Pediatr Orthop*. 2012;32(4):346–351.
45. Ernat J, Ho C, Wimberly RL, et al. Fracture classification does not predict functional outcomes in supracondylar humerus fractures: a prospective study. *J Pediatr Orthop*. 2017;37(4):e233–e237.
46. Etier BE Jr, Doyle JS, Gilbert SR. Avascular necrosis of trochlea after supracondylar humerus fractures in children. *Am J Orthop (Belle Mead NJ)*. 2015;44(10):E390–E393.
47. Fatemi MJ, Habibi M, Pooli AH, et al. Delayed radial nerve laceration by the sharp blade of a medially inserted Kirschner-wire pin: a rare complication of supracondylar humerus fracture. *Am J Orthop (Belle Mead NJ)*. 2009;38(2):E38–E40.
48. Feng C, Guo Y, Zhu Z, et al. Biomechanical analysis of supracondylar humerus fracture pinning for fractures with coronal lateral obliquity. *J Pediatr Orthop*. 2012;32(2):196–200.
49. Fitzgibbons PG, Bruce B, Got C, et al. Predictors of failure of nonoperative treatment for type-2 supracondylar humerus fractures. *J Pediatr Orthop*. 2011;31(4):372–376.
50. Fleuriau-Chateau P, McIntyre W, Letts M. An analysis of open reduction of irreducible supracondylar fractures of the humerus in children. *Can J Surg*. 1998;41(2):112–128.
51. Fletcher ND, Sirmon BJ, Mansour AS, et al. Impact of insurance status on ability to return for outpatient management of pediatric supracondylar humerus fractures. *J Child Orthop*. 2016;10(5):421–427.
52. Flynn K, Shah AS, Brusalis CM, et al. Flexion-type supracondylar humeral fractures: ulnar nerve injury increases risk of open reduction. *J Bone Joint Surg*. 2017;99(17):1485–1487.
53. Flynn JC, Zink WP. Fractures and dislocations of the elbow. In: MacEwen GD, Kasser JR, Heinrich SD, eds. *Pediatric Fractures: A Practical Approach to Assessment and Treatment*. Baltimore, MD: Lippincott Williams & Wilkins; 1993:133–164.
54. Gadgil A, Hayhurst C, Maffulli N, et al. Elevated, straight-arm traction for supracondylar fractures of the humerus in children. *J Bone Joint Surg Br*. 2005;87(1):82–87.
55. Garg S, Weller A, Larson AN, et al. Clinical characteristics of severe supracondylar humerus fractures in children. *J Pediatr Orthop*. 2014;34(1):34–39.
56. Gartland JJ. Management of supracondylar fractures of the humerus in children. *Surg Gynecol Obstet*. 1959;109(2):145–154.
57. Gaston RG, Cates TB, Devito D, et al. Medial and lateral pin versus lateral-entry pin fixation for type 3 supracondylar fractures in children: a prospective, surgeon-randomized study. *J Pediatr Orthop*. 2010;30(8):799–806.
58. Glotzbecker MP, Bae DS, Links AC, et al. Fishtail deformity of the distal humerus: a report of 15 cases. *J Pediatr Orthop*. 2013;33:592–597.
59. Gordon JE, Patton CM, Luhmann SJ, et al. Fracture stability after pinning of displaced supracondylar distal humerus fractures in children. *J Pediatr Orthop*. 2001;21(3):313–318.
60. Got C, Thakur N, Marcaccio EJ Jr, et al. Delayed presentation of a brachial artery pseudoaneurysm after a supracondylar humerus fracture in a 6-year-old boy: a case report. *J Pediatr Orthop*. 2010;30(1):57–59.
61. Gottschalk HP, Sagoo D, Glaser D, et al. Biomechanical analysis of pin placement for pediatric supracondylar humerus fractures: does starting point, pin size, and number matter? *J Pediatr Orthop*. 2012;32(5):445–451.
62. Griffin KJ, Walsh SR, Markar S, et al. The pink pulseless hand: a review of the literature regarding management of vascular complications of supracondylar humeral fractures in children. *Eur J Vasc Endovasc Surg*. 2008;36(6):697–702.
63. Gupta N, Kay RM, Leitch K, et al. Effect of surgical delay on perioperative complications and need for open reduction in supracondylar humerus fractures in children. *J Pediatr Orthop*. 2004;24(3):245–248.
64. Gurkan I, Bayrakci K, Tasbas B, et al. Posterior instability of the shoulder after supracondylar fractures recovered with cubitus varus deformity. *J Pediatr Orthop*. 2002;22(2):198–202.
65. Guven MF, Kaynak G, Inan M, et al. Results of displaced supracondylar humerus fractures treated with open reduction and internal fixation after a mean 22.4 years of follow-up. *J Shoulder Elbow Surg*. 2015;24(4):640–646.
66. Hadlow AT, Devane P, Nicol RO. A selective treatment approach to supracondylar fracture of the humerus in children. *J Pediatr Orthop*. 1996;16(1):104–106.
67. Hamdi A, Poitras P, Louati H, et al. Biomechanical analysis of lateral pin placements for pediatric supracondylar humerus fractures. *J Pediatr Orthop*. 2010;30(2):135–139.

68. Herman MJ, Boardman MJ, Hoover JR, et al. Relationship of the anterior humeral line to the capitellar ossific nucleus: variability with age. *J Bone Joint Surg Am*. 2009;91(9):2188–2193.
69. Higaki T, Ikuta Y. The new operation method of the domed osteotomy for 4 children with varus deformity of the elbow joint. *J Jpn Orthop*. 1982;31:300–335.
70. Holden CE. The pathology and prevention of Volkmann's ischaemic contracture. *J Bone Joint Surg Br*. 1979;61B(3):296–300.
71. Holt JB, Glass NA, Bedard NA, et al. Emerging U.S. national trends in the treatment of pediatric supracondylar humeral fractures. *J Bone Joint Surg*. 2017;99(8):681–687.
72. Howard A, Mulpuri K, Abel ML, et al. The treatment of pediatric supracondylar humerus fractures. *J Am Acad Orthop Surg*. 2012;20(5):320–327.
73. Iobst CA, Stillwagon M, Ryan D, et al. Assessing quality and safety in pediatric supracondylar humerus fracture care. *J Pediatr Orthop*. 2017;37(5):e303–e307.
74. Joiner ER, Skaggs DL, Arkader A, et al. Iatrogenic nerve injuries in the treatment of supracondylar humerus fractures: are we really just missing nerve injuries on preoperative examination? *J Pediatr Orthop*. 2014;34(4):388–392.
75. Kaewpornsawan K. Comparison between closed reduction with percutaneous pinning and open reduction with pinning in children with closed totally displaced supracondylar humeral fractures: a randomized controlled trial. *J Pediatr Orthop B*. 2001;10(2):131–137.
76. Kao H-K, Lee W-C, Yang W-E, et al. Clinical significance of anterior humeral line in supracondylar humeral fractures in children. *Injury*. 2016;47(10):2252–2257.
77. Karakurt L, Ozdemir H, Yilmaz E, et al. Morphology and dynamics of the ulnar nerve in the cubital tunnel after percutaneous cross-pinning of supracondylar fractures in children's elbows: an ultrasonographic study. *J Pediatr Orthop B*. 2005; 14(3):189–193.
78. Karalius VP, Stanfield J Ashley P, et al. The utility of routine postoperative radiographs after pinning of pediatric supracondylar humerus fractures. *J Pediatr Orthop*. 2017;37(5):e309–e312.
79. Kasser JR. Location of treatment of supracondylar fractures of the humerus in children. *Clin Orthop Relat Res*. 2005;(434):110–113.
80. Kay RM, Directo MP, Leathers M, et al. Complications of ketorolac use in children undergoing operative fracture care. *J Pediatr Orthop*. 2010;30(7):655–658.
81. Kim HT, Song MB, Conjares JN, et al. Trochlear deformity occurring after distal humeral fractures: magnetic resonance imaging and its natural progression. *J Pediatr Orthop*. 2002;22(2):188–193.
82. Kocher MS, Kasser JR, Waters PM, et al. Lateral entry compared with medial and lateral entry pin fixation for completely displaced supracondylar humeral fractures in children: a randomized clinical trial. *J Bone Joint Surg Am*. 2007;89(4):706–712.
83. Kocher T. *Beitrage zur Kenntniss einiger praktisch wichtiger Fracturformen*. Basel: Carl Sallman; 1896.
84. Konstantiniuk P, Fritz G, Ott T, et al. Long-term follow-up of vascular reconstructions after supracondylar humerus fracture with vascular lesion in childhood. *Eur J Vasc Endovasc Surg*. 2011;42(5):684–688.
85. Kurer MH, Regan MW. Completely displaced supracondylar fracture of the humerus in children: a review of 1708 comparable cases. *Clin Orthop Relat Res*. 1990;(256):205–214.
86. Kwak-Lee J, Kim R, Ebramzadeh E, et al. Is medial pin use safe for treating pediatric supracondylar humerus fractures? *J Orthop Trauma*. 2014;28(4):216–221.
87. Kzlay YO, Aktekin CN, Özsoy MH, et al. Gartland type 3 supracondylar humeral fractures in children: which open reduction approach should be used after failed closed reduction? *J Orthop Trauma*. 2017;31(1):e18–e23.
88. Lacher M, Schaeffer K, Boehm R, et al. The treatment of supracondylar humeral fractures with elastic stable intramedullary nailing (ESIN) in children. *J Pediatr Orthop*. 2011;31(1):33–38.
89. Ladenhauf HN, Schaffert M, Bauer J. The displaced supracondylar humerus fracture: indications for surgery and surgical options: a 2014 update. *Curr Opin Pediatr*. 2014;26(1):64–69.
90. Lal GM, Bhan S. Delayed open reduction for supracondylar fractures of the humerus. *Int Orthop*. 1991;15(3):189–191.
91. Lalanandham T, Laurence WN. Entrapment of the ulnar nerve in the callus of a supracondylar fracture of the humerus. *Injury*. 1984;16(2):129–130.
92. Lally KP, Foster CE III, Chwals WJ, et al. Long-term follow-up of brachial artery ligation in children. *Ann Surg*. 1990;212(2):194–196.
93. Larson, AN, Garg S, Weller A, et al. Operative treatment of type II supracondylar humerus fractures: does time to surgery affect complications? *J Pediatr Orthop*. 2014;34(4):382–387.
94. Larson L, Firoozbakhsh K, Passarelli R, et al. Biomechanical analysis of pinning techniques for pediatric supracondylar humerus fractures. *J Pediatr Orthop*. 2006;26(5):573–578.
95. Lee YH, Lee SK, Kim BS, et al. Three lateral divergent or parallel pin fixations for the treatment of displaced supracondylar humerus fractures in children. *J Pediatr Orthop*. 2008;28(4):417–422.
96. Lee SS, Mahar AT, Miesen D, et al. Displaced pediatric supracondylar humerus fractures: biomechanical analysis of percutaneous pinning techniques. *J Pediatr Orthop*. 2002;22(4):440–443.
97. Leitch KK, Kay RM, Femino JD, et al. Treatment of multidirectionally unstable supracondylar humeral fractures in children: a modified Gartland type-IV fracture. *J Bone Joint Surg Am*. 2006;88(5):980–985.
98. Louahem DM, Nebunescu A, Canavese F, et al. Neurovascular complications and severe displacement in supracondylar humerus fractures in children: defensive or offensive strategy? *J Pediatr Orthop B*. 2006;15(1):51–57.
99. Lyons JP, Ashley E, Hoffer MM. Ulnar nerve palsies after percutaneous cross-pinning of supracondylar fractures in children's elbows. *J Pediatr Orthop*. 1998;18(1):43–45.
100. Mahan ST, May CD, Kocher MS. Operative management of displaced flexion supracondylar humerus fractures in children. *J Pediatr Orthop*. 2007;27(5):551–556.
101. Mahan ST, Osborn E, Bae DS, et al. Changing practice patterns: the impact of a randomized clinical trial on surgeons preference for treatment of type 3 supracondylar humerus fractures. *J Pediatr Orthop*. 2012;32(4):340–345.
102. Mangat KS, Martin AG, Bache CE. The 'pulseless pink' hand after supracondylar fracture of the humerus in children. *J Bone Joint Surg Br*. 2009;91B(11):1521–1525.
103. Mapes RC, Hennrikus WL. The effect of elbow position on the radial pulse measured by Doppler ultrasonography after surgical treatment of supracondylar elbow fractures in children. *J Pediatr Orthop*. 1998;18(4):441–444.
104. Martin DF, Tolo VT, Sellers DS, et al. Radial nerve laceration and retraction associated with a supracondylar fracture of the humerus. *J Hand Surg Am*. 1989;14(3):542–545.
105. McGraw JJ, Akbarnia BA, Hanel DP, et al. Neurological complications resulting from supracondylar fractures of the humerus in children. *J Pediatr Orthop*. 1986;6(6):647–650.
106. Mehlman CT. Invited commentary related to: "Gartland type-3 supracondylar humeral fractures in children: which open reduction approach should be used after failed closed reduction?" *J Orthop Trauma*. 2017;31(1):e23–e24.
107. Mollon BG, McGuffin WS, Seabrook JA, et al. 198. Supracondylar humerus fractures in older children: treatment modalities and outcomes. *J Bone Joint Surg Br*. 2011;93-B(Suppl III):284.
108. Mooney JF III, Hosseinzadeh P, Oetgen M, et al. AAOS appropriate use criteria: management of pediatric supracondylar humerus fractures with vascular injury. *J Am Acad Orthop Surg*. 2016;24(2):e24–e28.
109. Mubarak SJ, Carroll NC. Volkmann's contracture in children: aetiology and prevention. *J Bone Joint Surg Br*. 1979;61B(3):285–293.
110. Muchow RD, Riccio AI, Garg S, et al. Neurological and vascular injury associated with supracondylar humerus fractures and ipsilateral forearm fractures in children. *J Pediatr Orthop*. 2015;35(2):121–125.
111. Mulpuri, K., A. Dobbe, E. Schaeffer, et al. Management of displaced supracondylar fractures of the humerus using lateral versus cross K wires: a prospective randomised trial. *Bone Joint J*. 2016;98(Suppl 21):93–93.
112. Nork SE, Hennrikus WL, Loncarich DP, et al. Relationship between ligamentous laxity and the site of upper extremity fractures in children: extension supracondylar fracture versus distal forearm fracture. *J Pediatr Orthop B*. 1999;8(2):90–92.
113. O'Driscoll SW, Spinner RJ, McKee MD, et al. Tardy posterolateral rotatory instability of the elbow due to cubitus varus. *J Bone Joint Surg Am*. 2001;83(9):1358–1369.
114. Oetgen ME, Mirick GE, Atwater L, et al. Complications and predictors of need for return to the operating room in the treatment of supracondylar humerus fractures in children. *Open Orthop J*. 2015;9:139–142.
115. Omid R, Choi PD, Skaggs DL. Supracondylar humeral fractures in children. *J Bone Joint Surg Am*. 2008;90(5):1121–1132.
116. Onwuanyi ON, Nwobi DG. Evaluation of the stability of pin configuration in K-wire fixation of displaced supracondylar fractures in children. *Int Surg*. 1998;83(3):271–274.
117. Or O, Weil Y, Simanovsky N, et al. The outcome of early revision of malaligned pediatric supracondylar humerus fractures. *Injury*. 2015;46(8):1585–1590.
118. Parikh SN, Lykissas MG, Roshdy M, et al. Pin tract infection of operatively treated supracondylar fractures in children: long-term functional outcomes and anatomical study. *J Child Orthop*. 2015;9(4):295–302.
119. Parikh SN, Wall EJ, Foad S, et al. Displaced type II extension supracondylar humerus fractures: do they all need pinning? *J Pediatr Orthop*. 2004;24(4):380–384.
120. Park MJ, Baldwin K, Weiss-Laxer N, et al. Composite playground safety measure to correlate the rate of supracondylar humerus fractures with safety: an ecologic study. *J Pediatr Orthop*. 2010;30(2):101–105.
121. Park MJ, Ho CA, Larson AN. AAOS appropriate use criteria: management of pediatric supracondylar humerus fractures. *J Am Acad Orthop Surg*. 2015;23(10):e52–e55.
122. Pennock AT, Charles M, Moor M, et al. Potential causes of loss of reduction in supracondylar humerus fractures. *J Pediatr Orthop*. 2014;34(7):691–697.
123. Peters CL, Scott SM, Stevens PM. Closed reduction and percutaneous pinning of displaced supracondylar humerus fractures in children: description of a new closed reduction technique for fractures with brachialis muscle entrapment. *J Orthop Trauma*. 1995;9(5):430–434.
124. Pirone AM, Graham HK, Krajbich JI. Management of displaced extension-type supracondylar fractures of the humerus in children. *J Bone Joint Surg Am*. 1988;70(5):641–650.
125. Ponce BA, Hedequist DJ, Zurakowski D, et al. Complications and timing of followup after closed reduction percutaneous pinning supracondylar humerus fractures. *J Pediatr Orthop*. 2004;24:610–614.
126. Pradhan A, Hennrikus W, Pace G, et al. Increased pin diameter improves torsional stability in supracondylar humerus fractures: an experimental study. *J Child Orthop*. 2016;10(2):163–167.
127. Prietto CA. Supracondylar fractures of the humerus: a comparative study of Dunlop's traction versus percutaneous pinning. *J Bone Joint Surg Am*. 1979;61(3):425–428.
128. Ramachandran M, Birch R, Eastwood DM. Clinical outcome of nerve injuries associated with supracondylar fractures of the humerus in children: the experience of a specialist referral centre. *J Bone Joint Surg Br*. 2006;88(1):90–94.
129. Ramachandran M, Skaggs DL, Crawford HA, et al. Delaying treatment of supracondylar fractures in children: has the pendulum swung too far? *J Bone Joint Surg Br*. 2008;90:1228–1233.
130. Rasool MN. Ulnar nerve injury after K-wire fixation of supracondylar humerus fractures in children. *J Pediatr Orthop*. 1998;18(5):686–690.
131. Ray SA, Ivory JP, Beavis JP. Use of pulse oximetry during manipulation of supracondylar fractures of the humerus. *Injury*. 1991;22(2):103–104.
132. Ring D, Waters PM, Hotchkiss RN, et al. Pediatric floating elbow. *J Pediatr Orthop*. 2001;4:456–459.
133. Robb JE. The pink, pulseless hand after supracondylar fracture of the humerus in children. *J Bone Joint Surg Br*. 2009;91(11):1410–1412.
134. Ryan DD, Lightdale-Miric NR, Joiner ERA, et al. Variability of the anterior humeral line in normal pediatric elbows. *J Pediatr Orthop*. 2016;36(2):e14–e16.
135. Sabharwal S, Tredwell SJ, Beauchamp RD, et al. Management of pulseless pink hand in pediatric supracondylar fractures of humerus. *J Pediatr Orthop*. 1997;17(3):303–310.
136. Sairyo K, Henmi T, Kanematsu Y, et al. Radial nerve palsy associated with slightly angulated pediatric supracondylar humerus fracture. *J Orthop Trauma*. 1997;11(3):227–229.

137. Sankar WN, Hebela NM, Skaggs DL, et al. Loss of pin fixation in displaced supracondylar humeral fractures in children: causes and prevention. *J Bone Joint Surg Am.* 2007;89(4):713–717.

138. Schroeder NO, Seeley MA, Hariharan A, et al. Utility of postoperative antibiotics after percutaneous pinning of pediatric supracondylar humerus fractures. *J Pediatr Orthop.* 2017;37(6):363–367.

139. Seehausen DA, Kay RM, Ryan DD, et al. Foam padding in casts accommodates soft tissue swelling and provides circumferential strength after fixation of supracondylar humerus fractures. *J Pediatr Orthop.* 2015;35(1):24–27.

140. Shaw BA, Kasser JR, Emans JB, et al. Management of vascular injuries in displaced supracondylar humerus fractures without arteriography. *J Orthop Trauma.* 1990;4(1):25–29.

141. Shore BJ, Gillespie BT, Miller PE, et al. Recovery of motor nerve injuries associated with displaced, extension-type pediatric supracondylar humerus fractures. *J Pediatr Orthop.* 2017. doi: 10.1097/BPO.0000000000001056. [Epub ahead of print]

142. Shrader MW, Campbell MD, Jacofsky DJ. Accuracy of emergency room physicians' interpretation of elbow fractures in children. *Orthopedics.* 2008;31(12).

143. Sibinski M, Sharma H, Bennet GC. Early versus delayed treatment of extension type-3 supracondylar fractures of the humerus in children. *J Bone Joint Surg Br.* 2006;88(3):380–381.

144. Silva M, Cooper SD, Cha A. The outcome of surgical treatment of multidirectionally unstable (type IV) pediatric supracondylar humerus fractures. *J Pediatr Orthop.* 2015;35(6):600–605.

145. Silva M, Pandarinath R, Farng E, et al. Inter- and intra-observer reliability of the Baumann angle of the humerus in children with supracondylar humeral fractures. *Int Orthop.* 2010;34(4):553–557.

146. Silva M, Wong TC, Bernthal NM. Outcomes of reduction more than 7 days after injury in supracondylar humeral fractures in children. *J Pediatr Orthop.* 2011;31(7):751–756.

147. Siriwardhane M, Siriwardhane J, Lam L, et al. Supracondylar fracture of the humerus in children: mechanism of injury. *J Bone Joint Surg Br.* 2012;94B(Suppl XXIII):141.

148. Skaggs DL, Cluck MW, Mostofi A, et al. Lateral-entry pin fixation in the management of supracondylar fractures in children. *J Bone Joint Surg Am.* 2004;86(4):702–707.

149. Skaggs DL, Glassman D, Weiss JM, et al. A new surgical technique for the treatment of supracondylar humerus fracture malunions in children. *J Child Orthop.* 2011;5(4):305–312.

150. Skaggs DL, Hale JM, Bassett J, et al. Operative treatment of supracondylar fractures of the humerus in children: the consequence of pin placement. *J Bone Joint Surg Am.* 2001;83(5):735–740.

151. Skaggs DL, Mirzayan R. The posterior fat pad sign in association with occult fracture of the elbow in children. *J Bone Joint Surg Am.* 1999;81(10):1429–1433.

152. Skaggs DL, Sankar WN, Albrektson J, et al. How safe is the operative treatment of Gartland type 2 supracondylar humerus fractures in children? *J Pediatr Orthop.* 2008;28(2):139–141.

153. Slobogean BL, Jackman H, Tennant S, et al. Iatrogenic ulnar nerve injury after the surgical treatment of displaced supracondylar fractures of the humerus: number needed to harm, a systematic review. *J Pediatr Orthop.* 2010;30(5):430–436.

154. Slongo T, Audigé L, Schlickewei W, et al. Development and validation of the AO pediatric comprehensive classification of long bone fractures by the Pediatric Expert Group of the AO Foundation in collaboration with AO clinical investigation and Documentation and the International Association for Pediatric Traumatology. *J Pediatr Orthop.* 2006;26(1):43–49.

155. Srikumaran U, Tan EW, Belkoff SM, et al. Enhanced biomechanical stiffness with large pins in the operative treatment of pediatric supracondylar humerus fractures. *J Pediatr Orthop.* 2012;32(2):201–205.

156. Swanson CE, Chang K, Schleyer E, et al. Postoperative pain control after supracondylar humerus fracture fixation. *J Pediatr Orthop.* 2012;32(5):452–455.

157. Takahara M, Sasaki I, Kimura T, et al. Second fracture of the distal humerus after varus malunion of a supracondylar fracture in children. *J Bone Joint Surg Br.* 1998;80(5):791–797.

158. Tripuraneni KR, Bosch PP, Schwend RM, et al. Prospective, surgeon-randomized evaluation of crossed pins versus lateral pins for unstable supracondylar humerus fractures in children. *J Pediatr Orthop B.* 2009;18(2):93–98.

159. Tuason D, Hohl JB, Levicoff E, et al. Urban pediatric orthopaedic surgical practice audit: implications for the future of this subspecialty. *J Bone Joint Surg Am.* 2009;91(12):2992–2998.

160. Voss FR, Kasser JR, Trepman E, et al. Uniplanar supracondylar humeral osteotomy with preset Kirschner wires for posttraumatic cubitus varus. *J Pediatr Orthop.* 1994;14(4):471–478.

161. Wang YL, Chang WN, Hsu CJ, et al. The recovery of elbow range of motion after treatment of supracondylar and lateral condylar fractures of the distal humerus in children. *J Orthop Trauma.* 2009;23(2):120–125.

162. Weiss JM, Kay RM, Waters P, et al. Distal humerus osteotomy for supracondylar fracture malunion in children: a study of perioperative complications. *Am J Orthop (Belle Mead NJ).* 2010;39(1):22–25.

163. White L, Mehlman CT, Crawford AH. Perfused, pulseless, and puzzling: a systematic review of vascular injuries in pediatric supracondylar humerus fractures and results of a POSNA questionnaire. *J Pediatr Orthop.* 2010;30(4):328–335.

164. Williamson DM, Cole WG. Treatment of selected extension supracondylar fractures of the humerus by manipulation and strapping in flexion. *Injury.* 1993;24(4):249–252.

165. Wiltse LL. Valgus deformity of the ankle: a sequel to acquired or congenital abnormalities of the fibula. *J Bone Joint Surg Am.* 1972;54(3):595–606.

166. Wind WM, Schwend RM, Armstrong DG. Predicting ulnar nerve location in pinning of supracondylar humerus fractures. *J Pediatr Orthop.* 2002;22(4):444–447.

167. Wingfield JJ, Ho CA, Abzug JM, et al. Open reduction techniques for supracondylar humerus fractures in children. *J Am Acad Orthop Surg.* 2015;23(12):e72–e80.

168. Woratanarat P, Angsanuntsukh C, Rattanasiri S, et al. Meta-analysis of pinning in supracondylar fracture of the humerus in children. *J Orthop Trauma.* 2012;26(1):48–53.

169. Yang K, Willoughby R, Donald G. Radiological comparison of lateral entry compared with combined medial and lateral entry pin fixation for type IIIS supracondylar fractures in children with particular focus on rotational displacement. *J Bone Joint Surg Br.* 2012;94B(Suppl 23):142.

170. Young S, Fevang JM, Gullaksen G, et al. Deformity and functional outcome after treatment for supracondylar humerus fractures in children: a 5- to 10-year follow-up of 139 supracondylar humerus fractures treated by plaster cast, skeletal traction or crossed wire fixation. *J Child Orthop.* 2010;4(5):445–453.

171. Zaltz I, Waters PM, Kasser JR. Ulnar nerve instability in children. *J Pediatr Orthop.* 1996;16(5):567–569.

172. Zionts LE, McKellop HA, Hathaway R. Torsional strength of pin configurations used to fix supracondylar fractures of the humerus in children. *J Bone Joint Surg Am.* 1994;76(2):253–256.

173. Zionts LE, Woodson CJ, Manjra N, et al. Time of return of elbow motion after percutaneous pinning of pediatric supracondylar humerus fractures. *Clin Orthop Relat Res.* 2009;467(8):2007–2010.

174. Ziv N, Litwin A, Katz K, et al. Definitive diagnosis of fracture-separation of the distal humeral epiphysis in neonates by ultrasonography. *Pediatr Radiol.* 1996;26(7):493–496.

14

T-Condylar Fractures of the Distal Humerus

Carley Vuillermin and Peter M. Waters

INTRODUCTION TO T-CONDYLAR FRACTURES OF THE DISTAL HUMERUS

In T-condylar fractures, the fracture line most commonly originates in the central groove of the trochlea and courses proximal to the olecranon and coronoid fossae, where it divides and separates the medial and lateral bony columns of the distal humerus. If the proximal fracture lines are oblique, the fracture may be termed *Y-condylar*. T- and Y-condylar fractures are rare injuries in skeletally immature children and are often a transitional fracture seen in adolescents at the end of skeletal development.

The early modern literature reflects only reports by Blount[6] and Zimmerman,[37] who each described a case of a T-condylar distal humerus fracture in an 11-year-old patient. The average age of pediatric patients reported in four major case series[16,19,26,29] was 12.8 years. Three studies have found that the nondominant arm is more likely to be injured 2.5 times greater than the dominant arm.[8,21,25,29] Thus, Maylahn and Fahey,[22] who reported six patients near skeletal maturity, were accurate when they said, "the fractures (T-condylar) take on the characteristics of an adult fracture and should be treated as such."

The actual incidence in younger children is certainly low, but it may be under diagnosed because it is often confused with other fractures, such as those involving the lateral condylar physis or total distal humeral physis. Special imaging studies such as arthrograms or MRI scans may be necessary to demonstrate the intracondylar aspects in young children. The combination of an increased awareness of the possibility of this injury and a more aggressive diagnostic approach may result in more cases being recognized acutely and appropriately treated in this younger age group. The poorer outcomes from these relatively rare injuries are due to either failure to recognize the complex nature of the fracture or treat in a more comprehensive manner.

ASSESSMENT OF T-CONDYLAR FRACTURES OF THE DISTAL HUMERUS

MECHANISMS OF INJURY OF T-CONDYLAR FRACTURES OF THE DISTAL HUMERUS

The primary mechanism of this injury is the direct wedge effect of the articular surface of the olecranon on the distal end of the humerus. The sharp edge of the semilunar notch or coronoid process acts as a wedge to break the trochlea and split the condyles, which in turn separates the two columns of the distal humerus. Flexion and extension types of injuries have been described.

The most common mechanism producing a flexion injury is a direct blow to the posterior aspect of the elbow, usually when the child falls directly on the flexed elbow. This flexion mechanism in young children contributes to its rarity because most upper-extremity injuries in children result from a fall on an outstretched hand and have a component of elbow hyperextension. In these flexion injuries, the wedge effect is produced at the apex of the trochlea by the central portion of the trochlear notch. The condylar fragments usually lie anterior to the shaft in these flexion injuries (Fig. 14-1A,B).

A T-condylar fracture may also be caused by a fall on the outstretched arm with the elbow in only slight flexion. This

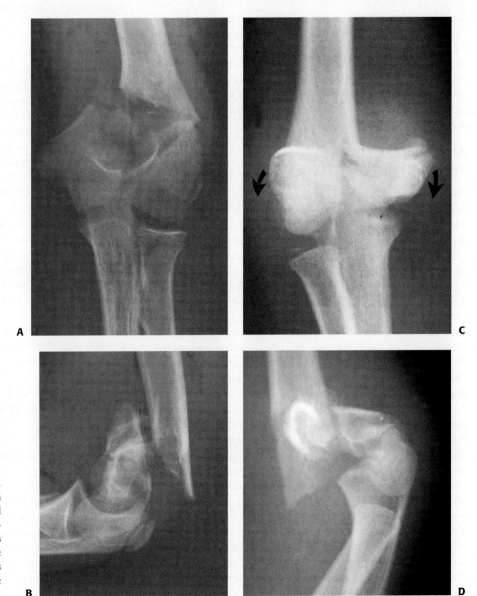

Figure 14-1. A–D: Mechanism patterns. **A, B:** The more common flexion pattern in which the condylar fragments are situated anterior to the distal shaft. **C, D:** An extensor pattern in which the condylar fragments are situated posterior to the distal shaft. The muscle origins on the respective condyles cause them to diverge in the coronal plane (*arrows*) and flex in the sagittal plane.

extension mechanism has been suggested by patients in their description of the dynamics of the fall and indirectly by the position of the distal fragments in relation to the diaphyses of the humerus—in other words, lying posterior (Fig. 14-1C,D). In the extension type of injury, the coronoid portion of the semilunar notch produces the wedge effect.

It has been suggested that the attachment of the forearm flexor and extensor muscles and their contraction during the injury may play a role in the displacement pattern of this fracture. Because of their origins on the epicondyles, they accentuate both the separation in the coronal plane and the forward displacement in the sagittal plane. This displacement pattern is often evident on the injury films (see Fig. 14-1C,D) and consideration will aid later reduction maneuvers.

INJURIES ASSOCIATED WITH T-CONDYLAR FRACTURES DISTAL OF THE HUMERUS

Very little has been written on the type of associated injuries seen with T-condylar fractures of the distal humerus in children. In general, these are high-velocity injuries which are typically the result of high-energy mechanisms, such as motor vehicle collisions, high-speed sporting accidents, or falls from significant heights.[15] Open wounds, other ipsilateral upper limb injuries, and general systemic injury can occur because of the heightened energy of the trauma that occurs. A recent series has documented in adolescents with intra-articular distal humerus fractures nearly a quarter were open injuries.[8]

SIGNS AND SYMPTOMS OF T-CONDYLAR FRACTURES OF THE DISTAL HUMERUS

The history should focus on the mechanism and time of injury and the identification of other sites of injury. It is important to recognize any prior elbow injury or upper extremity surgery. Rounding out the history would include gathering information on preexisting medical conditions, medication, and hand dominance.

In addition to a complete physical examination, a detailed head-to-toe trauma assessment should be completed, to rule out significant concomitant injuries to the axial and appendicular skeleton. Focused examination of the injured extremity should include inspection for bruising, swelling, deformity, and evidence of any open injuries. A thorough circumferential inspection of the elbow is critical to avoid missing open wounds, which commonly occur on the posterior aspect.[21] Careful examination of distal vascular status is performed, inspecting the distal extremity for color, turgor, and palpating the radial and ulnar pulses. If there is a questionable pulse in the setting of gross malalignment of the arm, gentle longitudinal traction can be used to realign the limb and often restore the distal pulse. A detailed and accurate distal neurologic examination including motor function, hand sensibility, and two-point discrimination or sweating pattern in younger children (median and ulnar nerves) should be performed to identify injury to the median, ulnar, radial, anterior, and posterior interosseous nerve. Documentation of this is very important as there is a high rate of associated nerve injuries and failure to document preoperatively may lead to attribution of the deficit

to the surgery rather than the injury. At the conclusion of the examination, the arm is splinted for comfort in a padded posterior, above-elbow splint.

IMAGING AND OTHER DIAGNOSTIC STUDIES FOR T-CONDYLAR FRACTURES OF THE DISTAL HUMERUS

Clinically, these fractures are most often confused with extension-type supracondylar fractures. The extended position of the elbow, along with the massive swelling, is almost identical to that of the displaced extension type of supracondylar fracture.

Plain radiographs are the cornerstone to the diagnosis. In older children, the differentiation must be made from that of a comminuted supracondylar fracture without intercondylar extension. Sometimes, the diagnosis is not obvious until the fragments have been partially reduced, which allows the vertical fracture lines splitting the trochlea to become more evident. In younger children, the diagnosis is much more difficult because the articular surface is cartilaginous and not visible on plain radiographs. In addition, because of its rarity, the possibility of a T-condylar fracture may not be considered in this age group.

The diagnosis must exclude common fracture patterns of either the isolated lateral or medial condyles and complete separation of the distal humeral physis. In these latter fractures, an important sign is the presence of a medial or lateral Thurstan Holland fragment in the metaphysis.[4] The key differential for the T-condylar fracture is the presence of a vertical fracture line extending down to the apex of the trochlea.

If the diagnosis is suspected after a careful evaluation of the static radiographs, it can be confirmed with a preoperative CT scan for adolescent children, MRI in younger children, or varus/valgus stress films made while the patient is under general anesthesia.[4] The use of contrast medium in the form of an arthrogram intraoperative can also be helpful to distinguish fracture lines and aid in the assessment of the quality of the articular reduction. This simple intervention is readily performed and should be included in the evaluation of a suspicious injury in a younger child due to the low morbidity and potential for treatment and outcome alteration. In the young, the additional arthrographic or MRI studies mostly aid in accurate diagnosis while in older patients with these complex injuries, the CT scans allow for proper surgical planning of fracture-specific fixation.

CLASSIFICATION OF T-CONDYLAR FRACTURES OF THE DISTAL HUMERUS

Fracture Pattern

The fracture pattern in adolescents is similar to that in adults. The condylar fragments are often separated, with the articular surface completely disrupted. In addition to separation of the condylar fragments by the force of the original injury, the muscles that originate on these condylar fragments rotate them in both the coronal and sagittal planes (see Fig. 14-1C,D). In the sagittal plane, the position of the condylar fragments in relation to the humeral shaft and metaphysis can either be anterior (flexor mechanism; see Fig. 14-1B) or posterior (extension mechanism; see Fig. 14-1D).

In skeletally immature patients, the central portions of the condylar fragments are usually separated, but the articular surface may remain intact because of its large cartilage component (Fig. 14-2).[26] Thus, the disruption and displacement are primarily in the osseous supracondylar area. The elasticity of the cartilage of the distal end of the humerus often acts as an opening hinge but protects the articular surface from being completely disrupted.

Classification Systems

Various classifications[16,31] for adult T-condylar fractures have been proposed, but there are problems with applying these classifications to children's injuries. For example, the number of young children with this fracture is so small that it limits the experience of any one clinician in treating all types of fracture patterns. In addition, there is no useful classification for younger patients, in whom the unossified intact articular cartilage is not visible on plain radiographs. Toniolo and Wilkins[34] proposed a simple classification based on the degree of displacement and comminution of the fracture fragments for pediatric T-condylar fractures. Type I fractures are minimally displaced (Fig. 14-3). Type II fractures are displaced but do not have comminution

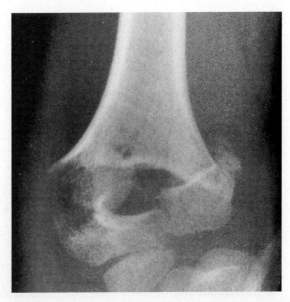

Figure 14-2. Intact articular surface. In this T-condylar fracture in a 7-year-old boy, the thick articular cartilage remains essentially intact, preventing separation of the condylar fragments. This fracture was secured with simple percutaneous pins.

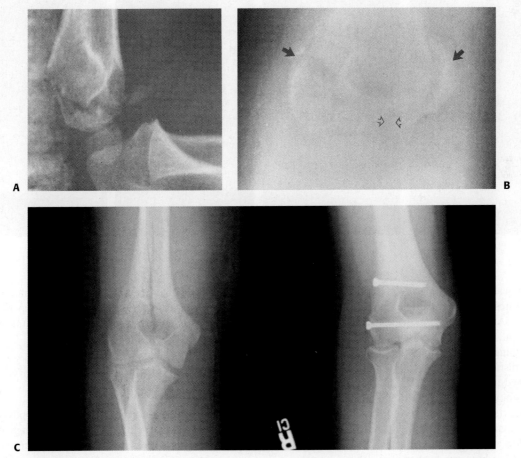

Figure 14-3. Examples of type I T-condylar fractures. **A:** Lateral view of type I undisplaced T-condylar fracture in a 6-year-old. **B:** AP of the T-condylar fracture line (*open arrows*) was not appreciated until it healed. There are both medial and lateral Thurstan Holland fragments (*solid arrows*) (Courtesy of Ruben D. Pechero, MD). **C:** Pre- and postoperative x-rays of minimally displaced intra-articular type I T-condylar fracture in a 16-year-old boy treated with closed reduction and percutaneous screw fixation.

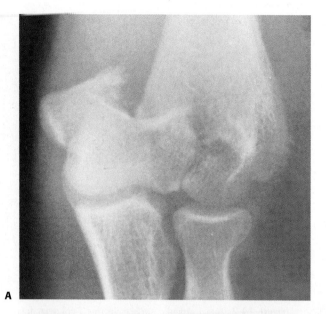

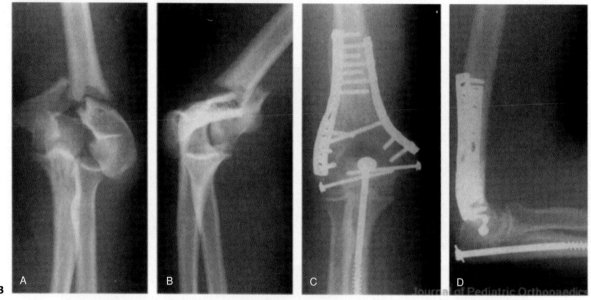

Figure 14-4. Type II displaced T-condylar factures. **A:** Type II displaced T-condylar fracture with very little metaphyseal comminution. **B:** Pre- and postoperative images of displaced type II T-condylar fracture with significant displacement but no comminution, treated with olecranon osteotomy and bicolumn rigid fixation to facilitate early range of motion.

of the metaphyseal fragments (Fig. 14-4). Type III fractures are displaced fractures with comminution of the metaphyseal fragments (Fig. 14-5A,B).

In a child, the integrity of the articular surface may be difficult to determine without using arthrography, ultrasound, or MRI. Because disruption of the articular surface is rare, this factor was not used in those general classification schemes. However, it is imperative to know the status of articular alignment before and after treatment.

In adolescents aged 12 years or older, classification and treatment follow similar patterns to those for adults. In general, intra-articular humerus fractures are defined by column (medial, lateral, or both) and degree of comminution. The Arbeitsgemeinschaft für Osteosynthesefragen (AO) classification is used most often (Fig. 14-6). T-condylar fractures in the adolescent are usually AO C1 and C2 injuries.[29] Fortunately,

C3 injuries with marked comminution are rare in the adolescent. Metaphyseal–diaphyseal fractures are separate entities and need to be recognized as such for proper treatment and fixation decisions.[11]

OUTCOME MEASURES FOR T-CONDYLAR FRACTURES OF THE DISTAL HUMERUS

Common clinical outcomes recorded in T-condylar fractures of the distal humerus include time to union, range of motion, and elbow strength as measured through Cybex testing. Functional outcome scores for both operative and nonoperative treatments such as the Mayo Elbow Performance Score[24] and the Disability of the Arm, Shoulder, and Hand[9] (DASH) are frequently used to measure functional improvement after upper extremity surgery.

(text continues on page 536)

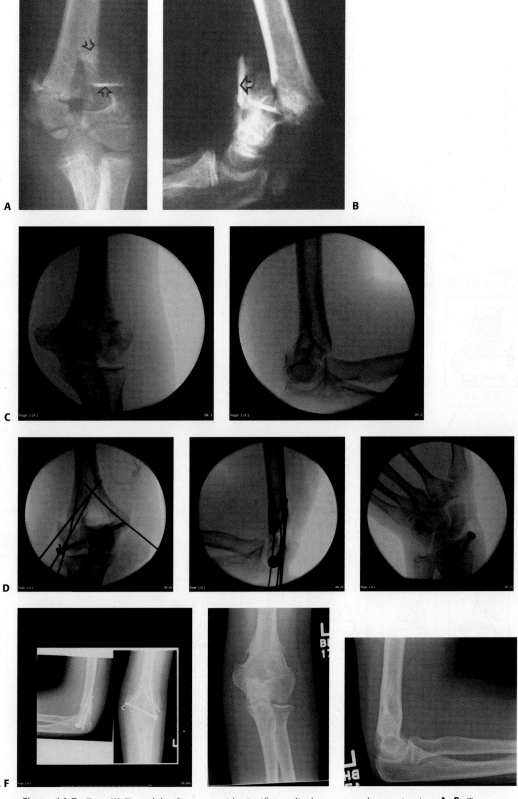

Figure 14-5. Type III T-condylar fractures with significant displacement and comminution. **A, B:** Type III—two views of markedly comminuted T-condylar fracture with multiple displaced fragments (*arrows*) in a 12-year-old. **C–F:** Pre-, intra-, postoperative, and final healed radiographs of a 12-year-old girl with displaced and severely comminuted distal humerus and ipsilateral distal radius fracture, treated with a combination of transarticular screw and cross-wire fixation. At 1 year she has made a complete recovery with comparable range of motion to her contralateral elbow.

Bone: humerus (1)

Location: Distal segment (13)

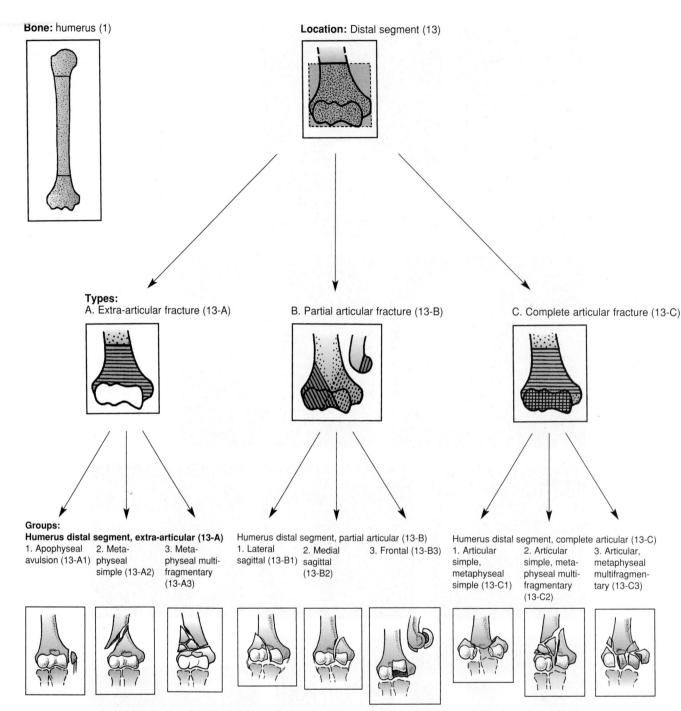

Types:

A. Extra-articular fracture (13-A)

B. Partial articular fracture (13-B)

C. Complete articular fracture (13-C)

Groups:

Humerus distal segment, extra-articular (13-A)

1. Apophyseal avulsion (13-A1)
2. Meta-physeal simple (13-A2)
3. Meta-physeal multi-fragmentary (13-A3)

Humerus distal segment, partial articular (13-B)

1. Lateral sagittal (13-B1)
2. Medial sagittal (13-B2)
3. Frontal (13-B3)

Humerus distal segment, complete articular (13-C)

1. Articular simple, metaphyseal simple (13-C1)
2. Articular simple, meta-physeal multi-fragmentary (13-C2)
3. Articular, metaphyseal multifragmen-tary (13-C3)

Figure 14-6. The AO classification of distal humerus fractures—fractures are classified as extra-articular, partial articular, and complete articular fracture and treatment can be tailored based on fracture classification. (Redrawn with permission from Marsh JL, Slongo TF, Agel J, et al. Fracture and dislocation classification compendium—2007: Orthopaedic Trauma Association classification, database, and outcomes committee. *J Orthop Trauma.* 2007;21(suppl 10):S1–S133.)

Humerus, distal complete, articular simple, metaphyseal simple (13-C1)

1. With slight displacement (13-C1.1)
(1) Y-shaped
(2) T-shaped
(3) V-shaped

2. With marked displacement
(13-C1.2)
(1) Y-shaped
(2) T-shaped
(3) V-shaped

3. T-shaped epiphyseal (13-C1.3)

C1

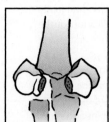
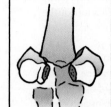
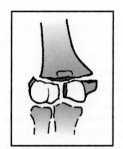

Humerus, distal, complete articular simple metaphyseal multifragmentary (13-C2)

1. With intact wedge (13-C2.1)
(1) metaphyseal lateral
(2) metaphyseal medial
(3) metaphysio-diaphyseal-lateral
(4) metaphysio-diaphyseal-medial

2. With a fragmented wedge (13-C2.2)
(1) metaphyseal lateral
(2) metaphyseal medial
(3) metaphysio-diaphyseal-lateral
(4) metaphysio-diaphyseal-medial

3. Complex (13-C2.3)

C2

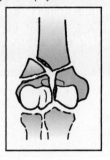
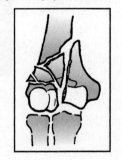
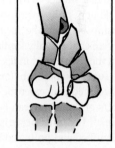

Humerus, distal, complete multifragmentary (13-C3)

1. Metaphyseal simple (13-C3.1)

2. Metaphyseal wedge (13-C3.2)
(1) intact
(2) fragmented

3. Metaphyseal complex (13-C3.3)
(1) localized
(2) extending into diaphysis

C3

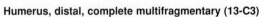
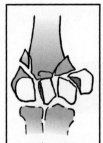
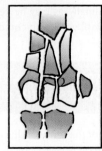

Figure 14-6. (*Continued*)

PATHOANATOMY AND APPLIED ANATOMY RELATING TO T-CONDYLAR FRACTURES OF THE DISTAL HUMERUS

The elbow is a complex joint composed of three individual joints contained within a common articular cavity. Ossification of the distal humerus proceeds in a predictable order. However, the rate of ossification in girls generally exceeds that of boys.[10,12,13,27] In some areas, such as the olecranon and lateral epicondyle, the difference between boys and girls in ossification age may be as great as 2 years.[12] Knowledge of the sequence and timing of ossification in the elbow will aid the treating physician in differentiating true intercondylar pathology from normal anatomic variant.

The bone of the distal humerus is triangular in shape. The medial and lateral columns of the distal humerus form the supracondylar region and are characterized by sharp and thin ridges of bone, respectively.[3] At the base of the triangle lies the trochlea, which represents the most distal portion of the humerus. It is important to realize that the lateral column of the distal humerus curves anteriorly along with the anteriorly translated articular surface of the distal humerus, but the medial column is straight in line with the humeral diaphysis. The spatial relationship between the medial column, lateral column, and trochlea are conceptually similar to a spool of thread being held between the thumb and index finger.[17]

The surgical approach for distal humerus fractures most widely accepted is an extensile posterior incision through which all aspects of the elbow can be exposed including the anterior structures.[28] The ulnar nerve is frequently a structure that needs to be identified and protected during open reduction and internal fixation. It passes through the cubital tunnel just posterior to the medial epicondyle and is held in close proximity to the distal humerus by Osborne's fascia. Higher on the lateral side the radial nerve pierces the intermuscular septum where it is vulnerable to injury by a fracture or a surgical exposure extending proximally, as may be necessary in the uncommon fracture with metaphyseal with comminution.

TREATMENT OPTIONS FOR T-CONDYLAR FRACTURES OF THE DISTAL HUMERUS

Because of the rarity of this injury, treatment recommendations are based on isolated case or small retrospective case series and/ or the application of adult treatment principles.[1,4,5,16,19,26,29,30,35] Regardless of the treatment method, certain basic principles must be considered in dealing with these fractures.

A treatment plan must be individualized for the specific fracture, patient age, and the surgeon's level of expertise and experience. The following principles must be considered in planning a treatment method:

- The T-condylar fracture is an articular fracture, so the first goal is to restore and stabilize the joint surface.
- Stability depends on the integrity of the lateral and medial supracondylar columns.

- Elbow articular mobility depends on articular congruity, correct alignment of the axis of motion, and debris- and bone-free fossae.
- Closed methods alone usually cannot produce an acceptable result because the muscle and collateral ligament forces applied to the fragments make the fracture unstable.
- Most patients are adolescents with minimal potential for bone remodeling and should be treated with bicolumn open reduction and internal fixation similar to an adult.
- Although surgical reduction may produce an acceptable reduction on radiograph, it may add to the already extensive damage to soft tissues; this in turn can contribute to postoperative stiffness. Stable internal fixation that allows for immediate postoperative movement is important in reducing the risk of contracture development.

NONOPERATIVE TREATMENT OF T-CONDYLAR DISTAL HUMERUS FRACTURES

Indications/Contraindications

Nonoperative Treatment of T-Condylar Fractures of the Distal Humerus:
INDICATIONS AND CONTRAINDICATIONS

Indications	Relative Contraindications
• Young children <8 years with intact periosteum • Simple fractures without comminution, displacement, or angulation	• Fracture displacement >2 mm • Fracture comminution • Ipsilateral arm injuries

Most T-condylar fractures of the distal humerus are best treated with some form of open reduction and internal fixation. However, there is a narrow range of fractures that are indicated for management of these injuries with closed treatment and casting. Children who are under 8 years of age with robust periosteum and essentially nondisplaced fractures may be candidates for closed treatment and casting.

Closed Treatment

A very small number of T-condylar fractures of the distal humerus can potentially be treated with immobilization exclusively. Nondisplaced fractures can be splinted or casted until healing with close radiographic follow-up. An above-elbow cast is applied for at least 3 weeks with repeat x-rays on a weekly interval to detect interval displacement. Some clinicians perform a closed reduction for very minimally displaced fractures, although this is not common. Reduction under conscious sedation or anesthesia with in-line traction and live fluoroscopy is necessary to ensure that acceptable reduction is maintained. Review of reduction may be necessary with three-dimensional (3D) imaging in the form of CT or MRI. To be honest, we rarely treat fractures with any displacement closed without fixation. If a reduction is required, we view this as an unstable injury and at a minimum and will use three percutaneous pins to stabilize the anatomic alignment of the articular surface and both columns.

Outcomes

Most T-condylar fractures of the distal humerus are treated operatively, and therefore it is very difficult to tease out the results of nonoperative management of these fractures. In our review of several series, only 4 of 48 combined fractures were treated nonoperatively.[19,26,29] In these limited cases, all patients achieved a full arc of motion without complications from their fracture or treatment. Good results can only be expected with very careful selection.

OPERATIVE TREATMENT OF T-CONDYLAR DISTAL HUMERUS FRACTURES

Indications/Contraindications

Adolescents with T-condylar fractures of the distal humerus are usually treated with bicolumn open reduction and internal fixation similar to an adult. Indications for open reduction and internal fixation include all displaced extra-articular fractures, displacement of the articular surface greater than 2 mm, comminution of the distal humerus with greater than two fracture fragments, and ipsilateral fracture(s) of the upper extremity. Open fractures, pending compartment syndromes, and avascular limbs are surgical emergencies. However, the majority of T-condylar fractures of the distal humerus can be treated electively within 72 hours from the initial injury.

In adolescents, most T-condylar fractures of the distal humerus are C1 according to the AO classification (see Fig. 14-6). Therefore, choosing either a triceps-splitting or triceps-reflecting approach is sufficient to facilitate access for open reduction and internal fixation. In the rare circumstances of C2 or C3 fractures, especially in the setting of anterior comminution, an olecranon osteotomy is warranted to facilitate visualization and fixation of the articular surface.

Closed Reduction and Percutaneous Pin/Screw Fixation

In young children (<8 years) with robust periosteum, the T-condylar distal humerus fracture may represent isolated hinging of the periosteum with minimal displacement of the intercondylar fracture. Careful preoperative imaging will demonstrate merely hinging of the articular surface without significant displacement. In younger children with minimal displacement, it is not unreasonable to perform a fluoroscopic guided reduction and stabilization with multiple percutaneous pins. Generally three smooth, appropriate-sized wires are used: One horizontally from the lateral to medial to stabilize the joint surface and two to stabilize the medial and lateral columns. These pins can either be divergent lateral entry or both medial and lateral entry pins.

In older children with minimal displacement, percutaneous reduction and cannulated column screw fixation are acceptable. This, to some degree, violates standard adult principles of open reduction internal fixation, it relies on the adolescent periosteum and rapid healing potential. However, if anatomic articular alignment and stable internal fixation can be achieved percutaneously, then less invasive treatment is appropriate. It is critical to have superior fluoroscopic images intraoperatively to prevent the realization of persistent fracture fragment displacement and/or inadvertent screw malposition on follow-up radio-

graphs. An arthrogram can be very helpful to confirm reduction at the articular surface.

Preoperative Planning

✔ Closed Reduction and Percutaneous Pin/Screw Fixation of T-Condylar Fractures of the Distal Humerus: PREOPERATIVE PLANNING CHECKLIST	
OR table	☐ Flat Jackson with addition of radiolucent hand table
Position/positioning aids	☐ Supine on hand table
Fluoroscopy location	☐ C-arm can come in from the head or foot of the bed when necessary
Equipment	☐ Large AO pelvic reduction clamps, C- or K-wires, cannulated screws (4 or 4.5 mm)
Tourniquet	☐ Sterile tourniquet can be used but not necessary

Surgical planning includes decisions on percutaneous pin versus screw fixation and patient positioning in the operative room. Careful scrutiny of preoperative radiographs and 3D imaging (usually CT scans) is imperative. Sometimes, intraoperative fluoroscopy images with traction realignment are essential in final decision-making about surgical approach and fixation methods. These should be performed before final positioning and prepping and draping as changing course intraoperative is difficult. Percutaneous treatment should only be chosen if anatomic reduction and stable fixation can be achieved with limited postoperative immobilization to lessen the risk of elbow contracture.

Similar principles for displaced adult distal humerus intra-articular fractures are employed, with reduction and stabilization of the articular surface first, followed by stabilization of the medial and lateral columns. If percutaneous reduction and fixation is performed, a large, external bone holding the reduction clamp is used to facilitate interfragmentary reduction and compression of the joint, prior to pin or screw fixation. Accurate placement of a transverse pin to hold the articular segments in an anatomic position is critical. Depending on the degree of displacement and fracture fragment configuration, provisional or definitive fixation can be achieved with standard medial and lateral column pins as in a supracondylar humerus fracture. As noted above, in limited scenarios, these fractures can be treated definitively with closed reduction and percutaneous fixation using either smooth wires or cannulated screws.

Positioning

Percutaneous fixation of T-condylar fractures of the distal humerus is usually performed in the supine position, but can be facilitated also in the lateral or prone position. Most commonly, the patient is positioned supine with arm on a hand table. The arm is elevated on a stack of towels to facilitate easier screw insertion. Bringing the shoulder into abduction and elbow into extension can improve the quality of visualization of the fracture with C-arm imaging. Generally the young have enough rotatory motion about the shoulder to allow for proper visualization in the supine position.

An alternative approach is to position the patient in the lateral position with an axillary roll to protect the brachial plexus on the nonoperative limb. In this position, a large bump is fashioned or a specialized arm holder is used to hold the arm in internally rotated position at the shoulder with 90 degrees of flexion at the elbow. The C-arm machine can obtain acceptable images coming from the head or feet parallel to the bed. Finally, patients can be positioned in the prone position with the operative limb exposed on a separate small arm board/table or hanging off the side of the bed. In this position, bolsters are used in a standard fashion similar to a spinal procedure to decompress the abdomen and protect the neurovascular structures. The arm is held similar to the lateral position, with internal rotation of the shoulder and 90 degrees of flexion at the elbow with minimal tension. Again, C-arm imaging is accessible from the head or foot of the bed. Prone positioning is most useful in obese patients. Positioning should always be selected to enable the fluoroscopy machine to be maneuvered around the patient, avoid operating directly on the fluoroscopy tube.

Surgical Approach

In closed reduction and percutaneous pin/screw fixation, limited surgical exposure is performed. In some settings, small stab incisions are made to ensure that the large bone reducing forceps can be placed directly on bone (medial and lateral epicondyles most commonly) to generate the desired compressive effect. In general, wires are placed percutaneously from the lateral column of the distal humerus. On the medial side, small 1- to 2-cm incisions can be made to prevent inadvertent injury to the ulnar nerve, there is a much higher incidence of ulnar nerve instability in children than adults. In addition, the arm is placed in a semi-extended position when passing wires/screws from the medial to lateral, to decrease the risk of iatrogenic ulnar nerve injury.

Technique

> ✔ **Closed Reduction and Percutaneous Pin/Screw Fixation of T-Condylar Fractures of the Distal Humerus:**
> KEY SURGICAL STEPS
>
> ❑ Begin with performance of accurate AP/lateral and oblique fluoroscopic images of the distal humerus.
> ❑ Make small stab incisions, to facilitate bone clamp application.
> ❑ Under dynamic fluoroscopy verify that fracture reduction is being achieved with dynamic compression.
> ❑ Consider the use of an arthrogram.
> ❑ Once the fracture is in an acceptable position.
> ❑ Place appropriate wires to achieve provisional stability.
> ❑ Fix the articular fragment first.
> ❑ Address column stability second.
> ❑ Once the wires are in the correct position, confirm with live fluoroscopy to ensure adequate reduction and wire placement.
> ❑ Measure screw lengths when appropriate and then overdrill guide wires.
> ❑ Place the screw across the articular fragment first and then stabilize the medial/lateral columns.
> ❑ Test stability with flexion and extension.

OPEN REDUCTION AND INTERNAL FIXATION

Preoperative Planning

> ✔ **ORIF of T-Condylar Fractures of the Distal Humerus:**
> PREOPERATIVE PLANNING CHECKLIST

OR table	❑ Flat Jackson with fluoroscopic arm board extension
Position/positioning aids	❑ Prone position on bolsters to decompress abdomen and protect neurovascular structures
Fluoroscopy location	❑ C-arm can come in from the head or foot of the bed when necessary
Equipment	❑ Large AO pelvic reduction clamps, K-wires, cannulated screws and precontoured distal humerus plates or pelvic reconstruction plates, Penrose drain and vessel loop to isolate the ulnar nerve
Tourniquet	❑ Sterile tourniquet used but can be let down if necessary because of timing
Other	❑ Monopolar and bipolar cautery to facilitate dissection of the ulnar nerve

The surgical treatment of T-condylar fractures of the distal humerus involves consideration of three critical components: (1) surgical approach—triceps splitting, paratricipital, triceps reflecting, or olecranon osteotomy; (2) type of fixation—single column, bicolumn orthogonal, or parallel plating; and (3) body positioning—prone, lateral decubitus, or supine.

Positioning

Fixation of distal humerus fractures can be facilitated in the supine, lateral, or prone positions with the choice determined primarily based on the anticipated exposure, presence of concomitant injuries, and surgeon experience.

In the setting of polytrauma, patients may be positioned in supine/sloppy lateral position with a large bump placed under the ipsilateral shoulder. Surgery can be performed with the arm across the chest, held in place by an assistant or a towel clamp. Bringing the arm into abduction and extension can aid with visualization of the fracture and improve the quality of C-arm imaging.

An alternative approach is to position the patient in the lateral position with an axillary roll to protect the brachial plexus on the nonoperative limb. In this position, a large bump is fashioned or a specialized arm holder is used to hold the arm in internally rotated position at the shoulder with 90 degrees of flexion at the elbow. The C-arm machine can obtain acceptable images coming from the head or feet parallel to the bed.

Finally, patients can be positioned in the prone position with the operative limb exposed on a separate small arm board/table. In this position, bolsters are used in standard fashion similar to a spinal procedure to decompress the abdomen and protect neurovascular structures. The arm is held similar to the lateral position, with internal rotation of the shoulder and 90 degrees

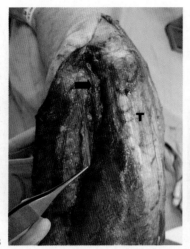 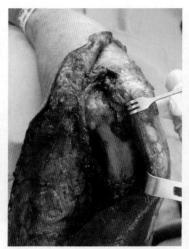 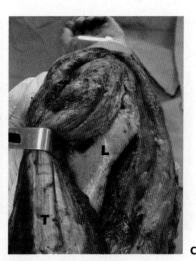

A, B   C

Figure 14-7. Paratricipital approach. The paratricipital approach is done through a longitudinal posterior skin incision. Medially (**A**) the ulnar nerve (*black arrow*) is identified. The medial intermuscular septum (forceps) is excised and the triceps muscle is elevated off the posterior aspect of the distal humerus (**B**). Laterally the triceps muscle is elevated off the posterolateral aspect of the distal humerus, allowing exposure of the lateral column, olecranon fossa, and posterior aspect of the trochlea (**C**). L, lateral column; T, triceps. (Reprinted with permission from Bucholz RW, Court-Brown CM, Heckman JD, et al. *Rockwood and Green's Fractures in Adults.* 7th ed. Philadelphia, PA: Lippincott Williams & Wilkins; 2010.)

of flexion at the elbow with minimal tension. Again, C-arm imaging is accessible from the head or foot of the bed.

Surgical Approach

A universal skin approach is used for most surgical approaches associated with T-condylar fractures of the distal humerus. A long curvilinear posterior skin incision is used, with the distal extension lateral to the olecranon and then back to the midline onto the proximal ulna. By avoiding the tip of the olecranon, this prevents an irritating posterior scar. Skin and subcutaneous fasciocutaneous flaps are elevated extensively at the level of the fascia. The ulnar nerve requires careful attention, protection, mobilization, and decompression at this stage and throughout the remainder of the operation. An elastic loop is placed around the nerve, and the nerve is handled gently for the entire surgical procedure.

Triceps-Splitting Approach

- Achieved either via a direct posterior incision in the triceps fascia (Fig. 14-7)[23]
- Or using long oblique fascial incisions from the medial and lateral epicondyles, to a more proximal connecting point in the midline and reflect the resultant tongue of fascia from proximal to distal down to its insertion on the olecranon, separating the tendon from the muscle, while protecting the ulnar nerve on the medial side.[35]
- The triceps muscle is split in the midline and is retracted beyond the medial and lateral columns, respectively, with broad retractors.
- The radial and ulnar nerves are protected behind retractors during exposure, reduction, and fixation. The radial nerve proximally limits this approach in fractures with metaphyseal comminution.

Flexion of the elbow allows for visualization and fixation of the articular fragments.

Triceps-Reflecting Approach (Bryan and Morrey)

- The medial aspect of the triceps is elevated from the humerus along the intermuscular septum to the level of the posterior capsule. In children and adolescents, this can be achieved with subperiosteal elevation (Fig. 14-8).[7,30]
- The superficial fascia of the forearm is incised distally for about 6 cm to the periosteum of the medial aspect of the proximal ulna.
- The periosteum and fascia are carefully elevated as a single layer from the medial to lateral, distal to proximal. Care must be taken to maintain the continuity of the triceps, periosteum, and fascia. The medial aspect of the junction between the triceps insertion and the superficial fascia and periosteum of the ulna is the weakest portion of the reflected tissue. Elevation off the apophysis is also delicate as buttonholing can occur here which will limit the length and strength of the triceps fascial flap and risk destabilizing the triceps insertion into the olecranon.
- At the conclusion of skeletal fixation, the triceps insertion periosteal sleeve is repaired directly to the bone with transosseus sutures or suture anchors.
- This approach is contraindicated in open fractures, where a portion of the triceps may become avascular secondary to the initial trauma from the fracture and further dissection increases this risk.

Olecranon Osteotomy

- The olecranon osteotomy has been described as a standard approach for adult T-condylar distal humerus fractures (Fig. 14-9).

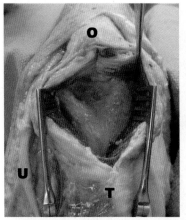
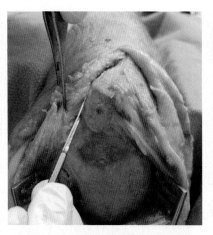
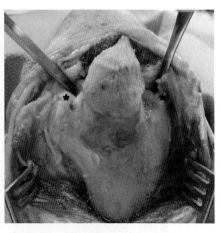

Figure 14-8. Triceps split. A midline approach is made through the center of the triceps tendon and medial head (**A**). The approach can be extended distally by splitting the triceps insertion to the olecranon and raisin medial and lateral full-thickness fasciotendinous flaps (**B, C**). To gain further exposure of the posterior trochlea, the elbow is flexed and the olecranon tip may be excised. (Reprinted with permission from Bucholz RW, Court-Brown CM, Heckman JD, et al. *Rockwood and Green's Fractures in Adults*. 7th ed. Philadelphia, PA: Lippincott Williams & Wilkins; 2010.)

- In our hands, we reserve this approach in children and adolescents for complex T-condylar fractures of the distal humerus with significant intra-articular comminution (AO C3 T-condylar fractures).
- Similar to the paratricipital approach, the triceps is mobilized from the medial and lateral septa and followed distally to the elbow joint.
- A longitudinal cancellous screw is predrilled down the olecranon from the tip or apophysis.
- This screw is removed, and a chevron-type osteotomy is performed at the deepest portion of the trochlear notch of the olecranon process and corresponding with the area devoid of articular cartilage (bare area).
- The chevron osteotomy points distally, and is initiated with a fine oscillating saw and completed with a thin osteotome.
- The triceps muscle and the osteotomized proximal half of the olecranon are then reflected superiorly.
- The osteotomy can alternatively be fixed with a precontoured olecranon plate or parallel K-wires and tension band technique.
- At the end of the reduction, the osteotomy is reduced and fixed with compression fixation with cancellous screw and washer fixation.

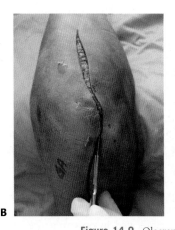
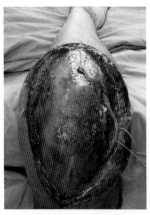
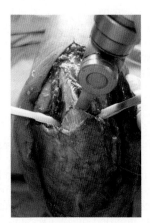
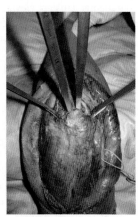

Figure 14-9. Olecranon osteotomy. The olecranon osteotomy is approached via a longitudinal posterior skin incision (**A**). The ulnar nerve is exposed and may be prepared for anterior subcutaneous transposition (**B**). The subcutaneous border of the proximal ulnar is exposed and the nonarticular portion of the greater sigmoid notch between the olecranon articular facet and the coronoid articular facet is clearly defined. Medial and lateral retractors are then placed into the ulnohumeral joint and an apex distal chevron osteotomy entering into the bare area is marked on the subcutaneous border of the ulna. A microsagittal saw is used to complete two-thirds of the osteotomy (**C**) and two osteotomes, placed into each arm of the chevron, apply controlled leverage to fracture the remaining third (**D**). (Reprinted with permission from Bucholz RW, Court-Brown CM, Heckman JD, et al. *Rockwood and Green's Fractures in Adults*. 7th ed. Philadelphia, PA: Lippincott Williams & Wilkins; 2010.)

Technique

> ### ✔ ORIF of T-Condylar Fractures of the Distal Humerus:
> #### KEY SURGICAL STEPS
>
> ❑ Longitudinal posterior midline skin incision, avoiding the tip of the olecranon
> ❑ Elevation of medial and lateral fasciocutaneous flaps as necessary
> ❑ Identification of the ulnar nerve, decompression, and mobilization for protection during the remainder of the procedure
> ❑ Surgical approach dictated by
> • Fracture type
> • Presence of associated injuries
> • Degree of soft tissue injury
> • Surgeon preference
> ❑ Exposure of fracture fragments, removal of intervening soft tissues and fracture hematoma
> ❑ Temporarily stabilize the joint anatomically with guide wires from the cannulated screw set (4 or 4.5 depending on the patient)
> ❑ Stabilize the anatomic joint fixation to columns temporarily
> ❑ Confirm anatomic alignment under direct visualization and fluoroscopically
> ❑ Replace temporary cannulated pin fixation with compressive screw fixation across the joint
> ❑ Convert the column fixation to orthogonal plates
> • Medial 3.5 pelvic reconstruction or precontoured anatomic specific plate
> • Posterolateral 3.5 reconstruction, dynamic compression, or precontoured anatomic specific plate
> ❑ Test stability and flexion and extension arc of motion
> ❑ Decide where the ulnar nerve should lie, in its original position or in a transposed position

Reconstruction of the Articular Surface

Our first priority is to reestablish the integrity of the articular fragments—in other words, to convert it to a supracondylar fracture (Fig. 14-10). The olecranon and coronoid fossae must be cleared of bony fragments or debris to eliminate the chance of bony impingement against their respective processes with motion. The best way to stabilize the condyles is with a screw passed transversely through the center of the axis of rotation in such a manner as to apply transverse compression. This stabilization method may require a small temporary secondary transverse pin proximal to the screw to prevent rotation of the fragments as the guide hole is drilled or when the compression screw is being applied. This pin can be removed after the fragments are secured.

In most adolescents, this is essentially an adult type of fracture pattern. Direct visualization of the reduction of all fracture fragments is mandatory. It is critical to get the joint surface anatomic and rigidly fixed. Regardless of surgical exposure (Bryan–Morey, Triceps splitting, Olecranon osteotomy), it is imperative the surgeon visualize the articular fracture reduction completely. A single, short-threaded cancellous screw and washer is most commonly used. A 3.5- to 4.5-mm diameter screw is placed from lateral to medial depending on the size of the bone and the available space between the articular surface and the olecranon fossa. Open physes further complicate the delicacy of exact screw placement in this region. The ulnar nerve is protected on the medial side. Once anatomic reduction and fixation of the articular surface are achieved, secure fixation of the columns is performed next. However, do not rush to column fixation

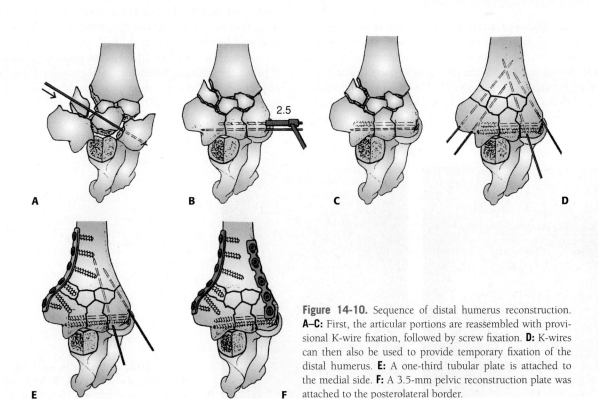

A   **B**   **C**   **D**

E   **F**

Figure 14-10. Sequence of distal humerus reconstruction. **A–C:** First, the articular portions are reassembled with provisional K-wire fixation, followed by screw fixation. **D:** K-wires can then also be used to provide temporary fixation of the distal humerus. **E:** A one-third tubular plate is attached to the medial side. **F:** A 3.5-mm pelvic reconstruction plate was attached to the posterolateral border.

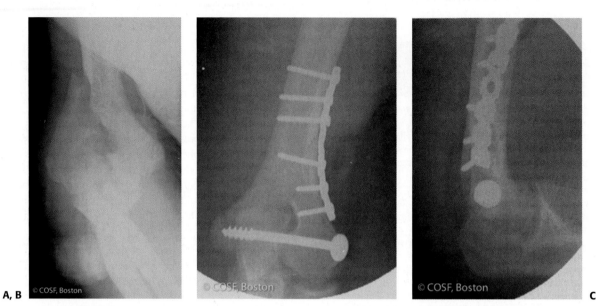

Figure 14-11. A–C: Type II displaced T-condylar fracture. This fracture was initially treated with distal transarticular compression screw for stability and then followed by single lateral column fixation.

unless the joint surface is reduced correctly. In younger teenagers, the joint cartilage can buckle and tear and this can make the anatomic alignment harder to discern than in more skeletally mature patients in which the bony fragments interdigitate nicely (Fig. 14-11). Fortunately, rarely do adolescent injuries have the same degree of extensive periarticular bony comminution like the more complex adult fracture–dislocations.

Stabilization of the Supracondylar Columns

Once the condylar and articular integrity has been reestablished, the distal fragments must be secured to the proximal fragment by stabilizing the supracondylar fragment columns. A factor in the column fixation decision is how important is it to initiate early motion. In a younger child with rapid bony healing, pin fixation is often satisfactory; the pins can be removed after 3 to 4 weeks to allow for protected motion. In an older adolescent nearer to skeletal maturity, we prefer rigid fixation— usually plates or less commonly, screws—that allows early motion (Figs. 14-10E,F and 14-12). Before applying the plates, the supracondylar columns can be stabilized temporarily with pin fixation (see Fig. 14-12).

Principles of Plate Fixation

The plates must be strong; thin semitubular plates can be inadequate and may break.[36] However, double stacking semitubular plates can be used in younger or thinner teenagers. Proper rotational bending is harder in these plates. Usually the reinforced malleable reconstructive type of plates used for fixation of pelvic fractures can be anatomically contoured and provide very secure fixation of the distal humerus. It is best to place the plates at 90 degrees to each other, which provides for a more stable construct.[14,20,32,33]

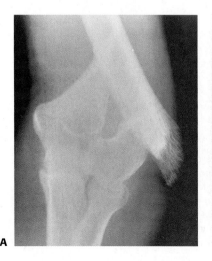
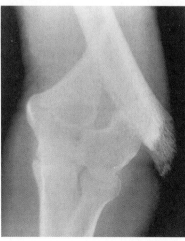

Figure 14-12. T-condylar humeral fracture with plate and screw fixation. **A, B:** Injury films of a type II flexion pattern in a 16-year-old boy.

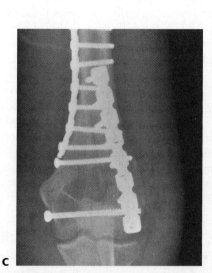
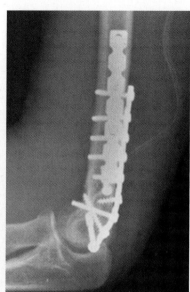

C

D

Figure 14-12. (*Continued*) **C, D:** Articular integrity was first restored with a transcondylar compression screw. The condyles were secured to the metaphysis and distal shaft using pelvic reconstruction plates placed at 90 degrees to each other.

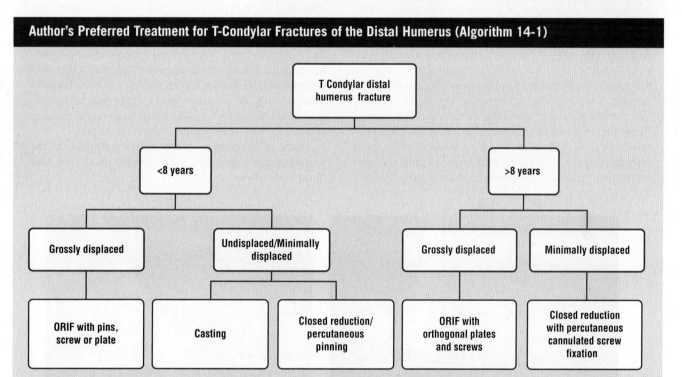

Algorithm 14-1 Author's preferred treatment of T-condylar fractures of the distal humerus according to age and displacement.

Because this fracture is rare in children, there are limited standard recommendations for treatment. Our suggestions are based on a combination of our clinical experience and the experience of others in a few series.[5,11,16,19,26,29,30,35] Our first imperative in these fractures is to reestablish the integrity of the articular surface to maintain the congruity of the joint. Rarely in the young, this can be achieved percutaneously and confirmed arthrographically. Usually, anatomic articular reduction cannot be achieved adequately by closed methods, so we proceed with an open surgical technique.

In the young child, we use the simple classification of Toniolo and Wilkins[34] separating the fractures into three types based on the degree of displacement or comminution to be helpful in guiding the aggressiveness of our treatment. In adolescents, we guide our treatment according to the AO classification.

Type I (Undisplaced or Minimally Displaced)

In type I injuries, there is little displacement of the bony supracondylar columns. In children, the periosteum is often intact and can provide some intrinsic stability. In addition, the thicker articular and epiphyseal cartilage in skeletally immature children may still be intact, even if the bony epiphysis appears severed by a vertical fracture line. Because of this condition, we have found two methods to be successful for these types of fractures.

Closed Treatment

Cast Application

Truly nondisplaced fractures can be treated in a cast. Again, it is imperative to judge completely stable fractures from injuries that can displace. Initial 3D imaging and careful radiographic follow-up are necessary to avoid an articular malunion. Because of the rapid healing in these nondisplaced fractures, the cast can be removed in 4 weeks and a hinged elbow brace initiated to permit early protected motion.

Percutaneous Pin Fixation or Screw Fixation

The minimally displaced fractures in the young require manipulation under general anesthesia and radiographic control to reestablish the supracondylar columns and articular surface anatomy. If there is minor anterior or posterior rotation in the sagittal plane of the metaphyseal portion of the column, a pin placed into that column can be used as a "joystick" to manipulate the fragment into a satisfactory position. Once a satisfactory reduction is achieved, the pin can then be advanced across the fracture site for fixation. These fractures usually require multiple pins placed percutaneously, such as those used in comminuted supracondylar fractures (Fig. 14-13). Because of the rapid healing, the pins can be removed at 3 to 4 weeks to allow early active motion.

In the setting of mild intra-articular displacement, we employ the use of a large bone reducing forceps to help facilitate with our reduction. Often this can be applied percutaneously or through small stab incisions to ensure that the tines of the clamp are placed directly onto the bone (usually medial and lateral epicondyles) of the distal humerus without injury to the neighboring neurovascular structures. Once the articular diastasis is corrected, guide wires from the cannulated screw set are placed with bicortical fixation perpendicular to the fracture line. Appropriate length screws with washers are placed over the guide wires. Compression is applied sequentially, alternating between screws to ensure optimal and balanced compression. This percutaneous technique can only be used when anatomic articular reduction is achieved.

Type II (Displaced Without Comminution)

Open Reduction and Internal Fixation

If there is wide separation of the condylar fragments with marked disruption of the articular surface, stability and articular congruity can be established only with an open surgical procedure. We prefer a triceps-splitting approach for C1 distal humerus fractures and a triceps-sparing Bryan–Morrey approach for C2 distal humerus fractures. Olecranon osteotomy is reserved for comminuted C3 articular fractures in adolescents. We place the patient supine in a "sloppy lateral" position to allow for easier lateral fluoroscopic imaging. A sterile tourniquet is used throughout the surgery.

Initial reconstruction is directed to restoration of the articular surface and then stable fixation of the articular block to the shaft.

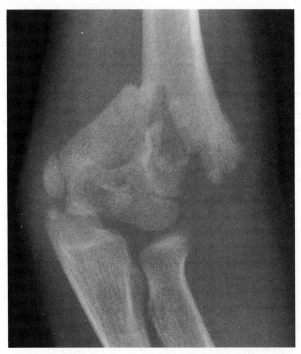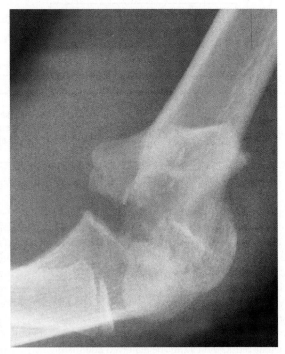

Figure 14-13. Closed reduction and pin fixation. **A, B:** Two views of a type II T-condylar fracture in a 15-year-old.

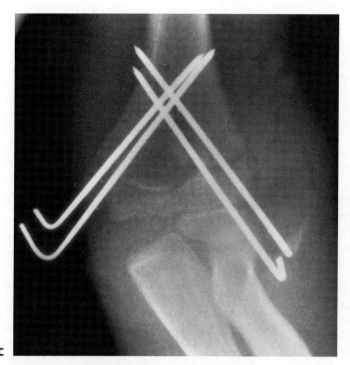
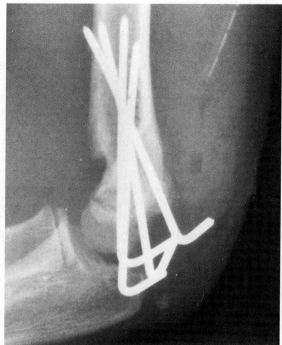

Figure 14-13. (*Continued*) **C, D:** Because an anatomic reduction was achieved by manipulative closed reduction, it was secured with simple multiple pin fixation placed percutaneously. The articular surface was minimally displaced. The pins were removed at 3 weeks. At this age, healing was rapid enough to pull the pins at 3 weeks to allow active motion. Ultimately, the patient was deficient only 10 degrees from achieving full extension.

Some of the plates specifically designed for distal humerus fracture fixation in the adult either do not fit anatomically or are too prominent for many pediatric patients. In these smaller patients, choosing an appropriate sized plate that provides rigid fixation is necessary. In the larger, skeletally mature adolescent, use of adult distal humerus specific plates is appropriate. Later plate removal may be necessary though.

Type III (Displaced With Comminution)

Limited Open Reduction Followed by Traction

Occasionally, the supracondylar columns are too fragmented or contaminated by an open fracture to allow adequate definitive fixation acutely. In such cases, we have found that the best initial treatment method in children involves reestablishing the articular surface and joint congruity with a limited open reduction. The separated condyles are secured with a transverse screw providing compression through the axis of rotation. This procedure can usually be done with minimal soft tissue dissection. Once this is stabilized, the supracondylar columns are then reestablished by placing the extremity in olecranon traction and allowing them to reconstitute with callus formation. The rotational displacement of the condyles created by the origins of the forearm muscles can be neutralized with olecranon traction, in which the elbow is suspended at 90 degrees of flexion. There is usually

adequate stability from the callus around the fracture site at 2 to 3 weeks to discontinue the traction. While in traction, motion can be initiated. This technique can also be used in patients seen late with contaminated soft tissue abrasions or severe soft tissue problems. In selected patients, such as an adolescent with severe bone loss, plating followed by bone grafting may be indicated. Following 3 weeks of traction, the elbow is then immobilized in a hinged cast brace for an additional 2 to 3 weeks. This immobilization allows the initiation of protected active motion. With the present emphasis on short hospitalization, however, we find that skeletal traction is less acceptable for both social and financial reasons.

Multiple Pin Fixation Treatment

In this time of extreme sports even in the young, there are instances of severely comminuted fractures in which the patient's bone will not allow for screw or plate fixation but the fracture is too displaced and/or comminuted to be successfully treated closed. In these instances, open reduction and pin fixation of each fracture fragment is a treatment option. There are times when even suture repair of fractures is required. The fixation does not allow for immediate motion but is started as soon as feasible (see Fig. 14-5, Alg. 14-1). The very distal comminuted injury, especially if there is an open physis, is amenable to this treatment and relies on the rapid healing biology of the younger patient.

Postoperative Care

In situations in which closed reduction and pin fixation is performed, a well-padded circumferential cast is applied for a total of 3 to 6 weeks depending on the degree of healing appreciated on the postreduction radiographs. Patients are then transitioned into a hinged elbow brace and physical therapy is initiated until full range of motion is achieved. Wires are removed when appropriate healing is appreciated.

Children treated with closed reduction and percutaneous screw fixation are transitioned from their circumferential cast at 7 to 10 days and placed into a hinged elbow brace. Increasing motion is permitted over time and healing. Physical therapy is initiated at the first postoperative visit and protected therapy is continued until full range of motion is achieved. Return to sports is dependent on bony healing, restoration of strength, and maximum motion, usually at 3 months.

If plate fixation is used, we place the extremity in a well-padded soft dressing and hinged brace. Continuous passive motion (CPM) initiated in hospital followed by home CPM for complex T-condylar fractures treated with ORIF can aid in regaining elbow motion sooner. The active motion of postoperative therapy is performed in a hinged elbow brace with full motion allowed. A mild 10-degree extension contracture in these patients is anticipated in the best results.

Potential Pitfalls and Preventative Measures

T-Condylar Fractures of the Distal Humerus: POTENTIAL PITFALLS AND PREVENTIONS

Pitfall	Prevention
Articular malreduction	• Appropriate skin and soft tissue exposure, with visualization of critical articular components. • Begin with joint reduction and stabilization, convert from three- or four-part fracture to a two-part supracondylar type fracture.
Inadequate stabilization to allow for early range of motion	• In most T-condylar fractures, rigid fixation is necessary to allow for early range of motion. • Use rigid plate fixation for both medial and lateral columns to facilitate early mobilization.
Ulnar nerve irritation	• At the end of the case, examine the ulnar nerve with flexion and extension. Ensure that it is not irritated by contact with the plate. • Consider ulnar nerve transposition if there is evidence of tether or impingement of the nerve during an arc of motion.

Outcomes

The literature reflects good results with surgical management of displaced distal humerus articular fractures. Zimmerman[37] advocated establishing an anatomic reduction with internal fixation so that early motion could facilitate a more rapid rehabilitation. In the two young children described by Beghin et al.,[4] operative intervention was necessary to achieve a satisfactory reduction. A review of four series[16,19,26,29] supports surgical management: 44 of the 48 elbows in these combined series were treated operatively. The investigators of these series maintained that open reduction and internal fixation was the best way to restore the integrity of the articular surface and stabilize the fracture sufficiently to allow early mobilization. All but one of the patients in this combined series who were treated surgically had good or very good results at follow-up.

Kanellopoulos and Yiannakopoulos[18] described closed reduction of the intra-articular component, with fixation by partially threaded pins for interfragmentary compression. Two elastic titanium intramedullary nails were used for stabilizing the supracondylar component. The T-condylar fractures in two adolescents healed without complications after using this technique. Both patients returned to sports with full elbow range of motion at 6 weeks after surgery.

The triceps-splitting approach, as described by Campbell, was first advocated by Van Gorder.[35] Kasser et al.[19] has demonstrated in children that the triceps-splitting approach did not appear to cause significant muscle dysfunction according to Cybex testing, and concluded that an olecranon osteotomy was unnecessary. The authors concluded that this approach gives adequate exposure of the fracture and the articular surface and does not seem to produce any loss of strength from splitting the triceps. Although one reported patient had radiographic evidence of osteonecrosis of the trochlea,[26] another had a nonunion,[19] and many had some loss of range of motion; none of these surgically treated patients demonstrated any significant loss of elbow function or discomfort.

Alonso-Llames[2] described a paratricipital approach for the treatment of supracondylar and intracondylar fractures in children. A recent series[8] suggests caution using this approach due to less optimal outcome. Bryan and Morrey[7] described a triceps-sparing approach in which the extensor mechanism is reflected laterally, exposing the whole distal humerus. Re et al.[29] found that both the Bryan–Morrey (Triceps Reflecting) and olecranon osteotomy approaches yielded improved extension compared to the triceps-splitting approach. Remia et al.[30] evaluated triceps function and elbow motion in nine patients with T-condylar fractures treated with open reduction through a Bryan and Morrey triceps-sparing approach and compared them to those reported after a triceps-splitting approach. No statistically significant differences were found in function or range of motion.

Recent literature additions support the treatment algorithms outlined in this chapter and prior study findings. Bell[5] has published retrospectively a large series of adolescent distal humerus fractures with 37 of 81 being intra-articular fractures. They found that younger children were more likely to have fractures amenable to management by percutaneous reduction and older adolescents by open reduction. Open reduction was associated with higher complications. However, this may be a product of the original injury rather than the management. Regardless, families should be counseled accordingly. Cook[8] in a retrospective review of 31 type C distal humeral fractures found that C2 and C3 fractures had significantly less motion postoperatively.

The surgeon must choose the surgical approach that allows for the best exposure with the least risk. The priority is adequate visualization of all fracture fragments, especially the joint surface, to achieve rigid anatomic fixation. Early motion is desired to lessen the risk of post-injury contractures about the elbow.

MANAGEMENT OF EXPECTED ADVERSE OUTCOMES AND UNEXPECTED COMPLICATIONS RELATED TO T-CONDYLAR FRACTURES OF THE DISTAL HUMERUS

T-Condylar Fractures of the Distal Humerus:
COMMON ADVERSE OUTCOMES AND COMPLICATIONS

- Postoperative elbow stiffness
- Fracture malunion
- Fracture nonunion and hardware failure
- Osteonecrosis of trochlea
- Hardware impingement and irritation

It is important to emphasize to the parents initially that this is a serious fracture. Because of the considerable soft tissue injury and the involvement of the articular surface of the distal humerus, stiffness and loss of motion of the elbow can be expected regardless of the treatment mode.[16,22,26] In adolescents, failure to provide solid internal fixation that facilitates early motion (i.e., using only pin fixation) can result in a satisfactory radiographic appearance but considerable dysfunction because of residual loss of elbow motion.

Although neurovascular complications have not been mentioned in the few cases reported in the literature, the incidence is probably about equal to that of supracondylar fractures. A recent paper[8] has documented a 16% incidence of preoperative neurologic injuries with these fractures in adolescents. Nerve injuries are predominantly of the ulnar nerve but have also involved the radial and median nerves. Because these fractures occur late in the growth process, partial or total growth arrest caused by the injury or internal fixation has not been a major complication. Likewise, because these are older children, little remodeling of a malunion can be expected. Nonunion,[19] osteonecrosis of the trochlea,[26] and failure of internal fixation have also been reported as complications.

Aside from stiffness, the biggest risk is fracture malunion caused by inadequate reduction and/or fixation. Extra-articular malunion may be tolerated if there is not a block to motion. Intra-articular malunion is clearly a real risk for pain, loss of motion and function, and eventually arthritis. Intra-articular malreduction should be avoided.

Hardware irritation and/or impingement can occur. Obviously, all smooth wires need to be removed after the fracture is healed. Hardware that contributes to impingement pain and/or loss of motion needs to be similarly removed.

Nerve injuries may be associated with the injury or fracture. However they have also been documented during surgical fixation[8]. The ulnar nerve is most at risk both during exposure of fracture fragments and with internal fixation. Ulnar nerve transposition should be considered when either nerve instability is noted with flexion–extension elbow motion or there is concern for hardware impingement on the nerve.

ACKNOWLEDGMENT

The authors thank Benjamin Shore, MD, as a previous co-author of this chapter for contributions that have been carried forward to this edition.

Annotated References

Reference	Annotation
Bell P, Scannell BP, Loeffler BJ, et al. Adolescent distal humerus fractures: ORIF versus CRPP. *J Pediatr Orthop*. 2017;37(8):511–520.	A recent series of distal humeral fractures managed operatively contrasting the outcomes of extra-articular and intra-articular distal humerus fractures.
Bryan RS, Morrey BF. Extensive posterior exposure of the elbow. A triceps-sparing approach. *Clin Orthop Relat Res*. 1982;166:188–192.	Seminal paper describing the triceps sparing approach to the elbow.
Cheung EV, Steinmann SP. Surgical approaches to the elbow. *J Am Acad Orthop Surg*. 2009;17(5):325–333.	This article outlines contemporaneous approaches to the elbow joint. It provides a discussion of their uses and limitations.
Cook JB, Riccio AI, Anderson T, et al. Outcomes after surgical treatment of adolescent intra-articular distal humerus fractures. *J Pediatr Orthop*. 2016;36(8):773–779.	This article provides a comprehensive audit of a recent series of adolescent intra articular distal humerus fractures, their associated injuries, and the expected outcomes.
Toniolo RM, Wilkins KE. *T-Condylar Fractures*. Philadelphia, PA: Lippincott-Raven; 1996.	Original description of the pediatric intra-articular distal humeral fracture types.

REFERENCES

1. Abraham E, Gordon A, Abdul-Hadi O. Management of supracondylar fractures of humerus with condylar involvement in children. *J Pediatr Orthop.* 2005;25(6):709–716.
2. Alonso-Llames M. Bilaterotricipital approach to the elbow: its application in osteosynthesis of supracondylar fractures of the humerus in children. *Acta Orthop Scand.* 1972;43(6):479–490.
3. Bareri P, Hanel D. *Fractures of the Distal Humerus, Green's Operative Hand Surgery,* 7th ed. In: Scott W, Hotchkiss Robert H, William P, et al., eds. Philadelphia, PA: Elsevier; 2017:697–733.
4. Beghin JL, Bucholz RW, Wenger DR. Intercondylar fractures of the humerus in young children: a report of two cases. *J Bone Joint Surg Am.* 1982;64(7):1083–1087.
5. Bell P, Scannell BP, Loeffler BJ, et al. Adolescent distal humerus fractures: ORIF versus CRPP. *J Pediatr Orthop.* 2017;37(8):511–520.
6. Blount WP, Schulz I, Cassidy RH. Fractures of the elbow in children. *J Am Med Assoc.* 1951;146(8):699–704.
7. Bryan RS, Morrey BF. Extensive posterior exposure of the elbow. A triceps-sparing approach. *Clin Orthop Relat Res.* 1982;(166):188–192.
8. Cook JB, Riccio AI, Anderson T, et al. Outcomes after surgical treatment of adolescent intra-articular distal humerus fractures. *J Pediatr Orthop.* 2016;36(8):773–779.
9. Ek ET, Goldwasser M, Bonomo AL. Functional outcome of complex intercondylar fractures of the distal humerus treated through a triceps-sparing approach. *J Shoulder Elbow Surg.* 2008;17(3):441–446.
10. Elgenmark O. Relationship between ossification and age. *Acta Paediatr Scand.* 1946; 33(Suppl 1):31–52.
11. Fayssoux RS, Stankovits L, Domzalski ME, et al. Fractures of the distal humeral metaphyseal-diaphyseal junction in children. *J Pediatr Orthop.* 2008;28(2):142–146.
12. Francis C. The appearance of centers of ossification from 6–15 years. *Am J Phys Antropol.* 1940;27:127–138.
13. Haraldsson S. The intra-osseous vasculature of the distal end of the humerus with special reference to capitulum: preliminary communication. *Acta Orthop Scand.* 1957;27–2:81–93.
14. Helfet DL, Hotchkiss RN. Internal fixation of the distal humerus: a biomechanical comparison of methods. *J Orthop Trauma.* 1990;4(3):260–264.
15. Henley MB, Bone LB, Parker B. Operative management of intra-articular fractures of the distal humerus. *J Orthop Trauma.* 1987;1(1):24–35.
16. Jarvis JG, D'Astous JL. The pediatric T-supracondylar fracture. *J Pediatr Orthop.* 1984;4(6):697–699.
17. Jupiter JB, Mehne DK. Fractures of the distal humerus. *Orthopedics.* 1992;15(7):825–833.
18. Kanellopoulos AD, Yiannakopoulos CK. Closed reduction and percutaneous stabilization of pediatric T-condylar fractures of the humerus. *J Pediatr Orthop.* 2004;24(1):13–16.
19. Kasser JR, Richards K, Millis M. The triceps-dividing approach to open reduction of complex distal humeral fractures in adolescents: a Cybex evaluation of triceps function and motion. *J Pediatr Orthop.* 1990;10(1):93–96.
20. Kirk P, Goulet J, Freiberg A, et al. A biomechanical evaluation of fixation methods for fractures of the distal humerus. *Orthop Trans.* 1990;14:674.
21. Landin LA, Danielsson LG. Elbow fractures in children: an epidemiological analysis of 589 cases. *Acta Orthop Scand.* 1986;57(4):309–312.
22. Maylahn DJ, Fahey JJ. Fractures of the elbow in children: review of three hundred consecutive cases. *J Am Med Assoc.* 1958;166(3):220–228.
23. McKee MD, Wilson TL, Winston L, et al. Functional outcome following surgical treatment of intra-articular distal humeral fractures through a posterior approach. *J Bone Joint Surg Am.* 2000;82-A(12):1701–1707.
24. Morrey BF, An KN, Chao EYS. Functional evaluation of the elbow. In: Morrey BF, ed. *The Elbow and Its Disorders.* 2nd ed. Philadelphia, PA: WB Saunders Co; 1993:95
25. Mortensson W, Thonell S. Left-side dominance of upper extremity fracture in children. *Acta Orthop Scand.* 1991;62(2):154–155.
26. Papavasiliou VA, Beslikas TA. T-condylar fractures of the distal humeral condyles during childhood: an analysis of six cases. *J Pediatr Orthop.* 1986;6(3):302–305.
27. Patel B, Reed M, Patel S. Gender-specific pattern differences of the ossification centers in the pediatric elbow. *Pediatr Radiol.* 2009;39(3):226–231.
28. Patterson SD, Bain GI, Mehta JA. Surgical approaches to the elbow. *Clin Orthop Relat Res.* 2000;370:19–33.
29. Re PR, Waters PM, Hresko T. T-condylar fractures of the distal humerus in children and adolescents. *J Pediatr Orthop.* 1999;19(3):313–318.
30. Remia LF, Richards K, Waters PM. The Bryan-Morrey triceps-sparing approach to open reduction of T-condylar humeral fractures in adolescents: Cybex evaluation of triceps function and elbow motion. *J Pediatr Orthop.* 2004;24(26):615–619.
31. Riseborough EJ, Radin EL. Intercondylar T fractures of the humerus in the adult. A comparison of operative and non-operative treatment in twenty-nine cases. *J Bone Joint Surg Am.* 1969;51(1):130–141.
32. Sanders RA, Raney EM, Pipkin S. Operative treatment of bicondylar intraarticular fractures of the distal humerus. *Orthopedics.* 1992;15(2):159–163.
33. Schemitsch EH, Tencer AF, Henley MB. Biomechanical evaluation of methods of internal fixation of the distal humerus. *J Orthop Trauma.* 1994;8(6):468–475.
34. Toniolo RM, Wilkins KE. *T-Condylar Fractures.* Philadelphia, PA: Lippincott-Raven; 1996.
35. Van Gorder GW. Surgical approach in supracondylar "T" fractures of the humerus requiring open reduction. *J Bone Joint Surg.* 1940;22:278–292.
36. Wildburger R, Mahring M, Hofer HP. Supraintercondylar fractures of the distal humerus: results of internal fixation. *J Orthop Trauma.* 1991;5(3):301–307.
37. Zimmerman H. *Fractures of the Elbow.* New York: Springer-Verlag; 1980.

15

Dislocations of the Elbow and Medial Epicondylar Humerus Fractures

Anthony Stans and Todd Milbrandt

INTRODUCTION TO ELBOW DISLOCATIONS AND MEDIAL EPICONDYLE FRACTURES

Disruptions of the elbow joint represent a spectrum of injuries involving three separate articulations: the radiocapitellar, the ulnohumeral, and the proximal radioulnar joints. Dislocations of the elbow joint in children are not common. Of all elbow injuries in skeletally immature patients, Henrikson[62] found that only about 3% of all were dislocations. The peak incidence of pediatric elbow dislocations typically occurs in the second decade of life, usually between 13 and 14 years of age when the physes begin to close.[62,77] Based on the National Electronic Injury Surveillance System database, the calculated incidence of elbow dislocations in adolescents aged 10 to 19 years old was 6.87 dislocations per 100,000 person-years with an almost 2:1 ratio of injuries in males compared to females (incidence 8.91 vs. 4.72 per 100,000 person-years).[167] The largest proportion of elbow dislocations (44.5%) occur in conjunction with sports activities; football/rugby, wrestling, and basketball being the most common sports for males and gymnastics and skating being the most common sports for females.[167] A recent report of the epidemiology of elbow dislocations in athletes showed that, elbow dislocations occurred in 0.38 per 100,000 athletic exposures.[193] Almost 60% of medial epicondyle fractures are associated with elbow dislocations in this age group.[86] As with all joint dislocations, the principles of treatment include promptly obtaining a concentric reduction of the elbow joint while identifying and treating all associated injuries. The ultimate goal is allowing protected motion and rehabilitation with the goal of restoring full elbow motion without recurrent instability.

ASSESSMENT OF ELBOW DISLOCATIONS AND MEDIAL EPICONDYLE FRACTURES

Because of the location of critical stabilizing factors and surrounding neurovascular structures, elbow dislocations should be considered based on the direction of dislocation and the associated fractures which may be present. As the mechanism of injury, the associated injuries, and imaging differ based on the nature of the injury, these factors should be considered for each dislocation pattern.

PATHOANATOMY AND APPLIED ANATOMY RELATING TO ELBOW DISLOCATIONS AND MEDIAL EPICONDYLE FRACTURES

Constraints about the elbow preventing dislocation can be considered as either dynamic or static. Dynamic elbow stabilizers consist of the elbow musculature, over which the patient has conscious control, which change depending on the degree of muscular contraction. Unlike the shoulder, dynamic stabilizers play only a modest role in elbow stability.

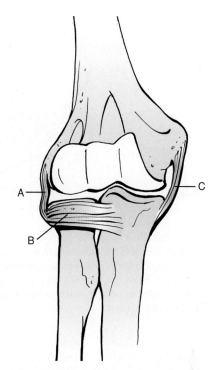

Figure 15-1. Anteroposterior view of the elbow illustrates the bone and ligamentous structures which contribute to elbow stability. (*A*, lateral collateral ligament; *B*, annular ligament; *C*, medial collateral ligament.)

Static constraints are of greater importance and can be divided into osseous and ligamentous restraints (Figs. 15-1 to 15-3). The bony geometry of the elbow creates a relatively constrained hinge. The coronoid and olecranon form a semicircle of approximately 180 degrees into which the trochlea of the humerus securely articulates. The concave surface of the radial head matches the convex capitellum and provides stability to the lateral aspect of the elbow joint. The bony configuration of the medial and lateral aspects of the elbow complement each other with the ulnohumeral articulation providing stability against medial–lateral or longitudinal translation, whereas the radiocapitellar joint provides resistance to axial compression.

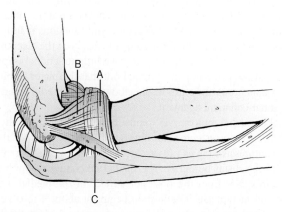

Figure 15-2. The annular ligament and lateral collateral ligament complex provides stability to the proximal radioulnar joint and radial capitellar articulation. (*A*, annular ligament; *B*, lateral collateral ligament insertion on annular ligament; *C*, lateral collateral ligament insertion on ulna.)

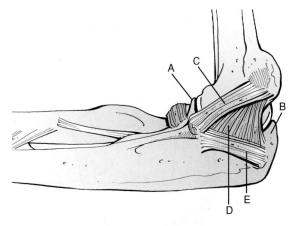

Figure 15-3. The medial elbow is stabilized by the hinge articulation between the proximal ulna and the humerus. Three components of the ulnar collateral ligament provide additional elbow stability. (*A*, coronoid process; *B*, olecranon process; *C*, anterior oblique medial collateral ligament; *D*, posterior oblique medial collateral ligament; *E*, transverse medial collateral ligament.)

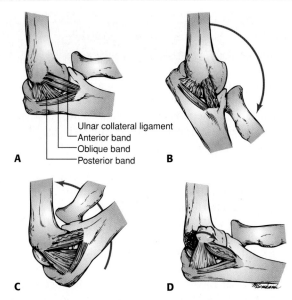

Figure 15-4. Ligamentous structures. **A:** The ulnar collateral ligament is divided into anterior, posterior, and oblique bands. **B:** On extension, the anterior fibers of the anterior band are taut. The posterior fibers of the anterior band and the entire posterior band are loose in this position. **C:** In flexion, the posterior fibers of the anterior band and the posterior band become taut. The anterior fibers of the anterior band become loose. **D:** When the epicondyle is rotated anteriorly, the entire anterior band can become loose. (Reprinted by permission from Woods GW, Tullos HS. Elbow instability and medial epicondyle fractures. *Am J Sports Med.* 1977;5(1):23–30. Copyright © 1977 SAGE Publications.)

The circular nature of the proximal radius allows for nearly 180 degrees of rotation through the full range of flexion and extension allowing for maintenance of these relationships with forearm rotation.

Lateral ligamentous constraints include the annular ligament that is attached to proximal ulna and encircles the radial neck and the lateral collateral ligaments that originate from the lateral epicondyle and insert into the annular ligament and the lateral aspect of the proximal ulna. The primary role of the annular ligament and the lateral collateral ligament complex is to provide stability to the radiocapitellar and proximal radioulnar joints by resisting varus stress.

The medial ulnar collateral ligament is the primary ligamentous restraint to valgus stress, resisting pathologic opening of the medial aspect of the elbow. Having its origin from the inferior aspect of the medial epicondyle, the medial collateral ligament has two primary components that contribute to elbow stability, the anterior and the posterior bands. The band's anterior portion is taut in extension and the posterior fibers are taut in flexion (Fig. 15-4). There is also a fan-shaped posterior oblique ligament that inserts on the olecranon and functions mainly in flexion and a small transverse ligament runs from the olecranon to the coronoid that is thought to have little functional importance. Woods and Tullos[183] pointed out that the major stabilizing ligamentous structure in the elbow is the anterior band of the ulnar collateral ligament.

The medial epicondyle represents a traction apophysis because the forces across its physis are in tension rather than the compressive forces present across the other condylar physes of the distal humerus. The medial epicondylar apophysis actually arises from the posterior surface of the medial distal humeral metaphysis. Ossification begins at about 4 to 6 years of age and fuses at about 15 years of age, making it the last secondary ossification center to fuse with the distal humeral metaphysis (Fig. 15-5). The ossification center starts as a small eccentric oval nucleus (see Fig. 15-5A). As it matures, parallel sclerotic margins develop along both sides of the physis (see Fig. 15-5B). There may be some irregularity of the ossification process, which gives the ossific nucleus a fragmented appearance. This fragmentation may be falsely interpreted as a fracture (see Fig. 15-5E).

Superficially the flexor–pronator mass, which includes the origin of the flexor carpi radialis, flexor carpi ulnaris, flexor digitorum superficialis, palmaris longus, and part of the pronator teres, originates from the anterior aspect of the medial epicondylar apophysis (Fig. 15-6).[156] Part of the flexor carpi ulnaris also originates on the posterior aspect of the epicondyle. Deep to these muscular insertions, the medial ulnar collateral ligament originates from the medial epicondyle. In younger children, some of the capsule's origin extends up to the physeal line of the epicondyle. In older children and adolescents, as the epicondyle migrates more proximally, the capsule is attached only to the medial crista of the trochlea.[12] Thus, in older children, if there is a pure muscular avulsion force on the epicondyle, the capsule and part of the medial ligamentous complex may remain attached to the trochlea's outer border and relative elbow stability preserved. However if the medial epicondyle is avulsed via the medial ulnar collateral ligament, given the importance of this ligament in elbow stability, relative elbow instability usually results.

In general, flexion and supination are usually regarded as positions of stability, whereas extension and pronation are positions of relative instability (Fig. 15-7).

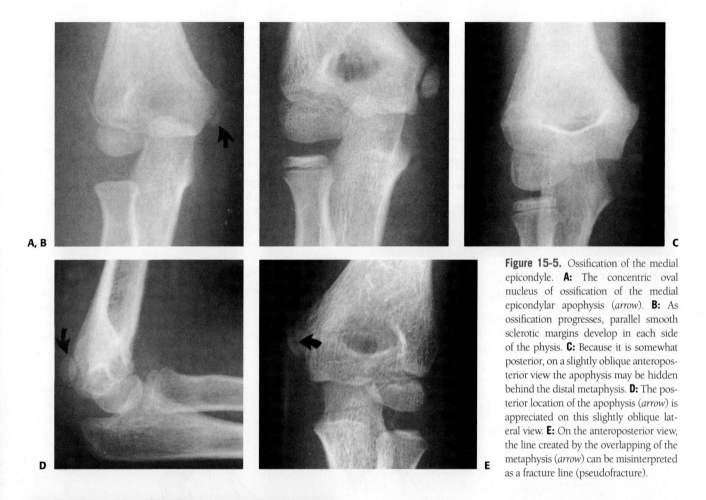

Figure 15-5. Ossification of the medial epicondyle. **A:** The concentric oval nucleus of ossification of the medial epicondylar apophysis (*arrow*). **B:** As ossification progresses, parallel smooth sclerotic margins develop in each side of the physis. **C:** Because it is somewhat posterior, on a slightly oblique anteroposterior view the apophysis may be hidden behind the distal metaphysis. **D:** The posterior location of the apophysis (*arrow*) is appreciated on this slightly oblique lateral view. **E:** On the anteroposterior view, the line created by the overlapping of the metaphysis (*arrow*) can be misinterpreted as a fracture line (pseudofracture).

CLASSIFICATION OF ELBOW DISLOCATIONS AND MEDIAL EPICONDYLE FRACTURES

Elbow dislocations are described by the position of the proximal radioulnar joint relative to the distal humerus: posterior, anterior, medial, or lateral. Posterior dislocations are typically further subdivided into posterolateral and posteromedial injuries. Occasionally, the proximal radioulnar joint is disrupted. When this happens, the radius and ulna can diverge from each other. Rarely, the radius and ulna translocate, with the radius medial and the ulna lateral. Isolated dislocations of the radial head must be differentiated from congenital dislocations. Isolated dislocations of the proximal ulna are exceedingly rare and

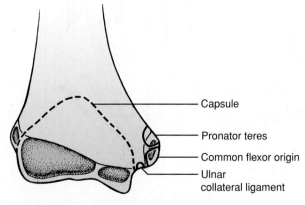

Figure 15-6. Soft tissue attachments. The AP view of the distal humerus demonstrates the relationship of the apophysis to the origins of the medial forearm muscles. The origin of the ulnar collateral ligament lies outside the elbow capsule. The margin of the capsule is outlined by the dotted line.

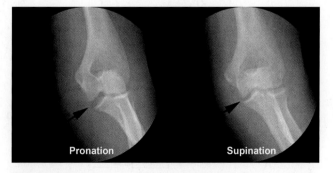

Figure 15-7. Assessment of elbow stability based on forearm rotation. Following closed reduction of a posterior elbow dislocation in a 15-year-old, stability was assessed. With the forearm in mild pronation, note the significant medial joint space opening (*arrow*) with only mild valgus stress. With the forearm slightly supinated a concentric elbow reduction was maintained through a greater range of motion. Stability should be assessed on an individual case by case basis.

have not been reported in children. Included in this chapter is a discussion of the commonly occurring subluxation of the radial head, or "nursemaid's elbow." This is not a true subluxation but rather a partial entrapment of the annular ligament in the radiocapitellar joint. Monteggia fracture–dislocations are discussed in detail in Chapter 11.

Posterior Elbow Dislocations

ASSESSMENT OF POSTERIOR ELBOW DISLOCATIONS

MECHANISMS OF INJURY FOR POSTERIOR ELBOW DISLOCATIONS

O'Driscoll et al.[121] have proposed that most posterior elbow dislocations begin with disruption of the lateral ligaments and proceed along the anterior capsular structures to the medial ligaments. Although this is likely the mechanism for the more rarely seen posteromedial elbow dislocation, for the more common posterior and posterolateral elbow dislocations, this notion has been challenged. Clinical and magnetic resonance imaging (MRI)-based studies noting that medial ulnar collateral ligament injuries occur more frequently than lateral ulnar collateral injuries[73,74,76,140] have led to the competing theory[140] that most posterior elbow dislocations initiate from a valgus force at the elbow leading to failure of the medial ulnar collateral ligament or the medial epicondyle apophysis, to which it is attached, creating a medial epicondyle fracture. As the proximal radius and ulna displace laterally, the coronoid disengages with the intact biceps tendon acting as the center of rotation for the displaced forearm (Fig. 15-8). Application of both an abduction and an extension force leads to forearm external rotation and, with anterior soft tissue disruption, the result is a posterior or posterolateral elbow dislocation.[121,140]

INJURIES ASSOCIATED WITH POSTERIOR ELBOW DISLOCATIONS

Fractures

Concomitant fractures occur in over one-half of posterior elbow dislocations.[87,117,143,146] Recent evaluations have found that number to be very high 78%.[211] The most common fractures

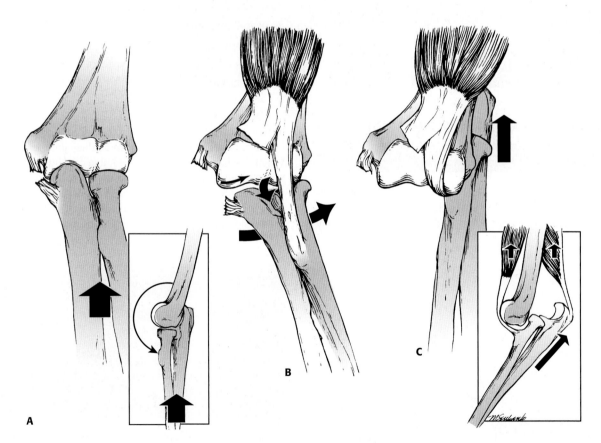

Figure 15-8. Mechanism of injury producing a posterior elbow dislocation. **A:** The elbow is forced into extension that ruptures the medial collateral ligaments. The normal valgus alignment of the elbow accentuates the valgus force at the elbow. **B:** The lateral slope of the medial crista of the trochlea forces the proximal ulna posterolaterally (*small arrow*). The biceps tendon serves as a fulcrum for rotation (*medium arrow*) leading to valgus hinging (*large arrow*) of the forearm. **C:** The proximal ulna and radius are then impacted posteriorly and held against the distal articular surface by the contraction of the biceps and triceps (*arrows*).

involve the medial epicondyle (55%), the coronoid process, and the radial head and neck. Fractures involving the lateral epicondyle, lateral condyle, olecranon, capitellum, and trochlea occur less frequently.[23,203] Given the significant association between fractures of the medial epicondyle, the coronoid process, and the proximal radius (especially markedly displaced radial neck fractures), and posterior elbow dislocations, evaluating for elbow stability when these fractures are noted is important.

Soft Tissue Injuries

Posterior dislocations normally produce moderate soft tissue injury and can be associated with neurovascular injuries in addition to concomitant fractures (Fig. 15-9). The anterior capsule fails in tension, opening the joint cavity. Radial head displacement strips the capsule from the posterolateral aspect of the lateral condyle with the adjacent periosteum. Because of the large amount of cartilage on the posterolateral aspect of the lateral condyle, the posterior capsule may not reattach firmly with healing. This lack of a strong reattachment is believed to be a factor in the rare recurrent elbow dislocation.[122] In a series of 62 adults and adolescents with elbow dislocations requiring surgical treatment, McKee et al.[107] reported that disruption of the lateral collateral ligament complex occurred in all 62 elbows.

Medially, the ulnar collateral ligament complex is disrupted either by an avulsion of the medial epicondyle or a direct tear of the ligament.[153,161] Cromack[28] found that with medial epicondylar fractures, the origins of the ulnar collateral ligaments and the medial forearm flexor muscles remain as a unit, along with most of the pronator teres, which is stripped from its humeral origin proximal to the epicondyle. These structures are then displaced posterior to the medial aspect of the distal humerus. The ulnar collateral ligaments and the muscular origins of the common flexor muscles tear if the epicondyle remains attached to the humerus. With posterolateral displacement of the forearm, the medial aspect of the distal humerus most often passes into the intermuscular space between the pronator teres posteriorly and the brachialis anteriorly. The brachialis, because it has little distal tendon, is easily ruptured. The rent in the anterior capsule usually is in this same area.

The structure most commonly torn on the lateral aspect of the elbow is the annular ligament.[161] On occasion, the lateral collateral ligament either avulses a small osteochondral fragment from the lateral epicondyle or tears completely within its substance.

Neurovascular Injuries

When the elbow is dislocated, the medial aspect of the distal humerus typically protrudes between the pronator teres posteriorly and the brachialis anteriorly. The median nerve and brachial artery lie directly over the distal humerus in the

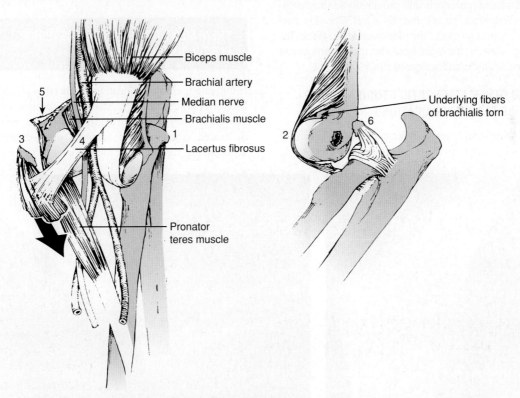

Figure 15-9. Injuries associated with elbow dislocation. (*1*) The radial head and olecranon are displaced posterolaterally. (*2*) The brachialis muscle is stretched across the articular surface of the distal humerus. (*3*) The origins of the medial forearm flexion muscles are either torn or avulsed with the medial epicondyle from the medial condyle. (*4*) The median nerve and brachial artery are stretched across the medial condyle and held firmly by the lacertus fibrosus. (*5*) The medial condyle lies in the subcutaneous tissue between the brachialis anteriorly and the pronator teres posteriorly. (*6*) The lateral (radial) collateral ligaments often avulse a piece of cartilage or bone from the lateral condyle.

subcutaneous tissues. In a cadaver and clinical study by Louis et al.,[91] there was a consistent pattern of disruption of the anastomosis between the inferior ulnar collateral artery and the anterior ulnar recurrent artery. If the main brachial arterial trunk also is compromised, the loss of this collateral system can result in the loss of circulation to the forearm and hand.

The ulnar nerve is at risk in posterior elbow dislocation because of its position posterior to the medial epicondyle. In clinical cases, the ulnar nerve is the most common neurovascular injury.[203] The injury is usually a stretch neurapraxia that resolves but at times the ulnar can be tethered or entrapped by the medial epicondyle displaced fracture. The median nerve is at risk for entrapment in the elbow with hyperextension reduction.

SIGNS AND SYMPTOMS OF POSTERIOR ELBOW DISLOCATIONS

Posterior elbow dislocations must be differentiated from extension-type supracondylar or physeal fractures of the distal humerus. With all these injuries, the elbow is held semiflexed and swelling may be considerable. Swelling initially is usually less with a dislocation than with a type III supracondylar humeral fracture. Crepitus is usually absent in children with a dislocation and the forearm appears shortened. The prominence produced by the distal humeral articular surface is more distal and is palpable as a blunt articular surface. The tip of the olecranon is displaced posteriorly and proximally so that its triangular relationship with the epicondyles is lost. The skin may have a dimpled appearance over the olecranon fossa. If the dislocation is posterolateral, the radial head also may be prominent and easily palpable in the subcutaneous tissues.

IMAGING AND OTHER DIAGNOSTIC STUDIES FOR POSTERIOR ELBOW DISLOCATIONS

Anteroposterior (AP) and lateral x-rays usually are diagnostic of a posterior elbow dislocation. There is a greater superimposition of the distal humerus on the proximal radius and ulna in the AP view. The radial head may be proximally and laterally displaced, or it may be directly behind the middistal humerus, depending on whether the dislocation is posterolateral, posterior, or posteromedial (Fig. 15-10). The normal valgus angulation between the forearm and the arm usually is increased with the most common posterolateral dislocation. On the lateral view, the coronoid process lies posterior to the condyles. Prereduction and postreduction x-rays must be examined closely for associated fractures. The medial epicondyle should be identified on the postreduction films. If it should be present based on the patient's age and elbow ossification pattern and it is not visible, the medial epicondyle is likely fractured and may be entrapped in the joint. Additional radiographs may be necessary to further evaluate an associated medial epicondyle fracture. In the young, contralateral elbow radiographs to confirm the presence or absence of the medial epicondyle on the normal elbow can assist in the radiographic evaluation for fractures. Postreduction radiographs should be carefully scrutinized for a congruent reduction and for subtle osteochondral fracture fragments that can become entrapped in the joint (Fig. 15-11). If reduction is not anatomic or is noncongruent or if osteochondral fragments are visualized, further evaluation with CT tomography or MRI is utilized. MRI also may be used to further define the extent of soft tissue injury in complex injury patterns.

TREATMENT OPTIONS FOR POSTERIOR ELBOW DISLOCATIONS

If untreated, elbow dislocation predictably results in dramatic loss of elbow function characterized by loss of motion and eventually pain (Fig. 15-12). In comparison, reduction of the dislocated elbow usually achieves marked improvement of acute pain as well as restoration of long-term function.

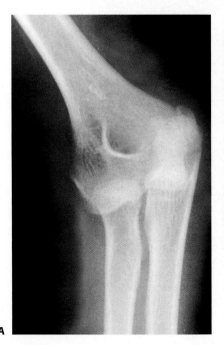

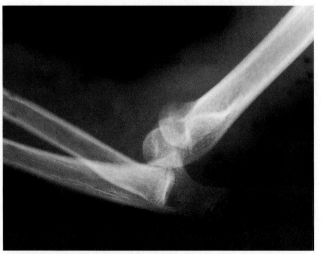

Figure 15-10. Radiographic findings. **A:** Anteroposterior radiograph. The radial head is superimposed behind the distal humerus. There is increased cubitus valgus. The medial epicondyle has not been avulsed. **B:** Lateral radiograph demonstrating that the proximal radius and ulna are both displaced posteriorly to the distal humerus.

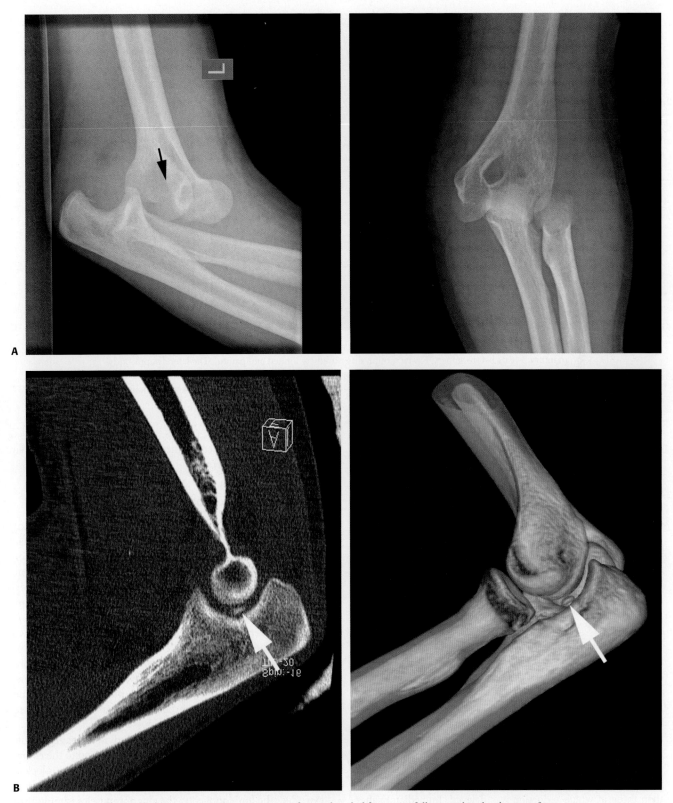

Figure 15-11. Intra-articular entrapment of osteochondral fragments following closed reduction of a posterior elbow dislocation. **A:** A 15-year-old female presented with a posterior elbow dislocation. **B:** Following successful closed reduction, fluoroscopic images suggested an entrapped intra-articular osteochondral fragment (*arrow*). This was confirmed with a CT scan. She subsequently underwent early open removal of these fragments via a medial approach. Significant damage was noted to the brachialis musculature.

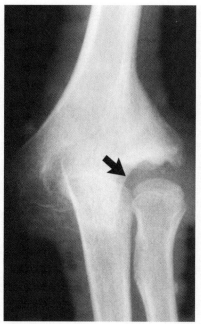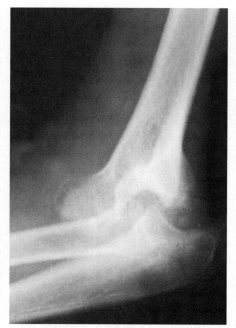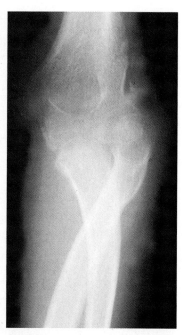

A, B   C

Figure 15-12. Unreduced dislocation. **A:** Preoperative anteroposterior radiograph. The elbow sustained an injury 3 years before surgery. Elbow motion was extremely limited and painful. The lateral supracondylar ridge had been eroded by the radial head (*arrow*). **B:** Lateral radiograph. The posterior position of the olecranon is apparent. **C:** Anteroposterior radiograph 3 months postoperatively. Total elbow motion was 30 degrees, but there was less pain and more stability.

NONOPERATIVE TREATMENT OF POSTERIOR ELBOW DISLOCATIONS

Indications/Contraindications

Nonoperative Treatment Following Successful Closed Reduction of Posterior Elbow Dislocation: INDICATIONS AND CONTRAINDICATIONS	
Indications	**Relative Contraindications**
• Stable concentric elbow reduction obtained following closed treatment	• Unable to obtain a concentric and stable elbow reduction • Intra-articular entrapment of fracture fragments • Vascular injury • Change in neurologic status following reduction or other indication of nerve entrapment

Expected progressive elbow swelling secondary to the soft tissue injury associated with an elbow dislocation makes it imperative that all acute elbow dislocations be promptly reduced under adequate sedation or anesthesia. Royle[146] found that dislocations reduced soon after the injury had better outcomes than those in which reduction was delayed. Immediately after reduction, the surgeon should determine and document the stability of the elbow by examination under anesthesia or sedation. Definitive nonoperative treatment following closed reduction can be considered if the elbow is stable through a functional range of motion, a concentric anatomic reduction can be obtained and maintained, and there is no evidence to suggest a vascular injury, nerve entrapment, or significant intra-articular osteochondral fragments.

Closed Reduction of Posterior Elbow Dislocations

All methods of closed reduction must overcome the deforming muscle forces so that the coronoid process and the radial head can slip past the distal end of the humerus. Adequate sedation or anesthesia is necessary to permit muscle relaxation. Before the primary reduction forces are applied, the forearm is hypersupinated to dislodge the coronoid process and radial head from their position behind the distal humerus and to reduce tension on the biceps tendon.[122] The reducing forces are applied in two major directions (Fig. 15-13). The first reducing force must be along the long axis of the humerus to overcome the contractions of the biceps and brachialis anteriorly and the triceps posteriorly. Once these forces are neutralized, the proximal ulna and radius must be passed from posterior to anterior. Combined pusher–puller techniques are also possible.[56,178]

Several authors[87,178] have strongly advised against initial hyperextension before reduction forces are applied to the elbow. Loomis[88] demonstrated that when the coronoid process is locked against the posterior aspect of the humerus and the elbow is extended, the force applied to the anterior muscles is multiplied by as much as five times because of the increased leverage. This places a marked strain on the injured structures in the antecubital fossa including the anterior capsule, the brachialis muscle, and the neurovascular structures (Fig. 15-14). By contrast, when force is applied to the proximal forearm with the elbow flexed, the force exerted against the muscles across the elbow is equal

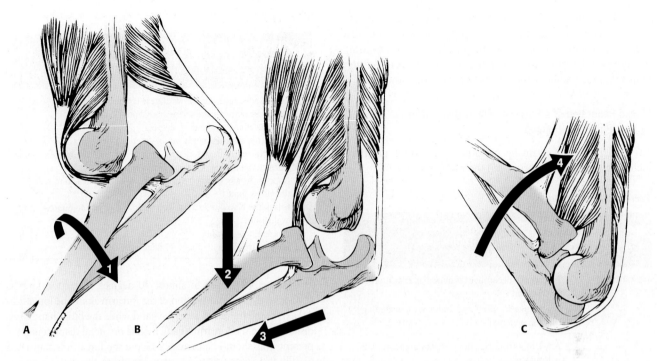

Figure 15-13. Forces required to reduce posterior elbow dislocations. **A:** The forearm is hypersupinated (*arrow 1*) to unlock the radial head. **B:** Simultaneous forces are applied to the proximal forearm along the axis of the humerus (*arrow 2*) and distally along the axis of the forearm (*arrow 3*). **C:** The elbow is then flexed (*arrow 4*) to stabilize the reduction once the coronoid is manipulated distal to the humerus.

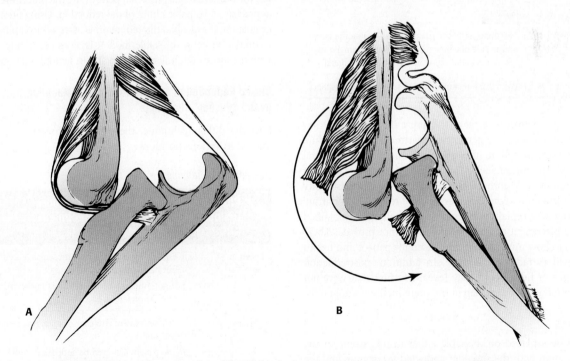

Figure 15-14. Hyperextension forces. **A:** The brachialis is stretched across the distal humerus. **B:** Hyperextending the elbow before it is reduced greatly increases the arc of motion and leverage placed across the brachialis. This can result in rupture of large portions of the muscle. (Reprinted from Loomis LK. Reduction and after-treatment of posterior dislocation of the elbow. *Am J Surg.* 1944;63(1):56–60. Copyright © 1944 Elsevier Inc. With permission.)

to the distracting force. For patients with posterolateral dislocations, the lateral displacement of the proximal radius and ulna must first be corrected to prevent the median nerve from being entrapped or injured during reduction.[16,20] Hyperextension reduction puts the median nerve more at risk for entrapment.

Closed Reduction of a Posterior Elbow Dislocation by the "Puller" Technique

The puller technique can be performed in various positions including the supine position and the prone position.

Prereduction Planning

✔ **Closed Reduction of a Posterior Elbow Dislocation by the "Puller" Technique:**
PREPROCEDURE PLANNING CHECKLIST

Location	❑ Emergency department if muscular relaxation can be obtained. ❑ If not, under general anesthesia in the operating room is preferred.
OR table	❑ Any supportive stretcher or operating room table will suffice.
Position/ positioning aids	❑ For supine technique, the patient is placed supine with the shoulder abducted 90 degrees and the elbow over the edge of the bed. ❑ For the prone technique, the patient is placed prone with the shoulder abducted 90 degrees and the elbow draped over the side of the table. ❑ Proper padding of all peripheral pressure points is critical.
Fluoroscopy location	❑ The image intensifier is placed alongside the table on the side of elbow dislocation and arranged to assess a lateral x-ray once the elbow is reduced.
Equipment	❑ Postreduction immobilization supplies (cast or splint)

If adequate sedation to achieve full muscular relaxation cannot be achieved in the emergency department, the procedure should be performed in the operating room under general anesthesia. An assistant who can provide adequate stabilizing force is required. Fluoroscopy can help assess elbow stability and provide a more dynamic assessment of reduction congruity that postreduction plain radiographs, especially those obtained following placement of immobilization, cannot provide. There are limits to how much fluoroscopy used for patient and health care providers radiation safety.[209] In addition, postreduction radiographs or fluoroscopy may reveal fractures that were not visible with the boney overlap in the prereduction radiographs.

Positioning

The patient is placed on the table either in the supine or the prone position with the shoulder abducted 90 degrees and the elbow off the side of the table. An assistant is positioned on the opposite side of the patient to provide the counterforce. A sheet can be placed around the patient for stabilization purposes if desired. If this is done, an additional assistant may be required to stabilize the upper arm during the reduction.

Technique

✔ **Closed Reduction of a Posterior Elbow Dislocation by the "Puller" Technique:**
KEY STEPS

❑ Ensure adequate sedation with near-complete muscular relaxation
❑ Have assistant to stabilize the body and the humerus
❑ Flex the elbow to about 90 degrees
❑ "Milk" the distal humerus out of anterior soft tissues
❑ Apply force on the anterior forearm in line with the humeral shaft
❑ Correct any medial or lateral displacement
❑ Apply a distally directed force in line with the forearm to reduce the elbow joint
❑ Check the elbow reduction with static and dynamic fluoroscopic evaluation
❑ Assess elbow stability
❑ Immobilize elbow in about 90 degrees of flexion

With the elbow flexed to almost 90 degrees, a traction force is applied to the anterior portion of the forearm along the longitudinal axis of the humerus with one hand while the other hand pulls distally along the forearm. If any medial or lateral displacement is present, this should be corrected before the forearm is translated distally to release soft tissue structures from the distal humerus and prevent entrapment of tissue around the distal humerus. Gently "milking" the anterior soft tissue out from around the distal humerus, by gently pinching and pulling the tissues enveloping the distal humerus forward, as the reduction is performed can also help the reduction. During the procedure, a counterforce is applied by an assistant to offset the manipulating forces and stabilize the humerus. The physician performing the procedure usually appreciates a palpable clunk of the reduction. Using fluoroscopic evaluation, if available, the reduction is assessed in multiple projections. The range of stable motion is assessed, noting stability with the forearm in full supination and in neutral rotation.

Closed Reduction of a Posterior Elbow Dislocation by the "Pusher" Technique

Like the puller technique, the pusher technique can be performed in various positions.

Prereduction Planning

✔ **Closed Reduction of a Posterior Elbow Dislocation by the "Pusher" Technique:**
PREPROCEDURE PLANNING CHECKLIST

Location	❑ Emergency department if muscular relaxation can be obtained. ❑ If not, under general anesthesia in the operating room is preferred.
OR table	❑ Any supportive stretcher or operating room table will suffice. ❑ The patient can even be supported in the arms of a parent or an assistant.
Position/ positioning aids	❑ For Lavine's method (Fig. 15-15A), the child is held by the parent while the elbow is draped over the edge of the chair. The back of the chair must be well padded.

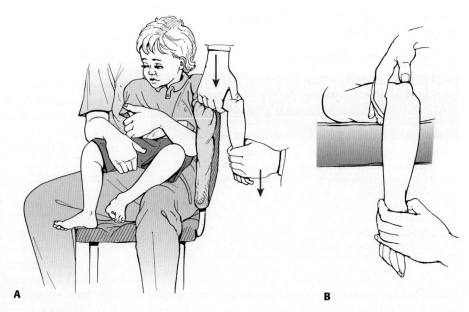

Figure 15-15. Reduction by "pusher" techniques. **A:** Lavine's method. The child is held by the parent while the elbow is draped over the edge of the chair. The olecranon is pushed distally past the humerus by the thumb of the physician while the other arm pulls distally along the axis of the forearm. **B:** Meyn's technique with patient lying prone on the table. (Adapted with permission from Meyn MA, Quigley TB. Reduction of posterior dislocation of the elbow by traction on the dangling arm. *Clin Orthop.* 1974;103:106–107.)

A   **B**

	❏ For Meyn's technique (Fig. 15-15B), the patient is placed prone with the shoulder abducted 90 degrees and the elbow draped over the side of the table.
	❏ Proper padding of all peripheral pressure points is critical.
Fluoroscopy location	❏ The image intensifier is placed alongside the table on the side of elbow dislocation and arranged to assess a lateral x-ray once the elbow is reduced.
Equipment	❏ Postreduction immobilization supplies (cast or splint).

Again, like the pusher technique, adequate sedation is required and fluoroscopy can be helpful for postreduction evaluation.

Positioning

The patient is positioned with the distal humerus over a fixed surface, either the back of a chair or the edge of the bed.

Technique

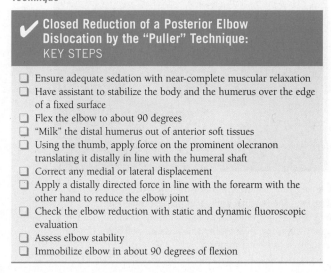

✔ **Closed Reduction of a Posterior Elbow Dislocation by the "Puller" Technique:** KEY STEPS

❏ Ensure adequate sedation with near-complete muscular relaxation
❏ Have assistant to stabilize the body and the humerus over the edge of a fixed surface
❏ Flex the elbow to about 90 degrees
❏ "Milk" the distal humerus out of anterior soft tissues
❏ Using the thumb, apply force on the prominent olecranon translating it distally in line with the humeral shaft
❏ Correct any medial or lateral displacement
❏ Apply a distally directed force in line with the forearm with the other hand to reduce the elbow joint
❏ Check the elbow reduction with static and dynamic fluoroscopic evaluation
❏ Assess elbow stability
❏ Immobilize elbow in about 90 degrees of flexion

With the elbow flexed to almost 90 degrees, the thumb is used to push the olecranon distally past the humerus. The other arm then pulls distally along the axis of the forearm affecting the reduction. Again, if any medial or lateral displacement is present, this should be corrected before the forearm is translated distally. Fluoroscopic evaluation, if available, can then be performed as with the puller technique. Elbow stability should be assessed and the elbow then immobilized in a position of stability.

Postreduction Care

Some type of immobilization, usually a posterior splint or circumferential cast, is advocated by most investigators. A frequently recommended period of immobilization is 3 weeks,[87,88,126,154] although some have advocated early motion.[145,146,183] Murphy et al. evaluated 145 pediatric dislocations and found that immobilization greater than 2 weeks led to loss of extension. O'Driscoll et al.[121] suggested that if the elbow was stable in response to valgus stress with the forearm pronated then the anterior portion of the medial collateral ligament was intact and the patient could begin early motion. Ninety degrees of elbow flexion appears to be the standard position of immobilization. Hinged elbow braces with adjustable blocks to motion are very useful for obtaining progressive, protected motion.

Outcomes

Closed reduction of posterior elbow dislocations is successful in most cases. In the combined series of 317 dislocations,[87,117,143,146] only two cases[87] could not be reduced by closed methods. In the Carlioz and Abols[23] series, two dislocations reduced spontaneously and closed reduction was successful in 50 cases, but failed in six cases (10%). Josefsson et al.[75] reported that all 25 dislocations without associated fractures were successfully reduced. In the largest reported series of pediatric elbow dislocations to date, Murphy et al. reported that only 1 of 145 cases required open treatment to obtain reduction.[203]

OPERATIVE TREATMENT OF POSTERIOR ELBOW DISLOCATIONS

Indications/Contraindications

Operative Treatment of Posterior Elbow Dislocation: INDICATIONS AND CONTRAINDICATIONS	
Indications	**Contraindications**
• Unable to obtain a concentric and stable elbow reduction • Intra-articular entrapment of fracture fragments • Vascular injury • Change in neurologic status following reduction or other indication of nerve entrapment	• Stable concentric elbow reduction obtained following closed treatment

Indications for primary open reduction include an inability to obtain or maintain a concentric closed reduction, an open dislocation, a displaced osteochondral fracture with entrapment in the joint, a vascular injury, or a neurologic injury for which there is any indication that there may be entrapment of the nerve.

Primary ligament repair is not routinely indicated. Adults with posterior elbow dislocations without concomitant fracture have no better function or stability following a primary ligamentous repair than those treated nonoperatively.[73,74] There was a recent report of more aggressive ligamentous repair if instability persisted following reduction with good clinical results.[202] However, this report is difficult to interpret as it did not have a control group where the ligaments were treated without repair. All fractures preventing concentric reduction need to be repaired with an open reduction of an elbow dislocation. Beware of elbow dislocations in children less than age 10 as they often have associated osteochondral fractures that can block reduction. More detailed examination and imaging may be required in the young.

Open Dislocations

Open dislocations have a high incidence of associated arterial injury.[60,79,87,91] Operative intervention is necessary in open posterior dislocations to irrigate and debride the open wound and elbow and to evaluate the brachial artery (Fig. 15-16). If there is vascular disruption, most advocate vascular repair or reconstruction with a vein graft even in the presence of adequate capillary refill. This may lessen the risk of late cold intolerance, dysesthesias, or dysvascularity.

Fractures

Children with an elbow dislocation usually have an associated fracture of the coronoid, lateral condyle, olecranon (Fig. 15-17), radial neck, or medial epicondyle (Fig. 15-18). In the Murphy et al. series of 145 pediatric dislocations, 80% had an associated fracture, 60% of which involved the medial epicondyle.[203] Fractures of the anteromedial facet of the coronoid have been recognized as an important injury associated with elbow dislocations in adolescents and adults.[33,34] The presence of a concomitant displaced fracture is a common indication for surgical intervention.[23,179] Surgery for associated fractures produced better results than nonoperative treatment of fracture–dislocations in the series of Carlioz and Abols,[23] and similar results were reported by Wheeler and Linscheid.[179] Repair of an associated medial epicondylar fracture may also improve elbow stability in throwing athletes when the injury is in the dominant arm.[153,183] Entrapment of any fracture fragments within the joint is an absolute indication for surgical treatment. Displaced medial epicondyle fractures can be entrapped within the joint after reduction and are often overlooked on the radiographs (Fig. 15-19). Because of the high association of this fracture with elbow dislocations, the location of the medial epicondyle should be confirmed in every case. Ultimately, the surgical treatment for fractures associated with an elbow dislocation is based on the circumstances surrounding each individual patient. Factors favoring operative treatment include older patient age, instability of the elbow during examination under sedation at

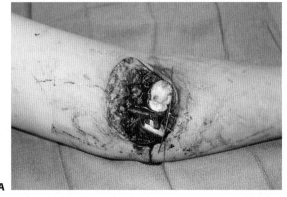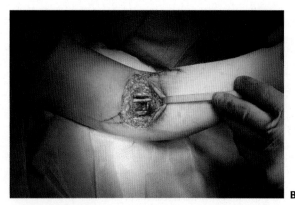

Figure 15-16. A: A 13-year-old male presented to the emergency department following a roll-over ATV injury with a contaminated, open posterior elbow dislocation. The brachial artery can be seen traversing the articular cartilage of the distal humerus. **B:** Following debridement and elbow reduction the brachial artery and median nerve are seen in the traumatic wound. Intra-operative assessment revealed palpable radial pulse and Doppler ultrasound studies found no evidence of vascular injury.

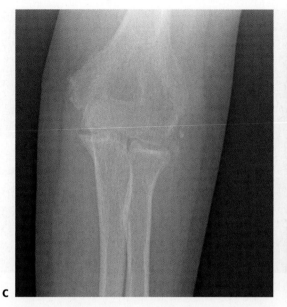
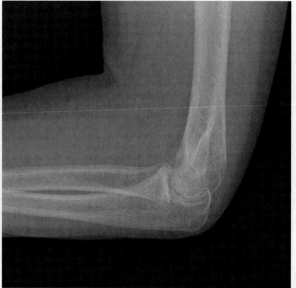

Figure 15-16. (*Continued*) **C, D:** Three months following injury elbow range of motions is from −20 extension to 130 degrees flexion with no pain and minimal functional limitations. Periarticular calcification is present with worrisome joint space irregularity.

the time of reduction, the presence of a displaced intra-articular fracture, injury to multiple elbow stabilizers, injury to the patient's dominant arm, and anticipated high-demand sports, especially overhead sports, or activities on the elbow. Murphy reported a high rate of fixation of the medial epicondyle fractures (79%) when associated with an elbow dislocation.[203] This may be a reflection of increased national trends in both operative fixation rates and youth sports participation.

Vascular Injuries

With initial evidence of vascular compromise, treatment should consist of urgent reduction of the elbow dislocation which usually returns the displaced brachial vessels to their normal position[61,180] followed by reassessment of the vascular status. With prompt normalization of the vascular status, serial observation is still recom-

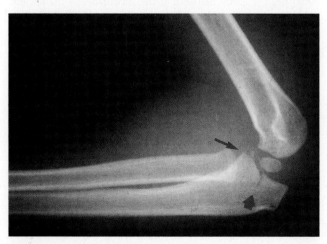

Figure 15-17. Lateral radiograph of a 4-year-old child who sustained an elbow dislocation with a concomitant olecranon fracture (*large arrow*) and a coronoid fracture (*small arrow*).

mended to evaluate for evolving circulatory compromise. If there is evidence of persistent vascular compromise after reduction, vascular exploration followed by operative repair of those structures that are ruptured or severely damaged should be pursued emergently. Even though collateral vessels may provide adequate vascular flow to give a warm hand with good capillary refill, if there has been a significant vascular injury, failure to repair the injury may predispose the patient to late ischemic changes such as claudication, cold sensitivity, or even late amputation.

Neurologic Injuries

As with vascular injuries, initial evidence of neurologic compromise should prompt urgent reduction. A significant negative change in the neurologic status following closed reduction may indicate intra-articular nerve entrapment and should prompt exploration. If missed, this may have significant consequences for hand function if not repaired and require cable nerve grafting.[188]

Open Reduction of an Irreducible Posterior Elbow Reduction

Preoperative Planning

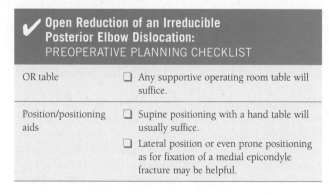

✔ Open Reduction of an Irreducible Posterior Elbow Dislocation: PREOPERATIVE PLANNING CHECKLIST	
OR table	❑ Any supportive operating room table will suffice.
Position/positioning aids	❑ Supine positioning with a hand table will usually suffice.
	❑ Lateral position or even prone positioning as for fixation of a medial epicondyle fracture may be helpful.

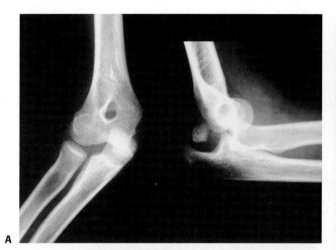

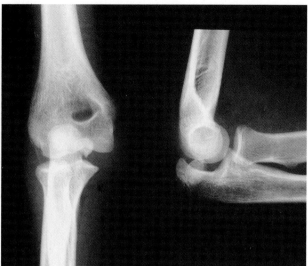

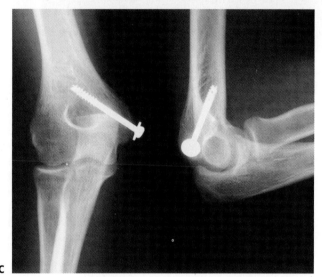

Figure 15-18. A: Anteroposterior and lateral radiograph of a 14-year-old male who sustained an elbow dislocation with an ipsilateral medial epicondyle fracture. **B:** Anteroposterior radiographs after a closed reduction. Note the entrapment of the medial epicondyle in the joint. **C:** This patient was treated with an open reduction to extract the medial epicondyle from the joint and an internal fixation using a cannulated screw that allowed rapid mobilization of his elbow.

Fluoroscopy location	❑ The image intensifier is placed alongside the table on the side of elbow dislocation, on the side opposite the anticipated surgical approach.
Equipment	❑ Loup magnification may facilitate identification of neurovascular structures in the surgical field. ❑ Bipolar electrocautery is preferred around neurovascular structures for hemostasis. ❑ A headlamp greatly facilitates visualization.
	❑ Suture anchors may be employed to resecure ligamentous avulsions and should be available.

The surgical approach will be dictated by the goals of the procedure and based on an estimation of the structures that may be blocking the reduction. The most common structures preventing reduction via closed means include the distal humerus being buttonholed through the brachialis musculature, the radial head being buttonholed through the capsule and lateral collateral ligament, and entrapment of fracture fragments, especially the medial epicondyle, with their attached ligamentous or muscular structures wedging them in place. If the distal humerus or the radial head is easily palpable in the subcutaneous tissues and not able to be milked out of these tissues through closed means, an operative approach to perform this will be necessary. For the distal humerus in the brachialis, a medial approach should be performed. For the radial head block, a lateral approach has been described.[52,81] If a fracture fragment, especially the medial epicondyle, can be visualized and is thought to be responsible for the block, the medial approach should be employed to facilitate fracture fixation. Loose osteochondral fracture fragments can block a congruent reduction and computed tomography (CT) and/or MRI scanning may be required to visualize the fragments and determine operative approach.

Positioning

Supine positioning with a hand table will usually suffice. With an associated medial epicondyle fracture, the lateral position or the prone position may be employed as well. (See the section on medial epicondyle fractures.)

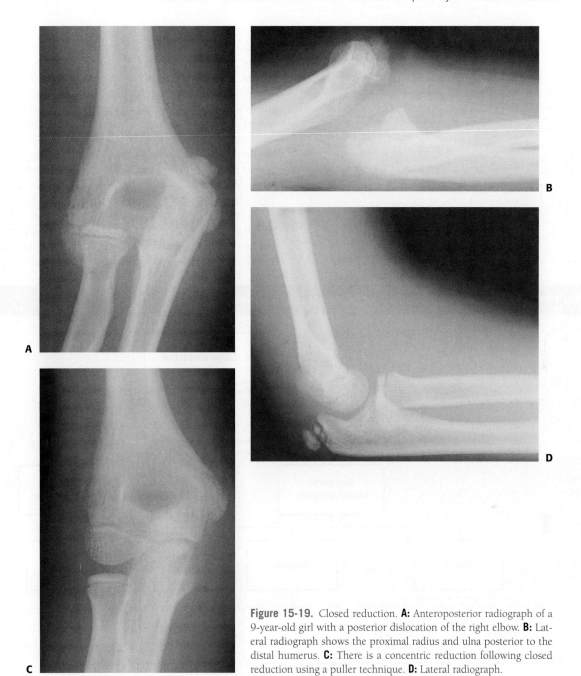

Figure 15-19. Closed reduction. **A:** Anteroposterior radiograph of a 9-year-old girl with a posterior dislocation of the right elbow. **B:** Lateral radiograph shows the proximal radius and ulna posterior to the distal humerus. **C:** There is a concentric reduction following closed reduction using a puller technique. **D:** Lateral radiograph.

Approach

Lateral approach is best if radial head noted to be subcutaneous indicating possible block to reduction because of buttonholing through the lateral capsule and around the lateral collateral ligaments. Medial approach is best if the distal humerus is noted to be subcutaneous indicating a block to reduction because of buttonholing through the brachialis or if an associated medial epicondyle fracture is present and surgical fixation is planned. With the lateral approach, the radial nerve needs to be protected; with the medial approach, the ulnar needs protection. The median nerve and brachial artery are of concern either way.

Open Reduction

✔ **Open Reduction of an Irreducible Posterior Elbow Dislocation:** KEY SURGICAL STEPS

- ☐ Make a medially based incision just anterior to the humerus curving distally at the elbow (note that the neurovascular structures may be very subcutaneous because of the injury).
- ☐ Identify the median and ulnar nerves and the brachial artery. Protect medial antebrachial cutaneous nerves.
- ☐ Remove any tissue or any other intervening structures.
- ☐ Visually inspect the joint surfaces and remove any loose osteochondral fragments.
- ☐ Flex the elbow to about 90 degrees.

- ❏ Apply force on the forearm in line with the humerus translating it distally in line with the humeral shaft and opening the joint surface.
- ❏ Correct any medial or lateral displacement.
- ❏ Apply a distally directed force in line with the forearm, or directly posteriorly translate the distal humerus to reduce the elbow joint.
- ❏ Check the elbow reduction with visual evaluation as well as dynamic fluoroscopic evaluation.
- ❏ Assess elbow stability through range of motion.
- ❏ Assess the extent of capsular and ligamentous damage and repair critical elements such as the medial ulnar collateral ligament and/or the medial epicondyle (see below separate medial epicondyle section).
- ❏ Reassess elbow stability through range of motion if repairs are performed.
- ❏ Be certain there is no neurovascular impingement or entrapment.
- ❏ Immobilize elbow in about 90 degrees of flexion

For a medial approach, an incision is made just anterior to the predicted midhumeral line and curved distally just anterior the medial epicondyle. With gentle spreading of the subcutaneous tissues, the significant soft tissue trauma is evident. The buttonholed distal humerus, the median and ulnar nerves, and the brachial artery should be identified. Any intervening tissue or osteochondral fragments are removed from the interval between the joint surfaces. The joint is then reduced through a similar set of distraction and translational forces as described for the closed reduction techniques. Once reduced, joint stability is evaluated and a thorough assessment of the capsular and ligamentous structures is performed. Primary repair or reattachment of the medial collateral ligament complex with small suture anchors or transosseous drill holes may be performed to improve stability. The elbow is stabilized in a posterior splint, bivalve cast, or hinged elbow brace in a position of stability.

Author's Preferred Method of Treatment for Posterior Elbow Dislocations (Algorithm 15-1)

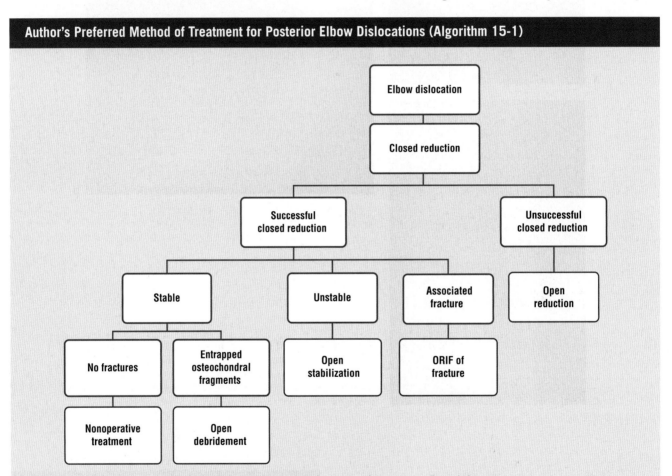

Algorithm 15-1. Author's preferred treatment for posterior elbow dislocation.

The "pusher" technique of reduction of an elbow dislocation is preferred in children 9 years of age or younger. In this age group, the child often can be seated comfortably in the parent's lap (see Fig. 15-15). Hanging the arm over the back of a well-padded chair may provide some stabilization.

For a child 10 years of age and older, the puller technique advocated by Parvin[126] is used (see Figs. 15-13 and 15-20). The forearm must remain supinated during the process of

reduction. Occasionally, it is necessary to hypersupinate the forearm to unlock the coronoid process and the radial head before reduction. Closed reduction is done with either heavy sedation or general anesthesia. The range of stable elbow motion is assessed. Fluoroscopy can be helpful during and after the reduction to assess stability as well. Formal x-rays are obtained after the manipulation to assess the adequacy of the reduction (see Fig. 15-19), to be certain the joint is

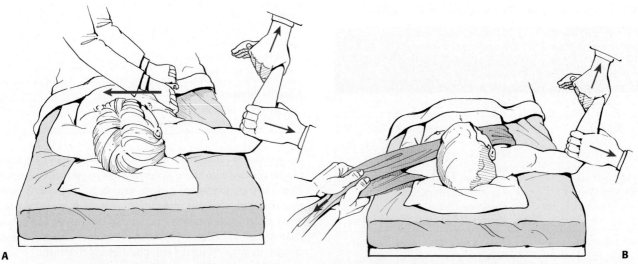

Figure 15-20. Reduction by "puller" techniques in a supine position. **A:** With the elbow flexed to almost 90 degrees, a force is applied to the anterior portion of the forearm with one hand while the other hand pulls distally along the forearm. A counterforce is applied to offset the manipulating forces by direct stabilization of the patient by a second medical person. **B:** The counterforce is applied with a sheet around the chest in the ipsilateral axilla. (Redrawn from Parvin RW. Closed reduction of common shoulder and elbow dislocations without anesthesia. *Arch Surg.* 1957;75(6):972–975.)

congruently reduced and to assess for the presence of any intra-articular fragments. If the elbow is stable through a functional range of motion, the elbow is immobilized in a posterior splint, hinged brace, or a split cast with the elbow flexed 90 degrees. If there is a question of persistent relative instability, the forearm is held in full supination. If the elbow is absolutely stable following reduction, the forearm can be immobilized in midpronation to allow the patient to be more functional with early progressive motion.

Entrapped intra-articular fragments should be removed before mobilizing the elbow (see Fig. 15-18). With the capsule disrupted and the joint full of blood clot, early arthroscopic removal of loose bodies is not recommended. Thus, we prefer to perform loose body removal with an open arthrotomy in the early postreduction period. Given the extensive medial soft tissue disruption, a medial approach with visualization of the joint through the windows created by the injury allows for easy access to all aspects of the joint.

Be certain to locate the ulnar nerve and medial antebrachial cutaneous nerves with operative exposure.

Persistent significant elbow instability should prompt a thorough investigation for associated fractures or incongruity of the reduction suggesting incarceration of soft tissue or chondral fragments in the joint. In the postreduction examination, an estimation of the direction of instability should be performed: valgus, varus, or posterolateral rotatory instability. In these circumstances, evaluation with a postreduction MRI to assess the extent of the soft tissue injury may help direct treatment.

Fractures associated with elbow dislocations may necessitate reduction and fixation as dictated by the guiding principles for the individual fracture. Failure to reduce and fix fractures associated with an elbow dislocation may lead to persistent instability. As is discussed at length in the second half of this chapter, we prefer to reduce and fix medial epicondyle fractures associated with elbow dislocations.

POSTOPERATIVE CARE

Immobilization after surgery depends on the procedure performed. After open reduction, management is similar to that after satisfactory closed reduction.

Because the major complication of elbow dislocations is stiffness, the initial full-time immobilization is removed after approximately 1 week and the patient transitioned to a removable splint or the hinged brace is unlocked for progressive motion. The patient begins intermittent protected active elbow motion out of the splint multiple times a day as limited by pain. In a reliable patient with minimal risk of additional trauma, the patient can usually dispense with the splint after

10 to 14 days and use a sling. If there are times at high risk for another fall, the splint can be continued up till about 5 to 6 weeks post injury during these times (i.e., during school), but should be removed at other times of the day when there is minimal risk (i.e., meal time) to promote range of motion. The emphasis is on early active motion in a safe environment to prevent stiffness that often occurs after this injury. Before reduction, it is important to emphasize to the parents that there may be some loss of motion, especially extension, regardless of the treatment. This is usually less than 30 degrees and not of functional or aesthetic significance. If open reduction is required, mobilization is begun after wounds have healed (1 to 2 weeks) as described above.

POTENTIAL PITFALLS AND PREVENTIVE MEASURES

Reduction of Posterior Elbow Dislocation:
POTENTIAL PITFALLS AND PREVENTIONS.

Pitfall	Prevention
• Stiffness	• Early mobilization
• Inadequate analgesia	• Perform the reduction in the OR if adequate analgesia for muscular relaxation is not available in the emergency setting
• Median nerve entrapment	• Correct lateral displacement before translating anteriorly • Hyperextension, pronation reduction
• Coronoid fracture during reduction	• Attempt reduction with the elbow in flexion

Closed reduction of pediatric elbow dislocations should always be done with adequate analgesia, sedation, or anesthesia. In addition to making the experience much less frightening and traumatic for the child, adequate analgesia, sedation, or anesthesia will achieve sufficient muscle relaxation for the reduction to be obtained more effectively with less force, thereby reducing the risk of creating an iatrogenic fracture (such as fracture of the radial neck) during reduction.

A careful neurologic examination must be done before and after the reduction with special attention to the median nerve in terms of entrapment. This same careful examination must be made at all follow-up evaluations. Persistent median nerve motor–sensory loss associated with severe pain and resistance with elbow flexion–extension arc of motion may be indicative of entrapment. Of note, ulnar neuropathy is not uncommon and usually resolves spontaneously.

OUTCOMES

Di Gennaro et al. evaluated elbow dislocations in children at an average of 15 years of follow-up and found that the majority of patients had a good prognosis.[192] Murphy et al. noted less than excellent outcomes with dislocations associated with multiple fractures, need for operative intervention, and immobilization greater than two weeks.

MANAGEMENT OF EXPECTED ADVERSE OUTCOMES AND UNEXPECTED COMPLICATIONS RELATED TO POSTERIOR ELBOW DISLOCATIONS

Posterior Elbow Dislocations:
COMMON ADVERSE OUTCOMES AND COMPLICATIONS

Early
- Neurologic injuries: Ulnar and median nerve are injured most commonly
- Vascular injuries: Injury to the brachial artery is most common

Late
- Loss of elbow range of motion
- Heterotopic bone formation
- Radioulnar synostosis
- Cubitus recurvatum

Special Problems
- Recurrent posterior dislocations
- Unreduced posterior elbow dislocations

Complications associated with posterior elbow dislocations can be divided into those occurring early and those occurring later. Early complications include neurologic and vascular injuries. Late complications include loss of motion, myositis ossificans, recurrent dislocations, radioulnar synostosis, and cubitus recurvatum. The special problems of chronic, unreduced dislocations are not considered complications of treatment.

NEUROLOGIC INJURIES

Ulnar Nerve Lesions

In a combined series of 317 patients,[87,117,143,146,203] the most commonly injured nerve was the ulnar nerve. Of the 32 patients (10%) who had nerve symptoms after reduction, 21 had isolated ulnar nerve injuries, seven had isolated median nerve injuries, and in four patients both the median and ulnar nerves were involved. During open reduction of elbow fracture dislocations, the ulnar nerve needs to be identified and protected.[87] Ulnar nerve transposition is recommended if there is concern about the nerve instability or impingement on the fixation screw.

Radial Nerve Lesions

Radial nerve injury with posterior elbow dislocation is very rare. Watson-Jones[178] reported two radial nerve injuries associated with elbow dislocation; in both the symptoms rapidly resolved after reduction. Rasool[138] reported a third case.

Median Nerve Lesions

The most serious neurologic injury involves the median nerve, which can be damaged directly by the dislocation or can be entrapped within the joint. Median nerve injuries occur most commonly in children 5 to 12 years of age. These injuries, either isolated median nerve (7 out of 317 total dislocations) or combined median and ulnar nerve injuries (4 out of 317 total dislocations), were present in only 3% of dislocations.[87,117,143,146] These injuries can present late[188] and can present after spontaneous elbow reduction.[208]

Types of Median Nerve Entrapment

Fourrier et al.[41] in 1977 delineated three types of medial nerve entrapment (Fig. 15-21).

Type 1

The child has an avulsion fracture of the medial epicondyle or has a rupture of the origin of the flexor–pronator muscle and ulnar collateral ligament (see Fig. 15-21A). This allows the median

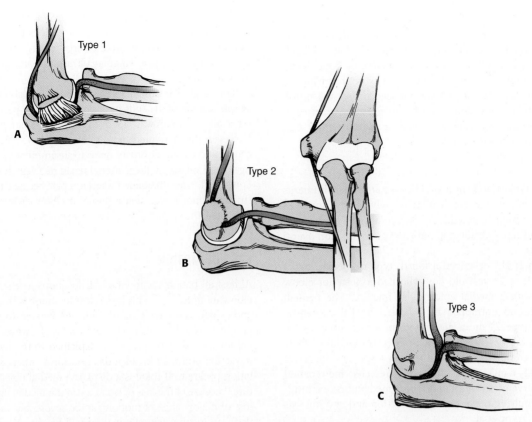

Figure 15-21. Median nerve entrapment. **A:** Type 1. Entrapment within the elbow joint with the median nerve coursing posterior to the distal humerus. **B:** Type 2. Entrapment of the nerve between the fracture surfaces of the medial epicondyle and the medial condyle. **C:** Type 3. Simple kinking of the nerve into the anterior portion of the elbow joint. (Redrawn from Hallett J. Entrapment of the median nerve after dislocation of the elbow. A case report. *J Bone Joint Surg Br.* 1981;63-B(3):408–412, with permission.)

nerve, with or without the brachial artery, to displace posteriorly, essentially wrapping posteriorly around the medial aspect of the humerus and then coursing distally around the articular surface of the distal humerus. With the deep groove of the trochlea acting like a hook for the nerve and catching it out of the anterior soft tissues, if the lateral displacement of the proximal radius and ulna is not corrected before reduction, the nerve may become entrapped in the joint, wrapped around the distal humerus alongside or even in the ulnotrochlear articulation during the process of reduction. Hallett[55] demonstrated in cadavers that pronation of the forearm while the elbow is hyperextended forces the median nerve posteriorly during the process of reduction making it vulnerable to entrapment. This type of entrapment also has been reported by other authors.[13,16,20,41,51,134,137,165] If median nerve dysfunction is present prior to reduction, it is often difficult to identify nerve entrapment postreduction. Certainly any significant decrease in median nerve function following a closed reduction or incongruity in the reduction should prompt evaluation for this injury pattern. In some patients with an associated medial epicondyle fracture, the nerve can be so severely damaged after being entrapped that neuroma resection, nerve transposition, and direct repair or grafting is necessary.[16,51] Good recovery of nerve function has been reported after operative decompression and repair.

If the nerve has been entrapped for a considerable period, the Matev sign may be present on the x-rays. This represents a depression on the posterior surface of the medial epicondylar ridge where the nerve has been pressed against the bone.[13,29,51,55,134,137,165] This groove is seen on x-ray as two sclerotic lines parallel to the nerve (Fig. 15-22). This sign disappears when the nerve has been decompressed.

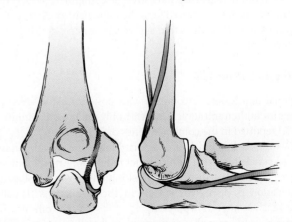

Figure 15-22. The Matev sign suggesting entrapment of the median nerve in the elbow joint and impingement of the nerve against the posterior surface of the medial condyle. This produces a depression with sclerotic margins. (Redrawn from Matev I. A radiological sign of entrapment of the median nerve in the elbow joint after posterior dislocation. A report of two cases. *J Bone Joint Surg Br.* 1976;58(3):353–355, with permission.)

Type 2

The nerve is entrapped between the fracture surfaces of the medial epicondyle and the distal humerus (see Fig. 15-21B). The fracture heals and the nerve is surrounded by bone, forming a neuroforamen.[134,141,165] This may or may not be visible on x-ray. The medial epicondyle is osteomized to free the nerve. Again, decompression alone may be an adequate treatment, although neuroma resection and repair or reconstruction with nerve grafts may be necessary.

Type 3

The nerve is kinked and entrapped between the distal humerus and the olecranon (see Fig. 15-21C). Only three injuries of this type have been reported.[13,133,136] Decompression, neuroma resection, and repair resulted in return of good function over 6 to 24 months.

Al-Qattan et al.[6] described a fourth type of median nerve entrapment in a 14-year-old boy who had a posterior elbow dislocation with a medial epicondylar fracture. The median nerve was found entrapped in a healed medial epicondylar fracture (type 2) in an anterior to posterior direction 18 months after injury. The nerve then passed through the elbow joint in a posterior to anterior direction (type 1). The nerve was so severely damaged that it had to be resected and repaired with sural nerve grafts. A second type 4 median nerve entrapment also requiring nerve segment resection and grafting was reported by Ozkoc et al.[123]

The combination of an associated fracture of the medial epicondyle and significant median nerve dysfunction was cited by Rao and Crawford[137] as an absolute indication for surgical exploration of the nerve because of the frequency of median nerve entrapment with fractures of the medial epicondyle. This has been reviewed recently by Simon et al.,[208] who came to the same conclusion. MRI may be helpful in defining the course of the median nerve if entrapment is suspected.[3] Electromyography and nerve conduction studies have been utilized to assist in operative decision-making. Painful dysesthesias with arc of motion is usually indicative of entrapment. Once the entrapped nerve is removed from the joint, neurologic function typically improves. Resection and repair or nerve grafting may be necessary.

ARTERIAL INJURIES

Arterial injuries are uncommon with posterior elbow dislocations in children and adolescents with only eight vascular injuries (3%) reported in the combined series of 317 patients.[87,117,143,146] However, Carlioz and Abols[23] reported four patients with diminished radial pulses that resolved after reduction. Arterial injuries have been associated with open dislocations in which collateral circulation is disrupted.[60,79,91,147] In these situations, usually the brachial artery is ruptured,[54,60,65,79,91,147] but it can also be thrombosed[180] as well as entrapped in the elbow joint.[61,129,180] Pearce[129] reported an entrapped radial artery in which there was a high bifurcation of the brachial artery. When there is a complete rupture, there usually is evidence of ischemia distally. However, the presence of good capillary circulation to the hand or a Doppler pulse at the wrist does not always mean the artery

is intact.[54,65] Arteriograms usually are not necessary because the arterial injury is at the site of the dislocation. If imaging is indicated to evaluate possible arterial injury, its minimal risk and invasiveness make vascular ultrasound an attractive initial imaging choice.

For surgical treatment of vascular injuries about the elbow, simple ligation of the ends has been done in the past with adults, especially if there was good capillary circulation distally.[60,79] However, this may predispose to late ischemic changes such as claudication, cold sensitivity, or even late amputation. Most investigators recommend direct arterial repair or a vein graft.[54,65,91,99,147] Louis et al.[91] recommended arterial repair because their cadaver studies demonstrated that a posterior elbow dislocation usually disrupted the collateral circulation necessary to maintain distal blood flow.

LOSS OF MOTION

Almost all patients with elbow dislocations lose some range of elbow motion.[23,73–75] This loss is less in children than in adults[75] and usually is no more than 10 degrees of extension. This rarely is of functional or aesthetic significance. However, the potential for loss of motion must be explained to the parents before reduction and may be an indication for a supervised rehabilitation program. If there is a displaced medial epicondylar fracture, because of the loss of isometry in the medial ligaments, the loss of major range of motion can be severe and limiting. Similarly, an incongruent elbow joint will have marked limitations of motion. In situations where the loss of motion is greater than 45 to 60 degrees, late operative release may be indicated for an elbow release. Successful release requires high level of patient cooperation with extensive therapy.

MYOSITIS OSSIFICANS VERSUS HETEROTOPIC CALCIFICATION

True myositis ossificans should be differentiated from heterotopic calcification, which is a dystrophic process. Myositis ossificans involves ossification within the muscle sheath that can lead to a significant loss of range of motion of the elbow. Disruption of the brachialis muscle is believed to be a contributory factor.[88] Fortunately, myositis ossificans is rare in children.[75,171] Although heterotopic calcification in the ligaments and capsule of the elbow is common,[75,143] it rarely results in loss of elbow function (Fig. 15-23).

In Neviaser and Wickstrom's[117] series of 115 patients, 10 had x-ray evidence of myositis ossificans; all, however, were asymptomatic. Roberts[143] differentiated true myositis ossificans from heterotopic calcification in his series of 60 elbow dislocations, and noted that only three patients had true myositis ossificans. Linscheid and Wheeler[87] reported that the incidence of some type of heterotopic calcification was 28%, which was most common around the condyles. Only in five patients was it anterior to the capsule (which probably represented true myositis ossificans in the brachialis muscle). Four of these patients had some decrease in elbow function. Josefsson et al.[75] reported that 61% of 28 children with posterior dislocations had periarticular calcification, but this did not appear to be functionally significant.

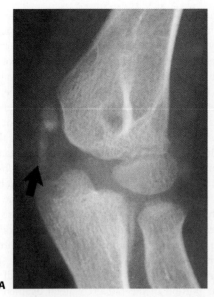
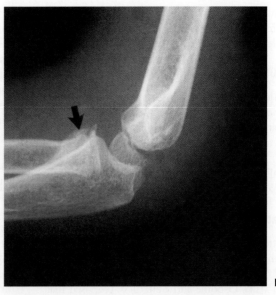

Figure 15-23. A: Heterotopic calcification of the ulnar collateral ligaments in an elbow that had been dislocated for 2 months (*arrow*). **B:** Lateral view of the same elbow. Some myositis ossification has occurred where the brachialis inserts into the coronoid process (*arrow*).

RADIOULNAR SYNOSTOSIS

In dislocations with an associated fracture of the radial neck, the incidence of a secondary proximal radioulnar synostosis is increased (Fig. 15-24). This can occur regardless of whether the radial neck fracture is treated operatively or nonoperatively[20,23,121] and likely occurs because of the extensive periosteal stripping that occurs along the anterior aspect of the forearm between the proximal radius and ulna. Carlioz and

Abols[23] reported a synostosis in one of three patients with posterior elbow dislocations associated with radial neck fractures.

CUBITUS RECURVATUM

Occasionally, a severe elbow dislocation results in significant tearing of the anterior capsule. As a result, after reduction, when all the stiffness created by the dislocation has subsided, the patient may have some hyperextension (cubitus

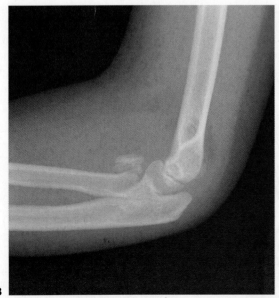
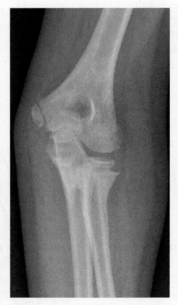
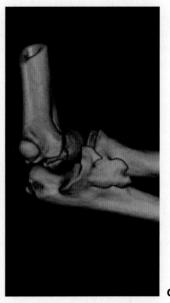

Figure 15-24. Radioulnar synostosis. An 11-year-old male fell injuring his nondominant left elbow. An elbow dislocation was reduced by emergency personnel prior to arrival at the hospital. **A:** Initial radiographs demonstrated a significantly displaced radial neck fracture. This was reduced using percutaneous techniques. **B:** Five months later radiographs and (**C**) a CT scan noted a complete radioulnar synostosis.

recurvatum) of the elbow. This is usually minimally symptomatic but if asymmetric, may be aesthetically disturbing to the parents and adolescent.

RECURRENT POSTERIOR DISLOCATIONS

Recurrent posterior elbow dislocation is rare. In the combined series of dislocations, only 2 of 317 patients (0.6%) experienced recurrent dislocations.[87,117,143,146] Approximately 80% of recurrent dislocations are in males. Three investigators have reported bilateral cases.[78,112,139] The pathology of recurrent dislocation involves any or all of a combination of collateral ligament instability, capsular laxity, and bone and articular cartilage defects.

Contributing Pathology

Osborne and Cotterill[122] suggested that articular changes are secondary and that the primary defect is a failure of the posterolateral ligamentous and capsular structures to become reattached after reduction (Fig. 15-25). Osborne and Cotterill[122] proposed that the extensive articular cartilage covering the surface of the distal humerus leaves little surface area for soft tissue reattachment and the presence of synovial fluid further inhibits soft tissue healing. With recurrent dislocations, the radial head impinges against the posterolateral margin of the capitellum, creating an osteochondral defect (Fig. 15-26). In addition to the defect in the capitellar articular surface, a similar defect develops in the anterior articular margin of the radial head. When these two defects oppose each other, recurrence of the dislocation is more likely. Subsequent studies have confirmed these findings in almost all recurrent dislocations, especially in children.[35,59,120,168,173,182]

O'Driscoll et al.[120] described posterolateral instability in five patients, including two children, in whom laxity of the ulnar part of the radial collateral ligament allowed a transitory rotary subluxation of the ulnohumeral joint and a secondary dislocation of the radiohumeral joint. This was confirmed with a report of another nine pediatric patients, most of whom had posterior elbow dislocation.[201] Patients with posterolateral instability often complain of a feeling of apprehension with certain activities or describe a history of recurrent temporary dislocation

of the elbow but, when examined, exhibit no unusual clinical findings. They also may present with contracture. The instability is diagnosed with a posterolateral rotary instability test, which is done by holding the patient's arm over the head while applying proximal axial compression plus a valgus and supination force to the forearm (Fig. 15-27). As the elbow is slowly flexed from an extended position, the radial head, which is initially posteriorly subluxated, reduces producing the appreciation of a "clunk" or "shift." In some cases the only positive finding is that of apprehension with the examination and in others, posterolateral rotary instability can be detected only with the patient completely relaxed under general anesthesia. The prone push-up test (performed with the forearms maximally supinated) or the chair push-up test (also performed with the arms maximally supinated) can often reproduce the patient's symptoms of pain or a feeling of subluxation or apprehension in the office setting, and thus can often help establish the diagnosis. O'Driscoll et al.[120] reported that surgical repair of the lax ulnar portion of the radial collateral ligament eliminated the posterolateral rotary instability. In children and adolescents, the same instability can occur from cartilage nonunion of the origin of the radial collateral ligament.

In addition to the osteochondral defects in the capitellum and radial head, bone defects may include a shallow semilunar notch resulting from a coronoid fossa process fracture or multiple recurrent dislocations.

Treatment Options

There is only one report of successful nonsurgical management of recurrent elbow dislocations. Herring and Sullivan[63] used an orthosis that blocked the last 15 degrees of extension. After his patient wore this orthosis constantly for 2 years and with vigorous activities for another 6 months, there were no further dislocations, but the follow-up period was only 1 year. Beaty and Donati[14] emphasized that physical therapy and the use of an orthosis should be tried before surgery is considered.

Because nonsurgical management is so often unsuccessful, the treatment of recurrent posterior elbow dislocations is predominately

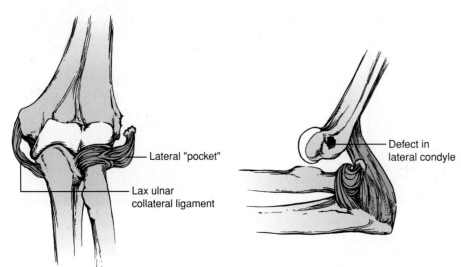

Figure 15-25. Pathology associated with recurrent elbow dislocations. The three components that allow the elbow to dislocate: A lax ulnar collateral ligament, a "pocket" in the radial collateral ligament, and a defect in the lateral condyle. (Adapted from Osborne G, Cotterill P. Recurrent dislocation of the elbow. *J Bone Joint Surg Br.* 1966;48(2):340–346.)

Lateral "pocket"

Lax ulnar collateral ligament

Defect in lateral condyle

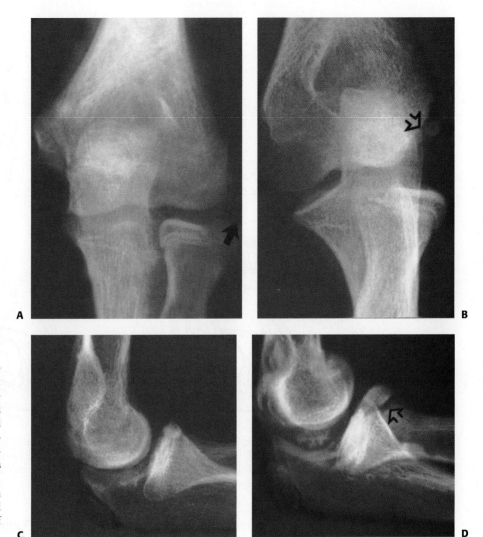

Figure 15-26. Radiographic changes associated with recurrent elbow dislocation. **A:** Anteroposterior radiograph of a 13-year-old who had recurrent dislocations. An osteochondral fragment (*arrow*) is attached to the lateral ligament. **B:** An oblique radiograph shows the defect (*arrow*) in the posterolateral condylar surface. **C:** Radiographs of an 11-year-old after his first dislocation. **D:** One year later, after recurrent dislocation and subluxations, blunting of the radial head has developed (*arrow*). (Courtesy of Marvin E. Mumme, MD.)

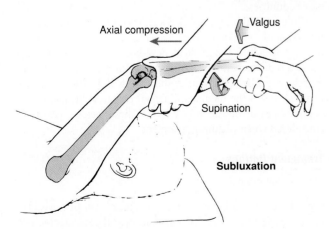

Figure 15-27. Posterolateral rotary instability. Posterolateral rotational instability is best demonstrated with the upper extremity over the head with the patient supine. The radial head can be subluxated or dislocated by applying a valgus and supination force to the forearm at the same time proximal axial compression is applied along the forearm. (Reprinted with permission from O'Driscoll SW, Bell DF, Morrey BF. Posterolateral rotary instability of the elbow. *J Bone Joint Surg Am.* 1991;73(3):440–446.)

surgical. Various surgical procedures have been described to correct bone and soft tissue abnormalities (Fig. 15-28).

Bone Procedures

These are directed toward correcting dysplasia of the semilunar notch of the olecranon. Milch[112] inserted a boomerang-shaped bone block. Others[49,108,176] found that a simple bone block was all that was necessary (see Fig. 15-28A). Mantle[100] increased the slope of the semilunar notch in two patients with an opening wedge osteotomy of the coronoid process (see Fig. 15-28B).

Soft Tissue Procedures

Reichenheim[139] and King[82] transferred the biceps tendon just distal to the coronoid process to reinforce it (see Fig. 15-28C). Kapel[78] developed a cruciate ligament-type reconstruction in which distally based strips of the biceps and triceps tendon were passed through the distal humerus (see Fig. 15-28D). Beaty and Donati[14] modified this technique by transferring a central slip of the triceps through the humerus posterior to anterior and attaching it to the proximal ulna.

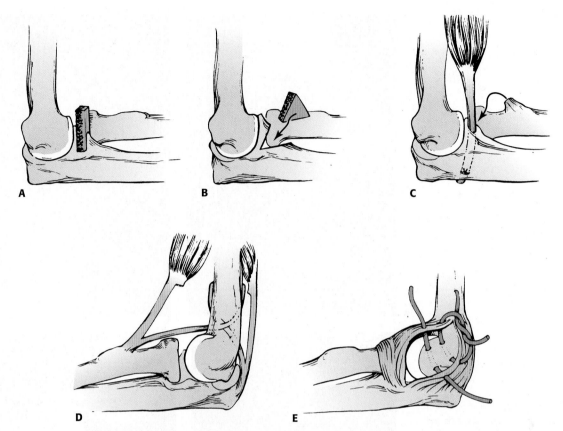

Figure 15-28. Surgical procedures for recurrent dislocation. **A:** Simple coronoid bone block. **B:** Open wedge coronoid osteotomy. **C:** Biceps tendon transfer to coronoid process. **D:** Cruciate ligament reconstruction. **E:** Lateral capsular reattachment of Osborne and Cotterill. (Adapted from Osborne G, Cotterill P. Recurrent dislocation of the elbow. *J Bone Joint Surg Br.* 1966;48(2):340–346.)

The most widely accepted technique is that described by Osborne and Cotterill,[122] in which the lateral capsule is reattached to the posterolateral aspect of the capitellum with sutures passing through holes drilled in the bone (see Fig. 15-28E). The joint should be inspected at surgery because osteocartilaginous loose bodies may be present.[59,98,168] Since Osborne and Cotterill's[122] initial report of eight patients, successful use of this technique has been reported in numerous others.[35,59,98,120,168,173,182] Zeier[186] and O'Driscoll et al.[120] reinforced the lateral repair with strips of fascia lata, triceps fascia, or palmaris longus tendon.

Postoperative Care

Postoperatively, especially after the repair described by Osborne and Cotterill,[122] the arm is immobilized in a long arm cast with the elbow flexed 90 degrees for 4 to 6 weeks. Protected active range-of-motion exercises are performed for an additional 4 to 6 weeks. Strenuous activities are avoided for 12 weeks postoperative.

Complications

Major complications after correction of recurrent dislocations include loose osteocartilaginous fragments and destruction of the articular surface of the joint (Fig. 15-29), elbow stiffness, or recurrent instability.

UNREDUCED POSTERIOR ELBOW DISLOCATIONS

Untreated posterior dislocations of the elbow in children are extremely rare in North America. Most reported series are from other countries.[42]

Children with untreated dislocations typically have pain and limited midrange of motion (see Fig. 15-12). Pathologically, there is usually subperiosteal new bone formation that produces a radiohumeral horn, myositis ossificans of the brachialis muscle, capsular contractures, shortening of the triceps muscle, contractures of the medial and lateral collateral ligaments, and compression of the ulnar nerve.[41,42] These factors have to be considered when planning treatment.

Treatment Options

Closed Reduction

Closed reduction of dislocations recognized within 3 weeks of injury may be possible.[5,42] If this fails or if the dislocation is of longer duration, open reduction is necessary.

Open Reduction

Open reduction through a posterior approach, as described by Speed,[164] involves lengthening of the triceps muscle and decompression or transposition of the ulnar nerve.[42] Satisfactory

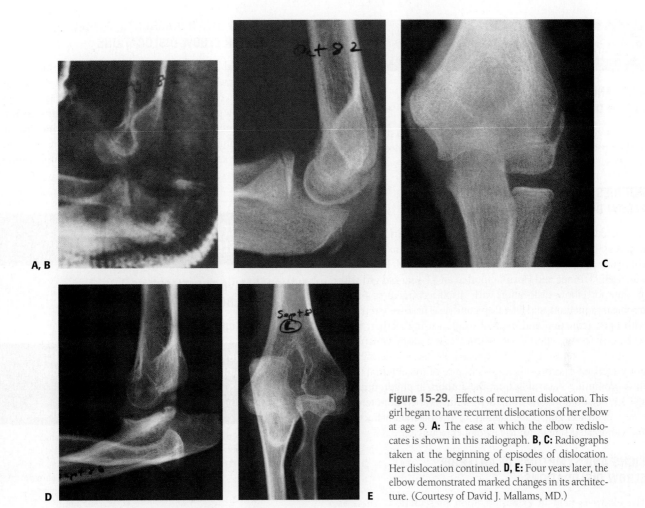

Figure 15-29. Effects of recurrent dislocation. This girl began to have recurrent dislocations of her elbow at age 9. **A:** The ease at which the elbow redislocates is shown in this radiograph. **B, C:** Radiographs taken at the beginning of episodes of dislocation. Her dislocation continued. **D, E:** Four years later, the elbow demonstrated marked changes in its architecture. (Courtesy of David J. Mallams, MD.)

results usually can be obtained if a stable concentric reduction is achieved within 3 months of the initial dislocation.[5] Results after surgical reconstruction decline thereafter but still may produce some improvement in function.[31,42,96,111,114] Fixation of the elbow joint to maintain reduction with one or two large smooth pins for 2 to 4 weeks followed by vigorous but protected physical therapy has been recommended.[42,114] Consideration may be given to hinged external fixation instead of transarticular pins.

Mahaisavariya et al.[97] reported improved extension and better functional results 1 to 3 months after injury in 34 patients with chronic elbow dislocation reconstruction in whom the triceps tendon was not lengthened compared with 38 patients who had the triceps lengthened at surgery.

CONGENITAL ELBOW DISLOCATIONS

Chronic elbow dislocation may be congenital in origin. Altered anatomy and limited motion predispose these patients to injury. The key to differentiating a congenital from an acute traumatic elbow dislocation is examination of the x-ray architecture of the articulating surfaces. In a congenitally dislocated elbow, there is atrophy of the humeral condyles and the semilunar notch of the olecranon. The radial head and neck may be hypoplastic, and the articular surface of the radial head may be dome shaped instead of concave. Unfortunately, these same changes can result from chronic recurrent dislocation after trauma, making the differentiation between congenital and chronic traumatic dislocation difficult. If other congenital anomalies are present or the child has an underlying syndrome, such as Ehlers–Danlos or Larsen syndrome, the dislocation is likely to be nontraumatic. Obtaining comparison x-rays of the asymptomatic, contralateral elbow often reveals identical anatomy, confirming the etiology of the dislocation as congenital or nontraumatic acquired.

Anterior Elbow Dislocations

INTRODUCTION TO ANTERIOR ELBOW DISLOCATIONS

Anterior elbow dislocations are rare. Of the 317 elbows in the combined series,[87,117,143,146] only five were anterior, for an incidence of slightly over 1%. They are associated with an increased incidence of complications, such as brachial artery disruption and associated fractures, compared with posterior dislocations.[70]

ASSESSMENT OF ANTERIOR ELBOW DISLOCATIONS

MECHANISMS OF INJURY FOR ANTERIOR ELBOW DISLOCATIONS

Anterior elbow dislocations usually are caused by a direct blow to the posterior aspect of the flexed elbow.[68] Hyperextension of the elbow also has been implicated in one study.

INJURIES ASSOCIATED WITH ANTERIOR ELBOW DISLOCATIONS

Associated fractures are common. In children, the triceps insertion may be avulsed from the olecranon with a small piece of cortical bone[181] or even a displaced fracture through the olecranon itself.[197] Inoue and Horii[68] reported an 11-year-old girl with an anterior elbow dislocation with displaced fractures of the trochlea, capitellum, and lateral epicondyle. These were repaired with open reduction and internal fixation using Herbert bone screws. A recent report reviews three cases, all of which had fractures.[189] Interestingly, the displaced olecranon fracture was not visualized in one of the cases because of the children's age, thus prompting a warning from the authors in children under age 10. Fixation options from these studies varied from tension band constructs and plate fixation for the olecranon fractures and cannulated screws for the medial epicondyle.

SIGNS AND SYMPTOMS OF ANTERIOR ELBOW DISLOCATIONS

The elbow is held in extension upon presentation. There is fullness in the antecubital fossa. Swelling usually is marked because of the soft tissue disruption associated with this type of dislocation. There is severe pain with attempted motion. A careful neurovascular examination is mandatory.

IMAGING AND OTHER DIAGNOSTIC STUDIES FOR ANTERIOR ELBOW DISLOCATIONS

Routine AP and lateral x-rays are diagnostic. In most cases, the proximal radius and ulna dislocate in an anteromedial direction (Fig. 15-30). As with posterior dislocations, postreduction radiographs should be carefully scrutinized for a congruent reduction and for subtle osteochondral fracture fragments. Evaluation with CT or MRI cap be used to further define the extent of soft tissue injury in complex injury patterns.

TREATMENT OPTIONS FOR ANTERIOR ELBOW DISLOCATIONS

NONOPERATIVE TREATMENT OF ANTERIOR ELBOW DISLOCATIONS

Indications/Contraindications

Nonoperative Treatment Following Successful Closed Reduction of Anterior Elbow Dislocation: INDICATIONS AND CONTRAINDICATIONS

Indications	Relative Contraindications
• Stable concentric elbow reduction obtained following closed treatment	• Unable to obtain a concentric and stable elbow reduction • Intra-articular entrapment of fracture fragments • Vascular injury • Change in neurologic status following reduction or other indication of nerve entrapment

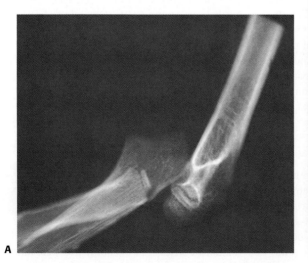 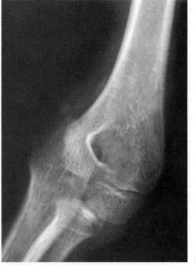

Figure 15-30. Anterior dislocation of the elbow. **A:** Initial anteroposterior radiograph. The olecranon lies anterior to the distal humerus. **B:** Initial lateral radiograph. The proximal ulna and radial head lie anteromedial, and the elbow carrying angle is in varus. (Courtesy of Hilario Trevino, MD.)

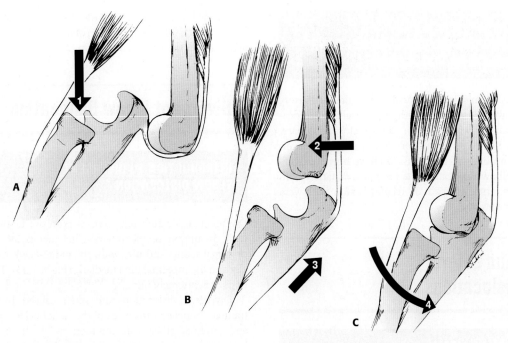

Figure 15-31. Reduction of anterior dislocation. **A:** With the elbow semiflexed, a longitudinal force is applied along the long axis of the humerus (*arrow 1*). Pulling distally on the forearm may be necessary to initially dislodge the olecranon. **B:** Once the olecranon is distal to the humerus, the distal humerus is pushed anteriorly (*arrow 2*) whereas a proximally directed force is applied along the long axis of the forearm (*arrow 3*). **C:** Finally, the elbow is immobilized in some extension (*arrow 4*).

As with posterior elbow dislocations, because of the significant amount of soft tissue swelling and potential for neurovascular compromise, all anterior elbow dislocations should be reduced with adequate analgesia and relaxation as soon as possible. Consideration for nonoperative treatment following closed reduction can only be considered if the elbow is stable through close to a functional range of motion, a concentric anatomic reduction can be obtained and maintained, and there is no evidence to suggest a vascular injury, nerve entrapment, or significant intra-articular osteochondral fragments.

Surgery usually is not required unless the dislocation is open, there is a brachial artery injury, or there is an associated fracture that does not realign satisfactorily after closed reduction. Open reduction and internal fixation of the fracture may then be necessary.[68]

Closed Reduction of Anterior Elbow Dislocations

Reduction usually is accomplished by flexing the elbow and pushing the forearm proximally and downward at the same time.[181] As with posterior dislocations, a force must first be applied longitudinally along the axis of the humerus with the elbow semiflexed to overcome the forces of the biceps and triceps. The longitudinal force along the axis of the forearm is directed toward the elbow (Fig. 15-31). To make reduction easier, the distal humerus can be forced in an anterior direction by pushing on the posterior aspect of the distal arm.

Because most anterior dislocations occur in flexion, the elbow should be immobilized in some extension for 1 to 3 weeks, followed by protected active range-of-motion exercises. Early motion after open reduction and internal fixation of an associated olecranon fracture usually can be allowed.[68]

Author's Preferred Method of Treatment for Anterior Elbow Dislocations (see Algorithm 15-1)

Closed reduction (see Fig. 15-31) is the initial procedure of choice. A distal force must be applied in line with and parallel to the long axis of the humerus first. Once the length has been reestablished, a posteriorly directed force along the axis of the forearm is applied until the elbow is reduced. The same principles that were discussed for posterior elbow dislocations apply to anterior elbow dislocations as well. There should be a thorough and systematic evaluation of the elbow stability following reduction, postreduction radiographs should be carefully scrutinized for a concentric reduction and associated fractures or entrapped loose bodies, and, if appropriate, a brief period of immobilization followed by an early protected motion program should be employed. Stable fixation of associated fractures is also necessary as dictated by the treatment principles for those fractures.

There appears to be an increased incidence of brachial artery rupture or thrombosis associated with anterior elbow dislocations.[70,163] As discussed with posterior elbow dislocations, early and persistent vigilance for circulatory issues should be exercised. When compromised, as discussed above in more detail with posterior elbow dislocations, a prompt evaluation with consideration for arterial repair or reconstruction with vein grafting may be necessary.

Medial and Lateral Elbow Dislocations

INTRODUCTION TO MEDIAL AND LATERAL ELBOW DISLOCATIONS

These are rare dislocations. In the recent series of 145 pediatric elbow dislocations, Murphy reported 10 medial dislocations and no lateral dislocations.[203]

ASSESSMENT OF MEDIAL AND LATERAL ELBOW DISLOCATIONS

SIGNS AND SYMPTOMS OF MEDIAL AND LATERAL ELBOW DISLOCATIONS

In an incomplete lateral dislocation, the semilunar notch articulates with the capitulotrochlear groove, and the radial head appears more prominent laterally. There is often good flexion and extension of the elbow, increasing the likelihood that a lateral dislocation will be overlooked. In a complete lateral dislocation, the olecranon is displaced lateral to the capitellum. This gives the elbow a markedly widened appearance. Similarly, in a medial dislocation, the forearm appears translated medially relative to the humerus.

IMAGING AND OTHER DIAGNOSTIC STUDIES FOR MEDIAL AND LATERAL ELBOW DISLOCATIONS

AP x-rays of the elbow usually are diagnostic. On the lateral view, the elbow may appear reduced.

TREATMENT OPTIONS FOR MEDIAL AND LATERAL ELBOW DISLOCATIONS

These rare dislocations can be treated by closed reduction in virtually all patients.[184] A longitudinal force is applied along the axis of the humerus to distract the elbow, and then direct medial or lateral pressure (opposite the direction of the dislocation) is applied over the proximal forearm (Fig. 15-32).

Divergent Elbow Dislocation

INTRODUCTION TO DIVERGENT ELBOW DISLOCATION

Divergent dislocation represents a posterior elbow dislocation with disruption of the interosseous membrane between the proximal radius and ulna with the radial head displaced laterally and the proximal ulna medially (Fig. 15-33). These dislocations are extremely rare.[10,21,30,46,66,67,106,115,154,162,175]

Divergent dislocations are often caused by high-energy trauma. Associated fractures of the radial neck, proximal ulna, and coronoid process are common.[2,21,38,175] It has been speculated that, in addition to the hyperextension of the elbow that produces the dislocation, a strong proximally directed force is applied parallel to the long axis of the forearm, disrupting the annular ligament and interosseous membrane and allowing the divergence of the proximal radius and ulna. In a cadaveric study, Altuntas et al.[7] confirmed that only after release of all the ligamentous stabilizers of the elbow and release of the intraosseous membrane from the elbow to the distal third of the forearm could a divergent dislocation be replicated.

TREATMENT OPTIONS FOR DIVERGENT ELBOW DISLOCATIONS

CLOSED REDUCTION IN DIVERGENT ELBOW DISLOCATIONS

Divergent dislocations are typically easily reduced using closed reduction under general anesthesia. Reduction is achieved by applying longitudinal traction with the elbow semiextended and at the same time compressing the proximal radius and ulna together.

After successful closed reduction, the elbow is immobilized in 90 degrees of flexion and the forearm in neutral. Postreduction CT scan may be useful to confirm the anatomic relationships have been restored between the humerus, radius, and ulna, as well as to evaluate for possible fracture displacement.[211] Active range-of-motion exercises are then begun after approximately 2 to 3 weeks following the injury. Most patients regain full elbow motion, including forearm pronation and supination.

OPEN REDUCTION IN DIVERGENT ELBOW DISLOCATIONS

Very few divergent dislocations reported in the literature have required open reduction.[38,106,116] Failure of closed reduction[106,116] and displaced associated fracture[38] are indications for

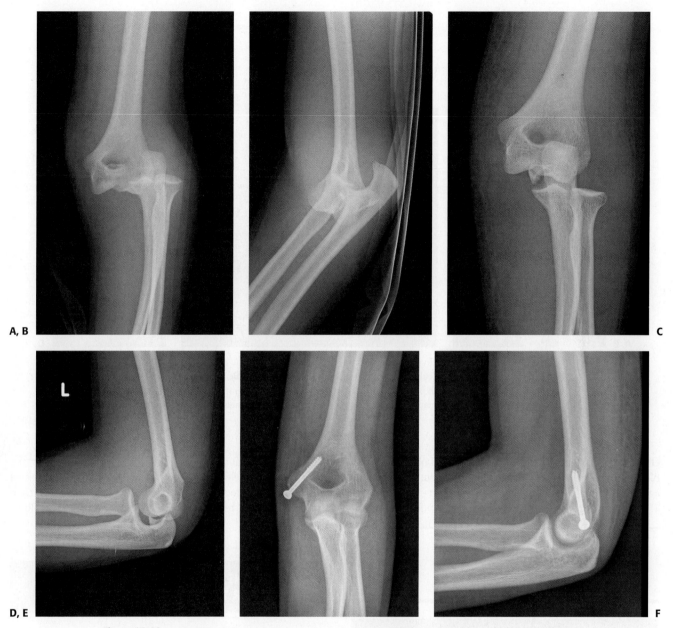

Figure 15-32. A 12-year-old female experienced a lateral elbow dislocation while playing basketball. **A, B:** AP and lateral radiographs demonstrate lateral translation of radius and ulna. Soft tissue shadows reflect visible clinical deformity in which forearm is laterally displaced relative to the arm. **C, D:** Images following attempted close reduction under general anesthesia confirm incarceration of the fractured medial epicondyle fragment within the elbow joint and incomplete reduction. **E, F:** Three months following open reduction and internal fixation of the medial epicondyle fragment, the elbow joint is concentrically reduced, and elbow range of motion is slightly restricted from −20 degrees of extension to 125 degrees of flexion.

open reduction. After failed attempted closed reduction was unsuccessful, Nanno et al.[116] performed surgical exploration and identified the avulsed anterior band of the medial collateral ligament complex of the elbow interposed between the medial condyle of the humerus and the olecranon. After removing and repairing the interposed ligament, stable reduction was achieved. van Wagenberg et al.[174] describes a patient with divergent elbow dislocation with associated distal radius and coronoid fractures. After anatomic reduction of the fractures a stable reduction of the divergent elbow dislocation was achieved.

MANAGEMENT OF EXPECTED ADVERSE OUTCOMES AND UNEXPECTED COMPLICATIONS RELATED TO DIVERGENT ELBOW DISLOCATIONS

A case of symptomatic radiocapitellar instability 7 years following a transverse, mediolateral divergent dislocation has been reported.[185] No discussion of treatment for this complication was provided, but knowledge of the difficulty treating chronic

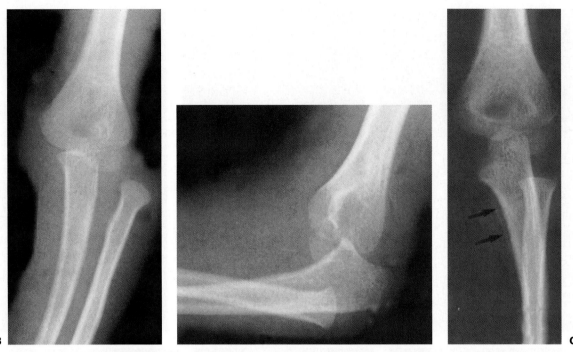

A, B   **C**

Figure 15-33. Medial–lateral divergent dislocation. **A:** Anteroposterior view demonstrating disruption of the proximal radioulnar joint with the radius lateral and the ulna medial. **B:** Lateral radiograph confirms that the radius and ulna are both posterior to the distal humerus. **C:** A radiograph taken 4 weeks after injury shows periosteal new bone formation (*arrows*), indicating where the soft tissues were extensively torn away from the proximal ulna.

elbow instability emphasizes the importance of obtaining a stable, congruent reduction during the time of acute injury management.

Proximal Radioulnar Translocations

INTRODUCTION TO PROXIMAL RADIOULNAR TRANSLOCATIONS

Translocation of the proximal radius and ulna is another extremely rare injury with only case reports being described in the English literature.[11,21,22,26,37,48,58,69,94] Radioulnar translocation is commonly missed on the AP x-ray unless the proximal radius and ulna are noted to be completely reversed in relation to the distal humerus. Translocations are believed to be caused by a fall onto the pronated hand with the elbow in full or nearly full extension, producing an axial force on the proximal radius. The anterior radial head dislocation occurs first, followed by the posterior dislocation of the olecranon. Combourieu et al.[26] suggests that avulsion of the brachialis insertion is necessary for the radial head to translate medially. The radial head, depending on the degree of pronation, can be lodged in the coronoid fossa or dislocated posteriorly. As a consequence, fractures of the

radial head, radial neck, or coronoid process may occur.[21,22,37,94] Harvey and Tchelebi[58] reported a case in which the cause of radioulnar translocation may have been iatrogenic: the result of inappropriate technique used to reduce a posterior elbow dislocation.

ASSESSMENT OF PROXIMAL RADIOULNAR TRANSLOCATIONS

Swelling and pain may obscure the initial examination, and minimal deformity may be apparent. Once pain has been adequately managed with analgesics, the most consistent finding on clinical examination is limited elbow range of motion, especially in supination.

INJURIES ASSOCIATED WITH PROXIMAL RADIOULNAR TRANSLOCATIONS

Radial neck fracture is the most common fracture associated with proximal radioulnar translocation.[22,37,69,94] Eklof et al.[37] also reported one patient who sustained a fracture of the tip of the coronoid. Proposed soft tissue injuries include radial collateral ligament, medial collateral ligament, annular ligament, interosseous ligament, and avulsion of the brachialis.[26,37,69] Transient ulnar nerve paresthesia that resolved after reduction of the translocation has been reported in several patients.[26,69] Osteonecrosis of the radial head was noted in one patient after open reduction of a proximal radioulnar translocation and premature closure of the proximal radial physis has been reported.[26,58]

TREATMENT OPTIONS FOR PROXIMAL RADIOULNAR TRANSLOCATIONS

CLOSED REDUCTION IN PROXIMAL RADIOULNAR TRANSLOCATIONS

Successful closed reduction of proximal radioulnar translocation has been reported.[26,69,94] The patient must be completely relaxed under general anesthesia, as sedation or regional anesthesia is unlikely to provide sufficient relaxation. With the elbow flexed approximately 90 degrees, longitudinal traction is applied to the elbow while the forearm is supinated (Fig. 15-34). If the radial head can be palpated, gentle anterior-directed pressure may help slide the radial head and neck over the coronoid process, allowing the proximal radius and ulna to resume their normal configuration. As always, just the right amount of force should be used; excessive force risks iatrogenic fracture to the proximal radius. Successful closed reduction should be confirmed on x-ray, and the elbow should be immobilized for approximately 3 to 4 weeks with the forearm supinated and the elbow flexed 90 to 100 degrees.

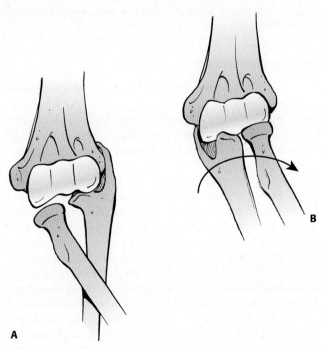

Figure 15-34. Proximal radioulnar translocation. **A:** Position of the proximal radius and ulna with a proximal radioulnar translocation. **B:** Closed reduction is rarely successful, but may be attempted under general anesthesia using gentle longitudinal traction while supinating the forearm. (Redrawn with permission from Harvey S, Tchelebi H. Proximal radioulnar translocation. A case report. *J Bone Joint Surg Am.* 1979;61(3):447–449.)

OPEN REDUCTION IN PROXIMAL RADIOULNAR TRANSLOCATIONS

Radioulnar translocations may require open reduction.[21,22,37,48,58,69] A lateral approach provides adequate exposure to the translocation and radial neck fracture if present. At surgery, the radial head and neck are typically found trapped beneath the trochlea of the distal humerus. Elbow extension tightens the biceps tendon, making reduction more difficult. With the elbow flexed, a freer or joker elevator can be placed beneath the radial head and neck facilitating delivery over the coronoid process as the forearm is supinated. If present, a radial neck fracture may now be treated in standard fashion. Internal fixation also may be necessary for an unstable displaced fracture.

Harvey and Tchelebi[58] used an osteotomy of the proximal ulna to expose and reduce the radius that was complicated by a postoperative ulnar nerve paralysis that recovered completely over 2 months. Just like after successful closed reduction, following open reduction the upper extremity is immobilized for approximately 3 to 4 weeks with the forearm supinated and the elbow flexed 90 to 100 degrees, followed by active elbow range-of-motion exercises.

Medial Epicondyle Apophysis Fractures

INTRODUCTION TO MEDIAL EPICONDYLE APOPHYSIS FRACTURES

In the early 1900s, it was recognized that the medial epicondyle fracture was often associated with elbow dislocation and the apophyseal fragment could become entrapped within the joint.[177] The reported incidence of medial epicondyle fracture associated with dislocation of the elbow in children and adolescents has varied from as low as 30% to as high as 60% in many of the reported series.[203] Two bilateral injuries associated with bilateral elbow dislocations have been reported,[40] both patients having sustained their injuries while participating in gymnastics (Table 15-1). Fractures involving the medial epicondylar apophysis constitute approximately 14% of fractures involving the distal humerus and 11% of all fractures in the elbow region.[24] The youngest reported patient with this injury was 3.9 years.[24] In the large series of fractures of the medial epicondylar apophysis, most occurred between ages 9 and 14, and the peak

TABLE 15-1. Incidence of Fractures of the Medial Epicondylar Apophysis

Overall incidence: Fractures of the elbow region, 11.5%
Age: peak, 11–12 yrs
Sex: males, 79% (4:1, male:female)
Association with elbow dislocation: approximately 50% (15–18% of these involve incarceration of the epicondylar apophysis)

age incidence was 11 to 12 years.[64,80,113,124,157] Fractures of the epicondylar apophysis preferentially affect males by a ratio of almost 4 to 1 over females. In six large series in the literature, boys constituted 79% of the patients.[44,102,144,177]

ASSESSMENT OF MEDIAL EPICONDYLE APOPHYSIS FRACTURES

MECHANISMS OF INJURY FOR MEDIAL EPICONDYLE APOPHYSIS FRACTURES

Injuries to the medial epicondylar apophysis most commonly occur as acute injuries in which a distinct event produces a partial or a complete separation of the apophyseal fragment. Three theories have been proposed about the mechanism of acute medial epicondylar apophyseal injuries: a direct blow, avulsion mechanisms, and association with elbow dislocation.

Direct Blow

Stimson[166] speculated that this type of injury could occur as a result of a direct blow on the posterior aspect of the epicondyle. Among more recent investigators, however, only Watson-Jones[178] described this injury as being associated with a direct blow to the posterior medial aspect of the elbow. In rare patients in whom the fragment is produced by a direct blow to the medial aspect of the joint, the medial epicondylar fragment is often fragmented (Fig. 15-35). In these injuries, there may also be more superficial ecchymosis in the skin.

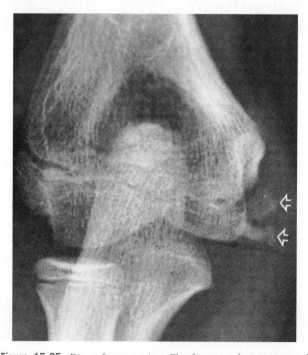

Figure 15-35. Direct fragmentation. The fragmented appearance of the medial epicondyle (*arrows*) in a 13-year-old who sustained a direct blow to the medial aspect of the elbow. (From Wilkins KE. Fractures of the medial epicondyle in children. *Instr Course Lect.* 1991;40:1–8, with permission.)

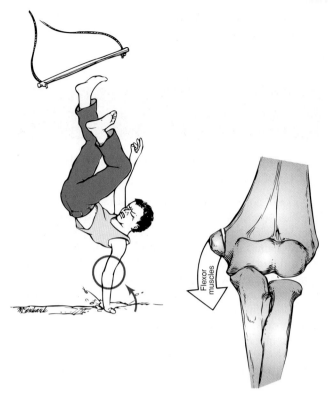

Figure 15-36. Hyperextension forces. When a person falls on the outstretched upper extremity, the wrist and fingers are forced into hyperextension (*solid arrow*), which places tension on the forearm flexor muscles. This sudden tension along with the normal valgus carrying angle tends to place a strong avulsion force on the medial epicondyle (*open arrow*).

Avulsion Mechanisms

Various investigators have suggested that some of these injuries are due to a pure avulsion of the epicondyle by the flexor–pronator muscles of the forearm.[80,128] This muscle avulsion force can occur in combination with a valgus stress in which the elbow is locked in extension, or as a pure musculature contraction that may occur with the elbow partially flexed.

Smith[157] proposed that when a child falls on his outstretched upper extremity with the elbow in extension, the wrist and fingers are often hyperextended as well, placing an added tension force on the epicondyle by the forearm flexor muscles (Fig. 15-36). The normal valgus carrying angle tends to accentuate these avulsion forces when the elbow is in extension. Many proponents of this theory point to the other associated elbow fractures that have been seen with this injury as evidence to confirm that a valgus force is applied across the elbow at the time of the injury. These associated injuries include radial neck fractures with valgus angulation and greenstick valgus fractures of the olecranon.[80]

Isolated avulsion can also occur in adolescents with the simple act of throwing a baseball. In this instance, the sudden contracture of the forearm flexor muscles may be sufficient to cause the epicondyle to fail[191] (Fig. 15-37). The literature has reflected a high incidence of medial epicondylar apophyseal avulsions occurring with arm wrestling in patients near skeletal

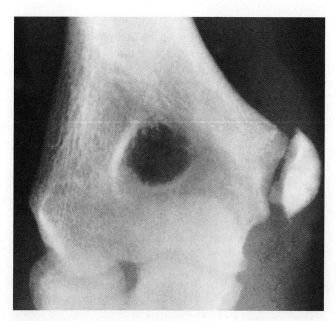

Figure 15-37. Muscle avulsion. Isolated avulsion of the medial epicondyle occurred suddenly in this 14-year-old Little League pitcher after throwing a curve ball. (From Wilkins KE. Fractures of the medial epicondyle in children. *Instr Course Lect.* 1991;40:1–8, with permission.)

maturity.[92,119] The largest series, reported by Nyska et al.[119] from Israel, involved eight boys of 13 to 15 years of age, all of whom were treated conservatively with good results.

Medial Epicondyle Fractures Associated With Elbow Dislocation

Avulsion fractures of the medial epicondyle may be associated with elbow dislocation in which the ulnar collateral ligament provides the avulsion force. If the patient presents with the elbow dislocated, there is no doubt that the dislocation is the major factor causing this fracture. If the patient presents with the elbow located, it is less clear as to whether the medial epicondyle fracture may have been caused by an occult or partial elbow dislocation that has reduced spontaneously. Some investigators have noticed calcification development in the lateral collateral ligaments and adjacent lateral periosteum after fracture. They believed this calcification was evidence that the ligament had been stretched during the process of elbow dislocation. Marion and Faysse[102] found that most elbow dislocations associated with medial epicondyle fractures were posterolateral, but some pure lateral, posterior, and posteromedial dislocations were also observed. A question has also arisen as to whether incarceration of the epicondylar fragment into the joint can occur without a dislocation. Patrick[128] believed that when an extreme valgus stress was applied to the joint, a vacuum was created within the joint that "sucks in" the avulsed epicondylar fragment.

It appears that any of these mechanisms can produce an acute apophyseal injury of the distal humerus. The direct blow mechanism appears to occur only rarely. Many of these injuries may be associated with an elbow dislocation that may or may not have reduced spontaneously.

SIGNS AND SYMPTOMS OF MEDIAL EPICONDYLE AVULSION FRACTURES

Medial epicondyle fractures associated with elbow dislocation are associated with gross deformity of the elbow, swelling, and distracting injuries so that the medial epicondyle fracture can be easily overlooked. A careful and focused evaluation looking specifically at the medial epicondyle is necessary to avoid missing this injury. If a fracture of the medial epicondyle has occurred, then tenderness to palpation will be present.

Because the anterior oblique band of the ulnar collateral ligament may be attached to the medial epicondylar apophysis, the elbow may exhibit some instability after injury. To evaluate the medial stability of the elbow, Woods and Tullos[183] and Schwab et al.[153] advocated a simple valgus stress test. This test is performed with the patient supine and the arm abducted 90 degrees. The shoulder and arm are externally rotated 90 degrees. The elbow must be flexed at least 15 degrees to eliminate the stabilizing force of the olecranon. If the elbow is unstable, simple gravity forces will open the medial side. A small additional weight or sedation may be necessary to acquire an accurate assessment of the medial stability with this test.

Ulnar nerve function must be carefully tested before initiating treatment and documented in the medical record.

IMAGING AND OTHER DIAGNOSTIC STUDIES OF MEDIAL EPICONDYLE AVULSION FRACTURES

Good quality AP and lateral radiographs are essential. Oblique radiographs as well as comparison radiographs of the opposite elbow are often helpful when the interpretation of initial images is not conclusive. Widening or irregularity of the apophyseal line may be the only clue in fractures that are slightly displaced or nondisplaced. If the fragment is significantly displaced, the radiographic diagnosis is usually obvious. If the fragment is totally incarcerated in the joint, however, it may be hidden by the overlying ulnar or distal humerus. The clue here is the total absence of the epicondyle from its normal position just medial and posterior to the medial metaphysis. Knowledge of the order and approximate age of appearance of elbow ossification centers is necessary to appreciate the absence of the epicondyle when it should be present. CT scans can be diagnostic in confusing situations.

Potter[132] suggested that properly performed MRI might disclose acute or chronic injury to the medial epicondylar apophysis, recommending pulse sequences for evaluating the apophysis include fat-suppressed gradient-echo imaging. On MRI, increased signal intensity and abnormal widening of the medial epicondylar physis are seen, typically with surrounding soft tissue edema.

Fractures of the medial epicondyle, even if displaced, may not produce positive fat pad signs.[57,156] If the fracture is only minimally displaced and if it is the result of an avulsion injury, there may be no effusion because all the injured tissues remain extra-articular. In fractures associated with elbow dislocation, there is rupture of the capsule, so its ability to confine the hemarthrosis is lost. In minimally displaced fractures of the medial epicondyle with significant hemarthrosis, the evaluation must be especially thorough to ensure that an unrecognized fracture involving the medial condylar physis is not present.

The ability to accurately measure medial epicondyle fracture displacement has been questioned by several authors who have published work regarding this concern. In a study of medial epicondyle fracture radiographs in 38 patients, Pappas et al.[125] reported poor intraobserver and interobserver agreement with regard to fracture displacement measurement, and questioned the value of perceived fracture displacement as a criterion for choosing surgical versus nonsurgical treatment. In a separate publication, a series of 11 patients judged to have nondisplaced or minimally displaced medial epicondyle fractures had their fractures imaged by both standard radiography and CT.[36] Medial and anterior displacement were then measured on standard radiographs and CT images and compared. Edmonds reported statistically significant differences between standard radiographs and CT images in all measurements with marked increased displacement appreciated on CT scan including six fractures with greater than 10 mm of displacement. To improve our ability to accurately measure fracture displacement on standard radiographs, Klatt and Aoki[83] performed a review of 171 normal AP and lateral elbow radiographs describing the relationship between the medial epicondyle center and reproducible local anatomic landmarks. On the AP radiographs the medial epicondyle center was located 0.5 mm inferior to a line based on the inferior olecranon fossa and on the lateral radiograph the medial epicondyle center was located 1.2 mm anterior to the posterior humeral line.

DIFFERENTIAL DIAGNOSIS OF MEDIAL EPICONDYLE AVULSION FRACTURES

The major injuries to differentiate from isolated medial epicondyle fractures are those fractures involving the medial condylar physis. This is especially true if secondary ossification centers are not present (see Chapter 17 "Fractures Involving the Medial Condylar Physis"). If there is a significant hemarthrosis or a significant piece of metaphyseal bone accompanying the medial epicondylar fragment, arthrography or MRI may be indicated to determine if there is an intra-articular component to the fracture (Fig. 15-38). Other elbow fractures that can be associated with this injury include fracture of the radial neck, olecranon, or coronoid process.

Better implants, improved surgical technique, greater appreciation of the importance of the ulnar collateral ligament inserting on the medial epicondyle, and increased understanding of the degree of displacement in fractures previously thought to be nondisplaced all contribute to a general trend toward more frequent surgical treatment of medial epicondyle fractures.[50] In a 2012 article, Mehlman and Howard[110] acknowledged the dearth of high-level evidence in the published literature on this topic but reports that meta-analysis of clinical research with a particular focus on harm supports surgical treatment for most patients. Independent of whether a nonoperative or operative approach is chosen for the management of a particular medial epicondyle fracture, treatment goals remain to obtain fracture healing and to promote the return of motion, strength, and stability to the elbow.[127]

Even though our ability to measure fracture displacement may be less accurate than we believed in the past, displacement remains an important fracture to consider when making treatment decisions. Additional factors to consider include intra-articular fragment entrapment, ulnar nerve symptoms, dominant arm, and patient activity level.

UNDISPLACED OR MINIMALLY DISPLACED FRACTURES

The apophyseal line remains intact in undisplaced medial epicondyle fractures. The clinical manifestations usually consist only of swelling and local tenderness over the medial

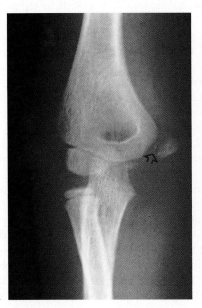 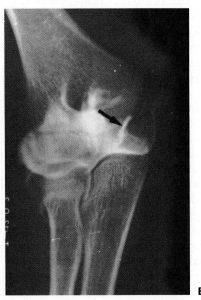

A **B**

Figure 15-38. Intra-articular extension. **A:** Injury film in a 7-year-old girl who was initially suspected of having only a fracture of the medial epicondyle. In addition to moderate displacement, there was a significant metaphyseal fragment (*arrow*). **B:** An arthrogram revealed intra-articular components (*arrow*), which defined this injury instead as a fracture involving the medial condylar physis. (Courtesy of Carl McGarey, MD.)

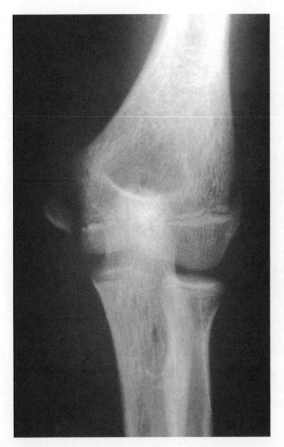

Figure 15-39. AP radiograph shows loss of normal smooth margins of the physis.

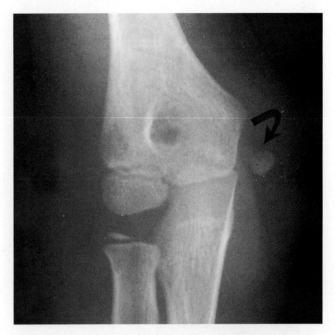

Figure 15-40. Displaced medial epicondylar fracture. AP view of an elbow in which the epicondyle (*arrow*) is significantly displaced both distally and medially. In addition, the fragment is rotated medially.

epicondyle. Crepitus and motion of the epicondyle are usually not present. On radiographs, the smoothness of the edge of the apophyseal line remains intact. Although there may be some loss of soft tissue planes medially on the radiograph, displacement of the elbow fat pads may not be present because the pathology is extra-articular.[57]

Fractures with displacement usually result from a stronger avulsion force, so there is often more soft tissue swelling. Palpating the fragment may elicit crepitus because the increased displacement allows motion of the fragment. On radiographs, there is a loss of parallelism of the smooth sclerotic margins of the physis (Fig. 15-39).[156] The radiolucency in the area of the apophyseal line is usually increased in width.

SIGNIFICANTLY DISPLACED FRACTURES

In significantly displaced fractures, the fragment may be palpable and freely movable. When displaced a considerable distance from the distal humerus, crepitus between the fragments may not be present. Significantly displaced fractures may be associated with an elbow dislocation that reduced spontaneously and there may be no documentation of the original dislocation. On radiograph, the long axis of the epicondylar apophysis is typically rotated medially (Fig. 15-40). The displacement often exceeds 5 mm, but the fragment remains proximal to the true joint surface.

ENTRAPMENT OF THE EPICONDYLAR FRAGMENT IN THE JOINT

Without Elbow Dislocation

In many instances, the elbow appears reduced. The key clinical finding is a block to motion, especially extension. The epicondylar fragment is usually between the joint surfaces of the trochlea and the semilunar notch of the olecranon. On a radiograph, any time the fragment appears at the level of the joint, it must be considered to be totally or partially within the elbow joint until proven otherwise.[128] If the radiograph is examined carefully, the elbow is usually found to be incompletely reduced. Because of an impingement of the fragment within the joint, a good AP view may be difficult to obtain because of the inability to extend the elbow fully. If the fracture is old, the fragment may be fused to the coronoid process, and widening of the medial joint space may be the only clue that the fragment is lying in the joint. The epicondylar ossification center may become fragmented and mistaken for the fragmented appearance of the medial crista of the trochlea.[24,144] Absence of the apophyseal center on the radiograph may be further confirmatory evidence that the fragment is within the joint. Comparison radiographs of the opposite elbow may be necessary to delineate the true pathology.

With Elbow Dislocation

If the elbow is dislocated, the fragment will occasionally lie within the joint and prevent reduction (Fig. 15-41). Recognition of this fragment as being within the joint before a manipulation should alert the physician to the possible need for open reduction. There should be adequate relaxation during the manipulative process.

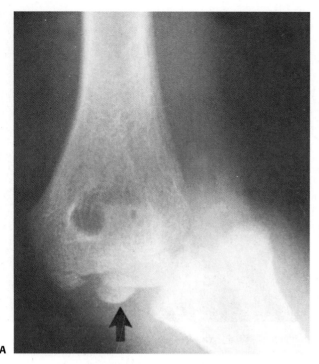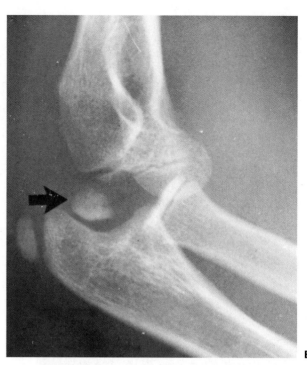

Figure 15-41. Dislocation with incarceration. **A:** AP view showing a posterolateral elbow dislocation. The presence of the medial epicondyle within the elbow joint (*arrow*) prevented a closed reduction. **B:** The lateral view of the same elbow demonstrates the fragment (*arrow*) between the humerus and olecranon.

FRACTURES THROUGH THE EPICONDYLAR APOPHYSIS

Fractures through the body of the epicondyle can result from either a direct blow or avulsion of only part of the apophysis. In either case, the fragments may or may not be displaced. The normal lucent line formed by the overlying metaphyseal border should not be confused with this injury. Although described by Silberstein et al.,[156] this intrafragment fracture is a rare presentation usually seen with throwing athletes.

TREATMENT OPTIONS FOR MEDIAL EPICONDYLE AVULSION FRACTURES

NONOPERATIVE TREATMENT OF MEDIAL EPICONDYLE AVULSION FRACTURES

Indications/Contraindications

Nonoperative Treatment of Medial Epicondyle Fractures: INDICATIONS AND CONTRAINDICATIONS	
Indications	**Relative Contraindications**
• Displacement less than 2 mm	• Displacement greater than 10 mm
• Low-to-moderate activity demands	• Displaced fracture involving the dominant arm in a throwing athlete; either arm in gymnast or wrestler
	• Incarcerated fragment within joint

There appears to be consensus that fractures that are undisplaced or minimally displaced less than 2 mm should be treated nonoperatively. Minimally displaced fractures may be treated using simple immobilization for comfort or cast immobilization for 2 to 3 weeks. Some investigators have recommended initiation of motion early to prevent stiffness, which is the most common complication of this injury.[157] Likewise, there is agreement that if the medial epicondyle fragment is irreducible and is incarcerated within the elbow joint, the accepted treatment is surgical extraction and stable internal fixation.

However, controversy remains as to the optimal treatment method for patients with displacement more than 2 mm.

Outcomes

Josefsson and Danielsson[72] reported 35-year follow-up results in 56 isolated fractures treated nonoperatively. Although more than 60% of their patients demonstrated nonunion on radiograph, these investigators reported a high percentage of good and excellent results. Other reports in the literature[4,124] also demonstrated overall good results with nonoperative management. Knapik and co-authors performed a meta-analysis to compare nonoperative treatment of medial epicondyle fractures in patients with, and without associated elbow dislocation.[198] While patients with associated elbow dislocation had a higher fracture nonunion rate, both groups had minimal clinical or functional limitations at final follow-up.

OPERATIVE TREATMENT OF MEDIAL EPICONDYLE AVULSION FRACTURES

Recent literature describes excellent results obtained with surgical treatment. Louahem et al.[90] from Montpellier, France, report excellent results in 130 and good results in 9 of 139 displaced medial epicondyle fractures treated surgically. Hines et al.,[64] whose practice was to surgically repair all fractures displaced more than 2 mm, found that 96% of their patients had good-to-excellent results. Poor results were attributed mainly to technical errors. Using contemporary outcome measures Canavese and co-authors describe good and excellent results following surgical treatment of medial epicondyle fractures.[190]

Indications/Contraindications

Operative Treatment Indications for Medial Epicondyle Fractures	
Absolute Indication	**Relative Indications**
• Incarceration of the epicondylar fragment	• Ulnar nerve dysfunction • Presence of elbow instability • Desire to avoid symptomatic nonunion

Indications for operative intervention in acute injuries are divided into two categories: absolute and relative. The single absolute indication is incarceration of the epicondylar fragment within the joint. The relative indications include ulnar nerve dysfunction, a need for elbow stability, and a desire to avoid symptomatic nonunion.

Incarceration of the Epicondylar Fragment

If the epicondylar fragment is found in the joint acutely, it must be removed. There are proponents of nonsurgical and surgical techniques for extraction.

Various methods of extracting the fragment by nonoperative methods have been proposed. The success rate of extracting the fragment successfully from the joint by manipulation alone at best has been reported at approximately 40%.[128] All the nonoperative methods require either heavy sedation or light general anesthesia.

The manipulative technique most commonly used is the method popularized by Roberts.[39,142] It involves placing a valgus stress on the elbow while supinating the forearm and simultaneously dorsiflexing the wrist and fingers to place the forearm muscles on stretch; theoretically, this maneuver should extract the fragment from the joint. To be effective, this procedure should be carried out within the first 24 hours after injury.

Failure to extract the fragment by manipulative techniques is an indication to proceed with open surgical extraction. Once open extraction and reduction have been performed, many methods have been advocated to stabilize the fragment, including screw fixation, smooth pins or suture fixation in comminuted fractures. Excision has also been advocated, especially if the fragment is comminuted.

Ulnar Nerve Dysfunction

Ulnar nerve dysfunction occurs more frequently when the medial epicondyle is incarcerated within the joint[194,210] is a relative indication for operative intervention. If there are mild-to-moderate ulnar nerve symptoms at the time of the injury, there is usually no need to explore the nerve, because most of these mild symptoms resolve spontaneously.[32] If the dysfunction is complete, then the ulnar nerve may be directly impinged upon by the fracture or entrapped within the fracture site and should be explored surgically.

There has been some question as to whether delayed ulnar nerve symptoms can occur after fractures of the epicondyle that are not associated with elbow dislocation. However, in a review of more than 100 patients with uncomplicated fractures involving the medial epicondylar apophysis, Patrick[128] could not find any instance in which a delayed ulnar neuritis developed.

Joint Stability

Woods and Tullos[183] suggested that even minor forms of valgus instability after elbow injuries involving the medial epicondylar apophysis can cause significant disability in athletes. This condition is especially true in athletes who must have a stable upper extremity, such as baseball pitchers, gymnasts, or wrestlers. In younger adolescents (younger than 14 years of age), the anterior band of the ulnar collateral ligament often displaces with the apophyseal fragment. In older individuals (15 years or older), large fragments may be avulsed without a ligamentous injury. Rather than depending on arbitrary measurements of fracture displacement, Woods and Tullos[183] recommended using the gravity valgus stress test to determine the presence or absence of valgus instability. They believed that demonstration of a significant valgus instability, using this simple gravity test, was an indication for surgical intervention in patients who require a stable elbow for their athletic activities.

Open Reduction and Internal Fixation of Medial Epicondyle Fractures

Preoperative Planning

✔ ORIF of Medial Epicondyle Fractures: PREOPERATIVE PLANNING CHECKLIST	
OR table	❑ Spine table or flat radiolucent table ❑ Hand table extension
Position/positioning aids	❑ Prone, "sloppy lateral," or supine position
Fluoroscopy location	❑ C-arm and monitor may be positioned on the same side or side opposite the surgeon
Equipment	❑ 4- or 4.5-mm diameter cannulated or solid screws
Tourniquet	❑ Nonsterile tourniquet high on the affected arm

Technique

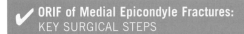

> **✔ ORIF of Medial Epicondyle Fractures:**
> KEY SURGICAL STEPS

- ❏ Position patient prone or "sloppy lateral" allowing the arm to be positioned in a "figure 4" configuration with the forearm resting behind the back.
- ❏ Make a longitudinal 5-cm incision just posterior to the anatomic location of the medial epicondyle.
- ❏ Expose the ulnar nerve and release the fascia.
- ❏ Anatomically reduce the medial epicondyle to the distal humeral metaphysis.
- ❏ Under fluoroscopic guidance, place a cannulated guide pin or solid drill through the center of the medial epicondyle fragment into the center of the medial column of bone in the distal humerus and confirm anatomic reduction of the fracture.
- ❏ Drill and tap into the medial column of the distal humeral metaphysis.
- ❏ Place a single screw within the dense cancellous bone of the medial column.
- ❏ Confirm anatomic reduction of the fracture and position of the implant with fluoroscopy before wound closure.

Our preferred operative technique involves positioning the patient prone position on a radiolucent table (Fig. 15-42). The arm is placed in a "figure 4" position with the forearm resting across the patient's back. This position places a varus stress on the elbow which facilitates fracture reduction while allowing a direct medial approach to the fracture site. Glotzbecker and colleagues describe a similar method for positioning the patient prone to repair the fracture.[196]

A longitudinal 5-cm incision is made just posterior to the anatomic location of the medial epicondyle. The fragment is usually displaced distally and anteriorly. Interposed periosteum and soft tissue are removed from the fracture site, and clot is extracted by irrigation. Expose the ulnar nerve and ensure that it is not trapped within the fracture. Transposition of the nerve is not necessary. Release the fascia overlying the ulnar nerve as the nerve travels in its groove behind the medial epicondyle. This allows mobilization of the nerve and gentle retraction. Exposure of the ulnar nerve will also expose the fracture site. The medial epicondyle fragment will typically be displaced distally and rotated anteriorly.

Preserve soft tissue attachments to the medial epicondyle and elevate just enough soft tissue at the fracture site to allow adequate visualization to achieve an anatomic reduction. Identify and protect the ulnar nerve along with medial antebrachial cutaneous nerves. If not already disrupted by the fracture, we typically release the cubital tunnel retinaculum, but a complete

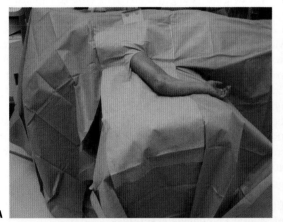
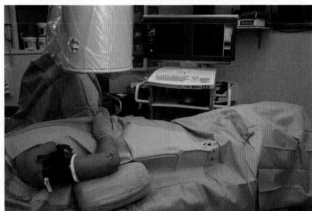
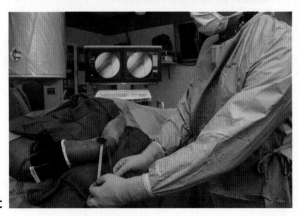
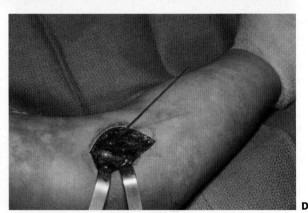

Figure 15-42. The patient is positioned prone on a radiolucent table with the shoulder internally rotated. The arm can be positioned on a hand table (**A**) or the arm can be positioned on a radiolucent table with a radiolucent support placed beneath the elbow (**B**). **C:** When using a radiolucent table, fluoroscopy can be positioned on the opposite side of the table, allowing excellent visualization of the fracture and the fluoroscopy monitor. **D:** A cannulated guide pin maintains the medial epicondyle fracture reduction with the ulnar nerve in close proximity.

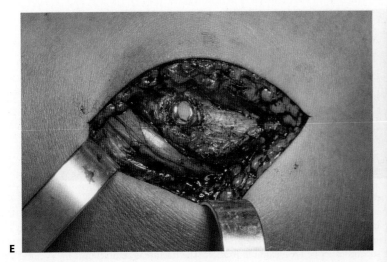

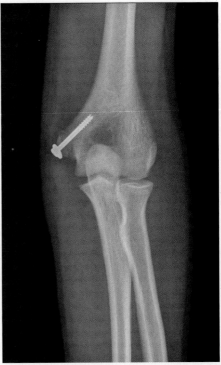

Figure 15-42. (*Continued*) **E:** A 4.5-mm cannulated screw with washer securely holds the medial epiconyle fragment. Bone wax is placed into the head of the cannulated screw to minimize intra-osseous bleeding and postoperative swelling. **F**

dissection of the nerve is usually unnecessary. A small towel clip or clamp is used to grasp the fascia and tendinous origin of the flexor–pronator group, avoiding fragmentation of the medial epicondyle, and the fracture is reduced while the elbow is flexed and the forearm is pronated. A dental instrument also work well to manipulate and position the fracture fragment. The medial epicondyle is reduced under direct vision to its anatomic position on the posterior aspect of the distal medial humerus. Temporarily stabilization with one or two small K-wires, or the guide pin for a cannulated screw, is performed under fluoroscopic guidance.

Final fixation is achieved using a partially threaded screw to compress the medial epicondyle fragment against the humeral metaphysic. Do not use a screw so long that it ends within the central intramedullary canal where screw purchase is poor. In large male patients, a 4.5-mm diameter screw is used, and a 4-mm diameter screw is appropriate for smaller elbows. Because cannulation increases the core diameter of the screw shaft, small-diameter cannulated screws have less coarse threads and less secure fixation. For this reason we will often use a solid 4-mm diameter screw. Fixations depend on a single screw which must be strong enough to allow early motion. Therefore every effort should be made to optimize its strength. Bicortical fixation has been used but injury to the radial nerve when penetrating the opposite cortex with a cannulated screw has been reported.[101] Dense cancellous bone of the medial condyle provides excellent fixation and care should be taken to avoid using a longer screw with threads solely within the hollow central intramedullary canal proximal to the olecranon fossa where fixation is less secure (Fig. 15-43).

A washer may be added to increase fixation surface area and reduce the risk of fragmenting the medial epicondyle with

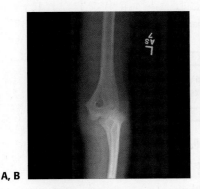

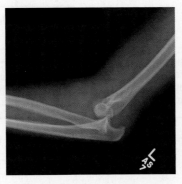

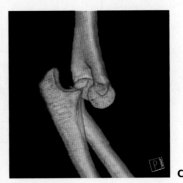

Figure 15-43. A 13-year-old boy is referred for treatment following posterolateral elbow dislocation. **A, B:** Notice on the AP and lateral radiographs that a medial epicondyle fracture cannot be easily seen but the medial epicondyle ossification center is absent from its normal anatomic position at the distal medial posterior humerus.

(*continues*)

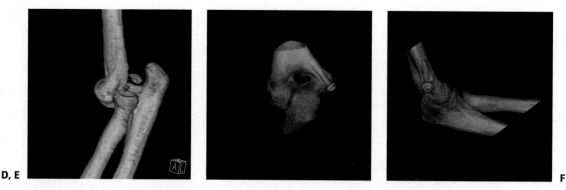

D, E   **F**

Figure 15-43. (*Continued*) **C, D:** A prereduction CT scan was obtained at the outside facility clearly demonstrating the medial epicondyle fragment within the elbow joint. **E, F:** Four months following surgical removal of the incarcerated medial epicondyle fragment and internal fixation of the fracture, a follow-up CT scan demonstrates anatomic reduction and excellent position of the single screw (with washer) within the medial column of bone, engaging subcortical bone for maximum fixation. The fracture is completely healed and the patient has returned to virtually all activities.

compression but this does make the implant slightly more prominent. After removal of the guide pin or K-wires, the elbow is assessed to ensure valgus stability and reestablishment of a full range of motion. After the surgical incision is closed, the extremity is placed in a well-padded posterior splint which is removed 5 to 10 days postoperatively and replaced with a removable splint or hinged brace, allowing initiation of early active range-of-motion exercise.

If the epicondyle is fragmented and if there is a need to achieve elbow stability, a spiked washer can be used to secure the multiple pieces to the metaphysis. If a washer is used, a second procedure may be necessary to remove the spike washer once the epicondyle is securely united to the metaphysis. If internal fixation is impossible, simply excise the fragments and reattach the ligament to the bone and periosteum at the base of the epicondylar defect.

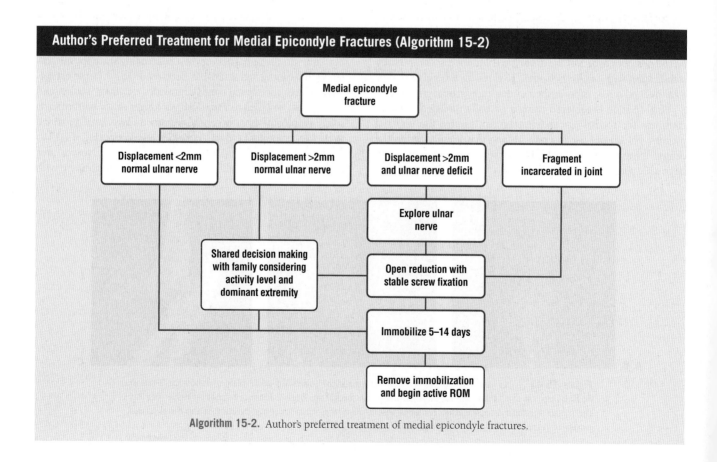

Author's Preferred Treatment for Medial Epicondyle Fractures (Algorithm 15-2)

Algorithm 15-2. Author's preferred treatment of medial epicondyle fractures.

Determining the appropriate treatment for each patient involves a process of shared decision-making in which the benefits and risks of each treatment alternative are discussed with the family. We use the general treatment guidelines outlined in Table 15-2 as a starting point for discussion with the patient and family. We strongly consider the expected activity of the patient and extremity in deciding with the patient and family on nonoperative or operative treatment.

For uncomplicated fractures of less than 2 mm of displacement, we recommend nonoperative treatment. The elbow is immobilized for 5 to 14 days and then range of motion is initiated. A removable splint is then used to protect the elbow at school and outside the home but is not worn indoors.

Redislocation or instability is rare but elbow stiffness is common, so early motion is important. Physical therapy should be used only if voluntary active motion is difficult to obtain. The therapist should emphasize modalities designed to decrease swelling and pain, and to reestablish strength. Range of motion should be achieved only by active means, not by passive stretching.

Our three primary indications for operative intervention are: (1) reduction of any medial epicondyle fragment incarcerated within the elbow joint, and (2) significant ulnar nerve deficit, and (3) stabilization of the elbow in patients anticipated to place significant stress on the medial epicondyle and its associated structures. We realize that it is difficult to predict the athletic potential of a young child but most parents do see great possibilities for their offspring. We are more likely to treat with internal fixation if the injury involves the dominant extremity of baseball pitchers, tennis players, or football quarterbacks. In wrestlers and gymnasts, the stability of the nondominant extremity also must be considered.

POTENTIAL PITFALLS AND PREVENTIVE MEASURES

Medial Epicondyle Fractures: POTENTIAL PITFALLS AND PREVENTIONS

Pitfalls	Prevention
• Failure to recognize a medial epicondyle fragment entrapped within the joint following elbow dislocation	• All children older than age 5 years should have a medial epicondyle ossification center which must be visualized in its normal anatomic location following elbow dislocation reduction.
• Fragmentation of the medial epicondyle during ORIF	• Instead of grasping the medial epicondyle bone with a clamp, grasp the flexor–pronator fascia where it attaches to the medial epicondyle. • Avoid overtightening the screw which is fixing the medial epicondyle in place. • Consider using a washer to distribute pressure over greater surface area.
• Injury to the radial nerve	• Do not obtain bicortical fixation in the lateral cortex of the distal humerus with the medial epicondyle screw.

TABLE 15-2. Author's Preferred Treatment for Medial Epicondyle Fractures

Nonoperative Treatment Indications
Nondisplaced or minimally displaced
Displaced in patients with low-demand upper extremity function
Operative Treatment Indications
Absolute: Irreducible incarcerated fragment in the elbow joint
Relative: Ulnar nerve dysfunction
Relative: Patient with high-demand upper extremity function

MANAGEMENT OF EXPECTED ADVERSE OUTCOMES AND UNEXPECTED COMPLICATIONS RELATED TO MEDIAL EPICONDYLE FRACTURES

Fractures of the Medial Epicondylar Apophysis: ADVERSE OUTCOMES AND COMPLICATIONS

Major
• Failure to recognize incarceration in the elbow
• Ulnar nerve dysfunction
• Symptomatic nonunion
• Valgus instability
• Radial nerve injury

Minor
• Slight loss of motion
• Myositis ossificans
• Calcification of the collateral ligaments
• Irritation from prominent implants
• Cosmetic appearance
• Nonunion in the high-performance athlete

Although much has been written about fractures involving the medial epicondylar apophysis, few complications are attributed to the fracture itself. The major complications that result in loss of function are failure to recognize incarceration in the joint and ulnar or median nerve dysfunction. Most of the other complications are minor and result in only minimal functional or cosmetic sequelae.

MAJOR COMPLICATIONS

Failure to Recognize Fragment Incarceration

Failure to recognize incarceration of the epicondylar fragment into the joint can result in significant loss of elbow motion and premature arthritis, especially if it remains incarcerated for any length of time. Fowles et al.[43] challenged the opinion that surgery is detrimental in patients with late incarceration, and the idea remains controversial. In their patients in whom the fragment was surgically extracted, an average of 14 weeks after injury, 80% more elbow motion was regained. In addition, the patients' preoperative pain was relieved, and the ulnar nerve dysfunction resolved. Lopez et al.[89] described a case report of an incarcerated fragment treated 12 weeks following injury by excision of the fragment. Twelve months following surgery, the ulnar neuropathy had resolved, the patient had minimal symptoms and excellent motion.

The long-term outcome following intra-articular retention of the medial epicondyle fragment is unpredictable. Rosendahl[144] reported an 8-year follow-up of a fragment retained within the joint. The epicondyle had fused to the semilunar surface of the ulna, producing a large bony prominence clinically. There was only minor loss of elbow motion, with little functional disability. Potenza et al.[131] described a case report of a neglected intra-articular medial epicondyle fracture with 48-year follow-up resulting in minimal symptoms. Similar to the case reported by Rosendahl, the fragment had fused to the olecranon where it caused minimal problems.

Ulnar Nerve Dysfunction

The other major complication associated with this injury is the development of ulnar nerve dysfunction. The incidence of ulnar nerve dysfunction varies from 10% to 16%.[102] If the fragment is entrapped in the joint, the incidence of ulnar nerve dysfunction may be as high as 50%.[40] More profound ulnar nerve injury has been reported after manipulative procedures.[128] Thus, in patients with fragments incarcerated in the joint, manipulation may not be the procedure of choice if a primary ulnar nerve dysfunction is present. Patients in whom the fragment was left incarcerated in the joint for a significant time have experienced poor recovery of the primary ulnar nerve injury.[102] A consistent finding noted by surgeons when exploring the ulnar nerve and removing the incarcerated fragment from the joint has been a thick fascial band binding the ulnar nerve to the underlying muscle.[12,128] Constriction by this band has been noted to cause immediate or late dysfunction of the ulnar nerve.

Delayed ulnar nerve palsy has also been reported following surgical treatment. Anakwe et al.[9] described two cases in which open reduction of a medial epicondyle was performed. Patients presented at 1- and 2-week follow-up with complete ulnar nerve palsy despite normal neurologic examination immediately postoperatively. In both patients, on reexploration the ulnar nerve was found to be compressed by scar tissue between two heads of the flexor carpi ulnaris just distal to the medial epicondyle. Both patients experienced a complete recovery following ulnar nerve decompression.

Symptomatic Nonunion

Nonunion of the medial epicondyle fragment with the distal metaphysis occurs in up to 50% of fractures with significant displacement treated nonoperatively. Although the majority of the nonunions cause minimal problems, symptomatic nonunions do occur (Fig. 15-44). Kulkarni and colleagues described 14 patients with symptomatic medial epicondyle nonunions experiencing symptoms including medial-sided

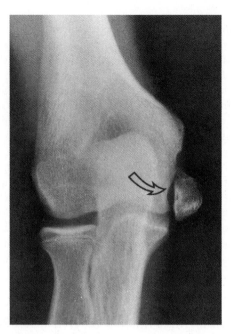

Figure 15-44. Nonunion in an athlete. This 15-year-old baseball pitcher had an untreated medial epicondyle fracture 1 year before this radiograph. He developed a fibrous union, but the epicondyle was shifted distally (*arrow*). His elbow was unstable enough to prevent him from pitching.

elbow pain, ulnar nerve dysfunction, valgus instability, and limited motion.[200] Smith et al.[158] from Boston Children's Hospital reviewed 137 patients treated for medial epicondyle fracture at their institution. Of the 42 fractures which were treated non-operatively, nonunion occurred in 19 fractures and 8 of those fracture nonunion patients experienced symptoms significant enough to warrant surgical treatment at a mean of 12 months following their initial injury. All patients were treated with open reduction and internal fixation of the ununited fragment, three of whom underwent grafting of the nonunion site. Successful fracture union was achieved in seven of the eight fractures and all patients experienced significant symptomatic improvement. Shukla and Cohen[155] described the treatment results of five patients with chronic medial epicondyle nonunion using a tension band construct. At a mean follow-up of 31 months all fractures were healed, patients reported being satisfied with their surgery and measurable outcome measures were significantly improved.

Valgus Instability

Valgus instability following displaced medial epicondyle fracture nonunion is a very challenging problem and has been used as an argument for surgical treatment. Gilcrist and McKee[47] reported good and excellent treatment results following excision of the ununited fragment and advancement of the medial collateral ligament complex with fixation to the distal humerus with suture anchors in five patients with symptomatic valgus elbow instability. Mayo Elbow Performance Score improved from 66 preoperatively to 91 postoperatively, and all patients were satisfied with the result.

Radial Nerve Injury

When fixing a medial epicondyle fragment, the operating surgeon must decide whether to accept fixation within the cancellous bone of the medial column or achieve bicortical fixation by gaining purchase in the lateral cortex of the proximal humeral metaphysis. Unfortunately the radial nerve travels on the surface of the humerus at the location where a bicortical screw penetrates the cortex. Marcu et al.[101] have reported two cases of radial nerve injury with cannulated screw fixation.

MINOR COMPLICATIONS

The most common minor complication is loss of the final degrees of elbow extension. A loss of 5% to 10% can be expected to develop in about 20% of these fractures. Minimal functional deficit is attributed to this loss of elbow motion. Prolonged immobilization seems to be the key factor contributing to loss of elbow extension. It is important to discuss with parents before treatment is begun that loss of motion is common after this injury, regardless of the treatment method used. Sufficient fracture stability to allow for early motion is paramount to lessening the risk of functional loss of motion.

Myositis ossificans is a rare occurrence following vigorous and repeated manipulation to extract the fragment from the joint. As with many other elbow injuries, myositis may be a result of the treatment rather than the injury itself. Myositis ossificans must be differentiated from ectopic calcification of the collateral ligaments, which involves only the ligamentous structures. This condition may occur after repeated injuries to the epicondyle and ligamentous structures (Fig. 15-45). Often, this calcified ligament is asymptomatic and does not seem to create functional disability. The cosmetic effects are minimal. In some patients, an accentuation of the medial prominence of the epicondyle creates a false appearance of an increased carrying angle of the elbow. In his extensive review, Smith[157] recognized a slight decrease in the carrying angle in only two patients.

Finally, following open reduction and internal fixation, the implants are sometimes prominent and cause discomfort. Pace and Hennrikus found that using a washer with a screw was more likely to cause discomfort significant enough for patients to undergo implant removal, compared to patients who underwent medial epicondyle fixation with a screw alone.[205]

CHRONIC TENSION STRESS INJURIES (LITTLE LEAGUE ELBOW)

This chronic injury is related to overuse in skeletally immature baseball pitchers. Brogdon and Crow[19] described the original radiographic findings in 1960. Later, Adams[1] demonstrated that the radiographic changes were due to excessive throwing and emphasized the need for preventive programs. This injury is thought to be due to excessive tension on the medial epicondyle with secondary tendinitis. There can also be a repeated compression on the lateral condyle, producing an osteochondritis. In chronic tension stress injuries, the history is usually quite characteristic. It is found in young baseball pitchers who are throwing an excessive number of pitches or who are just starting to throw curve pitches.[44] Clinically, this syndrome is manifested by a decrease in elbow extension. Medial epicondylar pain is accentuated by a valgus stress to the elbow in extension. There is usually significant local tenderness and swelling over the medial epicondyle. On radiographs, the density of the bone of the distal humerus is increased because of the chronicity of the stress. The physeal line is irregular and widened. If the stress has been going on for a prolonged period, there may be hypertrophy of the distal humerus with accelerated bone growth.

Previous authors have suggested that as long as the rules outlined by the Little League are followed (i.e., pitch counts of 50 to

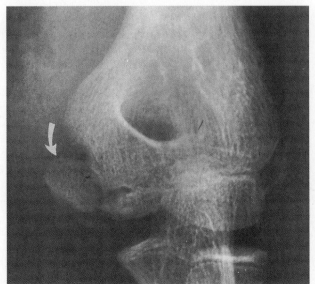
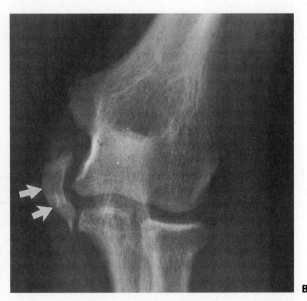

A   **B**

Figure 15-45. Heterotopic calcification. **A:** Injury to an 11-year-old who had moderate displacement of the medial epicondyle (*arrow*). **B:** One year later, she had considerable calcification of the ulnar collateral ligament (*arrows*). Other than mild instability with valgus stress, the patient had full range of motion and was asymptomatic. (Courtesy of Mark R. Christofersen, MD.)

75 pitches per game depending on age), the incidence of these chronic tension stress injuries is fairly low.[44] Exceeding the Little League guidelines does appear to increase the risk for acute and chronic injuries to medial elbow structures. Osbar et al. reported on eight youth baseball pitchers who presented with medial epicondyle avulsion fractures, five of whom acknowledged not conforming to Little League guidelines.[204] Exceeding Little League pitch count recommendations have also been shown in increase in the likelihood of undergoing ulnar collateral ligament surgery as an adult.[7,195] However recent research suggests that even in pitchers who are compliant with the Little League pitching guidelines, 28% experience pain during the season and 48% had abnormal MRI findings at the end of the season.[206] Throwing mechanics may also play a factor in developing medial elbow tension stress injuries. Albright et al.[4] found a greater incidence in pitchers who had improper pitching techniques.

A multifaceted approach that involves educating the parents, coaches, and player is recommended. Once symptoms develop, all pitching activities must cease until the epicondyle and adjacent flexor muscle origins become nontender. In addition, local and systemic measures to decrease the inflammatory response are used. Once the initial pain and inflammation have decreased, a program of forearm and arm muscle strengthening is initiated. The pitching technique is also examined to see if any corrections need to be made. Once strength has been reestablished in the muscles in the upper extremity and motion has been fully reestablished, the patient is gradually returned to pitching with careful monitoring of the number of innings and pitches within a specified time period.

In cases of chronic nonunion due to a chronic medial epicondylar stress fracture in older pitchers, open reduction with a compression screw and washer may be necessary to achieve union, stop pain, and allow return to full function.

Pulled Elbow Syndrome

INTRODUCTION TO PULLED ELBOW SYNDROME

Subluxation of the annular ligament, or pulled elbow syndrome, is a common elbow injury in young children.[8,25,67,71,159] The term "nursemaid's elbow" and other synonyms have been used to describe this condition. The demographics associated with subluxation of the radial head have been well described.[8,25,67,71,159] The mean age at injury is 2 to 3 years, with the youngest reported patient 2 months of age. It rarely occurs after 7 years of age; 60% to 65% of the children affected are girls, and the left elbow is involved in approximately 70%. It is difficult to determine the actual incidence because many subluxations are treated in primary care physician's offices, by parents, or resolve spontaneously before being seen by a physician.

MECHANISMS OF INJURY FOR PULLED ELBOW SYNDROME

Longitudinal traction on the extended elbow is the usual mechanism of injury (Fig. 15-46). Cadaver studies have shown that longitudinal traction on the extended elbow can produce a partial slippage of the annular ligament over the head of the

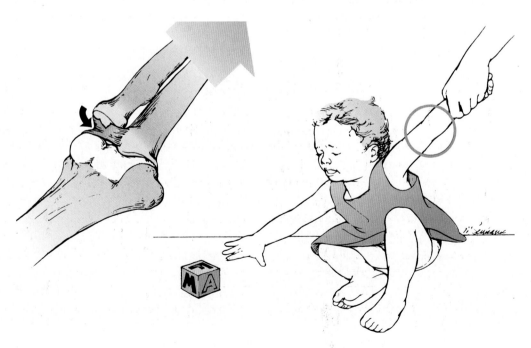

Figure 15-46. The injury most commonly occurs when a longitudinal pull is applied to the upper extremity. Usually the forearm is pronated. There may be a partial tear in the subannular membrane, allowing the annular ligament to subluxate into the radiocapitellar joint.

radius and into the radiocapitellar joint, sometimes tearing the subannular membrane.[104,111,150] Displacement of the annular ligament occurs most easily with the forearm in pronation. In this position, the lateral edge of the radial head, which opposes the main portion of the annular ligament, is narrow and round at its margin.[95,104] In supination, the lateral edge of the radial head is wider and more square at its margin, thereby restricting slippage of the annular ligament. McRae and Freeman[109] demonstrated that forearm pronation maintained the displacement of the annular ligament.

After 5 years of age, the distal attachments of the subannular membrane and annular ligament to the neck of the radius have strengthened sufficiently to prevent its tearing and subsequent displacement.[150] Previously, the theory was proposed that the radial head diameter was less in children than in adults and this contributed to subluxation of the annular ligament. However, cadaver studies of infants, children, and adults have shown that the ratio of the head and neck diameters is essentially the same.[148,150] Griffin[53] suggested that the lack of ossification of the proximal radial epiphysis in children less than 5 years of age made it more pliable, thereby facilitating slippage of the annular ligament.

Amir et al.[8] performed a controlled study comparing 30 normal children with 100 who had pulled elbow syndrome. They found an increased frequency of hypermobility or ligamentous laxity among children with pulled elbows. Also, there was an increased frequency of hypermobility in one or both parents of the involved children compared with noninvolved children, suggesting that hypermobility could be a factor predisposing children to this condition.

Thus, the most widely accepted mechanism is that the injury occurs when the forearm is pronated, the elbow extended, and longitudinal traction is applied to the patient's wrist or hand (see Fig. 15-46).[105,109,152] Such an injury typically occurs when a young child is lifted or swung by the forearm or when the child suddenly steps down from a step or off a curb while one of the parents is holding the hand or wrist.

Unusual Mechanisms

Newman[118] reported that five of six infants under 6 months of age with a pulled elbow sustained the injury when rolling over in bed with the extended elbow trapped under the body. It was believed that this maneuver, especially if the infant was given a quick push to turn over by an older sibling or a parent, provided enough longitudinal traction to displace the annular ligament proximally.

SIGNS AND SYMPTOMS OF PULLED ELBOW SYNDROME

The history is usually that of an episode of a longitudinal pull on the elbow of the young child. The initial pain usually subsides rapidly, and the child does not appear to be in distress except that he or she is reluctant to use the involved extremity. The upper extremity is typically held at the side with the forearm pronated. A limited painless arc of flexion and extension may be present; however, any attempt to supinate the forearm produces pain and is met with resistance. Although there is no evidence of an elbow effusion, local tenderness may be present over the radial head

and annular ligament. In some patients, the pain may be referred proximally to the shoulder and many complain of pain distally toward the wrist, usually on the dorsal forearm.[8,67]

Unfortunately, the classic history is not always present.[25,130,135,149,152] In some studies, 33% to 49% of patients had no clear history of longitudinal traction to the elbow.[149,152] In patients without a witnessed longitudinal traction injury, other causes, such as occult fracture or early septic arthritis, must be carefully ruled out.

IMAGING AND OTHER DIAGNOSTIC STUDIES FOR PULLED ELBOW SYNDROME

Radiography

Should x-rays be taken of every child before manipulation is attempted? If there is a reliable history of traction to the elbow, the child is 5 years of age or younger, and the clinical findings strongly support the diagnosis, x-rays are not necessary.[8,25,135,150,172] However, if there is an atypical history or clinical examination, x-rays should be obtained to be certain that there is not a fracture before manipulation is attempted.

AP and lateral x-rays usually are normal,[18,25,53,135,150,152,160] but subtle abnormalities may be present. Normally, the line down the center of the proximal radial shaft should pass through the center of the ossification center of the capitellum (radiocapitellar line).[45,160] Careful review of x-rays may demonstrate the radial capitellar line to be lateral to the center of the capitellum in up to 25% of patients.[45,160] Determination of this subtle change requires a direct measurement on the x-ray. Interestingly, the pulled elbow can be reduced by the radiology technician because the elbow x-rays are usually taken with the forearm supinated. The subluxation is reduced inadvertently when the technician places the forearm into supination to position it for the x-ray. Bretland[17] suggested that if the best x-ray that can be obtained is an oblique view with the forearm in pronation, pulled elbow syndrome is the likely diagnosis.

Ultrasonography

When the diagnosis is not evident, ultrasonography may be helpful,[85,95] although not always reliable.[151] The diagnosis is made by demonstrating an increase in the echo-negative area between the articular surfaces of the capitellum and the radial head and increased radial capitellar distance. Kosuwon et al.[85] found that this distance is normally about 3.8 mm with forearm pronated. With a subluxated radial head, this measured 7.2 mm. A difference of 3 mm between the normal and affected sides, therefore, suggests radial head subluxation.

MRI

While MRI is rarely indicated, if the source of elbow pain and disability is in doubt, and diagnoses such as fracture or infection are being considered, MRI may be helpful. Richardson described such a case in which subluxation of the annular ligament was revealed on MRI, reduction of the annular ligament performed while the patient was sedated in the MRI scanner, and additional images were obtained to confirm restoration of the annular ligament to its anatomically correct position.[207]

NONOPERATIVE TREATMENT OF PULLED ELBOW SYNDROME

Closed Reduction

Virtually all annular ligament subluxations are successfully treated by closed reduction. The traditional reduction maneuver has been to supinate the forearm.[25,53,67,135,152,159] Some authors have recommended that supination be done with the elbow flexed, and others have found that supination alone with the elbow extended can affect a reduction. In many patients, a snapping sensation can be both heard and palpated when the annular ligament reduces.

More recently there has been significant interest in forearm hyperpronation as a reduction maneuver. Macias reported that reduction was successful in 40 of 41 patients (98%) in the hyperpronation group compared with 38 of 44 patients (86%) in the supination group. They concluded that the hyperpronation technique was more successful, required fewer attempts, and was often successful when supination failed. More than one prospective randomized study has reported that hyperpronation is more successful than supination.[15,93,187,199]

Prereduction Planning

It is important to elicit a reliable history as to whether or not the child had a traction force applied across the extended elbow. The entire extremity is then carefully examined. Focal tenderness should be present directly over the radiocapitellar joint. If the history or physical examination is not entirely consistent with annular ligament subluxation, then x-rays of the upper extremity are obtained to assess for other injuries before manipulating the elbow.

Technique

✔ **Closed Reduction of Annular Ligament Subluxation:** KEY STEPS

- ❏ Obtain accurate history for evidence of appropriate injury mechanism.
- ❏ Examination should demonstrate the elbow to be held in extension with no visible deformity, but with tenderness at radiocapitellar joint.
- ❏ Perform AP and lateral elbow radiographs if history or examination is not consistent with annular ligament subluxation.
- ❏ Perform initial reduction maneuver by hyperpronating forearm with elbow in extension.
- ❏ After 10 minutes, if no resolution of symptoms then perform alternative reduction maneuver with forearm supination and elbow flexion.

Once the diagnosis of annular ligament subluxation is clearly established, reduction is performed. It is first explained to the parents that there will be a brief episode of pain followed by relief of the symptoms. The patient usually is seated on the parent's

lap. The patient's forearm is held with the elbow extended while the thumb of the surgeon's opposite hand is placed over the lateral aspect of the elbow. The forearm is hyperpronated with the elbow in extension. Gentle side-to-side pronation–supination in this position may help the annular ligament slip back in place over the radial head. A palpable or audible "click" may be appreciated as the annular ligament reduces. If no improvement is noted after 10 minutes, perform the alternative supination–flexion reduction maneuver (Fig 15-47).

What should be done if a definite snap or pop is not felt or if the patient fails to use the extremity after manipulation? In a subgroup of patients, discomfort may persist despite successful annular ligament reduction. If the subluxation has occurred more than 12 to 24 hours before the child is seen, there often is a mild secondary synovitis, and recovery may not be immediate and dramatic. One must confirm that the initial diagnosis was correct. If not taken before the manipulation, x-rays should be obtained and the entire extremity carefully reexamined. If the x-ray results are normal and the elbow can be fully flexed with free supination and pronation, the physician can be assured that the subluxated annular ligament has been reduced. Reexamination clinically and by x-ray in 5 to 10 days may be appropriate.

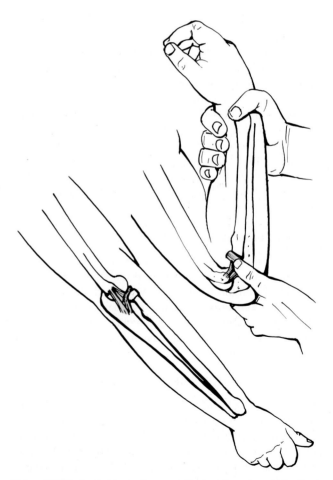

Figure 15-47. Supination reduction technique for nursemaid's elbow. **Left:** The forearm is first supinated. **Right:** The elbow is then hyperflexed. The surgeon's thumb is placed laterally over the radial head to feel the characteristic snapping as the ligament is reduced.

Postreduction Care

The value of immobilizing the elbow following reduction has been debated. Taha[169] reported a decreased rate of recurrence during the 10 days following reduction if the elbow was splinted in a flexed supinated position for 2 days following reduction. Salter and Zaltz[150] recommended the use of a sling, mainly to prevent the elbow from being pulled a second time. Kohlhaas and Roeder[84] recommended a T-shirt technique for flexed elbow stabilization in very young children. This provides adequate immobilization without the use of a sling by pinning the sleeve of the long sleeve T-shirt to the opposite chest. In general, after a successful closed reduction of a first-time annular ligament subluxation, immobilization of the extremity is not necessary if the child is comfortable and using the arm normally. After the reduction, it is important to explain to the parents the mechanism of injury and to emphasize the need to prevent longitudinal pulling on the upper extremities.

Picking the child up under the axillae and avoiding games such as "ring around the rosees" involving longitudinal traction to the arm are stressed. However, recurrence rate is high even with the most diligent parents. Therefore, instruction in home reduction of the pulled elbow is useful and reduces the number of visits to the emergency department and primary care physician.

OPERATIVE TREATMENT OF PULLED ELBOW SYNDROME

Even if untreated, most annular ligament subluxations eventually reduce spontaneously. There are no reported cases of negative long-term sequelae following untreated annular ligament subluxation. Therefore, open reduction is rarely, if ever, indicated for annular ligament subluxation. An indication for surgery might be the chronic, symptomatic, irreducible subluxation.[27,172] In such a circumstance, the annular ligament may need to be partially transected to achieve reduction.

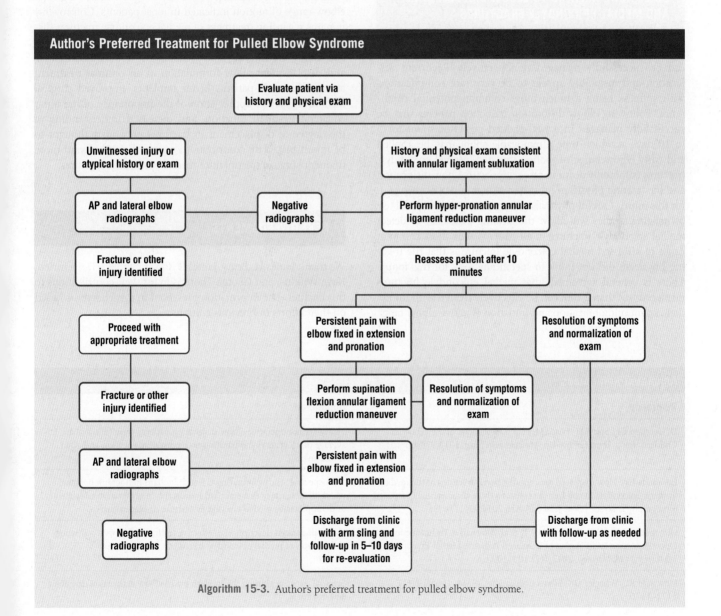

Author's Preferred Treatment for Pulled Elbow Syndrome

Algorithm 15-3. Author's preferred treatment for pulled elbow syndrome.

Management of Expected Adverse Outcomes and Unexpected Complications Related to Pulled Elbow Syndrome

There are no reports of long-term sequelae from unrecognized and unreduced subluxations (Algorithm 15-3). Almost all subluxations reduce spontaneously. The only problem seems to be discomfort to the patient until the annular ligament reduces.

Recurrent Subluxations

The reported incidence of recurrent subluxation has varied from 5% to 39%.[25,53,67,135,152,159,170] Children 2 years of age or younger appear to be at greatest risk for recurrence.[152,172] Recurrent subluxations usually respond to the same manipulative procedure as the initial injury. They eventually cease after 4 to 5 years when the annular ligament strengthens and ligament laxity lessens. Recurrences do not lead to any long-term sequelae. If recurrent annular ligament subluxation significantly impacts a patient's quality of life because of pain or limited activity, immobilization in an above-elbow cast with the forearm in supination or neutral position for 2 to 3 weeks is usually effective at preventing recurrence.

SUMMARY, CONTROVERSIES, AND FUTURE DIRECTIONS RELATED TO ELBOW DISLOCATIONS AND MEDIAL EPICONDYLE FRACTURES

Most dislocations about the elbow in children and adolescents can be successfully managed nonoperatively. Recurrent dislocation and instability appear to be very rare complications with stiffness being a much more common potential occurrence. Following elbow dislocation reduction patients may be successfully managed in a well-padded posterior splint for 5 to 10 days at which time a removable splint may be applied and early elbow range of motion initiated. Medial epicondyle fractures commonly occur in association with elbow dislocation and the treating physician must have a high index of suspicion for this injury. Careful physical examination and thoughtful use of imaging studies will allow the treating physician to detect medial epicondyle fractures in all patients. The most common cause of a missed medial epicondyle fracture is that the treating physician did not think to specifically look for this injury. There is general agreement that medial epicondyle fractures displaced less than 2 mm can be effectively treated with immediate splint immobilization and initiation of active elbow range of motion 5 to 10 days following the injury. Medial epicondyle fractures entrapped within the elbow joint must be extracted, with open reduction and stable internal fixation allowing early elbow range of motion indicated in most patients. Controversy remains regarding treatment of medial epicondyle fractures displaced more than 2 mm. Shared decision-making with patient and family, considering activity demands, dominant extremity, and displacement allow formulation of an optimal treatment strategy for each patient. Better implants, improved surgical technique, greater appreciation of the importance of the ulnar collateral ligament function, and increased understanding of the degree of displacement in fractures previously thought to be nondisplaced all contribute to a general trend toward more frequent surgical treatment of medial epicondyle fractures.

ACKNOWLEDGMENTS

We thank James H. Beaty, James R Kasser, Stephen D. Heinrich, Kaye Wilkins, and George Thompson for their contributions to this chapter. The information presented in this chapter is based on their efforts in previous editions.

Annotated References

Reference	Annotation
Di Gennaro GL, Spina M, Fosco M, et al. Dislocations of the Elbow in Children: Long-Term Follow-Up. *Musculoskelet Surg.* 2013;97(Suppl 1):3–7.	Thirty-six nonoperative elbow dislocation patients were followed an average of 15 years demonstrating no recurrent dislocation and good results overall.
Edmonds EW. How displaced are "nondisplaced" fractures of the medial humeral epicondyle in children? Results of a three-dimensional computed tomography analysis. *J Bone Joint Surg Am.* 2010;92(17):e33.	A prospective study comparing CT and standard radiograph imaging which demonstrates that standard radiograph interpretation consistently underappreciates medial epicondyle fracture displacement.
Glotzbecker MP, Shore B, Matheney T, et al. Alternative Technique for Open Reduction and Fixation of Displaced Pediatric Medial Epicondyle Fractures. *J Child Orthop.* 2012;6(2):105–109.	Nicely illustrated description of effective technique for open reduction and fixation of medial epicondyle fractures.
Linscheid RL, Wheeler DK. Elbow dislocations. *JAMA.* 1965;194(11):1171–1176.	Seminal paper beginning the modern era of elbow dislocation diagnosis and treatment.

Annotated References

Reference	Annotation
Murphy RF, Vuillermin C, Naqvi M, et al. Early Outcomes of Pediatric Elbow Dislocation-Risk Factors Associated With Morbidity. *J Pediatr Orthop*. 2017;37(7):440–446.	Analysis of this contemporary large series of pediatric elbow dislocation demonstrated a relatively high percentage of concomitant elbow fractures which may benefit from surgical treatment. Early mobilization was associated with improved elbow range of motion.
O'Driscoll SW, Bell DF, Morrey BF. Posterolateral rotatory instability of the elbow. *J Bone Joint Surg Am*. 1991;73:440–446.	O'Driscoll and co-authors introduced the concept of posterolateral elbow instability.

REFERENCES

1. Adams JE. Injury to the throwing arm. A study of traumatic changes in the elbow joints of boy baseball players. *Calif Med*. 1965;102:127–132.
2. Afshar A. Divergent dislocation of the elbow in an 11-year-old child. *Arch Iranian Med*. 2007;10(3):413–416.
3. Akansel G, Dalbayrak S, Yilmaz M, et al. MRI demonstration of intra-articular median nerve entrapment after elbow dislocation. *Skel Radiol*. 2003;32(9):537–541.
4. Albright JA, Jokl P, Shaw R, et al. Clinical study of baseball pitchers: correlation of injury to the throwing arm with method of delivery. *Am J Sports Med*. 1978;6(1):15–21.
5. Allende G, Freytes M. Old dislocation of the elbow. *J Bone Joint Surg Am*. 1944;26:692–706.
6. Al-Qattan MM, Zuker RM, Weinberg MJ. Type 4 median nerve entrapment after elbow dislocation. *J Hand Surg Am*. 1994;19(5):613–615.
7. Altuntas AO, Balakumar J, Howells RJ, et al. Posterior divergent dislocation of the elbow in children and adolescents: a report of three cases and review of the literature. *J Pediatr Orthop*. 2005;25(3):317–321.
8. Amir D, Frankl U, Pogrund H. Pulled elbow and hypermobility of joints. *Clin Orthop Relat Res*. 1990;(257):94–99.
9. Anakwe RE, Watts AC, McEachan JE. Delayed ulnar nerve palsy after open reduction and internal fixation of medial epicondylar fractures. *J Pediatr Orthop B*. 2010;19(3):239–241.
10. Andersen K, Mortensen AC, Gron P. Transverse divergent dislocation of the elbow. A report of two cases. *Acta Orthop Scand*. 1985;56(5):442–443.
11. Antonis K, Leonidou OA, Sbonias G, et al. Convergent type proximal radioulnar translocation complicating posterior elbow dislocation: watch out for dual dislocations in children's elbows. *J Pediatr Orthop B*. 2011;20(3):138–141.
12. Ashurst APC. *An Anatomical and Surgical Study of Fractures of the Lower End of the Humerus*. Philadelphia, PA: Lea & Febiger; 1910.
13. Ayala H, De Pablos J, Gonzalez J, et al. Entrapment of the median nerve after posterior dislocation of the elbow. *Microsurgery*. 1983;4(4):215–220.
14. Beaty JH, Donati NL. Recurrent dislocation of the elbow in a child: case report and review of the literature. *J Pediatr Orthop*. 1991;11(3):392–396.
15. Bek D, Yildiz C, Kose O, et al. Pronation versus supination maneuvers for the reduction of 'pulled elbow': a randomized clinical trial. *Eur J Emerg Med*. 2009;16(3):135–138.
16. Boe S, Holst-Nielsen F. Intra-articular entrapment of the median nerve after dislocation of the elbow. *J Hand Surg Br*. 1897;12(3):356–358.
17. Bretland PM. Pulled elbow in childhood. *Br J Radiol*. 1994;67(804):1176–1185.
18. Broadhurst BW, Buhr AJ. The pulled elbow. *Br Med J*. 1959;1(5128):1018–1019.
19. Brogdon BG, Crow NE. Little leaguer's elbow. *AJR Am J Roentgenol*. 1960;83:671–675.
20. Capo SR, Tito AV, Cuesta FJG. Median nerve paralysis following elbow fractures and dislocations. Apropos of a series of 12 cases [article in French]. *Ann Chir*. 1984;38:270–273.
21. Carey RP. Simultaneous dislocation of the elbow and the proximal radio-ulnar joint. *J Bone Joint Surg Br*. 1984;66(2):254–256.
22. Carl A, Prada S, Teixeira K. Proximal radioulnar transposition in an elbow dislocation. *J Orthop Trauma*. 1992;6(1):106–109.
23. Carlioz H, Abols Y. Posterior dislocation of the elbow in children. *J Pediatr Orthop*. 1984;4(1):8–12.
24. Chessare JW, Rogers LF, White H, et al. Injuries of the medial epicondylar ossification center of the humerus. *AJR Am J Roentgenol*. 1977;129(1):49–55.
25. Choung W, Heinrich SD. Acute annular ligament interposition into the radiocapitellar joint in children (nursemaid's elbow). *J Pediatr Orthop*. 1995;15(4):454–456.
26. Combourieu B, Thevenin-Lemoine C, Abelin-Genevois K, et al. Pediatric elbow dislocation associated with proximal radioulnar translocation: a report of three cases and a review of the literature. *J Bone Joint Surg Am*. 2010;92(8):1780–1785.
27. Corella F, Horna L, Villa A, et al. Irreducible 'pulled elbow' report of two cases and review of the literature. *J Pediatr Orthop B*. 2010;19(4):304–306.
28. Cromack PI. The mechanism and nature of the injury in dislocations of the elbow and a method of treatment. *Aust N Z J Surg*. 1960;30:212–216.
29. Danielsson LG. Median nerve entrapment in elbow dislocation. A case report. *Acta Orthop Scand*. 1986;57(5):450–452.
30. DeLee JC. Transverse divergent dislocation of the elbow in a child. Case report. *J Bone Joint Surg Am*. 1981;63(2):322–323.
31. Devnani AS. Outcome of longstanding dislocated elbows treated by open reduction and excision of collateral ligaments. *Singapore Med J*. 2004;45(1):14–19.
32. Dias JJ, Johnson GV, Hoskinson J, et al. Management of severely displaced medial epicondyle fractures. *J Orthop Trauma*. 1987;1(1):59–62.
33. Doornberg JN, Ring D. Coronoid fracture patterns. *J Hand Surg Am*. 2006;31(1):45–52.
34. Ring DC, Doornberg JN. Fracture of the anteromedial facet of the coronoid process. Surgical technique. *J Bone Joint Surg Am*. 2007;89(Suppl 2)267–283.
35. Dürig M, Gauer EF, Muller W. [The operative treatment of recurrent and simple traumatic dislocations of the elbow by the method of Osborne and Cotterill (author's transl)]. *Arch Orthop Unfall Chir*. 1976;86:141–156.
36. Edmonds EW. How displaced are "nondisplaced" fractures of the medial humeral epicondyle in children? Results of a three-dimensional computed tomography analysis. *J Bone Joint Surg Am*. 2010;92(17):2785–2791.
37. Eklöf O, Nybonde T, Karlsson G. Luxation of the elbow complicated by proximal radio-ulnar translocation. *Acta Radiol*. 1990;31(2):145–146.
38. el Bardouni A, Mahfoud M, Ouadghiri M, et al. [Divergent dislocation of the elbow. Apropos of a case]. *Rev Chir Orthop Reparatrice Appar Mot*. 1994;80(2):150–152.
39. Fahey JJ, O'Brien ET. Fracture-separation of the medial humeral condyle in a child confused with fracture of the medial epicondyle. *J Bone Joint Surg Am*. 1971;53(6):1102–1104.
40. Fairbank HA, Buxton JD. Displacement of the internal epicondyle into the elbow joint. *Lancet*. 1934;2:218.
41. Fourrier P, Levai JP, Collin JP. [Median nerve entrapment in elbow dislocation]. *Rev Chir Orthop Reparatrice Appar Mot*. 1977;63(1):13–16.
42. Fowles JV, Kassab MT, Douik M. Untreated posterior dislocation of the elbow in children. *J Bone Joint Surg Am*. 1984;66(6):921–926.
43. Fowles JV, Kassab MT, Moula T. Untreated intra-articular entrapment of the medial humeral epicondyle. *J Bone Joint Surg Br*. 1984;60:562–565.
44. Frances R, Bunch T, Chandler B. Little league elbow: a decade later. *Phys Sports Med*. 1978;6(4):88–94.
45. Frumkin K. Nursemaid's elbow: a radiographic demonstration. *Ann Emerg Med*. 1985;14(7):690–693.
46. George HL, Unnikrishnan PN, Bass A, et al. Transverse divergent dislocation of elbow in a child: a case report and review of current literature. *Pediatr Emerg Care*. 2011;27(5):411–413.
47. Gilcrist AD, McKee MD. Valgus instability of the elbow due to medial epicondyle nonunion: treatment by fragment excision and ligament repair—a report of five cases. *J Shoulder Elbow Surg*. 2002;11:493–497.
48. Gillingham BL, Wright JG. Convergent dislocation of the elbow. *Clin Orthop Relat Res*. 1997;(340):198–201.
49. Gosman JA. Recurrent dislocation of the ulna at the elbow. *J Bone Joint Surg*. 1943;2544.
50. Gottschalk HP, Eisner E, Hosalkar HS. Medial epicondyle fractures in the pediatric population. *J Am Acad Orthop Surg*. 2012;20(4):223–232.
51. Green NE. Entrapment of the median nerve following elbow dislocation. *J Pediatr Orthop*. 1983;3(3):384–386.
52. Grelss M, Messias R. Irreducible posterolateral elbow dislocation. A case report. *Acta Orthop Scand*. 1987;58:421–422.
53. Griffin ME. Subluxation of the head of the radius in young children. *Pediatrics*. 1955;15(1):103–106.
54. Grimer RJ, Brooks S. Brachial artery damage accompanying closed posterior dislocation of the elbow. *J Bone Joint Surg Br*. 1985;67(3):378–381.
55. Hallett J. Entrapment of the median nerve after dislocation of the elbow. A case report. *J Bone Joint Surg Br*. 1981;63-B(3):408–412.
56. Hankin FM. Posterior dislocation of the elbow. A simplified method of closed reduction. *Clin Orthop Relat Res*. 1984;(190):254–256.
57. Harrison RB, Keats TE, Frankel CJ, et al. Radiographic clues to fractures of the unossified medial humeral condyle in young children. *Skeletal Radiol*. 1984;11(3):209–212.
58. Harvey S, Tchelebi H. Proximal radio-ulnar translocation. A case report. *J Bone Joint Surg Am*. 1979;61(3):447–449.
59. Hassmann GC, Brunn F, Neer CS. Recurrent dislocation of the elbow. *J Bone Joint Surg Am*. 1975;57(8):1080–1084.
60. Henderson RS, Roberston IM. Open dislocation of the elbow with rupture of the brachial artery. *J Bone Joint Surg Br*. 1952;34:636–637.
61. Hennig K, Franke D. Posterior displacement of brachial artery following closed elbow dislocation. *J Trauma*. 1980;20(1):96–98.
62. Henrikson B. Supracondylar fracture of the humerus in children. A late review of end-results with special reference to the cause of deformity, disability and complications. *Acta Chir Scand Suppl*. 1966;369;1–72.
63. Herring JA, Sullivan JA. Recurrent dislocation of the elbow. *J Pediatr Orthop*. 1989;9(4):483–484.

64. Hines RF, Herndon WA, Evans JP. Operative treatment of medial epicondyle fractures in children. *Clin Orthop Relat Res.* 1987;223:170–174.
65. Hofammann KE, Moneim MS, Omer GE, et al. Brachial artery disruption following closed posterior elbow dislocation in a child—assessment with intravenous digital angiography. A case report with review of the literature. *Clin Orthop Relat Res.* 1984;(184):145–149.
66. Holbrook JL, Green NE. Divergent pediatric elbow dislocation. A case report. *Clin Orthop Relat Res.* 1988;(234):72–74.
67. Illingsworth CM. Pulled elbow: a study of 100 patients. *Br Med J.* 1975;2:672–674.
68. Inoue G, Horii E. Combined shear fractures of the trochlea and capitellum associated with anterior fracture-dislocation of the elbow. *J Orthop Trauma.* 1992;6(3):373–375.
69. Isbister ES. Proximal radioulnar translocation in association with posterior dislocation of the elbow. *Injury.* 1991;22(6):479–482.
70. Jackson JA. Simple anterior dislocation of the elbow joint with rupture of the brachial artery. Case report. *Am J Surg.* 1940;47:479–486.
71. Jongschaap HC, Youngson GG, Beattie TF. The epidemiology of radial head subluxation ('pulled elbow') in the Aberdeen city area. *Health Bull.* 1990;48(2):58–61.
72. Josefsson PO, Danielsson LG. Epicondylar elbow fracture in children. 35-year follow-up of 56 unreduced cases. *Acta Orthop Scand.* 1986;57(4):313–315.
73. Josefsson PO, Gentz CF, Johnell O, et al. Surgical versus non-surgical treatment of ligamentous injuries following dislocation of the elbow joint. A prospective randomized study. *J Bone Joint Surg Am.* 1987;69(4):605–608.
74. Josefsson PO, Gentz CF, Johnell O, et al. Surgical versus nonsurgical treatment of ligamentous injuries following dislocations of the elbow joint. *Clin Orthop Relat Res.* 1987;(214):165–169.
75. Josefsson PO, Johnell O, Gentz CF. Long-term sequelae of simple dislocation of the elbow. *J Bone Joint Surg Am.* 1984;66(6):927–930.
76. Josefsson PO, Johnell O, Wendeberg B. Ligamentous injuries in dislocations of the elbow joint. *Clin Orthop Relat Res.* 1987;221:221–225.
77. Josefsson PO, Nilsson BE. Incidence of elbow dislocation. *Acta Orthop Scand.* 1986;57(6):537–538.
78. Kapel O. Operation for habitual dislocation of the elbow. *J Bone Joint Surg Am.* 1951;33-A(3):707–710.
79. Kilburn P, Sweeney JG, Silk FF. Three cases of compound posterior dislocation of the elbow with rupture of the brachial artery. *J Bone Joint Surg Br.* 1962;44:119–121.
80. Kilfoyle RM. Fractures of the medial condyle and epicondyle of the elbow in children. *Clin Orthop Relat Res.* 1965;41:43–50.
81. Kim SJ, Ji JH. Irreducible posteromedial elbow dislocation: a case report. *J Shoulder Elbow Surg.* 2007;16(6):e1–e5.
82. King T. Recurrent dislocation of the elbow. *J Bone Joint Surg Br.* 1953;35:50–54.
83. Klatt JB, Aoki SK. The location of the medial humeral epicondyle in children: position based on common radiographic landmarks. *J Pediatr Orthop.* 2012;32(5):477–482.
84. Kohlhaas AR, Roeder J. Tee shirt management of nursemaid's elbow. *Am J Orthop (Belle Mead NJ).* 1995;24(1):74.
85. Kosuwon W, Mahaisavariya B, Saengnipanthkul S, et al. Ultrasonography of pulled elbow. *J Bone Joint Surg Br.* 1993;75(3):421–422.
86. Lee HH, Shen HC, Chang JH, et al. Operative treatment of displaced medial epicondyle fractures in children and adolescents. *J Shoulder Elbow Surg.* 2005;14(2):178–185.
87. Linscheid RL, Wheeler DK. Elbow dislocations. *JAMA.* 1965;194(11):1171–1176.
88. Loomis LK. Reeducation and after-treatment of posterior dislocation of the elbow. With special attention to the brachialis muscle and myositis ossificans. *Am J Surg.* 1944;63:56–60.
89. Lopez JT, Vilches Fernandez JM, Dominguez Amador JJ, et al. Chronic incarceration of the medial epicondyle: a case report. *J Shoulder Elbow Surg.* 2012;21(5):e12–e15.
90. Louahem DM, Bourelle S, Buscayret F, et al. Displaced medial epicondyle fractures of the humerus: surgical treatment and results. A report of 139 cases. *Arch Orthop Trauma Surg.* 2010;130(5):649–655.
91. Louis DS, Ricciardi JE, Spengler DM. Arterial injury: a complication of posterior elbow dislocation. A clinical and anatomical study. *J Bone Joint Surg Am.* 1974;56(8):1631–1636.
92. Low BY, Lim J. Fracture of humerus during armwrestling: report of 5 cases. *Singapore Med J.* 1991;32(1):47–49.
93. Macias CG, Bothner J, Wiebe R. A comparison of supination/flexion to hyperpronation in the reduction of radial head subluxations. *Pediatrics.* 1998;102(1):e10.
94. MacSween WA. Transposition of radius and ulna associated with dislocation of the elbow in a child. *Injury.* 1978;10:314–316.
95. Magill HK, Aitken AP. Pulled elbow. *Surg Gynecol Obstet.* 1954;98(6):753–756.
96. Mahaisavariya B, Laupattarakasem W. Neglected dislocation of the elbow. *Clin Orthop Relat Res.* 2005;(431):21–25.
97. Mahaisavariya B, Laupattarakasem W, Supachutikul A, et al. Late reduction of dislocated elbow. Need triceps be lengthened?. *J Bone Joint Surg Br.* 1993;75(3):426–428.
98. Malkawi H. Recurrent dislocation of the elbow accompanied by ulnar neuropathy: a case report and review of the literature. *Clin Orthop Relat Res.* 1981;(161):270–274.
99. Manouel M, Minkowitz B, Shimotsu G, et al. Brachial artery laceration with closed posterior elbow dislocation in an eight year old. *Clin Orthop Relat Res.* 1993;(296):109–112.
100. Mantle JA. Recurrent posterior dislocation of the elbow. *J Bone Joint Surg Br.* 1966;4:85–90.
101. Marcu DM, Balts J, McCarthy JJ, et al. Iatrogenic radial nerve injury with cannulated fixation of medial epicondyle fractures in the pediatric humerus: a report of 2 cases. *J Pediatr Orthop.* 2011;31(2):e13–e16.
102. Marion J, Faysse R. Fractures de l'épitrochlea. *Rev Chir Orthop.* 1962;48:447–469.
103. Matev I. A radiological sign of entrapment of the median nerve in the elbow joint after posterior dislocation. A report of two cases. *J Bone Joint Surg Br.* 1976;58(3):353–355.
104. Matles AL, Eliopoulos K. Internal derangement of the elbow in children. *Int Surg.* 1967;48(3):259–263.

105. Maylahn DJ, Fahey JJ. Fractures of the elbow in children; review of three hundred consecutive cases. *J Am Med Assoc.* 1958;166(3):220–228.
106. McAuliffe TB, Williams D. Transverse divergent dislocation of the elbow. *Injury.* 1988;19(4):279–280.
107. McKee MD, Schemitsch EH, Sala MJ, et al. The pathoanatomy of lateral ligamentous disruption in complex elbow instability. *J Shoulder Elbow Surg.* 2003;12(4):391–396.
108. McKellar Hall R. Recurrent posterior dislocation of the elbow joint in a boy. Report of a case. *J Bone Joint Surg Br* 1953;35-B(1):56.
109. McRae R, Freeman PA. The lesion of pulled elbow. *J Bone Joint Surg Br.* 1965;47:808.
110. Mehlman CT, Howard AW. Medial epicondyle fractures in children: clinical decision making in the face of uncertainty. *J Pediatr Orthop.* 2012;32(Suppl 2):S135–S142.
111. Mehta S, Sud A, Tiwari A, et al. Open reduction for late-presenting posterior dislocation of the elbow. *J Orthop Surg.* 2007;15(1):15–21.
112. Milch H. Bilateral recurrent dislocation of the ulna at the elbow. *J Bone Joint Surg Am.* 1936;18:777–780.
113. Murakami Y, Komiyama Y. Hypoplasia of the trochlea and the medial epicondyle of the humerus associated with ulnar neuropathy. Report of two cases. *J Bone Joint Surg Br.* 1978;60-B(2):225–227.
114. Naidoo KS. Unreduced posterior dislocations of the elbow. *J Bone Joint Surg Br.* 1982;64(5):603–606.
115. Nakano A, Tanaka S, Hirofuji E, et al. Transverse divergent dislocation of the elbow in a six-year-old boy: case report. *J Trauma.* 1992;32(1):118–119.
116. Nanno M, Sawaizumi T, Ito H. Transverse divergent dislocation of the elbow with ipsilateral distal radius fracture in a child. *J Orthop Trauma.* 2007;21(2):145–149.
117. Neviaser JS, Wickstrom JK. Dislocation of the elbow: a retrospective study of 115 patients. *South Med J.* 1977;70(2):172–173.
118. Newman J. "Nursemaid's elbow" in infants six months and under. *J Emerg Med.* 1985;2(6):403–404.
119. Nyska M, Peiser J, Lukiec F, et al. Avulsion fracture of the medial epicondyle caused by arm wrestling. *Am J Sports Med.* 1992;20(3):347–350.
120. O'Driscoll SW, Bell DF, Morrey BF. Posterolateral rotatory instability of the elbow. *J Bone Joint Surg Am.* 1991;73:440–446.
121. O'Driscoll SW, Morrey BF, Korinek S, et al. Elbow subluxation and dislocation. A spectrum of instability. *Clin Orthop Relat Res.* 1992;(280):186–197.
122. Osborne G, Cotterill P. Recurrent dislocation of the elbow. *J Bone Joint Surg Br.* 1966;48(2):340–346.
123. Ozkoc G, Akpinar S, Hersekli MA. Type 4 median nerve entrapment in a child after elbow dislocation. *Arch Orthop Trauma Surg.* 2003;123:555–557.
124. Papavasilou VA. Fracture-separation of the medial epicondylar epiphysis of the elbow joint. *Clin Orthop Relat Res.* 1982;171:172–174.
125. Pappas N, Lawrence JT, Donegan D, et al. Intraobserver and interobserver agreement in the measurement of displaced humeral medial epicondyle fractures in children. *J Bone Joint Surg Am.* 2010;92(2):322–327.
126. Parvin RW. Closed reduction of common shoulder and elbow dislocations without anesthesia. *AMA Arch Surg.* 1957;75(6):972–975.
127. Patel NM, Ganley TJ. Medial epicondyle fractures of the humerus: how to evaluate and when to operate. *J Pediatr Orthop.* 2012;32(Suppl 1)S10–S13.
128. Patrick J. Fracture of the medial epicondyle with displacement into the elbow joint. *J Bone Joint Surg Am.* 1946;28:143–147.
129. Pearce MS. Radial artery entrapment. A rare complication of posterior dislocation of the elbow. *Int Orthop.* 1993;17(2):127–128.
130. Piroth P, Gharib M. Traumatic subluxation of the head of the radius [article in German]. *Deutsche Med Wochenschr.* 1976;101(42):1520–1523.
131. Potenza V, Farsetti P, Caterini R, et al. Neglected fracture of the medial humeral epicondyle that was entrapped into the elbow joint: a case report. *J Pediatr Orthop.* 2010;19B(6):542–544.
132. Potter HG. Imaging of posttraumatic and soft tissue dysfunction of the elbow. *Clin Orthop Relat Res.* 2000;(370):9–18.
133. Pritchard DJ, Linscheid RL, Svien HJ. Intra-articular median nerve entrapment with dislocation of the elbow. *Clin Orthop Relat Res.* 1973;(90):100–103.
134. Pritchett JW. Entrapment of the median nerve after dislocation of the elbow. *J Pediatr Orthop.* 1984;4(6):752–753.
135. Quan L, Marcuse EK. The epidemiology and treatment of radial head subluxation. *Am J Dis Child.* 1985;139(12):1194–1197.
136. Rana NA, Kenwright J, Taylor RG, et al. Complete lesion of the median nerve associated with dislocation of the elbow joint. *Acta Orthop Scand.* 1974;45(3):365–369.
137. Rao SB, Crawford AH. Median nerve entrapment after dislocation of the elbow in children. A report of 2 cases and review of literature. *Clin Orthop Relat Res.* 1995;(312):232–237.
138. Rasool MN. Dislocations of the elbow in children. *J Bone Joint Surg Br.* 2004;86(7):1050–1058.
139. Reichenheim PP. Transplantation of the biceps tendon as a treatment for recurrent dislocation of the elbow. *Br J Surg.* 1947;35(138):201–204.
140. Rhyou IH, Kim S. New mechanism of the posterior elbow dislocation. *Knee Surg Sports Traumatol Arthrosc.* 2012;20(12):2535–2541.
141. Roaf R. Foramen in the humerus caused by the median nerve. *J Bone Joint Surg Br.* 1957;39:748–749.
142. Roberts NW. Displacement of the internal epicondyle into the joint. *Lancet.* 1934;2:78–79.
143. Roberts PH. Dislocation of the elbow. *Br J Surg.* 1969;56(11):806–815.
144. Rosendahl B. Displacement of the medial epicondyle into the elbow joint: the final result in a case where the fragment has not been removed. *Acta Orthop Scand.* 1959;28(3):212–219.
145. Ross G, McDevitt ER, Chronister R, et al. Treatment of simple elbow dislocation using an immediate motion protocol. *Am J Sports Med.* 1999;27(3):308–311.
146. Royle SG. Posterior dislocation of the elbow. *Clin Orthop Relat Res.* 1991;(269):201–204.

147. Rubens MK, Aulicino PL. Open elbow dislocation with brachial artery disruption: case report and review of the literature. *Orthopedics.* 1986;9(4):539–542.
148. Ryan JR. The relationship of the radial head to radial neck diameters in fetuses and adults with reference to radial-head subluxation in children. *J Bone Joint Surg Am.* 1969;51(4):781–783.
149. Sacchetti A, Ramoska EE, Glascow C. Nonclassic history in children with radial head subluxations. *J Emerg Med.* 1990;8(2):151–153.
150. Salter RB, Zaltz C. Anatomic investigations of the mechanism of injury and pathologic anatomy of "pulled elbow" in young children. *Clin Orthop Relat Res.* 1971;77:134–143.
151. Scapinelli R, Borgo A. Pulled elbow in infancy: diagnostic role of imaging. *Radiol Med.* 2005;110(5–6):655–664.
152. Schunk JE. Radial head subluxation: epidemiology and treatment of 87 episodes. *Ann Emerg Med.* 1990;19(9):1019–1023.
153. Schwab GH, Bennett JB, Woods GW, et al. Biomechanics of elbow instability: the role of the medial collateral ligament. *Clin Orthop Relat Res.* 1980;(146):42–52.
154. Shankarappa YK. Transverse divergent dislocation of the elbow with ipsilateral distal radius epiphyseal injury in a seven year old. *Injury.* 1998;29(10):798–802.
155. Shukla SK, Cohen MS. Symptomatic medial epicondyle nonunion: treatment by open reduction and fixation with a tension band construct. *J Shoulder Elbow Surg.* 2011;20(3):455–460.
156. Silberstein MJ, Brodeur AE, Graviss ER, et al. Some vagaries of the medial epicondyle. *J Bone Joint Surg Am.* 1981;63(4):524–528.
157. Smith FM. Medial epicondyle injuries. *JAMA.* 1950;142(6):396–402.
158. Smith JT, McFeely ED, Bae DS, et al. Operative fixation of medial humeral epicondyle fracture nonunion in children. *J Pediatr Orthop.* 2010;30(7):644–648.
159. Snellman O. Subluxation of the head of the radius in children. *Acta Orthop Scand.* 1959;28:311–315.
160. Snyder HS. Radiographic changes with radial head subluxation in children. *J Emerg Med.* 1990;8(3):265–269.
161. Sojbjerg JO, Helmig P, Kjaersgaard-Andersen P. Dislocation of the elbow: an experimental study of the ligamentous injuries. *Orthopedics.* 1987;12:461–463.
162. Sovio OM, Tredwell SJ. Divergent dislocation of the elbow in a child. *J Pediatr Orthop.* 1986;6(1):96–97.
163. Spear HC, Janes JM. Rupture of the brachial artery accompanying dislocation of the elbow or supracondylar fracture. *J Bone Joint Surg Am.* 1951;33-A(4):889–894.
164. Speed JS. An operation for unreduced posterior dislocation of the elbow. *South Med J.* 1925;18:193–197.
165. Steiger RN, Larrick RB, Meyer TL. Median-nerve entrapment following elbow dislocation in children. A report of two cases. *J Bone Joint Surg Am.* 1969;51(2):381–385.
166. Stimson LA. *A Practical Treatise on Fractures and Dislocations.* Philadelphia, PA: Lea Brothers & Co; 1900.
167. Stoneback JW, Owens BD, Sykes J, et al. Incidence of elbow dislocations in the United States population. *J Bone Joint Surg Am.* 2012;94(3):240–245.
168. Symeonides PP, Paschaloglou C, Stavrou Z, et al. Recurrent dislocation of the elbow. Report of three cases. *J Bone Joint Surg Am.* 1975;57(8):1084–1086.
169. Taha AM. The treatment of pulled elbow: a prospective randomized study. *Arch Orthop Trauma Surg.* 2000;120(5–6):336–337.
170. Teach SJ, Schutzman SA. Prospective study of recurrent radial head subluxation. *Arch Pediatr Adolesc Med.* 1986;150:164–166.
171. Thompson HC, Garcia A. Myositis ossificans: aftermath of elbow injuries. *Clin Orthop Relat Res.* 1967;50:129–134.
172. Triantafyllou SJ, Wilson SC, Rychak JS. Irreducible "pulled elbow" in a child. A case report. *Clin Orthop Relat Res.* 1992;(284):153–155.
173. Trias A, Comeau Y. Recurrent dislocation of the elbow in children. *Clin Orthop Relat Res.* 1974;(100):74–77.
174. van Wagenberg JM, van Huijstee PJ, Verhofstad MH. Pediatric complex divergent elbow dislocation. *J Orthop Trauma.* 2011;25(1):e5–e8.
175. Vicente P, Orduna M. Transverse divergent dislocation of the elbow in a child. A case report. *Clin Orthop Relat Res.* 1993;(294):312–313.
176. Wainwright D. Recurrent dislocation of the elbow-joint. *Proc R Soc Med.* 1947;40(14):885.
177. Walker HB. A case of dislocation of the elbow with separation of the internal epicondyle and displacement of the latter into the joint. *Br J Surg.* 1928;15:667–679.
178. Watson-Jones R. Primary nerve lesions in injuries of the elbow and wrist. *J Bone Joint Surg Am.* 1930;12:121–140.
179. Wheeler DK, Linscheid RL. Fracture-dislocations of the elbow. *Clin Orthop Relat Res.* 1967;50:95–106.
180. Wilmshurst AD, Millner PA, Batchelor AG. Brachial artery entrapment in closed elbow dislocation. *Injury.* 1989;20(4):240–241.
181. Winslow R. A case of complete anterior dislocation of both bones of the forearm at the elbow. *Surg Gynecol Obstet.* 1913;16:570–571.
182. Witvoet J, Tayon B. [Recurrent dislocation of the elbow. Apropos of 6 cases]. *Rev Chir Orthop Reparatrice Appar Mot.* 1974;60(6):485–495.
183. Woods GW, Tullos HS. Elbow instability and medial epicondyle fractures. *Am J Sports Med.* 1977;5(1):23–30.
184. Zaraa M, Saied W, Bouchoucha S, et al. [Purely lateral elbow dislocation in a child, case report and literature review]. *Chir Main.* 2012;31(1):38–40.
185. Zaricznyj B. Transverse divergent dislocation of the elbow. *Clin Orthop Relat Res.* 2000;373:146–152.
186. Zeier FG. Recurrent traumatic elbow dislocation. *Clin Orthop Relat Res.* 1982;(169):211–214.
187. Bexkens R, Washburn FJ, Evgendaal D, et al. Effectiveness of reduction maneuvers in the treatment of nursemaid's elbow: a systematic review and meta-analysis. *Am J Emerg Med.* 2017;35(1):159–163.
188. Bono KT, Popp JE. Intraosseous median nerve entrapment following pediatric posterior elbow dislocation. *Orthopedics.* 2012;35(4):e592–e594.
189. Butler MA, Martus JE, Schoenecker JG. Pediatric variants of the transolecranon fracture dislocation: recognition and tension band fixation: report of 3 cases. *J Hand Surg Am.* 2012;37(5):999–1002.
190. Canavese FM, Marengo L, Tiris A, et al. Radiological, clinical and functional evaluation using the quick disabilities of the arm, shoulder and hand questionnaire of children with medial epicondyle fractures treated surgically. *Int Orthop.* 2017;41(7):1447–1452.
191. Cruz AI, Steere JT, Lawrence JT. Medial epicondyle fractures in the pediatric overhead athlete. *J Pediatr Orthop.* 2016;36(Suppl 1):S56–62.
192. Di Gennaro GL, Spina M, Fosco M, et al. Dislocations of the elbow in children: long-term follow-up. *Musculoskel Surg.* 2013;97(Suppl 1):3–7.
193. Dizdarevic I, Low S, Currie DW, et al. Epidemiology of elbow dislocations in high school athletes. *Am J Sports Med.* 2016;44(1):202–208.
194. Dodd SD, Flanagin BA, Bohl DD, et al. Incarcerated medial epicondyle fracture following pediatric elbow dislocation: 11 cases. *J Hand Surg Am.* 2014;39(9):1739–1745.
195. Erickson BJ, Chalmers PN, Axe MJ, et al. Exceeding pitch count recommendations in Little League baseball increases the chance of requiring Tommy John surgery as a professional baseball pitcher. *Orthop J Sports Med.* 2017;5(3): eCollection 2017.
196. Glotzbecker MP, Shore B, Matheney T, et al. Alternative technique for open reduction and fixation of displaced pediatric medial epicondyle fractures. *J Child Orthop.* 2012;6(2):105–109.
197. Guitton TG, Albers RG, Ring D. Anterior olecranon fracture-dislocations of the elbow in children. A report of four cases. *J Bone Joint Surg.* 2009;91A:1487–1490.
198. Knapik DM, Fausett CL, Gilmore A, et al. Outcomes of nonoperative pediatric medial humeral epicondyle fractures with and without associated elbow dislocation. *J Pediatr Orthop.* 2017;37(4):e224–e228.
199. Krul M, van der Wouden JC, Kruijhof EJ, et al. Manipulative interventions for reducing pulled elbow in young children. *Cochrane Database Syst Rev.* 2017;7:CD007759.
200. Kulkarni VS, Arora N, Gehlot H, et al. Symptomatic medial humeral epicondylar fracture non-union- rare presentation of a relatively common injury. *Injury.* 2017;48(Suppl 2):S50–S53.
201. Lattanza LL, Goldfarb CA, Smucny M, et al. Clinical presentation of posterolateral rotatory instability of the elbow in children. *J Bone Joint Surg Am.* 2013;95(15):e105.
202. Lieber J, Zundel SM, Luithle T, et al. Acute traumatic posterior elbow dislocation in children. *J Pediatr Orthop B.* 2012;21(5):474–481.
203. Murphy RF, Vuillermin C, Naqvi M, et al. Early outcomes of pediatric elbow dislocation: risk factors associated with morbidity. *J Pediatr Orthop.* 2017;37:440–446.
204. Osbar DC, Chalmers PN, Frank JS, et al. Acute, avulsion fractures of the medial epicondyle while throwing in youth baseball players: a variant of Little League elbow. *J Shoulder Elbow Surg.* 2010;19(7):951–957.
205. Pace GI, Hennrikus WL. Fixation of displaced medial epicondyle fractures in adolescents. *J Pediatr Orthop.* 2017;37(2):e80–e82.
206. Pytiak AV, Stearns P, Bastrom TP, et al. Are the current Little League pitching guidelines adequate? A single-season prospective MRI study. *Orthop J Sports Med.* 2017;5(5), eCollection 2017.
207. Richardson M, Kuester VG, Hoover K. The usefulness of MRI in atypical pulled/nursemaid's elbow: a case report. *J Pediatr Orthop.* 2012;32(5):e20–e22.
208. Simon D, Masquijo JJ, Duncan MJ, et al. Intra-articular median nerve incarceration after spontaneous reduction of a pediatric elbow dislocation: case report and review of the literature. *J Pediatr Orthop.* 2010;30(2):125–129.
209. Sumko MJ, Hennrikus W, Slough J, et al. Measurement of radiation exposure when using mini c-arm to reduce pediatric upper extremity fractures. *J Pediatric Orthop.* 2016;36:122–125.
210. Vuillermin C, Donohue KS, Miller P, et al. Incarcerated medial epicondyle fractures with elbow dislocation: risk factors associated with morbidity. *J Pediatr Orthop.* 2017. [Epub ahead of print]
211. Wu Y, Jiang H, Miao W. A case report of children's divergent dislocation of the elbow and review of literature. *Medicine (Baltimore).* 2016;95(44):e4772.

16

Lateral Condylar and Capitellar Fractures of the Distal Humerus

Derek M. Kelly and Jeffrey R. Sawyer

Lateral Condylar Physeal Fractures

INTRODUCTION TO LATERAL CONDYLAR PHYSEAL FRACTURES

All the physes of the distal humerus are vulnerable to injury, each with a distinct fracture pattern. Next to those of the distal radius, injuries to the distal humeral physes are the most common physeal injuries. The vulnerability of the various physes to injury is altered by age and injury mechanism.[1,3] Fractures involving the total distal humeral physis may occur in neonates or within the first 2 to 3 years of life.[15,58] Fractures involving the lateral condylar physis occur later, with the average age around 6 years.[27,34,37,43] Fractures concerning the medial condylar physis are rare and occur most often in children 8 to 12 years of age.[9,27,28,37,43] Obesity and a larger varus carrying angle have been cited as indicators of the likelihood of a lateral condylar fracture rather than a supracondylar fracture.[25,41]

ASSESSMENT OF LATERAL CONDYLAR PHYSEAL FRACTURES

Fractures involving the lateral condyle in the immature skeleton can either cross the physis or follow it for a short distance into the trochlear cartilage. Fractures of the lateral condylar physis, which are less common than supracondylar fractures, constitute 17% of distal humeral fractures.

Fractures of the lateral condylar physis rarely are associated with injuries outside the elbow region[32,35,54] and unlike supracondylar humeral fractures, fractures of the lateral condyle rarely are associated with neurovascular injuries. Within the elbow region, the associated injuries that uncommonly occur with this fracture include dislocation of the elbow, radial head fractures, and fractures of the olecranon, which are often greenstick fractures.[40] Fractures with an associated elbow dislocation, which may be the result of loss of bony stability from the fracture itself, have been associated with slower return of range of motion than fractures without a dislocation.[79] Although nonaccidental trauma is a rare cause of these injuries, this must always be considered in the differential diagnosis, especially in young children.[45] Acute fractures involving only the capitellum are rare in skeletally immature patients but are serious injuries that need to be recognized and treated appropriately.

The diagnosis of lateral condylar physeal injury may be less obvious both clinically and on radiographs than that of supracondylar fracture (Fig. 16-1), especially if the fracture is minimally displaced. Internal oblique views of the distal humerus are very helpful in making accurate diagnosis and defining the extent of fracture displacement for treatment decisions.

MECHANISMS OF INJURY FOR LATERAL CONDYLAR PHYSEAL FRACTURES

Two mechanisms have been suggested: "push-off" and "pull-off." The pull-off or avulsion theory has more advocates than the push-off mechanism.[38,92] In early studies,[92] this injury was consistently produced in young cadavers by adducting the forearm with the elbow extended and the forearm supinated. The

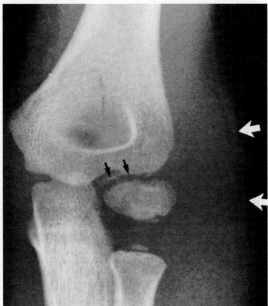
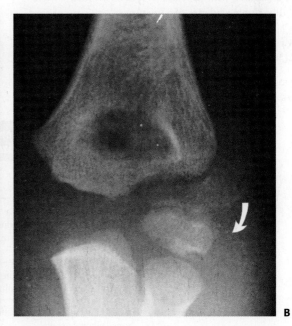

Figure 16-1. A: Injury film of a 7 year old with a nondisplaced fracture of the lateral condyle (*small arrows*). Attention was drawn to the location of the fracture because of extensive soft tissue swelling on the lateral aspect (*white arrows*). **B:** Because of the extensive soft tissue injury, there was little intrinsic stability, allowing the fracture to become displaced at 7 days (*arrow*).

push-off mechanism has also been reproduced in cadavers by applying a sharp blow to the palm with the elbow flexed, causing the radial head to push off the lateral condyle. This push-off injury also can result from a direct blow to the olecranon.

It is likely that both mechanisms can produce this injury. The more common type of fracture, which extends to the apex of the trochlea, probably is a result of avulsion forces on the condyle, with the olecranon's sharp articular surface serving to direct the force along the physeal line into the trochlea. When a child falls forward on his or her palm with the elbow flexed, the radial head is forced against the capitellum and may cause the less common physeal fracture that courses through the ossific nucleus of the capitellum.

SIGNS AND SYMPTOMS OF LATERAL CONDYLAR PHYSEAL FRACTURES

Compared with the marked distortion of the elbow that occurs with displaced supracondylar fractures, little distortion of the elbow, other than that produced by the fracture hematoma, may be present with lateral condylar fractures. The key to the clinical evaluation of this fracture is the location of soft tissue swelling and pain concentrated over the lateral aspect of the distal humerus.[50] Nondisplaced or minimally displaced fractures may produce only local tenderness at the condylar fracture site, which may be increased by flexing the wrist, placing the wrist extensors, which are attached to the fracture fragment, on stretch. The benign appearance of the elbow with some stage I displacements may account for the delay of parents seeking treatment for a child with a minimally displaced fracture. With more displaced fractures, there often is a hematoma present laterally, and attempted manipulation may result in local crepitus with motion of the lateral condylar fragment. This obviously would be associated with pain and should be avoided if there is a clear radiographic evidence of a fracture.

IMAGING AND OTHER DIAGNOSTIC STUDIES FOR LATERAL CONDYLAR PHYSEAL FRACTURES

The radiographic appearance varies according to the fracture line's anatomic location and the displacement stage. On standard anteroposterior and lateral radiographs, the metaphyseal fragment or "flake" may be small and seemingly minimally displaced. In determining whether the articular hinge is intact (i.e., stage I vs. stage II), the relationship of the proximal ulna to the distal humerus is evaluated for the presence of lateral translocation, which is suggestive of instability.

Internal oblique views are especially helpful in patients in whom displacement is suspected but not evident on AP and lateral views. To determine the importance of the internal oblique view in the radiographic evaluation of nondisplaced or minimally displaced lateral condylar fractures, Song et al.[85] compared the oblique view to standard AP views and found that the amount of displacement differed between the two views in 75% of children. They recommended routine use of an internal oblique view to evaluate the amount of fracture displacement and to assess stability if a lateral condylar fracture was suspected.

Three groups of nondisplaced and minimally displaced fractures of the lateral condyle have been described and correlated with the risk of late displacement: stable fractures, fractures with an undefinable risk, and fractures with a high risk of later displacement (Table 16-1).[21]

Arthrography, MRI, and more recently ultrasound evaluation[5] have been suggested to identify unstable fractures in the acute setting and to aid in preoperative planning for those with late displacement, delayed union, or malunion. Although not used with all fractures, MRI can be a very useful diagnostic aid to guiding treatment, especially with delayed unions, but often requires sedation in younger patients.

A major diagnostic difficulty lies in differentiating a lateral condylar fracture from a fracture of the entire distal humeral physis. In a young child in whom the condyle is unossified, an arthrogram or MRI may be helpful (Figs. 16-2 to 16-4).[12,32] Ultrasonography, which often can avoid MRI sedation issues, can be used to distinguish occult elbow fractures including lateral condyle from transphyseal separations in young patients.[11]

In fractures of the entire distal humeral physis, the proximal radius and ulna usually are displaced posteromedially (Fig. 16-5A). The relationship of the lateral condylar ossification center to the proximal radius remains intact. In true fractures involving only the lateral condylar physis, the relationship

TABLE 16-1. Risk of Subsequent Displacement of Lateral Humeral Condylar Fractures Immobilized in a Cast			
Fracture Type	Description	Risk Ratio	95% Confidence Interval
Group A (stable)	No gap or small gap in radial or radiodorsal aspect of metaphyseal fracture; fracture could not be followed all the way to epiphyseal cartilage	0	0–5.52
Group B (undefinable risk)	Same as group A, but fracture could be clearly observed all the way to epiphyseal cartilage	0.17	6.56–33.65
Group C (high risk)	Gap in fracture as wide, or almost as wide, medially as laterally	0.42	15.17–72.33

Modified with permission from Finnbogason T, Karlsson G, Lindberg L, et al. Nondisplaced and minimally displaced fractures of the lateral humeral condyle in children: A prospective radiographic investigation of fracture stability. *J Pediatr Orthop.* 1995;15(4):422–425.

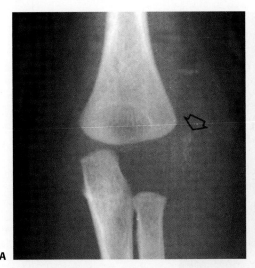
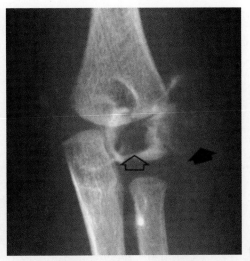

Figure 16-2. Unossified lateral condyle. **A:** AP view. A small ossific nucleus can barely be seen (*arrow*) in the swollen lateral soft tissues. **B:** An arthrogram shows the defect left by the displaced lateral condyle (*closed arrow*). The displaced condyle is outlined in the soft tissues (*solid arrow*). Note the large cartilaginous fragment that is not visible on radiograph.

of the condylar ossification center to the proximal radius is disrupted (Fig. 16-5B). In addition, displacement of the proximal radius and ulna is more likely to be lateral because of the loss of stability provided by the lateral crista of the distal humerus.

CLASSIFICATION OF LATERAL CONDYLAR PHYSEAL FRACTURES

Lateral condylar physeal fractures can be classified by either the fracture line's anatomic location or by the amount of displacement.

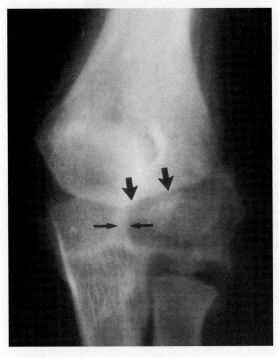

Figure 16-3. Arthrogram of stage I fracture of the lateral condyle (*large arrows*). Articular surface is intact with no displacement (*small arrows*).

Classification by Anatomic Location

The Milch classification, based on whether or not the fracture extends through (type I) or around (type II) the capitellar ossific nucleus, is used infrequently because of its poor reliability and predictive value[99] and is primarily of historic interest. Salter and Harris[73] classified lateral condylar physeal injuries as a form of type IV injuries. Because the fracture line starts in the metaphysis and then courses along the physeal cartilage, a lateral condylar humeral fracture has some of the characteristics of both type II and IV injuries. A true Salter–Harris type IV injury through the ossific nucleus of the lateral condyle is rare. Although lateral condylar fractures are similar to Salter–Harris type II and IV fractures, treatment guidelines follow those of a type IV injury: open reduction and internal fixation of displaced intra-articular fractures. The Salter–Harris classification is of little clinical use and is debatable as to the accuracy of terminology, because the fracture exits the joint in the not-yet-ossified cartilage of the trochlea.

Classification by Stage of Displacement

Lateral Condylar Physeal Fractures:
JAKOB'S CLASSIFICATION BY STAGE
OF FRACTURE DISPLACEMENT

- Stage I: Fracture relatively nondisplaced, articular surface intact
- Stage II: Articular surface disrupted; fragment and olecranon displaced
- Stage III: Fragment rotated and displaced

The amount of fracture displacement was described by Jakob et al.[38] in three stages (Fig. 16-6).[95] In the first stage, the fracture is relatively nondisplaced, and the articular surface is intact (see Fig. 16-6A,B). Because the trochlea is intact, there is no lateral shift of the olecranon. In the second stage, the fracture extends completely through the articular surface (see Fig. 16-6C,D). This allows the proximal fragment to become more displaced and can allow lateral displacement. In the third stage, the

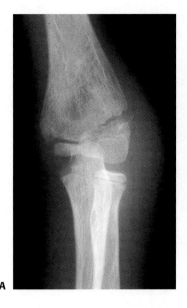
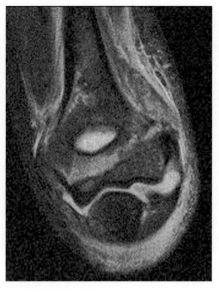

Figure 16-4. A: Radiograph of what appears to be a stable type II fracture of the lateral condyle in a 10-year-old child. **B:** Gradient-echo MRI clearly shows that this is a fracture of the entire distal humeral physis.

condylar fragment is rotated and totally displaced laterally and proximally, which allows translocation of both the olecranon and the radial head (see Fig. 16-6E,F).

Lateral Condylar Physeal Fractures:
WEISS CLASSIFICATION BY FRACTURE DISPLACEMENT AND CARTILAGINOUS HINGE

- Type I: <2 mm-displacement
- Type II: >2-mm displacement with intact cartilaginous hinge
- Type III: >2-mm displacement with nonintact cartilaginous hinge

---

Weiss et al.[99] modified this classification based on fracture displacement and disruption of the cartilaginous hinge (Fig. 16-7). Type I fractures are displaced less than 2 mm, type II fractures are displaced more than 2 mm but have an intact cartilaginous hinge, and type III fractures are displaced more than 2 mm and do not have an intact cartilaginous hinge. In their series of 158 type II and III fractures, they found that all type II fractures had less than 4 mm of displacement on initial radiographs and all type III fractures had more than 4 mm of displacement. This classification was found to be predictive of complications with type III fractures having a 3 times higher rate than type II fractures.

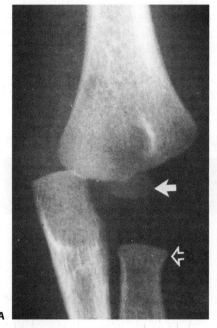
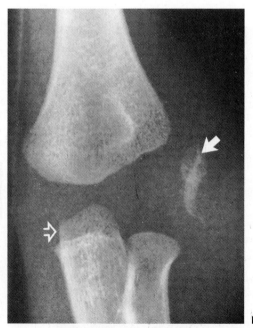

Figure 16-5. A: Total distal humeral physeal fracture in a 2 year old. The lateral condyle (*closed arrow*) has remained in line with the proximal radius. The proximal radius, ulna, and lateral condyle have all shifted medially (*open arrow*). **B:** Displaced fracture of the lateral condyle in a 2 year old. The relationship of the lateral condyle (*closed arrow*) to the proximal radius is lost. Both the proximal radius and ulna (*open arrow*) have shifted slightly laterally.

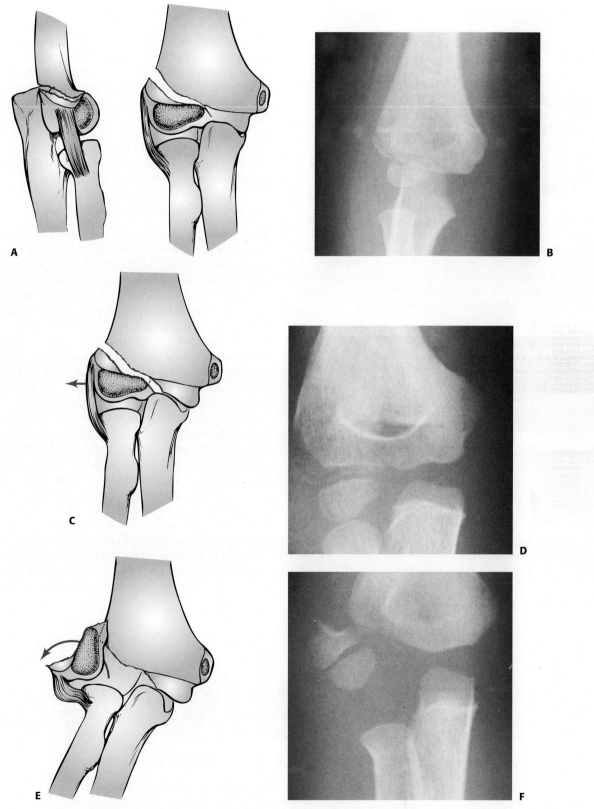

Figure 16-6. Stages of displacement. **A, B:** Stage I displacement—articular surface intact. **C, D:** Stage II displacement—articular surface disrupted. **E, F:** Stage III displacement—fragment rotated.

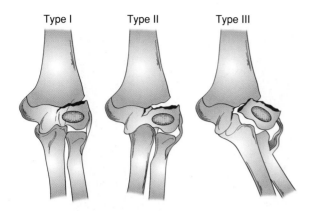

Figure 16-7. Classification of lateral humeral condylar fractures. Type I, less than 2 mm of displacement; type II, 2 mm or more of displacement and congruity of the articular surface; type III, more than 2 mm of displacement and lack of articular congruity. (Reprinted with permission from Weiss JM, Graves S, Yang S, et al. A new classification system predictive of complications in surgically treated pediatric humeral lateral condyle fractures. *J Pediatr Orthop.* 2009;29(6):602–605.)

Lateral Condylar Physeal Fractures:
SONG ET AL. CLASSIFICATION BY FRACTURE DISPLACEMENT AND FRACTURE PATTERN[85]

Stage	Displacement (mm)	Fracture Pattern	Stability
1	≤2	Limited to metaphysis	Stable
2	≤2	Indefinable; extends to epiphyseal articular cartilage	Indeterminate
3	≤2	Medial and lateral displacement of distal fragment	Unstable
4	>2	No rotation of fragment	Unstable
5	>2	Rotation of fragment	Unstable

Finally, Song et al.[85] proposed a five-stage system based on fracture stability where stage 1 (≤2-mm displacement) is limited to the metaphysis and therefore inherently stable. Stage 2 (≤2-mm displacement), in which the fracture line is indefinable because of the cartilaginous nature of the epiphysis, extends to the epiphyseal articular cartilage and carries an indeterminate risk of displacement. Stage 3 (≤2-mm displacement) is unstable and at higher risk of displacement because of the medial and lateral displacement of the distal fragment. Stage 4 (>2-mm displacement) and stage 5 (>2 mm displaced and rotated) are unstable fractures which by definition are displaced (Fig. 16-8). This classification helps refine surgical indications.

Displacement of the Fracture and Elbow Joint

The fracture line usually begins in the posterolateral metaphysis, with a soft tissue tear in the area between the origins of the extensor carpi radialis longus and the brachioradialis muscle. The extensor carpi radialis longus and brevis muscles remain attached to the distal fragment, along with the lateral collateral ligaments of the elbow. If there is much displacement, both the anterior and posterior aspects of the elbow capsule are usually torn. This soft tissue injury, however, usually is localized to the lateral side and may help identify a minimally displaced fracture. More extensive soft tissue swelling at the fracture site may indicate more severe soft tissue injury,[50,67] and predict that the fracture is unstable and prone to late displacement.

The degree of displacement varies according to the magnitude of the force applied and whether the cartilaginous hinge of the articular surface remains intact.[36] If the articular surface is intact, the condylar fragment may be either nondisplaced or tilted, hinging on the intact medial articular surface. If the fracture is complete, the fragment can be rotated and displaced in varying degrees; in the most severe fractures, rotation is almost full 180 degrees, so that the lateral condylar articular surface opposes the denuded metaphyseal fracture surface. In addition to this coronal rotation of the distal fragment, rotation can also occur in the horizontal plane.[101] The lateral margin is carried posteriorly, and the medial portion of the distal fragment rotates anteriorly.

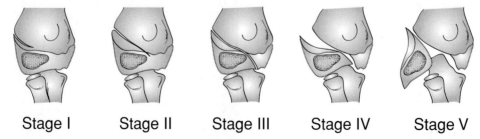

Stage I   Stage II   Stage III   Stage IV   Stage V

Figure 16-8. Stages of displacement of fractures of the lateral humeral condyle in children. Stage I, stable fracture with 2 mm or less of displacement and fracture line limited to within the metaphysis. Stage II, indefinable fracture with 2 mm or less of displacement and fracture line extending to the epiphyseal articular cartilage; there is a lateral gap. Stage III, unstable fracture with 2 mm or less of displacement and a gap that is wide laterally as medially. Stage IV, unstable fracture with displacement of more than 2 mm. Stage V, unstable fracture with displacement of more than 2 mm with rotation. (Reproduced with permission from Song KS, Kang CH, Min BW, et al. Closed reduction and internal fixation of displaced unstable lateral condylar fractures of the humerus in children. *J Bone Joint Surg Am.* 2008;90(12):2673–2681.)

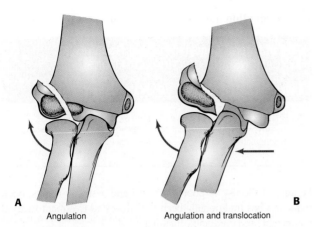

Figure 16-9. Angular deformities. **A:** Capitellar fracture. **B:** Fracture extending into the trochlea.

Because the usual fracture line disrupts the lateral crista of the trochlea, the elbow joint may be unstable, creating the possibility of posterolateral subluxation of the proximal radius and ulna. Thus, the forearm rotates along the coronal plane into valgus, and there may also be lateral translocation of the lateral condyle with the radius and ulna (Fig. 16-9). This concept of lateral translocation is important in the late reconstruction of untreated fractures.

When the fracture line traverses the lateral condylar epiphysis, the elbow remains reasonably stable because the trochlea remains intact. Total coronal rotation of the condylar fragment can occur with this injury. The axial deformity that results is pure valgus without translocation.

This posterolateral elbow instability with the lateral condyle fracture has led to a mistaken concept that this injury is associated with a primary dislocation of the elbow,[13] which is rarely the case. The posterolateral instability of the elbow is usually a result of the injury, not a cause of it, as the displacement of the joint is through the fracture.[3,70]

TREATMENT OPTIONS FOR LATERAL CONDYLAR PHYSEAL FRACTURES

Fractures involving the lateral condylar physis can be treated with immobilization alone, closed reduction and percutaneous pinning, or open surgical reduction depending on the degree of displacement and amount of instability.[87]

NONOPERATIVE TREATMENT OF LATERAL CONDYLAR PHYSEAL FRACTURES

Immobilization

Nonoperative Treatment of Lateral Condylar Fractures Following Successful Closed Reduction: INDICATIONS AND CONTRAINDICATIONS	
Indication	**Relative Contraindication**
• Stable articular reduction with <2 mm of displacement	• Inability to obtain acceptable reduction

Minimally displaced fractures (<2 mm) are stable and have intact soft tissue attachments that prevent displacement of the distal fragment. About 40% of lateral condylar physeal fractures are nondisplaced, are not at risk for late displacement, and can be treated with immobilization alone.[38] If the fracture line is barely perceptible on the original radiographs, including internal oblique views (stage I displacement), the chance for subsequent displacement is low. Immobilization of nondisplaced or minimally displaced (less than 2 mm) fractures in a posterior splint or cast is adequate.[4,5,7,10,86,88] Radiographs are important during the first 3 weeks after injury to ensure that late displacement does not occur.

OPERATIVE TREATMENT OF LATERAL CONDYLAR PHYSEAL FRACTURES

Closed Reduction and Percutaneous Pinning

Closed Reduction and Percutaneous Pinning of Lateral Condylar Physeal Fractures: INDICATIONS AND CONTRAINDICATIONS	
Indications	**Contraindications**
• Anatomic reduction with closed reduction	• Inability to obtain adequate reduction
• Arthrographic confirmation of articular congruity	• Unstable fracture that cannot be maintained with percutaneous pins

When a lateral condylar fracture is displaced more than 2 mm, closed or open reduction is required to restore anatomic alignment of the joint and physis. Unfortunately, it is difficult to maintain reduction of a displaced lateral condylar fracture with closed techniques, so closed reduction alone is not recommended for treating displaced lateral condylar fractures. Several techniques have been described for initial closed reduction, with the recommended elbow position ranging from hyperflexion to full extension. However, clinical experience and experimental studies indicate that closed reduction is best achieved with the forearm supinated and the elbow extended. Placing a varus stress on the extended elbow allows easier manipulation of the fragment. Fractures that are found to be stable with an intact cartilaginous hinge, either by stress maneuvers, arthrography, or other imaging modality, can be percutaneously pinned with the elbow in flexion, similar to a supracondylar humeral fracture. Several studies including that of Mintzer et al.[55] have shown good results with percutaneous reduction and fixation for unstable, moderately displaced lateral condylar fractures, which can then be stabilized with Kirschner (K-) wires or a cannulated screw.[66,78,102] A percutaneous pin from the lateral column also can be used as a "joystick" to maneuver the distal fragment and aid in reduction. The smooth pins or cannulated screw is then advanced across the fracture site to the opposite cortex to obtain stability.[53,55]

A comparison study of displaced lateral condylar fractures (>2 mm) treated with percutaneous or open reduction found that patients treated with percutaneous fixation had shorter operating room times and fewer complications (13% vs. 26%)

with equal healing times compared to patients treated with open reduction and internal fixation.[42] Anatomic alignment of the joint and fracture stability are confirmed by stress testing and/or arthrography. If a satisfactory reduction cannot be obtained, then reduction can be achieved and maintained by open reduction and internal fixation.

Technique

> ✔ **Closed Reduction and Percutaneous Pinning of Lateral Condylar Physeal Fractures:**
> KEY SURGICAL STEPS
>
> ❑ Always be prepared in terms of equipment, personnel, setup to do an open reduction
> ❑ Use general anesthesia with endotracheal tube and muscular paralysis
> ❑ Use C-arm receiver when open reduction is unlikely; use radiolucent table when the possibility of open reduction is unclear or likely
> ❑ Perform arthrogram/stress radiographs to assess stability
> ❑ Reduce the fracture with the elbow extended, forearm supinated, and wrist extended using thumb pressure and varus elbow stress
> ❑ Use smooth K-wire "joystick" to help reduction if necessary
> ❑ Pin with 2 or 3 smooth (0.62 or 5/64) K-wires in divergent fashion depending on stability of fracture
> ❑ Consider 4.0- or 4.5-mm cannulated screw as alternative
> ❑ Assess reduction and stability with stress radiographs and arthrography
> ❑ Cut and bend pins outside skin. Repeat radiographs to ensure cutting/bending did not change pin position
> ❑ If stable, place patient in long-arm bivalved cast. If unstable or poor reduction, proceed with open reduction and internal fixation

Outcomes

Song et al.[85] reported good results in 46 (73%) of 63 unstable lateral condylar fractures, 53 of which were treated with closed reduction and percutaneous pinning. Closed reduction was attempted in all fractures, regardless of the amount of displacement. If closed reduction was successful ($n = 53$), then percutaneous fixation was used. If closed reduction failed to achieve less than 2 mm of displacement, open reduction and internal fixation was performed ($n = 10$). They listed three elements as essential to obtaining good results with percutaneous reduction and pinning treatment: (1) accurate interpretation of the amount and direction of fracture displacement (mainly posterolaterally), (2) routine intraoperative confirmation of the reduction on both AP and internal oblique radiographs, and (3) maintenance of the reduction with two parallel percutaneous, smooth K-wires. More recently, Song et al.[86] described closed percutaneous manipulation of 24 completely displaced and rotated fractures (Jakob type III), followed by percutaneous pinning. In this series, closed reduction was successful in 18 (75%). Excellent results were obtained in 17 of the 18 patients; one patient had a good result. It should be noted that this technique is technically difficult, and the authors admit that it has a difficult learning curve; these results have not yet been reproduced at any other institution.

Open Reduction and Internal Fixation

ORIF of Lateral Condylar Physeal Fractures:
INDICATIONS AND CONTRAINDICATIONS

Indication	Contraindication
• Displaced, unstable fracture with articular malangulation and malrotation	• Able to obtain an adequate reduction and stabilize it with percutaneous reduction and pinning

Because of the risk of poor functional and aesthetic results, open reduction has traditionally been the advocated treatment method for unstable and irreducible fractures.[9,10,13,34,38,39,53,56,61,75,82,86,95,100,104] About 60% of all fractures involving the lateral condylar physis have at least 2 mm of displacement and are potentially unstable.[38,99]

Preoperative Planning

✔ **ORIF of Lateral Condylar Physeal Fractures:**
PREOPERATIVE PLANNING CHECKLIST

OR table	❑ Radiolucent table, seated
Position/positioning aids	❑ Patient supine
Fluoroscopy location	❑ At end of table to allow surgeon and assistant to work
Equipment	❑ Hohmann and metacarpal retractor reduction clamp, K-wire/4.0-/4.5-mm cannulated screws
Tourniquet	❑ Nonsterile if possible
[Other]	❑ Patient with endotracheal tube and muscular paralysis
	❑ Consider headlamp

Surgical Approach

The standard lateral Kocher approach is most commonly used because it is familiar to most surgeons and allows direct joint visualization while protecting the blood supply to the distal fragment posteriorly. Often, a tear in the aponeurosis of the brachioradialis muscle laterally leads directly to the fracture site. Alternatively, a posterolateral approach has been proposed because of proposed advantages of excellent exposure with minimal dissection and improved cosmetic results because of more posterior placement of the surgical scar.[47] This approach requires special care to avoid excessive dissection of the posterior soft tissue attachments and for this reason, it is less commonly used. Finally, some surgeons are now approaching displaced lateral condylar via an anterior incision, similar to open supracondylar fracture care. An anterior approach enters the joint and fracture site via the torn capsule and periosteum and protects the posterior blood supply to the fragment. The comparative benefit and risk of this approach have yet to be defined.

Technique

> ✔ **ORIF of Lateral Condylar Physeal Fractures:**
> KEY SURGICAL STEPS

- ☐ General anesthesia with muscular paralysis and nonsterile tourniquet
- ☐ Kocher approach and keep all dissection anterior to allow intra-articular visualization and protect posterior blood supply
- ☐ Use traumatic capsulotomy (if present) and extend proximally to end of proximal fragment and distally to the radial head
- ☐ Place blunt Hohmann or metacarpal retractor across joint medially to visualize joint. Be careful of ulnar nerve
- ☐ Obtain anatomic articular reduction which may leave lateral metaphysis with small amount of displacement due to plastic deformation
- ☐ Use bone reduction clamp to obtain compression and temporary fixation
- ☐ Stabilize fracture with 2 to 3 divergent smooth K-wires (0.62 or 5/64) or 4.0-/4.5-mm cannulated screws
- ☐ Manipulate elbow and perform stress maneuvers to confirm stability
- ☐ Cut and bend K-wires and reassess stability
- ☐ Layered wound closure and long-arm bivalved cast

The elbow is exposed through a 3- to 4-cm lateral approach, placing two-thirds of the incision proximal and one-third distal to the joint line (Fig. 16-10). In the interval between the brachioradialis and the triceps, the dissection is carried down to the lateral humeral condyle. The joint's anterior surfaces are exposed by separating the fibers of the common extensor muscle mass. An arthrotomy, placed slightly anteriorly, can be made from the radiocapitellar joint to the distal humeral shaft. With widely displaced fractures, these soft tissues often are already stripped and

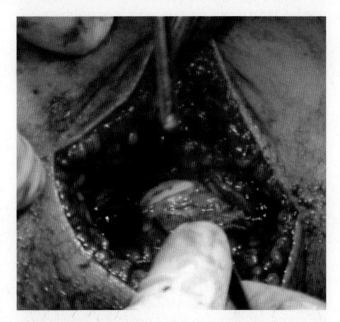

Figure 16-10. Lateral approach for open reduction and internal fixation of a lateral humeral condylar fracture of the left elbow. The approach is made through the brachioradialis–triceps interval; an anterior retractor is used to expose the joint surface. Note the large unossified articular fragment.

the surgeon can follow the fracture hematoma directly into the joint. Care must be taken to prevent injury to the distal humeral articular surface, which often is rotated into the wound and right underneath the capsule. Retracting the antecubital structures exposes the anterior joint surface. To protect the brachial artery and medial nerve, a small metacarpal or blunt Hohmann retractor can be passed across the joint to the opposite side, taking care to protect the ulnar nerve during its placement. The trochlea and fracture site are inspected. The displacement and the size of the fragment are always greater than is apparent on the radiographs because much of the fragment is cartilaginous. The fragment usually is rotated as well as displaced. The joint is irrigated to remove blood clots and debris, the articular surface and the metaphyseal fragment are reduced anatomically, and the reduction is confirmed by observing the articular surface, particularly at the trochlea. A headlamp can be helpful for visualization. It is important to assess the quality of the reduction on the articular surface and not the lateral humeral cortex, because often there is plastic deformation of the lateral cortex. Reducing the lateral cortex may lead to a nonanatomic articular reduction. In some cases, when mobilizing the distal fragment, the tourniquet will need to be released to remove tethering of the soft tissues, especially in young children. The reduction is held with a small tenaculum, bone holder, towel clip, or percutaneous pins as "joysticks." Two smooth K-wires are inserted in a parallel or slightly divergent configuration, across the physis, and into the humeral metaphysis, penetrating the medial cortex of the humerus. Occasionally a third lateral pin, more parallel to the joint surface, is used if greater stability is required. The pins should start in the metaphysis if the metaphyseal fragment is large enough and diverge as much as possible to enhance the stability of fixation. When there is only a small metaphyseal fragment, the pins can be safely placed across the physis. Alternatively, a cannulated screw can be placed instead of smooth K-wires for fracture stabilization.

The reduction and the position of the internal fixation are checked by direct observation as well as by AP, lateral, and oblique radiographs before wound closure. If used, the ends of the wires are cut off outside the skin to allow easy removal. There is evidence that pins left out of the skin have less complications than buried pins.[14] The arm is placed in a posterior splint or bivalved long-arm cast with the elbow flexed 90 degrees.

The cast is worn for 4 to 6 weeks after surgery until the fracture is healed. The pins can be removed at 4 to 6 weeks if union is progressing. Gentle active motion of the elbow usually is then resumed and continued until full range of motion returns.

Outcomes

Several large series have reported generally good results with open reduction and internal fixation of lateral condylar fractures, with complications such as delayed union or nonunion (1%) and osteonecrosis (1%) being infrequent.[8,48,66,80] Elbow stiffness is more common after open reduction than after closed treatment, but resolves in most patients by 24 to 48 months after injury.[8] While most authors advocate early surgical treatment of these injuries, Silva et al.[80] reported a series of 181 children (mean age 5 years, mean follow-up 38 weeks) who had either early (0 to 7 days) or late (8 to 14 days) fixation. There were no major neurovascular injuries in either group, and the complication rate, surgical time, range of motion, and patient satisfaction were similar between the two groups. A small study of 16 patients treated at a mean of 7.4 weeks (3 to 15.6 weeks) after fracture found that approximately half the patients developed a partial fishtail deformity but none developed osteonecrosis.[48] Yang et al.[103] described the use of an olecranon osteotomy to obtain anatomic reduction in 6 patients (mean age, 4.5 years) who had delayed treatment almost 4 months after injury. The optimal timing of surgery remains controversial because of its multifactorial nature, based on patient and fracture characteristics, the degree of soft tissue injury, and the exact definition of when delayed/nonunion occurs. Risk factors for delayed/nonunion include >1 mm of residual displacement after fixation and increased intraoperative fluoroscopy time.[11] Pin-related complications and infections are more common (1% to 2%), but are decreasing because of the increased use of cannulated screw fixation. Surgery alone does not ensure a good result unless an anatomic reduction is obtained and the fixation is secure enough to maintain the reduction.

Smooth pins are the most frequently used method of fragment fixation.[7,24,38,88,100,101,104] The passage of a smooth wire through the physis does not result in any growth disturbance,[20,49] which may be due to the fact that the cross-sectional area of the pins is small relative to the surface area of the physis and because only 20% of humeral growth occurs through the distal humeral physis. The effects of a transphyseal screw are unknown, but the risk of growth arrest following screw fixation of these fractures is extremely low, most likely due to reasons stated above.

Several studies comparing pins left outside or below the skin found that, while exposed pins had a slightly higher or no different initial infection rate, buried pins had higher rates of pin migration, symptomatic implants, and protrusion through the skin (up to 40%) causing late infection and increased treatment cost.[14,61]

Because of the issues related to pin fixation, as well as a biomechanical in vitro study showing increased rigidity of screw fixation compared to pin fixation,[74] there has been increased use of cannulated screws in this setting.[77,90] In a series of 62 patients, Li and Xu[46] found lower rates of infection (0% vs. 17%), lateral prominence (13% vs. 37%), and loss of motion (6% vs. 30%) in patients treated with open reduction and fixation with cannulated screws compared to those treated with K-wires. Although the two groups were similar, the type of fixation was not randomized. Gilbert et al.[30] in a similar-sized series found a higher rate of union, shorter cast time, and greater postoperative range of motion in patients treated with cannulated screws compared to wires; however, they did note that those with screw fixation did require a second surgical procedure to remove the screw.

Authors' Preferred Treatment for Lateral Condylar Physeal Fractures (Algorithm 16-1)

Immobilization

If the fracture is minimally displaced on all three radiographic views (i.e., the metaphyseal fragment is less than 2 mm from the proximal fragment on AP, lateral, and internal oblique views) and the clinical signs also indicate there is reasonable soft tissue integrity, the elbow is immobilized in a long-arm cast with the forearm in neutral rotation and the elbow flexed 80 to 90 degrees. Radiographs, including internal oblique views, are taken within the first week after the fracture with the cast removed and the elbow extended. If there is no displacement, the radiographs are repeated once again during the next 1 to 2 weeks. Immobilization is continued until fracture union is apparent, usually between 4 and 6 weeks after injury.

In some fractures with more than the allowable 2 mm of displacement (type II injury), the fracture pattern is such that the articular cartilage appears intact. If there is any question about the stability at the time of the fracture and it is believed that the fracture may be stable and not require pinning, an MRI is obtained. If the stability is questionable and it is believed that the fracture is likely to displace, or that the patient's family will not comply with close follow-up, the patient is examined under general anesthesia using arthrography and stress maneuvers to determine fracture stability. Usually in these circumstances, percutaneous pins are placed to maintain articular alignment until healed.

Percutaneous Pinning

For fractures with stage II displacement (2 to 4 mm), reduction and percutaneous pin fixation are attempted because open reduction often is not necessary (Fig. 16-11). We use a lateral entry pin to joystick the fracture into the correct alignment. If there are concerns about reduction or stability after percutaneous pinning, varus stress radiography and elbow arthrography are performed. Most commonly for these fractures, due to more stable soft tissue attachments, we use two to three smooth divergent K-wires left outside the skin to be removed in the office but occasionally use a cannulated screw; however, this does require a return to the operating room for removal. If these tests show residual or indeterminate malalignment, we proceed with open reduction and internal fixation to directly visualize the articular surface.

Open Reduction and Internal Fixation

If the fracture is completely displaced, malrotated, and/or grossly unstable (stage III), open reduction and internal fixation is indicated. We prefer open reduction and internal fixation within a few days of injury if the soft tissues will allow for all fractures with stage III displacement. We use a nonsterile tourniquet when possible and find a headlamp or illuminated suction tip to be helpful, especially in obese or extremely swollen patients. In fractures with significant displacement and soft tissue injury, we prefer a single

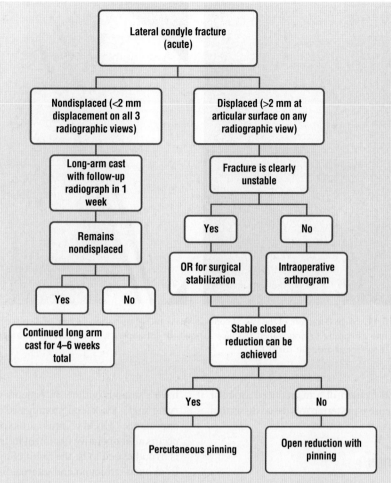

Algorithm 16-1. Authors' preferred treatment for lateral condylar physeal fractures.

cannulated screw (Fig. 16-12) to K-wires, which allows earlier mobilization and faster return of motion, especially in patients with higher-energy injuries such as fracture–dislocations. Patients are placed in a bivalved long-arm cast which is then removed at approximately 4 to 6 weeks to start range of motion.

Lateral Condyle Fractures:
PITFALLS AND PREVENTIONS

Pitfall	Prevention
Difficulty visualizing articular surface reduction	• Head lamp • Extend capsular incision to radiocapitellar joint
Difficulty mobilizing fragment	• Release tourniquet
Difficulty maintaining reduction with pins	• Use cannulated screw
Capitellar osteonecrosis	• Avoid all posterior dissection of displaced fragment
Elbow stiffness	• Use cannulated screw instead of pins
Pin complications	• Pins left outside the skin, removed in clinic

LATERAL CONDYLAR FRACTURE ADVERSE OUTCOMES AND COMPLICATIONS

If an adequate reduction is obtained promptly and maintained with solid fixation, results are uniformly good. With supracondylar fractures, an incomplete reduction may result in an aesthetic deformity, but functional results are generally good. In contrast, with displaced fractures of the lateral condylar physis and joint surface, a marginal reduction can result in both aesthetic deformities and functional loss of motion.[89] The complications that affect the outcome are numerous and can result from both biologic and technical problems. Lateral spur formation, stiffness, physeal arrest, and fishtail deformities may occur even when stable anatomic reduction is obtained. Osteonecrosis of the capitellar fragment, delayed neurologic injury, malunion, and nonunion are all more often related to technical problems, which may include failure to recognize a displaced fracture, immobilization treatment of an unstable fracture that

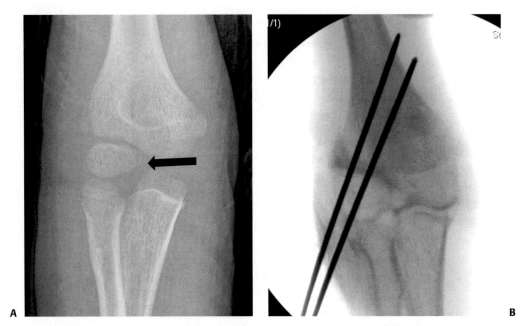

Figure 16-11. Stage II fracture of the lateral condyle. **A:** AP radiograph shows 4 mm of displacement with fracture line extending to nonossified trochlea (*arrow*). **B:** Intraoperative fluoroscopic arthrogram after pinning shows intact articular surface.

displaces in a cast, internal fixation of a malreduced articular fracture fragment, and extensive posterior soft tissue dissection that results in osteonecrosis.

LATERAL SPUR FORMATION

Lateral condylar spur formation is one of the most common sequelae after a fracture involving the lateral condylar physis.[42,99] The spur occurs after both nonoperative and operative treatment. Rates of lateral spur formation are high, approximately 75%. More severe initial fragment displacement and the need for surgical intervention both increase the risk of spur formation.[42,69]

After nonoperative treatment, lateral spurs result from the minimal displacement of the metaphyseal fragment and usually have a smooth outline. In patients with no real change in carrying angle, the lateral prominence of the spur may produce an appearance of mild cubitus varus (pseudovarus). The spur that occurs after operative treatment has a more irregular outline and is hypothesized to be the result of hypertrophic bone formation from open reduction and internal fixation (Fig. 16-13). During open reduction, care should be taken to limit the amount of dissection and to carefully replace the lateral periosteal flap of the metaphyseal fragment to lessen the size of lateral spur formation. Before treatment of lateral condylar fractures, the parents should be told that a lateral spur with pseudovarus is very likely to develop, regardless of the treatment method. They should be told that this mild deformity usually is not of functional significance and can resolve over the subsequent 1 to 2 years.

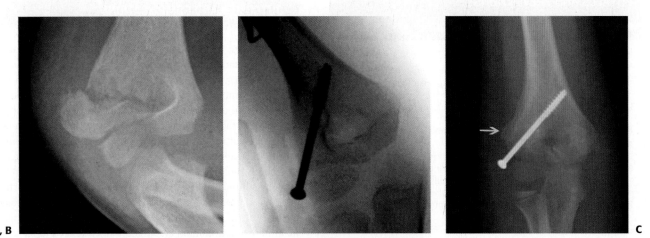

Figure 16-12. A: Lateral condylar fracture–dislocation in a 5-year-old boy. **B:** Intraoperative fluoroscopy showing placement of a cannulated screw. **C:** At final follow-up; note lateral overgrowth (*arrow*).

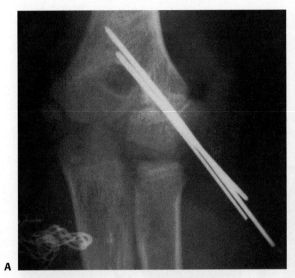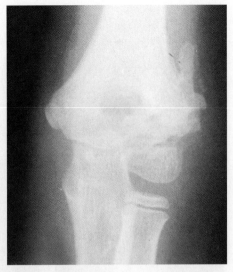

Figure 16-13. A: Considerable soft tissue dissection was performed in the process of open reduction of this lateral condylar fracture. **B:** At 2 months after surgery, there is a large irregular spur formation secondary to periosteal new bone formation from the extensive dissection. (From Wilkins KE. Residuals of elbow fractures. *Orthop Clin North Am.* 1990;21:289–312, with permission.)

ELBOW STIFFNESS

Elbow stiffness can occur after lateral condylar fractures, but most patients regain nearly full elbow range of motion within 4 to 6 months after cast removal.[47,96] Older patients, those requiring longer immobilization, and those requiring surgical treatment can be expected to have a greater loss of motion. Physiotherapy and dynamic splinting are both options for treating early persistent stiffness. Elbow release is rarely needed if fracture and joint alignment are anatomic in healing.

CUBITUS VARUS

Reviews of lateral condylar fractures show that a surprising number heal with some residual cubitus varus angulation (Fig. 16-14).[26,35,53,57,71,81,83,94] In some series, the incidence of

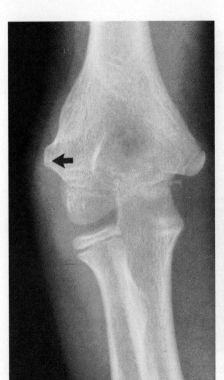

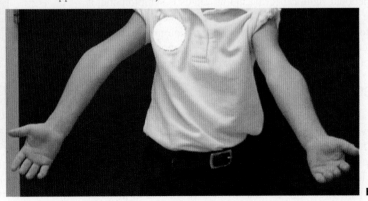

Figure 16-14. Cubitus varus. **A:** Follow-up radiograph of a boy whose lateral condylar fracture was treated nonoperatively and healed with a mild varus angulation. **B:** Clinical appearance of deformity.

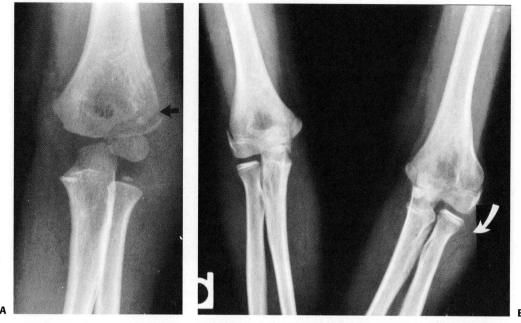

Figure 16-15. True varus. **A:** The injury film with a minimally displaced fracture (*arrow*). This 5-year-old child was treated with immobilization until the fracture was healed. **B:** Five years later, the patient had a persistent cubitus varus (*arrow*) that remained clinically apparent. The carrying angle of the uninjured right elbow measured 5 degrees of valgus; the injured elbow had 10 degrees of varus. (From Wilkins KE. Residuals of elbow trauma in children. *Orthop Clin North Am.* 1990;21:289–312, with permission.)

cubitus varus is as high as 40%,[26,83] and the deformity seems to be as frequent after operative treatment as after nonoperative treatment.[71,83] The exact cause is not completely understood. It can be due to an inadequate reduction, growth stimulation of the lateral condylar physis from the fracture insult, or a combination of both (Fig. 16-15).[83] The cubitus varus deformity rarely is severe enough to cause concern or require further treatment, but, like lateral spur formation and stiffness, families should be warned of the risk of cubitus varus so that this common adverse outcome is not a surprise.

CUBITUS VALGUS

Cubitus valgus (not associated with nonunion) is much less common after united lateral condylar fractures than is cubitus varus. It has rarely been reported to result from premature epiphysiodesis of the lateral condylar physis.[95] As with cubitus varus, cubitus valgus usually is minimal and rarely of clinical or functional significance. If cubitus valgus is symptomatic, it can be treated with a medial closing wedge osteotomy or dome osteotomy and internal fixation or with osteotomy and gradual distraction through an external fixator.[68] The more difficult type of cubitus valgus is associated with nonunions.

PHYSEAL ARREST

Physeal arrest may merely be premature fusion of the various secondary ossification centers with little or no deformity. Because only 20% of humeral growth occurs in the distal physis, complete physeal arrest seldom causes any clinically significant angular or length deformities; however, partial physeal arrest may be the cause of cubitus valgus or fishtail deformity in some patients.

GROWTH DISTURBANCE: FISHTAIL DEFORMITY

Two types of "fishtail deformity" of the distal humerus may occur. The first is more common and is a sharp-angled wedge (Fig. 16-16). It is believed that this type of malformation is caused

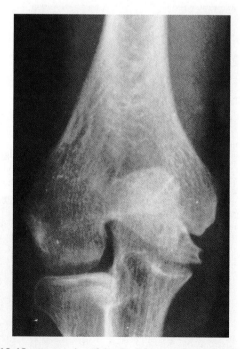

Figure 16-16. An angular "fishtail" deformity that persisted in this 14-year-old boy after operative treatment of a lateral condylar fracture, which occurred 6 years previously.

by persistence of a gap between the lateral condylar physis ossification center and the medial ossification of the trochlea.[95,100] Because of this gap, the lateral crista of the trochlea may be underdeveloped, which may represent a small "bony bar" in the distal humeral physis.[35] Thus, this may be both an articular malunion and minor growth disturbance problem. Despite some reports of loss of elbow motion and functional pain with this type of fishtail deformity,[54,95] most investigators[4,7,16,26] have not found this type of radiographic deformity to cause major functional deficiencies. Arthroscopic debridement of the articular flap has been used in symptomatic individuals.[97] The second type of fishtail deformity is a gentler, smoother curve. It is believed to be associated with osteonecrosis or larger growth arrest of the lateral part of the medial crista of the trochlea.[57]

OSTEONECROSIS

Osteonecrosis of the condylar fragment may be iatrogenic and is most commonly associated with the extensive dissection necessary to effect a late reduction or from loss of the blood supply at the time of injury.[34,38,53] Partial osteonecrosis has been described in an essentially nondisplaced fracture of the lateral condylar physis that had a radiographic appearance and clinical course similar to those of osteochondritis dissecans.[100] Osteonecrosis is rare in fractures of the lateral condylar physis that receive little or no initial treatment and result in nonunion.[38,101]

Overly vigorous dissection of fresh fractures can result in osteonecrosis of either the lateral condylar ossification center[26,64] (Fig. 16-17) or, rarely, the metaphyseal portion of

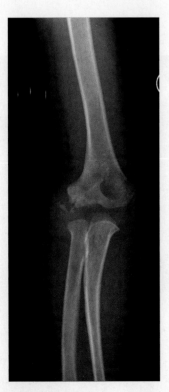

Figure 16-17. Radiographic appearance of capitellar fragment osteonecrosis 6 months after open reduction and internal fixation of a severely displaced lateral condylar fragment; extensive surgical dissection and multiple reduction attempts were the likely cause.

the fragment, leading to nonunion (Fig. 16-18). If the fracture unites, osteonecrosis of the lateral condyle reossifies over many years, much like Legg–Calvé–Perthes disease in the hip. Residual deformity can result in loss of motion, deformity, and/or pain. Central osteonecrosis that is extensive can be quite problematic; the proximal forearm subluxes into the defect resulting in bony impingement, osteochondral injury, loss of motion, and pain. There is no complete anatomic solution. Growth arrest of the columns to lessen deformity progression and arthroscopic debridement of loose bodies have been used with positive short-term results.[31]

NEUROLOGIC COMPLICATIONS

Neurologic complications can be divided into two categories: acute nerve problems at the time of the injury and/or treatment and delayed neuropathy involving the ulnar nerve (the so-called tardy ulnar nerve palsy).

Acute Nerve Injuries

Reports of acute nerve injuries associated with this injury are rare. McDonnell and Wilson[53] reported a case of transient radial nerve paralysis after an acute injury. Smith and Joyce,[82] reported two patients with posterior interosseous nerve injury after open reductions of the lateral condylar fragment, both of whom recovered spontaneously.

Tardy Ulnar Nerve Palsy

Tardy ulnar nerve palsy is a well-known late complication of fractures of the lateral condylar physis, especially after the development of cubitus valgus from malunion or nonunion of fractures of the lateral condylar physis.[29] The symptoms usually are gradual in onset. Motor loss occurs first, with sensory changes developing somewhat later.[29] The average interval of onset of symptoms has been reported as long as two decades from the time of injury. Various treatment methods have been advocated, ranging from anterior transposition of the ulnar nerve (originally the most commonly used procedure) to simple in situ decompression of the cubital tunnel. We prefer subcutaneous anterior transposition of the nerve. As noted in the following nonunion section, there are times when the nerve surgery is part of a more extensive reconstruction.

MALUNION

If not properly reduced and stabilized, the fragment can unite in an undesirable position. Cubitus valgus has been reported to occur as a result of malunion of the fracture fragments.[95] Malunion can result in the development of a bifid lateral condyle that may not be symptomatic if the malalignment is minor (Fig. 16-19). However, more severe articular malunion is problematic short and long term. Late osteotomy is complicated but can improve the situation if there is marked articular malalignment, loss of motion, and pain.[6,103]

DELAYED UNION AND NONUNION

Some of these fractures may go unrecognized or untreated for a prolonged period. Even in modern medical settings, elbow

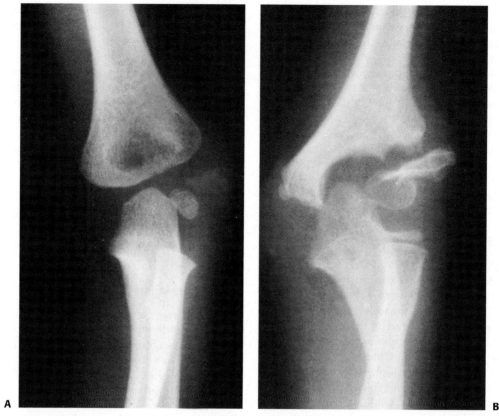

Figure 16-18. Osteonecrosis and nonunion developed in this child after extensive dissection and difficulty in obtaining a primary open reduction. **A:** Injury film. **B:** Two years later, there was extensive bone loss in the metaphysis and a nonunion of the condyle.

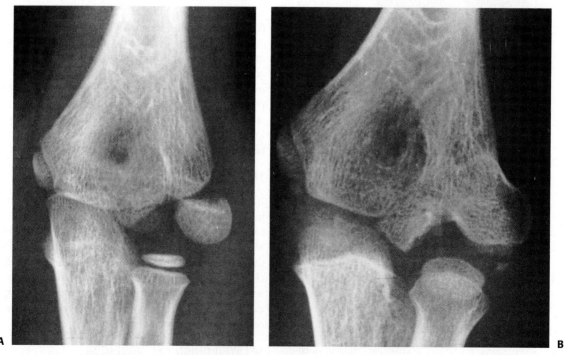

Figure 16-19. A: Injury film of a 7 year old who sustained a fracture of the capitellum that spared the trochlea and was treated with cast immobilization alone. **B:** Radiograph taken 2 years later showed complete fusion of the condylar epiphysis to the metaphysis, with the development of a "bifid" condyle.

injuries may be treated as "sprains," and the diagnosis of a displaced lateral condylar fracture is not made, especially in young children. Thus, patients can present weeks later with a delayed union or months or even years later with a nonunited or malunited fracture fragment.

Delayed Union

Delayed union, in contrast to nonunion or malunion, occurs in a fracture in which the fracture fragments are in satisfactory position but union of the lateral condylar fragment to the metaphysis is delayed. Various reasons have been suggested for delayed union of lateral condylar fractures, including poor circulation to the metaphyseal fragment[23] and bathing of the fracture site by articular fluid, which inhibits fibrin formation and subsequent callus formation.[33] It is most likely that a combination of these two factors, in addition to the constant tension forces exerted by the extensor musculature arising from the condylar fragment, is responsible for delayed union.

This complication is most common in patients treated nonoperatively. The symptoms and clinical examination determine the appropriate treatment. If on clinical examination the fragment is stable, the elbow is nontender, the range of elbow motion increases progressively, and the position of the fragment remains unchanged on radiographs, the fracture usually heals (Fig. 16-20). Lateral spur formation or cubitus varus is relatively common with these late healing fractures. The need for further treatment depends on the presence of significant symptoms, limited motion, or risk of further displacement that may disrupt the joint surface and cause functional impairment. If there is any question as to the integrity of the joint surface, an MRI or arthrogram may help determine any loss of continuity and the need for surgical treatment.

Most minimally displaced fractures will ultimately unite with long-term immobilization.[23,34] Percutaneous pinning or

screw fixation can expedite the healing. For fractures treated with initial surgical management, delayed healing is more likely if there is residual displacement of more than 1 mm after fixation or if longer-than-usual intraoperative fluoroscopy time was required for reduction.[72]

Controversy exists as to whether elbow function can be improved by a late open reduction and internal fixation of the malaligned fracture fragment with delayed union. Delayed open reduction (more than 3 weeks after injury) has a risk of osteonecrosis and further loss of elbow motion.[16,38,88,105] As previously discussed, osteonecrosis of the fragment is believed to result from the extensive soft tissue dissection necessary to replace the fragment anatomically (Fig. 16-21). The key to preventing osteonecrosis is recognition of the course of the blood supply to the lateral condyle. Only a small portion of the condyle is extra-articular, and the vessels that supply the lateral condylar epiphysis penetrate the condyle in a small posterior nonarticular area.[33] Careful late open reduction through a lateral approach generally is recommended to prevent displaced, painful nonunion and/or malunion.

Nonunion

True nonunion occurs most commonly in patients with progressive displacement of the fragment following initiation of nonoperative treatment or in patients with late presentation of a displaced fracture. If the fracture is displaced and is not united by 12 weeks, it is considered a nonunion.[22,23]

Nonunion can occur with or without angular deformity. Many patients with nonunions and minimal fragment displacement have no angulation and remain relatively asymptomatic for many activities of daily living (Fig. 16-22). Weakness or pain can occur when the arm is used for high-performance activities. Because they are not significantly displaced, these fractures often can be stabilized with minimal extra-articular dissection

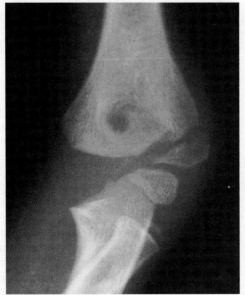
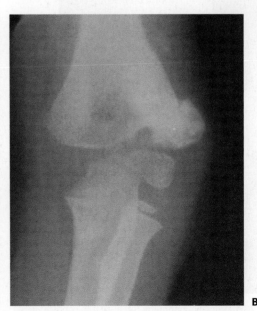

A   **B**

Figure 16-20. Delayed union and cubitus varus. **A:** Stage III lateral condylar fracture in a 7-year-old boy was treated in a cast. **B:** Seven months later, delayed union with malunion of the fracture and cubitus varus deformity was present.

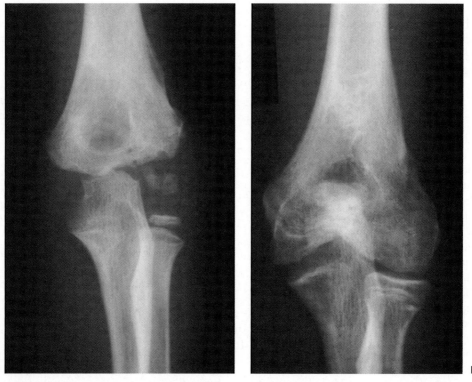

A   B

Figure 16-21. Osteonecrosis of the lateral condyle after lateral condylar fracture in a 10-year-old boy. Early (**A**) and long-term (**B**) follow-up.

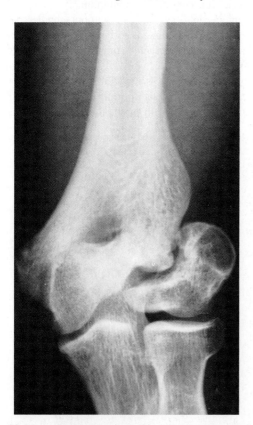

Figure 16-22. Asymptomatic nonunion of a lateral condyle in a 19-year-old military recruit. Because the patient had a completely normal and asymptomatic range of motion in his nondominant extremity, operative stabilization two not thought to be necessary.

using a combination of screw fixation and a laterally placed bone graft.

Nonunion with subsequent fragment displacement is more common after nonoperative treatment of unstable fractures with stages II and III displacement (Fig. 16-23). If the fragment is mobile, it tends to migrate proximally with a subsequent valgus elbow deformity. Nonunion can lead to a cubitus valgus deformity, which in turn, is associated with the development of tardy ulnar nerve palsy (Fig. 16-24). All of these nonunions have articular incongruity.

Nonunion seems to occur when the distal fragment is displaced enough to allow the condylar fragment's cartilaginous articular surface to oppose the bony surface of the humeral metaphysis. In such a situation, union is impossible. Stable internal fixation with percutaneously placed pins or cannulated screws has been recommended for impending, minimally displaced nonunions.[22,63] For late displaced nonunions, staged procedures have been described[63]: (1) ulnar nerve transposition and bone grafting and fixation in situ of the lateral condyle, followed by (2) distal humeral osteotomy to correct angulation once the nonunion is healed and elbow range of motion is regained.

The most common sequela of nonunion with displacement is the development of a progressive cubitus valgus deformity. The fragment migrates both proximally and laterally, producing not only an angular deformity but also lateral translocation of the proximal radius and ulna (Fig. 16-24). Lateral translocation is not as likely to develop in the more lateral type of these fractures because the lateral crista of the trochlea is intact (Fig. 16-25).

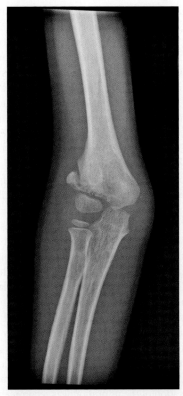

Figure 16-23. Minimally displaced lateral condylar fracture was treated nonoperatively and lost to follow-up. Patient returned 6 months later with a displaced nonunion.

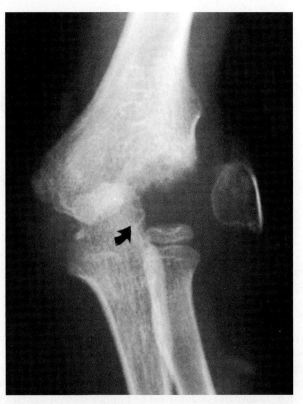

Figure 16-25. Nonunion without translocation. Despite nonunion, elbow stability was maintained because the lateral crista of the trochlea had remained intact (*arrow*). Valgus angulation also developed.

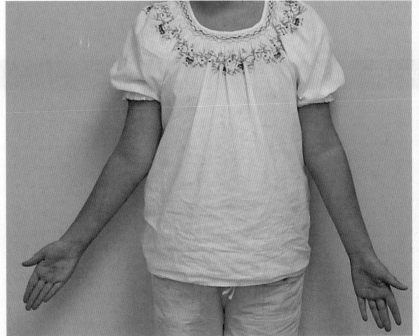

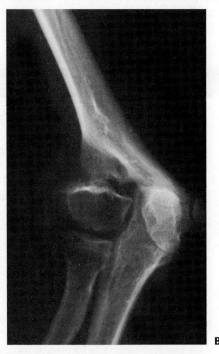

A   **B**

Figure 16-24. A: An 11-year-old girl with cubitus valgus resulting from a fracture of the lateral condylar physis with nonunion. **B:** Nonunion with cubitus valgus. Radiograph showing both angulation and translocation secondary to nonunion of the condylar fragment.

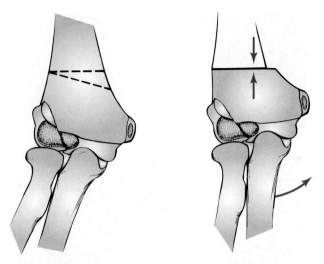

Figure 16-26. With fracture through the capitellum sparing the trochlea, an angular deformity can be corrected with a closing wedge osteotomy.

Surgical treatment of the nonunion deformity of the lateral condylar fragment is difficult and requires correcting two problems. First, articular cartilage of the displaced fragment may be opposing the distal humeral metaphysis, with resulting articular incongruity. Restoring articular alignment in this situation can be challenging and may not be possible without significant risk of osteonecrosis that comes with the extensive soft tissue dissection required to mobilize the fragment. The second problem is correcting the long-standing valgus angular deformity (Fig. 16-26).

To prevent progression of cubitus valgus deformity and subsequent ulnar nerve dysfunction, Shimada et al.[76] recommended osteosynthesis for nonunion of lateral humeral condylar fractures in children because union is easily achieved, the range of motion is maintained, ulnar nerve function remains intact, and remodeling of the articular surfaces can be expected. They noted that bone grafting is essential to bridge the defect, to obtain congruity of the joint, and to promote union; damage to the blood supply should be avoided to prevent osteonecrosis. To avoid the development of osteonecrosis after delayed open reduction and internal fixation of acute fractures, Wattenbarger et al.[98] accepted malreduction rather than stripping the soft tissue off the lateral condylar fragment to achieve a more anatomic reduction. For fractures with more than 1 cm of displacement, the position of the fragment often was improved very little by surgery, but all fractures were united, alignment of the arm was good, and no child had developed osteonecrosis at an average 6-year follow-up.

Tien et al.[93] described a technique that includes in situ compression fixation of the lateral condylar nonunion and a dome-shaped supracondylar osteotomy of the distal humerus through a single posterior incision. They recommended this procedure for minimally displaced, established lateral condylar nonunions with a cubitus valgus deformity of 20 degrees or more, especially when the deformity is progressing, is complicated by a concurrent ulnar neuropathy, or is in a patient with elbow instability or elbow pain during sports activities. They listed as a contraindication to the procedure a lateral condylar nonunion associated with radiographic evidence of prominent displacement and rotation. In situ fixation of the nonunion was recommended because the extensive soft tissue stripping required for mobilization and reduction of the fracture fragments results in devascularization of the fragment, which can cause osteonecrosis, loss of motion, and persistent nonunion. Another study recommended fixation for in situ displaced nonunions,[65] touting good functional results, but cosmetic varus and valgus malalignment was common, necessitating corrective osteotomy in some.

Authors' Preferred Treatment of Nonunion (Algorithm 16-2)

We distinguish between fractures seen late (2 to 12 weeks after injury) and established nonunions (usually from 3 months to several years after injury).[80] In all late-presenting fractures, we strive to obtain fracture union without loss of elbow motion and try to avoid osteonecrosis of the lateral condyle through a careful open reduction and internal fixation.

Treating an established nonunion of a lateral humeral condylar fracture poses a more difficult dilemma. If no treatment is rendered, a progressive cubitus valgus deformity may occur with growth. Patients usually are asymptomatic initially, except for those with high-demand athletic or labor activities. A mild flexion contracture of the elbow is present, but the cubitus valgus deformity initially can be more aesthetic than functional. The danger in this approach is failure to recognize that late deformity and tardy ulnar nerve palsy can occur. If surgery is performed for an established nonunion, the potential risks of osteonecrosis and loss of elbow motion must be carefully considered. We believe the criteria outlined by Flynn et al.[22,23] are helpful in determining if surgical treatment is appropriate for an established nonunion:

- A large metaphyseal fragment
- Displacement of less than 1 cm from the joint surface
- An open, viable lateral condylar physis

It is also helpful to distinguish between three distinct clinical situations. First, for an established nonunion with a large metaphyseal fragment, minimal migration, and an open lateral condylar physis, we recommend modified open reduction, screw fixation, and a lateral extra-articular bone graft. This technique is markedly different from the surgical treatment of an acute lateral condylar fracture. The metaphyseal fragment of the lateral condyle and the distal humeral metaphysis are exposed, but no attempt is made to anatomically realign the articular surface. Intra-articular dissection and posterior dissection should be avoided to help prevent osteonecrosis and any further loss of elbow motion. The metaphyseal fragments

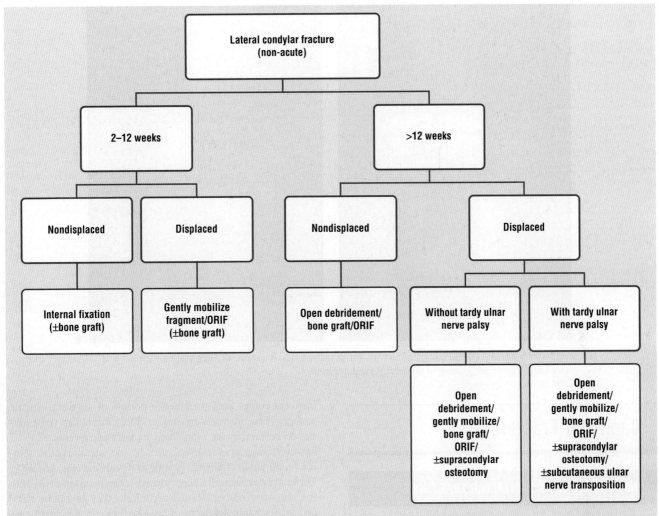

Algorithm 16-2. Authors' preferred treatment of nonunion.

are debrided by gently removing any interposed fibrous tissue. The lateral condylar fragment usually can be moved distally a small distance for improved apposition and alignment. The metaphyseal fragments are firmly apposed, and a screw is used to fix the fragments with interfragmentary compression. Bone graft can be placed between the metaphyseal fragments before compression and then laterally after fixation. The elbow is immobilized in 80 to 90 degrees of flexion until motion is no longer a risk for displacement (Fig. 16-27).

Second, in patients with a nonunion who have aesthetic concerns because of their malalignment but no functional complaints, treatment is similar to that for cubitus varus deformity after a supracondylar humeral fracture. If the patient and family desire, a supracondylar osteotomy can be performed.[52] Rigid internal fixation should be used if possible to allow early motion.

Third, patients with asymptomatic nonunion, cubitus valgus deformity, and symptomatic tardy ulnar nerve palsy can be treated with anterior transposition of the ulnar nerve; however, isolated ulnar nerve transposition rarely is done alone and usually is done in conjunction with corrective osteotomy.

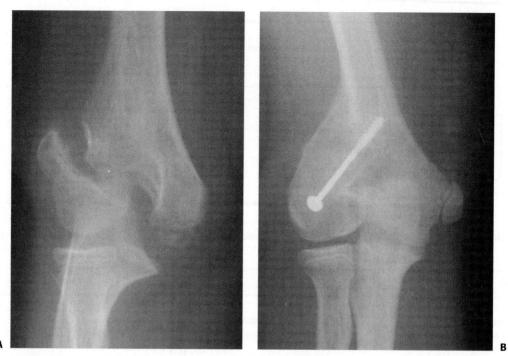

Figure 16-27.   A: Established nonunion with a large metaphyseal fragment. **B:** After fixation with a cancellous screw and bone grafting of the metaphyseal fragment.

Capitellar Fractures

INTRODUCTION TO CAPITELLAR FRACTURES

Fractures of the capitellum involve only the true articular surface of the lateral condyle. This includes, in some instances, the articular surface of the lateral crista of the trochlea. Generally, this fragment comes from the anterior portion of the distal articular surface. These fractures are rare in children.[51] When these injuries do occur, they are more likely in older adolescents[27,40,49,51,62]; however, anterior sleeve fractures of the lateral condyle have been reported in children as young as 8 years old (Fig. 16-28).[2,17] These anterior sleeve fractures involve a good portion of the anterior articular surface, although technically they are not be classified as pure capitellar fractures because they contain nonarticular epicondylar and metaphyseal portions in the fragment.

Capitellar fractures often are difficult to diagnose because there is little ossified tissue. The fragment is composed mainly

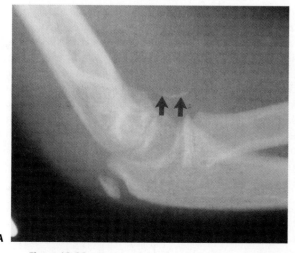
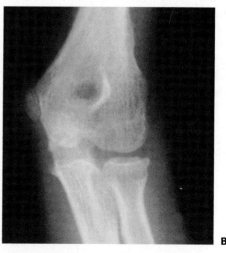

Figure 16-28.   Fracture of the capitellum. **A:** Osteochondral fracture of the capitellum in an 8-year-old girl. Note the small fleck of bone (*arrows*), which indicates possible osteochondral fragment. **B:** Healed fracture with articular congruity, restoration of cartilage space, and no osteonecrosis. (Reprinted with permission from Drvaric DM, Rooks MD. Anterior sleeve fracture of the capitellum. *J Orthop Trauma.* 1990;4(2):188–192.)

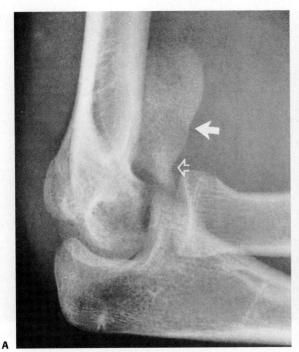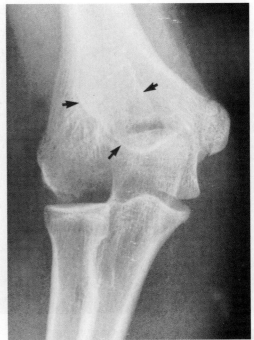

Figure 16-29. Fracture of the capitellum in a 13-year-old girl. **A:** Injury film, lateral view, shows the large capitellar fragment lying anterior and proximal to the distal humerus. Both the radiocapitellar (*solid arrow*) and trochlear grooves (*open arrow*) are seen in the fragment. **B:** In the AP view, only a faint outline of the fragment is seen (*arrows*).

of pure articular surface from the capitellum and essentially nonossified cartilage from the secondary ossification center of the lateral condyle.

CLASSIFICATION OF CAPITELLAR FRACTURES

Two fracture patterns have been described. The first is the more common Hahn–Steinthal type,[91] which usually contains a rather large portion of cancellous bone of the lateral condyle. The lateral crista of the trochlea also is often included (Fig. 16-29). The second, or Kocher–Lorenz, type is more of a pure articular fracture with little, if any, subchondral bone attached and may represent a piece of articular cartilage from an underlying osteochondritis dissecans. This type of fracture is rare in children.[2,84] Most recently, Murthy et al.[59] proposed a classification system to guide treatment: type I (anterior shear), nondisplaced (1A) or displaced (1B); type II (posterolateral shear), often associated with elbow dislocations; and type III, acute chondral shear injuries.

MECHANISMS OF INJURY FOR CAPITELLAR FRACTURES

The most commonly accepted mechanism is shearing of the anterior articular surface of the lateral condyle by the radial head.[27] The presence of cubitus hyperextension or cubitus valgus seems to predispose the elbow to this fracture pattern. Because the mechanism is postulated to be a pushing off of the capitellum by the radial head, it stands to reason that there may be an associated radial head or neck fracture[40]; associated injuries of the proximal radius were reported in 31% of adults and children with capitellar fractures.[62] Elbow dislocations are clearly causative, especially with posterolateral shear fractures.[59]

ASSESSMENT OF CAPITELLAR FRACTURES

Often, swelling is minimal, and the presence of the fragment restricts flexion. If the fragment is large, it may be readily apparent on a lateral radiograph (Fig. 16-30). On an AP radiograph, however, the fragment may be obliterated by the overlying distal metaphysis (see Fig. 16-29B). If the fragment is small, it often is difficult to see on plain radiographs. Oblique views may be necessary to show the fragment. A high index of suspicion is needed to make the diagnosis. In younger children, arthrography or MRI may be required to diagnose this rare fracture. Often, CT or MRI scans are used to confirm the diagnosis and plan operative fixation.

TREATMENT OPTIONS FOR CAPITELLAR FRACTURES

Nondisplaced fractures can be treated closed with immobilization, especially nondisplaced anterior shear fractures.[59] Excising the fragment and open reduction and reattachment are the two most common forms of treatment. Closed reduction is not likely to be successful as the fracture often is not reducible or is unstable after reduction.

Excision of the Fragment

The fragment can be excised through an open arthrotomy. Excision can be successful in very young patients, late-presenting small fractures, and osteochondritis dissecans lesions that no longer fit back in place.[27,51] In these circumstances, motion and rehabilitation can be initiated early. Even when large fragments are excised, joint instability does not appear to be a problem.[27]

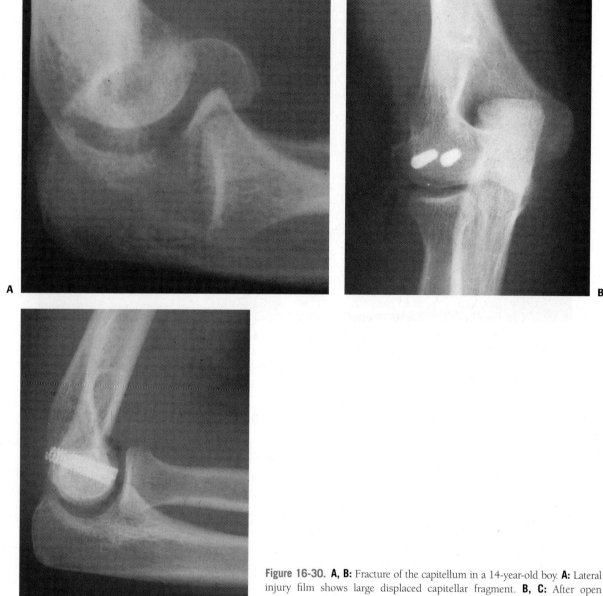

Figure 16-30. A, B: Fracture of the capitellum in a 14-year-old boy. **A:** Lateral injury film shows large displaced capitellar fragment. **B, C:** After open reduction and fixation with two small cannulated screws through a lateral approach.

However, currently, acute chondral fractures (type III) are most often repaired with bioabsorbable nails or buried interosseous screws. If excised, microfracture is added. In patients in whom treatment is delayed, although the results are not as good as when treatment is provided immediately after injury, improvement in function can be expected, even with late excision. In poor late results, osteoarticular transplant (OATS) is considered for reconstruction.

Reattachment of the Fragment

A large shear fracture fragment (types I and II) in an older child or adolescent is indicative of an intra-articular fracture, for which reduction is recommended. The stability of the fracture is provided by wires or screws inserted through the posterior surface of the lateral condyle. The major risk of open reduction and internal fixation is osteonecrosis of the reattached fragment. Satisfactory results have been reported with fixation with K-wires, Herbert screws, cannulated screws,[44] compression screws,[18,19] and even sutures.[84] An advantage of interosseous compression screw fixation is that it may not require later removal and allows earlier motion. Advantages cited for suture fixation include a low risk of growth arrest, sufficient stability to allow immediate postoperative motion, avoidance of implant removal, and facilitation of the acquisition of high-quality postoperative MR images to evaluate healing.

Authors' Preferred Treatment for Capitellar Fractures (Algorithm 16-3)

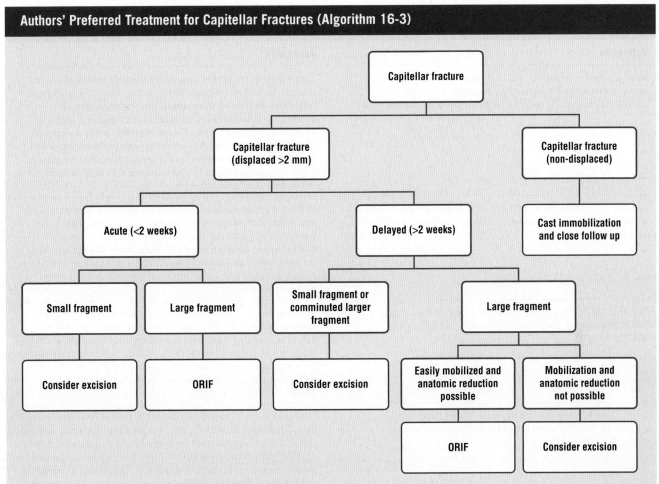

Algorithm 16-3. Authors' preferred treatment for capitellar fractures.

If the fragment is large, if the fracture is acute, and if an anatomic reduction can be achieved with a minimum of open manipulation or dissection, we prefer to reattach the fragment with two small cannulated screws inserted from posterior to anterior through a lateral approach if enough bone is present in the capitellar fragment to engage the screw threads. If the amount of bone in the capitellar fragment is limited, the screws can be placed from anterior to posterior, in which case, countersunk, headless screws are preferred. If the fracture is old, if there is any comminution of the fragment, or if there is little bone in which to engage the screw threads, we excise the fragment, perform microfracture of the bony surface, and start early motion.

MANAGEMENT OF EXPECTED ADVERSE OUTCOMES AND UNEXPECTED COMPLICATIONS RELATED TO CAPITELLAR FRACTURES

The major complication is osteonecrosis of the fragment. This occurs only in fractures in which the capitellar fragment is retained. Posttraumatic degenerative arthritis can occur whether the fragments are excised or retained. Many patients who are treated operatively or nonoperatively can expect to lose some range of motion, but this loss is not always of functional or aesthetic significance. It is important to emphasize to the parents before the onset of treatment that some motion may be lost regardless of the treatment method. Late reconstruction with OATS may be an option in very poor results.

Annotated References

Reference	Annotation
Bauer AS, Bae DS, Brustowicz KA, et al. Intra-articular corrective osteotomy of humeral lateral condyle malunions in children: early clinical and radiographic results. *J Pediatr Orthop*. 2013;33(1):20–25.	Lateral humeral condylar malunions are relatively uncommon. When present, the treatment is controversial. In this report of seven patients with elbow dysfunction due to lateral condylar malunions, the investigators describe their surgical technique, which includes intra-articular corrective osteotomy. They recommend careful preservations of soft-tissue attachments to preserve the capitellar blood supply and suggest that Milch I fractures (those that extend lateral to the trochlea) might be more appropriate for this technique than Milch II fractures (those that extend into the trochlea).
Bernthal NM, Hoshino CM, Dichter D, et al. Recovery of elbow motion following pediatric lateral condylar fractures of the humerus. *J Bone Joint Surg Am*. 2011;93(9):871–877.	In this prospective study of 141 lateral humeral condylar fractures, the total arc of elbow motion was limited in patients treated operatively for the first 18 weeks after injury as compared to those treated nonoperatively; however, beyond 18 weeks, range of motion between the two groups was statistically similar. Older patients with more severe injuries and those with longer periods of immobilization recovered motion more slowly.
Das De S, Bae DS, Waters PM. Displaced humeral lateral condyle fractures in children: should we bury the pins? *J Pediatr Orthop*. 2012;32:573–578.	In a series of 235 children treated with smooth pins, 41 (17%) had exposed pins and 194 (83%) had buried pins. While there was no difference in healing rates, there was a higher rate of superficial wound infection with exposed pins (9.8% vs. 3.1%); however, buried pins had an overall higher complication rate including implant migration, skin breakdown, and pain. The mean cost savings for exposed pins was $3,442.
Gay JR, Love JG. Diagnosis and treatment of tardy paralysis of the ulnar nerve; based on a study of 100 cases. *J Bone Joint Surg Am*. 1947;29(4):1087–1097.	This "classic" article presents a series of 100 cases of tardy ulnar nerve palsy, 57 of which were attributed to sequelae of an "old fracture of the elbow." The authors discussed the diagnosis of the condition and the need for "prophylaxis" to identify and treat these injuries in childhood to prevent the progressive palsy. In this review, the authors also present 10 detailed case reports and discuss eight possible surgical treatments for this condition. The most common surgical technique used in this patient population was anterior transposition of the ulnar nerve.
Gilbert SR, MacLennan PA, Schlitz RS, et al. Screw versus pin fixation with open reduction of pediatric lateral condyle fractures. *J Pediatr Orthop B*. 2016;25:148–152.	Forty-three patients with displaced lateral condyle fractures fixed with pins were compared to 43 with displaced fractures fixed with screws. Screw fixation led to a lower rate of nonunion (0) and faster return to motion. Screw fixation did require a second operative procedure to remove the screw.
Koh KH, Seo SW, Kim KM, et al. Clinical and radiographic results of lateral condylar fracture of distal humerus in children. *J Pediatr Orthop*. 2010;30(5):425–429.	A review of 175 patients with longer than 1 year of follow-up demonstrated that union can be reliably achieved with a variety of treatment options, and clinical outcomes are generally good. Cubitus varus and lateral overgrowth (spurring) were the most common residual deformities. Lateral spurring was more common with type 3 fractures and in those requiring ORIF.
Pennock AT, Salgueiro L, Upasani VV, et al. Closed reduction and percutaneous pinning versus open reduction and internal fixation for type II lateral condyle humerus fractures in children displaced >2 mm. *J Pediatr Orthop*. 2016;36:780–786.	A retrospective comparison of 74 patients treated with closed reduction and percutaneous pinning and open reduction internal fixation found that, while the time to union was the same in both groups, patients treated with closed reduction and pinning had shorter operating room times and lower complication rates than those treated with open reduction and internal fixation.
Pribaz JR, Bernthal NM, Wong TC, et al. Lateral spurring (overgrowth) after pediatric lateral condyle fractures. *J Pediatr Orthop*. 2012;32(5):456–460.	Retrospective analysis of 212 consecutive lateral condylar fractures revealed that lateral spurring, defined as "an overgrowth of bone over the lateral aspect of the lateral condyle resulting in an irregularity of the metaphyseal flare," is extremely common after lateral humeral condylar fractures in children regardless of fracture type or treatment modality. Final outcome seems to be unaffected by the presence of the spurring aside from cosmetic concerns.

Annotated References

Reference	Annotation
Song KS, Kang CH, Min BW, et al. Closed reduction and internal fixation of displaced unstable lateral condylar fractures of the humerus. *J Bone Joint Surg Am.* 2008;90:2673–2681.	Pediatric lateral condyle fractures that were classified into five groups based on fracture pattern and displacement were used to develop a treatment algorithm. The use of the internal oblique radiograph provides the most accurate assessment of displacement. A prospective study of 63 unstable fractures was performed using this algorithm and found displaced fractures can be reduced closed and recommended open reduction and internal fixation if there was >2 mm residual displacement after attempted closed reduction.
Weiss JM, Graves S, Yang S, et al. A new classification system predictive of complications in surgically treated pediatric humeral lateral condyle fractures. *J Pediatr Orthop.* 2009;29:602–605.	The authors developed a classification system based on the amount of fracture displacement. They found that patients with >2-mm displacement with a disrupted cartilaginous hinge (type III fractures) had a threefold higher complication rate than those with >2-mm displacement and an intact cartilaginous hinge (type II fractures) as demonstrated on arthrogram.

REFERENCES

1. Adams JE. Injury to the throwing arm. A study of traumatic changes in the elbow joints of boy baseball players. *Calif Med.* 1965;102:127–132.
2. Agins HJ, Marcus NW. Articular cartilage sleeve fracture of the lateral humeral condyle capitellum: a previously undescribed entity. *J Pediatr Orthop.* 1984;4:620–622.
3. Albright JA, Jokl P, Shaw R, et al. Clinical studies of baseball players: correlation of injury to throwing arm with method of delivery. *Am J Sports Med.* 1978;6:15–21.
4. Badelon O, Bensahel H, Mazda K, et al. Lateral humeral condylar fractures in children: a report of 47 cases. *J Pediatr Orthop.* 1988;8:31–34.
5. Bast SC, Hoffer MM, Aval S. Nonoperative treatment for minimally and nondisplaced lateral humeral condyle fractures in children. *J Pediatr Orthop.* 1998;18:448–450.
6. Bauer AS, Bae DS, Brustowicz KA, et al. Intra-articular corrective osteotomy of humeral lateral condyle malunions in children: early clinical and radiographic results. *J Pediatr Orthop.* 2013;33:20–25.
7. Beaty JH, Wood AB. Fractures of the lateral humeral condyle in children. *Paper Presented at the Annual Meeting of the American Academy of Orthopaedic Surgeons.* Las Vegas, NV: 1985.
8. Bernthal NM, Hoshino CM, Dichter D, et al. Recovery of elbow motion following pediatric lateral condylar fractures of the humerus. *J Bone Joint Surg Am.* 2011;93:871–877.
9. Blount WP, Schulz I, Cassidy RH. Fractures of the elbow in children. *JAMA.* 1951;146:699–704.
10. Böhler L. *The Treatment of Fractures.* New York: Grune & Stratton; 1956.
11. Burnier M, Buisson G, Ricard A, et al. Diagnostic value of ultrasonography in elbow trauma in children: prospective study of 34 cases. *Orthop Traumatol Surg Res.* 2016;102:839–843.
12. Chessare JW, Rogers LF, White H, et al. Injuries of the medial epicondyle ossification center of the humerus. *AJR Am J Roentgenol.* 1977;129:49–55.
13. Conner AN, Smith MG. Displaced fractures of lateral humeral condyle in children. *J Bone Joint Surg Br.* 1970;52:460–464.
14. Das De S, Bae DS, Waters PM. Displaced humeral lateral condyle fractures in children: should we bury the pins? *J Pediatr Orthop.* 2012;32:573–578.
15. DeLee JC, Wilkins KE, Rogers LF, et al. Fracture separation of the distal humeral epiphysis. *J Bone Joint Surg Am.* 1980;67:46–51.
16. Dhillon KS, Sengupta S, Singh BJ. Delayed management of fracture of the lateral humeral condyle in children. *Acta Orthop Scand.* 1988;59:419–424.
17. Drvaric DM, Rooks MD. Anterior sleeve fracture of the capitellum. *J Orthop Trauma.* 1990;4:188–192.
18. Elkowitz SJ, Kubiak EN, Polatsch D, et al. Comparison of two headless screw designs for fixation of capitellum fractures. *Bull Hosp Jt Dis.* 2003;61:123–126.
19. Elkowitz SJ, Polatsch DB, Egol KA, et al. Capitellum fractures: a biomechanical evaluation of three fixation methods. *J Orthop Trauma.* 2002;16:503–506.
20. Fahey JJ, O'Brien ET. Fracture-separation of the medial humeral condyle in a child confused with fracture of the medial epicondyle. *J Bone Joint Surg Am.* 1971;53:1102–1104.
21. Finnbogason T, Karlsson G, Lindberg L, et al. Nondisplaced and minimally displaced fractures of the lateral humeral condyle in children: a prospective radiographic investigation of fracture stability. *J Pediatr Orthop.* 1995;15:422–425.
22. Flynn JC, Richards JF Jr. Nonunion of minimally displaced fractures of the lateral condyle of humerus in children. *J Bone Joint Surg Am.* 1971;53:1096–1101.
23. Flynn JC, Richards JF Jr, Saltzman RI. Prevention and treatment of nonunion of slightly displaced fractures of the lateral humeral condyle in children. *J Bone Joint Surg Am.* 1975;57:1087–1092.
24. Fontanetta P, Mackenzie DA, Rosman M. Missed, maluniting, and malunited fractures of the lateral humeral condyle in children. *J Trauma.* 1978;18:329–335.
25. Fornari ED, Suszter M, Roocroft J, et al. Childhood obesity as a risk factor for lateral condyle fractures over supracondylar humerus fractures. *Clin Orthop Relat Res.* 2013;471:1193–1198.
26. Foster DE, Sullivan JA, Gross RH. Lateral humeral condylar fractures in children. *J Pediatr Orthop.* 1985;5:16–22.
27. Fowles JV, Kassab MT. Fracture of the capitulum humeri, treatment by excision. *J Bone Joint Surg Am.* 1974;56:794–798.
28. Fowles JV, Kassab MT. Displaced fracture of medial humeral condyle in children. *J Bone Joint Surg Am.* 1980;62:1159–1163.
29. Gay JR, Love JG. Diagnosis and treatment of tardy paralysis of the ulnar nerve. *J Bone Joint Surg.* 1947;29:1087–1097.
30. Gilbert SR, MacLennan PA, Schlitz RS, et al. Screw versus pin fixation with open reduction of pediatric lateral condyle fractures. *J Pediatr Orthop B.* 2016;25:148–152.
31. Glotzbecker MP, Bae DS, Links AC, et al. Fishtail deformity of the distal humerus: a report of 15 cases. *J Pediatr Orthop.* 2013;33:592–597.
32. Griffith JF, Roebuck DJ, Cheng JC, et al. Acute elbow trauma in children: spectrum of injury revealed by MR imaging not apparent on radiographs. *AJR Am J Roentgenol.* 2001;176:53–60.
33. Haraldsson S. Osteochondrosis deformans juvenilis capituli humeri including investigation of intra-osseous vasculature in distal humerus. *Acta Orthop Scand Suppl.* 1959;38:1–232.
34. Hardacre JA, Nahigian SH, Froimson AI, et al. Fracture of the lateral condyle of humerus in children. *J Bone Joint Surg Am.* 1971;53:1083–1095.
35. Herring JA, Fitch RD. Lateral condylar fracture of the elbow. *J Pediatr Orthop.* 1986;6:724–727.
36. Horn BD, Herman MJ, Crisci K, et al. Fractures of the lateral humeral condyle: role of the cartilage hinge in fracture stability. *J Pediatr Orthop.* 2002;22:8–11.
37. Houshian S, Mehdi B, Larsen MS. The epidemiology of elbow fracture in children: analysis of 355 fractures, with special reference to supracondylar humerus fractures. *J Orthop Sci.* 2001;6:312–315.
38. Jakob R, Fowles JV, Rang M, et al. Observations concerning fractures of the lateral humeral condyles in children. *J Bone Joint Surg Br.* 1975;57(4):430–436.
39. Jeffrey CC. Nonunion of epiphysis of the lateral condyle of the humerus. *J Bone Joint Surg Br.* 1958;40:396–405.
40. Johansson J, Rosman M. Fracture of the capitulum humeri in children: a rare injury, often misdiagnosed. *Clin Orthop Relat Res.* 1980;146:157–160.
41. Kang S, Park SS. Predisposing effect of elbow alignment on the elbow fracture type in children. *J Orthop Trauma.* 2015;29:3253–3258.
42. Koh SH, Seo SW, Kim KM, et al. Clinical and radiographic results of lateral condylar fracture of the distal humerus in children. *J Pediatr Orthop.* 2010;30:425–429.
43. Landin LA, Danielsson LG. Elbow fractures in children. An epidemiological analysis of 589 cases. *Acta Orthop Scand.* 1986;57:309–312.
44. Letts M, Rumball K, Bauermeister S, et al. Fractures of the capitellum in adolescents. *J Pediatr Orthop.* 1997;17:315–320.
45. Levin H, Sangha G, Carey TP, et al. Fracture and nonaccidental injury: a case report of a lateral condylar fracture in a 13 months old. *Pediatr Emerg Care.* 2016;32:865–867.
46. Li WC, Xu RJ. Comparison of Kirschner wires and AO cannulated screw internal fixation for displaced lateral humeral condyle fracture in children. *Int Orthop.* 2012;36:1261–1266.
47. Liu CH, Kao HK, Lee WC, et al. Posterolateral approach for humeral lateral condyle fractures in children. *J Pediatr Orthop B.* 2016;25:153–158.
48. Liu TJ, Wang EB, Dai Q, et al. Open reduction and internal fixation for the treatment of fractures of the lateral humeral condyle with an early delayed presentation in children: a radiological and clinical prospective study. *Bone Joint J.* 2016;98-B:244–248.
49. Ma YZ, Zheng CB, Zhou TL, et al. Percutaneous probe reduction of frontal fractures of the humeral capitellum. *Clin Orthop Relat Res.* 1984;183:17–21.
50. Major NM, Crawford ST. Elbow effusions in trauma in adults and children: is there an occult fracture? *AJR Am J Roentgenol.* 2002;178:413–418.
51. Marion J, Faysse R. Fracture du capitellum. *Rev Chir Orthop.* 1962;48:484–490.

52. Masada K, Kawai H, Kawabata H, et al. Osteosynthesis for old, established nonunion of the lateral condyle of the humerus. *J Bone Joint Surg Am.* 1990;72:32–40.

53. McDonnell DP, Wilson JC. Fracture of the lower end of the humerus in children. *J Bone Joint Surg Am.* 1948;30:347–358.

54. Menkowitz M, Flynn JM. Floating elbow in an infant. *Orthopedics.* 2002;25:185–186.

55. Mintzer CM, Waters PM, Brown DJ, et al. Percutaneous pinning in the treatment of displaced lateral condyle fractures. *J Pediatr Orthop.* 1994;14:462–465.

56. Morin B, Fassier F, Poitras B, et al. Results of early surgical treatment of fractures of the lateral humeral condyle in children. *Rev Chir Orthop Reparatrice Appar Mot.* 1988;74:129–131.

57. Morrissey RT, Wilkins KE. Deformity following distal humeral fracture in childhood. *J Bone Joint Surg Am.* 1984;66(4):557–562.

58. Moucha CS, Mason DE. Distal humeral epiphyseal separation. *Am J Orthop.* 2003;32:497–500.

59. Murthy PG, Vuillermin C, Naqvi MN, et al. Capitellar fractures in children and adolescents: classification and early results of treatment. *J Bone Joint Surg Am.* 2017;99:1282–1290.

60. Nwakama AC, Peterson HA, Shaughnessy WJ. Fishtail deformity following fracture of the distal humerus in children: historical review, case presentations, discussion of etiology, and thoughts on treatment. *J Pediatr Orthop B.* 2000;9:309–318.

61. Ormsby NM, Walton RD, Robinson S, et al. Buried versus unburied Kirschner wires in the management of paediatric lateral condyle elbow fractures: a comparative study from a tertiary centre. *J Pediatr Orthop B.* 2016;25:69–73.

62. Palmer I. Open treatment of transcondylar T fracture of the humerus. *Acta Chir Scand.* 1961;121:486–490.

63. Papandrea R, Waters PM. Posttraumatic reconstruction of the elbow in the pediatric patient. *Clin Orthop Relat Res.* 2000;370:115–126.

64. Papavasiliou VA, Beslikas TA. Fractures of the lateral humeral condyle in children—an analysis of 39 cases. *Injury.* 1985;16:364–366.

65. Park H, Hwang JH, Kwon YU, et al. Osteosynthesis in situ for lateral condyle nonunion in children. *J Pediatr Orthop.* 2015;35:334–340.

66. Pennock AT, Salgueiro L, Upasani VV, et al. Closed reduction and percutaneous pinning versus open reduction and internal fixation for type II lateral condyle humerus fractures in children displaced >2 mm. *J Pediatr Orthop.* 2016;36:780–786.

67. Petit P, Sapin C, Henry G, et al. Rate of abnormal osteoarticular radiographic findings in pediatric patients. *Am J Roentgenol.* 2001;176:987–990.

68. Piskin A, Tomak Y, Sen C, et al. The management of cubitus varus and valgus using the Ilizarov method. *J Bone Joint Surg Br.* 2007;89:1615–1619.

69. Pribaz JR, Bernthal NM, Wong TC, et al. Lateral spurring (overgrowth) after pediatric lateral condyle fractures. *J Pediatr Orthop.* 2012;32:456–460.

70. Rovinsky D, Ferguson C, Younis A, et al. Pediatric elbow dislocations associated with a Milch type I lateral condyle fracture of the humerus. *J Orthop Trauma.* 1999;13:458–460.

71. Rutherford AJ. Fractures of the lateral humeral condyle in children. *J Bone Joint Surg Am.* 1985;67:851–856.

72. Salgueiro L, Roocroft JH, Bastrom TP, et al. Rate and risk factors for delayed healing following surgical treatment of lateral condyle humerus fractures in children. *J Pediatr Orthop.* 2017;37:1–6.

73. Salter RB, Harris WR. Injuries involving the epiphyseal plate. *J Bone Joint Surg.* 1963;45:587–632.

74. Schlitz RS, Schwertz JM, Eberhardt AW, et al. Biomechanical analysis of screws versus K-wires for lateral humeral condyle fractures. *J Pediatr Orthop.* 2015;35:e93–e97.

75. Sharma JC, Arora A, Mathur NC, et al. Lateral condylar fractures of the humerus in children: fixation with partially threaded 4.0-mm AO cancellous screws. *J Trauma.* 1995;39:1129–1133.

76. Shimada K, Masada K, Tada K, et al. Osteosynthesis for the treatment of nonunion of the lateral humeral condyle in children. *J Bone Joint Surg Am.* 1997;79:234–240.

77. Shirley E, Anderson M, Neal K, et al. Screw fixation of lateral condyle fractures: results of treatment. *J Pediatr Orthop.* 2015;35:821–824.

78. Silva M, Cooper SD. Closed reduction and percutaneous pinning of displaced pediatric lateral condyle fractures of the humerus: a cohort study. *J Pediatr Orthop.* 2015;35:661–665.

79. Silva M, Cooper SD, Cha A. Elbow dislocation with an associated lateral condyle fracture of the humerus: a rare occurrence in the pediatric population. *J Pediatr Orthop.* 2015;35:329–333.

80. Silva M, Paredes A, Sadlik G. Outcomes of ORIF >7 days after injury in displaced pediatric lateral condyle fracture. *J Pediatr Orthop.* 2017;37:234–238.

81. Skak SV, Olsen SD, Smaabrekke A. Deformity after fracture of the lateral humeral condyle in children. *J Pediatr Orthop B.* 2001;10:142–152.

82. Smith FM, Joyce JJ 3rd. Fracture of lateral condyle of humerus in children. *Am J Surg.* 1954;87:324–329.

83. So YC, Fang D, Orth MC, et al. Varus deformity following lateral humeral condylar fracture in children. *J Pediatr Orthop.* 1985;5:569–572.

84. Sodl JF, Ricchetti ET, Huffman GR. Acute osteochondral shear fracture of the capitellum in a twelve-year-old patient. A case report. *J Bone Joint Surg Am.* 2008;90:629–633.

85. Song KS, Kang CH, Min BW, et al. Closed reduction and internal fixation of displaced unstable lateral condylar fractures of the humerus. *J Bone Joint Surg Am.* 2008;90:2673–2681.

86. Song KW, Shin YW, Oh CW, et al. Closed reduction and internal fixation of completely displaced and rotated lateral condylar fractures of the humerus in children. *J Orthop Trauma.* 2010;24:434–438.

87. Song KS, Waters PM. Lateral condylar humerus fractures: which ones should we fix? *J Pediatr Orthop.* 2012;32(Suppl 1):S5–S9.

88. Speed JS, Macey HB. Fracture of humeral condyles in children. *J Bone Joint Surg.* 1933;15:903–919.

89. Stans AA, Maritz NG, O'Driscoll SW, et al. Operative treatment of elbow contracture in patients 21 years of age or younger. *J Bone Joint Surg Am.* 2002;84-A:382–387.

90. Stein BE, Ramji AF, Hassanzadeh H, et al. Cannulated lag screw fixation of displaced lateral humeral condyle fractures is associated with lower rates of open reduction and infection than pin fixation. *J Pediatr Orthop.* 2017;37:7–13.

91. Steinthal D. Die isolirte fraktur der eminentia capitata im ellenbogengelenk. *Zentralbl F Chir.* 1898;15:17–20.

92. Stimson LA. *A Practical Treatise on Fractures and Dislocations.* Philadelphia, PA: Lea Brothers & Co; 1900.

93. Tien YC, Chen JC, Fu YC, et al. Supracondylar dome osteotomy for cubitus valgus deformity associated with a lateral condylar nonunion in children. Surgical technique. *J Bone Joint Surg Am.* 2006;88(Suppl 1 Pt 2):191–201.

94. van Vugt AB, Severijnen RV, Festern C. Fractures of the lateral humeral condyle in children: late results. *Arch Orthop Trauma Surg.* 1988;107:206–209.

95. Wadsworth TG. Premature epiphyseal fusion after injury of capitulum. *J Bone Joint Surg Br.* 1964;46:46–49.

96. Wang YL, Chang WN, Hsu CJ, et al. The recovery of elbow range of motion after treatment of supracondylar and lateral condylar fractures of the distal humerus in children. *J Orthop Trauma.* 2009;23:120–125.

97. Waters PM, Bae DS. *Pediatric Hand and Upper Limb Surgery: A Practical Guide.* Philadelphia, PA: Lippincott Williams & Wilkins; 2012:316–337.

98. Wattenbarger JM, Gerardi J, Johnson CE. Late open reduction internal fixation of lateral condyle fractures. *J Pediatr Orthop.* 2002;22:394–398.

99. Weiss JM, Graves S, Yang S, et al. A new classification system predictive of complications in surgically treated pediatric humeral lateral condyle fractures. *J Pediatr Orthop.* 2009;29:602–605.

100. Wilson JN. Fracture of the external condyle of the humerus in children. *Br J Surg.* 1955;43:88–94.

101. Wilson PD. Fracture of the lateral condyle of humerus in children. *J Bone Joint Surg.* 1936;18:299–316.

102. Wirmer J, Kruppa C, Fitze G. Operative treatment of lateral humeral condyle fractures in children. *Eur J Pediatr Surg.* 2012;22:289–294.

103. Yang WE, Shih CH, Lee ZL, et al. Anatomic reduction of old displaced lateral condylar fractures of the humerus in children via a posterior approach with olecranon osteotomy. *J Trauma.* 2008;64:1281–1289.

104. Zeir FG. Lateral condylar fracture and its many complications. *Orthop Rev.* 1981;10:49–55.

105. Zionts LE, Stolz MR. Late fracture of the lateral condyle of the humerus. *Orthopedics.* 1984;7:541–545.

17

Distal Humeral Physeal, Medial Condyle, Lateral Epicondylar, and Other Uncommon Elbow Fractures

Michael Glotzbecker

INTRODUCTION

There are rare injuries about the elbow that can be underappreciated or missed acutely that have serious long-term implications for patients. We have labeled these TRASH (*the radiographic appearance seemed harmless*) lesions about the elbow. Most commonly these occur in the very young before secondary centers of ossification would make the acute diagnosis and treatment easier. Examples of TRASH lesion include distal humeral physeal fractures before the capitellum ossifies, medial condylar fractures before the trochlea ossifies, and osteochondral fractures in children less than 10 years old that lead to joint incongruity and instability. Often additional radiographic evaluation with ultrasound, arthrography, and/or MRI scans is necessary to make the diagnosis acutely and intervene appropriately for the best long-term outcome. This chapter will cover many of the rare, potentially problematic injuries about the elbow.

Fractures Involving the Entire Distal Humerus

INTRODUCTION TO FRACTURES INVOLVING THE ENTIRE DISTAL HUMERUS

From 1960 to 1978, many individual patients who suffered a distal humeral physeal separation were reported.[40,69,77] Once the presence of this injury became recognized, larger series appeared. Subsequently, 12 separate series reported a total of 71 fractures.[3,14,15,35,48,54] Abe et al.[1] and Supakul et al.[76] reported a series of 21 and 16 fractures, respectively. Originally thought to be a rare injury, it appears that fractures involving the entire distal humeral physis occur frequently in children as they now have become more commonly reported. The major problem is the initial recognition of this injury and a recent ultrasound study showed that 56% may be missed on plain radiographs.[76] Delay in diagnosis even up to one week is not uncommon[2] and prolonged delay can have serious concerns to the child's long-term elbow function.

Most fractures involving the entire distal humeral physis occur before the age of 6 or 7 and are most common under the age of 3.[2] The younger the child is, the greater the relative volume of the distal humerus epiphysis. As the humerus matures, the physeal line progresses more distally, with a central V forming between the medial and lateral condylar physes (Fig. 17-1). Ashurst[3a] believed that this V-shaped configuration of the

physeal line helps protect the more mature distal humerus from physeal fractures.

ASSESSMENT OF FRACTURES INVOLVING THE ENTIRE DISTAL HUMERUS

MECHANISMS OF INJURY FOR FRACTURES INVOLVING THE ENTIRE DISTAL HUMERUS

The exact mechanism of this injury is unknown and probably varies with the age group involved. A few consistent factors are evident. First, many fractures of the entire distal humeral

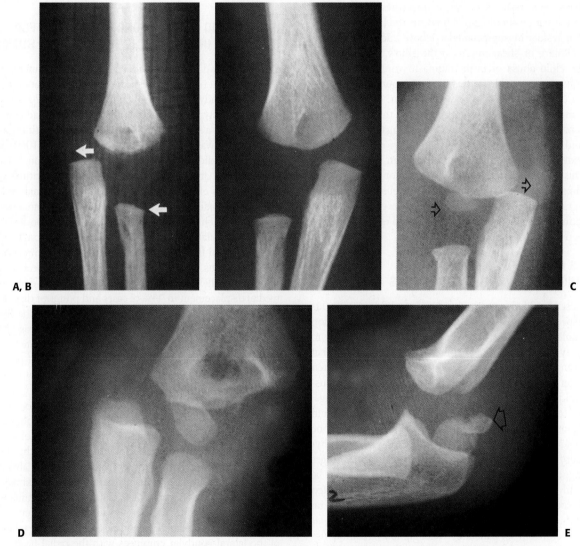

Figure 17-1. A: Group A—AP view of a small infant who had a swollen left elbow after a difficult delivery. The displacement medially of the proximal radius and ulna (*arrows*) helps to make the diagnosis of a displaced total distal humeral physis. **B:** Normal elbow for comparison. **C:** Group B—AP view showing the posteromedial displacement of the distal fragment (*arrows*). The relationship between the ossification center of the lateral condyle and the proximal radius has been maintained. **D:** Group C—AP view with marked medial displacement of the distal fragment. **E:** Group C—lateral view of the same patient showing posterior displacement of the distal fragment. There is also a large metaphyseal fragment associated with the distal fragment (*arrow*).

physis have occurred as birth injuries associated with difficult deliveries.[2–4,17,24,39,81] Siffert[72a] noted that the clinical appearance of these injured elbows at the time of delivery was not especially impressive. There was only moderate swelling and some crepitus.

Second, DeLee et al.[15] noted a high incidence of confirmed or suspected child abuse in their very young patients. Other reports[3,14,50,59] have confirmed the frequency of child abuse in infants and young children with these fractures, and up to 50% of these fractures in children under the age of 2 may be the result of abuse. Therefore, clinicians should have a high index of suspicion for nonaccidental trauma, especially in the setting of a history of multiple injuries or an inconsistent history of the mechanism of injury.[2]

Bright[8] showed that a physis is more likely to fail with rotary shear forces than with pure bending or tension forces. Young infants have some residual flexion contractures of the elbow from intrauterine positioning; this prevents the hyperextension injury that results in supracondylar elbow fractures in older children. Rotary or shear forces on the elbow, which can be caused by child abuse or birth trauma in young infants, are probably more responsible for this injury in young children. As it is often confused with an elbow dislocation, elbow dislocations are rare in this young age group because the cartilaginous physis is mechanically weaker than the bone ligament interface that would fail with an elbow dislocation.[2] In older children, a hyperextension force on an outstretched arm may cause the injury. This may occur from a fall from height or when an older child jumps on top of a younger child.[2,76] Abe et al.[1] reported 21 children, ranging in age from 1 to 11 years (average: 5 years), with fracture separations of the distal humeral epiphysis, all of which were sustained in falls.

INJURIES ASSOCIATED WITH FRACTURES INVOLVING THE ENTIRE DISTAL HUMERUS

Child abuse should always be considered in children with this injury, especially a type A fracture pattern (see classification below), unless it occurs at birth. A young infant is unlikely to incur this type of injury spontaneously from the usual falls that occur during the first year of life. Of the 16 fractures reported by DeLee et al.,[15] six resulted from documented or highly suspected child abuse, all in children younger than 2 years of age. Therefore, other injuries commonly found in cases of child abuse should be considered. If child abuse is suspected, a bone scan and a skeletal survey are warranted, to look for metaphyseal corner fractures, rib fractures, or fractures at various stages of healing, and the possibility of head trauma should not be ignored. In a series of 16 patients with this injury evaluated with ultrasound, 10 (63%) had one or more additional humeral fractures (bucket handle fractures in five patients and condylar avulsion fractures in six patients).[76] Recognition of child abuse and proper intervention can be life altering or even life saving for these children.

SIGNS AND SYMPTOMS OF FRACTURES INVOLVING THE ENTIRE DISTAL HUMERUS

In an infant less than 18 months of age, whose elbow is swollen secondary to trauma or suspected trauma, a fracture involving the entire distal humeral physis should be considered. The newborn may be irritable or inconsolable. Swelling, instability, limited range of motion, and/or lack of spontaneous movement (pseudoparalysis) all may suggest this injury.[2,76] In a young infant or newborn, swelling may be minimal with little crepitus. Poland[66a] described the crepitus as "muffled" crepitus because the fracture ends are covered with softer cartilage than the firm osseous tissue in other fractures about the elbow. Because of the large, wide fracture surfaces, there are fewer tendencies for tilting with distal fragment rotation, and the angular deformity is less severe than that with supracondylar fractures. In older children, the elbow is often so swollen that a clinical assessment of the bony landmarks is impossible, and only radiographic evaluation can provide confirmation of the diagnosis.

IMAGING AND OTHER DIAGNOSTIC STUDIES FOR FRACTURES INVOLVING THE ENTIRE DISTAL HUMERUS

Confirming radiographic evidence of a distal humeral physeal separation can be difficult, especially if the ossification center of the lateral condyle is not visible in an infant. Radiographs of the entire extremity not centered on the elbow may lead to a missed diagnosis.[2] In a series of 16 patients evaluated with ultrasound, the diagnosis was missed in 9 (56%) patients, and 10/16 patients in this series did not have a true lateral radiograph.[76] The only relationship that can be determined is that of the primary ossification centers of the distal humerus to the proximal radius and ulna. The proximal radius and ulna maintain an anatomic relationship to each other but are usually displaced posteriorly and medially in relation to the distal humerus. Although theoretically, the distal fragment can be displaced in any direction, with rare exceptions, most fractures reported have been displaced posteromedially. One recent series of 16 patients demonstrated medial displacement in 94% of cases and posterior displacement of the radius and ulna in 38%.[76] In a review of the literature including 33 cases, posteromedial displacement was identified in 64% of cases.[68] Comparison views of the opposite uninjured elbow may be helpful to determine the presence of posteromedial displacement (see Fig. 17-1A,B). A posterior fat pad sign is generally present while an anterior one is not.[2,25]

Distinguishing the injury from an elbow dislocation may be challenging. It should be remembered that elbow dislocations are rare in the peak age group for fractures of the entire distal humeral physis. With elbow dislocations, the displacement of the proximal radius and ulna is almost always posterolateral, and the relationship between the proximal radius and lateral condylar epiphysis is disrupted.[2] Unfortunately, this can be especially difficult to assess in young children when the capitellum is not ossified. In contrast, the anatomic relationship of the lateral condylar epiphysis with the radial head is maintained with a transphyseal separation, even though the distal humeral epiphysis is displaced posterior and medial in relation to the metaphysis of the humerus. Once the lateral condylar epiphysis becomes ossified, displacement of the entire distal epiphysis is much more obvious.

Because they have a large metaphyseal fragment, type C fractures may be confused with either a low supracondylar fracture or a fracture of the lateral condylar physis. The key diagnostic point is the smooth outline of the distal metaphysis in fractures involving the total distal physis. With supracondylar fractures, the distal portion of the distal fragment has a more irregular border.

Differentiation from a fracture of the lateral condylar physis in an infant can be made on radiograph. With a displaced fracture of the lateral condylar physis, the relationship between the lateral condylar epiphysis and the proximal radius can be disrupted but may remain normal (Fig. 17-2). If the lateral crista of the trochlea is involved, the proximal radius and ulna may be displaced posterolaterally. Oblique radiographs or other advanced imaging may be needed to distinguish these injuries.

If differentiation of this injury from an intra-articular fracture is uncertain, arthrography or MRI may be helpful (Fig. 17-3).[59] In neonates and infants in whom ossification has not begun, ultrasonography can be used to identify the displaced epiphysis of the humerus (Fig. 17-4).[16,58,76,81]

In a series of 16 patients in which 56% of the injuries were not identified on radiographs, ultrasound was performed in 12 of the patients and the diagnosis was made in all of them.[76] If the diagnosis is delayed, new periosteal bone forms around the distal humerus that will be seen on subsequent radiographs, and the whole epiphysis may remain displaced posteriorly and medially (Fig. 17-5).

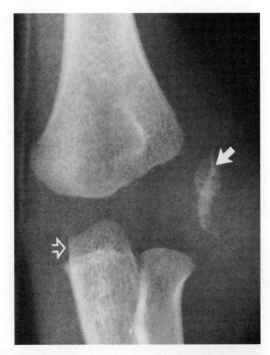

Figure 17-2. Displaced fracture of the lateral condyle in a 2-year-old. The relationship of the lateral condyle (*closed arrow*) to the proximal radius is lost. Both the proximal radius and ulna (*open arrow*) have shifted slightly laterally.

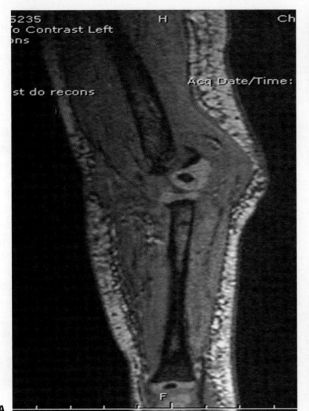
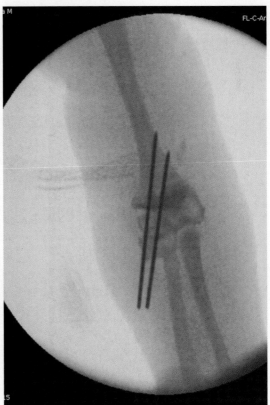

Figure 17-3. MRI (**A**) demonstrating transphyseal separation of the distal humerus and arthrogram (**B, C**) demonstrating realignment after pin fixation.

(continues)

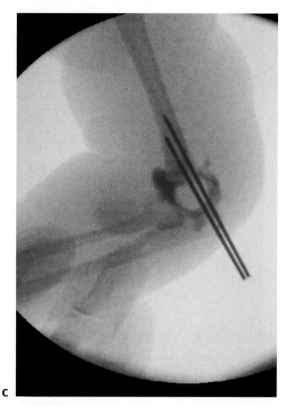

c

Figure 17-3. *(Continued)*

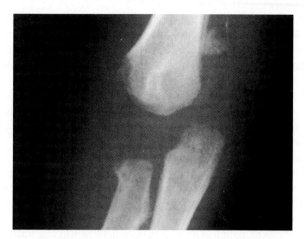

Figure 17-5. The true nature of this injury as involving the entire distal humeral physis was not appreciated until periosteal new bone became visible 3 weeks after injury.

CLASSIFICATION OF FRACTURES INVOLVING THE ENTIRE DISTAL HUMERUS

DeLee et al.[15] classified fractures of the entire distal humeral physis into three groups based on the degree of ossification of the lateral condylar epiphysis (see Fig. 17-1). Group A fractures occur in infants up to 12 months of age, before the secondary ossification center of the lateral condylar epiphysis appears (see Fig. 17-1A). They are usually Salter–Harris type I physeal injuries. This injury may be missed because of the lack of an ossification center in the lateral condylar epiphysis. Group B fractures occur most often in children of 12 months to 3 years of age in whom there is definite ossification of the lateral condylar epiphysis (see Fig. 17-1C). Although there may be a small flake of metaphyseal bone (Salter–Harris II fracture), this essentially behaves as a type I Salter–Harris physeal injury. Group C fractures occur in older children, from 3 to 7 years of age and result in a large metaphyseal fragment (Salter–Harris II fracture), that is most commonly lateral but can be medial or posterior (see Fig. 17-1D,E).

These fractures are almost always extension-type injuries with the distal epiphyseal fragment displacing posterior to the metaphysis. A rare flexion type of injury can occur in which the epiphyseal fragment is displaced anteriorly. Stricker et al.[74] reported a coronal plane transcondylar (Salter–Harris type IV) fracture in a 3-year-old child that was initially diagnosed as a fracture of the lateral humeral condyle. No growth disturbance was evident 3 years after open reduction and pin fixation.

PATHOANATOMY AND APPLIED ANATOMY RELATING TO FRACTURES INVOLVING THE ENTIRE DISTAL HUMERUS

Distal humeral physeal injuries have similar anatomic considerations as supracondylar humerus fractures. However, because the patients who suffer this injury are often very young, diagnosis and treatment can be more challenging.

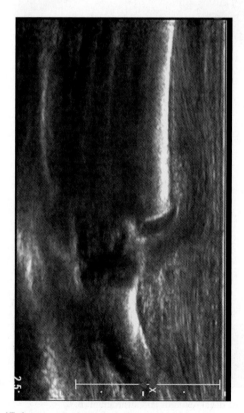

Figure 17-4. Sagittal ultrasound demonstrating posterior displacement of the distal humeral epiphysis.

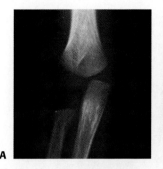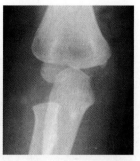

Figure 17-6. A: At 5 months of age, the metaphysis has advanced only to the supracondylar ridges. **B:** By 4 years of age, the edge of the metaphysis has advanced well into the area of the epicondyles.

Because the fracture is distal, the fracture surfaces are broader than those proximally through the supracondylar fractures. This broader surface area of the fracture line may help prevent tilting of the distal fragment. Because the fracture lines do not involve the articular surface, development of joint incongruity with resultant loss of elbow motion is unlikely if malunion occurs.

The distal humeral epiphysis extends across to include the secondary ossification of the medial epicondyle until about 6 to 7 years of age in girls and 8 to 9 years in boys. Thus, fractures involving the entire physeal line include the medial epicondyle up to this age. In older children, only the lateral and medial condylar physeal lines are included.

Finally, part of the blood supply to the medial crista of the trochlea courses directly through the physis. The blood supply to this area is vulnerable to injury, which may cause osteonecrosis in this part of the trochlea.

Because the physeal line is more proximal in young infants, it is nearer the center of the olecranon fossa (Fig. 17-6). A hyperextension injury in this age group is more likely to result in a physeal separation than a bony supracondylar fracture.[12]

TREATMENT OPTIONS FOR FRACTURES INVOLVING THE ENTIRE DISTAL HUMERUS

Treatment is first directed toward prompt injury recognition. Because this damage may be associated with child abuse, the parents may delay seeking treatment. The goal of treatment is to obtain acceptable alignment until the fracture heals over 2 to 3 weeks post-injury.

Simple splint or cast immobilization has been suggested by several authors.[4,15,48,63] In some small children, this may be the only treatment option that is reasonable. However, some investigators have shown cubitus varus after nonoperative treatment of these fractures.[1,14,15,35] The rate of varus was noted in 3/12,[15] 15/21,[1] and 5/7[35] in these series. De Jager and Hoffman[14] reported 12 fracture separations of the distal humeral epiphysis, three of which were initially diagnosed as fractures of the lateral condyle and one as an elbow dislocation. Because of the frequency of cubitus varus after this injury in young children, they recommended closed reduction and percutaneous pinning in

children younger than 2 years of age so that the carrying angle can be evaluated immediately after reduction and corrected if necessary. Arthrography may be helpful for diagnostic reasons and to assess reduction after fixation. In a review of 33 cases identified in the literature, 12% underwent surgical treatment, 88% were treated nonoperatively, and 23 cases (69%) had an attempted reduction. In this review, 88% recovered the carrying angle, and 80% range of motion and no differences in outcomes could be found between types of treatment.[68]

Several investigators have reported open reduction, usually performed owing to misdiagnosis as a displaced fracture of the lateral humeral condyle.[3,35,69] Mizuno et al.,[54] however, recommended primary open reduction because of their poor results with closed reduction. They approached the fracture posteriorly by removing the triceps insertion from the olecranon with a small piece of cartilage. If the fracture is old (more than 5 to 6 days) and the epiphysis is no longer mobile, manipulation should not be attempted, and the elbow should be splinted for comfort. Many essentially untreated fractures remodel completely without any residual deformity if the distal fragment is only medially translocated and not tilted (Fig. 17-7). In the more displaced three-dimensional malunions, a later osteotomy may be indicated.

NONOPERATIVE TREATMENT OF FRACTURES INVOLVING THE ENTIRE DISTAL HUMERUS

Indications/Contraindications

Nonoperative Treatment of Fractures Involving the Entire Distal Humerus: INDICATIONS AND CONTRAINDICATIONS	
Indications	**Relative Contraindications**
• Minimal displacement	• Markedly displaced fractures with prompt diagnosis
• Neonate/small infants where anesthesia or pin fixation difficult	

In neonates and very small infants in whom general anesthesia or percutaneous pin fixation may be difficult, splint or cast immobilization can be used to treat these fractures but does carry a risk of extra-articular malunion.

Technique

The arm is simply immobilized in splint or cast with up to 90 degrees of flexion with the forearm pronated. The extremity is then externally stabilized with a swathe or figure-of-eight splint.

Outcomes

Outcome and function is usually good; however, some investigators have shown cubitus varus after nonoperative treatment of these fractures.[1,14,15,35] The rate of varus was noted in 3/12,[15] 15/21,[1] and 5/7[35] in these series. In the series by Gilbert, 4

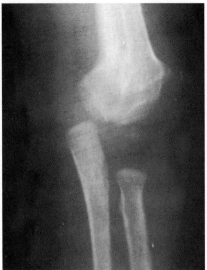
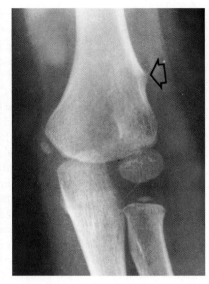
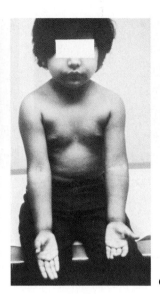

A, B   **C**

Figure 17-7. Remodeling of untreated fractures. **A:** AP view of a 2-year-old who had an unrecognized and untreated fracture of the distal humeral physis. The medial translocation is apparent. There was no varus or valgus tilting. **B:** Four years later, there had been almost complete remodeling of the distal humerus. A small supracondylar prominence (*arrow*) remains as a scar from the original injury. **C:** Clinical appearance 4 years after injury shows no difference in elbow alignment.

patients were treated with immobilization alone, with 3 of them having residual deformity.[25] In a review of 33 cases identified in the literature, 88% were treated nonoperatively, and 23 cases (69%) had an attempted reduction. In this review, 88% recovered the carrying angle, and 80% range of motion and no differences in outcomes could be found between types of treatment.[68]

OPERATIVE TREATMENT OF FRACTURES INVOLVING THE ENTIRE DISTAL HUMERUS

Indications/Contraindications

In most infants and young children with a displaced fracture, external immobilization is usually not dependable in maintaining the reduction, and therefore, operative intervention is indicated.

Closed Reduction and Percutaneous Pin Fixation

Preoperative Planning

✔ ORIF of Fractures Involving the Entire Distal Humerus: PREOPERATIVE PLANNING CHECKLIST	
OR table	☐ Regular OR table with C-arm used as table vs. radiolucent table
Position/positioning aids	☐ Position on edge of bed with arm free over side if using C-arm, position to opposite edge of table if using radiolucent table
	☐ For small infants, may need to position head and body on radiolucent table
Fluoroscopy location	☐ Parallel to table from head or from below
Equipment	☐ K-wires or C-wires, needle for arthrography

Planning is similar to that of treating a supracondylar humerus fracture. In cases where the elbow is largely unossified, one must prepare for arthrography to help with diagnosis and to assess reduction.

Positioning

The patient can be positioned two ways—on the edge of the table with the affected extremity free over the side of the table and with the base of the C-arm used as the operative surface, or on a radiolucent table on the edge opposite the affected extremity. The C-arm can be brought underneath the table so that you can use the radiolucent table as the operative surface rather than the C-arm. In the very young, the head and body may also need to be on the radiolucent table due to the small overall size of the child.

Technique

✔ Closed Reduction and Pinning of Fractures Involving the Entire Distal Humerus: KEY SURGICAL STEPS
☐ Assess arm under fluoroscopy
☐ If anatomy not clear, perform arthrogram to determine direction of displacement
☐ In extension, correct medial or lateral displacement
☐ Flex elbow up while pronating arm
☐ Secure fracture with two divergent lateral entry pins
☐ If medial pin is needed for stability, make small incision over medial epicondyle and visualize directly, and pull back ulnar nerve to avoid injury
☐ If difficult to assess reduction, perform arthrogram to assess alignment. Arthrogram can be performed by injecting posteriorly into olecranon fossa or posterolaterally into soft spot of elbow
☐ Bend and cut pins, and place xeroform and drain sponge under underneath pins
☐ Place well-padded bivalved long-arm cast in comfortable amount of flexion (approximately 60–80 degrees)

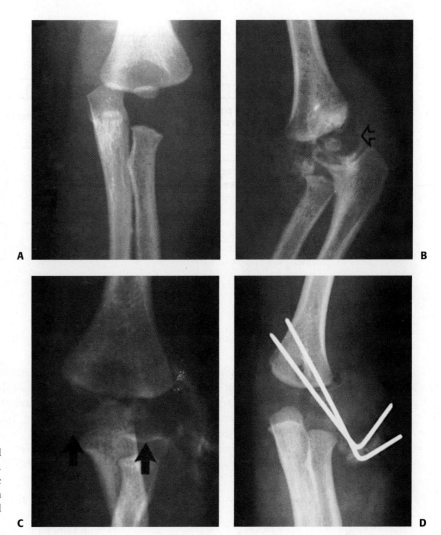

Figure 17-8. A: Injury film of a 20-month-old showing medial displacement of the distal fragment. **B, C:** The medial and posterior displacement of the condylar fragment (*arrows*) is better defined after an arthrogram. **D:** Fixation is achieved by two lateral pins placed percutaneously.

Under general anesthesia, the elbow is initially manipulated while extension to correct the medial displacement, and then the fragment is stabilized by flexing the elbow and pronating the forearm. When the forearm is supinated with the elbow flexed, the distal fragment tends to displace medially. This displacement is usually a pure medial horizontal translocation without mediolateral coronal tilting. The fragment is secured with two lateral entry pins (Fig. 17-8).

Because of the swelling and immaturity of the distal humerus, the medial epicondyle is difficult to define as

a distinct landmark, making it risky to attempt the percutaneous placement of a medial pin through the medial epicondyle. If a medial pin is necessary for stable fracture fixation, a medial incision can be made to allow direct observation of the medial epicondyle and the ulnar nerve. Usually two or lateral small, smooth lateral pins are used. In small infants and young children with minimal ossification of the epiphyseal fragment, an intraoperative arthrogram may be obtained to help determine the quality of the reduction.

Author's Preferred Treatment for Fractures Involving the Entire Distal Humerus (Algorithm 17-1)

In neonates and very small infants in whom general anesthesia and percutaneous pin fixation is contraindicated, we typically simply immobilize the extremity in 90 degrees of flexion with the forearm pronated. The extremity is then externally stabilized with a figure-of-eight splint.

In most older infants and young children, external immobilization is usually not dependable in maintaining the reduction. As a rule, in these patients, we perform the manipulation with the patient under general anesthesia and the fragment is

secured with two lateral pins (see Fig. 17-8). If a medial pin is necessary for stable fracture fixation, a medial incision should be made. An intraoperative arthrogram may be obtained to help determine the quality of the reduction in patients with limited ossification. We do closed reduction, pinning, and arthrographic assessment surgery in neonates and very young children who can tolerate anesthesia safely.

If treatment is delayed more than 3 to 5 days and if the epiphysis is not freely movable and at risk of growth arrest

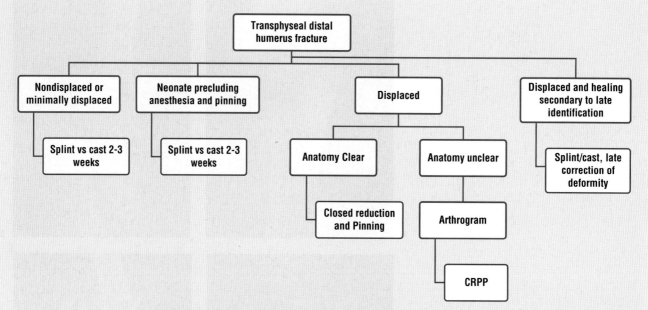

Algorithm 17-1. Author's preferred treatment for fractures involving the entire distal humerus.

if manipulated, the elbow is simply immobilized in a splint or cast. It is probably better to treat any resulting deformity later with a supracondylar osteotomy rather than to risk the complication of physeal injury or osteonecrosis of the epiphysis by performing a delayed manipulation or open reduction. Only occasionally does an untreated patient have a deformity severe enough to require surgical correction at a later date. Because the articular surface is intact, complete functional recovery can usually be expected.

Postoperative Care

A cast or splint is maintained for 3 weeks. At 3 weeks, the patient's cast is removed, imaging is obtained, and the pins are removed in the office. The patient is discharged without immobilization and active elbow motion is resumed. The patient is then followed until full motion is regained and until there is radiographic evidence of normal physeal and epiphyseal growth.

Potential Pitfalls and Preventive Measures

Fractures Involving the Entire Distal Humerus:
POTENTIAL PITFALLS AND PREVENTIONS

Pitfall	Prevention
• Use medial pin, inaccurate placement, or iatrogenic ulnar nerve palsy	• Lateral entry pin placement • If medial pin absolutely needed, make incision over medial epicondyle and visualize directly, pull ulnar nerve posteriorly during pinning
• Difficulty gauging reduction because of elbow being largely unossified	• Perform arthrogram to assess reduction

Because of the swelling and immaturity of the distal humerus, the ulnar nerve is at risk with placement of a medial pin. Making an incision and by visualizing and pulling ulnar nerve out of the way helps prevent iatrogenic injury. Quality of reduction is difficult to assess in small infants and young children and an intraoperative arthrogram can ensure adequate reduction.

MANAGEMENT OF EXPECTED ADVERSE OUTCOMES AND UNEXPECTED COMPLICATIONS IN FRACTURES INVOLVING THE ENTIRE DISTAL HUMERUS

Fractures Involving the Entire Distal Humerus:
COMMON ADVERSE OUTCOMES AND COMPLICATIONS

- Malunion/cubitus varus
- Neurovascular injuries (rare)
- Osteonecrosis of lateral condyle or trochlear epiphysis (rare)

MALUNION

Significant cubitus varus deformity can occur after this injury (see Fig. 17-7C).[48,51] Because the fracture surfaces are wider with this injury than with supracondylar fractures, the distal fragment tends to tilt less, which seems to account for the lower incidence or severity of cubitus varus after this injury than after untreated supracondylar fractures; however, reduction and percutaneous pinning are recommended for acute fractures with displacement to prevent this complication. Oh et al. reported on 12 cases treated with operative and nonoperative treatment and 7/12 had residual cubitus varus.[61] Late supracondylar humerus osteotomy may be indicated when there is insufficient remodeling. (See Chapter 13 for details of surgical techniques for osteotomies.)

NEUROVASCULAR INJURIES

Neurovascular injuries, either transient or permanent, are rare with this fracture. This is probably because the fracture fragments are covered with physeal cartilage and do not have sharp edges. In addition, the fracture fragments are usually not as markedly displaced as supracondylar humerus. Finally, the fracture displacement is usually posteromedial rather than posterolateral, which would put tension on median nerve and brachial artery.

NONUNION

Only one nonunion after this fracture has been reported; it occurred in a patient seen 3 months after the initial injury.[54] Because of the extreme vascularity and propensity for osteogenesis in this area, union is rapid even in patients who receive essentially no treatment.

OSTEONECROSIS

Osteonecrosis of the epiphysis of the lateral condyle or the trochlear epiphysis has rarely been reported after fractures of the entire distal humeral physis. Yoo et al.[85] reported eight patients with osteonecrosis of the trochlea after fracture separations of the distal end of the humerus. Six of the eight fractures were diagnosed initially as medial condylar fractures, lateral condylar fractures, or traumatic elbow dislocation. All eight patients had rapid dissolution of the trochlea within 3 to 6 weeks after injury, followed by the development of a medial or central condylar fishtail defect. Oh et al. reported on 12 cases, and of the seven cases that had cubitus varus, six had a partial defect of the medial condyle related to avascular necrosis.[61] Further discussion regarding the etiology of this complication is discussed in the section on osteonecrosis of the trochlea.

SUMMARY, CONTROVERSIES, AND FUTURE DIRECTIONS FOR FRACTURES INVOLVING THE ENTIRE DISTAL HUMERUS

Transphyseal injuries of the distal humerus are rare. In young children, child abuse should be suspected and the patient should be evaluated for associated injuries. This is imperative. The injury should be distinguished from an elbow dislocation, which may be difficult in the unossified elbow. In neonates or children in which anesthesia is difficult, simple immobilization can be used, but patients may heal in varus. In children who can tolerate anesthesia, closed reduction and pin fixation should be performed to improve alignment and minimize complications of cubitus varus. An arthrogram is often needed to assess reduction.

Fractures Involving the Medial Condyle

INTRODUCTION TO FRACTURES INVOLVING THE MEDIAL CONDYLE

Fractures of the medial condyle can be thought of as the mirror image of lateral condyle fractures, which are more commonly encountered (see Chapter 16). Fractures involving the medial condyle have two components. The intra-articular component involves, in some manner, the trochlear articular surface. The extra-articular portion includes the medial metaphysis and medial epicondyle. Because the fracture line extends into the articular surface of the trochlea, these often are called *trochlear fractures*. For purposes of description in this chapter, fractures of the trochlea are those that include only the articular surface.

Fractures involving the medial condyle are rare in skeletally immature children, accounting for less than 1% of fractures involving the distal humerus.[36] Many of the large series of elbow fractures in the literature and early fracture texts do not mention these fractures as a separate entity. Blount[7] described only one such fracture in his classic text. In Faysse and Marion's[19a] review of more than 2,000 fractures of the distal humerus in children, only 10 fractures involved the medial condyle. Although it has been reported in a child as young as 2 years of age, this fracture pattern is generally considered to occur during later childhood. These rare injuries are very problematic as they can occur before the trochlear secondary center of ossification appears. A high index of suspicion is necessary to avoid missing a displaced, intra-articular fracture in the young (Fig. 17-9). Resultant malunion of the trochlear articular surface is problematic.

Most series[64] show medial condylar fractures occurring somewhat later than lateral condylar fractures. A review of 40 patients in 11 series[11,19,23,29,62,64,67,75,82] in which the specific ages were given showed that 38 patients were in the age range of 8 to 14 years. Thus, this fracture seems to occur most often after the ossification centers of the medial condylar epiphysis begin to appear. As mentioned, a medial condylar fracture can occur as early as 6 months of age; however, before any ossification of the distal humerus has appeared,[5,13] making the diagnosis extremely difficult and outcome poor if missed and not treated acutely.

ASSESSMENT OF FRACTURES INVOLVING THE MEDIAL CONDYLAR PHYSIS

MECHANISMS OF INJURY FOR FRACTURES INVOLVING THE MEDIAL CONDYLAR PHYSIS

Two separate mechanisms can produce physeal fractures of the medial condyle. Ashurst's patients described falling directly on the point of the flexed elbow. This mechanism was also implicated in other reports.[5,11,31,67] In this mechanism, it is

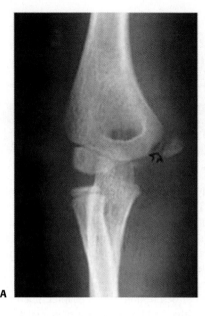
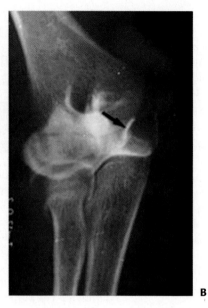

Figure 17-9. Intra-articular extension. **A:** Injury film in a 7-year-old girl who was initially suspected of having only a fracture of the medial epicondyle. In addition to moderate displacement, there was a significant metaphyseal fragment (*arrow*). **B:** An arthrogram revealed intra-articular components (*arrow*), which defined this injury instead as a fracture involving the medial condylar physis. (Courtesy of Carl McGarey, MD.)

speculated that the semilunar notch's sharp edge of the olecranon splits the trochlea directly (Fig. 17-10A). This mechanism is also supported by recent case reports of a medial condyle fracture in the setting of a pre-existing fishtail deformity.[56,62]

In three more recent series,[10,22,23] many patients sustained this injury when they fell on their outstretched arms. The theory is that this is an avulsion injury caused by a valgus strain at the elbow (Fig. 17-10B). Fowles and Kassab[22] reported a patient with a concomitant valgus greenstick fracture of the olecranon associated with a fracture of the medial condyle. They believed this fracture provided further evidence that this was a valgus avulsion type of injury. Once the fragment becomes

disassociated from the distal humerus, the forearm flexor muscles produce a sagittal anterior rotation of the fragment.

INJURIES ASSOCIATED WITH FRACTURES INVOLVING THE MEDIAL CONDYLAR PHYSIS

As this fracture is rare, studies describing associated injuries are rare. Medial condylar physeal fractures have been reported in association with greenstick fractures of the olecranon and with true posterolateral elbow dislocations (Fig. 17-11).[5,13,22] Some investigators[5,13] found that child abuse was more common in their younger patients with these fractures than with other elbow

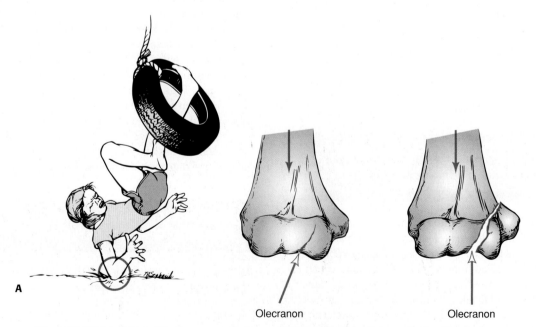

Olecranon   Olecranon

Figure 17-10. Medial condylar fracture mechanisms of injury. **A:** A direct force applied to the posterior aspect of the elbow causes the sharp articular margin of the olecranon to wedge the medial condyle from the distal humerus.

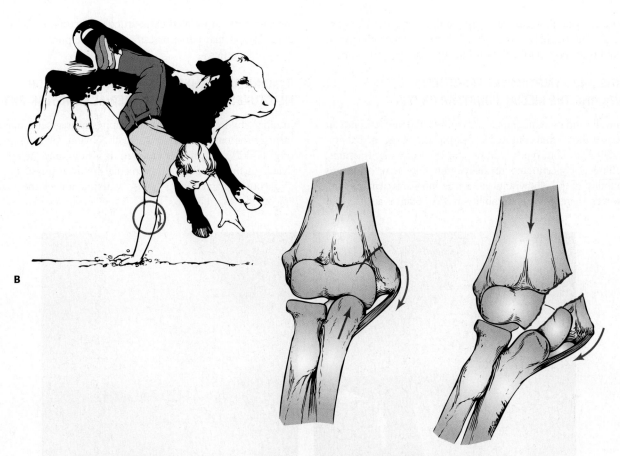

Figure 17-10. (*Continued*) **B:** Falling on the outstretched arm with the elbow extended and the wrist dorsiflexed causes the medial condyle to be avulsed by both ligamentous and muscular forces.

Figure 17-11. Lateral (**A**) and AP (**B**) injury films of a 10-year-old girl who sustained a type III displaced fracture of the medial condyle associated with a posterolateral elbow dislocation. (A, Courtesy of Elizabeth A. Szalay, MD.)

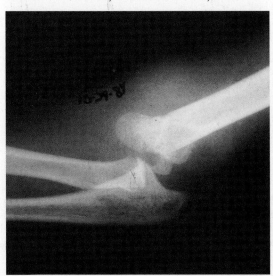

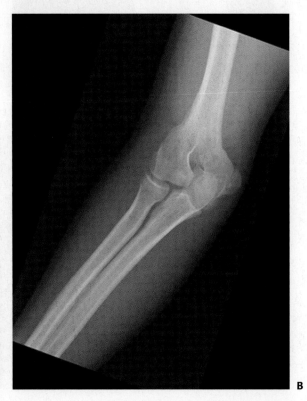

fractures. Regardless, the extremity should be evaluated for concomitant injuries of forearm, wrist, or hand, and the radiographs should be inspected for additional fractures about the elbow.

SIGNS AND SYMPTOMS OF FRACTURES INVOLVING THE MEDIAL CONDYLAR PHYSIS

Clinically and on radiographs, a fracture of the medial condylar physis is most often confused with a fracture of the medial epicondyle.[43] In both types of intra- and extra-articular fractures, swelling is concentrated medially, and there may be valgus instability of the elbow joint. In a true intra-articular fracture, however, there is varus instability as well. Such is usually not the case with an isolated extra-articular fracture of the medial epicondyle. Ulnar nerve paresthesia may be present with both types of fractures.

IMAGING AND OTHER DIAGNOSTIC STUDIES FOR FRACTURES INVOLVING THE MEDIAL CONDYLAR PHYSIS

In older children with a large metaphyseal fragment, involvement of the entire condyle is usually obvious on radiographs (Fig. 17-12A); in younger children, in whom only the epicondyle is ossified, fracture of the medial condylar physis may be erroneously diagnosed as an isolated fracture of the medial epicondyle (Fig. 17-12B,C).[19,22]

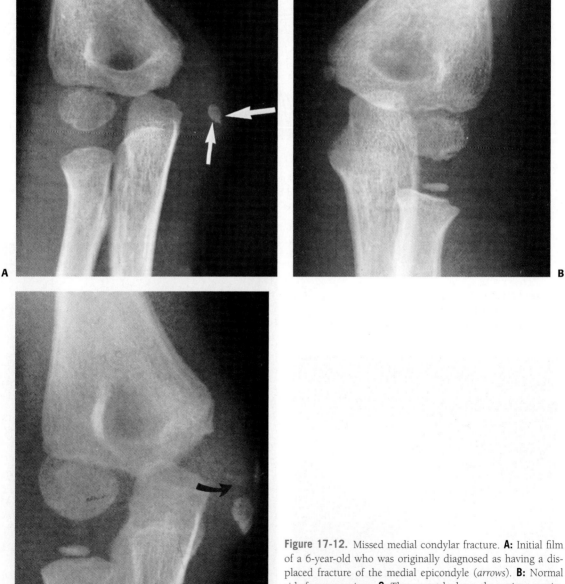

Figure 17-12. Missed medial condylar fracture. **A:** Initial film of a 6-year-old who was originally diagnosed as having a displaced fracture of the medial epicondyle (*arrows*). **B:** Normal side for comparison. **C:** Three months later, the patient continued to have a painful elbow, and there was ossification of the metaphysis (*arrow*) adjacent to the epicondyle.

In differentiating these two fractures, it is helpful to remember that medial epicondylar fractures are often associated with elbow dislocations, usually posterolateral, and that elbow dislocations are rare before ossification of the medial condylar epiphysis begins. With medial condylar physeal fractures, the elbow tends to subluxate posteromedially because of the loss of trochlear stability.

Any metaphyseal ossification with the epicondylar fragment suggests the presence of an intra-articular fracture of the medial condyle and is an indication for further evaluation. Often, the medial condyle and the medial epicondyle are markedly displaced as a unit. A positive fat pad sign indicates that the injury has entered the elbow joint and a fracture of the medial condyle is likely.[32,73] Isolated fractures of the medial epicondyle are extra-articular and usually do not have positive fat pad signs.

If the true location of the fracture line is questionable in a child younger than 8 to 10 years of age with significant medial elbow ecchymosis, arthrography or MRI of the elbow should be performed.

CLASSIFICATION OF FRACTURES INVOLVING THE MEDIAL CONDYLAR PHYSIS

Classification, as with fractures of the lateral condylar physis, is based on the fracture line's location and the degree of the fracture's displacement.

Location of the Fracture Line

Milch[52] classified fractures of the medial condylar physis in adults into two types. In type I fractures, the fracture line traverses the apex of the trochlea. In type II fractures, it traverses more laterally through the capitulotrochlear groove. He believed that the origin of the fracture line depended on whether the radial head, as in type II, or the semilunar notch of the olecranon, as in type I, served as the impinging force for the abduction injury. Both fracture patterns occur in children (Fig. 17-13A), but type I fractures seem to be more common because the common physeal line, which serves as a point of weakness, ends in the apex of the trochlea.

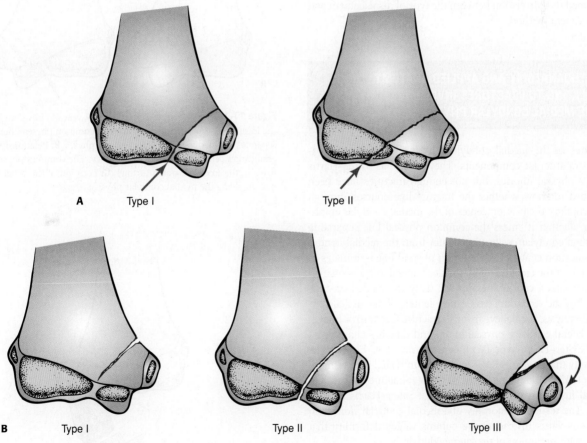

Figure 17-13. A: Medial condylar fracture patterns. In the Milch type I injury, the fracture line terminates in the trochlear notch (**left,** *arrow*). In the Milch type II injury, the fracture line terminates more laterally in the capitulotrochlear groove (**right,** *arrow*). **B:** Kilfoyle classification of displacement patterns. Degrees of displacement for fracture type I is an incomplete fracture that does not violate the joint but may hinge open; type II is a fracture that enters the joint but has less than 2 mm displacement; type III enters the joint and results in malangulation, malrotation, and articular displacement. (**A:** Adapted with permission from Milch H. Fractures and fracture–dislocations of the humeral condyles. *J Trauma.* 1964;4(5):592–607; **B:** Adapted with permission from Kilfoyle RM. Fractures of the medial condyle and epicondyle of the elbow in children. *ClinOrthop.* 1965;41(1):43–50.)

Displacement of the Fracture

Kilfoyle[41] described three fracture displacement patterns that can be helpful in determining appropriate treatment (Fig. 17-13B). In type I, the fracture line in the medial condylar metaphysis extends down to the physis. He noted that some of these might represent incomplete supracondylar fractures. Unless there is a greenstick crushing of the medial supracondylar column, these fractures are usually nondisplaced, stable, and of no clinical significance. In type II, the fracture line extends into the medial condylar physis. The intra-articular portion, as it is in preosseous cartilage, is often not recognized. In this second type, the medial condylar fragment usually remains undisplaced. In type III, the condylar fragment is both rotated and displaced. Some authors use a modification of Kilfoyle's classification based on the amount of displacement and describe it as nondisplaced (<2 mm), minimally displaced (2 to 4 mm), and displaced (>4 mm).[34] Bensahel et al.[5] and Papavasiliou et al.[64] found that type III displacement fractures, which accounted for only 25%, were more likely to occur in older adolescents, and type I fractures were more common in younger children. These studies also confirmed the correlation between the type of displacement and the treatment method.

PATHOANATOMY AND APPLIED ANATOMY RELATING TO FRACTURES INVOLVING THE MEDIAL CONDYLAR PHYSIS

Fractures of the medial condylar physis involve both intra- and extra-articular components. They behave as Salter–Harris type IV physeal injuries, but not enough fractures have been described to show whether the fracture line courses through the secondary ossification center of the medial condylar epiphysis or whether it enters the common physeal line separating the lateral condylar ossification center from the medial condylar ossification center. This common physeal line terminates in the notch of the trochlea. The trochlea's lateral crista is ossified from the lateral condylar epiphysis. Only the medial crista is ossified by the secondary ossification centers of the medial condylar epiphysis. We believe that this fracture is a "mirror image" of the lateral condylar physeal injury and thus has characteristics of Salter–Harris type IV physeal injuries (Fig. 17-14). The deformity that develops if the fracture is untreated is nonunion, similar to that after lateral condylar physeal fracture, rather than physeal fusion, as occurs after a typical Salter–Harris type IV injury. The resultant deformity of a medial condylar nonunion is cubitus varus instead of the cubitus valgus deformity that occurs with nonunion of the lateral condyle.

Characteristically, the metaphyseal fragment includes the intact medial epicondyle along with the common flexor origin of the muscles of the forearm. These flexor muscles cause the loosened fragment to rotate so that the fracture surface is facing anteriorly and medially and the articular surface is facing posteriorly and laterally (Fig. 17-15).[11] Rotation of the fragment is especially accentuated when the elbow is extended. Chacha[11] also noted that often the lateral aspect of the common flexor

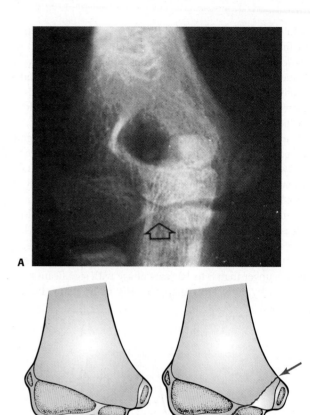

Figure 17-14. A: The AP radiograph of a 9-year-old boy demonstrates the location of the ossification centers. A common physeal line (*arrow*) separates the medial and lateral condylar physes. **B:** Relationship of the ossification centers to the articular surface. The common physis terminates in the trochlear notch (*arrow*). **C:** Location of the usual fracture line involving the medial condylar physis (*arrows*).

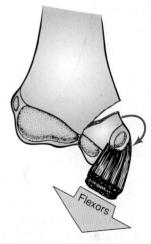

Figure 17-15. Displacement of the medial condyle. The pull of the forearm flexor muscles rotates the fragment so that the fracture surface is facing anteromedially and the articular surface is posterolateral. (Adapted with permission from Chacha PB. Fractures of the medial condyle of the humerus with rotational displacement. *J Bone Joint Surg Am.* 1970;52(7):1453–1458.)

origin and the anterior capsule of the joint were torn and the fracture surface could usually be reached through this anterior opening into the joint.

The blood supply to the medial epicondyle and medial metaphysis courses extra-articularly along with the medial flexor muscle groups. The blood supply to the lateral ossification center of the medial crista of the trochlea, however, must traverse the surface of the medial condylar physis. If the fracture line disrupts these small intra-articular vessels, disruption and subsequent circulation loss to the lateral portion of the medial crista can result, leading to the development of a fishtail deformity.

TREATMENT OPTIONS FOR FRACTURES INVOLVING THE MEDIAL CONDYLAR PHYSIS

In Kilfoyle's displacement types I and II fracture patterns, enough residual internal stability is usually present to allow the fracture to be simply immobilized in a cast or posterior splint.[5,26,41,64] As with fractures of the lateral condylar physis, union may be slow. In fractures treated promptly, results have been satisfactory.[11,19,22] Because there is usually more displacement in older children, the results in this age group are not as satisfactory with closed treatment as those in younger children, who tend to have relatively nondisplaced fractures.[5]

For displaced fractures, open reduction with internal fixation is the most often used treatment method.[5,10,22,23,41,64,66,67] The fracture fragment can be approached by a posteromedial incision that allows good exposure of both the fracture site and the ulnar nerve. Fixation is easily achieved with smooth K-wires or with screws in older adolescents (Fig. 17-16A,B). Two wires are

necessary because of the sagittal rotation forces exerted on the fracture fragment by the common flexor muscles. El Ghawabi[23] reported frequent delayed union and nonunion in fractures that were not rigidly stabilized.

NONOPERATIVE TREATMENT OF FRACTURES INVOLVING THE MEDIAL CONDYLAR PHYSIS

Indications/Contraindications

Nonoperative Treatment of Medial Condyle Fractures: INDICATIONS AND CONTRAINDICATIONS	
Indications	**Relative Contraindications**
• Nondisplaced fractures (Kilfoyle type I)	• Displaced fractures (Kilfoyle type III)
• Minimally displaced fractures (some) (Kilfoyle type II)	

Nondisplaced or minimally displaced fractures (Kilfoyle types I and II) can be treated nonoperatively with either splint or cast immobilization.

OPERATIVE TREATMENT OF FRACTURES INVOLVING THE MEDIAL CONDYLAR PHYSIS

Indications/Contraindications

For displaced fractures (Kilfoyle type III) operative fixation is recommended, as well as minimally displaced fractures (Kilfoyle type II) that demonstrate instability and/or progressive displacement.

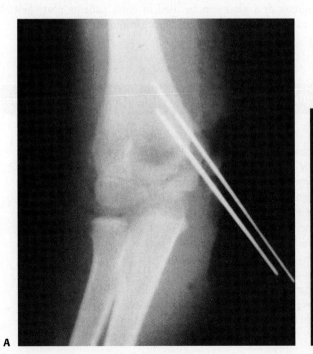
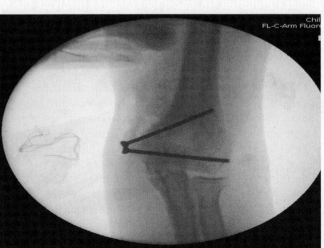

Figure 17-16. A: Medial condyle fracture in an adolescent fixed with wires. **B:** Medial condyle fracture fixed with cannulated screws to allow early range of motion.

Open Reduction Internal Fixation of Medial Condyle Fracture

Preoperative Planning

> ✔ **ORIF of Fractures Involving the Medial Condylar Physis:**
> PREOPERATIVE PLANNING CHECKLIST

OR table	☐ Regular table with hand table vs. radiolucent table in young child
Position/positioning aids	☐ Supine
Fluoroscopy location	☐ From head of bed under hand table
Equipment	☐ K-wires, cannulated screws (for patients near skeletal maturity)

Adequate radiographs, including oblique views, should be obtained to assess fracture morphology.

Positioning

Although medial epicondyle fractures may be approached supine or prone,[27] typically the patient is positioned supine to approach a medial condyle fracture. You attach a hand table on the affected side. The arm can be externally rotated through the shoulder to access the medial condyle, and the elbow is flexed to relax the flexor mass.

Surgical Approach

A posteromedial approach to the elbow is used that allows good exposure of both the fracture site and the ulnar nerve.

Technique

> ✔ **ORIF of Fractures Involving the Medial Condyle:**
> KEY SURGICAL STEPS

- ☐ Posteromedial incision over medial condyle
- ☐ Identify and protect ulnar nerve
- ☐ Clean fracture hematoma and identify fracture and joint surface
- ☐ Reduce fracture by taking tension of flexor mass by flexing elbow and wrist and pronating forearm
- ☐ Reduce joint and fracture
- ☐ Stabilize fracture with divergent K-wires (cannulated screws in older patients/adolescents)
- ☐ Apply bivalved long-arm cast

An incision is centered over the medial condyle/epicondyle. Often there is significant soft tissue swelling and displacement. Dissection is carefully carried out to the level of the bony condyle and usually the fracture hematoma is quickly encountered. The medial brachial and antebrachial cutaneous nerves that transverse the field are protected. Care in the dissection avoids injury to the ulnar nerve, which sits posterior to the fragment but may be displaced by the fracture. The ulnar nerve is identified and protected to ensure that it is not entrapped in the reduced fracture and it is not iatrogenically injured by a fixation pin or screw. The fracture is cleared out of hematoma. The entire fracture line and joint surface should be identified to ensure accurate reduction of the joint surface. The fracture is reduced. The flexor–pronator soft tissue attachments are left intact to lessen the risk of avascular necrosis. In the supine position, this requires flexion of the elbow and wrist with pronation of the forearm, which takes tension off of the condyle. The condyle is held in place, and K-wires are passed in a divergent manner to hold the fracture in place. Alternatively, cannulated screws or a plate can be used in older patients near skeletal maturity to allow more rigid fixation and early motion.

Author's Preferred Treatment for Fractures Involving the Medial Condylar Physis (Algorithm 17-2)

We generally treat Kilfoyle type I nondisplaced fractures with simple observation and a posterior splint or long-arm cast. Follow-up radiographs including oblique views at weekly intervals are taken to ensure there is no late displacement. When there is good callus at the metaphyseal portion of the fracture line by 4 to 6 weeks, the splint is removed and early active motion is initiated. We continue to follow the patient until there is a full range of motion and obliteration of the fracture line. Some type II fractures that maintain alignment can also be treated nonoperatively; however, careful follow-up on weekly intervals are required to document that the fragment has not moved.

Unstable Kilfoyle type II and type III displaced fractures must be reduced and stabilized. This is usually difficult to do by closed methods because the swelling associated with this injury makes it hard to accurately identify the landmarks for pin placement. We proceed with an open reduction through a medial approach with identification and protection of the ulnar nerve. The posterior surface of the condylar fragment and the medial aspect of the medial crista of the trochlea should be avoided in the dissection because these are the blood supply sources to the ossific nuclei of the trochlea. Fixation with two parallel pins should be in the metaphyseal segment if possible. We prefer cannulated screw fixation in adolescents near skeletal maturity to allow early protected range of motion.

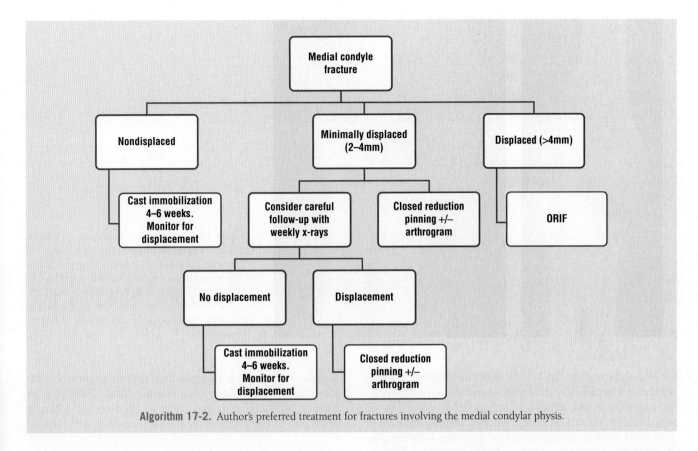

Algorithm 17-2. Author's preferred treatment for fractures involving the medial condylar physis.

Postoperative Care

Patients will be immobilized largely dependent upon age, fracture pattern, and type of fixation. Nonoperatively treated fractures may be casted for 4 to 6 weeks, in a similar fashion to the treatment of lateral condyle fractures based on age, displacement, and amount of healing. Those treated with pin fixation similarly will be casted for 4 to 6 weeks depending on healing, and the pins are often removed at 4 weeks if exposed, and can be removed any time after 6 weeks if buried. In patients treated with more rigid fixation, early (10 to 14 days) transition to a hinged elbow brace with protected range of motion is recommended.

Potential Pitfalls and Preventive Measures

Fractures Involving the Medial Condylar Physis: POTENTIAL PITFALLS AND PREVENTIONS	
Pitfall	**Prevention**
• Progressive displacement of minimally displaced fracture leading to delayed union or malunion	• Monitor fractures treated nonoperatively with careful radiographic follow-up
• Disruption of blood supply leading to osteonecrosis	• Avoid dissection posteriorly on the fragment on the medial aspect of the medial crista of the trochlea
• Iatrogenic ulnar nerve injury	• Perform adequate exposure to identify and protect ulnar nerve during reduction and pin fixation

Nondisplaced or minimally displaced fractures should be monitored closely to ensure that progressive displacement does not occur, which could lead to malunion, delayed union, or nonunion. When treating patients operatively, the posterior surface of the condylar fragment and the medial aspect of the medial crista of the trochlea should be avoided in the dissection because these are the blood supply sources to the ossific nuclei of the trochlea. The ulnar nerve should be identified to avoid iatrogenic injury.

MANAGEMENT OF EXPECTED ADVERSE OUTCOMES AND UNEXPECTED COMPLICATIONS IN FRACTURES INVOLVING THE MEDIAL CONDYLAR PHYSIS

Fractures Involving the Medial Condylar Physis: COMMON ADVERSE OUTCOMES AND COMPLICATIONS
• Stiffness
• Ulnar neuropathy
• Delayed union
• Nonunion
• Cubitus varus

The major complication is failure to make the proper diagnosis. This is especially true in younger children, in whom a medial condylar fracture can be confused with a displaced fracture of

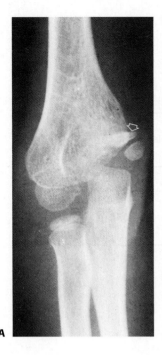
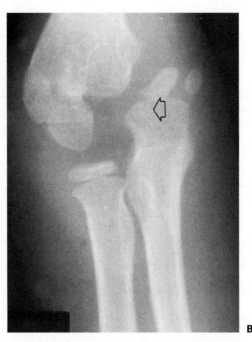

A

B

Figure 17-17. Nonunion in addition to cubitus varus deformity. **A:** Original film of a 5-year-old girl who sustained an injury 1 year previously. The metaphyseal fragment (*arrow*) is attached to the medial epicondyle. **B:** Film taken 2 years later. Some ossification has developed in the medial condylar epiphysis (*arrow*). (Courtesy of Roy N. Davis, MD.)

the medial epicondyle (Fig. 17-12). When the diagnosis is a real possibility, especially in a child with no ossification of the trochlea, examination with anesthesia, arthrography, and/or MRI is required (Fig. 17-9). Leet et al.[44] reported complications after 33% of 21 medial condylar fractures, including osteonecrosis of the trochlea, nonunion, and loss of reduction leading to malunion. Untreated displaced fractures usually result in nonunion or malunion with cubitus varus deformity (Fig. 17-17).[22,82] Sugiura reported on a child age 4 who was treated nonoperatively, and re-presented at age 10 with severe varus deformity secondary to a medial condyle nonunion.[75] These patients are at high risk for loss of motion, function, pain, and eventual arthrosis. Ryu et al.[71] described a painful nonunion of the medial condyle in an adolescent that apparently resulted from a fracture when he was 3 years old. An osteotomy was made to remove the nonunited section of bone, and an iliac bone graft was inserted and fixed with two malleolar screws. Union was obtained, and the patient was able to participate in sports without pain short term. Delayed union has been reported in patients treated with insecure fixation or simply placed in a cast.[23,41]

Some disturbance of the vascular supply to the medial condylar fragment may occur during open reduction and internal fixation or at the time of initial injury. Several investigators have reported subsequent avascular changes in the medial crista of the trochlea.[22,23,41,64] Hanspal[29] reviewed Cothay's[11a] original patient 18 years after delayed open reduction and found that despite some minimal loss of motion, the patient was asymptomatic. Radiographs, however, showed changes compatible with osteonecrosis of the medial condyle.

Both cubitus varus and valgus deformities have been reported in patients whose fractures united uneventfully. The valgus deformity appears to be caused by secondary stimulation or overgrowth of the medial condylar fragment. Some simple stimulation of the medial epicondyle's prominence may also produce the false appearance of a cubitus valgus deformity.

Cubitus varus appears to result from decreased growth of the trochlea, possibly caused by a vascular insult. Principles for treating nonunion of lateral condylar fractures are generally applicable to nonunions of the medial condyle (Fig. 17-18).

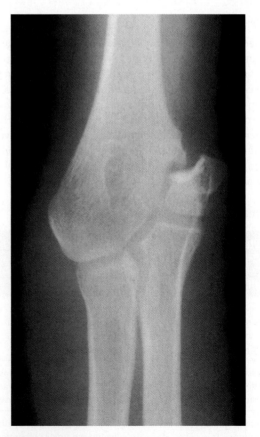

Figure 17-18. Nonunion of a medial condylar fracture in a 10-year-old girl. Note medial subluxation of the radius and ulna.

El Ghawabi[23] described one partial ulnar neuropathy occurring after this type of injury. The neuropathy almost completely recovered after anterior transposition of the ulnar nerve.

SUMMARY, CONTROVERSIES, AND FUTURE DIRECTIONS IN FRACTURES INVOLVING THE MEDIAL CONDYLAR PHYSIS

Medial condyle fractures are rare. The key is identifying them and making the proper diagnosis. The classification, radiographic assessment, and treatment goals are similar to lateral condyle fractures which are encountered much more commonly. Although nondisplaced or minimally displaced fractures can be treated nonoperatively in a cast, careful monitoring is required to identify further displacement and delayed union. When displaced, open treatment with identification of the ulnar nerve and direct visualization of the joint surface are needed. The rate of complications is relatively high and may include osteonecrosis, elbow stiffness, malunion, or delayed union.

Fractures Involving the Lateral Epicondylar Apophysis

INTRODUCTION TO FRACTURES INVOLVING THE LATERAL EPICONDYLAR APOPHYSIS

Fracture of the lateral epicondylar apophysis is a rare injury, with only a few isolated injuries described, mostly in textbooks.[49,72,79] In a review of 5,228 fractures of the distal humerus.

ASSESSMENT OF FRACTURES INVOLVING THE LATERAL EPICONDYLAR APOPHYSIS

MECHANISMS OF INJURY FOR FRACTURES INVOLVING THE LATERAL EPICONDYLAR APOPHYSIS

In adults, the most common etiology is that of a direct blow to the lateral side of the elbow. In children, because the forearm extensor muscles originate from this area, it is believed that avulsion forces from these muscles can be responsible for some of these injuries. Hasner and Husby[32a] suggested that the location of the fracture line in relation to the origins of the various extensor muscles determines the degree of displacement that can occur (Fig. 17-19). If the proximal part of the fracture line lays between the origin of the common extensors and the extensor carpi radialis longus, there is usually little displacement. If the fracture lines enter the area of origin of the extensor carpi radialis longus, then considerable displacement can occur.

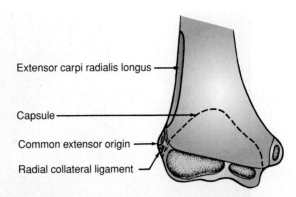

Figure 17-19. Soft tissue attachments. The origins of the forearm and wrist extensor muscles, radial collateral ligament, and outline of the capsule are shown in relation to the lateral epicondylar apophysis. (Redrawn from Hasner E, Husby J. Fracture of the epicondyle and condyle of humerus. *Acta Chir Scand.* 1951;101:195–202.)

SIGNS AND SYMPTOMS OF FRACTURES INVOLVING THE LATERAL EPICONDYLAR APOPHYSIS

Patients will present similar to other elbow fractures, with pain and swelling in the elbow, with pain often localized to the lateral aspect of the distal humerus. As this fracture is so rare, associated injuries are not well described.

IMAGING AND OTHER DIAGNOSTIC STUDIES FOR FRACTURES INVOLVING THE LATERAL EPICONDYLAR APOPHYSIS

Fractures can often be confused with normal anatomy of the lateral epicondyle.[72] The distal part of the epiphysis fuses with the capitellum before the proximal part unites with the adjacent humerus. This frequently results in the physis appearing like a fracture. Also, ossification of the epiphysis begins at the level of the capitellar physis and proceeds first to a typical sliver shape and then to a triangular shape. This natural separation can be confused with an avulsion fracture.[72] The key to determining true separation is looking beyond the osseous tissues for the presence of associated soft tissue swelling (Fig. 17-20). If the ossification center lies distal to the osteochondral border of the lateral condylar epiphysis, it should be considered displaced (Fig. 17-21). Comparing radiographs of the contralateral elbow can be used to aid in diagnosis.

PATHOANATOMY AND APPLIED ANATOMY RELATING TO FRACTURES INVOLVING THE LATERAL EPICONDYLAR APOPHYSIS

Because the presence of the lateral epicondylar apophysis is often misinterpreted as a small chip fracture, a thorough understanding of the anatomy and ossification process is essential for evaluating injuries in this area and distinguishing normal from pathoanatomy.

The lateral epicondylar apophysis is present for a considerable period but does not become ossified until the second

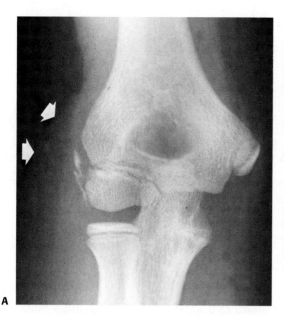 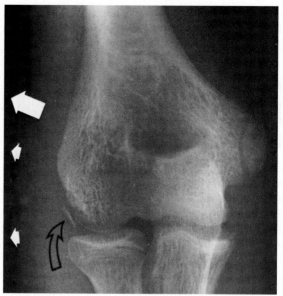

Figure 17-20. Lateral swelling. **A:** Soft tissue swelling in the area of the lateral epicondylar apophysis (*arrows*) suggests an undisplaced fracture involving the apophysis. The fragmentation of the apophysis is caused by irregular ossification. **B:** A small avulsion of the lateral epicondyle (*open arrow*) in an adolescent who is almost skeletally mature. There was considerable soft tissue swelling in this area (*solid arrows*).

decade. The best discussion of the anatomy of the ossification process is in a report by Silberstein et al.,[72] and much of the following discussion is paraphrased from their work. Just before ossification of the apophysis, the ossification margin of the lateral supracondylar ridge of the distal metaphysis curves abruptly medially toward the lateral condylar physis (Fig. 17-22). This process causes the osseous borders on the lateral aspect of the distal humerus to take the shape of the number 3. The central wedge of this defect contains the cartilaginous lateral epicondylar apophysis, which begins to ossify around 10 to 11 years of age. Ossification begins at the level of the lateral condylar physeal line and proceeds proximally and distally to

form a triangle, with the apex directed toward the physeal line. The shape of the epicondylar apophyseal ossification center may also be in the form of a long sliver of bone with an irregular ossification pattern. Silberstein et al.[72] noted that the fracture line involving the lateral condylar physis often involves the proximal physeal line of the lateral epicondylar apophysis. Thus, this apophysis is almost always included with the lateral condylar fragment.

TREATMENT OPTIONS FOR FRACTURES INVOLVING THE LATERAL EPICONDYLAR APOPHYSIS

Unless the fragment is incarcerated within the joint,[49] treatment usually consists of simple immobilization for comfort. Although nonunion of the fragment can occur, this radiographic finding usually does not affect elbow function. There are lateral column osteochondral nonunions that represent chronic lateral ligament instability. Those patients are symptomatic, have functional limitations, and benefit from open repair.

MANAGEMENT OF EXPECTED ADVERSE OUTCOMES AND UNEXPECTED COMPLICATIONS IN FRACTURES INVOLVING THE LATERAL EPICONDYLAR APOPHYSIS

Only one rare major complication has been described with fractures involving the lateral epicondylar apophysis: Entrapment of the fragment, either within the elbow joint[49] or between the capitellum and the radial head.[21]

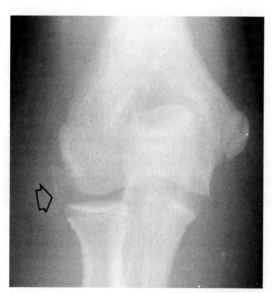

Figure 17-21. Avulsion injury. Avulsion of a portion of the lateral epicondyle in an adolescent (*arrow*). (Courtesy of R. Chandrasekharan, MD.)

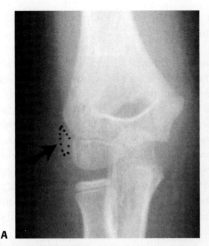
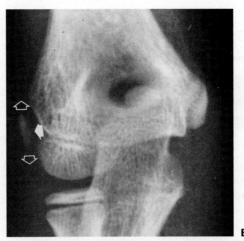

Figure 17-22. Lateral epicondylar apophysis. **A:** The cartilaginous apophysis occupies the wedge-shaped defect at the margin of the lateral condyle and metaphysis (*arrow*). The *dotted line* shows the margin of the cartilaginous apophysis. **B:** Ossification of the apophysis begins at the central portion of the wedge defect (*solid arrow*) and progresses both proximally and distally (*open arrows*) to form a triangular center.

SUMMARY, CONTROVERSIES, AND FUTURE DIRECTIONS RELATED TO FRACTURES INVOLVING THE LATERAL EPICONDYLAR APOPHYSIS

Fractures of the lateral epicondyle are extremely rare. The radiographic appearance of the lateral epicondyle during growth can be confused with what appears to be a fracture. Unless there is entrapment in the joint, treatment is nonoperative. Late nonunions with posterolateral instability will require open repair.

Fractures Involving the Trochlea

Osteochondral fractures involving only the articular portion of the trochlea are extremely rare in skeletally immature children. Grant and Miller[28] reported on a 13-year-old boy who had a posterolateral dislocation of the elbow with marked valgus instability and fractures of the medial epicondyle and radial neck. When the elbow was explored to secure the epicondyle, a large osteochondral fragment from the medial crista of the trochlea was found lying between the two articular surfaces. The fragment was replaced and fixed, and a satisfactory result was obtained, although the presence of the fragment was not detected preoperatively. Yano et al. describe a coronal shear fracture in a 7-year-old boy who at a trochlear shear fracture in the setting of a previously treated lateral epicondyle fracture at the age of 5.[83]

Patel and Weiner[65] described osteochondritis dissecans (OCD) in two patients (three elbows) aged 12 and 14 years. In one patient, open biopsy was done because the osteochondral lesion was thought to be a neoplastic lesion. The other patient with bilateral lesions was treated conservatively with good results. Matsuura et al.[46a] evaluated 1,802 young baseball players, 717 (40%) of whom had elbow pain. Of the 150 who

had bilateral elbow radiographic examination, osteochondral lesions of the elbow were identified in 121 (81%); trochlear lesions accounted for 0.5% of these. More recently, Marshall et al.[46] reported osteochondral lesions of the trochlea in 18 young athletes ranging in age from 6 to 17 years; 10 of the 18 were throwing athletes and two were gymnasts. Based on MRI and MR arthrogram findings, injuries were classified as chondral/osteochondral injury/OCD lesions (13 patients) or trochlear osteonecrosis (five patients). Ten of the 13 osteochondral lesions involved the lateral trochlea and were described as classic OCD; the three medial trochlear lesions were small (<6 mm) and were located on the posterior articular surface of the medial trochlea. Trochlear osteonecrosis in five patients was characterized by growth disturbance involving the ossification centers of the trochlea. The affected trochleas were misshapen and underdeveloped, and radiographs showed the secondary ossification centers to be fragmented, small, and sclerotic, or absent entirely. All five of the patients with osteonecrosis had histories of distal humeral fractures treated with K-wire fixation earlier in childhood (two lateral condylar fractures and one each supracondylar, medial epicondylar, and medial condylar fracture). The authors suggested that the athletic demands placed on the adolescent elbow revealed osteonecrosis from these earlier fractures.[46] The OCD lesions consistently occurred in the posteroinferior aspect of the lateral trochlea corresponding to a watershed zone of diminished vascularity, and the authors hypothesized that the lesions were caused by repeated forced elbow extension/hyperextension that led to impingement of the normal blood supply.[46] Small osteochondral lesions on the posteromedial trochlea were suggested to result from olecranon abutment occurring in an elbow with collateral ligament laxity or insufficiency.

In an older child who sustains an elbow dislocation and in whom there is some widening of the joint after reduction, an intra-articular osteochondral or chondral fracture of the trochlea, capitellum, or radial head should be suspected. Arthrography, MRI, or computed tomography–arthrography should be used for confirmation.

Osteonecrosis of the Trochlea

INTRODUCTION TO OSTEONECROSIS OF THE TROCHLEA

Toniolo and Wilkins[80] reported a series of 30 cases collected over the past 20 years from various sources and suggested that osteonecrosis of the trochlea is probably one of the most unrecognized sequelae of injuries to the distal humerus. A recent systematic review of Hegemann's disease and fishtail deformity identified 15 studies including 58 patients with fishtail deformity.[20] These patients had an average age of 7.8 and were predominantly male (74%).[20] Because avascular necrosis of the trochlea is rare, or often unrecognized, the true incidence is unknown. Bronfen reported six cases in 288 displaced supracondylar humerus fractures.[9] McDonnell and Wilson reported four cases in a series of 53 supracondylar humerus fractures.[47] Narayanan recently described seven cases of which five children had type 3 supracondylar humerus fractures, one had a medial condyle fracture, and the other a lateral condyle fracture.[57] Etier et al. describe five additional cases after supracondylar humerus fractures.[18] We recently examined 15 cases of osteonecrosis of the trochlea, and during the same time period, more than 3,500 patients were treated operatively for a supracondylar or humeral condylar fracture at our institution.[26] This gives an incidence of less than 0.5% and does not include fractures treated nonoperatively, although some mild osteonecrosis cases may have been missed.

Three theories have been proposed to account for the posttraumatic changes that occur in the distal humerus after fractures in the vicinity of the trochlea: malunion, partial growth arrest, and vascular injury. The most common form follows some type of elbow trauma. In some cases, the trauma is occult or poorly defined.[6,7,38,47,55,85] It can occur after displaced or minimally displaced supracondylar humerus fractures, lateral condylar fractures, physeal separations, or medial condylar fractures, or may occur iatrogenically from excessive soft tissue stripping during operative exposure.[60,80] Posttraumatic trochlear osteonecrosis results in a spectrum from simply a small defect of the trochlea (fishtail deformity) to complete destruction of the medial aspect of the distal humerus with a progressive varus deformity, decreased range of motion, and associated instability of the elbow.

ASSESSMENT OF OSTEONECROSIS OF THE TROCHLEA

SIGNS AND SYMPTOM OF OSTEONECROSIS OF THE TROCHLEA

Early there are often minimal, if any symptoms. It often may be 4 to 8 years after initial injury when symptoms related to the complication begin.[57] When symptoms are present, they can include pain and loss of motion secondary to joint incongruity and locking, which is related to loose body formation and joint instability.[9,18,42,55,60,80]

The clinical signs and symptoms differ considerably between the two patterns of necrosis. Patients who have the type A (central defect) fishtail deformity usually do not develop any angular deformities. The severity of the fishtail deformity is related to the degree of necrosis and seems to dictate the severity of the symptoms. In children who have a pattern of total osteonecrosis of the trochlea, including part of the nonarticular surface, a progressive varus deformity usually develops. Because the total medial trochlear surface is disrupted, significant loss of range of motion also develops. These deformities usually worsen aesthetically and functionally as the child matures. Early degenerative joint disease with a loss of range of motion is the most common sequela in severe cases.

Some children with osteonecrosis of the trochlea develop late-onset ulnar neuropathy,[53,70,78,84] thought to be due to a multiplicity of factors, including joint malalignment, abnormal position of the ulnar nerve and triceps tendon, loss of protection by a deep ulnar groove, and the acute angle of entrance of the two heads of the flexor carpi ulnaris. Rarely, a patient may present with fracture (Fig. 17-23).[45]

CLASSIFICATION OF OSTEONECROSIS OF THE TROCHLEA

Osteonecrosis of the trochlea can appear as either a central defect (type A) or total hypoplasia manifest by complete absence of the trochlea (type B), depending on the extent of the vascular injury.

Type A—Fishtail Deformity

In the type A deformity, only the lateral portion of the medial crista or apex of the trochlea becomes involved in the necrotic process, which produces the typical fishtail deformity (Fig. 17-24). This more common pattern of necrosis seems to occur with very distal supracondylar fractures or with fractures involving the lateral condylar physis.

Type B—Malignant Varus Deformity

The type B deformity involves osteonecrosis of the entire trochlea and sometimes part of the metaphysis (Fig. 17-25). This type of necrosis has occurred as a sequela of fractures involving the entire distal humeral physis or fractures of the medial condylar physis[82] and can lead to a cubitus varus deformity in which the angulation progresses as the child matures.

IMAGING AND OTHER DIAGNOSTIC STUDIES FOR OSTEONECROSIS OF THE TROCHLEA

Radiographically, in our series, loss of motion is associated with subluxation of the radial head.[26] With proximal migration of the ulna, the coronoid impinges anteriorly and olecranon impinges posteriorly, leading to progressive loss of motion.[33] Proximal migration of the ulna, radial head escape, or the combination of both may all lead to loss of motion and osteochondral impingement. Plain radiographs can be used for diagnosis, but advanced imaging including the use of MRI or CT can better characterize the deformity, assess osteochondral surfaces, and

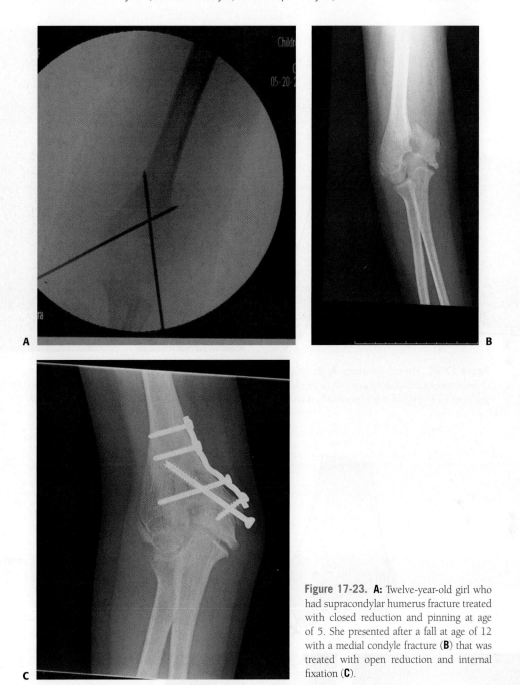

Figure 17-23. A: Twelve-year-old girl who had supracondylar humerus fracture treated with closed reduction and pinning at age of 5. She presented after a fall at age of 12 with a medial condyle fracture (**B**) that was treated with open reduction and internal fixation (**C**).

identify osteochondral loose bodies and arthrosis.[33,37,42] Because the trochlea generally ossifies between ages 7 and 10 with fusion around age 12 to 17, early diagnosis is often not possible after the initial fracture, and explains why often the diagnosis is not made until several years after the initial injury on radiographs.[57]

PATHOANATOMY AND APPLIED ANATOMY RELATING TO OSTEONECROSIS OF THE TROCHLEA

In Haraldsson's classic studies[30,31] of the blood supply of the distal humerus, it was demonstrated that the medial crista of the trochlea had two separate blood supply sources (Fig. 17-26). Neither has anastomoses with each other or with the other metaphyseal vessels. In the young infant, the vessels are small and lie on the surface of the perichondrium.

The lateral vessels supply the apex of the trochlea and the lateral aspect of the medial crista. These vessels cross the physis to enter the posterior aspect of the lateral trochlear ossification center. Their terminal branches lie just under the articular surface. Thus, they are particularly vulnerable to injury when the fracture line occurs through this area, as is typical in fractures of the medial condylar physis, lateral condyle, or a T-condylar fracture. By the same token, a fracture in the supracondylar area in which the fracture line is very distal or a total

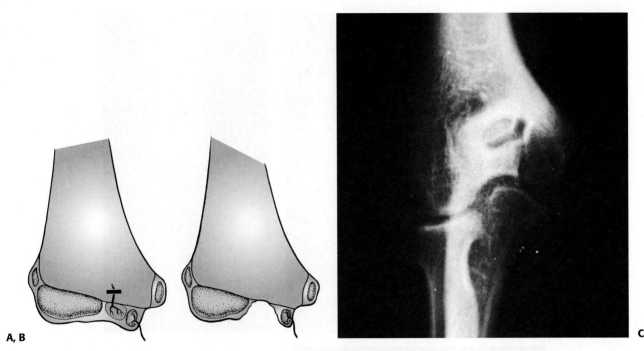

Figure 17-24. Fishtail deformity. **A, B:** Type A deformity. Osteonecrosis of only the lateral ossification center creates a defect in the apex of the trochlear groove. **C:** The typical fishtail deformity is seen in a radiograph of a 14-year-old boy who sustained an undisplaced distal supracondylar fracture 5 years previously.

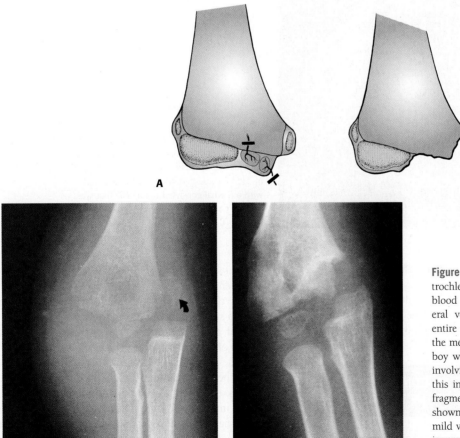

Figure 17-25. Osteonecrosis of the entire trochlea. **A:** In this type B deformity, loss of blood supply from both the medial and lateral vessels results in osteonecrosis of the entire medial crista along with a portion of the metaphysis. **B:** Radiograph of a 4-year-old boy who sustained a type II physeal fracture involving the entire distal humeral physis. In this injury film, there is a large metaphyseal fragment on the medial side (*arrow*). **C:** As shown by the appearance 5 months later, a mild varus deformity is present because of an incomplete reduction. The ossification in the medial metaphyseal fragment has disappeared.

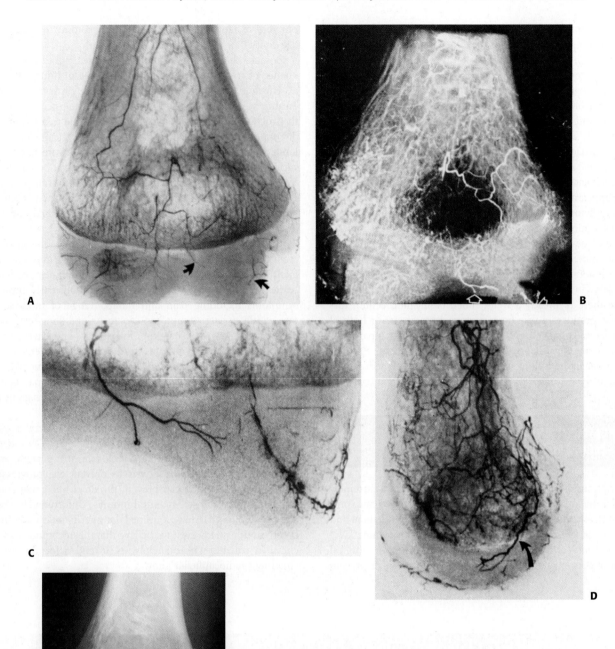

Figure 17-26. Blood supply of the trochlea. **A:** Intraosseous vasculature in a 3-year-old boy. Only two small vessels supply the medial crista of the trochlea (*arrows*). The central portion of the crista appears avascular. **B:** In the lateral view through the medial crista of the trochlea, note that the vessels penetrate the physis posteriorly (*arrow*) to enter the epiphyseal cartilage. **C:** Close-up view showing the extent of the vascular supply of the trochlea. Note that no anastomoses are seen between these medial and lateral vessels. **D:** Lateral view through the medial crista of the trochlea. Note that the vessels penetrate the physis posteriorly (*arrow*) to enter the epiphyseal cartilage. **E:** Radiograph of a 12-year-old boy. The persistence of the two separate ossification centers (*arrows*) of the media crista is seen. The area supplied by the lateral vessel. (**A–D:** Reprinted from Haraldsson S. On osteochondritis deformans juvenilis capituli humeri including investigation of intraosseous vasculature in distal humerus. *Acta Orthop Scand Suppl.* 1959;38:1–232, with permission.)

distal humeral physeal displacement can also disrupt the lateral trochlear epiphyseal vessels as they course along the surface of the metaphysis or at their entrance into the physeal plate. In a systematic review of 58 patients, 48% of patients had a preceding lateral condyle fracture, 31% had a supracondylar fracture, 3 patients had a capitellum fracture, 3 had a medial condyle fracture, and four patients had an unknown fracture.[20]

Another set of vessels enters medially through the nonarticulating surface of the trochlea. This set of vessels supplies the most medial aspect of the medial crista or the medial portion of the trochlear epiphysis. As shown in Haraldsson's studies,[30,31] there appear to be no anastomoses between the two sets of vessels supplying the trochlear epiphysis.

Ossification centers need blood supply for their appearance and development. Before these centers appear, the vessels are more superficial and less well defined. It is speculated that a lesion in these immature vessels in children leads only to a delay in the appearance of the centers. In older children, where there is already a well-defined ossification center, disruption produces a true bony osteonecrosis of one or both of the trochlea's ossification centers. This can result in a partial or total absence of further epiphyseal ossification, leading to either hypoplasia of the central or whole medial aspect of the trochlea, respectively.

TREATMENT OPTIONS FOR OSTEONECROSIS OF THE TROCHLEA

Descriptions of treatment options in the literature are extremely limited. In addition to observation and nonoperative care, proposed treatment options include arthroscopic debridement and removal of loose bodies, capsulotomy for contracture,[18,47,55] interposition arthroplasty for advanced arthrosis, surgical arrest of the remaining medial and/or lateral physis to prevent progressive fishtail deformity,[60] and/or osteotomy for persistent deformity.[60]

Because the osteonecrosis of the trochlea is a direct consequence of trauma to the vessels at the time of injury, there is no effective prevention or treatment of the primary necrosis. Treatment is aimed at only the sequelae of the osteonecrosis of the trochlea. If a loss of range of motion is due to a significant disruption of the articular surface itself, the surgical options are limited. If the osteonecrosis of the trochlea has resulted in a varus deformity of the elbow, this deformity can be corrected by a supracondylar osteotomy with ulnar nerve transposition. The correction of the carrying angle may be aesthetic without functional improvement. Surgical treatment carries the risk of increased stiffness to the already limited elbow.

In our experience, small defects with minimal joint involvement can be observed.[26] In patients with extensive joint involvement, associated with loss of motion, elbow stiffness, or loose bodies, arthroscopic debridement may help transiently improve symptoms including pain and limited range of motion. As one would expect, symptoms can recur and long-term outcomes are unknown. Therefore, in patients who have limited deformity and mild symptoms, arthroscopic debridement can prove to be useful, particularly if there is limited medial and lateral growth of the distal humerus remaining. It may be the only salvage option for symptomatic patients with significant deformity and subluxation of the radial head.

If there is growth remaining in the medial or lateral physis, physeal closure may be of benefit in some patients. Nwakama et al.[60] have suggested that surgical closure of the lateral and/or medial portions of the physis to prevent the progressive intracondylar notching can prevent proximal ulnar migration, impingement, and osteochondral injuries. Unfortunately, there are no studies that have outlined long-term follow-up from epiphysiodesis. However, we believe that this technique is beneficial in patients with open physes, a mild deformity, and a congruent radiocapitellar joint.

Annotated References

Reference	Annotation
Claessen FM, Louwerens JK, Doornberg JN, et al. Hegemann's disease and fishtail deformity: aetiopathogenesis, radiographic appearance and clinical outcome. *J Child Orthop.* 2015;9:1–8.	A systematic review of 15 articles[58] was conducted. Patient characteristics as well as clinical and radiologic evaluation for these patients were discussed. Outcome and treatment data are limited and generally not reported for these patients.
Glotzbecker MP, Bae DS, Links AC, et al. Fishtail deformity of the distal humerus: a report of 15 cases. *J Pediatr Orthop.* 2013;33(6):592–597.	14 patients with a mean age of 10 years old presented with osteonecrosis of the trochlea over a 15-year period. Mean age of presentation was 10 years and average time from index injury to presentation was 4.7 years. 80% presented with pain and mechanical symptoms. 7 patients underwent arthroscopic debridement and one patient had an open debridement. 6/7 who had arthroscopic debridement had initial relief of their symptoms. 5 of these required a second surgery for mechanical symptoms. One patient had an epiphysiodesis to maintain radiographic alignment. At latest follow-up, 40% had persistent pain, and only 13% had normal elbow motion. Patients with radial head subluxation or dislocation had the worst outcomes with regard to motion.

Annotated References

Reference	Annotation
Kilfoyle RM. Fractures of the medial condyle and epicondyle of the elbow in children. *Clin Orthop Relat Res.* 1965;41:43–50.	Three fracture displacement patterns for medial condyle fractures are described that can be helpful in determining appropriate treatment In type I, the fracture line in the medial condylar metaphysis extends down to the physis. Unless there is a greenstick crushing of the medial supracondylar column, these fractures are usually of no clinical significance. In type II, the fracture line extends into the medial condylar physis. The intra-articular portion, as it is in preosseous cartilage, is often not recognized. In this second type, the medial condylar fragment usually remains undisplaced. In type III, the condylar fragment is both rotated and displaced.
Leet AI, Young C, Hoffer MM. Medial condyle fractures of the humerus in children. *J Pediatr Orthop.* 2002;22(1):2–7.	Retrospective review of 21 medial condylar fractures revealed a 33% complication rate with these fractures. Operative treatment indicated for greater than 2 mm displacement. Most of minimally displaced fractures healed uneventfully, but one patient developed AVN and another developed a nonunion.
Marshall KW, Marshall DL, Busch MT, et al. Osteochondral lesions of the humeral trochlea in the young athlete. *Skeletal Radiol.* 2009;38(5):479–491.	18 patients with trochlear lesions were described. This included 3 medial lesions, 10 lateral lesions, and 5 cases of AVN. AVN occurred exclusively in athletes with a history of remote humeral fracture. 7/18 patients required arthroscopy. Trochlear lesions should be considered in throwing athletes presenting with medial elbow pain and flexion contracture/extension block.
Narayanan S, Shailam R, Grottkau BE, et al. Fishtail deformity—a delayed complication of distal humeral fractures in children. *Pediatr Radiol.* 2015;45:814–819.	Seven children aged 7–14 with AVN of the trochlea are presented after grade III supracondylar humerus fracture,[5] medial condyle[1] and lateral condyle[1] fractures. All patients had a central defect and demonstrated joints space narrowing, synovitis, and/or subluxation of the radial head.
Oh CW, Park BC, Ihn JC, et al. Fracture separation of the distal humeral epiphysis in children younger than 3 years old. *J Pediatr Orthop.* 2000;20(2):173–176.	12 cases of fracture separation of distal humerus analyzed, posteromedial displacement seen in all. Patients were treated with either closed reduction and pinning, closed reduction and casting, or cast without reduction, 7/12 developed cubitus varus and 6 had AVN of the medial condyle. Method of treatment, age of injury, and type of injury did not influence outcome.
Ratti C, Guidani N, Riva G, et al. Transphyseal elbow fracture in newborn: review of literature. *Musculoskelet Surg.* 2015;99(Suppl 1):S99–S105.	A review of the literature identified 33 cases from 20 case reports describing a transphyseal elbow fracture. Posteromedial displacement was identified in 21 elbows (64%). 4 patients were treated nonoperatively but 29 (88%) were treated operatively. At follow-up, 88% recovered the carrying angle and 80% range of motion. A relationship to type of treatment and results at follow-up could not be demonstrated.
Supakul N, Hicks RA, Caltoum CB, et al. Distal humeral epiphyseal separation in young children: an often-missed fracture-radiographic signs and ultrasound confirmatory diagnosis. *AJR Am J Roentgenol.* 2015;204(2):W192–W198.	16 patients with distal humeral epiphyseal separation were identified. 15 (94%) had medial and 6 (38%) had posterior displacement of the radius and ulna. The diagnosis was missed on radiographs in 9 (58%) of patients. Ultrasound in 12 patients identified the diagnosis in all cases. In 10 (63%) of the cases, one or more additional humeral fractures were identified. Birth trauma and nonaccidental trauma were common causes. All patients had full range of motion and 2 had mild varus deformities

REFERENCES

1. Abe M, Ishizu T, Nagaoka T, et al. Epiphyseal separation of the distal end of the humeral epiphysis: a follow-up note. *J Pediatr Orthop.* 1995;15(4):426–434.
2. Abzug JM, Ho CA, Ritzman TF, et al. Transphyseal fracture of the distal humerus. *J Am Acad Orthop Surg.* 2016;24:e39–e44.
3. Akbarnia BA, Silberstein MJ, Rende RJ, et al. Arthrography in the diagnosis of fractures of the distal end of the humerus in infants. *J Bone Joint Surg Am.* 1986; 68(4):599–602.
3a. Ashurst APC. *An Anatomical and Surgical Study of Fractures of the Lower End of the Humerus.* Philadelphia, PA: Lee & Febiger; 1910.
4. Barrett WP, Almquist EA, Staheli LT. Fracture separation of the distal humeral physis in the newborn. *J Pediatr Orthop.* 1984;4(5):617–619.
5. Bensahel H, Csukonyi Z, Badelon O, et al. Fractures of the medial condyle of the humerus in children. *J Pediatr Orthop.* 1986;6(4):430–433.
6. Beyer WF, Heppt P, Gluckert K, et al. Aseptic osteonecrosis of the humeral trochlea (Hegemann's disease). *Arch Orthop Trauma Surg.* 1990;110(1):45–48.
7. Blount WP. *Fractures in Children.* Baltimore, MD: Williams & Wilkins; 1955.
8. Bright RW, Burstein AH, Elmore SM. Epiphyseal-plate cartilage. A biomechanical and histological analysis of failure modes. *J Bone Joint Surg Am.* 1974;56(4): 688–703.
9. Bronfen CE, Geffard B, Mallet JF. Dissolution of the trochlea after supracondylar fracture of the humerus in childhood: an analysis of six cases. *J Pediatr Orthop.* 2007;27(5):547–550.
10. Case SL, Hennrikus WL. Surgical treatment of displaced medial epicondyle fractures in adolescent athletes. *Am J Sports Med.* 1997;25(5):682–686.

11. Chacha PB. Fractures of the medial condyle of the humerus with rotational displacement. Report of two cases. *J Bone Joint Surg Am.* 1970;52:1453–1458.

11a. Cothay DM. Injury to the lower medial epiphysis of the humerus before development of the ossific centre. Report of a case. *J Bone Joint Surg Am.* 1967;49:766–767.

12. Dameron TB, Jr. Transverse fractures of distal humerus in children. *Instr Course Lect.* 1981;30:224–235.

13. De Boeck H, Casteleyn PP, Opdecam P. Fracture of the medial humeral condyle. Report of a case in an infant. *J Bone Joint Surg Am.* 1987;69(9):1442–1444.

14. de Jager LT, Hoffman EB. Fracture-separation of the distal humeral epiphysis. *J Bone Joint Surg Br.* 1991;73(1):143–146.

15. DeLee JC, Wilkins KE, Rogers LF, et al. Fracture-separation of the distal humeral epiphysis. *J Bone Joint Surg Am.* 1980;62(1):46–51.

16. Dias JJ, Lamont AC, Jones JM. Ultrasonic diagnosis of neonatal separation of the distal humeral epiphysis. *J Bone Joint Surg Br.* 1988;70(5):825–828.

17. Downs DM, Wirth CR. Fracture of the distal humeral chondroepiphysis in the neonate. A case report. *Clin Orthop Relat Res.* 1982;(169):155–158.

18. Etier BE, Jr, Doyle S, Gilbert SR. Avascular necrosis of trochlea after supracondylar humerus fractures in children. *Am J Orthop.* 2015;44:E390–E393.

19. Fahey JJ, O'Brien ET. Fracture-separation of the medial humeral condyle in a child confused with fracture of the medial epicondyle. *J Bone Joint Surg Am.* 1971;53(6):1102–1104.

19a. Faysse R, Marion J. Fractures du condyle interne. *Rev Chir Orthop.* 1962;48:473–477.

20. Femke FM, Louwerens JK, Doornberg JN, et al. Hegemann's disease and fishtail deformity: aetiopathogenesis, radiographic appearance and clinical outcome. *J Child Orthop.* 2015;9:1–8.

21. Fowles JV, Kassab MT. Fracture of the capitulum humeri. Treatment by excision. *J Bone Joint Surg Am.* 1974;56(4):794–798.

22. Fowles JV, Kassab MT. Displaced fractures of the medial humeral condyle in children. *J Bone Joint Surg Am.* 1980;62(7):1159–1163.

23. Ghawabi MH. Fracture of the medial condyle of the humerus. *J Bone Joint Surg Am.* 1975;57(5):677–680.

24. Gigante C, Kini SG, Origo C, et al. Transphyseal separation of the distal humerus in newborns. *Chin J Traumatol.* 2017;20:183–186.

25. Gilbert SR, Conklin MJ. Presentation of distal humerus physeal separation. *Pediatr Emerg Care.* 2007;23(11):816–819.

26. Glotzbecker MP, Bae DS, Links AC, et al. Fishtail deformity of the distal humerus: a report of 15 cases. *J Pediatr Orthop.* 2013;33(6):592–597.

27. Glotzbecker MP, Shore B, Matheney T, et al. Alternative technique for open reduction and fixation of pediatric medial epicondyle fractures. *J Child Orthop.* 2012;6:105–109.

28. Grant IR, Miller JH. Osteochondral fracture of the trochlea associated with fracture-dislocation of the elbow. *Injury.* 1975;6(3):257–260.

29. Hanspal RS. Injury to the medial humeral condyle in a child reviewed after 18 years. Report of a case. *J Bone Joint Surg Br.* 1985;67(4):638–639.

30. Haraldsson S. The intra-osseous vasculature of the distal end of the humerus with special reference to capitulum; preliminary communication. *Acta Orthop Scand.* 1957;27(2):81–93.

31. Haraldsson S. On osteochondrosis deformans juvenilis capituli humeri including investigation of intra osseous vasculature in distal humerus. *Acta Orthop Scand Suppl.* 1959;38:1–232.

32. Harrison RB, Keats TE, Frankel CJ, et al. Radiographic clues to fractures of the unossified medial humeral condyle in young children. *Skeletal Radiol.* 1984;11(3):209–212.

32a. Hasner E, Husby J. Fracture of epicondyle and condyle of humerus. *Acta Chir Scand.* 1951;101(3):195–202.

33. Hayter CL, Giuffre BM, Hughes JS. Pictorial review: 'fishtail deformity' of the elbow. *J Med Imaging Radiat Oncol.* 2010;54(5):450–456.

34. Herring JA, ed. Upper extremity injuries. *Tachdjian's Pediatric Orthopaedics: From the Texas Scottish Rite Hospital for Children.* 5th ed. Philadelphia, PA: Saunders; 2008: 2483–2572.

35. Holda ME, Manoli A, 2nd, LaMont RI. Epiphyseal separation of the distal end of the humerus with medial displacement. *J Bone Joint Surg Am.* 1980;62(1):52–57.

36. Ingersoll RE. Fractures of the humeral condyles in children. *Clin Orthop Relat Res.* 1965;41:32–42.

37. Ito K, Ogino T, Aoki M, et al. Growth disturbance in aseptic osteonecrosis of the humeral trochlea (Hegemann's Disease): a case report with developmental distal radioulnar joint incongruency. *J Pediatr Orthop.* 2004;24(2):201–204.

38. Jakob R, Fowles JV, Rang M, et al. Observations concerning fractures of the lateral humeral condyle in children. *J Bone Joint Surg Br.* 1975;57(4):430–436.

39. Kamaci S, Danisman M, Marangoz S. Neonatal physeal separation of the distal humerus during cesarean section. *Am J Orthop.* 2014;43(11):E279–E281.

40. Kaplan SS, Reckling FW. Fracture separation of the lower humeral epiphysis with medial displacement. Review of the literature and report of a case. *J Bone Joint Surg Am.* 1971;53(6):1105–1108.

41. Kilfoyle RM. Fractures of the medial condyle and epicondyle of the elbow in children. *Clin Orthop Relat Res.* 1965;41:43–50.

42. Kim HT, Song MB, Conjares JN, et al. Trochlear deformity occurring after distal humeral fractures: magnetic resonance imaging and its natural progression. *J Pediatr Orthop.* 2002;22(2):188–193.

43. Lee HH, Shen HC, Chang JH, et al. Operative treatment of displaced medial epicondyle fractures in children and adolescents. *J Shoulder Elbow Surg.* 2005;14(2):178–185.

44. Leet AI, Young C, Hoffer MM. Medial condyle fractures of the humerus in children. *J Pediatr Orthop.* 2002;22(1):2–7.

45. Luqman I, Kurup H. Post-traumatic fishtail deformity of the distal humerus—is there a risk for refracture?. *BMJ Case Rep.* 2016;1–3.

46. Marshall KW, Marshall DL, Busch MT, et al. Osteochondral lesions of the humeral trochlea in the young athlete. *Skeletal Radiol.* 2009;38(5):479–491.

46a. Matsuura T, Kashiwaguchi S, Iwase T, et al. Epidemiology of elbow osteochondral lesions in young baseball players. *Presented at: 75th Annual Meeting of the American Academy of Orthopaedic Surgeons.* San Francisco, CA: 2008.

47. McDonnell DP, Wilson JC. Fractures of the lower end of the humerus in children. *J Bone Joint Surg Am.* 1948;30A(2):347–358.

48. McIntyre WM, Wiley JJ, Charette RJ. Fracture-separation of the distal humeral epiphysis. *Clin Orthop Relat Res.* 1984;(188):98–102.

49. McLeod GG, Gray AJ, Turner MS. Elbow dislocation with intra-articular entrapment of the lateral epicondyle. *J R Coll Surg Edinb.* 1993;38(2):112–113.

50. Merten DF, Kirks DR, Ruderman RJ. Occult humeral epiphyseal fracture in battered infants. *Pediatr Radiol.* 1981;10(3):151–154.

51. Micheli LJ, Santore R, Stanitski CL. Epiphyseal fractures of the elbow in children. *Am Fam Physician.* 1980;22(5):107–116.

52. Milch H. Fractures and fracture dislocations of the humeral condyles. *J Trauma.* 1964;4:592–607.

53. Minami A, Sugawara M. Humeral trochlear hypoplasia secondary to epiphyseal injury as a cause of ulnar nerve palsy. *Clin Orthop Relat Res.* 1988;(228):227–232.

54. Mizuno K, Hirohata K, Kashiwagi D. Fracture-separation of the distal humeral epiphysis in young children. *J Bone Joint Surg Am.* 1979;61(4):570–573.

55. Morrissy RT, Wilkins KE. Deformity following distal humeral fracture in childhood. *J Bone Joint Surg Am.* 1984;66(4):557–562.

56. Namba J, Tsujimoto T, Temporin K, et al. Medial condyle fracture of the distal humerus in an adolescent with pre-existing fishtail deformity. A case report. *Emerg Radiol.* 2011;18(6):507–511.

57. Narayanan S, Shailam R, Grottkau BE, et al. Fishtail deformity—a delayed complication of distal humeral fractures in children. *Pediatr Radiol.* 2015;45:814–819.

58. Navallas M, Diaz-Ledo F, Ares J, et al. Distal humeral epiphysiolysis in the newborn: utility of sonography and differential diagnosis. *Clin Imaging.* 2013;37:180–184.

59. Nimkin K, Kleinman PK, Teeger S, et al. Distal humeral physeal injuries in child abuse: MR imaging and ultrasonography findings. *Pediatr Radiol.* 1995;25(7):562–565.

60. Nwakama AC, Peterson HA, Shaughnessy WJ. Fishtail deformity following fracture of the distal humerus in children: historical review, case presentations, discussion of etiology, and thoughts on treatment. *J Pediatr Orthop B.* 2000;9(4):309–318.

61. Oh CW, Park BC, Ihn JC, et al. Fracture separation of the distal humeral epiphysis in children younger than three years old. *J Pediatr Orthop.* 2000;20(2):173–176.

62. Otsuka J, Horii E, Koh S, et al. Unusual humeral medial condyle fracture in an adolescent because of a previous post-traumatic fishtail deformity: a case report. *J Pediatr Orthop B.* 2015;24:408–411.

63. Paige ML, Port RB. Separation of the distal humeral epiphysis in the neonate. A combined clinical and roentgenographic diagnosis. *Am J Dis Child.* 1985; 139(12):1203–1205.

64. Papavasiliou V, Nenopoulos S, Venturis T. Fractures of the medial condyle of the humerus in childhood. *J Pediatr Orthop.* 1987;7(4):421–423.

65. Patel N, Weiner SD. Osteochondritis dissecans involving the trochlea: report of two patients (three elbows) and review of the literature. *J Pediatr Orthop.* 2002;22(1):48–51.

66. Pimpalnerkar AL, Balasubramaniam G, Young SK, et al. Type four fracture of the medial epicondyle: a true indication for surgical intervention. *Injury.* 1998;29(10):751–756.

66a. Poland J. *A Practical Treatise on Traumatic Separation of the Epiphyses.* London: Smith, Elder & Co.; 1898.

67. Potter CM. Fracture-dislocation of the trochlea. *J Bone Joint Surg Br.* 1954;36-B(2):250–253.

68. Ratti C, Guidani N, Riva G, et al. Transphyseal elbow fracture in newborn: review of literature. *Musculoskelet Surg.* 2015;99(Suppl 1):S99–S105.

69. Rogers LF, Rockwood CA, Jr. Separation of the entire distal humeral epiphysis. *Radiology.* 1973;106(2):393–400.

70. Royle SG, Burke D. Ulna neuropathy after elbow injury in children. *J Pediatr Orthop.* 1990;10(4):495–496.

71. Ryu K, Nagaoka M, Ryu J. Osteosynthesis for nonunion of the medial humeral condyle in an adolescent: a case report. *J Shoulder Elbow Surg.* 2007;16(3):e8–e12.

72. Silberstein MJ, Brodeur AE, Graviss ER. Some vagaries of the lateral epicondyle. *J Bone Joint Surg Am.* 1982;64(3):444–448.

72a. Siffert RS. Displacement of distal humeral epiphysis in newborn infant. *J Bone Joint Surg Am.* 1963;45:165–169.

73. Skaggs DL, Mirzayan R. The posterior fat pad sign in association with occult fracture of the elbow in children. *J Bone Joint Surg Am.* 1999;81(10):1429–1433.

74. Stricker SJ, Thomson JD, Kelly RA. Coronal-plane transcondylar fracture of the humerus in a child. *Clin Orthop Relat Res.* 1993;294:308–311.

75. Sugiura H, Horii E, Koh S. Malunion of medial condyle fracture of the humerus: a case report. *J Pediatr Orthop B.* 2017;26:437–440.

76. Supakul N, Hicks RA, Caltoum CB, et al. Distal humeral epiphyseal separation in young children: an often-missed fracture-radiographic signs and ultrasound confirmatory diagnosis. *AJR Am J Roentgenol.* 2015;204(2):W192–W198.

77. Sutherland DH. Displacement of the entire distal humeral epiphysis. *J Bone Joint Surg Am.* 1974;56:206.

78. Tanabu S, Yamauchi Y, Fukushima M. Hypoplasia of the trochlea of the humerus as a cause of ulnar-nerve palsy. Report of two cases. *J Bone Joint Surg Am.* 1985;67(1):151–154.

79. Toniolo RM, Wilkins KE. Apophyseal injuries of the distal humerus. In: Rockwood CA, Wilkinis KE, Beaty HB, eds. *Fractures in Children.* Philadelphia, PA: Lippincott Williams & Wilkins; 1996:819.

80. Toniolo RM, Wilkins KE. Avascular necrosis of the trochlea. In: Rockwood CA, Wilkinis KE, Beaty HB, eds. *Fractures in Children.* Philadelphia, PA: Lippincott Williams & Wilkins; 1996:822–830.

81. Varghese J, Teng M, Huang M, et al. Birth injuries to growth plates: a sheep in wolves' clothing. *J Clin Ultrasound.* 2017;45:511–514.

82. Varma BP, Srivastava TP. Fractures of the medial condyle of the humerus in children: a report of four cases including the late sequelae. *Injury.* 1972;4:171–174.

83. Yano K, Kaneshiro Y, Sakanaka H. Isolated osteochondral fracture of the trochlea in the coronal plane in a child before ossification of the trochlea: a case report and literature review. *J Hand Surg Am.* 2018;43:190.e1–190.e5.

84. Yngve DA. Distal humeral epiphyseal separation. *Orthopedics.* 1985;8(1):100, 102–103.

85. Yoo CI, Suh JT, Suh KT, et al. Avascular necrosis after fracture-separation of the distal end of the humerus in children. *Orthopedics.* 1992;15(8):959–963.

18

Shoulder Dislocation and Fractures of the Proximal Humerus and Humeral Shaft

Donald S. Bae

Shoulder Dislocation

Proximal Humerus Fractures

Humerus Shaft Fractures

Shoulder Dislocation

INTRODUCTION TO SHOULDER DISLOCATION

Historically, glenohumeral joint dislocations in skeletally imma-ture patients were thought to be a rare occurrence.[135,141,353] Rowe's classic series of 500 glenohumeral joint dislocations from 1956 contained only eight patients under 10 years of age, though 99 patients were reportedly between 10 and 20 years old.[291] Other published series similarly have docu-mented shoulder instability in adolescents without specific ref-erence to physeal status.[115,223,228,253,287] Prior studies in collegiate athletes have documented the incidence of shoulder instabil-ity to be approximately 1 per 10,000 athlete-exposures, and the incidence of dislocations has been reported to be 1.69 per 1,000 person-years in young adult military personnel.[260,261] A recent study of administrative databases in Ontario, Canada documented an incidence of 1.64 per 1,000 person-years among patients between the ages of 10 and 16 years.[203] Although these demographic data are limited, they do provide some insight into the expected range of glenohumeral joint instability rates in young, active people.

While the exact incidence of traumatic glenohumeral joint instability in skeletally immature patients remains unknown,

there appears to be a rising frequency with which these injuries are occurring in older children and adolescents. Potential etiol-ogies for this trend include increasing participation in higher-demand and higher-energy activities, younger age at first sports participation, and greater awareness among patients, families, and care providers. It is important to remember, however, that ligamentous laxity and shoulder subluxation may be a normal, nonpathologic finding in otherwise asymptomatic children and adolescents.[35] Indeed, there is published information to suggest that physical examination signs of glenohumeral joint instability may be seen in up to 50% of otherwise asymptomatic adolescents.[93]

ASSESSMENT OF SHOULDER DISLOCATION

MECHANISMS OF INJURY FOR SHOULDER DISLOCATION

In general, both traumatic and atraumatic glenohumeral joint instability may be seen. In traumatic instability, the predom-inant direction of humeral head dislocation is anterior. Typi-cally, an anteriorly directed force applied to the abducted and externally rotated shoulder results in anterior dislocation. These injury mechanisms may be seen with sports participation, alter-cations, motor vehicle collisions, and even simple falls onto an outstretched upper extremity.[148] The spectrum of injury includes an anterior labral tear (Bankart lesion), glenohumeral joint cap-sular stretch, compression injury to the posterior humeral head (Hill–Sachs lesion), and/or anterior glenoid rim fracture.

Posterior dislocations are less common, representing 5% or less of all traumatic glenohumeral instability. Typically patients dislocate with the affected shoulder forward flexed, internally rotated, and adducted. More commonly associated with high-er-energy injury, posterior instability events may be seen after falls, sports collisions, motor vehicle collisions, seizures, or electroconvulsive therapy. As in adults, the diagnosis of poste-rior dislocation is often subtle, and a high index of suspicion is needed to avoid untimely or missed diagnosis.[133,346]

Atraumatic shoulder instability is common in children and adolescents. These situations are characterized by initially pain-less glenohumeral dislocation without antecedent or causative trauma, and may be more commonly seen in patients with systemic ligamentous laxity and multidirectional instability.[43] Often patients will report instability symptoms of other parts of the body, including the patellofemoral, ankle, and hip joints. Associations with connective tissue disorders may be seen, such as Ehlers–Danlos or Marfan syndrome, although that diagnosis has yet to be made when they consult the orthopaedic surgeon. Atraumatic instability may be voluntary or involuntary, and both are thought to arise from selective firing of shoulder girdle muscles with inhibition of their antagonists (Fig. 18-1). Spon-taneous reduction is common, and if sedation or anesthesia is used, the glenohumeral joint typically reduces without need for manipulation.[287]

Finally, there are some pediatric patients who sustain gle-nohumeral joint dislocation due to neuromuscular pathology. In cases of arthrogryposis, brachial plexus birth injury, stroke,

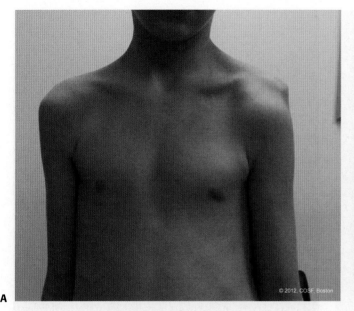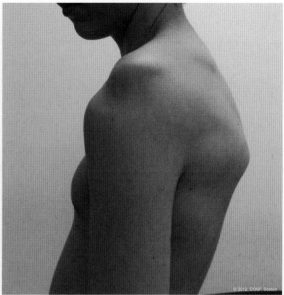

Figure 18-1. Clinical photographs of a preadolescent child with atraumatic multidirectional instability. **A:** Anterior view demonstrates obvious anteroinferior position of the humeral head. **B:** View of the lateral aspect depicts inferior humeral head position and the "sulcus" sign. (Courtesy of Children's Orthopaedic Surgery Foundation.)

or cerebral palsy, muscle imbalance with or without glenohumeral joint dysplasia can lead to atraumatic dislocations, even in neonates or young children.[58,115,361] These situations must be distinguished from neonatal pseudodislocation, in which a traumatic displaced physeal fracture and radiographically unossified proximal humeral epiphysis may give the radiographic appearance of glenohumeral dislocation.

ASSOCIATED INJURIES WITH SHOULDER DISLOCATIONS

The axillary nerve is commonly injured in association with shoulder dislocations. Because of its circuitous course around the proximal humerus and inferior to the glenohumeral joint, as well as its relative tethering at the quadrilateral space, the axillary nerve is usually stretched at the time of humeral head dislocation. As these are usually neuropraxic injuries, spontaneous recovery is typically seen, though recovery may take many months. In the event of complete axillary nerve injuries without spontaneous recovery after the expected period of time, the axillary nerve may be explored, repaired, grafted, or most often now treated with a partial radial to axillary motor nerve transfer to provide return of deltoid motor function.[8,60,91] Similarly, injuries to the axillary artery, though rare, have been reported in association with shoulder dislocation.[8] Prompt fracture reduction with or without arterial reconstitution should be performed in cases of vascular insufficiency and ischemia.

While less common than in adults, concomitant fractures of the proximal humerus (e.g., lesser tuberosity, greater tuberosity) or scapula (e.g., coracoid process, glenoid) may be seen with shoulder dislocation[57,85,286,350] (Fig. 18-2). Careful inspection of plain radiographs is needed to assess for associated bony injuries. While nondisplaced fractures may be effectively treated nonoperatively, displaced fractures may predispose to recurrent instability.[194]

SIGNS AND SYMPTOMS OF SHOULDER DISLOCATIONS

In cases of traumatic anterior glenohumeral joint dislocations, patients will present with pain, swelling, and limited shoulder motion. Typically the limb is held in slight abduction and external rotation, and often the patient will support the affected extremity with the contralateral hand. Careful inspection will reveal abnormal contour of the shoulder, with a prominent acromion, flattened or concavity to the posterolateral shoulder girdle, and obvious prominence or fullness anteriorly in the area of the dislocated humeral head. Careful and comprehensive physical examination is critical to rule out concomitant neurologic injury. The axillary nerve is most commonly affected; sensation over the lateral aspect of the shoulder and deltoid muscle function is checked to assess axillary nerve function (Fig. 18-3). In cases in which there has been spontaneous reduction after an anterior instability event, the shoulder appears more normal in contour and glenohumeral motion is typically preserved, although usually painful and with some anxiety. Patients will be guarded in active motion especially above the shoulder line, resist extremes of abduction and external rotation, and the apprehension test will be positive.[95,211,299,343]

Conversely, patients with traumatic posterior dislocations will present with a painful adducted and internally rotated shoulder. There is often flattening or concavity to the anterior aspect of the shoulder girdle, with palpable fullness posteriorly. Prominence of the superomedial scapular angle (the so-called Putti sign) is often seen, and patients will resist attempts at passive shoulder motion, especially external rotation. Inability to passively externally rotate the shoulder or supinate the forearm should alert the examiner to the possibility of a posterior glenohumeral joint dislocation. Again, a comprehensive examination is performed to evaluate for associated neurovascular deficits.

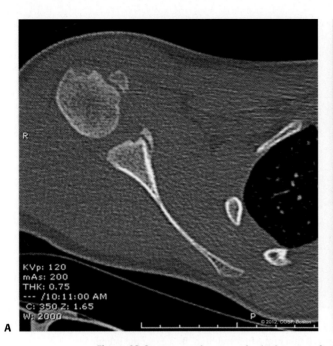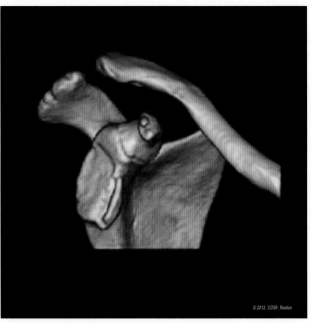

Figure 18-2. Computed tomography (CT) images of a 13-year-old male after traumatic anterior shoulder dislocation. Axial images (**A**) and three-dimensional reconstruction with subtraction of the humeral head (**B**) depict an anterior glenoid fracture (bony Bankart lesion). (Courtesy of Children's Orthopaedic Surgery Foundation.)

In neonates and infants, pseudodislocation may similarly present with pain, reluctance to move the affected upper limb, swelling, and asymmetric contour of the shoulder girdle. Occasionally crepitus due to motion at the fracture site may be appreciated with gentle, small arc range of motion.

Children and adolescents with atraumatic and/or multidirectional instability present quite differently. In addition to the lack of causative or antecedent trauma, these patients may not have pain with joint subluxation or dislocation (see Fig. 18-1).

Even with discomfort, patients will frequently report rapid resolution of pain after reduction. Examination will often elicit diffuse signs of ligamentous laxity, including hyperextension of the elbow, knee, and metacarpophalangeal joints.[246] Abnormally hyperelasticity and striae of the skin may be seen. Focused examination of the shoulder will demonstrate a positive sulcus sign and increased translation with anterior and posterior load-and-shift testing.[337] The sulcus sign refers to a concavity or indentation noted of the skin inferior to the acromion with

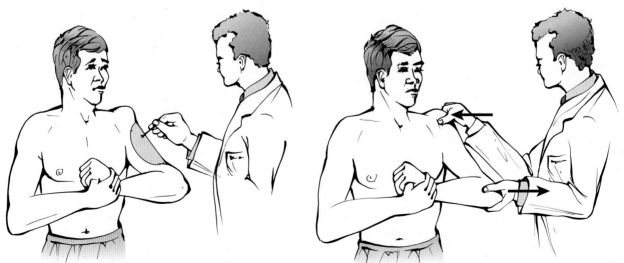

Figure 18-3. **A:** Sensory distribution for the axillary nerve important in anterior dislocation. **B:** Deltoid muscle can be tested in acute anterior dislocation by grabbing the muscle belly with the right hand (*arrow*) while supporting the elbow with the left. The patient then can actively contract the deltoid by pushing the elbow against the examiner's hand (*arrow*) while the examiner feels the muscle contraction.

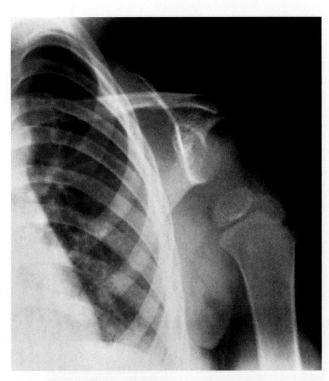

Figure 18-4. Dramatic demonstration of inferior subluxation of the glenohumeral joint in a patient with multidirectional instability. The clinical correlate is the sulcus sign.

manual longitudinal traction applied to the adducted arm (Fig. 18-4). Anterior and posterior load-and-shift tests are performed with the examiner standing behind or alongside the patient. While stabilizing the scapula with one hand, the humeral head is grasped and translated anteriorly and/or posteriorly with the examiner's other hand; translation of greater than 5 mm from center is thought to be an indicator of multidirectional instability. Though some patients are truly unstable in all directions, posterior-inferior dislocations are most common. This pattern may be elicited with forward flexion and slight adduction, with joint reduction achieved with abduction. Patients with voluntary instability may demonstrate their condition by contracting the anterior deltoid and internal rotators while inhibiting the antagonistic muscles.

IMAGING AND OTHER DIAGNOSTIC STUDIES FOR SHOULDER DISLOCATION

Radiographic evaluation should include orthogonal views of the shoulder to assess for direction of dislocation, congruency of subsequent joint reduction, and presence of associated bony injuries. Anteroposterior (AP) and axillary views are preferred (Fig. 18-5). In the acutely injured or anxious, uncomfortable child, alternative views including the transthoracic scapular Y, West Point lateral, or apical oblique projections may be performed.[110,120,322] AP views with the shoulder in internal rotation are not routinely required, but may allow for visualization of Hill–Sachs lesions of the humeral head.

In patients with recurrent instability or in whom the extent of injury needs to be assessed after the initial traumatic

dislocation, advanced imaging may be performed. Magnetic resonance imaging (MRI) will provide visualization of chondral, labral, capsular, and musculotendinous pathology. The addition of intra-articular contrast improves sensitivity for labral pathology and provides more detailed information regarding capsular patulousness; this is particularly helpful in patients with persistent, functionally limiting multidirectional instability in whom surgical treatment is being considered (Fig. 18-6). While computed tomography (CT) and CT-arthrography are less helpful for soft tissue evaluation, they do provide the best modality to identify and quantify bony defects in the glenoid and humeral head[56,79,183] (Fig. 18-7). In children and adolescents in whom a large portion of the glenoid is incompletely ossified, careful inspection of the glenoid contour is needed to avoid missing bony lesions. Loss of the normal sclerotic margin of the glenoid has been proposed as a sign of bony defects of the anterior glenoid rim.[168]

Radiographic evaluation of patients with atraumatic multidirectional instability is similar, though a few points deserve mention. Though plain radiographs are typically normal, patients with congenital glenoid hypoplasia will have subtle rounding or convexity to the glenoid fossa, with or without scapular neck dysplasia.[58,67] As cited above, MRI-arthrography is a useful tool in assessing the capsular laxity and presence of pathologic lesions of the labrum in these patients.

CLASSIFICATION OF SHOULDER DISLOCATION

Classification of Shoulder Instability				
	Mechanism	**Direction**	**Chronicity**	**Associated Conditions**
Classification	Traumatic Atraumatic	Anterior Posterior Inferior Multidirectional	Acute Recurrent Chronic	None Neuromuscular Connective tissue

In general, shoulder dislocations in children and adolescents are described according to the association with trauma, direction of instability, chronicity, and presence of underlying local or systemic disorders. Characterizing shoulder dislocations according to these categories is important and influences treatment decision-making.

Shoulder dislocations may be traumatic or atraumatic in etiology. Direction of humeral instability may be anterior, posterior, inferior (luxatio erecta), or multidirectional. As in adults, perhaps 90% of traumatic dislocations in children and adults is anterior, with posterior dislocations occurring much less commonly and luxatio erecta described in case reports.[141,230,287] Furthermore, pathologic instability may include both subluxation or true dislocation. Dislocation refers to situations in which the humeral head moves completely out of the glenoid fossa, with no articular contact and often with locking of the humeral head on the anterior or medial rim of the glenoid. Subluxation is defined as an incomplete dislocation characterized by pain, a feel of "looseness" or "slipping," and/or a "dead" feeling to the affected limb. Even traumatic subluxations have been

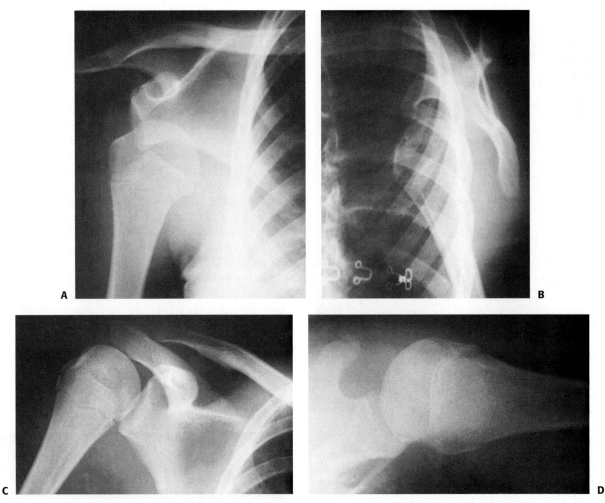

Figure 18-5. Anterior dislocation of the right shoulder in a 15-year-old girl. **A:** Note the typical sub-coracoid position on the AP film. **B:** On a true scapular lateral film, note the anterior displacement of the humeral head. **C:** Postreduction film demonstrates a Hill–Sachs compression fracture in the posterolateral aspect of the humeral head. **D:** On the postreduction axillary film, note the posterolateral compression fracture of the humeral head.

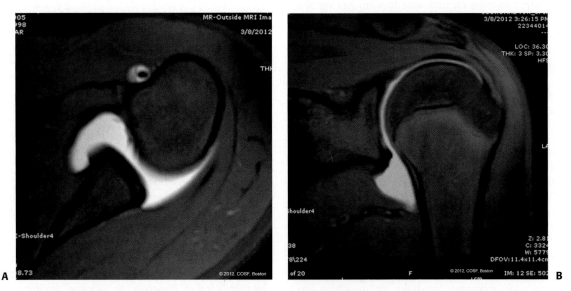

Figure 18-6. MRI arthrogram of the left shoulder in a 14-year-old female with multidirectional instability. Axial (**A**) and coronal (**B**) images depict an intact labrum with a patulous capsule. (Courtesy of Children's Orthopaedic Surgery Foundation.)

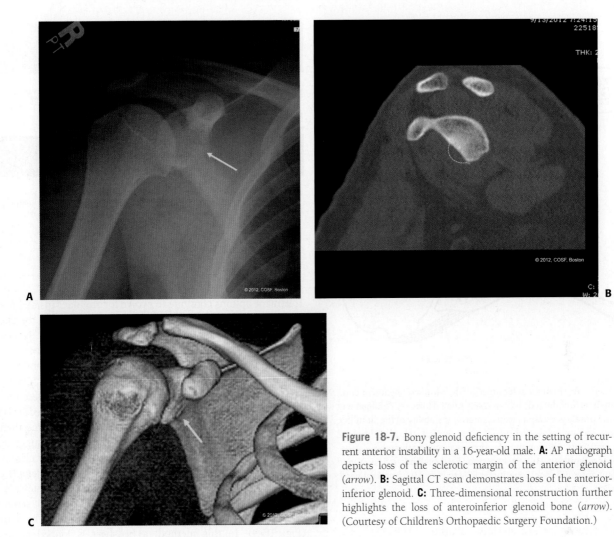

Figure 18-7. Bony glenoid deficiency in the setting of recurrent anterior instability in a 16-year-old male. **A:** AP radiograph depicts loss of the sclerotic margin of the anterior glenoid (*arrow*). **B:** Sagittal CT scan demonstrates loss of the anterior-inferior glenoid. **C:** Three-dimensional reconstruction further highlights the loss of anteroinferior glenoid bone (*arrow*). (Courtesy of Children's Orthopaedic Surgery Foundation.)

associated with structural injury to the glenoid labrum and Hill–Sachs lesions of the humeral head.[262] These conditions must be distinguished from ligamentous laxity, which is typically asymptomatic.

Chronicity is generally classified as being acute, recurrent, or chronic. While a single episode of dislocation denotes acute instability, recurrent instability refers to multiple episodes. Chronic instability refers to unrecognized or untreated shoulder dislocations in which the humeral head is not reduced, and may be seen with congenital or neuromuscular conditions in children.

The presence or absence of associated systemic conditions—including collagen disorders such as Ehlers–Danlos syndrome, or congenital/neuromuscular syndromes such as cerebral palsy—is also a key consideration in diagnosis and management.

PATHOANATOMY AND APPLIED ANATOMY RELATING TO SHOULDER DISLOCATION

The anatomic development, structure, and growth of the proximal humerus are described in the section on proximal humerus

fracture. The glenoid is a shallow, concave fossa with which the humeral head articulates. The radius of curvature of the humeral head is approximately three times that of the glenoid. As the glenohumeral articulation lacks substantial bony constraint, the shoulder is afforded near global range of motion, facilitating placement of the hand in space and holding it there for upper limb function.

Given the relatively unconstrained bony architecture, the glenohumeral joint relies primarily on soft tissue capsuloligamentous structures for stability. The cartilaginous labrum runs along the rim of the glenoid, deepening the concavity and conferring stability. The glenohumeral ligaments are confluent with the labrum and are thickenings of the joint capsule. The inferior glenohumeral ligament has both anterior and posterior components. The anteroinferior glenohumeral ligament is taught and biomechanically contributes most stability in shoulder abduction and external rotation. Disruptions of the anteroinferior glenohumeral ligament or anteroinferior labrum (Bankart lesion) are most commonly seen with anterior traumatic instability (Fig. 18-8). Furthermore, traumatic instability may also cause elevation of the anterior labrum with the periosteum of the anterior glenoid neck, resulting in the so-called anterior

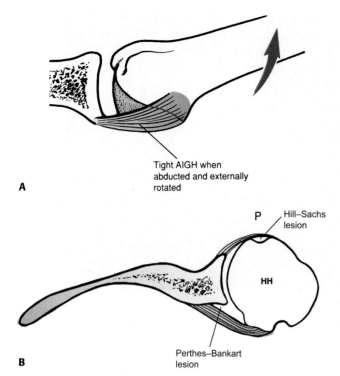

Tight AIGH when abducted and externally rotated

A

P — Hill–Sachs lesion

HH

Perthes–Bankart lesion

B

Figure 18-8. **A:** The tight anteroinferior glenohumeral ligament complex with the arm abducted and externally rotated (*arrow*). This ligament sling is the primary restraint against anterior instability of the shoulder. **B:** A cross section in the transverse plane through the glenohumeral joint demonstrates the common lesions associated with anterior instability of the shoulder: Hill–Sachs lesion, Perthes–Bankart lesion, and redundant anteroinferior glenohumeral ligaments. HH, humeral head; P, posterior.

labroligamentous periosteal sleeve avulsion (ALPSA).[248] The middle glenohumeral ligament is primarily responsible for stability in midabduction and external rotation, whereas the superior glenohumeral ligament resists inferior translation of the humeral head.

On the humeral side, the joint capsule inserts along the anatomic neck of the humerus, except for medially where the insertion lies more inferiorly along the proximal humeral metaphysis. Thus the proximal humeral physis is predominantly extracapsular, with exception of the very medial extent. Shoulder dislocation may result in detachment of the capsule from its humeral insertion, resulting in the so-called humeral avulsion of the glenohumeral ligament (HAGL) lesions.[367] Failure of recognition and repair of these HAGL lesions is a common cause of recurrent instability after surgical treatment.[274]

The glenohumeral joint is surrounded by the rotator cuff muscles, comprising the supraspinatus, infraspinatus, teres minor, and subscapularis. While rotator cuff tears are uncommon in children, these musculotendinous units form a force couple with the larger surrounding shoulder girdle muscles (deltoid, pectoralis major, teres major, and latissimus dorsi) and serve as important dynamic secondary stabilizers of the shoulder. The dynamic stabilizing effects of the rotator cuff muscles are largely the focus of nonoperative rehabilitative programs for young patients with glenohumeral instability.[32]

TREATMENT OPTIONS FOR SHOULDER DISLOCATIONS

NONOPERATIVE TREATMENT OF SHOULDER DISLOCATIONS
Indications/Contraindications

Nonoperative Treatment for Shoulder Instability: INDICATIONS AND CONTRAINDICATIONS

Indications
• Primary dislocation in patients willing to undergo physical therapy and accept risks of recurrent instability
• Multidirectional instability in setting of ligamentous laxity

Relative Contraindications
• Large bony glenoid fracture

Treatment options continue to evolve for shoulder instability in children and adolescents, though remain based upon the classification system and considerations described above. Nonoperative treatment is typically recommended for acute traumatic dislocations as well as atraumatic multidirectional instability.

Closed reduction is performed for acute traumatic dislocations, and a host of reduction maneuvers have been described. Adequate analgesia and relaxation facilitates closed reduction, and both conscious sedation and intra-articular anesthetic injection have been advocated. Multiple reports have suggested that intra-articular lidocaine injection is as safe and effective as intravenous sedation, with less cost and shorter length of stays.[55,227,238,243,354] Portable ultrasound makes accurate injection easier in the urgent care or emergency department setting. The method of traction–countertraction is advocated by many (Fig. 18-9). In this method, a bedsheet is looped around the axilla of the affected shoulder and passed superiorly and laterally to the contralateral shoulder. Longitudinal traction is

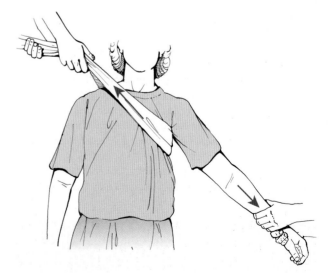

Figure 18-9. Techniques for closed shoulder reduction. A modification of the Hippocratic method uses a handheld sheet around the thorax (*arrow*) to provide countertraction (*arrow*).

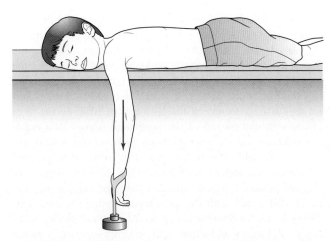

Figure 18-10. The Stimson technique for closed shoulder reduction. With the patient in prone position, weight is hung from the wrist to distract the shoulder joint (*arrow*). Eventually, with sufficient fatigue in the shoulder musculature, the joint can be easily reduced.

applied to the affected upper extremity in line with the deformity, with countertraction provided by pull of the bedsheet. Steady, continuous traction will ultimately overcome the spasm of the shoulder girdle muscles, and the humeral head may be disimpacted and reduced. Others advocate modifications of the Milch maneuver.[74,236,237,252,321] In this technique, the patient is positioned supine and the affected limb supported. Gradual abduction and external rotation is used to achieve glenohumeral reduction. As this technique does not employ traction to overcome muscle spasm, it may be successfully performed without sedation.[297] Still others use the Stimson technique of reduction (Fig. 18-10).[332] With the patient in prone position and the affected limb hanging free over the edge of the stretcher, longitudinal traction is applied to the extremity by means of a weight attached to the wrist. As the spasm of the shoulder girdle muscles fatigues and is overcome, reduction is achieved spontaneously and relatively atraumatically. Additional scapular mobilization may assist with reduction using the Stimson technique.[187,229]

Posterior dislocations may be similarly reduced with traction–countertraction maneuvers. Furthermore, the addition of a laterally directed force on the proximal humeral diaphysis may assist in achieving reduction.[241] In the rare inferior dislocations (or luxatio erecta), a two-step closed reduction maneuver has been advocated.[249] An anterior-directed force is applied to the humeral shaft, converting the inferior dislocation to an anterior one. Subsequent external rotation will then achieve glenohumeral reduction. Closed reduction is the definitive management of luxatio erecta in the majority of cases.[264]

Outcomes

Following closed reduction, patients are typically immobilized with a sling for comfort. There is no evidence that longer duration of sling immobilization with the shoulder in internal rotation reduces the risk of recurrent instability.[265] Recent work, however, has raised the question of whether immobilization with the shoulder in adduction and external rotation is

preferred. Anatomically, 30 degrees or more of external rotation of the shoulder may tension the anterior soft tissues and "reduce" the torn anterior capsulolabral structures to a more anatomic position on the glenoid.[164,239] Dynamic MRI have demonstrated improved position of the displaced labrum with external rotation.[165,307,311,320] Subsequent clinical studies have demonstrated up to a 40% reduction in recurrent instability rates when external rotation bracing was used for 4 or more weeks.[162,163,336] These findings have not been universally reproducible; other investigators have failed to demonstrate reduction in recurrent instability with external rotation immobilization.[99,206,208,265,335] Regardless of the type or time of immobilization after reduction of acute dislocation, physical therapy is typically recommended to improve the dynamic stability conferred by the rotator cuff and adjacent shoulder girdle muscles.[32]

Despite successful closed reduction and subsequent rehabilitation, there is a high risk of recurrent instability, particularly in young, active patients.[215] The available literature, however, is limited in quantifying the true recurrent dislocation rates in children and adolescents. Much of the previously published information consists of retrospective case series of both adult and pediatric patients with limited follow-up.

Rowe[292] previously reported recurrent anterior instability in 100% of children less than 10 years of age and 94% of patients between 11 and 20 years. Marans et al.[223] similarly reported universal recurrent instability in their series of 21 children following traumatic dislocations. Wagner and Lyne[353] reported an 80% recurrence in 10 patients with open physes. In a series of nine patients who sustained traumatic instability at a mean age of 12.3 years, Elbaum et al.[91] similarly reported recurrent instability in 71%. In their review of 154 traumatic dislocations, Vermeiren et al.[349] found a 68% recurrence rate in patients less than 20 years of age. Most recently, Longo et al. reported the results of a systematic review of 693 patients aged 18 years or younger.[215] Recurrent instability was seen in 71% of shoulders with nonoperative care. Higher rates of recurrent instability have been reported in higher-energy injuries as well as those associated with bony glenoid injuries.[235,280,285] Younger patients involved in overhead or contact sports have similarly been noted to have higher recurrent instability rates.[298]

Other reports, however, cite lower recurrence rates in younger patients. Rockwood[287] documented a 50% recurrence rate in patients between 13.8 and 15.8 years of age. Cordischi et al.[64] published their study of 14 patients between 10.9 and 13.1 years of age and reported that only three patients (21%) went on to surgical treatment for recurrent instability. In perhaps the largest study with the longest follow-up, Hovelius et al.[149] reported 25-year follow-up on 229 shoulders in 227 patients who sustained their first traumatic dislocation between 12 and 40 years of age. Of the 58 patients who sustained their primary dislocation between 12 and 19 years of age, 26% reported a single recurrence, and an additional 16% of shoulders stabilized over time (defined as no instability events in the last 10 years). Only 43% of patients underwent surgical stabilization procedures. Additional case reports and small case series exist of young patients without recurrent instability at midterm follow-up.[94,135]

OPERATIVE TREATMENT OF SHOULDER DISLOCATIONS

Arthroscopic Bankart Repair

Indications/Contraindications

Surgical treatment is considered in patients with functionally limiting recurrent instability as well as in high-demand, overhead, or contact athletes in whom the risk of recurrent instability after their primary event is unacceptably high. In general, patients considered for surgery should have failed attempts at physical therapy and rehabilitation. In patients with traumatic anterior shoulder dislocations, recurrent instability is due to injury to the anterior-inferior labrum and adjacent glenohumeral joint capsule and ligaments. Surgical treatment is focused on repairing the torn labrum to its anatomic location on the glenoid rim.

Preoperative Planning

✔ **Bankart Repair for Shoulder Instability:** PREOPERATIVE PLANNING CHECKLIST	
OR table	❑ Standard table
Position/positioning aids	❑ Bean bag and distraction apparatus for lateral decubitus positioning; bean bag and arm holder for beach chair positioning
Fluoroscopy location	❑ Not needed
Equipment	❑ 4-mm 30-degree arthroscope, arthroscopic cannulae, arthroscopic shaver, arthroscopic instruments to prepare tissue and pass sutures, bioabsorbable suture anchors, shoulder immobilizer

Arthroscopic labral repair is the standard treatment for post-traumatic shoulder instability. Preoperative imaging should include plain radiographs of the affected shoulder to rule out associated bony lesions (e.g., glenoid fractures, Hill–Sachs lesions). MRI, with or without intra-articular contrast, is also helpful in determining the extent of labral injury and assessing for concomitant soft tissue injuries. Typical equipment required includes a standard 4-mm 30-degree arthroscope, arthroscopic cannulae, and surgical instruments used to mobilize and prepare the capsulolabral tissue (e.g., arthroscopic shavers, elevators, rasps, and suture passing devices). While a host of commercially available instruments are available, all provide the same fundamental arthroscopic capabilities. Suture anchors are also invaluable for arthroscopic labral repairs, and increasingly the standard is to use bioabsorbable suture anchors for intra-articular procedures.

Positioning

In general, arthroscopic stabilization may be performed in either the beach chair or lateral decubitus position (Fig. 18-11). Advantages of lateral decubitus position include ease of longitudinal and lateral distraction to assist in visualization and access to the axillary recess of the glenohumeral joint. Patients are placed with the unaffected shoulder down, allowing the thorax to fall posteriorly about 10 degrees, which will place the glenoid parallel to the ground. Care is taken to place an axillary roll for the unaffected down side and pad all bony prominences (e.g., contralateral fibular head) to avoid excessive or prolonged compression of the peripheral nerves. The entire affected limb and shoulder girdle are prepped and draped into the surgical field. The limb is placed in balanced suspension with about 40 degrees of abduction and 10 to 20 degrees of forward flexion, typically with 7 to 10 lb of longitudinal and lateral distraction with the assistance of a limb holder. This allows for circumferential access to the shoulder girdle. Additional abduction–adduction and internal–external rotation may be employed during surgery for selective access and tensioning of soft tissues.

The modified beach chair position is also effective and commonly used. After placement of a roll or bump behind the patient between the scapulae, patients may be positioned with the affected limb and shoulder girdle off the edge of the table to allow circumferential access. The use of commercially available beach chairs, limb holders, and/or bean bags will assist with positioning.

Surgical Approach

The procedure begins with examination under anesthesia to assess pathologic instability anteriorly, posteriorly, and inferiorly. After the glenohumeral joint is insufflated with sterile saline solution through the posterior soft spot, a standard posterosuperior, anterosuperior, and anteroinferior arthroscopy portals are established. Viewing is traditionally performed from the posterosuperior portal, but moving the camera to the anterosuperior portal will allow for improved visualization of the anterior glenoid neck and anterior soft tissues, particularly in cases of long-standing instability where the labrum and capsule have scarred in a more medial position.

Technique

✔ **Bankart Repair for Shoulder Instability:** KEY SURGICAL STEPS
❑ Examination under anesthesia
❑ Establish arthroscopic portals
❑ Arthroscopic survey
❑ Mobilization of torn labrum and associated capsule
❑ Preparation of glenoid rim and glenoid neck
❑ Suture anchor placement in most inferior position of labral tear, just onto the chondral face of the glenoid
• Shuttle sutures through the adjacent capsulolabral tissue, effectuating an inferior-to-superior and medial-to-lateral shift
❑ Tie arthroscopic knot
❑ Repeat anchor placement, suture passage, and knot tying sequentially in more superior positions along the glenoid
❑ Minimum of three anchors are used
❑ Skin closure of portals with simple sutures
❑ Application of sling-and-swathe

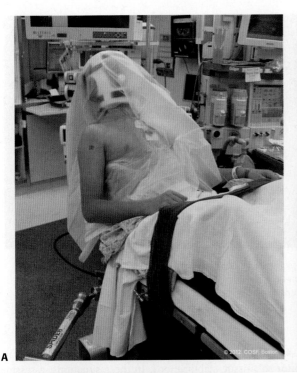
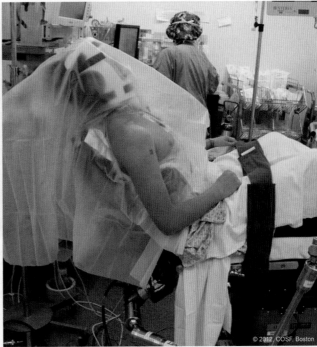
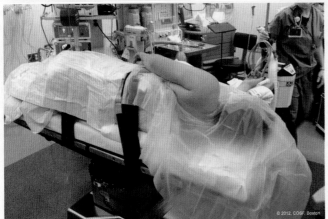
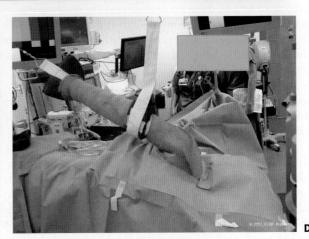

Figure 18-11. Patient positioning for surgical procedures. **A, B:** Beach chair positioning allows for near circumferential access to the shoulder girdle. **C:** Lateral decubitus positioning with assistance of a bean bag. **D:** Use of longitudinal and/or lateral distraction will facilitate arthroscopic visualization. (Courtesy of Children's Orthopaedic Surgery Foundation.)

Arthroscopic survey is performed to assess the extent of labral, capsular, and/or bony injury (Fig. 18-12). After confirmation of labral pathology, the capsulolabral complex is mobilized from its typical medial position using arthroscopic elevators. The glenoid rim and medial glenoid neck in the region of the labral tear is similarly prepared with arthroscopic rasps or shavers in efforts to debride fibrinous tissue and prepare a bleeding bony bed for biologic healing. In a sequential fashion, arthroscopic suture anchors are placed from inferior to superior and sutures are shuttled through the capsulolabral complex.[278,312,345] Knots are tied in a sequential fashion, reapproximating the labrum to its anatomic location and retensioning the soft tissues. While a host of commercially available devices and techniques may be used, all conform to the standard principles of soft tissue mobilization, glenoid preparation, and repair of the soft tissue to the glenoid rim, thus tensioning the anteroinferior capsule.

Latarjet Reconstruction

Indications/Contraindications

In patients with traumatic anterior shoulder dislocations, recurrent instability may also be due to bony fracture or bony insufficiency of the anteroinferior glenoid.[235,285] In these cases, soft tissue procedures alone may not address

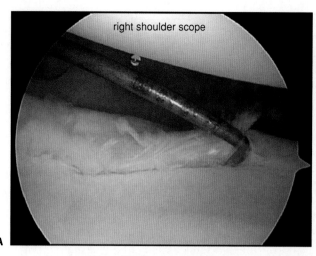 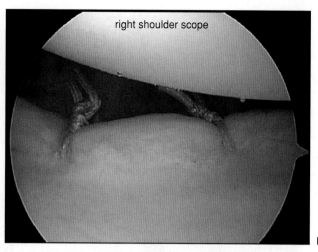

Figure 18-12. Arthroscopic Bankart repair. **A:** Arthroscopic image of an anterior labral tear in the right shoulder of a 16-year-old male. The patient is positioned in the lateral decubitus position. **B:** Arthroscopic appearance after anterior labral repair, demonstrating reapproximation of the labral tissue to the glenoid rim. (Courtesy of Children's Orthopaedic Surgery Foundation.)

the underlying pathoanatomy and are prone to failure. Surgical treatment in these situations typically involves restoring or augmenting the bony deficit of the glenoid. While several techniques have been advocated, transferring the coracoid process with its soft tissue attachments to the glenoid (the so-called Latarjet procedure) has increasingly become the standard of care.[266,270] Bony reconstructions such as the Latarjet procedure have also been advocated in patients with recurrent instability after prior failed soft tissue reconstruction.[176]

In addition to providing additional bony support for the articulating humeral head, the Latarjet procedure also stabilizes the glenohumeral joint by virtue of the fact that the conjoined tendon remains attached to the tip of the coracoid during transfer. These soft tissues act as a "sling" and provide additional anteroinferior stability. Stability is further conferred by preservation of the musculotendinous fibers of the subscapularis. This "triple effect" has been touted by Patte and Debeyre.[77,266,355]

Preoperative Planning

✔ **Latarjet Reconstruction for Shoulder Instability:** PREOPERATIVE PLANNING CHECKLIST	
OR table	☐ Standard table
Position/positioning aids	☐ Modified beach chair position
Fluoroscopy location	☐ Not needed
Equipment	☐ 90-degree oscillating saw, 3.5- or 4-mm cannulated screws

Though MRI is helpful in identifying and qualitatively assessing the extent of labral injury, Latarjet reconstructions are typically reserved for recurrent posttraumatic instability with

associated glenoid loss or in those patients who have failed prior soft tissue stabilizations. In these situations, assessment of glenoid bone loss and possible engaging Hill–Sachs lesions is best done with CT with three-dimensional reconstructions (see Fig. 18-7).

Most Latarjet reconstructions are performed via open deltopectoral approaches. Aside from the standard instruments and retractors used for open shoulder surgery, a few additional items are useful. A 90-degree oscillating saw blade will facilitate accurate and efficient coracoid osteotomy. Appropriate-sized cannulated screws—typically 4 mm in diameter and 34 to 40 mm in length—are used for fixation of the coracoid process to the anterior glenoid.

Positioning

The modified beach chair position is effective and commonly used. A roll or bump is placed behind the patient between the scapulae, to allow for scapular positioning and improved access to the glenoid neck. Patients are positioned with the affected limb and shoulder girdle off the edge of the table to allow circumferential access. The use of commercially available beach chairs, limb holders, and/or bean bags assist with positioning.

Surgical Approach

A standard deltopectoral approach is used. The incision is placed slightly more medial and superior than traditional deltopectoral approaches to the shoulder because of the need to expose the coracoid and medial glenoid neck. A vertical incision in Langer skin lines will maximize the aesthetics of the resultant scar. Superficial dissection will allow visualization of the deltopectoral interval, which is developed taking the cephalic vein laterally with the deltoid. Deep dissection will allow visualization of the coracoid process, conjoined tendon, clavipectoral fascia, and subscapularis muscles.

Technique

> ✔ **Latarjet Reconstruction for Shoulder Instability:**
> KEY SURGICAL STEPS
>
> ❑ Deltopectoral approach
> ❑ Expose coracoid process
> ❑ Release CA ligament with shoulder in abduction, external rotation
> ❑ Release pectoralis minor with shoulder in adduction, internal rotation
>   • Protect neurovascular structures deep to the pectoralis minor
> ❑ Osteotomize coracoid process
> ❑ Prepare undersurface of coracoid bone block and predrill holes
>   • Avoid excessive retraction of coracoid to protect musculocutaneous nerve
> ❑ Split subscapularis at superior 2/3–inferior 1/3 interval
> ❑ Make glenohumeral joint arthrotomy
> ❑ Expose and prepare anterior-inferior glenoid neck
> ❑ Approximate coracoid bone block to prepared glenoid neck
> ❑ Avoid lateral overhang
> ❑ Screw fixation of bone block
> ❑ Wound closure in layers

After initial dissection is performed, a spiked Hohmann retractor is placed superiorly over the coracoid process, with its tip just anterior to the origin of the coracoclavicular (CC) ligaments. The shoulder is abducted and externally rotated, placing the coracoacromial (CA) ligament under tension. The CA ligament is then divided approximately 1 to 2 cm from the coracoid, leaving a cuff of tissue which will be used later for capsular reconstruction. The shoulder is then adducted and internally rotated. The pectoralis minor insertion is then released off the coracoid process, being careful to protect the brachial plexus which lies deep to the pectoralis minor. Following this, the coracoid is osteotomized at its flexure, or "knee," from medial to lateral. The use of commercially available 90-degree microsagittal saws will facilitate coracoid osteotomy. The coracoid is then freed from the remaining surrounding soft tissue

attachments, including the deep coracohumeral ligament, and mobilized while protecting the origin of the conjoined tendon. The undersurface of the coracoid is decorticated to expose bleeding cancellous bone. Two drill holes (typically 3.5 to 4 mm) are made in the coracoid to facilitate subsequent screw placement. Overzealous mobilization or retraction of the freed coracoid process is avoided, as the musculocutaneous nerve enters the coracobrachialis approximately 4 to 5 cm distal.

Direction is then turned to glenoid preparation. With the shoulder in adduction and external rotation, the subscapularis is split in line with its muscle fibers between the superior two-thirds and inferior one-third. This muscle splitting technique preserves subscapularis integrity, contributing stability and minimizing iatrogenic injury to the axillary nerve. The plane between the subscapularis and underlying capsule is developed bluntly, and the glenohumeral joint line is identified. With the shoulder in neutral rotation, a vertical capsulotomy is made in the glenohumeral joint; this may be extended with a medial horizontal incision (in the shape of a sideways "T") for improved exposure of the anterior-inferior glenoid. With the shoulder internally rotated, a Fukuda or humeral head retractor is then placed into the glenohumeral joint. Exposure of the anterior-inferior glenoid neck is then performed via subperiosteal elevation or debridement of the scar tissue and prior bony Bankart fragments. The recipient bed on the glenoid is then decorticated until punctate bleeding is seen.

The coracoid process is then passed through the subscapularis split and its previously decorticated deep surface is approximated to the anterior-inferior glenoid neck. Care is made to position the coracoid bone block precisely; lateral overhang may result in joint incongruity and subsequent degenerative arthrosis or pain. After the coracoid is positioned, the previously placed drill holes are identified. Through these holes, the glenoid neck is drilled anterior to posteriorly in the path of anticipated screw passage. Measurements are taken, and screw fixation of the coracoid process to the glenoid is achieved with 3.5- or 4-mm screws (Fig. 18-13). Screws are typically

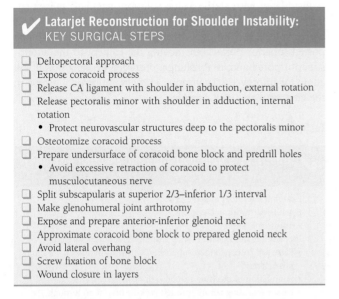
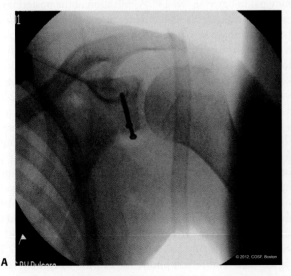
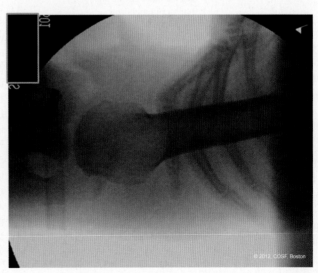

Figure 18-13. Intraoperative fluoroscopy images of the left shoulder following Latarjet reconstruction. **A:** Anteroposterior and (**B**) axillary projections depict screw fixation of the coracoid process, with care made not to lateralize the bone block. (Courtesy of Children's Orthopaedic Surgery Foundation.)

32 to 34 mm in older adolescents, though the size will vary according from patient to patient. The lateral portion of the glenohumeral capsule is then reapproximated to the cuff of prior CA ligament still attached to the coracoid, completing a capsular reconstruction. Wound closure is performed in layers including pectoralis major repair, though the subscapularis split need not be closed. Patients are placed in a sling and swathe postoperatively.

Arthroscopic Capsulorrhaphy

Indications/Contraindications

In patients with multidirectional instability which is painful and/or functionally limiting and has failed nonoperative treatment, arthroscopic capsulorrhaphy may be considered. As cited above, careful patient selection and preoperative counseling is critical, given the risk of recurrent instability and importance of postoperative therapy. Relative contraindications include patients with poorly controlled neuromuscular conditions, or those with cognitive or developmental delays limiting understanding and compliance with postoperative care.

Preoperative Planning

✔ Arthroscopic Capsulorrhaphy for Shoulder Instability: PREOPERATIVE PLANNING CHECKLIST

OR table	☐ Standard table
Position/positioning aids	☐ Bean bag and distraction apparatus for lateral decubitus positioning; bean bag and arm holder for beach chair positioning
Fluoroscopy location	☐ Not needed
Equipment	☐ 4-mm 30-degree arthroscope, arthroscopic cannulae, arthroscopic shaver, arthroscopic instruments to prepare tissue and pass sutures, bioabsorbable suture anchors, shoulder immobilizer

Preoperative planning and equipment is similar to arthroscopic Bankart repair, as described above. MRI-arthrography is particularly useful, as it may demonstrate areas of capsular redundancy and guide selective capsulorrhaphy.

Positioning

Arthroscopic capsulorrhaphy may be performed either in the lateral decubitus or modified beach chair positions. Given the need for circumferential access around the glenoid and glenohumeral joint, the addition of laterally directed distraction is useful. This may be facilitated with the use of lateral traction, commercially available arm holders, or placement of a bump beneath the axilla.

Surgical Approach

Similar to arthroscopic Bankart repairs, the procedure begins with examination under anesthesia to assess pathologic instability

anteriorly, posteriorly, and inferiorly. After glenohumeral joint is insufflated with sterile saline solution, standard posterosuperior, anterosuperior, and anteroinferior arthroscopy portals are established. Viewing is traditionally performed from the posterosuperior portal, but moving the camera to the anterosuperior portal and establishing a posterior working portal will allow for improved visualization and circumferential access to the glenohumeral joint capsule.

Technique

✔ Arthroscopic Capsulorrhaphy for Shoulder Instability: KEY SURGICAL STEPS

- ☐ Examination under anesthesia
- ☐ Establish arthroscopic portals
- ☐ Arthroscopic survey
- ☐ Preparation and imbrication of posterior glenohumeral joint
  - Place arthroscope anterosuperiorly with working portal posteriorly
  - Stimulation of bleeding response in posterior capsule
  - Pass imbricating suture through capsule first, then through chondrolabral junction, beginning in most inferior position
  - May store sutures in anteroinferior portal to ease visualization and subsequent suture management
  - Pass additional plication sutures from inferior to superior
  - After all posterior sutures have been placed, tie in sequential fashion from inferior to superior
- ☐ Preparation and imbrication of anterior glenohumeral joint
  - Place arthroscope posteriorly and establish accessory portal anterosuperiorly
  - Stimulate redundant anterior capsule until bleeding response seen
  - Pass imbricating sutures through capsule and then chondrolabral junction, placating redundant tissue
  - Tie sutures as they are placed, inferiorly to superiorly
- ☐ Skin closure with simple sutures
- ☐ Application of sling-and-swathe

Arthroscopic survey is performed to assess the extent of capsular patulousness and rule out unrecognized labral and/or bony pathology (Fig. 18-14). As plication of the posterior capsule is typically more challenging, direction is first turned to the posterior aspect of the shoulder. The arthroscope is placed in the anterosuperior portal and a working portal established posteriorly. The redundant capsule adjacent to the glenoid rim is prepared using arthroscopic rasps or shavers until punctate bleeding is seen, in efforts to stimulate a healing response; care is made to avoid overzealous tissue preparation, as the tissue is thin and undesirable rents in the capsule may be created. Following this, imbricating sutures may be placed, beginning in the most inferior aspect of the joint. Typically this is performed by passing a suture through capsular tissue approximately 1 cm from the labrum, and then passing the suture a second time from the capsule through the chondrolabral junction. (Prior biomechanical studies have demonstrated that sutures passed through the chondrolabral junction of patients with an intact labrum are as strong as suture anchors.[275]) This "pinch-tuck" suture will plicate the capsule when tied, reducing overall capsular volume. If knots are tied as the sutures are passed, the reduced capsular volume will often make subsequent suture placement more difficult; for this reason, consideration is made to pass all posterior sutures first before tying. After all posterior sutures are placed, they may be tied in sequential fashion from inferior to superior, completing the posterior capsulorrhaphy.

The arthroscope is then repositioned posteriorly and an accessory portal reestablished anterosuperiorly. The anteroinferior capsule is similarly prepared with rasps, shavers, or other instruments until punctate bleedings is seen. Plicating sutures are again passed in a "pinch-tuck" fashion, imbricating the redundant capsule to the intact glenoid labrum. These may be tied in series, completing the circumferential repair.

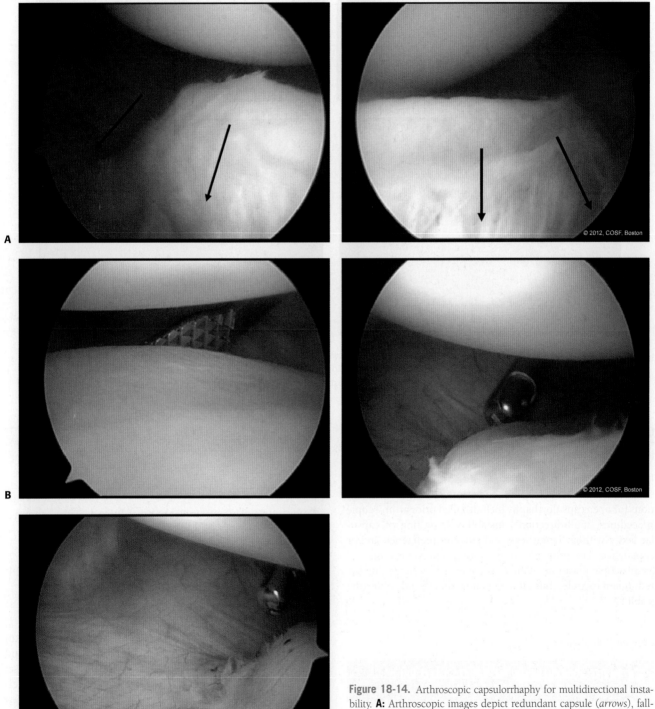

Figure 18-14. Arthroscopic capsulorrhaphy for multidirectional instability. **A:** Arthroscopic images depict redundant capsule (*arrows*), falling away from the glenoid rim and labrum. **B:** Tissue preparation may be performed with either rasps, shavers, or other devices to stimulate a bleeding response (**C**).

(continues)

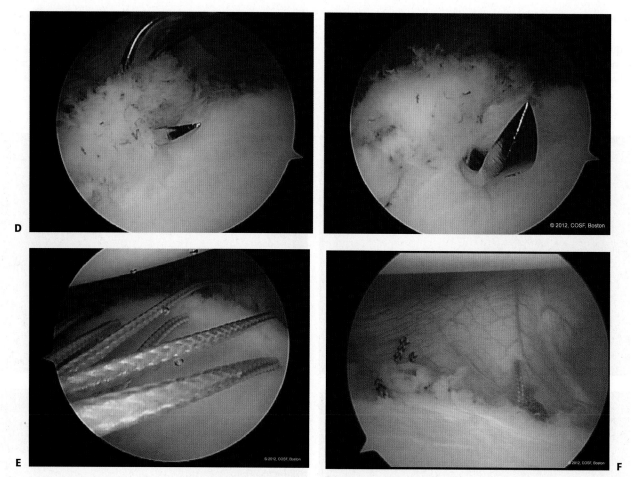

Figure 18-14. (*Continued*) **D:** Suture passing devices are used in a "pinch-tuck" fashion to imbricate the redundant tissue. **E:** Arthroscopic view after posterior plication sutures have been passed. **F:** After sutures have been tied, note is made of plication of the capsule and loss of the capsular redundancy. (Courtesy of Children's Orthopaedic Surgery Foundation.)

Open Capsulorrhaphy

Indications/Contraindications

Despite advances in arthroscopic surgical techniques, open soft tissue procedures may still be performed. Relative indications for open capsulorrhaphy include failed prior arthroscopic procedures, multidirectional instability in setting of capsular laxity without labral tear, and surgeon preference and/or experience. The principles of these procedures are similar to arthroscopic plication: Stability is conferred by tightening the redundant capsule, thus reducing joint volume and conferring stability.

Preoperative Planning

✔ **Open Capsulorrhaphy for Shoulder Instability:** PREOPERATIVE PLANNING CHECKLIST	
OR table	☐ Standard table
Position/positioning aids	☐ Modified beach chair position, limb holder if available
Fluoroscopy location	☐ Not needed
Equipment	☐ Shoulder retractors, nonabsorbable braided sutures

Preoperative planning similar to procedures described above.

Positioning

The modified beach chair position is used. Intraoperative positioning is aided by a limb holder.

Surgical Approach

A standard deltopectoral approach is used, with the skin incision beginning just lateral to the coracoid process and extending within Langer skin lines toward the axillary crease. The cephalic vein is typically retracted laterally with the deltoid. After the clavipectoral fascia is excised, the conjoined tendon is carefully retracted medially to avoid excessive traction to the musculocutaneous nerve. This will allow direct visualization of the subscapularis and underlying glenohumeral joint capsule.

Technique

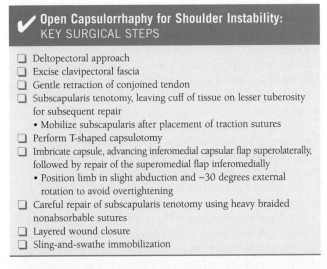

Open Capsulorrhaphy for Shoulder Instability:
KEY SURGICAL STEPS

☐ Deltopectoral approach
☐ Excise clavipectoral fascia
☐ Gentle retraction of conjoined tendon
☐ Subscapularis tenotomy, leaving cuff of tissue on lesser tuberosity for subsequent repair
 • Mobilize subscapularis after placement of traction sutures
☐ Perform T-shaped capsulotomy
☐ Imbricate capsule, advancing inferomedial capsular flap superolaterally, followed by repair of the superomedial flap inferomedially
 • Position limb in slight abduction and ~30 degrees external rotation to avoid overtightening
☐ Careful repair of subscapularis tenotomy using heavy braided nonabsorbable sutures
☐ Layered wound closure
☐ Sling-and-swathe immobilization

After the subscapularis is exposed, the limb is placed in adduction and external rotation. The lesser tuberosity is palpated and identified. A subscapularis tenotomy may then be performed 2 to 3 cm medial to its insertion on the lesser tuberosity, leaving a cuff of tissue laterally to allow for subsequent repair. Traction sutures are placed on the subscapularis tendon, which may then be mobilized and separated from the underlying glenohumeral joint capsule. In some situations, the upper two-thirds of the subscapularis may be divided, leaving a portion of the inferior musculotendinous unit intact. Final option is a subscapularis muscle splitting approach.

Next, a T-shaped capsulotomy is created; a vertical incision is made laterally, with a subsequent transverse extension medially. The superomedial and inferomedial capsular flaps are then mobilized with suture tags. With the limb in the desired position of slight abduction and external rotation, the inferomedial limb is advanced and shifted superolaterally, repaired to the lateral capsule with multiple interrupted nonabsorbable sutures. This positioning preserves normal capsular laxity and lessens risk of degenerative arthrosis that can occur with surgical over-tightening. The superomedial limb is then similarly advanced inferomedially and sewn to the lateral capsule, completing the capsulorrhaphy. Meticulous repair of the subscapularis tenotomy is performed with multiple braided nonabsorbable sutures. The subcutaneous tissues and skin are closed in layers, followed by application of a sling and swathe.

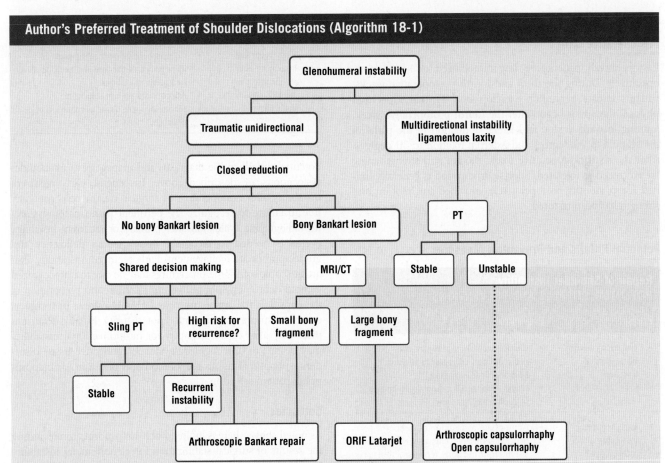

Author's Preferred Treatment of Shoulder Dislocations (Algorithm 18-1)

Algorithm 18-1. Author's preferred treatment for shoulder dislocation.

Children and adolescents with traumatic, anterior shoulder dislocations are treated with prompt closed reduction and sling immobilization. Radiographs are obtained to confirm adequacy of glenohumeral reduction and evaluate for possible bony glenoid fractures. In the majority of patients with purely soft tissue injuries—likely anterior-inferior labral tears—physical therapy is initiated following brief immobilization. Return to sports is limited until patients have restoration of motion, strength, and proprioception.

Early in the postinjury period, patients and families are counseled regarding the risk of recurrent instability. In high-risk patients (e.g., contact or overhead athletes) or patients for whom the risk of recurrent instability is judged to be unacceptable, arthroscopic Bankart repair may be performed after primary dislocation.[129,257] In rare circumstances where patients wish to continue with high-risk activities despite known risk of recurrent instability (e.g., in-season contact athlete), functional bracing with orthoses limiting abduction and external rotation may be used.

Patients with bony Bankart lesions are further assessed with CT, and quantification is made of glenoid deficiency. Given the high risk of recurrent instability in the setting of glenoid bone loss, patients with small marginal lesions are offered arthroscopic repair. Patients with larger bony glenoid lesions are treated with open reduction and internal fixation (ORIF) versus Latarjet reconstruction, depending upon the integrity of the bony fragment.

Surgical stabilization of adolescents with recurrent unidirectional instability is typically performed via arthroscopic capsulolabral repair. Preoperative imaging with MRI-arthrography will better define the extent of labral injury and rule out unrecognized or attritional glenoid insufficiency. Latarjet reconstructions are performed in cases of glenoid bone loss or recurrent instability failing prior arthroscopic stabilizations.

Patients with atraumatic multidirectional instability in the setting of ligamentous laxity or other systemic conditions (e.g., hypermobility, Ehlers–Danlos, etc.) are treated with physical therapy, emphasizing strength, proprioception, biofeedback, and neuromuscular retraining of the entire shoulder girdle. In select patients where there is persistent, painful or functionally limiting instability refractory to or precluding physical therapy, surgical treatment is considered. MRI-arthrography is obtained to characterize the extent and magnitude of capsular redundancy. Stabilization is performed via arthroscopic capsulorrhaphy, with appropriate postoperative immobilization and therapy.

Postoperative Care

Postoperatively, patients are sling immobilized for 4-week postoperatively. During the third and fourth postoperative weeks, patients initiate pendulum exercises only. Formal supervised physical therapy is begun after the fourth postoperative week, limiting forward flexion and lateral abduction in the plane of the scapula to 90 degrees and external rotation to 30 degrees. After the sixth postoperative week, motion and strengthening are advanced as tolerated. Sports participation is generally limited for 6 months postoperatively, provided full motion and strength has been restored.

Potential Pitfalls and Preventive Measures

Repair of Shoulder Instability: POTENTIAL PITFALLS AND PREVENTIONS	
Pitfall	**Prevention**
• Failure to identify bony glenoid fractures	• Careful evaluation of injury and postreduction radiographs including MRI and/or CT imaging • Use of orthogonal radiographic images, including axillary view
• Early recurrent instability after arthroscopic stabilization	• Appropriate recognition of glenoid deficiency or large, engaging Hill–Sachs lesion requiring bony reconstruction • Meticulous preparation, mobilization of capsulolabral tissue, particularly in the setting of an ALPSA lesion • Appropriate suture passage and knot security • Appropriate recognition of HAGL lesions
• Early recurrent instability after stabilization for multidirectional instability	• Comprehensive counseling regarding importance of therapy and nonoperative treatment modalities • Appropriate patient selection • Meticulous soft tissue preparation and plication

Potential pitfalls in the diagnosis and management of shoulder dislocations are described above. In general, early recurrent instability after nonoperative or surgical treatment is generally due to failure to recognize the pertinent pathoanatomy. Careful radiographic evaluation after primary or recurrent instability events is needed to recognize bony glenoid deficiency and guide appropriate management. Early recurrent instability after arthroscopic soft tissue procedures may be due to unrecognized glenoid deficiency, suboptimal mobilization and preparation of the capsulolabral tissue, untreated HAGL lesions, or technical errors in suture passage and knot security. Finally, recurrent instability after capsulorrhaphy for multidirectional instability may be due to unrecognized systemic connective tissue disorders, suboptimal tissue preparation and plication, or inappropriate patient selection.

Outcomes

As noted above, there is limited published information regarding the results of surgical stabilization for glenohumeral instability in children and adolescents. Much of the current understanding of the treatment outcomes is derived from applications of the adult experiences. A number of general observations may be gleaned from review of the existing retrospective case series. First, there has been an increase in the incidence of glenohumeral instability in younger patients, perhaps because of increasing activities and younger age of first sports participation, with expectation for high recurrence rates with nonoperative treatment alone.[78,116,149,338] Second, arthroscopic repairs have become increasingly common and preferred over open stabilization procedures.[222,280] Third, surgical stabilization of Bankart lesions safely and effectively improves shoulder stability, with the risk of recurrence reduced to 5% to 25%.[1,44,200] Castagna et al.[44] reported the results of 65 patients between 13 and 18 years of age, treated with arthroscopic capsulolabral repair, all of whom were overhead or contact athletes. At mean 5-year follow-up, shoulder motion was restored and 81% had returned to their preinjury level of sports participation. Recurrent instability was reported in 21%, and recurrence was associated with choice of sports participation. In a report of 32 arthroscopic stabilizations in 30 patients under 18 years of age, Jones et al.[172] similarly reported high functional outcomes, though recurrent instability was noted in 12% to 19% of patients. Shymon et al. corroborated these results in a series of 99 patients treated with either open or arthroscopic Bankart repairs. Recurrent instability or need for secondary surgery was noted in 21% of patients, and no difference was seen based upon surgical technique.[319] Finally, bony procedures including the Latarjet coracoid transfer are safe and effective, with low risk of recurrent instability.[10,151,153]

MANAGEMENT OF ADVERSE OUTCOMES AND UNEXPECTED COMPLICATIONS RELATED TO SHOULDER DISLOCATIONS

Shoulder Dislocations:
COMMON ADVERSE OUTCOMES AND COMPLICATIONS

- Recurrent instability
- Neurovascular injury
- Chondrolysis
- Arthrosis

Adverse outcomes and complications occur infrequently with glenohumeral instability. As noted above, vascular injury is exceedingly rare, and the majority of neurologic injuries associated with traumatic dislocations represent neurapraxic traction injuries to the axillary nerve more commonly than brachial plexus, with expectation of spontaneous resolution over time. Nerve repairs or reconstructions are rarely needed and reserved for patients who fail to demonstrate progressive spontaneous recovery.

Chondrolysis has been increasingly reported in patients undergoing arthroscopic stabilizations for glenohumeral instability. Reports suggest that use of intra-articular analgesics (e.g., indwelling intra-articular pain catheters) are associated with chondrolysis, and for this reason are currently contraindicated.[306,309,325,364] Similarly, unexpected joint degeneration has been reported after thermal capsulorrhaphy and loose metallic suture anchors, likely related to thermal injury and third body wear of the articular cartilage, respectively.[63,83,117,174] Cartilage loss in a young, skeletally immature shoulder is a disastrous and yet unsolved complication. Avoidance of excessive heat and proper placement of bioabsorbable suture anchors may

minimize these adverse events. Judicious placement of bone grafts and internal fixation, such as in the Latarjet procedure, is also critically important to minimize risk of early arthrosis.[152]

SUMMARY, CONTROVERSIES, AND FUTURE DIRECTIONS RELATED TO SHOULDER DISLOCATIONS

In summary, glenohumeral instability is common in children and adolescents. While closed reduction is easily performed after acute dislocations, there is a high risk of recurrent instability. In appropriately selected patients, arthroscopic or open soft tissue and/or bony stabilization procedures are safe and effective.

There is ongoing debate and controversy surrounding the indications for surgical stabilization after primary traumatic dislocation in the child or adolescent. Proponents of primary surgery point to the safety and efficacy of predominantly arthroscopic procedures in reducing recurrence risk and restoring stability and return of function. Furthermore, there is some evidence suggesting recurrent dislocations may lead to more extensive labral tears, development of glenoid insufficiency, and even arthrosis.[150,179] Many argue that surgical stabilization should be performed in higher-risk patients (e.g., young athletes involved in contact sports).[49,190] An expected-value decision analysis supports primary arthroscopic stabilization if recurrence risk above 32% and utility value of surgical intervention remains above 6.6.[19] Further investigation of the natural history of recurrent glenohumeral instability as well as prospective randomized trials of surgical versus nonoperative treatment is needed in the pediatric patient population.

Finally, as more information regarding the frequency and clinical significance of bony glenoid and humeral head defects becomes available, clarification of the indications for bony augmentation procedures (e.g., coracoid transfer, bone grafting) is needed. This is particularly relevant given the persistent risks of recurrent instability after arthroscopic Bankart repairs and the promising longer-term studies regarding the results of bony procedures.[56,151,153,168,183]

Proximal Humerus Fractures

INTRODUCTION TO PROXIMAL HUMERUS FRACTURES

Proximal humeral fractures are relatively uncommon injuries, with an estimated annual incidence of 1.2 to 4.4 per 1,000, and representing less than 5% of all childhood fractures.[195,196,289] Given the metaphyseal location, thick periosteum, and proximity to the proximal humeral physis, there is tremendous healing and remodeling potential of proximal humerus fractures. Furthermore, given the robust, near-universal motion about the glenohumeral joint, little functional impairment may be seen even in cases of considerable bony malalignment. For these reasons, most proximal humeral fractures are amenable to nonoperative treatment.[263]

MECHANISMS OF INJURY FOR PROXIMAL HUMERUS FRACTURES

Proximal humerus fractures occur through a number of characteristic injury mechanisms. Birth-related fractures of the proximal humerus are not uncommon.[202] In general, hyperextension and/or rotational forces imparted on the upper limb during labor and delivery result in failure through the proximal humeral physis or metaphysis (Fig. 18-15).[73,131,202,220] Risk factors include difficult delivery, macrosomia, and breech presentation, but are not entirely predictive.[36,170] Indeed, proximal humerus fractures may occur during vaginal delivery of infants of all weights and sizes, implicating other maternal and perinatal factors.

In older children and adolescents, proximal humerus fractures are typically sustained from traumatic mechanisms, such as sports-related activities or motor vehicle collisions (Fig. 18-16). Direct trauma to the anterior or posterior aspect of the proximal humerus may result in fracture.[73,247,323] More commonly, indirect trauma via forces imparted on the upper limb during falls or nonphysiologic positioning may result in a proximal humeral fracture.[323] Indeed, Williams[366] postulated six distinct mechanisms by which proximal humerus fractures may be sustained: forced extension, forced flexion, forced extension with lateral or medial rotation, and forced flexion with lateral or medial rotation. Fractures may occur at the level of the proximal metaphysis or physis.

Furthermore, the proximal humerus is a common location of pathologic fractures in children. Benign lesions—such as unicameral or aneurysmal bone cysts—and much less often malignant lesions (osteogenic sarcoma), commonly involve the proximal humerus and may first present in the setting of pathologic fracture.[2,258,284] Neuropathic conditions including Arnold–Chiari malformation, myelomeningocele, or syringomyelia have also been implicated in pathologic fractures of the proximal

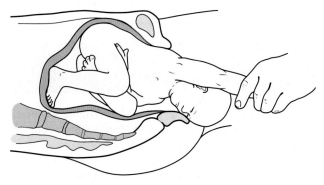

Figure 18-15. Hyperextension or rotation of the ipsilateral arm may result in a proximal humeral or physeal injury during birth.

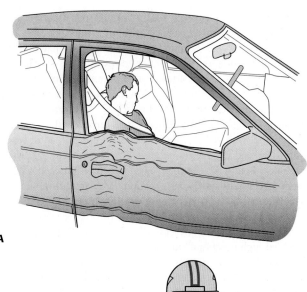

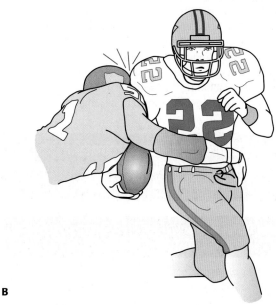

Figure 18-16. A: Motor vehicle crashes may result in proximal humeral fracture due to blunt trauma to the shoulder region. **B:** Blunt trauma from contact sports may result in fracture of the proximal humerus in children.

humerus.[9,212] Finally, radiation therapy to the shoulder girdle may result in bony abnormalities predisposing to proximal humerus fracture.[88]

Finally, proximal humerus fractures may be seen in the setting of nonaccidental trauma and child abuse.[233,316] For this reason, careful assessment including comprehensive history and physical examinations are needed when assessing infants and young children with proximal humerus fractures.

INJURIES ASSOCIATED WITH PROXIMAL HUMERUS FRACTURES

Fractures of the proximal humerus may have concomitant dislocations of the glenohumeral joint, particularly with high-energy mechanisms of injury.[61,119,187,251,358,346] Glenohumeral joint dislocation may be anterior, posterior, or inferior, and concomitant intra-articular or apophyseal avulsion fractures may be seen.[244,290] All patients with proximal humerus fractures should be evaluated for concomitant glenohumeral joint reduction with appropriate radiographic imaging. A high index of suspicion is needed to avoid delayed or missed diagnosis. Ipsilateral fractures of the upper limb have also been reported, emphasizing the importance of a comprehensive physical examination and imaging of the entire humerus or upper limb as appropriate.[123,167,217]

Given the proximity to the brachial plexus and axillary vessels, proximal humerus fractures may be associated with neurovascular injury. Axillary nerve, radial nerve, and total brachial plexus palsies have been reported in the setting of displaced proximal humerus fractures.[5,87,158,346,351] These are typically seen in valgus injuries, in which the distal diaphyseal segment displaces medially and proximally into the region of the brachial plexus. While spontaneous neurologic recovery is seen in the majority of patients within 9 to 12 months, patients may develop a profound neurogenic pain syndrome.[158] Proximal humerus fractures associated with arterial injury and vascular insufficiency require emergent reduction and/or stabilization and vascular repair.[132,363] Associated injuries to the thorax, including rib fractures and pneumothorax, have also been reported.

SIGNS AND SYMPTOMS OF PROXIMAL HUMERUS FRACTURES

In neonates, the signs and symptoms of proximal humerus fractures may be subtle. Rarely will ecchymosis, swelling, or deformity be clinically apparent. Care providers will often report irritability or "fussiness" with handling or motion of the affected extremity. Often the absence of spontaneous movement of the upper limb—so-called "pseudoparalysis"—will alert the examiner to an underlying fracture. It is imperative to rule out undiagnosed septic arthritis or proximal humeral osteomyelitis in the neonate as infections put the important proximal humerus physis at risk for growth arrest and glenohumeral joint of deformity.

In older children and adolescents, the clinical diagnosis is more obvious. Patients will present with pain, swelling, ecchymosis, and/or limited shoulder motion after traumatic injury. The limb is typically held against the body in adduction and internal rotation, and patients will guard against passive or active movement. Inspection will reveal asymmetry in the contour of the shoulder girdle compared with the contralateral, uninjured extremity. Subtle skin puckering may be seen, suggestive of soft tissue interposition in severely displaced fractures.[75] Careful evaluation of neurovascular status is critical to rule out concomitant nerve or vessel injury. Even in patients with considerable pain and guarding, axillary nerve function (sensation over the lateral deltoid, abduction of the shoulder) may be adequately assessed. Similarly brachial plexus integrity may be assessed by distal motor sensory function without moving the injured limb.

Patients with associated posterior glenohumeral joint dislocation will posture with internal rotation and have limited or extremely painful passive external rotation. Associated fracture–dislocations involving the greater tuberosity and luxation erecta will present with extreme abduction of the shoulder and elbow flexion.[186] Fractures of the lesser tuberosity and/or subscapularis

disruption may be more subtle in presentation, though patients will have weak internal rotation, a positive lift-off sign, and often increased passive external rotation.[205,290,318,350]

IMAGING AND OTHER DIAGNOSTIC STUDIES FOR PROXIMAL HUMERUS FRACTURES

The proximal humeral epiphysis is not radiographically apparent until approximately 6 months of age, limiting the diagnostic utility of plain radiographs in the evaluation of neonates and infants.[191,256] In these very young patients, ultrasonography may provide meaningful diagnostic information.[27,101,154] MRI may also help distinguish between proximal humeral fracture and other potential causes of pseudoparalysis, such as osteomyelitis, septic arthritis, or glenohumeral joint instability in the setting of brachial plexus birth palsy, though MRI requires conscious sedation or general anesthesia.

Subtle radiographic signs of proximal humerus fracture in infants include asymmetric positioning of the proximal humeral metaphysis in relationship to the scapula and acromion, particularly when compared to images of the contralateral shoulder. In patients with posteriorly displaced physeal fractures, the so-called "vanishing epiphysis" sign has been used to describe the apparent absence of the small epiphyseal ossification center, which lies behind the proximal metaphysis (Fig. 18-17).[182]

In older patients and adolescents, plain radiographs will confirm the diagnosis and characterize fracture pattern and displacement. Orthogonal views are necessary, and ideally AP and axillary views are obtained to assess for concomitant lesser tuberosity fracture or glenohumeral joint dislocation.[334] In appropriate axillary images, the humeral head normally resides between the acromion and coracoid process, concentrically reduced within the glenoid. Standardized assessment of plain radiographs will provide reliable measures of displacement and angulation, particularly when the epiphyseal margins of the humeral head

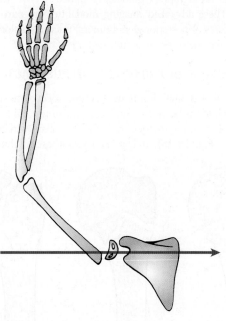

Figure 18-17. Vanishing epiphysis sign. The *arrow* depicts the direction of the x-ray beam.

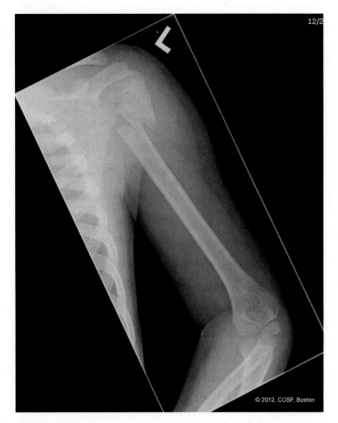

12/2

© 2012. COSF, Boston

Figure 18-18. Proximal humeral metaphyseal fracture in a 5-year-old male. (Courtesy of Children's Orthopaedic Surgery Foundation.)

fragment are identified and used.[31] Given the difficulty in obtaining axillary radiographs in the acutely injured child, a host of alternative radiographic views have been proposed, including the transthoracic scapular Y view, apical oblique view, and other variations.[110,322] In unusual situations in which adequate plain radiographs cannot be obtained, CT or MRI may be used. These advanced imaging modalities are particularly useful in cases of posterior glenohumeral fracture–dislocations, intra-articular fractures, or occult fractures.[119,296,341,342]

CLASSIFICATION OF PROXIMAL HUMERUS FRACTURES

Metaphyseal proximal humerus fractures occur most commonly in children between 5 and 12 years of age, and may be described according to their radiographic displacement and angulation (Fig. 18-18). It has been hypothesized that rapid

metaphyseal growth and thus relative porosity of the proximal humeral metaphysis contributes to the predilection to fracture in this age group.[73]

Physeal fractures are classified according to the Salter–Harris classification (Fig. 18-19).[300] Salter–Harris I injuries denote fractures through the physis and most commonly occur in patients under 5 years of age.[73,268] Salter–Harris II fractures exit through the metaphysis, often associated with an anterolateral bony fragment, and are more commonly seen in older children and adolescents.[30,73,101,268] Salter–Harris III fractures are relatively rare and have been associated with concomitant glenohumeral dislocation. Salter–Harris IV fractures have not been reported in children.

Neer and Horwitz[247] proposed a classification system for pediatric proximal humerus fractures based upon the amount of fracture displacement. In grade I fractures, there is up to 5 mm of displacement. Grade II fractures are displaced up to one-third of the cortical diameter of the humeral diaphysis. Grade III injuries have up to two-third displacement. Grade IV fractures have greater than two-thirds cortical diameter displacement. Angulation and malrotation are not specifically categorized in this classification system.

PATHOANATOMY AND APPLIED ANATOMY RELATING TO PROXIMAL HUMERUS FRACTURES

Care of proximal humerus fractures in children and adolescents is challenging for a number of reasons. First, given the robust remodeling potential in skeletally immature patients, there are variations in what is deemed "acceptable" deformity. Fracture reduction is often difficult, owing to the small size and deep location of the humeral head as well as the deforming muscle insertions on both the proximal and distal fracture fragments. Multiple reduction maneuvers and fixation options have been proposed, adding complexity to nonoperative or surgical decision making. Finally, the proximity of the zone of injury to adjacent neurovascular structures results in the potential for associated injuries and surgical risks. All of these considerations must be reconciled with evolving patient and family expectations regarding pain control, healing time, and functional return. For these reasons, understanding of the applied anatomy and pathoanatomy of proximal humerus fractures is critical.

The proximal humeral epiphysis does not become radiographically apparent until approximately 6 months of age.[191,256]

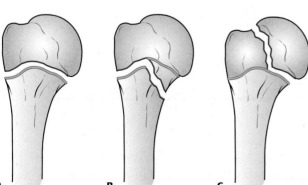

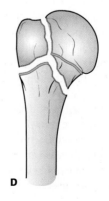

A   B   C   D

Figure 18-19. Physeal fractures of the proximal humerus. **A:** Salter–Harris type I. **B:** Salter–Harris type II. **C:** Salter–Harris type III. **D:** Salter–Harris type IV.

Furthermore, the greater and lesser tuberosities have their own distinct secondary centers of ossification, which become visible at 1 to 3 years and 4 to 5 years of age, respectively.[256,302] The greater and lesser tuberosities coalesce between 5 and 7 years of age, and subsequently fuse to the rest of the humeral head between 7 and 13 years of age.

The proximal humeral physis ultimately contributes 80% of the longitudinal growth of the humerus.[23,272,273] There is some variation over time, however, as the proximal humeral physis contributes 75% of longitudinal growth of the humerus prior to 2 years of age, but up to 90% of growth after the age of 11 years. Generally, the proximal humeral physis closes at 14 to 17 years of age in females and between 16 and 18 years of age in males.[23,272,273,327]

The articular surface of the humeral head encompasses the medial aspect of the epiphysis as well as the proximal medial corner of the metaphysis (Fig. 18-20). The capsule of the glenohumeral joint correspondingly surrounds the articular surface. However, the proximal humeral physis is extracapsular and thus susceptible to injury. Indeed, most fractures of the proximal humerus involve the physis.[30,73,268] As with other growth plate injuries, proximal humeral physeal fractures typically occur through the zone of hypertrophy and provisional calcification, sparing the resting and proliferative zones. For these reasons, the typical Salter–Harris I and II injuries have tremendous remodeling potential and have a low risk of subsequent growth disturbance.[11,73,300]

The periosteum is thick and strong along the posteromedial aspect of the proximal humerus, but relatively weak anterolaterally, allowing for fracture fragment displacement. In cases of displaced fractures, interposed periosteum may block reduction attempts.[73,86,216]

A number of muscles insert on the proximal humerus, influencing fracture pattern, location, and characteristic displacement. Understanding of these dynamic influences is critical for successful fracture reduction. The subscapularis inserts anteriorly on the lesser tuberosity, whereas the supraspinatus, infraspinatus, and teres minor attach to the greater tuberosity and

posterosuperior epiphysis. The deltoid tubercle lies more distally along the lateral aspect of the humeral diaphysis, and the pectoralis major and latissimus dorsi muscles insert along the anteromedial aspect of the metaphysis. In patients with physeal or metaphyseal fractures proximal to the pectoralis major insertion, the humeral head is abducted, flexed, and externally rotated by the action of the rotator cuff muscles, whereas the distal humeral diaphyseal segment is typically displaced proximally, medially, and into internal rotation. In metaphyseal fractures between the pectoralis major and deltoid insertions, the proximal fragment is adducted by the pull of the pectoralis major and the distal segment is pulled proximally and into abduction by the deltoid. For diaphyseal fractures distal to the deltoid insertion, the proximal fracture fragment is abducted by the deltoid and flexed by the pectoralis major, and the distal fragment is displaced proximally and medially by the biceps and triceps. Rarely, the subscapularis muscle may lead to displacement of an isolated fracture of the lesser tuberosity.

The vascularity of the proximal humerus arises from the axillary artery and its branches. In particular, the anterior and posterior humeral circumflex arteries supply the proximal humerus, whereas the humeral head derives most of its vascular supply from the arcuate artery, a branch of the ascending branch of the anterior humeral circumflex artery.[108,193] The posterior humeral circumflex artery supplies only a portion of the greater tuberosity and posteroinferior humeral head.[108]

Of the neurologic structures, the axillary nerve is the closest and most at risk in fractures and fracture–dislocations of the proximal humerus.[5,346] The axillary nerve arises from the posterior cord of the brachial plexus before it traverses the anterior aspect of the subscapularis muscle and passes just inferior to the glenohumeral joint. From there it passes through the quadrilateral space to innervate the deltoid and teres minor muscles and to supply sensation to the lateral aspect of the shoulder.

TREATMENT OPTIONS FOR PROXIMAL HUMERUS FRACTURES

NONOPERATIVE TREATMENT OF PROXIMAL HUMERUS FRACTURES

Indications/Contraindications

Nonoperative Treatment of Proximal Humerus Fractures: INDICATIONS AND CONTRAINDICATIONS
Indications
• Birth-related fractures
• Younger patients with stable or minimally displaced fractures
• Stress fractures
Relative Contraindications
• Open fractures
• Fractures with vascular or severe soft tissue injury
• Displaced intra-articular fractures
• Displaced tuberosity fractures
• Irreducible or unstable fractures in older adolescents with unacceptable alignment

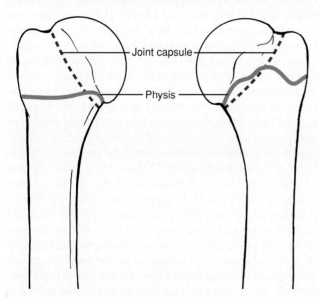

Figure 18-20. The anatomy of the proximal humerus.

Given their tremendous remodeling potential as well as the robust compensatory motion afforded by the shoulder joint, the vast majority of proximal humerus fractures may be treated by nonoperative means. Birth-related fractures of the proximal humerus may be successfully treated with simple pinning of the sleeve to the body or stockinette sling-and-swathe immobilization. Closed reduction is rarely needed in infants, and while ultrasonography may be used to confirm alignment, advanced imaging is almost always unnecessary. In these infants, healing is rapid and robust, typically within 2 to 3 weeks, and there is little concern for long-term aesthetic differences or functional limitations.[73,170]

Nondisplaced or minimally displaced fractures (Neer–Horwitz grades I and II) in older children and adolescents may also be treated with simple sling-and-swathe immobilization, with or without additional splinting (Fig. 18-21). As late fracture displacement is uncommon, recent reports suggest that serial radiographic evaluations are unnecessary and may impart additional cost and radiation exposure without clinical utility.[114] After confirmation of healing, patients may advance to motion and strengthening, with anticipation of excellent long-term results.[33,73] Similarly, stress fractures of the metaphysis or physis—such as seen from repetitive overuse sports activities, neurologic conditions, metabolic bone disease, or local radiation therapy—may be successfully treated with rest, activity modification, and/or simple sling immobilization.[26,71,88]

With increasing age and skeletal maturity, remodeling capacity diminishes; therefore, the amount of "acceptable" deformity changes with age. Given the remodeling potential in patients less than 11 years of age, good-to-excellent results have been reported with nonoperative treatment regardless of fracture displacement.[73,197,247,323] Immobilization options include sling-

TABLE 18-1. Acceptable Alignment of Proximal Humerus Fractures		
Age	Angulation	Displacement
<5 yrs	70 degrees	100%
5–11 yrs	40–70 degrees	50–100%
>12 yrs	<40 degrees	<50%

and-swathe, Velpeau thoracobrachial bandages, hanging arm casts, and shoulder spica casts in the "saluting" and "Statue of Liberty" positions.[33,73,197]

There continues to be controversy, however, regarding what constitutes "acceptable" alignment in pediatric proximal humerus fractures, particularly in older children and adolescents. Much of the available information comes from historic retrospective case series, with little or no comparative outcome data available. Traditional recommendations have divided treatment recommendations according to patient age and fracture displacement (Table 18-1).[12,86,316] In patients less than 5 years of age, up to 70 degrees of angulation and 100% displacement is deemed acceptable. In patients between 5 and 11 years of age, 40 to 70 degrees of angulation and 50% to 100% displacement may be accepted. And in patients greater than 12 years of age with less growth and remodeling potential, less than 40 degrees and 50% translation should be accepted. Though these guidelines are generally accepted, appropriate clinical judgment weighing individual patient and provider factors should be made on a case-by-case basis.[12,73,86,197] For example, in overhead athletes requiring maximal shoulder abduction and forward flexion, less varus or apex anterior angulation may be tolerable, given concerns regarding acromial impingement and bony blocks to glenohumeral motion.

In patients older than 12 years, fracture reduction and immobilization is recommended for Neer–Horwitz grade III and IV injuries with unacceptable alignment.[12,50,73,197,247] Indeed a recent matched cohort analysis by Chaus et al. suggested incremental increased likelihood of suboptimal function with nonoperative management for each year over 12 years of age.[51] While a host of reduction maneuvers have been described, all adhere to the fundamental principles of reversing the deformity and counteracting the deforming forces. Most fractures may be reducing by applying longitudinal traction to the distal brachium, followed by abduction, flexion, and external rotation; this technique essentially brings the distal diaphyseal segment to the displaced humeral head. Often, initial adduction and internal rotation to relax the pectoralis major, followed by posteriorly directed pressure on the humeral diaphysis to correct the apex anterior angulation, will facilitate reduction.[166] Alternatively, reduction may be achieved by abduction, flexion to 90 degrees, and external rotation.[247] Still others advocate placing the limb in 135 degrees abduction and slight (30 degrees) flexion, followed by longitudinal traction and manual manipulation of the fracture fragments.[170] In cases of physeal fractures, gentle manipulation with the assistance of conscious sedation or general anesthesia should be considered to avoid excessively forceful manipulation and minimize the risk of iatrogenic physeal disturbance. After reduction, fracture stability needs to be assessed. Often the intact periosteum will stabilize the reduction and allow for immobilization at the

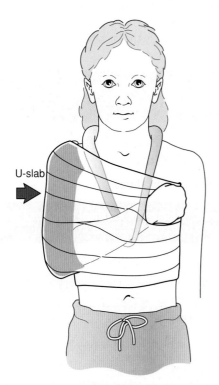

Figure 18-21. Sling-and-swathe for immobilization of proximal humeral fracture. A plaster U-slab (*arrow*) may be added for additional splinting.

patient's side. Typically, immobilization with sling-and-swathe or Velpeau thoracobrachial bandage is sufficient.[73]

Some fractures may not be reducible because of soft tissue interposition at the fracture site. Potential structural barriers to fracture realignment include the adjacent periosteum, glenohumeral joint capsule, and long head of biceps tendon.[12,86,166,216] In these situations, open reduction via a limited anterior deltopectoral approach may be needed to obtain appropriate reduction. Even in cases in which the bony alignment is improved to "acceptable" parameters but not anatomic, fracture healing and functional return may be expected; indeed, good functional results have been reported in patients with Neer–Horwitz grade III and IV injuries who were reduced to grade I or II displacement.[86,157]

There is additional controversy regarding the optimal management of the older adolescent who undergoes successful fracture reduction. Loss of reduction following initial manipulation has been reported to be as high as 50% in older adolescents, suggesting that internal fixation should be considered when caring for older patients with severely displaced injuries.[73,86,247] Again, there is no prospective or comparative data to inform us regarding the utility or cost effectiveness of internal fixation in these situations.

OPERATIVE TREATMENT OF PROXIMAL HUMERUS FRACTURES

Indications/Contraindications

Surgical indications include open fractures, fractures associated with vascular injury, fractures in the multitrauma patient, displaced intra-articular fractures, displaced tuberosity fractures, and irreducible or unstable fractures in unacceptable alignment.[12,68,86,157,213,224,268,310,331,358]

A host of surgical treatment options have been advocated in these situations, and in general may be divided according to manner of reduction (closed vs. open) and type of fixation (pin fixation, intramedullary fixation, and plate-and-screw constructs).[12,52,53,68,73,86,98,166,247,277,293,308,368]

Percutaneous Pin Fixation

Preoperative Planning

✔ Reduction and Percutaneous Pinning of Proximal Humerus Fractures: PREOPERATIVE PLANNING CHECKLIST	
OR table	☐ Radiolucent
Position/positioning aids	☐ Modified beach chair vs. supine with bump
Fluoroscopy location	☐ From head of table vs. contralateral side
Equipment	☐ Smooth K-wires

Percutaneous pin fixation is a common technique for the treatment of unstable proximal humerus fractures.[53,86,157] Appropriate preoperative planning includes orthogonal radiographic views of the proximal humerus—preferably AP and axillary views—to characterize the fracture pattern and displacement. Careful radiographic assessment should be made to identify associated bony lesions, as pathologic fractures due to unicameral bone cysts, aneurysmal bone cysts, and other benign and malignant lesions commonly occur in the proximal humerus. Preoperative evaluation should also include a careful neurovascular examination to rule out concomitant nerve palsy or vascular injury.

While terminally threaded pins are commonly used in adults, smooth pins are sufficient in pediatric patients given the bone quality, rapid healing, ease of implant removal, and typical simple extra-articular fracture patterns. The appropriate-sized implants should be determined in advance; typically smooth Kirschner (K)-wires between 0.0625 and 3/32 in diameter are used. Cannulated screw fixation has been advocated by some, citing its minimal invasiveness, improved stability, and avoidance of complications commonly seen with smooth K-wires. However, given the concerns regarding potential physeal disturbance and need for staged implant removal, cannulated screw fixation is not typically used or necessary.[53,362]

Positioning

Patient positioning should be predicated upon access to the shoulder girdle and upper limb and ease of fluoroscopic imaging. Use of the modified beach chair position will allow for easy manipulation, implant placement, and intraoperative imaging. In these cases, the fluoroscopy unit may be brought in from the head of the bed, allowing the surgeon to stand in the axilla or lateral to the affected shoulder and facilitating both AP and axillary views of the proximal humerus (Fig. 18-22). Alternatively, patients may be positioned supine on a radiolucent table with a bump placed under the ipsilateral pelvis or between the scapulae. With supine positioning, the fluoroscopy unit may be brought in from the ipsilateral or contralateral side of the table.

Surgical Approach

After adequate induction of general anesthesia, closed reduction is performed. Adequate muscle relaxation will facilitate fracture manipulation. In cases where closed reduction does not allow for adequate bony alignment, open reduction may be performed via a deltopectoral approach. As most physeal and metaphyseal fractures are extracapsular, the incision and deep dissection should be biased more inferiorly than standard approaches to the glenohumeral joint.

Technique

✔ Reduction and Percutaneous Pinning of Proximal Humerus Fractures: KEY SURGICAL STEPS
☐ Closed reduction
☐ Skin incisions at or proximal to deltoid tubercle
☐ Spreading through subcutaneous tissues to lateral humeral cortex
☐ Smooth K-wire fixation
☐ Fluoroscopic confirmation of alignment and implant placement
☐ Placement of additional K-wire(s)
☐ Final fluoroscopic evaluation
☐ Bent and cut pins beneath or outside the skin
☐ Sling-and-swathe immobilization

After appropriate positioning, the shoulder girdle and ipsilateral upper limb is prepped and draped into the surgical field. Care is

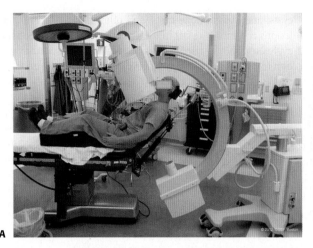
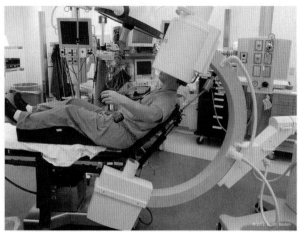

A   **B**

Figure 18-22. Intraoperative fluoroscopic visualization in the beach chair position. **A:** Anteroposterior and (**B**) axillary views may be obtained. (Courtesy of Children's Orthopaedic Surgery Foundation.)

made to provide circumferential access to the shoulder region. Closed reduction maneuvers are performed, as described above. For most injuries, initial adduction and internal rotation will relax the deforming forces of the pectoralis major muscle, and subsequent posterior translation of the diaphyseal fragment will correct the apex anterior angulation. Following this, longitudinal traction and increasing abduction and flexion will reduce the angulation and displacement (Fig. 18-23). In cases of marked fracture instability, the reduction achieved may be lost when the arm is brought into an adducted and internally rotated position. In these situations, it may be advantageous to preplace the pins into the distal humeral fracture fragment first, and then perform the appropriate reduction maneuver. Once the fracture is realigned, the pins may be simply passed across the fracture site into the proximal fragment, even with the shoulder abducted, external rotated, and/or flexed.

Once an adequate closed reduction has been achieved, the fracture is fixed with percutaneous smooth K-wires. Small stab incisions are made at or just proximal to the level of the deltoid tubercle, and careful blunt dissection is performed down to the lateral cortex of the humerus using a hemostat or narrow dissecting scissors. Injury to the axillary nerve may be avoided by placing the entry points for percutaneous pinning two times the height of the articular surface distal to the most proximal edge of the humerus.[293] Data from computer modeling studies of pediatric proximal humerus fractures suggest that pins entering laterally 4.4 and 8 cm distal to the superior aspect of the humeral head at a coronal angle of 21 degrees allow for optimal pin placement.[232]

After the first pin is placed, multiplanar fluoroscopic views are obtained to confirm appropriate alignment and implant placement. Following this one or two additional pins are placed, again in a distal-lateral to proximal-medial direction. Care is made not to violate the subchondral surface of the humeral head and enter the glenohumeral joint. A drill hole at the entry site may make pin adjustment and placement easier and avoid inadvertent joint and/or adjacent soft tissue (brachial plexus) penetration. Once the desired alignment, depth, and stability are achieved, the pins are bent and cut either below the skin or outside the skin.[157] The limb is placed in a sling-and-swathe.

Implants may be removed after radiographic evidence of healing is confirmed, typically 4 weeks after surgery.

Occasionally, additional fixation or assistance with closed reduction is needed. An antegrade pin entering the greater tuberosity and directed distally and medially may be considered, though is rarely necessary. These pins should be placed with the limb in external rotation and directed to a point at least 2 cm inferior to the most medial aspect of the articular surface.[293] As cited earlier, if closed reduction is not successful, open reduction via a deltopectoral approach can be used, with pinning techniques performed in a similar fashion.

Intramedullary Fixation

Preoperative Planning

✔ **Intramedullary Fixation of Proximal Humerus Fractures:** PREOPERATIVE PLANNING CHECKLIST	
OR table	❑ Radiolucent
Position/positioning aids	❑ Modified beach chair vs. supine
Fluoroscopy location	❑ From head of table vs. contralateral side
Equipment	❑ Appropriately sized intramedullary nails

Intramedullary nailing is a common technique in the treatment of pediatric proximal humerus fractures.[37,52,53,175,271,277,308,368] Unlike adults, in whom solid reamed antegrade nails have been used, intramedullary fixation in children and adolescents typically involves retrograde passage of multiple flexible titanium elastic nails, Rush rods, or Enders nails. Adequate AP and lateral radiographs of the proximal humerus should be reviewed to assess fracture location, pattern, and displacement. Again, careful preoperative evaluation should be made to document neurovascular status, given the known risks of associate nerve injury. Appropriately sized flexible stainless steel or titanium intramedullary nails should be available. Similar to intramedullary fixation techniques

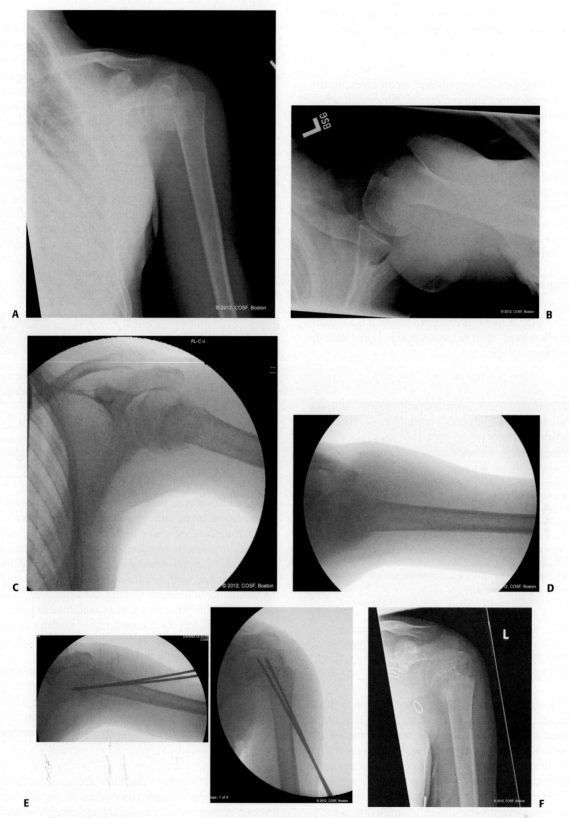

Figure 18-23. Percutaneous pin fixation. Injury AP (**A**) and views (**B**) of a proximal humerus fracture in a 12-year-old female. Note is made of excessive apex anterior angulation. Intraoperatively, the fracture is closed reduced with traction, abduction (**C**) and correction of the apex anterior angulation (**D**). **E:** Postoperative alignment after percutaneous pinning. **F:** Follow-up radiograph demonstrates improved alignment and bony healing. (Courtesy of Children's Orthopaedic Surgery Foundation.)

of pediatric femur fractures, the selected nail diameter should be approximately 40% of the intramedullary canal dimension.

Positioning

Patient positioning should be predicated upon access to the shoulder girdle and upper limb and ease of fluoroscopic imaging. Use of the modified beach chair position will allow for easy manipulation, implant placement, and intraoperative imaging. In these cases, the fluoroscopy unit may be brought in from the head of the bed, allowing the surgeon to stand in the axilla or lateral to the affected shoulder and facilitating both AP and axillary views of the proximal humerus. Alternatively, patients may be positioned supine on a radiolucent table with a bump placed under the ipsilateral pelvis or between the scapulae. With supine positioning, the fluoroscopy unit may be brought in from the ipsilateral or contralateral side of the table.

Surgical Approach

Again, closed reduction of the proximal humerus fracture is performed using the maneuvers described above. If inadequate realignment is achieved, open reduction may be performed via a limited deltopectoral approach.

Technique

> ✔ **Intramedullary Fixation of Proximal Humerus Fractures:**
> KEY SURGICAL STEPS
>
> ☐ Closed (or open) fracture reduction
> ☐ Incision along lateral column of distal humerus, at or proximal to olecranon fossa
> ☐ Alternatively, may use additional medial or posterior incisions and entry sites
> ☐ Blunt dissection to lateral humeral cortex
> ☐ Create cortical entry site with drill bit
> ☐ Precontour intramedullary nails
> ☐ Pass nails into intramedullary canal, across fracture site, and into proximal humeral fracture fragment
> ☐ Nail rotation to effectuate additional correction of translation/displacement
> ☐ Fluoroscopic confirmation of alignment and implant placement
> ☐ Bend and cut nails, leaving 2–3 cm flush along metaphyseal flare to allow subsequent removal
> ☐ Sling-and-swathe immobilization

Following fracture reduction, a longitudinal incision is made along the lateral column of the distal humerus at the level of the superior aspect of the olecranon fossa. Alternatively, medial column or posterior approaches may be used, splitting the triceps in the latter situation to gain access to the distal humerus and intramedullary canal above the olecranon fossa. Blunt dissection is performed through the subcutaneous tissues to the level of the distal humeral cortex (Fig. 18-24). Using a drill guide to protect the adjacent soft tissues, a 3.2- or 4.5-mm drill bit is used to create a cortical window in the lateral column; care is made to create this starting hole obliquely from distal-lateral to proximal-medial to facilitate subsequent nail passage. Appropriately sized intramedullary nails (typically 3 to 4 mm in diameter) are then prebent; if both nails are to be passed via a lateral

entry point, one nail is bent in the shape of a gentle "C" and the other in the shape of a lazy "S" to allow for some divergence of the nail ends in the proximal fracture fragment. Nails are then passed into the lateral column entry site, through the intramedullary canal of the humerus, across the fracture site, and into the proximal fracture fragment. Typically, the nails must be gently impacted into the proximal humerus, with care to avoid distraction or further displacement at the fracture site. Fracture translation or angulation may be further corrected with nail rotation once the proximal fragment is engaged. Intraoperative fluoroscopy is used to confirm fracture alignment, stability, and implant placement. Nails are then cut beneath the skin with the distal ends flush against the metaphyseal flare to allow for subsequent removal but lessen the risk of nail irritation during fracture healing. Wound is then closed, the dressing applied, and the upper extremity placed in sling-and-swathe immobilization.

Open Reduction and Internal Fixation

Preoperative Planning

> ✔ **ORIF of Humerus Shaft Fractures:**
> PREOPERATIVE PLANNING CHECKLIST

OR table	☐ Standard
Position/positioning aids	☐ Modified beach chair position
Fluoroscopy location	☐ From head of table
Equipment	☐ Appropriately sized small fragment implants or site-specific implants; shoulder retractors if desired

Open reduction and plate fixation is rarely necessary in the pediatric population, and typically reserved for cases of intra-articular extension, extensive fracture comminution, pathologic injuries, or severely displaced fractures in skeletally mature adolescents. Surgical principles follow established tenets of fracture fixation, with particular attention to preservation of the vascularity to the humeral head and avoidance of iatrogenic neurologic injury. Though a host of anatomically precontoured plates are available, these commercially available implants do not often fit the adolescent patient, and standard small fragment plate-and-screw constructs will suffice.

Appropriate preoperative planning includes orthogonal radiographic views of the proximal humerus—preferably AP and axillary views—to characterize the fracture pattern and displacement. A careful neurovascular examination to rule out concomitant nerve palsy or vascular injury is imperative.

Positioning

Similar to the procedures described above, patient positioning should allow near circumferential access to the shoulder girdle and ease of fluoroscopic imaging. Use of the modified beach chair position will allow for easy manipulation, implant placement, and intraoperative imaging. This semirecumbent position will also facilitate venous drainage and visualization. In these cases, the fluoroscopy unit may be brought in from the head of the bed, allowing the surgeon to stand in the axilla or lateral to the affected shoulder and facilitating both AP and axillary views of the proximal humerus.

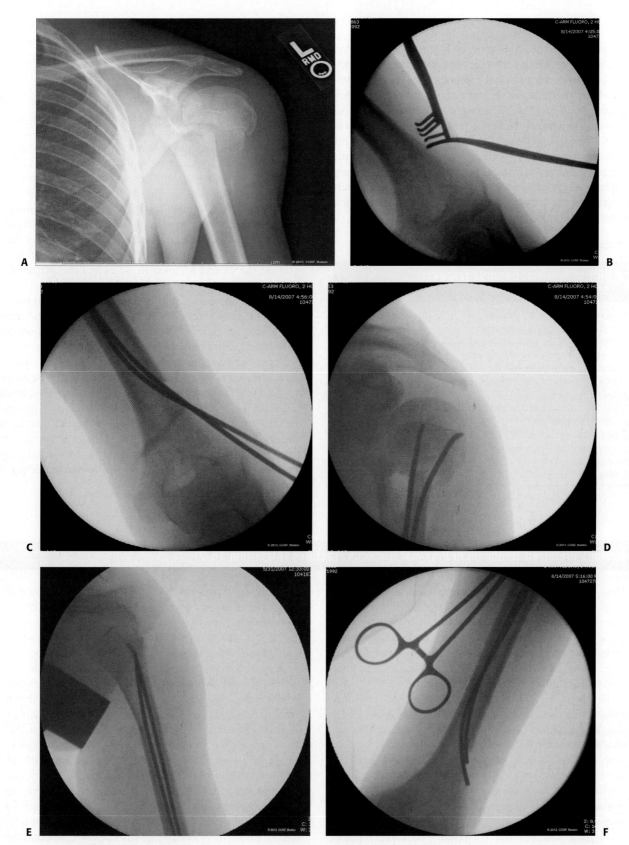

Figure 18-24. Intramedullary fixation. **A:** Displaced proximal humerus fracture in an adolescent female. **B:** Blunt spreading is performed via a lateral incision along the distal humeral metaphysis. **C:** Precontoured flexible intramedullary nails are passed into the medullary canal. **D:** The implants traverse the fracture site and engage the humeral head. **E:** Rotation of the nails may be used to improve translation or angulation. **F:** Implants are cut beneath the skin. (Courtesy of Children's Orthopaedic Surgery Foundation.)

Surgical Approach

A standard deltopectoral approach is typically used, as described above. As this procedure targets the proximal humeral metaphysis and diaphysis, rather than the glenohumeral joint, the incision is often biased distally. The approach is extensile and may be carried distally into an anterolateral or Henry approach to the proximal and middle humerus. Careful subperiosteal elevation of the deltoid and pectoralis major insertions will allow for adequate exposure of the metadiaphyseal humerus. Overzealous lateral retraction is avoided to prevent iatrogenic axillary neurapraxis. Great care should be taken to protect the ascending branch of the anterior humeral circumflex artery, which runs just lateral to the long head of biceps tendon.

Technique

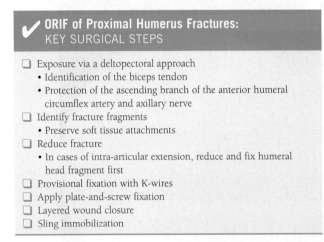

✔ ORIF of Proximal Humerus Fractures:
KEY SURGICAL STEPS

☐ Exposure via a deltopectoral approach
 • Identification of the biceps tendon
 • Protection of the ascending branch of the anterior humeral circumflex artery and axillary nerve
☐ Identify fracture fragments
 • Preserve soft tissue attachments
☐ Reduce fracture
 • In cases of intra-articular extension, reduce and fix humeral head fragment first
☐ Provisional fixation with K-wires
☐ Apply plate-and-screw fixation
☐ Layered wound closure
☐ Sling immobilization

After appropriate exposure is obtained, the fracture site is identified and cleared of fracture hematoma or any interposed soft tissue. Unlike adults, adolescent proximal humerus fractures tend not to be comminuted, and osteopenia is rare. The biceps tendon is a useful anatomic landmark, as the greater and lesser tuberosities lie lateral and medial to the biceps tendon, respectively. Anatomic fracture reduction may be achieved, and if needed provisional fracture fixation using smooth K-wires or fracture reduction clamps may be obtained. Following fracture realignment, internal fixation using appropriate plate-and-screw constructs is achieved. Careful intraoperative imaging will assist in proper screw placement within the humeral head and avoidance of intra-articular implant penetration. Typically six cortices of fixation into the distal fracture fragment are sufficient. After direct and fluoroscopic confirmation of appropriate alignment and stability, the wound is closed in layers and the affected limb placed in a sling.

As noted above, avulsion fractures of the lesser tuberosity may occur in adolescents. ORIF is recommended in patients with displaced injuries.[106,130,181,350] Similar patient positioning and surgical deltopectoral approach may be used. In general, the lesser tuberosity fracture fragment is easily identified, and the attachment of the subscapularis tendon and muscle are preserved. Once fracture site on the proximal humerus is defined and debrided, bioabsorbable suture anchors may be placed in the donor site. Heavy, nonabsorbable sutures are then passed through the undersurface of the lesser tuberosity fracture fragment, exiting superficially. The fracture is then reduced, and the previously passed sutures are tied down completing the repair.

Author's Preferred Treatment of Proximal Humerus Fractures (Algorithm 18-2)

Most proximal humerus fractures in children and adolescents can be successfully treated nonoperatively. In infants with birth-related fractures, immobilization with a stockinette or pinning of the sleeve to the trunk is simple and effective. Radiographic assessment of healing is performed at 4 to 6 weeks of age; immobilization is discontinued with evidence of clinical and radiographic healing.

In children and adolescents with closed proximal humerus fractures in acceptable deformity (see Table 18-1), simple sling immobilization is used. Serial radiographs are obtained to confirm adequate alignment. Bony union is typically obtained in 4 to 6 weeks, though clinically improvement and pain relief typically precedes radiographic healing. After confirmation of clinical and radiographic healing, range of motion and strengthening is advanced as tolerated.

In older children and adolescents with unacceptable radiographic alignment, initial closed reduction is performed with conscious sedation or general anesthesia. Careful radiographic evaluation of bony alignment and assessment of frac-

ture stability is performed. Given the data suggesting that late displacement is a frequent occurrence following closed manipulation alone of severely displaced proximal humerus fractures in adolescents, a low threshold exists for fracture stabilization. For unstable injuries with deformity beyond what is anticipated to remodel with continued skeletal growth, fracture fixation is performed. Physeal fractures are treated with closed reduction and percutaneous smooth pin fixation; typically two retrograde pins will suffice. Pins may be bent and cut outside the skin, which facilitates subsequent removal and obviates the need for additional anesthesia. If pins are left outside the skin, patients are immobilized with sling-and-swathe to prevent pin migration or pin-tract complications. In patients with metaphyseal fractures—in which there is still some metaphyseal bone on the proximal fracture fragment—intramedullary nailing is preferred (Fig. 18-25). Using the technique described above, appropriate flexible titanium intramedullary implants are prebent and inserted via a lateral entry point. Intramedullary nails are cut and left beneath the skin; attention to the trajectory and

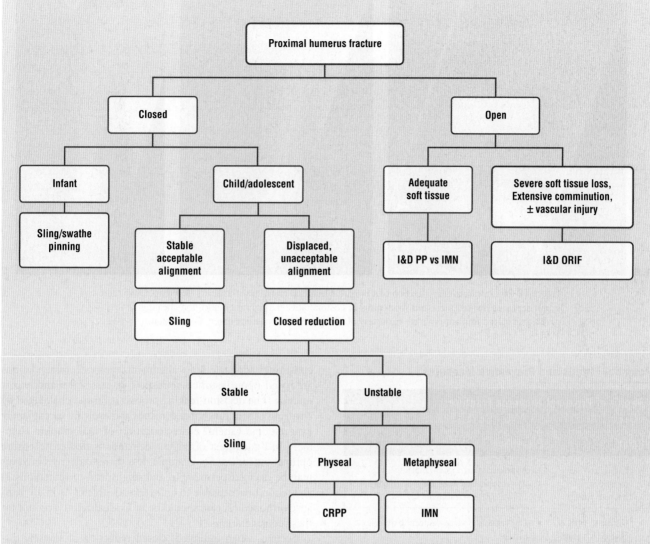

Algorithm 18-2. Author's preferred treatment for humeral shaft fracture.

location of nail entry will allow the ends of the nails to lie flush against the metaphyseal flare of the distal humerus, avoiding unnecessary soft tissue irritation. Patients are placed in sling-and-swathe immobilization.

In cases of open fractures with adequate soft tissue coverage, open reduction and either pin or intramedullary nail fixation is performed after thorough irrigation and debridement of the open wound. In cases associated with excessive fracture comminution, vascular insufficiency, or severe soft tissue loss, internal fixation with plate-and-screw constructs are considered. Open reduction is similarly performed in closed injuries in which an acceptable reduction may not be achieved with manipulation, typically because of interposed soft tissue.[7,68,86]

Postoperative Care

Patients receiving nonoperative treatment of proximal humeral fractures are followed weekly with radiographs to ensure confirm maintenance of alignment. Once there is evidence of clinical and radiographic healing, gentle shoulder pendulum and elbow range-of-motion exercises are begun. Immobilization is typically discontinued after 4 to 6 weeks. Sports participation is restricted until there is return of motion and strength, and patients/families are counseled regarding the risk of refracture.

Following surgical reduction and stabilization, sling immobilization is usually sufficient and continued until radiographic healing. With plate fixation, gentle pendulum and elbow range-of-motion exercises may be initiated once adequate comfort is achieved. In cases of intramedullary nail fixation, implants are typically removed at 6 months postoperatively.

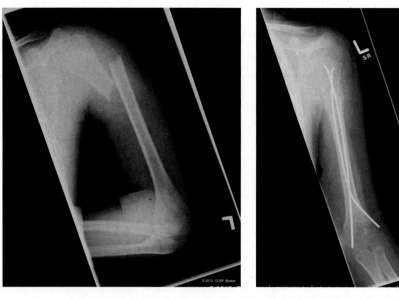

Figure 18-25. Intramedullary fixation of a proximal humeral metaphyseal fracture. **A:** Preoperative radiograph depicting displacement and shortening. **B:** Postoperative radiographs depict bony healing. **C:** Radiograph after staged implant removal. (Courtesy of Children's Orthopaedic Surgery Foundation.)

Potential Pitfalls and Preventive Measures

Repair of Proximal Humerus Fractures: POTENTIAL PITFALLS AND PREVENTIONS	
Pitfall	**Prevention**
• Failure to recognize fracture pattern	• Appropriate orthogonal imaging • Avoid varus and apex anterior angulation • Individualized treatment
• Difficulty with closed reduction	• Understand, reverse deforming muscle actions • Adequate analgesia/anesthesia • Orthogonal fluoroscopic imaging • Transition to open reduction if interposed soft tissue
• Loss of alignment after reduction	• Routine fracture fixation after closed reduction of severely displaced injuries in adolescents • Preset pins into the distal fracture fragment first, then perform the reduction, then pass the pins across the fracture site with the shoulder abducted and/or externally rotated
• Implant-related complications	• Correct insertion of percutaneous pins • Sling-and-swathe immobilization if percutaneous pins left out of skin

While the principles of treatment are seemingly straightforward, proximal humerus fractures present a number of challenges and potential pitfalls, particularly in the adolescent with severe displacement. First, assessment of what constitutes "acceptable deformity" can be challenging in the older pediatric patient population. Though guidelines exist on what

constitutes adequate bony alignment, these recommendations are based upon historical retrospective case series and expert opinion. The decision-making process is further challenged by changing patient functional demands and evolving parent/family expectations. Careful characterization of radiographic alignment in the context of patient demands is needed to ensure optimal outcomes. For example, less than 40 degrees of varus may be deemed permissible, but might lead to limitations in abduction unacceptable to an overhead athlete. As in all pediatric orthopedics, care should be individualized to account for these considerations.

Second, when indicated, closed reduction of severely displaced proximal humerus fractures is challenging. Awareness of the deforming muscular forces, adequate analgesia or anesthesia, and appropriate fluoroscopic imaging will facilitate successful closed manipulations. In cases where acceptable reduction cannot be achieved, open reduction should be pursued, and any interposed periosteum or soft tissue extricated from the fracture site.

In addition, loss of reduction and further fracture displacement is common in older adolescents with severely displaced injuries. Careful assessment of fracture stability at the time of reduction and with serial radiographs is recommended. A low threshold should exist for percutaneous pin fixation or intramedullary nailing of severely displaced fractures to maintain bony alignment.

Furthermore, there are a number of potential pitfalls commonly encountered during surgical stabilization. Judicious percutaneous pin placement is imperative to avoid iatrogenic axillary nerve injury or inadvertent intra-articular penetration of the glenohumeral joint. Given the frequency with which pins cause soft tissue or infectious complications, adequate immobilization of the affected limb and timely pin removal are needed. Conversely, if intramedullary devices are used, appropriate entry point(s) and trajectory will prevent soft tissue irritation or migration of the implants.

Outcomes

Multiple published reports have suggested that surgical reduction and stabilization of displaced proximal humerus fractures is safe and effective in obtaining radiographic healing with improved bony alignment and minimal complications.[15,52,86,185] In patients with Neer–Horwitz grade III and IV injuries, improvement to grade I and II displacement may be expected.[86,157]

Kohler and Trillaud[185] have previously reported the clinical and radiographic outcomes of 52 patients at a mean of 5 years following proximal humerus fractures. Clinical results were "good" or "very good" in all cases, with little correlation to longer-term radiographic parameters. While the authors suggest that surgical intervention offers no advantages over non-operative treatment, it should be noted that all surgical patients in their series underwent formal ORIF, with fixation including staples, pins, screws, and plate-and-screw constructs.

Beringer et al.[15] similarly advocated a nonoperative approach in their report of 48 patients with displaced proximal humerus fractures. All patients with longer-term follow-up reported no activity restrictions or limitations, and functional results did not correlate with radiographic findings. As three of the nine patients treated surgically had complications, the authors recommended nonsurgical treatment in the majority of cases.

Dobbs et al.[86] published their series of 29 patients treated for Neer–Horwitz grade III and IV fractures, of which 25 were treated with closed versus open reduction and pin or screw fixation. The majority of patients were greater than 15 years of age. Postoperatively, all patients improved to a grade I or II deformity, and there were no surgical complications. At a mean follow-up of 4 years, normal or near-normal motion and strength was seen in all patients. These findings support the efficacy and safety of surgical intervention for severely displaced injuries in older patients.

Chee et al.[52] presented their series of 14 patients, mean age 13 years, treated with single intramedullary flexible nail fixation for displaced proximal humerus fractures. All patients had full range of shoulder motion at final follow-up, supporting the authors' assertion that intramedullary fixation is effective in select patients.

More recently, Kraus et al. reported on 40 adolescents treated with either percutaneous pinning or intramedullary fixation. At mean 5.8 years, functional outcomes as measured by DASH and Constant–Murley scores were excellent and radiographic alignment markedly improved.[189]

To date, much of the available data comes from retrospective case series or limited comparative cohort studies, heavily weighted toward radiographic and/or physician-derived results. Little patient-derived functional outcomes data is available, and future prospective investigation assessing long-term results using validated outcomes instruments is needed to provide better insight into optimal management and potential adverse sequelae.

MANAGEMENT OF EXPECTED ADVERSE OUTCOMES AND UNEXPECTED COMPLICATIONS RELATED TO PROXIMAL HUMERUS FRACTURES

Proximal Humerus Fractures:
COMMON ADVERSE OUTCOMES AND COMPLICATIONS

- Neurovascular injury
- Malunion/humerus varus
- Upper limb length discrepancy
- Osteonecrosis
- Hypertrophic scar formation

While uncommon, complications of proximal humerus fractures may have considerable effect on shoulder girdle and upper limb function. Neurologic injury of the brachial plexus or peripheral nerves may be seen, particularly in severely displaced valgus injuries and the rare fracture–dislocation.[5,87,158,346,351] Most nerve palsies are diagnosed at the time of injury and represent neurapraxic injuries rather than true nerve transections. In general, these neurologic deficits will resolve spontaneously over 6 to 12 months but may be associated with neurogenic pain in the affected limb during recovery.[158] In patients with persistent nerve deficits without clinical signs of spontaneous recovery in the expected period of time, electrodiagnostic studies (electromyography and nerve conduction velocities) may be considered to characterize the location and severity of neurologic deficit. In rare situations, exploration with neurolysis, nerve repair, nerve grafting, or nerve transfers (i.e., radial motor branch of long head of triceps to axillary motor) may be necessary.[5,60] In chronic or late-presenting situations, salvage procedures such as tendon transfers or proximal humeral osteotomies may be considered to improve shoulder and upper limb function.[65,143,180,269]

Vascular insufficiency is a rare but potentially devastating complication of proximal humerus fractures. Treatment is predicated on prompt reduction, fracture stabilization, and reassessment of vascularity. In cases of persistent distal ischemia, appropriate exploration and vascular repair or reconstruction is needed.[158]

Humerus varus is another potential complication of proximal humerus fractures in children and adolescents. Humerus varus is characterized by a humeral neck-shaft angle of less than 140 degrees, a greater tuberosity cephalad to the superior aspect of the humeral head, and a reduced distance between the articular surface of the humeral head and the lateral cortex of the humerus.[184] The resultant varus angulation and prominent greater tuberosity leads to limitations in shoulder forward flexion and lateral abduction. Potential etiologies include varus malunion as well as partial physeal arrest following proximal humeral physeal fracture. In cases of functionally limiting humerus varus, corrective osteotomy to restore more anatomic proximal humeral morphology may be performed (Fig. 18-26).[92,112,344]

Upper limb length discrepancy may similarly be seen as a late sequela of physeal fractures.[11,73] Though more commonly reported in patients following operative reduction, physeal disturbance is

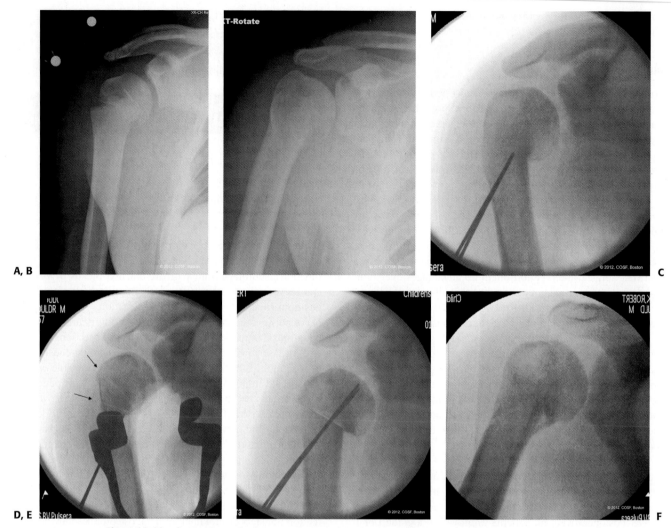

Figure 18-26. **A:** AP radiograph of a minimally displaced right proximal humeral physeal fracture in a 14-year-old male. **B:** Follow-up radiographs depicting humerus varus, characterized by a decreased neck-shaft angle and high-riding greater tuberosity resulting in limited shoulder abduction and bony impingement. **C:** Intraoperative image during corrective osteotomy, depicting percutaneous pin placement. **D:** Converging osteotomies (*arrows*) are made to create a lateral closing wedge osteotomy. **E:** Osteotomy fixed using percutaneous pins and a tension-band fixation construction. **F:** Follow-up radiographs demonstrating bony healing and restoration of more normal proximal humeral alignment. (Courtesy of Children's Orthopaedic Surgery Foundation.)

likely due to the trauma associated with the initial injury rather than surgical intervention. Furthermore, prior reports have suggested that limb length discrepancy is not correlated with the quality of initial fracture reduction.[11,247] Limb-length inequality has similarly been reported in patients with pathologic fractures of the proximal humerus through unicameral bone cysts.[142,242] In patients with functional limitations or predicted upper limb length discrepancies of greater than 6 cm at skeletal maturity, limb-lengthening procedures may be considered.[147,201,267]

Osteonecrosis of the humeral head is much less common in children than adults.[225] In setting of confirmed osteonecrosis, revascularization and humeral head remodeling may be seen in skeletally immature patients, leading to satisfactory clinical outcomes.[358]

Finally, hypertrophic scar formation is commonly seen after surgical treatment of proximal humerus fractures, particularly following open reduction via a deltopectoral approach. Prior

investigation has suggested this aesthetic difference may be psychologically troubling to adolescent patients.[111] For this reason, alternative, more aesthetic incisions in the axilla have been proposed.[121] Patients and families should be counseled about the possibility of hypertrophic scar formation from deltopectoral incisions or percutaneous pin sites prior to surgical intervention.

SUMMARY, CONTROVERSIES, AND FUTURE DIRECTIONS RELATED TO PROXIMAL HUMERUS FRACTURES

In summary, the majority of proximal humeral fractures may be effectively treated nonoperatively. In older adolescent patients with greater angulation and displacement, reduction and surgical stabilization is safe and effective in restoring radiographic alignment and shoulder motion. Future prospective, comparative investigation is needed to determine the criteria for reduction and fixation in older children and adolescents and characterize the patient-derived functional outcomes of these injuries in the long term.

Humerus Shaft Fractures

INTRODUCTION TO HUMERUS SHAFT FRACTURES

The humeral diaphysis is the location of 20% or less of all pediatric humerus fractures and 5% or less of all childhood skeletal injuries.[54,289] The incidence is estimated to be between 12 and 30 per 100,000 per year, and more recent epidemiologic information from the United States suggests that this incidence has remained relatively constant despite population changes.[178,195] There is a bimodal distribution of ages of children who sustain humeral diaphyseal fractures, with the greatest frequency seen in infants and adolescents.[12]

ASSESSMENT OF HUMERUS SHAFT FRACTURES

MECHANISMS OF INJURY FOR HUMERUS SHAFT FRACTURES

Humeral shaft fractures may be due to a variety of injury mechanisms, each with its own set of clinical considerations.

Birth-related trauma is a frequent cause of humeral diaphyseal injury, with a reported incidence between 0.035% and 0.34%.[36,220] Macrosomia, breech presentation, and/or difficult delivery are thought to be potential risk factors. The humerus is at particular risk in situations where the upper limb is abducted above the newborn's head and must be delivered inferiorly after version and extraction.[220] Similarly, humerus fractures may occur in cases of shoulder dystocia with rotational maneuvers or posterior arm delivery.[204] Cesarean section delivery is not necessarily protective, and any forceful extraction may impart enough energy to cause a humerus fracture.[16,40,282]

Nonaccidental trauma may also manifest as humerus fracture in a child. Indeed, 12% of all fractures and up to 60% of new fractures stemming from nonaccidental trauma affect the humerus.[214,316] While child abuse must be considered within the differential diagnosis of humeral diaphyseal fractures—particularly in children less than 3 years of age—only a minority of humeral shaft injuries in children are due to nonaccidental trauma.[316]

The most common mechanism of injury is direct or indirect force imparted upon the upper limb in the older child or adolescent. Direct blows to the brachium, falls onto an outstretched upper limb, motor vehicle collisions, and sports-related trauma may all result in diaphyseal fractures. Indeed, humeral shaft fractures have even been noted from throwing and other overuse activities, because of the rotational forces imparted upon the humerus during the throwing motion.[3,107,139,209,255]

INJURIES ASSOCIATED WITH HUMERUS SHAFT FRACTURES

Radial nerve palsies are commonly associated with humeral diaphyseal fractures and raise a number of treatment considerations and controversies.[12,72,90,136,218,221,288] Because of the anatomic proximity of the radial nerve to the mid- and distal humerus, the nerve may be contused, stretched, kinked, entrapped, or rarely transected with the initial injury and/or fracture displacement.[347] Furthermore, a delayed palsy may occur due to compression secondary to scar tissue, fracture callus, and even bone formation. It has been estimated that up to 20% of adult and 5% of pediatric humeral diaphyseal fractures will have associated radial nerve palsies.[22,218]

Clinically, radial nerve palsies may be categorized into the time of presentation. Primary radial nerve palsies occur at the time of injury and are clinically apparent at first evaluation. Secondary radial nerve palsies refer to deficits presumably sustained at the time of fracture reduction or manipulation, in patients in whom radial nerve function was initially intact.

Most published information suggests that the potential for spontaneous nerve recovery is high, with 78% to 100% of patients regaining radial nerve function with observation alone.[22,24,25,29,84,90,113,210,301] Indeed, in cases in which the primary radial nerve palsies were treated with immediate or early exploration, the vast majority of the time the nerve is found to be intact, though contused or tented over the displaced fracture fragments (Fig. 18-27).[118,218,314] In children, it has been hypothesized that the thicker periosteum may confer a protective effect on the radial nerve, reducing the risk of traumatic laceration or incarceration within the fracture site.

Radial nerve exploration should be performed in instances of open humeral diaphyseal fractures in which surgical debridement and stabilization is to be performed. If a true radial nerve laceration is encountered, options include tagging the nerve ends for subsequent identification and repair versus immediate primary neurorrhaphy.[102,333,340] Given the distance to reinnervation from a high radial nerve palsy, earlier repair allows for the best anatomic and functional potential.[18]

In cases of primary radial nerve palsy, recommendations have been made for observation and exploration at 8 weeks to 6 months if there is failure of adequate recovery.[72,84,146] While these time-based guidelines are helpful, each patient must be considered individually, adhering to fundamental principles.[20] In general, if there is failure of adequate recovery after the anticipated time—based upon the distance from the injury to distal points of reinnervation—surgical exploration should be considered. Physiologic studies have determined that following wallerian degeneration, nerve growth will occur at a rate on an average of 1 mm per day.[333] For high radial nerve palsies, spontaneous resolution should entail an advancing Tinel sign, with sequential return of radial wrist extensors, central wrist extensors, digital extensors, and thumb extensors. In cases of late exploration where radial nerve lacerations are encountered,

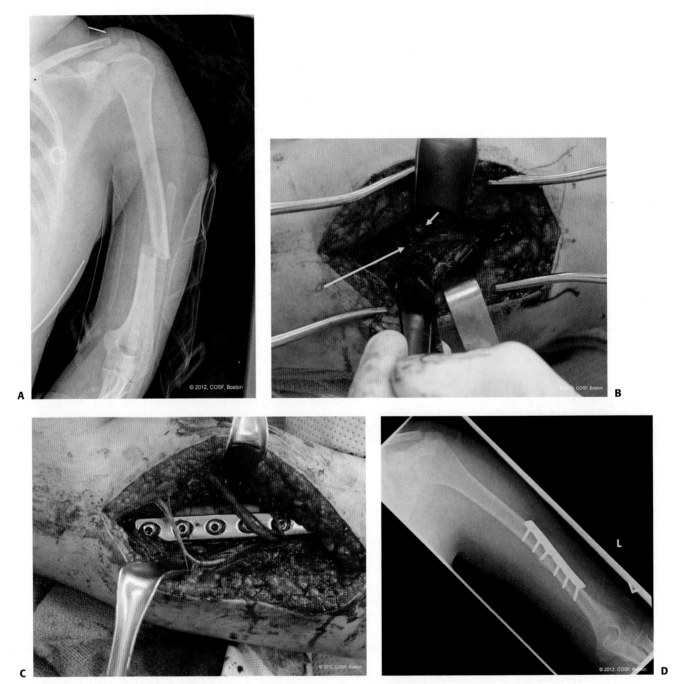

Figure 18-27. **A:** AP radiograph of a 15-year-old female with an open humeral diaphyseal fracture and radial nerve palsy. **B:** Intraoperative radiograph depicting exposure via a lateral approach. The kinked and contused radial nerve (*long arrow*) displaced by the proximal fracture fragment (*short arrow*). **C:** After irrigation, debridement, and plate fixation of the fracture, the nerve can be seen decompressed overlying the implant. **D:** Postoperative radiograph depicting bony healing and implant placement. (Courtesy of Children's Orthopaedic Surgery Foundation.)

sural nerve grafting may be performed, with anticipation of functional return.[18,100,254,348]

There continues to be controversy regarding the optimal management of secondary radial nerve palsy. If nerve function is lost after fracture manipulation, observation alone is still supported by published data suggesting that spontaneous recovery will occur in the majority of patients.[22,25,84,192] Others advocate early exploration because of liability concerns and late extraction

from fracture callus is much more difficult than early decompression. If radial nerve function is lost during the later period of fracture healing, careful consideration should be made regarding whether the nerve is entrapped within scar tissue, fracture callus, or bone.[89,370] Radiographs may depict an oval lucency corresponding to the bony foramen through which the nerve is running, the so-called Matev sign.[155,352] In these situations, surgical exploration and decompression should be performed.

SIGNS AND SYMPTOMS OF HUMERUS SHAFT FRACTURES

Clinical signs and symptoms will vary considerably depending upon the patient age and mechanism of injury.

In infants in whom a birth-related humerus fracture is suspected, a careful pre- and perinatal history should be obtained, specifically evaluating for macrosomia, prolonged or difficult labor and delivery, and history of shoulder dystocia. Additional historical information—such as whether the newborn will nurse from each breast—may guide the care provider to the correct diagnosis. Clinically, these infants will exhibit pseudoparalysis of the affected limb, holding or splinting the arm against the side. As distal neurologic function is intact, the infant will spontaneously grasp and move the digits and wrist. There will be reproducible tenderness, motion, and crepitus at the fracture site, though often little swelling or ecchymosis.

In older children who sustain traumatic or sports-related fractures, a careful history will provide insight into the mechanism of injury and any associated trauma. Details regarding the position of the upper limb, direction of forces imparted, and energy of injury will aid in clinical diagnosis. Patients will typically present with pain, swelling, ecchymosis, and guarding of the affected limb, with or without obvious deformity. The arm is typically held tightly against the body as the patient guards and protects the injured limb. Physical examination should include careful inspection of the overlying skin to assess for open wounds, ecchymosis, and skin tenting or dimpling. A thorough neurovascular examination is critical, particularly to assess potential injury of the radial nerve.[24,25,250,254]

IMAGING AND OTHER DIAGNOSTIC STUDIES FOR HUMERUS SHAFT FRACTURES

Plain radiographs of the humerus will confirm the diagnosis and should be performed in all cases of suspected humeral diaphyseal fractures (Figs. 18-28 and 18-29). Orthogonal views should be obtained, as nondisplaced or incomplete greenstick

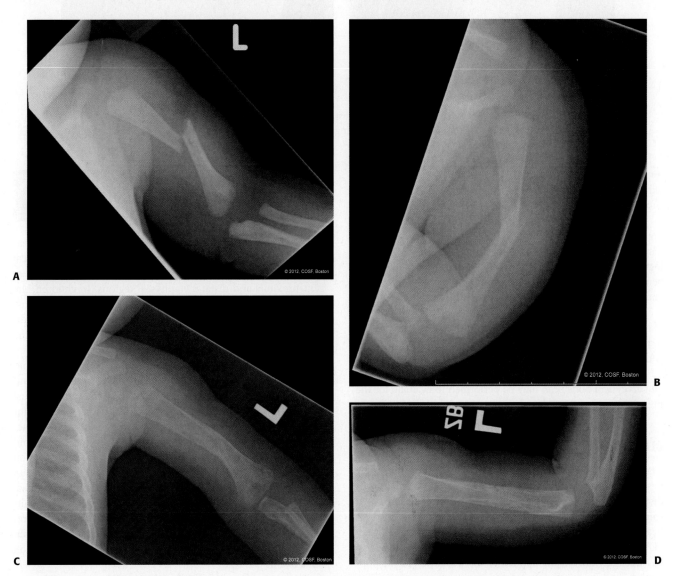

Figure 18-28. A, B: Radiographs depicting a humeral diaphyseal fracture in a 4-day-old infant with displacement and angulation. **C, D:** By 3 months of age, there is excellent bony healing and early remodeling. (Courtesy of Children's Orthopaedic Surgery Foundation.)

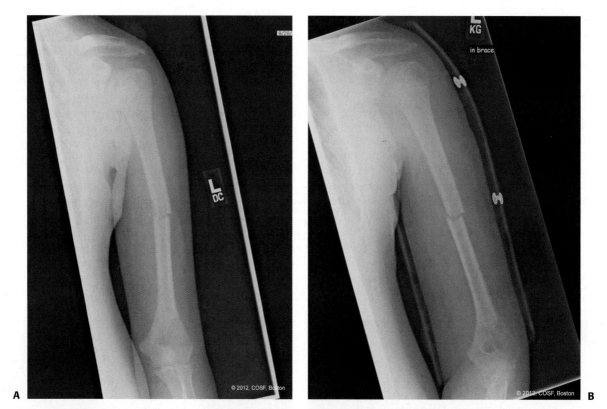

Figure 18-29. A: AP radiograph of a minimally displaced humeral diaphyseal fracture in a 13 year old male. **B:** Radiograph in fracture brace, demonstrating maintenance of alignment. (Courtesy of Children's Orthopaedic Surgery Foundation.)

fractures may occur in children. Appropriate lateral radiographs will demonstrate overlap or superimposition of the posterior supracondylar ridges of the medial and lateral epicondyles.[118]

In addition to confirming the diagnosis and characterizing its anatomic location and pattern, radiographs should be inspected for associated lesions to evaluate for possible pathologic fractures.[258,330,339] The humerus is a common site for both benign and malignant lesions in skeletally immature patients, and care should be taken to identify an associated condition.

"Floating elbow" injuries may occur, particularly in the setting of higher-energy mechanisms.[329] In patients with ipsilateral wrist or forearm pain or swelling, radiographic evaluation of the elbow and forearm will allow for diagnosis of these associated injuries.

Finally, in cases of suspected nonaccidental trauma, a skeletal survey and bone scan may be performed to evaluate for the presence of other fractures at various stages of healing.

CLASSIFICATION OF HUMERUS SHAFT FRACTURES

Classification of humeral diaphyseal fractures remains largely descriptive. Anatomic location, fracture pattern, direction of displacement and/or angulation, and the presence of associated soft tissue or ipsilateral skeletal injuries are used. While a classification system has been proposed by the Association for Study of Internal Fixation for humeral shaft fractures in adults, this has not been universally applied to the pediatric patient population, and questions persist over its interobserver reliability and clinical utility.[171,244]

PATHOANATOMY AND APPLIED ANATOMY RELATING TO HUMERUS SHAFT FRACTURES

While the humerus is a long, tubular bone, a number of anatomic features are worthy of note. First, the middiaphyseal region is triangular in cross section and narrower than the adjacent proximal and distal metaphyseal regions. In children, the humerus is enveloped in thick periosteum and has a rich vascular supply; the primary nutrient artery enters at the middiaphyseal level, though abundant accessory vessels supply the humeral shaft anteriorly and posteriorly.[42,118]

The deltoid tuberosity serves as the insertion of the deltoid and is located in the middiaphysis. The latissimus dorsi and teres major insert on the proximal aspect of the humerus, just medial to the bicipital groove. Conversely, the pectoralis major inserts along the anterior humerus lateral and distal to the bicipital groove. The coracobrachialis arises from the coracoid process and inserts along the middle third–distal third junction anteromedially. Distal and posterior to the deltoid tuberosity lies the so-called spiral groove, adjacent to which runs the radial nerve and from which the most proximal fibers of the brachialis originate. Similar to fractures of the proximal humerus, awareness of these muscle and soft tissue relationships help explain typical fracture displacement patterns and guide reduction maneuvers.

The anatomic path of the radial nerve deserves special attention, given the frequency with which the nerve is injured with humeral diaphyseal fractures. While much of the published literature is derived from cadaveric data in adults, a few principles may be applied to the pediatric population. First, as the radial nerve arises from the posterior cord of the brachial plexus, it passes through the triangular interval, bounded by the teres major superiorly and the lateral and long heads of the triceps medially and laterally. The radial nerve is typically accompanied by the profunda brachii artery as it passes through the upper arm. The nerve travels along the spiral groove, but is typically not in direct contact with the posterior humeral cortex; instead, it is separated from the bone by muscular fibers.[41] In general, the radial nerve is located directly posterior to the humeral diaphysis at the level of the deltoid tuberosity, a useful anatomic relationship in cases of surgical fracture treatment. The radial nerve continues distally and laterally, where it pierces the lateral intermuscular septum to enter the anterior compartment. Distally at the elbow, it may be found reliably in the brachialis–brachioradialis intermuscular interval.

The ulnar nerve runs in the medial aspect of the posterior compartment and does not give off any motor branches above the elbow. The median nerve travels just medial to the brachial artery in the distal half of the brachium.

TREATMENT OPTIONS FOR HUMERUS SHAFT FRACTURES

NONOPERATIVE TREATMENT OF HUMERUS SHAFT FRACTURES

Indications/Contraindications

Nonoperative Treatment of Humerus Shaft Fractures:
INDICATIONS AND CONTRAINDICATIONS

Indications
- Birth-related fractures
- Diaphyseal fractures with acceptable alignment
- Stress fractures
  - Benign pathologic fractures

Relative Contraindications
- Open fractures
- Associated vascular injury
- Diaphyseal fractures with unacceptable alignment

Most humeral diaphyseal fractures in children are amenable to nonoperative care.[38,81] As the upper limb is not weight bearing, anatomic alignment of the humerus is not necessary for functional restoration. Furthermore, shoulder motion, elbow flexion–extension, and forearm rotation may effectively compensate for mild-to-moderate humeral deformity. Finally, there is considerable remodeling potential for humeral deformity in skeletally immature patients; indeed, even up to 30 degrees may remodel in the adolescent population.[72] For these reasons, up to 20 to 30 degrees of varus, 20 degrees of apex anterior angulation, 15 degrees of internal rotation, and bayonet apposition with 1 to 2 cm of shortening is deemed acceptable.[72,279] As with all guidelines, these parameters for "acceptable deformity"

must be taken into their historical context, and individualized decisions should be made regarding the function demands and treatment goals of each patient. While limited information is available, recent comparisons of nonoperative and surgical treatment suggest that functional outcomes and return to activities are similar, though surgical stabilization may allow for less duration of immobilization.[38,39]

Birth-related fractures of the humeral diaphysis heal robustly and demonstrate profound remodeling potential. Indeed, 50% or greater remodeling may be seen within 1 to 2 years.[17] For this reason, simple immobilization to maximize comfort is sufficient, and no effort to achieve or maintain anatomic alignment is necessary.[144,156,317] A host of different treatment options have been proposed—ranging from sling-and-swathe, splinting, casting, traction, or simply pinning the sleeve of the affected arm to the body.[144,156,317] Concerns regarding immobilization and bony healing in excessive internal rotation may be addressed by immobilization of the upper extremity with elbow extension. This is particularly relevant in patients with concomitant brachial plexus birth palsies, in whom internal rotation contractures and external rotation weakness of the shoulder are common.[126,188,360]

Stress fractures of the humerus do occur and almost universally heal with appropriate rest, time, and activity modification.[3,107,209] Failure to allow for symptom-free healing may result in fracture completion and displacement.[3]

Sling-and-Swath Immobilization

Sling-and-swath immobilization is simple, safe, and effective for incomplete and minimally displaced fractures.[279] It may also be used for displaced fractures, though does not control apex anterior or varus angulation well, particularly in active and/or obese patients.[279,326] While the weight of the upper limb may be well supported, some patients find sling-and-swathe immobilization uncomfortable because of persistent motion at the fracture site.

Coaptation Splinting

Coaptation splinting (also referred to as U-plaster or sugartong splinting) has also been advocated in the treatment of humeral diaphyseal fractures.[371] The application of a coaptation splint is straightforward and is similar to that of sugartong splinting of the forearm (Fig. 18-30). A plaster splint, corresponding to the width of the brachium, is applied in a well-padded fashion from the acromion superolaterally, around the olecranon distally, and back up to the level of the axilla medially. The splint may be gently molded to the upper arm and secured in place with an elastic bandage or wrap. Efforts should be made to advance the superolateral extension of the splint to the level of the neck, in efforts prevent distal migration with gravity.[313] Others have recommended application of benzoin to the skin prior to splint placement and the use of a collar-and-cuff to prevent slippage.[144] Coaptation splinting has proven effective in children, and is particularly useful in the acute setting as the plaster slab may be molded comfortably to the swollen limb.[72] However, as the initial swelling subsides, refitting or transitioning to other methods of immobilization may be needed. Furthermore, coaptation splinting is not as effective as other forms of immobilization

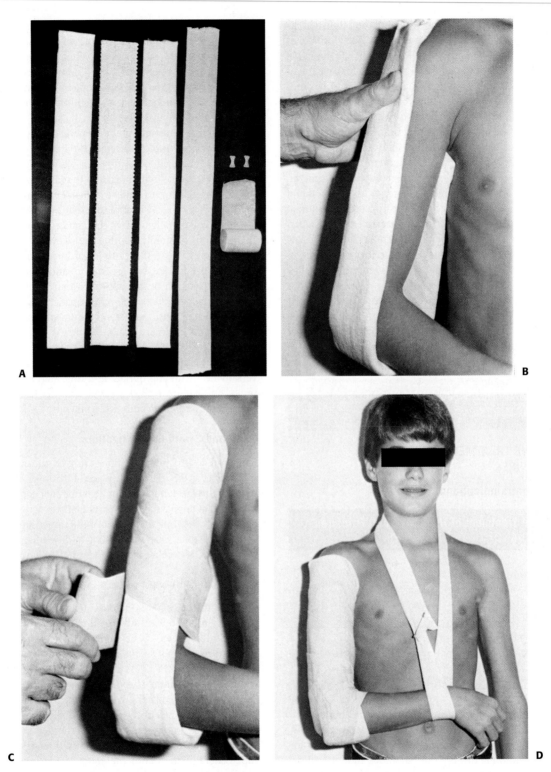

Figure 18-30. Coaptation splints with collar and cuff. **A:** The material used for a sugartong arm splint is two pieces of cast padding rolled out to the length of the plaster-of-Paris splint and applied to each side of the splint after it is wet. The splint is then brought into the tubular stockinette of the same width but 4 in longer than the splint. **B:** The plaster splint is applied to the arm from the axilla up to the tip of the acromion. **C:** As the plaster is setting, the splint is molded to the arm. An elastic bandage holds the splint in place. **D:** Stockinette is applied and attached to the wrist to form a collar-and-cuff sling.

at effectuating or maintaining reduction in cases of severe initial displacement.[144]

Traction

Both overhead and side-arm traction have been described for the treatment of humeral diaphyseal fractures.[144] Skin traction may be applied to the elbow, forearm, or hand. Alternatively, skeletal traction via an olecranon wingnut or transolecranon traction pin may be used.[6,14] Excessive or prolonged traction includes nonunion and elbow dislocation.[140] At present, because of patient and family demands, economic pressures, and wealth of alternative treatment options, the use of traction remains primarily of historic importance and is rarely used.

Hanging Casting

Hanging arm casts use both immobilization and gravity to impart stability and longitudinal traction to humerus fractures.[33] Long above-elbow casts are applied to the affected limb and supported by a sling or collar-and-cuff. Adjustments in sling/cuff placement may allow for correction of coronal and sagittal plane deformity, though rotational alignment is poorly controlled. While reported results demonstrate efficacy with this technique, compliance may be limited due to pain and difficulty maintaining an upright position, particularly in very young patients.[331] Furthermore, concerns regarding shoulder and elbow stiffness and internal rotation contractures persist.[59,283]

Functional Bracing

First described by Sarmiento et al.[304] in 1977, functional bracing of humeral diaphyseal fractures has been increasingly used in both children and adults.[48,125,315,356,357] In general, these functional braces confer a number of advantages over other nonoperative treatment options. In addition to providing external support via their clamshell design, when properly applied functional braces may effectuate and maintain fracture reduction due to the hydraulic effect to the surrounding soft tissues (see Fig. 18-29). Furthermore, functional braces allow for elbow motion, minimizing the risk of late elbow contractures. While limited comparative information is available, there is data to suggest that functional bracing is superior to coaptation splinting and equally effective as locked intramedullary nailing in appropriately selected patients.[315,357]

Prefabricated or custom-fit functional braces are used early in the course of treatment. Many patients will not tolerate functional bracing immediately, and are temporarily supported in a sling-and-swathe or coaptation splint until the initial swelling subsides. Serial clinical visits and radiographic assessment are needed to ensure adequate brace fit and maintenance of radiographic alignment. Functional braces may even be used for comminuted extra-articular fractures of the distal third of the humerus, though occasionally brace extensions may need to assist in coronal plane control.[169,303] By design, functional braces for humerus fractures are not as effective in controlling apex anterior angulation, nor are they meant to support weight bearing of the affected upper limb.

OPERATIVE TREATMENT OF HUMERUS SHAFT FRACTURES

Indications/Contraindications

In general, indications for surgical treatment of humeral diaphyseal fractures include open fractures, fractures with vascular injury, floating elbow injuries (Fig. 18-31), and failure to achieve adequate alignment with nonoperative means. In addition, multitrauma and secondary radial nerve palsies (i.e., those occurring after closed fracture manipulation in patients in whom radial nerve function was initially intact) are deemed by many as relative indications for surgical exploration and fracture fixation. A host of options exist for surgical fracture fixation, including ORIF using plate-and-screw constructs, intramedullary nailing, and external fixation.[82,137,259]

Open Reduction and Internal Fixation

Preoperative Planning

✔ ORIF of Humerus Shaft Fractures: PREOPERATIVE PLANNING CHECKLIST	
OR table	☐ Radiolucent table or regular table with radiolucent hand table extension
Position/positioning aids	☐ Supine
Fluoroscopy location	☐ From head of table as needed
Equipment	☐ 4.5 mm, 3.5 mm, or semitubular plates and screws
Tourniquet	☐ Sterile if needed

Preoperative planning for open reduction and plate-and-screw fixation includes appropriate AP and lateral radiographs of the humerus to assess fracture location, pattern, and displacement. The appropriate-sized implants should be determined in advance. While broad 4.5-mm dynamic compression plates are commonly used in adults, smaller 3.5 mm or semitubular plates are often used and sufficient for fixation of humeral diaphyseal fractures in children and adolescents, given the smaller size of the bone.[69,138,171,294] Furthermore, careful preoperative evaluation should be made to document neurovascular status, given the known risks of traumatic and iatrogenic radial nerve palsy associated with humeral diaphyseal fractures.

Positioning

Patient positioning is dependent in part on the planned surgical approach. In most instances, supine positioning is sufficient. In older children and adolescents, the affected limb may be placed on a radiolucent hand table to provide adequate access to both the surgeon and fluoroscopy unit. In the very young child, the patient and injured extremity may be positioned on a radiolucent fracture table. Even in cases in which a posterior surgical approach is to be used, supine positioning may be used with the limb adducted across the body. The fluoroscopy unit may be best positioned coming in from the head of the patient, allowing the surgeon to sit in the axilla and access the limb at all times.

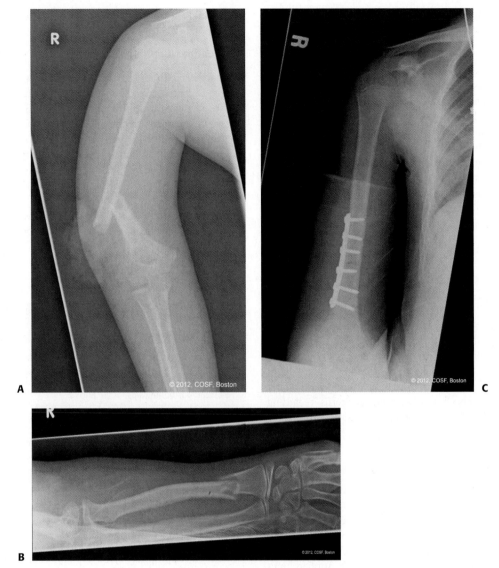

Figure 18-31. Floating elbow injury. **A:** AP radiograph depicting an open humeral diaphyseal fracture in a 10-year-old female. **B:** An ipsilateral radius fracture is also seen, consistent with a floating elbow injury. **C:** Postoperative radiograph after open irrigation and plate fixation of the humeral fracture. The radius fracture was also stabilized with internal fixation. (Courtesy of Children's Orthopaedic Surgery Foundation.)

Surgical Approach

A variety of different surgical approaches can be used. For distal humeral fractures, a posterior, triceps-splitting approach may be used.[145,245,365,372] Prone or lateral decubitus positioning may be helpful for this approach. After a posterior midline incision is made, dissection is performed down to the level of the triceps fascia, through the deep fascia. Skin flaps are elevated, exposing the triceps. The triceps tendon is split longitudinally in the midline, and this may be extended proximally in the interval between the long and lateral heads of the triceps. The deeper, medial head of the triceps may then be split and careful subperiosteal elevation is performed, exposing the humeral cortex. This approach is not extensile, and more proximal exposure is limited by the course of the radial nerve.

A traditional anterolateral approach is familiar to most surgeons and provides more extensile exposure.[13,145] In the supine position, a proximal deltopectoral incision is extended distally along the lateral aspect of the biceps. Proximally, the deltopectoral intermuscular interval is developed, retracting the cephalic vein laterally. More distally, the brachialis–brachioradialis interval is developed. Proximally, subperiosteal elevation will allow bony exposure. Distally, the brachialis muscle may be split longitudinally in the distal humeral shaft region, taking advantage of its dual innervation. The brachial artery and median and ulnar nerves are protected within the medial soft tissues. This exposure will not allow visualization or access to the radial nerve, which must be protected from overzealous retractor placement or drill/screw insertion posterior to the humerus.[369]

Alternatively, an extensile lateral or posterolateral approach will provide access to most of the humeral diaphysis as well as the radial nerve.[41,109,240] In the supine position, a lateral or posterolateral incision is created centered on the fracture site. Dissection is performed down to the level of the deep fascia and subcutaneous flaps elevated. The triceps fascia is incised just posterior to the lateral intermuscular septum, entering the posterior compartment of the brachium. The lateral head of the triceps is then elevated off the lateral intermuscular septum from distal to proximal. The radial nerve may then be identified, often surrounded by perineural fat, as it passes from the posterior to anterior compartments. Often the posterior antebrachial cutaneous nerve may be identified as it travels from proximal-posterior to distal-anterior more superficially; following this nerve proximally will allow for easy identification of the radial nerve proper. Other anatomic landmarks, including the apex of the triceps aponeurosis, have been used for radial nerve identification.[4] After the radial nerve is circumferentially dissected free, it may be isolated with a vessel loop and carefully retracted. Subperiosteal dissection will then allow for exposure of the humeral diaphysis.

Technique

> ### ✔ ORIF of Humerus Shaft Fractures:
> #### KEY SURGICAL STEPS
>
> ❑ Expose humeral diaphysis
> ❑ Identify and retract radial nerve, when applicable
> ❑ Anatomic reduction of humeral fracture
> ❑ Apply lateral plate, with care to protect the radial nerve
> ❑ Six cortices of fixation above and below the fracture site
> ❑ Layered wound closure
> ❑ Splint or cast immobilization

After the diaphysis is exposed and radial nerve identified and retracted, the fracture site is identified. Fracture hematoma is evacuated and the cortical fracture edges defined. Reduction may be performed under direct visualization, with interdigitation of the fracture edges restoring longitudinal alignment and proper rotation. The fracture is then fixed using appropriately sized plates for age and size of patient (3.5-mm compression plates, single or double-stacked semitubular plates), ideally obtaining six cortices of fixation above and below the fracture site using 3.5-mm cortical screws. Intraoperative fluoroscopy may be used to confirm anatomic reduction and appropriate implant placement. If the fracture site occurs adjacent to the radial nerve, care must be made to slide the plate beneath the nerve and avoid iatrogenic injury or kinking.

Intramedullary Fixation

Preoperative Planning

> ### ✔ Intramedullary Nailing of Humerus Shaft Fractures:
> #### PREOPERATIVE PLANNING CHECKLIST

OR table	❑ Radiolucent table or regular table with radiolucent hand table extension
Position/positioning aids	❑ Supine
Fluoroscopy location	❑ From head of table
Equipment	❑ Stainless steel or flexible titanium intramedullary nails, ideally 40% of intramedullary canal diameter

Preoperative planning for intramedullary nailing includes appropriate AP and lateral radiographs of the humerus to assess fracture location, pattern, and displacement. Again, careful preoperative evaluation should be made to document neurovascular status, given the known risks of traumatic and iatrogenic radial nerve palsy associated with humeral diaphyseal fractures. (In cases of radial nerve palsy, consideration should be given for formal open reduction and plate fixation, given the ability to simultaneously explore and decompress the radial nerve.) Appropriately sized flexible stainless steel or titanium intramedullary nails should be available. Similar to intramedullary fixation techniques of pediatric femur fractures, the selected nail diameter should be approximately 40% of the intramedullary canal dimension.

Positioning

In most cases, supine positioning is sufficient. In older children and adolescents, the affected limb may be placed on a radiolucent hand table to provide adequate access to both the surgeon and fluoroscopy unit. In the very young child, the patient and injured extremity may be supported by a radiolucent fracture table. The fluoroscopy unit may be best positioned coming in from the head of the patient, allowing the surgeon to sit in the axilla and access the limb at all times.

Surgical Approach

A theoretical advantage of intramedullary nailing of humeral diaphyseal fractures is the ability to achieve stable realignment via closed or indirect fracture reduction and minimally invasive implant placement. Reduction and stabilization may be achieved with efficiently, without need for extensive surgical dissection.[62,80,128] A host of surgical approaches may be used. Intramedullary implants (Enders nails, Rush rods, flexible titanium nails) may be inserted via a posterior approach. Through a small posterior incision and triceps-splitting approach to the posterior humeral cortex just proximal to the olecranon fossa, an oval corticotomy may be made, large enough to accommodate passage of two nails. Nails may then be inserted retrograde through this combined entry point. While two nails may be sufficient, some have advocated the Hackethal or "bouquet" technique, in which the canal is progressively filled with multiple pins to confer additional rigidity (Fig. 18-32).[124] This may be particularly useful in cases of segmental, comminuted, or pathologic fractures.

Alternatively, intramedullary nails may be placed via the lateral and/or medial columns of the distal humerus.[207,234] Small incisions may be made overlying the distal lateral and/or medial columns, at or above the level of olecranon fossa. Oval corticotomies are created at the site of nail entry to facilitate implant passage. Others have proposed insertion through the lateral and medial epicondyles via small drill holes. Care is made to retract and protect the posteromedial soft tissues—including the ulnar nerve—if a medial entry point is chosen. Nails may then be passed into the intramedullary canal and in a retrograde fashion to the fracture site.

Once fracture reduction is achieved, intramedullary nails may be atraumatically passed into the canal of the proximal fragment.

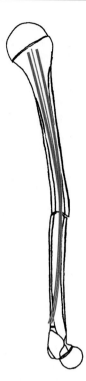

Figure 18-32. The Hackethal technique involves multiple smooth pins placed up the humeral shaft through a cortical window just above the olecranon fossa. The pins are placed until the canal is filled.

Fluoroscopic guidance is helpful, and efforts should be made to avoid repeated false passage of the nails into the adjacent soft tissues. In general, two nails are sufficient, provided they are of appropriate diameter and symmetrically contoured to allow for appropriate angular correction and rotational control.[198,199,234]

While the experience in adults is well documented, at present there are limited indications for solid reamed intramedullary nailing of humeral diaphyseal fractures in skeletally immature patients. This is in part because of the risks of physeal disturbance, shoulder impingement, and the relative narrow dimensions of the intramedullary canal in younger patients.[66,127,161,226,281,288]

Technique

✔ **Intramedullary Nailing of Humerus Shaft Fractures:**
KEY SURGICAL STEPS

- ❏ Measure anticipated diameter and length of intramedullary nails
- ❏ Precontour intramedullary nails
- ❏ Create entry sites along lateral (and medial) column(s) of distal humerus
- ❏ Create cortical entry points for subsequent nail passage
- ❏ Introduce intramedullary nails and pass proximally to level of fracture site
- ❏ Closed reduction of humerus
  - • Fluoroscopic assistance
- ❏ Pass nails into intramedullary canal of proximal fragment, avoiding excessive false passage and trauma to the adjacent soft tissues
- ❏ Pass nails up to 1 to 2 cm distal to the proximal humeral epiphysis
- ❏ Bent and cut intramedullary nails beneath the skin
- ❏ Application of splint or sling after wound closure

Patients are positioned in the supine position. The appropriate-sized intramedullary implants (titanium elastic nails, Enders nails, Rush rods) are placed over the brachium, and fluoroscopy is used to determine the anticipated length of the intramedullary nail. The nails are then prebent into a gentle bow, with the apex centered at the level of the fracture site. If lateral column entry site only is to be used, the nails should be contoured into the shape of a "C" and "S" to maximize spread (and thus stability) at the level of the fracture site while still allowing for medial and lateral engagement of the proximal humeral metaphysis. If both medial and lateral column entry sites are planned, each nail will be prebent into the shape of a "C."

A longitudinal incision is then created over the palpable lateral (and medial) column, just proximal to the olecranon fossa. Tourniquet control is not typically necessary. While epicondylar entry sites have been described, these have been associated with more frequent nail back-out.[128] Dissection is performed down to the level of the cortex. A small periosteal window may be elevated. Drill bits or awls may be used to create a cortical entry point, with care taken to orient the obliquity of the cortical tunnel along the anticipated trajectory of the nail. The intramedullary devices are then passed into the intramedullary canal of the distal fracture fragment to the level of the fracture. Fracture reduction is achieved through gentle closed manipulation, restoring length and correcting the angular deformity in the coronal and sagittal planes. Once fracture reduction is achieved, intramedullary nails may be atraumatically passed into the canal of the proximal fragment. A small bend at the leading tip of the intramedullary implant will facilitate engagement of the proximal fracture fragment. Fluoroscopic guidance is helpful, and efforts should be made to avoid repeated false passage of the nails into the adjacent soft tissues. In general, two nails are sufficient, provided they are of appropriate diameter and symmetrically contoured to allow for appropriate angular correction and rotational control.[198,199,234]

The implants are passed proximally into the proximal fragment until they lie 1 to 2 cm from the proximal humeral physis. At this time, the nails may be cut distally, leaving approximately 2 cm of length outside the cortex. If the nails were inserted with appropriate obliquity, the cut distal end of the nail will lie flush against the flare of the distal humeral metaphysis, avoiding symptomatic implant prominence yet still allowing for reliable implant retrieval. The entry wounds are closed in layers, and a long posterior splint, coaptation splint, or simple sling is applied.

External Fixation

Preoperative Planning

✔ **External Fixation of Humerus Shaft Fractures:**
PREOPERATIVE PLANNING CHECKLIST

OR table	❏ Radiolucent table
Position/positioning aids	❏ Supine
Fluoroscopy location	❏ Ipsilateral side of table
Equipment	❏ Appropriate-sized external fixation pins, bars, rings

External fixation remains a treatment option for humeral shaft fractures, particularly in critically ill multitrauma patients or patients with severe open fractures associated with extensive soft tissue injury and/or bone loss.[45,76,177,276,295,324] Preoperative planning includes appropriate AP and lateral radiographs of the humerus to assess fracture location, pattern, displacement, and/or bone loss. Thorough documentation of preoperative neurovascular status is needed. For the multitrauma patient, communication with other care providers is important for care coordination and prioritization of injury treatment. In cases of severe soft tissue injury, appropriate consultation with plastic surgeons is recommended; this will allow for guidance regarding appropriate pin placement and planning of ultimate soft tissue coverage, if needed. Appropriately sized external fixator pins and bars should be available. While unilateral constructs are sufficient in most situations to provide stability, multiplanar or ring fixators may be employed, particular if there are plans for subsequent lengthening, bone transport, or deformity correction.

Positioning

Patients may be positioned supine with the limb supported by a radiolucent table or hand table. Fluoroscopy units may be positioned on the ipsilateral side of the table, coming from the head or foot. Coordination should be made with other care providers in the multitrauma patient to allow adequate access to all anatomic regions necessitating care.

Surgical Approach

Surgical approaches are dictated by fracture characteristics, concomitant wounds and soft tissue injuries, and plans for future interventions. For a standard unilateral construct, pins may be inserted using percutaneous approaches via small incisions and careful spreading through the underlying soft tissues. Understanding of the cross-sectional anatomy of the brachium is important to avoid potential neurovascular injury.

Technique

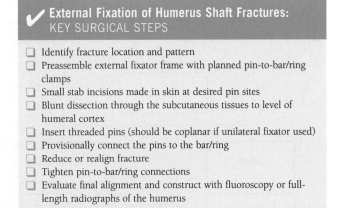

External Fixation of Humerus Shaft Fractures: KEY SURGICAL STEPS

- ☐ Identify fracture location and pattern
- ☐ Preassemble external fixator frame with planned pin-to-bar/ring clamps
- ☐ Small stab incisions made in skin at desired pin sites
- ☐ Blunt dissection through the subcutaneous tissues to level of humeral cortex
- ☐ Insert threaded pins (should be coplanar if unilateral fixator used)
- ☐ Provisionally connect the pins to the bar/ring
- ☐ Reduce or realign fracture
- ☐ Tighten pin-to-bar/ring connections
- ☐ Evaluate final alignment and construct with fluoroscopy or full-length radiographs of the humerus

Once the patient is positioned and the fracture location and pattern identified, the configuration of the ultimate external fixator construct is determined. Biomechanically, maximal spread of pins in both the proximal and distal fracture fragments will allow for the most rigid construct. If a unilateral frame is to be applied, preassembly of the bar with pin-to-bar clamps may facilitate coplanar placement of pins; indeed, the pin-to-bar clamps may be used as a "drill guide" during pin placement.

In a sequential fashion, the skin is incised at the site of pin placement and gentle, blunt dissection is performed through the subcutaneous tissues to the level of the humeral cortex. Appropriately sized threaded pins may then be drilled into the humerus, and use of cannulae or drill guides will protect the adjacent soft tissues and minimize the risk of iatrogenic neurovascular injury. This is particularly true for the radial nerve when lateral pins are placed in the mid- to distal diaphysis.

After pins are placed and connected to the external fixator bar, the fracture may be aligned in the desired position and stabilized. The addition of a second bar, while not always necessary, will improve bending rigidity of the construct.

Author's Preferred Treatment of Humerus Shaft Fractures (Algorithm 18-3)

The majority of humeral shaft fractures in children and adolescents may be successfully treated nonoperatively. In infants with birth-related fractures, immobilization with a stockinette or pinning of the sleeve to the trunk is simple and effective. Radiographic assessment of healing is performed at 4 to 6 weeks of age; immobilization is discontinued after confirmation of clinical and radiographic healing.

In children and adolescents with closed humeral diaphyseal fractures, stable injuries (e.g., torus or minimally displaced greenstick fractures) may be treated with simple sling immobilization. Patients with displaced fractures typically present with considerable pain, swelling, and ecchymosis. In these situations, gentle fracture realignment of the fracture may be performed with conscious sedation or general anesthesia, followed by application of a well-molded coaptation

splint. Patients may be transitioned to a fracture brace at 1 to 2 weeks postinjury, after the initial swelling and discomfort has subsided. Serial radiographs are obtained to monitor fracture alignment and bony healing. Bony union is typically obtained by 6 weeks, after which immobilization is discontinued and activities advanced.

Similar nonoperative treatment is advocated for patients with closed injuries and acceptable alignment who present with radial nerve palsies. Even after bony union is achieved, serial clinical checks are performed monthly to monitor nerve recovery. An advancing Tinel sign and sequential motor recovery, beginning with wrist extension and progressing to digital and thumb extension, portend a favorable prognosis and spontaneous recovery. In general, nerve regeneration progresses 1 mm per day, and calculation of the

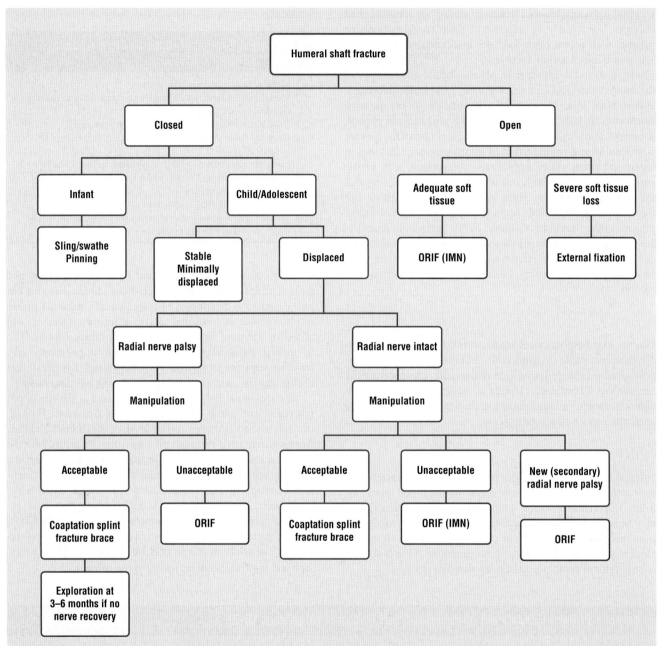

Algorithm 18-3. Author's preferred treatment for humeral shaft fractures.

distance from the fracture site to the sites of distal muscle innervation will allow for prediction of time to motor recovery. Surgical exploration with radial nerve decompression, repair, or reconstruction is considered after 3 to 6 months without evidence of any neurologic recovery.

Surgical intervention is indicated in cases of open fractures, fractures with vascular or severe soft tissue injury, and fractures in unacceptable alignment. Surgery is also considered for patients with failure of appropriate radial nerve recovery or new radial nerve palsies after fracture manipulation.

For most humeral diaphyseal fractures proximal to the distal metadiaphysis and without intercondylar extension

that are treated surgically, formal open reduction and plate fixation is preferred. An extensile lateral or posterolateral approach is used, as it allows safe access to up to 90% of the humeral diaphysis.[109] As surgery is often performed in the setting of radial nerve palsy, the lateral approach confers the additional advantage of allowing identification, mobilization, and/or repair of the radial nerve.[41,109,240]

Intramedullary nailing may be considered in patients without preoperative radial nerve palsy and transverse or short oblique (i.e., "length stable") fracture patterns. While the principles of intramedullary fixation are well established and the results well documented, closed nailing does not allow for visualization or decompression of the radial nerve.

Postoperative Care

Patients receiving nonoperative treatment of humeral diaphyseal fractures are followed weekly with radiographs in splint or fracture brace to ensure adequate fit, monitor neurovascular function, and confirm radiographic alignment. In patients with associated radial nerve palsies, evaluation for an advancing Tinel sign and sequential motor recovery is performed. Once there is evidence of clinical and radiographic healing, gentle shoulder pendulum and elbow range-of-motion exercises are begun. Immobilization is typically discontinued after 6 weeks. Sports participation is restricted until there is return of motion and strength, and patients/families are counseled regarding the risk of refracture.

Following surgical reduction and stabilization, sling immobilization is usually sufficient and continued until radiographic healing. With plate fixation, gentle elbow range-of-motion exercises may be initiated once adequate comfort is achieved. In cases of intramedullary nail fixation, implants are typically removed at 6 months postoperatively.

Potential Pitfalls and Preventative Measures

Repair of Humerus Shaft Fractures: POTENTIAL PITFALLS AND PREVENTIONS

Pitfall	Prevention
• Malalignment of distal fractures (nonoperative)	• Extensions of fracture brace • Use of long-arm casts/splints
• Malalignment of distal fractures (surgical)	• Avoid percutaneous pinning • Use of plates or IM nails • Bicolumnar fixation • Supplement with cast/splint immobilization
• Radial nerve injury during ORIF	• Careful dissection and mobilization • Position plate beneath nerve • Direct visualization of plate/screws
• Complications of IM nailing	• Lateral entry above olecranon fossa • Appropriate vector for nail insertion

While the techniques described above are well established, a number of potential pitfalls may be encountered during the treatment of diaphyseal fractures. First, nonoperative treatment of distal diaphyseal fractures may be challenging, given the anatomic location and relative limited amount of distal humerus that may be incorporated into a fracture brace or splint.[97] In these situations, use of medial and lateral extensions of conventional fracture brace may be needed to provide better control of coronal plane and rotational alignment. Alternatively, long-arm casts or long posterior splints may be used to provide stability and maintain alignment until clinical and radiographic healing occurs. Careful clinical and radiographic monitoring is needed, due to the tendency for varus malalignment and the limited capacity for remodeling of very distal humeral deformity.[28]

Similarly, surgical treatment of distal diaphyseal fractures may provide several challenges (Fig. 18-33).[97] Closed reduction and percutaneous pinning techniques commonly used

for supracondylar humerus fractures may not provide adequate stability, as the more proximal fracture location results in medial and lateral entry pins that cross at the fracture site (Fig. 18-34). This may result in longer operative times, loss of fixation with late deformity, and loss of motion. Alternative treatments include open plating or intramedullary nailing via medial and lateral epicondyle entry sites (Fig. 18-35). With a medial epicondylar entry, the ulnar nerve needs to be identified and protected. When open plate or intramedullary nail fixation is chosen, consideration should be made for stabilization of both the medial and lateral columns to provide maximal control and minimize risk for late instability. In cases where bicolumnar fixation is not possible, supplementation with long-arm casts or other external immobilization is suggested.

During ORIF via a lateral or posterolateral approach, care of the radial nerve is paramount. Identification of the posterior brachial cutaneous nerve and/or the characteristic fat stripe along the lateral aspect of the triceps will enable radial nerve identification during surgical exposures. Often the radial nerve must be mobilized to allow for implant placement between the humeral cortex below and the radial nerve above. Adequate direct visualization of plate placement and screw insertion is imperative to minimize the risk of iatrogenic nerve injury (Fig. 18-36).

Finally, a few maneuvers may aid in the intramedullary nailing of humeral diaphyseal fractures. Lateral column entry provides easy surgical access and minimizes risk to the ulnar nerve. If this is chosen, nails should be precontoured into the shape of a "C" and "S" to allow for maximal spread at the fracture site and engagement of the proximal humeral fracture fragment. Creating the cortical entry point above the olecranon fossa with the appropriate distal-lateral to proximal-medial vector will allow the nail to sit against the metaphyseal flare of the lateral column when cut; this will facilitate subsequent retrieval and minimize the soft tissue irritation commonly caused by epicondylar entry points.

Outcomes

Overall, reported clinical results are good after surgical treatment of humeral diaphyseal fractures using both intramedullary nailing and open plate fixation techniques.[13,66,128,137,161,288,331]

MANAGEMENT OF EXPECTED ADVERSE OUTCOMES AND UNEXPECTED COMPLICATIONS RELATED TO HUMERUS SHAFT FRACTURES

Humerus Shaft Fractures: COMMON ADVERSE OUTCOMES AND COMPLICATIONS

• Radial nerve palsy
• Malunion
• Nonunion
• Limb length discrepancy
• Stiffness

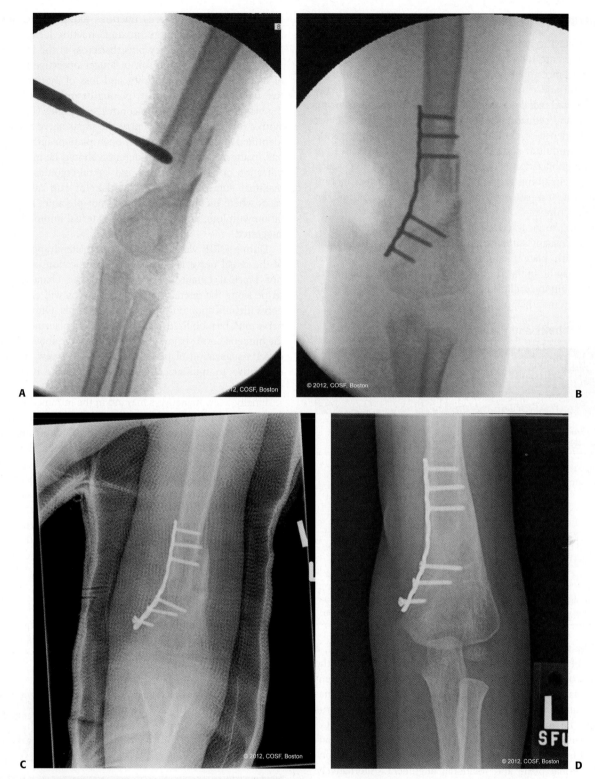

Figure 18-33. **A:** Intraoperative image depicting a comminuted, open distal humerus fracture in a 3-year-old male after a motorcycle injury. **B:** Intraoperative image after lateral column plate fixation, sparing the distal humeral physes. **C:** Given single column fixation, some loss of fixation is seen. Internal fixation was supplemented with spica cast immobilization. **D:** Final radiographs demonstrate appropriate bony healing and alignment. (Courtesy of Children's Orthopaedic Surgery Foundation.)

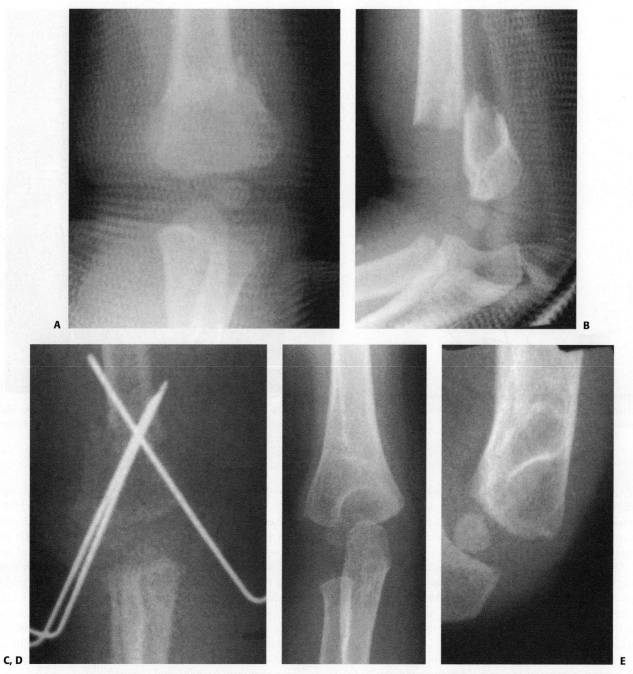

Figure 18-34. A, B: Distal humeral diaphyseal fracture in an 18-month-old treated with closed reduction and percutaneous pinning. **C:** The pins cross at the fracture site with decreased stability and some loss of position. **D, E:** The ultimate outcome was good.

Radial nerve palsies are commonly seen with humeral diaphyseal fractures. As discussed above, these nerve injuries may be primary or secondary. Secondary radial nerve injuries may result from a host of mechanisms, including excessive fracture manipulation resulting in neurapraxia, nerve incarceration within the fracture site or subsequent fracture callus, or rarely direct nerve injury or transection during fracture manipulation or implant placement. These inadvertent neurologic complications may be seen with both nonoperative and surgical treatment. There continues to be controversy regarding the initial management of immediate secondary nerve palsies, though it is clear that failure of spontaneous recovery after an appropriate period of observation should prompt surgical exploration, decompression, and/or nerve reconstruction.[103,359] In addition to radial nerve injuries, ulnar and median nerve injuries have been reported.[219,328]

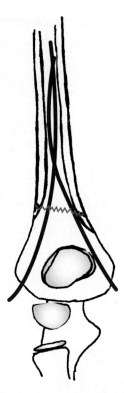

Figure 18-35. Ideally, pin fixation for distal humeral diaphyseal–metaphyseal junction fractures involves pins placed in intramedullary fashion up the medial and lateral columns.

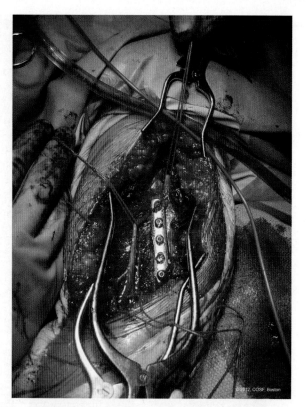

Figure 18-36. Intraoperative radiograph depicting radial nerve placement beneath a previously applied lateral plate. (Courtesy of Children's Orthopaedic Surgery Foundation.)

Compartment syndrome of the brachium is relatively rare, in part because of anatomic differences in fascial strength, ability to avoid extreme positioning during fracture immobilization, and fracture characteristics.[21,34,104,122] Patients with associated ipsilateral upper extremity fractures or vascular injuries are at highest risk.

Vascular injuries, including brachial artery transection, are uncommon but mandate prompt evaluation and intervention to restore vascularity to the upper limb.[231] In cases in which vascular repair or reconstruction is needed, fracture stability with external or internal fixation is needed to protect and facilitate vascular repair.

Functionally limiting malunion is uncommon in pediatric humeral diaphyseal fractures. As cited previously, 20 to 30 degrees of varus and 20 degrees of apex anterior angulation may be accepted, with often little aesthetic differences and functional consequence.[72,92,279,329] Up to 15 degrees of internal rotation is also well tolerated.[72] Patients younger than 6 years of age will remodel most angular deformity, and obese patients—though more prone to malunion given the challenges of immobilization—may hide their resultant deformity better.[146,294] Because of the remodeling potential, compensatory motion at the shoulder, elbow, and forearm, and lack of functional deficits, corrective osteotomies for humeral diaphyseal malunions are rarely necessary.

While more commonly reported in adults, nonunion of humeral diaphyseal fractures may rarely occur in children and adolescents (Fig. 18-37).[105] Risk factors may include excessive soft tissue injury, vascular insufficiency, segmental bone defects,

or underlying bone abnormalities, such as osteogenesis imperfecta. Treatment principles for humeral nonunion in children have been extrapolated from adult orthopedics.[96,134,244] In cases of hypertrophic nonunions, treatment is predicated on provision of bony stability, typically with ORIF. In cases of atrophic nonunions, ORIF with debridement of the pseudarthrosis back to bleeding bone and use of autogenous bone grafting is advised.[140] Alternative treatments include external fixation and the Ilizarov technique.[46,159,160] In cases of pathologic fractures or systemic bone abnormalities—such as osteogenesis imperfecta—intramedullary implants are preferred.[105] In rare situations, a vascularized fibula graft is appropriate to provide bony alignment, stability, and healing.[173]

Limb length discrepancy may result from prior humeral diaphyseal fracture, though clinically up to 6 to 8 cm of shortening may be well tolerated without functional loss. As with other long bone fractures, overgrowth may occur following humerus fracture, though the magnitude is often minimal (less than 1 cm).[305] In cases of considerable limb length discrepancy and functional compromise, humeral lengthening via distraction osteogenesis using unilateral or multiplanar ring fixators may be performed.[46,47,70,267]

Finally, while loss of shoulder and/or elbow motion is common with both nonoperative and surgical treatment of humeral diaphyseal fractures in adults, persistent stiffness is uncommon in pediatric patients.[140] Judicious initiation of early range of motion will aid to minimize the risk of this complication.

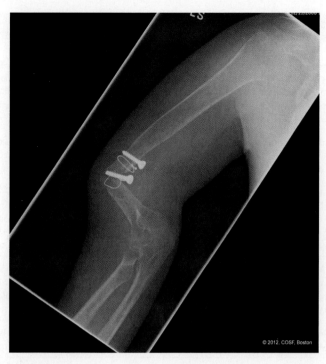

Figure 18-37. Radiograph depicting an atrophic humeral diaphyseal nonunion in a skeletally mature adolescent previously treated with screw and cerclage wire fixation of an open humeral diaphyseal fracture. (Courtesy of Children's Orthopaedic Surgery Foundation.)

SUMMARY, CONTROVERSIES, AND FUTURE DIRECTIONS RELATED TO HUMERUS SHAFT FRACTURES

In summary, most humeral diaphyseal fractures may be effectively treated nonoperatively. In older patients with greater deformity, surgical reduction and stabilization will result in reliable bony healing and improved radiographic alignment. Controversy continues regarding the optimal management of secondary radial nerve palsies as well as the relative indications for intramedullary nailing versus open reduction and plate fixation of displaced humeral shaft fractures. Future prospective, comparative investigation is needed to determine the optimal surgical management of these injuries.

Annotated References

Reference	Annotation
Beaty JH. Fractures of the proximal humerus and shaft in children. *Instr Course Lect.* 1992;41:369–372.	Instructional course lecture with guidelines regarding parameters of acceptable radiographic alignment for pediatric proximal humerus fractures.
Canavese F, Marengo L, Cravino M, et al. Outcome of conservative versus surgical treatment of humeral shaft fracture in children and adolescents: comparison between nonoperative treatment (Desault's bandage), external fixation and elastic stable intramedullary nailing. *J Pediatr Orthop.* 2017;37(3):e156–e163.	Comparative retrospective analysis of 36 patients treated with simple immobilization, external fixation, or flexible intramedullary nailing of humeral diaphyseal fractures. While surgical patients required less duration of immobilization and improved radiographic alignment, DASH scores and return to sports rates were similar among treatment groups.
Dobbs MB, Luhmann SL, Gordon JE, et al. Severely displaced proximal humeral epiphyseal fractures. *J Pediatr Orthop.* 2003;23(2):208–215.	Retrospective case series of children and adolescents with severely displaced (Neer–Horwitz 3 or 4) proximal humeral fractures. The authors identify risk of late displacement after initial closed reduction in adolescents, as well as soft tissue impediments to closed reduction.
Handoll HH, Almaiyah MA, Rangan A. Surgical versus non-surgical treatment for acute anterior shoulder dislocation. *Cochrane Database Syst Rev.* 2004;(1):CD004325.	Cochrane database review regarding the treatment of acute traumatic shoulder dislocation, suggesting surgical stabilization after primary dislocation may be beneficial in young male contact athletes.

Annotated References

Reference	Annotation
Hovelius L, Olofsson A, Sandstrom B, et al. Nonoperative treatment of primary anterior shoulder dislocation in patients forty years of age and younger: a prospective twenty-five-year follow-up. *J Bone Joint Surg Am.* 2008;90(5):945–952.	Long-term follow-up of young patients treated nonoperatively for traumatic shoulder dislocations, characterizing risk of recurrent instability and rates of subsequent surgical stabilization.
Khan A, Samba A, Pereira B, Canavese F. Anterior dislocation of the shoulder in skeletally immature patients: comparison between non-operative treatment versus open Latarjet's procedure. *Bone Joint J.* 2014;96-B(3):354–359.	In this retrospective case series of skeletally immature patients, surgical stabilization with the Latarjet procedure was effective in reducing risk of recurrent instability and allowing patients to return to pre-injury activities.
Kraus T, Hoermann S, Ploder G, et al. Elastic stable intramedullary nailing versus Kirschner wire pinning: outcome of severely displaced proximal humeral fractures in juvenile patients. *J Shoulder Elbow Surg.* 2014;23(10):1462–1467.	Excellent functional outcomes and radiographic alignment were achieved with either percutaneous pinning or elastic intramedullary nails for juvenile proximal humeral fractures.
Longo UG, van der Linde JA, Loppini M, et al. Surgical versus nonoperative treatment in patients up to 18 years old with traumatic shoulder instability: a systematic review and quantitative synthesis of the literature. *Arthroscopy.* 2016;32(5):944–952.	Systematic review from 15 published articles of 705 shoulders in patients 18 years of age or younger. Overall recurrent dislocation rate with nonoperative and surgical treatment was 71.3% vs. 17.5%, respectively.
Neer CS II, Horwitz BS. Fractures of the proximal humeral epiphysial plate. *Clin Orthop Relat Res.* 1965;41:24–31.	Classic paper with description of classification of proximal humeral fractures in pediatric and adolescent patients.

REFERENCES

1. Ahmed I, Ashton F, Robinson CM. Arthroscopic Bankart repair and capsular shift for recurrent anterior shoulder instability: functional outcomes and identification of risk factors for recurrence. *J Bone Joint Surg Am.* 2012;94:1308–1315.
2. Ahn JI, Park JS. Pathological fractures secondary to unicameral bone cysts. *Int Orthop.* 1994;18:20–22.
3. Allen ME. Stress fracture of the humerus. A case study. *Am J Sports Med.* 1984;12:244–245.
4. Arora S, Goel N, Cheema GS, et al. A method to localize the radial nerve using the "apex of triceps aponeurosis" as a landmark. *Clin Orthop Relat Res.* 2011;469:2638–2644.
5. Artico M, Salvati M, D'Andrea V, et al. Isolated lesion of the axillary nerve: surgical treatment and outcome in 12 cases. *Neurosurgery.* 1991;29:697–700.
6. Badhe NP, Howard PW. Olecranon screw traction for displaced supracondylar fractures of the humerus in children. *Injury.* 1998;29:457–460.
7. Bahrs C, Zipplies S, Ochs BG, et al. Proximal humeral fractures in children and adolescents. *J Pediatr Orthop.* 2009;29:238–242.
8. Baratta JB, Lim V, Mastromonaco E, et al. Axillary artery disruption secondary to anterior dislocation of the shoulder. *J Trauma.* 1983;23:1009–1011.
9. Barber DB, Janus RB, Wade WH. Neuroarthropathy: an overuse injury of the shoulder in quadriplegia. *J Spinal Cord Med.* 1996;19:9–11.
10. Barry TP, Lombardo SJ, Kerlan RK, et al. The coracoid transfer for recurrent anterior instability of the shoulder in adolescents. *J Bone Joint Surg Am.* 1985;67:383–387.
11. Baxter MP, Wiley JJ. Fractures of the proximal humeral epiphysis. Their influence on humeral growth. *J Bone Joint Surg Br.* 1986;68:570–573.
12. Beaty JH. Fractures of the proximal humerus and shaft in children. *Instr Course Lect.* 1992;41:369–372.
13. Bell MJ, Beauchamp CG, Kellam JK, et al. The results of plating humeral shaft fractures in patients with multiple injuries. The Sunnybrook experience. *J Bone Joint Surg Br.* 1985;67:293–296.
14. Berghausen T, Leslie BM, Ruby LK, et al. The severely displaced pediatric supracondylar fracture of humerus treated by skeletal traction with olecranon pin. *Orthop Rev.* 1986;15:510–515.
15. Beringer DC, Weiner DS, Noble JS, et al. Severely displaced proximal humeral epiphyseal fractures: a follow-up study. *J Pediatr Orthop.* 1998;18:31–37.
16. Bhat BV, Kumar A, Oumachigui A. Bone injuries during delivery. *Indian J Pediatr.* 1994;61:401–405.
17. Bianco AJ, Schlein AP, Kruse RL, et al. Birth fractures. *Minn Med.* 1972;55:471–474.
18. Birch R. Lesions of peripheral nerves: the present position. *J Bone Joint Surg Br.* 1986;68:2–8.
19. Bishop JA, Crall TS, Kocher MS. Operative versus nonoperative treatment after primary traumatic anterior glenohumeral dislocation: expected-value decision analysis. *J Shoulder Elbow Surg.* 2011;20:1087–1094.
20. Bishop J, Ring D. Management of radial nerve palsy associated with humeral shaft fracture: a decision analysis model. *J Hand Surg Am.* 2009;34:991–996.
21. Blakemore LC, Cooperman DR, Thompson GH, et al. Compartment syndrome in ipsilateral humerus and forearm fractures in children. *Clin Orthop Relat Res.* 2000;(376):32–38.
22. Bleeker WA, Nijsten MW, ten Duis HJ. Treatment of humeral shaft fractures related to associated injuries. A retrospective study of 237 patients. *Acta Orthop Scand.* 1991;62:148–153.
23. Bortel DT, Pritchett JW. Straight-line graphs for the prediction of growth of the upper extremities. *J Bone Joint Surg Am.* 1993;75:885–892.
24. Bostman O, Bakalim G, Vainionpaa S, et al. Immediate radial nerve palsy complicating fracture of the shaft of the humerus: when is early exploration justified?. *Injury.* 1985;16:499–502.
25. Bostman O, Bakalim G, Vainionpaa S, et al. Radial palsy in shaft fracture of the humerus. *Acta Orthop Scand.* 1986;57:316–319.
26. Boyd KT, Batt ME. Stress fracture of the proximal humeral epiphysis in an elite junior badminton player. *Br J Sports Med.* 1997;31:252–253.
27. Broker FH, Burbach T. Ultrasonic diagnosis of separation of the proximal humeral epiphysis in the newborn. *J Bone Joint Surg Am.* 1990;72:187–191.
28. Brug E, Winckler S, Klein W. Distal diaphyseal fracture of the humerus. *Unfallchirurg.* 1994;97:74–77.
29. Bumbasirevic M, Lesic A, Bumbasirevic V, et al. The management of humeral shaft fractures with associated radial nerve palsy: a review of 117 cases. *Arch Orthop Trauma Surg.* 2010;130:519–522.
30. Burgos-Flores J, Gonzalez-Herranz P, Lopez-Mondejar JA, et al. Fractures of the proximal humeral epiphysis. *Int Orthop.* 1993;17:16–19.
31. Burke MC, Minnock C, Robbins CB, et al. Intraobserver and interobserver reliability of radiographic analysis of proxima humerus fractures in adolescents. *J Pediatr Orthop.* 2017. doi: 10.1097/BPO.0000000000001083. [Epub ahead of print]
32. Burkhead WZ, Jr., Rockwood CA, Jr. Treatment of instability of the shoulder with an exercise program. *J Bone Joint Surg Am.* 1992;74:890–896.
33. Caldwell JA. Treatment of fractures in the Cincinnati General Hospital. *Ann Surg.* 1933;97:161–176.
34. Cameron SE. Acute compartment syndrome of the triceps. A case report. *Acta Orthop Scand.* 1993;64:107–108.
35. Cameron KL, Duffey ML, DeBerardino TM, et al. Association of generalized joint hypermobility with a history of glenohumeral joint instability. *J Athl Train.* 2010;45:253–258.
36. Camus M, Lefebvre G, Veron P, et al. Obstetrical injuries of the newborn infant. Retrospective study apropos of 20,409 births. *J Gynecol Obstet Biol Reprod (Paris).* 1985;14:1033–1043.
37. Canavese F, Athlani L, Marengo L, et al. Evaluation of upper-extremity function following surgical treatment of displaced proximal humerus fractures in children. *J Pediatr Orthop B.* 2014;23:144–149.
38. Canavese F, Marengo L, Cravino M, et al. Outcome of conservative versus surgical treatment of humeral shaft fracture in children and adolescents: comparison between nonoperative treatment (Desault's bandage), external fixation and elastic stable intramedullary nailing. *J Pediatr Orthop.* 2017;37:e156–e163.
39. Canavese F, Marengo L, Samba A, et al. Evaluation of upper extremity function of displaced diaphyseal humeral fractures in children treated by elastic stable intramedullary nailing: preliminary results. *J Pediatr Orthop B.* 2016;25:399–405.
40. Canpolat FE, Kose A, Yurdakok M. Bilateral humerus fracture in a neonate after cesarean delivery. *Arch Gynecol Obstet.* 2010;281:967–969.
41. Carlan D, Pratt J, Patterson JM, et al. The radial nerve in the brachium: an anatomic study in human cadavers. *J Hand Surg Am.* 2007;32:1177–1182.

42. Carroll SE. A study of the nutrient foramina of the humeral diaphysis. *J Bone Joint Surg Br.* 1963;45-B:176–181.
43. Carter C, Sweetnam R. Recurrent dislocation of the patella and of the shoulder. Their association with familial joint laxity. *J Bone Joint Surg Br.* 1960;42-R:721–727.
44. Castagna A, Delle Rose G, Borroni M, et al. Arthroscopic stabilization of the shoulder in adolescent athletes participating in overhead or contact sports. *Arthroscopy.* 2012;28:309–315.
45. Catagni MA, Lovisetti L, Guerreschi F, et al. The external fixation in the treatment of humeral diaphyseal fractures: outcomes of 84 cases. *Injury.* 2010;41:1107–1111.
46. Cattaneo R, Catagni MA, Guerreschi F. Applications of the Ilizarov method in the humerus. Lengthenings and nonunions. *Hand Clin.* 1993;9:729–739.
47. Cattaneo R, Villa A, Catagni MA, et al. Lengthening of the humerus using the Ilizarov technique. Description of the method and report of 43 cases. *Clin Orthop Relat Res.* 1990;(250):117–124.
48. Caviglia H, Garrido CP, Palazzi FF, et al. Pediatric fractures of the humerus. *Clin Orthop Relat Res.* 2005;(432):49–56.
49. Chahal J, Marks PH, Macdonald PB, et al. Anatomic Bankart repair compared with nonoperative treatment and/or arthroscopic lavage for first-time traumatic shoulder dislocation. *Arthroscopy.* 2012;28:565–575.
50. Chan D, Petricciuolo F, Maffulli N. Fracture of the humeral diaphysis with extreme rotation. *Acta Orthop Belg.* 1991;57:427–429.
51. Chaus GW, Carry PM, Pishkenari AK, et al. Operative versus nonoperative treatment of displaced proximal humeral physeal fractures: a matched cohort. *J Pediatr Orthop.* 2015;35:234–239.
52. Chee Y, Agorastides I, Garg N, et al. Treatment of severely displaced proximal humeral fractures in children with elastic stable intramedullary nailing. *J Pediatr Orthop B.* 2006;15:45–50.
53. Chen CY, Chao EK, Tu YK, et al. Closed management and percutaneous fixation of unstable proximal humerus fractures. *J Trauma.* 1998;45:1039–1045.
54. Cheng JC, Shen WY. Limb fracture pattern in different pediatric age groups: a study of 3,350 children. *J Orthop Trauma.* 1993;7:15–22.
55. Cheok CY, Mohamad JA, Ahmad TS. Pain relief for reduction of acute anterior shoulder dislocations: a prospective randomized study comparing intravenous sedation with intra-articular lidocaine. *J Orthop Trauma.* 2011;25:5–10.
56. Cho SH, Cho NS, Rhee YG. Preoperative analysis of the Hill-Sachs lesion in anterior shoulder instability: how to predict engagement of the lesion. *Am J Sports Med.* 2011;39:2389–2395.
57. Choi YS, Potter HG, Scher DM. A shearing osteochondral fracture of the humeral head following an anterior shoulder dislocation in a child. *HSS J.* 2005;1:100–102.
58. Chung SM, Nissenbaum MM. Congenital and developmental defects of the shoulder. *Orthop Clin North Am.* 1975;6:381–392.
59. Ciernik IF, Meier L, Hollinger A. Humeral mobility after treatment with hanging cast. *J Trauma.* 1991;31:230–233.
60. Coene LN, Narakas AO. Operative management of lesions of the axillary nerve, isolated or combined with other nerve lesions. *Clin Neurol Neurosurg.* 1992;94 (Suppl):S64–S66.
61. Cohn BT, Froimson AI. Salter 3 fracture dislocation of glenohumeral joint in a 10-year-old. *Orthop Rev.* 1986;15:403–404.
62. Confalonieri N, Simonatti R, Ramondetta V, et al. Intramedullary nailing with a Rush pin in the treatment of diaphyseal humeral fractures. *Arch Putti Chir Organi Mov.* 1990;38:395–403.
63. Coobs BR, LaPrade RF. Severe chondrolysis of the glenohumeral joint after shoulder thermal capsulorrhaphy. *Am J Orthop (Belle Mead NJ).* 2009;38:E34–E37.
64. Cordischi K, Li X, Busconi B. Intermediate outcomes after primary traumatic anterior shoulder dislocation in skeletally immature patients aged 10 to 13 years. *Orthopedics.* 2009;32(9).
65. Covey DC, Riordan DC, Milstead ME, et al. Modification of the L'Episcopo procedure for brachial plexus birth palsies. *J Bone Joint Surg Br.* 1992;74:897–901.
66. Crolla RM, de Vries LS, Clevers GJ. Locked intramedullary nailing of humeral fractures. *Injury.* 1993;24:403–406.
67. Currarino G, Sheffield E, Twickler D. Congenital glenoid dysplasia. *Pediatr Radiol.* 1998;28:30–37.
68. Curtis RJ, Jr. Operative management of children's fractures of the shoulder region. *Orthop Clin North Am.* 1990;21:315–324.
69. Dabezies EJ, Banta CJ, 2nd, Murphy CP, et al. Plate fixation of the humeral shaft for acute fractures, with and without radial nerve injuries. *J Orthop Trauma.* 1992;6:10–13.
70. Dalldorf PG, Bryan WJ. Displaced Salter-Harris type I injury in a gymnast. A slipped capital humeral epiphysis?. *Orthop Rev.* 1994;23:538–541.
71. Dal Monte A, Andrisano A, Manfrini M, et al. Humeral lengthening in hypoplasia of the upper limb. *J Pediatr Orthop.* 1985;5:202–207.
72. Dameron TB, Jr., Grubb SA. Humeral shaft fractures in adults. *South Med J.* 1981;74:1461–1467.
73. Dameron TB, Jr., Reibel DB. Fractures involving the proximal humeral epiphyseal plate. *J Bone Joint Surg Am.* 1969;51:289–297.
74. Danzl DF, Vicario SJ, Gleis GL, et al. Closed reduction of anterior subcoracoid shoulder dislocation. Evaluation of an external rotation method. *Orthop Rev.* 1986;15:311–315.
75. Davarinos N, Ellanti P, Khan Bhambro KS, et al. Skin puckering an uncommon sign of underlying humeral neck fracture: a case report. *Ir J Med Sci.* 2011;180:731–733.
76. De Bastiani G, Aldegheri R, Renzi Brivio L. The treatment of fractures with a dynamic axial fixator. *J Bone Joint Surg Br.* 1984;66:538–545.
77. de Beer J, Burkhart SS, Roberts CP, et al. The congruent-arc Latarjet. *Tech Shoulder Surg.* 2009;10:62–67.
78. Deitch J, Mehlman CT, Foad SL, et al. Traumatic anterior shoulder dislocation in adolescents. *Am J Sports Med.* 2003;31:758–763.
79. d'Elia G, Di Giacomo A, D'Alessandro P, et al. Traumatic anterior glenohumeral instability: quantification of glenoid bone loss by spiral CT. *Radiol Med.* 2008;113:496–503.
80. DeLong WG, Jr., Born CT, Marcelli E, et al. Ender nail fixation in long bone fractures: experience in a level I trauma center. *J Trauma.* 1989;29:571–576.
81. Denard A, Jr., Richards JE, Obremskey WT, et al. Outcome of nonoperative vs operative treatment of humeral shaft fractures: a retrospective study of 213 patients. *Orthopedics.* 2010;33(8).
82. Denies E, Nijs S, Sermon A, et al. Operative treatment of humeral shaft fractures. Comparison of plating and intramedullary nailing. *Acta Orthop Belg.* 2010;76:735–742.
83. Dhawan A, Ghodadra N, Karas V, et al. Complications of bioabsorbable suture anchors in the shoulder. *Am J Sports Med.* 2012;40:1424–1430.
84. Di Filippo P, Mancini GB, Gillio A. Humeral fractures with paralysis of the radial nerve. *Arch Putti Chir Organi Mov.* 1990;38:405–409.
85. Dimakopoulos P, Panagopoulos A, Kasimatis G, et al. Anterior traumatic shoulder dislocation associated with displaced greater tuberosity fracture: the necessity of operative treatment. *J Orthop Trauma.* 2007;21:104–112.
86. Dobbs MB, Luhmann SL, Gordon JE, et al. Severely displaced proximal humeral epiphyseal fractures. *J Pediatr Orthop.* 2003;23:208–215.
87. Drew SJ, Giddins GE, Birch R. A slowly evolving brachial plexus injury following a proximal humeral fracture in a child. *J Hand Surg Br.* 1995;20:24–25.
88. Edeiken BS, Libshitz HI, Cohen MA. Slipped proximal humeral epiphysis: a complication of radiotherapy to the shoulder in children. *Skeletal Radiol.* 1982;9:123–125.
89. Edwards P, Kurth L. Postoperative radial nerve paralysis caused by fracture callus. *J Orthop Trauma.* 1992;6:234–236.
90. Ekholm R, Ponzer S, Tornkvist H, et al. Primary radial nerve palsy in patients with acute humeral shaft fractures. *J Orthop Trauma.* 2008;22:408–414.
91. Elbaum R, Parent H, Zeller R, et al. Traumatic scapulo-humeral dislocation in children and adolescents. Apropos of 9 patients. *Acta Orthop Belg.* 1994;60:204–209.
92. Ellefsen BK, Frierson MA, Raney EM, et al. Humerus varus: a complication of neonatal, infantile, and childhood injury and infection. *J Pediatr Orthop.* 1994;14:479–486.
93. Emery RJ, Mullaji AB. Glenohumeral joint instability in normal adolescents. Incidence and significance. *J Bone Joint Surg Br.* 1991;73:406–408.
94. Endo S, Kasai T, Fujii N, et al. Traumatic anterior dislocation of the shoulder in a child. *Arch Orthop Trauma Surg.* 1993;112:201–202.
95. Farber AJ, Castillo R, Clough M, et al. Clinical assessment of three common tests for traumatic anterior shoulder instability. *J Bone Joint Surg Am.* 2006;88:1467–1474.
96. Fattah HA, Halawa EE, Shafy TH. Non-union of the humeral shaft: a report on 25 cases. *Injury.* 1982;14:255–262.
97. Fayssoux RS, Stankovits L, Domzalski ME, et al. Fractures of the distal humeral metaphyseal-diaphyseal junction in children. *J Pediatr Orthop.* 2008;28:142–146.
98. Fernandez FF, Eberhardt O, Langendorfer M, et al. Treatment of severely displaced proximal humeral fractures in children with retrograde elastic stable intramedullary nailing. *Injury.* 2008;39:1453–1459.
99. Finestone A, Milgrom C, Radeva-Petrova DR, et al. Bracing in external rotation for traumatic anterior dislocation of the shoulder. *J Bone Joint Surg Br.* 2009;91:918–921.
100. Fisher TR, McGeoch CM. Severe injuries of the radial nerve treated by sural nerve grafting. *Injury.* 1985;16:411–412.
101. Fisher NA, Newman B, Lloyd J, et al. Ultrasonographic evaluation of birth injury to the shoulder. *J Perinatol.* 1995;15:398–400.
102. Foster RJ, Swiontkowski MF, Bach AW, et al. Radial nerve palsy caused by open humeral shaft fractures. *J Hand Surg Am.* 1993;18:121–124.
103. Friedman RJ, Smith RJ. Radial-nerve laceration twenty-six years after screw fixation of a humeral fracture. A case report. *J Bone Joint Surg Am.* 1984;66:959–960.
104. Gaffney D, Slabaugh M. Deltoid compartment syndrome after antegrade humeral nailing. *J Orthop Trauma.* 2009;23:229–231.
105. Gamble JG, Rinsky LA, Strudwick J, et al. Non-union of fractures in children who have osteogenesis imperfecta. *J Bone Joint Surg Am.* 1988;70:439–443.
106. Garrigues GE, Warnick DE, Busch MT. Subscapularis avulsion of the lesser tuberosity in adolescents. *J Pediatr Orthop.* 2013;33:8–13.
107. Garth WP, Jr., Leberte MA, Cool TA. Recurrent fractures of the humerus in a baseball pitcher. A case report. *J Bone Joint Surg Am.* 1988;70:305–306.
108. Gerber C, Schneeberger AG, Vinh TS. The arterial vascularization of the humeral head. An anatomical study. *J Bone Joint Surg Am.* 1990;72:1486–1494.
109. Gerwin M, Hotchkiss RN, Weiland AJ. Alternative operative exposures of the posterior aspect of the humeral diaphysis with reference to the radial nerve. *J Bone Joint Surg Am.* 1996;78:1690–1695.
110. Geusens E, Pans S, Verhulst D, et al. The modified axillary view of the shoulder, a painless alternative. *Emerg Radiol.* 2006;12:227–230.
111. Giebel G, Suren EG. Injuries of the proximal humeral epiphysis. Indications for surgical therapy and results. *Chirurg.* 1983;54:406–410.
112. Gill TJ, Waters P. Valgus osteotomy of the humeral neck: a technique for the treatment of humerus varus. *J Shoulder Elbow Surg.* 1997;6:306–310.
113. Gjengedal E, Slungaard U. Treatment of humeral fractures with and without injury to the radial nerve. A follow-up study. *Tidsskr Nor Laegeforen.* 1981;101(31):1746–1749.
114. Gladstein AZ, Schade AT, Howard AW, et al. Reducing resource utilization during non-operative treatment of pediatric proximal humerus fractures. *Orthop Traumatol Surg Res.* 2017;103:115–118.
115. Goldberg BJ, Nirschl RP, McConnell JP, et al. Arthroscopic transglenoid suture capsulolabral repairs: preliminary results. *Am J Sports Med.* 1993;21:656–664.
116. Good CR, MacGillivray JD. Traumatic shoulder dislocation in the adolescent athlete: advances in surgical treatment. *Curr Opin Pediatr.* 2005;17:25–29.
117. Good CR, Shindle MK, Kelly BT, et al. Glenohumeral chondrolysis after shoulder arthroscopy with thermal capsulorrhaphy. *Arthroscopy.* 2007;23:797.

118. Gray DJ, Gardner E. The prenatal development of the human humerus. *Am J Anat.* 1969;124:431–445.
119. Gregg-Smith SJ, White SH. Salter-Harris III fracture-dislocation of the proximal humeral epiphysis. *Injury.* 1992;23:199–200.
120. Gudinchet F, Naggar L, Ginalski JM, et al. Magnetic resonance imaging of nontraumatic shoulder instability in children. *Skeletal Radiol.* 1992;21:19–21.
121. Guibert L, Allouis M, Bourdelat D, et al. Fractures and slipped epiphyses of the proximal humerus in children. Place and methods of surgical treatment. *Chir Pediatr.* 1983;24:197–200.
122. Gupta A, Sharma S. Volar compartment syndrome of the arm complicating a fracture of the humeral shaft. A case report. *Acta Orthop Scand.* 1991;62:77–78.
123. Guven M, Akman B, Kormaz T, et al. "Floating arm" injury in a child with fractures of the proximal and distal parts of the humerus: a case report. *J Med Case Rep.* 2009;3:9287.
124. Hackethal KH. *Die Bundel-Nagelung. Experimentelle und Klinische Studie über eine Neuartige Methode der Markraum-Schienung Langer Röhrenknochen.* Berlin: Springer-Verlag; 1961.
125. Hackstock H. Functional bracing of fractures. *Orthopade.* 1988;17:41–51.
126. Hale HB, Bae DS, Waters PM. Current concepts in the management of brachial plexus birth palsy. *J Hand Surg Am.* 2010;35:322–331.
127. Hall RF, Jr. Closed intramedullary fixation of humeral shaft fractures. *Instr Course Lect.* 1987;36:349–358.
128. Hall RF, Jr., Pankovich AM. Ender nailing of acute fractures of the humerus. A study of closed fixation by intramedullary nails without reaming. *J Bone Joint Surg Am.* 1987;69:558–567.
129. Handoll HH, Almaiyah MA, Rangan A. Surgical versus non-surgical treatment for acute anterior shoulder dislocation. *Cochrane Database Syst Rev.* 2004; CD004325.
130. Harper DK, Craig JG, van Holsbeeck MT. Apophyseal injuries of the lesser tuberosity in adolescents: a series of five cases. *Emerg Radiol.* 2013;20:33–37.
131. Harris BA, Jr. Shoulder dystocia. *Clin Obstet Gynecol.* 1984;27:106–111.
132. Hasan SA, Cordell CL, Rauls RB, et al. Brachial artery injury with a proximal humerus fracture in a 10-year-old girl. *Am J Orthop (Belle Mead NJ).* 2009;38: 462–466.
133. Hawkins RJ, Koppert G, Johnston G. Recurrent posterior instability (subluxation) of the shoulder. *J Bone Joint Surg Am.* 1984;66:169–174.
134. Healy WL, White GM, Mick CA, et al. Nonunion of the humeral shaft. *Clin Orthop Relat Res.* 1987;(219):206–213.
135. Heck CC. Anterior dislocation of the glenohumeral joint in a child. *J Trauma.* 1981;21:174–175.
136. Heckler MW, Bamberger HB. Humeral shaft fractures and radial nerve palsy: to explore or not to explore…That is the question. *Am J Orthop (Belle Mead NJ).* 2008;37:415–419.
137. Heim D, Herkert F, Hess P, et al. Surgical treatment of humeral shaft fractures—the Basel experience. *J Trauma.* 1993;35:226–232.
138. Henley MB, Monroe M, Tencer AF. Biomechanical comparison of methods of fixation of a midshaft osteotomy of the humerus. *J Orthop Trauma.* 1991;5: 14–20.
139. Hennigan SP, Bush-Joseph CA, Kuo KN, et al. Throwing-induced humeral shaft fracture in skeletally immature adolescents. *Orthopedics.* 1999;22:621–622.
140. Hermichen HG, Pfister U, Weller S. Influence of the treatment of fractures on the development of pseudoarthroses of the humerus shaft. *Aktuelle Traumatol.* 1980;10:137–142.
141. Hernandez A, Drez D. Operative treatment of posterior shoulder dislocations by posterior glenoidplasty, capsulorrhaphy, and infraspinatus advancement. *Am J Sports Med.* 1986;14:187–191.
142. Herring JA, Peterson HA. Simple bone cyst with growth arrest. *J Pediatr Orthop.* 1987;7:231–235.
143. Hoffer MM, Phipps GJ. Closed reduction and tendon transfer for treatment of dislocation of the glenohumeral joint secondary to brachial plexus birth palsy. *J Bone Joint Surg Am.* 1998;80:997–1001.
144. Holm CL. Management of humeral shaft fractures. Fundamental nonoperative technics. *Clin Orthop Relat Res.* 1970;71:132–139.
145. Hoppenfeld S, deBoer P, Buckley R. The humerus. In: *Surgical Exposures in Orthopaedics: The Anatomic Approach.* 4th ed. Philadelphia, PA: Lippincott Williams & Wilkins; 2009:74–110.
146. Hosner W. Fractures of the shaft of the humerus. An analysis of 100 consecutive cases. *Reconstr Surg Traumatol.* 1974;14(0):38–64.
147. Hosny GA. Unilateral humeral lengthening in children and adolescents. *J Pediatr Orthop B.* 2005;14:439–443.
148. Hovelius L. Anterior dislocation of the shoulder in teen-agers and young adults. Five-year prognosis. *J Bone Joint Surg Am.* 1987;69:393–399.
149. Hovelius L, Olofsson A, Sandstrom B, et al. Nonoperative treatment of primary anterior shoulder dislocation in patients forty years of age and younger: a prospective twenty-five-year follow-up. *J Bone Joint Surg Am.* 2008;90:945–952.
150. Hovelius L, Saeboe M. Neer Award 2008: Arthropathy after primary anterior shoulder dislocation: 223 shoulders prospectively followed up for twenty-five years. *J Shoulder Elbow Surg.* 2009;18:339–347.
151. Hovelius L, Sandstrom B, Olofsson A, et al. The effect of capsular repair, bone block healing, and position on the results of the Bristow-Latarjet procedure (study III): long-term follow-up in 319 shoulders. *J Shoulder Elbow Surg.* 2012;21: 647–660.
152. Hovelius L, Sandstrom B, Saebo M. One hundred eighteen Bristow-Latarjet repairs for recurrent anterior dislocation of the shoulder prospectively followed for fifteen years: study II-the evolution of dislocation arthropathy. *J Shoulder Elbow Surg.* 2006;15:279–289.
153. Hovelius L, Vikerfors O, Olofsson A, et al. Bristow-Latarjet and Bankart: a comparative study of shoulder stabilization in 185 shoulders during a seventeen-year follow-up. *J Shoulder Elbow Surg.* 2011;20:1095–1101.
154. Howard CB, Shinwell E, Nyska M, et al. Ultrasound diagnosis of neonatal fracture separation of the upper humeral epiphysis. *J Bone Joint Surg Br.* 1992;74:471–472.
155. Hugon S, Daubresse F, Depierreux L. Radial nerve entrapment in a humeral fracture callus. *Acta Orthop Belg.* 2008;74:118–121.
156. Husain SN, King EC, Young JL, et al. Remodeling of birth fractures of the humeral diaphysis. *J Pediatr Orthop.* 2008;28:10–13.
157. Hutchinson PH, Bae DS, Waters PM. Intramedullary nailing versus percutaneous pin fixation of pediatric proximal humerus fractures: a comparison of complications and early radiographic results. *J Pediatr Orthop.* 2011;31:617–622.
158. Hwang RW, Bae DS, Waters PM. Brachial plexus palsy following proximal humerus fracture in patients who are skeletally immature. *J Orthop Trauma.* 2008;22:286–290.
159. Ilizarov GA. *Transosseous Osteosynthesis.* Berlin: Springer-Verlag; 1992.
160. Ilizarov GA, Shevtsov VI. Bloodless compression-distraction osteosynthesis in the treatment of pseudarthroses of the humerus. *Voen Med Zh.* 1974;(6):27–31.
161. Ingman AM, Waters DA. Locked intramedullary nailing of humeral shaft fractures: implant design, surgical technique, and clinical results. *J Bone Joint Surg Br.* 1994;76:23–29.
162. Itoi E, Hatakeyama Y, Kido T, et al. A new method of immobilization after traumatic anterior dislocation of the shoulder: a preliminary study. *J Shoulder Elbow Surg.* 2003;12:413–415.
163. Itoi E, Hatakeyama Y, Sato T, et al. Immobilization in external rotation after shoulder dislocation reduces the risk of recurrence. A randomized controlled trial. *J Bone Joint Surg Am.* 2007;89:2124–2131.
164. Itoi E, Hatakeyama Y, Urayama M, et al. Position of immobilization after dislocation of the shoulder. A cadaveric study. *J Bone Joint Surg Am.* 1999;81:385–390.
165. Itoi E, Sashi R, Minagawa H, et al. Position of immobilization after dislocation of the glenohumeral joint. A study with use of magnetic resonance imaging. *J Bone Joint Surg Am.* 2001;83-A:661–667.
166. Jaberg H, Warner JJ, Jakob RP. Percutaneous stabilization of unstable fractures of the humerus. *J Bone Joint Surg Am.* 1992;74:508–515.
167. James P, Heinrich SD. Ipsilateral proximal metaphyseal and flexion supracondylar humerus fractures with an associated olecranon avulsion fracture. *Orthopedics.* 1991;14:713–716.
168. Jankauskas L, Rudiger HA, Pfirrmann CW, et al. Loss of the sclerotic line of the glenoid on anteroposterior radiographs of the shoulder: a diagnostic sign for an osseous defect of the anterior glenoid rim. *J Shoulder Elbow Surg.* 2010;19:151–156.
169. Jawa A, McCarty P, Doornberg J, et al. Extra-articular distal-third diaphyseal fractures of the humerus. A comparison of functional bracing and plate fixation. *J Bone Joint Surg Am.* 2006;88:2343–2347.
170. Jeffery CC. Fracture separation of the upper humeral epiphysis. *Surg Gynecol Obstet.* 1953;96:205–209.
171. Johnstone DJ, Radford WJ, Parnell EJ. Interobserver variation using the AO/ASIF classification of long bone fractures. *Injury.* 1993;24:163–165.
172. Jones KJ, Wiesel B, Ganley TJ, et al. Functional outcomes of early arthroscopic Bankart repair in adolescents aged 11 to 18 years. *J Pediatr Orthop.* 2007;27: 209–213.
173. Jupiter JB. Complex non-union of the humeral diaphysis. Treatment with a medial approach, an anterior plate, and a vascularized fibular graft. *J Bone Joint Surg Am.* 1990;72:701–707.
174. Kaar TK, Schenck RC, Jr., Wirth MA, et al. Complications of metallic suture anchors in shoulder surgery: a report of 8 cases. *Arthroscopy.* 2001;17:31–37.
175. Khan A, Athlani L, Rousset M, et al. Functional results of displaced proximal humerus fractures in children treated by elastic stable intramedullary nail. *Eur J Orthop Surg Traumatol.* 2014;24:165–172.
176. Khan A, Samba A, Pereira B, et al. Anterior dislocation of the shoulder in skeletally immature patients: comparison between non-operative treatment versus open Latarje's procedure. *Bone Joint J.* 2014;96-B:354–359.
177. Kim NH, Hahn SB, Park HW, et al. The Orthofix external fixator for fractures of long bones. *Int Orthop.* 1994;18:42–46.
178. Kim SH, Szabo RM, Marder RA. Epidemiology of humerus fractures in the United States: nationwide emergency department sample, 2008. *Arthritis Care Res (Hoboken).* 2012;64:407–414.
179. Kim DS, Yoon YS, Yi CH. Prevalence comparison of accompanying lesions between primary and recurrent anterior dislocation in the shoulder. *Am J Sports Med.* 2010;38:2071–2076.
180. Kirkos JM, Papadopoulos IA. Late treatment of brachial plexus palsy secondary to birth injuries: rotational osteotomy of the proximal part of the humerus. *J Bone Joint Surg Am.* 1998;80:1477–1483.
181. Klasson SC, Vander Schilden JL, Park JP. Late effect of isolated avulsion fractures of the lesser tubercle of the humerus in children. Report of two cases. *J Bone Joint Surg Am.* 1993;75:1691–1694.
182. Kleinman PK, Akins CM. The "vanishing" epiphysis: sign of Salter type I fracture of the proximal humerus in infancy. *Br J Radiol.* 1982;55(659):865–867.
183. Kodali P, Jones MH, Polster J, et al. Accuracy of measurement of Hill-Sachs lesions with computed tomography. *J Shoulder Elbow Surg.* 2011;20:1328–1334.
184. Kohler L. *Roentgenology.* 2nd ed. London: Balliere, Tindall, and Cox; 1935.
185. Kohler R, Trillaud JM. Fracture and fracture separation of the proximal humerus in children: report of 136 cases. *J Pediatr Orthop.* 1983;3:326–332.
186. Kothari K, Bernstein RM, Griffiths HJ, et al. Luxatio erecta. *Skeletal Radiol.* 1984;11:47–49.
187. Kothari RU, Dronen SC. Prospective evaluation of the scapular manipulation technique in reducing anterior shoulder dislocations. *Ann Emerg Med.* 1992;21:1349–1352.
188. Kozin SH. Correlation between external rotation of the glenohumeral joint and deformity after brachial plexus birth palsy. *J Pediatr Orthop.* 2004;24:189–193.
189. Kraus T, Hoermann S, Ploder G, et al. Elastic stable intramedullary nailing versus Kirschner wire pinning: outcome of severely displaced proximal humeral fractures in juvenile patients. *J Shoulder Elbow Surg.* 2014;23:1462–1467.

190. Kuhn JE. Treating the initial anterior shoulder dislocation—an evidence-based medicine approach. *Sports Med Arthrosc Rev*. 2006;14:192–198.
191. Kuhns LR, Sherman MP, Poznanski AK, et al. Humeral-head and coracoid ossification in the newborn. *Radiology*. 1973;107:145–149.
192. Kwasny O, Maier R, Kutscha-Lissberg F, et al. Treatment procedure in humeral shaft fractures with primary or secondary radial nerve damage. *Unfallchirurgie*. 1992;18:168–173.
193. Laing PG. The arterial supply of the adult humerus. *J Bone Joint Surg Am*. 1956;38-A:1105–1116.
194. Lal H, Bansal P, Sabharwal VK, et al. Recurrent shoulder dislocations secondary to coracoid process fracture: a case report. *J Orthop Surg (Hong Kong)*. 2012;20:121–125.
195. Landin LA. Fracture patterns in children. Analysis of 8,682 fractures with special reference to incidence, etiology and secular changes in a Swedish urban population 1950–1979. *Acta Orthop Scand Suppl*. 1983;202(Suppl):1–109.
196. Landin LA. Epidemiology of children's fractures. *J Pediatr Orthop B*. 1997;6:79–83.
197. Larsen CF, Kiaer T, Lindequist S. Fractures of the proximal humerus in children. Nine-year follow-up of 64 unoperated on cases. *Acta Orthop Scand*. 1990;61: 255–257.
198. Lascombes P, Haumont T, Journeau P. Use and abuse of flexible intramedullary nailing in children and adolescents. *J Pediatr Orthop*. 2006;26:827–834.
199. Lascombes P, Nespola A, Poircuitte JM, et al. Early complications with flexible intramedullary nailing in childhood fracture: 100 cases managed with precurved tip and shaft nails. *Orthop Traumatol Surg Res*. 2012;98:369–375.
200. Lawton RL, Choudhury S, Mansat P, et al. Pediatric shoulder instability: presentation, findings, treatment, and outcomes. *J Pediatr Orthop*. 2002;22:52–61.
201. Lee FY, Schoeb JS, Yu J, et al. Operative lengthening of the humerus: indications, benefits, and complications. *J Pediatr Orthop*. 2005;25:613–616.
202. Lemperg R, Liliequist B. Dislocation of the proximal epiphysis of the humerus in newborns. *Acta Paediatr Scand*. 1970;59:377–380.
203. Leroux T, Ogilvie-Harris D, Veillette C, et al. The epidemiology of primary anterior shoulder dislocations in patients aged 10 to 16 years. *Am J Sports Med*. 2015;43:2111–2117
204. Leung TY, Stuart O, Suen SS, et al. Comparison of perinatal outcomes of shoulder dystocia alleviated by different type and sequence of manoeuvers: a retrospective review. *BJOG*. 2011;118:985–990.
205. Levine B, Pereira D, Rosen J. Avulsion fractures of the lesser tuberosity of the humerus in adolescents: review of the literature and case report. *J Orthop Trauma*. 2005;19:349–352.
206. Liavaag S, Brox JI, Pripp AH, et al. Immobilization in external rotation after primary shoulder dislocation did not reduce the risk of recurrence: a randomized controlled trial. *J Bone Joint Surg Am*. 2011;93:897–904.
207. Ligier JN, Metaizeau JP, Prevot J. Closed flexible medullary nailing in pediatric traumatology. *Chir Pediatr*. 1983;24:383–385.
208. Limpisvasti O, Yang BY, Hosseinzadeh P, et al. The effect of glenohumeral position on the shoulder after traumatic anterior dislocation. *Am J Sports Med*. 2008;36: 775–780.
209. Linn RM, Kriegshauser LA. Ball thrower's fracture of the humerus. A case report. *Am J Sports Med*. 1991;19:194–197.
210. Liu GY, Zhang CY, Wu HW. Comparison of initial nonoperative and operative management of radial nerve palsy associated with acute humeral shaft fractures. *Orthopedics*. 2012;35:702–708.
211. Lo IK, Nonweiler B, Woolfrey M, et al. An evaluation of the apprehension, relocation, and surprise tests for anterior shoulder instability. *Am J Sports Med*. 2004;32:301–307.
212. Lock TR, Aronson DD. Fractures in patients who have myelomeningocele. *J Bone Joint Surg Am*. 1989;71:1153–1157.
213. Loder RT. Pediatric polytrauma: orthopaedic care and hospital course. *J Orthop Trauma*. 1987;1:48–54.
214. Loder RT, Bookout C. Fracture patterns in battered children. *J Orthop Trauma*. 1991;5:428–433.
215. Longo UG, van der Linde JA, Loppini M, et al. Surgical versus nonoperative treatment in patients up to 18 years old with traumatic shoulder instability: a systematic review and quantitative synthesis of the literature. *Arthroscopy*. 2016;32: 944–952.
216. Lucas JC, Mehlman CT, Laor T. The location of the biceps tendon in completely displaced proximal humerus fractures in children: a report of four cases with magnetic resonance imaging and cadaveric correlation. *J Pediatr Orthop*. 2004;24: 249–253.
217. Macfarlane I, Mushayt K. Double closed fractures of the humerus in a child. A case report. *J Bone Joint Surg Am*. 1990;72:443.
218. Machan FG, Vinz H. Humeral shaft fracture in childhood. *Unfallchirurgie*. 1993;19:166–174.
219. Macnicol MF. Roentgenographic evidence of median-nerve entrapment in a greenstick humeral fracture. *J Bone Joint Surg Am*. 1978;60:998–1000.
220. Madsen ET. Fractures of the extremities in the newborn. *Acta Obstet Gynecol Scand*. 1955;34:41–74.
221. Mahabier KC, Vogels LM, Punt BJ, et al. Humeral shaft fractures: retrospective results of non-operative and operative treatment of 186 patients. *Injury*. 2013;44:427–430.
222. Malhotra A, Freudmann MS, Hay SM. Management of traumatic anterior shoulder dislocation in the 17- to 25-year age group: a dramatic evolution of practice. *J Shoulder Elbow Surg*. 2012;21:545–553.
223. Marans HJ, Angel KR, Schemitsch EH, et al. The fate of traumatic anterior dislocation of the shoulder in children. *J Bone Joint Surg Am*. 1992;74:1242–1244.
224. Markel DC, Donley BG, Blasier RB. Percutaneous intramedullary pinning of proximal humeral fractures. *Orthop Rev*. 1994;23:667–671.
225. Martin RP, Parsons DL. Avascular necrosis of the proximal humeral epiphysis after physeal fracture. A case report. *J Bone Joint Surg Am*. 1997;79:760–762.
226. Marty B, Kach K, Candinas D, et al. Results of intramedullary nailing in humerus shaft fractures. *Helv Chir Acta*. 1993;59:681–685.
227. Matthews DE, Roberts T. Intraarticular lidocaine versus intravenous analgesic for reduction of acute anterior shoulder dislocations. A prospective randomized study. *Am J Sports Med*. 1995;23:54–58.
228. Matton D, Van Looy F, Geens S. Recurrent anterior dislocations of the shoulder joint treated by the Bristow-Latarjet procedure. Historical review, operative technique and results. *Acta Orthop Belg*. 1992;58:16–22.
229. McNamara RM. Reduction of anterior shoulder dislocations by scapular manipulation. *Ann Emerg Med*. 1993;22:1140–1144.
230. McNeil EL. Luxatio erecta. *Ann Emerg Med*. 1984;13:490–491.
231. McQuillan WM, Nolan B. Ischemia complicating injury. A report of thirty-seven cases. *J Bone Joint Surg Br*. 1968;50:482–492.
232. Mehin R, Mehin A, Wickham D, et al. Pinning technique for shoulder fractures in adolescents: computer modelling of percutaneous pinning of proximal humeral fractures. *Can J Surg*. 2009;52:E222–E228.
233. Merten DF, Kirks DR, Ruderman RJ. Occult humeral epiphyseal fracture in battered infants. *Pediatr Radiol*. 1981;10:151–154.
234. Metaizeau JP, Ligier JN. Surgical treatment of fractures of the long bones in children. Interference between osteosynthesis and the physiological processes of consolidation. Therapeutic indications. *J Chir (Paris)*. 1984;121(8–9):527–537.
235. Milano G, Grasso A, Russo A, et al. Analysis of risk factors for glenoid bone defect in anterior shoulder instability. *Am J Sports Med*. 2011;39:1870–1876.
236. Milch H. Treatment of dislocation of the shoulder. *Surgery*. 1934;3:732–740.
237. Milch H. The treatment of recent dislocations and fracture-dislocations of the shoulder. *J Bone Joint Surg Am*. 1949;31A:173–180.
238. Miller SL, Cleeman E, Auerbach J, et al. Comparison of intra-articular lidocaine and intravenous sedation for reduction of shoulder dislocations: a randomized, prospective study. *J Bone Joint Surg Am*. 2002;84-A:2135–2139.
239. Miller BS, Sonnabend DH, Hatrick C, et al. Should acute anterior dislocations of the shoulder be immobilized in external rotation? A cadaveric study. *J Shoulder Elbow Surg*. 2004;13:589–592.
240. Mills WJ, Hanel DP, Smith DG. Lateral approach to the humeral shaft: an alternative approach for fracture treatment. *J Orthop Trauma*. 1996;10:81–86.
241. Mimura T, Mori K, Matsusue Y, et al. Closed reduction for traumatic posterior dislocation of the shoulder using the "lever principle": two case reports and a review of the literature. *J Orthop Surg (Hong Kong)*. 2006;14:336–339.
242. Moed BR, LaMont RL. Unicameral bone cyst complicated by growth retardation. *J Bone Joint Surg Am*. 1982;64:1379–1381.
243. Moharari RS, Khademhosseini P, Espandar R, et al. Intra-articular lidocaine versus intravenous meperidine/diazepam in anterior shoulder dislocation: a randomised clinical trial. *Emerg Med J*. 2008;25:262–264.
244. Muller M, Allgower M, Schneider R, et al. *Manual of Internal Fixation*. 3rd ed. Berlin: Springer-Verlag; 1991.
245. Nauth A, McKee MD, Ristevski B, et al. Distal humeral fractures in adults. *J Bone Joint Surg Am*. 2011;93:686–700.
246. Neer CS, 2nd. Involuntary inferior and multidirectional instability of the shoulder: etiology, recognition, and treatment. *Instr Course Lect*. 1985;34:232–238.
247. Neer CS, 2nd, Horwitz BS. Fractures of the proximal humeral epiphysial plate. *Clin Orthop Relat Res*. 1965;41:24–31.
248. Neviaser TJ. The anterior labroligamentous periosteal sleeve avulsion lesion: a cause of anterior instability of the shoulder. *Arthroscopy*. 1993;9:17–21.
249. Nho SJ, Dodson CC, Bardzik KF, et al. The two-step maneuver for closed reduction of inferior glenohumeral dislocation (luxatio erecta to anterior dislocation to reduction). *J Orthop Trauma*. 2006;20:354–357.
250. Noaman H, Khalifa AR, El-Deen MA, et al. Early surgical exploration of radial nerve injury associated with fracture shaft humerus. *Microsurgery*. 2008;28:635–642.
251. Obremskey W, Routt ML, Jr. Fracture-dislocation of the shoulder in a child: case report. *J Trauma*. 1994;36:137–140.
252. O'Connor DR, Schwarze D, Fragomen AT, et al. Painless reduction of acute anterior shoulder dislocations without anesthesia. *Orthopedics*. 2006;29:528–532.
253. O'Driscoll SW, Evans DC. Contralateral shoulder instability following anterior repair. An epidemiological investigation. *J Bone Joint Surg Br*. 1991;73:941–946.
254. Ogawa BK, Kay RM, Choi PD, et al. Complete division of the radial nerve associated with a closed fracture of the humeral shaft in a child. *J Bone Joint Surg Br*. 2007;89:821–824.
255. Ogawa K, Yoshida A. Throwing fracture of the humeral shaft. An analysis of 90 patients. *Am J Sports Med*. 1998;26:242–246.
256. Ogden JA, Conlogue GJ, Jensen P. Radiology of postnatal skeletal development: the proximal humerus. *Skeletal Radiol*. 1978;2:153–160.
257. Olds M, Donaldson K, Ellis R, et al. In children 18 years and under, what promotes recurrent shoulder instability after traumatic anterior shoulder dislocation? A systematic review and meta-analysis of risk factors. *Br J Sports Med*. 2016;50:1135–1141.
258. Ortiz EJ, Isler MH, Navia JE, et al. Pathologic fractures in children. *Clin Orthop Relat Res*. 2005;(432):116–126.
259. Ouyang H, Xiong J, Xiang P, et al. Plate versus intramedullary nail fixation in the treatment of humeral shaft fractures: an updated meta-analysis. *J Shoulder Elbow Surg*. 2013;22:387–395.
260. Owens BD, Agel J, Mountcastle SB, et al. Incidence of glenohumeral instability in collegiate athletics. *Am J Sports Med*. 2009;37:1750–1754.
261. Owens BD, Dawson L, Burks R, et al. Incidence of shoulder dislocation in the United States military: demographic considerations from a high-risk population. *J Bone Joint Surg Am*. 2009;91:791–796.
262. Owens BD, Nelson BJ, Duffey ML, et al. Pathoanatomy of first-time, traumatic, anterior glenohumeral subluxation events. *J Bone Joint Surg Am*. 2010;92:1605–1611.
263. Pahlavan S, Baldwin KD, Pandya NK, et al. Proximal humerus fractures in the pediatric population: a systematic review. *J Child Orthop*. 2011;5:187–194.

264. Patel DN, Zuckerman JD, Egol KA. Luxatio erecta: case series with review of diagnostic and management principles. *Am J Orthop (Belle Mead NJ)*. 2011;40:566–570.
265. Paterson WH, Throckmorton TW, Koester M, et al. Position and duration of immobilization after primary anterior shoulder dislocation: a systematic review and meta-analysis of the literature. *J Bone Joint Surg Am*. 2010;92:2924–2933.
266. Patte D, Debeyre J. Luxations recidivantes de l'epaule. *Encycl Med Chir Paris-Technique chirurgicale Orthopedie*. 1980;44265(4).
267. Peterson HA. Surgical lengthening of the humerus: case report and review. *J Pediatr Orthop*. 1989;9:596–601.
268. Peterson HA, Madhok R, Benson JT, et al. Physeal fractures: Part 1. Epidemiology in Olmsted County, Minnesota, 1979–1988. *J Pediatr Orthop*. 1994;14:423–430.
269. Phipps GJ, Hoffer MM. Latissimus dorsi and teres major transfer to rotator cuff for Erb's palsy. *J Shoulder Elbow Surg*. 1995;4:124–129.
270. Piasecki DP, Verma NN, Romeo AA, et al. Glenoid bone deficiency in recurrent anterior shoulder instability: diagnosis and management. *J Am Acad Orthop Surg*. 2009;17:482–493.
271. Pogorelic Z, Kadic S, Milunovic KP, et al. Flexible intramedullary nailing for treatment of proximal humerus and humeral shaft fractures in children: a retrospective series of 118 cases. *Orthop Traumatol Surg Res*. 2017;103:765–770.
272. Pritchett JW. Growth and predictions of growth in the upper extremity. *J Bone Joint Surg Am*. 1988;70:520–525.
273. Pritchett JW. Growth plate activity in the upper extremity. *Clin Orthop Relat Res*. 1991;(268):235–242.
274. Provencher MT, Ghodadra N, Romeo AA. Arthroscopic management of anterior instability: pearls, pitfalls, and lessons learned. *Orthop Clin North Am*. 2010;41:325–337.
275. Provencher MT, Verma N, Obopilwe E, et al. A biomechanical analysis of capsular plication versus anchor repair of the shoulder: can the labrum be used as a suture anchor?. *Arthroscopy*. 2008;24:210–216.
276. Putnam MD, Walsh TM, 4th. External fixation for open fractures of the upper extremity. *Hand Clin*. 1993;9:613–623.
277. Rajan RA, Hawkins KJ, Metcalfe J, et al. Elastic stable intramedullary nailing for displaced proximal humeral fractures in older children. *J Child Orthop*. 2008;2:15–19.
278. Randelli P, Ragone V, Carminati S, et al. Risk factors for recurrence after Bankart repair a systematic review. *Knee Surg Sports Traumatol Arthrosc*. 2012;20: 2129–2138.
279. Rang M. *Children's Fractures*. Philadelphia, PA: JB Lippincott; 1983.
280. Rhee YG, Cho NS, Cho SH. Traumatic anterior dislocation of the shoulder: factors affecting the progress of the traumatic anterior dislocation. *Clin Orthop Surg*. 2009;1:188–193.
281. Riemer BL, Foglesong ME, Burke CJ, 3rd, et al. Complications of Seidel intramedullary nailing of narrow diameter humeral diaphyseal fractures. *Orthopedics*. 1994;17:19–29.
282. Rijal L, Ansari T, Trikha V, et al. Birth injuries in caesarian sections: cases of fracture femur and humerus following caesarian section. *Nepal Med Coll J*. 2009;11:207–208.
283. Ristic V, Maljanovic M, Arsic M, et al. Comparison of the results of treatment of humeral shaft fractures by different methods. *Med Pregl*. 2011;64:490–496.
284. Robin GC, Kedar SS. Separation of the upper humeral epiphysis in pituitary gigantism. *J Bone Joint Surg Am*. 1962;44-A:189–192.
285. Robinson CM, Kelly M, Wakefield AE. Redislocation of the shoulder during the first six weeks after a primary anterior dislocation: risk factors and results of treatment. *J Bone Joint Surg Am*. 2002;84-A:1552–1559.
286. Robinson CM, Shur N, Sharpe T, et al. Injuries associated with traumatic anterior glenohumeral dislocations. *J Bone Joint Surg Am*. 2012;94:18–26.
287. Rockwood CA, Jr. The shoulder: facts, confusions and myths. *Int Orthop*. 1991;15:401–405.
288. Rommens PM, Verbruggen J, Broos PL. Retrograde locked nailing of humeral shaft fractures. A review of 39 patients. *J Bone Joint Surg Br*. 1995;77:84–89.
289. Rose SH, Melton LJ, 3rd, Morrey BF, et al. Epidemiologic features of humeral fractures. *Clin Orthop Relat Res*. 1982;(168):24–30.
290. Ross GJ, Love MB. Isolated avulsion fracture of the lesser tuberosity of the humerus: report of two cases. *Radiology*. 1989;172:833–834.
291. Rowe CR. Prognosis in dislocations of the shoulder. *J Bone Joint Surg Am*. 1956;38-A:957–977.
292. Rowe CR. Anterior dislocations of the shoulder: prognosis and treatment. *Surg Clin North Am*. 1963;43:1609–1614.
293. Rowles DJ, McGrory JE. Percutaneous pinning of the proximal part of the humerus. An anatomic study. *J Bone Joint Surg Am*. 2001;83-A:1695–1699.
294. Ruedi T, Moshfegh A, Pfeiffer KM, et al. Fresh fractures of the shaft of the humerus: conservative or operative treatment?. *Reconstr Surg Traumatol*. 1974;14(0):65–74.
295. Ruland WO. Is there a place for external fixation in humeral shaft fractures?. *Injury*. 2000;31(Suppl 1):27–34.
296. Runkel M, Kreitner KF, Wenda K, et al. [Nuclear magnetic tomography in shoulder dislocation]. *Unfallchirurg*. 1993;96:124–128.
297. Russell JA, Holmes EM, 3rd, Keller DJ, et al. Reduction of acute anterior shoulder dislocations using the Milch technique: a study of ski injuries. *J Trauma*. 1981;21:802–804.
298. Sachs RA, Lin D, Stone ML, et al. Can the need for future surgery for acute traumatic anterior shoulder dislocation be predicted?. *J Bone Joint Surg Am*. 2007;89: 1665–1674.
299. Safran O, Milgrom C, Radeva-Petrova DR, et al. Accuracy of the anterior apprehension test as a predictor of risk for redislocation after a first traumatic shoulder dislocation. *Am J Sports Med*. 2010;38:972–975.
300. Salter RB, Harris WR. Injuries involving the epiphyseal plate. *J Bone Joint Surg Am*. 1963;45:587–622.
301. Samardzic M, Grujicic D, Milinkovic ZB. Radial nerve lesions associated with fractures of the humeral shaft. *Injury*. 1990;21:220–222.
302. Samilson RL. Congenital and developmental anomalies of the shoulder girdle. *Orthop Clin North Am*. 1980;11:219–231.
303. Sarmiento A, Horowitch A, Aboulafia A, et al. Functional bracing for comminuted extra-articular fractures of the distal third of the humerus. *J Bone Joint Surg Br*. 1990;72:283–287.
304. Sarmiento A, Kinman PB, Galvin EG, et al. Functional bracing of fractures of the shaft of the humerus. *J Bone Joint Surg Am*. 1977;59:596–601.
305. Sattel W. Effect of dia- and percondylar humeral fractures on the growth of the carpal bones in children. *Handchir Mikrochir Plast Chir*. 1982;14:103–105.
306. Scheffel PT, Clinton J, Lynch JR, et al. Glenohumeral chondrolysis: a systematic review of 100 cases from the English language literature. *J Shoulder Elbow Surg*. 2010;19:944–949.
307. Scheibel M, Kuke A, Nikulka C, et al. How long should acute anterior dislocations of the shoulder be immobilized in external rotation?. *Am J Sports Med*. 2009;37:1309–1316.
308. Senes FM, Catena N. Intramedullary osteosynthesis for metaphyseal and diaphyseal humeral fractures in developmental age. *J Pediatr Orthop B*. 2012;21:300–304.
309. Serrato JA, Jr., Fleckenstein CM, Hasan SS. Glenohumeral chondrolysis associated with use of an intra-articular pain pump delivering local anesthetics following manipulation under anesthesia: a report of four cases. *J Bone Joint Surg Am*. 2011;93:e99(1–8).
310. Sessa S, Lascombes P, Prevot J, et al. Centro-medullary nailing in fractures of the upper end of the humerus in children and adolescents. *Chir Pediatr*. 1990;31:43–46.
311. Seybold D, Schliemann B, Heyer CM, et al. Which labral lesion can be best reduced with external rotation of the shoulder after a first-time traumatic anterior shoulder dislocation?. *Arch Orthop Trauma Surg*. 2009;129:299–304.
312. Shah AS, Karadsheh MS, Sekiya JK. Failure of operative treatment for glenohumeral instability: etiology and management. *Arthroscopy*. 2011;27:681–694.
313. Shantharam SS. Tips of the trade #41. Modified coaptation splint for humeral shaft fractures. *Orthop Rev*. 1991;20:1033, 1039.
314. Shao YC, Harwood P, Grotz MR, et al. Radial nerve palsy associated with fractures of the shaft of the humerus: a systematic review. *J Bone Joint Surg Br*. 2005;87:1647–1652.
315. Sharma VK, Jain AK, Gupta RK, et al. Non-operative treatment of fractures of the humeral shaft: a comparative study. *J Indian Med Assoc*. 1991;89:157–160.
316. Shaw BA, Murphy KM, Shaw A, et al. Humerus shaft fractures in young children: accident or abuse?. *J Pediatr Orthop*. 1997;17:293–297.
317. Sherr-Lurie N, Bialik GM, Ganel A, et al. Fractures of the humerus in the neonatal period. *Isr Med Assoc J*. 2011;13:363–365.
318. Shibuya S, Ogawa K. Isolated avulsion fracture of the lesser tuberosity of the humerus. A case report. *Clin Orthop Relat Res*. 1986;(211):215–218.
319. Shymon SJ, Roocroft J, Edmonds EW. Traumatic anterior instability of the pediatric shoulder: a comparison of arthroscopic and open Bankart repairs. *J Pediatr Orthop*. 2015;35:1–6.
320. Siegler J, Proust J, Marcheix PS, et al. Is external rotation the correct immobilisation for acute shoulder dislocation? An MRI study. *Orthop Traumatol Surg Res*. 2010;96:329–333.
321. Singh S, Yong CK, Mariapan S. Closed reduction techniques in acute anterior shoulder dislocation: modified Milch technique compared with traction-countertraction technique. *J Shoulder Elbow Surg*. 2012;21:1706–1711.
322. Sloth C, Just SL. The apical oblique radiograph in examination of acute shoulder trauma. *Eur J Radiol*. 1989;9:147–151.
323. Smith FM. Fracture-separation of the proximal humeral epiphysis; a study of cases seen at the Presbyterian Hospital from 1929–1953. *Am J Surg*. 1956;91: 627–635.
324. Smith DK, Cooney WP. External fixation of high-energy upper extremity injuries. *J Orthop Trauma*. 1990;4:7–18.
325. Solomon DJ, Navaie M, Stedje-Larsen ET, et al. Glenohumeral chondrolysis after arthroscopy: a systematic review of potential contributors and causal pathways. *Arthroscopy*. 2009;25:1329–1342.
326. Spak I. Humeral shaft fractures. Treatment with a simple hand sling. *Acta Orthop Scand*. 1978;49:234–239.
327. Stahl EJ, Karpman R. Normal growth and growth predictions in the upper extremity. *J Hand Surg Am*. 1986;11:593–596.
328. Stahl S, Rosen N, Moscona R. Ulnar nerve palsy following fracture of the shaft of the humerus. *J Orthop Trauma*. 1998;12:363–364.
329. Stanitski CL, Micheli LJ. Simultaneous ipsilateral fractures of the arm and forearm in children. *Clin Orthop Relat Res*. 1980;(153):218–222.
330. Stephenson RB, London MD, Hankin FM, et al. Fibrous dysplasia. An analysis of options for treatment. *J Bone Joint Surg Am*. 1987;69:400–409.
331. Stewart MJ, Hundley JM. Fractures of the humerus; a comparative study in methods of treatment. *J Bone Joint Surg Am*. 1955;37-A:681–692.
332. Stimson LA. An easy method of reducing dislocations of the shoulder and hip. *Med Record*. 1900;57:356–357.
333. Szalay E, Rockwood C. Fractures of the distal shaft of the humerus associated with radial nerve palsy. *Orthop Trans*. 1982;6:455.
334. Szalay EA, Rockwood CA, Jr. Injuries of the shoulder and arm. *Emerg Med Clin North Am*. 1984;2:279–294.
335. Tanaka Y, Okamura K, Imai T. Effectiveness of external rotation immobilization in highly active young men with traumatic primary anterior shoulder dislocation or subluxation. *Orthopedics*. 2010;33:670.
336. Taskoparan H, Kilincoglu V, Tunay S, et al. Immobilization of the shoulder in external rotation for prevention of recurrence in acute anterior dislocation. *Acta Orthop Traumatol Turc*. 2010;44:278–284.
337. Tennent TD, Beach WR, Meyers JF. A review of the special tests associated with shoulder examination. Part II: laxity, instability, and superior labral anterior and posterior (SLAP) lesions. *Am J Sports Med*. 2003;31:301–307.
338. te Slaa RL, Brand R, Marti RK. A prospective arthroscopic study of acute first-time anterior shoulder dislocation in the young: a five-year follow-up study. *J Shoulder Elbow Surg*. 2003;12:529–534.

339. Thomas IH, Chow CW, Cole WG. Giant cell reparative granuloma of the humerus. *J Pediatr Orthop.* 1988;8:596–598.

340. Thomsen NO, Dahlin LB. Injury to the radial nerve caused by fracture of the humeral shaft: timing and neurobiological aspects related to treatment and diagnosis. *Scand J Plast Reconstr Surg Hand Surg.* 2007;41:153–157.

341. Tirman PF, Stauffer AE, Crues JV, 3rd, et al. Saline magnetic resonance arthrography in the evaluation of glenohumeral instability. *Arthroscopy.* 1993;9:550–559.

342. Troum S, Floyd WE, 3rd, Waters PM. Posterior dislocation of the humeral head in infancy associated with obstetrical paralysis. A case report. *J Bone Joint Surg Am.* 1993;75:1370–1375.

343. Tzannes A, Paxinos A, Callanan M, et al. An assessment of the interexaminer reliability of tests for shoulder instability. *J Shoulder Elbow Surg.* 2004;13:18–23.

344. Ugwonali OF, Bae DS, Waters PM. Corrective osteotomy for humerus varus. *J Pediatr Orthop.* 2007;27:529–32.

345. van der Linde JA, van Kampen DA, Terwee CB, et al. Long-term results after arthroscopic shoulder stabilization using suture anchors: an 8- to 10-year follow-up. *Am J Sports Med.* 2011;39:2396–2403.

346. Vastamaki M, Solonen KA. Posterior dislocation and fracture-dislocation of the shoulder. *Acta Orthop Scand.* 1980;51:479–484.

347. Venouziou AI, Dailiana ZH, Varitimidis SE, et al. Radial nerve palsy associated with humeral shaft fracture. Is the energy of trauma a prognostic factor?. *Injury.* 2011;42:1289–1293.

348. Verga M, Peri Di Caprio A, Bocchiotti MA, et al. Delayed treatment of persistent radial nerve paralysis associated with fractures of the middle third of humerus: review and evaluation of the long-term results of 52 cases. *J Hand Surg Eur Vol.* 2007;32:529–533.

349. Vermeiren J, Handelberg F, Casteleyn PP, et al. The rate of recurrence of traumatic anterior dislocation of the shoulder. A study of 154 cases and a review of the literature. *Int Orthop.* 1993;17:337–341.

350. Vezeridis PS, Bae DS, Kocher MS, et al. Surgical treatment for avulsion injuries of the humeral lesser tuberosity apophysis in adolescents. *J Bone Joint Surg Am.* 2011;93:1882–1888.

351. Visser CP, Coene LN, Brand R, et al. Nerve lesions in proximal humeral fractures. *J Shoulder Elbow Surg.* 2001;10:421–427.

352. Vural M, Arslantas A. Delayed radial nerve palsy due to entrapment of the nerve in the callus of a distal third humerus fracture. *Turk Neurosurg.* 2008;18:194–196.

353. Wagner KT, Jr., Lyne ED. Adolescent traumatic dislocations of the shoulder with open epiphyses. *J Pediatr Orthop.* 1983;3:61–62.

354. Wakai A, O'Sullivan R, McCabe A. Intra-articular lignocaine versus intravenous analgesia with or without sedation for manual reduction of acute anterior shoulder dislocation in adults. *Cochrane Database Syst Rev.* 2011;CD004919.

355. Walch G, Boileau P. Latarjet-Bristow procedure for recurrent anterior instability. *Tech Shoulder Elbow Surg.* 2000;1:256–261.

356. Wallny T, Sagebiel C, Westerman K, et al. Comparative results of bracing and interlocking nailing in the treatment of humeral shaft fractures. *Int Orthop.* 1997;21:374–379.

357. Wallny T, Westermann K, Sagebiel C, et al. Functional treatment of humeral shaft fractures: indications and results. *J Orthop Trauma.* 1997;11:283–287.

358. Wang P, Jr., Koval KJ, Lehman W, et al. Salter-Harris type III fracture-dislocation of the proximal humerus. *J Pediatr Orthop B.* 1997;6:219–222.

359. Wang JP, Shen WJ, Chen WM, et al. Iatrogenic radial nerve palsy after operative management of humeral shaft fractures. *J Trauma.* 2009;66:800–803.

360. Waters PM, Monica JT, Earp BE, et al. Correlation of radiographic muscle cross-sectional area with glenohumeral deformity in children with brachial plexus birth palsy. *J Bone Joint Surg Am.* 2009;91:2367–2375.

361. Waters PM, Smith GR, Jaramillo D. Glenohumeral deformity secondary to brachial plexus birth palsy. *J Bone Joint Surg Am.* 1998;80:668–677.

362. Watford KE, Jazrawi LM, Eglseder WA, Jr. Percutaneous fixation of unstable proximal humeral fractures with cannulated screws. *Orthopedics.* 2009;32:166.

363. Wera GD, Friess DM, Getty PO, et al. Fracture of the proximal humerus with injury to the axillary artery in a boy aged 13 years. *J Bone Joint Surg Br.* 2006;88:1521–1523.

364. Wiater BP, Neradilek MB, Polissar NL., et al. Risk factors for chondrolysis of the glenohumeral joint: a study of three hundred and seventy-five shoulder arthroscopic procedures in the practice of an individual community surgeon. *J Bone Joint Surg Am.* 2011;93:615–625.

365. Wilkinson JM, Stanley D. Posterior surgical approaches to the elbow: a comparative anatomic study. *J Shoulder Elbow Surg.* 2001;10:380–382.

366. Williams DJ. The mechanisms producing fracture-separation of the proximal humeral epiphysis. *J Bone Joint Surg Br.* 1981;63-B:102–107.

367. Wolf EM, Cheng JC, Dickson K. Humeral avulsion of glenohumeral ligaments as a cause of anterior shoulder instability. *Arthroscopy.* 1995;11:600–607.

368. Xie F, Wang S, Jiao Q, et al. Minimally invasive treatment for severely displaced proximal humeral fractures in children using titanium elastic nails. *J Pediatr Orthop.* 2011;31:839–846.

369. Yam A, Tan TC, Lim BH. Intraoperative interfragmentary radial nerve compression in a medially plated humeral shaft fracture: a case report. *J Orthop Trauma.* 2005;19:491–493.

370. Yang KH, Han DY, Kim HJ. Intramedullary entrapment of the radial nerve associated with humeral shaft fracture. *J Orthop Trauma.* 1997;11:224–226.

371. Zehms CT, Balsamo L, Dunbar R. Coaptation splinting for humeral shaft fractures in adults and children: a modified method. *Am J Orthop (Belle Mead NJ).* 2006;35:452–454.

372. Zlotolow DA, Catalano LW, 3rd, Barron OA, et al. Surgical exposures of the humerus. *J Am Acad Orthop Surg.* 2006;14(13):754–765.

19

Clavicle and Scapula Fractures and Acromioclavicular and Sternoclavicular Injuries

Benton E. Heyworth and Joshua M. Abzug

Midshaft Clavicle Fractures

Distal Clavicle Fractures

Midshaft Clavicle Fractures

INTRODUCTION

The clavicle is one of the most commonly fractured bones in children, representing 5% to 15% of all pediatric fractures.[114] The most common location for a clavicle fracture is the midshaft of the bone, accounting for up to 80% of fractures.[114,117,121,129] Despite this high incidence, literature is limited regarding management and outcomes of pediatric clavicle fractures. Much of the literature cited throughout this chapter is therefore extrapolated from scientific studies performed in adult clavicle fracture populations. However, there is a clear increasing trend for operative fixation in adults and older children.[143,162] Therefore, more scientific investigations regarding the management of clavicle fractures in children are being performed, the results of which are of utmost importance to elucidation of future treatment algorithms for this younger population. Until a more methodologically rigorous and comprehensive body of evidence emerges regarding the optimal treatment approach in children and, in particular, adolescents, this remains one of the most controversial areas in pediatric orthopedics and sports medicine.

ASSESSMENT OF MIDSHAFT CLAVICLE FRACTURES

MECHANISMS OF INJURY FOR MIDSHAFT CLAVICLE FRACTURES

Clavicle fractures are common in children of all ages, from birth to skeletal maturity, with different mechanisms of injury resulting in the fracture based on age.

Neonates can sustain a clavicle fracture during the birthing process, especially those babies who are large for gestational age or those involved in difficult deliveries.[15,63,82] Additional risk factors include a lower mean head-to-abdominal circumference ratio and a prior history of the mother having a previous child with macrosomia.[63] Neonatal clavicular fractures have been cited as one of the most frequent complications of natural delivery.[30,70,75,86,118,128] However, there is no uniform screening method for determining whether or not a fracture occurred. Therefore, the exact incidence of neonatal clavicle fractures remains unknown. The incidence has been reported to be as high as 4.4%, but the true incidence may be even higher, as some are diagnosed postdischarge from nursery.[86] Clavicle fractures due to birth trauma need to be distinguished from the rarer congenital pseudarthrosis of the clavicle, which is generally seen on the right side, except in dextrocardia (Fig. 19-1).

Based on the child's neonatal position in the uterus, the anterior shoulder, typically the right side, is the most likely location of the clavicle fracture, as the left occiput anterior (LOA) position is the most common.[63] In addition, this is the most common side of injury in neonatal brachial plexus palsy. Therefore, when an infant sustains a clavicle fracture during the birthing process and limited motion is present about the affected extremity, it is often unknown if the child has a concomitant brachial plexus injury or is not moving their arm secondary to the pain associated with the fracture, a so-called pseudopalsy. Once the fracture heals, typically in 1 to 3 weeks in a newborn, repeat assessment of the brachial plexus must be performed to distinguish pseudopalsy from a true nerve injury.

The exact mechanism for sustaining the clavicle fracture during the birthing process remains unknown. It is likely related to lateral compression of the shoulder girdle against the pelvis. However, neonatal clavicle fractures have also been shown to occur during cesarean sections.[63]

Toddlers who sustain clavicle fractures may sustain the injury due to a fall from a height or injuries sustained during child abuse.[22,75,119] In a series of children aged 4 years or

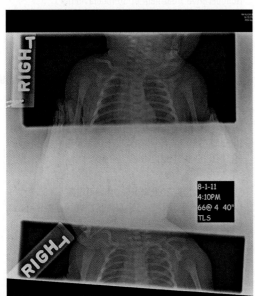

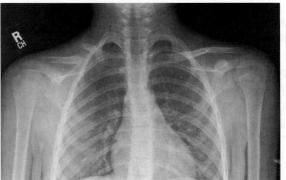

Figure 19-1. A: Radiograph of a left midshaft clavicular fracture in an infant sustained during the birthing process. **B:** Neonatal pseudarthrosis of the clavicle. (**B:** reprinted with permission from Waters PM, Bae DS, eds. *Pediatric Hand and Upper Limb Surgery: A Practical Guide.* 1st ed. Philadelphia, PA: Wolters Kluwer Health/Lippincott Williams & Wilkins; 2012.)

younger, children abused had an incidence of clavicle fractures of approximately 4% compared with only about 1% in the control group.[119]

School age clavicle fractures occurring in children are typically the result of a fall where the child sustains a lateral compressive force to the shoulder.[140] Typical activities include falls off of playground equipment, falls from bicycles, and during sporting activities. Alternatively, a direct blow to the clavicle can lead to fracture in a child; however, this mechanism is less common. The common fall onto an outstretched hand does not typically transmit enough force to the clavicle to sustain a fracture,[67] but is another reported mechanism of injury in some cases.

Adolescents sustain clavicle fractures due to similar mechanisms as school age children as well as due to high-energy mechanisms or competitive athletics. Motor vehicle and all-terrain vehicle (ATV) accidents are common high-energy mechanisms in adolescents that can result in either isolated clavicular fractures or clavicular fractures associated with polytrauma similar to adults.[77,121] High-level competitive athletes also commonly sustain clavicle fractures due to collision sports, such as football, or much less commonly, due to repetitive, high-intensity training, leading to a stress fracture, though this has only emerged in case reports.[1] Specific sporting activities that can lead to stress fractures include rowing, diving, baseball, and gymnastics, among others.[1,153,160]

The proposed mechanism leading to a clavicular stress fracture is excessive cyclic scapular protraction and retraction leading to clavicular fatigue.[1] Excessive motion at the sternoclavicular and acromioclavicular (AC) joints transfers the forces to the clavicle itself, with the end result being these forces exceeding the ultimate tensile strength of the clavicle.[1] This most commonly occurs in athletes who rapidly increase their training program.

INJURIES ASSOCIATED WITH MIDSHAFT CLAVICLE FRACTURES

Injuries that are associated with clavicle fractures depend on the age of the child and violence of trauma with the fracture. Neonates can have a concomitant neonatal brachial plexus palsy. The most common type of neonatal brachial plexus palsy is an injury affecting C5 and C6 (Erb's palsy) or C5, C6, and C7 with resultant limited shoulder movement, elbow flexion, forearm supination, and wrist extension.[48] Differentiation between a pseudopalsy, the child not moving their arm secondary to the clavicle fracture itself, and a concomitant l brachial plexus birth palsy can be made by 3 to 4 weeks of age, as the pain from the fracture will be markedly decreased. Toddlers who sustain clavicle fractures as a result of nonaccidental trauma are likely to sustain concomitant fractures, such as fractures of the rib, tibia/fibula, humerus, or femur, intracranial bleeding, eye contusions, retinal hemorrhage, and burns.[28,119] Finally, adolescents involved in high-energy mechanisms of injury can have associated polytrauma including injury to surrounding structures or vital organs. Concomitant rib fractures, scapula fractures, pneumothorax, brachial plexus injury, or subclavian vessel injury may be present.[67] Abdominal, head, spine, and/or lower extremity trauma can also occur.

SIGNS AND SYMPTOMS OF MIDSHAFT CLAVICLE FRACTURES

Clavicle fractures in neonates commonly present after difficult deliveries with decreased active movement about the shoulder region, crying upon passive movement of the shoulder and entire upper extremity, swelling, crepitation, and an asymmetrical bony contour. The Moro (startle) reflex (a newborn reflex in which a noise or sudden movement causes the baby to extend their neck, arms, and legs followed by pulling the arms and legs back in) may be decreased as well.[63] Presence of limited digit motion or Horner syndrome (ptosis, miosis, and anhydrosis) indicates the presence of a more serious concomitant brachial plexus birth palsy with injury affecting the lower portions of the brachial plexus.

Toddlers who sustain clavicle fractures associated with suspected abuse should undergo a complete head-to-toe survey, as if they were a trauma patient, looking for concomitant injuries and/or signs of abuse. This includes a thorough neurologic evaluation, an ophthalmologic examination, and a skeletal survey to look for corner fractures or additional fractures in various stages of healing.

Examination of an older child or adolescent with a clavicle fracture includes looking for deformity, swelling, and ecchymosis about the affected clavicle. Any tenting of the skin (Fig. 19-2) or open wounds should be noted. In addition, one should look at the lateral aspect of the shoulder for an abrasion or erythema, as this is most commonly the site of impact. Inspection may also demonstrate some drooping of the involved side as the scapula appears internally rotated and the shoulder appears shortened compared with the contralateral side. If significant swelling is present, this may be difficult to recognize.[67]

Pain about the entire shoulder girdle is typically present; however, significant tenderness to palpation is present overlying the fracture itself. Crepitus, with palpation or any attempt of active or passive range of motion, may be present. As noted above, concomitant injury to the brachial plexus may occur, especially in the medial cord-ulnar nerve because of its location adjacent to the middle third of the clavicle. Therefore, a thorough neurologic examination is required for all patients who sustain clavicular fractures. This includes assessing motor and sensory function throughout the entire upper extremity. It may be difficult to have a child in pain perform certain functions necessary to complete the neurologic evaluation; however, it is imperative to be patient and repeat the examination as often as necessary to obtain the necessary information.

Because of the location of the subclavian vessel, a thorough vascular examination is also necessary, especially in patients involved in high-energy mechanisms of injury. The vessel can spasm, have a thrombosis from blunt trauma, or rarely have a penetrating injury. Assessment of the radial pulse should be symmetric and if there is any concern for injury of the vessel, further diagnostic evaluation with advanced imaging should be performed.

IMAGING AND OTHER DIAGNOSTIC STUDIES FOR MIDSHAFT CLAVICLE FRACTURES

Initial imaging of a suspected clavicle fracture includes plain radiographs of the clavicle in two projections. Typically, a standard anteroposterior (AP) radiograph and a cephalic tilt

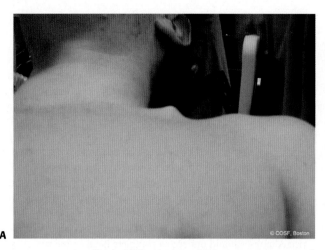 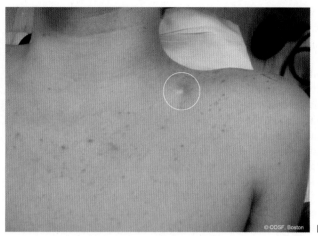

Figure 19-2. Photographs depicting skin tenting from a displaced, segmental left diaphyseal clavicle fracture. (Reprinted with permission from Waters PM, Bae DS, eds. *Pediatric Hand and Upper Limb Surgery: A Practical Guide.* 1st ed. Philadelphia, PA: Wolters Kluwer Health/Lippincott Williams & Wilkins; 2012.)

view, ranging from 15-degree cephalad to 45-degree cephalad, are obtained (Fig. 19-3). These images provide visualization of the shoulder girdle region as well as the upper lung fields, both of which should be assessed for additional injuries. However, if clinical suspicion is present for additional injuries, dedicated series of the suspected part(s) should be obtained.

Clavicle fractures are often detected on chest x-rays obtained for trauma patients, and rarely require additional imaging, if the general fracture pattern and approximate shortening can be assessed for completely displaced fractures. Advanced imaging is rarely needed to evaluate clavicle fractures, as the fracture pattern, displacement, and presence of comminution can almost always be assessed on plain films. As described in greater detail below, fractures or suspected dislocations about the sternoclavicular joint are frequently assessed with CT scans, but midshaft fractures, which are much more common, benefit from such imaging only in the case of a suspected or possible fracture nonunion or possible

refracture through a healing fracture. Distal fractures are assessed by CT scans at times to decide on degree and direction of displacement that might indicate need for operative intervention.

CLASSIFICATION OF MIDSHAFT CLAVICLE FRACTURES

Clavicle fractures are usually described based on the location of the fracture, the fracture pattern, and the presence or absence of displacement. Thus, clavicle fractures are either medial, midshaft, or lateral; nondisplaced or displaced; open or closed; comminuted or simple. Displaced fractures can be qualified as partially displaced, when the two fracture fragments of a two-part fracture are still in contact, with or without angulation, whereas completely displaced fractures have fracture fragments that are not in contact with each other, or are three-part or four-part fractures with comminution. The description of partially displaced fractures with angulation benefit from a measurement of the degree of angulation, as increasing angulation has been associated with a greater risk of refracture in some studies.[46,95] For completely displaced fractures, a measurement of the degree of "shortening," as measured in millimeters (mm), has been used more commonly in adult clavicle fracture studies. For example, some authors have contended that shortening greater than 14 or 20 mm may be associated with poorer outcomes with nonoperative treatment, when compared with lesser degrees of shortening. As a result, many have considered 20 mm as a potential threshold or an indication for surgery. However, important studies by Schulz et al.[134a] and Bae et al.[8] have suggested that even fractures with greater than 15 to 20 mm of shortening are not associated with functional limitations in adolescents treated nonoperatively. Moreover, new research suggests that traditional measurement techniques may grossly overestimate the 'true' shortening of the clavicle, by not accounting for the oblique nature of clavicle fractures.[87a] Thus, we believe that additional research is warranted before adult-based metrics are applied to the young who have greater healing and remodeling capacity. Classifications that go beyond this descriptive scheme, such as the AO classification,[44] have been proposed to evaluate clavicle fractures, but none are widely utilized, as they are either purely descriptive of fracture location[3] or cumbersome with multiple types and subtypes.[44,129]

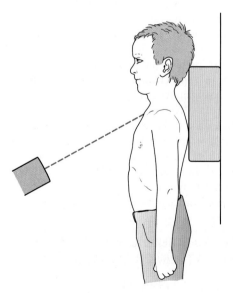

Figure 19-3. Depiction of a 45-degree cephalic tilt to obtain an additional view of the clavicle.

OUTCOME MEASURES FOR MIDSHAFT CLAVICLE FRACTURES

No specific outcome scores have been widely used to assess results following pediatric clavicle fractures, though the American Shoulder and Elbow Society (ASES) score, the Disability of the Arm, Shoulder, and Hand (DASH) Score, the QuickDASH, and the Constant Shoulder Score have been utilized in some studies. The creation of a novel Pediatric & Adolescent Shoulder & Elbow Survey (Pedi-ASES) has stemmed from research demonstrating that adult shoulder outcome scores are associated with poor validity and comprehensibility. The Pedi-ASES may represent a future standard for use in pediatric and adolescent shoulder research.[60]

PATHOANATOMY AND APPLIED ANATOMY RELATED TO MIDSHAFT CLAVICLE FRACTURES

The clavicle, also referred to as the collar bone, is an S-shaped bone that lies along the subcutaneous border of the anterior aspect of the shoulder girdle. An anterior convexity is present medially to permit the passage of the brachial plexus and axillary vessels from the neck region into the upper arm, whereas laterally there is an anterior concavity.

Development of the clavicle begins at five and a half weeks' gestation via intramembranous ossification, and by 8 weeks, the bone has developed into its S-shaped configuration.[47] Postnatally, the clavicle continues to grow at a steady rate until age 12, increasing approximately 8.4 mm per year.[99] After 12 years of age, the clavicle grows approximately 2.6 mm per year in females and 5.4 mm per year in males. Thus, 80% of the final clavicle length is reached by age 9 in females and age 12 in males.[99] However, because the clavicle is the last bone in the body to complete its ossification process, continuing up to the age of 25 in some patients, continued remodeling capacity may exist up through adolescence and into young adulthood.

Medially the clavicle articulates with the sternum, forming the sternoclavicular joint, whereas laterally the bone ends in an articulation with the acromion, forming the AC joint. The medial inferior aspect of the clavicle is the site of attachment of the costoclavicular ligament, whereas laterally on the inferior aspect there is the conoid tubercle and trapezoid line, the sites of attachment for the conoid and trapezoid ligaments, respectively. All of these ligaments slant posteriorly as they approach the clavicle, and therefore when the clavicle elevates and the ligaments are put on stretch, the clavicle rotates posteriorly. In addition, these ligaments provide significant stability at both ends of the clavicle, thus making fractures in the middle third of the clavicle more likely.

The pectoralis major originates from the medial aspect of the clavicle as well as the sternum and inserts onto the humerus at the intertubercular groove, whereas the deltoid originates from the lateral aspect of the clavicle as well as the acromion and scapular spine to insert onto the humerus at the deltoid tuberosity. In addition, the sternocleidomastoid and sternohyoid muscles originate from the clavicle whereas the trapezius and subclavius insert onto the clavicle.

TREATMENT OPTIONS FOR MIDSHAFT CLAVICLE FRACTURES

The mainstay of treatment of pediatric and adolescent clavicle fractures is nonoperative, allowing the fracture to form callous and heal in situ, even if significant displacement is present (Fig. 19-4).[8] It is well agreed upon that nondisplaced or minimally displaced fractures should be treated nonoperatively. Fractures that should proceed directly to operative intervention include open fractures, fractures with skin at risk of necrosis

Figure 19-4. A: Radiograph of a moderately displaced diaphyseal right clavicular fracture. **B:** Radiograph of the healed fracture with abundant callus formation, demonstrating the potential of remodeling with growth. (Reprinted with permission from Waters PM, Bae DS, eds. *Pediatric Hand and Upper Limb Surgery: A Practical Guide.* 1st ed. Philadelphia, PA: Wolters Kluwer Health/Lippincott Williams & Wilkins; 2012.)

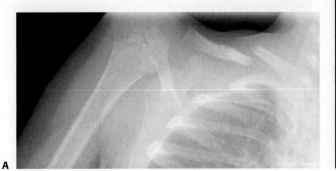

A

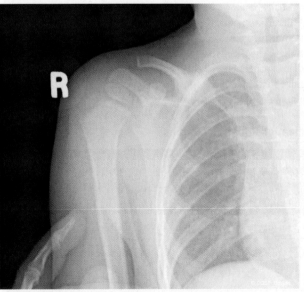

B

(i.e., skin with pallor or clear dysvascularity), and fractures with associated neurovascular injuries clearly affecting motor function or blood supply to the upper extremity. Decreased sensation in the skin of the chest wall distal to the fracture may be reported, and likely stems from contusions or stretch injuries to the superficial supraclavicular sensory nerves. While case reports of supraclavicular nerve branches entrapped in fracture callus have been published,[71] and may benefit from surgical exploration and neurolysis, these represent the minority of cases, and chest wall numbness does not represent an independent indication for surgery. Of note, these nerves are at risk for injury during primary surgical fixation.

NONOPERATIVE TREATMENT

Nonoperative treatment of clavicle fractures is performed by immobilizing the child's shoulder girdle, typically with a sling. Younger children may benefit from a sling and swath, at least in the first several days postinjury, primarily to improve comfort levels. While more traditional figure-of-eight dressings or shoulder immobilizers can be utilized, these are more cumbersome and have not been shown to provide improved results. Neonates who sustain a clavicular fracture during the birthing process can be immobilized with a swath technique, such as placing Webril or an soft elastic bandage around the torso and arm, but, due to the speed of callus formation, can usually be discontinued within 1 week.

Follow-up radiographs are obtained at typical intervals until fracture union occurs. A two-week postinjury radiograph allows for confirmation of maintenance of the fracture alignment or degree of shortening seen at the time of injury, as some nondisplaced fractures can displace in the early postinjury phase. Such a visit will also allow for a progression to use of the sling only when ambulating or at school, while the sling can often be discontinued when at home, as comfort allows from the 2-week to the 6-week period. A 6-week visit frequently shows significant callus formation stabilizing the fracture, which can allow for discontinuation of the sling, with an understanding that refractures can occur with falls or premature return to sports.[25] However, noncontact fitness activities can usually be allowed at 6 weeks, provided there is advanced healing. Return to contact sports only after the 3-month radiographs has confirmed a healed fracture with clear bony bridging. Calder et al. have suggested that follow-up radiographs are unnecessary in pediatric patients, given the near-universal expected fracture healing rate in a child. However, we routinely obtain radiographs until union is clearly established.

Indications/Contraindications

Nonoperative Treatment of Midshaft Clavicle Fractures: INDICATIONS AND CONTRAINDICATIONS	
Indications	**Relative Contraindications**
• Nondisplaced fractures	• Open fractures
• Minimally displaced fractures	• Fractures at risk of skin necrosis • Fractures associated with neurovascular injury

OPERATIVE TREATMENT OF MIDSHAFT CLAVICLE FRACTURES

Absolute indications for operative treatment of clavicle fractures in the pediatric and adolescent population include open fractures, fractures with skin tenting severe enough to risk skin necrosis (Fig. 19-5), and fractures associated with neurovascular injury. Additional relative indications may include floating shoulder injuries and fractures associated with polytrauma. Floating shoulder injuries involving midshaft clavicle fractures and fractures of the glenoid neck treated by open reduction internal fixation (ORIF) of the clavicle alone can be sufficient as ligamentotaxis can reduce the other fracture via the coracoclavicular (CC) ligament.[9]

Fractures with significant displacement that are treated nonoperatively in adults have been shown to subsequently heal with a malunion that can cause changes to shoulder mechanics. These alterations have been shown, at times, to lead to pain with overhead activities, decreased strength, and decreased endurance.[61,100] Therefore, multiple studies have investigated the benefit of operative fixation versus nonoperative management of displaced midshaft clavicle fractures. The most impactful of such studies was randomized controlled trial of an adult Canadian population with a mean age of 33.5 years, in which the operative cohort was shown to have improved functional outcome measures and lower rates of nonunion and symptomatic malunion than the nonoperative cohort.[26] A recent meta-analysis evaluating the results of randomized clinical trials that compared nonoperative and operative treatment in adults confirmed a significantly higher nonunion and symptomatic malunion rate in the nonoperative group. In addition, patients treated with operative intervention had earlier functional return.[101] Not only is it unclear whether these data are transferable to adolescents, but more recent randomized controlled trials in other adult populations[132,152] have suggested that the indications for surgery are more limited in adult populations than suggested by the McKee Canadian study. Clearly, younger children, especially less than age 13 years, have the potential to remodel even a foreshortened, displaced fracture. The approach to older adolescents has evolved into a shared decision-making process with families of young athletes, with considerations toward the

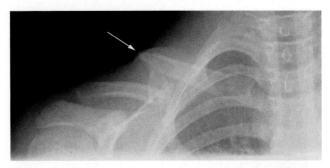

Figure 19-5. Radiograph of a segmental right diaphyseal clavicle fracture causing skin tenting and subsequent compromise. Note the vertical nature of the segmental fragment. (Reprinted with permission from Waters PM, Bae DS, eds. *Pediatric Hand and Upper Limb Surgery: A Practical Guide.* 1st ed. Philadelphia, PA: Wolters Kluwer Health/Lippincott Williams & Wilkins; 2012.)

laterality of the fracture, the sports played, and the tolerance level for a malunion that is likely to demonstrate a full return to function, but perhaps along an unpredictable timeline. To date, no studies in adolescent populations have demonstrated clear superiority of operative treatment over nonoperative treatment, given the significantly lower rates of nonunion and symptomatic malunion in adolescents relative to adults.

Open Reduction and Internal Fixation or Intramedullary Fixation

Preoperative Planning

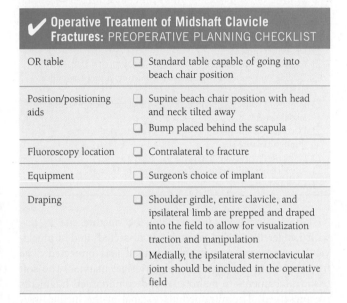

✔ Operative Treatment of Midshaft Clavicle Fractures: PREOPERATIVE PLANNING CHECKLIST	
OR table	❑ Standard table capable of going into beach chair position
Position/positioning aids	❑ Supine beach chair position with head and neck tilted away
	❑ Bump placed behind the scapula
Fluoroscopy location	❑ Contralateral to fracture
Equipment	❑ Surgeon's choice of implant
Draping	❑ Shoulder girdle, entire clavicle, and ipsilateral limb are prepped and draped into the field to allow for visualization traction and manipulation
	❑ Medially, the ipsilateral sternoclavicular joint should be included in the operative field

As with any procedure that will use implants, it is imperative to have the desired hardware available before proceeding to the operating room. Options for treatment of pediatric and adolescent clavicle fractures include anatomically designed clavicle plates, standard nonlocking and locking plates, and intramedullary devices including pins, wires, screws, and elastic nails.

Intramedullary fixation has the potential benefits of requiring less soft tissue stripping at the fracture site, better aesthetics with smaller skin incisions, easier hardware removal, less potential for hardware irritation, and less bony weakness following hardware removal compared with plate fixation. However, the ability to resist torsional forces is less with intramedullary fixation compared with plating which can result in fracture of the intramedullary implant (Fig. 19-6). Furthermore, the potential for the intramedullary device to migrate is a major concern for many surgeons, thus limiting its usage. More modern intramedullary devices with locking potential have decreased concerns regarding migration of traditional Kirschner-wire (K-wire) constructs, but are more likely to require secondary hardware removal surgeries to avoid soft tissue irritation at the posterior lateral clavicle entry sites.

If plate fixation is being planned, one must determine what the preferred location of the plate will be, anteroinferior or superior. Anteroinferior plates have the advantage of performing drilling in a posterosuperior direction, and thus the drill is not directed toward the surrounding neurovascular structures.

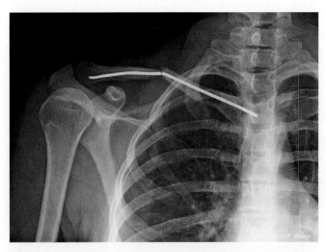

Figure 19-6. Radiograph of a right midshaft clavicular fracture treated with an intramedullary elastic nail, which subsequently went on to fracture. (Reprinted with permission from Waters PM, Bae DS, eds. *Pediatric Hand and Upper Limb Surgery: A Practical Guide.* 1st ed. Philadelphia, PA: Wolters Kluwer Health/Lippincott Williams & Wilkins; 2012.)

In addition, the plate is less prominent in this location. Superior placement of the plate is technically easier and allows for better resistance of the biomechanical forces acting to displace the fracture.

Positioning

Options for positioning during ORIF of clavicle fractures include using the beach chair position (i.e., ~60 degrees), having the patient supine, or different degrees of torso elevation in between the two, that is, "sloppy beach chair" positioning (e.g., ~45 degrees). With either position, a bump may be placed behind the scapula to bring the fracture fragments forward for ease of dissection.

Surgical Approach

ORIF is performed via a direct surgical approach to the clavicle using a skin incision that follows Langer lines. In an attempt to avoid problems, by having the incision directly over the plate, and to improve aesthetics, incise the skin on the inferior aspect of the clavicle,[32] or even up to 1 to 2 cm distal to the clavicle, with proximal dissection to the fracture site. Once the skin is incised, the platysma is dissected, revealing the underlying cutaneous supraclavicular nerves as they cross the clavicle, which should be identified and protected to avoid chest wall numbness, dysesthesias, or neuromas. Meticulous subperiosteal dissection is then carried out to expose the fracture site while ensuring maintenance of the soft tissue attachments to any malrotated or segmental fracture fragments. Preservation of the integrity of the periosteum, which may be torn at the site of the fracture, is critical to the postfixation closure of this layer, which will aid in optimization of bone healing and minimization of hardware irritation. The posterior periosteal sleeve also protects the underlying neurovascular structures.

Intramedullary fixation is performed by making a similar approach using a small incision over the fracture site to expose only the ends of fracture fragments. An additional percutaneous incision is placed over the superolateral part of the clavicle to place the intramedullary device in an antegrade manner.

Technique

Open Reduction and Internal Fixation

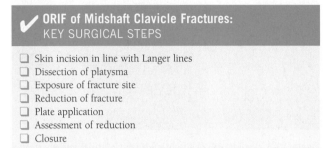

✔ **ORIF of Midshaft Clavicle Fractures:**
KEY SURGICAL STEPS

- ☐ Skin incision in line with Langer lines
- ☐ Dissection of platysma
- ☐ Exposure of fracture site
- ☐ Reduction of fracture
- ☐ Plate application
- ☐ Assessment of reduction
- ☐ Closure

We use the sloppy beach chair position at 45 degrees and make our skin incision approximately 1 to 1.5 cm inferior to the clavicle. Following exposure of the fracture fragments, reduction is performed utilizing bone holding forceps. It is imperative to restore the length and contour of the clavicle during the reduction process. This may require utilization of smooth wires, suture, or interfragmentary screws. Because comminuted fractures are among the more common fractures that, overall, undergo operative fixation, interfragmentary fixation of a free fragment with a 2.0- or 2.7-mm lag screw is helpful in turning a three-part or four-part fracture into a two-part fracture amenable to optimal plate placement. Once the reduction is near-anatomic, the plate is applied on the superior aspect of the clavicle. During drilling and screw placement, we protect the underlying neurovascular structures by placement of a malleable retractor inferior to the clavicle. Following provisional plate placement, fluoroscopic imaging and/or direct visualization is utilized to assess the plate position to ensure avoidance of far-medial or far-distal eccentric screw or plate position, which can increase the change of peri-implant fracture and hardware irritation. Compression techniques with eccentric drilling within the oblique holes of the plate are considered critical to an anatomic final reduction and optimization of healing rates. Final biplanar fluoroscopic views are used to confirm optimal screw length and establish a radiographic postoperative baseline for future assessment of healing of the fracture. The wound is then thoroughly irrigated and the periosteum closed. We

favor closure of the overlying fascial layer and platysma layer, to optimize soft tissue coverage over the subcutaneous plate. Final assessment of the supraclavicular nerves is performed to be certain they are intact and without entrapment. A meticulous dermal layer and subcuticular closure is then performed to obtain the best cosmetic result possible and decrease the chance of wound complications. Sterile dressings are applied followed by placement of the patient into a sling.

Intramedullary Fixation

✔ **Intramedullary Fixation of Midshaft Clavicle Fractures:** KEY SURGICAL STEPS

- ☐ Skin incision in line with Langer lines
- ☐ Dissection of platysma
- ☐ Exposure of fracture site
- ☐ Drilling of the medial segment of the fracture in preparation for device placement
- ☐ Drilling of distal fragment medullary canal and then posterior lateral cortex
- ☐ Placement of intramedullary device in a retrograde manner through fracture site
- ☐ Reduction of fracture fragments
- ☐ Advancement of device antegrade across the fracture
- ☐ Closure

A skin incision is made overlying the fracture site in line with Langer lines. The platysma is dissected, and supraclavicular cutaneous nerves are identified and protected. The fracture site is exposed in a subperiosteal manner. The soft tissue attachments to malrotated and comminuted fragments are preserved. The intramedullary canal of the medial fracture fragment is drilled in preparation for device placement, with care taken to ensure no violation of the anterior medial cortex occurs. The distal fragment medullary canal and then the posterior lateral cortex are drilled so that the drill can be visualized just beneath the skin. A percutaneous skin incision is made where the drill is tenting the skin. The intramedullary device is placed in a retrograde manner through fracture site to exit through posterior lateral skin incision. Fracture fragments are reduced, and the device is advanced in an antegrade manner across the fracture. If available, device-specific mechanisms are placed to prevent migration or permit compression. The periosteum, overlying fascial layers, platysma layer, and skin are closed. A sling or shoulder immobilizer is applied.

Author's Preferred Treatment for Midshaft Clavicle Fractures (Algorithm 19-1)

Most pediatric and adolescent clavicle fractures are treated nonoperatively with immobilization for 6 weeks. Patients then undergo home or formal rehabilitation to restore range of motion and strength before resuming full activities. Operative treatment is performed for open fractures, fractures at risk for skin necrosis, and fractures associated with neurologic or vascular injury (Fig. 19-7). For completely displaced

fractures with significant shortening clearly greater than 20 mm, or severely comminuted fractures, a shared decision-making process is pursued with the patient and family. Based on research demonstrating exceedingly low nonunion rates and symptomatic malunion rates in adolescents, even in the face of significant shortening, nonoperative treatment is generally recommended. For such fractures in the dominant

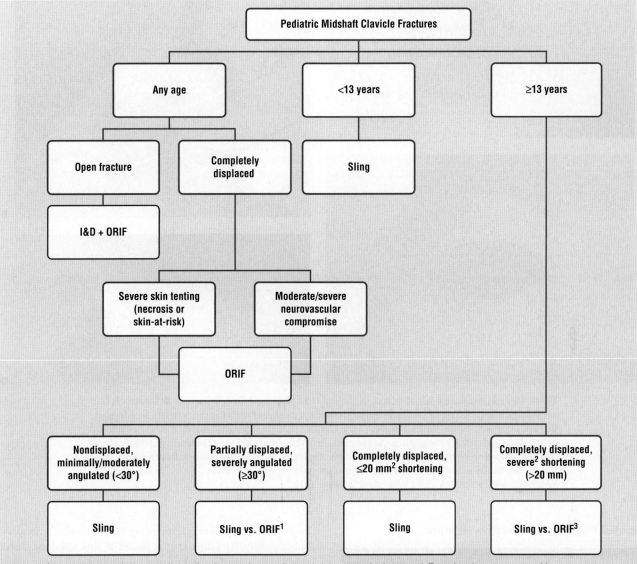

Algorithm flow chart content:

Pediatric Midshaft Clavicle Fractures

- **Any age**
  - **Open fracture** → **I&D + ORIF**
  - **Completely displaced**
    - **Severe skin tenting (necrosis or skin-at-risk)**
    - **Moderate/severe neurovascular compromise**
    - → **ORIF**
- **<13 years** → **Sling**
- **≥13 years**
  - **Nondisplaced, minimally/moderately angulated (<30°)** → **Sling**
  - **Partially displaced, severely angulated (≥30°)** → **Sling vs. ORIF[1]**
  - **Completely displaced, ≤20 mm² shortening** → **Sling**
  - **Completely displaced, severe[2] shortening (>20 mm)** → **Sling vs. ORIF[3]**

[1]Shared decision-making approach, based on latest evidence, including slightly increased refracture risk;[95] may be relevant to contact athletes
[2]Assessment of true shortening should be achieved with 'cortex to corresponding cortex' technique, rather than 'end to end' technique[87a]
[3]Shared decision-making approach, based on latest evidence, including a low risk of symptomatic malunion; may be relevant

Algorithm 19-1. Authors' preferred treatment for midshaft clavicle fractures.

arm of high-level baseball pitchers and other overhead or throwing athletes, consideration of the low risk of a potential symptomatic malunion, which may alter the short-term biomechanics of the throwing motion, may be discussed.

When families favor operative treatment, plate fixation is recommended over intramedullary fixation, provided there is awareness of a relatively high (~18%) rate of potential plate irritation and the need for secondary removal surgery.

Postoperative Care

Whether ORIF or intramedullary fixation is performed, the patient is placed in a sling for 2 weeks, after which a wound check is performed, elbow and wrist range of motion recommended, and an emphasis on sling use when out of the house and at school. Patients are permitted to discontinue sling use while in the home from 2 to 6 weeks. At 6 weeks, a clinical examination is utilized to assess tenderness at the fracture site and radiographs in two planes are obtained to assess bone healing. If the examination and radiographs are consistent with healing, the sling is discontinued and the patient is encouraged to begin range of motion and strengthening. Provided there is adequate healing, noncontact athletes are permitted return to sports activities around 6 to 8 weeks postoperatively. For contact athletes, return to contact activities are permitted at 3 months, provided there is advanced bony bridging.

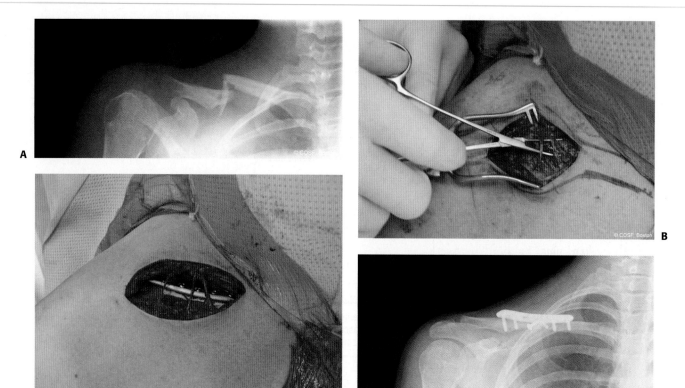

Figure 19-7. A: Radiograph of a displaced, segmental right diaphyseal clavicle fracture. **B:** Incision in line with Langer lines, ensuring protection of the supraclavicular cutaneous nerves as the exposure is performed. **C:** Plate placement on the superior aspect of the clavicle while preserving the supraclavicular cutaneous nerves. **D:** Postoperative radiograph of the anatomically reduced fracture. Note the interfragmentary screw that was utilized to convert this fracture from three fragments to two. (Reprinted with permission from Waters PM, Bae DS, eds. *Pediatric Hand and Upper Limb Surgery: A Practical Guide.* 1st ed. Philadelphia, PA: Wolters Kluwer Health/Lippincott Williams & Wilkins; 2012.)

Potential Pitfalls and Preventive Measures

Midshaft Clavicle Fractures: SURGICAL PITFALLS AND PREVENTIONS	
Pitfall	**Prevention**
• Neurovascular injury/ pneumothorax	• Utilize subperiosteal dissection • Place retractors inferiorly when drilling from superior to inferior direction
• Delayed union/ nonunion	• Maintain soft tissue attachments to comminuted or malrotated fragments
• Malunion	• Maintain soft tissue attachments to comminuted or malrotated fragments • Anatomically reduce and stabilize segmental fractures

The most dreaded intraoperative complication would be damage to a neurovascular structure or creation of a pneumothorax. Both of these exceedingly rare iatrogenic complications can be prevented by utilizing meticulous technique during the exposure of the fracture fragments and drilling/screw placement during the plate application. When exposing the fracture fragments, it is imperative to stay subperiosteal to create a layer between the bone and surrounding neurovascular structures. Subsequently, retractors can be placed in this layer and direct visualization can be used during the drilling and screw placement process to avoid damaging the neurovascular structures.

Maintenance of soft tissue attachments to comminuted or malrotated small fragments will aid the surgeon in the reduction process. Furthermore, if these fragments are completely devoid of soft tissue attachments, devitalization may cause bony union to be delayed or not occur.

Wound complications can be prevented by utilizing the inferior skin incision rather than a direct approach to the clavicle. In addition, a meticulous layered closure at the end of the procedure will permit the best cosmetic outcome while minimizing the chance of wound issues.

Outcomes

Despite the high incidence of pediatric clavicle fractures and the fact that the vast majority of these fractures are treated nonoperatively, limited data exist regarding the outcomes of these injuries. Generally, union rates from 95% to 100% have been reported with nonoperative treatment.[54,78,150] A recent study of 185 adolescent clavicle fractures with a median age of 14.4 years, 38% of which were completely displaced, demonstrated only 1 case of nonunion and 1 delayed union, with the majority demonstrating good-to-excellent functional outcomes measure scores.[123]

In addition, several small series have recently emerged regarding operative treatment. Mehlman et al. performed a retrospective review of 24 children in China with a mean age of 12 years who underwent operative treatment of completely displaced clavicle shaft fractures. In their series, there were no nonunions and no infections. Twenty-one of the 24 patients were able to return to unrestricted sports activity. Three complications were reported including two patients who had scar sensitivity and one patient who had a transient ulnar nerve neurapraxia. However, all patients underwent hardware removal on an elective basis, so the implications or sequellae of retained hardware could not be ascertained.[102] Namdari et al. also performed a retrospective review of 14 skeletally immature patients who underwent ORIF of displaced midshaft clavicle fractures. No nonunions occurred in the cohort, but 8 patients had numbness about the surgical site, and 4 patients underwent hardware removal.[107]

Vander Have et al. retrospectively reviewed 43 fractures, 25 of which were treated nonoperatively and 17 were treated operatively. The authors reported that five symptomatic malunions occurred in the nonoperative group, four of which were treated with a corrective osteotomy. All complications in the operative group were related to prominence of the hardware.[150]

A recent comparative study of over 650 clavicle fractures in patients 10 to 18 years old retrospectively reviewed at a large regional pediatric trauma center demonstrated a nonunion rate of 0.2% in fractures treated nonoperatively, and a symptomatic malunion rate of 2%.[60] The authors demonstrated a significantly higher complication rate (16.2%) in fractures treated operatively, compared with those treated nonoperatively (5.2%). The results of Li et al. corroborated these findings in a smaller, single-site study, in which there was a 43% major complication rate in 37 adolescents treated with plate fixation, the most common of which was secondary surgery for symptomatic plate removal.[88]

Most nondisplaced fractures have union by 4 to 8 weeks of time, whereas displaced fractures may take longer, approximately 10 weeks.[150] A retrospective multicenter investigation of all nonunion cases reported at 9 pediatric hospitals over an 11-year-period was performed by an adolescent clavicle fracture study group. The investigation yielded only 25 total cases, all of which were successfully treated with surgery, which speaks to about the ability to effectively treat this exceedingly rare complication, should it arise following nonoperative treatment. Thus, the vast majority of pediatric patients treated with a simple sling have excellent outcomes and are able to return to their activities without limitations. A small percentage of patients treated nonoperatively with significant fracture displacement may have subjective complaints of pain with prolonged activity, easy fatigability, axillary pain, or drooping shoulders with bony prominence.[150] However, Bae et al. evaluated a group of 16 patients with displaced (>2 cm) mid-diaphyseal clavicle fractures treated nonoperatively. All fractures united with no meaningful loss of shoulder motion or abduction–adduction strength by isokinetic testing. The vast majority of patients had low DASH and pain Visual Analog Scores (VAS) that were very low, means of

4.9 and 1.6, respectively. Only one patient out of 16 required a corrective osteotomy.[8] The authors concluded that routine surgical fixation for displaced, nonsegmental clavicle fractures may not be justified based upon concerns regarding shoulder motion and strength alone in the face of shortening. A similar study by Schulz et al. demonstrated no functional outcome deficits, when compared with the uninjured limb, in 16 adolescent patients with a minimum of 1 cm shortening and a mean of 14 mm shortening of a displaced clavicle fracture, when assessed more than 2 years following nonoperative treatment. Clearly, further investigation, including prospective comparative cohort studies, is required to better determine the risk factors for possible pain or functional compromise in the minority of pediatric patients who develop nonunion, symptomatic malunion, or other complications following clavicle shaft fractures, based on the two different treatment options.

MANAGEMENT OF EXPECTED ADVERSE OUTCOMES AND UNEXPECTED COMPLICATIONS RELATED TO MIDSHAFT CLAVICLE FRACTURES

Midshaft Clavicle Fractures: COMMON ADVERSE OUTCOMES AND COMPLICATIONS

- Hardware prominence
- Malunion
- Nonunion
- Wound complications

Patients who have prominence of their hardware can be successfully treated by removal of their hardware.[102,107,150] If a patient initially treated by nonoperative measures develops a symptomatic malunion, corrective osteotomy has been shown to be successful in eliminating symptoms (Fig. 19-8).[150] In the Vander Have series, all patients who underwent corrective osteotomy of their malunion went on to union and resolution of their symptoms.[150] As previously described in the above multicenter study of 25 cases, clavicle nonunion in adolescents can be successfully treated by subsequent ORIF, with most cases utilizing only local bone grafting from clavicle callus, as most cases are hypertrophic nonunions.

SUMMARY, CONTROVERSIES, AND FUTURE DIRECTIONS RELATED TO MIDSHAFT CLAVICLE FRACTURES

Most pediatric and adolescent midshaft clavicle fractures can be treated successfully with nonoperative measures. ORIF should be performed for the rare open fracture, fractures with skin at risk of necrosis, and fractures with nerve or vascular injury. Future prospective studies are underway to better determine the potential benefits and complications of operative fixation versus nonoperative treatment in adolescents.

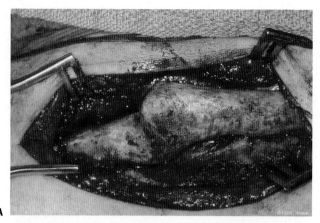

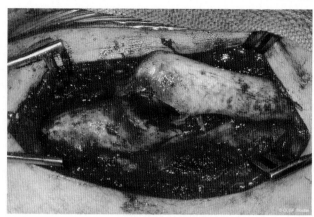

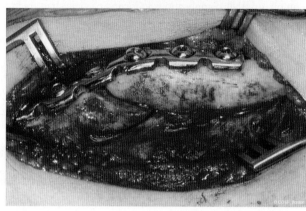

Figure 19-8. A: Intraoperative photograph depicting the mid-diaphyseal malunion. **B:** Intraoperative photograph showing the osteotomy has been performed in the plane of maximal deformity. **C:** Intraoperative photograph following reduction and plating of the malunion. (Reprinted with permission from Waters PM, Bae DS, eds. *Pediatric Hand and Upper Limb Surgery: A Practical Guide.* 1st ed. Philadelphia, PA: Wolters Kluwer Health/Lippincott Williams & Wilkins; 2012.)

Distal Clavicle Fractures

INTRODUCTION TO DISTAL CLAVICLE FRACTURES

Distal clavicle fractures account for 10% to 30% of all clavicle fractures, thus making it the second most common site for a clavicle fracture, after midshaft clavicle fractures.[130] Minimal studies exist regarding the treatment and outcomes of these fractures for pediatric and adolescent patients. Therefore, the information presented here will mainly be extrapolated from the adult literature and our experience.

ASSESSMENT OF DISTAL CLAVICLE FRACTURES

MECHANISMS OF INJURY FOR DISTAL CLAVICLE FRACTURES

Akin to midshaft clavicle fractures, distal clavicle fractures are typically the result of a direct blow to the shoulder girdle or a fall onto the distal aspect of the clavicle.[130,140] Direct blows typically occur in adolescents involved in collision-type sports such as football or lacrosse. When a fall is the mechanism of injury, direct contact from the ground is made against the acromion with the arm typically held in an adducted position. The force is transmitted from the acromion across the AC joint to the distal end of the clavicle.

INJURIES ASSOCIATED WITH DISTAL CLAVICLE FRACTURES

Common injuries associated with distal clavicle fractures include additional fractures about the shoulder girdle including proximal humerus and scapular fractures, thus constituting a floating shoulder-type injury. In addition, rib fractures, lung injuries including contusions, and brachial plexus injuries may occur concomitantly. Finally, cervical spine injuries must be ruled out in collision or high-energy mechanisms of injury.

SIGNS AND SYMPTOMS OF DISTAL CLAVICLE FRACTURES

Patients who sustain distal clavicle fractures present with pain about the involved shoulder especially with any attempt at movement of the arm. Paresthesias may be present if a concomitant brachial plexus injury has occurred.

Physical examination should begin by observing for obvious swelling, ecchymosis, and/or bony prominence or skin tenting, which may be present if there is a completely displaced fracture with superior displacement of the medial fragment and drooping of the unsupported shoulder girdle due to disruption of the strut function of the clavicle. The area posterior to the AC joint should be palpated, as a posteriorly displaced proximal fragment may be felt entrapped in the trapezius muscle, and is critical to treatment decision-making. In addition, palpation of the entire upper extremity, hemithorax, and cervical spine should be performed to identify the location of maximal tenderness as well as additional areas that may have sustained a concomitant injury. A complete neurovascular examination should be performed to evaluate for rare brachial plexus injury. Patients involved in high-energy mechanisms should have a complete head-to-toe survey performed by the orthopedic physician as well as either a member of the trauma team or the emergency room physician.

IMAGING AND OTHER DIAGNOSTIC STUDIES FOR DISTAL CLAVICLE FRACTURES

Initial imaging should be performed by obtaining plain radiographs of the shoulder including a true AP view and a cephalic tilt view, which may be performed most commonly with a 15-degree cephalic or 45-degree cephalic tilt.[163] Due to the significance of assessing posterior displacement of the medial fragment relative to the acromion or distal fragment, the axillary lateral view is of critical importance, and should be pursued, even if it requires assistance from a member of the clinical team, with gentle, gradual abduction of the arm to facilitate a clear view of the shoulder. A CT scan may be diagnostic for intra-articular fractures, which may require operative intervention for best results, and can be helpful to assess the precise degree and direction of the displaced medial fragment, the position of which will determine the need for surgery when physical examination and the axillary view do not allow for a clear assessment.

CLASSIFICATION OF DISTAL CLAVICLE FRACTURES

The most commonly used classification scheme for distal clavicle fractures is that proposed by Neer and modified by Craig.[33,110] This classification scheme includes five types based on the relationship of the fracture line to the CC ligaments, the AC ligaments, and the physis. Most lateral clavicle fractures in the skeletally immature patients are periosteal disruptions in which the bone displaces away from the periosteal sleeve whereas the CC ligaments remain attached to the intact inferior portion of the periosteum.

Type I fractures occur distal to the CC ligaments but do not involve the AC joint. Minimal displacement occurs due to the proximal fragment being stabilized by the intact CC ligaments and the distal fragment being stabilized by the AC joint capsule, the AC ligaments, and the deltotrapezial fascia.

Type II fractures are subdivided into type IIA and type IIB fractures, with type IIA fractures occurring medial to the CC ligaments and type IIB fractures occurring between the CC ligaments with concomitant injury to the conoid ligament. In type IIA injuries, the proximal fragment loses the stability provided by the CC ligaments and displaces superiorly out of the periosteal sleeve. In contrast, the distal fragment remains stable because of the attachments of the AC joint capsule, AC ligaments, and the CC ligament(s). This remains true for type IIB fractures as well, because even though the conoid ligament is disrupted, the trapezoid ligament remains attached.

Type III fractures occur distal to the CC ligaments and extend into the AC joint. As these fractures do not disrupt the ligamentous structures, minimal displacement is the norm.

Type IV fractures occur in skeletally immature patients and involve a fracture medial to the physis. The epiphysis and physis remain uninjured and attached to the AC joint. However, significant displacement can occur between the physis and metaphyseal fragment, as the CC ligaments are attached to the physis. This is especially true if the periosteal sleeve is disrupted. In essence, this is analogous to a type IIA fracture.

Type V fractures have a fracture line that leaves a free-floating inferior cortical fragment attached to the CC ligaments with an additional fracture line dividing the distal clavicle from the remainder of the clavicle. Therefore, neither the proximal nor distal fragment is attached to the CC ligaments. The end result is instability with the potential for significant displacement of the distal end of the proximal fragment.

OUTCOME MEASURES FOR DISTAL CLAVICLE FRACTURES

No outcome measures have been specifically applied to pediatric distal clavicle fractures. Commonly utilized measures for adult distal clavicle fractures include the ASES score, the DASH Score, the QuickDASH, and the Constant Shoulder Score. The recent publication of a novel Pedi-ASES demonstrated that adult shoulder outcome scores such as the DASH and ASES surveys are associated with poor validity and comprehensibility in pediatric populations, and this new metric, when more comprehensively validated, may emerge as a future standard for use in pediatric and adolescent shoulder research.[60]

PATHOANATOMY AND APPLIED ANATOMY RELATED TO DISTAL CLAVICLE FRACTURES

The distal aspect of the clavicle forms the articulation with the scapula via the AC joint. Ligamentous connections between this portion of the clavicle and the scapula include the AC ligaments and CC ligaments. The CC ligaments include the trapezoid ligament, located more laterally with an attachment to the distal clavicle approximately 2 cm from the AC joint, and the conoid ligament, located more medially with an attachment to the distal clavicle approximately 4 cm from the AC joint.[126] The presence of these ligamentous attachments and the acromioclavicular joint capsule permits fluid scapulothoracic motion.[11]

Stability of the clavicle in the horizontal/AP plane is provided by the AC ligaments, whereas stability in the vertical/superoinferior plane is provided by the CC ligaments.[45] This stability permits the definition of the CC space, the space between the coracoid process and the undersurface of the clavicle, which should be 1.1 to 1.3 cm.[16]

TREATMENT OPTIONS FOR DISTAL CLAVICLE FRACTURES

NONOPERATIVE TREATMENT OF DISTAL CLAVICLE FRACTURES

Indications/Contraindications

Nonoperative Treatment of Distal Clavicle Fractures: INDICATIONS AND CONTRAINDICATIONS	
Indications	**Relative Contraindications**
• Nondisplaced and minimally displaced fractures (type I and type III fractures)	• Open fractures • Fractures with associated skin compromise • Fractures with concomitant neurovascular injury requiring surgical intervention

Most distal clavicle fractures in the pediatric and adolescent population can be managed nonoperatively with immobilization alone as long as significant displacement is not present. Typically, this is universally true for type I and type III fractures. However, types II, IV, and V fractures may have significant displacement with subsequent skin tenting, bony prominence, or instability present about the shoulder girdle. Contraindications to nonsurgical management include open fractures, fractures associated with skin necrosis, and fractures with concomitant neurovascular injury requiring surgical intervention. Due to the relative thickness of the soft tissues overlying the AC joint region, skin tenting causing skin at risk of necrosis associated with distal clavicle fractures is rare, compared to that of the more subcutaneous position of the bone in the diaphyseal region. Displaced fractures in the pediatric and adolescent population (types II, IV, and V) should be treated on an individual basis depending on the patient's age, the amount of displacement, and the patient's activities.

Technique

The standard approach to nonoperative treatment includes use of a sling for approximately 6 weeks or sling and swath for the first 1 to 2 weeks, with progression to a simple sling when comfort levels allow. After 4 to 6 weeks, active range of motion may begin. Radiographs are taken at the 6-week follow-up visit to assess healing and progress to functional activities, though full contact in sports such as ice hockey, football, and lacrosse should generally be delayed until 2 to 3 months, after advanced bony bridging is observed radiographically.

Outcomes

Nonoperative treatment of nondisplaced or minimally displaced distal clavicle fractures typically has excellent outcomes with successful union occurring and patients able to return to full activities. While types I and III fractures have been shown to go on to delayed-onset symptomatic AC joint arthrosis in the adult literature,[109] this has not been replicated in pediatric studies.

Treatment of significantly displaced distal clavicle fractures is somewhat controversial, due to a relatively high nonunion rate reported in the adult literature. In a retrospective review performed by Neer,[108] he documented that all patients with type II distal clavicle fractures treated nonoperatively had either a delayed union (67%) or a nonunion (33%). Edwards et al.[37] treated 20 patients with type II distal clavicle fractures nonoperatively and had a 45% delayed union rate and a 30% nonunion rate. Additional studies have shown similar nonunion rates ranging from 25% to 44% for type II fractures treated nonoperatively.[115,130,131,134] In contrast, all type II fractures treated surgically with ORIF have gone on to union.[37,108,134] While nonunion of significantly displaced pediatric distal clavicle fractures may be considered to be a more common occurrence than nonunion of pediatric midshaft clavicle fractures, it still represents a rare event, and operative considerations revolve more around concerns of symptomatic malunion and altered shoulder biomechanics with overhead sports or activities.

OPERATIVE TREATMENT OF DISTAL CLAVICLE FRACTURES

Indications/Contraindications

Absolute indications for operative treatment of distal clavicle fractures include open fractures, fractures with significant skin compromise, displaced intra-articular extension, and fractures with associated neurovascular injuries that require operative intervention. Additional relative indications may include significantly displaced fractures in competitive athletes and adolescents, entrapment in the trapezius muscle, floating shoulder-type injuries, and patients with polytrauma. The most common indication for surgical treatment of distal clavicle fractures in the pediatric population is significant posterior displacement that suggests complete discontinuity of the proximal fragment and/or trapezial entrapment, in which case diffuse soft tissue swelling may be seen over the AC joint region with severe pain with any attempted shoulder motion. Children and younger adolescents are unlikely to experience disruption of the CC ligaments, given that the thick periosteum generally remains attached to the underlying ligamentous complex. Nevertheless, the proximal fragment may alternatively tear through the superior periosteum with enough force to generate severe superior displacement and bony prominence.

Open Reduction and Internal Fixation

Preoperative Planning

✔ ORIF of Distal Clavicle Fractures: PREOPERATIVE PLANNING CHECKLIST	
OR table	☐ Standard table capable of going into beach chair position
Position/positioning aids	☐ Beach chair position with head and neck tilted away or supine ☐ Bump placed behind the scapula ☐ Leave plenty of sterile standing space above the shoulder adjacent to the head

Fluoroscopy location	☐ Contralateral side of fracture
Equipment	☐ Nonabsorbable suture, anatomic distal clavicle plates, hook plates, mini-fragment, or modular hand locking plates
Draping	☐ Entire shoulder girdle region and ipsilateral limb are prepped and draped into the field to allow for traction and manipulation
	☐ Medially, the ipsilateral sternoclavicular joint should be included in the operative field

It is necessary to determine preoperatively what the plan for fixation is going to be as numerous techniques can be performed to stabilize the distal clavicle. Ideally, multiple options are available at the time of surgical intervention including various nonabsorbable suture options, specialty distal clavicle locking plates, and hook plates. The position the patient will be in during the procedure needs to be discussed with the anesthesiologist and operating room staff, especially if the beach chair position is being used.

Positioning

The patient can be positioned in either the beach chair position (i.e., ~60 degrees of head elevation) with the head and neck tilted away, a "sloppy beach chair" position (i.e., 45 degrees of head elevation), or supine on a radiolucent table. With either position, a bump should be placed behind the scapula. The entire shoulder girdle, beginning at the medial edge of the clavicle, and the entire limb should be prepped and draped in the operative field to allow for movement of the limb which facilitates fracture reduction and fixation. A sterile area above the shoulder adjacent to the head is maintained to allow for the surgeon to work both inferior and superior to the clavicle and shoulder.

Surgical Approach

An incision in Langer skin lines over the distal third of the clavicle and AC joint should be made. Once the skin is divided, the subcutaneous tissue, fascia, and periosteum are incised to maintain a thick flap. Subperiosteal dissection is then carried out from nonfractured clavicle out to the fracture site to expose the fracture fragments.

Technique

> ✔ **ORIF of Distal Clavicle Fractures:**
> KEY SURGICAL STEPS
>
> ☐ Skin incision over distal 1/3 of clavicle and acromion in line with Langer lines
> ☐ Electrocautery through subcutaneous tissue, fascia, and periosteum directly onto the clavicle
> ☐ Expose fracture site in a subperiosteal manner while preserving the acromioclavicular and CC ligaments
> ☐ Reduce fracture fragments with reduction clamps and temporary K-wire fixation if necessary
> ☐ Apply distal clavicle plate on superior aspect of distal clavicle

☐ Assess reduction and screw lengths with direct visualization and/or fluoroscopic imaging in multiple planes
☐ Repair periosteum to tighten CC and acromioclavicular ligaments. Rarely apply supplemental fixation to CC ligaments utilizing suture around coracoid and clavicle if fixation is marginal
☐ Irrigate wound and close periosteum
☐ Meticulous skin closure with absorbable suture
☐ Apply sling or shoulder immobilizer

The implant choice will depend on the age and size of the patient, as well as the size and location of the fracture fragments. Fixation with low-profile anatomic distal locking plates can be used for older adolescents with fractures that have a distal fracture fragment large enough to accommodate multiple screws, which may be locking screws, or a combination of cortical and locking screws. If there is not adequate bone on the distal fragment or in the rare case of a complete AC joint dislocation with no distal bony fragment, a hook plate may be used (Fig. 19-9), but has the disadvantage of requiring secondary surgery for hardware removal once healing is confirmed. Younger adolescents or preadolescents with robust periosteum may require only suture-based fixation, with three potential fixation constructs: (1) suture repair of the periosteum only, in cases in which a thick enough cuff of superior periosteum can provide adequate stabilization of the proximal fragment; (2) suture repair in which high-strength nonabsorbable figure-of-eight sutures are placed through the thick inferior periosteum/CC ligament complex and wrapped around the clavicle or through small superior-to-inferior drill holes through the distal aspect of the proximal fragment, with overlying superior periosteal repair; or (3) suture repair through small drill holes in the distal and proximal bone fracture fragments, with overlying superior periosteal repair. For younger patients with smaller clavicle sizes who undergo plate fixation, utilization of modular hand instrumentation or mini-fragment locking plates (Synthes, Inc., West Chester, PA) may be warranted. Distal radius plate fixation has also been suggested by placement of the 2.4-mm locking screws in the distal clavicle fragment.[72]

K-wire fixation is rarely utilized, but should be supplemented with a dorsal tension band, utilizing either suture or wire. Threaded wires are also rarely used, but have been described to lessen the risk of K-wire migration.[6,73,87,93]

Additional fixation of the CC ligaments has been suggested to decrease the chance of nonunion in adults, and may be applicable to the older adolescent. This has been performed utilizing suture or soft tissue tendon grafts.[49,156] In addition, arthroscopic techniques, utilizing suture, the Tightrope system (Arthrex, Naples, FL), or a double-button device, to stabilize the CC ligaments have also been reported in adults.[14,29,116,122] Some authors have proposed placement of a screw between the coracoid and clavicle; however, this requires screw removal following fracture union.[10,37,40,68,92,161] Neither of these techniques are used very often in children or adolescents.

Operative treatment of distal clavicle fractures has excellent results with regard to union rates, especially in children and adolescents. The most common postoperative complication is hardware irritation requiring secondary removal surgery. Because utilization of smooth wires about this region can lead to

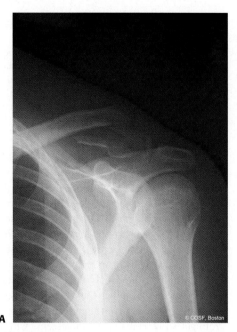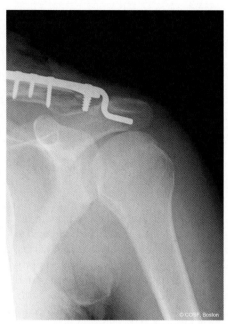

Figure 19-9. A: Radiograph of a displaced intra-articular lateral clavicle fracture where the lateral aspect of the medial fragment was entrapped in the trapezius muscle. **B:** Postoperative radiograph demonstrating fixation utilizing a hook plate. Removal of the implant is planned. (Reprinted with permission from Waters PM, Bae DS, eds. *Pediatric Hand and Upper Limb Surgery: A Practical Guide.* 1st ed. Philadelphia, PA: Wolters Kluwer Health/Lippincott Williams & Wilkins; 2012.)

migration of the wires into areas including the lung, abdomen, spine, trachea, and vascular structures, smooth K-wires should be avoided if possible; or, can be left outside of the skin and removed at 4 weeks.[91,124,149] Tension band wiring is particularly prone to symptoms requiring a second procedure for removal. Using nonabsorbable suture as a tension band can lessen the risk of hardware irritation but suture granulomas can also be irritating and require subsequent removal at times.[83]

Union rates with plate fixation have been reported to be as high as 100%.[25,47] Two studies have found that hook plate usage in adults yielded higher rates of return to work and sports participation and a lower complication rate than other techniques,[43,83] but a more recent study showed superior outcomes and lower complications with distal locking plates, compared with hook plates.[39] We advocate removal of the hook plate in an adolescent when the fracture is healed to avoid secondary complications.

Authors' Preferred Treatment for Distal Clavicle Fractures

Our preferred technique is to treat nearly all distal clavicle fractures in the pediatric and adolescent populations with nonoperative measures. Patients are placed into a sling for 6 weeks and then advanced to active range of motion, presuming union has occurred. Operative intervention is reserved for open fractures, fractures with skin compromise, fractures with associated neurovascular injury requiring operative intervention, displaced intra-articular fractures, and significantly displaced fractures, especially those displaced posteriorly with entrapment in trapezius muscle.

A direct approach to the fracture site is performed using a Langer skin line. Following sharp incision of the skin, electrocautery is utilized to divide the subcutaneous tissue, fascia, and periosteum. A periosteal elevator or scalpel is then used to elevate the periosteum off of the clavicle while preserving the AC and CC ligament attachments. The fracture fragments are then exposed and irrigated free of hematoma and debris in preparation for reduction.

For younger adolescents and preadolescents, if the superior periosteum is found to be robust enough, reduction of the proximal fragment and suture repair of the periosteum is preferred. If the stability of this construct appears questionable, high-strength nonabsorbable figure-of-eight sutures are placed through the thick inferior periosteum/CC ligament complex and wrapped around the clavicle or placed through small superior-to-inferior drill holes through the distal aspect of the proximal fragment, with additional overlying superior periosteal repair. For older adolescents, fixation of a distal clavicle fracture is ideally performed using an anatomically contoured distal clavicular locking plate and screw construct, assuming there is enough bone laterally for stable fixation. If the fragment is too small for these implants, we attempt to perform fixation utilizing mini-fragment or modular hand locking plates (Synthes, Inc., West Chester, PA).

If plate fixation is not an option, interosseous suture fixation of the fracture fragments can be performed, with the suture through the distal fragment also brought through the strong AC ligament complex, to provide additional stability (Fig. 19-10). Hook plates are utilized as a last resort in the setting of an older adolescent without adequate distal fragment bone to accommodate screws, as they require a second procedure for removal. However, all implant options are made available during all procedures, in case adequate fixation is unable to be obtained without them.

Postoperative Care

Postoperatively, patients are placed in a sling 6 weeks. When suture-only fixation is pursued in the younger adolescent or pre-adolescent, a sling and swath is generally favored. When solid rigid plate fixation is achieved, immobilization is removed several times a day for pendulum exercises. Following union of the fracture, active shoulder range of motion and strengthening is initiated. Contact sports participation is usually avoided for 3 months.

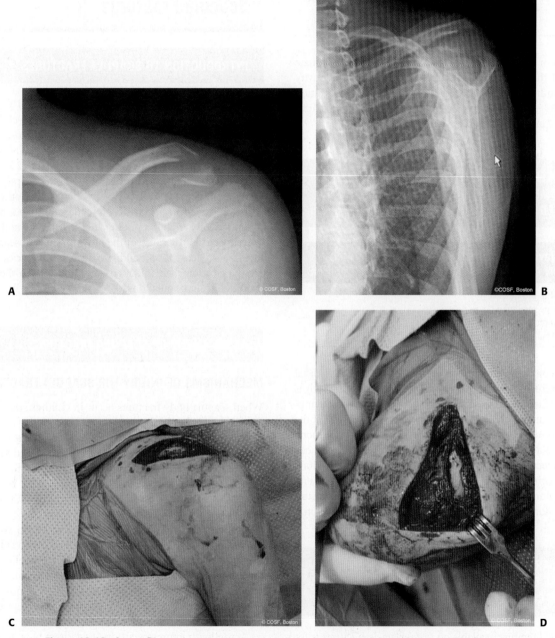

Figure 19-10. A and **B:** Preoperative AP and Scapula Y views of a displaced lateral clavicle fracture. **C:** Intraoperative photograph depicting the incision along Langer skin lines overlying the distal part of the clavicle and acromion. **D:** Intraoperative photograph showing fixation of the fracture utilizing interosseous suture. (Reprinted with permission from Waters PM, Bae DS, eds. *Pediatric Hand and Upper Limb Surgery: A Practical Guide.* 1st ed. Philadelphia, PA: Wolters Kluwer Health/Lippincott Williams & Wilkins; 2012.)

Potential Pitfalls and Preventive Measures

Nonunion or hardware failure can occur if there is inadequate fixation of the distal clavicular fragment or excessive activity early. In addition, it is imperative to avoid screw penetration into the AC joint, which can be assessed with direct visualization and/or utilizing fluoroscopy in multiple planes.

MANAGEMENT OF EXPECTED ADVERSE OUTCOMES AND UNEXPECTED COMPLICATIONS RELATED TO DISTAL CLAVICLE FRACTURES

Distal Clavicle Fractures: COMMON ADVERSE OUTCOMES AND COMPLICATIONS
• Hardware prominence • Hardware migration • Nonunion • Symptomatic malunion

The most common complication of treatment of operative distal clavicle fractures is related to symptomatic hardware, which is easily remedied by removal of hardware. Nonunion and symptomatic malunions are best managed by performing ORIF of the fracture. In rare cases of minimal distal fragment bone or bony erosion, the distal fragment can be excised and the AC joint can be reconstructed utilizing a modified Weaver–Dunn procedure, where the coracoacromial ligament is transferred to the distal end of the remaining clavicle.[5] However, this represents a more historical option for adults rarely applied in this younger population.

SUMMARY, CONTROVERSIES, AND FUTURE DIRECTIONS RELATED TO DISTAL CLAVICLE FRACTURES

Most of the literature available on distal clavicle fractures is for the adult population. Typically, if a child or adolescent sustains a fracture in this region, immobilization alone is sufficient to obtain a successful outcome. In older adolescents, highly competitive athletes, or instances of severe posterior or superior displacement, operative intervention may be warranted. Suture-based periosteal repair or fixation in younger adolescents or preadolescents avoids hardware-related complications, but adequate stability must be ensured through meticulous technique. Utilization of a plate and screw construct also typically yields excellent results with a rapid return to function, a very high union rate, and a low complication rate. Further studies evaluating the treatment and outcomes of these fractures in the pediatric and adolescent are needed.

Scapula Fractures

INTRODUCTION TO SCAPULA FRACTURES

Scapula fractures are uncommon accounting for 1% of all fractures in adults with an even lower incidence in children.[53,145] Fractures involving the scapular body are most common, accounting for approximately 45% of scapula fractures. The remainder of fractures involve the glenoid neck (25%), glenoid cavity (10%), acromion process (8%), coracoid process (7%), and scapular spine (5%).[98,145] Very rarely, scapulothoracic dissociation can occur and has been reported in two separate case reports involving children, one child 8 years old and the other 11 years old.[4,112] Because of the low incidence of scapular fractures, mostly case report and retrospective small case series literature exist on their treatment and outcomes in the pediatric and adolescent populations.

ASSESSMENT OF SCAPULA FRACTURES

MECHANISMS OF INJURY FOR SCAPULA FRACTURES

When scapula body fractures occur in children, they are likely the result of either high-energy mechanisms, such as a fall from a height, ATV accidents or motor vehicle accidents, or the result of nonaccidental injury.[22,135] Bullock et al.[22] showed that scapula fractures had the highest risk of abuse for any fracture other than rib/sternum fractures, and when they were present, they were more than twice as likely to be associated with child abuse than not.

Glenoid fractures most commonly occur due to a direct force on the lateral shoulder, such as that occur during a fall or a collision sport. The force is transmitted to the humeral head, which then is driven into the glenoid surface.[24] An alternative mechanism of injury is a fall onto a flexed elbow.[90] The position of the arm at the time of injury will determine whether an anterior or posterior rim fracture occurs.[105]

Acromion fractures occur due to a direct blow to the lateral aspect of the shoulder, which typically occurs during a fall or a collision in sport.[98] It is imperative to recognize that complete failure of the epiphyses to fuse is a normal anatomic variant known as os acromiale, and should not be mistaken for a fracture.[89] If necessary, comparison radiographs of the contralateral side can be obtained to confirm this.

Coracoid fractures occur due to the pull of either the AC ligaments or the conjoint tendon. When the AC ligaments avulse the coracoid from the remainder of the scapula, the fracture occurs at the physis through the base of the coracoid and upper quarter of the glenoid.[58] In contrast, when the conjoint tendon avulses the coracoid from the scapula, the fracture occurs through the tip of the coracoid.[34]

INJURIES ASSOCIATED WITH SCAPULA FRACTURES

Whether scapula fractures occur due to high-energy mechanisms or nonaccidental trauma, associated injuries are common, including life-threatening injuries. Such injuries include closed head injuries, pneumo- or hemothorax, rib fractures, ruptured viscera, and concomitant long-bone fractures.[53,65,145] A recent analysis of high-energy pediatric scapula fractures due to motorized vehicle accidents found a higher Injury Severity Score (ISS) in the scapula fracture patients compared with a cohort of patients with similar high-energy motor vehicle accidents that did not have scapula fractures.[136] Almost half of all children admitted to the hospital for nonaccidental trauma have at least one fracture and approximately one-third had a diagnosis of contusion.[22] Concomitant neurovascular injury may also occur involving the brachial plexus, subclavian artery/vein, or axillary vessels. Finally, additional fractures or dislocations can occur about the shoulder girdle, particularly clavicle fractures, leading to a floating shoulder.[136]

SIGNS AND SYMPTOMS OF SCAPULA FRACTURES

Because of the large amount of force required to sustain a scapula fracture, a complete head-to-toe survey should be performed by either the trauma team or emergency room physician. Associated rib fractures or lung injury may cause difficulty breathing, whereas ruptured viscera will lead to an acute abdomen. In cases of suspected nonaccidental trauma, a complete evaluation needs to be performed including a head CT scan, an ophthalmologic examination, a skeletal survey, and a social work consultation.

Patients with scapula fractures will often complain of significant pain about their chest, back, and shoulder region. Numbness may be present because of concomitant brachial plexus injury or significant swelling. Observation for significant swelling and ecchymosis should begin the examination. Subsequently, a complete neurovascular examination of the involved upper extremity is necessary. Palpation should then be performed to determine the location of maximal tenderness as well as additional areas of tenderness, as concomitant shoulder girdle fractures can be present. A secondary survey should be performed by the orthopedic surgeon to ensure there are no additional musculoskeletal injuries.

IMAGING AND OTHER DIAGNOSTIC STUDIES FOR SCAPULA FRACTURES

Scapula fractures may initially be discovered on the chest x-ray obtained during the trauma work-up; however, additional imaging is necessary to fully evaluate the fracture. Plain radiographs including true AP and lateral scapula views as well as a glenohumeral axillary view should be obtained when a scapula fracture is suspected. In addition, because of the significant amount of overlying bony and soft tissue structures, a CT scan will enable the surgeon to fully understand the fracture pattern. The addition of reconstructions, including three-dimensional reconstructions, will aid in preoperative planning if operative intervention is being considered.

CLASSIFICATION OF SCAPULA FRACTURES

Scapula fractures are classified according to the fracture location within the scapula: body, glenoid cavity, glenoid neck, acromion, and coracoid. In addition, scapulothoracic dissociation is a term utilized to describe complete separation of the scapula from the posterior chest wall.

Glenoid Neck Fractures: CLASSIFICATION	
Type I	• Displaced <1 cm and angulated <40 degrees
Type II	• Displaced >1 cm and angulated >40 degrees

Glenoid neck fractures are further classified based on their displacement and angulation. A type I fracture is displaced less than 1 cm and angulated less than 40 degrees, whereas a type II fracture has more than 1 cm of displacement and is angulated greater than 40 degrees.[52] Type I fractures account for 90% of glenoid neck fractures.[2,164]

Glenoid Cavity Fractures: CLASSIFICATION	
Type Ia	• Fracture involving the anterior glenoid rim
Type Ib	• Fracture involving the posterior glenoid rim
Type II	• Transverse fracture line that divides the superior and inferior aspects of the glenoid and then exits inferiorly through the lateral scapular border
Type III	• Fracture line dividing the superior and inferior aspects of the glenoid, but exits superiorly near or through the scapular notch
Type IV	• Fracture line dividing the superior and inferior aspects of the glenoid, but exits medially through the medial border of the scapula
Type Va	• More than one fracture line involving a combination of types II and IV fractures
Type Vb	• More than one fracture line involving a combination of types III and IV fractures
Type Vc	• More than one fracture line involving a combination of types II, III, and IV fractures
Type VI	• Severely comminuted fractures

Glenoid cavity fractures are classified into six types based on the location of the fracture within the glenoid cavity and their severity (Fig. 19-11).[51,64] Type I fractures involve either the

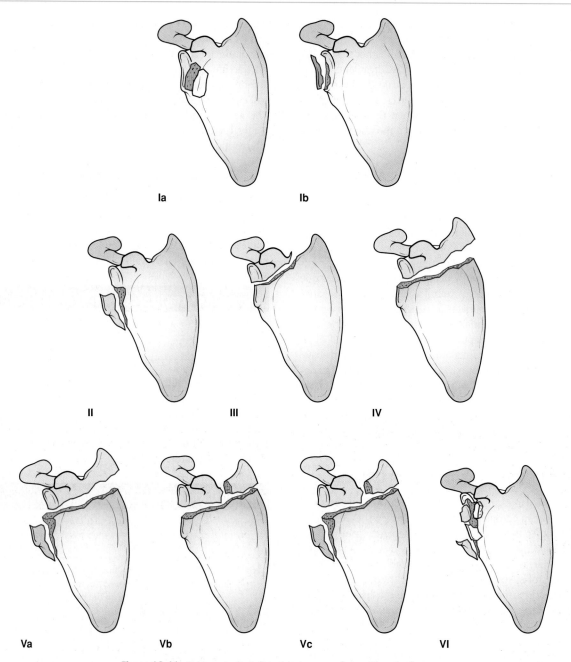

Figure 19-11. Schematic depicting the six types of glenoid cavity fractures.

anterior (type Ia) or posterior (type Ib) aspect of the glenoid rim. Type II fractures have a transverse fracture line that divides the superior and inferior aspects of the glenoid and then exits inferiorly through the lateral scapular border. Types III and IV fractures also begin with a fracture line dividing the superior and inferior aspects of the glenoid, but type III fractures exit superiorly near or through the scapular notch and type IV fractures exit medially through the medial border of the scapula. Type V fractures have more than one fracture line involving a combination of types II to IV and are further subclassified into a, b, and c. Type Va fractures are a combination of type II and IV fractures; type Vb fractures are a combination of types III and IV fractures; and type Vc fractures are a combination of types

II, III, and IV fractures. Finally, type VI fractures are severely comminuted fractures.

OUTCOME MEASURES FOR SCAPULA FRACTURES

No specific outcome measures exist for the evaluation of scapula fractures. Results in the adult literature utilize subjective complaints of pain, fracture displacement, residual deformity, nonunion, and development of posttraumatic arthritis as determinants for success.[38,76,81,96,113] Specific pediatric outcomes have not been developed but the goals of outcome are the same: restoration of motion, function, and strength without long-term limitations and/or pain.

PATHOANATOMY AND APPLIED ANATOMY RELATED TO SCAPULA FRACTURES

The scapula is a flat bone on the posterior aspect of the chest wall, covered almost entirely by muscle due to it having 17 muscular attachments on it. Only the dorsal aspect of the scapular spine and acromion are subcutaneous, and thus the remainder of the bone is deep and well protected from low-energy mechanisms of injury. Three articulations occur with the scapula; the acromion articulates with the clavicle at the AC joint; the proximal humerus articulates with the glenoid at the glenohumeral joint; and the posterior chest wall articulates with the anterior scapula to make up the scapulothoracic articulation.

TREATMENT OPTIONS FOR SCAPULA FRACTURES

NONOPERATIVE TREATMENT OF SCAPULA FRACTURES

Indications/Contraindications

Nonoperative Treatment of Scapula Fractures: INDICATIONS AND CONTRAINDICATIONS	
Indications	**Relative Contraindications**
• Nondisplaced or minimally displaced scapula body fractures	• Open fractures
• Acromion fractures	• Fractures with associated neurovascular injuries requiring surgical intervention
• Coracoid fractures with <2 cm of displacement	• Glenoid cavity fractures with >5 mm of intra-articular displacement
• Glenoid fractures with <1 cm of displacement and 40 degrees of angulation	• Large glenoid rim fractures with associated proximal humerus subluxation/dislocation
• Glenoid cavity fractures with <5 mm of intra-articular displacement	• Type II glenoid neck fractures
• Severely comminuted glenoid fractures unable to support stable fixation	

Most scapula fractures can be treated nonoperatively with immobilization alone, no matter what part of the scapula the fracture involves. Exceptions include open fractures, fractures with associated neurovascular injuries requiring operative intervention, scapulothoracic dissociation, large glenoid rim fractures with associated proximal humerus subluxation/dislocation, type II glenoid neck fractures, and glenoid cavity fractures with displacement greater than 5 mm.[2,4,76,112] All of these are very rare in children but need not be missed.

Techniques

A sling or shoulder immobilizer is used for 3 to 6 weeks depending on patient, injury severity, and healing. When there is sufficient healing and reduction in pain, rehabilitation progresses from pendulum exercises to full range of motion and strengthening. Return to sports is usually 8 to 12 weeks after injury.

Outcomes

No large studies exist regarding the outcomes of children treated for scapula fractures. In the adult literature, the vast majority of patients obtain fracture union and have minimal to no pain with good functional outcomes expected.[53,113] Similarly, most reports indicate children do well with this rare injury.

OPERATIVE TREATMENT OF SCAPULA FRACTURES

Indications/Contraindications

Operative indications for scapula fractures are limited in the pediatric and adolescent populations but include open fractures, fractures with associated neurovascular injuries requiring operative intervention, scapulothoracic dissociation, large glenoid rim fractures with associated proximal humerus subluxation/dislocation, type II glenoid neck fractures, coracoid process fractures with greater than 2 cm of displacement, and glenoid cavity fractures with displacement greater than 5 mm.[2,4,76,112] Floating shoulder injuries involving the midshaft of the clavicle and the glenoid neck can be treated by ORIF of the clavicle as the glenoid neck will reduce via ligamentotaxis provided by the intact CC ligament.[9] Similarly, floating shoulder injuries involving fractures of the glenoid neck, midshaft of the clavicle, and scapula spine will heal by ORIF of the clavicle and scapula spine due to ligamentotaxis provided by the intact CC and/or coracoacromial ligaments.[9] Nonoperative management with immobilization should be used for the remainder of injuries.

Open Reduction and Internal Fixation

Preoperative Planning

✔ ORIF of Scapula Fractures: PREOPERATIVE PLANNING CHECKLIST	
OR table	☐ Flattop Jackson table or standard OR table with the ability to go into beach chair position depending on the approach being utilized
Position/positioning aids	☐ Lateral decubitus in bean bag or beach chair
Fluoroscopy location	☐ Contralateral side of fracture
Equipment	☐ 2.7-mm or 3.5-mm plate/screw constructs; heavy nonabsorbable suture
Draping	☐ U-drapes

The position of the patient and necessary implants will depend on which part of the scapula is fractured. Typically, it is necessary to utilize plates that can be bent and twisted to match the shape of the scapula. Advanced imaging with three-dimensional reconstruction is helpful in planning for ORIF of scapula fractures.

Positioning

Patient positioning will depend on the location of the fracture within the scapula and subsequently the approach being used. If anterior exposure is necessary, the patient is placed in the beach chair position and a standard deltopectoral approach is performed. Posterior exposure is performed by having the patient in the lateral decubitus position in a bean bag, allowing the shoulder and trunk to droop slightly forward.

Surgical Approach

Anterior access to the glenoid and coracoid is performed through a standard deltopectoral approach. An incision is made along the deltopectoral groove from the coracoid proximally and carried 10 to 15 cm distally. Sharp dissection is carried out through the skin and the cephalic vein is identified in the deltopectoral groove. Subsequently, the deltoid is retracted laterally and the pectoralis major medially. The cephalic vein can be taken in either direction. Deep, the short head of the biceps and the coracobrachialis are identified and retracted in a medial direction. Access to the anterior aspect of the shoulder joint is now easily obtained. Typically, to have adequate exposure of the glenoid, the subscapularis must be taken down and a retractor placed in the glenohumeral joint to retract the humeral head.

If a posterior approach to the glenoid is being performed, a vertical incision is made overlying the posterior glenoid and full-thickness skin flaps are raised. Exposure of the glenoid is performed by splitting the deltoid longitudinally in line with its fibers. The infraspinatus and teres minor are now visible. These muscles can be partially or completely detached, or the interval between them can be utilized, depending on the amount of exposure necessary. Alternatively, a transverse incision can be performed along the length of the scapula spine, extending to the posterior corner of the acromion. The deltoid is then detached from its origin on the scapular spine and the plane between the deltoid and infraspinatus is identified and developed. Identification of the teres minor is now performed and the plane between the teres minor and infraspinatus is developed. By retracting the infraspinatus superiorly and the teres minor inferiorly, the posterior aspect of the glenoid and scapula neck is now exposed. The glenohumeral joint capsule can be incised longitudinally along the edge of the scapula to gain access to the joint.

Technique

✔ ORIF of Scapula Fractures:
KEY SURGICAL STEPS

Posterior Glenoid Cavity Fractures and Glenoid Neck Fractures
- [ ] Lateral decubitus position using bean bag
- [ ] Prep and drape entire upper extremity and hemithorax
- [ ] Posterior approach with arm abducted

- [ ] Retract posterior part of deltoid superolaterally without detaching its origin or insertion—the muscle can be detached if needed for improved visualization
- [ ] Identify and explore interval between the teres minor and infraspinatus by retracting the teres minor inferiorly and infraspinatus superiorly
- [ ] Detach infraspinatous insertion if necessary and incise capsule if fixing a glenoid cavity fracture
- [ ] Reduce fragment utilizing K-wires as joysticks and provisional fixation
- [ ] Fix fragment with either interfragmentary screws or plate/screw construct

Anterior Glenoid Cavity Fractures
- [ ] Beach chair position with Mayfield headrest
- [ ] Prep and drape entire upper extremity and hemithorax
- [ ] Standard deltopectoral approach
- [ ] Place stay sutures in subscapularis and detach muscle from humerus
- [ ] Longitudinal incision to enter glenohumeral joint
- [ ] Place Fuduka retractor on humeral head to expose glenoid
- [ ] Reduce fragment utilizing intact labrum or K-wires as joysticks and provisional fixation
- [ ] Fix fragment with either interfragmentary screws or plate/screw construct

Displaced Coracoid Process Fractures
- [ ] Beach chair position with Mayfield headrest
- [ ] Prep and drape entire upper extremity and hemithorax
- [ ] Standard deltopectoral approach
- [ ] Identify and protect musculocutaneous nerve
- [ ] Fix large coracoid process fractures with interfragmentary screw fixation
- [ ] Fix small coracoid process fractures using heavy nonabsorbable suture through the conjoint tendon and passed through a drill hole in the intact coracoid process

Displaced glenoid neck fractures are approached through the posterior approach with placement of a plate along the posterior aspect of the glenoid and extending down along the lateral angle of the scapula. Operative treatment of type Ib, type II, and type IV glenoid cavity fractures is also performed via a posterior approach. The infraspinatus can remain attached during fixation of type Ib fractures, whereas detachment is necessary for types II and IV fractures. Fixation of type Ib fragments is typically performed using two interfragmentary screws, whereas types II and IV fractures typically require plate and screw fixation.

An anterior deltopectoral approach is used to perform ORIF of type Ia and III glenoid cavity fractures as well as coracoid fractures displaced greater than 2 cm. Fixation is achieved with interfragmentary screws for type Ia and large coracoid process fractures if the fragment is large enough, whereas plate and screw fixation is typically necessary for type III fractures. Alternatively, suture anchors can be used to stabilize type Ia fragments and small coracoid process fractures can be reattached with the conjoint tendon utilizing heavy nonabsorbable suture placed in a Bunnell fashion through the tendon and passed through a drill hole in the intact coracoid process. Arthroscopic fixation of type Ia fractures can also be performed by using suture anchor fixation to the intact labral attachment of the fragment.[142]

Authors' Preferred Treatment for Scapula Fractures (Algorithm 19-2)

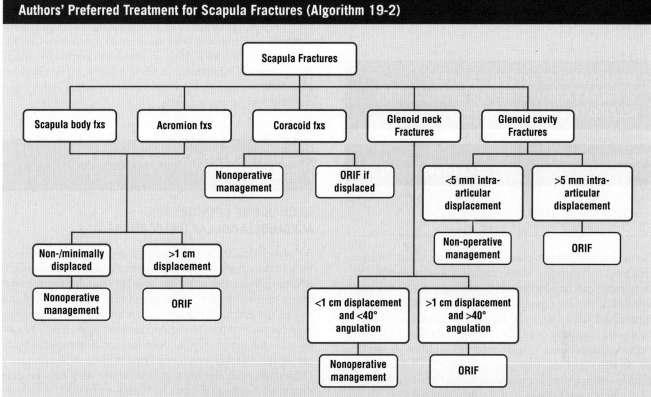

Algorithm 19-2. Authors' preferred treatment for scapula fractures.

Most pediatric and adolescent scapula fractures are treated nonoperatively with immobilization for 3 to 4 weeks followed by pendulum exercises and progressed to active range of motion as tolerated. This includes scapula body fractures, acromion fractures, coracoid process fractures, and glenoid neck and cavity fractures without significant displacement. Operative treatment is reserved for open fractures and glenoid cavity fractures with significant size and/or displacement leading to glenohumeral subluxation/dislocation.

Coracoid process fractures displaced greater than 2 cm are also treated with ORIF.

Our preference is to perform arthroscopic reduction of type Ia glenoid cavity fractures and ORIF for the remainder of glenoid cavity fractures and glenoid neck fractures requiring operative fixation. We routinely obtain three-dimensional CT scans to aid in preoperative planning and determination of the best surgical approach to utilize based on the fracture pattern.

Postoperative Care

Postoperatively, patients are placed in a sling or shoulder immobilizer for 3 to 6 weeks. Subsequently, pendulum exercises are performed followed by advancement to active range of motion based on radiographic union and pain. Strengthening and contact sports are not permitted for a minimum of 3 months postoperatively.

Potential Pitfalls and Preventive Measures

Scapula Fractures:
SURGICAL PITFALLS AND PREVENTIONS

Pitfall	Prevention
• Neurovascular injury	• Avoid overly vigorous retraction
• Persistent glenohumeral subluxation/dislocation	• Obtain near-anatomic (<2 mm incongruity) of glenoid cavity fragments

Care must be taken during ORIF when retracting structures about the shoulder region, as vigorous retraction can damage neurovascular structures. For example, the musculocutaneous nerve is at risk during excessive medial retraction about the glenohumeral joint/coracoid.

It is necessary to obtain a near-anatomic reduction of the articular surface during ORIF of glenoid cavity fractures as residual displacement greater than 2 mm leads to poorer outcomes.[76,96] Furthermore, failure to reduce large glenoid cavity fragments may lead to persistent glenohumeral subluxation/dislocation.

Outcomes

No data exist regarding the outcomes of pediatric and adolescent patients treated with ORIF for scapula fractures. The adult literature has demonstrated that the results of operative fixation of glenoid cavity fractures depend on near-anatomic restoration of joint alignment. If residual incongruity is less than 2 mm, good-to-excellent results can be expected for 80% to

90% of patients. Furthermore, posttraumatic arthritis will be minimal.[76,96]

Nonunion and symptomatic malunion can occur following treatment of scapular body fractures nonoperatively.[41,94,104] Nonunions can be addressed by performing ORIF with good-to-excellent results expected. In addition, significant displacement associated with glenoid neck fractures has been shown to be a poor prognostic indicator. Therefore, fixation of fractures with more than 1 cm of displacement or angulation greater than 40 degrees will yield improved outcomes.[38,81,113] Finally, large glenoid rim fractures should be addressed operatively to prevent subluxation/dislocation of the glenohumeral joint.

SUMMARY, CONTROVERSIES, AND FUTURE DIRECTIONS RELATED TO SCAPULA FRACTURES

Scapula fractures are rare injuries that occur due to high-energy mechanisms or nonaccidental trauma. Conservative treatment with immobilization yields excellent outcomes in the vast majority of cases. However, it is important to recognize fractures that can potentially lead to adverse outcomes and complications. Advanced imaging with CT scans, including three-dimensional reconstruction, can aid the surgeon by providing better understanding of the fracture pattern. Operative fixation should be performed for fractures about the glenoid with significant displacement or those leading to glenohumeral subluxation/dislocation. Because of the rarity of these fractures, it is likely that future multicenter studies will be necessary to provide information regarding the best treatments and their outcomes for pediatric and adolescent scapula fractures.

Acromioclavicular Dislocations

INTRODUCTION TO ACROMIOCLAVICULAR DISLOCATIONS

While AC dislocations are common in adults, they are rare in children. Injuries that appear to disrupt the AC joint in a child may actually be an epiphyseal separation of the distal clavicle termed a "pseudodislocation," rather than a true AC joint disruption.[133] However, older adolescents can sustain true AC dislocations, especially those involved in competitive sports participation.[35,74] Treatment of these injuries, especially complete dislocations, remains somewhat controversial and is based on individual patient demands.

ASSESSMENT OF ACROMIOCLAVICULAR DISLOCATIONS

MECHANISMS OF INJURY FOR ACROMIOCLAVICULAR DISLOCATIONS

Acromioclavicular joint injuries typically occur due to a direct blow to the acromion with the shoulder adducted, as can occur during collision sports, or due to a fall onto the superolateral aspect of the shoulder. The result of this blow is inferior and medial movement of the acromion while the clavicle remains stable because of the sternoclavicular joint ligaments.[127] Propagation of the force to the CC ligaments and deltotrapezial fascia can occur following complete disruption of the AC ligaments.[133] Indirect force can also result in injury to the AC joint, as occurs during a fall onto an outstretched hand or elbow.[137]

INJURIES ASSOCIATED WITH ACROMIOCLAVICULAR DISLOCATIONS

As with any injury to the shoulder region, the entire shoulder girdle must be examined for a concomitant injury. Anterior sternoclavicular dislocations or additional scapula, humerus, or clavicle fractures can occur simultaneously if enough force was present at the time of impact. In addition, brachial plexus or cervical spine injuries may be present, especially if the injury occurred during a collision sport, such as football.

SIGNS AND SYMPTOMS OF ACROMIOCLAVICULAR DISLOCATIONS

Patients with AC dislocations usually complain of pain in the shoulder region localized to the AC joint area. Numbness and tingling may be present because of swelling or concomitant cervical spine/brachial plexus injury. Sometimes, they only complain of a "bump" in the region.

The physical examination should begin by observation of the shoulder region with the patient in an upright position, which permits the weight of the arm to make any deformity more apparent. Swelling, ecchymosis, abrasions, and skin tenting should be noted. Palpation overlying the AC joint will cause significant discomfort and should be reserved until the end of the examination. Additional areas that should be palpated first include the proximal humerus, the midshaft and medial clavicle, the sternoclavicular joint, and the cervical spine. A thorough neurologic examination should be performed to assess for concomitant brachial plexus or cervical spine injury. Most displaced distal clavicle fractures are malpositioned superiorly and have both visual and palpable deformities. However, some displace posteriorly, get entrapped in the trapezius muscle, and have a palpable prominence and tenderness medial and posterior to the acromion. These type IV injuries may be hard to diagnose unless examined specifically.

Once an AC injury is suspected, the joint should be assessed for stability if possible. Typically, this needs to be done after the acute pain has subsided, approximately 5 to 7 days following the injury. Horizontal and vertical stabilities can be assessed and potentially the joint can be reduced by closed means. This is performed by stabilizing the clavicle with one hand and using the other hand to place an upward force under the ipsilateral elbow. Once the joint is reduced in the coronal plane, the midshaft of the clavicle can be grasped and translated in an anterior and posterior direction to assess horizontal stability.[137]

IMAGING AND OTHER DIAGNOSTIC STUDIES FOR ACROMIOCLAVICULAR DISLOCATIONS

Plain radiographs are the initial imaging modality of choice and should include a true AP view of the shoulder, an axillary lateral view of the shoulder, and a Zanca view to better visualize the AC joint. The Zanca view is performed with the patient in an upright position, allowing the injured arm to hang by the weight of gravity, and aiming the x-ray beam 10 to 15 degrees cephalad.[163] In addition, stress views can be performed, to differentiate between types II and III injuries, by having the patient hold a weight in each hand, with a single radiograph of the bilateral clavicles obtained. The posterior fracture dislocation (type IV) is often difficult to recognize by plain radiographs and may require a CT scan for accurate diagnosis.

CLASSIFICATION OF ACROMIOCLAVICULAR DISLOCATIONS

The classic description of acromioclavicular injuries for adults is that of Tossy et al.[148] and Allman[3] which was subsequently modified by Rockwood and colleagues (Fig. 19-12).[157] Type I injuries have normal radiographs with the only finding being tenderness to palpation over the AC joint due to a sprain of the AC ligaments. Type II injuries have disruption of the AC ligaments and a sprain of the CC ligaments. The radiographs show a widened AC joint with slight vertical displacement demonstrated by a mild increase in the CC space. Type III injuries have disruption of the AC and CC ligaments with the radiographs showing the clavicle displaced superiorly relative to the acromion by 25% to 100% the width of the clavicle. Type IV injuries have disruption of the AC and CC ligaments as well as the deltopectoral fascia which allows for the clavicle to be posteriorly displaced into or through the trapezius muscle. Type V injuries have disruption of the AC and CC ligaments as well as the deltopectoral fascia with concomitant injury to the deltoid and trapezius muscle attachments to the clavicle. These injuries present with the clavicle displaced greater than 100% and lying in the subcutaneous tissue. Type VI injuries have disruption of the AC ligaments and deltopectoral fascia, but the CC ligaments remain intact. This occurs due to a high-energy mechanism of injury that causes the shoulder to be hyperabducted and externally rotated. The end result is that the clavicle lies subacromial

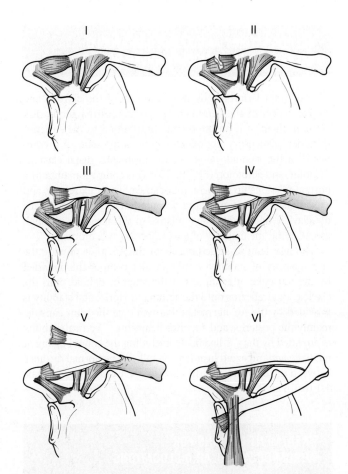

Figure 19-12. Schematic depicting the Rockwood classification of acromioclavicular joint injuries.

or subcoracoid, with a resultant decrease in the CC distance seen on radiographs.

The classification mentioned above has been modified for the pediatric and adolescent populations as true AC injuries are rare during skeletal immaturity compared with fractures of the distal clavicle.[35] Typically, the clavicle itself displaces out of the periosteal sleeve, leaving the periosteum attached to the CC and AC ligaments. The resultant clavicle injuries are then analogous to the six types described for the adult classification.

OUTCOME MEASURES FOR ACROMIOCLAVICULAR DISLOCATIONS

Typically, results of AC injuries have been reported based on subjective outcomes, the development of AC osteoarthritis, and range of motion. No outcome measures have been specifically applied to pediatric acromioclavicular injuries. Commonly utilized measures for adult AC joint injuries include the ASES score, the DASH Score, the QuickDASH, and the Constant Shoulder Score. The recent publication of a novel Pedi-ASES demonstrated that adult shoulder outcome scores such as the DASH and ASES surveys are associated with poor validity and comprehensibility in pediatric populations, and this new metric, when more comprehensively validated, may emerge as a future standard for use in pediatric and adolescent shoulder research.[59]

PATHOANATOMY AND APPLIED ANATOMY RELATED TO ACROMIOCLAVICULAR DISLOCATIONS

The AC joint is formed by the distal end of the clavicle and medial aspect of the acromion with a fibrocartilaginous disk between them. It is an important contribution to the superior shoulder suspensory complex, a bone–soft tissue ring composed of the glenoid, coracoid, CC ligaments, distal clavicle, AC joint, and acromion (Fig. 19-13). This complex maintains a normal relationship between the scapula, upper extremity, and axial skeleton to permit fluid scapulothoracic motion. While the clavicle does rotate some relative to the acromion through the AC joint, the majority of motion occurs synchronously.[42]

The ligamentous structures about the AC joint provide the vast majority of stability with a smaller component provided by the muscular attachments of the anterior deltoid onto the clavicle and trapezius onto the acromion. Horizontal stability is provided by the AC ligaments that reinforce the joint capsule, mainly the posterior and superior ligaments.[79] Vertical stability is provided by the CC ligaments, including the conoid ligament medially and trapezoid ligament laterally.[45] The normal distance between the coracoid and the clavicle, the CC space, should be 1.1 to 1.3 cm.[16]

TREATMENT OPTIONS FOR ACROMIOCLAVICULAR DISLOCATIONS

NONOPERATIVE TREATMENT OF ACROMIOCLAVICULAR DISLOCATIONS

Nonoperative treatment of types I and II AC injuries is uniformly accepted. However, treatment of type III injuries remains somewhat controversial. The vast majority of types IV, V, and VI injuries should be treated surgically to reduce the AC joint and restore stability to the superior shoulder suspensory complex. Absolute contraindications to nonoperative treatment include open injuries and injuries with associated neurovascular injury requiring operative intervention.

Techniques

Nonoperative treatment is performed using immobilization in a sling or shoulder immobilizer for 2 to 4 weeks. Following the period of immobilization and resolution of the pain, patients are gradually progressed from pendulum exercises to active range of motion. Strengthening is begun once range of motion is equal to the uninjured side. Contact sports are avoided for 6 to 12 weeks following injury to allow for complete ligamentous healing and for prevention of converting an incomplete injury (type II) to a complete injury (type III).[137]

Little published data exist regarding the nonoperative treatment of types I and II injuries in the pediatric and adolescent populations. The adult literature has demonstrated a 9% to 30% rate of pain and limitation of activities with closed treatment of type I injuries and a 23% to 42% rate for closed treatment of type II injuries, some of which required surgical intervention.[17,106] Children and adolescents seem to do better in terms of pain and restoration of function but it has not been studied extensively.

Treatment of type III injuries remains controversial because of the outcomes demonstrated in the adult literature. Bannister et al.[12] found that injuries with 2 cm or more of displacement treated nonsurgically had 20% good or excellent results compared with 70% in the surgically treated group. However, a study involving athletes and laborers with type III injuries treated nonoperatively showed that they were able to recover adequate strength and endurance to return to their preinjury activities.[159] A meta-analysis by Phillips et al.[120] supported nonoperative treatment of type III injuries as patients treated surgically had a higher complication rate, with patients treated nonoperatively able to return to work and preinjury activities faster.

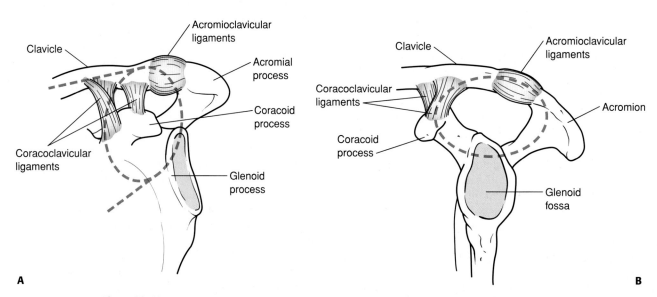

A   **B**

Figure 19-13. Schematic of the superior shoulder suspensory complex. **A:** Frontal view. **B:** Lateral view.

Indications/Contraindications

Nonoperative Treatment of Acromioclavicular Dislocations: INDICATIONS AND CONTRAINDICATIONS

Indications	Relative Contraindications
• Type I injuries	• Open injuries
• Type II injuries	• Injuries with associated neurovascular injuries requiring operative treatment

OPERATIVE TREATMENT OF ACROMIOCLAVICULAR DISLOCATIONS

Indications/Contraindications

Indications for operative treatment of AC injuries include complete disruptions of the joint, leading to true dislocations in adolescents or fracture dislocations in the pediatric population, mainly types IV, V, and VI injuries. The most common operative indication in the young is a type IV injury with displacement and entrapment in the trapezius muscle posteriorly. In addition, an injury that is open or has a concomitant neurovascular injury requiring operative intervention should be treated operatively. As noted above, the treatment of type III injuries is somewhat controversial.

Open Reduction and Internal Fixation

Preoperative Planning

ORIF of Acromioclavicular Dislocations: PREOPERATIVE PLANNING CHECKLIST

OR table	☐ Standard table capable of going into beach chair position
Position/positioning aids	☐ Beach chair position with adequate sterile space above the shoulder adjacent to the head
Fluoroscopy location	☐ Contralateral side
Equipment	☐ Implants may include hook plate, cannulated screws, K-wires, heavy nonabsorbable suture, hamstring autograft, allograft

Treatment of AC injuries surgically requires planning to ensure that the appropriate equipment is available. If implants are being utilized, these may include a hook plate, cannulated screws, K-wires, or heavy nonabsorbable suture. Reconstruction of the ligaments, however, requires either planning to obtain hamstring autograft or having allograft available.

Positioning

Whether open reduction or ligament reconstruction is being performed, the beach chair position is utilized. A bump is placed behind the scapula to bring the acromion into a more anterior position.

Surgical Approach

A direct approach to the AC joint is used by making an incision along the lateral clavicle and anterior aspect of the joint in Langer skin lines. Sharp dissection is carried out through the skin only. Subsequently, electrocautery is utilized the remainder of the way down to bone so that hemostasis and dissection can occur simultaneously. It is easiest to incise the periosteum of the distal clavicle and acromion before entering the joint. It is imperative to avoid disruption of the CC ligaments in type VI injuries as they are intact. The AC and CC ligaments as well as the deltopectoral fascia are disrupted in types II, IV, and V injuries in the skeletally mature patients; they are attached to the periosteum in younger patients.

Technique

ORIF of Acromioclavicular Dislocations: KEY SURGICAL STEPS

☐ Skin incision in Langer line directly anterior to acromioclavicular joint
☐ Electrocautery down to distal clavicle and acromion
☐ Reduce acromioclavicular joint
☐ Repair periosteum and ligamentous structures and assess stability
☐ Use hook plate if joint remains unstable for segmental fractures or intra-articular fractures
☐ Place lateral end of hook plate under acromion and facilitate AC joint reduction by placing medial part of plate on clavicle
☐ Place bicortical screws in medial part of hook plate
☐ Irrigate wound and close
☐ Plate removal 2–3 months postoperatively

Once the dissection has exposed the AC joint, an open reduction of the joint is performed. Type IV injuries necessitate carefully extracting the distal clavicle from the trapezius muscle, type V injuries require reducing the distal clavicle from the subcutaneous tissue, and type VI injuries require removing the distal clavicle from beneath the coracoid process. Once the distal clavicle is reduced to the level of the acromion, temporary pin fixation may be necessary to hold the reduction. As the periosteum is torn but still attached to the acromion, once the clavicle is reduced, simple repair of the periosteum and ligamentous structures may be all that is required in the pediatric population.

If the patient is older and a hook plate is being utilized, the lateral end of the plate is placed deep to the acromion and the medial side is placed on the clavicle, which will facilitate joint reduction and maintenance of the reduction. Bicortical screws are now placed into the clavicle to hold the plate in place.

Ligament reconstruction and/or augmentation have been performed, via various methods, as the primary method of treatment for the injury in adults. Fortunately, these operations are rare in the acute setting for adolescents. More often these reconstructions are in chronic, painful AC separations in adults. Both semitendinosus autograft and allograft can be used as a loop around the coracoid and clavicle[69] or placed through bone tunnels in the coracoid and clavicle and secured with interference screws.[97] The interference screws are placed at the locations of the CC ligaments in an attempt to restore normal anatomy.

Coracoclavicular screw placement or loops of heavy nonabsorbable suture/Dacron tape around the coracoid and clavicle has also been described to treat AC injuries, either by itself or in conjunction with ligament reconstruction.[19] Screw placement requires removal whereas the loop technique can lead to suture cutout or aseptic foreign body reactions.[18,141] The modified Weaver Dunn procedure has been performed in arthritic situations by resecting the distal end of the clavicle, detaching the coracoacromial ligament from the deep surface of the acromion, and transferring it to the distal end of the clavicle. Again, this is very rarely performed in children and adolescents.

Author's Preferred Treatment for Acromioclavicular Dislocations

We treat all types I and II AC injuries as well as most type III injuries nonoperatively, with immobilization in a sling or shoulder immobilizer for 2 to 4 weeks followed by early restoration of range of motion. Contact sports are avoided for at least 6 to 12 weeks. The vast majority of types IV, V, and VI injuries are treated operatively. Once the distal clavicle is exposed, we determine whether repair of the periosteum and ligamentous structures surrounding the clavicle is sufficient or if a plate is required. The vast majority can be treated with periosteal repair over the reduced clavicle. Most often operative repair is for type IV fracture–dislocations with entrapment in the trapezius. Hook plates are most commonly utilized in older patients with fractures that are either segmental or intra-articular. Following plate placement, the periosteum and ligamentous structures are repaired.

Postoperative Care

Postoperatively, patients are placed in either a sling or shoulder immobilizer for 4 to 6 weeks. Pendulum exercises are then begun followed by gentle active range of motion below shoulder level for 6 to 8 weeks. At 8 weeks, full active range of motion is permitted. If a hook plate or CC screw was placed, it is removed with sufficient healing, usually at approximately 12 weeks. Contact sports are avoided for a minimum of 3 months following operative intervention.

Potential Pitfalls and Preventive Measures

Acromioclavicular Dislocations:
SURGICAL PITFALLS AND PREVENTIONS

Pitfall	Prevention
• Missing a type IV injury	• Careful assessment of the radiographs • Adequate lateral radiograph • Utilize physical examination to aid in the diagnosis • CT scan

One of the biggest pitfalls when treating AC injuries is failure to recognize a type IV injury. Although types V and VI injuries are fairly obvious on AP plain radiographs, type IV injuries, because of their posterior displacement, may not be readily apparent. Furthermore, lateral views may be inadequate or difficult to obtain, thus making it easy to miss a type IV injury. A high index of clinical suspicion, careful examination, and often a CT scan are necessary for accurate diagnosis and appropriate surgical treatment.

Outcomes

No studies have specifically evaluated the treatment of AC injuries in the pediatric and adolescent populations. In our experience, operative treatment of types IV, V, and VI injuries has yielded excellent outcomes in the majority of patients. Restoration of joint congruity and stability permits rapid return to function. However, we do not have long-term data to determine how many patients develop degenerative arthritis.

MANAGEMENT OF EXPECTED ADVERSE OUTCOMES AND UNEXPECTED COMPLICATIONS RELATED TO ACROMIOCLAVICULAR DISLOCATIONS

Acromioclavicular Dislocations:
COMMON ADVERSE OUTCOMES AND COMPLICATIONS

- Posttraumatic arthritis
- Persistent instability
- Symptomatic hardware
- Pin migration
- Persistent pain
- Suture cutout
- Aseptic foreign body reaction

Development of degenerative arthritis can be treated by distal clavicle resection. However, the results of this are not favorable if the CC ligaments are disrupted as instability will ensue.[31] Persistent instability following closed treatment of an AC joint injury can be treated with ligament reconstruction or augmentation.

Complications related to open reduction include migration of pins, symptomatic hardware, and persistent pain. As noted earlier, usage of synthetic material can lead to suture cutout or aseptic foreign material reaction. Any technique that passes material around the coracoid may lead to coracoid fracture or injury to the musculocutaneous nerve.

SUMMARY, CONTROVERSIES, AND FUTURE DIRECTIONS RELATED TO ACROMIOCLAVICULAR DISLOCATIONS

AC injuries are relatively rare in the pediatric and adolescent populations. The injury patterns are classified similar to the adult population. However, in the young, the periosteum tears permitting the clavicle to displace while the periosteal attachment to the acromion and coracoid remains intact.

Treatment can be immobilization alone for injuries that are not widely displaced, but operative intervention should be performed for significantly displaced injuries. Restoration of normal anatomy by reduction of the AC joint, suture repair of the periosteum, and ligamentous repair as needed can yield excellent outcomes in the pediatric population while avoiding utilization of metal implants. Future studies are necessary to assess outcomes of these injuries in the pediatric and adolescent populations.

Sternoclavicular Fracture–Dislocations

INTRODUCTION TO STERNOCLAVICULAR FRACTURE–DISLOCATIONS

Injuries to the sternoclavicular joint are rare, representing less than 5% of shoulder girdle injuries.[27,66] These injuries occur secondary to high-energy mechanisms and therefore can be associated with life-threatening complications. Historically, treatment by observation has occurred in the pediatric and adolescent populations. More recent trends are to operatively reduce and stabilize acute posterior fracture–dislocations to restore anatomy and improve functional outcomes.

ASSESSMENT OF STERNOCLAVICULAR FRACTURE–DISLOCATIONS

MECHANISMS OF INJURY FOR STERNOCLAVICULAR FRACTURE–DISLOCATIONS

A significant amount of force is required to disrupt the sternoclavicular joint because of the numerous surrounding ligaments as well as the stability provided by the rib cage. Therefore, high-energy mechanisms, such as motor vehicle accidents and sports participation, result in greater than 80% of injuries.[21,111,154] Sports injuries are the most common mechanism of injury (71%), with football, rugby, and wrestling being the most commonly involved sports.[144] Motor vehicle collisions may result in either an anterior or posterior force across the joint with a resultant anterior or posterior dislocation or fracture/dislocation.[57,103] A direct lateral blow to the shoulder with the shoulder extended will result in the more common anterior dislocation. Posterior dislocations can result from indirect force transferred to the shoulder girdle when the shoulder is adducted and flexed. Alternatively, a direct anterior-to-posterior blow to the medial clavicle is another mechanism for posterior sternoclavicular dislocation during sports participation.[55] Of note, most cases of anterior sternoclavicular instability are atraumatic and associated with ligamentous laxity.

INJURIES ASSOCIATED WITH STERNOCLAVICULAR FRACTURE–DISLOCATIONS

Because of the high-energy mechanisms that cause posterior sternoclavicular injuries, associated chest wall injuries do occur such as rib fractures. In addition, the trachea, esophagus, lungs, or great vessels may be compressed. Dysphagia or dyspnea is present in up to 30% of patients.[144] Patients may also experience a brachial plexopathy. Life-threatening injuries, including vessel laceration, stroke, pneumomediastinum, or even death can occur but are rare. Very rarely, the entire clavicle may dislocate from both the sternoclavicular joint and AC joint, thus constituting a floating shoulder. It is imperative to carefully evaluate the entire shoulder girdle for concomitant fractures or dislocations.

SIGNS AND SYMPTOMS OF STERNOCLAVICULAR FRACTURE–DISLOCATIONS

Patients who sustain sternoclavicular joint injuries present with complaints of pain localized to the sternoclavicular joint. Additional subjective complaints may include shortness of breath, dyspnea, dysphagia, odynophagia, or hoarseness.[155] If an associated brachial plexopathy is present, patients may report the presence of paresthesias and/or weakness in the ipsilateral arm.

Objective evaluation will demonstrate a significant amount of swelling and ecchymosis present, so much so, that it may be difficult to determine the direction of the dislocation.[55] Anterior dislocations may exhibit prominence of the medial clavicle, which is more easily appreciated with the patient supine (Fig. 19-14).[55] In contrast, the corner of the sternum may be palpable in cases of posterior dislocation, as the medial clavicle is displaced posteriorly.[111] However, at times, the posterior fracture dislocation can be more subtle than expected as the swelling can mimic normal sternoclavicular alignment on cursory examination.

Passive range of motion of the ipsilateral shoulder will cause pain and may elicit the sensation of instability. It is imperative that a formal trauma team or emergency room physician

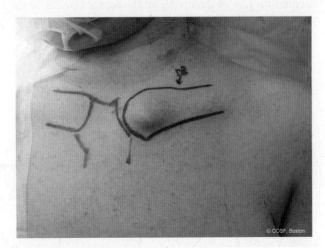

Figure 19-14. Clinical photograph demonstrating an anterior sternoclavicular dislocation. This was more easily identified once the patient was lying supine. (Reprinted with permission from Waters PM, Bae DS, eds. *Pediatric Hand and Upper Limb Surgery: A Practical Guide.* 1st ed. Philadelphia, PA: Wolters Kluwer Health/Lippincott Williams & Wilkins; 2012.)

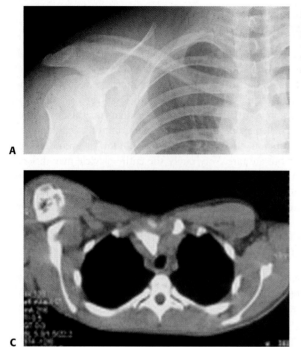

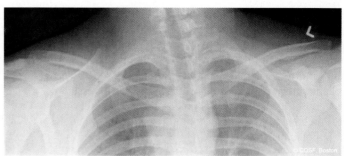

Figure 19-15. A: Apparent normal anteroposterior (AP) view of the clavicle. **B:** Serendipity view demonstrating asymmetry of the sternoclavicular joint with a posterior dislocation on the right. **C:** CT scan clearly showing the right posterior sternoclavicular dislocation. (Reprinted with permission from Waters PM, Bae DS, eds. *Pediatric Hand and Upper Limb Surgery: A Practical Guide.* 1st ed. Philadelphia, PA: Wolters Kluwer Health/Lippincott Williams & Wilkins; 2012.)

evaluation occurs to rule out associated life-threatening injuries. Signs of venous congestion and arterial insufficiency to the involved extremity or neck region may be present due to compression of vessels.

IMAGING AND OTHER DIAGNOSTIC STUDIES FOR STERNOCLAVICULAR FRACTURE–DISLOCATIONS

As with any injury, plain radiographs are the initial imaging modality performed. The routine AP chest radiograph may demonstrate asymmetry of the sternoclavicular articulations or clavicle lengths. However, these studies can be quite difficult to interpret because of the overlap of the medial clavicle, lungs, ribs, sternum, and spine (Fig. 19-15).

Specific radiographic views to evaluate the sternoclavicular joint have been described to overcome these obstacles. Heinig described a tangential view of the sternoclavicular joint which is obtained by laying the patient supine and placing the cassette behind the opposite shoulder. The beam is then angled coronally, parallel to the longitudinal axis of the opposite clavicle (Fig. 19-16A).[57] Hobbs[62] proposed taking a 90-degree cephalocaudal lateral view, by having the patient seated and flexed over a table while the beam is directed through the cervical spine (Fig. 19-16B). Finally, the serendipity view described by Rockwood is performed by placing the cassette behind the chest and angling the x-ray beam 40 degrees cephalad while it is centered on the sternum, thus providing a view of both sternoclavicular joints (Fig. 19-16C).[158] In cases of anterior dislocation, the

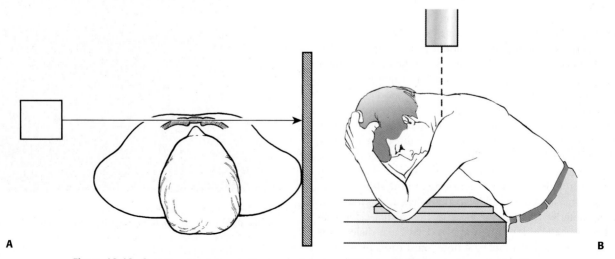

Figure 19-16. A: Schematic demonstrating tangential view of Heinig. **B:** Schematic demonstrating the 90-degree cephalocaudal lateral of Hobbs.

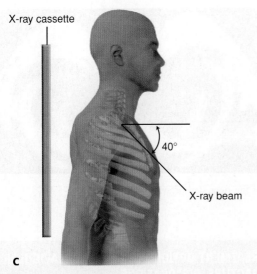

Figure 19-16. (*Continued*) **C:** Schematic demonstrating a serendipity view of Rockwood. (Reprinted with permission from Waters PM, Bae DS, eds. *Pediatric Hand and Upper Limb Surgery: A Practical Guide.* 1st ed. Philadelphia, PA: Wolters Kluwer Health/Lippincott Williams & Wilkins; 2012.)

affected side will appear superiorly displaced, whereas in cases of posterior dislocation, the affected side will appear inferiorly displaced (Fig. 19-17).

Despite these described plain radiographic views, the easiest way to evaluate the sternoclavicular joint is with computed tomography (CT) scan which provides a three-dimensional view of the joint (Fig. 19-18). In addition to assessment of the sternoclavicular joint, one can evaluate the adjacent soft tissue structures including the esophagus, trachea, lungs, and brachiocephalic vessels. Distinction between a physeal fracture and a true dislocation may also be possible if the secondary center has ossified.

Magnetic resonance imaging can also be utilized to evaluate the sternoclavicular joint as well as the surrounding soft tissues. The integrity of the costoclavicular ligaments and intra-articular disk may be possible.[55] Despite the potential

to gain additional information, CT scan is recommended over MRI scan to evaluate acute injuries because of its speed and availability.

CLASSIFICATION OF STERNOCLAVICULAR FRACTURE–DISLOCATIONS

Sternoclavicular dislocations are classified based on the direction of displacement, anterior or posterior, as well as the chronicity of the injury, acute or chronic. The injury needs to be defined as a dislocation (displacement between the epiphysis and the sternum) or a fracture (displacement through the physis with the epiphysis still articulating with sternum). In addition, a sprain, rather than a true dislocation, may occur leading to subluxation.

OUTCOME MEASURES FOR STERNOCLAVICULAR FRACTURE–DISLOCATIONS

No specific outcome scores exist that specifically evaluate sternoclavicular joint injuries. Results reported have assessed subjective complaints of pain, recurrence of instability, return to function, and utilization of adult shoulder outcome measures, such as the ASES score, the simple shoulder test, and Rockwood scores.

PATHOANATOMY AND APPLIED ANATOMY RELATED TO STERNOCLAVICULAR FRACTURE–DISLOCATIONS

The sternoclavicular joint is a true diarthrodial joint comprising the medial clavicle and clavicular notch of the sternum. Thus, this joint is the only connection between the axial skeleton and the upper extremity. However, less than 50% of the clavicular head articulates with the clavicular notch of the sternum, resulting in little bony congruity. Stability is therefore provided by the multiple ligamentous and muscular attachments, including the sternocleidomastoid, pectoralis major,

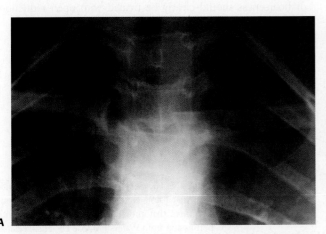
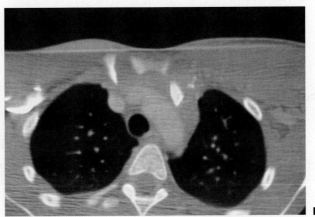

Figure 19-17. A: Serendipity radiograph showing a left posteriorly dislocated sternoclavicular joint. Note that the affected side appears inferiorly displaced. **B:** CT scan of the same patient clearly showing the left posterior dislocation.

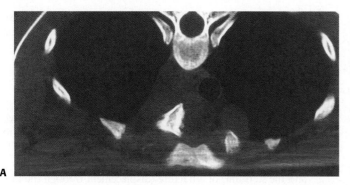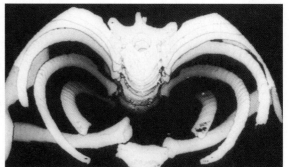

A   **B**

Figure 19-18. A: CT scan showing a posterior dislocation of the right sternoclavicular joint. **B:** Three-dimensional reconstruction makes the injury more apparent.

and sternohyoid muscles. The ligamentous structures include anterior and posterior sternoclavicular ligaments which reinforce the joint capsule as well as the interclavicular (connects both medial ends of the clavicle) and costoclavicular ligaments (between the inferior aspect of the clavicle and the superior costal cartilage of the adjacent rib). In addition, there is an intra-articular disk that is attached to the superior-posterior part of the clavicular articular surface and inferiorly to the costocartilaginous junction of the first rib (Fig. 19-19). The greatest amount of stability with regard to anterior translation is provided by the posterior capsule and sternoclavicular ligaments. The greatest stability with regard to posterior translation is provided by the posterior capsule.[138,139]

The medial epiphysis of the clavicle does not ossify until approximately 18 to 20 years of age, and closes between 22 and 25 years of age. Therefore, sternoclavicular injuries occurring in pediatric and adolescent patients are difficult to discern radiographically between fractures and dislocations. Operative treatment of posterior sternoclavicular injuries has taught us that dislocations and physeal fractures have near equivalent incidence rather than the previous teaching that most posterior sternoclavicular injuries were physeal fractures. Although the medial physis contributes approximately 80% of longitudinal growth of the clavicle, the degree of remodeling possible from a physeal fracture is uncertain. Clearly remodeling cannot occur with a dislocation.

TREATMENT OPTIONS FOR STERNOCLAVICULAR FRACTURE–DISLOCATIONS

NONOPERATIVE TREATMENT OF STERNOCLAVICULAR DISLOCATIONS

Indications/Contraindications

Nonoperative Treatment of Sternoclavicular Fracture–Dislocations: INDICATIONS AND CONTRAINDICATIONS	
Indications	**Relative Contraindications**
• Atraumatic anterior dislocations	• Acute posterior dislocations with associated neurovascular injury, dyspnea, dysphagia, odynophagia, or hoarseness

An atraumatic anterior dislocation should be treated nonoperatively. Some have advocated closed reduction maneuvers be performed for acute posterior fracture–dislocations due to potential stability of reduction and/or remodeling of the medial clavicle.[85,158] Acute posterior dislocations with associated neurovascular injury, dyspnea, dysphagia, odynophagia, or hoarseness should clearly be treated with open reduction.

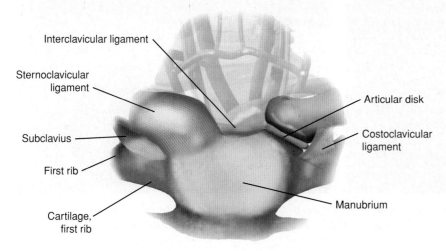

Interclavicular ligament

Sternoclavicular ligament

Subclavius

First rib

Cartilage, first rib

Articular disk

Costoclavicular ligament

Manubrium

Figure 19-19. Schematic drawing of the sternoclavicular joint. Note the numerous ligamentous structures that provide stability. (Reprinted with permission from Waters PM, Bae DS, eds. *Pediatric Hand and Upper Limb Surgery: A Practical Guide.* 1st ed. Philadelphia, PA: Wolters Kluwer Health/Lippincott Williams & Wilkins; 2012.)

We advocate that all posterior fracture–dislocations should be treated operatively.

Techniques

Closed treatment of a nondisplaced injury consists of sling immobilization for approximately 3 weeks followed by gradual return to activities. Attempted closed reduction of anterior dislocations can be performed by placing a posteriorly directed force over the medial clavicle as the scapula is retracted by utilization of a bump placed between the shoulders. Subsequently, the patient is placed in a figure-of-eight strap or Velpeau-type sling for 6 weeks.[55] Successful reduction can often be obtained; however, recurrent instability is common.

Closed reduction of a posterior dislocation is performed by placing the patient supine on an operating room table with a thick bump placed between the scapulae to extend the shoulders and the involved arm off the edge of the table. The ipsilateral arm is then abducted in line with the clavicle, with traction applied, while an assistant applies countertraction and stabilizes the patient. Traction is continued and increased and the arm is brought into extension as the joint reduces.[55] Alternatively, the arm can be placed in adduction while posterior pressure is applied to the shoulder which levers the clavicle over the first rib to permit reduction of the joint.[20] If these maneuvers fail, a sterile towel clip can be used to percutaneously grasp the medial clavicle and draw it anteriorly while traction is applied to the ipsilateral limb. An audible snap is typically noted as the joint reduces.[55]

Closed reductions of posterior sternoclavicular injuries are at risk for mediastinal hemorrhage and hemodynamic compromise. Therefore, closed reductions are performed in the controlled setting of the operating suite with vascular surgery standby. In addition, the orthopedic concern with closed reduction is recurrent instability.[50,56,155]

Outcomes

Most patients treated with immobilization alone for anterior dislocations yield good outcomes, despite the high rates of recurrent instability.[36] Those patients who develop symptoms following closed treatment of anterior dislocations may achieve relief of symptoms with physical therapy to promote scapular retraction and avoid provocative positions. If therapy is unsuccessful, ligament reconstruction can be performed with reasonable outcomes anticipated.[7,23,139]

Posterior fracture–dislocations that are reduced by closed means have been reported by some to be stable following reduction,[56] whereas others have shown recurrent instability does occur.[50,56,84,155] If the reduction is maintained over time, return to full activities can be expected in the majority of patients.[144]

OPERATIVE TREATMENT OF STERNOCLAVICULAR FRACTURE–DISLOCATIONS

Indications/Contraindications

Although many surgeons have attempted closed treatment of posterior fracture–dislocations with either immobilization alone or closed reduction followed by immobilization, recurrent instability can occur leading to symptomatic patients who require operative

intervention.[13] Therefore, the majority of patients with acute traumatic posterior sternoclavicular fracture–dislocations are currently treated operatively. Operative intervention provides symptomatic relief, restores anatomy, and decreases the chance of late complications including recurrent instability and degenerative arthritis.[155]

Additional indications for operative treatment include patients with symptomatic acute or chronic anterior dislocations who have failed conservative measures and symptomatic patients with chronic posterior dislocations. Contraindications to operative intervention include those patients with asymptomatic anterior dislocations or patients with atraumatic recurrent anterior instability.

Open Reduction and Internal Fixation

Preoperative Planning

✔ ORIF of Sternoclavicular Fracture–Dislocations: PREOPERATIVE PLANNING CHECKLIST	
OR table	☐ Standard table capable of going into beach chair position
Position/positioning aids	☐ Beach chair position with Mayfield head positioner and a bump behind the scapula
Fluoroscopy location	☐ Contralateral side, if used
Equipment	☐ Heavy nonabsorbable suture, drill
	☐ General surgery or thoracic surgery backup

It is imperative to be familiar with the anatomy surrounding the sternoclavicular joint as well as the bony articulation of the medial clavicle and clavicular notch of the sternum. Having a general surgeon or thoracic surgeon available to assist the orthopedic surgeon in case of hemodynamic compromise is essential during the reduction maneuver or open reduction.

Positioning

Patients undergoing any procedure involving the sternoclavicular joint are placed in the modified beach chair position with a large bump or rolled towel placed between the scapulae to provide scapular retraction. The entire limb and hemithorax including the contralateral sternoclavicular joint, medial clavicle, and chest is prepped and draped into the operative field. The sternum to upper abdomen is prepped and draped in case an emergency median sternotomy is required (Fig. 19-20).

Surgical Approach

A transverse incision is made through the skin from the medial aspect of the clavicle over the ipsilateral sternoclavicular joint in Langer lines. The subcutaneous tissue and platysma are divided, utilizing electrocautery. The supraclavicular nerves are protected if in the operative field. The periosteum of the mid portion of the clavicle is elevated and a bone clamp is applied to the clavicle for control. The anterior periosteum is delicately divided over the posteriorly displaced clavicle until either the epiphysis or sternum is reached depending on whether it is a dislocation or a physeal fracture (Fig. 19-21). Typically, the

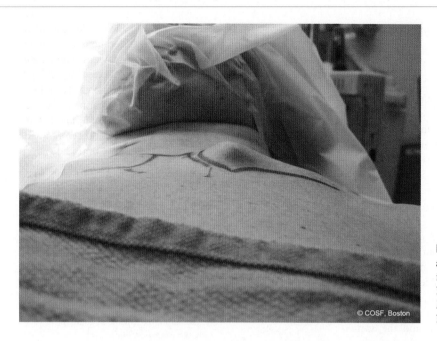

Figure 19-20. Intraoperative photograph showing the area that should be prepped and draped into the sterile field. (Reprinted with permission from Waters PM, Bae DS, eds. *Pediatric Hand and Upper Limb Surgery: A Practical Guide.* 1st ed. Philadelphia, PA: Wolters Kluwer Health/Lippincott Williams & Wilkins; 2012.)

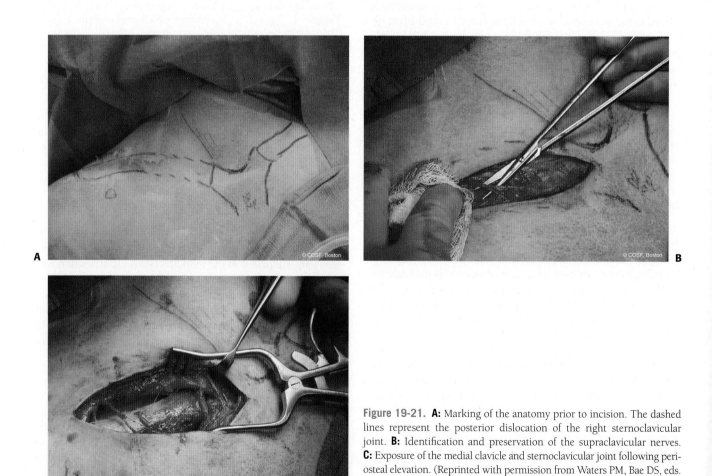

Figure 19-21. A: Marking of the anatomy prior to incision. The dashed lines represent the posterior dislocation of the right sternoclavicular joint. **B:** Identification and preservation of the supraclavicular nerves. **C:** Exposure of the medial clavicle and sternoclavicular joint following periosteal elevation. (Reprinted with permission from Waters PM, Bae DS, eds. *Pediatric Hand and Upper Limb Surgery: A Practical Guide.* 1st ed. Philadelphia, PA: Wolters Kluwer Health/Lippincott Williams & Wilkins; 2012.)

posterior periosteum of the clavicle and the posterior joint capsule are intact, providing a protective layer between the bony injury and mediastinal structures.

Technique

> **✔ ORIF of Sternoclavicular Fracture–Dislocations:**
> **KEY SURGICAL STEPS**
>
> ❏ Prep and drape the entire limb and hemithorax including contralateral sternoclavicular joint, chest, and upper abdomen
> ❏ Transverse skin incision in Langer lines from the diaphysis of the clavicle to the sternoclavicular joint
> ❏ Divide subcutaneous tissue and platysma in line with skin incision. Protect the supraclavicular nerves.
> ❏ Expose clavicle and sternum and incise periosteum working from lateral to medial on clavicle and from midline to lateral on sternum
> ❏ Evaluate the sternoclavicular joint to determine whether a true dislocation or physeal fracture occurred
> ❏ Reduce dislocation/fracture with aid of a fracture reduction clamp
> ❏ Converse with anesthesia to ensure hemodynamic stability of patient
> ❏ Place drill holes in anterior epiphysis and metaphysis for physeal fractures or anterior epiphysis and sternum for dislocations
> ❏ Pass heavy nonabsorbable suture in a figure-of-eight fashion and tie
> ❏ Reapproximate periosteum with heavy suture
> ❏ Irrigate and close wound in sequential layers
> ❏ Immobilize patient in sling and swathe or shoulder immobilizer

Following exposure of the physeal fracture or sternoclavicular dislocation, a gentle reduction is performed utilizing the aid of a fracture reduction clamp. Once the clavicle is brought anteriorly, it is important to converse with the anesthesiologist to ensure that the patient remained hemodynamically stable. An anatomic reduction is now performed ensuring that the clavicular head is anatomically seated in the clavicular notch of the sternum.

Following anatomic reduction of either the fracture or dislocation, drill holes are made in the anterior metaphysis and epiphysis of the clavicle in cases of a fracture or the anterior epiphysis and sternum in cases of a dislocation. Placement of malleable retractors between the bone and posterior periosteum is helpful in preventing the drill from entering the mediastinum. Heavy nonabsorbable suture is then passed in a figure-of-eight fashion to provide the necessary stability (Fig. 19-22). The periosteum is then reapproximated with heavy suture to provide added stability, especially with a true dislocation as it provides indirect repair of the costoclavicular and sternoclavicular ligaments. Stability is now assessed by ranging the ipsilateral shoulder and limb. Once stability is satisfactory, the wound is irrigated and closed in sequential layers.

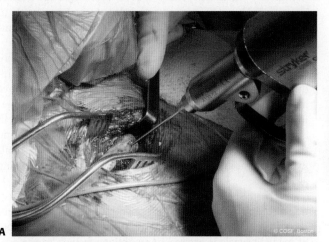
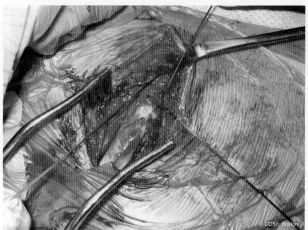
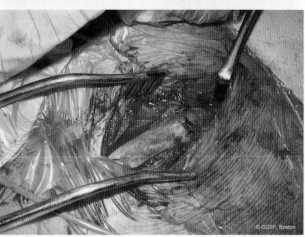

Figure 19-22. A: Drill holes created in the anterior medial clavicle and sternum in cases of true dislocations or anterior medial clavicular metaphysis and clavicular epiphysis in cases of physeal fracture. **B:** Heavy nonabsorbable suture placed through the drill holes in a figure-of-eight fashion. **C:** Anatomic joint reduction following tying of the sutures. (Reprinted with permission from Waters PM, Bae DS, eds. *Pediatric Hand and Upper Limb Surgery: A Practical Guide.* 1st ed. Philadelphia, PA: Wolters Kluwer Health/Lippincott Williams & Wilkins; 2012.)

We treat acute atraumatic anterior dislocations with immobilization alone for 1 to 4 weeks followed by gradual return to function. If patients experience recurrent instability, therapy is initiated. Operative intervention is reserved for patients with persistent symptoms and typically involves reconstruction of the ligaments.

Acute posterior dislocations are treated operatively with ORIF. Chronic posterior dislocations that are symptomatic are treated with ligament reconstruction utilizing allograft. At times, medial clavicle resection is required in painful chronic dislocations that have deformity of the bone and early arthritis of the joint.

Postoperative Care

Postoperatively, patients are placed in either a sling and swathe or shoulder immobilizer for 4 to 6 weeks. Subsequently, range-of-motion exercises are begun. Strengthening is permitted at 3 months postoperatively. Return to sports is dependent on full motion and strength, usually 3 to 6 months postoperatively.

Potential Pitfalls and Preventive Measures

Sternoclavicular Fracture–Dislocations:
SURGICAL PITFALLS AND PREVENTIONS

Pitfall	Prevention
• Overreduction of clavicle into clavicular notch of sternum	• Be knowledgeable about the bony anatomy of the sternoclavicular joint
• Osteolysis from Dacron	• Utilize heavy nonabsorbable suture
• K-wire migration	• Avoid K-wires

It is imperative to be familiar with the sternoclavicular bony alignment as overreduction of the clavicle into the clavicular notch of the sternum can occur. In addition, utilization of Dacron tape may cause osteolysis. Pins may migrate and therefore should be avoided.[91,125,151]

Outcomes

The outcomes following ORIF of posterior sternoclavicular dislocations or medial clavicle physeal fractures in pediatric and adolescent patients have been quite favorable in most reported cases.[13,50,80,147,155] In a retrospective review by Waters et al.,[155] all patients treated with open reduction and suture fixation of their posterior sternoclavicular joint fracture dislocation had restoration of joint stability and shoulder motion with full return to activities. Similar findings were reported by Goldfarb et al.[50] with all patients returning to their preinjury function including sports participation. Lee et al. recently published a series that included 40 patients treated operatively, of which one patient had a recurrent dislocation on postoperative day 1 that was addressed immediately. None of the other patients had a subsequent dislocation. It is important to note that none of the patients required reconstruction of the sternoclavicular or costoclavicular ligaments to maintain stability.[84]

The best evidence regarding these injuries is from a recent meta-analysis that showed that 96% of patients treated with ORIF had full pain-free range of motion without recurrence.[144]

Sternoclavicular Fracture–Dislocations:
COMMON ADVERSE OUTCOMES AND COMPLICATIONS

- Failure of closed treatment
- Persistent pain
- Recurrent instability

Attempts at closed reduction may be unsuccessful, leading to the necessity to perform an open reduction and internal fixation. Studies have shown that the success of closed reduction greatly reduces beyond 24 to 48 hours from the time of injury.[84,144] Therefore, one may consider proceeding directly to ORIF if the patient presents greater than 48 hours from the initial injury.

Recurrent instability following acute repair is relatively rare but can occur, especially if the sternoclavicular joint is overreduced. Patients will present with persistent pain and a sense of instability. Treatment with ligament reconstruction can be performed utilizing semitendinosus autograft or allograft passed in a figure-of-eight fashion similar to the suture utilized during the acute repair. Ideally, the tendon is passed on the "instability side" to minimize the risk of recurrent instability occurring again.

Alternatively, as a salvage procedure, medial clavicle resection arthroplasty can be performed with supplemental ligament reconstruction or soft tissue interposition. Approximately 1 cm of medial clavicle is excised in an oblique fashion to preserve the inferior ligamentous attachments. The intra-articular disk can be passed into the medullary canal of the clavicle by detaching its superior end while preserving the inferior attachments. Sutures are passed through drill holes in the superior clavicle and tied over a bony bridge (Fig. 19-23). Additional stability can be provided by sutures passed between the costoclavicular ligament and the clavicle. In a case series by Ting et al. of surgical care for patients, this rare complication revealed pain reduction and improved function.[146]

The results of treatment for recurrent anterior instability have been reported by Bae et al. in a retrospective review.[7] Sixty percent of patients had stable, pain-free joints following the procedure. No patients developed instability following their treatment. Many still had some minor limitations of function or persistent pain.

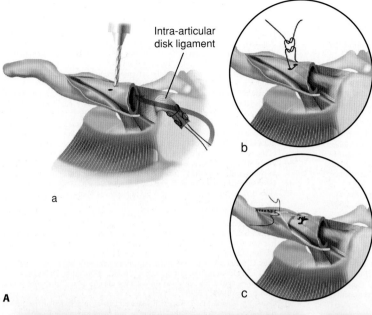

Figure 19-23. A: Schematic demonstrating the technique of medial clavicular resection arthroplasty. **B:** Intraoperative photograph of a patient with recurrent anterior sternoclavicular instability with resultant pain due to a deformed and irreducible clavicular head. **C:** Intraoperative photograph following medial clavicular head resection and intramedullary passage of the intra-articular disk ligament. (Reprinted with permission from Waters PM, Bae DS, eds. *Pediatric Hand and Upper Limb Surgery: A Practical Guide.* 1st ed. Philadelphia, PA: Wolters Kluwer Health/Lippincott Williams & Wilkins; 2012.)

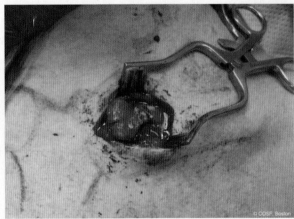

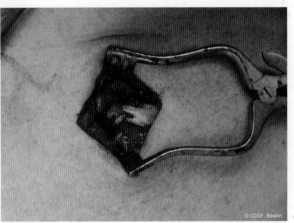

SUMMARY, CONTROVERSIES, AND FUTURE DIRECTIONS RELATED TO STERNOCLAVICULAR FRACTURE–DISLOCATIONS

Although sternoclavicular joint injuries are relatively rare, they do occur, even in the pediatric and adolescent populations. As high-energy mechanisms cause sternoclavicular injuries, associated damage to critical mediastinal structures can occur, and therefore, a thorough evaluation is necessary to avoid missing an associated life-threatening injury. The majority of anterior dislocations can be treated with immobilization alone, whereas acute posterior injuries are typically treated with operative intervention yielding excellent results.

Annotated References

Reference	Annotation
Lee JT, Nasreddine AY, Black EM, et al. Posterior sternoclavicular joint injuries in skeletally immature patients. *J Pediatr Orthop.* 2014;34(4);369–375.	Retrospective case series of 48 patients treated for a posterior sternoclavicular joint injury.
Shannon SF, Hernandez NM, Sems SA, et al. High-energy pediatric scapula fractures and their associated injuries. *J Pediatr Orthop.* 2017. doi: 10.1097/BPO.0000000000000969.	This is the largest series of pediatric scapula fractures that investigates the associated injuries, the morbidity, and the mortality.
Tepolt F, Carry PM, Heyn PC, et al. Posterior sternoclavicular joint injuries in the adolescent population: a meta-analysis. *Am J Sports Med.* 2014;42(10):2517–2524.	Meta-analysis reviewing associated injuries and outcomes of posterior sternoclavicular joint injuries in the adolescent population.

REFERENCES

1. Abbot AE, Hannafin JA. Stress fracture of the clavicle in a female lightweight rower: a case report and review of literature. *Am J Sports Med.* 2001;29:370–372.
2. Ada JR, Miller ME. Scapula fracture: analysis of 113 cases. *Clin Orthop Relat Res.* 1991;269:174–180.
3. Allman FL Jr. Fractures and ligamentous injuries of the clavicle and its articulation. *J Bone Joint Surg Am.* 1967;49:774–784.
4. An HS, Vonderbrink JP, Ebraheim NA, et al. Open scapulothoracic disassociation with intact neurovascular status in a child. *J Orthop Trauma.* 1988;2:36–38.
5. Anderson K. Evaluation and treatment of distal clavicle fractures. *Clin Sports Med.* 2003;22:319–326.
6. Badhe SP, Lawrence TM, Clark DI. Tension band suturing for the treatment of displaced type 2 lateral end clavicle fractures. *Arch Orthop Trauma Surg.* 2007;127:25–28.
7. Bae DS, Kocher MS, Waters PM, et al. Chronic recurrent anterior sternoclavicular joint instability: results of surgical management. *J Pediatr Orthop.* 2006;26:71–74.
8. Bae DS, Shah AS, Kalish LA, et al. Shoulder motion, strength, and functional outcomes in children with established malunion of the clavicle. *J Pediatr Orthop.* 2013;33(5):544–550.
9. Bahk MS, Kuhn JE, Galatz LM, et al. Acromioclavicular and sternoclavicular injuries and clavicular, glenoid, and scapular fractures. *J Bone Joint Surg Am.* 2009; 91:2492–2510.
10. Ballmer FT, Gerber C. Coracoclavicular screw fixation for unstable fractures of the distal clavicle: a report of five cases. *J Bone Joint Surg Br.* 1991;73:291–294.
11. Banerjee R, Waterman B, Padalecki J, et al. Management of distal clavicle fractures. *J Am Acad Orthop Surg.* 2011;19:392–401.
12. Bannister GC, Wallace WA, Stableforth PG, et al. The management of acute acromioclavicular dislocation: a randomized prospective controlled trial. *J Bone Joint Surg Br.* 1989;71:848–850.
13. Baumann M, Vogel T, Weise K, et al. Bilateral posterior sternoclavicular dislocation. *Orthopedics.* 2010;33:510.
14. Baumgarten KM. Arthroscopic fixation of a type II-variant, unstable distal clavicle fracture. *Orthopedics.* 2008;31.
15. Beall MH, Ross MG. Clavicle fracture in labor: risk factors and associated morbidities. *J Perinatol.* 2001;21:513–515.
16. Bearden JM, Hughston JC, Whatley GS. Acromioclavicular dislocation: method of treatment. *J Sports Med.* 1973;1:5–17.
17. Bergfield JA, Andrish JT, Clancy WG. Evaluation of the acromioclavicular joint following first- and second-degree sprains. *Am J Sports Med.* 1978;6:153–159.
18. Boldin C, Frankhauser F, Ratschek M, et al. Foreign-body reaction after reconstruction of complete acromioclavicular dislocation using PDS augmentation. *J Shoulder Elbow Surg.* 2004;12:99–100.
19. Bosworth BM. Acromioclavicular separation: new method of repair. *Surg Gynecol Obstet.* 1941;73:866–871.
20. Buckerfield CT, Castle ME. Acute traumatic retrosternal dislocation of the clavicle. *J Bone Joint Surg Am.* 1984;66:379–385.
21. Buckley BJ, Hayden SR. Posterior sternoclavicular dislocation. *J Emerg Med.* 2008;34:331–332.
22. Bullock DP, Koval KJ, Moen KY, et al. Hospitalized cases of child abuse in America: who, what, when, and where. *J Pediatr Orthop.* 2009;29:231–237.
23. Burrows HJ. Tenodesis of subclavius in the treatment of recurrent dislocation of the sterno-clavicualr joint. *J Bone Joint Surg Br.* 1951;33B:240–243.
24. Butters KP. Fractures and dislocations of the scapula. In: Rockwood CA Jr, Green DP, Bucholz RW, eds. *Fractures in Adults.* Philadelphia, PA: JB Lippincott; 1991:990–1019.
25. Calder JD, Solan M, Gidwani S, et al. Management of paediatric clavicle fractures: is follow-up necessary? An audit of 346 cases. *Ann R Coll Surg Engl.* 2002;84: 331–333.
26. Candian Orthopedic Trauma Society. Nonoperative treatment compared with plate fixation of displaced mishaft clavicular fractures: a multicenter, randomized clinical trial. *J Bone Joint Surg Am.* 2007;89A:1–10.
27. Cave EF. *Fractures and Other Injuries.* Chicago, IL: Year Book Medical Publishers; 1958.
28. Chang DC, Knight V, Ziegfeld S, et al. The tip of the iceberg for child abuse: the critical roles of the pediatric trauma service and its registry. *J Trauma.* 2004;57: 1189–1198.
29. Checcia SL, Doneux PS, Miyazaki AN, et al. Treatment of distal clavicle fractures using an arthroscopic technique. *J Shoulder Elbow Surg.* 2008;17:395–398.
30. Cohen AW, Otto SR. obstetric clavicular fractures: a three-year analysis. *J Reprod Med.* 1980;25:119–122.
31. Corteen DP, Teitge RA. Stabilization of the clavicle after distal resection: a biomechanical study. *Am J Sports Med.* 2005;33:61–67.
32. Coupe BD, Wimhurst JA, Indar R, et al. A new approach for plate fixation of midshaft clavicular fractures. *Injury.* 2005;36:1166–1171.
33. Craig EV. Fractures of the clavicle. In: Rockwood CA Jr, Green DP, Bucholz RW, Heckman JD, eds. *Rockwood and Green's Fractures in Adults.* 4th ed. Philadelphia, PA: Lippincott-Raven; 1996:1009–1193.
34. Curtis RJ, Rockwood CA. Fractures and dislocations of the shoulder in children. In: Rockwood CA Jr, Matsen FAI, eds. *The Shoulder.* Philadelphia, PA: WB Saunders; 1990:991–1032.
35. Dameron TB, Rockwood CA Jr. Fractures and dislocations of the shoulder. In: Rockwood CA Jr, ed. *Fractures in Children.* Philadelphia, PA: JB Lippincott; 1984:577–682.
36. de Jong KP, Sukul DM. Anterior sternoclavicular dislocation: a long-term follow-up study. *J Orthop Trauma.* 1990;4:420–423.
37. Edwards DJ, Kavanagh TG, Flannery MC. Fractures of the distal clavicle: a case for fixation. *Injury.* 1992;23:44–46.
38. Edwards SG, Whittle AP, Wood GW 2nd. Nonoperative treatment of ipsilateral fractures of the scapula and clavicle. *J Bone Joint Surg Am.* 2000;82:774–780.
39. Erdle B, Izadpanah K, Jaeger M, et al. Comparative analysis of locking plate versus hook plate osteosynthesis of Neer type IIB lateral clavicle fractures. *Arch Orthop Trauma Surg.* 2017;137(5):651–662.
40. Fazal MA, Saksena J, Haddad FS. Temporary coracoclavicular screw fixation for displaced distal clavicle fractures. *J Orthop Surg (Hong Kong).* 2007;15:9–11.
41. Ferraz IC, Papadimitriou NG, Sotereanos DG. Scapular body nonunion: a case report. *J Shoulder Elbow Surg.* 2002;11:98–100.
42. Flatow EL. The biomechanics of the acromioclavicular, sternoclavicular, and scapulothoracic joints. *Instr Course Lect.* 1993;42:237–245.
43. Flinkkila T, Ristiniemi J, Hyvonen P, et al. Surgical treatment of unstable fractures of the distal clavicle: a comparative study of Kirschner wire and clavicular hook plate fixation. *Acta Orthop Scand.* 2002;73:50–53.
44. Fracture and dislocation compendium. Orthopedic Trauma Association Committee for Coding and Classification. *J Orthop Trauma.* 1996;10(Suppl 1):1–154.
45. Fukada K, Craig EV, An KN, et al. Biomechanical study of the ligamentous system of the acromioclavicular joint. *J Bone Joint Surg Am.* 1986;68:434–440.
46. Furey MJ, Zdero R, McKee MD. Clavicular refracture at the site of angular malunion in young athletes. *J Orthop Trauma.* 2017;31(4):e130–e132.
47. Gardner E. The embryology of the clavicle. *Clin Orthop.* 1968;58:9–16.
48. Gilbert A, Whitaker I. Obstetrical brachial plexus lesions. *J Hand Surg Br.* 1991; 16:489–491.
49. Goldberg JA, Bruce WJ, Sonnabend DH, et al. Type 2 fractures of the distal clavicle: a new surgical technique. *J Shoulder Elbow Surg.* 1997;6:380–382.
50. Goldfarb CA, Bassett GS, Sullivan S, et al. Retrosternal displacement after physeal fracture of the medial clavicle in children treatment by open reduction and internal fixation. *J Bone Joint Surg Br.* 2001;83:1168–1172.
51. Goss TP. Fractures of the glenoid cavity. *J Bone Joint Surg Am.* 1992;74:299–305.
52. Goss TP. Fractures of the glenoid neck. *J Shoulder Elbow Surg.* 1994;3:42–52.
53. Goss TP. Scapular fractures and dislocations: diagnosis and treatment. *J Am Acad Orthop Surg.* 1995;3:22–33.
54. Grassi FA, Tajana MS, D'Angelo F. Management of midclavicular fractures: comparison between nonoperative treatment and open intramedullary fixation in 80 patients. *J Trauma.* 2001;50:1096–1100.
55. Groh GI, Wirth MA. Management of traumatic sternoclavicular injuries. *J Am Acad Orthop Surg.* 2011;19:1–7.
56. Groh GI, Wirth MA, Rockwood CA Jr. Treatment of traumatic posterior sternoclavicular joint dislocations. *J Shoulder Elbow Surg.* 2011;20:107–113.
57. Heinig CF. Retrosternal dislocations of the clavicle: early recognition, x-ray diagnosis and management. *J Bone Joint Surg Am.* 1968;50:830.
58. Heyse-Moore GH, Stoker DJ. Avulsion fractures of the scapula. *Skeletal Radiol.* 1982;9:27–32.
59. Heyworth BE, Cohen L, von Heideken J, et al. Validity and comprehensibility of outcome measures in children with shoulder and elbow disorders: creation of a new Pediatric and Adolescent Shoulder and Elbow Survey (Pedi-ASES). *J Shoulder Elbow Surg.* 2018;27:1162–1171.
60. Heyworth BE, May C, Carsen S, et al. Outcomes of operative and non-operative treatment of adolescent mid-diaphyseal clavicle fractures. Presented at 2014 POSNA Annual Meeting (unpublished).
61. Hill JM, McGuire MH, Crosby LA. Closed treatment of displaced middle-third fractures of the clavicle gives poor results. *J Bone Joint Surg Br.* 1997;79-B:537–539.
62. Hobbs DW. Sternoclavicular joint: a new axial radiographic view. *Radiology.* 1968;90:801.
63. Hsu TY, Hung FC, Lu YJ, et al. Neonatal clavicular fracture: clinical analysis of incidence, predisposing factors, diagnosis, and outcome. *Am J Perinatol.* 2002;19:17–21.
64. Ideberg R, Grevsten S, Larsson S. Epidemiology of scapular fractures: incidence and classification of 338 fractures. *Acta Orthop Scand.* 1995;66:395–397.
65. Imatani RJ. Fractures of the scapula: a review of 53 fractures. *J Trauma.* 1975; 15:473–478.
66. Jaggard MK, Gupte CM, Gulati V, et al. A comprehensive review of trauma and disruption to the sternoclavicular joint with the proposal of a new classification system. *J Trauma.* 2009;66:576–584.
67. Jeray KJ. Acute midshaft clavicular fracture. *J Am Acad Orthop Surg.* 2007;15:239–248.
68. Jin CZ, Kim HK, Min BH. Surgical treatment for distal clavicle fracture associated with coracoclavicular ligament rupture using a cannulated screw fixation technique. *J Trauma.* 2006;60:1358–1361.
69. Jones HP, Lemos MJ, Schepsis AA. Salvage of failed acromioclavicular joint reconstruction using autogenous semitendinosus tendon from the knee: surgical technique and case report. *Am J Sports Med.* 2001;29:234–237.
70. Joseph PR, Rosenfeld W. Clavicular fractures in neonates. *Am J Dis Child.* 1990; 144:165–167.
71. Jupiter JB, Leibman MI. Supraclavicular nerve entrapment due to clavicular fracture callus. *J Shoulder Elbow Surg.* 2007;16(5):e13–e14.
72. Kalamaras M, Cutbush K, Robinson M. A method for internal fixation of unstable distal clavicle fractures: early observations using a new technique. *J Shoulder Elbow Surg.* 2008;17:60–62.
73. Kao FC, Chao EK, Chen CH, et al. Treatment of distal clavicle fracture using Kirschner wires and tension-band wires. *J Trauma.* 2001;51:522–525.
74. Kaplan LD, Flanigan DC, Norwig J, et al. Prevalence and variance of shoulder injuries in elite collegiate football players. *Am J Sports Med.* 2005;33:1142–1146.
75. Kaplan B, Rabinerson D, Avrech OM, et al. Fracture of the clavicle in the newborn following normal labor and delivery. *Int J Gynaecol Obstet.* 1998;63:15–20.
76. Kavanagh BF, Bradway JK, et al. Open reduction and internal fixation of displaced intra-articular fractures of the glenoid fossa. *J Bone Joint Surg Am.* 1993;75: 479–484.
77. Kellum E, Creek A, Dawkins R, et al. Age-related patterns of injury in children involved in all-terrain vehicle accidents. *J Pediatr Orthop.* 2008;28(8):854–858.
78. Khan LA, Bradnock TJ, Scott C, et al. Fractures of the clavicle. *J Bone Joint Surg Am.* 2009;91:447–460.

79. Klimkiewicz JJ, Williams GR, Sher JS, et al. The acromioclavicular capsule as a restraint to posterior translation of the clavicle: a biomechanical analysis. *J Shoulder Elbow Surg*. 1999;8:119–124.
80. Koch MJ, Wells L. Proximal clavicle physeal fracture with posterior displacement: diagnosis, treatment, and prevention. *Orthopedics*. 2012;35:e108–e111.
81. Labler L, Platz A, Weishaupt D, et al. Clinical and functional results after floating shoulder injuries. *J Trauma*. 2004;57:595–602.
82. Lam MH, Wong GY, Lao TT. Reappraisal of neonatal clavicular fracture: relationship between infant size and risk factors. *J Reprod Med*. 2002;47:903–908.
83. Lee YS, Lau MJ, Tseng YC, et al. Comparison of the efficacy of hook plate versus tension band wire in the treatment of unstable fractures of the distal clavicle. *Int Orthop*. 2009;33:1401–1405.
84. Lee JT, Nasreddine AY, Black EM, et al. Posterior stenoclavicular joint injuries in skeletally immature patients. *J Pediatr Orthop*. 2014;34(4);369–375.
85. Leighton RK, Buhr AJ, Sinclair AM. Posterior sternoclavicular dislocations. *Can J Surg*. 1986;29:104–106.
86. Levin MG, Holroyde J, Wood JR Jr, et al. Birth trauma: incidence and predisposing factors. *Obstet Gynecol*. 1984;63:792–295.
87. Levy O. Simple, minimally invasive surgical technique for treatment of type 2 fractures of the distal clavicle. *J Shoulder Elbow Surg*. 2003;12:24–28.
87a. Li Y, Donohue KS, Robbins CB, et al; Function After Adolescent Clavicle Trauma and Surgery (FACTS) Multicenter Study Group. Reliability of radiographic assessments of adolescent midshaft clavicle fractures by the FACTS multicenter study group. *J Orthop Trauma*. 2017;31(9):479–484.
88. Li Y, Helvie P, Farley FA, et al. Complications after plate fixation of displaced pediatric midshaft clavicle fractures. *J Pediatr Orthop*. 2018;38(7):350–353.
89. Liberson F. Os acromiale: a contested anomaly. *J Bone Joint Surg*. 1937;19:683–689.
90. Liechti R. Fractures of the clavicle and scapula. In: Weber BG, Brenner C, Freuler F, eds. *Treatment of Fractures in Children and Adolescents*. New York: Springer-Verlag; 1980:87–95.
91. Lyons FA, Rockwood CA Jr. Migration of pins used in operations on the shoulder. *J Bone Joint Surg Am*. 1990;72:1262–1267.
92. Macheras G, Kateros KT, Savvidou OD, et al. Coracoclavicular screw fixation for unstable distal clavicle fractures. *Orthopedics*. 2005;28:693–696.
93. Mall JW, Jacobi CA, Philipp AW, et al. Surgical treatment of fractures of the distal clavicle with polydioxanone suture tension band wiring: an alternative osteosynthesis. *J Orthop Sci*. 2002;7:535–537.
94. Martin SD, Weiland AJ. Missed scapular fracture after trauma: a case report and a 23-year follow-up report. *Clin Orthop Relat Res*. 1994;299:259–262.
95. Masnovi ME, Mehlman CT, Eismann EA, et al. Pediatric refracture rates after angulated and completely displaced clavicle shaft fractures. *J Orthop Trauma*. 2014;28(11):648–652.
96. Mayo KA, Benirschke SK, Mast JW. Displaced fractures of the glenoid fossa: results of open reduction and internal fixation. *Clin Orthop Relat Res*. 1998;347:122–130.
97. Mazzocca AD, Santangelo SA, Johnson ST, et al. A biomechanical evaluation of an anatomical coracoclavicular ligament reconstruction. *Am J Sports Med*. 2006;34: 236–246.
98. McGahan JP, Rab GT, Dublin A. Fractures of the scapula. *J Trauma*. 1980;20: 880–883.
99. McGraw MA, Mehlman CT, Lindsdell CJ, et al. Postnatal growth of the clavicle: birth to 18 years of age. *J Pediatr Orthop*. 2009;29:937–943.
100. McKee MD, Wild LW, Schemitsch EH. Midshaft malunions of the clavicle. *J Bone Joint Surg Am*. 2003;85-A:790–797.
101. McKee RC, Whelan DB, Schemitsch EH, et al. Operative versus nonoperative care of displaced midshaft clavicular fractures: a meta-analysis of randomized clinical trials. *J Bone Joint Surg Am*. 2012;94A:675–684.
102. Mehlman CT, Yihua G, Bochang C, et al. Operative treatment of completely displaced clavicle shaft fractures in children. *J Pediatr Orthop*. 2009;29:851–855.
103. Mehta JC, Sachdev A, Collins JJ. Retrosternal dislocation of the clavicle. *Injury*. 1973;5:79–83.
104. Michael D, Fazal MA, Cohen B. Nonunion of a fracture of the body of the scapula: case report and literature review. *J Shoulder Elbow Surg*. 2001;10:385–386.
105. Mooney JF III, Webb LX. Fractures and dislocations about the shoulder. In: Green NE, Swiontkowski MF, eds. *Skeletal Trauma in Children*. Philadelphia, PA: Saunders Elsevier; 2009:283–312.
106. Mounshine E, Garofalo R, Crevoisier X, et al. Grade I and II acromioclavicular dislocations: results of conservative treatment. *J Shoulder Elbow Surg*. 2003;12: 599–602.
107. Namdari S, Ganley TJ Jr, Baldwin K, et al. Fixation of displaced midshaft clavicle fractures in skeletally immature patients. *J Pediatr Orthop*. 2011;31:507–511.
108. Neer CS 2nd. Fracture of the distal clavicle with detachment of the coracoclavicular ligaments in adults. *J Trauma*. 1963;3:99–110.
109. Neer CS 2nd. Fractures of the distal third of the clavicle. *Clin Orthop Relat Res*. 1968;58:43–50.
110. Neer C II. Fractures and dislocations of the shoulder. In: Rockwood CA Jr, Green DP, eds. *Fractures in Adults*. Philadelphia, PA: JB Lippincott; 1984:711–712.
111. Nettles JL, Linscheid RL. Sternoclavicular dislocations. *J Trauma*. 1968;8:158–164.
112. Nettrour LF, Krufky EL, Mueller RE, et al. Locked scapula: intrathoracic dislocation of the inferior angle. A case report. *J Bone Joint Surg Am*. 1972;54:413–416.
113. Nordqvist A, Petersson C. Fracture of the body, neck, or spine of the scapula: a long-term follow-up study. *Clin Orthop Relat Res*. 1992;283:139–144.
114. Nordqvist A, Petersson C. The incidence of fractures of the clavicle. *Clin Orthop Relat Res*. 1994;300:127–132.
115. Norqvist A, Petersson C, Redlund-Johnell I. The natural course of lateral clavicle fracture: 15 (11–21) year follow-up of 110 cases. *Acta Orthop Scand*. 1993;64: 87–91.
116. Nourissat G, Kakuda C, Dumontier C, et al. Arthroscopic stabilization of Neer type 2 fracture of the distal part of the clavicle. *Arthroscopy*. 2007;23:674.e1–e4.
117. Nowak J, Mallmin H, Larsson S. The aetiology and epidemiology of clavicular fractures: a prospective study during a two-year period in Uppsala, Sweden. *Injury*. 2000;31:353–358.
118. Oppenheim WL, Davis A, Growdon WA, et al. Clavicle fractures in the newborn. *Clin Orthop Res*. 1990;250:176–180.
119. Pandya NK, Baldwin K, Wolfgruber H, et al. Child abuse and orthopaedic injury patterns: analysis at a level I pediatric trauma center. *J Pediatr Orthop*. 2009;29: 618–625.
120. Phillips AM, Smart C, Groom AF. Acromioclavicular dislocation: conservative or surgical therapy. *Clin Orthop Relat Res*. 1998;353:10–17.
121. Postachhini F, Gumina S, De Santis P, et al. Epidemiology of clavicle fractures. *J Shoulder Elbow Surg*. 2002;11:452–456.
122. Pujol N, Philippeau JM, Richou J, et al. Arthroscopic treatment of distal clavicle fractures: a technical note. *Knee Surg Sports Traumatol Arthrosc*. 2008;16: 884–886.
123. Randsborg PH, Fuglesang HF, Røtterud JH, et al. Long-term patient-reported outcome after fractures of the clavicle in patients aged 10 to 18 years. *J Pediatr Orthop*. 2014; 34(4):393–399.
124. Regel JP, Pospiech J, Aalders TA, et al. Intraspinal migration of a Kirschner wire 3 months after clavicular fracture fixation. *Neurosurg Rev*. 2002;25:110–112.
125. Reilly P, Bruguera JA, Copeland SA. Erosion and nonunion of the first rib after sternoclavicular reconstruction with Dacron. *J Shoulder Elbow Surg*. 1999;8: 76–78.
126. Renfree KJ, Riley MK, Wheeler D, et al. Ligamentous anatomy of the distal clavicle. *J Shoulder Elbow Surg*. 2003;12:355–359.
127. Rios CG, Arciero RA, Mazzocca AD. Anatomy of the clavicle and coracoid process for reconstruction of the coracoclavicular ligaments. *Am J Sports Med*. 2007; 35:811–817.
128. Roberts S, Hernandez C, Adams M, et al. Neonatal clavicular fracture: an unpredictable event. *Am J Obset Gynecol*. 1993;168:433.
129. Robinson CM. Fractures of the clavicle in the adult: epidemiology and classification. *J Bone Joint Surg Br*. 1998;80:476–484.
130. Robinson CM, Cairns DA. Primary nonoperative treatment of displaced lateral fractures of the clavicle. *J Bone Joint Surg Am*. 2004;86:778–782.
131. Robinson CM, Court-Brown CM, McQueen MM, et al. Estimating the risk of nonunion following nonoperative treatment of a clavicular fracture. *J Bone Joint Surg Am*. 2004;86:1359–1365.
132. Robinson CM, Goudie EB, Murray IR, et al. Open reduction and plate fixation versus nonoperative treatment for displaced midshaft clavicular fractures: a multicenter, randomized, controlled trial. *J Bone Joint Surg Am*. 2013;95A: 1576–1584.
133. Rockwood CA Jr, Williams GR Jr, et al. Disorders of the acromioclavicular joint. In: Rockwood CA, Matsen FA, eds. *The Shoulder*. Philadelphia, PA: WB Saunders; 1998:483–553.
134. Rokito AS, Zuckerman JD, Shaari JM, et al. A comparison of nonoperative and operative treatment of type II distal clavicle fractures. *Bull Hosp Jt Dis*. 2002–2003; 61:32–39.
134a. Schulz J, Moor M, Roocroft J, et al. Functional and radiographic outcomes of nonoperative treatment of displaced adolescent clavicle fractures. *J Bone Joint Surg Am*. 2013;95:1159–1165.
135. Shannon SF, Hernandez NM, Sems SA, et al. Pediatric orthopaedic trauma and associated injuries of snowmobile, ATV, and dirtbike accidents: a 19-year experience at a level 1 pediatric trauma center. *J Pediatr Orthop*. 2018;38(8): 403–409.
136. Shannon SF, Hernandez NM, Sems SA, et al. High-energy pediatric scapula fractures and their associated injuries. *J Pediatr Orthop*. 2017. doi: 10.1097/ BPO.0000000000000969.
137. Simovitch R, Sanders B, Ozbaydar M, et al. Acromioclavicular joint injuries: diagnosis and management. *J Am Acad Orthop Surg*. 2009;17:207–219.
138. Spencer EE Jr, Kuhn JE. Biomechanical analysis of reconstructions for sternoclavicular joint instability. *J Bone Joint Surg Am*. 2004;86:98–105.
139. Spencer EE, Kuhn JE, Huston LJ, et al. Ligamentous restraints to anterior and posterior translation of the sternoclavicular joint. *J Shoulder Elbow Surg*. 2002;11: 43–47.
140. Stanley D, Trowbridge EA, Norris SH. The mechanism of clavicular fracture: a clinical and biomechanical analysis. *J Bone Joint Surg Br*. 1988;70:461–464.
141. Stewart AM, Ahmad CS. Failure of acromioclavicular reconstruction using Gore-Tex graft due to aseptic foreign-body reaction and clavicle osteolysis: a case report. *J Shoulder Elbow Surg*. 2004;13:558–561.
142. Sugaya H, Kon Y, Tsuchiya A. Arthroscopic repair of glenoid fractures using suture anchors. *Arthroscopy*. 2005;21:635.
143. Suppan CA, Bae DS, Donohue KS, et al. Trends in the volume of operative treatment of midshaft clavicle fractures in children and adolescents: a retrospective, 12-year, single-institution analysis. *J Pediatr Orthop B*. 2016;25(4):305–309.
144. Tepolt F, Carry PM, Heyn PC, et al. Posterior sternoclavicular joint injuries in the adolescent population: a meta-analysis. *Am J Sports Med*. 2014;42:2517–2524.
145. Thompson DA, Flynn C, Miller PW, et al. The significance of scapular fractures. *J Trauma*. 1985;25:974–977.
146. Ting BL, Bae DS, Waters PM. Chronic posterior sternoclavicular joint fracture dislocations in children and young adults: results of surgical management. *J Pediatric Orthop*. 2014;34:542–547.
147. Tompkins M, Bliss J, Villarreal R, et al. Posterior-sternoclavicular disruption with ipsilateral clavicle fracture in a nine-year-old hockey player. *J Orthop Trauma*. 2010; 24:e36–e39.
148. Tossy JD, Mead MC, Sigmond HM. Acromioclavicular separations: useful and practical classification for treatment. *Clin Orthop Relat Res*. 1963;28:111–119.
149. Tsai CH, Hsu HC, Huan CY, et al. Late migration of threaded wire (Schanz screw) from right distal clavicle to the cervical spine. *J Chin Med Assoc*. 2009;72:48–51.

150. Vander Have KL, Perdue AM, Caird MS, et al. Operative versus nonoperative treatment of midshaft clavicle fractures in adolescents. *J Pediatr Orthop.* 2010;30:307–312.

151. Venissac N, Alifano M, Dahan M, et al. Intrathoracic migration of Kirschner pins. *Ann Thorac Surg.* 2000;69:1953–1955.

152. Virtanen KJ, Remes V, Pajarinen J, et al. Sling compared with plate osteosynthesis for treatment of displaced midshaft clavicular fractures: a randomized clinical trial. *J Bone Joint Surg Am.* 2012;94A:1546–1553.

153. Waninger KN. Stress fracture of the clavicle in a collegiate diver. *Clin J Sport Med.* 1997;7:66–68.

154. Waskowitz WJ. Disruption of the sternoclavicular joint: an analysis and review. *Am J Orthop.* 1961;3:176–179.

155. Waters PM, Bae DS, Kadiyala RK. Short-term outcomes after surgical treatment of traumatic posterior sternoclavicular fracture-dislocations in children and adolescents. *J Pediatr Orthop.* 2003;23:464–469.

156. Webber MC, Haines JF. The treatment of lateral clavicle fractures. *Injury.* 2000; 31:175–179.

157. Williams GR Jr, Nguyen VD, Rockwood CA Jr. Classification and radiographic analysis of acromioclavicular dislocations. *Appl Radiol.* 1989;18:29–34.

158. Wirth MA, Rockwood CA Jr. Acute and chronic traumatic injuries of the sternoclavicular joint. *J Am Acad Orthop Surg.* 1996;4:268–278.

159. Wojtys EM, Nelson G. Conservative treatment of Grade III acromioclavicular dislocations. *Clin Orthop Relat Res.* 1991;268:112–119.

160. Wu CD, Chen YL. Stress fracture of the clavicle in a professional baseball player. *J Shoulder Elbow Surg.* 1998;7:164–167.

161. Yamaguchi H, Arakawa H, Kobayashi M. Results of the Bosworth method for unstable fractures of the distal clavicle. *Int Orthop.* 1998;22:366–368.

162. Yang S, Werner BC, Gwathmey FW Jr. Treatment trends in adolescent clavicle fractures. *J Pediatr Orthop.* 2015;35(3):229–233.

163. Zanca P. Shoulder pain: involvement of the acromioclavicular joint: analysis of 1,000 cases. *Am J Roentgenol Radium Ther Nucl Med.* 1971;112:493–506.

164. Zdravkovic D, Damholt VV. Comminuted and severely displaced fractures of the scapula. *Acta Orthop Scand.* 1974;45:60–65.

Section **Three**
SPINE

20

Cervical Spine Injuries in Children

William C. Warner and Daniel J. Hedequist

Burst Fracture

Spondylolysis and Spondylolisthesis

Cervical Spine Injury

INTRODUCTION TO CERVICAL SPINE INJURY

Cervical spine fractures in children are rare, accounting for only 1% of pediatric fractures and 2% of all spinal injuries.[15,17,56,147,159,160,183,192,215,240,310,349,392] The incidence is estimated to be 7.41 in 100,000 per year[270]; however, that may be misleading because some injuries are not detected or are detected only at autopsy. Aufdermaur[24] examined the autopsied spines of 12 juveniles who had spinal injuries. All 12 had cartilage endplates that were separated from the vertebral bodies in the zone of columnar and calcified cartilage, similar to a Salter–Harris type I fracture, although clinically and radiographically, a fracture was suggested in only one patient. Only radiographs at autopsy showed the disruption, represented by a small gap and apparent widening of the intervertebral space.[24]

Cervical spine injuries in children younger than 8 years of age occur in the upper cervical spine, whereas older children and adolescents tend to have fractures involving either the upper or lower cervical spine.[185,199,309,311,312] The upper cervical spine in children is more prone to injury because of the anatomic and biomechanical properties of the immature spine.[440,441] The immature spine is hypermobile because of ligamentous laxity, and the facet joints are oriented in a more horizontal position; both of these properties predispose children to more forward translation. Younger children also have a relatively large head compared to the body, which changes the fulcrum of motion of the upper cervical spine. All of these factors predispose younger children to injuries of the upper cervical spine; with age, the anatomic changes lead to an increased prevalence of lower cervical spine injuries.

Cervical spine injuries associated with neurologic deficits are infrequent in children, and when incomplete there tends to be a better prognosis for recovery in children than in adults.[33,88,111,112,299,418,428] Complete neurologic deficits, regardless of patient age, tend to have a poor prognosis for any recovery and may be indicative of the severity and magnitude of injury.[115,216,295,321] Death from cervical spine injuries tends to be related to the level of injury and the associated injuries. Higher cervical spine injuries (e.g., atlantooccipital dislocation) in younger children are associated with the highest mortality rate.[38,304,305] Children with significant cervical spine injuries also may have associated severe head injuries, leading to an increase in mortality. In a study of 61 pediatric deaths related to spinal cord injuries, 89% of fatalities occurred at the scene, and most were related to high cervical cord injuries in patients who had sustained multiple injuries.[164]

MECHANISMS OF INJURY FOR CERVICAL SPINE INJURY

The mechanism of injury in the cervical spine varies with age. Infants are at risk during birth and early development because of their lack of head control. Most cervical spine injuries in infants not related to birth trauma are caused by child abuse and often involve the spinal cord.[24] In young children, most cervical spine injuries result from motor vehicle accidents or being struck by a vehicle, although injuries have been reported after seemingly low-energy falls from heights less than 5 ft.[49,154,280] As children become adolescents, the prevalence of sporting injuries increases as does the prevalence of athletic-related spinal cord injury without radiographic abnormality (SCIWORA).[62,100,116,227,249]

INJURIES ASSOCIATED WITH CERVICAL SPINE INJURY

Patients with suspected cervical spine injuries need to be thoroughly evaluated for other injuries. Facial injuries as well as traumatic brain injuries are commonly seen with cervical spine injuries, due to the anatomical proximity of these body regions.[81,303,350] Vigilance must be high for noncontiguous spine fractures, as well as other orthopedic injuries. Inconsolable children need particular attention, with a thorough search for noncontiguous spine fractures or other associated injuries.

Spinal Cord Injury

Careful radiographic evaluation is helpful in the workup of these patients. Magnetic resonance imaging (MRI) may show a spinal cord lesion that often is some distance from the vertebral column injury. As many as 5% to 10% of children with spinal cord injuries have normal radiographic results.[79,159]

Spinal cord injuries are rare in children. Ranjith et al.[337] reviewed spinal injuries at the Toronto Hospital for Sick Children over 15 years and found that children constituted a small percentage of the patients with acquired quadriplegia or paraplegia. He found that paraplegia was three times more common than quadriplegia. When a spinal cord injury is suspected, the neurologic examination must be complete and meticulous. Several examinations of sensory and motor function may be necessary.

Spinal column and spinal cord injury can occur during birth, especially during a breech delivery.[235,298] Injuries associated with breech delivery usually are in the lower cervical spine or upper thoracic spine and are thought to result from traction, whereas injuries associated with cephalic delivery usually occur in the upper cervical spine and are thought to result from rotation. Skeletal spine injury from obstetric trauma is probably underreported because the infantile spine is largely cartilaginous and difficult to evaluate with radiographs, especially if the injury is through the cartilage or cartilage–bone interface.[24] A cervical spine injury should be considered in an infant who is floppy at birth, especially after a difficult delivery. Flaccid paralysis, with areflexia, usually is followed by a typical pattern of hyperreflexia once spinal cord shock is over. Brachial plexus palsy also may be present after a difficult delivery and warrants cervical spine radiographs and an MRI. It is unclear whether cesarean section reduces spinal injury in neonates[251]; however, Bresnan and Abroms[58] noted that neck hyperextension in utero (star-gazing fetus) in breech presentations is likely to result in an estimated 25% incidence of spinal cord injury with vaginal delivery and can be prevented by cesarean section delivery.

Immature neck musculature in infants and toddlers increases the risk for cervical spine injury. Distraction-type injuries to the upper cervical spine have been reported in infants in forward-facing car seats. During sudden deceleration maneuvers, the head continues forward while the remainder of the body is strapped in the car seat, resulting in injury.[87,151,208] Similar injuries have been reported in adults involved in motor vehicle accidents.[31,264] Child abuse is probably one of the most frequent causes of spinal injury in infants. Swischuk[400] in 1969 and Caffey[70] in 1974 described a form of child abuse they termed the shaken baby syndrome. This whiplash-type stress can cause not only fracture to the spinal column and spinal cord injury, but intracranial and intraocular hemorrhages as well. The cerebral and spinal insult can result in death or retardation and permanent visual and hearing defects. In autopsy

studies, Shulman et al.[380] found atlantooccipital and axial dislocations, and Tawbin[403] found a 10% incidence of brain and spinal injuries.

Spinal Cord Injury Without Radiographic Abnormality

SCIWORA, a syndrome first brought to the attention of the medical community by Pang and Wilberger,[310] is unique to children. This condition is defined as a spinal cord injury in a patient with no visible fracture or dislocation on plain radiographs, tomograms, or computed tomography (CT) scans.

A complete or incomplete spinal cord lesion may be present, and the injury usually results from severe flexion or distraction of the cervical spine. SCIWORA is believed to occur because the spinal column (vertebrae and disk space) in children is more elastic than the spinal cord and can undergo considerable deformation without being disrupted.[66,239,404] The spinal column can elongate up to 2 in. without disruption, whereas the spinal cord ruptures with only a quarter-inch of elongation.[309,310]

SCIWORA also may represent an ischemic injury in some patients, although most are believed to be due to a distraction-type injury in which the spinal cord has not tolerated the degree of distraction but the bony ligamentous elements have not failed. Aufdermaur[14] suggested another possibility: a fracture through a pediatric vertebral endplate reduces spontaneously (much like a Salter–Harris type I fracture), giving a normal radiograph appearance, although the initial displacement could have caused spinal cord injury.

SCIWORA abnormalities are more common in children under 8 years of age than in older children,[310,318,349,426] perhaps because of predisposing factors such as cervical spine hypermobility, ligamentous laxity, and an immature vascular supply to the spinal cord. The reported incidence of this condition varies from 7% to 66% of patients with cervical spine injuries.[309,310,452]

Delayed onset of neurologic symptoms has been reported in as many as 52% of patients in some series.[275,310] Pang and Pollack[309] reported 15 patients who had delayed paralysis after their injuries. Nine had transient warning signs such as paresthesia or subjective paralysis. In all patients with delayed onset of paralysis, the spine had not been immobilized after the initial trauma, and all were neurologically normal before the second event. This underlines the importance of diligent immobilization of a suspected spinal cord injury in a child. Approximately half of the young children with SCIWORA in reported series had complete spinal cord injuries, whereas the older children usually had incomplete neurologic deficit injuries that involved the subaxial cervical spine.[19,25,167,275]

SIGNS AND SYMPTOMS OF CERVICAL SPINE INJURY

The most common presenting symptom in patients with cervical spine injuries is pain localized to the cervical region. Other complaints, such as headache, inability to move the neck, subjective feelings of instability, and neurologic symptoms, all warrant complete evaluation. Infants may present with unexplained respiratory distress, motor weakness, or hypotonia, which warrant further evaluation. Patients with head and neck trauma, distraction injuries, or altered levels of consciousness are at high risk for a cervical spine injury and need to be thoroughly evaluated before obtaining cervical spine clearance.[62,273] The presence of an occult cervical spine injury in an uncooperative or obtunded patient needs to be considered because of the frequency of SCIWORA in the pediatric population.[310,349]

IMAGING AND OTHER DIAGNOSTIC STUDIES FOR CERVICAL SPINE INJURY

Plain Radiographs

Plain radiographs are the standard first step for evaluating the cervical spine in children.[294] Currently, there is no consensus regarding whether or not all pediatric trauma patients require cervical spine films. The presence of tenderness and association with a distracting injury (like facial fracture, humerus fracture) are clinical presentations that most commonly require cervical spine films.[422] While some studies have shown that plain radiographs are of low yield in patients without evidence of specific physical findings, the burden remains on the treating physician to clear the cervical spine.[16,103,238,244] Clearly, patients with tenderness, distracting injuries, neurologic deficits, head and neck trauma, and altered levels of consciousness need to have a complete set of cervical spine radiographs. Initial radiographs should include an anteroposterior view, open-mouth odontoid view, and lateral view of the cervical spine. Patients who are deemed unstable in the emergency room and are not able to tolerate multiple radiographs should have a cross-table lateral view of the cervical spine until further radiographs can be taken.[60] The false-negative rates for a single cross-table radiograph have been reported to be 23% to 26%, indicating that complete radiographs are necessary when the patient is stable.[27,368]

Flexion and extension radiographs may further aid the evaluation of the cervical spine, but these views are unlikely to be abnormal when standard views show no abnormalities. These views are helpful, however, in ruling out acute ligamentous injury.[335] We recommend flexion and extension views in an alert patient with midline tenderness who has normal plain films of the cervical spine. These views should be taken only with a cooperative and alert child; they should not be used in obtunded or uncooperative patients, nor should they be done by manually placing the child in a position of flexion and extension.

Evaluation of cervical spine radiographs should proceed with a knowledge of the anatomic ossification centers and variations that occur in children. Each vertebral level should be systematically evaluated, as should the overall alignment of the cervical spine with respect to the anterior and posterior aspects of the vertebral bodies, the spinolaminar line, and the interspinous distances. The absence of cervical lordosis, an increase in the prevertebral soft tissue space, and subluxation of C2 on C3 are all anatomic variations that may be normal in children.[70] Ossification centers also may be confused with fractures, most commonly in evaluation of the dens. The presence of a synchondrosis at the base of the odontoid can be distinguished from a fracture based on the age of the patient and the location of synchondrosis well below the facet joints. Knowledge of these normal variants is useful in evaluating plain radiographs of the cervical spine in children.

Normal Ossification Centers and Anomalies Frequently Confused With Injury

Avulsion Fracture

- Apical ossification center of the odontoid. Secondary ossification centers at the tips of the transverse and spinous processes

Fracture

- Persistence of the synchondrosis at the base of the odontoid
- Apparent anterior wedging of a young child's vertebral body
- Normal posterior angulation of the odontoid seen in 4% of normal children

Instability

- Pseudosubluxation of C2–C3 (Fig. 20-1)
- Incomplete ossification, especially of the odontoid process, with apparent superior subluxation of the anterior arch of C1
- Absence of the ossification center of the anterior arch of C1 in the first year of life may suggest posterior displacement of C1 on the odontoid
- Increase in the atlanto–dens interval (ADI) of up to 4.5 mm

Miscellaneous

- Physiologic variations in the width of the prevertebral soft tissue due to crying misinterpreted as swelling due to edema or hemorrhage
- Overlying structures such as ears, braided hair, teeth, or hyoid bone. Plastic rivets used in modern emergency cervical immobilization collars can simulate fracture line
- Horizontally placed facets in the younger child, creating the illusion of a pillar fracture
- Congenital anomalies such as os odontoideum, spina bifida, and congenital fusion or hemivertebrae

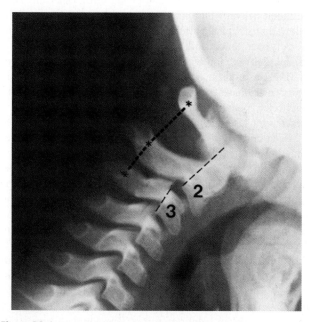

Figure 20-1. Pseudosubluxation of C2 on C3. In flexion, the posterior element of C2 should normally align itself with the posterior elements C1 and C3. The relationship of the body of C2 with the body of C3 gives the appearance of subluxation; however, the alignment of the posterior elements of C1 to C3 confirms pseudosubluxation.

Radiographic Evaluation of Specific Areas of the Spine

Atlantooccipital Junction

The atlantooccipital interval remains the most difficult to assess for abnormalities, partly because of the difficulty in obtaining quality radiographs and partly because of the lack of discrete and reproducible landmarks. The distance between the occipital condyles and the facet joints of the atlas should be less than 5 mm; any distance of more than this suggests an atlantooccipital disruption.[105,322] The foramen magnum and its relationship to the atlas also are useful in detecting injuries of the atlantooccipital region. The anterior cortical margin of the foramen magnum is termed the basion, whereas the posterior cortical margin of the foramen magnum is termed the opisthion. The distance between the basion and the tip of the dens should be less than 12 mm as measured on a lateral radiograph.[64] The Powers ratio (Fig. 20-2) is used to assess the position of the skull base relative to the atlas and is another way of evaluating the atlantooccipital region. To determine this ratio, a line is drawn from the basion to the anterior cortex of the posterior arch of C1, and this distance is divided by the distance of a line drawn from the opisthion to the posterior cortex of the anterior arch of C1. The value should be between 0.7 and 1; a higher value indicates anterior subluxation of the atlantooccipital joint and a lower value indicates a posterior subluxation. The problem lies in the fact that the basion is not always visible on plain radiographs and this ratio is not frequently used clinically. The Wackenheim line (Fig. 20-3), which is drawn along the posterior aspect of the clivus, probably is the most easily identified line to determine disruption of the atlantooccipital

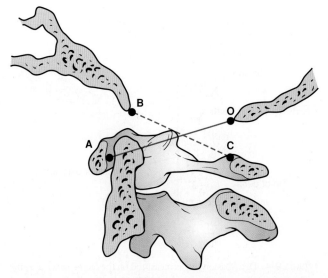

Figure 20-2. The Powers ratio is determined by drawing a line from the basion (*B*) to the posterior arch of the atlas (*C*) and a second line from the opisthion (*O*) to the anterior arch of the atlas (*A*). The length of the line BC is divided by the length of the line OA, producing the Powers ratio. (Reprinted with permission from Lebwohl NH, Eismont FJ. Cervical spine injuries in children. In: Weinstein SL, ed. *The Pediatric Spine: Principles and Practice.* 1st ed. New York, NY: Raven; 1994.)

joint. If the line does not intersect the tip of the odontoid tangentially and if this line is displaced anteriorly or posteriorly, disruption or increased laxity about the atlantooccipital joint should be suspected.

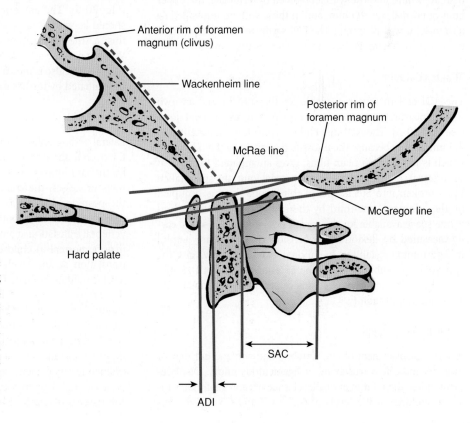

Figure 20-3. The ADI and the space available for cord are used in determining atlantoaxial instability. The Wackenheim clivus-canal line is used to determine atlantooccipital injury, while the McRae and McGregor lines are used in the measurement of basilar impression. (Modified from Copley LA, Dormans JP. Cervical spine disorders in infants and children. *J Am Acad Orthop Surg.* 1998;6(4):204–214. With permission.)

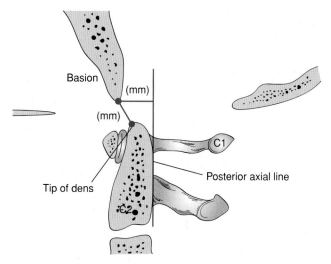

Figure 20-4. Dens-basion line is measured on the lateral cervical spine radiograph; a distance of more than 12.5 mm generally is considered indicative of AOD; however, this measurement is less reliable in children younger than the age of 5 years because of the variability in dens ossification.

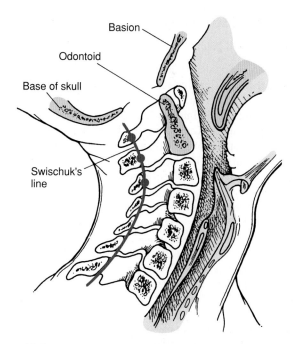

Figure 20-5. The spinolaminar line (Swischuk line) is used to determine the presence of pseudosubluxation of C2 on C3. (Reprinted from Copley LA, Dormans JP. Cervical spine disorders in infants and children. *J Am Acad Orthop Surg.* 1998;6(4):204–214. With permission.)

Measurement of the basion-dens interval (BDI) also is helpful in the diagnosis of atlantooccipital dissociation (Fig. 20-4). The BDI is measured on the lateral cervical spine radiograph, and a distance of more than 12.5 mm generally is considered indicative of atlanto occipital dissociation (AOD); however, this measurement is less reliable in children younger than the age of 5 years because of the variability in dens ossification.[48] Bertozzi et al.[40] determined that on MDCT 97% of 117 children had a BDI of less than 10.5 mm; in those with an ossified os terminale, the upper limit of normal was 9.5 mm, and in those with an unossified os terminale, it was 11.6 mm. The BDI seems to be more practical than other radiographic assessments such as the powers.

Atlantoaxial Joint

The ADI and the space available for the spinal canal are two useful measurements for evaluation of the atlantoaxial joint (see Fig. 20-3). The ADI in a child is considered normal up to 4.5 mm, partly because the unossified cartilage of the odontoid, which is not seen on plain films, gives an apparent increase in the interval. At the level of the atlantoaxial joint, the space taken up is broken into Steel's rule of thirds: one-third is occupied by the odontoid, one-third by the spinal cord, and one-third is free space available for the cord. These intervals also are easily measured on flexion and extension views and are helpful in determining instability. In children, extension views give the appearance of subluxation of the anterior portion of the atlas over the unossified dens, but this represents a pseudosubluxation and not instability.[75,97]

Upper Cervical Spine

Anterior displacement of one vertebral body on another may or may not indicate a true bony or ligamentous injury. Displacement of less than 3 mm at one level is a common anatomic variant in children at the levels of C2 to C3 and C3 to C4. This displacement is seen on flexion radiographs and reduces in extension. The posterior line of Swischuk and Rowe[338] has been described to differentiate pathologic subluxation from normal anatomic variation; this line is drawn from the anterior cortex of the spinous process of C1 to the spinous process of C3 (Fig. 20-5). The anterior cortex of the spinous process of C2 should lie within 3 mm of this line; if the distance is more than this, a true subluxation should be suspected (see Fig. 20-1). Widening of the spinous processes between C1 and C2 of more than 10 mm also is indicative of a ligamentous injury and should be evaluated by further imaging studies.[9]

Lower Cervical Spine

Lateral radiographs of the cervical spine should be evaluated for overall alignment. The overall alignment can be evaluated by the continuous lines formed by the line adjoining the spinous processes, the spinolaminar line, and the lines adjoining the posterior and anterior vertebral bodies (Fig. 20-6). These lines should all be smooth and continuous with no evidence of vertebral translation at any level. Loss of normal cervical lordosis may be normal in children, but there should be no associated translation at any level.[426] The interspinous distance at each level should be evaluated and should be no more than 1.5 times the distance at adjacent levels; if this ratio is greater, an injury should be suspected. There are calculated norms for the interspinous distances in children, and any value greater than two standard deviations above normal is indicative of a ligamentous injury.[235] The measurement of soft tissue spaces is important in evaluating any evidence of swelling or hemorrhage, which may be associated with an occult injury. The normal retropharyngeal soft tissue space should be less than 6 mm at C3 and less than

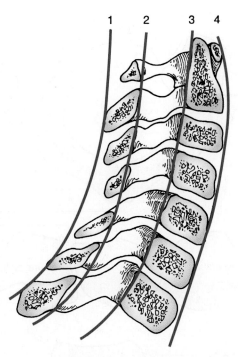

Figure 20-6. Normal relationships in the lateral cervical spine: *1*, spinous processes; *2*, spinolaminar line; *3*, posterior vertebral body line; *4*, anterior vertebral body line. (Reprinted from Copley LA, Dormans JP. Cervical spine disorders in infants and children. *J Am Acad Orthop Surg.* 1998;6(4):204–214. With permission.)

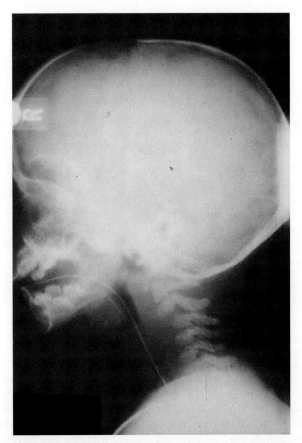

Figure 20-7. Anterior translation with patient on a spine board.

14 mm at C6. These spaces may be increased in children without an injury who are crying at the time of the radiograph, because the attachment of the pharynx to the hyoid bone results in its forward displacement with crying, producing an apparent increase in the width of these spaces. These radiographs must be taken with the patient quiet and repeated if there is any doubt.

Special Imaging Studies

Most cervical spine injuries in children are detected by plain radiographs.[10,236,266] Most ligamentous injuries can be identified on flexion and extension views of the cervical spine in a cooperative and alert patient. The roles of CT imaging and MRI continue to evolve in the evaluation of trauma patients.[78]

Plain radiographs remain the standard for initial evaluation of the pediatric cervical spine; CT imaging as an initial diagnostic study is associated with an increase in radiation with no demonstrable benefit over plain radiographs.[3] However, when CT imaging is used in children, a few salient points should be kept in mind. First, the proportion of a child's head to his/her body is greater than that of an adult, so care must be taken not to position the head in flexion to obtain the scan, which could potentiate any occult fracture not seen on plain films (Fig. 20-7). Second, the radiation doses for CT imaging are significantly higher than for plain radiographs, and CT protocols for children should be used to limit the amount of radiation. Although axial views are standard, coronal and sagittal formatted images and three-dimensional reconstruction views provide improved anatomic detail of the spine and can be obtained

without any additional radiation to the patient.[177,259] In patients with head injuries, the cervical spine can be included in the CT image of the head to reduce the number of plain films necessary to rule out an occult spinal injury.[213] CT imaging is particularly useful in evaluating occipital condyle fractures which are difficult to see on plain x-ray.

MRI has become increasingly useful in evaluating pediatric patients with suspected cervical spine injuries (Fig. 20-8), especially for ruling out ligamentous injuries in patients who cannot cooperate with flexion and extension views.[133,179] The advantages of an early MRI are the ability to allow mobilization if no injury is present and the early detection of an unrecognized spinal fracture to allow proper treatment. MRI is also useful in evaluating patients with SCIWORA. MR angiography (MRA) has replaced standard arteriography for evaluation of the vertebral arteries in patients with upper cervical spine injuries who have suspected arterial injuries.[314] MRI also remains the best imaging modality for evaluating injuries of the intervertebral disks and is especially useful to detect disk herniation in adolescent patients with facet joint injuries that may require operative reduction.

CLASSIFICATION OF CERVICAL SPINE INJURY

There is currently no fracture classification for pediatric cervical spine injuries. Fractures are defined by the level of injury as well as whether there is an associated bony injury or ligamentous

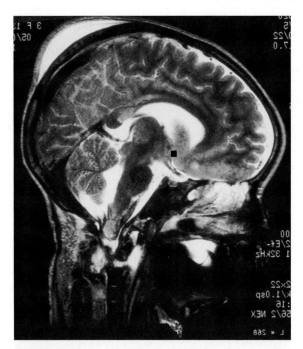

Figure 20-8. MRI depicts injury to the cervical cord and upper cervical spine.

injury. The presence of ligamentous injuries is more common in younger children whereas subaxial cervical injuries are more common toward skeletal maturity, and fractures may then be classified using adult fracture classifications. Classifications for specific fractures are discussed later in the chapter.

PATHOANATOMY AND APPLIED ANATOMY RELATED TO CERVICAL SPINE INJURY

Understanding the normal growth and development of the cervical spine is essential when treating a child with a suspected cervical spine injury. This will allow the physician to differentiate normal physes or synchondroses from pathologic fractures or ligamentous disruptions and will alert the physician to any possible congenital anomalies that may be mistaken for a fracture.[301]

UPPER CERVICAL SPINE

At birth, the atlas is composed of three ossification centers, one for the body and one for each of the neural arches (Fig. 20-9). In approximately 20% of individuals, the ossification center for the anterior arch is present at birth; in the remainder, they appear by 1 year of age. Occasionally, the anterior arch is bifid, and the body may be formed from two centers, or it may fail to completely form. The posterior arches usually fuse by 3 years of age; however, occasionally, the posterior synchondrosis between the two arches fails to fuse, resulting in a bifid arch. The neurocentral synchondroses that link the neural arches to the body close by 7 years of age. They are best seen on an open-mouth odontoid view and should not be mistaken for fractures.[70] The canal of the atlas is large enough to allow for the rotation that

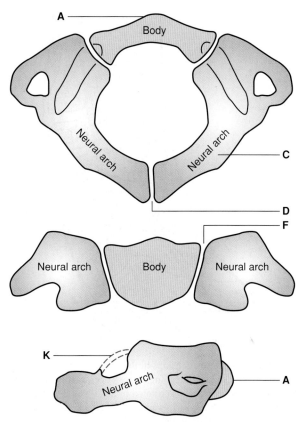

Figure 20-9. Diagram of C1 (atlas). The body (*A*) is not ossified at birth, and its ossification center appears during the first year of life. The body may fail to develop, and forward extension of neural arches (*C*) may take its place. Neural arches appear bilaterally about the seventh week (*D*), and the most anterior portion of the superior articulating surface usually is formed by the body. The synchondrosis of the spinous processes unites by the third year. Union rarely is preceded by the appearance of the secondary center within the synchondrosis. Neurocentral synchondrosis (*F*) fuses about the seventh year. The ligament surrounding the superior vertebral notch (*K*) may ossify, especially in later life. (With permission from Bailey DK. Normal cervical spine in infants and children. *Radiology*. 1952;59:713–714.)

is necessary at this joint as well as some forward translation.[78] The vertebral arteries are about 2 cm from the midline and run in a groove on the superior surface of the atlas. This must be remembered during lateral dissection at the occipital–cervical junction. The ring of C1 reaches about normal adult size by 4 years of age.[14]

The axis develops from at least four separate ossification centers: one for the dens, one for the body, and two for the neural arches (Fig. 20-10). Between the odontoid and the body of the axis is a synchondrosis or vestigial disk space that often is mistaken for a fracture line. This synchondrosis runs well below the level of the articular processes of the axis and usually fuses at 6 to 7 years of age, although it may persist as a sclerotic line until 11 years of age.[75,276] The most common odontoid fracture pattern in adults and adolescents is transverse and at the level of the articular processes. The normal synchondrosis should not be confused with this fracture; the synchondrosis is more cup-shaped and below the level of the articular processes. After

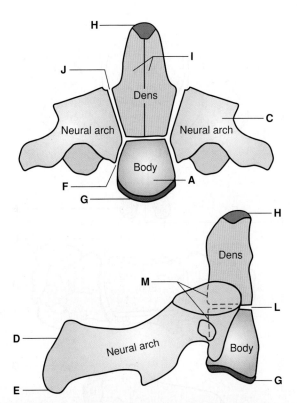

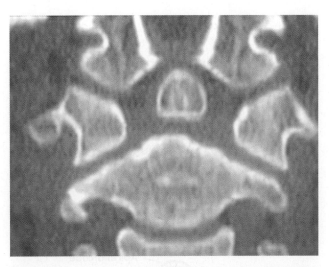

Figure 20-11. CT scan showing presence of an os odontoideum. Note the position of the os well above the C1 to C2 facets. The scan also shows the vestigial scar of the synchondrosis between the dens and the body below the C1 to C2 facet.

Figure 20-10. Diagram of C2 (axis). The body (*A*) in which one center (occasionally two) appears by the fifth fetal month. Neural arches (*C*) appear bilaterally by the seventh fetal month. Neural arches fuse (*D*) posteriorly by the second or third year. Bifid tip (*E*) of spinous process (occasionally a secondary center is present in each tip). Neurocentral synchondrosis (*F*) fuses at 3 to 6 years. The inferior epiphyseal ring (*G*) appears at puberty and fuses at about 25 years of age. The summit ossification center (*H*) for the odontoid appears at 3 to 6 years and fuses with the odontoid by 12 years. Odontoid (dens) (*I*). Two separate centers appear by the fifth fetal month and fuse with each other by the seventh fetal month. The synchondrosis between the odontoid and neural arch (*I*) fuses at 3 to 6 years. Synchondrosis between the odontoid and body (*L*) fuses at 3 to 6 years. Posterior surface of the body and odontoid (*M*). (With permission from Bailey DK. Normal cervical spine in infants and children. *Radiology*. 1952;59:713–714.)

7 years of age, the synchondrosis should not be present on an open-mouth odontoid view; a fracture should be considered if a lucent line is present after this age. The neural arches of C2 fuse at 3 to 6 years of age; these are seen as vertical lucent lines on the open-mouth odontoid view. Occasionally, the tip of the odontoid is V-shaped (dens bicornum), or a small separate summit ossification center may be present at the tip of the odontoid (ossiculum terminale). An os odontoideum is believed to result from a history of unrecognized trauma. The differentiation between an os odontoideum and the synchondrosis of the body is relatively easy because of their relationships to the level of the C1 to C2 facet (Fig. 20-11).

The arterial supply to the odontoid is derived from the vertebral and carotid arteries. The anterior and posterior ascending arteries arise from the vertebral artery at the level of C3 and ascend anterior and posterior to the odontoid, meeting superiorly to form an apical arcade. These arteries supply small penetrating branches to the body of the axis and the odontoid process. The internal carotid artery gives off cleft perforators that supply the superior portion of the odontoid. This arrangement of arteries and vessels is necessary for embryologic development and anatomic function of the odontoid. The synchondrosis prevents direct vascularization of the odontoid from C2, and vascularization from the blood supply of C1 is not possible because the synovial joint cavity surrounds the odontoid. The formation of an os odontoideum after cervical trauma may be related to this peculiar blood supply (Fig. 20-12).

LOWER CERVICAL SPINE

The third through seventh cervical vertebrae share a similar ossification pattern: a single ossification center for the vertebral body and an ossification center for each neural arch (Fig. 20-13). The neural arch fuses posteriorly between the second and third years, and the neurocentral synchondroses between the neural arches and the vertebral body fuse by 3 to 6 years of age. These vertebrae normally are wedge-shaped until 7 to 8 years of age.[24,239,334] The vertebral bodies, neural arches, and pedicles enlarge by periosteal appositional growth, similar to that seen in long bones. By 8 to 10 years of age, a child's spine usually reaches near adult size and characteristics. There are five secondary ossification centers that can remain open until 25 years of age.[238] These include one each for the spinous processes, transverse processes, and the ring apophyses about the vertebral endplates. These should not be confused with fractures.

The superior and inferior endplates are firmly bound to the adjacent disk. The junction between the vertebral body and the endplate is similar to a physis of a long bone. The vertebral body is analogous to the metaphysis and the endplate to the physis, where longitudinal growth occurs. The junction between the vertebral body and the endplate has been shown to be weaker than the adjacent vertebral body or disk, which can result in a fracture at the endplate in the area of columnar and calcified

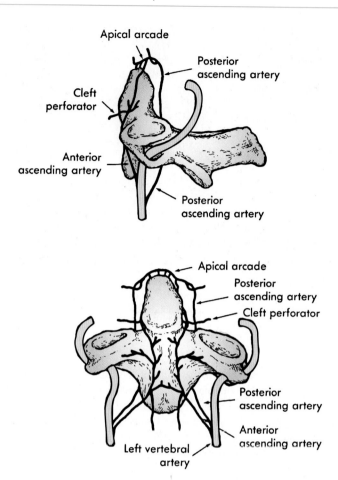

Figure 20-12. Blood supply to odontoid: posterior and anterior ascending arteries and apical arcade.[257] (Reprinted with permission from Schiff DC, Parke WW. The arterial supply of the odontoid process. *J Bone Joint Surg Am.* 1973;55(7):1450–1464.)

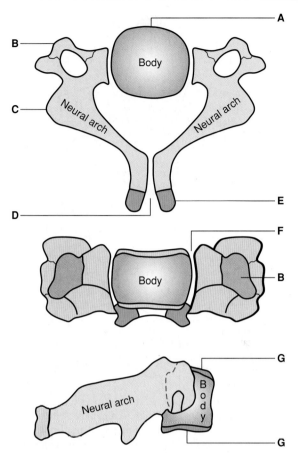

Figure 20-13. Diagram of typical cervical vertebrae, C3 to C7. The body (*A*) appears by the fifth fetal month. The anterior (costal) portion of the transverse process (*B*) may develop from a separate center that appears by the sixth fetal month and joins the arch by the sixth year. Neural arches (*C*) appear by the seventh to ninth fetal week. The synchondrosis between spinous processes (*D*) usually unites by the second or third year. Secondary centers for bifid spine (*E*) appear at puberty and unite with spinous process at 25 years. Neurocentral synchondrosis (*F*) fuses at 3 to 6 years. Superior and inferior epiphyseal rings (*G*) appear at puberty and unite with the body at about 25 years. The seventh cervical vertebra differs slightly because of a long, powerful, nonbifid spinous process. (With permission from Bailey DK. Normal cervical spine in infants and children. *Radiology.* 1952;59:713–714.)

cartilage of the growth zone, similar to a Salter–Harris type I fracture of a long bone.[24] The inferior end plate may be more susceptible to this injury than the superior endplate because of the mechanical protection afforded by the developing uncinate processes.[46]

The facet joints of the cervical spine change in orientation with age. The angle of the C1 to C2 facet is 55 degrees in newborns and increases to 70 degrees at maturity. In the lower cervical spine, the angle of the facet joints is 30 degrees at birth and 60 to 70 degrees at maturity. This may explain why the pediatric cervical spine may be more susceptible to injury from the increased motion or translation allowed by the facet joint orientation.

Increased ligamentous laxity in young children allows a greater degree of spinal mobility than in adults. Flexion and extension of the spine at C2 to C3 are 50% greater in children between the ages of 3 and 8 years than in adults. The level of the greatest mobility in the cervical spine descends with increasing age. Between 3 and 8 years of age, the most mobile segment is C3 to C4; from 9 to 11 years, C4 to C5 is the most mobile segment, and from 12 to 15 years, C5 to C6 is the most mobile segment.[10,322] This explains the tendency for craniocervical injuries in young children.

Several anomalies of the cervical spine may influence treatment recommendations. The atlas can fail to segment from the skull, a condition called occipitalization of the atlas, and can lead to narrowing of the foramen magnum, neurologic symptoms, and increased stresses to the atlantoaxial articulation, which often causes instability. Failure of fusion of the posterior arch of C1 is not uncommon and should be sought before any procedure that involves C1. Wedge-shaped vertebrae, bifid vertebrae, or a combination of these also can occur. Klippel–Feil syndrome is defined as congenital fusion of at least two cervical vertebrae, and may present with the classic triad of a short neck, low posterior hairline, and severe restriction of motion of the neck.[182,223] Congenital fusion of the cervical spine may predispose a child to injury from trauma by concentrating stresses in the remaining mobile segments.

Hensinger et al.[181] reported congenital anomalies of the odontoid, including aplasia (complete absence), hypoplasia (partial absence in which there is a stubby piece at the base of the odontoid located above the C1 articulation), and os odontoideum. Os odontoideum consists of a separate ossicle of the odontoid with no connection to the body of C2. The cause may be traumatic. These anomalies also may predispose a child to injury or instability.

TREATMENT OPTIONS FOR CERVICAL SPINE INJURY

INITIAL MANAGEMENT OF PATIENTS WITH SUSPECTED CERVICAL SPINE INJURY

The initial management of a child with a suspected cervical spine injury is paramount to avoiding further injury to the cervical spine and spinal cord.[108] The initial management of any child suspected of having a cervical spine injury starts with immobilization in the field. Extraction from an automobile or transport to the hospital may cause damage to the spinal cord in a child with an unstable cervical spine injury if care is not taken to properly immobilize the neck. The immobilization device should allow access to the patient's oropharynx and anterior neck if intubation or tracheostomy becomes necessary. The device should allow splintage of the head and neck to the thorax to minimize further movement.[85,217]

The use of backboards in pediatric trauma patients deserves special attention because of the anatomic differences between children and adults. Compared with adults, children have a disproportionately larger head with respect to the body. This anatomic relationship causes a child's cervical spine to be placed in flexion if immobilization is done on a standard backboard. Herzenberg et al.[184] reported 10 children under the age of 7 years whose cervical spines had anterior angulation or translation on radiograph when they were placed on a standard backboard (Fig. 20-14A,B). Unnecessary flexion can be avoided by using a backboard with a recess into which the head can be lowered or by supporting the body with two mattresses and the head with only one mattress, allowing the cervical spine to assume a neutral position (Fig. 20-14C,D). Children younger than 8 years of age should be immobilized on a backboard using one of these techniques.[83,300]

Cervical collars supplement backboards for immobilization in the trauma setting. While soft collars tend to be more comfortable and cause less soft tissue irritation, rigid collars are preferred for patients with acute injuries because they provide better immobilization. Even rigid collars may allow up to 17 degrees of flexion, 19 degrees of extension, 4 degrees of rotation, and 6 degrees of lateral motion.[92,279] Supplemental sandbags and taping on either side of the head are recommended in all children and have been shown to limit the amount of spinal motion to 3 degrees in any plane.[194]

Further displacement of an unstable cervical injury may occur if resuscitation is required. The placement of pediatric patients on an appropriate board with the neck in a neutral position makes recognition of some fractures difficult because

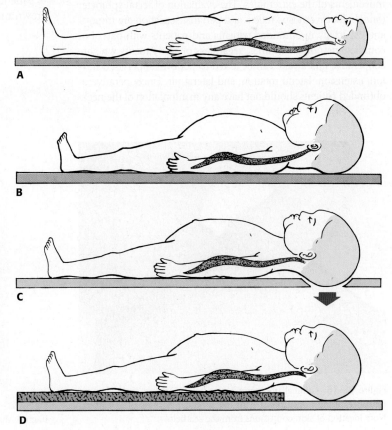

Figure 20-14. A: Adult immobilized on a standard backboard. **B:** Young child on a standard backboard. The relatively large head forces the neck into a kyphotic position. Such flexion can be avoided by using a modified backboard that has a cutout to the recess of the occiput, obtaining better supine cervical alignment (**C**) or by using a modified backboard that has a double-mattress pad (**D**) to raise the chest, obtaining better supine cervical alignment. (Reprinted with permission from Herzenberg JE, Hensinger RN, Dedrick DK, et al. Emergency transport and positioning of young children who have an injury of the cervical spine: the standard blackboard may be hazardous. *J Bone Joint Surg Am.* 1989;71(1):15–22.)

positional reduction may have occurred, especially with ligamentous injuries or endplate fractures. An apparently normal lateral radiograph in a patient with altered mental status or multiple injuries does not rule out a cervical spine injury. A study of four patients with unstable cervical spine injuries who had attempted resuscitation in the emergency department showed that axial traction actually increased the deformity.[46] Any manipulation of the cervical spine, even during intubation, must be done with caution and with the assumption that the patient has an unstable cervical spine injury until proven otherwise.

The physical evaluation of any patient with a suspected cervical spine injury should begin with inspection. Head and neck trauma is associated with a high incidence of cervical spine injuries.[10,24,306] Soft tissue abrasions or shoulder-harness marks on the neck from a seatbelt are clues to an underlying cervical spine injury (Fig. 20-15).[135,148,190] Unconscious patients should be treated as if they have a cervical spine injury until further evaluation proves otherwise. The next step in the evaluation is palpation of the cervical spine for tenderness, muscle spasm, and overall alignment. The most prominent levels should be the spinous processes at C2, C3, and C7. Anterior palpation should focus on the presence of tenderness or swelling. The entire spine should be palpated and thoroughly examined because 20% of patients with cervical spine injuries have other spinal fractures.

A thorough neurologic examination should be done, which can be difficult in pediatric patients. Strength, sensation, reflexes, and proprioception should be documented. In patients who are uncooperative because of age or altered mental status, repeat examinations are important; however, the initial neurovascular examination should be documented even if it entails only gross movements of the extremities. The evaluation of rectal sphincter tone, bulbocavernosus reflex, and perianal sensation are important, especially in obtunded patients and patients with partial or complete neurologic injuries, regardless of age. Patients who are cooperative and awake can be asked to perform supervised flexion, extension, lateral rotation, and lateral tilt. Uncooperative or obtunded patients should not have any manipulation of the neck.

NONOPERATIVE TREATMENT OF CERVICAL SPINE INJURY

Immobilization of the cervical spine may continue after the emergency setting if there is an injury that requires treatment. Specific injuries and their treatment are described later in this chapter. Further immobilization of some cervical spine injuries requires a cervical collar. A rigid collar can be used for immobilization if it is an appropriately fitting device with more padding than a standard cervical collar placed in the emergency department. More unstable or significant injuries can be treated with a custom orthosis, a Minerva cast, or a halo device.[218,369,402] An advantage of custom devices is the ability to use lightweight thermoplastic materials that can be molded better to each patient's anatomy and can be extended to the thorax (Fig. 20-16). These devices must be properly applied for effective immobilization, and skin breakdown, especially over the chin region, needs to be carefully monitored. Minerva casts tend to provide more immobilization than thermoplastic devices, but their use is not as common and their application requires attention to detail.

A halo device can be used for the treatment of cervical spine injuries even in children as young as 1 year old.[47,353,408] The halo can be used as either a ring alone to apply traction or with a vest for definitive immobilization of an unstable cervical spine injury. Prefabricated vests are available in sizes for infants, toddlers, and children, with measurements based on the circumference of the chest at the xiphoid process.

The fabrication of a halo for any patient needs to consider both the size of the ring and the size of the vest. Prefabricated rings and prefabricated vests are available for even the smallest of patients and are based on circumferential measurements at the crown and at the xiphoid process. If the size of the patient or the

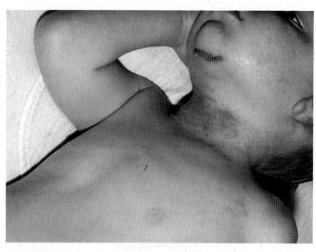

Figure 20-15. Clinical photograph of a patient with a cervical spine injury resulting from impact with the shoulder harness of a seatbelt. Note location of skin contusions from the seatbelt.

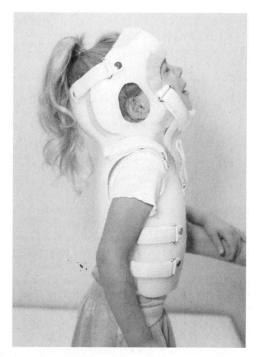

Figure 20-16. Custom-made cervicothoracic brace used to treat a C2 fracture that reduced in extension.

anatomy of the patient does not fit within these standard sizes, the fabrication of a custom halo may be necessary. Mubarak et al.[288] recommended the following steps in the fabrication of a custom halo for a child: (a) the size and configuration of the head are obtained with the use of the flexible lead wire placed around the head, (b) the halo ring is fabricated by constructing a ring 2 cm larger in diameter than the wire model, (c) a plaster mold of the trunk is obtained for the manufacture of a custom bivalved polypropylene vest, and (d) linear measurements are made to ensure appropriate length of the superstructure.

The placement of pins into an immature skull deserves special attention because of the dangers of inadvertent skull penetration with a pin. CT imaging before halo application aids in determining bone structure and skull thickness but is not always necessary and radiation exposure must be considered. It also aids in determining whether or not cranial suture interdigitation is complete and if the fontanels are closed. The thickness of the skull varies greatly up to 6 years of age and is not similar to that of adults until the age of 16 years.[244] Garfin et al.[138] evaluated the pediatric cranium by CT and determined that

the skull is thickest anterolaterally and posterolaterally, making these the optimal sites for pin placement.

The number of pins used for placement of a ring and the insertion torques used in younger children also deserve special mention. The placement of pins at the torque pressures used in adults will lead to penetration during insertion.[244] In infants and younger children, we recommend the placement of multiple pins (8 to 12) tightened to finger-tightness or 2- to 4-in. pounds to avoid unwanted skull penetration. In older children, six to eight pins are used and tightened to 4-in. pounds. In adolescents, four to eight pins can be tightened with a standard torque wrench to 6- to 8-in. pounds. The variability and reliability of pressures found with various torque wrenches during cadaver testing are great, and each pin must be inserted cautiously.[89] The use of 8 to 12 pins inserted at lower torque pressures aids in obtaining a stable ring with less chance of inadvertent penetration (Fig. 20-17). The insertion of each pin perpendicular to the skull also improves the pin–bone interface and the overall strength of the construct.[90] We have had success using halo vests even in children younger than 2 years of age

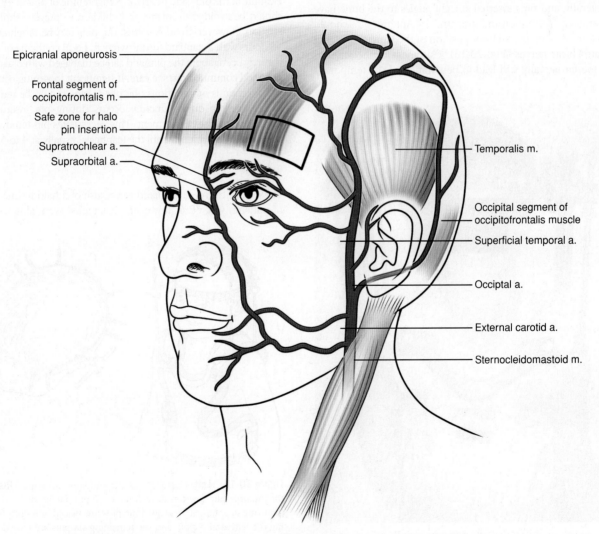

Figure 20-17. "Safe zone" for halo pin insertion.[184] (Adapted from Manson NA, An HS. Halo placement in the pediatric and adult patient. In: Vaccaro AR, Barton EM. *Operative Techniques in Spine Surgery.* 2nd ed. Philadelphia, PA: Saunders; 2008:13.)

by using multiple pins inserted to finger-tightness rather than relying on torque wrenches.

Halo Immobilization

A halo can be applied in older children and adolescents with a local anesthetic; however, in most younger children, a general anesthetic should be used. The patient is positioned on the operating table in a position that prevents unwanted flexion of the neck and maintains the proper relationship of the head and neck with the trunk. The area of skin in the region of pin insertion is cleaned with an antiseptic solution and appropriate areas are shaved as needed for pin placement posteriorly. The ring is placed while an assistant holds the patient's head; it should be placed just below the greatest circumference of the skull, which corresponds to just above the eyebrows anteriorly and 1 cm above the tips of the earlobes laterally. We recommend injection of local anesthetic into the skin and periosteum through the ring holes in which the pins will be placed. The pins are placed with sterile technique.

To optimize pin placement, a few points should be kept in mind. The thickest area of the skull is anterolaterally and posterolaterally, and pins inserted at right angles to the bone have greater force distribution and strength.[90,138] Anterior pins should be placed to avoid the anterior position of the supraorbital and supratrochlear nerves (Fig. 20-18). Placement of the anterior pins too far laterally will lead to penetration of the temporalis

muscle, which can lead to pain with mastication and talking, as well as early pin loosening. The optimal position for the anterior pins is in the anterolateral skull, just above the lateral two-thirds of the orbit and just below the greatest circumference of the skull. The posterior pins are best placed posterolaterally directly diagonal from the anterior pins. We also recommend placing the pins to finger-tightness originally and tightening two directly opposing pins simultaneously. During placement of the pins, meticulous attention should be paid to the position of the ring to have a circumferential fit on the patient's skull and to avoid any pressure of the ring on the scalp, especially posteriorly. The halo should not be touching the ears.

The number of pins used and the torque pressures applied vary according to the age of the patient as discussed above. Once the pins are tightened, they must be fastened to the ring by the appropriate lock nuts or set screws. The halo vest and superstructure are then applied, with care to maintain the position of the head and neck. Appropriate positioning of the head and neck can be done by adjusting the superstructure (Fig. 20-19).

Daily pin care should consist of hydrogen peroxide/saline cleaning at the pin–skin interface. Retightening of pins at 48 hours should be avoided in infants and children to prevent skull penetration; however, in adolescents, the pins can be retightened at 48 hours with a standard torque wrench. Local erythema or drainage may occur about the pins and can be managed with oral antibiotics and continued pin site care. If significant loosening occurs or the infection is more serious, the pin or pins should be removed. Occasionally, a dural puncture occurs during pin insertion or during the course of treatment. This necessitates pin removal and prophylactic antibiotics until the tear heals, usually at 4 to 5 days.

Outcomes

The complication rate related to the use of a halo in one series of patients was 68%; however, all patients were able to wear

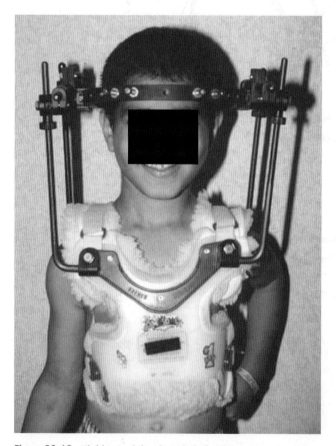

Figure 20-18. Child immobilized in a halo for C1 to C2 rotary subluxation. Note the position of the anterior pins, as well as the placement of the posterior pins at 180 degrees opposite the anterior pins.

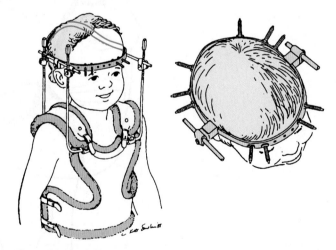

Figure 20-19. (**Left**) Custom halo vest and superstructure. (**Right**) In the multiple-pin, low-torque technique, 10 pins are used for an infant halo ring attachment. Usually, four pins are placed anteriorly, avoiding the temporal region, and the remaining six pins are placed in the occipital area. (Reprinted with permission from Mubarak SJ, Camp JF, Fuletich W, et al. Halo application in the infant. *J Pediatr Orthop.* 1989;9(5):612–613.)

the halo until fracture healing occurred or arthrodesis was achieved.[82] The most common complications in this series were superficial pin track infection and pin loosening. Other complications that occur less frequently include dural penetration, supraorbital nerve injury, unsightly pin scars, and deep infection.[34,106] Prefabricated halo vests are used in adults and are easily fitted to older adolescents. Because of the age and size ranges of children, however, a custom vest or even a cast vest may be needed. Improper fitting of a vest may allow unwanted movement of the neck despite the halo, and a significant size mismatch between the head and chest may require a custom vest or cast vest.

Methylprednisolone

If an acute spinal cord injury is determined by examination, the administration of methylprednisolone within the first 8 hours after injury has been shown to improve the chances of neurologic recovery in some early studies.[52–55] The initial loading dose of methylprednisolone is 30 mg/kg body weight, and then a maintenance infusion of 5.4 mg/kg is given for 24 to 48 hours after injury.

More recently, some studies have shown little or no benefit and increased complications with the use of methylprednisolone, and currently, it is most often recommended as a treatment option.[6,50,125] There are few studies on the use of methylprednisolone for spinal cord injury in pediatric patients.[21,71,74,323] Pettiford et al.[323] noted that data from adult studies remain controversial and concluded that, based on current evidence, the use of methylprednisolone is associated with an increased risk of infection and no neurologic improvements. In their review of 354 pediatric patients with acute spinal cord injuries, Caruso et al.[74] determined that methylprednisolone was not reliably administered according to protocol and those who received steroids were significantly more likely to have complications than those who did not. Based on these findings, Caruso et al. suggested removing high-dose methylprednisolone as a treatment option for pediatric acute spinal cord injury. Cage et al.[71] however, found infections more frequent in a control group than in those treated with methylprednisolone.

No clear evidence exists for the administration of steroids after spinal cord injury; however, a 2010 review on the subject revealed that many physicians continue to practice this in the face of an injury because of the perceived risks of litigation.[156] The potential side effects of steroids, namely pulmonary complications and wound complications, should be weighed against both the paucity of evidence regarding their therapeutic value and the institutional protocols that may be in place for spinal cord injury patients.

Once spinal cord injury is diagnosed, routine care includes prophylaxis for stress ulcers, routine skin care to prevent pressure sores, and initial Foley catheterization followed by intermittent catheterization and a bowel training program.

Outcomes

With incomplete lesions, children have a better chance than adults for useful recovery. Hadley et al.[159] noted that 89% of pediatric patients with incomplete spinal cord lesions improved, whereas only 20% of patients with complete injuries had evidence of significant recovery. Laminectomy has not been shown to be beneficial and can actually be harmful[374,450] because it increases instability in the cervical spine; for example, it can cause a swan neck deformity or progressive kyphotic deformity.[267,380] The risk of spinal deformity after spinal cord injury has been investigated by several researchers.[30,36,67,124,216,267] Mayfield et al.[267] found that patients who had a spinal cord injury before their growth spurt all developed spinal deformities, 80% of which were progressive. Ninety-three percent developed scoliosis, 57% kyphosis, and 18% lordosis. Sixty-one percent of these patients required spinal arthrodesis for stabilization of their curves. Orthotic management usually is unsuccessful, but in some patients it delays the age at which arthrodesis is necessary. Lower extremity deformities also may occur, such as subluxations and dislocations about the hip. Pelvic obliquity can be a significant problem and may result in pressure sores and difficulty in seating in a wheelchair.

Treatment of Neonatal Injury

Treatment of neonatal cervical spine injuries is nonoperative and should consist of careful realignment and positioning of the child on a bed with neck support or a custom cervical thoracic orthosis. Healing of bony injuries usually is rapid and complete.[392]

OPERATIVE TREATMENT OF CERVICAL SPINE INJURY

Preoperative Planning

The patient with an unstable cervical spine injury must be intubated and properly positioned to avoid further injury.

Stabilization

The injured cervical spine should be immobilized during transport. As discussed early in this chapter, in patients younger than 8 years of age, the use of a backboard with an occipital recess or having the trunk elevated approximately 2.5 cm is recommended. This will allow the cervical spine to remain in neutral alignment due to the relatively large head size compared with the trunk size in these younger patients. Soft cervical collars provide no significant stability to the cervical spine. Properly fitting hard cervical collars offer better support. The addition of sandbags and tape immobilization offers even more support.

Airway Management

In a patient with an unstable cervical spine, manipulation during intubation may injure the spinal cord. Axial traction, in particular, has been shown to result in increased distraction during intubation compared with either no immobilization or manual stabilization and is not recommended.[241] Manual in-line stabilization (MILS) is the most widely accepted technique for immobilization during intubation. This technique consists of grasping the mastoid processes with the fingertips with no traction being applied and then cupping the occiput in the palm of the hands.[146,257] Studies have confirmed the clinical safety of orotracheal intubation by direct laryngoscopy with MILS in patients with cervical spine injury.[357,371]

Several methods for intubation have been described for the patient with an unstable cervical spine. Awake intubation that is sometimes performed in adult patients is not feasible in the pediatric patient. Direct laryngoscopy with MILS is the method most often used. Fiberoptic intubation with MILS is a popular alternative. This causes minimal cervical movement and facilitates improved visualization of the vocal cords during intubation. However, the time to intubation with the fiberoptic technique is twice as long compared with direct laryngoscopy. The GlideScope videolaryngoscopy (Verathon, Bothell, WA) provides an indirect view of the glottis on a screen and has the potential for reduced motion. Nasotracheal intubation can be performed fiberoptically or without direct visualization. This technique is contraindicated in patients with basilar skull fractures or craniofacial trauma, which often is the case in pediatric cervical spine trauma.

Spinal Cord Monitoring

Spinal cord monitoring is usually used during surgical stabilization of the unstable cervical spine. Motor potential and somatosensory-evoked potentials (SSEP) are used for monitoring.

Spinal Cord Monitoring Techniques

Method	Function	Technique	Advantages	Disadvantages	Intraoperative Considerations
SSEPs 25% sensitive 100% specific	Monitor integrity of dorsal column sensory pathways	Signal initiation • LE: usually posterior tibial nerve • UE: usually ulnar nerve • Signal recording • Transcranial recording of somatosensory cortex	Reliable and unaffected by anesthetics	Not reliable for monitoring integrity of anterior spinal cord pathways	Loss of signal during distraction mandates immediate removal of device and assessment of monitoring signals
Motor-evoked potential (MEP) 100% sensitive 100% specific	Monitor integrity of lateral and ventral corticospinal tract	Signal initiation • Transcranial stimulation of motor cortex • Signal recording • Muscle contraction in extremity	Effective at detecting ischemic injury (loss of the anterior spinal artery in the anterior 2/3 of the spinal cord)	Often unreliable due to effects of anesthesia	

Data from Moore D. Spinal Cord Monitoring. 2016, November 6. Retrieved from https://www.orthobullets.com/spine/9023/spinal-cord-monitoring.

Positioning

The two primary techniques for prone positioning of patients with cervical spine injuries are manual turning using the log-roll technique or use of a spinal positioning table. Cadaver models have shown that turning using a spinal positioning table and a cervical collar results in the least amount of motion and is the preferred technique. If a spinal positioning table is not available, however, the log-roll technique with a cervical collar can be used. Once the patient is positioned, Gardner-Wells tongs or a halo ring is applied and attached to a Mayfield headrest attachment. Care must be taken when using these devices, because the head is in a fixed position and the torso is relatively free. Distraction and translation at the fracture site can occur, and fluoroscopy is recommended to verify proper alignment of the cervical spine when the patient is prone.

Surgical Approaches

The two most common approaches for surgical treatment of the unstable pediatric cervical spine are the posterior approach and anterior approach.[367] The posterior approach is the most commonly used and is most familiar to most orthopedic surgeon.[401]

Posterior Approach

This approach has been well described and can extend from the base of the occiput to the upper thoracic spine.

Technique

> ✔ **Posterior Approach to Cervical Spine Injury:** KEY SURGICAL STEPS
>
> ☐ Incision: Midline from suboccipital area to C3
> ☐ Dissect deep to ligamentum nuchae
> ☐ Release of cervical musculature from vertebrae

An incision is made in the midline from the suboccipital and can extend distally to C7 or T1. The dissection is extended deep within the relatively avascular intermuscular septum (also known as the ligamentum nuchae) and the cervical musculature is released from the spinous process. Bipolar cautery should be used judiciously and hemostatic products incorporated as needed to control bleeding from the perivertebral venous plexus, particularly at the C1 to C2 interlaminar space. Increased care must be taken when dissecting out laterally on C1 in younger patients, as the vertebral artery tends to be closer to the midline than has been described in adults. In patients under the age of 2 years, the artery could be as close as 8 mm from midline. In patients 2 to 8 years old, the artery was no closer than 10 mm, and in children over age 8, it was no closer than 12 mm.[154]

Potential Pitfalls and Preventive Measures

Posterior Approach to Cervical Spine Injury:
PITFALLS AND PREVENTIONS

Pitfall	Prevention
• Autofusion of all exposed vertebrae	• Avoid exposure of vertebrae not planned in fusion
• Vertebral artery injury with lateral dissection at C1	• Avoid over 8 mm lateral dissection at C1 in <2 year olds, 10 mm in 2–8 year olds, and 12 mm in older children
• Lordosis in posterior-only fusion	• May consider addition of anterior fusion

Anterior Approach

The anterior exposure is performed with the patient supine through a lateral retropharyngeal approach. The lateral retropharyngeal approach described by Whitesides and Kelly is an extension of the Henry approach to the vertebral artery. The sternocleidomastoid muscle is everted and retracted posteriorly, and the remainder of the dissection follows a plane posterior to the carotid sheath.

Technique

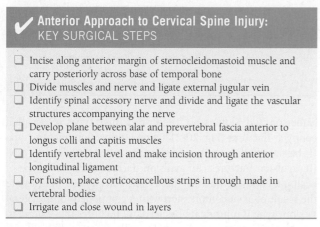

✔ Anterior Approach to Cervical Spine Injury:
KEY SURGICAL STEPS

- ☐ Incise along anterior margin of sternocleidomastoid muscle and carry posteriorly across base of temporal bone
- ☐ Divide muscles and nerve and ligate external jugular vein
- ☐ Identify spinal accessory nerve and divide and ligate the vascular structures accompanying the nerve
- ☐ Develop plane between alar and prevertebral fascia anterior to longus colli and capitis muscles
- ☐ Identify vertebral level and make incision through anterior longitudinal ligament
- ☐ For fusion, place corticocancellous strips in trough made in vertebral bodies
- ☐ Irrigate and close wound in layers

A longitudinal incision is made along the anterior margin of the sternocleidomastoid muscle. At the superior end of the muscle, the incision is carried posteriorly across the base of the temporal bone. If extensive exposure is needed, the muscle can be divided at its mastoid origin and the splenius capitis muscle can be partially divided at its insertion in the same area. At the superior pole of the incision is the external jugular vein, which crosses the anterior margin of the sternocleidomastoid; this vein should be divided and ligated. Branches of the auricular nerve also may be encountered and may require division. The sternocleidomastoid muscle is everted and the spinal accessory nerve is identified as it approaches and passes into the muscle. The vascular structures that accompany the nerve are divided and ligated. The approach posterior to the carotid sheath and anterior to the sternocleidomastoid muscle is developed (Fig. 20-20). The transverse processes of all the exposed cervical vertebrae are palpable in this interval. Using sharp and blunt dissection, the plane between the alar and prevertebral fascia is developed along the anterior aspect of the transverse processes of the vertebral bodies. The dissection

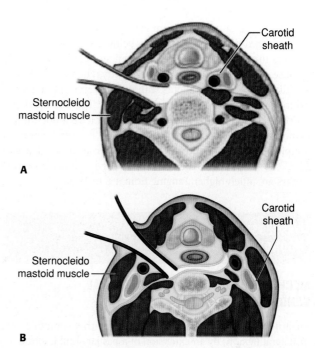

Figure 20-20. A and **B:** Anterior approach to the cervical spine. (Redrawn with permission from Canale ST, Beaty JH. *Campbell's Operative Orthopaedics.* 12th ed. Philadelphia, PA: Elsevier/Mosby; 2013.)

plane is anterior to the longus colli and capitis muscles and the overlying sympathetic trunk and superior cervical ganglion. (An alternative approach is to elevate the longus colli and capitis muscles from their bony insertion on the transverse processes, and retract the muscles anteriorly; however, this approach may disrupt the sympathetic rami communicantes and cause Horner syndrome.) When the vertebral level is identified, a longitudinal incision to bone is made through the anterior longitudinal ligament. The ligament and soft tissues are dissected subperiosteally to expose the vertebral bodies. Instrumentation and fusion can be performed as needed. The wound is irrigated and closed in layers over a suction drain in the retropharyngeal space.

The patient should be monitored closely for postoperative edema and airway obstruction. The patient may be immobilized in a cervical collar, cervicothoracic brace, halo vest, or halo cast depending on stability.

Occiput–C1 Injuries

OCCIPITAL CONDYLAR FRACTURES

INTRODUCTION TO OCCIPITAL CONDYLAR FRACTURES

Occipital condylar fractures are rare, and their diagnosis requires a high index of suspicion.[281,296] This fracture was described by

Bell in 1817 after a postmortem examination of a patient who fell backward off a wall, and upon being discharged from the hospital turned his head to bid farewell and died immediately because of the instability of his neck injury. The use of CT scan as a diagnostic tool in patients with cranial cervical trauma has led to increased recognition of this injury.[319] The true incidence of occipital condylar fractures in pediatric patients is not known, as most reported cases are in adult patients.[206] Several reports of occipital condylar fractures in children indicate an incidence of ≤1%[167,258,296]; however, prevalences reported in other CT-based studies are much higher, ranging from 4% to 19%.[43,44,247]

ASSESSMENT OF OCCIPITAL CONDYLAR FRACTURES

MECHANISMS OF INJURY FOR OCCIPITAL CONDYLAR FRACTURES

Fracture may be caused by axial loading with a component of ipsilateral flexion, by an extension of a basilar skull fracture, or by extreme rotation or lateral bending causing avulsion fracture of the inferomedial portion of the condyle that is attached to the alar ligament.

ASSOCIATED INJURIES AND SIGNS AND SYMPTOMS OF OCCIPITAL CONDYLAR FRACTURE

Most patients with occipital condylar fractures have associated head injuries.[7,281,414] Reports of associated cranial nerve deficits vary from 31% to 53% of patients with occipital condylar fractures.[14,167,412] Damage to the hypoglossal nerve (CN XII) can occur as the nerve passes through the hypoglossal canal that is located above the middle third of the occipital condyle.[207] The function of the hypoglossal nerve can be assessed by asking the patient to protrude the tongue. It will deviate to the paralyzed side.[51,82,384,453] When all four of the lower cranial nerves (IX–XII) are involved, this is known as Collet-Sicard syndrome. CN IX (glossopharyngeal nerve) is responsible for the ipsilateral gag reflex and sense of taste on the posterior third of the tongue. Impairment of CN X (vagus nerve) causes dysphagia and hoarseness, and damage of CN XI (accessory nerve) causes atrophy of the trapezius and ipsilateral sternocleidomastoid muscles. Almost all reports of Collet-Sicard syndrome associated with cervical fractures involve adult patients with high-impact injuries, including occipital condylar and Jefferson fractures.[86,104,118,173,231,370,417]

When cranial nerve deficits are noted, the presentation is acute in two-thirds of patient and delayed in one-third of the patients. Delayed cranial nerve palsies may be the result of migration of the fractured bony fragments or compression from proliferation of bone and fibrous tissue during the healing process. Vascular injuries involving the posteroinferior cerebellar artery and carotid arteries also have been reported with occipital condylar fracture.[77,203,209,229,242,248,406]

The clinical presentation is variable.[215,216] Pain and tenderness in the posterior occipitocervical region or torticollis may be the only complaints, whereas others may have significant neurologic deficits.[443]

IMAGING AND OTHER DIAGNOSTIC STUDIES FOR OCCIPITAL CONDYLAR FRACTURE

Plain radiographs often do not clearly show occipital condylar fractures, and CT with multiplanar reconstruction usually is necessary to establish the diagnosis.[17,51,233,262] The presence of a retropharyngeal hematoma on a lateral radiograph of the cervical spine may be the only clue to a fracture of the occipital condyle. Tuli et al.[412] recommended that a CT scan be obtained in the following circumstances: presence of lower cranial nerve deficits, associated head injury or basal skull fracture, or persistent neck pain despite normal radiographs.

CLASSIFICATION OF OCCIPITAL CONDYLAR FRACTURES

Occipital Condylar Fractures:
ANDERSON AND MONTESANO CLASSIFICATION

Type	Description	Biomechanics
I	Impaction	Results from axial loading; ipsilateral alar ligament may be compromised, but stability is maintained by contralateral alar ligament and tectorial membrane.
II	Skull base extension	Extends from occipital bone via condyle to enter foramen magnum; stability is maintained by intact alar ligaments and tectorial membrane.
III	Avulsion	Mediated via alar ligament tension; associated disruption of tectorial membrane and contralateral alar ligament may cause instability.

Anderson and Montesano[14] described three types of occipital condylar fractures (Fig. 20-21): type I, impaction fracture; type II, basilar skull fracture extending into the condyle; and type III, avulsion fractures. An avulsion fracture is the only type of occipital condylar fracture that is unstable. Type I injuries are the result of axial compression with a component of ipsilateral flexion. Type II injuries are basilar skull fractures that extend to involve the occipital condyle and usually are caused by a direct blow. Type III injuries are avulsion fractures of the inferomedial portion of the condyle that is attached to the alar ligament. Types I and II occipital condylar fractures usually are stable. Type III or avulsion fractures can be stable or unstable.[12]

Occipital Condylar Fractures:
CLASSIFICATION BY DISPLACEMENT AND STABILITY (Tuli et al.)

Type	Description	Biomechanics
1	Nondisplaced	Stable
2A	Displaced (≥2 mm of osseous separation)	Stable; no radiographic, CT, or MRI evidence of occipitoatlantoaxial instability of ligamentous disruption
2B	Displaced (≥2 mm of osseous separation)	Unstable; positive radiographic, CT, or MRI evidence of occipitoatlantoaxial instability or ligamentous disruption

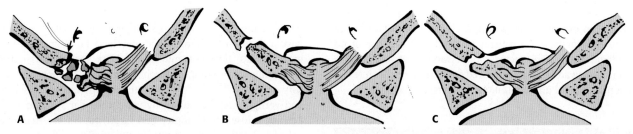

Figure 20-21. Classification of occipital condylar fractures according to Anderson and Monsanto. **A:** Type I fractures can occur with axial loading. **B:** Type II fractures are extensions of basilar cranial fractures. **C:** Type III fractures can result from an avulsion of the condyle during rotation, lateral bending, or a combination of mechanisms.[114] (From Hadley MN. Occipital condyle fractures. *Neurosurgery.* 2002;50(Suppl):S114–S119. Reproduced by permission of Oxford University Press.)

Tuli et al.[412] also classified occipital condylar fractures based on displacement and stability of the occiput/C1 to C2 complex. In their classification, type 1 fractures are nondisplaced and type 2 are displaced. They further subdivided type 2 fractures into type 2A, displaced but stable, and type 2B, displaced and unstable.

TREATMENT OPTIONS FOR OCCIPITAL CONDYLAR FRACTURES

NONOPERATIVE TREATMENT OF OCCIPITAL CONDYLAR FRACTURES

Nonoperative Treatment of Occipital Condylar Fractures: INDICATIONS AND CONTRAINDICATIONS	
Indications	**Relative Contraindications**
• Stable Anderson and Montesano types I and II occipital condylar fracture	• Anderson and Montesano type III fracture
• Tuli type 1 and type 2A	• Tuli type 2B fracture Cranial cervical instability

Most occipital condylar fractures are stable and can be treated with a cervical orthosis or halo immobilization.[253,263,289,443] Anderson and Montesano types I and II are stable fractures and can be treated with a cervical orthosis. Tuli type 1 and type 2A are stable and can be treated with a cervical orthosis.

OPERATIVE TREATMENT OF OCCIPITAL CONDYLAR FRACTURES

The decision for surgery is based on cranial cervical instability identified by CT or MRI.[262,319] Bilateral occipital condylar fractures usually are unstable and require occipital cervical fusion.[94,167,263,264,361,414] Type III may be unstable and require occipital cervical fusion. Type 2B will need an occipital cervical fusion.

See page 782 for occipital cervical fusion techniques.[12,13,17,19,23,24,26,29,34,35,41,46,415,416]

Atlantooccipital Instability

INTRODUCTION TO ATLANTOOCCIPITAL INSTABILITY

Atlantooccipital dislocation was once thought to be a rare fatal injury found only at the time of autopsy (Fig. 20-22).[24,45,53,63,379] This injury is now being recognized more often, and children are surviving.[106,114,121,313,390] Bulas et al.[64] reported 11 atlantooccipital

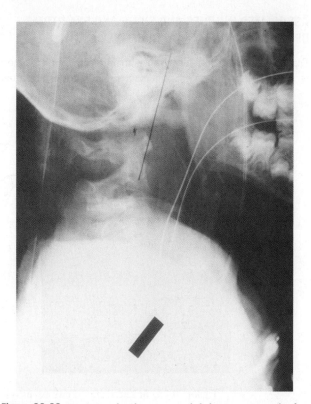

Figure 20-22. Patient with atlantooccipital dislocation. Note the forward displacement of the Wackenheim line and the significant anterior soft tissue swelling.

dislocations in 1,600 pediatric trauma patients (a 0.7% prevalence) seen over a 5-year period; 6 children died with severe neurologic deficits, but 5 patients survived with minimal or no neurologic sequela. This increase in the survival rate may be due to increased awareness and improved emergency care with resuscitation and spinal immobilization by emergency personnel.

ASSESSMENT OF ATLANTOOCCIPITAL INSTABILITY

MECHANISMS OF INJURY FOR ATLANTOOCCIPITAL INSTABILITY

Atlantooccipital dislocation occurs in sudden acceleration and deceleration accidents, such as motor vehicle or pedestrian–vehicle accidents. The head is thrown forward, and this can cause sudden craniovertebral separation.[5]

The atlantooccipital joint is a condylar joint that has little inherent bony stability. Stability is provided by the ligaments about the joint. The primary stabilizers are the paired alar ligaments, the articular capsule, and the tectorial membrane (a continuation of the posterior longitudinal ligament and the major stabilizer of the atlantooccipital joint). In children, this articulation is not as well formed as in adults and it is less cup-shaped. Therefore, there is less resistance to translational forces.[24,39,45,63,64,379,429] Sectioning of the tectorial membrane in biomechanical cadaver studies has resulted in instability from the occiput to C2.[172,203]

ASSOCIATED INJURIES AND SIGNS AND SYMPTOMS OF ATLANTOOCCIPITAL INSTABILITY

Diagnosis may be difficult because atlantooccipital dislocation is a ligamentous injury. Spontaneous reduction after initial immobilization may occur and up to 60% may be missed on initial examination.[203,394,397] Although patients with this injury have a history of trauma, some may have no neurologic findings. Others, however, may have symptoms such as cranial nerve injury, vomiting, headache, torticollis, or motor or sensory deficits.[63,69,84,169,188,313] Brain stem symptoms, such as ataxia and vertigo, may be caused by vertebrobasilar vascular insufficiency. Closed head injury and facial trauma are frequently associated with atlantooccipital instability. The high association of closed head injures may mask other physical findings. Unexplained weakness or difficulty in weaning off a ventilator after a closed head injury may be a sign of this injury.

IMAGING AND OTHER DIAGNOSTIC STUDIES FOR ATLANTOOCCIPITAL INSTABILITY

The treating physician must have a high index of suspicion in children with closed head injuries or associated facial trauma and must be aware of the radiographic findings associated with atlantooccipital dislocation. A significant amount of anterior soft tissue swelling usually can be seen on a lateral cervical spine radiograph. This increased anterior soft tissue swelling should be a warning sign that an atlantooccipital dislocation may have occurred.

Radiographic findings that aid in the diagnosis of atlantooccipital dislocation are the Wackenheim line, Powers ratio, dens–basion interval, and occipital condylar distance. The Wackenheim line is drawn along the clivus and should intersect tangentially the tip of the odontoid. A shift anterior or posterior of this line represents either an anterior or posterior displacement of the occiput on the atlas (Fig. 20-23). This line is probably the most helpful because it is reproducible and easy to identify on a lateral radiograph. The Powers ratio (see Fig. 20-2) is determined by drawing a line from the basion to the posterior arch of the atlas (BC) and a second line from the opisthion to

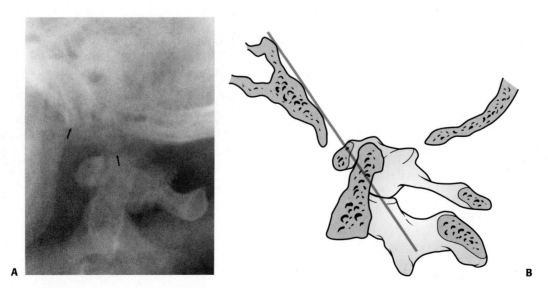

Figure 20-23. A: Lateral view shows extensive soft tissue swelling. The distance between the basion and the dense is 2.4 cm (*arrows*); normal is 1 cm. **B:** Abnormal relationship between the occiput and the upper cervical spine in craniovertebral dislocation. (With permission from El-Khoury GY, Kathol MH. Radiographic evaluation of cervical trauma. *Semin Spine Surg.* 1991;3:3–23.)[80]

the anterior arch of the atlas (OA). This measurement is best made on CT images but can be done on plain radiographic images. The length of line BC is divided by the length of the line OA, producing the Powers ratio. A ratio of more than 1.0 is diagnostic of anterior atlantooccipital dislocation. A ratio of less than 0.7 is diagnostic of posterior atlantooccipital dislocation. Values between 1.0 and 0.7 are considered normal.[214] The Powers ratio has the advantage of not being affected by magnification of the radiograph, but the landmarks may be difficult to define. Another radiographic measurement is the dens–basion interval. The distance is measured between the apex of the dens and the tip of the clivus (basion; see Fig. 20-3). If the interval measures more than 1.2 cm, disruption of the atlantooccipital joint has occurred.[64,330]

Kaufman et al.[211] described an occipital condylar facet distance of more than 5 mm from the occipital condyle to the C1 facet as indicative of atlantooccipital injury. They recommended measuring this distance from five reference points along the occipital condyle and the C1 facet. Harris et al.[171,172] described the basion–axial interval. A posterior axial line (PAL) is drawn tangential to the posterior wall of the C2 vertebra. A line parallel to the PAL is drawn through the basion. Normal values for children are from 0 to 12 mm. Sun et al.[397] proposed using an interspinous ratio that was sensitive and specific in detecting tectorial membrane injuries. The interspinous distance between C1 and C2 and between C2 and C3 is determined on lateral radiographs or CT scans. The ratio C1 to C2:C2 to C3 of more than 2.5 was indicative of injury to the tectorial membrane.[203,308,397]

MRI is useful in diagnosing atlantooccipital dislocation by showing soft tissue edema around the tectorial membranes and lateral masses and ligament injury or disruption.[65] Steinmetz et al.[394] and Sun et al.[397] suggested that the disruption of the tectorial membrane is the critical threshold for instability of the occipitoatlantal joint. Disruption of the tectorial membrane can best be identified by MRI.

CLASSIFICATION OF ATLANTOOCCIPITAL INSTABILITY

Atlantooccipital dislocation is classified radiographically into three types: longitudinal distraction with axial occipital separation, rotational injury, and anterior or posterior occipital displacement with respect to the atlas.[410]

TREATMENT OPTIONS FOR ATLANTOOCCIPITAL INSTABILITY

NONOPERATIVE TREATMENT OF ATLANTOOCCIPITAL INSTABILITY

Because atlantooccipital dislocation is a ligamentous injury, nonoperative treatment usually is unsuccessful. Although Farley et al.[123] reported successful stabilization in a halo, Georgopoulos et al.[145] found persistent atlantooccipital instability after halo immobilization. Immobilization in a halo should be used with caution: if the vest or cast portion is not fitted properly, displacement can increase (Fig. 20-24) because the head is fixed in the halo but movement occurs because of inadequate immobilization of the trunk in the brace or cast. Traction should be avoided because it can cause distraction of the skull from the atlas.

OPERATIVE TREATMENT OF ATLANTOOCCIPITAL INSTABILITY

Surgical stabilization is the recommended treatment.[186,202,399] Posterior arthrodesis can be performed in situ, with wire fixation or fixation with a contoured Luque rod and wires or with plate and screw fixation.[4,20,126,152,168,175,176,220,274,344,346,451,454] If the C1 to C2 articulation is stable, arthrodesis can be done only from the occiput to C1 so that C1 to C2 motion is preserved.[390,391,445] Stability of the C1 to C2 articulation often is questionable, and

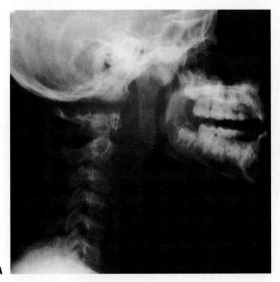 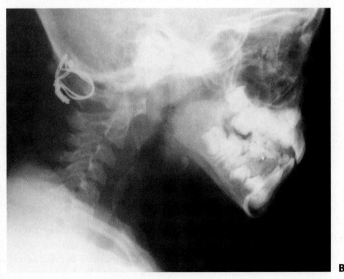

Figure 20-24. A: Lateral radiograph of a patient with atlantooccipital dislocation. Note the increase in the facet condylar distance. **B:** Lateral radiograph after occipital C1 arthrodesis.

arthrodesis may need to be extended to C2.[205] Most reports have expressed reservations about the chance of obtaining fusion in the narrow atlantooccipital interval and have recommended arthrodesis from the occiput to C2.[23,203]

Instability at the atlantooccipital joint is increased in patients with Down syndrome as well as in those with a high cervical arthrodesis below the axis. These patients may be at risk of developing chronic instability patterns and are at higher risk of having instability after trauma.

Several methods of obtaining an occiput to C2 arthrodesis are available to the treating surgeon. The decision of which technique is used usually is based on stability and anatomy of the upper cervical spine of the patient. Because of the inherent instability associated with traumatic injuries to the upper cervical spine, internal fixation is preferred. Instrumentation with rods and screws may not always be possible because of the patient's size and anatomy.[108,166,290] When instrumentation cannot be used, the surgeon must be aware of fusion and other stabilization techniques that may rely on stability obtained from the bone graft or wires and cables.[193,351] These techniques will usually need to be supplemented with external immobilization such as a halo vest or cast or a Minerva cast. Acute hydrocephalus can occur after this injury or in the early postoperative period because of changes in cerebrospinal fluid flow at the cranial–cervical junction. In a series of 14 patients with traumatic atlantooccipital dislocations treated at our institution, hydrocephalus was the most common complication, occurring in 4 patients. If there is neurologic decline after spinal fixation, obstructive hydrocephalus should be suspected.[23]

See page 776 for preoperative planning and surgical approaches for the surgical procedures that follow.

Occiput to C2 Arthrodesis Without Internal Fixation

In younger children in whom the posterior elements are absent at C1 or separation is extensive in the bifid part of C1 posteriorly, posterior cervical arthrodesis from the occiput to C2 with iliac crest bone graft can be done using a periosteal flap from the occiput to provide an osteogenic tissue layer for the bone graft.[228,237]

Positioning

The patient is placed in a prone position using Gardner-Wells tongs or a halo ring attached to a Mayfield headrest. A radiograph is obtained to evaluate the position of the head and cervical spine in the prone position. The radiograph also aids in identifying landmarks and levels; although once the skin incision is made, the occiput and spinous processes can be palpated.

Technique

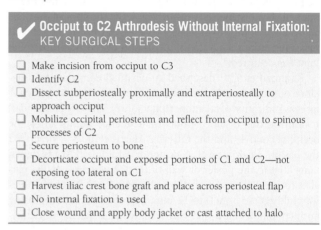

✔ **Occiput to C2 Arthrodesis Without Internal Fixation:** KEY SURGICAL STEPS

- ❑ Make incision from occiput to C3
- ❑ Identify C2
- ❑ Dissect subperiosteally proximally and extraperiosteally to approach occiput
- ❑ Mobilize occipital periosteum and reflect from occiput to spinous processes of C2
- ❑ Secure periosteum to bone
- ❑ Decorticate occiput and exposed portions of C1 and C2—not exposing too lateral on C1
- ❑ Harvest iliac crest bone graft and place across periosteal flap
- ❑ No internal fixation is used
- ❑ Close wound and apply body jacket or cast attached to halo

A straight posterior incision is made from the occiput to about C3, with care not to expose below C2 to avoid extension of the fusion to lower levels. An epinephrine and lidocaine solution is injected into the cutaneous and subcutaneous tissues to help control local skin and subcutaneous bleeding. The incision is deepened in the midline to the spinous processes of C2. Once identified, the level of the posterior elements of C1 or the dura is more easily found. After C2 is identified, subperiosteal dissection is carried proximally. Extraperiosteal dissection is used to approach the occiput (Fig. 20-25A). The dura is not completely exposed; if possible, any fat or ligamentous tissue present is left intact. The interspinous ligaments also should be left intact.

The occipital periosteum is mobilized by making a triangular incision directly on the posterior skull, with the apex

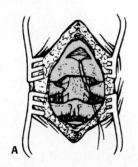
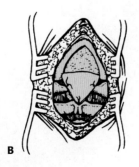
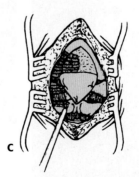
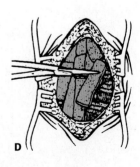

Figure 20-25. Technique of occipitocervical arthrodesis used when the posterior arch of C1 is absent. **A:** Exposure of the occiput, atlas, and axis. **B:** Reflection of periosteal flap to cover defect in atlas. **C:** Decortication of exposed vertebral elements. **D:** Placement of autogenous cancellous iliac bone grafts. (Reprinted with permission from Koop SE, Winter RB, Lonstein JE. The surgical treatment of instability of the upper part of the cervical spine in children and adolescents. *J Bone Joint Surg Am.* 1984;66(3):403–411.)

posteriorly and the broad base over the foramen magnum region. A flap of 3 or 4 cm at the base can be created. With subperiosteal elevation, the periosteum can be reflected from the occiput to the spinous processes of C2 (Fig. 20-25B). The apex of the flap is sutured to the spinous process of C2 and is attached laterally to any posterior elements that are present at C1 or other lateral soft tissues. After the periosteum is secured to the bone and any rudimentary C1 ring is exposed subperiosteally, a power burr is used to decorticate the occiput and any exposed portions of C1 and C2 (Fig. 20-25C).

Iliac crest bone graft is harvested, and struts of iliac bone are placed across the area on the periosteal flap (Fig. 20-25D). No internal fixation is used other than sutures to secure the periosteum. The wound is closed in a routine fashion, and a body jacket or cast is applied and attached to the halo.

Postoperative Care

The halo cast is worn until radiographs show adequate posterior arthrodesis, usually in 8 to 12 weeks.

Occiput to C2 Arthrodesis With Triple-Wire Fixation

In patients in whom the posterior elements of C1 and C2 are intact, a triple wire technique, as described by Wertheim and Bohlman,[438] can be used. The wires are passed through the outer table of the skull at the occipital protuberance. Because the transverse and superior sagittal sinuses are cephalad to the protuberance, they are not endangered by wire passage.

Positioning

The patient is placed prone, and a lateral radiograph is obtained to document proper alignment. The subcutaneous tissues are injected with an epinephrine solution (1:500,000).

Technique

> ✔ **Occiput to C2 Arthrodesis With Triple-Wire Fixation:**
> KEY SURGICAL STEPS
>
> ☐ Expose occiput and cervical laminae avoiding the paramedian venous plexus
> ☐ Create trough on either side of occipital protuberance and make a hole in the outer table of bone of the ridge created
> ☐ Pass three wires to secure bone graft
> ☐ Harvest bone graft from iliac crest and divide into two pieces
> ☐ Drill three holes in each graft
> ☐ Decorticate occiput and anchor grafts with the wires and pack with cancellous bone
> ☐ Close wound in layers

A midline incision is made extending from the external occipital protuberance to the spine of the third cervical vertebra. The paraspinous muscles are sharply dissected subperiosteally with a scalpel, and a periosteal elevator is used to expose the occiput and cervical laminae, with special care to stay in the midline to avoid the paramedian venous plexus.

At a point 2 cm above the rim of the foramen magnum, a high-speed diamond burr is used to create a trough on either side of the protuberance, making a ridge in the center (Fig. 20-26A). A towel clip is used to make a hole in this ridge through only the outer table of bone. A 20-gauge wire is looped through the hole and around the ridge; then, another 20-gauge wire is looped around the arch of the atlas. A third wire is passed through a hole drilled in the base of the spinous process of the axis and around this structure, giving three separate wires to secure the bone grafts on each side of the spine (Fig. 20-26B).

A thick, slightly curved graft of corticocancellous bone of premeasured length and width is removed from the posterior

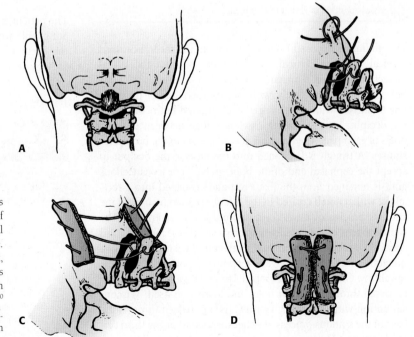

Figure 20-26. Technique of occipitocervical arthrodesis used in older adolescents with intact posterior elements of C1 and C2. **A:** A burr is used to create a ridge in the external occipital protuberance, and then a hole is made in the ridge. **B:** Wires are passed through the outer table of the occiput, under the arch of the atlas, and through the spinous process of the axis. **C:** Corticocancellous bone grafts are placed on the wires. **D:** Wires are tightened to secure grafts in place.[310] (Reprinted with permission from Wertheim SB, Bohlman HH. Occipitocervical fusion: indications, technique, and long-term results. *J Bone Joint Surg Am.* 1987;69(6):833–836.)

iliac crest. The graft is divided horizontally into two pieces, and three holes are drilled into each graft (Fig. 20-26C). The occiput is decorticated and the grafts are anchored in place with the wires on both sides of the spine (Fig. 20-26D). Additional cancellous bone is packed around and between the two grafts. The wound is closed in layers over suction drains.

Postoperative Care

Either a rigid cervical orthosis or a halo cast is worn for 6 to 12 weeks, followed by a soft collar that is worn for an additional 6 weeks.

Arthrodesis

Positioning

A halo ring is applied initially with the patient supine. The patient is carefully placed in the prone position, the halo is secured to the operating table with a halo positioning device, and the alignment of the occiput and the cervical spine is confirmed with a lateral radiograph.

Technique

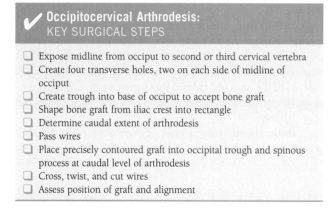

✔ **Occipitocervical Arthrodesis:**
KEY SURGICAL STEPS

❑ Expose midline from occiput to second or third cervical vertebra
❑ Create four transverse holes, two on each side of midline of occiput
❑ Create trough into base of occiput to accept bone graft
❑ Shape bone graft from iliac crest into rectangle
❑ Determine caudal extent of arthrodesis
❑ Pass wires
❑ Place precisely contoured graft into occipital trough and spinous process at caudal level of arthrodesis
❑ Cross, twist, and cut wires
❑ Assess position of graft and alignment

The midline is exposed from the occiput to the second or third cervical vertebra. Particular care is taken to limit the lateral dissection to avoid damaging the vertebral arteries.[127,154] Four holes, aligned transversely, with two on each side of the midline, are made with a high-speed drill through both cortices of the occiput, leaving a 1-cm osseous bridge between the two holes of each pair. The holes are placed caudal to the transverse sinuses. A trough is fashioned into the base of the occiput to accept the cephalad end of the bone graft. A corticocancellous graft is obtained from the iliac crest and is shaped into a rectangle, with a notch created in the inferior base to fit around the spinous process of the second or third cervical vertebra. The caudal extent of the intended arthrodesis (the second or third cervical vertebra) is determined by the presence or absence of a previous laminectomy, congenital anomalies, or the level of the instability. On each side, a looped 16- or 18-gauge Luque wire is passed through the burr holes and looped on itself. Wisconsin button wires (Zimmer, Warsaw, IN) are passed through the base of the spinous process of either the second or the third cervical vertebra. The wire that is going into the left arm of the graft

is passed through the spinous process from right to left. The graft is placed into the occipital trough superiorly and about the spinous process of the vertebra that is to be at the caudal level of the arthrodesis (the second or third cervical vertebrae). The graft is precisely contoured so that it fits securely into the occipital trough and around the inferior spinous process before the wires are tightened. The wires are subsequently crossed, twisted, and cut. An intraoperative radiograph is made at this point to assess the position of the graft and the wires as well as the alignment of the occiput and the cephalad–cervical vertebrae. Extension of the cervical spine can be controlled by positioning of the head with the halo frame, by adjustment of the size and shape of the graft, and to a lesser extent by appropriate tightening of the wires.

Atlantooccipital Arthrodesis

Although most patients with atlantooccipital dislocations are treated with fusion from the occiput to C2 or lower, Sponseller and Cass[390] described occiput–C1 fusion in two children with atlantooccipital arthrodesis who had complete or near-complete neurologic preservation. Their rationale was that rotation would be preserved by sparing the C1 to C2 articulation from fusion and that less stress would be concentrated on the lower cervical spine by fusing one level instead of two. In both of their patients, stable fusion was obtained and neurologic status was maintained.

Preoperative Planning

Before surgery, radiographs and CT scans should be reviewed to be sure a bifid or hypoplastic C1 arch is not present. A halo ring is applied before positioning the patient.

Positioning

The patient is placed prone, the halo ring is secured to the operating table with a halo positioning device, and the alignment of the occiput and the cervical spine is confirmed with a lateral radiograph, using a halo ring and attachment.

Technique

✔ **Atlantooccipital Arthrodesis:**
KEY SURGICAL STEPS

❑ Expose base of skull to ring of C1 and elevate periosteum to create flap
❑ Create unicortical trough in occiput at level directly cranial to ring of C1
❑ Drill two holes through occiput close to trough
❑ Pass wires
❑ Bridge occiput–C1 interval with periosteal flap
❑ Shape iliac crest bone graft to fit in trough and place graft in occiput–C1 interval
❑ Drill two more holes above distal end of graft and pass wires
❑ The two stands of wire are passed through the occiput
❑ Twist wires together and tighten
❑ Add additional cancellous bone to any available space

flap is turned down to bridge the occiput–C1 interval. A small, rectangular, bicortical, iliac crest bone graft approximately 1.5 cm wide and 1 cm high is shaped to fit the trough in the occiput; the graft is contoured to fit the individual patient's occiput–C1 interval. The inferior surface of the bone graft is contoured to fit snugly around the ring of C1 to keep it from migrating anteriorly into the epidural space. Two holes are drilled directly above the distal end of the graft, and the wire around C1 is passed through these holes, forming two distal strands; the wire passed through the occiput forms two proximal strands. These are twisted together and sequentially tightened to apply slight compression to the bone graft. This keeps the graft in the occipital trough and prevents migration into the canal by the occiput. Additional cancellous bone is added to any available space.

Postoperative Care

The halo vest is kept in place for 6 to 8 weeks in a young child and for as long as 12 weeks in an older child or adolescent. Union is confirmed by a lateral radiograph of the posterior occiput–C1 interval and by flexion–extension lateral views. A rigid cervical collar is used for an additional 2 to 4 weeks to protect the fusion and support the patient's cervical muscles while motion is regained.

Occipitocervical Arthrodesis With Contoured Rod and Segmental Wire

Occipitocervical arthrodesis using a contoured rod and segmental wire has the advantage of achieving immediate stability of the occipitocervical junction, which allows the patient to be immobilized in a cervical collar after surgery, avoiding the need for halo immobilization.[157]

Technique

> ✔ **Occipitocervical Arthrodesis With Contoured Rod and Segmental Wire:**
> KEY SURGICAL STEPS
>
> ❑ Expose base of occiput to spinous process of upper cervical vertebrae
> ❑ Create a template of intended shape of rod
> ❑ Make two burr holes on each side 2 cm lateral from midline and 2.5 cm above foramen magnum
> ❑ Pass wires or Songer cables
> ❑ Bend rod to match template
> ❑ Secure wires or cables to rod
> ❑ Decorticate spine and occiput and place autogenous cancellous bone graft

The base of the occiput and the spinous processes of the upper cervical vertebrae are approached through a longitudinal midline incision, which extends deep within the relatively avascular intermuscular septum. The entire field is exposed subperiosteally (Fig. 20-28).

A template of the intended shape of the stainless steel rod is made with the appropriate length of Luque wire. Two burr holes are made on each side, about 2 cm lateral to the midline and 2.5 cm above the foramen magnum. Care should be taken to avoid

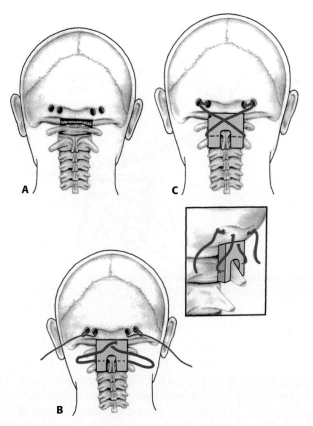

Figure 20-27. Occipitocervical arthrodesis. **A:** Four burr holes are placed into the occiput in transverse alignment, with two on each side of the midline, leaving a 1-cm osseous bridge between the two holes of each pair. A trough is fashioned into the base of the occiput. **B:** Sixteen- or 18-gauge Luque wires are passed through the burr holes and looped on themselves. Wisconsin button wires are passed through the base of the spinous process of either the second or third cervical vertebra. The graft is positioned into the occipital trough and spinous process of the cervical vertebra at the caudal extent of the arthrodesis. The graft is locked into place by the precise contouring of the bone. **C:** The wires are crossed, twisted, and cut. The extension of the cervical spine can be controlled by positioning of the head with the halo frame, by adjustment of the size and shape of the bone graft, and to a lesser extent by tightening of the wires.[72] (Reprinted with permission from Dormans JP, Drummond DS, Sutton LN, et al. Occipitocervical arthrodesis in children. *J Bone Joint Surg Am.* 1995;77(8):1234–1240.)

The base of the skull to the ring of C1 is exposed, and the periosteum of the skull is elevated so that it forms a flap from the foramen magnum located posterosuperiorly (Fig. 20-27).

The ring of C1 is carefully exposed, with care taken not to dissect more than 1 cm to either side of the midline to protect the vertebral arteries. Care also is taken not to expose any portion of C2 to prevent bridging of the fusion. The dissection of C1 should be done gently. A trough for the iliac crest bone graft is made in the occiput at a level directly cranial to the ring of C1. This trough is unicortical only and extends the width of the exposed portion of C1. Superior to this, two holes are drilled through the occiput as close to the trough as possible to avoid an anteriorly translating vector on the skull when tightening it down to C1. One 22-gauge wire is passed through the holes and another is placed around the ring of C1. The periosteal

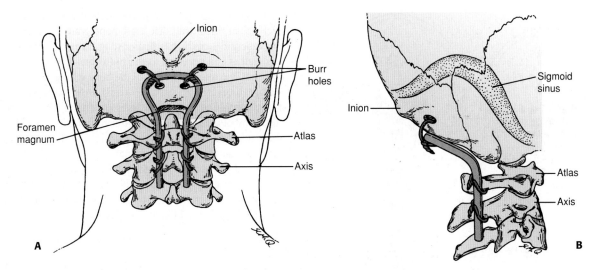

Figure 20-28. A and **B:** Occipitocervical arthrodesis using a contoured rod and segmental wire or cable fixation. (Reprinted with permission from Warner WC. Pediatric cervical spine. In: Canale ST, ed. *Campbell's Operative Orthopaedics*. St. Louis, MO: Mosby; 1998.)[307]

the transverse and sigmoid sinus when making these burr holes. At least 10 mm of intact cortical bone should be left between the burr holes to ensure solid fixation. Luque wires or Songer cables are passed in an extradural plane through the two burr holes on each side of the midline. The wires or cables are passed sublaminar in the upper cervical spine. The rod is bent to match the template; this usually will have a head–neck angle of about 135 degrees and slight cervical lordosis. A Bend Meister (Sofamor/Danek, Memphis, TN) may be helpful in bending the rod. The wires or cables are secured to the rod. The spine and occiput are decorticated, and autogenous cancellous bone grafting is performed.

Plate and Rod Fixation of Occiput to C2

This technique uses a contoured occipital plate that attaches to a rod for fixation.

Technique

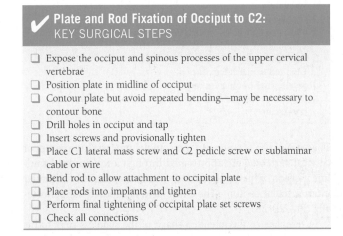

> ✔ **Plate and Rod Fixation of Occiput to C2:**
> KEY SURGICAL STEPS

- ☐ Expose the occiput and spinous processes of the upper cervical vertebrae
- ☐ Position plate in midline of occiput
- ☐ Contour plate but avoid repeated bending—may be necessary to contour bone
- ☐ Drill holes in occiput and tap
- ☐ Insert screws and provisionally tighten
- ☐ Place C1 lateral mass screw and C2 pedicle screw or sublaminar cable or wire
- ☐ Bend rod to allow attachment to occipital plate
- ☐ Place rods into implants and tighten
- ☐ Perform final tightening of occipital plate set screws
- ☐ Check all connections

Screw fixation is used in the occiput, and, if the anatomy allows, screw fixation may be used at C1 and C2. The occipital plate is

positioned in the midline (occipital keel) between the external occipital protuberance and the posterior border of the foramen magnum. The plate is contoured for an anatomic fit against the occiput. Avoid repeated bending of the plate because this may compromise its integrity. It may be necessary to contour the bone of the occiput to allow for an optimal fit of the plate. With an appropriate-size drill bit and guide that match the screw diameter, a hole is drilled into the occiput to the desired predetermined depth. Drilling must be done through the occipital plate to ensure proper drilling depth. Each hole should be completely tapped. The appropriate-size occipital screw is inserted and provisionally tightened. The rest of the screws are then inserted and hand-tightened.

If the anatomy allows, a C1 lateral mass screw and a C2 pedicle screw can be placed. If the anatomy does not allow placement of screws, then sublaminar wires or cables may be used for fixation at C1 and C2. The rods are bent to approximately 130 to 135 degrees to allow attachment to the occipital plate. The rods are placed into the implants and stabilized by tightening the set screws. If cables or sublaminar wires are used, these are tightened to secure the rods to the cervical spine. Final tightening of the occipital plate set screws is performed, and all connections of the final construct are checked before wound closure.

Postoperative Care

The cervical spine is immobilized in an orthosis for 8 to 12 weeks.

Pitfalls and Preventive Measures of Surgical Treatment of Atlantooccipital Instability

It is important to remember that acute hydrocephalus can occur after this injury or in the early postoperative period because of changes in cerebrospinal fluid flow at the cranial cervical junction.

C1–C2 Injuries

FRACTURES OF THE ATLAS

INTRODUCTION TO FRACTURES OF THE ATLAS

A fracture of the ring of C1 (Jefferson fracture) is a rare injury and accounts for less than 5% of all cervical spine fractures in children.[19,41]

ASSESSMENT OF FRACTURES OF THE ATLAS

MECHANISMS OF INJURY OF FRACTURES OF THE ATLAS

This fracture is caused by an axial load applied to the head.[29,42,201,205,261,341,407] The force is transmitted through the occipital condyles to the lateral masses of C1, causing a disruption in the ring of C1, usually in two places, with fractures occurring in both the anterior and posterior rings.[99] In children, an isolated single fracture of the ring can occur with the remaining fracture hinging on a synchondrosis.[35,225] This is an important distinction in children because fractures often occur through a normal synchondrosis. In addition, there can be plastic deformation of the ring with no evidence of a fracture.[26,205,337,405] This distinction can be seen on plain radiographs and CT scan, with fractures appearing through what appears to be normal physes. CT scan usually is the best imaging modality for making the diagnosis. As the lateral masses separate, the transverse ligament may be ruptured or avulsed, resulting in C1 and C2 instability.[278] If the two lateral masses are widened more than 7 mm beyond the borders of the axis on an anteroposterior radiograph, then an injury to the transverse ligament is presumed.[423] Two case reports have described C1 arch fractures with minor trauma after laminectomy.[8,28]

SIGNS AND SYMPTOMS OF FRACTURES OF THE ATLAS

The classic signs of an atlas fracture in a child are neck pain, cervical muscle spasm, decreased range of motion, and head tilt.[205] Children often hold their heads with their hands to relieve pain.

IMAGING AND OTHER DIAGNOSTIC STUDIES OF FRACTURES OF THE ATLAS

Injury to the transverse ligament may be from a rupture of the ligament or an avulsion of the ligament attachment to C1. Jefferson fractures may be evident on plain radiographs, but CT scans are superior at showing this injury (Fig. 20-29). CT scans also can be used to follow the progress of healing. MRI is useful in determining the integrity of the transverse atlantal ligament (TAL) and detecting fractures through the normal synchondroses of the atlas. With a fracture through a synchondrosis, associated edema and hemorrhage are seen on MRI.[230]

Other cervical spine fractures may be present with an atlas fracture, and MRI should be carefully scrutinized to identify other fractures.[163,268]

CLASSIFICATION OF FRACTURES OF THE ATLAS

Treatment algorithms for Jefferson fractures are based on the integrity of the TAL. These fractures are considered potentially unstable if the TAL is disrupted.

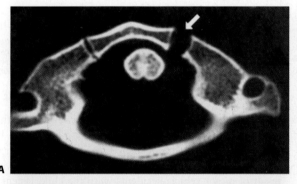

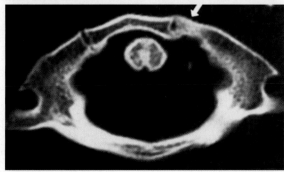

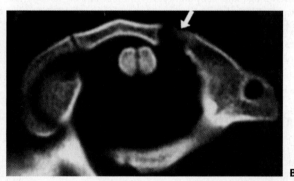

Figure 20-29. A: Initial CT scan through the atlas, demonstrating left anterior synchondrosis diastasis (*arrow*). **B:** CT scan 1 month after presentation with callus formation at the synchondrosis, demonstrating healing at the fracture site. **C:** CT scan 4 months after presentation, showing bony bridging across the fracture site. (From Judd D, Liem LK, Petermann G. Pediatric atlas fracture: A case of fracture through a synchondrosis and review of the literature. *Neurosurgery.* 2000;46(4):991–994. Reproduced by permission of Oxford University Press.)

Dickman Classification of Unstable Atlas Fractures Based on Transverse Atlantoaxial Ligament		
Type	Description	Treatment
Type I	Intrasubstance tear of the TAL	C1–C2 fusion
Type II	Bony avulsion at tubercle on C1 lateral mass	Halo vest successful in 75%

According to Spence et al.[387] a loss of structural properties of the TAL can occur when the combined overhang of the lateral masses of the atlas extends more than 7 mm beyond the lateral masses of the axis.

TREATMENT OPTIONS FOR FRACTURES OF THE ATLAS

NONOPERATIVE TREATMENT OF FRACTURES OF THE ATLAS

Nonoperative Treatment of Fractures of the Atlas: INDICATIONS AND CONTRAINDICATIONS	
Indication	Relative Contraindication
• Stable atlas fracture	• Intrasubstance tear of TAL

Most atlas fractures are stable fractures and treatment consists of immobilization in an orthosis (rigid collar or sternal occipital mandibular immobilizer), Minerva cast, or halo brace. The extent of this immobilization is debatable and should consider the patient's age and cooperation.[230] Immobilization usually is for 8 weeks but is based on documented healing by CT imaging and no instability on flexion and extension views. If there is excessive widening (7 mm), halo traction followed by halo brace or cast immobilization is recommended. Stability of C1 to C2 must be documented on flexion and extension lateral radiographs once the fracture is healed.

OPERATIVE TREATMENT OF FRACTURES OF THE ATLAS

Surgery rarely is necessary to stabilize these fractures but may be indicated if there is a documented intrasubstance tear of the TAL (Fig. 20-30).

Odontoid Fracture

INTRODUCTION TO ODONTOID FRACTURE

Odontoid (atlantoaxial) fracture is a relatively common fracture of the cervical spine in children,[127] occurring at an average

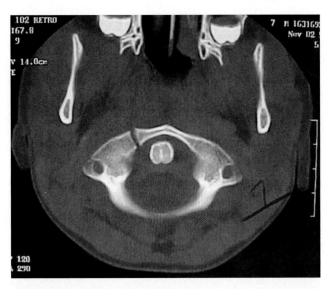

Figure 20-30. CT scan of an atlas fracture.

age of 4 years.[107,155,366] This fracture accounts for approximately 10% of all cervical spine fractures and dislocations in children. The unique feature of odontoid fractures in children is that the fracture most commonly occurs through the synchondrosis of C2 distally at the base of the odontoid. This synchondrosis is a cartilage line at the base of the odontoid and looks like a physeal or Salter–Harris type I injury. Most odontoid injuries are anteriorly displaced and usually have an intact anterior periosteal sleeve that provides some stability to the fracture when immobilized in extension and allows excellent healing of the fracture.[19,343,358,372] Growth disturbances are uncommon after this type of fracture. This synchondrosis normally closes at about 3 to 6 years of age and adds little to the longitudinal growth of C2.

ASSESSMENT OF ODONTOID FRACTURE

MECHANISMS OF INJURY OF ODONTOID FRACTURE

A fracture of the odontoid usually is associated with head trauma from a motor vehicle accident or a fall from a height, although it also can occur after trivial head trauma.[363] Odent et al.[302] reported that 8 of 15 fractures in children were the result of motor vehicle accidents, with the child fastened in a forward-facing seat. The sudden deceleration of the body as it is strapped into the car seat while the head continues to travel forward causes this fracture.

ASSOCIATED INJURIES AND SIGNS AND SYMPTOMS OF ODONTOID FRACTURE

Head and facial trauma may be associated with odontoid fracture. Children with odontoid fractures complain of neck pain and resist attempts to extend the neck. Radiographs should be obtained in any child complaining of neck pain.

IMAGING AND OTHER DIAGNOSTIC STUDIES FOR ODONTOID FRACTURE

Most often, the diagnosis is made by viewing the plain radiographs. Anteroposterior views usually appear normal, and the diagnosis must be made from lateral views because displacement of the odontoid usually occurs anteriorly. Plain radiographs sometimes can be misleading when the fracture occurs through the synchondrosis and has spontaneously reduced. When this occurs, the fracture has the appearance of a nondisplaced Salter–Harris type I fracture. CT scans with three-dimensional reconstruction views may be needed to fully delineate the injury.[373] MRI also may be useful to diagnose nondisplaced fractures by detecting edema around the injured area, indicating that a fracture may have occurred. Flexion and extension views to demonstrate instability may be obtained if a nondisplaced fracture is suspected. These studies should be done only in a cooperative child and under the direct supervision of the treating physician.

CLASSIFICATION OF ODONTOID FRACTURE

Odontoid fractures have been classified in adults by location.[13] Type I (<5%) occurs at the tip of dens at the insertion of alar ligament that connects the dens to the occiput. Type II (>60%) is a fracture at the base of the dens at its attachment to the body of C2. Type III (30%) does not actually involve the dens but is subdentate through the body of C2. Other fractures include a rare longitudinal fracture through dens and body of C2. This classification is useful in older children and adolescents after the C2 synchondrosis has fused. Most odontoid fractures in children occur through the synchondrosis. Hosalkar et al.[187] proposed a classification system based on the extent of displacement of the odontoid process from the vertebral body (Table 20-1).

OUTCOME MEASURES FOR ODONTOID FRACTURE

Odontoid fractures in children generally heal uneventfully and rarely have complications. Neurologic deficits rarely have been reported after this injury.[302,395] Odent et al.[302] described neurologic injuries in 8 of 15 patients, although most were stretch injuries to the spinal cord at the cervical thoracic junction and not at the level of the odontoid fracture.

TABLE 20-1. Classification of Odontoid Fractures[187]

Type I		At level of the synchondrosis
Type IA		Displacement less than 10%
Type 1B		Displacement 10%–100%
Type 1C		Displacement more than 100%
Type II		Fractures above the level of the synchondrosis

Adapted from Hosalkar HS, Greenbaum JM, Flynn DM, et al. Fractures of the odontoid in children with an open basilar synchondrosis. *Bone Joint J.* 2009;91(6):789–796.

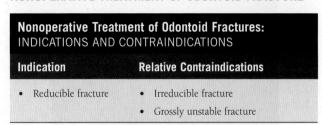

TREATMENT OPTIONS FOR ODONTOID FRACTURE

NONOPERATIVE TREATMENT OF ODONTOID FRACTURE

Nonoperative Treatment of Odontoid Fractures:
INDICATIONS AND CONTRAINDICATIONS

Indication	Relative Contraindications
• Reducible fracture	• Irreducible fracture
	• Grossly unstable fracture

Treatment of odontoid fractures is by closed reduction (usually extension or slight hyperextension of the neck), although complete reduction of the translation is not necessary. At least 50% apposition should be obtained to provide adequate cervical alignment, and then the patient should be immobilized in a Minerva or halo cast or custom orthosis. This fracture will heal in about 6 to 8 weeks. After bony healing, stability should be documented by flexion–extension lateral radiographs. Once the Minerva cast or halo is removed, a cervical collar is worn for 1 to 2 weeks. If an adequate reduction cannot be obtained by recumbency and hyperextension, then a head halter or halo traction is needed.

OPERATIVE TREATMENT OF ODONTOID FRACTURE

Rarely, manipulation under general anesthesia is needed for irreducible fractures (Fig. 20-31). Surgery with internal fixation rarely is needed due to the good results that are achieved with conservative treatment in children.[153,331,360,368,413] In a grossly unstable fracture, a posterior C1 to C2 fusion and instrumentation may be needed (see Table 20-2 for various fusion techniques).[427] Hosalkar et al.[187] recommended surgical stabilization of type IC fractures, and Fulkerson et al.[136] recommended surgical stabilization of fractures with significant displacement and >30 degrees of angulation.

Os Odontoideum

INTRODUCTION TO OS ODONTOIDEUM

Os odontoideum consists of a round ossicle that is separated from the axis by a transverse gap, which leaves the apical segment without support.

ASSESSMENT OF OS ODONTOIDEUM

MECHANISMS OF INJURY FOR OS ODONTOIDEUM

Fielding et al.[127–131] suggested that this was an unrecognized fracture at the base of the odontoid. Some studies have

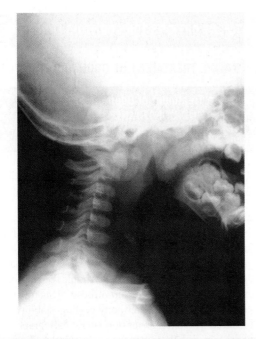

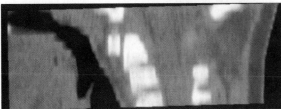

Figure 20-31. Lateral radiograph and CT reconstruction view of odontoid fracture through the synchondrosis of C2. Note the anterior displacement.

documented normal radiographs of the dens with abnormal radiographs after trivial trauma. This can be explained by a distraction force being applied by the alar ligaments, which pulls the tip of the fractured odontoid away from the base and produces a nonunion.[174,195,234,340,362,398,421] Other authors believe this to be of congenital origin because of its association with other congenital anomalies and syndromes.[149,272,374,377,448] Sankar et al.[355] reported that 6 of their 16 patients had associated congenital anomalies in the cervical spine and only 8 of the 16 reported any previous trauma.[22]

ASSOCIATED INJURIES AND SIGNS AND SYMPTOMS OF OS ODONTOIDEUM

Cerebellar infarctions due to vertebrobasilar artery insufficiency caused by an unstable os odontoideum were described by Sasaki et al.[355] The presentation of an os odontoideum can be variable. Instability from os odontoideum can mimic a spinal cord tumor.[150] Signs and symptoms can range from a minor to a frank compressive myelopathy or vertebral artery compression.[455] Presenting symptoms may be neck pain, torticollis, or headaches caused by local irritation of the atlantoaxial joint. Neurologic symptoms can be transient or episodic after trauma to complete myelopathy caused by cord compression.[110] Symp-

TABLE 20-2. Posterior Fusion Techniques

Atlantoaxial Fusion
Gallie[137]

Advantage: One wire passed beneath lamina of C1

Disadvantage: Wire may cause unstable C1 vertebra to displace posteriorly and fuse in dislocated position

Brooks and Jenkins[62]

Advantage: Greater resistance to rotational movement, lateral bending, and extension

Disadvantage: Requires sublaminar wires at C1 and C2

Harms and Melcher[170]

Advantage: Individual placement of polyaxial screws simplifies technique and involves less risk to C1–C2 facet joint and vertebral artery

Disadvantage: Possible irritation of the C2 ganglion from instrumentation

Magerl and Seeman[255]

Advantage: Significant improvement in fusion rates over traditional posterior wire stabilization and bone grafting techniques

Disadvantage: Technically demanding and must be combined with Gallie or Brooks fusion for maximum stability

Occipitocervical Fusion
Required when other bony anomalies occur at occipitocervical junction

Wertheim and Bohlman[438]

Wires passed through outer table of skull at occipital protuberance instead of through inner and outer tables near foramen magnum

Lessens risk of danger to superior sagittal and transverse sinuses (which are cephalad to occipital protuberance)

Koop et al.[228]

No internal fixation used

Autogenous corticocancellous iliac bone graft

Dormans et al.[107]

Stable fixation is achieved by exact fit of autogenous iliac-crest bone graft and fixation of the spinous process with button wire and fixation of the occiput with wires through burr holes

Can be used in high-risk patients (Down syndrome) with increased stabilization and shorter immobilization time

CONTOURED ROD, SCREW OR CONTOURED PLATE FIXATION

Has the advantage of achieving immediate stability of the occipitocervical junction

From Warner WC Jr. Pediatric cervical spine. In: Canale ST, Beaty JH, eds. *Campbell's Operative Orthopaedics.* 12th ed. Philadelphia, PA: Elsevier; 2013.[434]

toms may consist of weakness and loss of balance with upper motor neuron signs, although upper motor neuron signs may be completely absent. Proprioceptive and sphincter dysfunctions also are common.

IMAGING AND OTHER DIAGNOSTIC STUDIES OF OS ODONTOIDEUM

Os odontoideum usually can be diagnosed on routine cervical spine radiographs, which include an open-mouth odontoid view (Fig. 20-32). Lateral flexion and extension views should be obtained to determine if any instability is present. With os

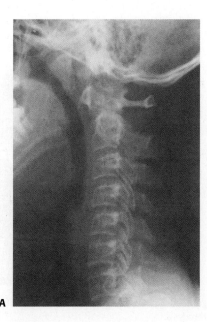
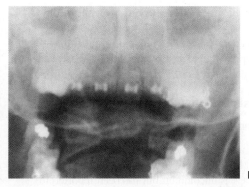

Figure 20-32. Lateral radiograph (**A**) and open-mouth odontoid radiograph (**B**) showing os odontoideum. (With permission from Warner WC. Pediatric cervical spine. In: Canale ST, ed. *Campbell's Operative Orthopaedics*. St. Louis, MO: A Mosby Year Book, 1998:2817.)

odontoideum, there is a space between the body of the axis and a bony ossicle. The free ossicle of the os odontoideum usually is half the size of a normal odontoid and is oval or round, with smooth sclerotic borders. The space differs from that of an acute fracture in which the space is thin and irregular instead of wide and smooth. The amount of instability should be documented on lateral flexion and extension plain radiographs that allow measurement of both the anterior and posterior displacement of the atlas on the axis. Because the ossicle is fixed to the anterior arch of C1 and moves as a unit with the anterior arch of C1 both in flexion and extension, measurement of the relationship of C1 to the free ossicle is of little value. A more meaningful measurement is made by projecting lines superiorly from the body of the axis to a line projected inferiorly from the posterior border of the anterior arch of the atlas. This gives more information as to the stability of C1 to C2. Another measurement that is very helpful is space available for the cord, which is the distance from the back of the dens to the anterior border of the posterior arch of C1.

Watanabe, Toyama, and Fujimura described two radiographic measurements that correlate with neurologic signs and symptoms.[435] They found that if there is a sagittal plane rotation angle of more than 20 degrees or an instability index of more than 40%, a patient is likely to have neurologic signs and symptoms. The instability index is measured from lateral flexion and extension radiographs. Minimal and maximal distances are measured from the posterior border of the C2 body to the posterior arc of the atlas. The instability index is calculated by the following equation:

$$\text{Instability Index (\%)} = \frac{\text{maximum distance} - \text{minimum distance}}{\text{maximum distance}} \times 100$$

The sagittal plane rotation angle is measured by the change in the atlantoaxial angle between flexion and extension. MRI can be useful in identifying reactive retrodental lesions that can occur with chronic instability. This reactive tissue is not seen on routine radiographs but can be responsible for a decrease in the space available for the spinal cord and compressive myelopathy.

CLASSIFICATION OF OS ODONTOIDEUM

Os odontoideum is radiographically classified as either orthotopic (in which the ossicle may appear free and in a relatively anatomic position) or dystopic (in which the ossicle may be fixed to the clivus or to the anterior ring of the atlas). See the above discussion on radiographic findings.

OUTCOMES MEASURES FOR OS ODONTOIDEUM

The prognosis of os odontoideum depends on the clinical presentation. The prognosis is good if only mechanical symptoms (torticollis or neck pain) or transient neurologic symptoms exist. It is poor if neurologic deficits slowly progress.

TREATMENT OPTIONS FOR OS ODONTOIDEUM

OPERATIVE TREATMENT OF OS ODONTOIDEUM

There is little role for nonoperative treatment because of the potential instability of this injury. Some authors, however, have recommended clinical and radiographic monitoring for patients who have no mechanical symptoms, neurologic signs, or documented instability.[1,93,222,378,388,395,442] Others, such as Dyck[110] and Klimo et al.[220,221] advocate posterior fusion for all children with os odontoideum because of the risk of significant instability that could be catastrophic.[91,98,191,431]

Absolute indications for surgical stabilization include: evidence of spinal instability, neurologic involvement, or intractable pain.[342,425,437] A general guideline for significant instability may include a posterior space available for the spinal cord of less than 13 mm, sagittal plane rotation angle greater than 20 degrees, and instability index of more than 40%, and C1 to C2 translation of more than 5 mm. Due to the abnormal anatomy and potential instability, the treating surgeon may still recommend instrumentation and fusion.

See page 777 for general preoperative planning, patient positioning, posterior approach, and potential pitfalls and preventions in cervical spine injury.

Posterior Arthrodesis of C1 to C2

Preoperative Planning

Before arthrodesis is attempted, the integrity of the arch of C1 must be documented by CT scan.[328] Incomplete development of the posterior arch of C1 is uncommon but has been reported to occur with increased frequency in patients with os odontoideum. This may necessitate an occiput to C2 arthrodesis for stability.

Technique

See page 794 for C1 to C2 arthrodesis. If a C1 to C2 arthrodesis is done, one must be careful not to overreduce the odontoid and cause posterior translation. Care also must be taken in positioning the neck at the time of arthrodesis and when tightening the wires if a Gallie or Brooks arthrodesis is performed to prevent posterior translation (Figs. 20-33 to 20-35).

Outcomes

Brockmeyer et al.[60] and Wang et al.[428] both reported good results with transarticular screw fixation and fusion in the treatment of children with os odontoideum (see Fig. 20-34). Wang et al.[305] reported the use of this technique in children as young as 3 years of age. This technique may be preferred depending on the patient's anatomy and the surgeon's experience. Harms and Melcher[170] and Brecknell and Malham[57] reported that a high-riding vertebral artery may make transarticular screw placement impossible in about 20% of patients.

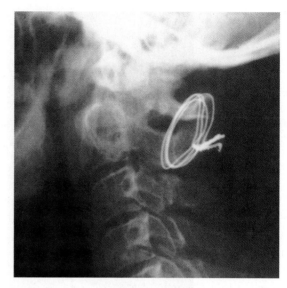

Figure 20-33. Posterior translation of atlas after C1 to C2 posterior arthrodesis.

Traumatic Transverse Ligamentous Disruption

INTRODUCTION TO TRAUMATIC TRANSVERSE LIGAMENTOUS DISRUPTION

The transverse ligament is the primary stabilizer of an intact odontoid against forward displacement. Secondary stabilizers

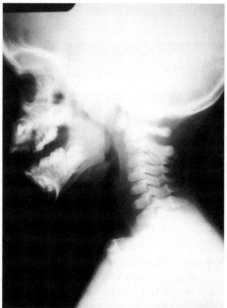
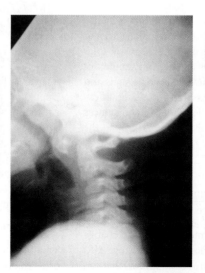
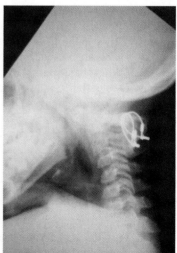

A, B   **C**

Figure 20-34. A: Lateral radiograph of traumatic C1 to C2 instability. **B:** Note the increase in the atlanto–dens interval. **C:** Lateral radiograph after C1 to C2 posterior arthrodesis.

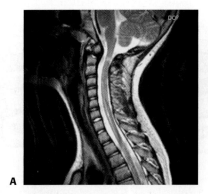
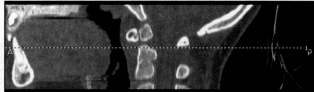
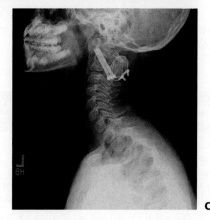

Figure 20-35. MRI (**A**) and CT scan (**B**) of a 9-year-old girl with os odontoideum. **C:** After Brooks posterior fusion and transarticular screw fixation.

consist of the apical and alar ligaments, which arise from the tip of the odontoid and pass to the base of the skull. These also stabilize the atlantooccipital joint indirectly.[154] The normal distance from the anterior cortex of the dens to the posterior cortex of the anterior ring of C1 is 3 mm in adults and 4.5 mm in children. In children, if the distance is more than 4.5 mm, disruption of the transverse ligament is presumed. The spinal canal at C1 is large compared with other cervical segments and accommodates a large degree of rotation and some degree of pathologic displacement without compromising the spinal cord. Steel[393] expressed this as a rule of thirds: the spinal canal at C1 is occupied equally by the spinal cord, odontoid, and a free space, which provides a buffer zone to prevent neurologic injury. Steel[393] found that anterior displacement of the atlas that exceeds a distance equal to the width of the odontoid may place the spinal cord at risk.

Acute rupture of the transverse ligament is rare and reportedly occurs in fewer than 10% of pediatric cervical spine injuries.[250,270] However, avulsion of the attachment of the transverse ligament to C1 may occur instead of rupture of the transverse ligament.

ASSESSMENT OF TRANSVERSE LIGAMENTOUS DISRUPTION

MECHANISMS OF INJURY FOR TRAUMATIC TRANSVERSE LIGAMENTOUS DISRUPTION

This injury may occur from a fall with a blow to the back of the head or other associated upper cervical spine trauma.

ASSOCIATED INJURIES AND SIGNS AND SYMPTOMS OF TRAUMATIC TRANSVERSE LIGAMENTOUS DISRUPTION

A patient with disruption of the transverse ligament usually has a history of cervical spine trauma and complaints of neck pain, often with notable muscle spasms.

IMAGING AND OTHER DIAGNOSTIC STUDIES FOR TRAUMATIC TRANSVERSE LIGAMENTOUS DISRUPTION

Diagnosis is confirmed on lateral radiographs that show an increased ADI. An active flexion view may be required to show instability in cooperative patients with unexplained neck pain or neurologic findings. CT scans are useful to demonstrate avulsion of the transverse ligament from its origins to the bony ring of C1. MRI is also useful in determining the integrity of the TAL.

TREATMENT OPTIONS FOR TRAUMATIC TRANSVERSE LIGAMENTOUS DISRUPTION

NONOPERATIVE TREATMENT OF TRAUMATIC TRANSVERSE LIGAMENTOUS DISRUPTION

Nonoperative treatment is not effective for ligamentous disruption. Nondisplaced avulsion injuries with a significant fragment may be treated nonoperatively to allow for bone healing. Stability and bone healing must be documented at the end of the nonoperative period with lateral flexion and extension views of the cervical spine.

OPERATIVE TREATMENT OF TRAUMATIC TRANSVERSE LIGAMENTOUS DISRUPTION

For acute injuries, reduction in extension is recommended, followed by surgical stabilization of C1 and C2. Depending on what type of instrumentation is feasible, immobilization for 8 to 12 weeks in a Minerva cast, a halo brace, or a cervical orthosis may be needed. Flexion and extension views should be obtained at the end of treatment to document stability.

See page 782 for general preoperative planning, patient positioning, posterior approach, and potential pitfalls and preventions in cervical spine injury.

Atlantoaxial Arthrodesis (Brooks and Jenkins)

Depending on the anatomy and size of the patient, wire or cables may be used to stabilize C1 and C2. If anatomy allows for placement of screws in C1 and C2, then a screw and rod construct can be used that will allow for more stable fixation.

Positioning

The patient is placed prone using Gardner-Wells tongs or a halo ring attached to a Mayfield headrest.[42]

Technique

> ✔ **Atlantoaxial Arthrodesis (Brooks and Jenkins):**
>   KEY SURGICAL STEPS
>
> ☐ Expose C1 and C2 through a midline incision
> ☐ Pass sublaminar wires or cables
> ☐ Harvest two full-thickness bone grafts from the iliac crest
> ☐ Bevel grafts to fit in the interval between arch of atlas and lamina of axis
> ☐ Create notches in upper and lower cortical surfaces to hold wires or cables
> ☐ Tighten wires or cables
> ☐ Close wound in layers

A lateral cervical spine radiograph is obtained to ensure proper alignment before surgery. The skin is prepared and draped in a sterile fashion and a solution of epinephrine (1:500,000) is injected intradermally to aid hemostasis. C1 and C2 are exposed through a midline incision.

With an aneurysm needle, a Mersiline suture is passed from cephalad to caudad on each side of the midline under the arch of the atlas and then beneath the lamina of C2. These serve as guides to introduce two doubled 20-gauge wires or Songer cables. Another technique is to pass the sublaminar wires or cables subperiosteally around the ring of C1 and lamina of C2. The periosteum can be easily elevated with a periosteal elevator and allows for some protection of the spinal cord when passing the wires or cables, since they do not pass directly into the epidural space with this technique. The size of the wire used may vary depending on the size and age of the patient. Two full-thickness bone grafts, approximately 1.25 × 3.5 cm, are harvested from the iliac crest and beveled so that the apex of the graft fits in the interval between the arch of the atlas and the lamina of the axis. Notches are fashioned in the upper and lower cortical surfaces to hold the circumferential wires or cables and prevent them from slipping. The doubled wires or cables are tightened over the graft. The wound is irrigated and closed in layers over suction drains (Fig. 20-36).

Postoperative Care

A halo cast or vest is used for postoperative immobilization for 6 to 8 weeks in a young child and for as long as 12 weeks in an older child or adolescent.

Atlantoaxial Arthrodesis (Gallie)

Positioning

The patient is placed prone using Gardner-Wells tongs or a halo ring attached to a Mayfield headrest.[137]

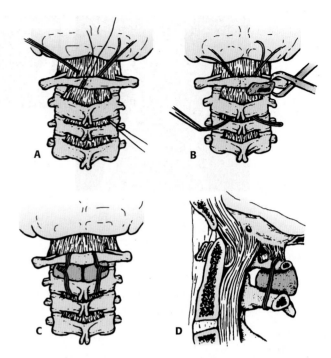
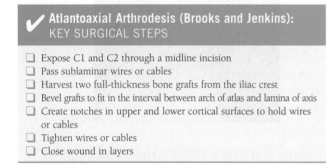
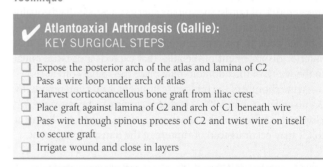

Figure 20-36. Technique of atlantoaxial arthrodesis (Brooks–Jenkins). **A:** Wires are inserted under the atlas and axis. **B:** Full-thickness bone grafts from the iliac crest are placed between the arch of the atlas and the lamina of the axis. **C** and **D:** The wires are tightened over the graft and twisted on each side. (Adapted with permission from Brooks AL, Jenkins EB. Atlantoaxial arthrodesis by the wedge compression method. *J Bone Joint Surg Am.* 1978;60(3):279–284.)

Technique

> ✔ **Atlantoaxial Arthrodesis (Gallie):**
>   KEY SURGICAL STEPS
>
> ☐ Expose the posterior arch of the atlas and lamina of C2
> ☐ Pass a wire loop under arch of atlas
> ☐ Harvest corticocancellous bone graft from iliac crest
> ☐ Place graft against lamina of C2 and arch of C1 beneath wire
> ☐ Pass wire through spinous process of C2 and twist wire on itself to secure graft
> ☐ Irrigate wound and close in layers

A lateral cervical spine radiograph is obtained to ensure proper alignment before surgery. The skin is prepared and draped in a sterile fashion, and a solution of epinephrine (1:500,000) is injected intradermally to aid hemostasis.

A midline incision is made from the lower occiput to the level of the lower end of the fusion, extending deeply within the relatively avascular midline structures, the intermuscular septum, or ligamentum nuchae. Care should be taken not to expose any more than the area to be fused to decrease the chance of spontaneous extension of the fusion.

By subperiosteal dissection, the posterior arch of the atlas and the lamina of C2 are exposed. The muscular and ligamentous attachments from C2 are removed with a curet. Care should be taken to dissect laterally along the atlas to prevent injury to the vertebral arteries and vertebral venous plexus that lie on the superior

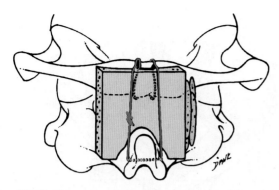

Figure 20-37. Wires are passed under the lamina of the atlas and through the spine of the axis and tied over the graft. This method is used most frequently. (Reprinted with permission from Fielding JW, Hawkins RJ, Ratzan SA. Spine fusion for atlanto-axial instability. *J Bone Joint Surg Am.* 1976;58(3):400–407.)

aspect of the ring of C1, less than 2 cm lateral to the midline. The upper surface of C1 is exposed no farther laterally than 1.5 cm from the midline in adults and 1 cm in children. Decortication of C1 and C2 generally is not necessary. From below, a wire loop of appropriate size is passed upward under the arch of the atlas either directly or with the aid of a Mersiline suture. The Mersiline suture can be passed with an aneurysm needle. The free ends of the wire are passed through the loop, grasping the arch of C1 in the loop.

A corticocancellous graft is taken from the iliac crest and placed against the lamina of C2 and the arch of C1 beneath the wire. One end of the wire is passed through the spinous process of C2, and the wire is twisted on itself to secure the graft in place (Fig. 20-37). The wound is irrigated and closed in layers with suction drainage tubes.

Postoperative Care

A halo cast or vest is used for postoperative immobilization for 6 to 8 weeks in a young child and for as long as 12 weeks in an older child or adolescent.

Atlantoaxial Arthrodesis With Posterior C1 to C2 Transarticular Screw Fixation

Posterior C1 to C2 transarticular screw fixation can be used to stabilize the atlantoaxial joint. This technique has the advantage of being biomechanically superior to posterior wiring techniques,[178] and postoperative halo vest immobilization usually is not required. The disadvantages of this technique are potential injury to the vertebral artery, its technical difficulty, and the requirement for sublaminar wire and fusion (Brooks or Gallie technique).

Preoperative Planning

Preoperative imaging should include plain radiographs, CT scan, MRI, and MRA of the cervical spine. Supervised dynamic lateral flexion and extension views must determine the reducibility of the atlantoaxial joint.[271] If an anatomic reduction cannot be obtained, transarticular screws cannot be safely used. MRA can delineate the course of the vertebral artery through the foramen transversarium and its relationship to the surrounding bony architecture. Approximately 20% of patients show anatomic

variations in the path of the vertebral artery and osseous anatomy that would preclude transarticular screw placement.[1,57,170]

Technique

> ✔ **Atlantoaxial Arthrodesis With Posterior C1–C2 Transarticular Screw Fixation:** KEY SURGICAL STEPS
>
> ☐ Expose the spine from C1 to C3
> ☐ Using C2 inferior facet as landmark, entry point for drill is 2 mm lateral to medial edge and 2 m above inferior border of C2 facet
> ☐ Tap hole and place 3.5-mm lag screw across C1–C2 joint on both sides
> ☐ Harvest bone graft from posterior iliac crest
> ☐ Perform C1–C2 fusion using either Brooks or Gallie technique

The patient is placed prone with the head held in a Mayfield skull clamp or with a halo ring attached to the Mayfield attachment. Under fluoroscopic guidance, proper alignment of the atlantoaxial joint is confirmed. The spine is prepared and draped from the occiput to the upper thoracic spine. The upper thoracic spine must be included in the surgical field to allow percutaneous placement of the transarticular screw. Percutaneous screw placement may be necessary because of the cephalad orientation of the C1 to C2 transarticular screw.

A midline posterior cervical exposure is made from C1 to C3.

The C2 inferior facet is used as the landmark for screw entry: the entry point is 2 mm lateral to the medial edge and 2 mm above the inferior border of the C2 facet (Fig. 20-38A). The drill trajectory is angled medially 5 to 10 degrees. On the lateral fluoroscopic radiograph, the drill trajectory is adjusted toward the posterior cortex of the anterior arch of C1. Percutaneous placement of the C1 to C2 facet screws may be necessary if the intraoperative atlantoaxial alignment precludes drilling or placement of screws through the operative incision. After tapping, a 3.5-mm lag screw is placed across the C1 to C2 joint (Fig. 20-38B). Another screw is then placed in exactly the same way on the other side. After placement of the C1 to C2 transarticular screw, a bone graft is harvested from the posterior iliac crest. A traditional posterior C1 to C2 fusion is done using either the Gallie or the Brooks technique (Fig. 20-39).

Postoperative Care

The patient is immobilized in a hard cervical collar only; no halo or Minerva cast is used postoperatively.

Potential Pitfalls and Preventive Measures

The disadvantages of this technique are potential injury to the vertebral artery, its technical difficulty, and the requirement for sublaminar wire and fusion (Brooks or Gallie technique).

Atlantoaxial Arthrodesis With Posterior C1 to C2 Polyaxial Screw and Rod Fixation

Harms and Melcher[170] described a technique of atlantoaxial stabilization using fixation of the C1 lateral mass and the C2 pedicle with polyaxial screws and rods (Fig. 20-40). This technique has the advantages of minimizing the risk of vertebral artery

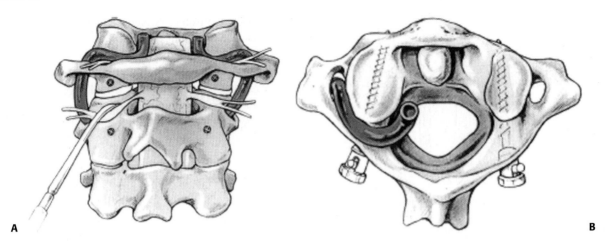

Figure 20-38. Posterior C1 to C2 transarticular screw fixation. **A:** Location of entry points in C1 and C2 for screw placement. **B:** Polyaxial screws placed bicortically into the lateral mass. (Reprinted with permission from Harms J, Melcher RP. Posterior C1–C2 fusion with polyaxial screw and rod fixation. *Spine.* 2001;26(22):2467–2471.)

injury, does not require the use of sublaminar wires, and does not require an intact posterior arch of C1.

Technique

> ✔ **Atlantoaxial Arthrodesis With Posterior C1–C2 Polyaxial Screw and Rod Fixation:**
> KEY SURGICAL STEPS

- ❑ Expose the spine from the occiput to C3
- ❑ Expose entry point for C1 screw
- ❑ Direct drill bit to midpoint of C1 lateral mass
- ❑ Tap drill hole and insert 3.5-mm polyaxial screw
- ❑ Drill pilot hole for C2 pedicle screw in superior and medial quadrant of C2 lateral mass
- ❑ Tap drill hole and insert a 3.5-mm polyaxial screw into CT
- ❑ Fix rods to polyaxial screws with locking nuts
- ❑ Decorticate C1 and C2 and insert cancellous bone from posterior iliac crest

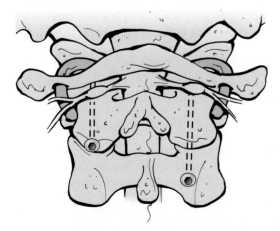

Figure 20-39. Position of vertebral arteries and position of screws across atlantoaxial joint. (Reprinted with permission from Menezes AH. Surgical approaches to the craniocervical junction. In: Weinstein SL, ed. *Pediatric Spine Surgery.* 2nd ed. Philadelphia, PA: Lippincott Williams & Wilkins; 2001.)

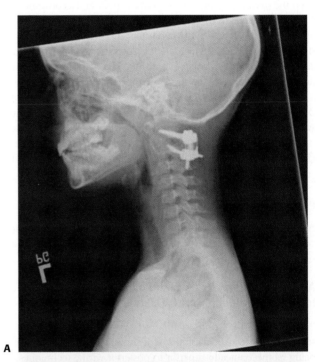

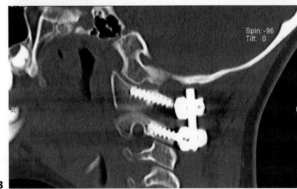

Figure 20-40. Radiograph (**A**) and MRI (**B**) after fixation with polyaxial screws and rods.

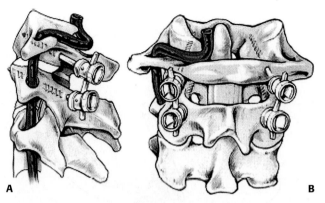

Figure 20-41. Lateral (**A**) and posterior (**B**) views after C1 to C2 fixation by the polyaxial screw and rod technique. (Reprinted with permission from Harms J, Melcher RP. Posterior C1–C2 fusion with polyaxial screw and rod fixation. *Spine.* 2001;26(22):2467–2471.)

The patient is placed prone with the head held in a Mayfield skull clamp or with a halo ring attached to the Mayfield attachment. Under fluoroscopic guidance, proper alignment of the atlantoaxial joint is confirmed. The cervical spine is exposed from the occiput to C3.

The C1 to C2 complex is exposed to the lateral border of the C1 to C2 articulation. The C1 to C2 joint is exposed and opened by dissection over the superior surface of the C2 pars interarticularis. The dorsal root ganglion of C2 is retracted in a caudal direction to expose the entry point for the C1 screw. This ganglion can be ligated, but this has been associated with an increased risk of neuralgic pain in adults.[452] This entry point is at the midpoint of the C1 lateral mass at its junction with the posterior arch of C1. A 2-mm high-speed burr is used to mark the starting point for the drill. The drill bit is directed in a straight to slightly convergent trajectory in the anteroposterior plane and parallel to the posterior arch of C1 in the sagittal plane. After determining the appropriate screw length, the drill hole is tapped and a 3.5-mm polyaxial screw is inserted. A number 4 Penfield elevator is used to define the medial border of the C2 isthmus or pedicle. The starting point for the C2 pedicle screw is in the superior and medial quadrant of the C2 lateral mass. A C2 pedicle pilot hole is drilled with a 2-mm drill in a 20- to 30-degree convergent and cephalad trajectory, using the superior and medial surface of the C2 pedicle as a guide. The hole is tapped, and a 3.5-mm polyaxial screw of appropriate length is inserted. Fixation of the rods to the polyaxial screws is obtained with locking nuts (Fig. 20-41). C1 and C2 are decorticated posteriorly and cancellous bone from the posterior iliac crest is used for bone graft.

Postoperative Care

Rigid cervical collar immobilization is used postoperatively.

Potential Pitfalls and Preventive Measures

Disadvantages of this technique are the anatomic limitations of the C1 lateral mass,[2,61] which may prevent the use of a 3.5-mm screw, and the potential risk of irritation or injury of the C2 ganglion.[142]

C1–C2 Injuries Associated With Other Conditions

ATLANTOAXIAL INSTABILITY ASSOCIATED WITH CONGENITAL ANOMALIES AND SYNDROMES

INTRODUCTION TO ATLANTOAXIAL INSTABILITY ASSOCIATED WITH CONGENITAL ANOMALIES AND SYNDROMES

Although acute atlantoaxial instability in children is rare, chronic atlantoaxial instability occurs in certain conditions such as juvenile rheumatoid arthritis, Reiter syndrome, Down syndrome, and Larsen syndrome. Bone dysplasia—such as Morquio polysaccharidosis, spondyloepiphyseal dysplasia, and Kniest syndrome—also may be associated with atlantoaxial instability, as well as os odontoideum, Klippel–Feil syndrome, and occipitalization of the atlas.[68,96,165,180,226,232,280] Certain cranial facial malformations have high incidences of associated anomalies of the cervical spine, such as Apert syndrome, hemifacial microsomy, and Goldenhar syndrome.[376] Treatment recommendations are individualized based on the natural history of the disorder and future risk to the patient. Minimal trauma may result in significant instability and neurologic compromise in patients with these conditions. There has been considerable interest in the incidence and treatment of atlantoaxial instability in children with Down syndrome.[11,35,332,333,386,419,446]

ASSESSMENT OF ATLANTOAXIAL INSTABILITY ASSOCIATED WITH CONGENITAL ANOMALIES AND OTHER CONDITIONS

MECHANISMS OF INJURY FOR ATLANTOAXIAL INSTABILITY ASSOCIATED WITH CONGENITAL ANOMALIES AND SYNDROMES

Generalized ligamentous laxity caused by the underlying collagen defect can result in atlantoaxial and atlantooccipital instability in children with Down syndrome. Pizzutillo and Herman[326] made a distinction between cervical instability and hypermobility in Down syndrome patients. Instability implies pathologic motion that jeopardizes neurologic integrity. Hypermobility refers to increased excursions that occur in the cervical spine of patients with Down syndrome compared with normal controls but do not result in loss of structural integrity of the anatomical restraints that protect neural tissues.[447]

Atlantoaxial instability has been reported to occur in 10% to 20% of children with Down syndrome.[387] Atlantooccipital instability may also occur in patients with Down syndrome. Despite reports of atlantoaxial and atlantooccipital instability in Down syndrome patients, the exact natural history related to this insta-bility is unknown. Differentiating between hypermobility and clinically significant instability in these patients may be difficult.

ASSOCIATED INJURIES AND SIGNS AND SYMPTOMS OF ATLANTOAXIAL INSTABILITY ASSOCIATED WITH CONGENITAL ANOMALIES AND SYNDROMES

Cervical instability usually is discovered on routine screening examination or cervical radiographs obtained for other reasons. Neurologic symptoms are present in 1% to 2.6% of patients with cervical instability. Progressive instability leading to neuro-logic symptoms is most common in boys older than 10.5 years of age. Involvement of the pyramidal tract usually results in gait abnormalities, hyperreflexia, and motor weakness. Other symptoms include neck pain, occipital headaches, and torticol-lis. Detailed neurologic examination often is difficult in patients with Down syndrome, and somatosensory-evoked potentials may be beneficial in documenting neurologic involvement.

IMAGING AND OTHER DIAGNOSTIC STUDIES FOR ATLANTOAXIAL INSTABILITY ASSOCIATED WITH CONGENITAL ANOMALIES AND SYNDROMES

Radiographic examination should include anteroposterior, flex-ion and extension lateral, and odontoid views. CT scans, MRI scans, or cineradiography in flexion and extension may be needed to evaluate the occipitoatlantal joint and the atlantoaxial joint for instability.[252] MRI may help to demonstrate spinal cord signal changes in suspected instability and neurologic compromise in patients in whom it is often difficult to obtain a detailed neurologic examination. MacKenzie et al. determined that, with adequate supervision, cervical spine flexion–extension MRI under seda-tion/anesthesia is safe in children with skeletal dysplasia and is essential for medical and surgical decision-making. Based on MRI findings, 14 of 31 children in their study had surgery and 17 had continued observation. Radiographic evidence of atlantooccipital instability is not as well defined as that for atlantoaxial instabil-ity, but measurements described by Wackenheim (see Fig. 20-3), Wiesel and Rothman (Fig. 20-42), Powers (see Fig. 20-2), and Tredwell et al.[411] are helpful. A Powers ratio of more than 1.0 is indicative of abnormal anterior translation of the occiput, and a ratio of less than 0.55 indicates posterior translation. However, some studies have reported the poor reliability and reproduc-ibility of these measurements in Down syndrome.[210,436] CT scans in flexion and extension or cineradiography may be needed to give better detail and information about possible atlantooccipital instability. An ADI of 4.5 to 5 mm indicates instability in normal pediatric patients. An increased ADI in patients with Down syn-drome has not been directly correlated with an increase in neuro-logic compromise. This suggests that radiographs of the cervical spine in Down syndrome must be evaluated by standards spe-cific to that population and not by standards for general pediatric patients because this may result in overdiagnosis of a pathologic process. Neurologic compromise occurs with a similar incidence in individuals with Down syndrome who have a normal ADI and those with an ADI from 4 to 10 mm. In Down syndrome, an ADI of less than 4.5 mm is normal; an ADI of 4.5 to 10 mm is con-

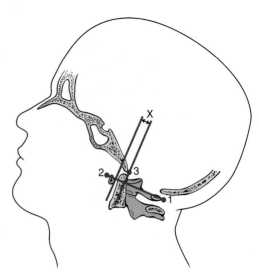

Figure 20-42. Atlantooccipital instability measurement according to Wiesel and Rothman. Lines are drawn on flexion and extension lateral radiographs. Translation should be no more than 1 mm. Atlantal line joins points 1 and 2. Line drawn perpendicular to atlantal line at pos-terior margin of anterior arch of atlas. Point 3 is basion. Distance from point 3 to perpendicular line is measured in flexion and extension. Dif-ferences represent anteroposterior translation. (Adapted from Warner WC Jr. Pediatric cervical spine. In: Canale ST, Beaty JH, eds. *Campbell's Operative Orthopaedics.* 12th ed. Philadelphia, PA: Elsevier; 2013.)

sidered hypermobile but not unstable unless there are neurologic findings; and an ADI of more than 10 mm is considered unstable; the patient is at risk for neurologic compromise because of the decrease in the space available for the spinal cord.

CLASSIFICATION OF ATLANTOAXIAL INSTABILITY ASSOCIATED WITH CONGENITAL ANOMALIES AND SYNDROMES

See page 787 for classification of atlantoaxial injuries.

> ### TREATMENT OPTIONS FOR ATLANTOAXIAL INSTABILITY ASSOCIATED WITH CONGENITAL ANOMALIES AND SYNDROMES

NONOPERATIVE TREATMENT OF ATLANTOAXIAL INSTABILITY ASSOCIATED WITH CONGENITAL ANOMALIES AND SYNDROMES

Nonoperative Treatment of Atlantoaxial Instability Associated With Down Syndrome:
INDICATIONS AND CONTRAINDICATIONS

Indication	Relative Contraindications
• ADI 4.5–10 mm with no neurologic symptoms	• Hypermobility • Neurologic deficit • Abnormal MRI signal change in spinal cord • ADI more than 10 mm

Hypermobility of the occipitoatlantal junction has been observed in more than 60% of patients with Down syndrome, but this usually is not associated with neurologic risk. If hypermobility of this joint is documented but the patient is neurologically normal, then high-risk activities should be restricted. When the ADI is less than 4.5 mm, no restriction of activities is necessary. In those who have an ADI of 4.5 to 10 mm, with no neurologic symptoms, high-risk activities also are restricted.

OPERATIVE TREATMENT OF ATLANTOAXIAL INSTABILITY ASSOCIATED WITH CONGENITAL ANOMALIES AND SYNDROMES

If there is hypermobility of the occipitoatlantal junction and a neurologic deficit or an abnormal signal change in the spinal cord on MRI, then an occiput to C2 or C3 fusion is recommended. If there is a neurologic deficit or spinal cord changes on MRI and hypermobility of just the atlantoaxial joint, then a C1 to C2 fusion is indicated (see page 794). If the ADI is 10 mm or more, posterior fusion and instrumentation are recommended (see page 794).

Surgical Procedures

See page 794 for surgical procedures for atlantoaxial instability. Before fusion and passage of the wire, the unstable C1 to C2 joint should be reduced by traction. If reduction cannot be obtained, an in situ fusion reduces the risk of neurologic compromise, which may occur if intraoperative reduction is performed and the wires are passed through a narrowed space available for the spinal cord.

Postoperative Care

Postoperative immobilization in a halo cast or halo vest should be continued for as long as possible because graft resorption 6 months after fusion has been reported. More stable fixation may decrease this complication. C1 to C2 transarticular screw fixation or occiput to C2 instrumentation with plates and rods can be used successfully.

Outcomes

Complications are relatively common after cervical fusions in children with Down syndrome. Segal et al.[365] reported frequent graft resorption after 10 posterior fusions and suggested as causes inadequate inflammatory response and collagen defects. Msall et al.[201] reported the frequent development of instability above and below C1 to C2 fusion in patients with Down syndrome.

Atlantoaxial Rotatory Subluxation

INTRODUCTION TO ATLANTOAXIAL ROTATORY SUBLUXATION

Atlantoaxial rotatory subluxation is a common cause of childhood torticollis.[329] This condition is known by several names,

such as rotatory dislocation, rotatory displacement, rotatory subluxation, and rotatory fixation. Atlantoaxial rotatory subluxation probably is the most accepted term used, except for long-standing cases (3 months), which are called rotatory fixation.

A significant amount of motion occurs at the atlantoaxial joint; half of the rotation of the cervical spine occurs there.[139] Through this range of motion at the C1 to C2 articulation, some children develop atlantoaxial rotatory subluxation. Differential diagnoses include torticollis caused by ophthalmologic problems, sternocleidomastoid tightness from muscular torticollis, brain stem or posterior fossa tumors or abnormalities, congenital vertebral anomalies, and infections of the vertebral column.[139]

ASSESSMENT OF ATLANTOAXIAL ROTATORY SUBLUXATION

MECHANISMS OF INJURY FOR ATLANTOAXIAL ROTATORY SUBLUXATION

The two most common causes are trauma and infection; the most common cause is an upper respiratory infection (Grisel syndrome).[32,325,439] Subluxation also can occur after a retropharyngeal abscess, tonsillectomy, pharyngoplasty, or trivial trauma. There is free blood flow between the veins and lymphatics draining the pharynx and the periodontoid plexus.[318] Any inflammation of these structures can lead to attenuation of the synovial capsule or transverse ligament or both, with resulting instability. Another potential etiologic factor is the shape of the superior facets of the axis in children. Kawabe et al.[212] showed that the facets are smaller and more steeply inclined in children than in adults. A meniscus-like synovial fold was found between C1 and C2 that could prohibit reduction after displacement has occurred. The normal rotation at the atlantoaxial joint is about 40 degrees to each side. Although atlantoaxial rotatory subluxation is most commonly seen from inflammatory syndromes, it also can occur after trauma. Villas et al.[424] reported uncovering of the C1–C2 facets (72% to 85% uncovering) through a normal range of motion documented on CT scans. Mönckeberg et al.[282] reported similar findings on CT scans in adults. Increased uncovering may allow rotatory subluxation and fixation.

ASSOCIATED INJURIES AND SIGNS AND SYMPTOMS OF ATLANTOAXIAL ROTATORY SUBLUXATION

If the cause is traumatic, other spine and head injuries may be associated. Clavicular fracture associated with atlantoaxial rotatory subluxation also has been described.[293]

Clinical findings include neck pain, headache, and a cockrobin position of rotating to one side, as well as lateral flexion to the other (Fig. 20-43). When rotatory subluxation is acute, the child resists attempts to move the head and has pain with any attempts at correction. Usually, the child is able to make the deformity worse but cannot correct it. Associated muscle spasms of the sternocleidomastoid muscle occur predominantly on the side of the long sternocleidomastoid muscle in an attempt to correct the deformity. If the deformity becomes fixed, the pain subsides but the torticollis and the decreased range of

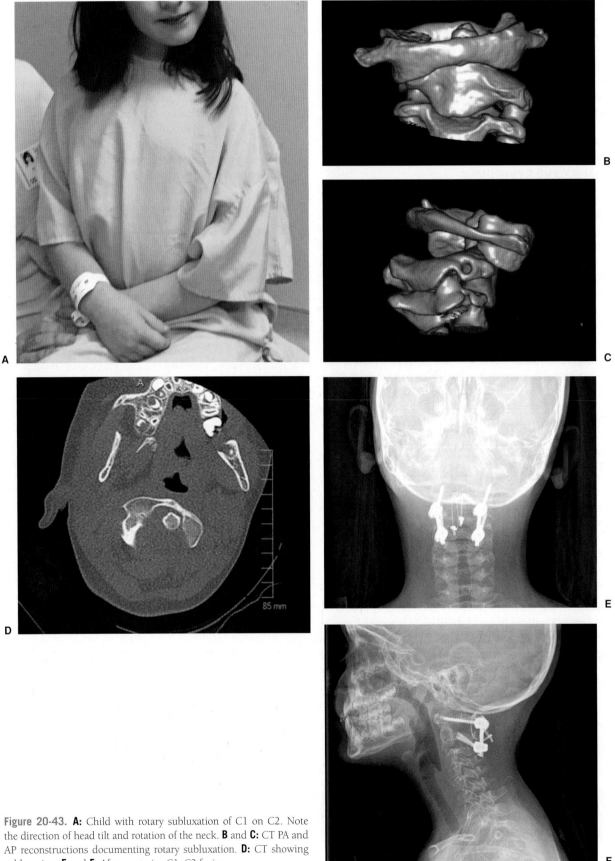

Figure 20-43. A: Child with rotary subluxation of C1 on C2. Note the direction of head tilt and rotation of the neck. **B** and **C:** CT PA and AP reconstructions documenting rotary subluxation. **D:** CT showing subluxation. **E** and **F:** After posterior C1–C2 fusion.

motion will persist.[129,196] If rotatory fixation has been present for a long time in a small child, plagiocephaly is sometimes noted. Neurologic abnormalities are extremely rare, although a few cases have been reported.

IMAGING AND OTHER DIAGNOSTIC STUDIES FOR ATLANTOAXIAL ROTATORY SUBLUXATION

Adequate radiographs may be difficult to obtain because of the associated torticollis and difficulty in positioning the head and neck. Anteroposterior and open-mouth odontoid views should be taken with the shoulders flat and the head in as neutral a position as possible.[181,325] Lateral masses that have rotated forward appear wider and closer to the midline, whereas the opposite lateral mass appears narrower and farther away from the midline on this view. One of the facet joints may be obscured because of apparent overlapping. The distance between the lateral mass and the dens also will be asymmetric. On the lateral view, the lateral facet appears anterior and usually appears wedge-shaped instead of the normal oval shape. The posterior arches of the atlas may fail to superimpose because of head tilt, giving the appearance of fusion of C1 to the occiput (occipitalization). Flexion and extension lateral views are recommended to exclude C1 to C2 instability.

CT should be performed with the head and body positioned as close to neutral as possible. This will show a superimposition of C1 on C2 in a rotated position and will allow the degree and amount of malrotation to be quantified. Some researchers have recommended dynamic CT scans taken with the patient looking to the right and the left to diagnose rotatory fixation.[324] McGuire et al.[271] classified findings on dynamic CT scans into three stages: stage 0, torticollis but a normal dynamic CT scan; stage 1, limitation of motion with less than 15 degrees difference between C1 and C2, but with C1 crossing the midline; and stage 2, fixed with C1 not crossing the midline. Duration of treatment and intensity of treatment were greater, the higher the stage. Three-dimensional CT scans also are helpful in identifying rotatory subluxation.[358] Ishii et al.[197] reported the use of the lateral inclination angle to grade the severity of subluxation: grade 1, no lateral inclination; grade 2, less than 20 degrees; and grade 3, more 20 degrees (Fig. 20-44). They

also noted adaptive changes in the superior facet joint of C2 in grade 3 subluxations and reported that grade 3 subluxations were more commonly irreducible. MRI demonstrates more soft tissue detail, such as associated spinal cord compression, integrity of the TAL, and underlying vertebral or soft tissue infections (Fig. 20-45).[345]

CLASSIFICATION OF ATLANTOAXIAL ROTATORY SUBLUXATION

Fielding and Hawkins[129] classified atlantoaxial rotatory displacements into four types based on the direction and degree of rotation and translation (Fig. 20-46).

Fielding and Hawkins Classification of Atlantoaxial Rotatory Subluxation	
Type I	• Unilateral facet subluxation with intact transverse ligament; no displacement between anterior arch of C1 and dens
Type II	• Unilateral facet subluxation with anterior displacement of 3–5 mm
Type III	• Bilateral anterior facet displacement; interval between C1 arch and dens is >5 mm
Type IV	• Atlas is displaced posteriorly

Type I is a unilateral facet subluxation with an intact transverse ligament. This is the most common and benign type. Type II is a unilateral facet subluxation with anterior displacement of 3 to 5 mm. The unilateral anterior displacement of one of the lateral masses may indicate an incompetent transverse ligament with potential instability. Type III is bilateral anterior facet displacement with more than 5 mm of anterior displacement. This type is associated with deficiencies of the transverse and secondary ligaments, which can result in significant narrowing of the space available for the cord at the atlantoaxial level. Type IV is an unusual type in which the atlas is displaced posteriorly. This usually is associated with a deficient dens. Although types III and IV are rare, neurologic involvement may be present. Both types must be managed with great care.

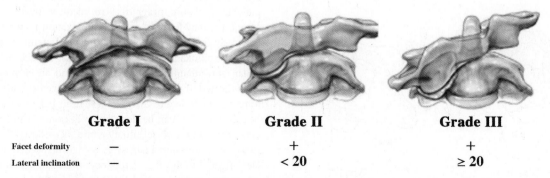

Grade I   **Grade II**   **Grade III**

Facet deformity	—	+	+
Lateral inclination	—	< 20	≥ 20

Figure 20-44. Classification of chronic atlantoaxial rotatory fixation: grade I, no lateral inclination; grade II, 20 degrees; grade III, 20 degrees. (With permission from Ishii K, Chiba K, Maruiwa H, et al. Pathognomonic radiological signs for predicting prognosis in patients with chronic atlantoaxial rotatory fixation. *J Neurosurg Spine.* 2006;5:385–391.)

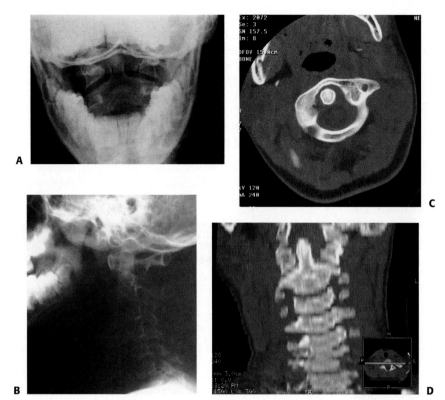

Figure 20-45. **A** and **B:** Odontoid view and lateral cervical spine radiograph of rotary subluxation of C1 on C2. **C:** Note the asymmetry on the open-mouth odontoid view. **D:** CT and CT reconstruction documenting rotary subluxation.

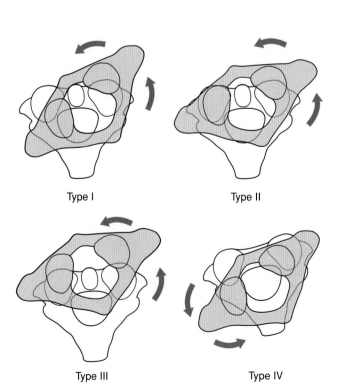

Figure 20-46. Classification of rotary displacement. (Reprinted with permission from Fielding JW, Hawkins RJ. Atlantoaxial rotary fixation. *J Bone Joint Surg Am.* 1977;59(1):37–44.)

TREATMENT OPTIONS FOR ATLANTOAXIAL ROTATORY SUBLUXATION

NONOPERATIVE TREATMENT OF ATLANTOAXIAL ROTATORY SUBLUXATION

Nonoperative Treatment of Atlanto-Rotatory Subluxation: INDICATIONS AND CONTRAINDICATIONS	
Indication	**Relative Contraindications**
• Reducible subluxation	• Irreducible subluxation • Instability • Neurologic deficits

Treatment depends on the duration of the symptoms.[37,324] Many patients probably never receive medical treatment because symptoms may be mild and the subluxation may reduce spontaneously over a few days before medical attention is sought. If rotary subluxation has been present for a week or less, a soft collar, anti-inflammatory medication, and an exercise program are indicated. If this fails to produce improvement and the symptoms persist for more than a week, head halter traction should be initiated. This can be done either at home or in the hospital, depending on the social situation and the severity of symptoms. Muscle relaxants and analgesics also may be needed. Phillips and Hensinger[324] found that if rotary subluxation was present for less than 1 month, head halter traction and bed rest were usually sufficient to relieve symptoms. If the subluxation has been present for longer than a month, successful reduction is not very likely.[69] However, halo traction can still be used to try to reduce the subluxation. The halo allows increased traction weight to be applied without interfering with opening of the jaw or causing skin pressure on the mandible. While the traction is being applied, active rotation to the right and left should be encouraged. Once the atlantoaxial rotatory subluxation has been reduced, motion has been restored, and the reduction is documented by CT scan, the patient is maintained in a halo vest for 6 weeks.[383]

A customized halo vest, known as a noninvasive halo, may also be used to reduce an acute or chronic atlantoaxial rotatory subluxation. In this technique, the noninvasive halo is placed with gentle pressure rotating the head toward the side lacking rotation. This may be adjusted every few days until the head can turn significantly past midline. A limited cut CT of C1 and C2 can confirm reduction. The noninvasive halo can be left in place to maintain the reduction for about 3 weeks, followed by a hard collar at 3 weeks.[383] In chronic subluxations, re-subluxations are not infrequent, and surgery is then indicated.

OPERATIVE TREATMENT OF ATLANTOAXIAL ROTATORY SUBLUXATION

If reduction cannot be maintained, posterior atlantoaxial arthrodesis is recommended.[307] Even though internal rotation and alignment of the atlas and axis may not be restored, successful fusion should result in the appearance of normal head alignment by relieving the muscle spasms that occurred in response to the malrotation. Posterior arthrodesis also is recommended if any signs of instability or neurologic deficits secondary to the subluxation are present, if the deformity has been present for more than 3 months, or if conservative treatment of 6 weeks of immobilization has failed. The editor has had experience of successful reduction of subluxations present for >3 months with a noninvasive halo. An alternative technique to an arthrodesis is to tie C1 and C2 together in the reduced position with a thick absorbable suture, such as no. 2 vicryl, in a sublaminar position bilaterally. In theory, the suture holds the reduction long enough for scarring to prevent re-subluxation, but decreased range of motion of a fusion is avoided.

Posterior Atlantoaxial Arthrodesis

See page 794 for this procedure.

C2–C3 Injuries

HANGMAN'S FRACTURE

INTRODUCTION TO HANGMAN'S FRACTURE

Bilateral spondylolisthesis of C2, or Hangman's fractures, also may occur in children.[327] This injury probably occurs more frequently in this age group because of the disproportionately large head, poor muscle control, and hypermobility. The possibility of child abuse also must be considered.[219,336,420]

ASSESSMENT OF HANGMAN'S FRACTURE

MECHANISMS OF INJURY FOR HANGMAN'S FRACTURE

The mechanism of injury is forced hyperextension and axial loading. Most reports of this injury have been in children under the age of 2 years.[131,134,189,219,317,327,337,338,348]

ASSOCIATED INJURIES AND SIGNS AND SYMPTOMS OF HANGMAN'S FRACTURE

Facial and head injuries may be associated. Patients present with neck pain and resist any movement of the head and neck.[283] There should be a history of trauma (Fig. 20-47).

IMAGING AND OTHER DIAGNOSTIC STUDIES FOR HANGMAN'S FRACTURE

Radiographs reveal a lucency anterior to the pedicles of the axis, usually with some forward subluxation of C2 on C3. One must be sure this is a fracture and not a persistent synchondrosis of the axis.[225,297,385,420,444] Differentiating a persistent synchondrosis from a fracture may be difficult. Several radiographic findings can help distinguish congenital spondylolysis from a Hangman's fracture. With congenital spondylolysis, there should be a symmetrical osseous gap with smooth, clearly defined cortical margins; no prevertebral soft tissue swelling should be observed; and there should be no signs of instability. Often, small foci of ossification are seen in the defect. CT scans show the defect to be at the level of the neurocentral chondrosis. MRI does not show any edema or soft tissue swelling that typically is present with a fracture.[283,420]

CLASSIFICATION OF HANGMAN'S FRACTURE

The classification by Effendi et al.,[113] which was modified by Levine and Edwards[245] and later by Müller,[291] is based on the severity of associated soft tissue injuries.

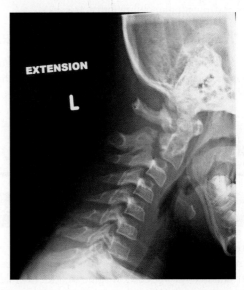

Figure 20-47. Lateral radiograph of patient with traumatic C2 spondylolisthesis (Hangman's fracture).

Classification of Hangman's Fracture (Edwards and Levine)			
Type	**Fracture Characteristics**	**Mechanism of Injury**	**Stability**
Type I	Bilateral pars fracture, <3 mm anterior C2 to C3 subluxation, intact C2 to C3 discoligamentous complex	Pure hyperextension-axial loading	Stable
Type II	Discoligamentous injury at C2 to C3 with displacement of the pars fracture and anterior translation of the C2 body	Combination hyperextension-axial loading with secondary anterior flexion-compression	Unstable
Type IIa	Minimal displacement, severe angulation (hinging from anterior longitudinal ligament)	Flexion-distraction	Unstable
Type III	Fracture of the pars interarticularis with C2 to C3 facet dislocations	Flexion-compression	Very unstable

Müller subclassified type II fractures as flexion, extension, and listhesis. Type III is a fracture of the pars interarticularis with C2 to C3 facet dislocations. This classification is for adult patients and may not be completely applicable to pediatric patients.[300]

TREATMENT OPTIONS FOR HANGMAN'S FRACTURE

NONOPERATIVE TREATMENT OF HANGMAN'S FRACTURE

Nonoperative Treatment of Hangman's Fracture: INDICATIONS AND CONTRAINDICATIONS	
Indication	**Relative Contraindications**
• Stable fracture	• Nonunion
	• Documented instability

Treatment of stable Hangman's fractures should be with immobilization in a Minerva cast, halo, or cervical orthosis for 8 to 12 weeks.[277,327] Pizzutillo et al.[327] reported that four of five patients healed with immobilization.

OPERATIVE TREATMENT OF HANGMAN'S FRACTURE

If union does not occur or there is documented instability, a posterior or anterior arthrodesis can be done to stabilize this fracture.

Subaxial (C3–C7) Injuries

INTRODUCTION TO SUBAXIAL (C3–C7) INJURIES

Fractures and dislocations involving C3 to C7 are rare in children and infants.[132,204,269,375] and usually occur in teenagers or older children. Lower cervical spine injuries in children as opposed to those in adults can occur through the cartilaginous endplate.[101] The endplate may break completely through the cartilaginous portion (Salter–Harris type I) or may exit through the bony edge (Salter–Harris type II). Usually, the inferior endplate fractures because of the protective effect of the uncinate processes of the superior endplate.[24,432]

Depending on the size and anatomy of the patient, adult posterior instrumentation techniques with screw and rods usually can be used in subaxial spine fractures.[200] Before these techniques are used, the size of the lateral masses must be evaluated to ensure that there is adequate room to place these screws. Occasionally, wire fixation may be needed for posterior stabilization of subaxial spine fractures. In appropriate-sized patients, anterior instrumentation techniques commonly used in adults also can be used to stabilize the pediatric cervical spine.

Posterior Ligamentous Disruptions

ASSESSMENT OF POSTERIOR LIGAMENTOUS DISRUPTIONS

MECHANISM OF INJURY FOR POSTERIOR LIGAMENTOUS DISRUPTION

Posterior ligamentous disruption can occur with a flexion or distraction injury to the cervical spine.

ASSOCIATED INJURIES AND SIGNS AND SYMPTOMS OF POSTERIOR LIGAMENTOUS DISRUPTION

Intervertebral disc disruption, facet fracture, and other ligamentous disruptions may be associated with this injury. The patient usually has point tenderness at the injury site and complaints of neck pain.

IMAGING AND OTHER DIAGNOSTIC STUDIES FOR POSTERIOR LIGAMENTOUS DISRUPTION

Initial radiographs may be normal except for loss of normal cervical lordosis. This may be a normal finding in young children but should be evaluated for possible ligamentous injury in an adolescent. Widening of the posterior interspinous distance is suggestive of this injury. Guidelines for instability in children have not been fully developed. Instability in adults has been defined as angulation between adjacent vertebrae in the sagittal plane of 11 degrees more than the adjacent normal segment or translation in the sagittal plane of 3.5 mm or more.[234,235,332,333] Brockmeyer and Aptelbaum[59] has suggested that more than 7 degrees of kyphotic angulation between adjacent vertebral bodies in the pediatric spine implies an unstable ligamentous injury.[285,287] MRI may be helpful in documenting ligamentous damage.

CLASSIFICATION OF POSTERIOR LIGAMENTOUS DISRUPTION

The Subaxial Injury Classification (SLIC) and severity score identifies three major injury characteristics to describe subaxial cervical injuries: injury morphology, discoligamentous complex integrity, and neurologic status.[320]

Subaxial Injury Classification (SLIC) System	
Characteristic	**Points**
Morphology	
No abnormality	0
Compression	1
Burst	+1 = 2
Distraction (e.g., facet perch, hyperextension)	3
Rotation/translation (e.g., facet dislocation, unstable teardrop, or advanced-stage flexion compression injury)	4
DLC	
Intact	0
Indeterminate (e.g., isolated interspinous widening, MRI signal change only)	1
Disrupted (e.g., widening of anterior disc space, facet perch or dislocation, kyphotic deformity)	2
Neurologic Status	
Intact	0
Root injury	1
Complete cord injury	2
Incomplete cord injury	3
Ongoing cord compression (in setting of a neurologic deficit)	+1

Reproduced with permission from Patel JC, Dailey A, Brodke DS, et al. Subaxial cervical spine trauma classification: The Subaxial Injury Classification system and case examples. *Neurosurg Focus.* 2008;25:E8.

TREATMENT OPTIONS FOR POSTERIOR LIGAMENTOUS DISRUPTION

NONOPERATIVE TREATMENT OF POSTERIOR LIGAMENTOUS DISRUPTION

Nonoperative Treatment of Posterior Ligamentous Disruption: INDICATIONS AND CONTRAINDICATIONS	
Indication	**Relative Contraindication**
• Stable posterior ligamentous disruption	• Instability

Posterior ligamentous injuries if stable should be protected with an extension orthosis, and patients should be followed closely for the development of instability. Stability should be documented by lateral flexion and extension radiographs at the end of treatment.

OPERATIVE TREATMENT OF POSTERIOR LIGAMENTOUS DISRUPTION

If signs of instability are present, a posterior arthrodesis should be performed (see page 763).

Compression Fracture

ASSESSMENT OF COMPRESSION FRACTURE

Compression fractures are stable injuries and heal in children in 3 to 6 weeks.

MECHANISMS OF INJURY FOR COMPRESSION FRACTURE

Compression fractures, the most common fractures of the subaxial spine in children, are caused by flexion and axial loading that results in loss of vertebral body height.

ASSOCIATED INJURIES AND SIGNS AND SYMPTOMS OF COMPRESSION FRACTURE

Associated injuries can include anterior teardrop, laminar, and spinous process fractures. Pain and neurologic symptoms may be present.[449]

IMAGING AND OTHER DIAGNOSTIC STUDIES FOR COMPRESSION FRACTURE

These injuries can be detected on a lateral radiograph. Because the vertebral disks in children are more resilient than the vertebral bodies, the bone is more likely to be injured. Many compression fractures may be overlooked because of the normal wedge shape of the vertebral bodies in young children. Flexion and extension films to confirm stability should be obtained 2 to 4 weeks after injury. In children under 8 years of age, the vertebral body may reconstitute itself with growth, although Schwarz et al.[364] reported that kyphosis of more than 20 degrees may not correct with growth.

CLASSIFICATION OF COMPRESSION FRACTURE

See page 804 for subaxial cervical spine injury classification.

TREATMENT OPTIONS FOR COMPRESSION FRACTURE

NONOPERATIVE TREATMENT OF COMPRESSION FRACTURE

Immobilization in a cervical collar is recommended for 3 to 6 weeks. Operative treatment is not usually necessary.

Unilateral and Bilateral Facet Dislocations

INTRODUCTION TO UNILATERAL AND BILATERAL FACET DISLOCATIONS

Unilateral facet dislocations and bilateral facet dislocations are the second most common injuries in the subaxial spine in children. Most occur in adolescents and are similar to adult injuries.

ASSESSMENT OF UNILATERAL AND BILATERAL FACET DISLOCATIONS

MECHANISMS OF INJURY FOR UNILATERAL AND BILATERAL FACET INJURY DISLOCATIONS

Facet dislocations can occur from a range of injury mechanisms that include hyperflexion, hyperextension, and/or axial rotation injuries from motor vehicle accidents, diving accidents, sports injuries, and falls.[18]

ASSOCIATED INJURIES AND SIGNS AND SYMPTOMS OF UNILATERAL AND BILATERAL FACET DISLOCATIONS

Cervical spine ligamentous injuries are often associated with bilateral dislocations as well as disc herniations. Bilateral facet dislocation has a high risk of cord damage.

Unilateral facet dislocation may have minimal localized pain or no symptoms; however, pain and neurologic symptoms are frequent in bilateral dislocations.

IMAGING AND OTHER DIAGNOSTIC STUDIES FOR UNILATERAL AND BILATERAL FACET DISLOCATIONS

The diagnosis usually can be made on anteroposterior and lateral radiographs. In children, the so-called perched facet is a true dislocation. The cartilaginous components are overlapped and locked. On the radiograph, the facet appears perched because the overlapped cartilage cannot be seen.

CLASSIFICATION OF UNILATERAL AND BILATERAL FACET DISLOCATIONS

See page 805 for subaxial spine injury classification.

TREATMENT OPTIONS FOR UNILATERAL AND BILATERAL FACET DISLOCATIONS

NONOPERATIVE TREATMENT OF UNILATERAL AND BILATERAL FACET DISLOCATIONS

Unilateral facet dislocation is treated with traction and reduction.

OPERATIVE TREATMENT OF UNILATERAL AND BILATERAL FACET DISLOCATIONS

If reduction cannot be easily obtained, open reduction and arthrodesis are indicated. Complete bilateral facet dislocation, although rare, is more unstable and has a higher incidence of neurologic deficit (Fig. 20-48). In a patient with bilateral jumped facets and motor-complete spinal cord injury, an emergent reduction followed by immediate MRI to evaluate for an epidural hematoma or herniated disk should be done. In a patient who is neurologically intact or has a motor-incomplete lesion with jumped facets, an urgent MRI is obtained to evaluate for a herniated disk or hematoma in the canal. In the absence of such a lesion, a closed reduction is obtained by traction. After reduction, treatment may consist of anterior or posterior instrumentation and arthrodesis. When there is gross instability and anterior disc injury, both anterior and posterior instrumentation and arthrodesis are usually needed.

Burst Fracture

ASSESSMENT OF BURST FRACTURE

MECHANISMS OF INJURY FOR BURST FRACTURE

Although rare, burst fractures can occur in children. These injuries are caused by an axial load after high-energy trauma.

SIGNS AND SYMPTOMS OF BURST FRACTURE

Patients may present with pain, deformity, and neurologic symptoms.

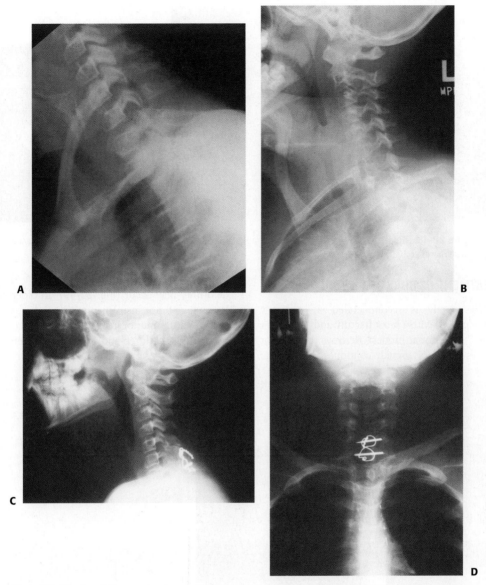

Figure 20-48. A and **B:** Lateral radiograph of a patient with the so-called perched facets, demonstrating a facet dislocation. **C** and **D:** Lateral and anteroposterior radiographs after reduction and posterior arthrodesis (Hall technique).

IMAGING AND OTHER DIAGNOSTIC STUDIES FOR BURST FRACTURE

Radiographic evaluation should consist of anteroposterior and lateral views. CT scans aid in detecting any spinal canal compromise from retropulsed fracture fragments and occult laminar fractures. The posterior aspect of the vertebral body can displace posteriorly, causing canal compromise and neurologic deficit. Loss of body height may be noted on radiographs.

CLASSIFICATION OF BURST FRACTURE

See page 804 for classification of subaxial injuries. Treatment decisions are based on the severity of deformity, canal compromise, degree of vertebral body height loss, and degree of neurologic deficit.

TREATMENT OPTIONS FOR BURST FRACTURE

NONOPERATIVE TREATMENT OF BURST FRACTURE

Nonoperative Treatment of Burst Fracture:
INDICATIONS AND CONTRAINDICATIONS

Indication	Relative Contraindication
• Burst fracture with no neurologic complications or canal compromise	• Significant canal compromise

If no neurologic deficit or significant canal compromise is present, treatment consists of traction followed by halo immobilization.

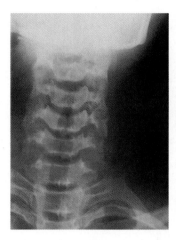
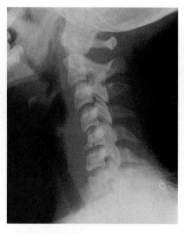
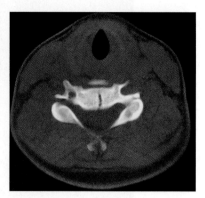

Figure 20-49. Anteroposterior and lateral radiographs and CT scan of patient with a minimally displaced burst fracture of C5.

OPERATIVE TREATMENT OF BURST FRACTURE

Anterior arthrodesis rarely is recommended in pediatric patients, except in a patient with a burst fracture and significant canal compromise.[366] Anterior arthrodesis destroys the anterior growth potential; as posterior growth continues, a kyphotic deformity may occur (Fig. 20-49). In older children and adolescents, anterior instrumentation can be used for stabilization (Fig. 20-50). Anterior instrumentation can be used for stabilization in older children and adolescents when there is significant canal compromise.

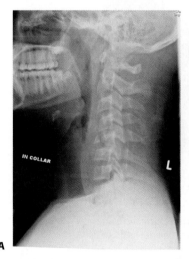

A

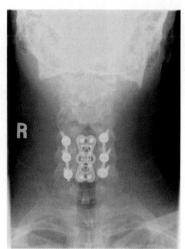

C

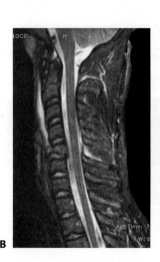

B

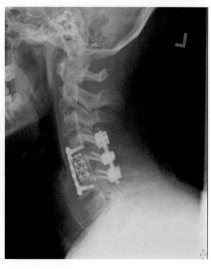

D

Figure 20-50. Radiograph (**A**) and MRI (**B**) of a 12-year-old boy with three-column injury sustained during football game. **C** and **D**: After anterior and posterior fusion and fixation with anterior plate and screws and posterior instrumentation.

Spondylolysis and Spondylolisthesis

ASSESSMENT OF SPONDYLOLYSIS AND SPONDYLOLISTHESIS

MECHANISMS OF INJURY FOR SPONDYLOLYSIS AND SPONDYLOLISTHESIS

Spondylolysis and spondylolisthesis of C2 to C6 have been reported. These injuries can occur from either a hyperextension or flexion axial loading injury.

ASSOCIATED INJURIES AND SIGNS AND SYMPTOMS OF SPONDYLOLYSIS AND SPONDYLOLISTHESIS

Associated anterosuperior avulsion or compression fractures of the vertebral body may occur. Patients may present with shoulder or localized neck pain.

IMAGING AND OTHER DIAGNOSTIC STUDIES FOR SPONDYLOLYSIS AND SPONDYLOLISTHESIS

The diagnosis usually is made on plain radiographs that show a fracture line through the pedicles. Oblique views may be necessary to better identify the fracture line. CT imaging and MRI may be useful in differentiating an acute fracture from a normal synchondrosis.

CLASSIFICATION OF SPONDYLOLYSIS AND SPONDYLOLISTHESIS

See page 805 for classification of subaxial injuries

TREATMENT OPTIONS FOR SPONDYLOLYSIS AND SPONDYLOLISTHESIS

NONOPERATIVE TREATMENT OF SPONDYLOLYSIS AND SPONDYLOLISTHESIS

Nonoperative Treatment of Spondylolysis and Spondylolisthesis: INDICATIONS AND CONTRAINDICATIONS

Indication	Relative Contraindication
• Stable spondylolysis and spondylolisthesis	• Instability • Nonunion

Treatment consists of immobilization in a cervical orthosis or halo brace.

OPERATIVE TREATMENT OF SPONDYLOLYSIS AND SPONDYLOLISTHESIS

Surgical stabilization is recommended only for truly unstable fractures or nonunions. Neurologic involvement is rare.

Posterior Arthrodesis for Subaxial Injuries

Positioning

The patient is placed prone using a Mayfield headrest or Gardner-Wells tongs or a halo ring attached to a Mayfield headrest.

Technique

> ✔ **Posterior Arthrodesis for Subaxial Injuries:** KEY SURGICAL STEPS
>
> ☐ Expose the chosen spinous processes with a midline incision
> ☐ Make a hole in the base of the spinous process and in spinous process of inferior vertebra to be fused
> ☐ Pass wire and tighten
> ☐ Place corticocancellous bone graft
> ☐ Close wound in layers

Radiographs are obtained to confirm adequate alignment of the vertebrae and to localize the vertebrae to be exposed. Extension of the fusion mass can occur when extra vertebrae or spinous processes are exposed in the cervical spine. A midline incision is made over the chosen spinous processes, and the spinous process and lamina are exposed subperiosteally to the facet joints.

If the spinous process is large enough, a hole is made in the base of the spinous process with a towel clip or Lewin clamp (Fig. 20-51). An 18-gauge wire is passed through this hole, looped over the spinous process, and passed through the hole again. A similar hole is made in the base of the spinous process of the inferior vertebra to be fused, and the wire is passed through this vertebra. The wire is then passed through this hole, looped under the inferior aspect of the spinous process, and then passed back through the same hole. The wire is tightened and corticocancellous bone grafts are placed along the exposed lamina and spinous processes. The wound is closed in layers. If the spinous process is too small to pass wires, then an in situ arthrodesis can be performed and external immobilization used.

Hall et al.[161] used a 16-gauge wire and threaded Kirschner wires. The threaded Kirschner wires are passed through the bases of the spinous processes of the vertebrae to be fused. This is followed by a figure-of-eight wiring with a 16-gauge wire (Fig. 20-52). After tightening the wire about the Kirschner wires, strips of corticocancellous and cancellous bone are packed over the posterior arches of the vertebrae to be fused.

Posterior Arthrodesis With Lateral Mass Screw Fixation

Several techniques of lateral mass screw fixation for the lower cervical spine have been described. They differ primarily in the entry points for the screws and in the trajectory of screw placement, which yield different exit points.[254,346]

Positioning

The patient is placed prone using a Mayfield headrest or Gardner-Wells tongs or a halo ring attached to a Mayfield headrest.

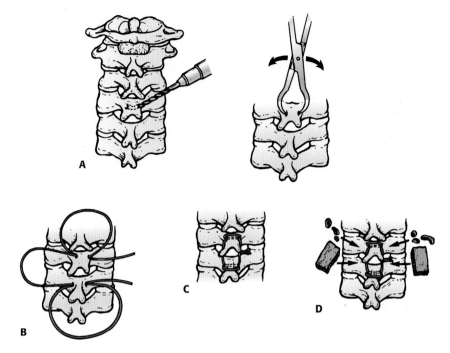

Figure 20-51. Technique of posterior arthrodesis in subaxial spine levels C3 to C7. **A:** A hole is made in the spinous process of the vertebrae to be fused. **B:** An 18-gauge wire is passed through both holes and around the spinous processes. **C:** The wire is tightened. **D:** Corticocancellous bone grafts are placed.[203] (Reprinted by permission from Murphy MJ, Southwick WO. Posterior approaches and fusions. In: Cervical Spine Research Society. *The Cervical Spine.* 2nd ed. Philadelphia, PA: JB Lippincott; 1983:506–507.)

Technique

Roy-Camille Technique[347]

> ✔ **Posterior Arthrodesis With Lateral Mass Screw Fixation (Roy-Camille):** KEY SURGICAL STEPS
>
> ❑ Place entry point for screw at center of rectangular posterior face of lateral mass
> ❑ Drill perpendicular to posterior wall to a safe depth
> ❑ Exit point should be at junction of lateral mass and transverse process for additional pullout strength

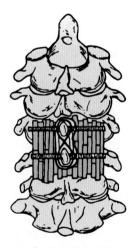

Figure 20-52. Alternative fixation method for posterior arthrodesis of C3 to C7. A 16-gauge wire is placed in a figure-of-eight pattern around two threaded Kirschner wires passed through the bases of the spinous processes of the vertebrae to be fused.[114] (Reprinted with permission from Hall JE, Simmons ED, Danylchuk K, et al. Instability of the cervical spine and neurological involvement in Klippel–Feil syndrome: A case report. *J Bone Joint Surg Am.* 1990;72(3):460–462.)

The entry point for the screw is at the center of the rectangular posterior face of the lateral mass or can be measured 5 mm medial to the lateral edge and midway between the facets included in the fusion joints (Fig. 20-53A). The drill is directed perpendicular to the posterior wall of the vertebral body with a 10-degree lateral angle (Fig. 20-53B). This trajectory establishes an exit point slightly lateral to the vertebral artery and below the exiting nerve root. The lateral mass depth from C3 to C6 ranges from 6 to 14 mm in men (average 8.7 mm) and 6 to 11 mm in women (average 7.9 mm). An adjustable drill guide set to a depth of 10 to 12 mm is used to prevent penetration beyond the anterior cortex. The depth can be gradually and safely increased if local anatomy permits. If the additional 20% of pullout strength with bicortical fixation is desired, the exit point should be at the junction of the lateral mass and the transverse process. Lateral fluoroscopic imaging makes it easier to choose the optimal trajectory and avoid penetration of the subjacent facet joint (Fig. 20-53C), which is especially important at the caudal level of fixation because this joint should be

Magerl and Seeman

> ✔ **Posterior Arthrodesis With Lateral Mass Screw Fixation (Magerl and Seeman):** KEY SURGICAL STEPS
>
> ❑ Place entry point for screw 1 mm medial and rostral to center point of posterior surface of lateral mass
> ❑ Drill at a 45- to 60-degree rostral angle parallel to adjacent fact joint articular surface and 25-degree lateral angle
> ❑ Depth of penetration is approximately 18 mm

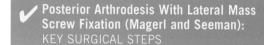

The entry point for the screw is 1 mm medial and rostral (proximal) to the center point of the posterior surface of the lateral mass (Fig. 20-54A). It is oriented at a 45- to 60-degree rostral angle, parallel to the adjacent facet joint articular surface, and at a

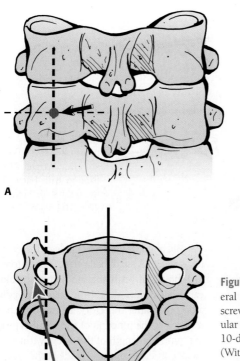

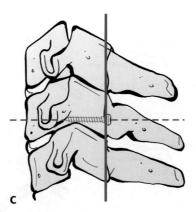

Figure 20-53. Roy–Camille technique of lateral mass screw insertion. **A:** Entry point for screw insertion. **B:** Drill is directed perpendicular to posterior wall of vertebral body with a 10-degree lateral angle. **C:** Final screw position. (With permission from Heller JG, Jeffords P. Internal fixation of the cervical spine. Posterior instrumentation of the lower cervical spine. In: Frymoyer JW, Wiesel SW, eds. *The Adult and Pediatric Spine*. 3rd ed. Philadelphia, PA: Lippincott Williams & Wilkins; 2004.)

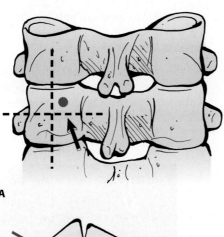

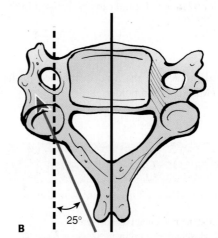

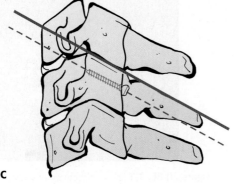

Figure 20-54. Magerl technique of lateral mass screw insertion. **A:** Entry point for screw insertion. **B:** Drill is directed at a 25-degree lateral angle. **C:** Final screw position. (With permission from Heller JG, Jeffords P. Internal fixation of the cervical spine. Posterior instrumentation of the lower cervical spine. In: Frymoyer JW, Wiesel SW, eds. *The Adult and Pediatric Spine*. 3rd ed. Philadelphia, PA: Lippincott Williams & Wilkins; 2004.)

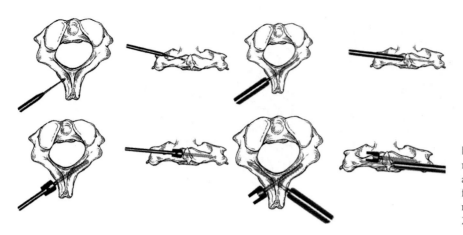

Figure 20-55. C2 translaminar screw placement (see text). (With permission from Leonard JR, Wright NM. Pediatric atlantoaxial fixation with bilateral, crossing C2 translaminar screws. Technical note. *J Neurosurg Pediatr.* 2006;104:59–63.)

25-degree lateral angle (Fig. 20-54B). This trajectory establishes an exit point lateral to the vertebral artery and above the exiting nerve root while engaging the lateral portion of the ventral cortex of the superior articular facet (Fig. 20-54C). The proper trajectory for this technique is more difficult to achieve than in the Roy-Camille technique. The prominence of the thorax can impede proper alignment of the drill and guide, risking injury to the nerve root if the second cortex is penetrated. The depth of penetration at this angle is approximately 18 mm, compared to 14 mm with the Roy-Camille technique, which has some implications for purchase strength and mode of screw failure.

Crossed Translaminar Screw Fixation of C2

Crossed translaminar screws may be used for posterior fixation if the lateral masses are not adequate for screw fixation. This has been described for fixation at C2 but can also be used in the lower cervical spine.[356,382]

Positioning

The patient is placed prone with the head maintained in the neutral position in a Mayfield head holder.

Technique

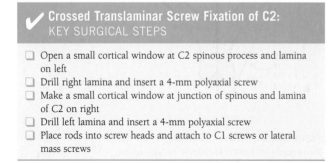

✔ Crossed Translaminar Screw Fixation of C2:
KEY SURGICAL STEPS

☐ Open a small cortical window at C2 spinous process and lamina on left
☐ Drill right lamina and insert a 4-mm polyaxial screw
☐ Make a small cortical window at junction of spinous and lamina of C2 on right
☐ Drill left lamina and insert a 4-mm polyaxial screw
☐ Place rods into screw heads and attach to C1 screws or lateral mass screws

The posterior arch of C1 and the spinous process, laminae, and medial–lateral masses of C2 are exposed. A high-speed drill is used to open a small cortical window at the junction of the C2 spinous process and the lamina on the left, close to the rostral margin of the C2 lamina (Fig. 20-55). With a hand drill, the contralateral (right) lamina is carefully drilled along its length, with the drill

visually aligned along the angle of the exposed contralateral laminar surface. A small ball probe is used to palpate the length of the drill hole and verify that no cortical breakthrough into the spinal canal has occurred. A 4-mm diameter polyaxial screw is inserted along the same trajectory. In the final position, the screw head remains at the junction of the spinous process and lamina on the left, with the length of the screw within the right lamina. Next, a small cortical window is made at the junction of the spinous process and lamina of C2 on the right, close to the caudal aspect of the lamina. Using the same technique, a 4-mm diameter screw is placed into the left lamina, with the screw head remaining on the right side of the spinous process (Fig. 20-56). Appropriate rods are then placed into the screw heads and attached to C1 screws or lateral mass screws below C2 (Fig. 20-57).[76,243]

Potential Pitfalls and Preventive Measures

See page 807 for potential pitfalls with posterior approaches.

Anterior Arthrodesis

In older pediatric patients and adolescents, adult anterior instrumentation and fusion techniques may be used. Anatomy of the vertebral body should be evaluated preoperatively to determine if anterior plates and screws may be used.[33]

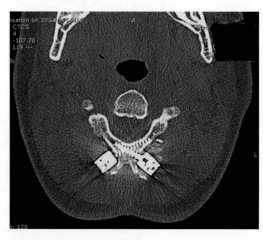

Figure 20-56. CT shows placement of screws.

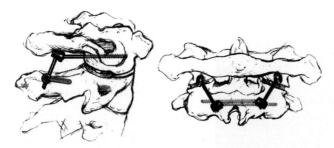

Figure 20-57. Lateral (**left**) and anteroposterior (**right**) views of completed C1 to C2 fixation with C1 lateral mass screws connected to C2 laminar screws (**lateral view**). (With permission from Leonard JR, Wright NM. Pediatric atlantoaxial fixation with bilateral, crossing C2 translaminar screws. Technical note. *J Neurosurg Pediatr.* 2006;104:59–63.)

Author's Preferred Treatment for Cervical Spine Injury

Occipital Condyle Fracture

Most occipital condyle fractures can be treated nonoperatively with an orthosis. A rigid occipital mandibular orthosis or cervical collar is the preferred method of immobilization.[73,207,208,253] In the rare case that surgical stabilization is needed (type III), fusion from the occiput to C2 with a Luque rod and wire instrumentation or an occipital plate with screw fixation are recommended.[233]

Atlantooccipital Instability

Atlantooccipital dislocation is an unstable ligamentous injury. The author recommends operative treatment in the vast majority of patients. Fusion with instrumentation of the occiput to C2 is the preferred treatment. Instrumentation will depend on the size of the patient and the anatomy of the upper cervical spine. In small children in whom placement of screws will be difficult, contoured Luque rods and cables will give adequate stabilization. This provides immediate stabilization, and the patient can be mobilized in a cervical collar. If the patient's anatomy allows, an occipital plate and C1 and C2 screw fixation can be used; this rod and screw fixation provides more secure fixation than Luque rods and cables. These injuries usually are in younger patients, and screw and plate instrumentation may not be possible. Instrumentation to C2 is preferred over ending instrumentation at C1. There are usually significant soft tissue injuries and associated injuries. Extending the fusion and instrumentation to C2 gives better fixation and more surface area for fusion but is at the expense of increased loss of motion of the upper cervical spine postoperatively.

Fractures of the Atlas

Most pediatric patients with an atlas fracture may be treated nonoperatively. Minimally displaced fractures or greenstick-type fractures through the synchondrosis often can be treated in a rigid collar. If there is significant displacement on plain radiographs (>7 mm overhang) or on CT scan, then a short period of traction followed by halo immobilization is recommended.

Odontoid Fracture

Most odontoid fractures can be treated nonoperatively in an extension Minerva cast or halo cast or brace. Closed reduction of an odontoid fracture can be performed on an anesthetized patient with neuromonitoring.[193] Gentle extension or flexion of the neck under live lateral fluoroscopy often reduces the fracture (Fig. 20-58). If the odontoid is anteriorly displaced or angulated, it can be reduced by the surgeon placing their finger into the patient's mouth and applying a posterior force directly to the odontoid with fluoroscopic visualization of reduction.[354]

If the patient cannot be managed nonoperatively, then a C1 to C2 fusion is the authors' preferred method. In older children, the Harms C1, C2 instrumentation is used. If the anatomy does not allow for screw fixation, then a Brooks-type fusion is performed, and patient is immobilized in a halo.

Atlantoaxial Instability

Atlantoaxial instability from rupture of the transverse ligament is rare in children. When an avulsion fracture of the transverse ligament occurs and is nondisplaced, nonoperative treatment may be considered in this special situation. Most injuries to the transverse ligament are unstable. The authors' preferred method of stabilization is with the Harms C1, C2 screw and rod technique and posterior fusion. Transarticular screw fixation is another acceptable stabilization method but is more difficult in a small child because of anatomical consideration. If the anatomy does not allow for safe placement of screws, then Brooks instrumentation and fusion are recommended. This will require halo or Minerva cast immobilization postoperatively.

Subaxial Injuries

Most subaxial injuries occur in older children and adult instrumentation and fusion techniques are appropriate. In unstable subaxial injuries, such as facet fracture dislocations, lateral mass screw and rod fixation usually can be performed in children. Anterior instrumentation and fusion may need to be performed in burst-type fractures or fracture-dislocation with disc herniation.

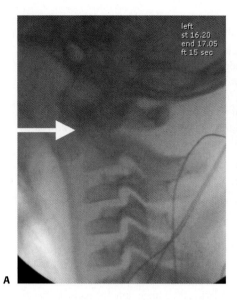

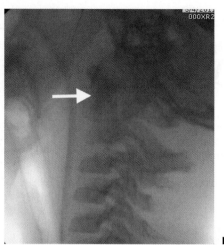

Figure 20-58. A: A 4-year-old with anteriorly displaced odontoid fracture (*arrow*) before reduction. **B:** With neuromonitoring under general anesthesia, gentle extension and traction reduces an anteriorly displaced odontoid fractures. Pushing posteriorly on the odontoid fragment with the surgeon's finger in the patient's mouth is also effective at reducing the fracture. *Arrow* points at reduced odontoid fracture. Halo vest immobilization is used postoperatively for 8 weeks. (Courtesy of the Children's Orthopaedic Center, Los Angeles.)

Annotated References

Reference	Annotation
Astur N, Klimo P Jr, Sawyer JR, et al. Traumatic atlanto-occipital dislocation in children: evaluation, treatment, and outcomes. *J Bone Joint Surg Am.* 2013;95:e194(1–8).	In their report of 14 patients who survived traumatic atlantoaxial dislocations, the authors recommended surgical stabilization, but noted the risk of postoperative hydrocephalus.
Beier AD, Vachhranji S, Bayerl SH, et al. Rotatory subluxation: experience from the Hospital for Sick Children. *J Neurosurg Pediatr.* 2012;9:144–148.	Of 40 patients with atlantoaxial rotatory subluxation, those with longer durations of symptoms required halo traction or surgical fixation and fusion.
Bono CM, Vaccaro AR, Fehlings M, et al. Measurement techniques for upper cervical spine injuries: consensus statement of the Spine Trauma Study Group. *Spine (Phila Pa 1976).* 2007;32:593–600.	This review described the technique for and importance of different radiographic measurements for diagnosis of upper cervical spine trauma.
Brown RL, Brunn MA, Garcia VF. Cervical spine injuries in children: a review of 103 patients treated consecutively at a level 1 pediatric trauma center. *J Pediatr Surg.* 2001;36(8):1107–1114.	This study is a review of 103 patients treated for a cervical spine injury at a level 1 pediatric trauma center. The mean age of the patients was 10 years of age with most common mechanism being motor vehicle collisions (52%) followed by sporting injuries (27%). The majority of injuries were of the upper cervical spine with predictors of mortality being younger age, mechanism, upper cervical injuries, and associated closed head injuries.
Cattell HS, Filtzer DL. Pseudosubluxation and other normal variations in the cervical spine in children. *J Bone Joint Surg Am.* 1965;47:1295–1309.	A classic reference which reviews the normal variations of the cervical spine radiographs in children. This article describes the variations seen which help determine normal variants on plain films which can be confused as fractures or ligamentous injuries in children.
Fielding JW, Hawkins RJ. Atlanto-axial rotatory fixation. (Fixed rotatory subluxation of the atlanto-axial joint). *J Bone Joint Surg Am.* 1977;59:37–44.	This classic article provided the definition of atlantoaxial rotatory fixation and the classification system that is currently used.
Flynn JM, Closkey RF, Mahboubi S, et al. Role of magnetic resonance imaging in the assessment of pediatric cervical spine injuries. *J Pediatr Orthop.* 2002;22:573–577.	A review of 74 children who underwent MRI as a screening tool for suspected cervical spine injury. MRI is the imaging study of choice for potential cervical spine injuries in children who are obtunded, unable to cooperate with an exam, or who have unexplained neurologic findings. MRI findings altered the diagnosis in 34% of patients.
Frank JM, Lim CK, Flynn JM, et al. The efficacy of magnetic resonance imaging in pediatric cervical spine clearance. *Spine (Phila Pa 1976).* 2002;27:1176–1179.	Time to cervical spine clearance, intensive care unit stay, hospital stay, and costs were all reduced, demonstrating that cervical spine MRI is effective and cost-efficient in cervical spine clearance in obtunded and intubated pediatric patients.
Hedequist D, Hresko T, Proctor M. Modern cervical spine instrumentation in children. *Spine (Phila Pa 1976).* 2008;33:379–383.	A retrospective review of 25 pediatric patients treated with modern cervical spine instrumentation determined that these devices are safe and feasible to use in children older than 6 years of age.

Annotated References

Reference	Annotation
Herzenberg JE, Hensinger RN, Dedrick DK, et al. Emergency transport and positioning of young children who have an injury of the cervical spine: the standard backboard may be hazardous. *J Bone Joint Surg Am.* 1989;71:15–22.	A retrospective study looking at trauma patients less than 7 years of age who were found to have anterior translation of a cervical spine injury on initial lateral radiographs on a standard backboard. This study showed that to prevent undesirable cervical flexion in younger children, it is necessary to either transport them with a specialized backboard that has an occipital recess or to use a double mattress pad to raise the body and allow the occiput to fall posteriorly.
Hosalkar HS, Greenbaum JN, Flynn JM, et al. Fractures of the odontoid in children with an open basilar synchondrosis. *J Bone Joint Surg Br.* 2009;91:789–796.	These authors described a new classification system and made treatment recommendations for odontoid fractures in children with open basilar synchondroses.
Knox JB, Schneider JE, Cage JM, et al. Spine trauma in very young children: a retrospective study of 206 patients presenting to a level 1 pediatric trauma center. *J Pediatr Orthop.* 2014;34:698–702.	This retrospective study compared injuries in two age groups: 0–3 years and 4–9 years. Children in the 0–3 years group had more ligamentous injuries, and 19% of them were caused by nonaccidental trauma.
Menezes AH. Craniocervical developmental anatomy and its implications. *Childs Nerv Syst.* 2008;24:1109–1122.	In-depth review of the important anatomy of the craniocervical junction in children.
Pang D, Pollack IF. Spinal cord injury without radiologic abnormality in children: the SCIWORA syndrome. *J Trauma.* 1989;29:654–664.	This is a study looking at the clinical experience of 55 children with SCIWORA. The study showed that more severe SCIWORA injuries were seen in younger children with propensity of recovery based on admission neurologic status. Treatment for these injuries revolves around ruling out injuries that require surgical stabilization and preventing recurrent injury.
Pang D, Pollock IF. Spinal cord injury without radiologic abnormality in children: the SCIWORA syndrome. *J Trauma.* 1989;29:654–664.	Review of clinical outcomes in 55 children showed that more SCIWORA injuries occurred in young children, with propensity for recovery based on admission neurologic status. Treatment focuses on ruling out injuries that require surgical stabilization and preventing recurrent injury.
Tull S, Tator CH, Fehlings MG, et al. Occipital condyle fractures. *Neurosurgery.* 1997;41:368–376.	This modification of the classification system of Anderson and Montesano (based on mechanism of injury) is based on stability of the occiput/C1-2 joint.

REFERENCES

1. Abd-El-Barr MM, Snyder BD, Emans JB, et al. Combined preoperative traction with instrumented posterior occipitocervical fusion for severe ventral brainstem compression secondary to displaced os odontoideum: technical report of 2 cases. *J Neurosurg Pediatr.* 2016;25:724–729.
2. Abou Madawi A, Solanki G, Casey AT, et al. Variation of the groove in the axis vertebra for the vertebral artery. Implications for instrumentation. *J Bone Joint Surg Br.* 1997;79:820–823.
3. Adlegais KM, Grossman DC, Langer SC, et al. Use of helical computed tomography for imaging the pediatric cervical spine. *Acad Emerg Med.* 2004;11:228–236.
4. Ahmadan A, Dakwar E, Vale FL, et al. Occipitocervical fusion via occipital condylar fixation: a clinical case series. *J Spinal Disord Tech.* 2014;27:232–236.
5. Ahmed R, Traynelis VC, Menezes AH. Fusions at the craniovertebral junction. *Childs Nerv Syst.* 2008;24:1209–1224.
6. Ahuja CS, Schroeder GD, Vaccaro AR, et al. Spinal cord injury-what are the controversies? *J Orthop Trauma.* 2017;31(Suppl 4):S7–S13.
7. Alcelik I, Manik KS, Sian PS, et al. Occipital condylar fractures. Review of the literature and case report. *J Bone Joint Surg Br.* 2006; 88:665–669.
8. Allam E, Zhou Y. Bipartite atlas or Jefferson fracture? A case series and literature review. *Spine (Phila Pa 1976).* 2015;40:E661–E664.
9. Allington JJ, Zembo M, Nadell J, et al. C1–C2 posterior soft tissue injuries with neurologic impairment in children. *J Pediatr Orthop.* 1990;10:596–601.
10. American Academy of Orthopaedic Surgeons, Committee on Pediatric Orthopaedics. *Trauma of the Cervical Spine. Position Statement.* Rosemont, IL: Author; 1990.
11. American Academy of Pediatrics, Committee on Sports Medicine. Atlantoaxial instability in Down syndrome. *Pediatrics.* 1984;74:152–154.
12. American Academy of Pediatrics, Committee on Sports Medicine and Fitness. Atlantoaxial instability in Down syndrome: subject review. *Pediatrics.* 1995;96(1 Pt 1):151–154.
13. Anderson LD, D'Alonzo RT. Fractures of the odontoid process of the axis. *J Bone Joint Surg Am.* 1974;56(8):1663–1674.
14. Anderson PA, Montesano PX. Morphology and treatment of occipital condyle fractures. *Spine.* 1988;13:731–736.
15. Anderson JM, Schutt AH. Spinal injury in children: a review of 156 cases seen from 1950 through 1978. *Mayo Clin Proc.* 1980;55:499–504.
16. Anderson LD, Smith BL Jr, DeTorre J, et al. The role of polytomography in the diagnosis and treatment of cervical spine injuries. *Clin Orthop Relat Res.* 1982;165:64–68.
17. Annis JA, Finlay DB, Allen MJ, et al. A review of cervical-spine radiographs in casualty patients. *Br J Radiol.* 1987;60:1059–1061.
18. Annispour AK, Agel JH, Bellabara C, et al. Cervical facet dislocations in the adolescent population: a report of 21 cases at a Level 1 trauma center from 2004 to 2014. *Eur Spine J.* 2017;26:1266–1271.
19. Apple JS, Kirks DR, Merten DF, et al. Cervical spine fractures and dislocations in children. *Pediatr Radiol.* 1987;17:45–49.
20. Arlet V, Aebi M. Anterior and posterior cervical spine fusion and instrumentation. In: Weinstein SL, ed. *Pediatric Spine Surgery.* 2nd ed. Philadelphia, PA: Lippincott Williams & Wilkins; 2001:209–226.
21. Arora B, Suresh S. Spinal cord injuries in older children: is there a role for high-dose methylprednisolone? *Pediatr Emerg Care.* 2011;27:1192–1194.
22. Arvin B, Fournier-Gosselin MP, Fehlings MG. Os odontoideum: etiology and surgical management. *Neurosurgery.* 2010;66(3):22–31.
23. Astur N, Klimo P Jr, Sawyer JR, et al. Traumatic atlanto-occipital dislocation in children: evaluation, treatment and outcomes. *J Bone Joint Surg.* 2013;95(24):e194(1–8).
24. Aufdermaur M. Spinal injuries in juveniles: necropsy findings in 12 cases. *J Bone Joint Surg Br.* 1974;56:513–519.
25. Aulino JM, Tutt LK, Kaye JJ, et al. Occipital condyle fractures: clinical presentation and imaging findings in 76 patients. *Emerg Radiol.* 2005;11:342–347.
26. AuYong N, Piatt J Jr. Jefferson fractures of the immature spine. Report of 3 cases. *J Neurosurg Pediatr.* 2009;3:15–19.
27. Bachulis BL, Long WB, Hynes GD, et al. Clinical indications for cervical spine radiographs in the traumatized patient. *Am J Surg.* 1987;153:473–477.
28. Baghdassarian A, Piatt JH Jr, Giordano K. Fracture of the anterior arch of atlas after minor trauma in the immature spine postlaminectomy. *Pediatr Emerg Care.* 2014;30:340–342.
29. Bailey DK. Normal cervical spine in infants and children. *Radiology.* 1952;59: 713–714.
30. Banniza von Bazan UK, Paeslack V. Scoliotic growth in children with acquired paraplegia. *Paraplegia.* 1977;15:65–73.
31. Baranowska A, Baranowska J, Pydych A, et al. Brachial plexus root avulsion injury with occipital condyle fractures. Case study. *Ortop Traumatol Rehabil.* 2016;18: 359–365.

32. Barcelos AC, Patriota GC, Netto AU. Nontraumatic atlantoaxial rotatory subluxation: Grisel syndrome. Case report and literature review. *Global Spine J.* 2014; 4:179–186.
33. Baron EM, Loftus CM, Vaccaro AR, et al. Anterior approach to the subaxial cervical spine in children: a brief review. *Neurosurg Focus.* 2006;20:E4.
34. Baum JA, Hanley EN Jr, Pullekines J. Comparison of halo complications in adults and children. *Spine.* 1989;14:251–252.
35. Bayar MA, Erdem Y, Ozturk K, et al. Isolated anterior arch fracture of the atlas: child case report. *Spine.* 2002;27:E47–E49.
36. Bedbrook GM. Correction of scoliosis due to paraplegia sustained in pediatric age group. *Paraplegia.* 1977;15:90–96.
37. Beier AD, Vachhrajani S, Bayeri SH, et al. Rotatory subluxation: experience from the Hospital for Sick Children. *J Neurosurg Pediatr.* 2012;9:144-148.
38. Benzel EC, Zhang DH, Iannotti C, et al. Occipitocervical fusion in an infant with atlantooccipital dislocation. *World Neurosurg.* 2012;78(6):e17–e24. www.world-neurosurgery.org.
39. Bernini EP, Elefante R, Smaltino F, et al. Angiographic study on the vertebral artery in cases of deformities of the occipitocervical joint. *AJR Am J Roentgenol.* 1969;107:526–529.
40. Bertozzi JC, Rojas CA, Martinez CR. Evaluation of the pediatric craniocervical junction in MDCT. *AJR Am J Roentgenol.* 2009;192:26–31.
41. Birney TJ, Hanley EN Jr. Traumatic cervical spine injuries in childhood and adolescence. *Spine.* 1989;14:1277–1282.
42. Bivins HG, Ford S, Bezmalnovic Z, et al. The effect of axial traction during orotracheal intubation of the trauma victim with an unstable cervical spine. *Ann Emerg Med.* 1988;17:25–29.
43. Bloom AI, Neeman Z, Floman TY, et al. Occipital condyle fracture and ligament injury: imaging by CT. *Pediatr Radiol.* 1996;26:786–790.
44. Bloom AI, Neeman Z, Slasky BS, et al. Fracture of the occipital condyles and associated craniocervical ligament injury: incidence, CT imaging and implications. *Clin Radiol.* 1997;52:198–202.
45. Bohlman HH. Acute fractures and dislocations of the cervical spine. *J Bone Joint Surg Am.* 1969;61:1119–1142.
46. Bohn D, Armstrong D, Becker L, et al. Cervical spine injuries in children. *J Trauma.* 1990;30:463–469.
47. Bono CM. The halo fixator. *J Am Acad Orthop Surg.* 2007;15:728–737.
48. Bono CM, Vaccaro AR, Fehlings M, et al. Measurement techniques for upper cervical spine injuries: consensus statement of the Spine Trauma Study Group. *Spine (Phila Pa 1976).* 2007;32:593–600.
49. Booth TN. Cervical spine evaluation in pediatric trauma. *Am J Radiol.* 2012;198:W417–W425.
50. Bowers CA, Kundu B, Hawryluk GWJ. Methylprednisolone for acute spinal cord injury: an increasingly philosophical debate. *Neural Regen Res.* 2016;11: 882–885.
51. Bozkurt G, Hazer B, Yaman ME, et al. Isolated paralysis of glossopharyngeal and vagus nerve associated with type II occipital condyle fracture: case report. *Childs Nerv Syst.* 2010;26:719–722.
52. Bracken MB. Treatment of acute spinal cord injury with methylprednisolone: results of a multicenter randomized clinical trial. *J Neurotrauma.* 1991;8(Suppl 1):47–50.
53. Bracken MB. Pharmacological treatment of acute spinal cord injury: current status and future projects. *J Emerg Med.* 1993;11(Suppl 1):43–48.
54. Bracken MB, Shepard MJ, Collins WF Jr, et al. A randomized controlled trial of methylprednisolone or naloxone in the treatment of acute spinal cord injury: results of the Second National Spinal Cord Injury Study. *N Engl J Med.* 1990;322:1405–1411.
55. Bracken MB, Shepard MJ, Collins WF Jr, et al. Methylprednisolone or naloxone treatment after acute spinal cord injury: 1-year follow-up data. Results of the Second National Acute Spinal Cord Injury Study. *J Neurosurg.* 1992;76:23–31.
56. Bransford RJ, Alton TB, Patel AR, et al. Upper cervical spine trauma. *J Am Acad Orthop Surg.* 2014;22:718–729.
57. Brecknell JE, Malham GM. Os odontoideum: report of three cases. *J Clin Neurosci.* 2008;15:295–301.
58. Bresnan MJ, Abroms IF. Neonatal spinal cord transection secondary to intrauterine hyperextension of neck in breech presentation. *J Pediatr.* 1974;84:734–737.
59. Brockmeyer DL, Apfelbaum RI. A new occipitocervical fusion construct in pediatric patients with occipitocervical instability. Technical note. *J Neurosurg.* 1999;90(Suppl 2):271–275.
60. Brockmeyer DL, Ragel BT, Kestle JR. The pediatric cervical spine instability study. A pilot study assessing the prognostic value of four imaging modalities in clearing the cervical spine for children with severe traumatic injuries. *Childs Nerv Syst.* 2012;28:699–705.
61. Brockmeyer DL, York JE, Apfelbaum RI. Anatomic suitability of C1–C2 transarticular screw placement in pediatric patients. *J Neurosurg.* 2000;92(Suppl 1):7–11.
62. Brooks AL, Jenkins EB. Atlantoaxial arthrodesis by the wedge compression method. *J Bone Joint Surg Am.* 1978;60:279–290.
63. Bucholz RW, Burkhead WZ. The pathological anatomy of fatal atlanto-occipital dislocations. *J Bone Joint Surg Am.* 1979;61:248–250.
64. Bulas DI, Fitz CR, Johnson DL. Traumatic atlanto-occipital dislocation in children. *Radiology.* 1993;188:155–158.
65. Bundschuh CV, Alley JB, Ross M, et al. Magnetic resonance imaging of suspected atlanto-occipital dislocation. *Spine.* 1992;17:245–248.
66. Burke DC. Spinal cord trauma in children. *Paraplegia.* 1971;9:1–14.
67. Burke DC. Traumatic spinal paralysis in children. *Paraplegia.* 1971;9:268–276.
68. Burke SW, French HG, Roberts JM, et al. Chronic atlanto-axial instability in Down syndrome. *J Bone Joint Surg Am.* 1985;67:1356–1360.
69. Burkus JK, Deponte RJ. Chronic atlantoaxial rotatory fixation: correction by cervical traction, manipulation, and branching. *J Pediatr Orthop.* 1986;6:631–635.
70. Caffey J. The whiplash shaken infant syndrome. *Pediatrics.* 1974;54:396–403.
71. Cage JM, Knox JB, Wimberly RL, et al. Complications associated with high-dose corticosteroid administration in children with spinal cord injury. *J Pediatr Orthop.* 2015;35:687–692.
72. Capuano C, Costagliola C, Shamsaldin M, et al. Occipital condyle fractures: a hidden nosological entity. An experience with 10 cases. *Acta Neurochir (Wien).* 2004;146:779–784.
73. Caroli E, Rocchi G, Orlando ER, et al. Occipital condyle fractures: report of five cases and literature review. *Eur Spine J.* 2005;14:487–492.
74. Caruso MC, Daugherty MC, Moody SM, et al. Lessons learned from administration of high-dose methylprednisolone sodium succinate for acute pediatric spinal cord injuries. *J Neurosurg Pediatr.* 2017;20(6):1–8.
75. Cattell HS, Filtzer DL. Pseudosubluxation and other normal variations in the cervical spine in children. *J Bone Joint Surg Am.* 1965;47:1295–1309.
76. Chamoun RB, Relyea KM, Johnson KK, et al. Use of axial and subaxial translaminar screw fixation in the management of upper cervical spinal instability in a series of 7 children. *Neurosurgery.* 2009;64(4):734–739.
77. Chen JY, Soares G, Lambiase R, et al. A previously unrecognized connection between occipital condyle fractures and internal carotid injuries. *Emerg Radiol.* 2006;12(4):192–195.
78. Chern JJ, Chamoun RB, Whitehead WE, et al. Computed tomography morphometric analysis for axial and subaxial translaminar screw placement in the pediatric cervical spine. *J Neurosurg Pediatr.* 2009;3:121–128.
79. Chin K, Abzug JM, Bae DS, et al. Avoiding errors in the management of pediatric polytrauma patients. *Instr Course Lect.* 2016;65:345–352.
80. Chou CW, Huang WC, Shih YH, et al. Occult occipital condyle fracture with normal neurological function and torticollis. *J Clin Neurosci.* 2008;15:920–922.
81. Chu MW, Soleimani T, Evans TA, et al. C-spine injury and mandibular fractures: lifesaver broken in two spots. *J Surg Res.* 2016;206:386–390.
82. Chugh S, Kamian K, Depreitere B, et al. Occipital condyle fracture with associated hypoglossal nerve injury. *Can J Neurol Sci.* 2006;33:322–324.
83. Chung S, Mikrogianakis A, Wales PW, et al. Trauma Association of Canada Pediatric Subcommittee National Pediatric Cervical Spine Evaluation Pathway: consensus guidelines. *J Trauma.* 2011;70:873–884.
84. Collalto PM, DeMuth WW, Schwentker EP, et al. Traumatic atlanto-occipital dislocation. *J Bone Joint Surg Am.* 1986;68:1106–1109.
85. Colo D, Schlosser TP, Oostenbroek HJ, et al. Complete remodeling after conservative treatment of a severely angulated odontoid fracture in a patient with osteogenesis imperfecta: a case report. *Spine (Phila Pa 1976).* 2015;40:E1031–E1034.
86. Connolly B, Turner C, DeVine J, et al. Jefferson fracture resulting in Collet-Sicard syndrome. *Spine (Phila Pa 1976).* 2000;25:395–398.
87. Conry BG, Hall CM. Cervical spine fractures and rear car seat restraints. *Arch Dis Child.* 1987;62:1267–1268.
88. Copley LA, Dormans JP. Cervical spine disorders in infants and children. *J Am Acad Orthop Surg.* 1998;6:204–214.
89. Copley LA, Dormans JP, Pepe MD, et al. Accuracy and reliability of torque wrenches used for halo application in children. *J Bone Joint Surg Am.* 2003;85: 2199–2204.
90. Copley LA, Pepe MD, Tan V, et al. A comparison of various angles of halo pin insertion in an immature skull model. *Spine.* 1999;24:1777–1780.
91. Crostelli M, Mariani M, Mazza O, et al. Cervical fixation in the pediatric patient: our experience. *Eur Spine J.* 2009;18(Suppl 1):20–28.
92. Curran C, Dietrich AM, Bowman MJ, et al. Pediatric cervical-spine immobilization: achieving neutral position? *J Trauma.* 1995;39:729–732.
93. Dai L, Yuan W, Ni B, et al. Os odontoideum: etiology, diagnosis, and management. *Surg Neurol.* 2000;53:106–108.
94. Dashti R, Ulu MO, Albayram S, et al. Concomitant fracture of bilateral occipital condyle and inferior clivus: what is the mechanism of injury? *Eur Spine J.* 2007;16(Suppl 3):261–264.
95. Davidson RG. Atlantoaxial instability in individuals with Down syndrome: a fresh look at the evidence. *Pediatrics.* 1988;81:857–865.
96. Dawson EG, Smith L. Atlanto-axial subluxation in children due to vertebral anomalies. *J Bone Joint Surg Am.* 1979;61:582–587.
97. de Beer JD, Hoffman EB, Kieck CF. Traumatic atlantoaxial subluxation in children. *J Pediatr Orthop.* 1990;10:397–400.
98. De Iure F, Donthineni R, Boriani S. Outcomes of C1 and C2 posterior screw fixation for upper cervical spine fusion. *Eur Spine J.* 2009;18(Suppl 1):2–6.
99. Dettling SD, Morscher MA, Masin JS, et al. Cranial nerve IX and X impairment after a sport-related Jefferson (C1) fracture in a 16-year-old male: a case report. *J Pediatr Orthop.* 2013;33:e23–e27.
100. Deutsch RJ, Badawy MK. Pediatric cervical spine fracture caused by an adult 3-point seatbelt. *Pediatr Emerg Care.* 2008;24:105–108.
101. DiBenedetto T, Lee CK. Traumatic atlanto-occipital instability: a case report with follow-up and a new diagnostic technique. *Spine.* 1990;15:595–597.
102. Dickman CA, Greene KA, Sonntag UK. Injuries involving the transverse atlantal ligament: classification and treatment guidelines based on experience with 39 injuries. *Neurosurgery.* 1996;38:44–50.
103. Dietrich AM, Ginn-Pease ME, Bartkowski HM, et al. Pediatric cervical spine fractures: predominantly subtle presentation. *J Pediatr Surg.* 1991;26:995–1000.
104. Domenicucci M, Mancarella C, Dugoni E, et al. Post-traumatic Collet-Sicard syndrome: personal observation and review of the pertinent literature with clinical, radiological and anatomic considerations. *Eur Spine J.* 2015;24:663–670.
105. Donahue D, Maulbauer MS, Kaufman RA, et al. Childhood survival of atlanto-occipital dislocation: underdiagnosis, recognition, treatment, and review of the literature. *Pediatr Neurosurg.* 1994;21:105–111.
106. Dormans JP, Criscitiello AA, Drummond DS, et al. Complications in children managed with immobilization in a halo vest. *J Bone Joint Surg Am.* 1995;77:1370–1373.
107. Dormans JP, Drummond DS, Sutton LN, et al. Occipitocervical arthrodesis in children. *J Bone Joint Surg Am.* 1995;77:1234–1240.

108. Duhem R, Tonnelle V, Vinchon M, et al. Unstable upper pediatric cervical spine injuries: report of 28 cases and review of the literature. *Childs Nerv Syst.* 2008;24:343–348.
109. Dvorak J, Panjabi M, Gerber M, et al. CT-functional diagnostics of the rotatory instability of the cervical spine. 1. An experimental study on cadavers. *Spine.* 1987;12:197–205.
110. Dyck P. Os odontoideum in children: neurological manifestations and surgical management. *Neurosurgery.* 1978;2:93–99.
111. Easter JS, Barkin R, Rosen CL, et al. Cervical spine injuries in children, part I: mechanism of injury, clinical presentation, and imaging. *J Emerg Med.* 2011;41:142–150.
112. Easter JS, Barkin R, Rosen CL, et al. Cervical spine injuries in children, part II: management and special considerations. *J Emerg Med.* 2011;41(3):252–256.
113. Effendi B, Roy D, Cornish B, et al. Fracture of the rung of the axis. A classification based on the analysis of 131 cases. *J Bone Joint Surg Br.* 1981;63:319–327.
114. Ehlinger M, Charles YP, Adam P, et al. Survivor of a traumatic atlanto-occipital dislocation. *Orthop Traumatol Surg Res.* 2011;97:335–340.
115. Eleraky MA, Theodore N, Adams M, et al. Pediatric cervical spine injuries: report of 102 cases and review of the literature. *J Neurosurg.* 2000;92(Suppl 1):12–17.
116. Elgamal EA, Elwatidy S, Zakaria AM, et al. Spinal cord injury without radiological abnormality (SCIWORA). A diagnosis that is missed in unconscious children. *Neurosciences (Riyadh).* 2008;13:437–440.
117. El-Khoury GY, Kathol MH. Radiographic evaluation of cervical trauma. *Semin Spine Surg.* 1991;3:3–23.
118. Erol FS, Topsakal C, Kaplan M, et al. Collet-Sicard syndrome associated with occipital condyle fracture and epidural hematoma. *Yonsei Med J.* 2007;48:120–123.
119. Evaniew N, Noonan NK, Fallah N, et al. Methylprednisolone for the treatment of patients with acute spinal cord injuries: a propensity score-matched cohort study from a Canadian multi-center spinal cord injury register. *J Neurotrauma.* 2015;32:1674–1683.
120. Evans DL, Bethem D. Cervical spine injuries in children. *J Pediatr Orthop.* 1989;9:563–568.
121. Evarts CM. Traumatic occipito-atlanto dislocation. *J Bone Joint Surg Am.* 1970;52:1653–1660.
122. Fardon DF, Fielding JW. Defects of the pedicle and spondylolisthesis of the second cervical vertebra. *J Bone Joint Surg Br.* 1981;63:526–528.
123. Farley FA, Graziano GP, Hensinger RN. Traumatic atlanto-occipital dislocation in a child. *Spine.* 1992;17:1539–1541.
124. Farley FA, Hensinger RN, Herzenberg JE. Cervical spinal cord injury in children. *J Spinal Disord.* 1992;5:410–416.
125. Fehlings MG, Wilson JR. Methylprednisolone for the treatment of acute spinal cord injury: counterpoint. *Neurosurgery.* 2014;61(Suppl 1):36–42.
126. Ferri-de-Barros F, Little DG, Bridge C, et al. Atlantoaxial and craniocervical arthrodesis in children. A tomographic study comparing suitability of C2 pedicles and C2 laminae for screw fixation. *Spine.* 2010;35(3)291–293.
127. Fielding JW. Cineroentgenography of the normal cervical spine. *J Bone Joint Surg Am.* 1957;39:1280–1288.
128. Fielding JW, Griffin PP. Os odontoideum: an acquired lesion. *J Bone Joint Surg Am.* 1974;56:187–190.
129. Fielding JW, Hawkins RJ. Atlanto-axial rotary fixation (fixed rotary subluxation of the atlanto-axial joint). *J Bone Joint Surg Am.* 1977;59:37–44.
130. Fielding JW, Hensinger RN, Hawkins RJ. Os odontoideum. *J Bone Joint Surg Am.* 1980;62:376–383.
131. Fielding JW, Stillwell WT, Chynn KY, et al. Use of computed tomography for the diagnosis of atlanto-axial rotatory fixation. A case report. *J Bone Joint Surg Am.* 1978;60:1102–1104.
132. Finch GD, Barnes MJ. Major cervical spine injuries in children and adolescents. *J Pediatr Orthop.* 1998;18:811–814.
133. Flynn JM, Closkey RF, Mahboubi S, et al. Role of magnetic resonance imaging in the assessment of pediatric cervical spine injuries. *J Pediatr Orthop.* 2002;22:573–577.
134. Francis WR, Fielding JW, Hawkins RJ, et al. Traumatic spondylolisthesis of the axis. *J Bone Joint Surg Br.* 1981;63:313–318.
135. Fuchs S, Barthel MJ, Flannery AM, et al. Cervical spine fractures sustained by young children in forward-facing car seats. *Pediatrics.* 1989;84:348–354.
136. Fulkerson DH, Hwang SW, Patel AJ, et al. Open reduction and internal fixation for angulated, unstable odontoid synchondrosis fractures in children: a safe alternative to halo fixation? *J Neurosurg Pediatr.* 9:35–41.
137. Gallie WE. Fractures and dislocations of the cervical spine. *Am J Surg.* 1939;46:495–499.
138. Garfin SR, Roux R, Botte MJ, et al. Skull osteology as it affects halo pin placement in children. *J Pediatr Orthop.* 1986;6:434–436.
139. Garrett M, Consiglieri G, Kakarla UK, et al. Occipitoatlantal dislocation. *Neurosurgery.* 2010;66:48–55.
140. Geehr RB, Rothman SLG, Kier EL. The role of computed tomography in the evaluation of upper cervical spine pathology. *Comput Tomogr.* 1978;2:79–97.
141. Geisler FH, Dorsey FC, Coleman WP. Recovery of motor function after spinal cord injury—a randomized, placebo-controlled trial with GM-1 ganglioside. *N Engl J Med.* 1991;324:1829–1838.
142. Geisler FH, Dorsey FC, Coleman WP. Recovery of motor function after spinal cord injury—a randomized, placebo-controlled trial with GM-1 ganglioside [erratum]. *N Engl J Med.* 1991;325:1669–1670.
143. Geisler FH, Dorsey FC, Coleman WP. GM-1 ganglioside in human spinal cord injury. *J Neurotrauma.* 1992;9(Suppl 1):407–416.
144. Geisler FH, Dorsey FC, Coleman WP. Past and current clinical studies with GM-1 ganglioside in acute spinal cord injury. *Rev Ann Emerg Med.* 1993;22:1041–1047.
145. Georgopoulos G, Pizzutillo PD, Lee MS. Occipito-atlanto instability in children. A report of five cases and review of the literature. *J Bone Joint Surg Am.* 1987;69:429–436.
146. Gerling MC, Davis DP, Hamilton RS, et al. Effects of cervical spine immobilization technique and laryngoscope blade selection on an unstable cervical spine in a cadaver model of intubation. *Ann Emerg Med.* 2000;36:279–300.
147. Ghanem I, El Hage S, Rachkidi R, et al. Pediatric cervical spine instability. *J Child Orthop.* 2008;2:71–84.
148. Ghatan S, Ellenbogen RG. Pediatric spine and spinal cord injury after inflicted trauma. *Neurosurg Clin North Am.* 2002;13:227–233.
149. Giannestras NJ, Mayfield FH, Maurer J. Congenital absence of the odontoid process. *J Bone Joint Surg Am.* 1964;46:839–843.
150. Gigante PR, Feldstein NA, Anderson RC. C1-2 instability from os odontoideum mimicking intramedullary spinal cord tumor. *J Neurosurg Pediatr.* 2011;8:363–366.
151. Givens T, Polley KA, Smith GF, et al. Pediatric cervical spine injury: a 3-year experience. *J Trauma.* 1996;41:310–314.
152. Gluf WM, Brockmeyer DL. Atlantoaxial transarticular screw fixation: a review of surgical indications, fusion rate, complications, and lessons learned in 67 pediatric patients. *J Neurosurg Spine.* 2005;2:164–169.
153. Godard J, Hadji M, Raul JS. Odontoid fractures in the child with neurologic injury. Direct osteosynthesis with a cortico-spongious screw and literature review. *Childs Nerv Syst.* 1997;13:105–107.
154. Goldstein RY, Sunde CD, Assaad P, et al. Location of the vertebral artery at C1 in children: how far out laterally can one safely dissect? *J Bone Joint Surg Am.* 2014;96(18):1552–1556.
155. Grantham SA, Dick HM, Thompson RC, et al. Occipitocervical arthrodesis: indications, technique, and results. *Clin Orthop Relat Res.* 1969;65:118–129.
156. Griffiths SC. Fracture of the odontoid process in children. *J Pediatr Surg.* 1972;7:680–683.
157. Gupta R, Bathen ME, Smith JS, et al. Advances in the management of spinal cord injury. *J Am Acad Orthop Surg.* 2010;18(4):210–222.
158. Gupta R, Narayan S. Sublaminar wiring for odontoid synchondrotic fracture stabilization in a 4-year-old: a case report. *Childs Nerv Syst.* 2015;31:2185–2187.
159. Hadley MN. Occipital condyle fractures. *Neurosurgery.* 2002;50:S114–S119.
160. Hadley MN, Zabramski JM, Browner CM, et al. Pediatric spinal trauma: review of 122 cases of spinal cord vertebral column injuries. *J Neurosurg.* 1988;68:18–24.
161. Haffner DL, Hoffer MM, Wiedebusch R. Etiology of children's spinal injuries at Rancho Los Amigos. *Spine.* 1993;18:679–684.
162. Hall JE, Denis F, Murray J. Exposure of the upper cervical spine for spinal decompression by a mandible and tongue-splitting approach. Case report. *J Bone Joint Surg Am.* 1977;59:121–125.
163. Hall JE, Simmons ED, Danylchuk K, et al. Instability of the cervical spine and neurological involvement in Klippel-Feil syndrome: a case report. *J Bone Joint Surg Am.* 1990;72:460–462.
164. Halsey JN, Hoppe IC, Marano AA, et al. Characteristics of cervical spine injury in pediatric patients with facial fractures. *J Craniofac Surg.* 2016;27:109–111.
165. Hamilton MG, Myles ST. Pediatric spinal injury: review of 61 deaths. *J Neurosurg.* 1988;77:705–708.
166. Hammerschlag W, Ziv I, Wald U, et al. Cervical instability in an achondroplastic infant. *J Pediatr Orthop.* 1988;8:481–484.
167. Hamoud K, Abbas J. A new technique for stabilization of injuries at C2–C3 in young children. *Injury.* 2014;45:1791–1795.
168. Hanson JA, Deliganis AV, Baxter AB, et al. Radiologic and clinical spectrum of occipital condyle fractures: retrospective review of 107 consecutive fractures in 95 patients. *AJR Am J Roentgenol.* 2002;178:1261–1268.
169. Haque A, Price AV, Sklar FH, et al. Screw fixation of the upper cervical spine in the pediatric population. *J Neurosurg Pediatr.* 2009;3:529–533.
170. Harmanli O, Kaufman Y. Traumatic atlanto-occipital dislocation with survival. *Surg Neurol.* 1993;39:324–330.
171. Harms J, Melcher RP. Posterior C1–C2 fusion with polyaxial screw and rod fixation. *Spine.* 2001;26:2467–2471.
172. Harris JH Jr, Carson GC, Wagner LK, et al. Radiologic diagnosis of traumatic occipitovertebral dissociation: 2. Comparison of three methods of detecting occipitovertebral relationships on lateral radiographs of supine subjects. *AJR Am J Roentgenol.* 1994;162:887–892.
173. Harris MB, Duval MJ, Davis JA Jr, et al. Anatomical and roentgenographic features of atlantooccipital instability. *J Spinal Disord.* 1993;6:5–10.
174. Hashimoto T, Watanabe O, Takase M, et al. Collet-Sicard syndrome after minor head trauma. *Neurosurgery.* 1988;23:367–370.
175. Hawkins RJ, Fielding JW, Thompson WJ. Os odontoideum: congenital or acquired. *J Bone Joint Surg Am.* 1976;58:413.
176. Hedequist DJ, Emans JB. The correlation of preoperative three-dimensional computed tomography reconstructions with operative findings in congenital scoliosis. *Spine.* 2003;28:2531–2534.
177. Hedequist D, Hresko T, Proctor M. Modern cervical spine instrumentation in children. *Spine.* 2008;33:379–383.
178. Heller JG, Jeffords P. Internal fixation of the cervical spine. C. Posterior instrumentation of the lower cervical spine. In: Frymoyer JW, Wiesel SW, eds. *The Adult and Pediatric Spine.* Philadelphia, PA: Lippincott Williams & Wilkins; 2004:803–816.
179. Henriques T, Cunningham BW, Olerud C, et al. Biomechanical comparison of five different atlantoaxial posterior fixation techniques. *Spine.* 2000;25:2877–2883.
180. Henry M, Riesenburger RI, Kryzanski J, et al. A retrospective comparison of CT and MRI in detecting pediatric cervical spine injury. *Childs Nerv Syst.* 2013;29:1333–1338.
181. Hensinger RN, Fielding JW, Hawkins RJ. Congenital anomalies of the odontoid process. *Orthop Clin North Am.* 1978;9:901–912.
182. Hensinger RN, Lang JE, MacEwen GD. Klippel-Feil syndrome: a constellation of associated anomalies. *J Bone Joint Surg Am.* 1974;56:1246–1252.
183. Herzenberg JE, Hensinger RN. Pediatric cervical spine injuries. *Trauma Q.* 1989;5:73–81.

184. Herzenberg JE, Hensinger RN, Dedrick DK, et al. Emergency transport and positioning of young children who have an injury of the cervical spine: the standard backboard may be hazardous. *J Bone Joint Surg Am*. 1989;71:15–22.
185. Hofbauer M, Jaindi M, Höchtl LL, et al. Spine injuries in polytraumatized pediatric patients: characteristics and experience from a Level I trauma center over two decades. *J Trauma Acute Care Surg*. 2012;73:156–161.
186. Hohl M, Baker HR. The atlanto-axial joint: Roentgenographic and anatomical study of normal and abnormal motion. *J Bone Joint Surg Am*. 1964;46:1739–1752.
187. Hosalkar HS, Greenbaum JN, Flynn JM, et al. Fractures of the odontoid in children with an open basilar synchondrosis. *J Bone Joint Surg Br*. 2009;91:789–796.
188. Hosono N, Yonenobu K, Kawagoe K, et al. Traumatic anterior atlanto-occipital dislocation. *Spine*. 1993;18:786–790.
189. Howard AW, Letts RM. Cervical spondylolysis in children: is it posttraumatic? *J Pediatr Orthop*. 2000;20:677–681.
190. Hoy GA, Cole WG. The paediatric cervical seat belt syndrome. *Injury*. 1993;24:297–299.
191. Hu Y, Dong WX, Kepler CK, et al. A novel anterior odontoid screw plate for C1–C3 internal fixation: an in vitro biomechanical study. *Spine (Phila Pa 1976)*. 2016;41:E64–E72.
192. Hubbard DD. Injuries of the spine in children and adolescents. *Clin Orthop Relat Res*. 1974;100:56–65.
193. Huber H, Ramseier LE, Boos N. Open mouth digital reduction of an odontoid synchondrosis fracture: a case report. *J Pediatr Orthop*. 2010;30:115–118.
194. Huerta C, Griffith R, Joyce SM. Cervical spine stabilization in pediatric patients. Evaluation of current techniques. *Ann Emerg Med*. 1987;16:1121–1126.
195. Hukda S, Ota H, Okabe N, et al. Traumatic atlantoaxial dislocation causing os odontoideum in infants. *Spine*. 1980;5:207–210.
196. Hussain K, Abdo MM, AlNajjar FJ, et al. Not your typical torticollis: a case of atlantoaxial rotatory subluxation. *BMJ Case Rep*. 2014.
197. Ishii K, Chiba K, Maruiwa H, et al. Pathognomonic radiological signs for predicting prognosis in patients with chronic atlantoaxial rotatory fixation. *J Neurosurg Spine*. 2006;5:385–391.
198. Ishikawa M, Matsumoto M, Chiba K, et al. Long-term impact of atlantoaxial arthrodesis on the pediatric cervical spine. *J Orthop Sci*. 2009;14:274–278.
199. Jain A, Brooks JT, Rao SS, et al. Cervical fractures with associated spinal cord injury in children and adolescents: epidemiology, costs, and in-hospital mortality rates in 4418 patients. *J Child Orthop*. 2015;9:171–175.
200. Jea A, Johnson KK, Whitehead WE, et al. Translaminar screw fixation in the subaxial pediatric cervical spine. *J Neurosurg Pediatr*. 2008;2:386–390.
201. Jefferson G. Fracture of the atlas vertebra: report of four cases and a review of those previously recorded. *Br J Surg*. 1920;7:407–422.
202. Joaquim AF, Ghizoni E, Tedeschi H, et al. Upper cervical injuries—a rational approach to guide surgical management. *J Spinal Cord Med*. 2014;37:139–151.
203. Jones TM, Anderson PA, Noonan KJ. Pediatric cervical spine trauma. *J Am Acad Orthop Surg*. 2011;19:600–611.
204. Jones ET, Hensinger RN. Cervical spine injuries in children. *Contemp Orthop*. 1982;5:17–23.
205. Judd DB, Liem LK, Petermann G. Pediatric atlas fracture: a case of fracture through a synchondrosis and review of the literature. *Neurosurgery*. 2000;46:991–995.
206. Junewick JJ. Pediatric craniocervical junction injuries. *Am J Radiol*. 2011;196:1003–1010.
207. Kaiser R, Mehdian H. Permanent twelfth nerve palsy secondary to C0 and C1 fracture in patient with craniocervical pneumatisation. *Eur Spine J*. 2014.
208. Kapapa T, Tschan CA, König K, et al. Fracture of the occipital condyle caused by minor trauma in a child. *J Pediatr Surg*. 2006;41:1774–1776.
209. Karam YR, Traynelis VC. Occipital condyle fractures. *Neurosurgery*. 2010;66(3 Suppl):56–59.
210. Karol LA, Sheffield EG, Crawford K, et al. Reproducibility in the measurement of atlanto-occipital instability in children with Down's syndrome. *Spine*. 1996;21:2463–2468.
211. Kaufman RA, Carroll CD, Buncher CR. Atlanto-occipital junction: standards for measurement in normal children. *AJNR Am J Neuroradiol*. 1987;8:995–999.
212. Kawabe N, Hirotoni H, Tanaka O. Pathomechanism of atlanto-axial rotatory fixation in children. *J Pediatr Orthop*. 1989;9:569–574.
213. Keenan HT, Hollingshead MC, Chung CJ, et al. Using CT of the cervical spine for early evaluation of pediatric patients with head trauma. *AJR Am J Roentgenol*. 2001;177:1405–1409.
214. Kenter K, Worley G, Griffin T, et al. Pediatric traumatic atlanto-occipital dislocation: five cases and a review. *J Pediatr Orthop*. 2001;21:585–589.
215. Kewalramani LS, Kraus JF, Sterling HM. Acute spinal-cord lesions in a pediatric population: epidemiological and clinical features. *Paraplegia*. 1980;18:206–219.
216. Kilfoyle RM, Foley JJ, Norton PL. Spine and pelvic deformity in childhood and adolescent paraplegia. *J Bone Joint Surg Am*. 1965;47:659–682.
217. Kim W, O'Malley M, Kieser DC. Noninvasive management of an odontoid process fracture in a toddler: case report. *Global Spine J*. 2015;5:59–62.
218. Kinkpé CV, Dansokho AV, Coulibaly NF, et al. Fracture of the odontoid process in children: a case report. *Orthop Traumatol Surg Res*. 2009;95:234–236.
219. Kleinman PK, Shelton YA. Hangman's fracture in an abused infant: imaging. *Pediatr Radiol*. 1997;27:776–777.
220. Klimo P Jr, Astur N, Gabrick K, et al. Occipitocervical fusion using a contoured rod and wire construct in children: a reappraisal of a vintage technique. *J Neurosurg Pediatr*. 2013;11:160–169.
221. Klimo P Jr, Coon V, Brockmeyer D. Incidental os odontoideum: current management strategies. *Neurosurg Focus*. 2011;31:E10.
222. Kline DG. Atlanto-axial dislocation simulating a head injury: hypoplasia of the odontoid. Case report. *J Neurosurg*. 1996;24:1013–1016.
223. Klippel M, Feil A. Anomalies de la collone vertebrale par absence des vertebres cervicales; avec cage thoraque remontant jusqu'ala bas du crane. *Bull Soc Anat Paris*. 1912;87:185.
224. Knox JB, Schneider JE, Cage JM, et al. Spine trauma in very young children: a retrospective study of 206 patients presenting to a level 1 pediatric trauma center. *J Pediatr Orthop*. 2014;34:698–702.
225. Kobets AJ, Nakhla J, Biswas A, et al. Isolated synchondrosis fracture of the atlas presenting as rotatory fixation of the neck: case report and review of the literature. *Surg Neurol Int*. 2016;7(Suppl 42):S1092–S1095.
226. Kobori M, Takahashi H, Mikawa Y. Atlanto-axial dislocation in Down syndrome: report of two cases requiring surgical correction. *Spine*. 1986;11:195–200.
227. Kokoska ER, Keller MS, Rallo MC, et al. Characteristics of pediatric cervical spine injuries. *J Pediatr Surg*. 2001;36:100–105.
228. Koop SE, Winter RB, Lonstein JE. The surgical treatment of instability of the upper part of the cervical spine in children and adolescents. *J Bone Joint Surg Am*. 1984;66:403–411.
229. Kopelman TR, Berardoni NE, O'Neill PJ, et al. Risk factors for blunt cerebrovascular injury in children: do they mimic those seen in adults? *J Trauma*. 2011;71:559–564.
230. Korinth MC, Kapser A, Weinzierl MR. Jefferson fracture in a child—illustrative case report. *Pediatr Neurosurg*. 2007;43:526–530.
231. Kown HC, Cho DK, Jang YY, et al. Collet-Sicard syndrome in a patient with Jefferson fracture. *Ann Rehabil Med*. 2011;35:934–938.
232. Kransdorf MJ, Wherle PA, Moser RP Jr. Atlantoaxial subluxation in Reiter syndrome. *Spine*. 1988;13:12–14.
233. Krüger A, Oberkircher L, Frangen T, et al. Fractures of the occipital condyle clinical spectrum and course in eight patients. *J Craniovertebr Junction Spine*. 2013;4:49–55.
234. Kuhns LR, Loder RT, Farley FA, et al. Nuchal cord changes in children with os odontoideum: evidence for associated trauma. *J Pediatr Orthop*. 1998;18:815–819.
235. Kuhns LR, Strouse PJ. Cervical spine standards for flexion radiograph interspinous distance ratios in children. *Acta Radiol*. 2000;7:615–619.
236. Kuniyoshi Y, Kamura A, Yasuda S, et al. Laryngeal injury and pneummediastinum due to minor blunt neck trauma: case report. *J Emerg Med*. 2017;52:e145–e148.
237. Labbe JL, Peres O, Leclair O, et al. Posterior C1–C2 fixation using absorbable suture for type II odontoid fracture in 2-year-old child: description of a new technique and literature review. *J Pediatr Orthop*. 2016;36:e96–e100.
238. Lally KP, Senac M, Hardin WD Jr, et al. Utility of the cervical spine radiograph in pediatric trauma. *Am J Surg*. 1989;158:540–542.
239. Launay F, Leet AI, Sponseller PD. Pediatric spinal cord injury without radiographic abnormality: a metaanalysis. *Clin Orthop Relat Res*. 2005; (433):166–170.
240. Lawson JP, Ogden JA, Bucholz RW, et al. Physeal injuries of the cervical spine. *J Pediatr Orthop*. 1987;7:428–435.
241. Lebwohl NH, Eismont FJ. Cervical spine injuries in children. In: Weinstein SL, ed. *The Pediatric Spine: Principles and Practice*. Philadelphia, PA: Lippincott Williams & Wilkins; 2001:553–566.
242. Lennarson PJ, Smith D, Todd MM, et al. Segmental cervical spine motion during orotracheal intubation of the intact and injured spine with and without external stabilization. *J Neurosurg*. 2000;92:201–206.
243. Leonard JC, Kuppermann N, Olsen C, et al. Factors associated with cervical spine injury in children after blunt trauma. *Ann Emerg Med*. 2011;58:145–155.
244. Leonard JR, Wright NM. Pediatric atlantoaxial fixation with bilateral, crossing C2 translaminar screws. Technical note. *J Neurosurg Pediatr*. 2006;104:59–63.
245. Letts M, Kaylor D, Gouw G. A biomechanical study of halo fixation in children. *J Bone Joint Surg Br*. 1987;70:277–279.
246. Levine AM, Edwards CC. The management of traumatic spondylolisthesis of the axis. *J Bone Joint Surg Am*. 1985;67:217–222.
247. Lewis SJ, Canavese F, Keetbaas S. Intralaminar screw insertion of thoracic spine in children with severe spinal deformities: two case reports. *Spine (Phila Pa 1976)*. 2009;E251–E254.
248. Link TM, Schuierer G, Hufenbiek A, et al. Substantial head trauma: value of routine CT examination of the cervicocranium. *Radiology*. 1995;196:741–745.
249. Liu JK, Decker D, Tenner MS, et al. Traumatic arteriovenous fistula of the posterior inferior cerebellar artery treated with endovascular coil embolization: case report. *Surg Neurol*. 2004;61(3):255–261.
250. Loder RT, Schultz W, Sabatino M. Fractures from trampolines: results from a national database, 2002 to 2011. *J Pediatr Orthop*. 2014;34:683–690.
251. Lui TN, Lee ST, Wong CW, et al. C1–C2 fracture-dislocations in children and adolescents. *J Trauma*. 1996;40:408–411.
252. Lynch JM, Meza MP, Pollack IF, et al. Direct injury to the cervical spine of a child by a lap-shoulder belt resulting in quadriplegia: case report. *J Trauma*. 1996;41:747–749.
253. Mackenzie WG, Dhawale AA, Demczko MM, et al. Flexion-extension cervical spine MRI in children with skeletal dysplasia: is it safe and effective? *J Pediatr Orthop*. 2013;33:91–98.
254. Maddox JJ, Rodriguez-Feo JA 3rd, Maddox GE, et al. Nonoperative treatment of occipital condyle fractures: an outcomes review of 32 fractures. *Spine (Phila Pa 1976)*. 2012;37:E964–E968.
255. Maekawa K, Masaki T, Kokubun Y. Fetal spinal cord injury secondary to hyperextension of the neck: no effect of caesarean section. *Dev Med Child Neurol*. 1976;18:228–232.
256. Magerl F, Seeman P. Stable posterior fusion of the atlas and axis by transarticular screw fixation. In: Kehr P, Weidner A, eds. *Cervical Spine*. Vienna: Springer-Verlag; 1985:322–327.
257. Maheshwaran S, Sgouros S, Jeyapalan K, et al. Imaging of childhood torticollis due to atlanto-axial rotatory fixation. *Childs Nerv Syst*. 1995;11:667–671.
258. Majernick TG, Bieniek R, Houston JB, et al. Cervical spine movement during orotracheal intubation. *Ann Emerg Med*. 1986;15:417–420.
259. Malham GM, Ackland HM, Jones R, et al. Occipital condyle fractures: incidence and clinical follow-up at a level 1 trauma centre. *Emerg Radiol*. 2009;16:291–297.
260. Mannix R, Nigrovic LE, Schutzman SA, et al. Factors associated with the use of cervical spine computed tomography imaging in pediatric trauma patients. *Acad Emerg Med*. 2011;18:906–911.

261. Manson NA, An HS. Halo placement in the pediatric and adult patient. In: Vaccaro AR, Barton EM, eds *Operative Techniques in Spine Surgery*. Philadelphia, PA: Saunders; 2008:13.
262. Marlin AE, Gayle RW, Lee JF. Jefferson fractures in children. *J Neurosurg*. 1983; 58:277–279.
263. Martinez-Del-Campo E, Turner JD, Rangel-Castilla L, et al. Pediatric occipitocervical fixation: radiographic criteria, surgical technique, and clinical outcomes based on experience of a single surgeon. *J Neurosurg Pediatr*. 2016;18:452–462.
264. Maserati MB, Stephens B, Zohny Z, et al. Occipital condyle fractures: clinical decision rule and surgical management. *J Neurosurg Spine*. 2009;11:388–395.
265. Mathews MS, Owen CM, Hasso AN, et al. Traumatic retropharyngeal pseudomeningocele with atlanto-occipital dislocation in a neurologically intact patient. *Neuroradiol J*. 2007;20:694–698.
266. Matthews LS, Vetter LW, Tolo VT. Cervical anomaly stimulating Hangman's fracture in a child. *J Bone Joint Surg Am*. 1982;64:299–300.
267. Maxwell MJ, Jardine AD. Paediatric cervical spine injury but NEXUS negative. *Emerg Med J*. 2007;24:676.
268. Mayfield JK, Erkkila JC, Winter RB. Spine deformities subsequent to acquired childhood spinal cord injury. *Orthop Trans*. 1979;3:281–282.
269. Mazur JM, Loveless EA, Cummings RJ. Combined odontoid and Jefferson fracture in a child: a case report. *Spine*. 2002;27:E197–E199.
270. McClain RF, Clark CR, El-Khoury GY. C6–C7 dislocation in a neurologically intact neonate: a case report. *Spine*. 1989;14:125–126.
271. McGrory BJ, Klassen RA, Chao EY, et al. Acute fracture and dislocations of the cervical spine in children and adolescents. *J Bone Joint Surg Am*. 1993;75:988–995.
272. McGuire KJ, Silber J, Flynn JM, et al. Torticollis in children: can dynamic computed tomography help determine severity and treatment? *J Pediatr Orthop*. 2002;22: 766–770.
273. McKay SD, Al-Omari A, Tomlinson LA, et al. Review of cervical spine anomalies in genetic syndromes. *Spine (Phila Pa 1976)*. 2012;37:E269–E277.
274. McNamara C, Mironova I, Lehman E, et al. Predictors of intrathoracic injury after blunt torso trauma in children presenting to an emergency department as trauma activations. *J Emerg Med*. 2017;52:793–800.
275. Menezes AH. Surgical approaches to the craniocervical junction. In: Weinstein SL, ed. *Pediatric Spine Surgery*. 2nd ed. Philadelphia, PA: Lippincott Williams & Wilkins; 2001:127–148.
276. Menezes AH. Craniocervical developmental anatomy and its implications. *Childs Nerv Syst*. 2008;24:1109–1122.
277. Menezes AH, Ryken JC. Craniovertebral junction abnormalities. In: Weinsten SL, ed. *The Pediatric Spine: Principles and Practice*. 2nd ed. Philadelphia, PA: Lippincott Williams & Wilkins; 2001:219–238.
278. Mesfin A, Nesterenko SO, Al-Hourani KG, et al. Management of Hangman's fractures and a subaxial compression fracture in two children with osteogenesis imperfecta. *J Surg Orthop Adv*. 2013;22:326–329.
279. Mikawa Y, Watanabe R, Yamano Y, et al. Fractures through a synchondrosis of the anterior arch of the atlas. *J Bone Joint Surg Br*. 1987;69:483.
280. Millington PJ, Ellingsen JM, Hauswirth BE, et al. Thermoplastic Minerva body jacket–a practical alternative to current methods of cervical spine stabilization. *Phys Ther*. 1987;67:223–225.
281. Miz GS, Engler GL. Atlanto-axial subluxation in Larsen's syndrome: a case report. *Spine*. 1987;12:411–412.
282. Momjian S, Dehdashti AR, Kehrli P, et al. Occipital condyle fractures in children: case report and review of the literature. *Pediatr Neurosurg*. 2003;38:265–270.
283. Mönckeberg JE, Tomé CV, Matias A, et al. CT scan study of atlantoaxial rotatory mobility in asymptomatic adult subjects: a basis for better understanding C1–C2 rotatory fixation and subluxation. *Spine (Phila Pa 1976)*. 2009;34:1292–1295.
284. Mondschein J, Karasick D. Spondylolysis of the axis vertebra: a rare anomaly simulating Hangman's fracture. *AJR Am J Roentgenol*. 1999;172:556–557.
285. Montalbano M, Fisahn C, Loukas M, et al. Pediatric Hangman's fracture: a comprehensive review. *Pediatr Neurosurg*. 2017;52:145–150.
286. Mortazavi MM, Dogan S, Civelek R, et al. Pediatric multilevel spine injuries: an institutional experience. *Childs Nerv Syst*. 2011;27:1095–1100.
287. Mortazavi M, Gore PA, Chang S, et al. Pediatric cervical spine injuries: a comprehensive review. *Childs Nerv Syst*. 2011;27:705–717.
288. Msall ME, Reese ME, DiGaudio K, et al. Symptomatic atlantoaxial instability associated with medial and rehabilitative procedures in children with Down syndrome. *Pediatrics*. 1990;85:447–449.
289. Mubarak SJ, Camp JF, Vuletich W, et al. Halo application in the infant. *J Pediatr Orthop*. 1989;9:612–614.
290. Mueller FJ, Fuechtmeier B, Kinner B, et al. Occipital condyle fractures. Prospective follow-up of 31 cases within 5 years at a level 1 trauma centre. *Eur Spine J*. 2012;21:289–294.
291. Mueller OM, Gasser T, Hellwig A, et al. Instable cervical spine injury in a toddler: technical note. *Childs Nerv Syst*. 2010;26:1625–1631.
292. Müller EJ, Wick M, Muhr G. Traumatic spondylolisthesis of the axis: treatment rationale based on the stability of the different fracture types. *Eur Spine J*. 2000;9:123–128.
293. Murphy MJ, Southwick WO. Posterior approaches and fusions. In: *Cervical Spine Research Society. The Cervical Spine*. Philadelphia, PA: JB Lippincott; 1983:506–507.
294. Nannapaneni R, Nath FP, Papastefanou SL. Fracture of the clavicle associated with a rotatory atlantoaxial subluxation. *Injury*. 2001;32:71–73.
295. Nigrovic LE, Rogers AJ, Adelgais KM, et al. Utility of plain radiographs in detecting traumatic injuries of the cervical spine in children. *Pediatr Emerg Care*. 2012;28:426–432.
296. Nitecki S, Moir CR. Predictive factors of the outcome of traumatic cervical spine fracture in children. *J Pediatr Surg*. 1994;29:1409–1411.
297. Noble ER, Smoker WRK. The forgotten condyle: the appearance, morphology, and classification of occipital condyle fractures. *AJNR Am J Neuroradiol*. 1996;17: 507–513.
298. Nordström RE, Lahrendanta TV, Kaitila II, et al. Familial spondylolisthesis of the axis is vertebra. *J Bone Joint Surg Br*. 1986;68:704–706.
299. Norman MG, Wedderburn LC. Fetal spinal cord injury with cephalic delivery. *Obstet Gynecol*. 1973;42:355–358.
300. Nuckley DJ, Van Nausdle JA, Eck MP, et al. Neural space and biomechanical integrity of the developing cervical spine in compression. *Spine*. 2007;32:E181–E187.
301. Nypaver M, Treloar D. Neutral cervical spine positioning in children. *Ann Emerg Med*. 1994;23:208–211.
302. O'Brien WT Sr, Shen P, Lee P. The dens: normal development, developmental variants and anomalies, and traumatic injuries. *J Clin Imaging Sci*. 2015;5:38.
303. Odent T, Langlais J, Glorion C, et al. Fractures of the odontoid process: a report of 15 cases in children younger than 6 years. *J Pediatr Orthop*. 1999;19:51–54.
304. Oluigbo CO, Gan YC, Sgouros S, et al. Pattern, management and outcome of cervical spine injuries associated with head injuries in paediatric patients. *Childs Nerv Syst*. 2008;24:87–92.
305. Orenstein JB, Klein BL, Gotschall CS, et al. Age and outcome in pediatric cervical spine injury: 11-year experience. *Pediatr Emerg Care*. 1994;10:132–137.
306. Orenstein JB, Klein BL, Oschensclager DW. Delayed diagnosis of pediatric cervical spine injury. *Pediatrics*. 1992;89:1185–1188.
307. Panczykowski D, Nemecek AN, Selden NR. Traumatic type III odontoid fracture and severe rotatory atlantoaxial subluxation in a 3-year-old child: case report. *J Neurosurg Pediatr*. 2010;5:200–203.
308. Pang D. Atlantoaxial rotatory fixation. *Neurosurgery*. 2010;66(3):A161–A183.
309. Pang D, Nemzek WR, Zovickian J. Atlanto-occipital dislocation—part 2: the clinical use of (occipital) condyle-C1 interval, comparison with other diagnostic methods, and the manifestation, management, and outcome of atlanto-occipital dislocation in children. *Neurosurgery*. 2007;61:995–1015.
310. Pang D, Pollack IF. Spinal cord injury without radiologic abnormality in children: the SCIWORA syndrome. *J Trauma*. 1989;29:654–664.
311. Pang D, Wilberger JE. Spinal cord injury without radiologic abnormalities in children. *J Neurosurg*. 1982;57:114–129.
312. Panjabi MM, White AA III, Johnson RM. Cervical spine mechanics as a function of transection of components. *J Biomech*. 1975;8(5):327–336.
313. Panjabi MM, White AA III, Keller D, et al. Stability of the cervical spine under tension. *J Biomech*. 1978;11:189–197.
314. Papadopoulos SM, Dickman CA, Sonntag VK, et al. Traumatic atlanto-occipital dislocation with survival. *Neurosurgery*. 1991;28:574–579.
315. Parbhoo AH, Govender S, Corr P. Vertebral artery injury in cervical spine trauma. *Injury*. 2001;32:565–568.
316. Parent S, Dimar J, Dekutoski M, et al. Unique features of pediatric spinal cord injury. *Spine*. 2010;35(Suppl 21):S202–S208.
317. Parent S, Mac-Thiong JM, Roy-Beaudry M, et al. Spinal cord injury in the pediatric population: a systematic review of the literature. *J Neurotrauma*. 2011;28: 1515–1524.
318. Parisi M, Lieberson R, Shatsky S. Hangman's fracture or primary spondylolysis: a patient and a brief review. *Pediatr Radiol*. 1991;21:367–368.
319. Parke WW, Rothman RH, Brown MD. The pharyngovertebral veins: an anatomical rationale for Grisel syndrome. *J Bone Joint Surg Am*. 1984;66:568–574.
320. Passi Y, Sumathi P, Thota S. Occipital condyle fracture. *Anesthesiology*. 2016; 125:806.
321. Patel JC, Dailey A, Brodke DS, et al. Subaxial cervical spine trauma classification: the Subaxial Injury Classification system and case examples. *Neurosurg Focus*. 2008;25:E8.
322. Patel JC, Tepas JJ 3rd, Mollitt DL, et al. Pediatric cervical spine injuries: defining the disease. *J Pediatr Surg*. 2001;36:373–376.
323. Pennecot GF, Gourard D, Hardy JR, et al. Roentgenographical study of the stability of the cervical spine in children. *J Pediatr Orthop*. 1984;4:346–352.
324. Pettiford JN, Bikhchandani J, Ostlie DJ, et al. A review: the role of high dose methylprednisolone in spinal cord trauma in children. *Pediatr Surg Int*. 2012;28: 298–294.
325. Phillips WA, Hensinger RN. The management of rotatory atlantoaxial subluxation in children. *J Bone Joint Surg Am*. 1989;71:664–668.
326. Pilge H, Holzapfel BM, Lampe R, et al. A novel technique to treat Grisel's syndrome: results of a simplified, therapeutical algorithm. *Int Orthop*. 2013;37:1307–1313.
327. Pizzutillo PD, Herman MJ. Cervical spine issues in Down syndrome. *J Pediatr Orthop*. 2005;25:253–259.
328. Pizzutillo PD, Rocha EF, D'Astous J, et al. Bilateral fractures of the pedicle of the second cervical vertebra in the young child. *J Bone Joint Surg Am*. 1986;68: 892–896.
329. Plant JG, Ruff SJ. Migration of rod through skull, into brain following C1–C2 instrumental fusion for os odontoideum: a case report. *Spine (Phila Pa 1976)*. 2010;35:E90–E92.
330. Powell EC, Leonard JR, Olsen CS, et al. Atlantoaxial rotatory subluxation in children. *Pediatr Emerg Care*. 2017;33:86–91.
331. Powers B, Miller MD, Kramer RS, et al. Traumatic anterior occipital dislocation. *Neurosurgery*. 1979;4:12–17.
332. Price E. Fractured odontoid process with anterior dislocation. *J Bone Joint Surg Br*. 1960;42:410–413.
333. Pueschel SM. Atlantoaxial subluxation in Down syndrome. *Lancet*. 1983;1:980.
334. Pueschel SM, Scolia FH. Atlantoaxial instability in individuals with Down syndrome: epidemiologic, radiographic, and clinical studies. *Pediatrics*. 1987;4:555–560.
335. Rachesky I, Boyce WT, Duncan B, et al. Clinical prediction of cervical spine injuries in children: radiographic abnormalities. *Am J Dis Child*. 1987;141:199–201.
336. Ralston ME, Chung K, Barnes PD, et al. Role of flexion-extension radiographs in blunt pediatric cervical spine injury. *Acad Emerg Med*. 2001;8:237–245.
337. Ranjith RK, Mullett JH, Burke TE. Hangman's fracture cause by suspected child abuse. a case report. *J Pediatr Orthop B*. 2002;11:329–332.
338. Reilly CW, Leung F. Synchondrosis fracture in a pediatric patient. *Can J Surg*. 2005; 48:158.

339. Reinges MH, Mayfrank L, Rohde V, et al. Surgically treated traumatic synchondrotic disruption of the odontoid process in a 15-month-old girl. *Childs Nerv Syst.* 1998;14:85–87.

340. Riascos R, Bonfante E, Cotes C, et al. Imaging of atlanto-occipital and atlantoaxial traumatic injuries: what the radiologist needs to know. *Radiographics.* 2015; 35:2121–2134.

341. Ricciardi JE, Kaufer H, Louis DS. Acquired os odontoideum following acute ligament injury. *J Bone Joint Surg Am.* 1976;58:410–412.

342. Richards PG. Stable fractures of the atlas and axis in children. *J Neurol Neurosurg Psychiatry.* 1984;47:781–783.

343. Riebel M, Westrick R, Goss D. Unstable os odontoideum. *J Orthop Sports Phys Ther.* 2016;46:930.

344. Ries MD, Ray S. Posterior displacement of an odontoid fracture in a child. *Spine.* 1986;11:1043–1044.

345. Ringel F, Reinke A, Stüer C, et al. Posterior C1-2 fusion with C1 lateral mass and C2 isthmic screws: accuracy of screw position, alignment and patient outcome. *Acta Neurochir.* 2012;154:305–312.

346. Roche CJ, O'Malley M, Dorgan JC, et al. A pictorial review of atlantoaxial rotatory fixation: key points for the radiology. *Clin Radiol.* 2001;56:947–958.

347. Rodgers WB, Coran DL, Emans JB, et al. Occipitocervical fusions in children. Retrospective analysis and technical considerations. *Clin Orthop Relat Res.* 1999;364:125–133.

348. Roy-Camille R, Saillant G, Mazel C. Internal fixation of the unstable cervical spine by posterior osteosynthesis with plates and screws. In: Sherk HH, ed. *The Cervical Spine.* 2nd ed. Philadelphia, PA: JB Lippincott; 1989:390–412.

349. Ruff SJ, Taylor TKF. Hangman's fracture in an infant. *J Bone Joint Surg Br.* 1986;68:702–703.

350. Ruge JR, Sinson GP, McLone DG, et al. Pediatric spinal injury: the very young. *J Neurosurg.* 1988;69:25–30.

351. Rush JK, Kelly DM, Astur N, et al. Associated injuries in children and adolescents with spinal trauma. *J Pediatr Orthop.* 2013;33:393–397.

352. Rusin JA, Ruess L, Daulton RS. New C2 synchondrosal fracture classification system. *Pediatr Radiol.* 2015;45:872–881.

353. Samartzis D, Shen FH, Herman J, et al. Atlantoaxial rotatory fixation in the setting of associated congenital malformations: a modified classification system. *Spine (Phila Pa 1976).* 2010;35:E119–E127.

354. Sanborn MR, Diluna ML, Whitmore RG, et al. Fluoroscopically guided, transoral, closed reduction, and halo vest immobilization for an atypical C-1 fracture. *J Neurosurg Pediatr.* 2011;7:380–382.

355. Sankar WN, Wills BPD, Dormans JP, et al. Os odontoideum revisited: the case for a multifactorial etiology. *Spine.* 2006;31:979–984.

356. Sasaki H, Itoh T, Takei H, et al. Os odontoideum with cerebellar infarction: a case report. *Spine.* 2000;25:1178–1181.

357. Savage JG, Fulkerson DH, Sen AN, et al. Fixation with C-2 laminar screws in occipitocervical or C1-2 constructs in children 5 years of age or younger: a series of 18 patients. *J Neurosurg Pediatr.* 2014;14:87–93.

358. Scannell G, Waxman K, Tominaga G, et al. Orotracheal intubation in trauma patients with cervical fractures. *Arch Surg.* 1993;128(8):903–905.

359. Scapinelli R. Three-dimensional computed tomography in infantile atlantoaxial rotatory fixation. *J Bone Joint Surg Br.* 1994;76:367–370.

360. Schiff DC, Parke WW. The arterial supply of the odontoid process. *J Bone Joint Surg Am.* 1973;55:1450–1464.

361. Schippers N, Könings P, Hassler W, et al. Typical and atypical fractures of the odontoid process in young children. Report of two cases and a review of the literature. *Acta Neurochir (Wien).* 1996;138:524–530.

362. Schnake KJ, Pingel A, Scholz M, et al. Temporary occipito-cervical stabilization of a unilateral occipital condyle fracture. *Eur Spine J.* 2012;21:2198–2202.

363. Schuler TC, Kurz L, Thompson DE, et al. Natural history of os odontoideum. *J Pediatr Orthop.* 1991;11:222–225.

364. Schwartz GR, Wright SW, Fein JA, et al. Pediatric cervical spine injury sustained in falls from low heights. *Ann Emerg Med.* 1997;30:249–252.

365. Schwarz N, Genelin F, Schwarz AF. Posttraumatic cervical kyphosis in children cannot be prevented by nonoperative methods. *Injury.* 1994;25:173–175.

366. Segal LS, Drummond DS, Zanotti RM, et al. Complications of posterior arthrodesis of the cervical spine in patients who have Down syndrome. *J Bone Joint Surg Am.* 1991;73:1547–1560.

367. Seimon LP. Fracture of the odontoid process in young children. *J Bone Joint Surg Am.* 1977;59:943–948.

368. Shacked I, Ram Z, Hadani M. The anterior cervical approach for traumatic injuries to the cervical spine. *Clin Orthop Relat Res.* 1993;292:144–150.

369. Shaffer MA, Doris PE. Limitation of the cross-table lateral view in detecting cervical spine injuries: a retrospective review. *Ann Emerg Med.* 1981;10:508–513.

370. Shammassian B. Wright CH, Wright J, et al. Successful delayed non-operative management of C2 neurosynchondrosis fractures in a pediatric patient: a case report and review of management strategies and considerations for treatment. *Childs Nerv Syst.* 2016;32:163–168.

371. Sharma BS, Mahajan RK, Bhatia S, et al. Collet-Sicard syndrome after closed head injury. *Clin Neurol Neurosurg.* 1994;96:197–198.

372. Shatney CH, Brunner RD, Nguyen TQ. The safety of orotracheal intubation in patients with unstable cervical spine fracture or high spinal cord injury. *Am J Surg.* 1995;170:676–679.

373. Shaw BA, Murphy KM. Displaced odontoid fracture in a 9-month-old child. *Am J Emerg Med.* 1999;1:73–75.

374. Sherburn EW, Day RA, Kaufman BA, et al. Subdental synchondrosis fracture in children: the value of three-dimensional computerized tomography. *Pediatr Neurosurg.* 1996;25:256–259.

375. Sherk HH, Dawoud S. Congenital os odontoideum with Klippel-Feil anomaly and fatal atlantoaxial instability. *Spine.* 1981;6:42–45.

376. Sherk HH, Schut L, Lane J. Fractures and dislocations of the cervical spine in children. *Orthop Clin North Am.* 1976;7:593–604.

377. Sherk HH, Whitaker LA, Pasquariello PS. Facial malformations and spinal anomalies: a predictable relationship. *Spine.* 1982;7:526–531.

378. Shetty GM, Song HR, Unnikrishnan R, et al. Upper cervical spine instability in pseudoachondroplasia. *J Pediatr Orthop.* 2007;27:782–787.

379. Shirasaki N, Okada K, Oka S, et al. Os odontoideum with posterior atlantoaxial instability. *Spine.* 1991;16:706–715.

380. Shulman ST, Madden JD, Esterly JR, et al. Transection of the spinal cord. A rare obstetrical complication of cephalic delivery. *Arch Dis Child.* 1971;46:291–294.

381. Silva CT, Dorai AS, Traubici J, et al. Do additional views improve the diagnostic performance of cervical spine radiography in pediatric trauma? *AJR Am J Roentgenol.* 2010; 194:500–508.

382. Sim F, Svien HJ, Bickel WH, et al. Swan neck deformity following extensive cervical laminectomy. *J Bone Joint Surg Am.* 1974;56:564–580.

383. Singh B, Cree A. Laminar screw fixation of the axis in the pediatric population: a series of eight patients. *Spine J.* 2015;15:e17–e25.

384. Skaggs DL, Lerman D, Albrekston J, et al. Use of a noninvasive halo in children. *Spine (Phila Pa 1976).* 2008;33:1650–1654.

385. Smejkal K, Lochman P, Holecek, T. [Post-traumatic hypoglossal nerve paresis due to occipital condyle fracture]. *Acta Chir Orthop Traumatol Cech.* 2009;76:335–337.

386. Smith T, Skinner SR, Shonnard NH. Persistent synchondrosis of the second cervical vertebra simulating a Hangman's fracture in a child. *J Bone Joint Surg Am.* 1993;75:1228–1230.

387. Special Olympics, Inc. *Participation by Individuals with DS Who Suffer from Atlantoaxial Dislocation.* Washington, DC: Author; 1983.

388. Spence KF Jr, Decker S, Sell KW. Bursting atlantal fracture associated with rupture of the transverse ligament. *J Bone Joint Surg Am.* 1970;52(3):543–549.

389. Spierings EL, Braakman R. The management of os odointideum: analysis of 37 cases. *J Bone Joint Surg Br.* 1982;64:442–428.

390. Spitzer R, Rabinowitch JY, Wybar KC. A study of the abnormalities of the skull, teeth and lenses in Mongolism. *Can Med Assoc J.* 1961;84:567–572.

391. Sponseller PD, Cass J. Atlanto-occipital arthrodesis for instability with neurologic preservation. *Spine.* 1997;22:344–347.

392. Sponseller PD, Herzenberg JE. Cervical spine injuries in children. In: Clark CR, Dvorak J, Ducker TB, et al., eds. *The Cervical Spine.* Philadelphia, PA: Lippincott-Raven; 1998:357–371.

393. Stauffer ES, Mazur JM. Cervical spine injuries in children. *Pediatr Ann.* 1982;11:502–511.

394. Steel HH. Anatomical and mechanical consideration of the atlantoaxial articulation. *J Bone Joint Surg Am.* 1968;50:1481–1482.

395. Steinmetz MP, Lechner RM, Anderson JS. Atlantooccipital dislocation in children: presentation, diagnosis, and management. *Neurosurg Focus.* 2003;14:1–7.

396. Stevens JM, Chong WK, Barber C, et al. A new appraisal of abnormalities of the odontoid process associated with atlantoaxial subluxation and neurological disability. *Brain.* 1994;117:133–148.

397. Stillwell WT, Fielding W. Acquired os odontoideum. *Clin Orthop Relat Res.* 1978;135:71–73.

398. Sun PP, Poffenbarger GJ, Durham S, et al. Spectrum of occipitoatlantoaxial injury in young children. *J Neurosurg.* 2000;93(Suppl 1):28–39.

399. Swischuk LE. Spine and spinal cord trauma in the battered child syndrome. *Radiology.* 1969;92:733–738.

400. Swischuk EH Jr, Rowe ML. The upper cervical spine in health and disease. *Pediatrics.* 1952;10:567–572.

401. Syre P, Petrov D, Malhotra NR. Management of upper cervical injuries: a review. *J Neurosurg Sci.* 2013;57:219–240.

402. Tauchi R, Imagama S, Ito Z, et al. Complications and outcomes of posterior fusion in children with atlantoaxial instability. *Eur Spine J.* 2012;21:1346–1352.

403. Tavares JO, Frankovitch KF. Odontoid process fracture in children: delayed diagnosis and successful conservative management with a halo cast. A report of two cases. *J Bone Joint Surg Am.* 2007;89:170–176.

404. Tawbin A. CNS damage in the human fetus and newborn infant. *Am J Dis Child.* 1951;33:543–547.

405. Taylor AR. The mechanism of injury to the spinal cord in the neck without damage to the vertebral column. *J Bone Joint Surg Br.* 1951;33:453–547.

406. Thakar C, Harish S, Saifuddin A, et al. Displaced fracture through the anterior atlantal synchondrosis. *Skeletal Radiol.* 2005;34:547–549.

407. Tolhurst SR, Vanderhave KL, Caird MS, et al. Cervical arterial injury after blunt trauma in children: characterization and advanced imaging. *J Pediatr Orthop.* 2013;33:37–42.

408. Tolo VT, Weiland AJ. Unsuspected atlas fractures and instability associated with oropharyngeal injury: case report. *J Trauma.* 1979;19:278–280.

409. Tomaszewski R, Pyzinska M. Treatment of cervical spine fractures with halo vest method in children and young people. *Ortop Traumatol Rehabil.* 2014;16:449–454.

410. Tomaszewski R, Wiktor L. Occipital condyle fractures in adolescents. *Ortop Traumatol Rehabil.* 2015;17:219–227.

411. Traynelis VC, Marano GD, Dunker RO, et al. Traumatic atlanto-occipital dislocation: case report. *J Neurosurg.* 1986;65:863–870.

412. Tredwell SJ, Newman DE, Lockitch G. Instability of the upper cervical spine in Down syndrome. *J Pediatr Orthop.* 1990;10:602–606.

413. Tuli S, Tator CH, Fehlings MG, et al. Occipital condyle fractures. *Neurosurgery.* 1997;41:368–377.

414. Uchiyama T, Kawaji Y, Moriya K, et al. Two cases of odontoid fracture in preschool children. *J Spinal Disord Tech.* 2006;19:204–207.

415. Ueda S, Sasaki N, Fukuda M, et al. Surgical treatment for occipital condyle fracture, C1 dislocation, and cerebellar contusion with hemorrhage after blunt head trauma. *Case Rep Orthop.* 2016;2016:8634831.

416. Uribe JS, Ramos E, Baaj A, et al. Occipital cervical stabilization using occipital condyles for cranial fixation: technical case report. *Neurosurgery*. 2009;65:E1216–E1217.

417. Uribe JS, Ramos E, Vale F. Feasibility of occipital condyle screw placement for occipitocervical fixation: a cadaveric study and description of a novel technique. *J Spinal Disord Tech*. 2008;21:540–546.

418. Utheim NC, Josefsen R, Nakstad PH, et al. Occipital condyle fracture and lower cranial nerve palsy after blunt head trauma a literature review and case report. *J Tauma Manag Outcomes*. 2015;9:2.

419. Vanderhave KL, Chiravuri S, Caird MS, et al. Cervical spine trauma in children and adults: perioperative considerations. *J Am Acad Orthop Surg*. 2011;19:319–327.

420. Van Dyke DC, Gahagan CA. Down syndrome: cervical spine abnormalities and problems. *Clin Pediatr*. 1988;27:415–418.

421. van Rijn RR, Kool DR, de Witt Hamer PC, et al. An abused 5-month-old girl: Hangman's fracture or congenital arch defect? *J Emerg Med*. 2005;29:61–65.

422. Verska JM, Anderson PA. Os odontoideum. A case report of one identical twin. *Spine*. 1997;22:706–709.

423. Viccellio P, Simon H, Pressman BD, et al. A prospective multicenter study of cervical spine injury in children. *Pediatrics*. 2001;108:E20.

424. Vilela MD, Peterson EC. Atlantal fracture with transverse ligament disruption in a child. Case report. *J Neurosurg Pediatr*. 2009;4:196–198.

425. Villas C, Arriagada C, Zubieta JL. Preliminary CT study of C1–C2 rotational mobility in normal subjects. *Eur Spine J*. 1999;8:223–228.

426. Visocchi M, Fernandez E, Ciampini A, et al. Reducible and irreducible os odontoideum in childhood treated with posterior wiring, instrumentation and fusion. Past or present? *Acta Neurochir (Wien)*. 2009;151:1265–1274.

427. Walsh JW, Stevens DB, Young AB. Traumatic paraplegia in children without contiguous spinal fracture or dislocation. *Neurosurgery*. 1983;12:439–445.

428. Wang X, Fan CY, Liu ZH. The single transoral approach for os odontoideum with irreducible atlantoaxial dislocation. *Eur Spine J*. 2010;19(Suppl 2):S91–95.

429. Wang MY, Hoh DJ, Leary SP, et al. High rates of neurological improvement following severe traumatic pediatric spinal cord injury. *Spine*. 2004;29:1493–1497; discussion E1266.

430. Wang S, Passias PG, Cui L, et al. Does atlantoaxial dislocation influence the subaxial cervical spine. *Eur Spine J*. 2013;22:1603–1607.

431. Wang J, Vokshoor A, Kim S, et al. Pediatric atlantoaxial instability: management with screw fixation. *Pediatr Neurosurg*. 1999;30:70–78.

432. Wani MA, Tandon PN, Banerji AK, et al. Collet-Sicard syndrome resulting from closed head injury: case report. *J Trauma*. 1991;31:1437–1439.

433. Ware ML, Gupta N, Sun PP, et al. Clinical biomechanics of the pediatric craniocervical junction and the subaxial spine. In: Brockmeyer DL, ed. *Advanced Pediatric Craniocervical Surgery*. New York: Thieme; 2006:27–42.

434. Warner WC. Pediatric cervical spine. In: Canale ST, ed. *Campbell's Operative Orthopaedics*. St. Louis, MO: Mosby; 1998.

435. Warner WC Jr. Pediatric cervical spine. In: Canale ST, Beaty JH, eds. *Campbell's Operative Orthopaedics*. 12th ed. Philadelphia, PA; Elsevier; 2013.

436. Watanabe M, Toyama Y, Fujimura Y. Atlantoaxial instability in os odontoideum with myelopathy. *Spine*. 1996;21:1435–1439.

437. Wellborn CC, Sturm PF, Hatch RS, et al. Intraobserver reproducibility and interobserver reliability of cervical spine measurements. *J Pediatr Orthop*. 2000;20:66–70.

438. Weng C, Tian W, Li ZY, et al. Surgical management of symptomatic os odontoideum with posterior screw fixation performed using the Magerl and Harms techniques with intraoperative 3-dimensional fluoroscopy-based navigation. *Spine (Phila Pa 1976)*. 2012;37:1839–1846.

439. Wertheim SB, Bohlman HH. Occipitocervical fusion: indications, technique, and longterm results. *J Bone Joint Surg Am*. 1987;69:833–836.

440. Wetzel FT, Larocca H. Grisel syndrome. *Clin Orthop Relat Res*. 1989;240:141–152.

441. White AA III, Johnson RM, Panjabi MM, et al. Biomechanical analysis of clinical stability in the cervical spine. *Clin Orthop Relat Res*. 1975;109:85–96.

442. White AA III, Panjabi MM. The basic kinematics of the human spine. A review of past and current knowledge. *Spine*. 1978;3:12–20.

443. White D, Al-Mahfoudh R. The role of conservative management in incidental os odontoideum. *World Neurosurg*. 2016;88:695.e615–e697.

444. Wiktor L, Tomaszewski R. Occipital condyle fracture with accompanying meningeal spinal cysts as a result of cervical spine injury in 15-year-old girl. *Case Rep Orthop*. 2015;2015:627502.

445. Williams JP III, Baker DH, Miller WA. CT appearance of congenital defect resembling the Hangman's fracture. *Pediatr Radiol*. 1999;29:549–550.

446. Wills BPD, Jencikova-Celerin L, Dormans JP. Cervical spine range of motion in children with asymptomatic os odontoideum. *J Pediatr Orthop*. 2006;26(6):753–757.

447. Wind WM, Schwend RM, Larson J. Sports for the physically challenged child. *J Am Acad Orthop Surg*. 2004;12:126–137.

448. Windell J, Burke SW. Sports participation of children with Down syndrome. *Orthop Clin North Am*. 2003;34:439–443.

449. Wollin DG. The os odontoideum. *J Bone Joint Surg Am*. 1971;45:1459–1471.

450. Xu G, Li W, Bao G, et al. Tear-drop fracture of the axis in a child with an 8-year follow-up: case report. *J Pediatr Orthop B*. 2014;23:299–305.

451. Yasuoko F, Peterson H, MacCarty C. Incidence of spinal column deformity after multiple level laminectomy in children and adults. *J Neurosurg*. 1982;57:441–445.

452. Yeom JS, Buchowski JM, Kim HJ, et al. Postoperative occipital neuralgia with and without C2 nerve root transection during atlantoaxial screw fixation: a post-hoc comparative outcome study of prospectively collected data. *Spine J*. 2013;13(7):786–795.

453. Yin TYH, Yu XG, Qiao GY, et al. C1 lateral mass screw placement in occipitalization with atlantoaxial dislocation and basilar invagination: a report of 146 cases. *Spine (Phila Pa 1976)*. 2014;39:2013–2018.

454. Yngve DA, Harris WP, Herndon WA, et al. Spinal cord injury without osseous spine fracture. *J Pediatr Orthop*. 1988;8:153–159.

455. Yoon JW, Lim OK, Park KD, et al Occipital condyle fracture with isolated unilateral hypoglossal nerve palsy. *Ann Rehabil Med*. 2014;38:689–693.

456. Zhou F, Ni B, Li S, et al. C2 translaminar screw as the optimal choice for atlantoaxial dislocation with C2–C3 congenital fusion. *Arch Orthop Trauma Surg*. 2010;130:1505–1509.

457. Zygourakis CC, Cahill KS, Proctor MR. Delayed development of os odontoideum after traumatic cervical injury: support for a vascular etiology. *J Neurosurg Pediatr*. 2011;7:201–204.

21

Thoracolumbar Spine Fractures

Peter O. Newton and Vidyadhar V. Upasani

INTRODUCTION TO THORACOLUMBAR SPINE FRACTURES

Fractures of the thoracic and lumbar spine in pediatric patients are relatively uncommon[38,75] as the inherent elasticity and mobility of the pediatric spine protects children. The mechanisms of injury vary with age.[20,76] These fractures can be broadly grouped as compression, burst, flexion-distraction, and fracture-dislocations. The treatment principles are based on the mechanism of injury and the stability of the fracture. Clarifying the stability of any given fracture can be challenging, and controversy remains in determining which fractures require surgical stabilization. Understanding the mechanism of injury, the neurologic status[5,29] and associated injuries[7,36,41,53,57,72] are important to guide treatment of pediatric thoracolumbar fractures. The goals of treatment are to provide skeletal stability to protect against spinal cord injury (SCI) and to maximize the potential for recovery of spinal cord function if an SCI is present. These two goals may be analyzed separately when both instability and SCI exist.

ASSESSMENT OF THORACOLUMBAR SPINE FRACTURES

MECHANISMS OF INJURY OF THORACOLUMBAR SPINE FRACTURES

One of the most important aspects of treating pediatric thoracolumbar spinal fractures is understanding the mechanism of injury. In general, the mechanism of injury correlates with the age of the patient.[20] Spine trauma, just like appendicular trauma, should raise concern for child abuse or nonaccidental injury in infants and young children.[15,23,48]

Motor vehicle accidents may be the most common cause of spinal column injury in all age groups.[7] The type of seat belt restraint has clear implications in the mechanism of force transferred to the spine, with the lap belt a common cause of both intra-abdominal and spinal injuries.[36,53,72,77,86] Addition of a shoulder strap or child seat with a five-point frontal harness limits flexion of the torso with frontal impact accidents and protects the spine (and other vital organs) from injury.

Falls from a height generally result in axial loading of the spine, which may result in a compression fracture (anterior column injury) or burst fracture (anterior and middle column injury), depending on the degree of flexion of the trunk at the time of impact. These fracture patterns are possible with any mechanism associated with axial compression and can also occur with motor vehicle accidents and sporting injuries.[20] Compression of the vertebra when the trunk in flexed creates the greatest forces in the anterior aspect of the vertebra, leading more commonly to anterior column wedging (compression fracture). This is in contrast to axial compression when the trunk is in an extended position, which loads the vertebral body more symmetrically. Fractures in this case often collapse with radial expansion and fracture both the anterior and middle columns of the vertebral body (burst fracture). Displacement of the vertebral body fragments into the spinal canal may cause injury or compression of the neurologic elements (spinal cord or cauda equina).[39]

If the magnitude of injury sustained seems out of proportion to the force applied, the possibility of an insufficiency fracture due to weak bone should be considered. Osteoporotic insufficiency fractures, common in the elderly, are rare in children; however, several disease states may predispose children to these injury patterns. Chronic corticosteroid use associated with the management of many pediatric rheumatologic and oncologic diseases often leads to osteoporosis and increased risk of compression fractures. In addition, primary lesions of the bone, such as Langerhans histiocytosis or bone cysts, can weaken thoracic vertebrae.[6,30] Other tumors and infections warrant consideration when nontraumatic compression fractures are identified.[60,74]

INJURIES ASSOCIATED WITH THORACOLUMBAR SPINE FRACTURES

Just as the mechanism of injury should raise suspicion of a particular fracture pattern (e.g., lap belt injury and flexion-distraction lumbar fracture pattern), so should the presence of one injury

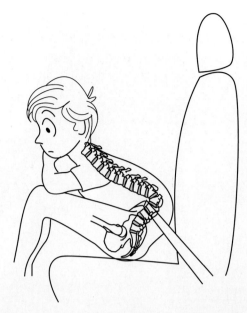

Figure 21-1. A lap belt used for a child can create a point of rotation about which the spine is flexed with an abrupt stop. This is a common mechanism for creating both intra-abdominal and flexion-distraction spinal injuries.

raise suspicion of a concomitant associated injury. First, any vertebral fracture should be considered a significant risk factor for a vertebral fracture at another level.[56] The traumatic force required to create one fracture is often enough to result in one or more additional fractures at other locations.

The lap belt mechanism of injury is well known to create flexion-distraction injuries of the spine, but also is associated with intra-abdominal injury (Fig. 21-1).[72] Compressed between the seat belt and the spinal column, the aorta, intestinal viscera, and abdominal wall musculature are at risk for laceration. Abdominal injuries are present in almost 50% of pediatric patients with Chance fractures.[62] Ecchymosis on the anterior abdomen is suggestive of intra-abdominal injury that warrants further evaluation with advanced imaging (Fig. 21-2).[7,86] A high index of suspicion is required, as missed injuries may be life-threatening.[53]

Associated injury to the spinal cord has obvious significance and may be present with many fracture patterns. Disruption of the stability of the spinal column or bony intrusion into the spinal canal may result in compromise of neurologic function (Fig. 21-3). All patients with a known spinal column fracture or dislocation warrant a careful neurologic examination.

Overall, most pediatric patients with thoracolumbar fractures are neurologically intact (85%), and less commonly present with SCIs (incomplete in 5% and complete in 10%).[25] Similarly, patients with a traumatic neurologic deficit require a careful evaluation of the spinal column integrity. There are, however, a subset of patients who present with SCI without radiographic abnormality.[63,64] The concept of spinal cord injury without radiographic abnormality (SCIWORA) was popularized by Pang and Wilberger[64] who described their experience at the University of Pittsburgh. They noted a series of patients presenting with traumatic SCIs that were not evident on plain

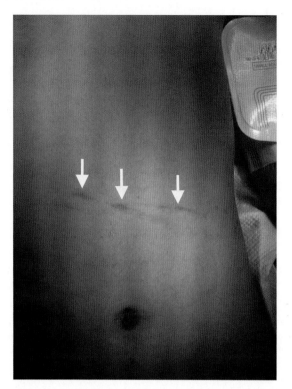

Figure 21-2. A seatbelt sign may be subtle, as in this example of horizontal ecchymosis in the setting of a soft tissue L2–L3 chance fracture. In this case, the injury was missed on the initial radiology reading, and the clinical picture helped establish the diagnosis. *Arrows* demonstrate horizontal ecchymosis across the abdomen consistent with a seatbelt sign. (Used with permission of Children's Orthopaedic Center, Los Angeles Children's Hospital.)

radiographs or tomograms. Several mechanisms to explain these findings have been proposed, including spinal cord stretch and vascular disruption/infarction. MRI studies have confirmed patterns of both cord edema and hemorrhage in such cases.[34,90,102] Important additional facts about SCIWORA include the finding that some patients had a delayed onset of their neurologic deficits. Transient neurologic symptoms were persistent in many who later developed a lasting deficit. In addition, the younger patients (less than 8 years old) had more severe neurologic involvement.[9] Although these injuries may not be visible on plain radiographs, nearly all will have some evidence of soft tissue injury of the spine on more sensitive magnetic resonance imaging (MRI) studies.[34] The term SCIWORA is less relevant in the era of routine MRI, which is now obtained in all patients with possible SCI.[45]

SIGNS AND SYMPTOMS OF THORACOLUMBAR SPINE FRACTURES

Careful evaluation of a patient with a potential traumatic spinal injury begins as with any serious trauma victim. The ABCs of resuscitation (airway, breathing, circulation) are performed while maintaining cervical and thoracolumbar spine precautions. The frequency of spinal injuries in the setting of major trauma (motor vehicle accident, fall, etc.) is particularly high. After stabilizing the cardiorespiratory systems, symptoms of pain, numbness, and tingling should be sought if the patient is old enough and alert enough to cooperate. Pain in the back is often not appreciated when other distracting injuries exist

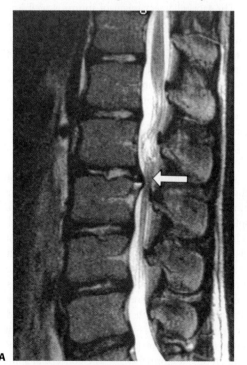

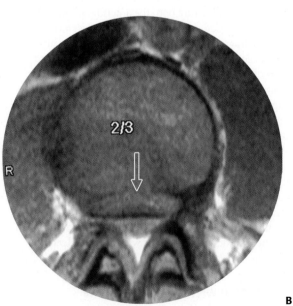

Figure 21-3. Ring apophyseal avulsion injuries. **A:** This lateral MRI image demonstrates displacement of the ring apophysis, which functionally acts as a disc herniation. This, however, represents largely a bony and cartilaginous fragment, which results in neural element compression. **B:** Transverse image demonstrating canal stenosis associated with this injury. *Arrow* indicates the apophyseal fracture resulting in central canal stenosis.

and the patient is immobilized on a backboard. Examination of the back must not be forgotten and is performed by logrolling the patient. Visual inspection, along with palpation, should seek areas of swelling, deformity, ecchymosis, and/or tenderness that may provide a clue to the presence of an injury. In trauma patients, thoracolumbar fractures are more common in older children and adolescents, and there is a low mortality rate and infrequent need for operative stabilization.[78] Clinically, the ability to diagnose a thoracolumbar spine fracture in pediatric trauma patients has been demonstrated to have an 87% sensitivity and average specificity.[43,78]

Hence, routine screening radiographs of any patients suspected of having a thoracolumbar spine injury should be performed, to minimize the likelihood of missing an injury.

Neurologic examination provides information on the integrity of the spinal cord. The age of the patient may limit the thoroughness of this assessment, but some indication of sensory and motor function should be sought. In cases of spinal cord deficit, a detailed examination of the strength of appropriate muscle group, sensory levels, and rectal tone will need to be serially compared over time and the quality of the documentation cannot be overemphasized. The prognosis for recovery is significantly better if the SCI is incomplete.[17,37,95] The status of the neurologic function over time may lead to important treatment decisions regarding the necessity and timing of surgical intervention. A progressive neurologic deficit warrants immediate surgical attention, whereas an improving status may suggest a less urgent approach.

IMAGING AND OTHER DIAGNOSTIC STUDIES FOR THORACOLUMBAR SPINE FRACTURES

Following a careful clinical examination of all patients with a suspected spinal injury, plain radiographs are obtained first. An alert, cooperative patient without pain or tenderness in the back can be cleared without radiographs. However, any patient with a significant mechanism or associated injury (motor vehicle accident, fall from greater than 10 foot, cervical or head injury) requires thoracolumbar spine radiographs if they have spinal tenderness, are obtunded, or have a distracting injury. Initial films should include supine anteroposterior (AP) and lateral views of the thoracic and lumbar spine. In addition, because of the strong association between cervical spine fractures and thoracolumbar spine fractures after blunt or vehicular trauma, routine imaging of the complete spine when a cervical fracture is identified is indicated.[99]

Plain radiographs often show relatively subtle findings. On AP radiographs, soft tissue shadows may be widened by paravertebral hematoma. The bony anatomy is viewed to evaluate for loss of height of the vertebral body as compared with adjacent levels. Similar comparisons can be made with regard to interpedicular distance and interspinous spacing.[12] Lateral radiographs give important information about the sagittal plane: anterior vertebral wedging or collapse or posterior element distraction or fracture. Careful scrutiny of the plain radiographs is always prudent; however, the computed tomography (CT) scan will nearly always be used to clarify any suspected fractures. Antevil et al.[3] reported the sensitivity of plain radiographs to be 70%

(14 of 20 patients) for spine trauma, whereas the sensitivity was 100% for CT scanning (34 of 34 patients).

CT is now a standard component of the evaluation of many trauma patients. Multidetector scanners allow rapid assessment with axial, coronal, and sagittal images for patients with plain radiographic abnormalities. The axial images are best for evaluating the integrity of the spinal canal in cases of a burst fracture, whereas the sagittal views will demonstrate vertebral body compression as well as posterior element distraction or fracture. In addition, major dislocations easily seen on plain radiographs will be better understood with regard to the space left in the spinal canal for the neurologic elements. The amount of spinal canal compromise has been correlated with the probability of neurologic deficit.[61]

MRI is the modality of choice for evaluating the discs, spinal cord, and posterior ligamentous structures.[45,52,88] Although more difficult to obtain in a multiply injured patient, this study is mandatory in patients with a neurologic deficit to assess the potential cause of cord dysfunction. The MRI is able to distinguish areas of spinal cord hemorrhage and edema. Assessment of the posterior ligamentous complex (PLC) is critical in differentiating stable and unstable burst fractures, as well as compression fractures and flexion-distraction injuries. Although subject to overinterpretation, MRI has been shown to modify the diagnosis made by plain radiographs and CT and correlates very well with intraoperative findings of the structural integrity of the posterior soft tissues.[52,69]

CLASSIFICATION OF THORACOLUMBAR SPINE FRACTURES

Several classification systems have been developed for thoracolumbar spine fractures. The most commonly used in practice today include: Denis—three column,[22] Thoracolumbar Injury Classification and Severity Score (TLICS),[92] and the AOSpine Thoracolumbar Spine Injury Classification System.[92]

Denis (Three-Column System): CLASSIFICATION
• Compression fracture
• Burst fracture
• Flexion-distraction injuries
• Fracture-dislocation

Designed primarily with the adult spine fracture patterns in mind, the Denis classification translates well for the categorization of most pediatric thoracolumbar injuries.[50] Based on theories of stability related to the three-column biomechanical concept of the spine (anterior, middle, posterior columns), the Denis classification in its simplest form includes compression, burst, flexion-distraction, and fracture-dislocations (Fig. 21-4).

Compression fractures are the most common thoracolumbar spine fracture pattern.[14,40] The vertebral body loses height anteriorly compared with the posterior wall. The anterior aspect of the vertebral body is involved, but the middle column (posterior wall) of the vertebral body is by definition intact. Axial load with flexion is the common mechanism. Depending on the degree and direction of flexion, the wedging may vary between

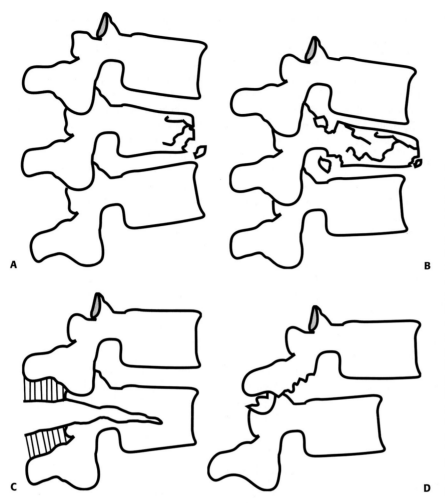

A

B

C

D

Figure 21-4. Denis classification of thoracolumbar fractures. **A:** Compression fracture: This injury results in mild wedging of the vertebra primarily involving the anterior aspects of the vertebral body. The posterior vertebral height and posterior cortex remain intact. **B:** Burst fracture: A burst fracture involves both the anterior and middle columns with loss of height throughout the vertebral body. There may be substantial retropulsion of the posterior aspect of the vertebra into the spinal canal. In addition, posterior vertebral fractures and/or ligamentous injury may occur. **C:** Flexion-distraction injuries: This fracture, which occurs commonly with a seat belt injury mechanism, results in posterior distraction with disruption of the ligaments and bony elements of the posterior column, commonly extending into the anterior columns with or without compression of the most anterior aspects of the vertebra. **D:** Fracture-dislocation: These complex injuries involve marked translation of one vertebra on another with frequently associated SCI as a result of translations through the spinal canal.

the coronal and sagittal planes (Fig. 21-5). The percentage of lost height defines the severity of compression fractures, which rarely have an associated neurologic deficit. However, the fractures are often associated with similar or occasionally more severe fractures at adjacent or distant levels. Contiguous compression fractures, each of a modest degree, together may result in a substantial kyphotic deformity. Because the cause of these injuries, such as a fall, is fairly common, it is at times necessary to determine if a wedged vertebra seen radiographically represents an acute compression fracture, sequelae of Scheuermann kyphosis, anatomic variant with delayed ossification, or a remote injury. Clinical examination can localize pain to the site of the fracture in acute injuries; however, MRI or bone scan can be used to confirm acute fracture based on signal changes and increased isotope uptake.

Burst fractures likely represent a more severe form of compression fracture that extends posteriorly in the vertebral body to include the posterior wall (middle column). Axial compression is the primary mechanism, although posterior element fractures may also occur. Laminar fractures have been known to entrap the dural contents. The fractures are most common in the lower thoracic and upper lumbar levels. Associated neurologic injury is related to the severity of injury (greater injury index scores correlate with greater frequency of SCI[55] and the degree

of spinal canal encroachment by retropulsed bony fragments).[39] SCI at the thoracolumbar junction may result in conus medullaris syndrome or cauda equina syndrome. Careful examination of the perineal area is required to identify these spinal lesions.

Flexion-distraction injuries are especially relevant to the pediatric population because this classic lap belt injury is more frequent in backseat passengers, particularly when a shoulder strap or five-point harness is lacking. Motor vehicle accidents are the primary cause of this injury. The lap belt, which restrains the pelvis in adults, may ride up onto the abdomen in children. Chance, and later Smith, described how with a frontal impact, the weight of the torso is driven forward, flexing over the restraining belt. With the axis of rotation in front of the spine, distractive forces are placed on the posterior elements, with variable degrees of anterior vertebral compression. This three-column injury is generally unstable. The disruption of the posterior elements may occur entirely through the bony (Chance; Fig. 21-6) or ligamentous (Smith; Fig. 21-7) elements, although many times the fracture propagates through both soft and bony tissues.

The injury is most obvious on lateral radiographs; however, if no fracture exists, widening of the intraspinous distance may be the only finding on an AP radiograph. A recent study demonstrated the difficulty in appropriately diagnosing this injury in

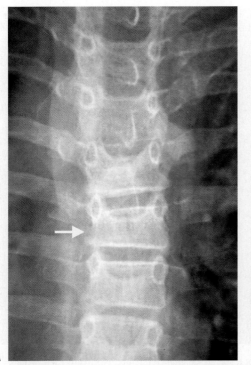
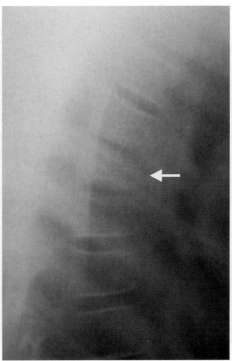

Figure 21-5. Compression fractures. **A:** This PA view demonstrates wedging in the coronal plane. **B:** The more commonly recognized compression fractures involve wedging primarily in the sagittal plane with loss of anterior vertebral height. *Arrow* indicates vertebral body wedging in the coronal and sagittal plane respectively.

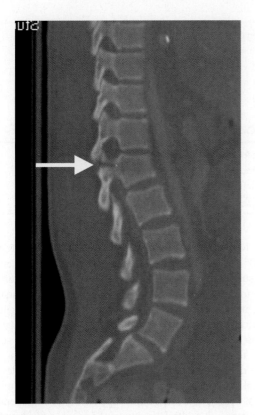

Figure 21-6. Bony chance fractures have distraction of the posterior elements through bone (*arrow*), not the interspinous ligament. This is much less common than a soft tissue chance fracture. (Used with permission of Children's Orthopaedic Center, Los Angeles Children's Hospital.)

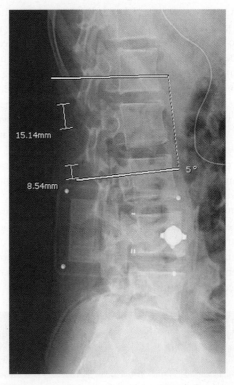

Figure 21-7. Soft tissue chance fractures can be easily missed on lateral x-rays, particularly when there is not too much compression anteriorly. Note the increased separation between the spinous processes suggesting a diagnosis of a chance fracture. (Used with permission of Children's Orthopaedic Center, Los Angeles Children's Hospital.)

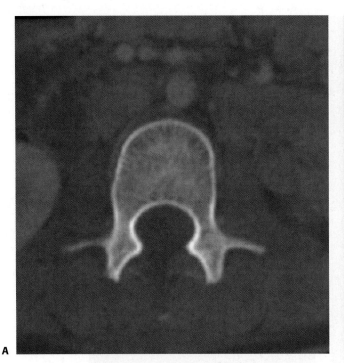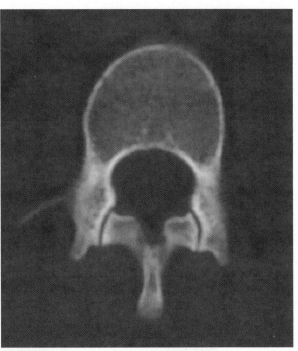

Figure 21-8. A: "Empty facet sign" characteristic of a soft tissue chance fracture. Normally, there would be both superior and inferior facets present in a transverse CT cut, but with separation of the posterior elements, only the superior facet is visualized. **B:** In contrast, this is an image of normal facet joints at an uninjured level in the same patient. (Used with permission of Children's Orthopaedic Center, Los Angeles Children's Hospital.)

children, with an average delayed diagnosis of 3 months at a level 1 pediatric trauma center.[1] Standard axial CT imaging may also miss this injury because the plane of injury lies within the plane of imaging. One classic finding in ligamentous flexion-distraction injuries is the "empty facet" sign (Fig. 21-8). When the inferior articular process of the superior vertebra is no longer in contact with the superior articular process of the inferior vertebra, the facet appears empty in the transverse CT image.[31] Sagittal reconstructions are most revealing and MRI will provide information about the integrity of the PLC. Identification of a purely intravertebral flexion-distraction fracture is important, as this may alter the treatment compared with those with severe ligamentous injury.

Fracture-dislocations of the spinal column result from complex severe loading mechanisms. These are by definition unstable injuries with a component of shearing and/or rotational displacement. A special note in the pediatric population is the documentation of this injury pattern in young patients exposed to nonaccidental trauma.[23,48,54]

Thoracolumbar Injury: CLASSIFICATION AND SEVERITY SCORE	
Category	**Points**
1. Injury morphology	
a. Compression/burst	1/+1
b. Translational/rotation	3
c. Distraction	4

2. Neurological status	
a. Intact	0
b. Nerve root injury	2
c. Cord/conus medullaris	
Incomplete	3
Complete	2
Cauda equine	3
3. Posterior ligamentous complex	
a. Intact	0
b. Injury suspected	2
c. Injured	3

The TLICS system, introduced by the Spine Trauma Study Group in 2005, was developed to streamline injury assessment and guide surgical decision-making.[92] The system assigns numerical values to each injury based on the categories of morphology of injury, integrity of the PLC, and neurologic involvement. The numerical scores are then summated to produce an injury severity score, which is, in turn, used to guide treatment. A score of greater than or equal to 5 suggests operative treatment of the patient due to significant instability, whereas a score of less than or equal to 3 suggests nonoperative treatment. A patient with a score of 4 may be treated either operatively or nonoperatively. In the setting of multiple fractures, the injury with the greatest TLICS score is used to guide treatment. This system has demonstrated good-to-excellent inter- and intra-observer reliability and has been shown to be easily taught, learned, and incorporated into clinical practice.[42,68,82] A recent multicenter evaluation of the validity of TLICS in children was performed demonstrating very good concordance with surgeon decision-making. The authors concluded that TLICS appeared to be an effective classification of thoracic and lumbar spine injuries and was able to appropriately guide treatment in these patients.[81]

AOSpine Thoracolumbar Spine Injury Classification System
Type A: Compression injury
A0: Minor injuries (transverse process/spinous process)
A1: Wedge compression
A2: Split or pincer type
A3: Incomplete burst
A4: Complete burst
Type B: Posterior or anterior tension band injury
B1: Monosegmental bony posterior tension band
B2: Posterior tension band disruption
B3: Hyperextension injury
Type C: Failure of all elements (dislocation)—translation or displacement type

The AOSpine Thoracolumbar Spine Injury Classification System was published in 2013 and has yet to be validated in a multicenter pediatric population.[91]

OUTCOME MEASURES FOR THORACOLUMBAR SPINE FRACTURES

SCIs in children have remarkable potential for recovery.[66,95] In a study from a major metropolitan trauma center, complete SCIs were associated with fatal injuries in one-third and no neurologic recovery in another third, whereas most of the remaining one-third of patients made improvements that ultimately allowed functional ambulation. Less surprisingly, nearly all patients with incomplete SCI made some improvement over time as well.[95] This ability to recover, even from complete injuries, has led some to suggest more aggressive attempts at spinal cord decompression in the early course of treatment,[28,65] whereas others have suggested a period of "spinal cord rest" with observation.[55] In adults, early fracture fixation has been shown to be beneficial, minimizing respiratory morbidity and decreasing days in the intensive care setting and length of hospital stay.[8] There are certainly no controlled series of pediatric patients treated by both approaches to support either hypothesis. The data do, however, suggest a more optimistic view regarding the potential recovery of traumatic SCIs in children compared with adults.

Spinal column structural integrity should be assessed in all cases of injury because the functional capacity of the vertebral elements to protect the spinal cord will continue to be required. This evaluation may be performed with functional radiographs, such as flexion–extension views (much more common in the cervical spine) or with an MRI evaluation of associated soft tissue injuries that may coexist with more obvious bony fractures. Several methods of estimating spinal column stability have been proposed including the three-column concept of Denis.[22] Based on division into anterior, middle, and posterior columns, injuries

to two and certainly three of these sagittal columns have been considered an unstable injury pattern. Plain radiography with a CT scan is appropriate for evaluating the bony elements. An MRI is often required to elucidate the nature of the disc and ligamentous injuries.[35,45,89] MRI is extremely sensitive and, given the brightness of edema fluid on T2 images, may be overinterpreted. A study correlating MRI and intraoperative surgical findings, however, demonstrated high levels of both sensitivity and specificity in the MRI evaluation of posterior soft tissue injuries (Fig. 21-9).[52]

The ultimate treatment goal is a stable spinal column. This often requires surgical treatment in unstable fracture patterns. In contrast, most stable injuries can be managed nonoperatively. There are particular exceptions to these generalizations, of course. At times, the associated SCI or a substantial associated deformity may alter the treatment approach to an otherwise mechanically stable injury. The presence of a complete SCI in a child younger than 10 years is also a determinant that may affect treatment strategies. The incidence of paralytic spinal deformity (scoliosis) is nearly 100% in such cases, and a long instrumented fusion will likely be required at some point.[2,51,67] Depending on the fracture pattern and age of the patient, it may be prudent to include much of the thoracic and lumbar spine in the initial instrumented fusion.[58] However, in the patient without neurologic deficit, there is evidence that the use of

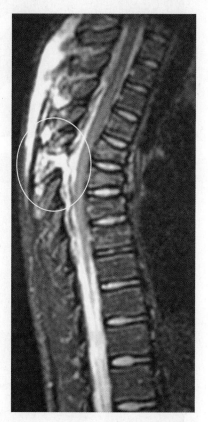

Figure 21-9. This sagittal MRI demonstrates marked increased signal in the posterior ligamentous complex. Anteriorly, a loss of height at the vertebra can be seen, suggesting a three-column spinal injury. Extensive posterior hematoma is also demonstrated, which is often a clinical sign of posterior ligamentous disruption. *Circle* depicts the area of increased signal in the posterior ligamentous complex.

posterior stabilization of thoracolumbar fractures using nonfusion methods followed by removal of metal implants within an appropriate period appears to be a safe, viable option.[21,47]

PATHOANATOMY AND APPLIED ANATOMY RELATED TO THORACOLUMBAR SPINE FRACTURES

The thoracic and lumbar spine links the upper and lower extremities through the torso. The 12 thoracic and 5 lumbar vertebrae are joined by intravertebral discs and strong ligaments, both anteriorly and posteriorly. The bony architecture of the vertebrae varies, with the smaller thoracic vertebrae having a more shingled overlapping configuration compared with the lumbar segments. The thoracic facets are oriented in the coronal plane, whereas those in the lumbar spine lie nearly in the sagittal plane (Fig. 21-10).

Mobility is less in the thoracic spine owing to the adjacent and linked rib cage as well as the smaller intervertebral discs. The ribs make an important connection between the vertebra with each rib head articulating across a given disc space. This is in contrast to the relatively mobile lumbar segments, which have thick intravertebral discs that permit substantial flexion–extension, lateral bending, and axial rotation motion. The junction between the stiffer thoracic spine and more flexible lumbar spine is a region of frequent injury because of this transition between two regions which have differing inherent flexibility.

Ligamentous components include the anterior and posterior longitudinal ligaments, facet capsules, ligamentum flavum, as well as the interspinous and supraspinous ligaments. Together, these structures limit the motion between vertebrae to protect the neurologic elements. The anterior longitudinal ligament is rarely disrupted in flexion injuries but may be rendered incompetent by extension loading or a severe fracture-dislocation. On

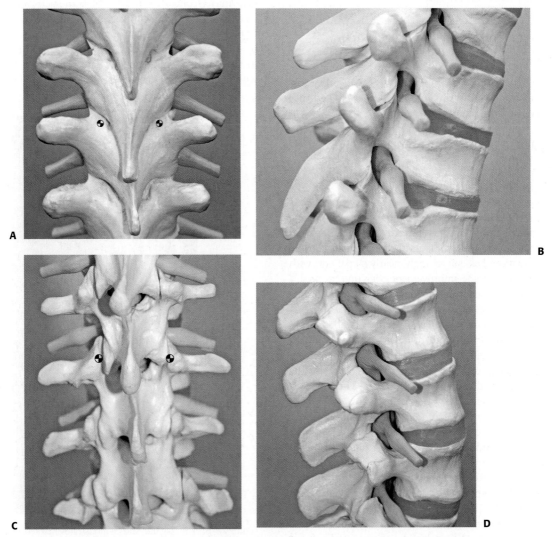

Figure 21-10. A and **B:** Thoracic spine posterior and lateral views demonstrating the overlapping lamina and spinous processes present in this region. The circles mark the location of the thoracic pedicles, which may be important in surgical reconstruction. **C** and **D:** Lumbar spine posterior and lateral projections demonstrating the differences in lumbar spine anatomy. Again, the circles mark locations of the lumbar pedicles relative to the facets and transverse processes.

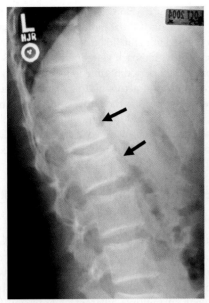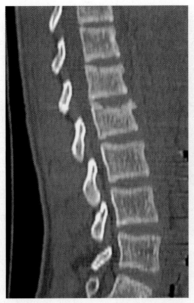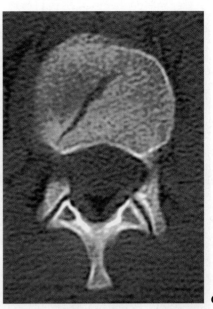

Figure 21-11. A: This lateral radiograph demonstrates two upper lumbar vertebrae with slight loss of height suggestive of compression fractures. *Arrows* demonstrate slight wedging of the vertebral bodies consistent with superior end plate compression fractures. **B** and **C:** The CT images confirm an intact posterior vertebral body wall. This injury, therefore, represents a compression fracture rather than a burst fracture injury.

the contrary, flexion is the primary mechanism of injury to the PLC—supraspinous and interspinous, facet capsule, and ligamentum flavum. The healing capacity of the completely torn PLC is limited, though substantially better in the pediatric population compared with adults, whereas bony fractures are more likely to heal with resultant stability.

The neural anatomy varies over the length of the thoracolumbar spine as well. The space within the canal is largest in the lumbar spine. The spinal cord traverses the entirety of the thoracic spine and typically terminates as the conus medullaris at the L1 or L2 level. The cauda equina occupies the dural tube below this level, and injuries below L1 are generally less likely to lead to permanent neurologic deficit. This is not to say that compression at this level cannot be serious, and careful examination of the perineum for sensation as well as rectal tone is important in the evaluation of potential conus medullaris and cauda equina syndromes.

Treatment Options for Thoracolumbar Spine Fractures

COMPRESSION FRACTURES

NONOPERATIVE TREATMENT OF COMPRESSION FRACTURES

Indications/Contraindications

These are nearly always stable injuries, although examination of the posterior soft tissues is required to rule out any more

severe flexion-distraction injury. If there is concern for a higher energy injury, a CT scan is required to rule out a burst fracture (Fig. 21-11). Indications for nonoperative treatment are intact posterior soft tissues and kyphosis less than 40 degrees. The presence of disrupted posterior soft tissues implies the injury is more significant, such as a chance fracture, which is more likely to require operative intervention.

Techniques

An isolated compression fracture without neurologic involvement is the most common thoracolumbar fracture pattern and can nearly always be treated with immobilization with rest and activity modification. Molding a thoracolumbosacral orthosis (TLSO) into slight hyperextension at the fracture site will limit flexion, provides pain relief, and reduces further loading of the fracture. Alternatively, a less-constricting hyperextension brace is often well tolerated (Fig. 21-12).

Outcomes

Most fractures heal in 4 to 6 weeks without significant additional collapse, and radiographs should be obtained to follow the sagittal alignment. Long-term studies have suggested modest remodeling capacity of compression fractures occurring in childhood.[44,70,85] Asymmetric growth at the end plates seems to allow some correction in the wedged alignment over time in the skeletally immature patient. Long-term results of compression fractures have been generally favorable, although fractures of the end plates can be associated with later disc degeneration.[46]

Osteoporosis of a variety of etiologies may affect children and adolescents to a degree that predisposes them to insufficiency fractures that are most often compression fractures (Fig. 21-13). Multiple-level fractures are more frequent in this setting, and

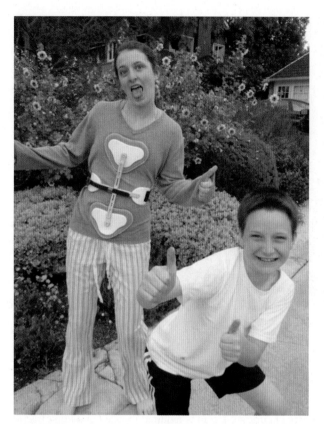

Figure 21-12. The editor's (DLS) daughter demonstrates good patient acceptance of a hyperextension brace for a two-level lumbar compression fracture treated for 6 weeks. (Used with permission of Children's Orthopaedic Center, Los Angeles Children's Hospital.)

problematic kyphosis may develop. Differentiating new from old fractures can be difficult if serial radiographs are not available. An MRI can be used to define fracture acuity based on the amount edema present within each vertebral body. A TLSO or hyperextension brace for a period of time longer than typically used for simple compression fracture healing may be necessary to prevent progressive kyphosis, though treating the primary cause of the osteopenia is critical to maintaining normal alignment in such cases. Evaluation by a Pediatric Endocrinologist and possibly assessment of bone density by dual-energy x-ray absorptiometry (DEXA) are advised.

OPERATIVE TREATMENT OF COMPRESSION FRACTURES

Indications/Contraindications

If the kyphosis associated with compression fractures markedly alters local sagittal alignment, surgical treatment may be considered. For example, 30 to 40 degrees of additional relative kyphosis than would be anticipated for that region of the spine. This is most frequent in multiple adjacent compression fractures that together create unacceptable focal region of relative kyphosis. Single-level compression fractures rarely require surgical stabilization.

Surgical Procedures

The preferred surgical treatment of such fractures is generally a posterior compression instrumentation construct that spans one or two levels above and below the affected vertebrae. Anterior surgical treatment is rarely required. The intact posterior vertebral wall provides a fulcrum to achieve kyphosis correction.

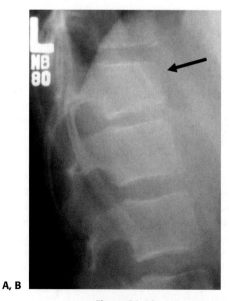
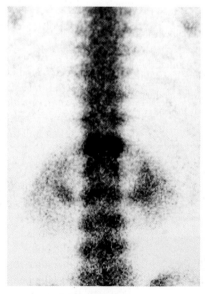
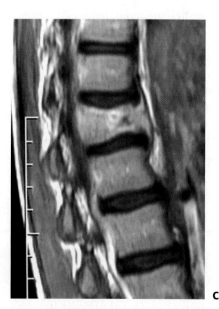

A, B   C

Figure 21-13. A: Lateral radiograph demonstrating what appears to be a routine compression fracture. The patient did not have a significant history of trauma; however, pain was present and a bone scan was obtained to further evaluate this site. *Arrow* demonstrates slight wedging of the vertebral body. **B:** The bone scan demonstrated markedly increased uptake, confirming an acute process and prompting additional study. **C:** An MRI was obtained, which demonstrated loss of height and a lesion within the anterior aspect of the vertebral body, which was later confirmed to be an infectious process.

The method of posterior fixation may be either hooks or pedicle screws. A posterior fusion over the instrumented segments ensures a lasting stable correction. Cadaver studies and clinical studies on the use of balloon vertebroplasty with calcium phosphate cement in adult patients are encouraging, as this technique may be a potentially viable option to treat compression fractures with significant angulation.[49,93,94]

BURST FRACTURES

NONOPERATIVE TREATMENT OF BURST FRACTURES

The treatment and classification of this fracture pattern are controversial areas of spinal trauma management. There are clearly some burst fractures that can be easily managed nonoperatively in a brace and others that collapse further, resulting in increased deformity unless surgically stabilized. Defining the characteristics of stable and unstable burst fractures has been attempted by several authors.[19,22,32,59,92] An additional compounding variable in the treatment algorithm is SCI, which is more frequent with burst fractures than with compression fractures.

Indications/Contraindications

Assuming an intact neurologic system, defining stable and unstable burst fractures has been attempted based on the degree of comminution, loss of vertebral height, kyphotic wedging, and integrity of the PLC. A load-sharing classification system assigns points based on comminution, fragment apposition, and kyphosis.[59] Although the Denis classification suggests that all burst fractures are unstable because of the involvement of at least two columns, it is clear that in many cases the addition of a third-column injury (PLC) is required to result in a truly unstable condition. Vertebral body translation of greater than 3.5 mm has been demonstrated to predict PLC injury.[71] Some advocate differentiating stable and unstable burst fractures solely on the integrity of the PLC.[84,101]

Techniques

When a burst fracture is deemed stable, it must be done so on a presumptive basis. In these patients, an extension molded cast or TLSO can be used with the goal of allowing an upright position and ambulation.[84] Frequent radiographic and neurologic follow-up is necessary to identify early failures. Depending on the age of the patient and severity of the fracture, immobilization is suggested for a duration of 2 to 4 months.

Outcomes

Studies of immature patients treated for burst fractures are uncommon,[50] yet much of the adult literature provides valuable information about the outcomes to expect following nonoperative treatment. Most of these fractures in adults heal with little change in kyphosis and function and minimal, if any, residual pain.[33,97] It is reasonable to expect adolescent patients to heal at least as well and probably even faster. Wood et al.[101] compared operative and nonoperative treatment in a prospective randomized study of patients with burst fractures who were neurologically intact with a normal PLC. The radiologic and functional outcomes were not substantially different, and these authors concluded that nonoperative treatment should be considered when the PLC and neurologic function are intact.[101] Functional outcome does not appear to correlate with the degree of spinal kyphosis, although long-term studies of scoliosis treatment do suggest that an alteration of sagittal alignment may be detrimental (flat back syndrome) in the long term.

OPERATIVE TREATMENT OF BURST FRACTURES

Indications/Contraindications

Fractures with three-column involvement, neurologic deficit, concomitant musculoskeletal injury, and thoracic/abdominal injury precluding the use of a brace are all considered indications for surgical management of burst fractures. Contraindications mainly center on medical conditions (coexisting or new) which make surgical intervention too risky.

Surgical Procedure

When surgical treatment is selected, either an anterior or posterior approach can be used, although this also remains controversial. Anterior stabilization generally involves discectomy and strut grafting that spans the fractured vertebra. Stabilization with a plate or dual-rod system is appropriate. Posterior options include pedicle screw fixation one or two levels above and below the fractured vertebra. Advances in the application of posterior instrumentation for thoracolumbar fractures have demonstrated encouraging, early outcomes with fracture stabilization without fusion and in minimally invasive surgical techniques.[83,96,98] The presence of a dural tear due to the retropulsed posterior wall fragment may also play a role when deciding how to approach the fracture.

The decision to proceed anteriorly or posteriorly for the surgical treatment of a burst fracture is largely dictated by surgeon preference and, to some degree, the features of the fracture. Posterior approaches are familiar to all surgeons and can easily be extended over many levels. In addition, a transforaminal lumbar interbody fusion (TLIF) can be performed if anterior interbody support is deemed beneficial to construct stability. Decompression of the spinal cord can be achieved by indirect or direct methods. Restoration of the sagittal alignment frequently leads to spontaneous repositioning of the posteriorly displaced vertebral body fracture fragments. If additional reduction of posterior wall fragments is required, direct fracture reduction can be accomplished with a posterolateral or transpedicular decompression.[28] This also allows additional anterior column bone grafting that may add structural integrity and speed fracture healing.

The anterior approach allows direct canal decompression through a corpectomy of the fractured vertebra. Structural strut grafting restores the integrity of the anterior column. With this graft, a load-sharing anterior plate or rod system completes the reconstruction. This approach deals most directly with the

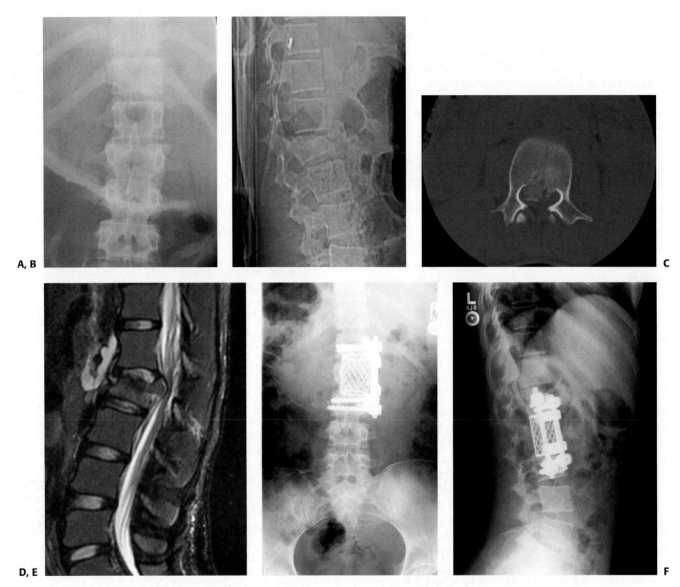

Figure 21-14. Burst fracture. **A:** This teenage patient presented with loss of vertebral body height associated with a motorcycle accident after jumping more than 20 ft. His neurologic examination was intact. **B:** CT scan confirmed a burst fracture component with very little retropulsion into the spinal canal. This appeared to be a stable injury and was initially managed with an orthosis. **C** and **D:** There was poor compliance with the orthosis and further collapse. **E** and **F:** Given the lack of compliance and progressive kyphosis, the patient underwent anterior reconstruction with an iliac crest strut graft and plating.

pathology, which in burst fractures lies within the anterior and middle vertebral columns (Fig. 21-14). Proponents of the anterior approach cite better biomechanical stabilization of the unstable spine, better correction of segmental kyphosis, and less loss of correction postoperatively.[79,80,100] In adults, a combined anterior and posterior approach may provide the best stability and sagittal alignment, especially in very unstable injuries. However, the increased morbidity with this approach is likely why it is not routinely in the pediatric/adolescent patient population.[73]

FLEXION-DISTRACTION INJURIES (CHANCE FRACTURES)

NONOPERATIVE TREATMENT OF FLEXION-DISTRACTION INJURIES (CHANCE FRACTURES)

Indications/Contraindications

The treatment of flexion-distraction injuries is dictated by the particular injury pattern and the associated abdominal injuries.

In general, these fractures are reduced by an extension moment that can be maintained with either a cast or internal fixation. A hyperextension cast or brace is ideal for younger patients (less than approximately 10 years) with a primary bony injury pattern and no significant intra-abdominal injuries as long as there is unacceptable kyphosis in the cast or brace. As described above, the posterior disruption may pass through ligaments or joint capsules in a purely soft tissue plane of injury or traverse an entirely bony path. The distinction is important, because bony fractures have the potential for primary bony union, whereas the severe ligamentous injuries are less likely to heal with lasting stability without surgical intervention.

Technique

Hyperextension cast or TLSO as detailed for compression and burst fractures.

Outcomes

Nonoperative treatment has been demonstrated to be effective in selected patients. The most frequent problem with the nonoperative approach has been progression of the kyphotic deformity.[1,4]

OPERATIVE TREATMENT OF FLEXION-DISTRACTION INJURIES (CHANCE FRACTURES)

Indications/Contraindications

The greater the degree of ligamentous/facet disruption, the more likely the need for stabilization with an arthrodesis of the injured motion segment. In addition, the greater the degree of injury

kyphosis, the more likely posttraumatic kyphosis will become a problem.[4] Healing of posterior ligamentous disruption is not reliable, though in very young children it may be possible.

Surgical Procedure

Options for internal fixation include posterior wiring in young children (supplemented with a cast) and segmental fixation in a primarily compressive mode (Fig. 21-15). This approach can decrease the injury kyphosis and maintain this alignment during the healing process. Operative treatment has been demonstrated to have a good clinical outcome in 84% of pediatric patients, compared with 45% in the nonoperative group.[4]

FRACTURE-DISLOCATIONS

OPERATIVE TREATMENT OF FRACTURE-DISLOCATIONS

Indications/Contraindications

These highly unstable injuries nearly always require surgical stabilization. When the spinal cord function remains intact, instrumented fusion gives the greatest chance for maintaining cord function. On the other hand, if a complete SCI has occurred, internal fixation will aid in the rehabilitation process, allowing early transfers and upright sitting.

Surgical Procedure

The typical procedure is a posterior instrumented fusion that extends at least two levels above and below the level of injury

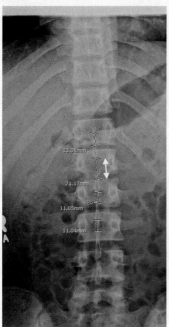
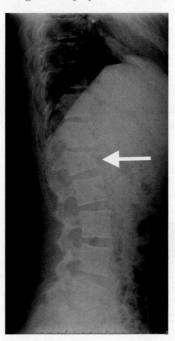
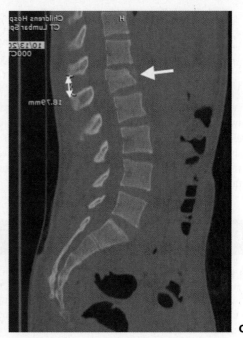

A, B   C

Figure 21-15. A: PA radiograph demonstrates increased distance between the spinous processes of T12 and L1 suggesting posterior ligamentous disruption. *Double headed arrow* indicates increased distance between spinous processes. **B:** Lateral x-ray demonstrates compression of L1. *Arrow* indicates anterior vertebral body compression fractures. **C:** CT demonstrates increased interspinous distance between T12 and L1 as well as compression of L1. *Double headed arrow* indicates increased distance between spinous processes. *Arrow* indicates anterior vertebral body compression fractures.   *(continues)*

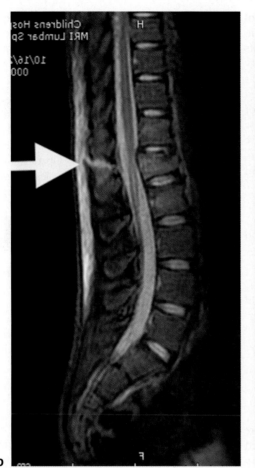
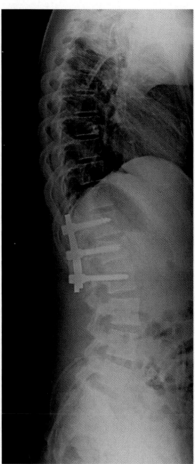

Figure 21-15. (*Continued*) **D:** Sagittal stir MRI shows increased signal at disrupted interspinous ligament (*arrow*). **E:** Posterior spinal fusion was performed with restoration of sagittal balance. Strong fixation obviated the need for postoperative bracing. Usually, only two-level fixation is necessary if the vertebral height has been maintained as in this case. (Used with permission of Children's Orthopaedic Center, Los Angeles Children's Hospital.)

to ensure restoration of alignment and stability. In cases of SCI below the age of 10 years (Fig. 21-16), a longer fusion may be considered to reduce the incidence and severity of subsequent paralytic scoliosis. Those injured after the adolescent growth spurt are at low risk for late deformity if the fracture is well aligned at the time of initial fixation (Fig. 21-17).

SPECIAL FRACTURES

End Plate Fractures

End plate fractures are essentially growth plate fractures similar to a Salter I fracture or Salter II fracture (with a tiny metaphyseal fragment) of long bones. It is thus a unique pediatric injury that does not occur in adults. There is almost always a history of a specific inciting event, such as kicking a soccer ball or landing in a gymnastics competition with sudden pain and sometimes hearing a "pop." The mechanism is thought to be related to flexion with a portion of the posterior corner of the vertebral body (ring apophysis) fracturing and displacing posteriorly into the

spinal canal. Symptoms may mimic disc herniation, although the offending structure is bone and cartilage rather than disc material.[24,26]

This injury is rarely noted on x-rays, and often misread on MRI as a bulging disc. The diagnosis is confirmed with CT, usually best visualized on a sagittal cut (Fig. 21-18).

On physical examination, the patients are in very significant pain, to the point where physicians at times wonder if they are exaggerating the pain. The pain is consistent with nerve roots being tented across the bony edge of a fresh fracture. While historically some have suggested observation will eventually lead to resolution, this is rarely if ever clinically tolerated. Injections are unlikely to help, and physical therapy is contraindicated as it is likely to exacerbate pain with little hope of benefit. Treatment is removal of the fracture fragment through a laminectomy. A TLSO for 4 to 6 weeks would allow rapid healing of this growth plate injury.

Facet Fractures

Lumbar and sacral facet fractures have been described as a likely underrecognized source of low back pain, particularly in

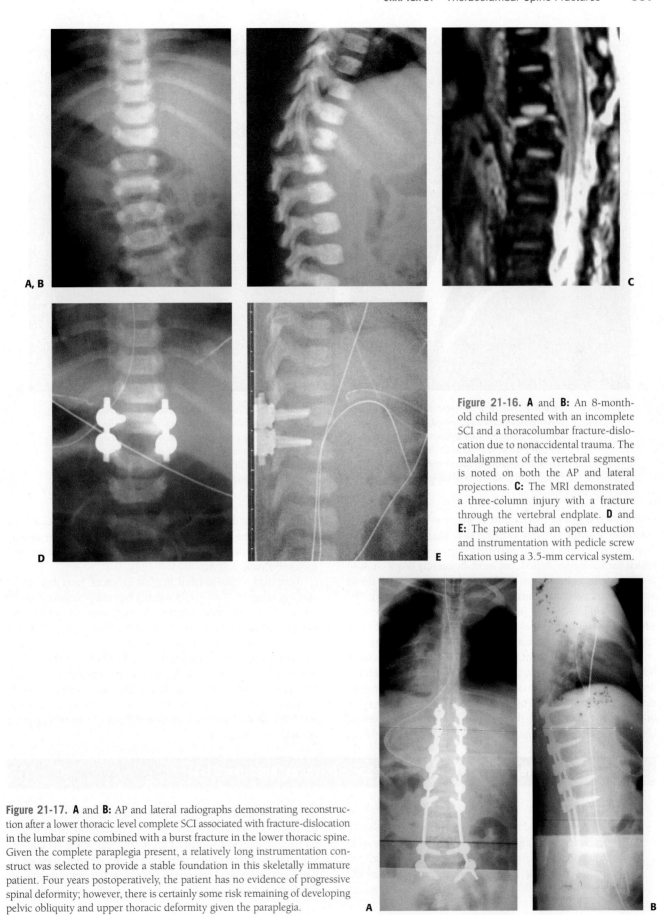

Figure 21-16. A and **B:** An 8-month-old child presented with an incomplete SCI and a thoracolumbar fracture-dislocation due to nonaccidental trauma. The malalignment of the vertebral segments is noted on both the AP and lateral projections. **C:** The MRI demonstrated a three-column injury with a fracture through the vertebral endplate. **D** and **E:** The patient had an open reduction and instrumentation with pedicle screw fixation using a 3.5-mm cervical system.

Figure 21-17. A and **B:** AP and lateral radiographs demonstrating reconstruction after a lower thoracic level complete SCI associated with fracture-dislocation in the lumbar spine combined with a burst fracture in the lower thoracic spine. Given the complete paraplegia present, a relatively long instrumentation construct was selected to provide a stable foundation in this skeletally immature patient. Four years postoperatively, the patient has no evidence of progressive spinal deformity; however, there is certainly some risk remaining of developing pelvic obliquity and upper thoracic deformity given the paraplegia.

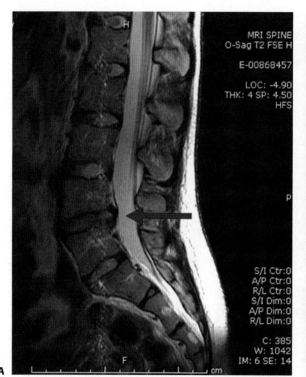 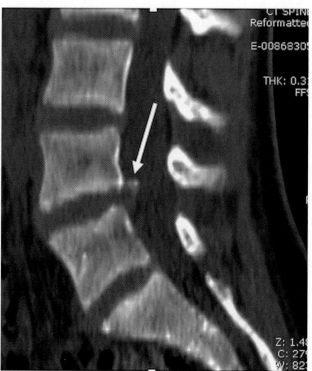

Figure 21-18. A: A 14-year-old girl felt a pop while kicking a soccer ball and had severe back pain. Months of steroid injections did nothing to relieve her pain. She was unable to walk or go to school. *Red arrow* demonstrates L4 inferior end plate fracture on MRI. **B:** CT scan confirmed diagnosis of an end plate fracture. Surgical removal of the intra-canal fragment adjacent to nerve roots relieved pain and the patient was able to return to soccer within a few weeks. *White arrow* more clearly demonstrates same injury on CT. (Used with permission of Children's Orthopaedic Center, Los Angeles Children's Hospital.)

young athletes.[87] The mechanism of injury is probably hyperextension with or without twisting that places stress on the facets. At times, the patient may remember a specific event in which the back pain started, but more frequently it is a chronic pain. An acute history tends to be more localized and those with chronic pain may have a wider distribution of pain. On physical examination, the pain is reproduced with hyperextension while standing. This should produce fairly localized back pain. If there is no back pain reproduced with hyperextension, one should be very hesitant to attribute the back pain to a facet fracture. The fractures are almost never seen on plane radiographs, and they are quite often missed by MRI. CT is the gold standard, and three-dimensional reconstructions are helpful both for identification of the fracture and surgical approach (Fig. 21-19). Injections or conservative care is highly unlikely

to help relieve the patient symptoms. An intra-articular fracture could cause joint damage, which would suggest removing this fragment sooner than later would help prevent arthritis and long-term pain.

Treatment of an isolated lumbar or sacral facet fracture is surgical removal. This could usually be accomplished through about a 16-mm incision using either a minimally invasive retractor set or standard retractors. Having the three-dimensional CT scan in the operating room is very helpful. At times, a bit of normal facet must be removed to see the fragment. At the time of surgery, the fragment is clearly mobile and usually surrounded by some inflammatory tissue. Removal tends to cause immediate pain relief and the patient may return to normal activities as tolerated. One may use the clinical analogy of removing a piece of sand from one's eye.

Authors' Preferred Treatment for Thoracolumbar Spine Fractures (Algorithm 21-1)

Compression Fractures

Nearly all are managed nonoperatively in an off-the-shelf TLSO brace. Occasionally, a fracture is too proximal for such an orthosis and an extension to the chin/occiput is required. For fractures proximal to T6, a Minerva brace is used. These fractures typically heal within 4 to 6 weeks, when

the immobilization can be discontinued. Activities should be limited for an additional 6 weeks. Compression fractures with more than 50% loss of anterior vertebral height are considered for either a closed reduction in an extension molded body cast or surgical correction with posterior instrumentation. The determination of which of these two approaches to

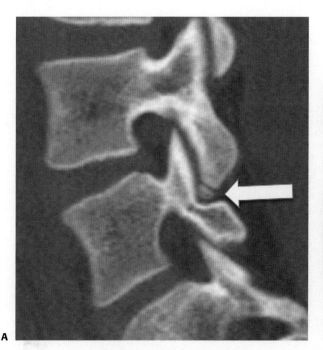

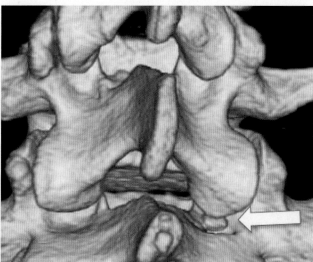

A

B

Figure 21-19. A: A 16-year-old year-round club soccer player had chronic pain eventually preventing him from playing soccer. He had localized pain on the right side of L4 with back extension. **A:** Sagittal image demonstrates fracture at the inferior facet of L4. **B:** 3D CT scan helps one determine the surgical approach and identify anatomic landmarks. Surgical removal offered immediate relief. Patient played soccer for many years afterwards without back pain. (Used with permission of Children's Orthopaedic Center, Los Angeles Children's Hospital.)

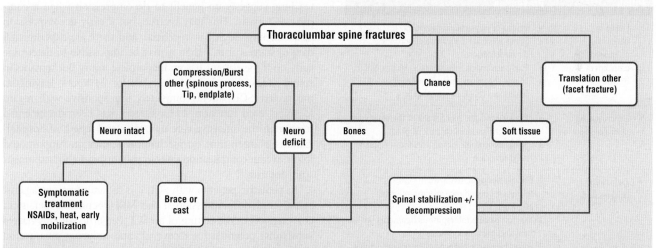

Algorithm 21-1. Authors' preferred treatment for thoracolumbar spine fractures.

choose is based on associated injuries and a discussion with the family. Compression fractures associated with neurologic injury are managed surgically to allow for early rehabilitation and optimize neurologic recovery.

Burst Fractures

Our preferred approach to neurologically intact patients with burst fractures is nonoperative in light of recent studies. If the neurologic status is normal and the posterior soft tissues are intact, a TLSO or cast is used for 3 months. A cast is used when

local kyphosis is more than 20 degrees, and the cast is placed in a hyperextension position in an attempt to restore sagittal alignment. An anterior decompression could be performed for canal compromise, especially when greater than 50% of spinal canal volume. In the lumbar spine, posterior instrumentation with the restoration of normal sagittal profile and some distraction can reduce the fracture and open up the canal assuming the posterior ligament is intact, which it should be for a compression fracture. In the lumbar spine, a small laminectomy can assist in decompression from the posterior approach.

Flexion-Distraction Injuries

Our treatment of Chance fractures is based on two findings: associated abdominal injuries and the presence of a ligamentous component to the fracture. If either exists, surgical treatment is the preferred approach. Casting or a well-molded brace in extension is appropriate for fractures that transverse an entirely bony plane without intra-abdominal pathology. A thigh extension may be incorporated into the cast for greater control of lumbar lordosis. Surgical treatment is by a posterior approach and includes only the involved vertebrae. Monosegmental pedicle screw fixation is generally preferred.

Fracture-Dislocations

Posterior surgery is the treatment of choice for all fracture-dislocations with or without neurologic injury (see Fig. 21-19). The timing of such intervention depends on the associated injuries and the ability of the patient to tolerate surgical intervention; however, stabilization as early as possible is preferred, with consideration to associated injuries and operating room team optimization. SCI nearly always complicates the management of these injuries, and a deteriorating neurologic examination makes surgical treatment of the spine an emergency that should be treated as quickly as possible.

Steroid Treatment

Methylprednisolone sodium succinate (MPSS) has been studied as a pharmacological adjunct that may be given to patients with acute SCI to improve neurological recovery. It became the standard of care in adults, despite a lack of evidence supporting clinical benefit.[10,11] Recent studies in adolescent and pediatric patients have demonstrated increased complication rates associated with steroid use including hyperglycemia and infection rates.[13,16,27] Additionally, a recent systematic review and consensus-based expert panel recommended that there was no evidence to support the use of neuroprotective approaches for the treatment of SCI in children.[66] As such, our current practice is to not use MPSS in the acute trauma setting.

POTENTIAL PITFALLS AND PREVENTIVE MEASURES FOR THORACOLUMBAR SPINE FRACTURE

Thoracolumbar Spine Fracture: PITFALLS AND PREVENTIONS	
Pitfall	**Prevention**
• Delay in diagnosis or missed associated injuries	• Through physical examination. • Serial physical examination with clear documentation. • Early advanced imaging (CT and/or MRI). • Image the entire spine to identify additional levels of spinal injury.
• Deteriorating neurologic status	• Understand the mechanics of the injury to develop a rational treatment plan. • Serial neurologic exams to monitor spinal cord function.
• Deformity progression	1. Follow nonoperative patients closely to ensure compliance and maintained alignment. 2. Do not assume interspinous ligaments will heal and prevent kyphosis. 3. Anticipate development of spinal deformity in SCI in patients <10 years and treat accordingly.

SUMMARY, CONTROVERSIES, AND FUTURE DIRECTIONS RELATED TO THORACOLUMBAR SPINE FRACTURES

Several areas of controversy remain with regard to the management of pediatric thoracolumbar fractures and associated SCI. These include both nonoperative and operative methods of treatment. Investigations into the benefits of steroids, cooling therapy, or other neuroprotective techniques in mitigating the effects of the secondary phase of SCI that follows the acute trauma have been mixed. The timing and necessity of spinal decompression for an SCI also remains debated. Traditional teaching suggests no benefit to decompression when a complete SCI exists. This may be true, but if early decompression of an incomplete SCI is beneficial, and there are experimental data to suggest it is,[65] then it may be impossible to determine early on if the patient has an incomplete injury but remains in spinal shock. Spinal shock may last for 24 hours, leaving an incomplete SCI patient completely unresponsive with regard to spinal cord function. Early surgery has been documented to shorten the intensive care unit stays and length of hospitalizations, shorten time on mechanical ventilation support, and lower overall complication rates in patients with thoracolumbar spine injuries.[18]

In pediatric patients with SCI, it is difficult to argue against spinal cord decompression if the MRI documents persistent compression in the setting of an SCI. Pediatric patients have a substantial potential for recovery,[66] and reducing pressure on the neural elements may be important in maximizing functional recovery. There is little controversy if spinal cord function is deteriorating in a patient with a known compressive lesion. This is an emergency that warrants decompression by either an anterior or posterior approach. Realignment of the spinal column and removal of fragments from the canal are required. The exact surgical approach depends on the location of offending structures and the nature of the instability.

Annotated References

Reference	Annotation
Bellabarba C, Fisher C, Chapman JR, et al. Does early fracture fixation of thoracolumbar spine fractures decrease morbidity and mortality? *Spine (Phila Pa 1976)*. 2010;35:S138–S145.	Systematic review of articles published from 1990 to 2008 that concluded that patients with unstable thoracic fractures should undergo early (<72 hours) stabilization of their injury to reduce morbidity, and possibly mortality.
Caruso MC, Daugherty MC, Moody SM, et al. Lesson learned from administration of high-dose methylprednisolone sodium succinate for acute pediatric spinal cord injuries. *J Neurosurg Pediatr*. 2017;20:567–574.	Single-center review of 354 patients concluding that pediatric patients who received high-dose methylprednisolone sodium succinate for acute spinal cord injury were significantly more likely to experience complications.
Denis F. The three column spine and its significance in the classification of acute thoracolumbar spinal injuries. *Spine (Phila Pa 1976)*. 1983;8:817–831.	Classic article that reviewed 412 thoracolumbar injuries to classify them into four different categories: compression fractures, burst fracture, seatbelt-type injuries, and fracture dislocations.
Lee HM, Kim HS, Kim DJ, et al. Reliability of magnetic resonance imaging in detecting posterior ligament complex injury in thoracolumbar spinal fractures. *Spine (Phila Pa 1976)*. 2000;25:2079–2084.	Prospective study of 34 patients with thoracolumbar spinal fractures that demonstrated that fat-suppressed T2-weighted sagittal sequence is a highly sensitive, specific, and accurate method of evaluating posterior ligamentous complex injury.
Mahan ST, Mooney DP, Karlin LI, et al. Multiple level injuries in pediatric spinal trauma. *J Trauma*. 2009;67:537–542.	Single-center retrospective review of 195 patients that found that pediatric spine injuries are more common in patients over age 8 and that these patients are more likely to have multiple levels of injury (similar to the adult population).
Pang D, Wilberger JE Jr. Spinal cord injury without radiographic abnormalities in children. *J Neurosurg*. 1982;57:114–129.	Retrospective review of 24 children treated between 1960 and 1980 with spinal cord injury without radiographic abnormality. This article reports on the proposed mechanism of injury and the grim long-term prognosis for neurologic recovery in their cohort.
Radcliff K, Su BW, Kepler CK, et al. Correlation of posterior ligamentous complex injury and neurological injury to loss of vertebral body height, kyphosis, and canal compromise. *Spine (Phila Pa 1976)*. 2012;37:1142–1150.	Retrospective case–control study which demonstrated that loss of vertebral body height and local kyphosis were not predictive of posterior ligamentous complex (PLC) injury. Translation greater than 3.5 mm was associated with PLC injury.
Vaccaro AR, Lehman RA JR, Hulbert RJ, et al. A new classification of thoracolumbar injuries: the importance of injury morphology, the integrity of the posterior ligamentous complex, and neurologic status. *Spine (Phila Pa 1976)*. 2005;30:2325–2333.	Proposed the Thoracolumbar Injury Classification and Severity Score (TLICS) to facilitate clinical decision-making and improve communication between providers regarding these complex injuries.
Weinstein JN, Collalto P, Lehmann TR. Thoracolumbar "burst" fractures treated conservatively: a long-term follow-up. *Spine (Phila Pa 1976)*. 1988;13:33–38.	Retrospective review of 42 patients followed for an average of 20 years concluding that nonoperative treatment of thoracolumbar burst fractures is a viable alternative in patients without neurologic deficit and can lead to acceptable long-term results.

REFERENCES

1. Andras LM, Skaggs KF, Badkoobehi H, et al. Chance fractures in the pediatric population are often misdiagnosed. *J Pediatr Orthop*. 2016. doi: 10.1097/BPO.0000000000000925.
2. Angelliaume A, Bouty A, Sales De Gauzy J, et al. Post-trauma scoliosis after conservative treatment of thoracolumbar spinal fracture in children and adolescents: results in 48 patients. *Eur Spine J*. 2016;25:1144–1152.
3. Antevil JL, Sise MJ, Sack DI, et al. Spiral computed tomography for the initial evaluation of spine trauma: a new standard of care? *J Trauma*. 2006;61:382–387.
4. Arkader A, Warner WC, Tolo VT, et al. Pediatric chance fractures: a multicenter perspective. *J Pediatr Orthop*. 2011;31:741–744.
5. Augutis M, Levi R. Pediatric spinal cord injury in Sweden: incidence, etiology and outcome. *Spinal Cord*. 2003;41:328–336.
6. Baghaie M, Gillet P, Dondelinger RF, et al. Vertebra plana: benign or malignant lesion? *Pediatr Radiol*. 1996;26:431–433.
7. Beaunoyer M, St-Vil D, Lallier M, et al. Abdominal injuries associated with thoracolumbar fractures after motor vehicle collision. *J Pediatr Surg*. 2001;36:760–762.
8. Bellabarba C, Fisher C, Chapman JR, et al. Does early fracture fixation of thoracolumbar spine fractures decrease morbidity and mortality? *Spine (Phila Pa 1976)*. 2010;35:S138–S145.
9. Bosch PP, Vogt MT, Ward WT. Pediatric spinal cord injury without radiographic abnormality (SCIWORA): the absence of occult instability and lack of indication for bracing. *Spine (Phila Pa 1976)*. 2002;27:2788–2800.
10. Bracken MB. Methylprednisolone in the management of acute spinal cord injuries. *Med J Aust*. 1990;153:368.
11. Bracken MB, Shepard MJ, Holford TR, et al. Administration of methylprednisolone for 24 or 48 hours or tirilazad mesylate for 48 hours in the treatment of acute spinal cord injury: results of the third national acute spinal cord injury randomized controlled trial. National Acute Spinal Cord Injury Study. *JAMA*. 1997;277:1597–1604.
12. Caffaro MF, Avanzi O. Can the interpedicular distance reliably assess the severity of thoracolumbar burst fractures? *Spine (Phila Pa 1976)*. 2012;37:E231–E236.
13. Cage JM, Knox JB, Wimberly RL, et al. Complications associated with high-dose corticosteroid administration in children with spinal cord injury. *J Pediatr Orthop*. 2015;35:687–692.
14. Carreon LY, Glassman SD, Campbell MJ. Pediatric spine fractures: a review of 137 hospital admissions. *J Spinal Disord Tech*. 2004;17:477–482.
15. Carrion WV, Dormans JP, Drummond DS, et al. Circumferential growth plate fracture of the thoracolumbar spine from child abuse. *J Pediatr Orthop*. 1996;16:210–214.
16. Caruso MC, Daugherty MC, Moody SM, et al. Lesson learned from administration of high-dose methylprednisolone sodium succinate for acute pediatric spinal cord injuries. *J Neurosurg Pediatr*. 2017;20:567–574.
17. Catz A, Thaleisnik M, Fishel B, et al. Recovery of neurologic function after spinal cord injury in Israel. *Spine (Phila Pa 1976)*. 2002;27:1733–1735.
18. Chipman JG, Deuser WE, Beilman GJ. Early surgery for thoracolumbar spine injuries decreases complications. *J Trauma*. 2004;56:52–57.

19. Chow GH, Nelson BJ, Gebhard JS, et al. Functional outcome of thoracolumbar burst fractures managed with hyperextension casting or bracing and early mobilization. *Spine (Phila Pa 1976)*. 1996;21:2170–2175.

20. Cirak B, Ziegfeld S, Knight VM, et al. Spinal injuries in children. *J Pediatr Surg*. 2004; 39:607–612.

21. Cui S, Busel GA, Puryear AS. Temporary percutaneous pedicle screw stabilization without fusion of adolescent thoracolumbar spine fracture. *J Pediatr Orthop*. 2016; 36:701–708.

22. Denis F. The three column spine and its significance in the classification of acute thoracolumbar spinal injuries. *Spine (Phila Pa 1976)*. 1983;8:817–831.

23. Diamond P, Hansen CM, Christofersen MR. Child abuse presenting as a thoracolumbar spinal fracture dislocation: a case report. *Pediatr Emerg Care*. 1994;10:83–86.

24. Dietemann JL, Runge M, Badoz A, et al. Radiology of posterior lumbar apophyseal ring fractures: report of 13 cases. *Neuroradiology*. 1988;30:337–344.

25. Dogan S, Safavi-Abbasi S, Theodore N, et al. Thoracolumbar and sacral spinal injuries in children and adolescents: a review of 89 cases. *J Neurosurg*. 2007;106:426–433.

26. Epstein NE, Epstein JA. Limbus lumbar vertebral fractures in 27 adolescents and adults. *Spine (Phila Pa 1976)*. 1991;16:962–966.

27. Galandiuk S, Raque G, Appel S, et al. The two-edged sword of large-dose steroids for spinal cord trauma. *Ann Surg*. 1993;218:419–425.

28. Gambardella G, Coman TC, Zaccone C, et al. Posterolateral approach in the treatment of unstable vertebral body fractures of the thoracic-lumbar junction with incomplete spinal cord injury in the paediatric age group. *Childs Nerv Syst*. 2003; 19:35–41.

29. Garcia RA, Gaebler-Spira D, Sisung C, et al. Functional improvement after pediatric spinal cord injury. *Am J Phys Med Rehabil*. 2002;81:458–463.

30. Garg S, Mehta S, Dormans JP. Langerhans cell histiocytosis of the spine in children. Long-term follow-up. *J Bone Joint Surg Am*. 2004;86-A:1740–1750.

31. Gellad FE, Levine AM, Joslyn JN, et al. Pure thoracolumbar facet dislocation: clinical features and CT appearance. *Radiology*. 1986;161:505–508.

32. Gertzbein SD, Court-Brown CM. Rationale for the management of flexion-distraction injuries of the thoracolumbar spine based on a new classification. *J Spinal Disord*. 1989;2:176–183.

33. Gnanenthiran SR, Adie S, Harris IA. Nonoperative versus operative treatment for thoracolumbar burst fractures without neurologic deficit: a meta-analysis. *Clin Orthop Relat Res*. 2012;470:567–577.

34. Grabb PA, Pang D. Magnetic resonance imaging in the evaluation of spinal cord injury without radiographic abnormality in children. *Neurosurgery*. 1994;35:406–414.

35. Green RA, Saifuddin A. Whole spine MRI in the assessment of acute vertebral body trauma. *Skeletal Radiol*. 2004;33:129–135.

36. Griffet J, Bastiani-Griffet F, El-Hayek T, et al. Management of seat-belt syndrome in children: gravity of 2-point seat-belt. *Eur J Pediatr Surg*. 2002;12:63–66.

37. Hadley MN, Zabramski JM, Browner CM, et al. Pediatric spinal trauma: review of 122 cases of spinal cord and vertebral column injuries. *J Neurosurg*. 1988;68:18–24.

38. Haffner DL, Hoffer MM, Wiedebusch R. Etiology of children's spinal injuries at Rancho Los Amigos. *Spine (Phila Pa 1976)*. 1993;18:679–684.

39. Hashimoto T, Kaneda K, Abumi K. Relationship between traumatic spinal canal stenosis and neurologic deficits in thoracolumbar burst fractures. *Spine (Phila Pa 1976)*. 1988;13:1268–1272.

40. Holmes JF, Miller PQ, Panacek EA, et al. Epidemiology of thoracolumbar spine injury in blunt trauma. *Acad Emerg Med*. 2001;8:866–872.

41. Inaba K, Kirkpatrick AW, Finkelstein J, et al. Blunt abdominal aortic trauma in association with thoracolumbar spine fractures. *Injury*. 2001;32:201–207.

42. Joaquim AF, de Almeida Bastos DC, Jorge Torres HH, et al. Thoracolumbar injury classification and injury severity score system: a literature review of its safety. *Global Spine J*. 2016;6:80–85.

43. Junkins EP Jr, Stotts A, Santiago R, et al. The clinical presentation of pediatric thoracolumbar fractures: a prospective study. *J Trauma*. 2008;65:1066–1071.

44. Karlsson MK, Moller A, Hasserius R, et al. A modeling capacity of vertebral fractures exists during growth: an up-to-47-year follow-up. *Spine (Phila Pa 1976)*. 2003;28:2087–2092.

45. Kerslake RW, Jaspan T, Worthington BS. Magnetic resonance imaging of spinal trauma. *Br J Radiol*. 1991;64:386–402.

46. Kerttula LI, Serlo WS, Tervonen OA, et al. Posttraumatic findings of the spine after earlier vertebral fracture in young patients: clinical and MRI study. *Spine (Phila Pa 1976)*. 2000;25:1104–1108.

47. Kim YM, Kim DS, Choi ES, et al. Nonfusion method in thoracolumbar and lumbar spinal fractures. *Spine (Phila Pa 1976)*. 2011;36:170–176.

48. Kleinman PK, Marks SC. Vertebral body fractures in child abuse: radiologic-histopathologic correlates. *Invest Radiol*. 1992;27:715–722.

49. Korovessis P, Repantis T, Petsinis G, et al. Direct reduction of thoracolumbar burst fractures by means of balloon kyphoplasty with calcium phosphate and stabilization with pedicle-screw instrumentation and fusion. *Spine (Phila Pa 1976)*. 2008;33:E100–E108.

50. Lalonde F, Letts M, Yang JP, et al. An analysis of burst fractures of the spine in adolescents. *Am J Orthop (Belle Mead NJ)*. 2001;30:115–120.

51. Lancourt JE, Dickson JH, Carter RE. Paralytic spinal deformity following traumatic spinal-cord injury in children and adolescents. *J Bone Joint Surg Am*. 1981;63:47–53.

52. Lee HM, Kim HS, Kim DJ, et al. Reliability of magnetic resonance imaging in detecting posterior ligament complex injury in thoracolumbar spinal fractures. *Spine (Phila Pa 1976)*. 2000;25:2079–2084.

53. Letts M, Davidson D, Fleuriau-Chateau P, et al. Seat belt fracture with late development of an enterocolic fistula in a child: a case report. *Spine (Phila Pa 1976)*. 1999;24:1151–1155.

54. Levin TL, Berdon WE, Cassell I, et al. Thoracolumbar fracture with listhesis: an uncommon manifestation of child abuse. *Pediatr Radiol*. 2003;33:305–310.

55. Limb D, Shaw DL, Dickson RA. Neurological injury in thoracolumbar burst fractures. *J Bone Joint Surg Br*. 1995;77:774–777.

56. Mahan ST, Mooney DP, Karlin LI, et al. Multiple level injuries in pediatric spinal trauma. *J Trauma*. 2009;67:537–542.

57. Mann DC, Dodds JA. Spinal injuries in 57 patients 17 years or younger. *Orthopedics*. 1993;16:159–164.

58. Mayfield JK, Erkkila JC, Winter RB. Spine deformity subsequent to acquired childhood spinal cord injury. *J Bone Joint Surg Am*. 1981;63:1401–1411.

59. McCormack T, Karaikovic E, Gaines RW. The load sharing classification of spine fractures. *Spine (Phila Pa 1976)*. 1994;19:1741–1744.

60. Meehan PL, Viroslav S, Schmitt EW Jr. Vertebral collapse in childhood leukemia. *J Pediatr Orthop*. 1995;15:592–595.

61. Meves R, Avanzi O. Correlation between neurologic deficit and spinal canal compromise in 198 patients with thoracolumbar and lumbar fractures. *Spine (Phila Pa 1976)*. 2005;30:787–791.

62. Mulpuri K, Reilly CW, Perdios A, et al. The spectrum of abdominal injuries associated with chance fractures in pediatric patients. *Eur J Pediatr Surg*. 2007;17:322–327.

63. Pang D, Pollack IF. Spinal cord injury without radiographic abnormality in children: the SCIWORA syndrome. *J Trauma*. 1989;29:654–664.

64. Pang D, Wilberger JE Jr. Spinal cord injury without radiographic abnormalities in children. *J Neurosurg*. 1982;57:114–129.

65. Papadopoulos SM, Selden NR, Quint DJ, et al. Immediate spinal cord decompression for cervical spinal cord injury: feasibility and outcome. *J Trauma*. 2002;52: 323–332.

66. Parent S, Mac-Thiong JM, Roy-Beaudry M, et al. Spinal cord injury in the pediatric population: a systematic review of the literature. *J Neurotrauma*. 2011;28:1515–1524.

67. Parisini P, Di Silvestre M, Greggi T. Treatment of spinal fractures in children and adolescents: long-term results in 44 patients. *Spine (Phila Pa 1976)*. 2002;27:1989–1994.

68. Patel AA, Vaccaro AR. Thoracolumbar spine trauma classification. *J Am Acad Orthop Surg*. 2010;18:63–71.

69. Pizones J, Izquierdo E, Alvarez P, et al. Impact of magnetic resonance imaging on decision making for thoracolumbar spine fracture diagnosis and treatment. *Eur Spine J*. 2011;20:390–396.

70. Pouliquen JC, Kassis B, Glorion C, et al. Vertebral growth after thoracic or lumbar fracture of the spine in children. *J Pediatr Orthop*. 1997;17:115–120.

71. Radcliff K, Su BW, Kepler CK, et al. Correlation of posterior ligamentous complex injury and neurological injury to loss of vertebral body height, kyphosis, and canal compromise. *Spine (Phila Pa 1976)*. 2012;37:1142–1150.

72. Reid AB, Letts RM, Black GB. Pediatric chance fractures: association with intra-abdominal injuries and seatbelt use. *J Trauma*. 1990;30:384–391.

73. Reinhold M, Knop C, Beisse R, et al. Operative treatment of 733 patients with acute thoracolumbar spinal injuries: comprehensive results from the second, prospective, internet-based multicenter study of the Spine Study Group of the German Association of Trauma Surgery. *Eur Spine J*. 2010;19:1657–1676.

74. Ribeiro RC, Pui CH, Schell MJ. Vertebral compression fracture as a presenting feature of acute lymphoblastic leukemia in children. *Cancer*. 1988;61:589–592.

75. Roche C, Carty H. Spine trauma in children. *Pediatr Radiol*. 2001;31:677–700.

76. Ruge JR, Sinson GP, McLone DG, et al. Pediatric spinal injury: the very young. *J Neurosurg*. 1988;68:25–30.

77. Rumball K, Jarvis J. Seat-belt injuries of the spine in young children. *J Bone Joint Surg Br*. 1992;74:571–574.

78. Santiago R, Guenther E, Carroll K, et al. The clinical presentation of pediatric thoracolumbar fractures. *J Trauma*. 2006;60:187–192.

79. Sasso RC, Best NM, Reilly TM, et al. Anterior-only stabilization of three-column thoracolumbar injuries. *J Spinal Disord Tech*. 2005;18:S7–S14.

80. Sasso RC, Renkens K, Hanson D, et al. Unstable thoracolumbar burst fractures: anterior only versus short-segment posterior fixation. *J Spinal Disord Tech*. 2006;19:242–248.

81. Satyarthee GD, Sangani M, Sinha S, et al. Management and outcome analysis of pediatric unstable thoracolumbar spine injury: large surgical series with literature review. *J Pediatr Neurosci*. 2017;12:209–214.

82. Sellin JN, Steele WJ 3rd, Simpson L, et al. Multicenter retrospective evaluation of the validity of the Thoracolumbar Injury Classification and Severity Score system in children. *J Neurosurg Pediatr*. 2016;18:164–170.

83. Shen WJ, Liu TJ, Shen YS. Nonoperative treatment versus posterior fixation for thoracolumbar junction burst fractures without neurologic deficit. *Spine (Phila Pa 1976)*. 2001;26:1038–1045.

84. Shen WJ, Shen YS. Nonsurgical treatment of three-column thoracolumbar junction burst fractures without neurologic deficit. *Spine (Phila Pa 1976)*. 1999;24:412–415.

85. Singer G, Parzer S, Castellani C, et al. The influence of brace immobilization on the remodeling potential of thoracolumbar impaction fractures in children and adolescents. *Eur Spine J*. 2016;25:607–613.

86. Sivit CJ, Taylor GA, Newman KD, et al. Safety-belt injuries in children with lap-belt ecchymosis: CT findings in 61 patients. *AJR Am J Roentgenol*. 1991;157:111–114.

87. Skaggs DL, Avramis I, Myung K, et al. Sacral facet fractures in elite athletes. *Spine (Phila Pa 1976)*. 2012;37(8):E514–E517.

88. Sledge JB, Allred D, Hyman J. Use of magnetic resonance imaging in evaluating injuries to the pediatric thoracolumbar spine. *J Pediatr Orthop*. 2001;21:288–293.

89. Smith AD, Koreska J, Moseley CF. Progression of scoliosis in Duchenne muscular dystrophy. *J Bone Joint Surg Am*. 1989;71:1066–1074.

90. Trigylidas T, Yuh SJ, Vassilyadi M, et al. Spinal cord injuries without radiographic abnormality at two pediatric trauma centers in Ontario. *Pediatr Neurosurg*. 2010; 46(4):283–289.

91. Vaccaro AR, Cumhur O, Kepler C, et al. AOSpine thoracolumbar spine injury classification system: fracture description, neurological status, and key modifiers. *Spine (Phila Pa 1976)*. 2013;38:2028–2037.

92. Vaccaro AR, Lehman RA Jr, Hulbert RJ, et al. A new classification of thoracolumbar injuries: the importance of injury morphology, the integrity of the posterior ligamentous complex, and neurologic status. *Spine (Phila Pa 1976)*. 2005;30: 2325–2333.

93. Verlaan JJ, van de Kraats EB, Oner FC, et al. Bone displacement and the role of longitudinal ligaments during balloon vertebroplasty in traumatic thoracolumbar fractures. *Spine (Phila Pa 1976)*. 2005;30:1832–1839.

94. Verlaan JJ, van de Kraats EB, Oner FC, et al. The reduction of endplate fractures during balloon vertebroplasty: a detailed radiological analysis of the treatment of burst fractures using pedicle screws, balloon vertebroplasty, and calcium phosphate cement. *Spine (Phila Pa 1976)*. 2005;30:1840–1845.

95. Wang MY, Hoh DJ, Leary SP, et al. High rates of neurological improvement following severe traumatic pediatric spinal cord injury. *Spine (Phila Pa 1976)*. 2004;29: 1493–1497.

96. Wang ST, Ma HL, Liu CL, et al. Is fusion necessary for surgically treated burst fractures of the thoracolumbar and lumbar spine? A prospective, randomized study. *Spine (Phila Pa 1976)*. 2006;31:2646–2652.

97. Weinstein JN, Collalto P, Lehmann TR. Thoracolumbar "burst" fractures treated conservatively: a long-term follow-up. *Spine (Phila Pa 1976)*. 1988;13:33–38.

98. Wild MH, Glees M, Plieschnegger C, et al. Five-year follow-up examination after purely minimally invasive posterior stabilization of thoracolumbar fractures: a comparison of minimally invasive percutaneously and conventionally open treated patients. *Arch Orthop Trauma Surg*. 2007;127:335–343.

99. Winslow JE 3rd, Hensberry R, Bozeman WP, et al. Risk of thoracolumbar fractures doubled in victims of motor vehicle collisions with cervical spine fractures. *J Trauma*. 2006;61:686–687.

100. Wood KB, Bohn D, Mehbod A. Anterior versus posterior treatment of stable thoracolumbar burst fractures without neurologic deficit: a prospective, randomized study. *J Spinal Disord Tech*. 2005;18:S15–S23.

101. Wood K, Buttermann G, Mehbod A, et al. Operative compared with nonoperative treatment of a thoracolumbar burst fracture without neurological deficit: a prospective, randomized study. *J Bone Joint Surg Am*. 2003;85:773–781.

102. Yucesoy K, Yuksel KZ. SCIWORA in MRI era. *Clin Neurol Neurosurg*. 2008; 110(5):429–433.

Pelvic and Acetabular Fractures

Wudbhav N. Sankar, James J. McCarthy, and Martin J. Herman

Introduction to Pelvic and Acetabular Fractures

INTRODUCTION TO PELVIC AND ACETABULAR FRACTURES

Pelvic and acetabular fractures in children vary from simple apophyseal avulsion and stress fractures to high-energy unstable pelvic ring injuries that are life-threatening. Pelvic and acetabular fractures in the pediatric population are quite uncommon. Pelvic fractures account for less than 1% of all pediatric fractures, but as many as 5% of children admitted to level 1 pediatric trauma centers with blunt trauma have pelvic fractures.[6,11,16,24,110] Although published studies focus on pelvic fractures from high-energy mechanisms, most pelvic fractures in children and adolescents occur from low-energy mechanisms and are stable ring injuries or avulsions of secondary ossification centers of the pelvis. Acetabular fractures, especially as isolated pelvic fractures, are rare in the pediatric age group.

Pediatric pelvic and acetabular fractures differ in important ways from adult pelvic fractures. Children in general have greater plasticity of the pelvic bones, increased elasticity of the sacroiliac (SI) joints and symphysis pubis, and thicker and stronger periosteum. Therefore, a relatively greater amount of energy can be dissipated before sustaining a pelvic fracture in a child as compared to an adult, and the relative force needed to sustain a pelvic fracture in a child is higher than in an adult.[14,91,95] The presence of the triradiate cartilage is another major difference. This critical physeal area is responsible for acetabular growth and development, acts as a stress riser in the pelvic ring, and is susceptible to permanent damage. These important differences correlate with clinical outcomes. Children involved in blunt trauma are less likely to sustain pelvic fractures, and those who do have generally less severe fractures, as compared with adults who sustain pelvic fractures blunt trauma.[97] Patients under 18 years of age tend to have better outcomes[111] and lower mortality rates associated with these injuries compared with adults and, when mortality occurs, it is more commonly related to associated injuries of the thorax, abdomen, and central nervous systems rather than direct blood loss from the pelvic injury.[6,11,16,24,31,39,55,74,91,103,110] When separating further the group of patients younger than 18 years of age who sustain pelvic fractures, however, overall adolescents have decreased mortality

and overall complication rates compared with both adults and children younger than 13 years of age.[52]

Most low-energy stable pelvic ring injuries and avulsions are treated through conservative measures. Unstable pelvic ring injuries may be a source of life-threatening hemorrhage in children. Coordinated management of a multidisciplinary trauma team and careful treatment of the associated head and thoracoabdominal injuries, in addition to pelvic ring fracture management, improve outcomes. Historically, most pelvic fractures, including unstable injuries, were treated nonoperatively. While many patients had satisfactory outcomes, some of those who healed with pelvic deformity had poor outcomes related to issues such as leg length inequality, low back and SI joint pain.

The experience extrapolated from the care of adults with pelvic fractures has led to a growing movement to treat selected cases surgically in an attempt to decrease long-term disability.[19,44,105] In addition, follow-up after acetabular fractures in children with at least 2 years of growth remaining is critical because damage to the triradiate cartilage may cause a long-term growth abnormality.[44,104] This may lead to hip dysplasia and subsequent hip pain and premature osteoarthritis.

ASSESSMENT OF PELVIC AND ACETABULAR FRACTURES

MECHANISMS OF INJURY FOR PELVIC AND ACETABULAR FRACTURES

Most pediatric pelvic fractures result from motor vehicle–related accidents.[6,11,74,91] These injuries are seen most commonly in children who are occupants of motor vehicles involved in collisions or who are struck by motor vehicles while riding a bicycle or other types of wheeled vehicles.[91] Other mechanisms include falls from motorized vehicles, such as all-terrain vehicles or motor bikes, falls from heights, and equestrian accidents. Sporting activities account for 4% to 11% of pelvic fractures, the majority of which are simple avulsion fractures of the secondary ossification centers of the growing pelvis. Avulsion injuries are the result of forceful contraction of large muscles, typically those which traverse both the hip and knee joints and have their origins on pelvic apophyses. Gymnasts typically sustain acute ischial tuberosity avulsion fractures from the violent pull of hamstring or adductor muscles, whereas soccer players more commonly sustain avulsions of the anterior-superior and anterior-inferior iliac apophyses, the result of contraction of the sartorius and rectus femoris muscles, respectively.[75] Iliac apophysitis is most frequently associated with long-distance running and is thought to result from repetitive muscle traction injury from the pull of the external oblique muscles of the abdomen.[12]

Much like pelvic ring fractures, acetabular fractures usually result from high-energy injuries, although sporadic cases of low-energy mechanisms from sports have been reported.[19,55] The mechanism of injury of acetabular fractures in children is similar to that in adults: the fracture occurs from a force transmitted through the femoral head to the articular surface

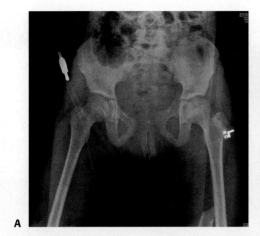
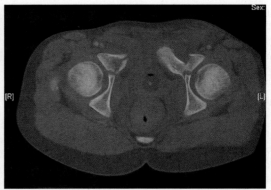

Figure 22-1. A: Pelvic radiograph showing a pelvic fracture with the left superior rami injury propagating toward the triradiate cartilage. **B:** CT scan showing the rami fractures propagating into the triradiate cartilage.

of the acetabulum. The position of the leg with respect to the pelvis and the direction of the impact determine the fracture pattern; the magnitude of the force determines the severity of the fracture or fracture-dislocation. For example, forces applied along the axis of the femur with the hip in a flexed position usually result in injury to the posterior aspect of the acetabulum. Fractures of the acetabulum are intimately associated with pelvic fractures. Some acetabular fractures involve only the hip socket. Others represent the exit point of a fracture of the pelvic ring. Pelvic fractures, particularly ramus fractures, may propagate into the triradiate cartilage (Fig. 22-1). Even fracture-dislocations of the SI joint have been associated with triradiate cartilage injuries.[47,84]

Child abuse is a rare cause of pelvic and acetabular fractures. The diagnosis of a pelvic fracture in infants and very young children, especially those without a reported history of high-energy injury, mandates a thorough investigation by the child protection team and child welfare services.

ASSOCIATED INJURIES WITH PELVIC AND ACETABULAR FRACTURES

While death rates in children who sustain pelvic fractures have been reported to be as high as 25%, most series report a mortality rate of 2% to 12% in children.[16,36,62,97] Significant hemorrhage that requires blood transfusion occurs in as many as 30% of patients with pelvic fractures and is most common in patients who sustain anterior and posterior pelvic ring fractures and those with unstable fractures. However, hemorrhage from pelvic fracture–related vascular injury is the cause of death in less than 1% of children as compared to 3.4% of adults who sustain pelvic ring and acetabular fractures.[30,39] One possible explanation for the low rate of hemorrhage relates to the lack of underlying atherosclerotic disease and the increased contractility of children's smaller arterial vessels, both of which result in greater vasoconstriction after injury.[36] In addition, children are injured typically in motor vehicle versus pedestrian accidents and therefore tend to sustain lateral compression forces,

or a combination of forces that yield mixed injury patterns, as opposed to anterior–posterior forces that cause the most common pelvic fractures patterns seen in adults. Injuries caused by laterally directed forces do not as commonly result in expansion of the pelvic ring or disruption of the SI joints, generally resulting in less intrapelvic hemorrhage.[31]

Associated injuries, rather than fractures about the pelvis, are more commonly the causes of morbidity and mortality in children and adolescents who are diagnosed with pelvic ring and acetabular fractures. Between 58% and 87% of children who sustain pelvic fractures have at least one associated injury and many have several.[11,24,30,74,91] The most common associated injuries are other fractures, particularly of the lower extremities and spine, which are identified in nearly half of children with pelvic fractures.[24,91,101] In one study of 79 children with pelvic fractures, patients with even one additional fracture demonstrated a significantly increased need for other nonorthopedic procedures.[106] The incidence of associated traumatic brain injuries varies from as little as 9% to nearly 50%[6,11,24,74,91] and clearly is the most important comorbidity that influences outcomes. Associated thoracoabdominal injuries occur at a rate between 14% and 33% in children with pelvic fractures.[4,11,14,25,80,83] These injuries are second only to head injuries as the primary cause of death in children with pelvic fractures and should be carefully ruled out in children who sustain serious pelvic ring or acetabular injuries.

Other less common injuries have been reported in children who sustain pelvic fractures. Vaginal and rectal lacerations are seen in 2% to 18% of children with pelvic fractures.[72,98] The incidence of these injuries is much higher in open fractures of the pelvis, a rare injury in children.[57] The surgeon must have a high index of suspicion for these types of injuries because early detection, appropriate irrigation and debridement, and repair of lacerations may prevent the development of infection. Genitourinary injuries, most commonly urethral tears and bladder disruptions, are diagnosed in 4% of patients who sustain fractures[24,98] but hematuria has been noted in up to 50% of children with pelvic fractures.[11,71,98] Female pediatric patients who have a pelvic fracture and have a vaginal laceration, disruption of the pelvic circle, multiple pelvic fractures, or a sacral spine injury are at higher risk for bladder and urethral injuries.[15] Peripheral nerve injury occurs in less than of 3% of children. Posterior or superior displacement of the hemipelvis or the iliac wing from severe pelvic ring disruption can cause tension on the lumbosacral plexus and sciatic nerve as they exit the pelvis.[72,93] A thorough neurologic examination of the lower extremities, including motor and sensory testing, and assessment of sphincter tone and perianal sensation should be routine in all patients with displaced fractures. Magnetic resonance imaging (MRI) is sometimes helpful to assess the integrity of the lumbosacral plexus. The superior gluteal nerve, the obturator nerve, sacral roots, and incomplete lumbosacral trunk injuries in particular are sometimes difficult to diagnose and may not be recognized until days to weeks after injury. Neurophysiologic studies are indicated in the recovery phase if deficits persist.

Thromboembolic events, including venous thromboembolism and pulmonary embolism, are uncommon in children, even in those with significant trauma. The current use of anticoagulation regimens varies greatly between institutions.[23,27,58] A clinical tool to predict the risk of developing venous thromboembolism (VTE) in pediatric trauma patients has been internally (not externally) validated, and may be an initial step toward the development of the specific VTE protocols for pediatric trauma patients.[13]

SIGNS AND SYMPTOMS OF PELVIC AND ACETABULAR FRACTURES

A full systematic examination of the child with a pelvic or acetabular injury is indicated. The patient will often be first seen in the trauma bay by a multidisciplinary trauma team. Other life-threatening issues may prevent a complete examination immediately, and the patient's mental status may be impaired. Secondary examinations after the patient is stabilized are critical to identify lesser injuries that may not have been as obvious initially.

Evaluation of a child with a suspected pelvic injury should begin with the assessment of the airway, breathing, and circulatory status, as with any polytraumatized patient.[100] The Glasgow Coma Score (GCS) is one method for assessing the patient's mental status; the reliability of the clinical exam is diminished for patients with a GCS less than 13 and aids in identifying patients with a closed injury. Aside from the primary pelvic evaluation, careful examination of the head, neck, and spine should be performed to assess for obvious spinal or head injury. A careful neurovascular examination, including evaluation of peripheral pulses in the lower extremities, should be part of the initial survey in all patients when possible. Documentation of the function of the muscles innervated by the lumbosacral plexus and the skin supplied by its sensory branches is sometimes difficult to fully assess in the acute setting but is especially important to perform for patients with possible severe pelvic trauma. A secondary survey, after stabilization of cardiovascular status and provisional treatment of obvious injuries, should include a careful repeat evaluation of

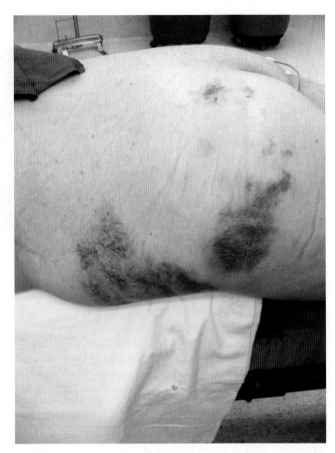

Figure 22-2. Clinical photograph of a Morel–Lavellee lesion, the result of an underlying unstable pelvic fracture. This is an internal degloving injury in which the skin and subcutaneous fat are sheared off the underlying muscle. (Reproduced with permission from Samir Mehta, MD.)

the axial skeleton and extremities as well a follow-up neurovascular evaluation.

After the primary survey, the evaluation specific to pelvic injuries begins with a complete inspection of the pelvis and perineum to evaluate for lacerations and ecchymosis. The child should be gently log-rolled to facilitate a complete inspection. The Morel–Lavellee lesion (a degloving injury in which the skin and subcutaneous fat is sheared from the underlying muscle, creating a large space where a hematoma can form) may be identified (Fig. 22-2). A careful genitourinary evaluation must be performed because of the intimate relationship between the pelvis, bladder, and urethra. Rectal examination has historically been recommended for children with significantly displaced fractures pelvic or if there is any blood in the perineal area. A more recent study, however, revealed that routine use of this examination for all patients may not be necessary, but should be reserved for patients at higher risk for more significant injury.[86,87]

Pelvic landmarks, including the anterior-superior iliac spine, crest of the ilium, SI joints, and symphysis pubis should be palpated. Manual manipulation should be performed carefully when needed. The maneuvers are often painful and if performed too vigorously may further displace the fracture or stimulate further intrapelvic bleeding. Pushing posteriorly on the anterior-superior iliac crest produces pain at the fracture site as the pelvic ring is opened. Compressing the pelvic ring by squeezing the right and left iliac wings together also causes pain, and crepitation may be felt if a pelvic fracture is present. Pressure downward on the symphysis pubis and posteriorly on the SI joints causes pain and possibly motion if there is a disruption. Pain with range of motion of the extremities, especially the hip joint, may indicate acetabular involvement or pelvic ring instability as well as other fractures or tendon and ligament injuries. Passive gentle flexion, abduction, and external rotation of the hip, known as the FABER test, will elicit pain in the posterior buttock and hip in cases of SI joint injury.

While classified as pelvic fractures, avulsion injuries present differently than the more serious pelvic ring disruptions and are seen in the outpatient setting more frequently than in the trauma bay. Avulsion fractures of the pelvis typically result in localized swelling and tenderness at the site of the avulsion fracture, often after a specific acute injury. Hip motion may be limited because of guarding, and pain may be mild or marked. In the case of repetitive stress injury, pain and limitation of motion are gradually progressive. In patients with

ischial avulsions, pain at the ischial tuberosity can be elicited by flexing the hip and extending the knee (straight-leg raising). Patients may also have pain while sitting or moving on the involved tuberosity. Avulsion fractures of the AIIS, ASIS, and iliac apophysis, in the acute setting, present with localized pain at these sites and tenderness to palpation over the affected apophysis.

IMAGING AND OTHER DIAGNOSTIC STUDIES FOR PELVIC AND ACETABULAR FRACTURES

Following initial stabilization of the child, all multitrauma patients and those with suspected pelvic or acetabular trauma should undergo an anteroposterior (AP) radiograph of the pelvis as part of the initial trauma series. Once the primary survey is completed and the patient is stable, region-specific radiographs should be obtained of any area with signs of trauma on secondary assessment.

Additional views, including the inlet/outlet and Judet views, are useful for further evaluation of pelvic ring injuries (Fig. 22-3). The inlet view is obtained by directing the x-ray beam caudally at an angle of 60 degrees to the x-ray plate. The inlet view is best for the determination of posterior displacement

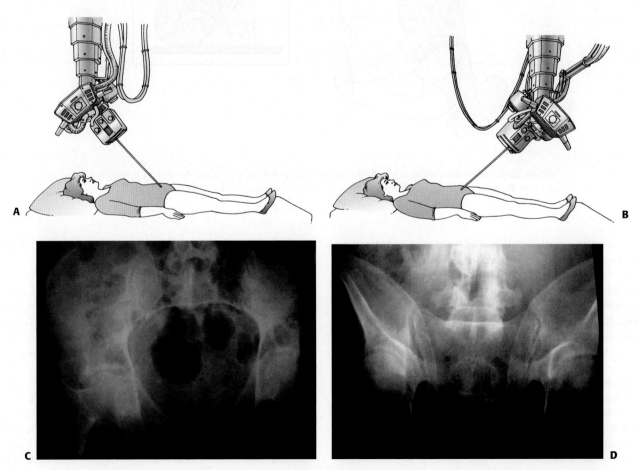

Figure 22-3. Schematic representing the direction of the incident x-ray beam for (**A**) inlet projection and (**B**) outlet projection of the pelvic ring. **C:** Inlet projection of the pelvic ring. **D:** Outlet projection of the pelvic ring.

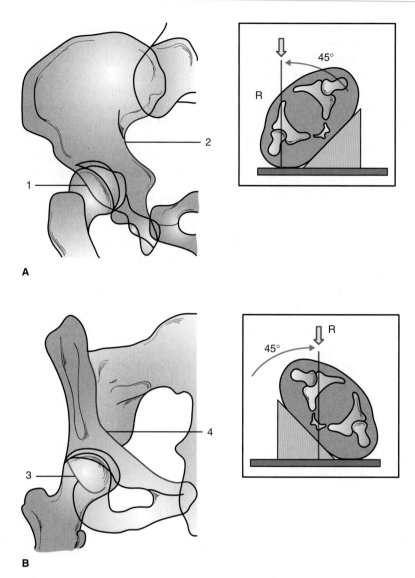

Figure 22-4. Judet views of the pelvis. **A:** Iliac Oblique (external) view. 1 is anterior wall, 2 is posterior column. **B:** Obturator Oblique (internal) view. 3 is posterior wall, 4 is anterior column.

of a hemipelvis or rami fractures. The outlet view is obtained by directing the x-ray beam in a cephalad direction at an angle of 45 degrees to the x-ray plate. The outlet view best demonstrates superior displacement of the hemipelvis or vertical shifting of the anterior pelvis.[100] Internal and external rotation views (also called Judet or oblique views) are primarily obtained when an acetabular fracture is identified (Fig. 22-4).

A number of studies have tried to identify clinical criteria which would effectively rule out the need for pelvic radiographs in childhood trauma patients.[32,43,45] Children being evaluated after blunt trauma who have a GCS score of 13 or higher but are without abdominal pain, an abnormal abdominal or pelvic examination, femur deformity, hematuria, or hemodynamic instability constitute a low-risk population for pelvic fracture, with less than 0.5% risk rate.[28] This population may not require routine pelvic imaging. The value of these criteria for avoiding radiation to the pelvis is a noble effort but its efficacy has not

yet been established and most polytraumatized children do not meet these criteria.

Computed tomography (CT) is the best modality to evaluate the bony pelvis, especially the details of potential injury of the SI joints, sacrum, and acetabulum. Most authors agree that CT is indicated if there is doubt about the diagnosis on the plain radiographs or if operative intervention is planned. Plain radiographs alone, however, allow classification of most pelvic fracture patterns routinely seen in children equally as well as CT.[3] For those with potential operative fractures, however, CT better defines the type of fracture and the degree and direction of displacement. CT imaging also can detect retained intra-articular bony fragments which may prevent concentric reduction of the hip joint for patients with concomitant hip dislocations or fracture patterns with intra-articular extension (Fig. 22-5).[9,10,26,55,90] This information is crucial for determining the best treatment option and selection of the operative approach.[51] Three-dimensional

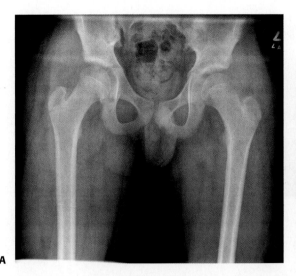
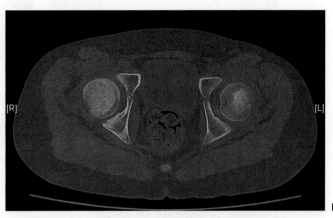

Figure 22-5. A: Postreduction anteroposterior pelvis radiograph of a 12-year-old with the left hip appearing nonconcentric. **B:** CT scan showing a bony fragment from the posterior wall impeding reduction.

CT reconstructions can give an excellent view of the overall bony fracture pattern but often underestimate the magnitude of cartilaginous fragments, especially of posterior wall fractures in children.[71] Many trauma centers routinely obtain CT scans of the abdomen and pelvis to assess patients for possible visceral injuries.

MRI currently has a minimal role in evaluation of the acute trauma patient, although this practice may evolve with quicker sequencing and better access. MRI is better than CT in delineating soft tissue injuries and does not emit ionizing radiation. Cartilaginous structures, such as posterior wall fractures associated with traumatic hip dislocations, or nonacute fractures, such as occult stress fractures or avulsion fractures, may be diagnosed more readily with MRI.[31,76] An MRI is recommended as an adjunctive imaging study for all pediatric acetabular fractures because MRI discloses the true size of largely cartilaginous posterior wall fragments in children (Fig. 22-6).[76] Particularly following a traumatic hip dislocation, any bony "fleck" visualized on postreduction CT scans or radiographs warrants an MRI, as it may represent a larger posterior labral osteochondral avulsion.[4]

Radioisotope bone scan is rarely indicated but may be useful for the identification of occult pelvic fractures or other acute injuries in children and adults with head injuries or multiple-system injuries.[34,91]

In children with avulsions of the pelvis, radiographs will usually show displacement of the affected apophysis. Avulsion injuries affect secondary centers of ossification before the center is fused with the pelvis, primarily in children of ages 11 to 17 years.[88] Comparison views of the contralateral apophysis, or the routine use of an AP pelvis x-ray instead of a view of the affected side only, help to ensure that what appears to be an avulsion fracture is not in reality a normal adolescent variant. Radiographs of children with delayed presentations of these injuries may demonstrate callus formation and these findings can occasionally mimic a malignant process. In this scenario,

MRI is helpful in distinguishing these pathologies from each other.

CLASSIFICATION OF PELVIC AND ACETABULAR FRACTURES

Pelvic Fracture Classification

Pediatric Classification

Pelvic Fractures in Children:
MODIFIED TORODE AND ZIEG CLASSIFICATION

I. Avulsion fractures
II. Iliac wing fractures
   a. Separation of the iliac apophysis
   b. Fracture of the bony iliac wing
III. Stable ring disruptions
   a. Simple anterior ring fractures involving pubic rami or pubic symphysis
   b. Stable anterior and posterior ring fractures
IV. Unstable ring disruptions
   a. "Straddle" fractures, characterized by bilateral inferior and superior pubic rami fractures
   b. Fractures involving the anterior pubic rami or pubic symphysis and the posterior elements (e.g., SI joint, sacral ala)
   c. Fractures that create an unstable segment between the anterior ring of the pelvis and the acetabulum

The original Torode and Zieg[103] classification based on plain radiographs, and its most recent modification based on radiographs and CT scans,[51] is the most commonly used classification of pediatric pelvic fractures. To create this classification, the authors reviewed the radiographs of 141 children with pelvic fractures and classified the injuries on the basis of the fracture pattern as well as their associated prognosis. The classification defines type I (avulsion fractures), type II (iliac wing fractures), type III (simple ring fractures), and type IV (ring disruptions) fracture patterns. The modified scheme,

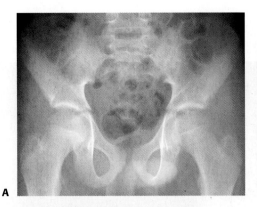

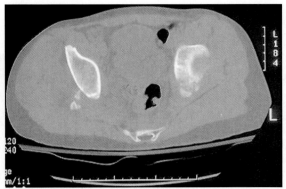

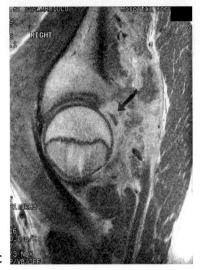

Figure 22-6. A: Postreduction radiograph of a left hip dislocation in a 12-year-old boy. **B:** CT scan demonstrates small ossified posterior wall fragments. **C:** Sagittal MRI demonstrates 90% posterior wall involvement with intra-articular step-off (*black arrow*). (Reprinted by permission from Springer: Rubel IF, Kloen P, Potter HG, et al. MRI assessment of the posterior acetabular wall fracture in traumatic dislocation of the hip in children. *Pediatr Radiol.* 2002;32(6):435–439. Copyright © 2002 Springer-Verlag.)

published 27 years after the original classification from the same institution, is identical to the earlier scheme but additionally divides type III "stable" simple ring injuries into IIIA (anterior only ring fractures) and IIIB (anterior and posterior ring fractures) (Fig. 22-7).[51] The morbidity, mortality, and complications are all greatest in the type IV group with "unstable" ring disruptions, but it should be emphasized that one "stable" pattern, type IIIB, also is associated with higher transfusion rates and morbidity compared with the other "stable" patterns. This classification does not include acetabular fractures.

Silber and Flynn[89] reviewed radiographs of 133 children and adolescents with pelvic fractures and classified them into two groups: immature (Risser 0 and all physes open) and mature (closed triradiate cartilage). These authors suggested that, in the immature group, management should focus on the associated injuries because the pelvic fractures rarely required surgical intervention compared with the group with mature pelvises. Fractures in the mature group were best classified utilizing adult pelvic fracture schemes and treated according to management principles utilized for adult patients.[7,63,91] This classification emphasizes the concept that pelvic ring injury patterns reflect the patient's skeletal maturity and not their chronologic age, an important factor to consider when evaluating and managing these injuries.

Adult Classifications

Pelvic Fractures in Adults:
TILE AND PENNAL CLASSIFICATION

A. Stable fractures
   A1. Avulsion fractures
   A2. Undisplaced pelvic ring or iliac wing fractures
   A3. Transverse fractures of the sacrum and coccyx
B. Partially unstable fractures
   B1. Open-book fractures
   B2. Lateral compression injuries (includes triradiate injury)
   B3. Bilateral type B injuries
C. Unstable fractures of the pelvic ring
   C1. Unilateral fractures
      C1-1. Fractures of the ilium
      C1-2. Dislocation or fracture-dislocation of the SI joint
      C1-3. Fractures of the sacrum
   C2. Bilateral fractures, one type B and one type C
   C3. Bilateral type C fractures

Pennal et al.[66] classified adult pelvic fractures according to the direction of force producing the injury: (a) AP compression, (b) lateral compression with or without rotation, and (c) vertical shear. This classification was modified and expanded by Tile et al.[99] Burgess et al.[9] further modified the Pennal system and incorporated subsets to the lateral compression and AP

Torode I

Torode II

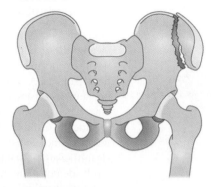

Torode III-A

Torode III-B

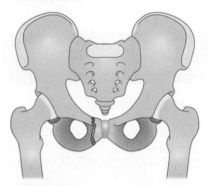
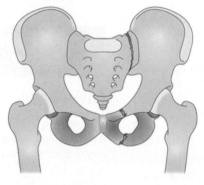

Torode IV

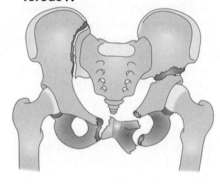

Figure 22-7. The modified Torode and Zieg classification. Torode I (avulsion fractures): avulsion of the bony elements of the pelvis, invariably a separation through or adjacent to the cartilaginous growth plate. Torode II (iliac wing fractures): resulting from a direct lateral force against the pelvis, causing a disruption of the iliac apophysis or an infolding fracture of the wing of the ilium. Torode III-A (simple anterior ring fractures): This group involved only children with stable anterior fractures involving the pubic rami or pubic symphysis. Torode III-B (stable anterior and posterior ring fractures): This new group involved children with both anterior and posterior ring fractures that were stable. Torode IV (unstable ring disruption fractures): This group of children had unstable pelvic fractures, including ring disruptions, hip dislocations, and combined pelvic and acetabular fractures. (Reprinted with permission from Shore BJ, Palmer CS, Bevin C, et al. Pediatric pelvic fracture: A modification of a preexisting classification. *J Pediatr Orthop.* 2012;32(2):162–168.)

compression groups to quantify the amount of force applied to the pelvic ring. These authors also created a fourth category, combined mechanical injury, to include injuries resulting from combined forces that may not be strictly categorized according to the classification scheme of Pennal.

Pelvic Fractures in Adults:
OTA/AO CLASSIFICATION

A. Stable fractures
B. Rotationally unstable fractures, vertically stable
C. Rotationally and vertically unstable fractures
 C1. Unilateral posterior arch disruption
  C1-1. Iliac fracture
  C1-2. Sacroiliac fracture-dislocation
  C1-3. Sacral fracture
 C2. Bilateral posterior arch disruption, one side vertically unstable
 C3. Bilateral injury, both unstable

The Tile classification has been incorporated into the Orthopaedic Trauma Association/AO classification, which is divided into bone segments, types, and groups.[69] The Orthopaedic Trauma Association/AO system classifies pelvic fractures on the basis of stability versus instability, and surgical indications are based on the fracture types. Surgery is rarely indicated for type A fractures, whereas anterior and/or posterior surgical stabilization may be indicated for type B and C fractures. Numerous subtypes are included, and are beyond the scope of this chapter.

In general, the basic classifications, (a) mature or immature pelvis and (b) stable or unstable fracture, are very useful for making treatment decisions. Hemodynamic parameters are a primary concern for management of pelvic injuries regardless of the specific pattern. From the standpoint of orthopedic management standpoint, however, if there is an extremely misshapen pelvic ring pelvis, a displaced posterior ring injury, or a displaced triradiate fracture, the injury should be considered

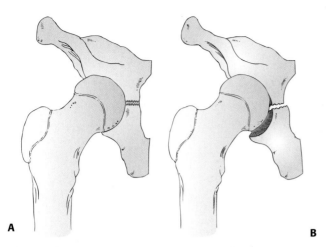

Figure 22-8. Types of triradiate cartilage fractures. **A:** Normal triradiate cartilage. **B:** Salter–Harris type I fracture.

unstable and will likely require surgical intervention regardless of the patient's age or the specific classification of the injury.

Acetabular Fracture Classification

Pediatric Classifications

Bucholz et al.[6] classified pediatric acetabular fractures based on the Salter–Harris classification (Fig. 22-8). Their classification system is used to help determine the prognosis of a triradiate cartilage injury that may result in a deformity of the acetabulum with growth. The anatomy of the triradiate is such that the superior weight-bearing portion of the acetabulum is separated from the inferior third by the superior arms of the triradiate cartilage. These superior arms are usually the ones involved in a fracture. In the Bucholz classification, a type I or II injury occurs from a traumatic force to the ischial ramus, pubic ramus, or proximal femur resulting in a shearing force through the superior arms of the triradiate cartilage. If there is a metaphyseal bone fragment, this is a type II fracture. A type V injury is a crush injury to the physis.[6,45] Watts[109] described four types of acetabular fractures in children: (i) small fragments that most often occur with dislocation of the hip, (ii) linear fractures that occur in association with pelvic fractures without displacement and usually are stable, (iii) linear fractures with hip joint instability, and (iv) fractures secondary to central fracture-dislocation of the hip.

Adult Acetabular Classification

Acetabular fractures in children can also be described similarly to those in adults, which are usually classified by the system of Judet et al.[40] and Letournel and Judet.[48] A more comprehensive system is the AO fracture classification, which groups all fractures into A, B, and C types with increasing severity. Type A acetabular fractures involve a single wall or column; type B fractures involve both columns (transverse or T-types) and a portion of the dome remains attached to the intact ilium; and type C fractures involve both columns and separate the dome fragment from the axial skeleton by a fracture through the ilium. Both of these classification systems are discussed in more detail in *Rockwood and Wilkins' Fractures in Adults.*[73]

OUTCOME MEASURES FOR PELVIC AND ACETABULAR FRACTURES

Outcome data have been assessed by several functional assessments; these outcome measure are not specific to pelvic fractures but are broadly applied outcome measures for traumatized patients. A national multicenter study is currently tracking outcomes using the WeeFim functional assessment.[62] Other measures used to evaluate the quality of life in trauma patients include the Child Health Questionnaire (CHQ), the Functional Independence Measure, the Impact of Family Scale,[76] and the Health-Related Quality of Life (HRQOL) scale.[75] Preliminary results demonstrate that 6-month functional scores after injury approach baseline levels,[62] despite the increased patient and family stress encountered.

PATHOANATOMY AND APPLIED ANATOMY RELATED TO PELVIC AND ACETABULAR FRACTURES

PELVIC AND ACETABULAR DEVELOPMENT

The pelvis of a child arises from three primary ossification centers: the ilium, ischium, and pubis. The three centers meet at the triradiate cartilage and fuse at approximately 12 to 14 years of age (Fig. 22-9).[70] The pubis and ischium fuse inferiorly at the pubic ramus at 6 or 7 years of age. Occasionally, at approximately the time of fusion of the ischium to the pubis, an asymptomatic lucent area is noted on radiographs in the midportion of the inferior pubic ramus, termed the ischiopubic synchondrosis. It is often bilateral, fuses completely in most children, and may be confused with an acute or stress fracture of the pelvis, or tumor or infection (see below) (Fig. 22-10).

Secondary centers of ossification arise in the iliac crest, ischium, anterior-superior iliac spine, anterior-inferior iliac spine, pubic tubercle, angle of the pubis, ischial spine, and the lateral wing of the sacrum; the first four centers listed are most important for understanding of pelvic avulsion fractures. Secondary ossification of the iliac crest is first seen at age 13 to 15 years and fuses to the ilium by age 15 to 17 years. This ossification pattern progresses from anterior to posterior (or lateral to medial when viewed on AP radiographs) and its time course of progression to fusion is the basis of Risser staging of skeletal maturity. The secondary ossification center of the ischium is first seen at 15 to 17 years and fuses at 19 years of age, although in some young adults it may fuse as late as 25 years of age. The ASIS develops as an apophysis of the anterior iliac crest at 13 years of age and fuses sometime around age 15. A center of ossification appears at the anterior-inferior iliac spine at approximately 14 years, fusing at 16 years of age.[63,70,109] Knowledge about the location, age of appearance, and fusion of the secondary centers are important in differentiating these centers from fractures and avulsion injuries. Chondro-osseous growth also occurs through "physes" in the pubis at the area adjacent to the symphysis pubis, in the ilium adjacent to the SI joint, and to a lesser extent in the lateral sacrum; symphyseal separations and SI joint injuries in children may represent fractures through these growth areas as opposed to ligamentous disruptions.[63]

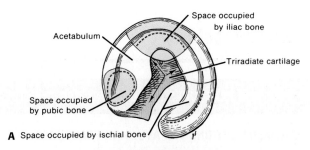

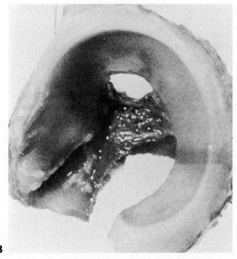

Figure 22-9. A: Triradiate-acetabular cartilage complex viewed from the lateral side, showing the sites occupied by the iliac, ischial, and pubic bones. **B:** Normal acetabular cartilage complex of a 1-day-old infant. The ilium, ischium, and pubis have been removed with a curette. The lateral view shows the cup-shaped acetabulum. (Reprinted with permission from Ponseti IV. Growth and development of the acetabulum in the normal child. Anatomical, histological, and roentgenographic studies. *J Bone Joint Surg Am.* 1978;60(5):575–585.)

The acetabulum contains the shared physes of the ilium, ischium, and pubis that merge to become the triradiate cartilage. Interstitial growth in the triradiate part of the cartilage complex causes the acetabulum to expand during growth and causes the pubis, ischium, and ilium to enlarge as well. The concavity of the acetabulum develops in response to the presence of a spherical head. The depth of the acetabulum increases during development as the result of interstitial growth in the acetabular cartilage, appositional growth of the periphery of this cartilage, and periosteal new bone formation at the acetabular margin.[70] The triradiate cartilage of the acetabulum closes at approximately 12 years of age in girls and 14 years of age in boys.[104] At puberty, three secondary centers of ossification appear in the hyaline cartilage surrounding the acetabular cavity. The os acetabuli, which is the epiphysis of the pubis, forms the anterior wall of the acetabulum. The epiphysis of the ilium, the acetabular epiphysis,[70,108] forms a large part of the superior wall of the acetabulum. The small secondary center of the ischium is rarely seen. The os acetabuli, the largest part, starts to develop at approximately 8 years of age and expands to form the major portion of the anterior wall of the acetabulum; it unites with the pubis at approximately 18 years of age. The acetabular epiphysis develops in the iliac acetabular cartilage at approximately 8 years and fuses with the ilium at 18 years of age, forming a substantial part of the superior acetabular joint surface (Fig. 22-11). The secondary center of the ischium, the smallest of the three, develops in the ninth year, unites with the acetabulum at 17 years, and contributes very little to acetabular development. These secondary centers are sometimes confused with avulsion fractures or loose bodies in the hip joint.

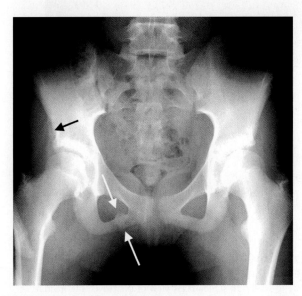

Figure 22-10. AP pelvis of 14-year-old girl demonstrating an asymptomatic ischiopubic synchondrosis (*white arrows*) and a healing ASIS avulsion (*black arrow*). (Used with permission of the Children's Orthopaedic Center, Los Angeles.)

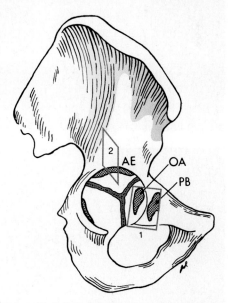

Figure 22-11. Right innominate bone of an adolescent. The os acetabuli (OA) is shown within the acetabular cartilage adjoining the pubic bone (PB); the acetabular epiphysis (AE), within the acetabular cartilage adjoining the iliac bone; and another small epiphysis (not labeled), within the acetabular cartilage adjoining the ischium (**left**). (Reprinted with permission from Ponseti IV. Growth and development of the acetabulum in the normal child. Anatomical, histological, and roentgenographic studies. *J Bone Joint Surg Am.* 1978;60(5):575–585.)

CHILD VERSUS ADULT PELVIS

As mentioned previously, there are important anatomic differences between the pelvis of a child and that of an adult:

- Greater bone plasticity and ligament elasticity that permit more bone deformation and greater mobility of the SI joints and symphysis pubis with trauma
- Thick periosteum, structural cartilage components, including the triradiate cartilage, that also permit more mobility of the ring but are susceptible to growth disturbance
- The presence of bone–cartilage apophyses toward the end of skeletal growth that are susceptible to avulsion fractures from violent contraction of attached muscles

Because of some of these differences, the pediatric pelvis is better able to absorb energy without significant displacement. Minimally displaced fractures and single breaks of the ring are frequently seen in pediatric pelvic fractures, a finding opposed to the traditional concept of a mandatory "double break" in the ring seen in adult fractures.[63] More importantly, a child may sustain a higher energy injury than suspected from the bony injury, making it crucial that the surgeon be aware that even minor pelvic fractures may be associated with other potentially serious injuries.

Pelvic Fractures

AVULSION FRACTURES (TORODE AND ZIEG TYPE I)

TREATMENT OPTIONS FOR AVULSION FRACTURES

Nonoperative Treatment of Avulsion Fractures

Of pelvic avulsion fractures reported in two large published series,[79] approximately 37% were avulsions of the anterior-inferior iliac spine, 31% were ischial tuberosity avulsions, 25% were avulsions of the anterior-superior iliac spine, and 6% were iliac crest avulsions. Some athletes experience more than one avulsion fracture over the course of their development. Most pelvic avulsion fractures in children heal satisfactorily with nonoperative management, including rest, careful extremity positioning to minimize muscle stretch, partial weight-bearing on crutches for 2 or more weeks, and physical therapy after symptoms improve. Typically, children resume normal activities by 6 to 8 weeks (Fig. 22-12). Two small series of adolescents with pelvic avulsion fractures treated

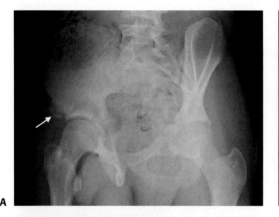

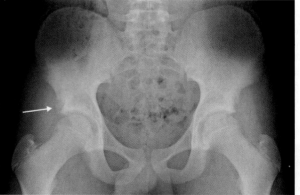

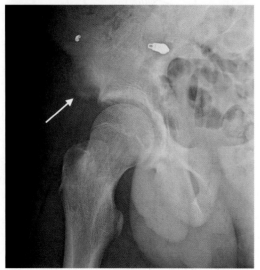

Figure 22-12. A: A 13-year-old who suffered an ASIS avulsion fracture while kicking a football. He experienced sudden pain and initially was unable to walk. On standard PA view of the pelvis, the fracture is difficult to visualize. **B:** The avulsion of the ASIS is much easier to appreciate on the iliac oblique view. **C:** One month after injury, there is significant healing present. (Used with permission of David L. Skaggs.)

conservatively concluded that nonsurgical treatment was successful in all patients, and all patients returned to preinjury activity levels.

Operative Treatment of Ischial Avulsion Fractures

Surgical treatment of ASIS and AIIS fractures has been described but is rarely indicated. While most pelvic avulsion fractures heal without surgical treatment, however, some fractures types, specifically, avulsion of the ischial tuberosity, and less so of the AIIS, require surgery. In one series of 198 competitive adolescent athletes with pelvic avulsion fractures, 3 were treated operatively,[75] corroborating the findings of another recent series of 228 fractures in which 3% required surgery.[79] In this later series, the authors reported that 14% of patients with avulsion fractures report pain greater than 3 months in duration and that AIIS avulsion fractures are 4.47 times more likely to have chronic pain greater than 3 months compared with all other types; additionally, 5 nonunions required surgery:

4 ischial tuberosity avulsions and 1 AIIS avulsion. Ischial avulsion fractures have been associated with a higher incidence of functional disability and inability to return to competitive athletic activity compared with other types.[96] In one long-term follow-up study of 12 patients with ischial avulsions, 8 reported significant reduction in athletic ability and 5 had persistent local symptoms.[78] Because many have satisfactory outcomes without surgery, indications for surgical management are not clear nor is the best operative technique established. Some authors have recommended consideration for open reduction and internal fixation of those rare acute avulsion fractures displaced more than 1 to 2 cm (Fig. 22-13)[50,79] because of concern for late complications but the authors have rarely found this necessary. Excision of the apophyseal fragment and takedown of nonunion and fixation are options in the chronic pain and disability. Other indications for late surgery include painful prominence after healing, concern for labral involvement,[38] and painful anterior hip impingement from heterotopic bone after healing.[53]

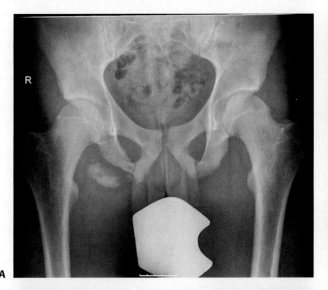

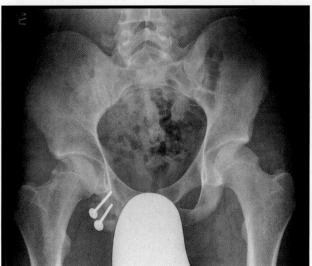

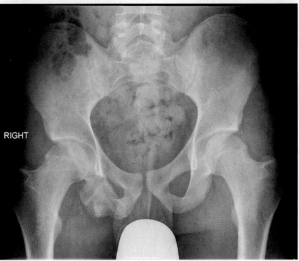

Figure 22-13. A: A painful ischial apophyseal nonunion in an athlete. **B:** Fixation of the apophysis. **C:** Healed apophysis after implant removal. (Courtesy of Dr. David C Scher, Hospital for Special Surgery, NY.)

Open Reduction and Internal Fixation of Avulsion Fractures

Preoperative Planning

✔ **Open Reduction and Internal Fixation of Ischial Avulsion Fractures:** PREOPERATIVE PLANNING CHECKLIST	
OR table	❏ Fluoroscopic table such as a Jackson table
Position/positioning aids	❏ Prone
Fluoroscopy location	❏ *Opposite the side of injury*
Equipment	❏ Screw set including 4.5- to 6.5-mm screws with washers ❏ Cables, wires, and/or suture anchors available as a backup

Technique

✔ **Open Reduction and Internal Fixation of Avulsion Fractures:** KEY SURGICAL STEPS
❏ Prone position with the hip and knee slightly flexed.   ❏ 7- to 10-cm incision is made along the gluteal crease.   ❏ The gluteus maximus/hamstrings plane is developed and the hamstring muscles are then traced to the fracture site.   ❏ Identify the bony fragment with the hamstrings attached.   ❏ The fragment is reduced more easily with the hip extended and the knee slightly flexed.   ❏ The fragment is stabilized with cancellous screws, with or without washers.   ❏ If necessary, additional fixation with suture anchors, cables, or wires can be used.

Postoperative Care

After surgery, the patient is permitted to sit up with the hips and knees slightly flexed to decrease stress on the hamstrings. Initially made nonweight-bearing, patients may progress to full weight-bearing in 3 to 6 weeks. At 12 weeks postoperatively, the patient may resume full activities.

ISOLATED ILIAC WING FRACTURES (TORODE AND ZIEG TYPE II)

Direct trauma may fracture the wing of the ilium, but isolated iliac wing fractures are relatively rare, with a reported incidence of 5% to 14% in children with fractures of the pelvis.[71,74,89] However, iliac wing fractures often occur in conjunction with other fractures of the pelvis, and thus the overall incidence of iliac wing fractures is significantly higher than the incidence of isolated iliac wing fractures.

The patient with an iliac wing fracture typically presents with pain that is located over the wing of the ilium, which worsens with trunk rotation or hip abduction. On examination, motion at the fracture site may be noted. A painful Trendelenburg gait may be

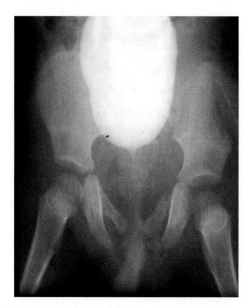

Figure 22-14 Stable fracture of the iliac wing.

present because of spasm of the hip abductor muscles. Plain radiographic diagnosis is sometimes difficult. A fracture of the wing of the ilium may be overlooked on an underexposed radiograph of the pelvis in which the ilium is poorly visualized, appearing only as a large area of radiolucency. CT is useful to delineate the fracture pattern and displacement in situations where surgery is being considered. Displacement of the fracture usually occurs laterally, but it may also occur medially or proximally. Severe displacement is rare because the iliac wing is tethered by the abdominal muscles, the hip abductors, and thick periosteum.

Treatment of an iliac wing fracture is mostly dictated by the associated injuries such as abdominal trauma. Symptomatic treatment is all that is necessary for most iliac wing fractures and typically includes pain management and partial weight-bearing on crutches for comfort until the symptoms are completely resolved. Regardless of comminution or displacement, these fractures usually unite without complications (Fig. 22-14). Open reduction and fixation with screws alone or plate-screw constructs are rarely indicated, except for large fragments with severe displacement. These fractures may also require fixation if the fracture extends into the acetabulum and is displaced.

OTHER STABLE FRACTURES

FRACTURES OF THE SACRUM

Sacral fractures constitute a very small fraction of pelvic fractures reported in children. Rieger and Brug[74] reported two sacral fractures and seven SI fracture-dislocations in 54 patients. Nine of 166 patients (5.4%) with pelvic fractures in the series by Silber et al.[91] had associated sacral fractures, none with nerve root involvement. Sacral fractures are probably more common than reported, but may be missed because these injuries are sometimes obscured by the anterior ring of the bony pelvis and the soft tissue shadows of the abdominal viscera on plain radiographs, and are rarely displaced.

There are two general types of sacral injuries. Spinal-type injuries may present as a crush or compression-type injury, with vertical foreshortening of the sacrum or horizontal fractures across the sacrum. These fractures may be significant because sacral nerve root injury may result in the loss of bowel and bladder function. Alar-type injuries are vertical fractures through the alae or sacral foraminae. It is important to note that these fractures may represent the posterior break of the double ring fracture, an indicator of potential pelvic ring instability. In cases where the pelvic ring is disrupted, small compression fractures or avulsion fragments of the sacral periphery at the SI joint may be seen but the body and ala are intact.

The presence of sacral fractures may be suggested clinically. Pain, swelling, and tenderness over the sacrum posteriorly are present in some injuries. Digital rectal examination performed in patients with sacral fractures may reveal stepoffs, fracture fragments, rectal tears, and urethral disruptions. Because digital rectal examination in pediatric trauma patients has a high false-negative rate, however, its usefulness is questionable and is not routinely performed in all centers.[87]

As suggested above, sacral fractures are sometimes difficult to diagnose on plain radiographs. AP and outlet views of the pelvis and a lateral view of the sacrum are best for identifying these injuries. Occasionally, the fracture line is oblique, but most are transverse with minimal displacement and occur through a sacral foramen, which is the weakest part of the body of the sacrum. Minimal disruption of the cortical rim of the foramen and offset of the lateral edge of the body of the sacrum are subtle indicators of a sacral fracture. Lateral views are helpful if there is anterior displacement, which is rare. CT and MRI scans are best for identification of sacral fractures missed on plain radiographic images.[26,85,90] In one study comparing radiographs with CT scans in a consecutive series of 103 pediatric trauma patients with pelvic radiographs and pelvic CT scans, only three sacral fractures were identified with plain radiographs whereas nine sacral fractures were identified with CT (Fig. 22-15).[26] Sacral fractures are generally managed nonsurgically with pain management and protected weight-bearing for comfort; weight-bearing as tolerated is generally permitted because most are stable patterns. In rare cases, sacral nerve roots encroached upon by fracture displacement or fracture

fragments may require surgical decompression. Sacral avulsion fractures and chondro-osseous injuries of the sacrum associated with SI joint fracture-dislocations generally are managed as part of the treatment for the SI joint injury with reduction of the SI joint and SI screw fixation. Open reduction and fixation of isolated sacral fractures, however, is rarely necessary in children.

FRACTURES OF THE COCCYX

Many children fall on the tailbone and have subsequent pain. The possibility of fracture must be entertained. Because the coccyx is made up of multiple small segments composed of cartilage and bone, is obscured by soft tissue, and naturally has a "crook" or apex posterior angulation of the distal segments, it is difficult to determine on radiographs whether a coccygeal fracture has occurred. These fractures rarely have associated injuries other than localized pain at the injury site. Clinically, patients describe immediate, severe pain in the area of the coccyx. Pain on defecation may be present as well as pain on rectal examination. Because radiographic identification is difficult, clinical confirmation of the diagnosis may be made by digital rectal examination though palpation outside of the rectum is usually sufficient. Exquisite pain may be elicited and an abnormal mobility of the coccygeal fragments may be noted. Acute, severe symptoms typically abate in 1 to 2 weeks, but chronic, mild-to-moderate discomfort can persist in some patients for weeks or even months. Lateral radiographs of the coccyx with the hips flexed maximally may reveal an obvious fracture in some cases (Fig. 22-16), but apex posterior angulation of the coccyx is a normal variant, and should not be falsely interpreted as a fracture or dislocation. CT and MRI may be helpful in differentiating between physeal plates and fracture lines[13] and also help to rule out other possible etiologies of the pain such as neoplasm or intrapelvic pathology. Treatment is symptomatic initially and consists of activity restriction and a pressure-relieving cushion for sitting, with an expectation of resolution in 4 to 6 weeks for acute fractures. Some rare pediatric patients have chronic pain that persists for several months, probably better described by the diagnosis of "coccydynia." Symptomatic treatments, injections, and coccygectomy are some management options with good results in adolescents.[25]

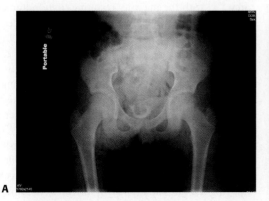
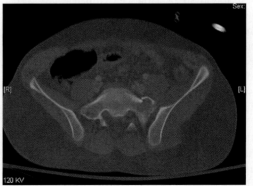

Figure 22-15. A: An example of an anterior–posterior pelvic radiograph where the sacral fracture is not well visualized. **B:** CT scan of the patient showing the sacral fracture.

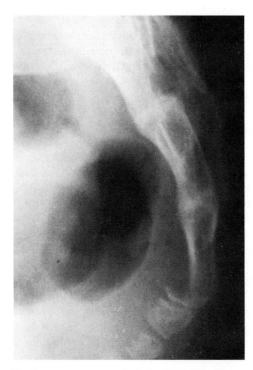

Figure 22-16. Lateral radiograph with the hips maximally flexed reveals a displaced coccygeal fracture in a 14-year-old boy.

STRESS FRACTURES OF THE PELVIS

Stress fractures of the pelvis are rare in children, but do occur in adolescents and young adults from chronic, repetitive stress, most commonly from sports activities such as running and during the last trimester of pregnancy. These may occur through the sacrum, and pubic rami and pelvic apophyses. Stress fractures of the sacrum have been described rarely in adolescent runners, volleyball players, and pregnant women who present primarily with low back pain.[59,85] Chronic low-grade groin and pubic pain that worsens with activities, especially distance running, are presenting signs of stress fractures of the pubic rami, most commonly at a site in the inferior ramus adjacent to the pubis.[61,65] Patients with hip dysplasia who undergo periacetabular osteotomies are also at greater risk for stress rami fractures after surgery.[29] Stress fractures of the iliac crest apophysis of adolescent athletes have also been reported.[32] Radiographs often reveal no evidence of fracture initially but a small amount of periosteal reaction may become obvious after 4 to 6 weeks of symptoms. MRI is the best test to identify stress fractures of the pelvis. Alternatively, technetium bone scan may reveal increased uptake early in the course of symptoms.[36] Treatment should consist of avoiding the stressful activity and limited weight-bearing for 4 to 6 weeks.

Stress fracture of the ischiopubic synchondrosis may also occur. This diagnosis is rare, however, and must be differentiated from ischiopubic osteochondritis, infections, and neoplasms. The ischiopubic synchondrosis usually closes between 4 and 7 years of age.[43] Caffey and Ross[42] noted that bilateral fusion of the ischiopubic synchondrosis is complete

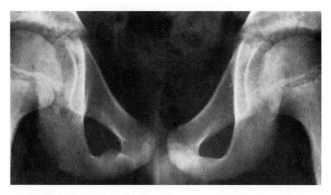

Figure 22-17. Radiograph of the pelvis of a 9-year-old child. Although the differentiation could not be made between a fracture and fusion of the right ischiopubic ossification at the time of radiograph, the patient was asymptomatic and the mass was considered a variant of normal development.

in only 6% of children at 4 years of age but is seen in 83% of children by 12 years of age. Children at an average of 7 years who present with vague groin or buttock pain, mild tenderness or fullness at the ischiopubic junction and radiographs that reveal hyperostosis at the junction likely have ischiopubic osteochondritis or van Neck disease, a self-limited process that resolves with fusion of the synchondrosis.[63,108] Remember that the ischiopubic older children, those with a history suggestive of infection or neoplasm, or those who participate in repetitive stress activities such as distance running, with findings of hyperostosis of the ischiopubic synchondrosis on radiographs, should be ruled out for other diagnoses such as osteomyelitis, tumors, and stress fractures. Further diagnostic evaluation includes MRI of the pelvis, technetium bone scan, and blood work based on the clinical setting (Fig. 22-17).

SIMPLE RING FRACTURES (TORODE AND ZIEG TYPE IIIA AND IIIB)

Using the original Torode and Zieg classification scheme, simple ring injuries constitute up to 56% of all pelvic fractures in children,[69,77] with the majority resulting from motor vehicles striking pedestrians.[89] Many of these reported injuries were breaks in the anterior pelvic ring and were single ramus fractures, most commonly fractures of the superior ramus (Fig. 22-18).[46] With the increased use of CT scans to define these injuries, however, it became apparent that not all stable pelvic ring injuries are the same with regard to fracture pattern, mechanism, associated injuries, or prognosis. To reflect important differences among the types of simple ring injuries, Shore et al.[84] modified the Torode and Zieg scheme. In the modified classification, type III stable or simple ring fractures are subdivided into types IIIA and IIIB. Type IIIA fractures are defined as simple anterior ring fractures and type IIIB fractures are stable anterior and posterior ring fractures. This distinction is critical because type IIIB injuries are associated with an increased need for blood

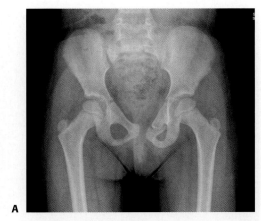 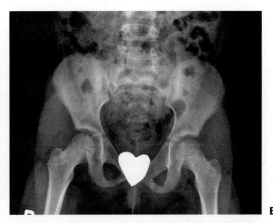

Figure 22-18. A: Stable superior pubic ramus fracture. The patient was allowed full weight-bearing as tolerated. **B:** Radiographs show complete fracture union and remodeling.

transfusions, an increased length of hospital stay, more frequent admissions to the ICU, and more associated injuries compared with type IIIB fractures.

NONOPERATIVE TREATMENT OF SIMPLE RING FRACTURES

Patients with these injuries typically present with pain and tenderness along the pubic rami. Weight-bearing is difficult or impossible secondary to pain, and hip range of motion is often limited because of muscle guarding around the hip. The pelvic ring is grossly stable to rocking and compression but, for patients with type IIIB injuries, tenderness along the sacrum and SI joints may be elicited with palpation. Pelvic inlet and outlet radiographic views, or more commonly a CT scan, are used to distinguish type IIIA from type IIIB fractures.

Most stable ring fractures require no surgical intervention for management of the pelvic ring injury because, by definition, the pelvic ring is stable. For patients with type IIIB fractures, monitoring of cardiovascular status and blood loss and management of associated injuries are priorities compared to pelvic fracture management. Most patients with type III fractures, however, require only symptomatic treatment. Pain control and mobilization out of bed with nonweight-bearing or protected weight-bearing, as dictated but the status of associated injuries when present, is important for the initial 1 to 2 weeks after injury. After pelvic ring healing has progressed and the pain has diminished, progressive weight-bearing is permitted. Most children with type III pelvic fractures return to full activities within 6 to 8 weeks of the initial injury, unless associated comorbidities influence recovery.

Special Situations

Fractures of the Two Ipsilateral Rami

Fractures of the ipsilateral superior and inferior pubic rami made up 18% of pediatric pelvic fractures in one series of 120 pediatric pelvic fractures.[11] Although these fractures are generally stable, they may be associated with injuries of the abdominal viscera, especially the genitourinary system (e.g., bladder

rupture).[11] A careful examination of the perineum, rectal examination, and a cystourethrogram may be indicated to fully assess these injuries. Because these fractures typically unite without surgical treatment, most are treated nonsurgically except when severe displacement has occurred.

Fractures of the Body of the Ischium

Fracture of the body of the ischium near the acetabulum is extremely rare in children. The fracture occurs from external force to the ischium, most commonly in a fall from a considerable height. The fracture usually is minimally displaced and management consists of symptomatic treatment and progressive weight-bearing (Fig. 22-19).

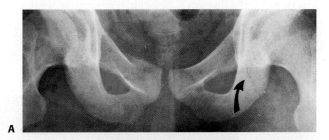
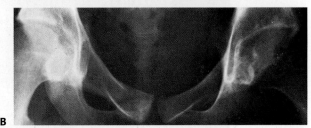

Figure 22-19. A: Nondisplaced fracture (*curved arrow*) through left ischium and contralateral pubic ramus fracture. **B:** Follow-up radiograph shows mild displacement and incongruity of the acetabulum and complete healing of the superior pubic ramus fracture. Either displacement of the fracture fragments or premature closure of the triradiate cartilage could have contributed to the incongruity of the femoral head in the acetabulum.

Widening of the Symphysis Pubis

Isolated injuries to the symphysis pubis are rare because these typically occur in association with disruption of the posterior ring, at or near the SI joint most commonly. Although significant force is necessary to disrupt or fracture the symphysis pubis in children, isolated disruption of the symphysis pubis can occur.[109] Clinically, exquisite pain is present anteriorly at the symphysis. The lower extremities may lie externally rotated when the patient is supine. Motion of the hips in flexion, abduction, external rotation, and extension is restricted and painful (FABER sign). Pain associated with a pubic diastasis is often improved by side-lying compared with supine positioning.[109]

Radiographs and CT imaging may reveal subluxation or widening of the symphysis or in the bone of the anterior ring just adjacent to it, and vertical or anterior–posterior offset of the two sides of the symphysis.[94] Although some elasticity of the pubic symphysis is normal in children and adolescents, diastasis greater than or equal to 2.5 cm or rotational deformity greater than 15 degrees suggests significant instability and is an indication for reduction.[19] There is a normal variation of the width of the symphysis in children as measured on radiographs because the pubic bones at the symphysis are composed of ischiopubic cartilage with a thickness that varies with age, making the extent of traumatic separation difficult to evaluate. Watts[109] suggested obtaining radiographs with and without lateral compression of the pelvis to detect abnormalities, with greater than 1 cm of difference in the width of the symphysis pubis between the two views indicating a symphyseal separation. Imaging must also be carefully scrutinized to detect SI joint disruptions and triradiate cartilage fractures, both of which may occur in association with symphysis pubis separation (Fig. 22-20).[59]

Treatment of an isolated injury of the symphysis pubis with less than 2 cm of diastasis is generally symptomatic, similar to that described above for other stable pelvic ring injuries. Wider diastasis is best treated with closed reduction and external fixation or open reduction and plating of the symphysis through an

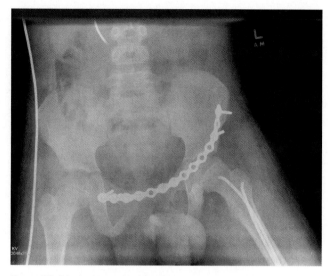

Figure 22-21. Radiograph of the pelvis after plating of the pubic symphysis that also includes acetabular fixation.

anterior Pfannenstiel incision (Fig. 22-21). Because this injury in children is often through the cartilage of the pubis at the symphysis, and not disruption of symphyseal ligaments, healing is more reliable and rapid compared with adults.

Fractures Near or Through the Sacroiliac Joint

The type IIIB fracture pattern is the most common injury pattern that is associated with stable, nondisplaced or minimally displaced fractures near or through the SI joints. The anatomy of the child's SI joint complex is different from that of an adult in several important ways. In children, disruptions tend to be incomplete because, while the anterior ligaments may tear, the thick posterior ligamentous complex prevents complete disruption in most cases. In addition, the SI joint may separate not through the joint but instead through the chondro-osseous "physis" of the medial ilium or, less commonly, the lateral sacrum

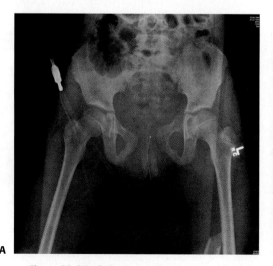 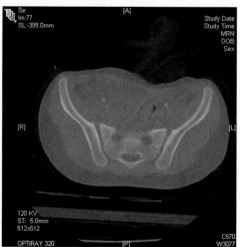

Figure 22-20. A: Fracture adjacent to the symphysis pubis with symphysis pubis separation. **B:** CT scan showing no posterior instability.

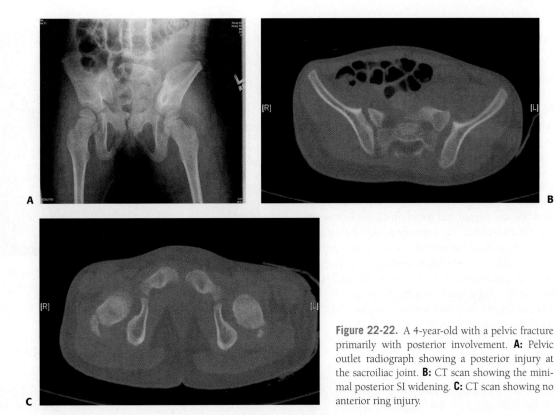

Figure 22-22. A 4-year-old with a pelvic fracture primarily with posterior involvement. **A:** Pelvic outlet radiograph showing a posterior injury at the sacroiliac joint. **B:** CT scan showing the minimal posterior SI widening. **C:** CT scan showing no anterior ring injury.

of the growing child.[63] These fractures are clinically impossible to separate from ligamentous SI joint disruption and often are not identified on radiographs, making this a CT diagnosis.[11] Axial imaging by CT reveals subtle asymmetry of the rotation of the iliac wings, SI joint space widening, and a metaphyseal fracture line or tiny avulsion fragments of the ilium where the physeal fracture line exits out of metaphyseal bone just adjacent to the SI joint.[63,64] The "crescent" fracture is a iliac wing fracture that also occurs adjacent to the SI joint and is characterized by a metaphyseal fracture that exits posteriorly out of the ilium from the SI joint creating a posterior iliac fragment that remains attached to the intact posterior ligaments; the surgeon must distinguish this pattern because it may reflect rotational instability of the injury.[92] Inlet/outlet pelvic views and coronal CT images reveal subtle distal SI joint stepoff (Fig. 22-22) and anterior SI joint widening. Minimally displaced SI joint injuries are rarely associated with vascular or nerve root injuries. These injuries are treated conservatively with a short period of bed-to-chair nonweight-bearing for comfort, typically 4 to 6 weeks or, in rare cases, with a spica cast.

RING DISRUPTION: UNSTABLE FRACTURE PATTERNS (TORODE AND ZIEG TYPE IV)

Unstable pelvic fractures in children and adolescents constitute a small percentage of all pelvic fractures in pediatric patients. These are classified as Torode and Zieg type IV injuries and may have multiple fracture patterns. In one series of pelvic ring fractures, type IV injuries represented 10% of all pelvic fractures seen.[88] Most of these injuries result from high-velocity trauma, such as motor vehicle collisions and pedestrians being struck by motor vehicles. Children older than 12 years of age and those with closed triradiate cartilages[89] are more likely to sustain these types of fractures compared with younger patients with open triradiate cartilages. Blood transfusions, intensive care unit lengths of stay, and surgical interventions, among other parameters, are generally increased in patients with type IV fractures compared with other types of pelvic fractures, as is the incidence of death.[88]

Type IV fractures are typically divided into three subcategories:

1. Double anterior ring disruptions. This injury subtype includes bilateral inferior and superior pubic rami fractures (the straddle or floating injury) and disruptions of the pubis with an associated second break in the anterior ring.
2. Anterior and posterior pelvic ring (double ring) disruptions with instability and displacement, including vertical displacement (Malgaigne type). The anterior disruptions may be rami fractures or symphysis pubis disruption. Posterior ring injuries include fractures of the sacrum or ilium and disruptions through or adjacent to the SI joints.
3. Multiple crushing injuries that produce at least two severely comminuted fractures located at any site in the pelvic ring. These fractures may also be associated with acetabular fractures.

BILATERAL FRACTURES OF THE INFERIOR AND SUPERIOR PUBIC RAMI

Bilateral fractures of the inferior and superior pubic rami may occur in a fall while straddling a hard object, bilateral compression of the pelvis, or by sudden impact while riding a motorized cycle. The floating fragment usually is displaced superiorly, pulled in this direction by the rectus abdominis muscles.[109] As with ipsilateral superior and inferior pubic rami fractures, which may occur by similar mechanisms, bladder or urethral disruptions[15,93] are commonly associated injuries that must be ruled out in patients with this type of pelvic fracture.

Radiographically, an inlet/outlet views or CT scan most accurately determine the degree and direction of displacement. Bilateral fractures of the inferior and superior pubic rami (straddle fractures) or disruption of the symphysis pubis with unilateral fractures of the rami are two fracture patterns that result in a floating anterior segment of the pelvic ring. Although this floating anterior arch is inherently unstable (Fig. 22-23), the posterior ring is usually not disrupted except, in some cases, by stable fractures of the sacrum or ilium.

Treatment

Because in most cases the posterior ring is intact and the anterior fractures are not displaced, treatment is similar to that described for type IIIB injuries. After associated injuries have been diagnosed and managed appropriately, treatment initially includes bed rest and pain control. Skeletal traction is unnecessary, and a pelvic sling is contraindicated because of the possibility that compression will cause medial displacement of the ilium.[63,109] Protected weight-bearing with progression to full weight-bearing and unrestricted activities is then permitted as pain improves. In children, pelvic ring healing occurs reliably in 6 to 8 weeks for most injuries. Bone remodeling can be expected over the ensuing months. Surgical treatment of the superior ramus fractures with reduction and fixation with cannulated screws or plating techniques are rarely necessary to treat children but may be indicated in adolescents with significant displacement.

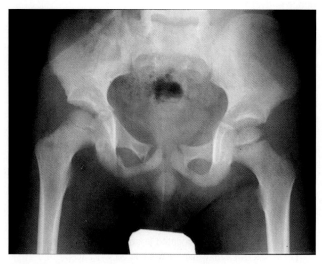

Figure 22-23. Example of a straddle fracture.

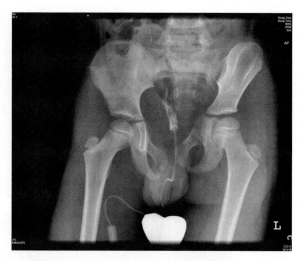

Figure 22-24. An unstable pelvis fracture with fractures in both the anterior and posterior ring of the pelvis. The left hemipelvis is displaced and rotated.

ANTERIOR AND POSTERIOR RING DISRUPTIONS

Double breaks in the pelvic ring, in which fractures occur both anterior and posterior to the acetabulum (Fig. 22-24), result in instability of the pelvis in many cases, especially when the posterior ring injury is displaced. These injuries result from a variety of mechanisms. In one report,[9] AP compression forces were suspected to be the mechanism of injury, although the exact forces were not readily defined in all patients. Other possible causes of injury are severe direct lateral compressive forces, indirect forces transmitted proximally along the femoral shaft with the hip fixed in extension and abduction, and combined mechanisms of injury in which the pelvis is subject to multiple forces from different directions.[60,63] The injury patterns are best classified according to the AO-OTA scheme which may be applied to children's injuries.[69,81]

Double breaks in the pelvic ring especially those with displacement represent the most dangerous type of pelvic fracture in children.[24,88,91,103] These unstable fractures are often accompanied by retroperitoneal and intraperitoneal bleeding and are most likely to be associated with severe, life-threatening hemorrhage. Concomitant abdominal injury is also significantly more likely to occur in patients with unstable pelvic fractures compared to those with stable pelvic fractures.[24,88,91,103]

Aside from the physical signs usually associated with pelvic fractures, leg length discrepancy and asymmetry of the pelvis may be present. Apparent leg length discrepancy is seen in patients with vertical or cephalad displacement of the fractured hemipelvis. Internal or external rotation of the unstable hemipelvis may appear as asymmetry of the iliac crests.

Inlet and outlet radiographs and CT scan reveal the degree and direction of pelvic displacement and determine the exact fracture pattern. Anterior ring disruption may be the result of rami fractures or symphyseal separation. The posterior ring disruption may occur through the SI joint, with the majority causing tearing of the anterior ligaments but sparing the stronger and thicker posterior complex, although complete ligamentous disruptions do occur. More commonly, however, especially in younger children, the posterior ring disruption occurs through the chondro-osseus junction of the ilium or sacrum adjacent to the SI joint, as mentioned above.

Treatment

Initial treatment is focused on cardiovascular resuscitation with fluids and blood products, and stabilization of the child's overall condition before treatment of the pelvic fractures.[37,92] Pelvic binders or sheets, placed circumferentially across the greater trochanters to limit pelvic ring expansion with severe hemorrhage, may be used safely in larger children and adolescents with similar indications and precautions as in adults. Some injuries caused predominantly by lateral compression forces, however, may not be amenable to this because compression may increase the pelvic deformity. Embolization of arterial vessels is also an option for uncontrolled bleeding. Evidence-based literature regarding the use of pelvic binders and embolization in younger children is lacking, however, predominantly because unstable ring injuries that contribute to hemodynamic instability are exceedingly rare. The search for other sites of hemorrhage must be undertaken before attributing hemodynamic instability to the pelvic trauma in these younger children.

Minimally Displaced Fractures

Treatment of the anterior–posterior pelvic ring injury varies based on the fracture pattern, degree of displacement, and the age and condition of the child. Most fractures with minimal displacement, some of which are type IV injuries, or more commonly type IIIB injuries, are treated symptomatically by pain control, weight-bearing restrictions, and close radiographic follow-up for displacement (Fig. 22-25). Spica casting can be used in the younger children to improve the comfort of the patient and to prevent weight-bearing, after cardiovascular parameters and associated injures have been stabilized. In some cases, older children and adolescents with minimally displaced

fractures benefit from fixation to lessen pain associated with the fracture and facilitate mobilization.

Displaced Fractures

Nonoperative Treatment

Historically, operative treatment of pelvic fractures in children has not been routinely used for the following reasons:[24,39,91]

- Severe hemorrhage from the pelvic fracture is unusual in children, making operative pelvic stabilization to control bleeding rarely necessary.
- The thick periosteum and ligaments about the pelvis in children limit displacement and stabilize the fracture to some degree, limiting fracture fragment mobility and facilitating healing so that nonsurgical treatment is well tolerated by patients, and prolonged immobilization is not necessary for fracture healing.
- Remodeling may occur in skeletally immature patients, reducing the need to achieve anatomic alignment of some fractures.
- With few exceptions, long-term morbidity after pelvic fractures is rare in children.

Techniques

Nonoperative treatment for unstable pelvic fractures includes bed rest and spica cast immobilization, neither of which significantly improves fracture alignment. For children younger than 8 years of age or so, closed reduction and spica casting may be used for symphyseal disruptions and SI joint injuries with small degrees of displacement. Skeletal traction is the only nonsurgical treatment that can be used to improve alignment of widely displaced fractures. Unstable fractures with vertical displacement of the hemipelvis may be reduced with this modality. Longitudinal traction is applied through a pin placed in the distal femur with weights similar to those utilized for femoral shaft reduction, typically 5 to 7 lb or one-eighth of body weight depending on the size of the child. Postreduction imaging is used to assess reduction and progression of healing. Traction is applied for a minimum of

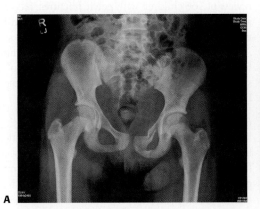
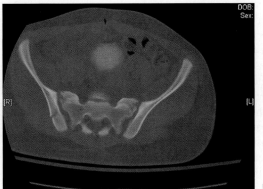

Figure 22-25. A potentially unstable pelvic fracture with anterior and posterior injury. **A:** The radiograph shows left superior and inferior rami fractures. **B:** The CT scan shows a minimally displaced fracture adjacent to the sacroiliac joint. This is also an example where both CT and plain radiographs can be used to evaluate the injury and help decide on displacement and treatment. This patient was treated nonoperatively with follow-up making sure there was no displacement.

2 to 4 weeks to achieve some stability of the injury, after which the child may be placed in a spica cast or kept on bed rest until further healing allows safe mobilization. Skeletal traction cannot improve alignment of symphyseal "open book" injuries, severe SI disruptions with widening or posterior displacement, or fractures with rotational deformities of the hemipelvis.

Outcomes

Despite the fact that the classic assumptions and observations regarding unstable pelvic fractures are generally correct, the published outcomes of nonsurgical treatments have not been uniformly satisfactory. Nierenberg et al.[59] reported excellent or good results after conservative treatment of 20 unstable pelvic fractures in children, despite radiographic evidence of deformity. These authors concluded that treatment guidelines for unstable pelvic fractures are not the same for children as for adults, and recommended that external or internal fixation should be used only when conservative methods fail.[59] In another study, however, the authors found that a third of 15 skeletally immature patients with unstable fractures treated nonoperatively had chronic pain at follow-up.[54a] Similar findings were shown in another large series of unstable pediatric pelvic fractures treated nonsurgically with a mean of 7.4 years follow-up. In this study, about one-fourth of patients had musculoskeletal complaints at follow-up, including leg length discrepancy, back pain, and SI ankylosis.[95] In addition, these authors identified important nonorthopedic complications, including 23 patients with genitourinary abnormalities, such as incontinence and erectile dysfunction, and 31 patients with psychiatric diagnoses such as posttraumatic stress disorder and major depression. These authors stressed the importance of minimizing prolonged hospital stays, addressing urologic needs fully, and anticipating the need for mental health support.

In addition to the advantages of improved mobilization, anatomic or near-anatomic realignment of pelvic fractures likely improves outcomes. Residual pelvic ring asymmetry, specifically vertical displacement of the hemipelvis and SI joint malalignment, and acetabular malrotation leading to altered hip coverage and mechanics do not reliably remodel after fracture healing and have been associated with poor long-term outcomes such as leg length discrepancy, hip pain, back pain, scoliosis, and SI arthrosis in children.[80,93] Pelvic obliquity and asymmetry has also been associated with pelvic floor dysfunction and pain. In one long-term follow-up study[80] of 17 children with unstable pelvic fractures treated nonoperatively, 8 patients had pelvic asymmetry at follow-up. Of these 8 patients, 5 had functional deformities, including scoliosis and leg length discrepancies that resulted in chronic back pain. In another study, Smith et al.[93] followed 20 patients with open triradiate cartilages who were treated for unstable pelvic fractures for a mean of 6.5 years. Pelvic asymmetry was quantified on an AP pelvis radiograph by measuring the difference in length (in centimeters) between two diagonal lines drawn from the border of the SI joint to the contralateral triradiate cartilage. Eighteen patients were treated operatively with external fixation, internal fixation, or a combination of both; pelvic asymmetry was less than 1 cm in 10 of 18 patients. At follow-up, the authors noted that pelvic asymmetry did not remodel to any significant degree, even in younger

patients. Based on the Short Musculoskeletal Function Assessment (SMFA) questionnaire, patients with 1 cm or less of pelvic asymmetry had significantly less back and SI pain, and better SMFA outcome scores than those patients with pelvic asymmetry greater than 1 cm. In addition, all patients with greater than 1.1 cm of pelvic asymmetry had three or more of the following: nonstructural scoliosis, lumbar pain, a Trendelenburg sign, or SI joint tenderness and pain. The authors concluded that fractures associated with at least 1.1 cm of pelvic asymmetry following closed reduction should be treated with open reduction and internal or external fixation to improve alignment and the long-term functional outcome.[93]

Operative Treatment

Because of concerns for poor outcomes based on prior experience with nonsurgical treatment of unstable pediatric pelvic fractures, modern evidence supports the safety and efficacy of surgical treatment for displaced and unstable pelvic fractures in children and adolescents. Karunaker et al.[42] surgically managed 18 unstable pelvic and acetabular fractures in children younger than 16 years of age using the principles of anatomic realignment and stable fixation routinely applied to adults. All patients healed by 10 weeks after surgery and had recovered full function with minimal residual pain at follow-up. No significant complications occurred, notably no cases of premature triradiate cartilage closure or SI joint abnormalities. They recommended operative intervention in skeletally immature patients with significant deformity of the pelvis at the time of injury to prevent late morbidities.[42] Others have drawn similar conclusions based on their experience with surgical management of unstable pediatric pelvic disruptions.[1,69,81,102]

Indications/Contraindications

The exact indications for surgical treatment are not clearly delineated in the literature but have become less controversial over time. Holden et al.[37] determined, after a review of the literature prior to 2006, that fractures with more than 2 cm of displacement must be reduced and stabilized in children. Others have suggested that pelvic asymmetry greater than or equal to 1.1 cm is an indication for reduction. Silber et al,[91] in one review of 166 children with pelvic fractures, recommended that all patients with closed triradiate cartilages, regardless of age, be treated as adults with anatomic realignment and stable fixation. Anatomic realignment and fixation is recommended by others for all displaced pelvic ring fractures regardless of age, utilizing similar parameters applied to adults with displaced and unstable pelvic ring injuries.[1,69,81,102]

Preoperative Planning

Because surgery for pelvic ring reduction and fixation in children is rare, one may consider including an experienced orthopedic traumatologist, in conjunction with a pediatric orthopedic surgeon, using techniques more commonly needed in adults but modified for children. These modifications include implants sized appropriately for children and techniques that preserve, as much as possible, the potential for growth. Perioperative care is best accomplished with a multidisciplinary team that is familiar with pediatric anesthesia and critical care and includes pediatric trauma nursing, child support services, and pediatric rehabilitation.

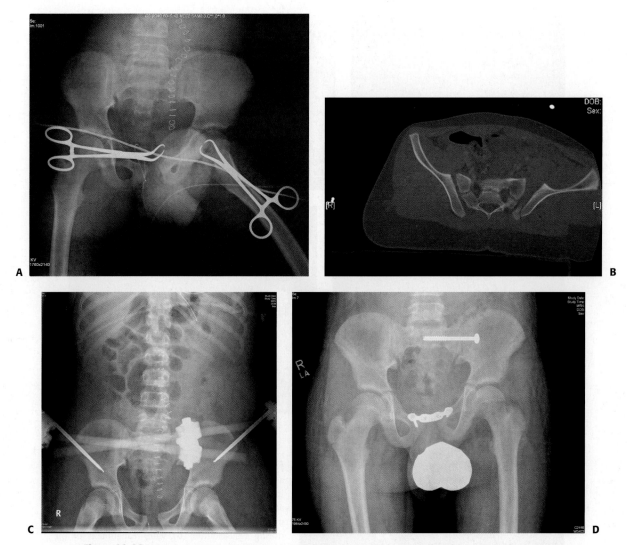

Figure 22-26. This radiographic series highlights treatment of an unstable pelvic fracture with hemodynamic instability. **A:** Anteroposterior pelvic radiograph of a 12-year-old boy who was a pedestrian hit by a car. There is a wide symphysis and a displaced fracture adjacent to the left sacroiliac joint. The towel clips seen on radiograph are to hold a sheet (sling) around the pelvis to help temporarily control hemorrhage. **B:** CT scan showing the displaced posterior injury. **C:** Pelvic radiograph after an anterior external fixation was placed urgently to stabilize the pelvis. This along with resuscitation stabilized the hemodynamic status. **D:** Once the patient had stabilized, the external fixation was converted to anterior internal fixation with a plate on the symphysis pubis and the posterior instability was treated with a sacroiliac screw.

The timing of surgery is based on the needs of the individual patient. Although uncommon, emergency placement of external or internal fixation may be necessary to achieve cardiovascular stability, such as with an open book pelvis fracture not stabilized by a pelvic binder. Complex surgery, however, represents a "second hit" to the traumatized patient that further incites inflammatory processes and challenges the body's ability to respond to the stress of surgery. Although not directly studied in children, the concept of "Damage Control Orthopedics"[21] favors delaying surgery until concomitant injuries have been managed and after a period of cardiovascular stability. Because of this, pelvic surgery is typically performed in a delayed fashion, typically 7 to 10 days after the initial injury.

The timing of surgery, however, is ultimately determined by a host of factors and is based on the condition of the patient and the team's judgment.

Many different surgical strategies and techniques may be utilized to achieve reduction and stability. The surgical team must carefully plan which technique or combination of techniques is best for the individual patient. Stabilization of the anterior ring may be accomplished with external fixation, symphyseal, and/or rami plate fixation, or screw fixation of the rami and anterior column (Fig. 22-26). Options for posterior stabilization include SI screw fixation and plate fixation (Fig. 22-27). Because these techniques are discussed in detail in the companion to this text, *Rockwood and Wilkins' Fractures in Adults*, this section will

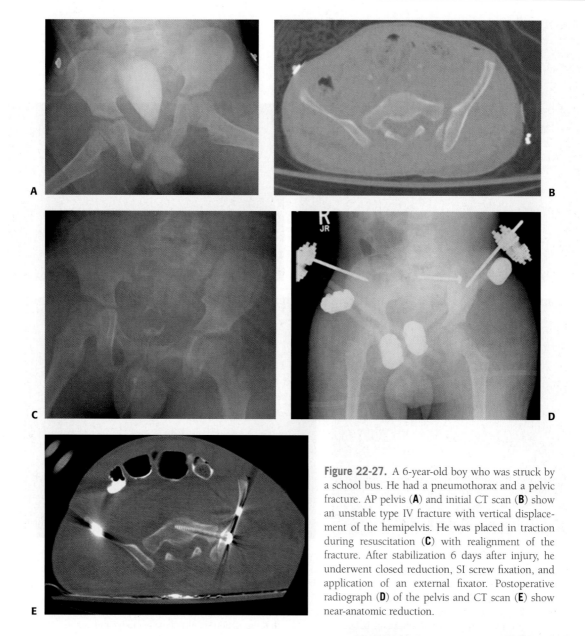

Figure 22-27. A 6-year-old boy who was struck by a school bus. He had a pneumothorax and a pelvic fracture. AP pelvis (**A**) and initial CT scan (**B**) show an unstable type IV fracture with vertical displacement of the hemipelvis. He was placed in traction during resuscitation (**C**) with realignment of the fracture. After stabilization 6 days after injury, he underwent closed reduction, SI screw fixation, and application of an external fixator. Postoperative radiograph (**D**) of the pelvis and CT scan (**E**) show near-anatomic reduction.

discuss only the two most commonly used techniques for children, external fixation and SI screw fixation.

External Fixation

External fixation is used to stabilize an unstable fracture with anterior ring separation or anterior fractures and for control of pelvic ring volume emergently in some anterior–posterior ring disruptions. This technique maintains reduction, decreases pain, facilitates mobilization out of bed, and may be better tolerated by older children than spica casting.[22,44] External fixation, however, may not effectively control the posterior ring[54] for all fracture patterns. Anterior external fixation may be achieved by placing one or two pins in the supra-acetabular bone on each side of the pelvis (Fig. 22-28)[77] or by placing one to two pins into each iliac crest and spanning these pin clusters with an external frame, ideally one that allows access to the abdomen.

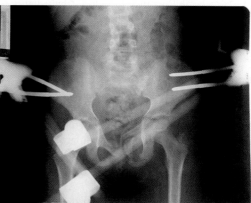

Figure 22-28. Fixation of an unstable pelvic fracture with external fixation. One or two pins are placed in the iliac wing. The starting point is 1 to 2 cm posterior to the anterior-superior iliac spine. An anterior-to-posterior supra-acetabular pin may also be used.

Preoperative Planning

> ✔ **Placement of Pelvic External Fixation in Children:**
> PRE-OPERATIVE PLANNING CHECKLIST

OR table	❑ Fluoroscopic table such as Flat top Jackson table
Position/positioning aids	❑ Supine with a small bolster under the sacrum
Fluoroscopy	❑ Position for either side of the table. Confirm ability to obtain AP, inlet, outlet, and oblique views of the pelvis
Equipment	❑ 4-, 4.5-, 5-mm half pins ❑ Radiolucent external fixation frame

Technique

> ✔ **Placement of Pelvic External Fixation in Children:**
> KEY SURGICAL STEPS

❑ Complete prep and drape of the abdomen above the umbilicus, pelvis, and lower extremities

❑ For placement of iliac crest pins:
  • Small transverse incision over iliac crest for each pin. The first incision is made 2 cm posterior to AIIS
  • Split the iliac apophysis and locate the metaphyseal bone between the iliac tables
  • Drill path between the tables perpendicular to the iliac crest; confirm position with fluoroscopy
  • Place pin (self-drilling screws may be placed directly through apophysis)
  • Place second pin 2 cm posterior to the first along the iliac crest; place a total of 2–3 pins per side
  • The inner or outer table of the pelvis may be palpated to ensure pin is wholly in bone
  • Construct frame that allows access to the abdomen

❑ For placement of supra-acetabular pins:
  • Small longitudinal incision 2 cm proximal to the joint just medial to an imaginary line drawn between AIIS and ASIS
  • Bluntly dissect to the supra-acetabular bone
  • Drill path perpendicular to the bone; confirm position with fluoroscopy
  • Place pin
  • A single pin may be placed per side or second pin may be placed just superior and in line with the first
  • Construct frame that allows access to the abdomen

❑ Loosen frame to allow for closed reduction under fluoroscopic guidance: provisional reduction held manually before pin placement may facilitate the process

❑ Confirm reduction and final tightening of the frame

Postoperative Care

After frame placement, patients may be out of bed to a chair if pelvic ring stability is acceptable and the associated injuries permit mobilization. Half-pin care is typically initiated within 4 to 7 days of surgery and continues until the frame is removed. Care regimens vary but daily cleaning is typically recommended. By 4 to 6 weeks after placement, limited weight-bearing is started. Weight-bearing in the frame may be possible for some patients but typically for children is not fully instituted until removal of the frame, which is typically done in the operating room 6 to 10 weeks after application.

Symphyseal Plating

Symphyseal plating is a good alternative to anterior ring fixation in some children and adolescents.[22] This fixation choice is less bulky than external fixation and can often be performed at the time of other procedures for associated urogenital or abdominal injuries. The approach and technique are identical to that utilized for adult symphyseal plating, except that the plate size must be selected appropriately based on the size of the child. The best choice is a rigid plate–screw construct, such as a 3.5-mm reconstruction plate, but small and less bulky choices may be indicated for smaller patients.

Sacroiliac Reduction and Screw Fixation

Posterior ring injuries in children are typically SI joint disruptions, either from a true joint disruption or from fractures of the ilium, fractures of the iliac, or sacral chondro-osseous zones that extend into or are adjacent to the SI joint, or sacral fractures. Indications for surgical treatment of these injuries are unstable ring injuries with combined anterior and posterior instability and posterior ring fractures with displacement greater than about 1 cm, although, as noted above, the amount of acceptable displacement is controversial. Closed reduction, or limited open reduction, with percutaneous stabilization is an important strategy for pelvic fracture management in children and is the first option when addressing displaced fractures.[1,81] Open reduction and plate fixation of posterior ring injuries is indicated when closed reduction and screw fixation techniques cannot achieve adequate realignment or stable fixation.

Preoperative Planning

> ✔ **Placement of SI Screw Fixation:**
> PRE-OPERATIVE PLANNING CHECKLIST

OR table	❑ Fluoroscopic table such as Flat top Jackson table
Position/positioning aids	❑ Supine with a small bolster under the sacrum ❑ Place leads for neuromonitoring of the lower extremity on the affected side
Fluoroscopy	❑ Position for either side of the table. Confirm ability to obtain AP, inlet, outlet, and oblique views of the pelvis
Equipment	❑ 4.5–6.5 mm fully threaded cannulated screws ❑ Pelvic plate system (as back up) ❑ Setup for femoral traction pin placement ❑ Setup to perform open reduction and fixation of the SI joint if necessary

Before considering this technique, the CT scan of the pelvis must be carefully scrutinized to determine if the fracture pattern is amenable to closed reduction. Specifically, it is important to determine if comminution or severe displacement may prevent reduction or risk soft tissue or neurovascular entrapment or injury. The CT scan is helpful to assess the sacral anatomy of the individual patient, which may vary widely, to determine the ideal entry position and safe trajectory. In the pediatric patient, the narrow corridor for safe screw placement makes the procedure difficult but safe placement of percutaneous SI screws can be achieved[81,95] and has been reported in children as young as 6 of age.[1] When a concomitant anterior pelvic injury is present, it may be necessary to stabilize it prior to fixation of the posterior injury, although the strategy varies based on the fracture pattern and displacement.

Technique

> #### ✔ Placement of SI Screws:
> ##### KEY SURGICAL STEPS
>
> ❑ Careful analysis of preoperative CT scan to review sacral anatomy and safe zones for screw placement
> ❑ Complete prep and drape of the abdomen above the umbilicus, pelvis, and lower extremities. Achieve provisional reduction of the SI joint
> ❑ Identify starting point:
> • Utilize the outlet view to obtain AP of the sacrum to provisionally mark skin incision start point
> • Obtain a perfect lateral view of the S1 body; the greater sciatic notches should overlap completely on the ideal lateral view of the sacrum. Mark the skin in the lateral plane along your first provisional line (the entry point is typically at the intersection of the long axis of the femur and a vertical line drawn posteriorly for the ASIS)
> ❑ Place the guidewire on to the lateral ilium and confirm position with fluoroscopy
> ❑ Advance guidewire, confirming position as you proceed to prevent entering the sacral foramen, the neural canal, and penetrating the anterior cortex of the S1 body: neuromonitoring is checked to assure safe passage
> ❑ After confirming the final position of the guidewire to the midline of the sacrum or just past the midline, the length is measured and the guidewire is over-drilled
> ❑ The screw is advanced over a washer to the level of the lateral ilium
> ❑ Multi-plane fluoroscopy is utilized to confirm reduction and stability. A second SI screw, in rare occasions, is indicated; the need for anterior ring fixation is then determined
> ❑ After completion of the procedure, neuromonitoring confirms that no injury has occurred to the lumbosacral plexus or L5 nerve
> ❑ Reduction techniques:
> • To reduce vertical displacement, longitudinal traction is applied through the leg manually or by a traction bow attached to a distal femoral traction pin
> • Posterior and rotational displacement may be reduced manually or by applying force through a T-handled chuck on a half-pin placed in the iliac crest away from potential incision sites
> • Open reduction may be required, most commonly anteriorly

Postoperative Care

If the pelvic ring is stable after fixation, cast immobilization is not necessary. The patient may be out of bed to a chair after surgery. Weight-bearing is restricted for a minimum of 6 weeks before gradual progression. Sacroiliac screws are not typically removed in adults. Although the growth consequences of SI joint fixation in younger children are not fully understood, it is our preference to remove screws after healing in this younger age group.

Open Reduction and Plate Fixation

Like adults, open reduction and plating of SI joint disruptions and fractures of the posterior ring are also sometimes indicated, most commonly when adequate reduction cannot be achieved with closed manipulative techniques, such as with large vertical displacement of the hemipelvis. This technique can be done either through an anterior retroperitoneal approach or via a posterior approach. The choice of implants is based on the size of the patient and the fracture type. Safe and effective plate fixation of unstable pelvic injuries has been reported in toddlers using 3.5-mm plating systems and adult techniques.[94]

SEVERE CRUSH INJURIES AND OPEN FRACTURES

Crush injuries of the pelvis and open fractures are relatively rare. In patients with crushing injuries, distortion of the pelvic ring is severe, resulting in multiple breaks in both the anterior and posterior pelvis as well as the acetabulum and triradiate cartilage. These uncommon injuries are nearly always associated with serious concomitant injuries, particularly thoracoabdominal and genitourinary abnormalities (Fig. 22-29). Neurologic injuries of the lumbosacral plexus and vascular injuries are also common associated findings. Risk of massive hemorrhage is highest for patients who sustain these types of fractures and, in one series, about 20% of children with crushed open pelvic fractures died within hours of admission secondary to uncontrolled hemorrhage.[57] Open fractures are more common than crush injuries, representing 13% of patients[57] with pelvic fractures, the result of motor vehicle trauma and gunshot wounds.

The principles of emergency management are similar to those applied for other unstable pelvic fractures. Surgical stabilization of the pelvic ring may be extremely challenging in the face of multiple fractures sites, comminution, and soft tissue

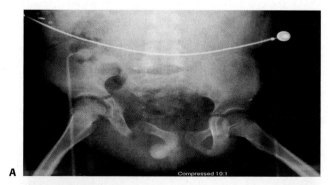

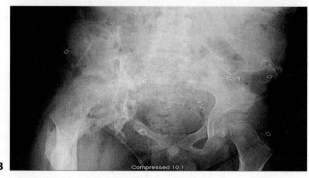

Figure 22-29. A: Open pelvic fracture with severe displacement. **B:** The soft tissue injury precluded pelvic reduction and fixation. This radiograph shows remarkable late deformity.

trauma. Lacerations of the vagina and rectum, bladder injuries, and urethral disruptions complicate management and increase the risk of infection. External fixation alone may not be sufficient to manage these complex injuries, making it frequently necessary to perform internal fixation or a combination of these techniques. Stable pelvic fixation, multiple debridements, soft tissue management, and careful surveillance for infection are recommended to improve the chances of successful outcomes.[57]

Acetabular Fractures

TREATMENT OPTIONS FOR ACETABULAR FRACTURES

Acetabular fractures constitute only 2% to 17% of pediatric pelvic fractures, making them very uncommon.[24,57,89,107] However, these injuries carry the potential for significant long-term morbidity. The goals of treatment for acetabular fractures in children are twofold. The first is to restore a congruent and stable joint with an anatomically reduced articular surface. The second is to preserve alignment of the triradiate cartilage in hopes of ensuring normal growth. Schlickewei et al.[77] noted that there are a variety of injury patterns and limited evidence of outcomes for any specific treatment. Thus, each fracture should be evaluated on an individual basis with the following guidelines: (i) Anatomic reduction will likely result in a good long-term outcome; (ii) MRI is the best tool for identifying closure of the triradiate cartilage; and (iii) patients should be informed about the possibility of growth arrest and secondary associated problems such as joint subluxation or dysplasia.[77]

NONOPERATIVE TREATMENT OF ACETABULAR FRACTURES

In general, conservative treatment is indicated for simple, nondisplaced fracture patterns. Short-term bed rest followed by non-weight bearing ambulation with crutches can be used for nondisplaced or minimally (≤2 mm) displaced fractures, particularly those that do not involve the superior acetabular dome. Because weight-bearing forces must not be transmitted across the fracture, crutch ambulation is appropriate only for older children who can reliably avoid weight-bearing on the injured limb. Nonweight-bearing usually is continued for 6 to 8 weeks. Radiographs should be obtained frequently in the first few weeks to confirm fracture alignment. For those younger children who cannot comply with nonweight-bearing ambulation, spica cast immobilization is preferred.

Skeletal traction is an option for those rare acetabular fractures that can be reduced to ≤2 mm of displacement or those with medical contraindications to surgical treatment. To avoid injury to the physis, the traction pin is usually inserted in the distal femur under anesthesia using fluoroscopic guidance. Follow-up radiographs should confirm fracture reduction and joint congruency, and traction is generally maintained for 4 to

6 weeks until fracture healing is sufficient to allow progressive weight-bearing.

There are few studies reporting the outcome of nonoperative treatment of acetabular fractures in children. Heeg et al.[34] reported on 23 patients with a variety of fracture patterns, with 18 being treated conservatively. The authors reported excellent functional and radiographic results of nonoperative treatment in those who were able to maintain congruent joints.

OPERATIVE TREATMENT OF ACETABULAR FRACTURES
Indications/Contraindications

The primary indication for operative treatment of pediatric acetabular fractures is either (1) an unstable joint or (2) an incongruent joint, regardless of fracture pattern. Instability usually results from posterior or anterior wall fractures, and, when present, must be remedied by operative reduction and fixation. Lack of congruency may result from bony fragments and/or soft tissue within the joint or from fracture displacement in the weight-bearing dome. In the former situation, open reduction is necessary to remove the offending agents and avoid premature osteoarthritis and, in the latter case, anatomic restoration of the articular surface with stable internal fixation is the operative goal. Gordon et al.[22] recommended accurate reduction and internal fixation of any displaced acetabular fracture in a child. They noted that the presence of incomplete fractures and plastic deformation may make accurate reduction difficult or impossible; they recommended that incomplete fractures be completed and that osteotomies of the pubis, ilium, or ischium be made if necessary to achieve accurate reduction of the acetabulum.[22] Improved outcomes with early (<24 hours) fixation of acetabular fractures in adults have been reported,[68] and Gordon et al.[22] noted that early fixation (before callus formation) is especially important to prevent malunion in young patients in whom healing is rapid (Fig. 22-30).

Another important indication for surgical treatment is malalignment of the triradiate cartilage, which can result in growth arrest and progressive acetabular dysplasia (Fig. 22-31). Linear growth of the acetabulum occurs by interstitial growth in the triradiate part of the cartilage complex, causing the pubis, ischium, and ilium to enlarge. The depth of the acetabulum develops in response to the presence of a spherical femoral head and interstitial growth of the acetabular cartilage.[70,82] Growth derangement of all or part of the triradiate cartilage as a result of poor fracture reduction may result in a dysplastic acetabulum. Since the ilioischial limb of the triradiate contributes the most to acetabular growth, injury to the ilioischial limb of the triradiate cartilage has a greater potential for late acetabular deformity than an anterior iliopubic limb injury.[20]

Outcomes

Sen et al.[83] reviewed a series of 38 adolescent acetabular fractures (patient ages 11 to 18 years) of which 37 were treated operatively. They reported generally good outcomes with 34/38 (89%) returning to full activity with 29 (76%) being pain-free at a mean follow-up of 38.2 months. Based on these results, the authors advocated a more aggressive surgical approach for any acetabular fracture with more than minimal displacement.

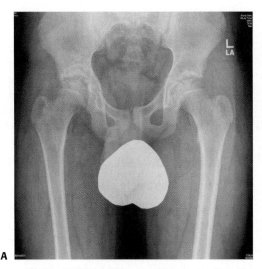
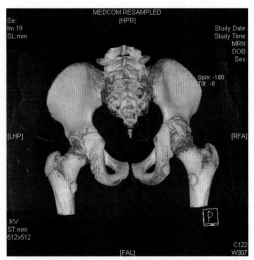

Figure 22-30. A: Pelvic radiograph of a 12-year-old 1 year after an acetabular fracture. The fracture is a malunion with subluxation of the hip joint. **B:** Three-dimensional CT scan showing the malunited fragment.

Open Reduction and Internal Fixation of Acetabular Fractures

Preoperative Planning

✔ Open Reduction and Internal Fixation of Acetabular Fractures: PREOPERATIVE PLANNING CHECKLIST	
OR table	☐ Fluoroscopic table such as a Jackson table
Fluoroscopy location	☐ Contralateral side of the table (opposite the injury)

Equipment	☐ Screw set including long 3.5- to 4.5-mm and various sized cannulated screws
	☐ Threaded Kirschner wires
	☐ Plate set including small fragment plates, pelvic reconstruction plates, and smaller "hook" plates
	☐ Pelvic retractors, clamps, and reduction instruments
	☐ Femoral distractor

The positioning and approach for ORIF of pediatric acetabular fractures varies according to the pattern of the fracture and the direction of the displacement as determined on the preoperative

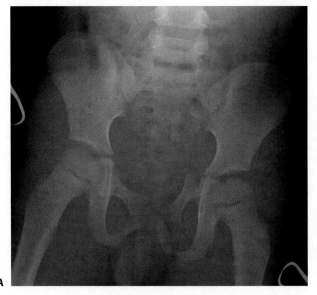
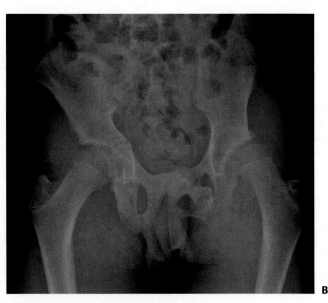

Figure 22-31. A: AP pelvis of a 4-year-old boy who was struck by a truck demonstrates left superior and inferior pubic rami fractures and involvement of the open triradiate cartilage. **B:** AP pelvis of the same patient 8 years later demonstrates premature closure of the left triradiate cartilage and posttraumatic acetabular dysplasia. (Reproduced with permission from Wudbhav N. Sankar, MD.)

TABLE 22-1. Surgical Exposure for Operative Fixation of Acetabular Fractures

Fracture Type	Exposure
Anterior column or wall	Ilioinguinal
Posterior column or wall	Kocher–Langenbeck
Transverse	Ilioinguinal (or extended lateral)
T-shaped	Ilioinguinal and Kocher–Langenbeck (or extended lateral)
Anterior column and posterior hemitransverse	Ilioinguinal
Both columns	Ilioinguinal (or extended lateral)

Reprinted from Gordon RG, Karpik K, Hardy S. Techniques of operative reduction and fixation of pediatric and adolescent pelvic fractures. *Oper Tech Orthop.* 1995;5(2):95–114. Copyright © 1995 Elsevier Inc. With permission.

radiographs and CT scans (Table 22-1).[22] Fractures of the posterior wall and/or posterior column can be approached through a Kocher–Langenbeck approach with the patient in either lateral decubitus or prone position (Fig. 22-32). Anterior column injuries can be approached through an ilioinguinal approach with the patient placed supine. Some transverse fractures may require an extended iliofemoral approach. The extended lateral approaches, which include the extended iliofemoral and triradiate approaches, should be avoided as much as possible because of the risk of devascularization of the ilium and heterotopic bone formation.

Technique

✔ Open Reduction and Internal Fixation of Acetabular Fractures: KEY SURGICAL STEPS

☐ Consider consultation with adult orthopedic traumatologist depending on experience level
☐ Careful preoperative planning requires advanced imaging (e.g., CT)
☐ Approach (i.e., iliofemoral, ilioinguinal, Kocher–Langenbach, etc.) and positioning (supine vs. prone) dictated by particular fracture pattern
☐ Obtain anatomic reduction via direct visualization or indirect reduction techniques
☐ Achieve stable fixation using screws or plates that can be contoured to specific anatomy
☐ Postoperative immobilization (e.g., Spica cast) for young children

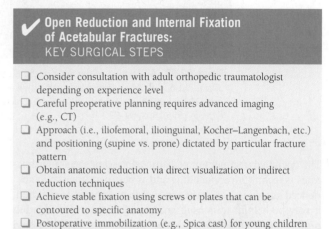

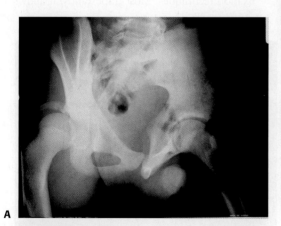

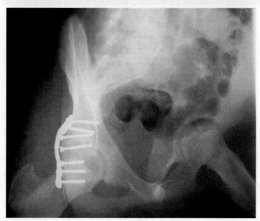

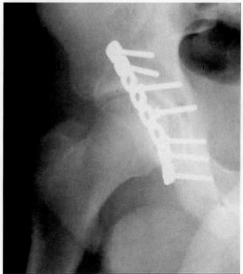

Figure 22-32. A: Radiograph of a football injury with posterior acetabular fracture and dislocation. **B** and **C:** Postoperative radiographs after a posterior approach and plating.

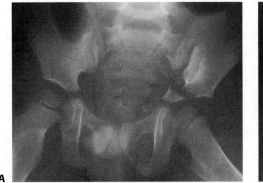
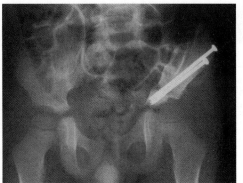

Figure 22-33. A: Fracture of the wing of the ilium with extension into the dome of the acetabulum in a 3-year-old boy. **B:** After reduction and fixation with two cannulated screws. (Reprinted with permission from Habacker TA, Heinrich SD, Dehne R. Fracture of the superior pelvic quadrant in a child. *J Pediatr Orthop.* 1995;15(1):69–72.)

The operative treatment of pediatric/adolescent acetabular fractures is technically demanding and is best performed by experienced surgeons. Given the rarity of these injuries in children, it may be helpful to consult and/or collaborate with an adult orthopedic traumatologist.[62] The operative surgeon should be familiar with the treatise by Judet et al.[40] on the operative reduction of acetabular fractures and with Letournel et al.[48] work before performing this surgery. For smaller children and smaller fragments, Watts[109] recommended threaded Kirschner wires for fixation. In larger children, cannulated screws can provide secure fixation (Figs. 22-33 and 22-34). Small-fragment

reconstruction plates, appropriately contoured, also can be used. Gordon et al.[22] described the addition of a small (two- or three-hole) "hook plate" for small or comminuted fragments (Fig. 22-35).

Brown et al.[7] described the use of CT image-guided fixation of acetabular fractures in 10 patients, including bilateral posterior wall fractures in a 14-year-old girl. They cite as advantages of image-guided surgery the reduced operating time (~20% reduction), less extensive surgical dissection, reduced fluoroscopic time, and compatibility with traditional fixation techniques. Most importantly, it allows accurate and

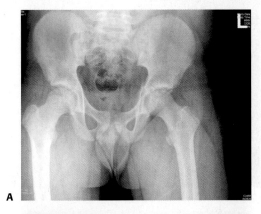
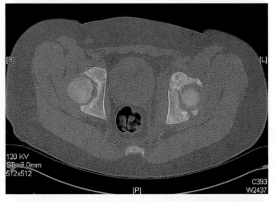
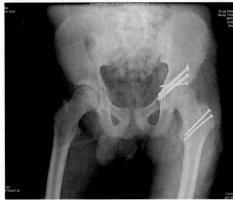

Figure 22-34. A: Radiograph of a 13-year-old with an acetabular fracture through the closing triradiate cartilage. **B:** CT scan showing the fracture in the region of the triradiate and posterior wall. **C:** Postoperative radiograph of the fracture fixed with cannulated screws via a surgical hip dislocation approach.

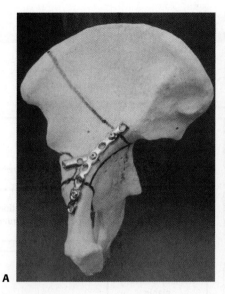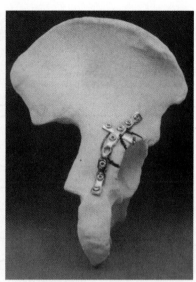

Figure 22-35. A: Anterior column plate and additional wall "hook" plate. **B:** Posterior wall buttress plate and hook plate. (Reprinted from Gordon RG, Karpik K, Hardy S. Techniques of operative reduction and fixation of pediatric and adolescent pelvic fractures. *Oper Tech Orthop.* 1995;5(2):95–114. Copyright © 1995 Elsevier Inc. With permission.)

safe placement of screws and pins for acetabular fixation. This technology is attractive, but anatomic reduction of the joint surface and secure fixation outweigh the benefits of surgical convenience.

Postoperative Care

Small children can be immobilized in a spica cast for 6 weeks after surgery depending on stability and patient compliance. If radiographs show adequate healing at that time, the cast is removed and free mobility is allowed. In an older child with stable fixation, crutches are used for protected weight-bearing for 6 to 8 weeks. If radiographs show satisfactory healing, weight-bearing is progressed as tolerated. Return to vigorous activities, especially competitive sports, is delayed for at least 3 months. For most children, some surgeons consider removal of metallic implants 6 to 18 months after surgery, assuming adequate healing, to facilitate future imaging and operative procedures about the hip.

Pelvic radiographs should be obtained for 2 years after an acetabular fracture to assess for triradiate closure. If the radiographs indicate a physeal bar, CT and MRI can be obtained to confirm the diagnosis.

Potential Pitfalls and Preventive Measures

Acetabular Fracture Surgery: PITFALLS AND PREVENTIONS	
Pitfalls	**Prevention**
• Avascular necrosis of the femoral head	• Urgent treatment of fracture-dislocations of the hip
• Posttraumatic arthrosis	• Anatomic or near-anatomic (≤2 mm) reduction of the articular surface
• Iatrogenic sciatic nerve injury (posterior approach)	• Consider intraoperative nerve monitoring; careful patient positioning; maintain knee flexion during posterior approach
• Iatrogenic lateral femoral cutaneous nerve injury (anterior approach)	• Careful retraction of LFCN; inform patient about potential for postoperative symptoms
• Heterotopic ossification	• Minimize stripping of gluteal muscles from outer table of ilium; careful choice of surgical approach; consider prophylaxis with indomethacin
• Fracture malunion	• Timely and accurate reduction and fixation of fractures
• Intra-articular placement of implants	• Use of intraoperative fluoroscopy supplemented by intraoperative portable radiographs when necessary. Consider postoperative CT scan to confirm appropriate implant position
• Venous thromboembolism	• Early mobilization; mechanical prophylaxis (e.g., compression boots, foot pumps); consider chemoprophylaxis

The potential complications following treatment of an acetabular fracture include avascular necrosis, posttraumatic arthritis, premature closure of the triradiate cartilage, infection, iatrogenic nerve injury, heterotopic ossification, fracture malunion, intra-articular penetration of implants, and venous thromboembolism. Although some of these outcomes may be unavoidable as a result of the initial injury, many can be prevented or at least mitigated by accurate decision-making, detailed surgical technique, and appropriate perioperative care.

Authors' Preferred Treatment of Pelvic and Acetabular Fractures (Algorithms 22-1 and 22-2)

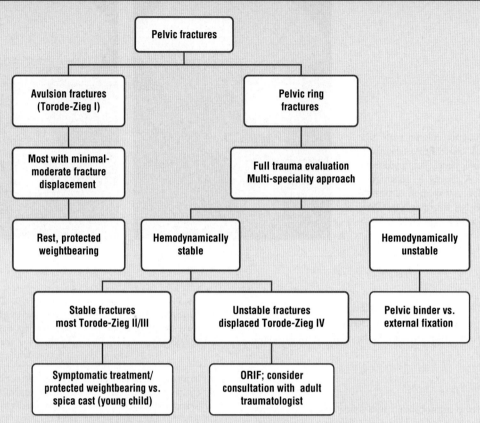

Algorithm 22-1. Authors' preferred treatment of pelvic fractures.

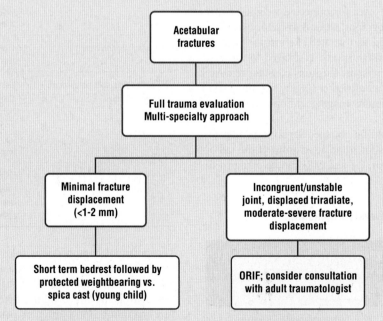

Algorithm 22-2. Authors' preferred treatment of acetabular fractures.

We almost always manage low-energy pelvic avulsion fractures (Torode and Zieg type I) conservatively with rest and partial weight-bearing on crutches for 2 or more weeks, followed by gradual resumption of normal activities after about 6 weeks. For those rare fractures with significant displacement (>2 cm) or persistent disability, fragment fixation or excision may be warranted.

For higher energy pelvic and acetabular fractures, a multispecialty approach is essential, especially at the time of initial presentation. The team should be aware of the large incidence of concomitant injuries to the head, thorax, and abdomen. The urogenital system should be carefully evaluated specifically looking for open fractures. If there is hemodynamic instability, the trauma surgeon, orthopedic surgeon, radiologist, and blood bank should work together to stabilize the patient. The orthopedic surgeon can provide temporary relief with pelvic wrapping, external fixation, or wound packing depending on the treatment of other injuries. If needed, operative fixation can be done in the same session as surgery for associated injuries or it can be timed later when the patient is stabilized.

Definitive treatment is usually conservative for isolated iliac wing fractures (Torode and Zieg type II), and simple pubis and ischium fractures (Torode and Zieg type III), and consists of symptomatic treatment and protected weight-bearing. For toddlers and younger school-age children, this treatment may include a spica cast for immobilization and comfort. For more involved pelvic and acetabular fractures, treatment is more likely to be conservative in children with an immature pelvis and operative in children with an unstable fracture pattern and a mature pelvis or closed triradiate cartilage.[81] In the younger, immature child with severe displacement, femoral traction on the displaced side of the hemipelvis may be indicated if operative reduction with implants is not technically feasible. There is mounting evidence, however, that unstable pelvic ring fractures and displaced acetabular fractures in children should be operatively reduced and stabilized using the same principles as in adults. Given the technically demanding nature of these operations, it is important that the surgeon has experience with these procedures and, if necessary, we recommend consultation and collaboration with an adult orthopedic traumatologist.

Torode and Zieg class IV injuries with displacement and/or pelvic ring fractures with displacement of more than 1 cm and anterior and posterior ring fractures should undergo reduction and fixation. Open reduction of the SI joint or a posterior iliac injury can be performed with a combination of plate and/or screws. The approach can be anterior in the iliac fossa or posterior depending on the fracture characteristics. Sacroiliac screws can be used in the immature pelvis, but the anatomy and size of S1 must be conducive for screw placement. Imaging, including the use of fluoroscopy for placement of the screws, is necessary. With a widened symphysis, anterior external fixation or plating is recommended along with posterior stabilization. Similarly, we advocate open reduction and internal fixation for any pediatric acetabular fracture that is associated with hip instability, incongruity of the joint, or significant displacement of the triradiate cartilage. The surgical approach and technique for fixation is dictated by the fracture pattern.

MANAGEMENT OF EXPECTED ADVERSE OUTCOMES AND UNEXPECTED COMPLICATIONS RELATED TO PELVIC AND ACETABULAR FRACTURES

Pelvic and Acetabular Fractures:
COMMON ADVERSE OUTCOMES AND COMPLICATIONS

- Malunion of the pelvic ring leading to leg length discrepancy, hip and spine arthrosis, SI joint pain or fusion, and distortion of the birth canal hindering vaginal delivery
- Premature triradiate closure after acetabular fractures leading to acetabular dysplasia and premature hip arthrosis
- Heterotopic ossification that causes pain at the site, hip impingement, and restricted hip range of motion
- Genitourinary complications including urethral and bladder injury, incontinence, chronic pelvic floor pain, and sexual dysfunction
- Disability related to associated injuries such as traumatic brain injury, thoracoabdominal trauma and lumbosacral plexus disruption
- Venous thromboembolism from the traumatic injury, immobilization, or as a complication of surgery

The major adverse outcomes following treatment of pediatric pelvic and acetabular fractures are malunion of the pelvic ring leading to long-term morbidity and premature triradiate closure after acetabular fracture. Because of the rapid healing in young children, loss of reduction and nonunion usually are not problems. Malunion of the pelvis can lead to leg length discrepancy, SI joint arthrosis, back pain, lumbar scoliosis, incompetency of the pelvic floor, and distortion of the birth canal. Because of the possibility of dystocia during childbirth, pelvimetry is recommended before pregnancy. Rieger and Brug[74] reported one female patient who required Caesarean section because of ossification of the symphysis pubis after nonoperative treatment of an open-book fracture. Schwarz et al.[80] reported leg length discrepancies of 1 to 5 cm in 10 of 17 patients after nonoperative treatment of unstable pelvic fractures; 5 had low back pain at long-term follow-up. Heeg and Klasen[33] reviewed 18 children with unstable pelvic fractures and reported that 9 had a leg length discrepancy greater than 1 cm and 3 had back pain. For those patients with growth remaining, an appropriately timed epiphysiodesis may be used to manage any residual leg length discrepancy. Of course, the best way to avoid the negative effects of pelvic malunion is to achieve and maintain an adequate initial reduction.

Acetabular dysplasia secondary to growth arrest of the triradiate cartilage is a concerning complication after trauma to the acetabulum. Premature closure of the triradiate cartilage has an overall incidence of less than 5% (range 0% to 11%) after pediatric acetabular fractures.[34,49,82,104] Heeg et al.[35] reported acetabular deformity and subluxation of the hip in two of three patients with premature fusion of the triradiate cartilage. Peterson and Robertson[67] reported formation of a physeal osseous bar in a 7-year-old boy 2 years after fracture of the lateral portion of the superior ramus at the junction with the triradiate cartilage. After excision of the osseous bridge, the physis remained open. Although the injured physis closed earlier than the contralateral side, there was only a slight increase in the thickness of the acetabular wall and lateral displacement of the femoral head. The authors emphasized that early recognition and treatment are essential before premature closure of the entire physis and development of permanent osseous deformity (Fig. 22-36).[67]

Bucholz et al.[8] noted two main patterns of physeal injury in nine patients with triradiate cartilage injury: A Salter–Harris type I or II injury, which had a favorable prognosis for continued normal acetabular growth, and a crush injury (Salter–Harris V), which had a poor prognosis with premature closure of the triradiate cartilage caused by formation of a medial osseous bridge. In either pattern, the prognosis depended on the child's age at the time of injury. In young children, especially those younger than 10 years of age, acetabular growth abnormality was common and resulted in a dysplastic acetabulum. By the time of skeletal maturity, disparate growth increased

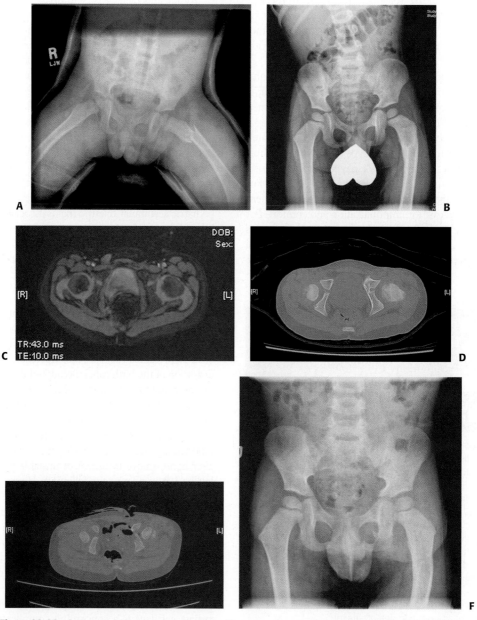

Figure 22-36. A: Radiograph of a 2-year-old child with a ramus fracture that involves the triradiate cartilage. **B:** Six months after the injury, there is indication of a physeal bar on the medial aspect of the triradiate cartilage. **C:** MRI confirming the presence of a physeal bar. **D:** CT scan confirming the physeal bar. **E:** CT scan confirming the physeal bar excision. This procedure was performed through an ilioinguinal approach and CT-guided excision. **F:** Radiograph of the pelvis after bar excision.

the incongruity of the hip joint and led to progressive sub-luxation. Triradiate injuries that occurred after the age of 10, however, generally did not result in significant changes to the acetabulum because of the diminished growth remaining in these patients. As a result, excision of a physeal bar is gen-erally recommended for patients younger than 10 years of age. Outcomes of triradiate physeal bar excision are limited to scattered case reports.[2,67] Badina et al. reported successful bar resection with methylmethacrylate or fat interposition through an extended Pfannenstiel approach in three patients aged 3, 4, and 5. All three patients demonstrated continued acetabular growth and no radiographic evidence of acetabular dysplasia at a mean follow-up of six years (one patient did require repeat bar excision). The typical dysplastic changes seen after prema-ture closure of the triradiate cartilage differ significantly from developmental dysplasia and include both lateralization of the hip joint and acetabular retroversion.[18,104] In severe cases, sub-luxation or dislocation can develop. Once present, this post-traumatic dysplasia often requires a complete redirectional acetabular osteotomy to improve femoral head coverage and correct the malorientation of the acetabulum.[8,104]

SUMMARY, CONTROVERSIES, AND FUTURE DIRECTIONS RELATED TO PELVIC AND ACETABULAR FRACTURES

Pelvic fractures are less common in the pediatric population, with only a small percentage of patients requiring operative treatment. In children, the overall long-term prognosis is gen-erally more favorable than in adults. Many children, however, have serious associated injuries including head trauma, and tho-racoabdominal and genitourinary injuries that contribute to the morbidity for these patients. Massive hemorrhage and death are rarely caused by the pelvic fracture itself and more commonly result from the concomitant injuries associated with unstable

fracture patterns, particularly those with vertical displacement of the hemipelvis and double breaks in the pelvic ring (modified Torode and Zieg types IIIb and IV). The goals of emergency treat-ment are to stabilize the hemodynamic status of the patient and to diagnose and treat serious, life-threatening associated inju-ries. Unstable pelvic fractures may initially require stabilization with a pelvic binder or external fixator. For most patients with displaced pelvic ring fractures, fracture realignment and stable fixation is utilized to reduce the risk of long-term complications such as leg length discrepancy, back pain, and SI joint arthrosis.

The future of pelvic fracture management has to address several important topics. Although much progress has been made regarding the delivery of specialized pediatric trauma care, the development of techniques and the knowledge gained from research at these specialized centers must continually be updated and disseminated to all who provide emergency trauma care for children. This is particularly important with regard to management of unstable pediatric pelvic fractures. Because of their rarity, few surgeons gain a broad experience managing these injuries at children's hospitals where most of these inju-ries initially presented. Collaboration with adult orthopedic traumatologists is, in our opinion, the solution to this problem. Together, principles of treatment and protocols for care can be refined including emergency management strategies, such as the use of embolization for massive bleeding, and the best indica-tions for surgery that are specific to pediatric patients.

From the standpoint of surgical techniques, pelvic fracture management must continue to improve so that procedures that are routinely performed on adults may be safely applied to children. Advances in implant development and the increased availability of intraoperative navigation may improve the outcomes of pel-vic fracture surgery for children of all ages with severe injuries. With advances in the care of the pediatric polytrauma patient and technical improvements for pelvic fracture management, the hope is that mortality will be greatly reduced and that the long-term complications may be eliminated or at least made more manage-able for patients as they progress into adulthood.

Annotated References

Reference	Annotation
Blasier RD, McAtee J, White R, et al. Disruption of the pelvic ring in pediatric patients. *Clin Orthop Relat Res.* 2000;(376):87–95.	The authors reviewed nearly 200 pediatric pelvic ring fractures, about ¼ were unstable, and of these, 43 were available for follow-up. Overall outcomes were slightly higher for the operative versus nonoperative treatment (92% vs. 80% good or excellent results) and both groups reported high patient satisfaction.
Chia JP, Holland AJ, Little D, et al. Pelvic fractures and associated injuries in children. *J Trauma.* 2004;56(1):83–88.	One hundred and twenty children with pelvic fractures from a single institution were identified. Associated injuries were identified in nearly 80%. Only 6% required surgery for their pelvic fractures, but over ¼ required surgery for their associated injuries. Five died and 27% had a poor outcome due to the associated injuries.
Greenwald LJ, Yost MT, Sponseller PD, et al. The role of clinically significant venous thromboembolism and thromboprophylaxis in pediatric patients with pelvic or femoral fractures. *J Pediatr Orthop.* 2012;32(4):357–361.	The records of 1,782 children with pelvic or femoral fractures admitted to a single institution were reviewed. Over 90% did not receive thromboprophylaxis. Only 3 (0.17%) of patients have a diagnosis of deep vein thrombosis, none were diagnosed with a pulmonary embolism and there was no related mortality.

Annotated References

Reference	Annotation
Holden CP, Holman J, Herman MJ. Pediatric pelvic fractures. *J Am Acad Orthop Surg.* 2007;15(3):172–177.	Pelvic and acetabular fractures are uncommon but often associated with life-threatening injuries. This article summarizes the assessment and care of these injuries in children.
Ismail N, Bellemare JF, Mollitt DL, et al. Death from pelvic fracture: children are different. *J Pediatr Surg.* 1996;31(1):82–85.	This article reviewed data on 23,700 children in the National Pediatric Trauma Registry (NPTR) and compared this to over 10,000 adults. The frequency of pelvic fractures was 50% less than adults and the mortality was less than 1/3 that of adults (5% vs. 17%).
McDonnell M, Schachter AK, Phillips DP, et al. Acetabular fracture through the triradiate cartilage after low-energy trauma. *J Orthop Trauma.* 2007;21(7):495–498.	This article presents an uncommon acetabular fracture through the triradiate cartilage, and describes the possible long-term complications.
Shore BJ, Palmer CS, Bevin C, et al. Pediatric pelvic fracture: a modification of a preexisting classification. *J Pediatr Orthop.* 2012;32(2):162–168.	One hundred and twenty-four children with pediatric pelvic fractures were identified and classified based on a modified Torode and Zieg classification. The classification was found to be predictive of increased hospital care and blood product use.
Silber JS, Flynn JM. Changing patterns of pediatric pelvic fractures with skeletal maturation: implications for classification and management. *J Pediatr Orthop.* 2002;22(1):22–26.	One hundred and sixty-six pelvic fractures were reviewed, 80% had radiographs adequate to evaluate the triradiate cartilage, which was used to determine maturity. Ninety-seven were determined to be immature (mean age 5.7) and 32 mature (mean age 14). The immature more commonly had isolated stable fractures while those in the mature group were more likely to have acetabular fractures and pubic or sacroiliac diastasis and all operative procedures were done in this group.
Swaid F, Peleg K, Alfici R, et al. A comparison study of pelvic fractures and associated abdominal injuries between pediatric and adult blunt trauma patients. *J Pediatr Surg.* 2017;52(3):386–389.	This study is a retrospective review of 7,621 patients in a national registry. They were classified as children (0–14) and adults (15–64 years old). There was a much lower incidence of these injuries in children (0.8 vs. 4.3%), and the severity of the pelvic injury was greater in adults, although in this study the morbidity was similar. The most common mechanism is pedestrian versus car in children versus motor vehicle accident in adults.
Tarman GJ, Kaplan GW, Lerman SL, et al. Lower genitourinary injury and pelvic fractures in pediatric patients. *Urology.* 2002;59(1):123–126.	Over 8,000 trauma patients presenting to a pediatric trauma center were reviewed, of which 212 patients had pelvic fractures. Seventeen percent were found to have genitourinary injuries, but of these, less than 3% had significant lower genitourinary injuries, and not found in stable pelvic fractures or in the absence of gross hematuria and a normal examination.

REFERENCES

1. Abdelgawad AA, Davey S, Salmon J, et al. Ilio-sacral (IS) screw fixation for sacral and sacroiliac joint (SIJ) injuries in children. *J Pediatr Orthop.* 2016;36(2):117–121.
2. Badina A, Vialle R, Fitoussi F, et al. Case reports: treatment of traumatic triradiate cartilage epiphysiodesis. What is the role of bridge resection? *Clin Orthop Relat Res.* 2013;471(11):3701–3705.
3. Bent MA, Hennrikus WL, Latorre JE, et al. Role of computed tomography in the classification of pediatric pelvic fractures-revisited. *J Orthop Trauma.* 2017;31(7):e200–e204.
4. Blanchard C, Kushare I, Boyles A, et al. Traumatic, posterior pediatric hip dislocations with associated posterior labrum osteochondral avulsion: recognizing the acetabular "fleck" sign. *J Pediatr Orthop.* 2016;36(6):602–607.
5. Blasier RD, McAtee J, White R, et al. Disruption of the pelvic ring in pediatric patients. *Clin Orthop Relat Res.* 2000;(376):87–95.
6. Bond SJ, Gotschall CS, Eichelberger MR. Predictors of abdominal injury in children with pelvic fracture. *J Trauma.* 1991;31(8):1169–1173.
7. Brown GA, Willis MC, Firoozbakhsh K, et al. Computed tomography image-guided surgery in complex acetabular fractures. *Clin Orthop Relat Res.* 2000;(370):219–226.
8. Bucholz RW, Ezaki M, Ogden JA. Injury to the acetabular triradiate physeal cartilage. *J Bone Joint Surg Am.* 1982;64(4):600–609.
9. Burgess AR, Eastridge BJ, Young JW, et al. Pelvic ring disruptions: effective classification system and treatment protocols. *J Trauma.* 1990;30(7):848–856.
10. Canale ST, Manugian AH. Irreducible traumatic dislocations of the hip. *J Bone Joint Surg Am.* 1979;61(1):7–14.
11. Chia JP, Holland AJ, Little D, et al. Pelvic fractures and associated injuries in children. *J Trauma.* 2004;56(1):83–88.
12. Clancy WG Jr, Foltz AS. Iliac apophysitis and stress fractures in adolescent runners. *Am J Sports Med.* 1976;4(5):214–218.
13. Connelly CR, Laird A, Barton JS, et al. A clinical tool for the prediction of venous thromboembolism in pediatric trauma patients. *JAMA Surg.* 2016;151(1):50–57.
14. Currey JD, Butler G. The mechanical properties of bone tissue in children. *J Bone Joint Surg Am.* 1975;57(6):810–814.
15. Delaney KM, Reddy SH, Dayama A, et al. Risk factors associated with bladder and urethral injuries in female children with pelvic fractures: an analysis of the National Trauma Data Bank. *J Trauma Acute Care Surg.* 2016;80(3):472–476.
16. Demetriades D, Karaiskakis M, Velmahos GC, et al. Pelvic fractures in pediatric and adult trauma patients: are they different injuries? *J Trauma.* 2003;54(6):1146–1151; discussion 1151.
17. Donoghue V, Daneman A, Krajbich I, et al. CT appearance of sacroiliac joint trauma in children. *J Comput Assist Tomogr.* 1985;9(2):352–356.
18. Dora C, Zurbach J, Hersche O, et al. Pathomorphologic characteristics of posttraumatic acetabular dysplasia. *J Orthop Trauma.* 2000;14(7):483–489.
19. Fitze G, Dahlen C, Zwipp H. Acetabular avulsion fracture in a 13-year-old patient after a minor trauma. *J Pediatr Surg.* 2008;43(3):E13–E16.
20. Gepstein R, Weiss RE, Hallel T. Acetabular dysplasia and hip dislocation after selective premature fusion of the triradiate cartilage. An experimental study in rabbits. *J Bone Joint Surg Br.* 1984;66(3):334–336.
21. Giannoudis PV, Pape HC. Damage control orthopaedics in unstable pelvic ring injuries. *Injury.* 2004;35(7):671–677.
22. Gordon R, Karpik K, Hardy S. Techniques of operative reduction and fixation of the pediatric adolescent pelvic fractures. *Oper Tech Ortho.* 1995;5:95–114.
23. Greenwald LJ, Yost MT, Sponseller PD, et al. The role of clinically significant venous thromboembolism and thromboprophylaxis in pediatric patients with pelvic or femoral fractures. *J Pediatr Orthop.* 2012;32(4):357–361.
24. Grisoni N, Connor S, Marsh E, et al. Pelvic fractures in a pediatric level I trauma center. *J Orthop Trauma.* 2002;16(7):458–463.
25. Grosso NP, Van Dam BE. Total coccygectomy for the relief of coccygodynia: a retrospective review. *J Spinal Disord.* 1995;8(4):328–330.
26. Guillamondegui OD, Mahboubi S, Stafford PW, et al. The utility of the pelvic radiograph in the assessment of pediatric pelvic fractures. *J Trauma.* 2003;55(2):236–239; discussion 239–240.

27. Guzman D, Sabharwal S, Zhao C, et al. Venous thromboembolism among pediatric orthopedic trauma patients: a database analysis. *J Pediatr Orthop B*. 2018;27(2):93–98.
28. Haasz M, Simone LA, Wales PW, et al. Which pediatric blunt trauma patients do not require pelvic imaging? *J Trauma Acute Care Surg*. 2015;79(5):828–832.
29. Hamai S, Nakashima Y, Akiyama M, et al. Ischio-pubic stress fracture after periacetabular osteotomy in patients with hip dysplasia. *Int Orthop*. 2014;38(10):2051–2056.
30. Hauschild O, Strohm PC, Culemann U, et al. Mortality in patients with pelvic fractures: results from the German pelvic injury register. *J Trauma*. 2008;64(2):449–455.
31. Hearty T, Swaroop VT, Gourineni P, et al. Standard radiographs and computed tomographic scan underestimating pediatric acetabular fracture after traumatic hip dislocation: report of 2 cases. *J Orthop Trauma*. 2011;25(7):e68–e73.
32. Hébert KJ, Laor T, Divine JG, et al. MRI appearance of chronic stress injury of the iliac crest apophysis in adolescent athletes. *AJR Am J Roentgenol*. 2008;190(6):1487–1491.
33. Heeg M, Klasen HJ. Long-term outcome of sacroiliac disruptions in children. *J Pediatr Orthop*. 1997;17(3):337–341.
34. Heeg M, Klasen HJ, Visser JD. Acetabular fractures in children and adolescents. *J Boint Joint Surg Br*. 1989;71(3):418–421.
35. Heeg M, Visser JD, Oostvogel HJ. Injuries of the acetabular triradiate cartilage and sacroiliac joint. *J Bone Joint Surg Br*. 1988;70(1):34–37.
36. Heinrich SD, Gallagher D, Harris M, et al. Undiagnosed fractures in severely injured children and young adults. Identification with technetium imaging. *J Bone Joint Surg Am*. 1994;76(4):561–572.
37. Holden CP, Holman J, Herman MJ. Pediatric pelvic fractures. *J Am Acad Orthop Surg*. 2007;15(3):172–177.
38. Hosalkar HS, Pennock AT, Zaps D, et al. The hip antero-superior labral tear with avulsion of rectus femoris (HALTAR)lesion: does the SLAP equivalent in the hip exist? *Hip Int*. 2012;22(4):391–396.
39. Ismail N, Bellemare JF, Mollitt DL, et al. Death from pelvic fracture: children are different. *J Pediatr Surg*. 1996;31(1):82–85.
40. Judet R, Judet J, Letournel E. Fractures of the acetabulum: classification and surgical approaches for open reduction. Preliminary report. *J Bone Joint Surg Am*. 1964;46:1615–1646.
41. Junkins EP Jr, Nelson DS, Carroll KL, et al. A prospective evaluation of the clinical presentation of pediatric pelvic fractures. *J Trauma*. 2001;51(1):64–68.
42. Karunakar MA, Goulet JA, Mueller KL, et al. Operative treatment of unstable pediatric pelvis and acetabular fractures. *J Pediatr Orthop*. 2005;25(1):34–38.
43. Keats T, Anderson M. *Atlas of Normal Roentgen Variants that May Stimulate Disease*. St. Louis, MO: Mosby; 2001:371.
44. Keshishyan RA, Rozinov VM, Malakhov OA, et al. Pelvic polyfractures in children. Radiographic diagnosis and treatment. *Clin Orthop Relat Res*. 1995;(320):28–33.
45. Kruppa CG, Khoriaty JD, Sietsema DL, et al. Pediatric pelvic ring injuries: how benign are they? *Injury*. 2016;47(10):2228–2234.
46. Kuhn J, Slovis T, Haller JO. *Caffey's Pediatric Diagnostic Imaging*. 10th ed. Philadelphia, PA: Mosby; 2004.
47. Lee DH, Jeong WK, Inna P, et al. Bilateral sacroiliac joint dislocation (anterior and posterior) with triradiate cartilage injury: a case report. *J Orthop Trauma*. 2011;25(12):e111–e114.
48. Letournel E, Judet R, Elson RA. *Fractures of the Acetabulum*. 2nd ed. New York: Springer-Verlag; 1993.
49. Liporace FA, Ong B, Mohaideen A, et al. Development and injury of the triradiate cartilage with its effects on acetabular development: review of the literature. *J Trauma*. 2003;54(6):1245–1249.
50. Lynch SA, Renstrom PA. Groin injuries in sport: treatment strategies. *Sports Med*. 1999;28(2):137–144.
51. Magid D, Fishman EK, Ney DR, et al. Acetabular and pelvic fractures in the pediatric patient: value of two- and three-dimensional imaging. *J Pediatr Orthop*. 1992;12(5):621–625.
52. Marmor M, Elson J, Mikhail C, et al. Short-term pelvic fracture outcomes in adolescents differ from children and adults in the National Trauma Data Bank. *J Child Orthop*. 2015;9(1):65–75.
53. Matsuda DK, Calipusan CP. Adolescent femoroacetabular impingement from malunion of the anteroinferior iliac spine apophysis treated with arthroscopic spinoplasty. *Orthopedics*. 2012;35(3):e460–e463.
54. Matta JM, Saucedo T. Internal fixation of pelvic ring fractures. *Clin Orthop Relat Res*. 1989;(242):83–97.
54a. McDonald G. Pelvic disruptions in children. *Clin Orthop Relate Res*. 1980;151:130–134.
55. McDonnell M, Schachter AK, Phillips DP, et al. Acetabular fracture through the triradiate cartilage after low-energy trauma. *J Orthop Trauma*. 2007;21(7):495–498.
56. Micheli LJ, Curtis C. Stress fractures in the spine and sacrum. *Clin Sports Med*. 2006;25(1):75–88, ix.
57. Mosheiff R, Suchar A, Porat S, et al. The "crushed open pelvis" in children. *Injury*. 1999;30(Suppl 2):B14–B18.
58. Murphy RF, Naqvi M, Miller PE. Pediatric orthopaedic lower extremity trauma and venous thromboembolism. *J Child Orthop*. 2015;9(5):381–384.
59. Nierenberg G, Volpin G, Bialik V. Pelvic fractures in children: a follow-up in 20 children treated conservatively. *J Pediatr Orthop B*. 1992;1:140–142.
60. Nieto LL, Camacho SG, Reinoso JP. [Treatment of Torode and Zieg type IV unstable pelvic fractures in children]. *Acta Ortop Mex*. 2010;24(5):338–344.
61. Noakes TD, Smith JA, Lindenberg G, et al. Pelvic stress fractures in long distance runners. *Am J Sports Med*. 1985;13(2):120–123.
62. Ochs BG, Marintschev I, Hoyer H, et al. Changes in the treatment of acetabular fractures over 15 years: analysis of 1266 cases treated by the German Pelvic Multicentre Study Group (DAO/DGU). *Injury*. 2010;41(8):839–851.
63. Ogden JA. *Skeletal Injury in the Child*. 3rd ed. New York: Springer-Verlag; 2000.
64. Oransky M, Arduini M, Tortora M, et al. Surgical treatment of unstable pelvic fracture in children: long term results. *Injury*. 2010;41(11):1140–1144.
65. Pavlov H, Nelson TL, Warren RF, et al. Stress fractures of the pubic ramus. A report of twelve cases. *J Bone Joint Surg Am*. 1982;64(7):1020–1025.
66. Pennal GF, Tile M, Waddell JP, et al. Pelvic disruption: assessment and classification. *Clin Orthop Relat Res*. 1980;(151):12–21.
67. Peterson HA, Robertson RC. Premature partial closure of the triradiate cartilage treated with excision of a physical osseous bar. Case report with a fourteen-year follow-up. *J Bone Joint Surg Am*. 1997;79(5):767–770.
68. Plaisier BR, Meldon SW, Super DM, et al. Improved outcome after early fixation of acetabular fractures. *Injury*. 2000;31(2):81–84.
69. Pohlemann T. Pelvic ring injuries: assessment and concepts of surgical management. In: Ruedi T, Murphy W, eds. *AO Principles of Fracture Management*. New York: Thieme; 2000.
70. Ponseti IV. Growth and development of the acetabulum in the normal child. Anatomical, histological, and roentgenographic studies. *J Bone Joint Surg Am*. 1978;60(5):575–585.
71. Reed MH. Pelvic fractures in children. *J Can Assoc Radiol*. 1976;27(4):255–361.
72. Reichard SA, Helikson MA, Shorter N, et al. Pelvic fractures in children—review of 120 patients with a new look at general management. *J Pediatr Surg*. 1980;15(6):727–734.
73. Reilly BR, Ma MC. Acetabulum fractures. In: Robert JDH, Bucholz W, Court-Brown Charles M, et al, eds. *Rockwood and Green's Fractures in Adults*. Philadelphia, PA: Lippincott Williams & Wilkins; 2010:1463–1524.
74. Rieger H, Brug E. Fractures of the pelvis in children. *Clin Orthop Relat Res*. 1997;(336):226–239.
75. Rossi F, Dragoni S. Acute avulsion fractures of the pelvis in adolescent competitive athletes: prevalence, location and sports distribution of 203 cases collected. *Skeletal Radiol*. 2001;30(3):127–131.
76. Rubel IF, Kloen P, Potter HG, et al. MRI assessment of the posterior acetabular wall fracture in traumatic dislocation of the hip in children. *Pediatr Radiol*. 2002;32(6):435–439.
77. Schlickewei W, Keck T. Pelvic and acetabular fractures in childhood. *Injury*. 2005;36(Suppl 1):A57–A63.
78. Schlonsky J, Olix ML. Functional disability following avulsion fracture of the ischial epiphysis. Report of two cases. *J Bone Joint Surg Am*. 1972;54(3):641–644.
79. Schuett DJ, Bomar JD, Pennock AT. Pelvic apophyseal avulsion fractures: a retrospective review of 228 cases. *J Pediatr Orthop*. 2015;35(6):617–623.
80. Schwarz N, Posch E, Mayr J, et al. Long-term results of unstable pelvic ring fractures in children. *Injury*. 1998;29(6):431–433.
81. Scolaro JA, Firoozabadi R, Routt ML. Treatment of pediatric and adolescent pelvic ring injuries with percutaneous screw placement. *J Pediatr Orthop*. 2018;38(3):133–137.
82. Scuderi G, Bronson MJ. Triradiate cartilage injury. Report of two cases and review of the literature. *Clin Orthop Relat Res*. 1987;(217):179–189.
83. Sen MK, Warner SJ, Sama N, et al. Treatment of acetabular fractures in adolescents. *Am J Orthop (Belle Mead NJ)*. 2015;44(10):465–470.
84. Sener M, Karapinar H, Kazimoglu C, et al. Fracture dislocation of sacroiliac joint associated with triradiate cartilage injury in a child: a case report. *J Pediatr Orthop B*. 2008;17(2):65–68.
85. Shah MK, Stewart GW. Sacral stress fractures: an unusual cause of low back pain in an athlete. *Spine (Phila Pa 1976)*. 2002;27(4):E104–E108.
86. Shlamovitz GZ, Mower WR, Bergman J, et al. Lack of evidence to support routine digital rectal examination in pediatric trauma patients. *Pediatr Emerg Care*. 2007;23(8):537–543.
87. Shlamovitz GZ, Mower WR, Bergman J, et al. Poor test characteristics for the digital rectal examination in trauma patients. *Ann Emerg Med*. 2007;50(1):25–33, 33.e1.
88. Shore BJ, Palmer CS, Bevin C, et al. Pediatric pelvic fracture: a modification of a preexisting classification. *J Pediatr Orthop*. 2012;32(2):162–168.
89. Silber JS, Flynn JM. Changing patterns of pediatric pelvic fractures with skeletal maturation: implications for classification and management. *J Pediatr Orthop*. 2002;22(1):22–26.
90. Silber JS, Flynn JM, Katz MA, et al. Role of computed tomography in the classification and management of pediatric pelvic fractures. *J Pediatr Orthop*. 2001;21(2):148–151.
91. Silber JS, Flynn JM, Koffler KM, et al. Analysis of the cause, classification, and associated injuries of 166 consecutive pediatric pelvic fractures. *J Pediatr Orthop*. 2001;21(4):446–450.
92. Smith WR, Oakley M, Morgan SJ. Pediatric pelvic fractures. *J Pediatr Orthop*. 2004;24(1):130–135.
93. Smith W, Shurnas P, Morgan S, et al. Clinical outcomes of unstable pelvic fractures in skeletally immature patients. *J Bone Joint Surg Am*. 2005;87(11):2423–2431.
94. Stiletto RJ, Baacke M, Gotzen L. Comminuted pelvic ring disruption in toddlers: management of a rare injury. *J Trauma*. 2000;48(1):161–164.
95. Subasi M, Arslan H, Necmioglu S, et al. Long-term outcomes of conservatively treated paediatric pelvic fractures. *Injury*. 2004;35(8):771–781.
96. Sundar M, Carty H. Avulsion fractures of the pelvis in children: a report of 32 fractures and their outcome. *Skeletal Radiol*. 1994;23(2):85–90.
97. Swaid F, Peleg K, Alfici R, et al; A comparison study of pelvic fractures and associated abdominal injuries between pediatric and adult blunt trauma patients. *J Pediatr Surg*. 2017;52(3):386–389.
98. Tarman GJ, Kaplan GW, Lerman SL, et al. Lower genitourinary injury and pelvic fractures in pediatric patients. *Urology*. 2002;59(1):123–126; discussion 126.
99. Tile M. Pelvic fractures: operative versus nonoperative treatment. *Orthop Clin North Am*. 1980;11(3):423–464.
100. Tile M, Helfet DL, Kellam JF. *Fractures of the Pelvis and Acetabulum*. 3rd ed. Baltimore, MD: Lippincott Williams & Wilkins; 2003.
101. Tolo VT. Orthopaedic treatment of fractures of the long bones and pelvis in children who have multiple injuries. *Instr Course Lect*. 2000;49:415–423.
102. Tomaszewski R, Gap A. Operative treatment of pediatric pelvic fractures—our experience. *Orthop Traumatol Rehabil*. 2011;13(3):241–252.
103. Torode I, Zieg D. Pelvic fractures in children. *J Pediatr Orthop*. 1985;5(1):76–84.

104. Trousdale RT, Ganz R. Posttraumatic acetabular dysplasia. *Clin Orthop Relat Res.* 1994;(305):124–132.
105. Upperman JS, Gardner M, Gaines B, et al. Early functional outcome in children with pelvic fractures. *J Pediatr Surg.* 2000;35(6):1002–1005.
106. Vazquez WD, Garcia VF. Pediatric pelvic fractures combined with an additional skeletal injury is an indicator of significant injury. *Surg Gynecol Obstet.* 1993;177(5):468–472.
107. Von Heyden J, Hauschild O, Strohm PC, et al. Paediatric acetabular fractures: data from the German Pelvic Trauma Registry Initiative. *Acta Orthop Belg.* 2012;78(5):611–618.
108. Wait A, Gaskill T, Sarwar Z, et al. Van neck disease: osteochondrosis of the ischiopubic synchondrosis. *J Pediatr Orthop.* 2011;31(5):520–524.
109. Watts HG. Fractures of the pelvis in children. *Orthop Clin North Am.* 1976;7(3):615–624.
110. Worlock P, Stower M. Fracture patterns in Nottingham children. *J Pediatr Orthop.* 1986;6(6):656–660.
111. Zwingmann J, Aghayev E, Südkamp NP, et al. Pelvic fractures in children results from the German pelvic trauma registry: a cohort study. *Medicine (Baltimore).* 2015;94(51):e2325.

23

Fractures and Traumatic Dislocations of the Hip in Children

Rachel Y. Goldstein and Young-Jo Kim

Hip Fractures

INTRODUCTION TO HIP FRACTURES

While hip fractures are common in adults, they are rare in children, comprising less than 1% of all pediatric fractures.[9,10,83] Pediatric hip fractures typically result from high-energy mechanisms, and may be associated with additional extremity, visceral, or head injuries in 30% of patients. This is in contrast to low-energy adult hip fractures common in elderly patients, whose fractures are typically associated with osteoporosis. Occasionally, pediatric hip fractures result from minor trauma superimposed upon bone that is weakened by tumor or metabolic bone disease. These fractures can occur through the physis, but more commonly occur through the femoral neck and the intertrochanteric region.

The presence of the proximal femoral physis is an important consideration when treating pediatric hip fractures. Injury to the greater trochanter apophysis can lead to coxa valga.[18] Damage to the proximal femoral physis from fracture or implant use can result in limb length discrepancies, coxa breva or coxa vara. The surgeon should generally place fixation across the physis in older children with poor bone quality, in adolescents who have little growth potential remaining, or if fracture location dictates that adequate fixation must cross the physis.

Pediatric hips are also at risk secondary to their limited blood supply. The physis may act as a barrier to potential interosseous blood supply to the femoral head. Because of this, and the fact that there is little blood supply to the femoral head from the ligamentum teres, an increased risk of osteonecrosis (ON) is present following hip fracture that may disrupt the important retinacular vessels.

Although they are less common than other pediatric fractures, pediatric hip fractures are important secondary to the high rate of complications and the potential lifetime morbidity that may result from complications. Potential complications from the fracture and its treatment include chondrolysis, ON, varus malunion, nonunion, physeal disruption, and growth abnormalities leading to leg length discrepancy or angular deformities.[18] Because the hip is developing in the growing child, deformities can progress and change with age. However, outcomes for these complex fracture can be significantly improved if certain treatment principles are consistently followed.[9]

ASSESSMENT OF HIP FRACTURES

MECHANISMS OF INJURY FOR HIP FRACTURES

Hip fractures in children can be caused by axial loading, torsion, hyperabduction, or a direct blow to the hip. Almost all hip fractures in children are caused by severe, high-energy trauma, such as those seen with motor vehicle and in accidents or falls from a height.[5,34] With the exception of the physis, the proximal femur in children is extremely strong, and significant force is necessary to cause fracture. If a child suffers a fracture as a result of insignificant trauma, then one should suspect an underlying etiology such as prior injury or surgery,[20] metabolic bone disease, or pathologic lesion of the proximal femur (Fig. 23-1).

Infants with hip fractures and without a plausible cause for fracture should be evaluated for nonaccidental trauma by a careful history and an examination of the skin, other extremities, trunk, and head. Further skeletal radiographic imaging is often indicated, and an evaluation by a child protective team is required to diagnose life-threatening head and visceral injuries that can be easily missed in this group.

INJURIES ASSOCIATED WITH HIP FRACTURES

Because these fractures are caused by high-energy trauma, they are frequently accompanied by associated injuries that can affect the patient's overall outcome. Pape et al.,[71] in a series of 28 patients with a mean follow-up of 11 years, found favorable outcomes in type II, III, and IV fractures according to Ratliff's criteria.[83] Poorer functional outcomes were attributed to associated head trauma, amputation, or peripheral neurologic damage.[71] In a series of 14 patients with hip fractures, all of which were caused by vehicular accidents or falls from height, 12 patients (86%) had associated injuries including head and facial injury, other fractures, and/or visceral injury.[65] In a series of hip fractures secondary to high-energy trauma, Bagatur and Zorer[4] similarly found associated injuries in 4 of their 17 patients.

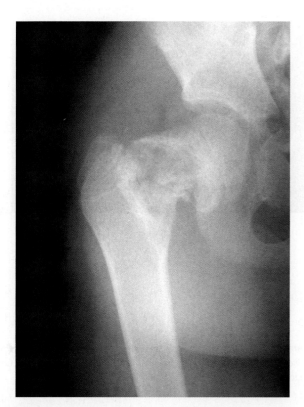

Figure 23-1. A 10-year-old boy with a fracture through a unicameral bone cyst sustained while running for a soccer ball.

SIGNS AND SYMPTOMS OF HIP FRACTURES

The diagnosis of hip fracture in a child is based on the history of high-energy trauma and the typical signs and symptoms of the shortened, externally rotated, and painful lower extremity. Clinical examination is usually obvious, and a patient with a complete fracture is unable to ambulate because of severe pain in the hip and has a shortened, externally rotated extremity. An infant with a hip fracture holds the extremity flexed, abducted, and externally rotated. Infants and newborns with limited ossification of the proximal femur can be challenging patients to diagnose with hip fractures as the differential diagnosis can include infection and congenital dislocation of the hip. In the absence of infection symptoms, pseudoparalysis, shortening, and a strong suspicion are the keys to a fracture diagnosis in this age group.

With an incomplete or stress fracture of the femoral neck, the patient may be able to bear weight with a limp and may demonstrate hip or knee pain only with extremes of range of motion, especially internal rotation. In a case series of six patients under the age of ten with femoral neck stress fractures, Boyle et al. found that patients presented with a limp that worsened with activity.[14] Only half of the patients experienced pain with the terminal flexion, while the other half had no pain with hip range of motion.

IMAGING AND OTHER DIAGNOSTIC STUDIES FOR HIP FRACTURES

A good-quality anteroposterior (AP) pelvic radiograph will provide a comparison view of the opposite hip if a displaced fracture is suspected. For the pelvic radiograph, the leg should be held in extension and in as much internal rotation as possible without causing extreme pain to the patient. A cross-table lateral radiograph should be considered to avoid further displacement and unnecessary discomfort to the patient from an attempt at a frog-leg lateral view.

Nondisplaced fracture or stress fractures may be difficult to detect on radiographs. Any break or offset of the bony trabeculae near Ward's triangle, the radiolucent area between the principle compressive, secondary compressive, and primary tensile trabeculae in the femoral neck, is an evidence of a nondisplaced or impacted fracture. Special studies may be required to reveal an occult fracture as case examples of further displacement of nondisplaced fracture have been reported.[36] Adjunctive studies for stress fracture diagnosis may include a magnetic resonance imaging (MRI), computed tomography (CT) scan, or a technetium bone scan which can demonstrate increased uptake at the fracture site.

The typical MRI appearance of a fracture is a linear black line (low signal) on all sequences surrounded by a high-signal band of bone marrow edema and hemorrhage. The low signal represents the trabecular impaction (Fig. 23-2). MRI may detect an occult hip fracture within the first 24 hours after injury.[48] In addition, pathologic fractures may require special imaging to aid diagnosis or to fully appreciate bone quality which would impact implant placement. MRI is also a useful test in planning treatment for a pathologic fracture; this test will delineate soft tissues in and around the fracture, which can provide insight into diagnosis and delineate high-yield areas for biopsy.

In infants, an ultrasound can be used to detect epiphyseal separation. In addition, an ultrasound can demonstrate the presence of an effusion, which may be aspirated to aid in diagnosis. A bloody aspirate is suggestive of fracture, whereas a serous or purulent aspirate suggests synovitis or infection, respectively. If performed in the operating room, an aspiration and confirmatory arthrogram of the hip can also be useful, especially if closed reduction and cast immobilization is chosen as treatment.

In a patient with posttraumatic hip pain without evidence of a fracture, other diagnoses must be considered, including Perthes disease, synovitis, spontaneous hemarthrosis, and infection. A complete blood count, erythrocyte sedimentation rate, C-reactive protein, and vital signs are helpful to evaluate for infection. When the presentation is unclear, MRI scan may be a useful test to diagnose aseptic ON as a result of Perthes disease or more remote causes of ON. In children under 5 years of age, developmental coxa vara can be confused with an old hip fracture.[18]

CLASSIFICATION OF HIP FRACTURES

Hip Fractures: DELBET CLASSIFICATION
• Type IA: Transepiphyseal fracture without dislocation from the acetabulum
• Type IB: Transepiphyseal fracture with dislocation from the acetabulum
• Type II: Transcervical fracture
• Type III: Cervicotrochanteric fracture
• Type IV: Intertrochanteric fracture

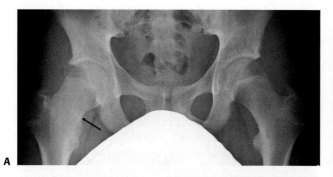

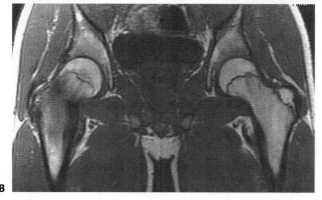

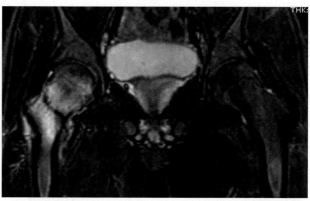

Figure 23-2. Right hip pain with nondisplaced stress fracture (**A**). The T1-weighted image shows the impacted cortex (**B**). The STIR sequence image shows surrounding bony edema (**C**).

Pediatric hip fractures generally are classified by the method of Delbet (Fig. 23-3).[24] This classification system continues to be useful because it is not only descriptive but also has prognostic significance.[61] In general, more significant rates of ON and growth arrest are noted in fractures in the proximal end of the femoral neck (type I and type II injuries), whereas lower rates of ON are noted in type III and type IV injuries. Conversely, the latter two groups tend to have higher rates of significant varus malunion if not treated appropriately. Subtrochanteric fractures have been included by some in the discussion of proximal femoral fractures but they are not included in the Delbet classification and are discussed elsewhere in this book.

Type I

Transphyseal fractures occur through the proximal femoral physis, with (type IA) or without (type IB) dislocation of the femoral head from the acetabulum (Fig. 23-4). Such fractures are rare, constituting 8% of hip fractures in children.[47] Approximately half of type I fractures are associated with a dislocation of the capital femoral epiphysis. True transphyseal fractures tend to occur in young children after high-energy trauma[19,31] and are different from unstable slipped capital femoral epiphysis (SCFE), which usually follows a prodromal period of activity-related hip or knee pain. Unstable SCFE differs from traumatic separation as it occurs following minor trauma, which is superimposed on a weakened physis while a true transphyseal fracture is secondary to a high-energy trauma.

Iatrogenic fracture of the physis in children and adolescents has been described as occurring during reduction of a hip dislocation (Fig. 23-5).[15,45] As true physeal fractures are high-

energy injuries, it is possible, and perhaps more likely, that these patients had unrecognized physeal injury at the time of dislocation and the epiphysis became displaced during reduction.

Transphyseal fractures without femoral head dislocation have a better prognosis than those with dislocation. Similarly, younger children with these fractures have a better prognosis than older children. Osteonecrosis in younger children is unlikely, although coxa vara, coxa breva, and premature physeal closure can cause subsequent leg length discrepancy.[18,20] In cases of femoral head dislocation in a type I fracture, the outcome is poor secondary to ON and premature physeal closure in virtually 100% of patients.[19,31]

Type II

Transcervical fractures are the most common fracture type (45% to 50% of all hip fractures).[47] These fractures occur between the proximal femoral physis and the intertrochanteric line. By definition, these fractures are considered intracapsular femoral neck fractures. Nondisplaced transcervical fractures have a better prognosis and a lower rate of ON than displaced fractures, regardless of treatment.[19,67,83] However, ON can still occur in minimally displaced fractures, and this may be secondary to the fact that it is difficult to document how much displacement and spontaneous reduction occurs at the time of trauma. Moon and Mehlman[61] performed a meta-analysis of available literature and documented a 28% incidence of ON in type II fractures. The occurrence of ON is thought by these and other investigators to be directly related to fracture displacement, which may lead to disruption or kinking of the blood supply to the femoral head. In addition, the meta-analysis demonstrated

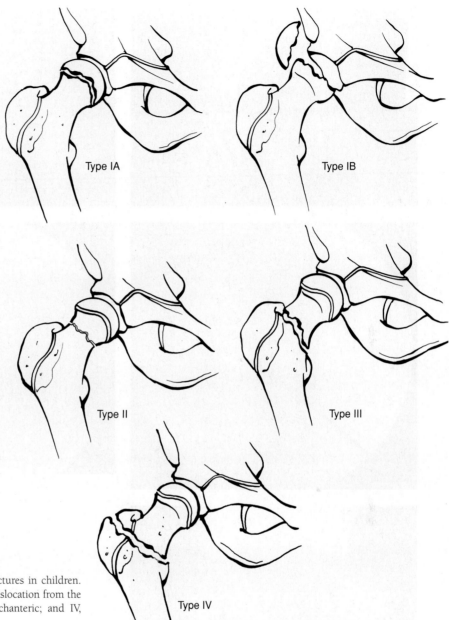

Figure 23-3. Delbet classification of hip fractures in children. I, transepiphyseal with (IB) or without (IA) dislocation from the acetabulum; II, transcervical; III, cervicotrochanteric; and IV, intertrochanteric.

higher rates of ON in children older than 10 years at the time of their injury.[67] Because the pediatric hip capsule is tough and less likely to tear, some have hypothesized that a possible etiology of vascular impairment in minimally displaced fractures is a result of intra-articular hemarthrosis leading to vessel compression from tamponade.[19,47]

Type III

Cervicotrochanteric fractures are located at or slightly above the anterior intertrochanteric line and are the second most common type of hip fracture in children, representing about 34% of fractures.[47] It is conceivable that a certain portion of these fractures may be intra- and extracapsular as a result of anatomic differences in capsule insertion. Nondisplaced type

III fractures also have a much lower complication rate than displaced fractures. Displaced type III are similar to type II fractures in the type of complications that can occur. The incidence of ON seen with this fracture pattern is 18%, slightly less than in type II fractures.[67] Similar to type II fractures, the risk of ON is directly related to the degree of displacement at the time of injury.[13] Premature physeal closure occurs in 25% of patients, and coxa vara occurs in approximately 14% of patients.[47]

Type IV

Intertrochanteric fractures account for only 12% of hip fractures in children.[47] This fracture is completely extracapsular and has the lowest complication rate of all four types. Nonunion in this

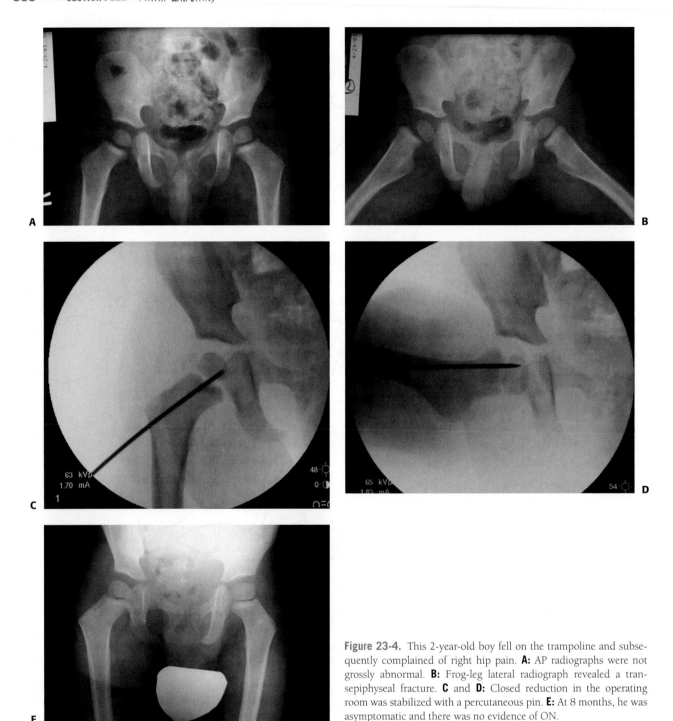

Figure 23-4. This 2-year-old boy fell on the trampoline and subsequently complained of right hip pain. **A:** AP radiographs were not grossly abnormal. **B:** Frog-leg lateral radiograph revealed a transepiphyseal fracture. **C** and **D:** Closed reduction in the operating room was stabilized with a percutaneous pin. **E:** At 8 months, he was asymptomatic and there was no evidence of ON.

fracture is rare. Moon and Mehlman[61] documented a rate of ON of only 5%, which is much lower than in the other types of hip fractures. Coxa vara and premature physeal closure have occasionally been reported.[19,47,56,82,83]

UNUSUAL FRACTURE PATTERNS

Rarely, proximal femoral physeal separation occurs during a difficult delivery and can be confused on radiographs with congenital dislocation of the hip.[14] Type I fracture in a neonate

deserves special attention. This injury is exceedingly rare and, because the femoral head is not visible on plain radiographs, the diagnosis can be difficult. The index of suspicion must be high in neonates, after a difficult delivery, who are not moving their leg. The differential diagnosis includes septic arthritis and developmental hip dislocation. Plain radiographs may show a high-riding proximal femoral metaphysis on the involved side, thus mimicking a developmental hip dislocation. Ultrasonography is useful in diagnosis of neonatal proximal femoral physeal fracture; with this test, the cartilaginous

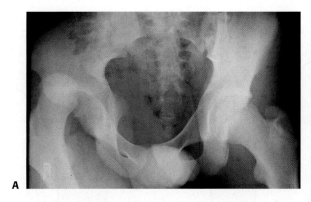

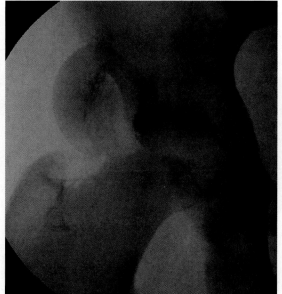

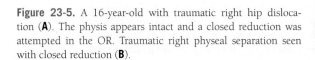

Figure 23-5. A 16-year-old with traumatic right hip dislocation (**A**). The physis appears intact and a closed reduction was attempted in the OR. Traumatic right physeal separation seen with closed reduction (**B**).

head remains in the acetabulum but its dissociation from the femoral shaft can be appreciated.[70] The diagnosis can be missed if there is no history of trauma or if there is an ipsilateral fracture of the femoral shaft.[2] In the absence of a known history of significant trauma in a young child, nonaccidental trauma should be ruled out.

Stress fractures are caused by repetitive injury and result in hip or knee pain and a limp. Pain associated with long-distance running, marching, or a recent increase in physical activity is suggestive of stress fracture. Though in a recent case study of young children with femoral neck fractures, no increase in activity was noted prior to the onset of symptoms.[14] Close scrutiny of high-quality radiographs may identify sclerosis, cortical thickening, or new bone formation. Nondisplaced fractures may appear as faint radiolucencies. If radiographs are inconclusive, adjunctive tests such as MRI, CT, or bone scintigraphy may be helpful.

An unstable SCFE can be mistaken for a traumatic type I fracture; however, SCFE is caused by an underlying abnormality of the physis and occurs after trivial trauma, usually in adolescents, while type I fractures typically occur with significant high-energy trauma in younger children. Often in a SCFE, there may be signs of remodeling or callus formation in the femoral metaphysis.

Fracture after minor trauma suggests weakened bone possibly from systemic disease, tumor, cyst, or infection. If the physical and radiographic evidence of trauma is significant but the history is not consistent, nonaccidental trauma must always be considered. In the multiply traumatized patient, it is easy to miss hip fractures that are overshadowed by more dramatic or painful injuries. Radiographs of the pelvis should be obtained and examined carefully in patients with femoral shaft fractures because ipsilateral hip fracture or dislocation can occur.[2] While the rate of ipsilateral femoral neck fracture is reported to be as high as 9% in adults with femoral shaft fractures, this rate is less than 1% in pediatric trauma patients.[27]

PATHOANATOMY AND APPLIED ANATOMY RELATED TO HIP FRACTURES

Ossification of the femur begins in the seventh fetal week.[31] In early childhood, only a single proximal femoral chondroepiphysis exists. During the first year of life, the medial portion of this physis grows faster than the lateral, creating an elongated femoral neck by 1 year of age. The capital femoral epiphysis begins to ossify at approximately 4 months in girls and 5 to 6 months in boys. The ossification center of the trochanteric apophysis appears at 4 years in boys and girls.[47] The proximal femoral physis is responsible for the metaphyseal growth in the femoral neck, whereas the trochanteric apophysis contributes to the appositional growth of the greater trochanter and, to a lesser extent, to the metaphyseal growth of the femur.[23] Fusion of the proximal femoral and trochanteric physis occurs at about the age of 14 in girls and 16 in boys.[42] The confluence of the greater trochanteric physis with the capital femoral physis along the superior femoral neck and the unique vascular supply to the capital femoral epiphysis makes the immature hip vulnerable to growth derangement and subsequent deformity after a fracture (Fig. 23-6).

VASCULAR ANATOMY

Because of the frequency and sequelae of ON of the hip in children, the blood supply of the femoral head has been studied extensively.[22,41,46,75] Postmortem injection and microangiographic studies have provided clues to the vascular changes with age. These observations are as follows:

- At birth, interosseous continuation of branches of the medial and lateral circumflex arteries (metaphyseal vessels) traversing the femoral neck predominantly supply the femoral head. These arteries gradually diminish in size as the cartilaginous

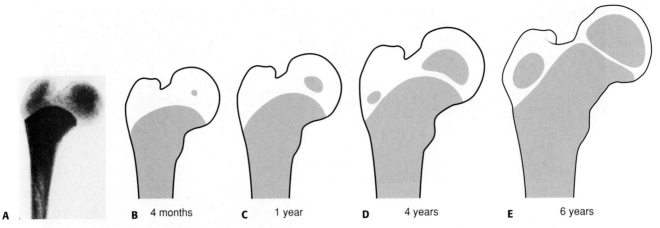

A

B 4 months   C 1 year   D 4 years   E 6 years

Figure 23-6. The transformation of the preplate to separate growth zones for the femoral head and greater trochanter. The diagram shows development of the epiphyseal nucleus. **A:** Radiograph of the proximal end of the femur of a stillborn girl, weight 325 g. **B–E:** Drawings made on the basis of radiographs. (Reprinted with permission from Edgren W. Coxa plana. A clinical and radiological investigation with particular reference to the importance of the metaphyseal changes for the final shape of the proximal part of the femur. *Acta Orthop Scand Suppl.* 1965;84:1–129.)

physis develops and forms a barrier, preventing transphyseal continuity of these vessels into the femoral head. As a result, the metaphyseal blood supply to the femoral head is virtually nonexistent by age 4.

- When the metaphyseal vessels diminish, the intracapsular lateral epiphyseal vessels predominate and the femoral head is primarily supplied by these vessels. The lateral epiphyseal vessels extend superiorly on the exterior of the neck, bypassing the physeal barrier, and continuing into the epiphysis.

- Ogden[69] noted that the lateral epiphyseal vessels consist of two branches: the posterosuperior and posteroinferior branches of the medial circumflex artery. At the level of the intertrochanteric groove, the medial circumflex artery branches into a retinacular arterial system (the posterosuperior and posteroinferior arteries). These arteries penetrate the capsule and traverse proximally (covered by the retinacular folds) along the neck of the femur to supply the femoral head peripherally and proximal to the physis. At about 3 to 4 years of age, the lateral posterosuperior vessels appear to predominate and supply the entire anterior lateral portion of the capital femoral epiphysis. The posteroinferior and posterosuperior arteries persist and supply the femoral head throughout life.

- The vessels of the ligamentum teres are of virtually no importance. They contribute little blood supply to the femoral head until age 8, and then only about 20% as an adult.

A thorough understanding of the vascular anatomy of the femoral head is needed for understanding pediatric hip fractures. The multiple small vessels of the young coalesce with age to a limited number of larger vessels. As a result, damage to a single vessel can have serious consequences; for example, occlusion of the posterosuperior branch of the medial circumflex artery can cause ON of the anterior lateral portion of the femoral head.[18]

It is also important for surgeons to recognize where capsulotomy should be performed to decrease iatrogenic injury to existing blood supply. It is suspected that anterior capsulotomy does not damage the blood supply to the femoral head as long as the intertrochanteric notch and the superior lateral ascending cervical vessels are avoided.

SOFT TISSUE ANATOMY

The pediatric hip joint is enclosed by a thick fibrous capsule that is considered less likely to tear than in adult hip fractures. Bleeding within an intact capsule may lead to a tense hemarthrosis after intracapsular fracture which can theoretically tamponade the ascending cervical vessels and may have implications in the development of ON. The hip joint is surrounded on all sides by a protective cuff of musculature; as such, open hip fracture is rare. In the absence of associated hip dislocation, neurovascular injuries are rare.

There is complex neurovascular anatomy throughout the soft tissue surrounding the hip joint. The sciatic nerve emerges from the sciatic notch beneath the piriformis and courses superficial to the external rotators and the quadratus femoris medial to the greater trochanter. The lateral femoral cutaneous nerve lies in the interval between the tensor and sartorius muscles and supplies sensation to the lateral thigh. This nerve must be identified and preserved during an anterolateral approach to the hip. The femoral neurovascular bundle is separated from the anterior hip joint by the iliopsoas. Thus, any retractor placed on the anterior acetabular rim should be carefully placed deep to the iliopsoas to protect the femoral bundle. Inferior and medial to the hip capsule, coursing from the deep femoral artery toward the posterior hip joint, is the medial femoral circumflex artery. Placement of a distal Hohmann retractor too deeply can tear this artery, and control of the bleeding may be difficult.

TREATMENT OPTIONS FOR HIP FRACTURES

Recent literature supports the concept that attempted conservative treatment can result in unacceptably high rates of coxa vara.[5] Subsequent authors have documented lower rates of ON, coxa vara, and nonunion in patients who were aggressively treated with anatomic reduction (open or closed) and internal fixation (with or without supplemental casting).[4,21,34,73] A study that followed 36 patients until healing concluded that patients treated with open reduction had a smaller complication rate and recommended open reduction and internal fixation (ORIF) over closed reduction and internal fixation (CRIF) whenever possible.[6] Current management is directed at early anatomic reduction of these fractures with stable internal fixation and selective use of supplemental external stabilization (casting), with the goal of minimizing devastating late complications.[21,83]

NONOPERATIVE TREATMENT OF HIP FRACTURES

Indications/Contraindications

Nonoperative Treatment of Hip Fractures: INDICATIONS AND CONTRAINDICATIONS	
Indications	**Relative Contraindications**
• Infants and toddlers 0–2 yr with stable minimally displaced type I fractures	• Type I fractures >2 yr
• Nondisplaced type II and III fractures in younger children (0–5 yr)	• Displaced fractures
• Nondisplaced stress fractures	• Older children (>5 yr with types II and III) fractures

Techniques

Nonoperative treatment in children less than 1 year may be either a Pavlik harness or abduction brace. In older children treated nonoperatively, a spica cast past the knee may be considered. There are no outcome studies on spica or brace treatment but a spica cast should only be considered in younger children up to 5 years with nondisplaced fractures. Nonoperative and spica cast treatment alone is not optimal in older children as the potential for nonunion is too great not to perform internal fixation.

OPERATIVE TREATMENT OF HIP FRACTURES

Indications/Contraindications

Internal fixation is indicated in children with displaced hip fractures. Internal fixation is also recommended for most acute nondisplaced fractures except in children where size limits the efficacy of internal fixation (0 to 5 years). Completely nondisplaced fractures may be treated with percutaneous screw placement with or without capsulotomy. Displaced fractures may be treated with attempted CRIF. However, if there is any residual displacement after an attempted closed reduction, an open reduction should be performed to decrease the incidence of ON and nonunion.

Watson-Jones (Anterior Lateral) Approach
Preoperative Planning

✔ **Watson-Jones (Anterior Lateral) Approach:** PREOPERATIVE PLANNING CHECKLIST	
OR table	☐ Fracture table/flattop table to allow adequate imaging
Position/positioning aids	☐ The patient should have a bump on the back and posterior pelvis to allow access to the region posterior to the greater trochanter
Fluoroscopy location	☐ On the side opposite the operative field ☐ If percutaneous fixation is indicated, two C-arms may be helpful
Equipment	☐ Deep retractors

Surgical Approach

If open reduction is necessary, the Watson-Jones approach is a useful, direct approach to the femoral neck. A lateral incision is made over the proximal femur, slightly anterior to the greater trochanter (Fig. 23-7A). The fascia lata is incised longitudinally (Fig. 23-7B). The innervation of the tensor muscle by the superior gluteal nerve is 2 to 5 cm above the greater trochanter, and care should be taken not to damage this structure. The tensor muscle is reflected anteriorly. The interval between the gluteus medius and the tensor muscles will be used (Fig. 23-7C). The plane is developed between the muscles and the underlying hip capsule (Fig. 23-7D). If necessary, the anterior-most fibers of the gluteus medius tendon can be detached from the trochanter for wider exposure. After clearing the anterior hip capsule, longitudinal capsulotomy is made along the anterosuperior femoral neck. A transverse incision can be added superiorly for wider exposure (Fig. 23-7E). Once the hip fracture is reduced, guidewires for cannulated screws can be passed perpendicular to the fracture along the femoral neck from the base of the greater trochanter.

Smith-Peterson (Anterior) Approach
Preoperative Planning

✔ **Smith-Petersen (Anterior) Approach:** PREOPERATIVE PLANNING CHECKLIST	
OR table	☐ Radiolucent
Position/positioning aids	☐ A bump under the thoracolumbar spine to the posterior-superior iliac spine to access the greater trochanter for screw insertion
Fluoroscopy location	☐ Opposite the surgeon
Equipment	☐ Long retractors

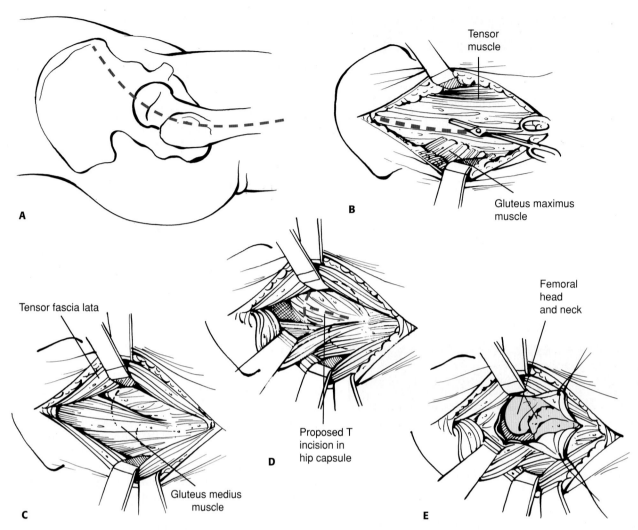

Figure 23-7. Watson-Jones lateral approach to the hip joint for open reduction of femoral neck fractures in children. **A:** Skin incision. **B:** Incision of the fascia lata between the tensor muscle (anterior) and gluteus maximus (posterior). **C:** Exposure of the interval between the gluteus medius and tensor fascia lata (retracted anteriorly). Development of the interval will reveal the underlying hip capsule. **D:** Exposure of the hip capsule. **E:** Exposure of the femoral neck after T incision of the capsule.

Surgical Approach

A longitudinal incision distal and lateral to the anterior-superior iliac spine or bikini approach can be used through the Smith-Petersen interval (Fig. 23-8). Care should be taken to identify and protect the lateral femoral cutaneous nerve. The fascia over the tensor fascia muscle is opened longitudinally. Blunt dissection is then done to expose the medial aspect of the muscle as far proximal as the iliac crest. The rectus muscle is seen and the lateral fascia of the rectus is incised and the rectus can then be retracted in a medial direction. The fascia on the floor of the rectus is incised longitudinally and the lateral iliopsoas is elevated off the hip capsule in a medial direction to expose the hip capsule. The sartorius and rectus muscles can be detached for greater exposure of the hip capsule if required. Medial and inferior retractors should be carefully placed around the femoral neck once the capsule is incised to avoid damage to the femoral neurovascular bundle and medial

femoral circumflex artery, respectively. Care must be taken not to violate the intertrochanteric notch and the lateral ascending vessels. Because the lateral aspect of the greater trochanter is not exposed, wires must be passed percutaneously once the hip fracture is reduced.

Lateral Approach for Decompression

In some cases, an adequate closed reduction can be obtained, thus avoiding the need to open the hip joint for reduction purposes. However, the surgeon may decide to perform a capsulotomy to decompress the hip joint. The authors prefer to do this from a lateral approach. With this method, a 4-cm incision is made distal and lateral to the greater trochanter. From this incision, the fascia lata is incised and guide pins for cannulated screws are placed and screws are inserted in the standard manner. The anterior fibers of the gluteus medius are elevated allowing incision of the anterior capsule with a Cobb elevator, knife, or osteotome.

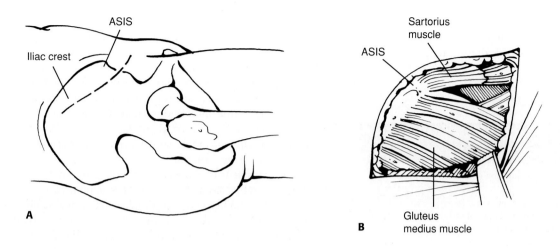

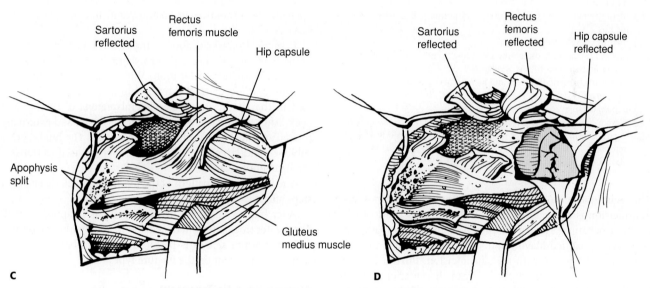

Figure 23-8. Smith-Petersen anterolateral approach to the hip joint. **A:** Skin incision. Incision is 1 cm below the iliac crest and extends just medial to the anterior-superior iliac spine. **B:** Skin is retracted, exposing the fascia overlying the anterior-superior iliac spine. The interval between the sartorius and the tensor fascia lata is identifiable by palpation. **C:** The sartorius is detached from the anterior-superior iliac spine. Splitting of the iliac crest apophysis and detachment of the rectus femoris (shown attached to anterior-inferior iliac spine) will facilitate exposure of the hip capsule. **D:** The hip capsule is exposed. A T incision is made to reveal the femoral head and neck.

Surgical Dislocation of the Hip

Preoperative Planning

✔ Surgical Dislocation of the Hip: PREOPERATIVE PLANNING CHECKLIST	
OR table	❏ Radiolucent
Position/positioning aids	❏ Patients are positioned in the lateral position. This can be accomplished with a pegboard, beanbag, or other available positioning devices
Fluoroscopy location	❏ Opposite the surgeon

Equipment	❏ Curved scissors are needed if the ligamentum teres is to be transected for dislocation
	❏ An oscillating saw or osteotomes are needed for the greater trochanteric osteotomy
	❏ 3.5- or 4.5-mm cannulated screws

Positioning

Patients are positioned in the lateral position on a radiolucent table. The opposite leg should be well padded so there is no pressure on the peroneal nerve. An axillary roll is needed and both upper extremities should be carefully positioned to avoid any pressure or tension on the upper extremity and brachial plexus. The complete hip and leg is draped free as high as the iliac crest.

Technique

> ✔ **Surgical Dislocation of the Hip:**
> KEY SURGICAL STEPS
>
> ❑ Lateral incision centered over junction of anterior and middle thirds of greater trochanter
> ❑ Split fascia lata in line with skin incision
> ❑ Continue proximal dissection through interval between anterior edge of gluteus maximus and the tensor OR split gluteus maximus
> ❑ Elevate proximal vastus lateralis just anterior to the gluteus maximus from posterior to anterior
> ❑ Identify and develop interval between piriformis and gluteus medius
> ❑ Identify capsule deep to medius
> ❑ Perform trochanteric osteotomy, extending from superoposterior corner of trochanter to vastus ridge
> ❑ Reflect trochanteric flip piece and its muscular attachments anteriorly
> ❑ Expose capsule
> ❑ Elevate capsular minimus anteriorly
> ❑ Expose capsule to the rim of the acetabulum both superiorly and anteriorly
> ❑ Make Z-shaped capsulotomy

The technique was originally described by Ganz et al.[35] A lateral incision is created centered on the anterior third of the greater trochanter. The leg can then be abducted by placing it on a sterile, padded Mayo stand. The tensor fascia is incised longitudinally in line with the skin incision. Proximally, the dissection may be carried out between the anterior edge of the gluteus maximus and the tensor (Gibson modification[66]), or the gluteus maximus may be split bluntly. This exposes the proximal vastus lateralis, gluteus medius, and greater trochanter.

The leg is then taken off of the Mayo and positioned with the hip in adduction and slight internal rotation to better visualize the anatomic landmarks. Identify and develop the interval between the piriformis and the gluteus medius. The piriformis is the thick, white tendon visualized deep to the posterior/distal aspect of gluteus medius. Once exposed, the tendon can be gently retracted distally to expose the inferior margin of the gluteus minimus fascia. The inferior fascia of the minimus is then opened to allow the muscle to be retracted in an anterior-superior direction off of the hip capsule. This should allow visualization of the hip capsule.

A greater trochanteric osteotomy is then performed from the posterior border of the vastus lateralis ridge to the anterior to the tip of the greater trochanter using either an oscillating saw or an osteotomy. The width of the osteotomy should be approximately 15 mm. The piriformis and short external rotators should remain attached to the stable trochanteric bed. Maintaining the piriformis tendon intact protects

the retinacular branch of the medial circumflex artery. The trochanteric flip piece with attached gluteus minimus, gluteus medius, vastus lateralis, and vastus intermedius is then reflected anteriorly.

Capsular exposure then continues anteriorly and superiorly. Gentle, progressive flexion and external rotation of the operative hip will facilitate the muscle dissection. Capsular muscular attachments are elevated anteriorly to the indirect head of the rectus tendon, superiorly to the superior rim of the acetabulum, and posteriorly to the piriformis.

The hip capsule is then opened in a Z-shaped fashion. The longitudinal limb is along the axis of the femoral neck in line with the iliofemoral ligament. The distal aspect is proximal but in line with the intertrochanteric ridge. The posterior limb of the capsule is opened in the capsular recess of the acetabulum as far posterior as the piriformis tendon, protecting the retinaculum as it pierces the hip capsule. Once the capsule is opened, the intra-articular anatomy and fracture pattern can be visualized.

If surgical hip dislocation is indicated, temporary fixation of the fracture with a threaded Kirschner wire (K-wire) is recommended for safe dislocation. Without temporary fixation, damage may occur to the retinaculum that is easily visualized in the lateral and posterolateral regions of the femoral neck. After temporary fixation, the leg is flexed and externally rotated and the leg placed in a sterile leg bag. The hip is gently subluxed and large, curved large scissors are used to transect the ligamentum teres.

The location and pattern of the hip fracture will dictate next steps after the capsulotomy.

After fracture fixation, the hip capsule is re-approximated. The greater trochanter is reduced and fixation with two to three 3.5- or 4.5-mm screws is performed. Weight-bearing restrictions are dependent on the fracture type.

Fracture-Specific Treatment

Type I

Fracture treatment is based on the age of the child, presence of femoral head dislocation, and fracture stability after reduction. In toddlers under 2 years of age with nondisplaced or minimally displaced fractures, simple spica cast immobilization is likely to be successful. Because the fracture tends to displace into varus and external rotation, the limb should be casted in mild abduction and neutral rotation to prevent displacement. Close follow-up in the early postinjury period is critical.

Displaced fractures in toddlers should be reduced closed by gentle traction, abduction, and internal rotation. If the fracture reduces and is stable, casting without fixation is indicated. If casting without fixation is performed, repeat radiographs should be taken in the early postoperative period to look for re-displacement. The likelihood of successful repeat reduction decreases rapidly with time and healing in a young child.

If the fracture is not stable, it should be fixed with small-diameter smooth pins that cross the femoral neck and into the epiphysis. Use of smooth pins will theoretically decrease risk of additional physeal injury in patients with a transphyseal fracture. An arthrogram *after* reduction and stabilization of the fracture may be indicated to ensure alignment is anatomic. An arthrogram *prior* to reduction and pinning may obscure bony detail and hinder assessment during reduction.

Children older than 2 years should have operative fixation, even if the fracture is nondisplaced, because the complications of late displacement are significant. Fixation must cross the physis into the capital femoral epiphysis in order to stabilize the fracture. Smooth pins can be used in young children, but cannulated screws are better for older, larger children, and adolescents. In this older group (>10 years), the effect of eventual limb length discrepancy is small and is a reasonable tradeoff for the superior fixation and stabilization needed to avoid complications in larger and older children.

Closed reduction of type IB fracture-dislocations may be attempted, but immediate open reduction is necessary if a single attempt at closed reduction is unsuccessful. Internal fixation is required to stabilize these injuries. The surgical approach should be dictated by the direction of the femoral head dislocation, most commonly posterolateral. Regardless of treatment technique chosen, parents must be advised in advance about the substantial risk of avascular necrosis (AVN) of the femoral head.

Postoperative spica cast immobilization is recommended for younger children if internal fixation stops distal to the epiphyseal physis, which makes it less stable.

Older, more reliable children may be immobilized in a hip abduction orthosis. Long-term follow-up is required in these patients to watch for growth disturbance and/or AVN. Smooth fixation should be removed shortly after fracture healing to enable further growth. Threaded fixation can be left in place or removed according to surgeon and patient preference.

Type II and Type III

Intra-capsular femoral neck fractures require anatomic reduction and, in most cases, internal fixation. In rare cases, children under 5 years of age with nondisplaced, completely stable transcervical or cervicotrochanteric fractures can be managed with spica casting and close follow-up to detect varus displacement in the cast.[47,56] However, in almost all cases, internal fixation is recommended by most investigators for nondisplaced transcervical fractures[36,47] because the risk of late displacement in such fractures far outweighs the risk of percutaneous screw fixation, especially in young children.[16]

Displaced neck fractures should be treated with anatomic reduction and stable internal fixation to minimize the risk of late complications. Coxa vara and nonunion were frequent in several large series of displaced transcervical fractures treated with immobilization but without internal fixation.[5,19,56] However, when an anatomic closed reduction or ORIF was used, the rates of these complications were much lower.[17,19,34,83]

Gentle closed reduction of displaced fractures is accomplished with the use of longitudinal traction, abduction, and internal rotation. Given the findings that reduction quality significantly impacts the risk for postoperative complications, open reduction frequently is necessary for displaced fractures and should be done through a Watson-Jones surgical approach.

Internal fixation with cannulated screws is performed through a small lateral incision with planned entry above the level of the lesser trochanter. Care should be taken to minimize drill holes or hardware placement in the subtrochanteric region as they create a stress riser, increasing the risk of subtrochanteric fracture. Two to three screws should be placed; if possible, the most inferior screw should skirt along the calcar with the remaining screws spaced as widely as possible.[15] Often, the small diameter of the child's femoral neck will accommodate only two screws.

In type II fractures, it may be necessary to cross the physis for fixation stability[47]; the sequelae of premature physeal closure and trochanteric overgrowth are much less than those of nonunion, pin breakage, and ON. Treatment of the fracture is the first priority, and any subsequent growth disturbance and leg length discrepancy are secondary. Consideration may be given to simultaneous capsulotomy or aspiration of the joint to eliminate pressure from a hemarthrosis at the time of surgery.

Displaced cervicotrochanteric (type III) fractures have been shown to have a complication rate similar to that for type II fractures and should be treated similarly. Whenever possible, screws should be inserted short of the physis in type III fractures. Given the more distal anatomic location, fixation generally does not need to cross the physis in these fractures. Alternatively, a pediatric hip compression screw or a pediatric locking hip plate[51] can be used to provide more secure fixation of distal cervicotrochanteric fractures in a child over 5 years of age. These plates can be particularly useful if there is a smaller region for screw purchase distal to the fracture. Spica casting is routine in most type II and III fractures in younger children.[34] Older children, whose screws can cross the physis, may use a hip abduction orthosis as external supplementation to their internal fixation.

Type IV

Good results can be obtained after closed treatment of most intertrochanteric (type IV) fractures in younger children, regardless of displacement. Traction and spica cast immobilization are effective.[15] Instability or failure to maintain adequate reduction and polytrauma are indications for internal fixation.

Older children (>10 years) or those with significant displacement should be treated with internal fixation (Fig. 23-9). A pediatric hip screw, blade plate, or pediatric hip locking plate provide rigid internal fixation for intertrochanteric fractures. Smaller hip devices have made ORIF an option in children younger than 10 years. This may avoid the period of spica cast treatment and allow for a more anatomic fracture reduction.

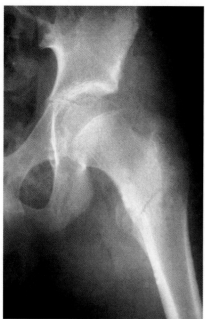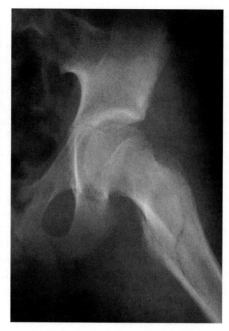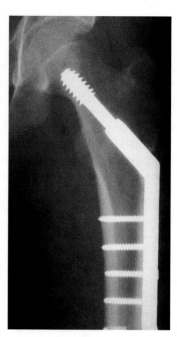

A, B   C

FIGURE 23-9. A: A 14-year-old boy who fell from a tree swing sustained this nondisplaced left intertrochanteric hip fracture. **B:** Lateral radiograph shows the long spiral fracture. **C:** Three months after fixation with an adult sliding hip screw.

Authors' Preferred Treatment for Hip Fractures

The choice of treatment modality for pediatric hip fractures is based on several key factors:

- The location of the fracture (i.e., Delbert classification)
- The proximity of the fracture to the physis and the need for fixation *across* the physis
- The age of the patient
- The amount of displacement present

The authors present their preferred techniques below based on fracture classification.

Type I

Nondisplaced or minimally displaced stable fractures in toddlers up to age 2 should be treated with a spica cast without internal fixation. The limb should be casted in a position of abduction and neutral rotation to prevent displacement into varus. If the fracture requires reduction or moves significantly during reduction or casting maneuvers, then internal fixation is mandatory. Two-millimeter smooth K-wires are inserted percutaneously to cross the physis. We recommend two or three wires. Wires should be cut off and bent below the skin for retrieval under a brief general anesthetic when the fractures healed. We do not recommend leaving the wires outside the skin secondary to the risk for infection. Frequent radiographs are necessary to check for migration of the pins into the joint space. A spica cast is always applied in this age group and should remain in place for at least 6 weeks.[34]

Even if type I fractures in children older than 2 years are anatomically reduced, these patients should always have stabilization with internal fixation. While K-wires are appropriate for small children, 4- to 7.3-mm cannulated screws crossing the physis can be considered in older, larger children after closed reduction. Fluoroscopically placing a guide pin from the femoral neck, across the physis, and into the femoral head allows one to locate the proper site for a small incision overlying the lateral femur in line with the femoral neck. Two guide pins are placed into the epiphysis, and the wires are overdrilled to the level of the physis (but not across to avoid growth arrest as much as possible). The hard metaphysis and lateral femoral cortex are tapped (in contrast to elderly patients with osteoporosis) to the level of the physis and stainless steel screws are placed.

If gentle closed reduction cannot be achieved, an open approach is preferred. The choice of approach is dictated by surgeon experience and position of the femoral epiphysis. For type IA fractures, an anterior approach or surgical dislocation approach is recommended. For type IB fractures, the choice of approach is dictated by the position of the femoral epiphysis. If it is anterior or inferior, a Watson-Jones approach should be used. On the other hand, most type IB fractures are displaced posteriorly, in which case a posterior approach should be selected. A surgical dislocation approach may also be used to give complete visualization of the hip and retinacular vessels.

Under direct vision, the fracture is reduced and guidewires are passed from the lateral aspect of the proximal femur up the neck perpendicular to the fracture; predrilling is necessary before the insertion of screws. All children are immobilized. A spica cast is utilized in younger, taller patients. A hip abduction orthosis may be considered in older, larger, more compliant patients.

Older children and adolescents will usually require similar reduction methods on a fracture table, and the fracture is stabilized after closed or, if needed, open reduction. Larger 6.5- or 7.3-mm screws are needed and are placed after predrilling over the guide pins. The screws are placed through a lateral incision, and an anterior capsulotomy is performed. Such stout fixation usually obviates the need for spica casting in an adolescent but, if future patient compliance or fracture stability is in doubt, some type of external stabilization may be used. The lateral position is utilized for the surgical dislocation approach. The fracture can be reduced without the need for a traction table in the surgical dislocation approach.

Types II and III

In all cases, we attempt a closed reduction. It is critical that the fracture be reduced anatomically to decrease the potential of nonunion and AVN. If unsuccessful, a reduction can be performed through a Watson-Jones approach. This approach provides direct exposure of the femoral neck for gentle fracture reduction. If there is experience with the surgical dislocation approach, this will give the surgeon visualization for fracture reduction and fixation. Both approaches allow the fracture to be anatomically reduced under direct vision.

Once the fracture is visualized and anatomically reduced, guidewires are then placed up the femoral neck perpendicular to the fracture. If possible, penetration of the physis should be avoided.[20,33] However, in most unstable type II fractures, crossing of the physis may be necessary to achieve stability and avoid the complications associated with late displacement.[15] Stable fixation of type III fractures generally is possible without crossing the physis.

If the surgeon selects a surgical dislocation approach, the reduction can usually be performed without dislocation of the femoral head from the acetabulum. If femoral head dislocation is required, the fracture and femoral head should be provisionally reduced and fixed prior to subluxation and transecting the ligamentum teres to prevent traction on the retinaculum with the dislocation. Once dislocated, a guidewire can be placed retrograde through the fovea.

Type II and III fractures should be stabilized with 4- to 4.5-mm cannulated screws in small children up to age 8. After the age of 8, fixation with 6.5-mm cannulated screws is appropriate. Two or three appropriately sized screws should be used, depending on the size of the child's femoral neck. As in type I fractures, we recommend placing at least two guide pins. Similarly, predrilling the femoral neck is necessary to avoid displacement of the fracture while advancing the screws. Finally, we believe that if the physis is not crossed with implants, supplementary spica casting is needed to prevent malunion or nonunion.

Type IV

Nondisplaced type IV fractures in children younger than 3 to 4 years are treated without internal fixation with immobilization in a spica cast for 6 to 12 weeks. Great care is needed to cast the limb in a position that best aligns the bone (Fig. 23-10A,B). Frequent radiographic examination is necessary to assess for late displacement, particularly into varus. In some cases, it may be difficult to assess reduction in a spica cast, and additional imaging like a limited CT scan may be useful (Fig. 23-10C,D).

Displaced type IV fractures in children over 3 years should be treated with internal fixation with a pediatric or juvenile compression hip screw or pediatric locking hip plate placed into femoral neck, with neck fixation stopping short of the physis. It is important to place an derotation wire prior to drilling and tapping the neck for the dynamic hip screw. Closed reduction often is possible with a combination of traction and internal rotation of the limb. If open reduction is necessary, a lateral approach with anterior extension to close reduce the fracture is preferred.

Postoperative Care

In general, we believe supplementary casting or bracing should be considered for most patients with proximal femoral fractures. For instance, casting is indicated in all type I fractures except in the rare adolescents who have been treated with two to three large screws that cross the physis and who will be compliant with restricted weight-bearing. For type II and III fractures, we recommend a hip spica cast to be used for at least 6 weeks in all patients whose implants do not cross the femoral physis. This recommendation makes sense when one considers that in children younger than 10, we try to avoid crossing the physis, and these patients usually do well with these casts. On the other hand, children older than 12 years can be treated with transphyseal fixation that will be stable enough to avoid casting, which coincidently also tends to be poorly tolerated in this age group. For children 10 to 12 years, the use of a postoperative cast depends on the stability of fracture fixation and the patient's compliance; if either is in doubt, a single hip spica cast is used.

Type IV fractures treated with a hip screw and side plate do not require cast immobilization. Formal rehabilitation usually is unnecessary unless there is a severe persistent limp, which may be due to abductor weakness. Stiffness is rarely a problem in the absence of ON.

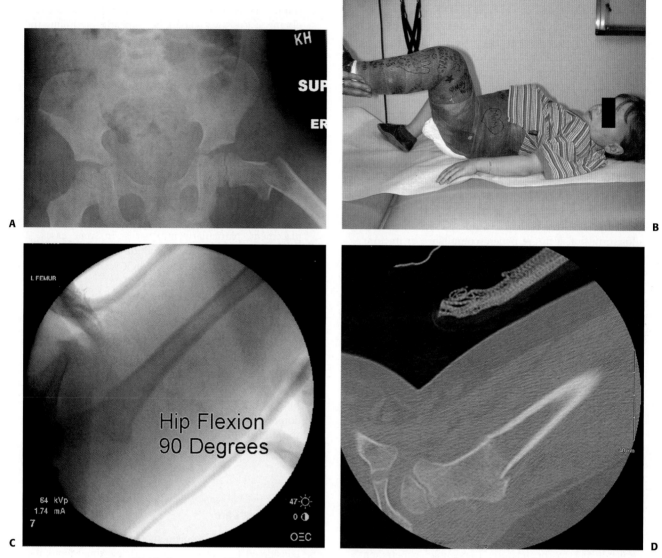

Figure 23-10. A: A 4-year-old boy fell from a window, causing a displaced type IV fracture. **B:** Positioning of the hip in a spica cast is usually in hip flexion and confirmed under fluoroscopy. **C:** Fluoroscopic radiographs in 90 degrees of hip flexion ensure anatomic correctness. **D:** At 1-week follow-up, radiographs were inconclusive; a CT scan assists in confirming the location.

Potential Pitfalls and Preventive Measures

Hip Fracture Repair:
POTENTIAL PITFALLS AND PREVENTION

Pitfall	Prevention
• Nonunion	• Anatomic reduction, open the fracture site if necessary
	• Stable internal fixation, cross the physis if necessary
	• Spica cast supplemental immobilization for children <10 or 10–12 years old if there is a concern for stabilization
• AVN	• Urgent reduction >24 hrs
	• Open reduction or capsulotomy if reduction is closed
	• Anatomic reduction
• Physeal arrest	• Stop the fixation distal to the physis but do not compromise stability. Most type III and IV fractures can achieve stable fixation without crossing the physis
	• If the stability of fracture fixation is not enough with implants distal to the physis, the surgeon must cross the physis
	• Consider removal of implants once the fracture has bony union

Management of Expected Adverse Outcomes and Unexpected Complications Related to Hip Fractures

OSTEONECROSIS

Osteonecrosis is the most serious and frequent complication of hip fractures in children and is the primary cause of poor results after fractures of the hip in children.[59] Its overall prevalence is approximately 30%, based on the literature.[21,47,83] The risk of ON is highest after displaced type IB, II, and III fractures (Fig. 23-11).[15,17,83] In the meta-analysis by Moon and Mehlman,[61] the incidence of ON in type I through type IV is 38%, 28%, 18%, and 5%, respectively. In addition to location of the fracture (as described by the Delbet classification), ON is believed to be increased with increased initial fracture displacement and older age at the time of injury.[17,89]

Several studies report lower rates of ON in their series of patients treated within 24 hours of injury with prompt reduction and internal fixation.[17,21,34,83] In contrast, other studies have demonstrated no association between early treatment and risk for AVN.[89] It is hypothesized that early reduction and stabilization may decrease ON by preventing further injury to the tenuous blood supply, and alleviating the tamponade effect, as open reduction or capsulotomy may decrease intra-articular pressure caused by fracture hematoma.[47,94] The efficacy of alleviating the "tamponade effect" has equivocal support in the literature, with some articles reporting that aspirating the hematoma may decrease the intracapsular pressure and increase blood flow to the femoral head[21] and others suggesting that this may have little effect.[47,61]

Perhaps, the most important modifiable factor in reducing ON is the quality of reduction. Schrader et al. found that better quality reduction and the use of modern cannulated implants reduced the risk of ON in their study population.[83] Timing to the operating room and the addition of a capsulotomy have not been previously associated with reducing osteonecrosis.

Osteonecrosis has been classified by Ratliff as follows: type I, involvement of the whole head; type II, partial involvement of the head; and type III, an area of necrosis of the femoral neck from the fracture line to the physis (Fig. 23-12).[83] Type I is the most severe, the most common form, and has the poorest prognosis. Type I most likely results from damage to all of the retinacular epiphyseal vessels. Type II is secondary to localized damage to one or more of the lateral epiphyseal vessels near their insertion into the anterolateral aspect of the femoral head. And type III ON is from damage to the superior

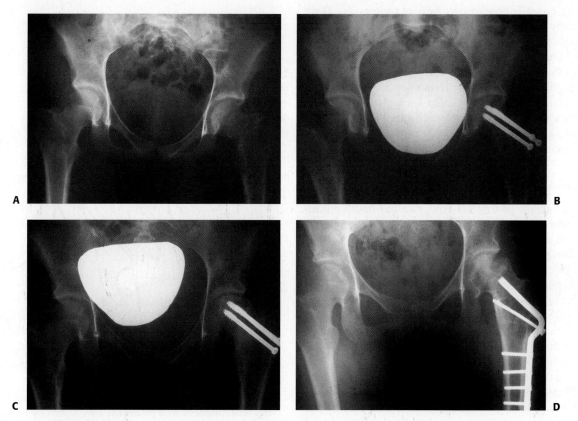

Figure 23-11. A: A 14-year-old girl with a type II fracture of the left femoral neck. **B:** After fixation with three cannulated screws. **C:** Osteonecrosis with collapse of the superolateral portion of the femoral head. **D:** After treatment with valgus osteotomy.

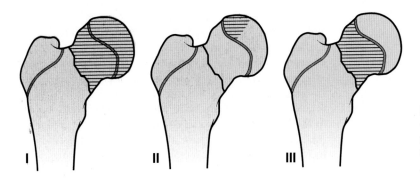

Figure 23-12. The three types of osteonecrosis. Type I, whole head; type II, partial head; and type III, femoral neck. (Reprinted with permission from Ratliff AH. Fractures of the neck of the femur in children. *J Bone Joint Surg Br.* 1962;44:528–542.)

metaphyseal vessels. Type III is rare, but has a good prognosis provided the fracture goes on to heal.[83] Signs and symptoms of ON usually develop within the first year after injury, with a mean time to presentation of just over 11 months, but patients may not become symptomatic for up to 2 years.[17,47,82] Some authors have utilized bone scan for early detection of ON to manage family expectations and guide potential treatment. Ramachandran et al.[75] treated 28 patients with early bone scan changes of ON from SCFE or femoral neck fracture. The group was treated with an intravenous bisphosphonate (pamidronate or zoledronate) for an average of 20 months, which greatly improved the outcome at 3-year follow-up. The long-term results of established ON are likely related to age of the patient and extent and location of the necrosis within the head, and results are typically poor in over 60% of patients.[19,73] There is no clearly effective treatment for established posttraumatic ON in children.[47,82] Older children (greater than 10 years old) tend to have worse outcomes than younger children. Treatment of ON is controversial and inconclusive and is beyond the scope of this text. Ongoing research includes the role of redirectional osteotomy,[58] distraction arthroplasty with external fixation, core decompression, vascularized fibular grafting (Fig. 23-13), injection of bone marrow concentrate, and direct bone grafting.

COXA VARA

The prevalence of postfracture coxa vara has been approximated between 20% and 30%[47,52]; however, it is significantly lower in series in which internal fixation was used after reduction of displaced fractures.[19] Coxa vara may be caused by malunion, ON of the femoral neck, premature physeal closure, or a combination of these problems (Fig. 23-14). Severe coxa vara results in the greater trochanter being higher than the center of the femoral head, leading to abductor weakness and shortening of the extremity. This may result in a significant limp and functional limitations.

Remodeling of an established malunion may occur if the child is less than 8 years old, or with a neck–shaft angle greater than 110 degrees. Older patients with progressive deformity may not remodel and subtrochanteric valgus osteotomy may be considered to recreate a more normal trochanter–femoral head relationship, improve limb length inequality, and restore the abductor moment arm (Fig. 23-15).[47,55]

PREMATURE PHYSEAL CLOSURE

Premature physeal closure occurs after approximately 28% of fractures.[47] The risk of premature physeal closure increases when the physis is violated by surgical technique or when ON occurs. It is most commonly seen in patients who have type II or III ON (see Fig. 23-14).[82,83]

The capital femoral physis contributes only 13% of the growth of the entire extremity (approximately 3 mm per year) and normally closes earlier than most of the other physes in the lower extremity. As a result, shortening secondary to premature physeal closure does not cause significant functional

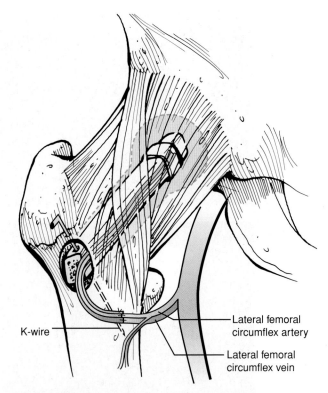

K-wire — Lateral femoral circumflex artery

Lateral femoral circumflex vein

Figure 23-13. Vascularized fibular grafting for osteonecrosis of the femoral head. (Redrawn with permission from Aldrich JM III, Berend KR, Gunneson EE, et al. Free vascularized fibular grafting for the treatment of postcollapse osteonecrosis of the femoral head. *J Bone Joint Surg Am.* 2004;86(suppl_1):87–101.)

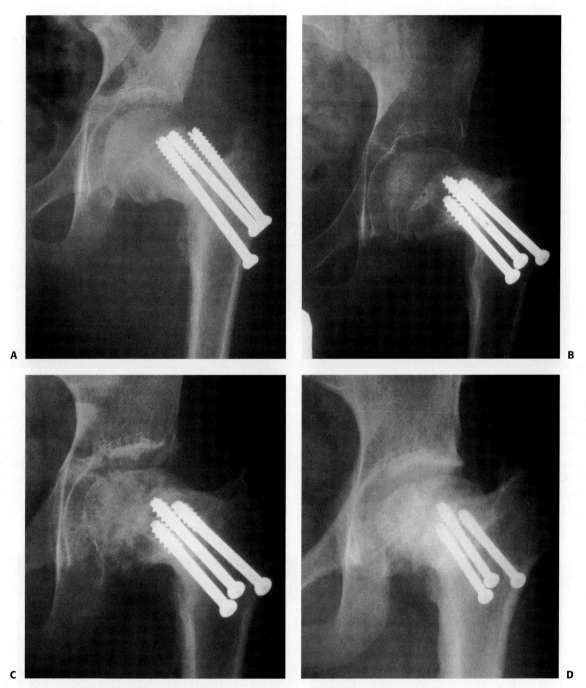

Figure 23-14. A: A 12-year-old boy with a type III left hip fracture. Poor pin placement and varus malposition are evident. **B:** The fracture united in mild varus after hardware revision. **C:** Fourteen months after injury, collapse of the weight-bearing segment is evident. **D:** Six years after injury, coxa breva and trochanteric overgrowth are seen secondary to osteonecrosis, nonunion, and premature physeal closure.

abnormalities except in very young children.[15,49] Treatment for leg length discrepancy is indicated only for significant discrepancy (2.5 cm or more projected at maturity).[47] If femoral growth arrest is expected because of the implant use or injury to the physis in children 8 and under, the surgeon may consider concomitant greater trochanteric epiphysiodesis to maintain a more normal articular trochanteric relationship (Fig. 23-16).

NONUNION

Nonunion occurs infrequently, with an overall incidence of 7% of hip fractures in children.[47] Nonunion is a complication seen more commonly in types II and III fractures and is rare after type I or type IV fractures. The primary cause of nonunion is failure to obtain or maintain an anatomic reduction.[15] After femoral neck fracture in a child, pain should resolve and bridging callus

Figure 23-15. A: A 10-year-old boy with a type III fracture treated without cast immobilization develops progressive varus deformity 4 months after surgery. Inset CT scan demonstrates delayed union. Valgus osteotomy is indicated for his progressive varus deformity and delayed healing. **B:** Three years after valgus osteotomy, the fracture is healed and the deformity corrected.

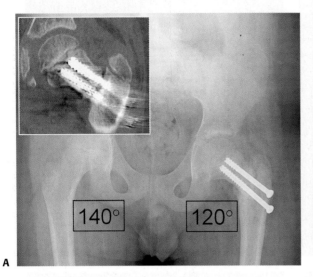

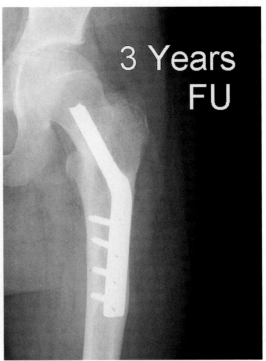

should be seen at the fracture site by 3 months after injury. If a delayed or nonunion is suspected, a CT scan may be helpful to look for bridging bone. If no or minimal healing is seen by 3 to 6 months, the diagnosis of nonunion is established. Nonunion should be treated operatively as soon as possible. If rigid fixation was not utilized initially, the fracture should be revised using rigid internal fixation. If stable fixation was obtained

in the initial procedure, a subtrochanteric valgus osteotomy should be performed to alter the orientation of the fracture and allow compression across the fracture site (Fig. 23-17).[55,56] Allograft bone graft may be used to supplement in these procedures. However, given the increased morbidity required for harvest, autograft should be reserved for persistent nonunions. Internal fixation should extend across the site of the nonunion,

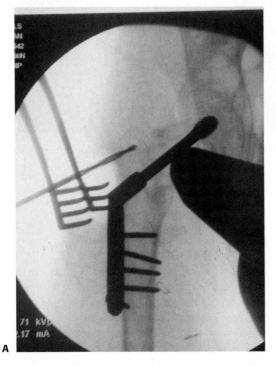

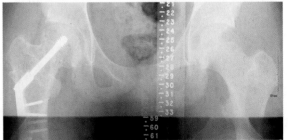

Figure 23-16. A: Greater trochanteric epiphysiodesis was performed at the time of open reduction and internal fixation of a pathologic femoral neck fracture (see Fig. 23-1) in a 10-year-old boy. Because the implant crosses the physis, growth arrest is expected and trochanteric arrest may minimize trochanteric overgrowth. **B:** Seven-year follow-up shows that growth arrest occurred and some trochanteric mismatch is present despite prior epiphysiodesis.

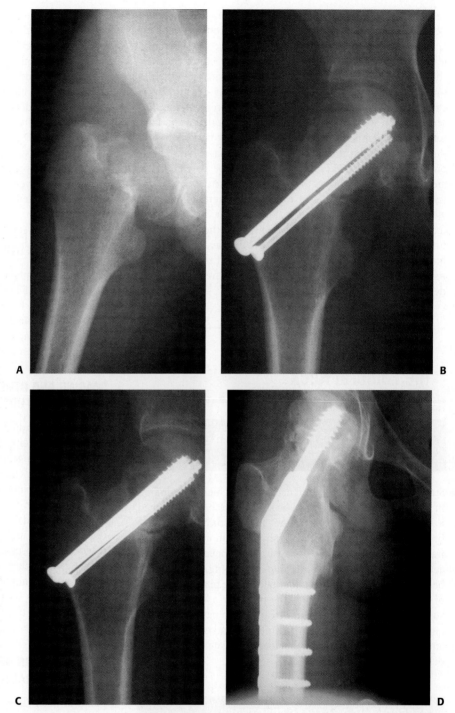

Figure 23-17. A: A 15-year-old girl with a markedly displaced type II femoral neck fracture. **B:** She underwent open reduction and internal fixation with two 7.3-mm cannulated screws and one 4.5-mm cannulated screw. Primary bone grafting of a large defect in the superior neck was also performed. **C:** Radiograph at 5 months showing a persistent fracture line. **D:** Six weeks after valgus intertrochanteric osteotomy. The fracture is healing.

and supplemental external forms of immobilization should be used in all but the most mature and cooperative adolescents.

LESS COMMON COMPLICATIONS

Infection is uncommon after hip fractures in children. The reported incidence of 1%[1,7,8] is consistent with the expected infection rate in any closed fracture treated surgically with ORIF. Chondrolysis is exceedingly rare.[4] Care must be taken to avoid persistent penetration of hardware into the joint, which can cause chondrolysis in conditions such as SCFE. Finally, SCFE

has been reported as a rare complication after fixation of an ipsilateral femoral neck fracture.[48]

Pediatric femoral neck fractures have a relatively small incidence compared with other lower extremity fractures, but the potential for complications is much greater. Except for very young children, the majority of these fractures should be treated with reduction and internal fixation to assure an anatomic reduction. For closed reduction to be successful, the fracture must be reduced nearly anatomic. Fracture reduction should be done early, but controversy persists as to whether this must be done within 24 hours. A variety of approaches exist for open reduction of pediatric hip fractures, and the chosen approach should be based on surgeon experience and fracture pattern. Surgical dislocation allows direct visualization of the fracture and the retinaculum, which may have some benefit on the incidence of AVN, but this is yet to be proven. There are a variety of fixation methods once the fracture is anatomically reduced. The goal is to avoid fixation across the physis when possible. However, if the patient is older (>10 years), or fixation would otherwise be inadequate, cross the physis. Fracture stability and union are more critical than avoiding physeal injury. Continued research is required to better understand the risk factors for AVN and to determine optimal treatment of this devastating complication.

Stress Fractures of the Femoral Neck

INTRODUCTION TO STRESS FRACTURES OF THE FEMORAL NECK

Stress fractures of the femoral neck are extremely uncommon in children, and only a few cases series have been published in the English-language literature. In one study of 40 stress fractures in children, there was only one femoral neck stress fracture.[28] Stress fractures are typically associated strenuous activities such as repetitive running or jumping, but have also been described in children under taking free play.[14] The rarity of such fractures underscores the need for a high index of suspicion when a child has unexplained hip pain. The differential can be long for hip pain in children, and early diagnosis and treatment are essential to avoid complete fracture with displacement.

ASSESSMENT OF STRESS FRACTURES OF THE FEMORAL NECK

MECHANISMS OF INJURY FOR STRESS FRACTURES OF THE FEMORAL NECK

Stress fractures of the femoral neck usually result from repetitive cyclic loading of the hip, such as that produced by a new or increased activity. A recent increase in the repetitive activity is highly suggestive of the diagnosis. An increase in intensity of soccer,[10] and an increase in distance running are examples of such activities. However, similar to previous

studies on this topic,[91] a recent case series of children under 10 with femoral neck stress fractures saw no evidence of increased activity level or elevated sporting volume before the onset of symptoms.[14]

Younger children may present with a limp or knee pain and may not have a clear history of increased activity. Underlying metabolic disorders or immobilizations that weaken the bone may predispose to stress fracture. There is an increased awareness of vitamin D deficiency in children who may predispose to a femoral neck stress fracture.[69] In adolescent female athletes, amenorrhea, anorexia nervosa, osteoporosis, and the "female athlete triad" have been implicated in the development of stress fractures of the femoral neck.[40]

SIGNS AND SYMPTOMS OF STRESS FRACTURES OF THE FEMORAL NECK

The usual presentation is that of progressive hip or groin pain with or without a limp. The pain may be perceived in the thigh or knee and may be mild enough so that it does not significantly limit activities. In the absence of displacement, examination may reveals slight limitation of hip motion with increased pain and hip pain with terminal hip flexion.[14]

IMAGING AND OTHER DIAGNOSTIC STUDIES FOR STRESS FRACTURES OF THE FEMORAL NECK

Usually, plain radiographs reveal the fracture, but in the first 4 to 6 weeks after presentation, plain films may be negative. If there are no changes or only linear sclerosis, a bone scan or MRI will help identify the fracture. MRI has been documented as a sensitive test for nondisplaced fractures of the femoral neck. If a sclerotic lesion is seen on plain radiographs, the differential diagnosis should include osteoid osteoma, chronic sclerosing osteomyelitis, bone infarct, and osteosarcoma. The differential diagnosis of hip pain in a child is broad, but includes SCFE, Legg–Calvé–Perthes disease, infection, avulsion injuries of the pelvis, eosinophilic granuloma, and bony malignancies. Untreated stress fractures may progress with continued activity to complete fracture with displacement.[95] For this reason, prompt diagnosis and treatment are important.

CLASSIFICATION OF STRESS FRACTURES OF THE FEMORAL NECK

Femoral neck stress fractures have been classified into two types: compression fractures and tension fractures.[28] The compression type appears as reactive bone formation on the inferior cortex without cortical disruption. This type rarely becomes completely displaced but may collapse into a mild varus deformity,[30] and compression types have been reported to progress to complete fracture without early treatment (Fig. 23-18).[95] The tension type is a transverse fracture line appearing on the superior portion of the femoral neck. This type is inherently unstable because the fracture line is perpendicular to the lines of tension. Tension stress fractures have not been reported in children but may occur in skeletally mature teenagers.[14,95]

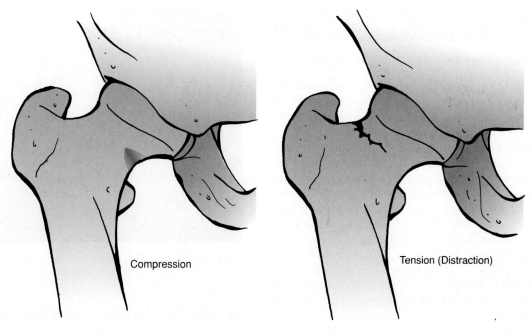

Figure 23-18. A line drawing of stress fractures, comparing compression (**A**) and tension (**B**) types.

TREATMENT OF STRESS FRACTURES OF THE FEMORAL NECK

Compression-type fractures generally can be treated with a period of nonweight-bearing on crutches. Partial weight-bearing can be allowed at 6 to 8 weeks with progression to full weight-bearing at 12 to 16 weeks provided that the pain is resolved and there is radiographic evidence of healing. Close follow-up and careful evaluation are mandatory to ensure that the fracture heals without propagation. Underlying conditions should be evaluated and addressed. In small or uncooperative children, spica casting may be necessary. Displacement into varus, however minimal, mandates internal fixation. Tension fractures are at high risk for displacement and should be treated with in situ compression fixation using cannulated screws.

Management of Expected Adverse Outcomes and Unexpected Complications Related to Stress Fractures of the Femoral Neck

Coxa vara is the most common complication of untreated compression-type fractures. Acute displacement of this type also has been described.[81] Once displaced, the stress fracture is subject to all the complications of type II and type III displaced femoral neck fractures.

Hip Dislocations

INTRODUCTION TO HIP DISLOCATIONS

Traumatic hip dislocations are uncommon injuries in children, constituting less than 5% of pediatric dislocations.[57] In one study, the author identified only 15 cases over a 20-year period at a large trauma center.[3] The character of the injury tends to vary with age. Children under age 6 commonly suffer isolated hip dislocation from a low-energy injury, whereas older children require a high-energy mechanism to dislocate the hip, and these injuries are often associated with more severe trauma.[3,7,39,74,87] Most hip dislocations in children can be reduced easily, and long-term outcome is generally good with prompt and complete reduction. Delay in reduction or neglected dislocations routinely do poorly, with a high incidence of AVN of the femoral head.[6,8] Incomplete reductions can occur from interposed soft tissue or bony fragments, and postoperative imaging is mandatory to ensure complete reduction.[60] Difficult reductions or hip dislocation that occurs in adolescents (with a widened proximal femoral physis) should be performed with anesthesia, muscle relaxation, and the use of fluoroscopy to ensure that physeal separation does not occur.[45,73] Open reduction may be needed if the hip cannot be reduced, or if there is a femoral head fracture or an incarcerated fragment. Incomplete reductions may be treated open or arthroscopically.[53] Complications, although uncommon, may occur, and these patients should be closely followed for recurrent subluxation, dislocation, and AVN.[3,39,87]

ASSESSMENT OF HIP DISLOCATION

MECHANISMS OF INJURY FOR HIP DISLOCATIONS

The mechanism of injury in children with hip dislocation varies. Posterior hip dislocations are the most common[7,87,91] and generally occur when a force is applied to the leg with the hip flexed and slightly adducted (Fig. 23-19). Anterior dislocations comprise fewer than 10% of pediatric hip dislocations (Fig. 23-20).[3,87] Anterior dislocations can occur superiorly or inferiorly and result from forced abduction and external rotation. If the hip is extended while undergoing forced abduction and external rotation, it will dislocate anteriorly and superiorly; if the hip is flexed while abducted and externally rotated, the femoral head tends to dislocate anteriorly and inferiorly. In very rare cases, the femoral head may dislocate directly inferiorly, a condition known as *luxatio erecta femoris* or infracotyloid dislocation. Although this condition is extremely rare, it tends to occur more commonly in children than in adults.[86]

In younger children, hip dislocations can occur with surprisingly little force, such as a fall while at play. The mechanism for hip dislocations in older children and adolescents is similar to that of adults in that significant trauma is needed. In a French study,[3] the authors assessed children with hip dislocations and divided them into two groups by age: those under 6 years (seven patients) and those aged 6 and older (seven patients). All of the children under age 6 had low-energy mechanisms and isolated hip dislocations without other injuries, but often had predisposing factors, such as hyperlaxity, coxa valga, or decreased acetabular coverage (Fig. 23-21). In the over 6-years-old group, all of the dislocations were a result of higher energy injuries and often had associated injuries.[3] American football and motor vehicle accidents are the most common etiologies, accounting for over 50% of the dislocations in older children and adolescents.[62,63]

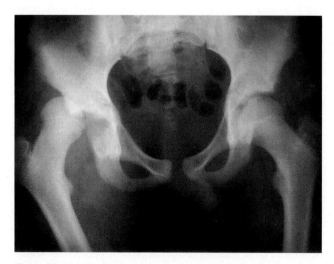

Figure 23-19. A typical posterior dislocation of the hip.

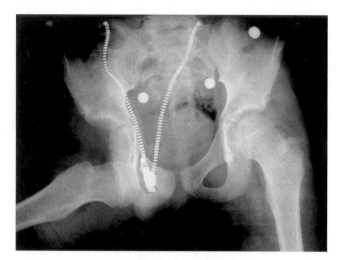

Figure 23-20. An anterior (inferior) dislocation of the hip.

INJURIES ASSOCIATED WITH HIP DISLOCATIONS

Older children with traumatic hip dislocations often present with associated injuries due to a high-energy mechanism of injury. In one study of 42 patients, there were 17 associated fractures in nine patients and one closed head injury. Of the 17 fractures, 6 were acetabular posterior wall factures and 1 required ORIF.[63] Careful evaluation of the posterior wall in children and adolescents who sustain a traumatic hip dislocation with MRI is important because standard radiographic assessments and CT may underestimate the amount of damage posteriorly.[85] Posterior dislocations of the femoral head can result in injury to the sciatic nerve in about 10% of adults and 5% of children. Partial recovery occurs in 60% to 70% of patients.[25] The function of the sciatic nerve should be specifically tested at the time of the initial assessment and after reduction.

Anterior dislocations can damage the femoral neurovascular bundle, and femoral nerve function and perfusion of the limb should be assessed. Tears of the capsule or acetabular labrum often occur and can prevent concentric reduction of the hip or lead to ongoing instability. Postreduction imaging must be carefully evaluated to ensure that there is no interposed soft tissue, such as the labrum or capsule, or osteochondral fragments. Rupture of the ligamentum teres is common in hip dislocations and can rarely be a cause of residual pain in some patients.

In addition, ipsilateral knee injuries commonly occur in high-energy injuries. One study evaluated the ipsilateral knees in 28 adults who had a traumatic hip dislocation and found that 75% had knee pain and 93% had MRI evidence of a knee injury, including effusion, bone bruise, or meniscal tears.[88]

SIGNS AND SYMPTOMS OF HIP DISLOCATIONS

A patient with a traumatic hip dislocation will generally present with hip pain and inability to ambulate after a trauma. Younger patients may localize the pain to the knee or thigh rather than in the hip. The hallmark of the clinical diagnosis of dislocation of

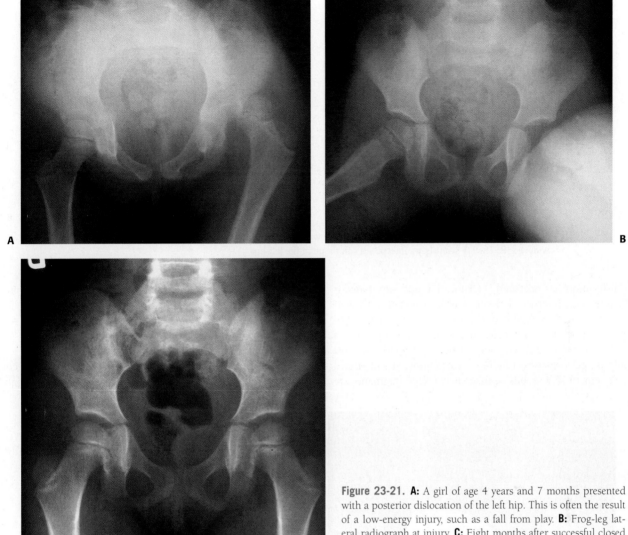

Figure 23-21. A: A girl of age 4 years and 7 months presented with a posterior dislocation of the left hip. This is often the result of a low-energy injury, such as a fall from play. **B:** Frog-leg lateral radiograph at injury. **C:** Eight months after successful closed reduction, radiographic appearance is normal.

the hip is abnormal positioning of the limb, which is not seen in fracture of the femur. Dislocations may spontaneously reduce, leaving the child with an incompletely reduced hip that may be misdiagnosed. Price et al.[74] reported on three children who presented with a history of trauma and an incongruous hip. In all cases, the diagnosis was originally missed.[80] A high index of suspicion is required for these injuries and all pelvic trauma imaging should be scrutinized for a concentric reduction of the hip joint.

IMAGING AND OTHER DIAGNOSTIC STUDIES FOR HIP DISLOCATIONS

Plain radiographs, combined with a thorough history and physical examination, usually confirms the diagnosis of a traumatic hip dislocation. Traumatic dislocations with spontaneous reductions may be more subtle, and are often missed. Radiographs should be examined for concomitant fracture of the acetabular rim, femoral head, and proximal femur, which

may be associated with dislocation. Any asymmetry of the joint space (Fig. 23-22), as compared with the contralateral hip, is suspicious for interposed tissue. MRI is useful for evaluating the acetabulum and may be useful in localizing intra-articular bony fragments or soft tissue interposition after reduction.[44,60,63] The identification of nonbony fragments is difficult by CT without the use of concomitant arthrography.[44] MRI is more useful for evaluating soft tissues that may be interposed between the femoral head and acetabulum and has an advantage over plain radiographs and CT scan to detect cartilage fractures and soft tissue and cartilage defects prior to complete ossification of the acetabulum.[43] MRI is especially helpful in nonconcentric reductions when the initial direction of dislocation is unknown, and in younger children with less ossification (Fig. 23-23).[60,85]

Spontaneous reduction can occur after a traumatic hip dislocation,[68,76,80] and the diagnosis may be missed if it is not considered. The presence of air in the hip joint, which may be detectable on CT scan of the pelvis, is evidence that a

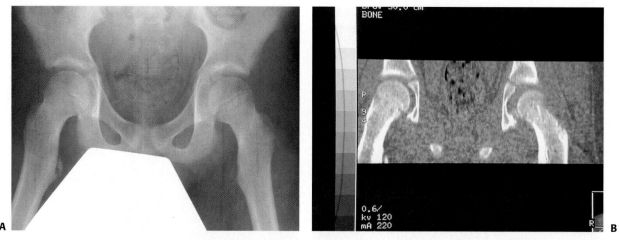

Figure 23-22. Spontaneously reduced left hip but with persistent pain. **A:** The joint space on the left is widened. **B:** The CT scan shows interposed soft tissue in the left hip.

hip dislocation has occurred.[33] Dislocation and spontaneous reduction with interposed tissue may lead to late arthropathy if untreated.[76] Widening of the joint space on plain radiographs suggests the diagnosis. In patients with hip pain, a history of trauma, and widening of the joint space, an MRI should be performed to rule out incarceration of soft tissue. If incarcerated soft tissues or osseous cartilage fragments are found, open or arthroscopic removal is necessary to obtain concentric reduction of the hip.[53]

CLASSIFICATION OF HIP DISLOCATIONS

Hip dislocations in children are generally classified according to the direction of dislocation in relation to the pelvis,

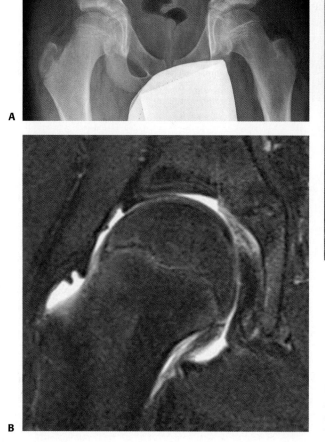

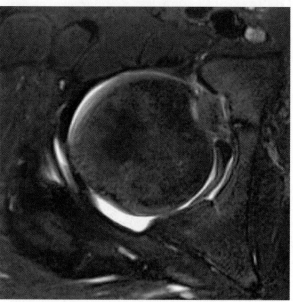

Figure 23-23. Right hip pain after a fall. The plain film shows no significant abnormality at time of injury (**A**). Persistent pain prompted an MRI 2 months after injury, which showed an interposed labrum in the joint (**B** and **C**).

namely posterior, anterior-superior, anterior-inferior, or infra-cotyloid.[50] Traumatic hip dislocations in children are posterior more than 90% of the time. The Stewart–Milford classification is based on associated fractures. Grade I is defined as dislocation without an associated fracture or only a small bony avulsion of the acetabular rim, grade II is a posterior rim fracture with a stable hip after reduction, grade III is a posterior rim fracture with an unstable hip (Fig. 23-24), and grade IV is a dislocation that has an associated fracture of the femoral head or neck.

Stewart-Milford Classification of Hip Dislocations

Grade	Associated Fracture
I	• No associated fracture or small avulsion of acetabular rim
II	• Posterior rim fracture, stable hip after reduction
III	• Posterior rim fracture, unstable hip after reduction
IV	• Femoral head or neck fracture

Pipkin Classification for Dislocations With Femoral Head/Neck Fractures

Type	Associated Fracture
1	• Head fracture caudal to the fovea (small fragment)
2	• Head fracture cranial to the fovea (large fragment)
3	• Combined head and neck fracture
4	• Combined neck and acetabular fracture

Fracture-dislocation of the hip involving the femoral head or the acetabulum is less common in children than in adults. Older adolescents generally sustain adult-type fracture-dislocations of the hip. Dislocations associated with femoral head or neck fractures are most commonly classified by the methods of Pipkin.[77] He classified the head fractures as occurring either caudal to the fovea with a resultant small fragment (type 1) (Fig. 23-25; also see Fig. 23-24), cranial to the fovea with a resultant large fragment (type 2), any combined femoral head and neck fracture (type 3), and any femoral neck fracture with an acetabular

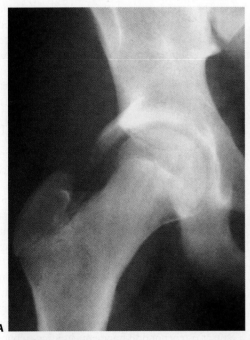
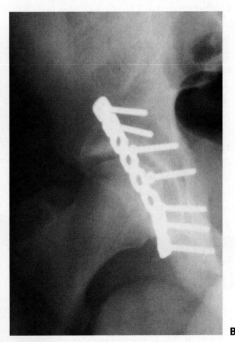
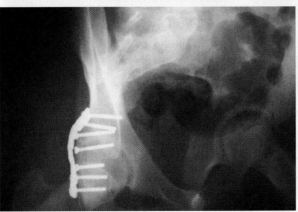

Figure 23-24. A: A 12-year-old boy was tackled from behind in football. The right hip was dislocated. Reduction was easily achieved, but the hip was unstable posteriorly as a result of fracture of the posterior rim of the acetabulum. This is the most common fracture, occurring with hip dislocation. **B:** The fracture and capsule were fixed via a posterior approach. **C:** Oblique view shows reconstitution of the posterior rim.

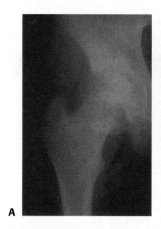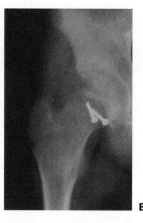

Figure 23-25. A: A posterior dislocation associated after reduction with a femoral head fracture caudal to the ligamentum teres (Pipkin type 2). This is uncommon in children. **B:** This was treated with open reduction and internal fixation, with follow-up radiographs taken 1 year after the injury.

fracture (type 4). *The youngest patient in his series from 1957 was 20, and most of these fractures were secondary to the relatively new phenomena of traffic accidents.*

Habitual dislocation of the hip has been described in children. In this condition, the child can actually voluntarily dislocate the hip. Many factors may contribute to this ability, including generalized ligamentous laxity or hyperlaxity disorders, excessive anteversion of the femur and acetabulum, and coxa valga.[93] A commonly confused condition is snapping of the iliotibial band over the greater trochanter, and often the patient will describe this as "dislocating their hip." Yet, the hip remains well seated both before and after the snap, which can be quite dramatic. The more common iliotibial band snapping can usually be differentiated from a true hip dislocation by examination, or if needed, radiographs with the hip "in" versus "out." A snapping iliotibial band will demonstrate a well-seated hip on both radiographs.

PATHOANATOMY AND APPLIED ANATOMY RELATED TO HIP DISLOCATIONS

The hip joint is a synovial ball and socket joint formed by the articulation of the round head of the femur and the cup-like acetabulum of the pelvis. If this is injured early in childhood, the growth of the acetabulum can be affected and this may result in acetabular dysplasia[13] or impingement.[37]

TREATMENT OPTIONS FOR HIP DISLOCATIONS

The immediate goal in the treatment of a traumatic hip dislocation is to obtain concentric reduction as soon as possible. Reduction of a pediatric or adolescent hip dislocation should be considered an orthopedic emergency. Generally, closed reduction should be attempted initially. Successful closed reduction can be achieved with intravenous or intramuscular sedation in the emergency room in most patients.[84] However, there is a risk of

separating the femoral epiphysis from the femoral neck. Hence, complete muscle relaxation and the ability to urgently open the hip is often helpful, and this is best provided in the operating room with a general anesthetic. Open reduction is indicated if closed reduction is unsuccessful or incomplete. In children, especially in their early teenage years, cases of proximal physeal separation with attempted closed reduction have been reported, and therefore, the use of fluoroscopy to assess the stability of the proximal femoral physis is highly recommended.[45,73]

Several methods of closed reduction have been described for reduction of posterior dislocations. With any type of dislocation, traction along the axis of the thigh coupled with gentle manipulation of the hip usually results in reduction after satisfactory relaxation of the surrounding muscles.

Allis[26] described a maneuver in which the patient is placed supine and the surgeon stands above the patient. For this reason, either the patient must be placed on the floor or the surgeon must climb onto the bed. The knee is flexed to relax the hamstrings. While an assistant stabilizes the pelvis, the surgeon applies longitudinal traction along the axis of the femur and gently manipulates the femoral head over the rim of the acetabulum and back into the acetabulum.

The gravity method of Stimson[90] entails placing the patient prone with the lower limbs hanging over the edge of a table. An assistant stabilizes the patient while the surgeon applies gentle downward pressure with the knee and hip flexed 90 degrees, in an attempt to pull the femoral head anteriorly over the posterior rim of the acetabulum and back into the socket. Gentle internal and external rotation may assist in the reduction.

OPERATIVE TREATMENT OF HIP DISLOCATION

If satisfactory closed reduction cannot be obtained using reasonable measures or the reduction is not concentric secondary to bone fragments or soft tissue interposition, it is appropriate to proceed with open reduction and inspection of the joint. The goal of an open reduction is to remove and potentially reconstruct any obstructing soft tissues and identify and remove intra-articular osteochondral fragments. The approach for open reduction includes the approaches discussed in the prior section (anterior, posterior, or surgical dislocation). The choice of approach depends on the direction of dislocation and surgeon experience. Surgeons with extensive hip arthroscopic experience may be able to arthroscopically extract interposed soft tissue or osteochondral fragments limiting a concentric reduction.

In an irreducible hip, imaging can be performed prior to reduction to aid in surgical planning, but it should not delay treatment. As mentioned previously, in children in their early teenage years, cases of proximal physeal separation with attempted closed reduction have been reported, and therefore, the use of fluoroscopy to assess the stability of the proximal femoral physis is highly recommended.[45,73]

Surgical Technique for Open Reduction of a Posterior Hip Dislocation Through a Posterolateral Approach

Open reduction of a posterior dislocation should be performed through a posterolateral (Kocher–Langenbeck) approach or surgical dislocation approach. For the Kocher–Langenbeck approach, the patient is positioned in the lateral decubitus position with the dislocated side facing up. The incision is centered on and just posterior to the greater trochanter and extends proximally into the buttock. Generally, a straight incision can be made when the hip is flexed approximately 90 degrees. Once the fascia lata is incised, the femoral head can be palpated beneath or within the substance of the gluteus maximus muscle. The fibers of the gluteus maximus can then be divided by blunt dissection, exposing the dislocated femoral head. The path of dislocation is followed through the short external rotator muscles and capsule down to the acetabulum. The sciatic nerve lies on the short external rotators and should be identified and inspected. The piriformis may be draped across the acetabulum, obstructing the view of the reduction. It may be necessary to detach the short external rotators to see inside the joint. After the joint is inspected, repair of the fracture of the posterior acetabular rim can be performed in the standard fashion.

Surgical Technique for Open Reduction of an Anterior Hip Dislocation

Anterior dislocations should be approached through an anterior approach. This can be performed through a bikini incision that uses the interval between the sartorius and the tensor fascia lata. The deep dissection follows the defect created by the femoral head down to the level of the acetabulum. In the anterior approach, the femoral head should be dislocated and any interposed soft tissue extracted. A Schanz screw or bone hook may be needed to displace the femur enough to see inside the joint in the anterior approach. Any bony fragments displaced from the femoral head or the acetabulum should have reduction and fixation if the size is significant. In younger hips, the cartilaginous labral–chondral junction may be displaced from the bony rim. Suture anchor repair through the base of the labrum should be performed.

Surgical Technique for Open Reduction of a Hip Dislocation Through a Surgical Dislocation Approach

A surgical dislocation approach is particularly useful for hips that are reduced but are not concentric, or in hips with ongoing instability after reduction. A lateral incision is created centered on the anterior third of the greater trochanter. The leg can then be abducted by placing it on a sterile, padded Mayo stand. The tensor fascia is incised longitudinally in line with the skin incision. Proximally, the dissection may be carried out between the anterior edge of the gluteus maximus and the tensor (Gibson modification[66]), or the gluteus maximus may be split bluntly. This exposes the proximal vastus lateralis, gluteus medius, and greater trochanter.

The leg is then taken off of the Mayo and positioned with the hip in adduction and slight internal rotation to better visualize the anatomic landmarks. Identify and develop the interval between the piriformis and the gluteus medius. The piriformis is the thick, white tendon visualized deep to the posterior/distal aspect of gluteus medius. Once exposed, the tendon can be gently retracted distally to expose the inferior margin of the gluteus minimus fascia. The inferior fascia of the minimus is then opened to allow the muscle to be retracted in an anterior-superior direction off of the hip capsule. This should allow visualization of the hip capsule.

A greater trochanteric osteotomy is then performed from the posterior border of the vastus lateralis ridge to the anterior to the tip of the greater trochanter using either an oscillating saw or an osteotomy. The width of the osteotomy should be approximately 15 mm. The piriformis and short external rotators should remain attached to the stable trochanteric bed. Maintaining the piriformis tendon intact protects the retinacular branch of the medial circumflex artery. The trochanteric flip piece with attached gluteus minimus, gluteus medius, vastus lateralis, and vastus intermedius is then reflected anteriorly.

Capsular exposure then continues anteriorly and superiorly. Gentle, progressive flexion and external rotation of the operative hip will facilitate the muscle dissection. Capsular muscular attachments are elevated anteriorly to the indirect head of the rectus tendon, superiorly to the superior rim of the acetabulum, and posteriorly to the piriformis.

The hip capsule is then opened in a Z-shaped fashion. The longitudinal limb is along the axis of the femoral neck in line with the iliofemoral ligament. The distal aspect is proximal but in line with the intertrochanteric ridge. The posterior limb of the capsule is opened in the capsular recess of the acetabulum as far posterior as the piriformis tendon, protecting the retinaculum as it pierces the hip capsule. Once the capsule is opened, the intra-articular anatomy can be visualized. The epiphysis should be provisionally pinned with a smooth K-wire if there is any concern of epiphysiolysis.

Flexion and external rotation of the leg will allow anterior dislocation of the femoral head. Complete dislocation may not be necessary if the majority of the soft tissue injury is located posteriorly, as is typically seen in a posterior hip dislocation. The femoral head and acetabulum should be inspected for damage. Frequently, the labrum or hip capsule is entrapped within the joint.

Surgical Technique for Treatment of Irreducible or Incomplete Hip Dislocation

Regardless of approach selected, any small intra-articular fragments should be removed. The labrum and capsule should be inspected for repairable tears. Labral fragments that cannot be securely replaced should be excised, but repair should be attempted. Any bony fragments displaced from the femoral head or the acetabulum should have reduction and fixation if the size allows. In younger hips, the cartilaginous labral–chondral junction may be displaced from the bony rim. Suture anchor repair through the base of the labrum should be performed. The hip joint is then reduced under direct vision. The capsule should be repaired and, in the case of a surgical dislocation approach, the greater trochanter should be reduced and secured with two or three 3.5- or 4.5-mm screws.

Postreduction radiographs should be taken to confirm concentric reduction. If the joint appears slightly widened, repeat investigation is indicated to rule out interposed tissue. Slight widening secondary to fluid in the hip joint or decreased muscle tone can occur, and this may improve over the next few days.

Treatment of Open Dislocations

Open injuries should be treated with immediate irrigation and debridement. The surgical incision should incorporate and enlarge the traumatic wound. Inspection should proceed as detailed above. Capsular repair should be attempted if the hip joint is not contaminated. The wound should be left open or should be well drained to prevent invasive infection. As in all open fractures, intravenous antibiotics should be administered and patients should be screened for tetanus.

Postoperative Management

After reduction, a short period of immobilization should be instituted. In younger children, a spica cast can be used for 4 to 6 weeks; older cooperative children can be treated with hip abduction orthosis. Range of motion precautions are dependent on the direction of the dislocation approach used in treatment. Patients with a posterior dislocation treated with a posterolateral approach should be restricted from excessive adduction, internal rotation, and flexion. Patients with an anterior dislocation treated with an anterior approach should be restricted from excessive extension and external rotation. And those patients treated with a surgical dislocation approach require limitations to active abduction and passive adduction past the midline. All patients may be touch down weight-bearing if developmentally appropriate.[39,84]

Authors' Preferred Treatment for Hip Dislocations

Urgent closed reduction by applying traction in line with the femur and gently manipulating the femoral head back into the acetabulum should be performed. A controlled reduction with sedation or general anesthesia and muscle relaxation in the operating room is preferable, and aggressive techniques should not be attempted without muscle relaxant. The use of fluoroscopy to monitor the reduction, especially in children over 12 with open physis, is important to ensure that proximal femoral epiphysiolysis does not occur. Surgery is indicated for dislocations that are irreducible or for nonconcentric reductions. We recommend an MRI should be considered after reduction to assess for interposing fragments of bone, cartilage, or soft tissue.

Potential pitfalls and preventive measures reduce the hip urgently. The most devastating outcome is ON, and prolonged time to reduction (more than 6 hours) appears

to be the greatest risk factor. In multitrauma patients, this concept needs to be expressed to the trauma team so that it can be prioritized properly.

Look for associated fractures and other injuries. In older children, it is important to evaluate the posterior rim of the acetabulum after posterior dislocation to rule out fracture. Relying on plain radiographs and CT may underestimate the extent of damage to the posterior wall of the acetabulum in children because of the incomplete ossification of the pediatric bone. MRI may be required to adequately assess the posterior wall of the acetabulum in children.[85]

Fractures at other sites in the femur must be considered. It is important to obtain radiographs that show the entire femur to rule out ipsilateral fracture. Careful evaluation of the entire patient is needed especially for high-energy injuries that result in a hip dislocation in older children and adults.

Separation of the capital femoral epiphysis and femoral neck fracture has been reported in association with dislocation of the hip and the attempted reduction. Children in their early teenage years, aged 12 to 16, should have reduction performed with fluoroscopy under general anesthesia when possible. This strategy may avoid the possibility of displacing the proximal femoral epiphysis (with attendant increased ON risk) during attempted closed reduction (Fig. 23-26). Spontaneous relocation of a dislocation of the hip may occur with subsequent soft tissue or osteocartilaginous interposition. Failure to appreciate the presence of hip dislocation may lead to inadequate treatment. Traumatic hip subluxation may go undetected or may be treated as a sprain or strain if the diagnosis is not considered.[68,80] After dislocation and spontaneous reduction, soft tissue may become interposed in the hip joint potentially resulting in chronic arthropathy. In a child with posttraumatic hip pain without obvious deformity, the possibility of dislocation–relocation must be considered.

Always image the hip for evaluation of interposed tissue after reduction. The incidence of widened joint space after hip reductions is as high as 26%.[60] After reduction, hemarthrosis may initially cause the hip joint to appear slightly wider on the affected side, but this should decrease after a few days. If the hip fails to appear concentric, the possibility of interposed soft tissue must be considered and MRI or CT scan should be performed.[76,84,92]

Long-term follow-up is important in children who undergo hip dislocation. Injury to the triradiate cartilage may cause acetabular dysplasia with growth.[11] ON, although uncommon, may lead to early arthrosis, and this may not be identified radiographically for several years. If there has been a significant delay in time to reduction or the patient is otherwise at higher risk for ON, then consideration of a bone scan or MRI to evaluate for ON may be warranted, especially if early treatment with bisphosphonates is considered.

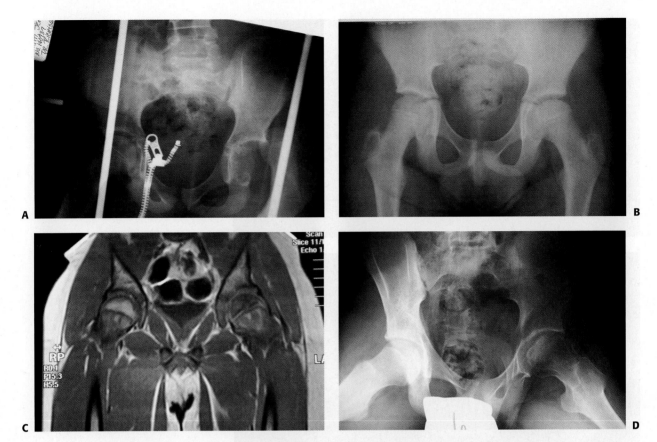

Figure 23-26. A: An 11-year-old boy dislocated his left hip while wrestling. **B:** The hip was easily reduced. **C:** After 5 months, hip pain led to an MRI, which shows osteonecrosis of the capital femoral epiphysis. **D:** At 10 months after injury, there are typical changes of osteonecrosis despite nonweight-bearing.

Management of Expected Adverse Outcomes and Unexpected Complications Related to Hip Dislocations in Children

Osteonecrosis occurs in about 10% of hip dislocations in children (Fig. 23-27).[38,63,71,91] Urgent reduction may decrease the incidence of this complication.[63,91] The risk of ON is most likely related to the severity of initial trauma.[91] If the force of the hip dislocation is so strong as to disrupt the obturator externus muscle, the posterior ascending vessels may simultaneously be torn.[71] In the rare case of dislocation with an intact capsule, increased intra-capsular pressure as a result of hemarthrosis may have a tamponade effect, resulting in ON.[84] The type of postreduction care has not been shown to influence the rate of ON.

Early technetium bone scanning with pinhole-collimated images can be used to detect osteonecrosis as an area of decreased uptake. Findings on T2-weighted MRI images are abnormal but of variable signal intensity, and the MRI may be falsely negative if performed within a few days of injury.[79] Conversely, many perfusion defects seen on MRI spontaneously resolve after several months.[79] As treatment for early osteonecrosis continues to develop, the utility of postreduction perfusion imaging may change, and early assessment may be considered for those at high risk of osteonecrosis. Currently, posttraumatic hips should be followed by serial radiographs even after healing to look for signs of osteonecrosis. It is recommended that these studies continue for at least 2 years following a traumatic dislocation, as radiographic changes may appear late.[7]

If osteonecrosis develops, pain, loss of motion, and deformity of the femoral head may occur.[8] The course of traumatic osteonecrosis in a young child resembles Legg–Calvé–Perthes disease and may be treated like Perthes disease.[8] The goals of treatment are to maintain mobility and containment of the femoral head to maximize congruity after resolution. Osteonecrosis in older children should be treated as in adults and may require osteotomy, reconstruction, or arthroplasty. If identified early, medical treatment with bisphosphonates or revascularization techniques, such as a vascularized fibular bone graft, may be considered.[1,90]

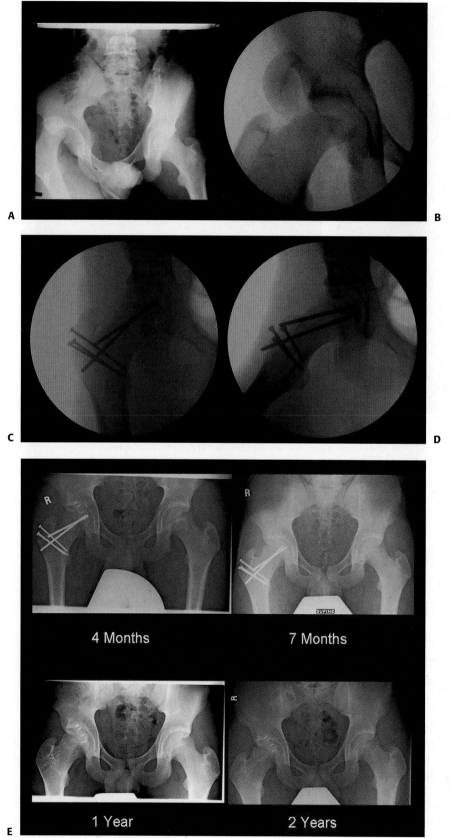

4 Months   7 Months

1 Year   2 Years

Figure 23-27. **A:** Anteroposterior radiograph of the pelvis, showing dislocation of the right hip. **B:** Anteroposterior radiograph of the right hip, showing the physeal separation after attempted closed reduction. Anteroposterior (**C**) and lateral (**D**) radiographs made after surgical dislocation, reduction, and fixation of the epiphysis through a trochanteric flip osteotomy. **E:** Anteroposterior radiographs made during the 2-year period after surgical reconstruction. (Reprinted with permission from Schoenecker JG, Kim Y, Ganz R. Treatment of traumatic separation of the proximal femoral epiphysis without development of osteonecrosis: A report of two cases. *J Bone Joint Surg Am.* 2010;92(4):973–977.)

CHONDROLYSIS

Chondrolysis has been reported after hip dislocation in up to 6% of children[38,74] and probably occurs as a result of articular damage at the time of dislocation. Chondrolysis cannot be reversed by medical or surgical techniques, and treatment is symptomatic. Anti-inflammatory medication and weight-relieving devices should be used as needed. One study suggests that hip joint distraction with a hinged external fixator may improve range of motion and decrease pain.[29] If the joint fails to reconstitute, fusion, reconstruction, or replacement should be considered.

COXA MAGNA

Coxa magna occasionally occurs after hip dislocation. The reported incidence varies widely and ranges from 0% to 47%.[38,74] It is believed to occur as a result of posttraumatic hyperemia.[74] In most children, this condition is asymptomatic and does not require any treatment.[74] There is no intervention that will prevent coxa magna.

HABITUAL DISLOCATION

Habitual or voluntary dislocation of the hip usually is unrelated to trauma. Many factors may contribute to this ability, including generalized ligamentous laxity, excessive anteversion of the femur and acetabulum, and coxa valga. Initial management should include counseling the child to cease the activity (with or without psychiatric counseling) and observation. If episodes of dislocation persist, permanent changes such as secondary capsular laxity or osteocartilaginous deformation of the hip may occur. These changes may lead to pain, residual subluxation, or degenerative joint disease. Conservative treatment should be initially attempted and may include simple observation with or without psychiatric counseling or immobilization with cast or brace.

Hip stabilization by surgical means may be indicated for persistent painful episodes of hip, despite conservative treatment or those with underlying medical conditions predisposing to habitual dislocation, such as Down syndrome.[75,93] Knight et al. reported their 10-year follow-up of Down syndrome patients with habitual subluxation treated with a varus/derotation intertrochanteric osteotomy. They recommend surgery in these patients before age 7 and attempting to get the neck/shaft angle to 105 degrees to prevent later hip abnormality.[50] Therefore, corrective surgery, if considered, should be performed only to correct specific anatomic abnormality and perhaps in patients with known ligamentous laxity. Surgery may include capsular plication, although bony correction with redirectional pelvic osteotomy, or osteotomy of the proximal femur, is required to treat the underlying pathology.[93]

HETEROTOPIC OSSIFICATION

Heterotopic ossification can result after closed reduction of hip dislocations in children, but is generally asymptomatic and rarely requires intervention. In one study, three children (all under 16 years of age) developed heterotopic ossification, one of which required surgical excision.[63]

INTERPOSED SOFT TISSUE

Interposed tissues may result in a nonconcentric reduction or a complete failure of closed reduction. Muscle, bone, articular cartilage, and labrum have been all been implicated.[80,92] An MRI can provide the most useful information on obstacles to complete concentric reduction.[92] Open reduction generally is necessary to clear impeding tissues from the joint.[74,80,92] Untreated, nonconcentric reduction may lead to permanent degenerative arthropathy.

LATE PRESENTATION

Not all hip dislocations in children cause severe or incapacitating symptoms. Ambulation may even be possible. As a result, treatment may be delayed or the diagnosis missed until shortening of the limb and contracture are well established, making reduction difficult. Nearly all patients with a delayed treatment of traumatic hip dislocation develop osteonecrosis.[6,54] Prolonged, heavy traction has been described as a method to effect reduction.[39] If this fails, preoperative traction, extensive soft tissue release, or primary femoral shortening should be considered in association with an open reduction. Open reduction will likely be difficult and may not always be successful. Even if a stable, concentric reduction is achieved, progressive arthropathy may lead to a stiff and painful hip. The likelihood of a good result decreases with the duration of dislocation.

NERVE INJURY

The sciatic nerve may be directly compressed by the femoral head after a posterior dislocation of the hip in 2% to 13% of patients.[32,87,91] If the hip is expediently reduced, nerve function returns spontaneously in most patients.[32] If the sciatic nerve palsy is present prior to reduction, the nerve does not need to be explored unless open reduction is required for other reasons. If sciatic nerve function is shown to be intact and is lost during the reduction maneuver, the nerve should be explored to ensure that it has not displaced into the joint. Other nerves around the hip joint are rarely injured at dislocation. Treatment is generally expectant unless laceration or incarceration is suspected; if so, exploration is indicated.

RECURRENT DISLOCATION

Recurrence after traumatic hip dislocation is rare but occurs most frequently after posterior dislocation in children under 8 years of age[6] or in children with known hyperlaxity (Down syndrome, Ehlers–Danlos disease, etc.). The incidence of recurrence is estimated to be less than 3%.[74] Recurrence can be quite disabling, and in the long term may result in damage to the articular surfaces as a result of shear damage to the cartilaginous hip. Prolonged spica casting (at least 3 months) may be effective in younger chidren.[64] Surgical exploration with capsulorrhaphy can be performed if conservative treatment fails.[6,50] Prior to hip reconstruction, an MRI or arthrography is recommended to identify soft tissue defects or capsular redundancy.[6]

In older children, recurrent dislocation can occur as a result of a bony defect in the posterior rim of the acetabulum similar to that in adults and may require posterior acetabular reconstruction (Fig. 23-28). Recent literature suggests a more

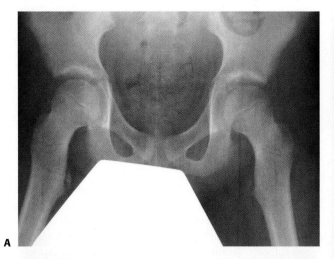

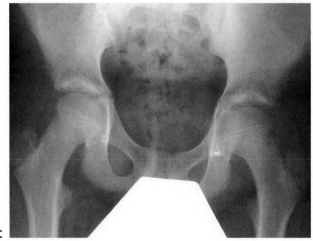

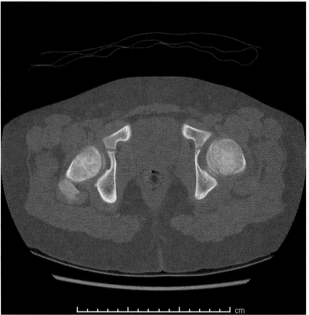

Figure 23-28. An 11-year-old who had left persistent pain after closed reduction of left hip after sledding accident. **A:** Anteroposterior radiograph of reduced hip preoperatively. **B:** Preoperative CT slice clearly demonstrating entrapped fragment. **C:** Anteroposterior radiograph postoperatively.

severe soft tissue injury associated with these fractures than had been previously appreciated.[72,78,96] These patients may have large labral tears that can contribute to ongoing issues if instability, with a near-complete or radial tear of the posterior labrum. MRI evaluation of the hip after reduction allows for evaluation of these potential findings without the risk of radiation exposure.[12]

VASCULAR INJURY

Impingement on the femoral neurovascular bundle has been described after anterior hip dislocation in children, and this may occur in up to 25% of patients.[91] The hip should be reduced as soon as possible to remove the offending pressure on the femoral vessels. If reduction of the hip fails to restore perfusion, immediate exploration of the femoral vessels is indicated.

SUMMARY, CONTROVERSIES, AND FUTURE DIRECTIONS RELATED TO HIP DISLOCATIONS

The treatment for hip disorders is evolving. We now have new surgical and medical treatment options for hip disorders such as surgical hip dislocation and hip arthroscopy. Although most do not directly apply to the urgent reduction of hip dislocations, they are applicable to the sequelae that may occur. The use of bisphosphonates and other medications that inhibit bone resorption is an active area of research and may have direct effects on limiting collapse of the femoral head if osteonecrosis occurs.[1] This could soon change our paradigm for the evaluation of a hip after reduction of a dislocation, and early perfusion MRI or bone scans may be indicated.

A host of surgical methods are available to manage deformity as a result of osteonecrosis or hip instability. Techniques to increase vascularity, such as vascularized bone grafting, remain a controversial method to improve the natural history. Hinged distraction across the hip may now play a role as a primary treatment for chondrolysis or as an adjunct to other techniques.[29] Hip arthroscopy is much more commonly performed and allows for a much less invasive approach for the removal of loose bodies in the hip, as well as assessing and treating chondral, labral, and capsular injuries.[15,53]

Together, these new techniques offer future opportunities to decrease the severity of known complications and potentially improve functional outcomes. Time and follow-up will be required to determine if these methods improve the natural history of these posttraumatic sequelae.

Annotated References

Reference	Annotation
Mehlman CT, Hubbard GW, Crawford AH, et al. Traumatic hip dislocation in children. *Clin Orthop Relat Res.* 2000;376:68–79.	Retrospective review of 46 pediatric patients with traumatic hip dislocation with long-term follow-up. Found that functional outcomes were generally good in these patients. Time to reduction was the only studied factor predictive of the risk for avascular necrosis.
Moon ES, Mehlman CT. Risk factors for avascular necrosis after femoral neck fractures in children: 25 Cincinnati cases and meta-analysis of 360 cases. *J Orthop Trauma.* 2006;20(5):323–329.	Meta-analysis of over 300 pediatric hip fractures, which identified fracture pattern and age at injury as the two most significant risk factors for the development of avascular necrosis of the femoral head.
Schrader MW, Jacofsky DJ, Stans AA, et al. Femoral neck fractures in pediatric patients: 30 years experience at a level 1 trauma center. *Clin Orthop Relat Res.* 2007;454:169–173.	Retrospective review of 20 patients with pediatric femoral neck fractures with medium-term follow-up. Found that quality of reduction and time to reduction were associated with good outcomes.
Spence D, DiMauro JP, Miller PE, et al. Osteonecrosis after femoral neck fractures in children and adolescents: analysis of risk factors. *J Pediatr Orthop.* 2016;36:111–116.	Retrospective review of 70 patients with pediatric femoral neck fractures, which identified factors associated with increased risk for avascular necrosis. Risk factors identified included fracture displacement, fracture location, and time to treatment.

REFERENCES

1. Agarwala S, Jain D, Joshi VR, et al. Efficacy of alendronate, a bisphosphonate, in the treatment of AVN of the hip: a prospective open-label study. *Rheumatology (Oxford).* 2005;44(3):352–359.
2. Alho A. Concurrent ipsilateral fractures of the hip and femoral shaft: a meta-analysis of 659 cases. *Acta Orthop Scand.* 1996;67:19–28.
3. Ayadi K, Trigui M, Gdoura F, et al. Traumatic hip dislocations in children. *Rev Chir Orthop Reparatrice Appar Mot.* 2008;94(1):19–25.
4. Bagatur AE, Zorer G. Complications associated with surgically treated hip fractures in children. *J Pediatr Orthop B.* 2002;11:219–228.
5. Bali K, Sudesh P, Patel S, et al. Pediatric femoral neck fractures: our 10 years of experience. *Clin Orthop Surg.* 2011;3(4):302–308.
6. Banskota AK, Spiegel DA, Shrestha S, et al. Open reduction for neglected traumatic hip dislocation in children and adolescents. *J Pediatr Orthop.* 2007;27(2):187–191.
7. Barquet A. Traumatic hip dislocation in childhood. A report of 26 cases and review of the literature. *Acta Orthop Scand.* 1979;50:549–553.
8. Barquet A. Natural history of avascular necrosis following traumatic hip dislocation in childhood: a review of 145 cases. *Acta Orthop Scand.* 1982;53:815–820.
9. Beaty JH. Fractures of the hip in children. *Orthop Clin North Am.* 2006;37:223–232.
10. Bettin D, Pankalla T, Böhm H, et al. Hip pain related to femoral neck stress fracture in a 12-year-old boy performing intensive soccer playing activities: a case report. *Int J Sports Med.* 2003;24:593–596.
11. Blair W, Hanson C. Traumatic closure of the triradiate cartilage: report of a case. *J Bone Joint Surg Am.* 1979;61:144–145.
12. Blanchard C, Kushare I, Boyles A, et al. Traumatic, posterior pediatric hip dislocations with associated posterior labrum osteochondral avulsion: recognizing the acetabular "fleck" sign. *J Pediatr Orthop.* 2016;36:602–607.
13. Boardman MJ, Herman MJ, Buck B, et al. Hip fractures in children. *J Am Acad Orthop Surg.* 2009;17(3):162–173.
14. Boyle MJ, Hogue GD, Heyworth BE, et al. Femoral neck stress fractures in children younger than 10 years of age. *J Pediatr Orthop.* 2017;37(2):e96–e99.
15. Bray TJ. Femoral neck fracture fixation. Clinical decision making. *Clin Orthop Relat Res.* 1997;(339):20–31.
16. Byrd JW, Jones KS. Traumatic rupture of the ligamentum teres as a source of hip pain. *Arthroscopy.* 2004;20(4):385–391.
17. Caldwell L, Chan CM, Sanders JO, et al. Detection of femoral neck fractures in pediatric patients with femoral shaft fractures. *J Pediatr Orthop.* 2017;37(3):e164–e167.
18. Canale ST, Bourland WL. Fracture of the neck and intertrochanteric region of the femur in children. *J Bone Joint Surg Am.* 1977;59(4):431–443.
19. Canale ST, Casillas M, Banta JV. Displaced femoral neck fractures at the bone-screw interface after in situ fixation of slipped capital femoral epiphysis. *J Pediatr Orthop.* 1997;17(2):212–215.
20. Cheng JC, Tang N. Decompression and stable internal fixation of femoral neck fractures in children can affect the outcome. *J Pediatr Orthop.* 1999;19:338–343.
21. Chun KA, Morcuende J, El-Khoury GY. Entrapment of the acetabular labrum following reduction of traumatic hip dislocation in a child. *Skeletal Radiol.* 2004;33(12):728–731.
22. Colonna PC. Fracture of the neck of the femur in childhood: a report of six cases. *Ann Surg.* 1928;88:902–907.
23. Cornawall R, Radomisli TE. Nerve injury in traumatic dislocation of the hip. *Clin Orthop Relat Res.* 2000;377:84–91.
24. Currey JD, Butler G. The mechanical properties of bone tissue in children. *J Bone Joint Surg Am.* 1975;57:810–814.
25. Davison BL, Weinstein SL. Hip fractures in children: a long-term follow-up study. *J Pediatr Orthop.* 1992;12:355–358.
26. De Yoe LE. A suggested improvement to the Allis' method of reduction of posterior dislocation of the hip. *Ann Surg.* 1940;112(1):127–129.
27. Diaz MJ, Hedlund GL. Sonographic diagnosis of traumatic separation of the proximal femoral epiphysis in the neonate. *Pediatr Radiol.* 1991;21(3):238–240.
28. Edgren W. Coxa plana. A clinical and radiological investigation with particular reference to the importance of the metaphyseal changes for the final shape of the proximal part of the femur. *Acta Orthop Scand Suppl.* 1965;84:1–129.
29. Egol KA, Koval KJ, Kummer F, et al. Stress fractures of the femoral neck. *Clin Orthop Relat Res.* 1998;(348):72–78.
30. Epstein HC. Traumatic dislocations of the hip. *Clin Orthop Relat Res.* 1973;(92):116–142.
31. Fairbairn KJ, Mulligan ME, Murphey MD, et al. Gas bubbles in the hip joint on CT: an indication of recent dislocation. *AJR Am J Roentgenol.* 1995;164(4):931–934.
32. Flynn JM, Wong KL, Yeh GL, et al. Displaced fractures of the hip in children. Management by early operation and immobilization in a hip spica cast. *J Bone Joint Surg Br.* 2002;84:108–112.
33. Forlin E, Guille JT, Kumar SJ, et al. Transepiphyseal fractures of the neck of the femur in very young children. *J Pediatr Orthop.* 1992;12:164–168.
34. Forster NA, Ramseier LE, Exner GU. Undisplaced femoral neck fractures in children have a high risk of secondary displacement. *J Pediatr Orthop B.* 2006;15(2):131–133.
35. Ganz R, Gill TJ, Gautier E, et al. Surgical dislocation of the adult hip a technique with full access to the femoral head and acetabulum without the risk of avascular necrosis. *J Bone Joint Surg Br.* 2001;83(8):1119–1124.
36. Ganz R, Parvizi J, Beck M, et al. Femoroacetabular impingement: a cause for early osteoarthritis of the hip. *Clin Orthop Relat Res.* 2003;(417):112–120.
37. Gennari JM, Merrot T, Bergoin V, et al. X-ray transparency interpositions after reduction of traumatic dislocations of the hip in children. *Eur J Pediatr Surg.* 1996;6:288–293.
38. Guevara CJ, Pietrobon R, Carothers JT, et al. Comprehensive morphologic evaluation of the hip in patients with symptomatic labral tear. *Clin Orthop Relat Res.* 2006;453:277–285.
39. Hamilton PR, Broughton NS. Traumatic hip dislocation in childhood. *J Pediatr Orthop.* 1998;18:691–694.
40. Hansman CF. Appearance and fusion of ossification centers in the human skeleton. *Am J Roentgenol Radium Ther Nucl Med.* 1962;88:476–482.
41. Hearty T, Swaroop VT, Gourineni P, et al. Standard radiographs and computed tomographic scan underestimating pediatric acetabular fracture after traumatic hip dislocation: report of 2 cases. *J Orthop Trauma.* 2011;25(7):e68–e73.
42. Herrera-Soto JA, Price CT, Reuss BL, et al. Proximal femoral epiphysiolysis during reduction of hip dislocation in adolescents. *J Pediatr Orthop.* 2006;26(3):371–374.
43. Hougard K, Thomsen PB. Traumatic hip dislocation in children. Follow-up of 13 cases. *Orthopedics.* 1989;12:375–378.
44. Hughes LO, Beaty JH. Fractures of the head and neck of the femur in children. *J Bone Joint Surg Am.* 1994;76:283–292.
45. Ingari JV, Smith DK, Aufdemorte TB, et al. Anatomic significance of magnetic resonance imaging findings in hip fracture. *Clin Orthop Relat Res.* 1996;(332):209–214.
46. Joeris A, Audigé L, Ziebarth K, et al. The locking compression paediatric hip plate: technical guide and critical analysis. *Int Orthop.* 2012;36(11):2299–2306.
47. Joseph B, Mulpuri K. Delayed separation of the capital femoral epiphysis after an ipsilateral transcervical fracture of the femoral neck. *J Orthop Trauma.* 2000;14(6):446–448.
48. Kashiwagi N, Suzuki S, Seto Y. Arthroscopic treatment for traumatic hip dislocation with avulsion fracture of the ligamentum teres. *Arthroscopy.* 2001;17(1):67–69.

49. Kirkos JM, Papavasiliou KA, Kyrkos MJ, et al. Multidirectional habitual bilateral hip dislocation in a patient with Down syndrome. *Clin Orthop Relat Res.* 2005;(435):263–266.

50. Knight DM, Alves C, Wedge JH. Femoral varus derotation osteotomy for the treatment of habitual subluxation and dislocation of the pediatric hip in trisomy 21: a 10-year experience. *J Pediatr Orthop.* 2011;31(6):638–643.

51. Kumar S, Jain AK. Neglected traumatic hip dislocation in children. *Clin Orthop Relat Res.* 2005;(431):9–13.

52. Lam SF. Fractures of the neck of the femur in children. *J Bone Joint Surg Am.* 1971;53:1165–1179.

53. Langenskiöld A, Salenius P. Epiphyseodesis of the greater trochanter. *Acta Orthop Scand.* 1967;38:199–219.

54. Maeda S, Kita A, Fujii G, et al. Avascular necrosis associated with fractures of the femoral neck in children: histological evaluation of core biopsies of the femoral head. *Injury.* 2003;34:283–286.

55. Magu NK, Singh R, Sharma A, et al. Treatment of pathologic femoral neck fractures with modified Pauwels' osteotomy. *Clin Orthop Relat Res.* 2005;(437):229–235.

56. Magu NK, Singh R, Sharma AK, et al. Modified Pauwels' intertrochanteric osteotomy in neglected femoral neck fractures in children: a report of 10 cases followed for a minimum of 5 years. *J Orthop Trauma.* 2007;21(4):237–243.

57. Maruenda JI, Barrios C, Gomar-Sancho F. Intracapsular hip pressure after femoral neck fracture. *Clin Orthop Relat Res.* 1997;(340):172–180.

58. Mehlman CT, Hubbard GW, Crawford AH, et al. Traumatic hip dislocation in children. Long-term followup of 42 patients. *Clin Orthop Relat Res.* 2000;(376):68–79.

59. Mirdad T. Fractures of the neck of the femur in children: an experience at the Aseer Central Hospital, Abha, Saudi Arabia. *Injury.* 2002;33:823–827.

60. Moed BR. The modified Gibson posterior surgical approach to the acetabulum. *J Orthop Trauma.* 2010;24(5):315–322.

61. Moon ES, Mehlman CT. Risk factors for avascular necrosis after femoral neck fractures in children: 25 Cincinnati cases and meta-analysis of 360 cases. *J Orthop Trauma.* 2006;20(5):323–329.

62. Moorman CT 3rd, Warren RF, Hershman EB, et al. Traumatic posterior hip subluxation in American football. *J Bone Joint Surg Am.* 2003;85:1190–1196.

63. Morsy HA. Complications of fracture of the neck of the femur in children. A longterm follow-up study. *Injury.* 2001;32:45–51.

64. Nagao S, Ito K, Nakamura I. Spontaneous bilateral femoral neck fractures associated with a low serum level of vitamin D in a young adult. *J Arthroplasty.* 2009;24(2):322.

65. Ng GP, Cole WG. Effect of early hip decompression on the frequency of avascular necrosis in children with fractures of the neck of the femur. *Injury.* 1996;27:419–421.

66. Nötzli HP, Siebenrock KA, Hempfing A, et al. Perfusion of the femoral head during surgical dislocation of the hip. Monitoring by laser Doppler flowmetry. *J Bone Joint Surg Br.* 2002;84:300–304.

67. Nötzli HP, Wyss TF, Stoecklin CH, et al. The contour of the femoral head–neck junction as a predictor for the risk of anterior impingement. *J Bone Joint Surg Br.* 2002;84(4):556–560.

68. Odent T, Glorion C, Pannier S, et al. Traumatic dislocation of the hip with separation of the capital epiphysis: 5 adolescent patients with 3 to 9 years of follow-up. *Acta Orthop Scand.* 2003;74(1):49–52.

69. Ogden JA. Changing patterns of proximal femoral vascularity. *J Bone Joint Surg Am.* 1974;56:941–950.

70. Ogden JA, Lee KE, Rudicel SA, et al. Proximal femoral epiphysiolysis in the neonate. *J Pediatr Orthop.* 1984;4(3):285–292.

71. Pape HC, Krettek C, Friedrich A, et al. Long-term outcome in children with fractures of the proximal femur after high-energy trauma. *J Trauma.* 1999;46:58–64.

72. Philippon MJ, Kuppersmith DA, Wolff AB, et al. Arthroscopic findings following traumatic hip dislocation in 14 professional athletes. *Arthroscopy.* 2009;25:169–174.

73. Poggi JJ, Callaghan JJ, Spritzer CE, et al. Changes on magnetic resonance images after traumatic hip dislocation. *Clin Orthop Relat Res.* 1995;(319):249–259.

74. Price CT, Pyevich MT, Knapp DR, et al. Traumatic hip dislocation with spontaneous incomplete reduction: a diagnostic trap. *J Orthop Trauma.* 2002;16:730–735.

75. Ramachandran M, Ward K, Brown RR, et al. Intravenous bisphosphonate therapy for traumatic osteonecrosis of the femoral head in adolescents. *J Bone Joint Surg Am.* 2007;89(8):1727–1734.

76. Ratliff AH. Complications after fractures of the femoral neck in children and their treatment. *J Bone Joint Surg Br.* 1970;52:175.

77. Rieger H, Pennig D, Klein W, et al. Traumatic dislocation of the hip in young children. *Arch Orthop Trauma Surg.* 1991;110:114–117.

78. Riley PM Jr, Morscher MA, Gothard MD, et al. Earlier time to reduction did not reduce rates of femoral head osteonecrosis in pediatric hip fractures. *J Orthop Trauma.* 2015;29:231–238.

79. Rubel IF, Kloen P, Potter HG, et al. MRI assessment of the posterior acetabular wall fracture in traumatic dislocation of the hip in children. *Pediatr Radiol.* 2002;32:435–439.

80. Salisbury RD, Eastwood DM. Traumatic dislocation of the hip in children. *Clin Orthop Relat Res.* 2000;(377):106–111.

81. Sanders S, Egol KA. Adult periarticular locking plates for the treatment of pediatric and adolescent subtrochanteric hip fractures. *Bull NYU Hosp Jt Dis.* 2009;67(4):370–373.

82. Schmidt GL, Sciulli R, Altman GT. Knee injury in patients experiencing a high-energy traumatic ipsilateral hip dislocation. *J Bone Joint Surg Am.* 2005;87:1200–1204.

83. Schrader MW, Jacofsky DJ, Stans AA, et al. Femoral neck fractures in pediatric patients: 30 years experience at a level 1 trauma center. *Clin Orthop Relat Res.* 2007;454:169–173.

84. Scientific Research Committee of the Pennsylvania Orthopaedic Society. Traumatic dislocation of the hip in children: final report. *J Bone Joint Surg Am.* 1968;50:79–88.

85. Scully SP, Aaron RK, Urbaniak JR. Survival analysis of hips treated with core decompression or vascularized fibular grafting because of avascular necrosis. *J Bone Joint Surg Am.* 1998;80(9):1270–1275.

86. Sener M, Karapinar H, Kazimoglu C, et al. Fracture dislocation of sacroiliac joint associated with triradiate cartilage injury in a child: a case report. *J Pediatr Orthop B.* 2008;17(2):65–68.

87. Song KS, Choi IH, Sohn YJ, et al. Habitual dislocation of the hip in children: report of eight additional cases and literature review. *J Pediatr Orthop.* 2003;23:178–183.

88. Song KS, Kim YS, Sohn SW, et al. Arthrotomy and open reduction of the displaced fracture of the femoral neck in children. *J Pediatr Orthop B.* 2001;10:205–210.

89. Spence D, DiMauro JP, Miller PE, et al. Osteonecrosis after femoral neck fractures in children and adolescents: analysis of risk factors. *J Pediatr Orthop.* 2016;36:111–116.

90. Stimson LA. An easy method of reduction dislocation of the shoulder and hip. *Med Rec.* 1900;57:356.

91. St Pierre P, Staheli LT, Smith JB, et al. Femoral neck stress fractures in children and adolescents. *J Pediatr Orthop.* 1995;15:470–473.

92. Thacker MM, Feldman DS, Madan SS, et al. Hinged distraction of the adolescent arthritic hip. *J Pediatr Orthop.* 2005;25(2):178–182.

93. Togrul E, Bayram H, Gulsen M, et al. Fractures of the femoral neck in children: long-term follow-up in 62 hip fractures. *Injury.* 2005;36:123–130.

94. Trueta J, Morgan JD. The vascular contribution to osteogenesis. I. Studies by the injection method. *J Bone Joint Surg Br.* 1960;42:97–109.

95. Vialle R, Odent T, Pannier S, et al. Traumatic hip dislocation in childhood. *J Pediatr Orthop.* 2005;25(2):138–144.

96. Yoo JH, Hwang JH, Chang JD, et al. Management of traumatic labral tear in acetabular fractures with posterior wall component. *Orthop Traumatol Surg Res.* 2014;100:187–192.

24

Femoral Shaft Fractures

John M. Flynn and David L. Skaggs

INTRODUCTION TO FEMORAL SHAFT FRACTURES

Femur fractures are common.[53,110] When subtrochanteric and supracondylar fractures are included, the femoral shaft represents about 1.6% of all bony injuries in children. Fractures are more common in boys (2.6:1), and occur in an interesting bimodal distribution with a peak during the toddler years (usually from simple falls) and then again in early adolescence (usually from higher-energy injury).[68,75,101] A 21st century Swedish incidence study[69] also showed a seasonal bimodal variation, with the peak in March and in August.

Although pediatric femoral shaft fractures create substantial short-term disability, with attention to detail and modern techniques, these major injuries can generally be treated successfully with few long-term sequelae. Over the past 20 years, there has been a dramatic and sustained trend toward the operative stabilization of femoral shaft fractures in school-aged children using flexible intramedullary nails, external fixation, locked intramedullary nails, and more recently, submuscular plate fixation. These advances have decreased the substantial early disability for the children as well as the family's burden of care during the recovery period. A sustained and well-documented trend towards operative management of pediatric femur fractures, including much younger children than in the past, is well documented in recent studies, and does not necessarily follow national guideline suggestions.[138,145,161]

ASSESSMENT OF FEMORAL SHAFT FRACTURES

The diagnosis of pediatric femoral shaft fractures is usually not subtle: There is a clear mechanism of injury, a deformity and swelling of the thigh, and obvious localized pain. The diagnosis is more difficult in patients with multiple trauma or head injury and in nonambulatory, severely disabled children. A physical examination is usually sufficient to document the presence of a femur fracture. In patients lacking sensation (e.g., paraplegic or myelomeningocele), the swelling and redness caused by a fracture may mimic the clinical findings of an infection.

In the setting of a femur fracture, a comprehensive physical examination should be performed looking for other sites of injury. Hypotension rarely results from an isolated femoral fracture. Waddell's triad of femoral fracture, intra-abdominal or intrathoracic injury, and head injury are associated with high-velocity automobile injuries. Multiple trauma may necessitate rapid stabilization of femoral shaft fractures[109,152] to facilitate overall care. This is particularly true with head injury and vascular disruption.

The hemodynamic significance of femoral fracture has been studied by two groups.[30,112] Hematocrit levels below 30% rarely occur without multisystem injury. A declining hematocrit should not be attributed to closed femoral fracture until other sources of blood loss have been eliminated.[30,112]

MECHANISMS OF INJURY OF FEMORAL SHAFT FRACTURES

The etiology of femoral fractures in children varies with the age of the child. Before walking age, up to 80% of femoral fractures may be caused by abuse.[11,15,60,195] In a study of over 5,000 children at a trauma center, Coffey et al.[32] found that abuse was the cause of only 1% of lower extremity fractures in children older than 18 months, but 67% of lower extremity fractures in children younger than 18 months.

Baldwin et al.[8] found three primary risk factors for abuse in young children presenting with a femur fracture: a history suspicious for abuse, physical or radiographic evidence of prior injury, and age under 18 months. Children with no risk factors had only a 4% chance of being a victim of abuse, whereas children with all three risk factors had a 92% chance that their femur fractures with result of abuse.

Murphy et al. showed that[137] transverse fractures of the femoral shaft are a better predictor of nonaccidental trauma in young children than spiral fractures.

Older children are unlikely to have a femoral shaft fracture caused by abuse because their bone is sufficiently strong to tolerate forceful blows, or is able to resist torque without fracture. In older children, femoral fractures are most likely to be caused by high-energy injuries; motor vehicle accidents account for over 90% of femur fractures in this age group.[38,68,109] Pathologic femur fractures are relatively rare in children, but may occur because of generalized osteopenia in infants or young children with osteogenesis imperfecta. Osteogenesis imperfecta should be considered when a young child, with no history suggestive of abuse or significant trauma, presents with a femoral shaft fracture.[100] Radiologic evaluation is often insufficient to diagnose osteogenesis imperfecta; skin biopsy, collagen analysis, and bone biopsy may be required to make a definitive diagnosis. Generalized osteopenia also may accompany neurologic diseases, such as cerebral palsy or myelomeningocele, leading to fracture with minor trauma in osteopenic bone.[92,100] Pathologic fractures may occur in patients with neoplasms, most often benign lesions such as nonossifying fibroma, aneurysmal bone cyst, unicameral cyst, or eosinophilic granuloma. Although pathologic femur fractures are rare in children, it is essential that the orthopedist and radiologists study the initial injury films closely for the subtle signs of primary lesions predisposing to fracture, particularly in cases of low-energy injury from running or tripping. Radiographic signs of a pathologic fracture may include mixed lytic–blastic areas disrupting trabecular architecture, break in the cortex and periosteal reaction in malignant lesions such as osteosarcoma, or better-defined sclerotic borders with an intact cortex seen in benign lesions such as nonossifying fibroma (Fig. 24-1).

Stress fractures may occur in any location in the femoral shaft.[24,88,123] In this era of high-intensity, year-round youth

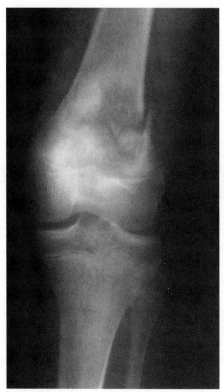
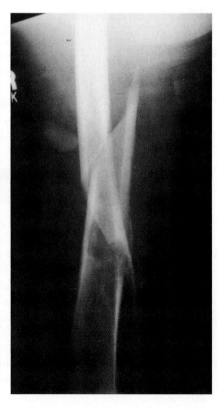

A   **B**

Figure 24-1. A: Femoral fracture through a poorly demarcated, mixed, osteoblastic, osteolytic lesion—an osteosarcoma. **B:** Sclerotic borders of this lesion in the distal femur are typical of a pathologic fracture through a nonossifying fibroma.

sports, orthopedists are more commonly encountering adolescents with femoral stress fractures from running, soccer, and basketball.[20] Although uncommon (4% of all stress fractures in children), femoral shaft or femoral neck stress fractures should be considered in a child with thigh pain because an unrecognized stress fracture may progress to a displaced femoral fracture. A high index of suspicion is important, because even nontraditional sports can lead to stress fractures with extreme overuse; a recent report of bilateral femoral stress fractures were reported in a Rollerblade enthusiast.[184]

IMAGING AND OTHER DIAGNOSTIC STUDIES FOR FEMORAL SHAFT FRACTURES

Radiographic evaluation should include the entire femur, including the hip and knee, because injury of the adjacent joints is common. An anteroposterior (AP) pelvis x-ray is a valuable supplement to standard femoral shaft views, because there may be associated intertrochanteric fractures of the hip, fractures of the femoral neck, or physeal injuries of the proximal femur.[13,25] Distal femoral fractures may be associated with physeal injury about the knee, knee ligament injury, meniscal tears,[187] and tibial fractures.[105]

Plain x-rays generally are sufficient for making the diagnosis. In rare circumstances, bone scanning and magnetic resonance imaging (MRI) may be helpful in the diagnosis of small buckle fractures in limping children or stress fractures in athletes. The orthopedist should carefully evaluate radiographs for comminution or nondisplaced "butterfly" fragments, second fractures, joint dislocations, and pathologic, as these findings can substantially alter the treatment plan.

CLASSIFICATION OF FEMORAL SHAFT FRACTURES

Femoral fractures are classified as: (a) transverse, spiral, or short oblique; (b) comminuted or noncomminuted; and (c) open or closed. Open fractures are classified according to Gustilo's system.[72] The presence or absence of vascular and neurologic injury is documented and is part of the description of the fracture. The most common femoral fracture in children (over 50%) is a simple transverse, closed, noncomminuted injury.

The level of the fracture (Fig. 24-2) leads to characteristic displacement of the fragments based on the attached muscles. With subtrochanteric fractures, the proximal fragment lies in abduction, flexion, and external rotation. The pull of the gastrocnemius on the distal fragment in a supracondylar fracture produces an extension deformity (posterior angulation of the femoral shaft), which may make the femur difficult to align.

PATHOANATOMY AND APPLIED ANATOMY RELATED TO FEMORAL SHAFT FRACTURES

Through remodeling during childhood, a child's bone changes from primarily weak woven bone to stronger lamellar bone.[167] Strength also is increased by a change in geometry (Fig. 24-3). The increasing diameter and area of bone result in a markedly increased area moment of inertia, leading to an increase

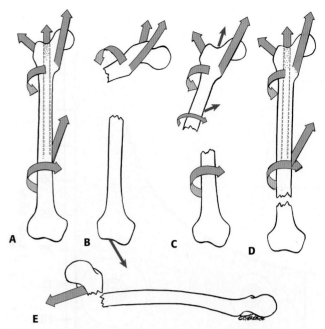

Figure 24-2. The relationship of fracture level and position of the proximal fragment. **A:** In the resting unfractured state, the position of the femur is relatively neutral because of balanced muscle pull. **B:** In proximal shaft fractures the proximal fragment assumes a position of flexion (iliopsoas), abduction (abductor muscle group), and lateral rotation (short external rotators). **C:** In midshaft fractures the effect is less extreme because there is compensation by the adductors and extensor attachments on the proximal fragment. **D:** Distal shaft fractures produce little alteration in the proximal fragment position because most muscles are attached to the same fragment, providing balance. **E:** Supracondylar fractures often assume a position of hyperextension of the distal fragment because of the pull of the gastrocnemius.

in strength. This progressive increase in bone strength helps explain the bimodal distribution of femoral fractures. In early childhood, the femur is relatively weak and breaks under load conditions reached in normal play. In adolescence, high-velocity trauma is required to reach the stresses necessary for fracture.

TREATMENT OPTIONS FOR FEMORAL SHAFT FRACTURES

Treatment of femoral shaft fractures in children depends on two primary considerations: age (Table 24-1) and fracture pattern. Secondary considerations, especially in operative cases, include the child's weight, associated injuries, mechanism of injury, availability of equipment, and the experience of the surgeon. Economic concerns,[35,52,140,143,179] the family's ability to care for a child in a spica cast or external fixator, and the advantages and disadvantages of any operative procedure also are important factors. A comprehensive decision-making model incorporating all of these factors has been designed, and will be discussed in more detail in the authors' preferred method section.[49] Kocher et al.[98] summarized the current evidence for pediatric femur fracture treatment in a clinical practice guideline summary.

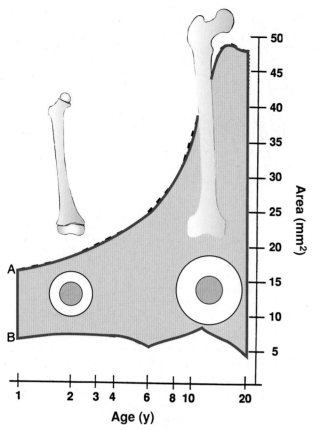

Figure 24-3. The *shaded area* represents cortical thickness by age-group. This rapid increase in cortical thickness may contribute to the diminishing incidence of femoral fractures during late childhood. (Redrawn from Netter FH. *The Ciba collection of medical illustrations. Musculoskeletal System. I. Anatomy, Physiology, and Metabolic Disorders.* Vol. 8. Summit, NJ: Ciba-Geigy; 1987.)

TABLE 24-1. Treatment Options for Isolated Femoral Shaft Fractures in Children and Adolescents

Age	Treatments
Birth to 24 mo	Pavlik harness (newborn to 6 mo) Early spica cast Traction → spica cast (very rare)
24 mo–5 yrs	Early spica cast Traction → spica cast External fixation (rare) Flexible intramedullary nails (rare)
6–11 yrs	Flexible intramedullary nails Traction → spica cast Submuscular plate External fixation
12 yrs to maturity	Trochanteric entry intramedullary rod Flexible intramedullary nails Submuscular plate External fixation (rare)

Treatment choices are influenced by fracture pattern, the child's weight, the presence of other injuries (head, chest, abdominal, etc.) and associated soft tissue trauma.

TREATMENT VARIATION WITH AGE

Infants

Femoral shaft fractures in infants are usually stable because their periosteum is thick. In fractures occurring in infancy, management should include evaluation for underlying metabolic bone abnormality or abuse. Once these have been ruled out, most infants with a proximal or midshaft femoral fracture are comfortably and successfully treated with simple splinting to provide some stability and comfort, with a Pavlik harness to improve the resting position of the fracture. For the rare unstable fracture, the Pavlik harness may not offer sufficient stabilization. Morris et al.[134] reported a group of eight birth-related femoral fractures in 55,296 live births. Twin pregnancies, breech presentation, and prematurity were associated with birth-related femur fractures. The typical fracture is a spiral fracture of the proximal femur with flexion of the proximal fragment. With thick periosteum, and remarkable remodeling potential, newborns rarely need a manipulative reduction of their fracture, nor rigid external immobilization. For femoral fractures with more shortening (1 to 2 cm) or angulation (>30 degrees), reduction and spica casting may be used. Traction rarely is necessary in this age group.

Preschool Children

In children 6 months to 5 years of age, early spica casting (Fig. 24-4) is the treatment of choice for isolated femur fractures with less than 2 cm of initial shortening (Fig. 24-5). In low-energy fractures, the "walking spica" is ideal (Fig. 24-6). Femur fractures with more than 2 cm of initial shortening or marked instability and fractures that cannot be reduced with early spica casting require 3 to 10 days of skin or skeletal traction. Internal or external fixation is rarely needed in children less than 5 years of age. Although internal fixation of femoral shaft fractures in toddlers can produce a very pleasing radiographic appearance, reduction, casting, and remodeling produces such consistently excellent results that operative methods cannot compete on safety and value, except in the rare, most displaced high-energy injuries. In rare circumstances, external fixation can be used for children with open fractures or multiple traumas. Intramedullary fixation is used in children with metabolic bone disease that predisposes to fracture or after multiple fractures, such as in osteogenesis imperfecta, or following multitrauma. Flexible nailing can be used in the normal-sized preschool child[17] but is rarely necessary. Larger children (in whom reduction cannot be maintained with a spica cast) occasionally may benefit from flexible intramedullary nailing, traction, or in rare cases, submuscular plating.

Children 5 to 11 Years of Age

In children 5 to 11 years of age, many different methods can be used successfully, depending on the fracture type, patient characteristics, and surgeon skill and experience.[53] In rare circumstances, a nondisplaced fracture might be treated in a walking spica cast in children less than 10 years old. Although traction and casting is still a successful method of managing femur fractures in young school-age children, the cost and the social problems related to school-age children in casts have resulted

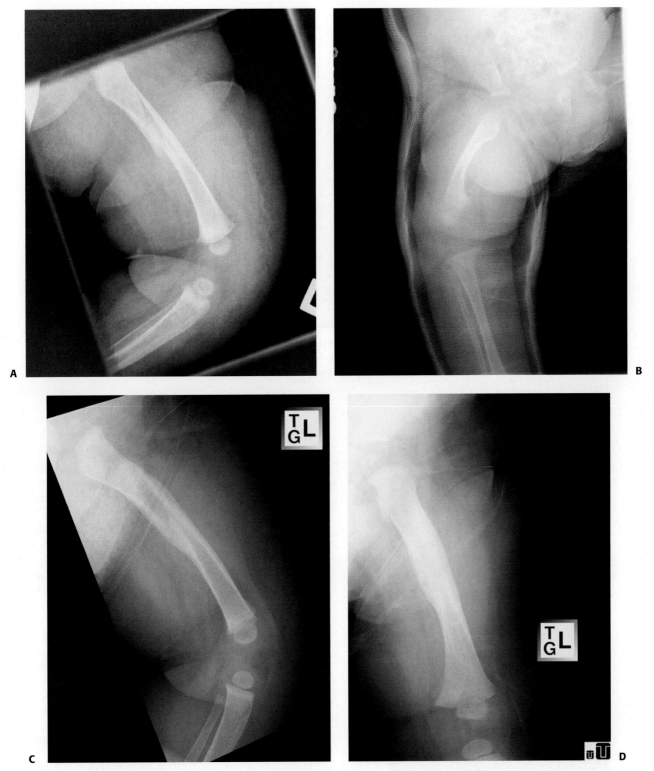

Figure 24-4. A: This 7-month-old sustained a low-energy spiral femoral shaft fracture. **B:** Treatment was in a spica cast. **C, D:** Excellent healing with abundant callus at only 4 weeks after injury.

in a strong trend towards internal fixation. Spica cast management is generally not used for children with multiple trauma, head injury, vascular compromise, floating knee injuries, significant skin problems, or multiple fractures. Flexible intramedullary nails are the predominant treatment for femur fractures in

5- to 11-year olds, although submuscular plating and external fixation[99] have their place, especially in length-unstable fractures, or in those difficult to manage fractures in the proximal and distal third of the femoral shaft (see Authors' Preferred Treatment section).

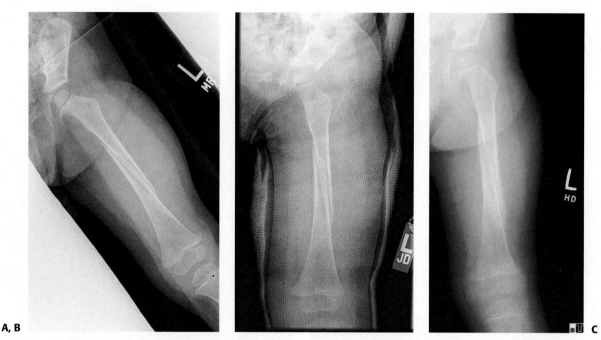

A, B   **C**

Figure 24-5. A: This 2-year-old sustained a low-energy spiral femoral shaft fracture, ideal for walking spica treatment. **B:** Immediately after reduction, note the lateral mold at the fracture site. **C:** Six weeks after injury, there is anatomic alignment, minimal shortening, and good callus formation.

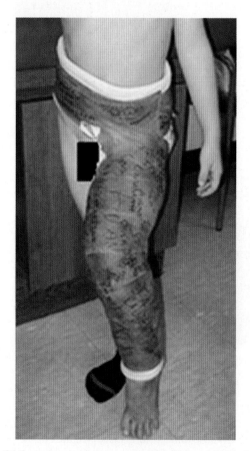

Figure 24-6. A 4-year-old with a minimally displaced midshaft femur fracture treated with a walking spica cast, shown here 4 weeks after injury.

Age 11 to Skeletal Maturity

Trochanteric entry, locked intramedullary nailing is the primary mode of treatment for femur fractures in the preadolescent and adolescent age groups.[36] Several studies designed to refine the indications for flexible intramedullary nailing have concluded that although most results are excellent or satisfactory in children older than 11, complications rise significantly when this popular technique is used for bigger and older children.[137] In an international multicenter, retrospective study, Moroz et al.[133] found a statistically significant relationship between age and outcome, with children older than 11 years or heavier than 49 kg faring worse. Sink et al.[172] found a much higher rate of complications in length-unstable fractures. Fortunately, surgeons can now select from several different trochanteric entry nails that allow a relatively safe, lateral entry point, with the stability of proximal and distal locking. With this new information and technology, locked intramedullary nailing is used commonly for obese children of ages 10 to 12, and most femoral shaft fractures in children of age 13 to skeletal maturity.

TREATMENT VARIATION WITH FRACTURE PATTERN

In addition to age, the treating surgeon should consider fracture pattern, especially when choosing implant. Elastic nailing is ideal for the vast majority of length-stable midshaft femur fractures in children between the ages of 5 and 11 years old. For length-unstable fractures, the risk of shortening and malunion increases substantially when elastic nailing is used.[171] Length-unstable fractures are best treated with locked trochanteric entry nailing in older children, external fixation in younger children, or submuscular plating in either of these age cohorts.

NONOPERATIVE TREATMENT OF FEMORAL SHAFT FRACTURES

Indications/Contraindications for Nonoperative Treatment		
Age	Indications for Nonoperative Treatment	Contraindications for Nonoperative Treatment
Birth to 4 yrs/o	The vast majority of fractures in this age group	The extremely rare, high energy, displaced fracture, esp. in the setting of multitrauma
5 yrs–10 yrs/o	Nondisplaced fractures	Displaced fractures (almost all fractures treated with fixation)
11 yrs/o to maturity	The very rare, nondisplaced fracture in family preferring nonop care. Insufficiency fracture in nonambulatory children	Displaced fractures (almost all fractures treated with fixation)

Pavlik Harness

Stannard et al.[178] popularized the use of the Pavlik harness for femur fractures in infants. This treatment is ideal for a proximal or midshaft femoral fracture that occurs as a birth-related injury. Pain can be reduced by loosely wrapping cotton cast padding around the thigh. In a newborn infant in whom a femur fracture is noted in the intensive care unit or nursery, the femur is immobilized with simple padding or a soft splint. For a stable fracture, this approach may be sufficient and will allow intravenous access to the feet if needed. The Pavlik harness can be applied with the hip in moderate flexion and abduction. This often helps align the distal fragment with the proximal fragment (Fig. 24-7). Evaluation of angulation in the coronal plane (varus–valgus) is difficult because of hyperflexion. Stannard et al.[178] reported acceptable alignment in all patients with less than 1 cm of shortening. Morris et al.[134] showed that all treatments, including traction, spica cast, and Pavlik harness, are effective and resulted in satisfactory outcome in all patients regardless of treatment.

Podeszwa et al.[150] reported infants treated with a Pavlik had higher pain scores when compared to an immediate spica cast; however, none of the Pavlik patients had skin problems but one-third of the spica patients did. Average overgrowth after Pavlik harness usage was 5 mm (1 to 18 mm) in a recent study.[113]

Spica Casting

Spica casting[85,177] is usually the best treatment option for isolated femoral shaft fractures in children under 5 years of age, unless there is (a) shortening of more than 2 cm, (b) massive swelling of the thigh, or (c) an associated injury that precludes

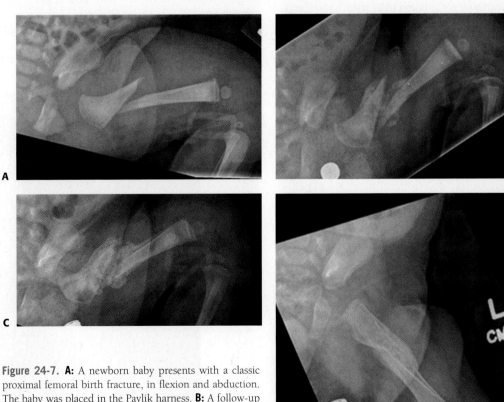

Figure 24-7. A: A newborn baby presents with a classic proximal femoral birth fracture, in flexion and abduction. The baby was placed in the Pavlik harness. **B:** A follow-up check 2 weeks after injury shows excellent alignment and early callous. **C:** A follow-up at 4 weeks shows a healed fracture. The Pavlik harness was removed. **D:** Follow-up 7 weeks after injury shows the dramatic early remodeling that is typical of these fractures.

cast treatment. Several centers have adopted spica application in the emergency department as their standard treatment for infants and toddlers. Mansour et al.[116] compared spica cast placement in the emergency department versus the operating room, and concluded that the outcome and complications were similar, but the children treated in the operating room had longer hospital stays and significantly higher hospital charges. Cassinelli et al.[28] treated 145 femur fractures, all in children younger than age 7, with immediate spica cast application in the emergency department. All children younger than 2 years of age, and 86.5% of children of ages 2 to 5 years old, met acceptable alignment parameters on final radiographs. Re-reduction in the operating room was needed in 11 patients. The investigators concluded that initial shortening was the only independent risk factor associated with lost reduction.

The advantages of a spica cast include low cost, excellent safety profile, and a very high rate of good results, with acceptable leg length equality, healing time, and motion.[47,84] Hughes et al.[79] evaluated 23 children ranging in age from 2 to 10 years who had femur fractures treated with early spica casting to determine the impact of treatment on the patients and their families. The greatest problems encountered by the family in caring for a child in a spica cast were transportation, cast intolerance by the child, and hygiene. In a similar study, Kocher[97] used a validated questionnaire for assessing the impact of medical conditions on families demonstrated that for family, having a child in a spica cast is similar to having a child on renal dialysis. They found that the impact was greatest for children older than 5 years, and when both parents are working. Such data should inform the decisions of orthopedic surgeons and families who are trying to choose among the many options for young school-age children.

Illgen et al.[83] in a series of 114 isolated femoral fractures in children under 6 years of age, found that 90-degree/90-degree spica casting was successful in 86% without cast change or wedging, based on tolerance of shortening less than 1.5 cm and angulation less than 10 degrees. Similar excellent results have been reported by Czertak and Hennrikus[37] using the 90/90 spica cast.

Thompson et al.[181] described the telescope test in which patients were examined with fluoroscopy at the time of reduction and casting. If more than 3 cm of shortening could be demonstrated with gentle axial compression, traction was used rather than immediate spica casting. By using the telescope test, these researchers decreased unacceptable results (>2.5 cm of shortening) from 18% to 5%. Shortening is acceptable, but should not exceed 2 cm. This is best measured on a lateral x-ray taken through the cast. If follow-up x-rays reveal significant varus (>10 degrees) or anterior angulation (>30 degrees), the cast may be wedged. However, Weiss et al.[193] noted that wedging of 90/90 spica casts can cause peroneal nerve palsy, especially during correction of valgus angulation (a problem that rarely occurs). For unacceptable position, the fracture can be manipulated and a new cast applied, or the cast can be removed and the patient placed in traction to regain or maintain length. Angular deformity of up to 15 degrees in the coronal plane and up to 30 degrees in the sagittal plane may be acceptable, depending on the patient's age (Table 24-2). Finally, if shortening exceeds 2 cm, traction or an external fixator can be used (Fig. 24-8).

TABLE 24-2. Acceptable Angulation

Age	Varus/Valgus (degrees)	Anterior/Posterior (degrees)	Shortening (mm)
Birth to 2 yrs	30	30	15
2–5 yrs	15	20	20
6–10 yrs	10	15	15
11 yrs to maturity	5	10	10

The position of the hips and knees in the spica cast is controversial. Some centers prefer a spica cast with the hip and knee flexed 90 degrees each. Studies have shown that the results from the sitting spica cast are good.[120,128] The child is placed in a sitting position with the legs abducted about 30 degrees on either side. The synthetic material used for the cast gives it sufficient strength so that no bar is required between the legs. This not only allows the child to be carried on the parent's hip but also aids in toiletry needs, making bedpans unnecessary. Also, a child who can sit upright during the day can attend school in a wheelchair. More recently, with reports about compartment syndrome of the leg after using the 90/90 spica cast, several centers now cast with the hip and knee are more extended (about 45 degrees each) and the bottom of the foot cut out to prevent excessive shortening. Varying the amounts of hip and knee flexion in the spica cast based on the position of the fracture also has been recommended: The more proximal the fracture, the more the hip should be flexed.[177]

Recently, there has been a resurgence of interest in the "walking spica cast" (see Fig. 24-6). Practitioners of the single leg,

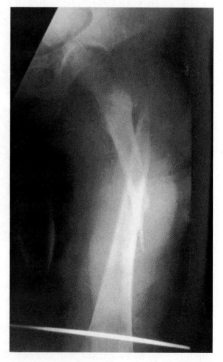

Figure 24-8. A proximal spiral femur fracture, which failed treatment with pins and plaster, and was salvaged with an external fixator.

or walking spica, apply the technique primarily for toddlers with very stable, low-energy fractures. The cast must be extensively reinforced at the hip. With the hip and knee much more extended, the single leg spica not only improves function and ease of care, but also avoids a technique that has been associated with compartment syndrome in several children (see below).[102,136] Increasingly, the walking spica is considered the best treatment for low-energy femur fractures in toddlers.[50,106]

Technique

The cast is applied in the operating room or, in some centers, the sedation unit or emergency department.[116] For the sitting spica cast technique, a long leg cast is placed with the knee and ankle flexed at 90 degrees (Fig. 24-9B). Knee flexion greater than 60 degrees improved maintenance of length and reduction.[83] However, if one applies excessive traction to maintain length (Fig. 24-10), the risk of compartment syndrome is unacceptably high. Less traction, less knee flexion, and accepting slightly more shortening is a reasonable compromise. Extra padding, or a felt pad, is placed in the area of the popliteal fossa. The knee should not be flexed after the padding is placed because the lump of material in the popliteal fossa may create vascular obstruction (Fig. 24-9A). Because most diaphyseal fractures lose reduction into varus angulation while in a spica cast, a valgus mold at the fracture site is strongly recommended

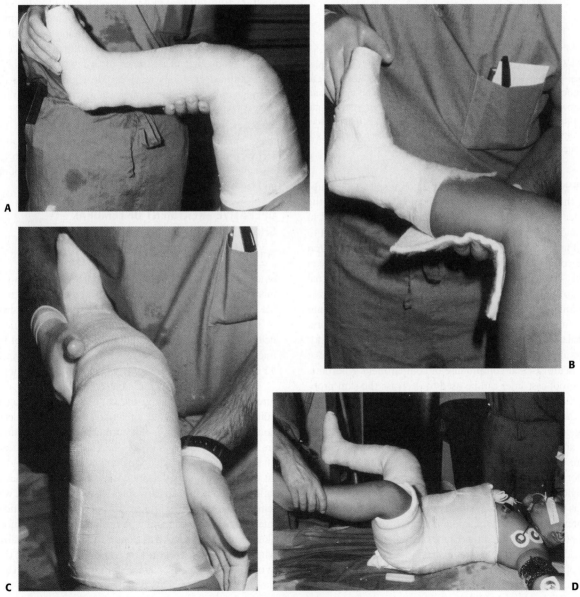

Figure 24-9. Application of a 90-degree/90-degree spica cast. **A:** Generous padding is applied over the foot, and a pad is placed on the popliteal fossa to prevent injury to the peroneal nerve and popliteal vessels. **B:** A long leg cast is applied with the knee flexed 90 degrees. **C:** A mold is placed over the apex of the fracture, generally correcting a varus deformity into slight valgus. **D:** Using a standard spica table, a 1½ spica cast is applied with the hip flexed 90 degrees and abducted 30 degrees.

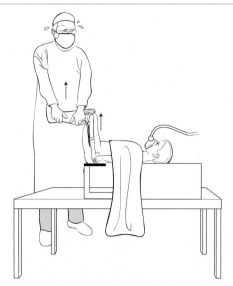

Figure 24-10. The dangers of pulling upward on the calf when applying a spica: This upward pull, which is used to reduce the fracture, can be dangerous, because it puts pressure on the gastrocnemius muscle and the other posterior leg structures, such as the femoral artery and femoral vein. (Reprinted with permission from Skaggs D, Flynn J. *Trauma about the pelvis/hip/femur. Staying Out of Trouble in Pediatric Orthopaedics.* 1st ed. Philadelphia, PA: Lippincott Williams & Wilkins; 2006:105.)

(Fig. 24-9C). The patient is then placed on a spica table, supporting the weight of the legs with manual traction, and the remainder of the cast is applied with the hips in 90 degrees of flexion and 30 degrees of abduction, holding the fracture out to length (Fig. 24-9D). It is mandatory to avoid excessive traction because compartment syndromes and skin sloughs have been reported. The leg should be placed in 15 degrees of external rotation to align the distal fragment with the external rotation of the proximal fragment. After the spica cast is in place, AP and lateral x-rays are obtained to ensure that length and angular and rotational alignment are maintained. We observe all patients for 24 hours after spica application to be sure that the child is not at risk for neurovascular compromise or compartment syndrome. A waterproof cast liner can be used to decrease the skin problems of diaper rash and superficial infection.

For the single leg spica or "walking spica" technique, the long leg cast is applied with approximately 45 degrees of knee flexion, and when the remaining cast is placed, the hip is flexed 45 degrees and externally rotated 15 degrees. The hip should be reinforced anteriorly with multiple layers of extra fiberglass. The pelvic band should be fairly wide so that the hip is controlled as well as possible. A substantial valgus mold is important to prevent varus malangulation. It is better to err on the side of mild posterior angulation, because the pull of the psoas generally leads to some procurvatum over time. We leave the foot out, stopping the distal end of the cast in the supramalleolar area, which is protected with plenty of extra padding. Seven to 10 days after injury, the child returns to clinic anticipating the need for cast wedging, if radiographs show the very common mild increase in shortening and varus angulation. Most toddlers pull to a stand and begin walking in their walking cast about 2 to 3 weeks after injury.

If excessive angulation occurs, the cast should be changed, with manipulation in the operating room. Casts can be wedged for less than 15 degrees of angulation. If shortening of more than 2 cm is documented, the child should be treated with cast change, traction, or conversion to external fixation, using lengthening techniques if the shortening is not detected until the fracture callus has developed. When conversion to external fixation is required, we recommend osteoclasis (either closed or open if needed) at the time of the application of the external fixator, with slow lengthening over a period of several weeks (1 mm per day) to reestablish acceptable length (see Fig. 24-8).

Generally, the spica cast is worn for 4 to 8 weeks, depending on the age of the child and the severity of the soft tissue damage accompanying the fracture. Typically, an infant's femoral shaft fracture will heal in 3 to 4 weeks; and a toddler's fracture will heal in 6 weeks. After the cast is been removed, parents are encouraged to allow their children to stand and walk whenever the child is comfortable; most children will need to be carried or pushed in a stroller for a few days until hip and knee stiffness gradually resolves. Most joint stiffness resolves spontaneously in children after a few weeks. It is unusual to need physical therapy. In fact, aggressive joint range-of-motion exercises with the therapist immediately after cast removal make children anxious, and may prolong rather than hasten recovery. A few follow-up visits are recommended in the first year after femur fracture, analyzing gait, joint range of motion, and leg lengths.

OPERATIVE TREATMENT OF FEMORAL SHAFT FRACTURES

Traction and Spica Casting

Since as early as the 18th century, traction has been used for management of femur fractures. Vertical overhead traction with the hip flexed 90 degrees and the knee straight was introduced by Bryant in 1873,[21,33] but this often resulted in vascular insufficiency,[141] and it is now rarely used for treatment of femoral fractures. Modified Bryant traction, in which the knee is flexed 45 degrees, increases the safety of overhead skin traction.[48]

Traction prior to spica casting is indicated when the fracture is length unstable and the family and surgeon agree that nonoperative measures are preferred. In general, skeletal traction then spica casting is not currently used for children who are older than 12 years of age, because of the significant risk of shortening and angular malunion; in children older than 12 years of age, internal fixation is recommended. Children who rapidly shortened in an early spica cast can be salvaged with cast removal and subsequent traction. The limit of skin traction is the interface between skin and tape or skin and foam traction boot. Skin complications, such as slough and blistering, usually occur when more than 5 lb of traction is applied. When more than 5 lb of traction is required, or simply for ease in patient management, skeletal traction can be used to maintain alignment.[5]

The distal femur is the location of choice for a traction pin.[5,164] Although proximal tibial traction pins have been recommended by some clinicians,[81] growth arrest in the proximal tibial physis and subsequent recurvatum deformity have been associated with their use (Fig. 24-11). Also, knee ligament and meniscal

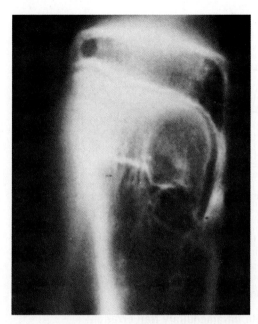

Figure 24-11. This tomogram shows a bony bridge caused by a tibial traction pin that was placed for femoral fracture.

injuries that sometimes accompany femoral fractures may be aggravated by the chronic pull of traction across the knee.

Technique

> ✔ **Traction and Spica Casting:**
> KEY SURGICAL STEPS

❏ A large Steinmann pin is placed in the distal femur, avoiding the distal femoral physis. The insertion should be on the medial side, to have full control adjacent to the femoral artery in Hunter's canal. Fluoroscopic controls recommended, to ensure optimal pin position. The pin should be placed parallel to the joint surface.

❏ Traction is applied, initially using 5 pounds, and increasing is necessary.

❏ Traction is applied in a 90/90 position. An x-ray should be taken once or twice per week to monitor alignment.

❏ When early callus is seen on x-ray (usually about three weeks), the child is returned to the operating room, the traction pin is removed, the pin site is dressed, and a spica cast is applied as described above.

In a child under 10 years of age, the ideal fracture position in traction should be less than 1 cm of shortening and slight valgus alignment to counteract the tendency to angulate into varus in the cast and the eventual overgrowth that may occur (average 0.9 cm). If this method is used for adolescents (11 years or older), normal length should be maintained.

Spica Casting With Traction Pin Incorporated

In rare circumstances, a child's femur fractures best treated by spica casting, incorporating a traction pin in the cast to maintain fracture length. This technique may be particularly useful in an environment where there are limited resources.

Complications

Traction and Spica Casting of Femoral Shaft Fractures: PITFALLS AND PREVENTIONS	
Pitfall	**Prevention**
• Compartment syndrome	• There is risk in placing an initial below knee cast, then using that cast to apply traction while immobilizing the child in the 90/90 position. Avoid traction on a short leg cast, leave the foot out, and use less hip and knee flexion.
• Malalignment and shortening	• Radiographs once or twice a week, with adjustments made based on alignment and fracture short

Outcomes

Epps et al.[44] reported on immediate single leg spica cast for pediatric femoral diaphyseal fracture. In a series of 45 children, 90% of the children pulled to stand and 62% of the children walked independently by the end of treatment. Fifty percent of patients were able to return to school or day care while in the cast. Only two children had unacceptable shortening, and two required repeat reduction. Flynn et al.[50] performed a prospective study of low-energy femoral shaft fractures in young children, comparing a walking spica cast to a traditional spica cast. Although the outcome with the two treatment method was similar, the walking spica cast resulted in substantially lower burden of care for the family. Children with a walking spica are more likely to have their cast wedged in clinic to correct early loss of reduction.

In a study by Gross et al.,[59] 72 children with femoral fractures were treated with early cast brace/traction management. In this technique, a traction pin is placed in the distal femur and then incorporated in a cast brace. The traction pin is left long enough to be used for maintaining traction while the patient is in the cast brace or traction is applied directly to the cast. The patient is allowed to ambulate in the cast brace starting 3 days after application. Radiographs are taken of the fracture in the cast brace to document that excessive shortening is not occurring. The patient then is returned to traction in the cast brace until satisfactory callus is present to prevent shortening or angular deformity with weight bearing. The technique was not effective in older adolescents with midshaft fractures but achieved excellent results in children 5 to 12 years of age. The average hospital stay was 17 days.

Comparative studies and retrospective reviews have demonstrated unsatisfactory results in a small, yet significant, percentage of patients treated with skeletal traction.[81,96,157] Recently, increased attention has been focused on the risk of compartment syndrome in children treated in 90/90 spica cast.[136] Mubarak et al.[136] presented a multicenter series of nine children with an average age of 3.5 years who developed compartment syndrome of the leg after treatment of a low-energy femur fracture in a 90/90 spica cast. These children had extensive muscle

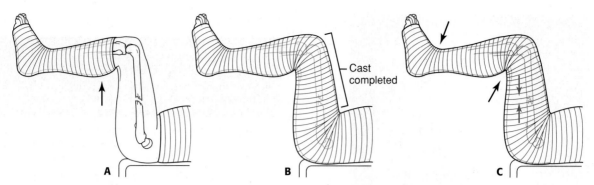

Figure 24-12. This drawing shows the pathogenesis of leg compartment syndrome caused by improper application of a spica cast. **A:** In the original description, a short leg cast was applied first, and used to pull the fracture out to length, as shown in this drawing. **B:** As the cast was completed, traction held on the short leg cast portion put pressure in the popliteal fossa. **C:** After the child awakens from general anesthesia, there is shortening of the femur from muscular contraction which causes the thigh and leg to slip somewhat back into the spica. This causes pressure to occur at the corners of the cast. (Reprinted with permission from Mubarak SJ, Frick S, Sink E, et al. Volkmann contracture and compartment syndromes after femur fractures in children treated with 90/90 spica casts. *J Pediatr Orthop.* 2006;26(5):570–572.)

damage and the skin loss around the ankle (Fig. 24-12). The authors emphasize the risk in placing an initial below knee cast, then using that cast to apply traction while immobilizing the child in the 90/90 position. The authors recommend avoiding traction on a short leg cast, leaving the foot out, and using less hip and knee flexion (Fig. 24-13).

Flexible Intramedullary Nail Fixation

In most centers, flexible intramedullary nailing is the standard treatment for midshaft femur fractures in children between the ages of 5 and 11 years old. The flexible intramedullary nailing technique can be performed with either stainless steel nails[156,168,169,191] or titanium elastic nails.

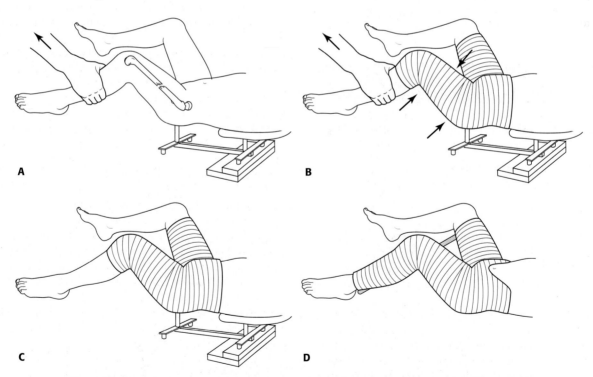

Figure 24-13. Authors recommended technique of spica cast application. **A:** The patient is placed on a child's fracture table. The leg is held in about 45-degree angle of flexion at the hip and knee with traction applied to the proximal calf. **B:** The 1½ spica is then applied down to the proximal calf. Molding of the thigh is accomplished during this phase. **C:** The x-rays of the femur are obtained and any wedging of the cast that is necessary can occur at this point in time. **D:** The leg portion of the cast and the cross bar are applied. The belly portion of the spica is trimmed to the umbilicus. (Reprinted with permission from Mubarak SJ, Frick S, Sink E, et al. Volkmann contracture and compartment syndromes after femur fractures in children treated with 90/90 spica casts. *J Pediatr Orthop.* 2006;26(5):570–572.)

The popularity of flexible intramedullary nailing results from its safety, efficacy, and ease of implant removal. The flexible nailing technique offers satisfactory fixation, enough stress at the fracture site to allow abundant callous formation, and relatively easy insertion and removal. The implants are inexpensive and the technique has a short learning curve. The primary limitation of flexible nailing is the lack of rigid fixation. Length-unstable fractures can shorten and angulate, especially in older and heavier children. Compared to children with rigid fixation, children who have their femur fracture treated with flexible nailing clearly have more pain and muscle spasm in the early postoperative period. The surgeon should take this into consideration in planning the early rehabilitation.

As the flexible nailing technique has become more popular, there have been many studies to refine the technique and indications,[169] and to elucidate the inherent limitations of fixation with flexible implants.[168] Mechanical testing of femoral fracture fixation systems showed that the greatest rigidity is provided by an external fixation device and the least by flexible intramedullary rodding.[104] Stainless steel rods are stiffer than titanium in bending tests. Recognizing this flexibility, the French pioneers[103,108] of elastic nailing stressed the critical importance of proper implant technique, including prebending the nails so that the apex of the bend was at the fracture site, and so that the two implants balance one another to prevent bending and control rotation. Frick et al.[54] found there to be greater stiffness and resistance to torsional deformation when retrograde nails are contoured into a double C pattern than with the antegrade C and S configuration. Sagan et al.[165] noted that apex anterior malunion is less likely if at least one nail has its shoe tip point anteriorly, such that the nail is in procurvatum.

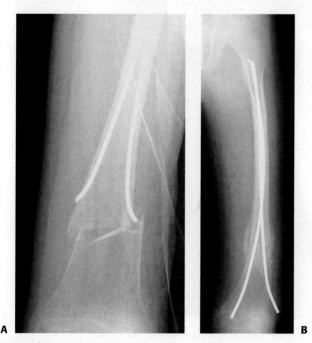

Figure 24-14. A: A few years after titanium lasting nailing, the nails have migrated proximally with growth, creating a stress riser and the subsequent insufficiency fracture. **B:** The refracture was treated with removal of the old nails and replacement with longer implants.

The prevailing technique for flexible nail insertion at most centers throughout the world has been retrograde, with small medial and lateral incisions just above the distal femoral physis. However, some prefer an antegrade technique, with entry in the subtrochanteric area. The primary advantages of a proximal insertion site are a fewer knee symptoms postoperatively

Flexible nails are removed after fracture union at most centers. However, some surgeons choose to leave the implants permanently. There is a theoretical concern that if flexible nails are left in young children, they will come to lie in the distal diaphysis as the child grows older. This may create a stress riser in the distal diaphysis, leading to a theoretical risk of fracture (Fig. 24-14).

Preoperative Planning

✔ **Flexible Intramedullary Nail Fixation:** PREOPERATIVE PLANNING CHECKLIST	
OR table	❏ Most surgeons prefer a fracture table, with the injured leg in traction bringing the fracture out to length, and the well leg positioned in maximum abduction, avoiding the lithotomy position in the risk of well leg compartment. Alternatively, the nails can be inserted prone on a radiolucent table, although this method makes it very difficult to both get the fracture out to length and pass the nails across the fracture site without a significant amount of surgical assistance
Fluoroscopy location	❏ Opposite the surgeon
Equipment	❏ Elastic nails, Bender, F-tool (for manipulative reduction)
Tourniquet	❏ None
[Other]	

The ideal patient for flexible intramedullary nailing is the child between the ages of 5 and 11 years old with a length-stable femur fracture, in the mid-80% of the diaphysis (Fig. 24-15), who has a body weight less than 50 kg.[133] Unstable fracture patterns can also be treated with flexible nailing, but the risk of shortening and angular malunion is greater,[172] and supplemental immobilization during early healing phase may be valuable.

Initial radiographs should be studied carefully for fracture lines that propagate proximally and distally, and might be otherwise unnoticed (Fig. 24-16). Although it is technically difficult to obtain satisfactory fixation with a retrograde technique when the fracture is near the distal metaphysis, a recent biomechanical study[124] demonstrated that retrograde insertion provides better stability than antegrade insertion for distal femoral shaft fractures. Nail size is determined by measuring the minimum diameter of the diaphysis, then multiplying by 0.4 to get nail diameter. For instance, if the minimum diameter of the diaphyseal canal is 1 cm, the 4-mm nails are used. Always choose the largest possible nail size that permits two nails to fit medullary canal.

Flexible nailing is most effectively performed on a fracture table, with a fracture reduced to near-anatomic position before

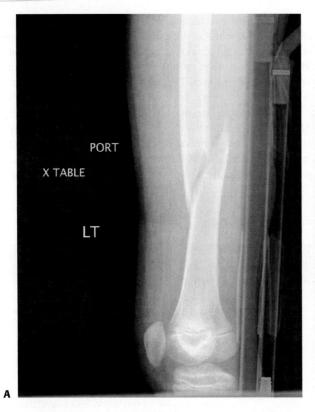
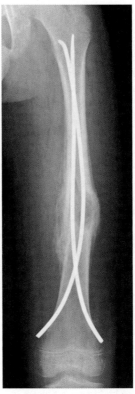

Figure 24-15. Titanium elastic nailing of the midshaft femur fracture through a benign lytic defect. **A:** Portable radiograph of a short oblique femur fracture through a benign lytic defect. **B:** AP radiograph taken several weeks after surgery that show the fracture well aligned with titanium elastic nail internal fixation and early callus at the fracture site.

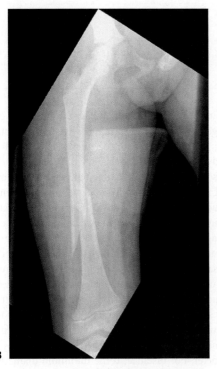
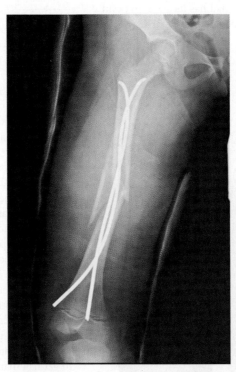
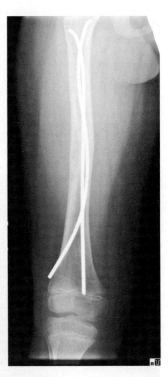

Figure 24-16. A: This high-energy, midshaft femur fracture was treated with titanium nails. **B:** A large butterfly fragment was dislodged during nail insertion. Because the fracture is now length-unstable, the surgeon wisely chose to protect the child for a few weeks in a one-leg spica cast. **C:** The fracture healed and excellent alignment. Note how the nails have wound around each other. This can make nail removal more difficult.

incisions are made. Alternatively, a fluoroscopic table can be used, but the surgeon should assure that a reduction can be obtained prior to the start of the procedure, and extra assistance may be necessary.

Technique

 Flexible Intramedullary Nail Fixation of Femoral Shaft Fractures:
KEY SURGICAL STEPS

❑ Most pediatric femur fractures are fixed with 4-mm diameter nails; in smaller children, 3.5-mm nails may be necessary. Two nails of similar size should be used, and they should be as large as possible.

❑ After the child is placed on the fracture table and the fracture reduced as much as possible, the leg is prepared and draped with the thigh (hip to knee) exposed. The image intensifier is used to localize the placement of skin incisions by viewing the distal femur in the AP and lateral planes.

Incisions are made on the medial and lateral side distal to the insertion site in the bone. The proximal end of the 2- to 3-cm incision should be at or just distal to the level of the insertion site, which is about 2.5 to 3 cm proximal to the distal femoral physis (Fig. 24-17). A 4.5-mm drill bit or awl is used to make a hole in the cortex of the bone. The distal femoral metaphysis is opened 2.5 cm proximal to the distal femoral physis using a drill or awl. The drill is then steeply angled in the frontal plane to facilitate passage of the nail through the dense pediatric metaphyseal bone.

❑ The distance from the top of the inserted rod to the level of the fracture site is measured, and a gentle 30-degree bend is placed in the nail

❑ A second bend is sometimes helpful near the entering tip of the nail to facilitate clearance of the opposite cortex during initial insertion

❑ Upon insertion the rod glances off the cortex as it advances toward the fracture site. Both medial and lateral rods are inserted to the level of the fracture. At this point, the fracture reduction is optimized if necessary with a radiolucent fracture reduction tool which holds the unstable femoral fracture in the appropriate position to allow fixation

❑ The surgeon judge which nail will be most difficult to get across the fracture site, and pass it first. If the easier nail is passed first, it may stabilize the two fragments such that the second, more difficult nail, cannot be passed easily. The two nails then are driven into the proximal end of the femur, with one driven toward the femoral neck and the other toward the greater trochanter.

❑ After the nails are driven across the fracture and before they are seated, fluoroscopy is used to confirm satisfactory reduction of the fracture and to ensure that the nails did not comminute the fracture as they were driven into the proximal fragment.

The nails are pulled back approximately 2 cm, the end of each nail is cut, then driven back securely into the femur. The end of the nail should lie adjacent to the bone of the distal femoral metaphysis, exposed just enough to allow easy removal once the fracture is healed. Do not bend the exposed to distal tip of the nail away from femoral metaphysis as this will irritate surrounding tissues.

The procedure described is with titanium elastic rods, but other devices are available and can be used with slight variations in procedure. The technique of elastic fixation of femoral fractures

as described by Ligier et al.[108] requires that a bend be placed in the midportion of the rod at the level of the fracture site. This produces a spring effect (Fig. 24-18) that adds to the rigidity of the fracture fixation. The spread of the rods in opposite directions provides a "prestressed" fixation, which increases resistance to bending. The opposite bends of the two rods at the level of the fracture significantly increase resistance to varus and valgus stress, as well as torsion. A second bend is sometimes helpful near the entering tip of the nail to facilitate clearance of the opposite cortex during initial insertion. Based on the report by Sagan et al.,[165] sagittal plane configuration should be considered as well. An apex-posterior bend in one of the nails, with the nail shoe pointing anteriorly in the proximal femur, resists apex-anterior malunion.

Using nails that are too small, or mismatched in size, increases the rate of complications.[139] It is very unusual to use nails smaller than 3.5 mm, except in the very youngest, smallest children.

On the lateral, one nail should have its tip pointing anteriorly. When passing the second nail across the fracture site and rotating it, care must be taken not to wind one rod around the other.

A proximal insertion site can also be used. An insertion site through the lateral border of the trochanter avoids creating the stress riser that results from subtrochanteric entry.

Technique Tip. Mazda et al.[119] emphasized that for insertion of titanium elastic nails, the nails have to be bent into an even curve over the entire length, and the summit of the curve must be at the level of the fracture or very close to it in comminuted fractures. The depth of curvature should be about three times the diameter of the femoral canal. Flynn et al.[51] also stressed the importance of contouring both nails with similar gentle curvatures, choosing nails that are 40% of the narrowest diaphyseal diameter and using medial and lateral starting points that are at the same level in the metaphysis.

In length-unstable fractures, an endcap has been shown to confer increased stability that might lessen the risk of shortening[190] and nail backout.

Postoperative Care

A knee immobilizer is beneficial in the early postoperative course to decrease knee pain and quadriceps spasm. When the flexible nailing technique is used for length-unstable fracture, walking (or one leg) spica is recommended, generally for about 4 to 6 weeks until callus is visible on radiographs. For length-stable fractures, touch-down weight bearing could begin as soon as the patient is comfortable. Gentle knee exercises and quadriceps strengthening can be begun, but there should be no aggressive passive motion of the knee, which increases the motion at the fracture site and increases quadriceps spasm. Postoperative knee motion does return to normal over time. Full weight bearing generally is tolerated by 6 weeks. Ozdemir et al.[148] recommended the use of postoperative functional bracing, demonstrating effectiveness in a group of patients treated with elastic rodding. Such postoperative support may occasionally be required, but in most cases it appears not to be needed.

The nails can be removed 6 to 12 months after injury when the fracture is fully healed, usually as an outpatient procedure.

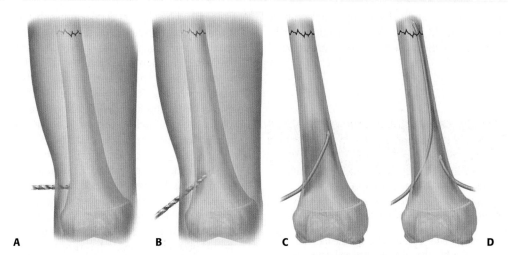

Figure 24-17. A: A drill bit slightly larger than the nail that will be implanted is used to broach the cortex. The drillbit can initially be placed in a perpendicular orientation. **B:** Once the cortex is broached, the drill bit is dropped to a sharply oblique angle and the medullary canal is entered. **C:** The contoured nails inserted following the track of the drillbit. The angle insertion is sharply oblique so that the nail tip bounces off the opposite cortex and precedes up the canal. **D:** After the first nail is just across the fracture site, the second nail is inserted in a similar fashion.

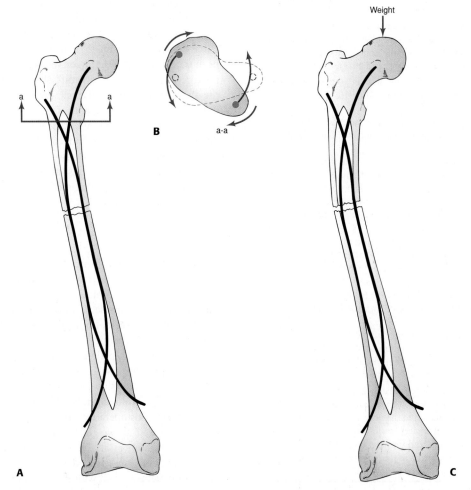

Figure 24-18. A: Stability from flexible rods comes from proper technique. **B:** Torsional stability results from divergence of the rods in the metaphysis. **C:** Resistance to sagittal and coronal bending results from spreading of the prebent rods through the diaphysis, as well as the size and material properties of the rods. Elastic rods return to their predetermined alignment when loaded unless plastic deformation occurs.

Complications

Flexible Intramedullary Nail Fixation of Femoral Shaft Fractures:
PITFALLS AND PREVENTIONS

Pitfall	Prevention
• Overgrowth in preschool children[134]	• The technique should be used infrequently in preschool children.
• Painful bursae and limited knee flexion[119]	• Do not leave rods too long.
• Malunion	• Obtain a proper reduction of the fracture, use nails of adequate size, contour the nails so that the maximum bend is at the fracture site and there is good canal fill.
• Shortening	• Use nails of adequate size, contour the nails properly, be sure that the proximal tip of the nail is embedded firmly in the strong metaphyseal bone of the proximal femur.

Outcomes

A study comparing steel to titanium flexible nails found a higher complication rate in the titanium group.[191] They reported that a typical 3.5-mm stainless steel nail has the same strength as a 4-mm diameter titanium nail. Lee et al.[104] analyzed a group of synthetic fractured femurs instrumented with Enders rods and determined that there was sufficient axial and torsional stiffness to allow "touch-down weight bearing" despite fracture type. Gwyn et al.[62] similarly showed that 4-mm titanium rods impart satisfactory torsional stability regardless of fracture pattern.

Bourdelat[18] compared retrograde and antegrade (ascending and descending) flexible intramedullary rodding in a group of 73 femoral fractures. An antegrade transtrochanteric approach was recommended by Carey and Galpin,[26] who reported excellent results in 25 patients without growth arrest of the upper femur and no osteonecrosis. Satisfactory alignment and fracture healing were obtained in all patients.

Retrograde intramedullary nailing with Ender nails or titanium nails has been reported by Ligier et al.,[108] Mann et al.,[115] Heinrich et al.,[70] Herscovici et al.,[74] and others.[26,91,121] Heinrich et al.[70] recommended a 3.5-mm Ender nail in children 6 to 10 years of age and a 4-mm nail in children over 10 years of age. Ligier et al.[108] used titanium nails ranging from 3 to 4 mm inserted primarily in a retrograde fashion. Heinrich et al.[71] recommended flexible intramedullary nails for fixation of diaphyseal femoral fractures in children with multiple system injury, head injury, spasticity, or multiple long bone fractures. Flynn et al.[51] published the first North American experience with titanium elastic nails. In this multicenter study, 57/58 patients had an excellent or satisfactory result, there was no loss of rotational alignment, but four patients healed with an angular malunion of more than 10 degrees. Narayanan et al.[139] looked at one center's learning curve with titanium elastic nails, studying

the complications of 79 patients over a 5-year period. Nails that were bent excessively away from the bone led to irritation at the insertion site in 41. The center also had eight malunions and two refractures. They noted that complications could be diminished by using rods with similar diameter and contour, and by avoiding bending the distal end of the nail way from the bone and out into the soft tissues. Luhmann et al.[111] reported 21 complications in 43 patients with titanium elastic nails. Most of the problems were minor, but a hypertrophic nonunion and a septic joint occurred in their cohort. They suggested that problems could be minimized by using the largest nail possible and leaving only 2.5 cm out of the femoral cortex.

Morshed et al.[135] performed a retrospective analysis of 24 children treated with titanium elastic nails and followed for an average of 3.6 years. The original plan with these children was to retain their implants. However, about 25% of the children had their nails removed for persistent discomfort.

Flynn et al.[52] compared traction and spica cast with titanium elastic nails for treatment of femoral fractures in 83 consecutive school-aged children. The three unsatisfactory results were treated with traction followed by casting. The overall complication rate was 34% in the traction group and 21% in the elastic nail group.

An international multicenter study focused on factors that predict a higher rate of complications after flexible nailing of pediatric femoral shaft fractures.[17] Analyzing 234 fractures in 229 patients from six different Level 1 trauma centers, the authors found significantly more problems in older, heavier children. A poor outcome was five times more likely in patients who weigh more than 108.5 lb. A poor outcome was also almost four times more likely in patients older than 11 years old. The authors concluded that results were generally excellent for titanium elastic nailing, but poor results were more likely in children older than 11 years and heavier than 50 kg. Ho et al.[76] reported a 34% complication rate in patients 10 years and older, but only a 9% complication rate in patients younger than 10 years, emphasizing the concept that complications of flexible nailing are higher in older, heavier children.

Salem and Keppler[166] noted a 47% incidence of torsional malunion of 15 degrees or more in the patients they treated at one center in Germany. These authors could not determine if the torsional malunion was due to instability after fixation, or faulty surgical technique. In either case, the findings call attention to the need for rotational assessment after fixation.

Complications are relatively infrequent after flexible intramedullary nailing. In 351 fractures reported in seven studies,[10,26,46,71,108,111,119] one nonunion, one infection, and no occurrence of osteonecrosis were reported. Approximately 12% of patients had malunions, most often mild varus deformities, and approximately 3% had clinically significant leg length discrepancies from either overgrowth or shortening. A recent study noted overgrowth of more than 1 cm in 8.2% of preschool children treated with titanium elastic nailing.[134] This is a much higher rate of overgrowth than seen in older children, suggesting the technique should be used infrequently in preschool children. Mazda et al.[119] pointed out a technique-related complication that occurred in 10 of their 34 patients: Rods were left too long and caused painful bursae and limited knee flexion. All 10 patients had the nails removed 2 to 5 months after surgery. Flexible nails inserted in a retrograde fashion may also penetrate into the knee joint, causing an acute synovitis.[162] In a multicenter study[51] that included 58 femoral fractures stabilized with titanium elastic nails, irritation of the soft tissue near the knee by the nail tip occurred in four patients (7%), leading to a deeper infection in two patients. This study also reported one refracture after premature nail removal, leading to a recommendation that nail removal be delayed until callus is solid around all cortices and the fracture line is no longer visible. Ozdemir et al.[148] measured overgrowth with a scanogram and found that the average increase in length was 1.8 mm, suggesting that significant femoral overgrowth is not seen with this method of treatment.

External Fixation

External fixation of femoral shaft fractures offers an efficient, convenient method to align and stabilize the fractured pediatric femur. It is particularly valuable when severe soft tissue injury precludes nailing or submuscular plating, when a fracture shortens excessively in a spica cast, or as part of a "damage-control" strategy.[132] In head-injured or multiply injured patients and those with open fractures, external fixation offers an excellent method of rapid fracture stabilization. It is also valuable for very proximal or distal fractures, where options for flexible nailing, plating, or casting are limited. External fixation may be valuable for the benign pathologic fracture (e.g., through a nonossifying fibroma)

at the distal metaphyseal–diaphyseal junction (Fig. 24-19), where the fracture will heal rapidly, but angular malunion must be avoided.

Following early enthusiasm for the use of external devices, interest waned in the 21st century, because of complications with pin track infections, pin site scarring, delayed union, and refracture. These complications, coupled with the very low complication rate from flexible nailing, led to a decline of external fixation for pediatric femoral shaft fractures. Data from comparison studies also contributed to the change.

Preoperative Planning

✔ **External Fixation of Femoral Shaft Fractures:** PREOPERATIVE PLANNING CHECKLIST	
OR table	❏ Either the fracture table or radiolucent table can be used
Fluoroscopy location	❏ Opposite surgeon
Equipment	❏ Ex fix of choice
Tourniquet	❏ None

During preoperative planning, the fracture should be studied carefully for comminution, or fracture lines that propagate proximally or distally. The surgeon should assure that the fixator devices available are long enough to span the distance between the optimal proximal and distal pin insertion sites.

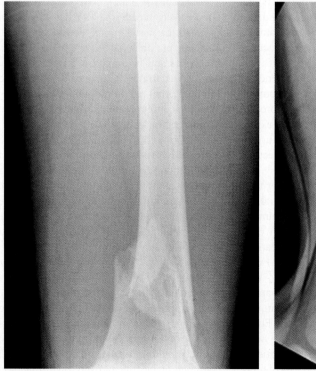
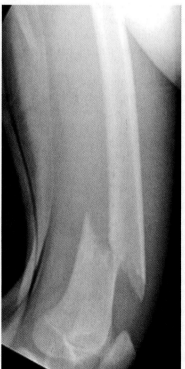

Figure 24-19. AP (**A**) and lateral (**B**) radiographs a low-energy short oblique fracture through a fibrous cortical defect in the distal femur; this type of fracture is not unusual. The surgeon judged that there was enough distance between the fracture site and the growth plate to allow external fixation.

If the fracture is open, it should be irrigated and debrided before application of the external fixation device. With the fracture optimally aligned, fixation is begun. The minimal and maximal length constraints characteristic of all external fixation systems must be kept in mind, and the angular adjustment intrinsic to the fixation device should be determined. Rotation is constrained with all external fixation systems once the first pins are placed. That is, if parallel pins are placed with the fracture in 40 degrees of malrotation, a 40-degree malalignment will exist (Fig. 24-20).

Technique

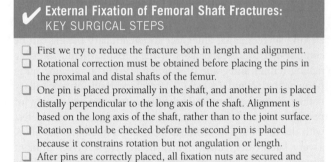

✔ External Fixation of Femoral Shaft Fractures:
KEY SURGICAL STEPS

❑ First we try to reduce the fracture both in length and alignment.
❑ Rotational correction must be obtained before placing the pins in the proximal and distal shafts of the femur.
❑ One pin is placed proximally in the shaft, and another pin is placed distally perpendicular to the long axis of the shaft. Alignment is based on the long axis of the shaft, rather than to the joint surface.
❑ Rotation should be checked before the second pin is placed because it constrains rotation but not angulation or length.
❑ After pins are correctly placed, all fixation nuts are secured and sterile dressings are applied to pins.

Technique Tips. Pin sizes vary with manufacturers, as do drill sizes. In general the pins are placed through predrilled holes to avoid thermal necrosis of bone. Sharp drills should be used. The manufacturer's recommendation for drill and screw sizes should be checked before starting the procedure. Some self-drilling and self-tapping pins are available. At least two pins should be placed proximally and two distally. An intermediate or auxiliary pin may be beneficial.

Postoperative Care

The key to preventing pin site irritation is avoiding tension at the skin–pin interface. We recommend that our patients clean their pin sites daily with soap and water, perhaps as part of regular bath or shower. Showering is allowed once the wound is stable and there is no communication between the pin and the fracture hematoma. Antibiotics are commonly used at some point while the fixator is in place, because pin site infections are common and easily resolved with antibiotic treatment, usually cephalosporin.

There are two general strategies regarding fixator removal. The external fixation device can be used as "portable traction." With this strategy, the fixator is left in place until early callus stabilizes the fracture. At this point, usually 6 to 8 weeks after injury, the fixator device is removed and a walking spica cast is placed. This minimizes stress shielding from the fixator, and allows time for the pin holes to fill in while the cast is on. The alternative, classic strategy, involves using the fixator until the fracture is completely healed. Fixator dynamization, which is difficult in small, young children, is essential for this classic strategy. The surgeon should not remove the device until three or four cortices show bridging bone continuous on AP and lateral x-rays, typically 3 to 4 months after injury.

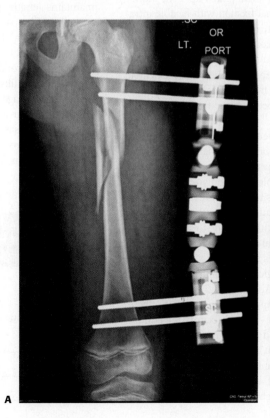
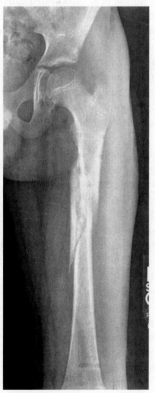

Figure 24-20. A: This proximal spiral femur fracture was deemed length unstable and a poor candidate for titanium elastic nails. The surgeon chose an external fixator, rather than a plate. **B:** Eight weeks after injury, the fracture is healing in excellent alignment and there is good early callous. Fixator removal is easier than plate removal. **A**   **B**

Complications

External Fixation: PITFALLS AND PREVENTIONS	
Pitfall	**Prevention**
• Malalignment	• Placement of the pins perpendicular to the shaft of the femur
• Pin site infection	• Release any skin that will move against the pin when the patient begins to ambulate
• Refracture after external fixator removal	• Be sure there is at least three cortices of bridging callus before external fixator is removed

Although joint stiffness has been noted in older patients treated with external fixation, it is relatively uncommon in children with femoral fractures unless major soft tissue injury is present.[45]

Outcomes

Aronson and Tursky[6] reported their early experience with 44 femoral fractures treated with primary external fixation and early weight bearing. Most patients returned to school by 4 weeks after fracture and had full knee motion by 6 weeks after the fixator was removed. In this early study, end-on alignment was the goal and overgrowth was minimal. Recently, Matzkin et al.[118] reported on a series of 40 pediatric femur fractures treated with external fixation. Seventy-two percent of their series were dynamized prior to external fixator removal, and their refracture rate was only 2.5%. They had no overgrowth, but one patient ended up 5 cm short.

Bar-On et al.[10] compared external fixation with flexible intramedullary rodding in a prospective randomized study. They found that the early postoperative course was similar but that the time to return to school and to resume full activity was less with intramedullary fixation. Muscle strength was better in the flexible intramedullary fixation group at 14 months after fracture. Parental satisfaction was also significantly better in the flexible intramedullary rodding group. Bar-On et al.[10] recommended that external fixation be reserved for open or severely comminuted fractures.

The most common complication of external fixation is pin track irritation/infection, which has been reported to occur in up to 72% of patients.[130] This problem generally is easily treated with oral antibiotics and local pin site care. Sola et al.[176] reported a decreased number of pin track infections after changing their pin care protocol from cleansing with peroxide to simply having the patient shower daily. Superficial infections should be treated aggressively with pin track releases and antibiotics. Deep infections are rare, but if present, surgical debridement and antibiotic therapy are usually effective. Any skin tenting over the pins should be released at the time of application or at follow-up.

In a study of complications of external fixators for femoral fractures, Gregory et al.[57] reported a 30% major complication rate and a high minor complication rate. Among the major complications were five refractures or fractures through pin sites. Another comprehensive study of external fixation complications[27] found an overall rate of refracture of 4.7%, with a pin

track infection rate of 33.1%. Skaggs et al.[174] reviewed the use of external fixation devices for femoral fractures and found a 12% rate of secondary fractures in 66 patients. Fractures with fewer than three cortices with bridging callus at the time of fixator removal had a 33% risk of refracture, whereas those with three or four cortices showing bridging callus had only a 4% rate of refracture. Other reports in the literature with smaller numbers, but still substantial experience, document refracture rates as high as 21.6% with more significant complications.[40,42,58,80,130,154] Despite the complications, patients and treating physicians have found wound care and ability to lengthen through the fracture to be of great benefit of external fixation.

Antegrade Transtrochanteric Intramedullary Nailing

With reports by Beaty et al.[12] and others in the early 1990s alerting surgeons that antegrade intramedullary nailing can be complicated by osteonecrosis of the proximal femur, flexible nailing (either antegrade or retrograde) quickly became more popular than standard locked, antegrade rigid intramedullary nailing. Recently, however, locked antegrade femoral nailing for pediatric femur fractures has enjoyed a resurgence of interest with the introduction of newer generation implants that allow a very lateral trochanteric entry point. These newer implant systems avoid a piriformis entry site, reducing (but perhaps not completely eliminating) the risk of osteonecrosis.[77,94] Antegrade-locked intramedullary fixation is particularly valuable for adolescent femur fractures.

Open fractures in older adolescents can be effectively treated with intramedullary rodding, either as delayed or primary treatment, including those caused by gunshot wounds and high-velocity injuries.[183] Antegrade intramedullary rod insertion maintains length, prevents angular malunion and nonunion, and allows the patient to be rapidly mobilized and discharged from the hospital. However, other techniques with fewer potential risks should be considered.

Retrograde rodding of the femur has become an accepted procedure in adults.[147,159] In a large patient approaching skeletal maturity (bone age >16 years) but with an open proximal femoral physis and an unstable fracture pattern, one might consider this treatment as a way to avoid the risk of osteonecrosis yet stabilize the fracture. If growth from the distal femur is predicted to be less than 1 cm, leg length inequality should not be a problem.

Preoperative Planning

✔ Antegrade Transtrochanteric Intramedullary Nailing of Femoral Shaft Fractures: PREOPERATIVE PLANNING CHECKLIST	
OR table	☐ Fracture table, with the fracture out to length before prepping and draping
Fluoroscopy location	☐ Opposite the surgeon
Equipment	☐ Trochanteric entry IM nail of choice
Tourniquet	☐ None
[Other]	

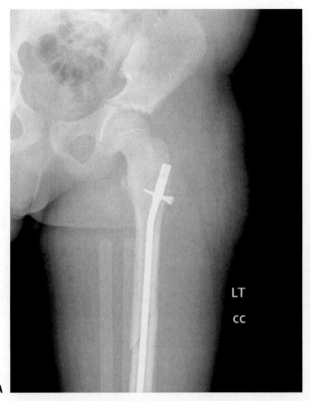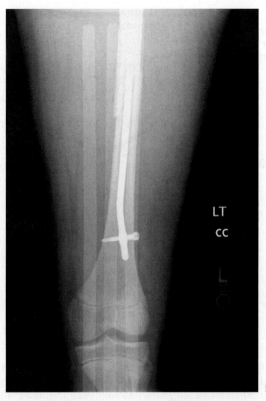

Figure 24-21. AP (**A**) and lateral (**B**) radiographs immediately after internal fixation of the midshaft femur fracture in a 13-year-old with a pediatric locking nail that permits easy lateral entry, and requires minimal reaming of the child's proximal femur.

The patient is placed either supine or in the lateral decubitus position on a fracture table. The upper end of the femur is approached through a 3-cm longitudinal incision proximal that allows access to the lateral trochanteric entry point. The skin incision can be precisely placed after localization on both the AP and lateral views.

Technique

> ✔ **Antegrade Transtrochanteric Intramedullary Nailing of Femoral Shaft Fractures:**
> KEY SURGICAL STEPS

- ❑ Dissection should be limited to the lateral aspect of the greater trochanter, avoiding the piriformis fossa. This prevents dissection near the origin of the lateral ascending cervical artery medial to the piriformis fossa.
- ❑ The rod should be inserted through the lateral aspect of the greater trochanter. In children and adolescents, it is preferable to choose the smallest implant, with the smallest diameter reaming, to avoid damage to the proximal femoral insertion area.
- ❑ The technique for reaming and nail insertion varies according to the specifics of the implant chosen.
- ❑ In general, the smallest rod that maintains contact with the femoral cortices is used (generally 9 mm or less) and is locked proximally and distally (Fig. 24-21). Rods that have an expanded proximal cross section should be avoided, as they require excessive removal of bone from the child's proximal femur.
- ❑ Only one distal locking screw is necessary, but two can be used.[93]

Technique Tips. Dissection should be limited to the lateral aspect of the greater trochanter (Fig. 24-23), without extending to the capsule or midportion of the femoral neck. Some systems provide a small diameter, semiflexible tube that can be inserted up to the fracture site after initial entry-site reaming. This tube is extremely valuable in manipulating the flexed, abducted proximal fragment in proximal-third femur fractures.

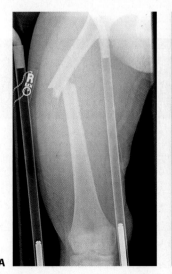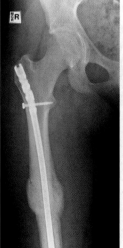

Figure 24-22. Preoperative (**A**) and postoperative (**B**) images showing the use of a newer generation lateral entry nail to treat a proximal third femur fracture in a 14-year-old girl.

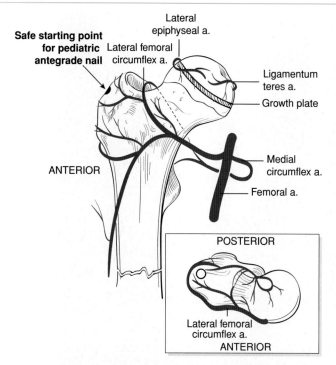

Figure 24-23. Trochanteric entry point for intramedullary nail indicated with *arrow*. Entry here with smaller diameter nails limits the risk of AVN and ensures no awl in the piriformis fossa. (Reprinted with permission from Skaggs D, Flynn J. *Trauma about the pelvis/hip/femur. Staying Out of Trouble in Pediatric Orthopaedics.* 1st ed. Philadelphia, PA: Lippincott Williams & Wilkins; 2006:109.)

Postoperative Care

Nails can be removed 9 to 18 months after radiographic union to prevent bony overgrowth over the proximal tip of the nail. We do not routinely remove locked antegrade nails from our teenage patients unless they are symptomatic or request removal for another reason. Dynamization with removal of the proximal or distal screw generally is not necessary.

Complications

Antegrade Transtrochanteric Intramedullary Nailing of Femoral Shaft Fractures: PITFALLS AND PREVENTIONS	
Pitfall	**Prevention**
• Avascular necrosis	• Use a far lateral, trochanteric entry point.
• Excessive reaming of a child's proximal femur	• Use the smallest diameter femoral nail possible.
• Postoperative shortening or loss of reduction	• Used proximal and distal interlocks.
• Irritation at the greater trochanter	• Do not leave an excessive amount of nail exposed proximally.
• Rotational malreduction	• Assure proper rotational alignment before placing the distal interlocks.

Outcomes

Comparative studies by Reeves et al.[157] and Kirby et al.[96] as well as retrospective reviews of traction and casting, suggest that femoral fractures in adolescents are better treated with intramedullary fixation[12,40,55,56,59,90,96,108,182,194,196] than with traditional traction and casting (Table 24-3). Keeler et al.[94] reported on 80 femur fractures in patients 8 to 18 years old treated with a lateral trochanteric entry starting point. There was no osteonecrosis, no malunion, and a 2.5% infection rate.

Length-unstable adolescent femur fractures benefit from interlocking proximally and distally to maintain length and rotational alignment.[64] Beaty et al.[12] reported the use of interlocking intramedullary nails for the treatment of 31 femoral shaft fractures in 30 patients 10 to 15 years of age. All fractures united, and the average leg length discrepancy was 0.51 cm. No angular or rotational malunions occurred. All nails were removed at an average of 14 months after injury; no refracture or femoral neck fracture occurred after nail removal. One case of osteonecrosis of the femoral head occurred, which was thought to be secondary to injury to the ascending cervical artery during nail insertion.

Reamed antegrade nailing in children with an open proximal femoral physis must absolutely avoid the piriformis fossa, because of the risk of proximal femoral growth abnormalities,[155] the risk of osteonecrosis of the femoral head,[12,127,153,180] the size of the proximal femur, and the relative success of other treatment methods. Beaty et al.[12] reported the use of pediatric "intermediate" interlocking nails for femoral canals with diameters as small as 8 mm. Townsend and Hoffinger[185] and Momberger et al.[131] published reviews of trochanteric nailing in adolescents with very good results. The combined series includes 82 patients of age 10 to 17+ 6 years with no reported cases of osteonecrosis and no significant alteration in proximal femoral anatomy.

Ricci et al.[159] have shown that the complication rate with this technique compares favorably to that of antegrade nailing, with a higher rate of knee pain but a lower rate of hip pain. The malunion rate was slightly lower with retrograde rodding than with antegrade rodding of the femur.

Although good results have been reported with locked intramedullary nails and patient satisfaction is high, problems with proximal femoral growth, osteonecrosis, and leg length discrepancy cannot be ignored. Fortunately, the osteonecrosis rate with newer lateral trochanteric entry nails is lower.

In a series of intramedullary nailing of 31 fractures, Beaty et al.[12] reported one patient with segmental osteonecrosis of the femoral head (Fig. 24-24), which was not seen on x-ray until 15 months after injury. Kaweblum et al.[93] reported a patient with osteonecrosis of the proximal femoral epiphysis after a greater trochanteric fracture, suggesting that the blood supply to the proximal femur may have been compromised by vascular disruption at the level of the greater trochanter during rod insertion. Other researchers have reported single patients with osteonecrosis of the femoral head after intramedullary nailing.[127,146,180] A poll of the members of the Pediatric Orthopaedic Society disclosed 14 patients with osteonecrosis in approximately 1,600 femoral fractures. Despite the use of a "safe" transtrochanteric

TABLE 24-3.   Results of Treatment of Femoral Shaft Fractures in Adolescents

Series	No. of Patients	Average Age (Range) in Years	Treatment	Results and Complications (n)
Kirby et al.[96]	13	12 + 7 (10 + 11–15 + 6)	Traction + cast	Short >2.5 cm (2) Significant residual angulation (4)
	12	12 + 0 (10 + 10–15 + 7)	Intramedullary nailing	No overgrowth No significant residual angulation
Ziv et al.[196]	17	8 + 3 (6–12)	Intramedullary nailing (9 Rush pins, 9 Kuntscher nails)	No leg length discrepancy >1 cm Change in AID 0.5–1 cm = 3 with Kuntscher nails
Reeves et al.[157]	41	12 + 4 (9 + 9–16 + 4)	Traction + cast	Delayed union (4) Malunion (5) Growth disturbance (4) Psychotic episodes (2)
	49	14 + 11 (11–16 + 10)	Intramedullary nailing	No infection, nonunion, or malunion
Beaty et al.[12]	30	12 + 3 (10–15)	Intramedullary nailing	Overgrowth >2.5 cm (2) AVN femoral head (1)
Aronson et al.[6]	42	9 + 7 (2 + 5–17 + 8)	External fixation	8.5% pin infection 10% cast or reapplication
Ligier et al.[108]	123	10 (5–16)	Flexible IM rods	1 infection 13 wound ulcerations 2 LLD >2 cm
Mazda et al.[119]	34	9.5 (6–17)	Flexible IM rods	1–1.5 cm overgrowth (3) 1–15-degree malalignment (2)

LLD, leg length discrepancy.

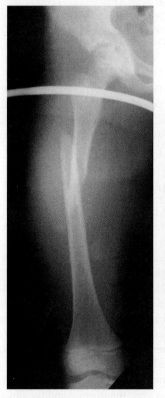
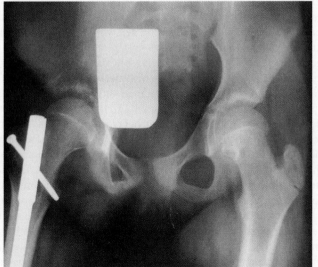

Figure 24-24. A: Isolated femoral shaft fracture in an 11-year-old. **B:** After fixation with an intramedullary nail, femoral head appears normal.

(continues)

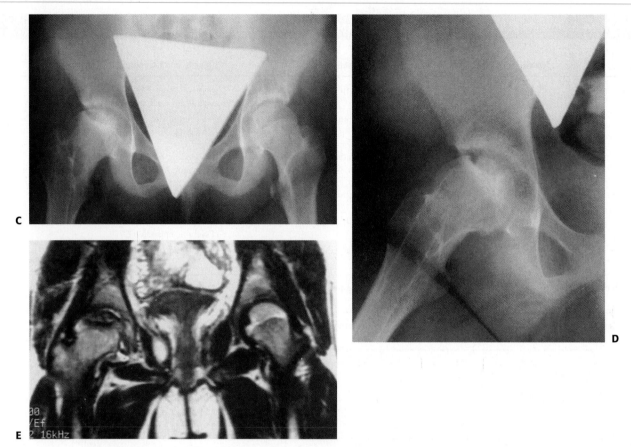

Figure 24-24. (*Continued*) **C:** Eight months after injury, fracture is healed; note early signs of osteonecrosis of right femoral head. **D:** Fifteen months after injury, segmental osteonecrosis of the femoral head is evident on x-rays. **E:** Magnetic resonance image shows extent of osteonecrosis of right femoral head. (**D:** reprinted with permission from Beaty JH, Austin SM, Warner WC, et al. Interlocking intramedullary nailing of femoral-shaft fractures in adolescents: Preliminary results and complications. *J Pediatr Orthop.* 1994;14(2):178–183.)

insertion site for antegrade femoral rodding, a case of osteonecrosis has been reported. Buford et al.[23] showed in their MRI study of hips after antegrade rodding that subclinical osteonecrosis may be present. Antegrade rodding through the trochanter or the upper end of the femur appears to be associated with a risk of osteonecrosis in children with open physes, regardless of chronologic age. Chung[29] noted the absence of transphyseal vessels to the proximal femoral epiphysis and demonstrated that the singular lateral ascending cervical artery predominantly supplies blood to the capital femoral epiphysis (Fig. 24-25). He stated that all of the epiphyseal and metaphyseal branches of the lateral ascending cervical artery originate from a single stem that crosses the capsule at the trochanteric notch. Because the space between the trochanter and the femoral head is extremely narrow, this single artery is vulnerable to injury and appears to be so until skeletal maturity, regardless of chronologic age.

The proximal femoral physis is a continuous cartilaginous plate between the greater trochanter and the proximal femur in young children. Interference with the physis may result in abnormal growth of the femoral neck, placing the child at a small risk for subsequent femoral neck fracture. Antegrade nailing with reaming of a large defect also may result in growth disturbance in the proximal femur as well as femoral neck fracture

(Fig. 24-26). Beaty et al.[12] reported no "thinning" of the femoral neck in their patients, which they attributed to an older patient group (10 to 15 years of age) and design changes in the femoral nail that allowed a decrease in the cross-sectional diameter of the proximal portion of the femoral rods.

Submuscular Bridge Plating

Submuscular bridge plating (Fig. 24-27)[66,89] allows for stable internal fixation with maintenance of vascularity to small fragments of bone, facilitating early healing.[107]

Modern techniques of femoral plating, limiting incisions, maintaining the periosteum, and using long plates and filling only a few select screw holes, have been adopted by many pediatric orthopedic trauma surgeons as a valuable tool to manage length-unstable femur fractures. Pathologic fractures, especially in the distal femoral metaphysis, create larger areas of bone loss that can be treated with open biopsy, plate fixation, and immediate bone grafting.

In very rare situations, such as when there is limited bone for fixation between the fracture and the physes, locked plating techniques may be valuable. This technique provides greater stability by securing the plate with a fixed-angle screw in which

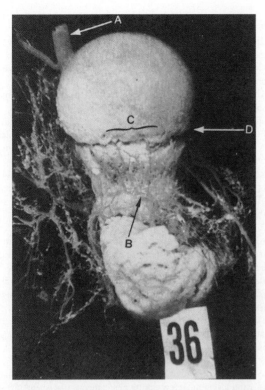

Figure 24-25. The single ascending cervical artery (*B*) is the predominant blood supply to the femoral head. The vessel is at risk during antegrade insertion of an intramedullary rod. (Reprinted with permission from Chung S. The arterial supply of the developing proximal end of the femur. *J Bone Joint Surg Am.* 1976;58(7):961–970.)

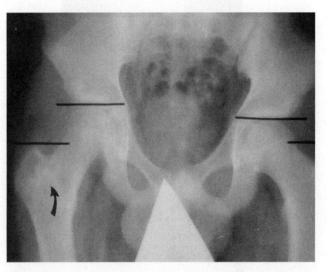

Figure 24-26. A 15-year-old boy 3 years after intramedullary nailing of the right femur. Articulotrochanteric distance increased by 1.5 cm; note partial trochanteric epiphysiodesis (*arrow*) with mild overgrowth of the femoral neck. (Reprinted with permission from Beaty JH, Austin SM, Warner WC, et al. Interlocking intramedullary nailing of femoral-shaft fractures in adolescents: Preliminary results and complications. *J Pediatr Orthop.* 1994;14(2):178–183.)

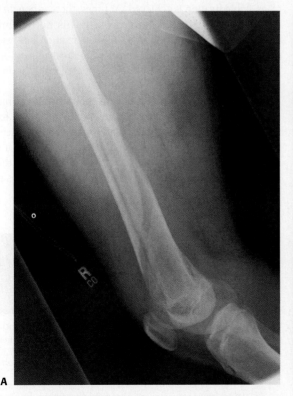

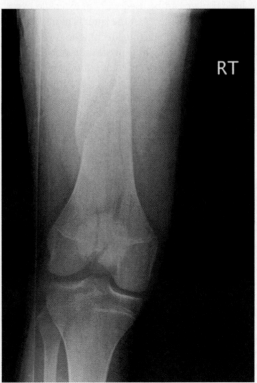

A   **B**

Figure 24-27. AP (**A**) and lateral (**B**) radiographs showing a complex spiral distal femur fracture that extends into the joint. This is a variation of Salter IV fracture.   (*continues*)

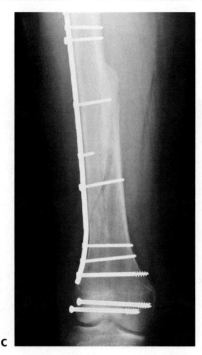

C

Figure 24-27. (*Continued*) **C:** The fracture was managed with submuscular plating, and percutaneous lag screw fixation of the distal femoral condyle fractures.

the threads lock to the plate as well as in the bone. This effectively converts the screw-plate to a fixed-angle blade plate device. In using this type of device, one should lock first, then compress, and finally lock the plate on the opposite side of the fracture. The locked plate can be used with an extensile exposure or with submuscular plating, but the latter is more difficult and should only be attempted when the technique is mastered.

We do not routinely use locking plates unless pathologic lesions, severe osteopenia, or severe comminution is present. Locking screws can "cold weld" to the plate, later turning a simple implant removal into a very difficult exercise involving large exposures, cutting of the implant, and possibly locally destructive maneuvers to remove the screws.

Technique

✔ **Submuscular Bridge Plating of Femoral Shaft Fractures:**
KEY SURGICAL STEPS

- ❑ Technique for submuscular bridge plating of pediatric femur fractures has been well described.[90,172,173]
- ❑ Patient is positioned on a fracture table, and a provisional reduction is obtained with gentle traction.
- ❑ In most cases, a 4.5-mm narrow, low-contact DCP plate is used. A very long plate, with 10 to 16 holes, is preferred.
- ❑ The plate selection is finalized by obtaining an image with the plate over the anterior thigh, assuring that there are six screw holes proximal and distal to the fracture (although in some more proximal and distal fractures, only three holes will be available).
- ❑ The table-top plate bender is used to create a small flare proximally for the plate to accommodate the contour of the greater trochanter, or a larger flare to accommodate the distal femoral metaphysis.

- ❑ A 2- to 3-cm incision is made over the distal femur, just above the level of the physis. Exposure of the periosteum just below the vastus lateralis facilitates the submuscular passage of the plate. A Cobb elevator is used to dissect the plane between the periosteum and the vastus lateralis.
- ❑ The plate is inserted underneath the vastus lateralis, and the femoral shaft is held to length by traction. The plate is advanced slowly, allowing the surgeon to feel the bone against the tip of the plate.
- ❑ Fluoroscopy is helpful in determining proper positioning of the plate. A bolster is placed under the thigh to help maintain sagittal alignment.
- ❑ Once the plate is in position and the femur is out to length, a Kirschner wire is placed in the most proximal and most distal hole of the plate to maintain length (Fig. 24-28).
- ❑ Fluoroscopy is used to check the AP and lateral views and be sure the bone is at appropriate length at this point.
- ❑ A third Kirschner wire may be used to provide a more stable reduction of the femoral shaft. Although screws can be used to facilitate angular reduction to the plate, length must be achieved before the initiation of fixation.
- ❑ Rather than using a depth gauge directly, because the bone will be pulled to the plate, the depth gauge is placed over the thigh itself to measure appropriate length of the screw.
- ❑ Place one screw through the distal incision under direct visualization. At the opposite end of the femur, the next most proximal screw is placed to fix length and provisionally improve alignment.
- ❑ Stab holes are made centrally for drill and screw insertion.
- ❑ When screws are inserted, a Vicryl tie is placed around the shank to avoid losing the screw during percutaneous placement.
- ❑ Self-tapping screws are required for this procedure. Six cortices are sought on either side of the fracture.

The postoperative management includes protected weight bearing on crutches with no need for cast immobilization, as long as stable fixation is achieved. At times, there is benefit to a knee immobilizer; however, in general, this is not required. Early weight bearing in some series of plate fixation has resulted in a low but significant incidence of plate breakage and nonunion. These complications should be decreased by a cautious period of postoperative management.

There are occasional cases with sufficient osteopenia or comminution to require a locked plate to provide secure fixation. In using a locked plate submuscularly, a large enough incision must be used to be sure the bone is against the plate when it is locked. The articular fragment is fixed first to ensure that the angular relationship between the joint surface and the shaft is perfect.

Complications

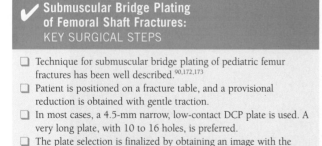

Submuscular Bridge Plating of Femoral Shaft Fractures:
PITFALLS AND PREVENTIONS

Pitfall	Prevention
• Refracture	• Remove the plate after satisfactory union, and about one year after injury.
• Failure fixation/plate bending	• Restrict weight-bearing until early callus is seen.
• Distal femur varus or valgus malunion	• Very carefully contour the plate distally.

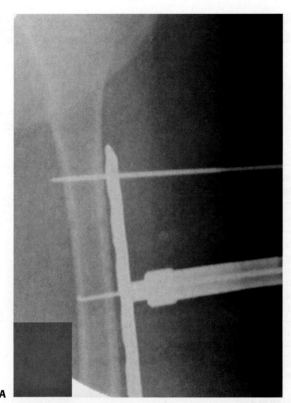
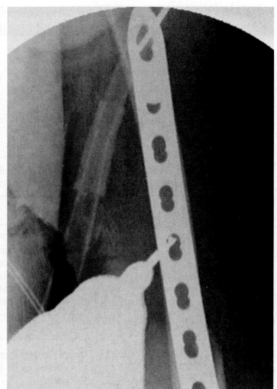

Figure 24-28. A: A Kirschner wire is inserted in the end holes of the plate to maintain length. **B:** Drill holes and screws are placed with fluoroscope imaging.

Outcomes

Kanlic et al.[90] reported a series of 51 patients using submuscular bridge plating with up to 10-year follow-up. Fifty-five percent had unstable fracture patterns. There were two significant complications: one plate breakage (3.5 mm) and one fracture after plate removal. Functional outcome was excellent with 8% significant leg length discrepancy. Hedequist et al.[65] reported on 32 patients aged 6 to 15 years old. Most fractures in their series were comminuted, pathologic, osteopenic, or in a difficult location. Rozbruch et al. described modern techniques of plate fixation popularized by the AO Association for the Study of Internal Fixation that include indirect reduction, biologic approaches to internal fixation, and greater use of blade plates and locked plates (Fig. 24-29).

Sink et al.[171] reported on their center's transition to treating unstable femur fractures with submuscular plating and trochanteric entry nails, and reserving elastic nailing for stable fractures. Their complication rate declined sharply with this change in treatment philosophy.

Plate removal can be difficult after submuscular plating; in fact, the problems with plate removal keep some surgeons from using the technique routinely. Pate et al.[149] reviewed a series of 22 cases of plate removal after submuscular plating for femoral shaft fracture. In 7 of the 22 cases, the incision and surgical dissection was more extensive in the plate removal than in the initial insertion. The authors alert the reader that bone can form on the leading edge of the plate, complicating plate removal.

Quadriceps strength after plate fixation appears not to be compromised, relative to intramedullary fixation or cast immobilization.

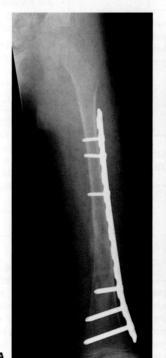
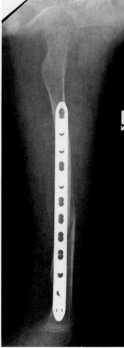

Figure 24-29. A: This child with an unstable femoral fracture in osteopenic bone was managed with a submuscular locking plate providing alignment and stability. **B:** The lateral bow of the femur may be partially preserved despite a straight plate.

Authors' Preferred Treatment for Femoral Shaft Fractures (Algorithm 24-1)

With many different treatment options, and several different factors that must be considered when choosing among the options, a comprehensive decision-making algorithm is needed; published guidelines are not being followed.[138,145,161] We have designed an algorithm modeled after the system used to rate rivers for Whitewater rafting.[49] In Whitewater rafting, class 1 rapids are easy, class 2 rapids are novice, class 3 rapids are intermediate, class 4 rapids are advanced, and class 5 rapids are expert.

A similar classification system can be made to describe the severity, risk, and optimal treatment option for pediatric femur fractures (Algorithm 24-1).

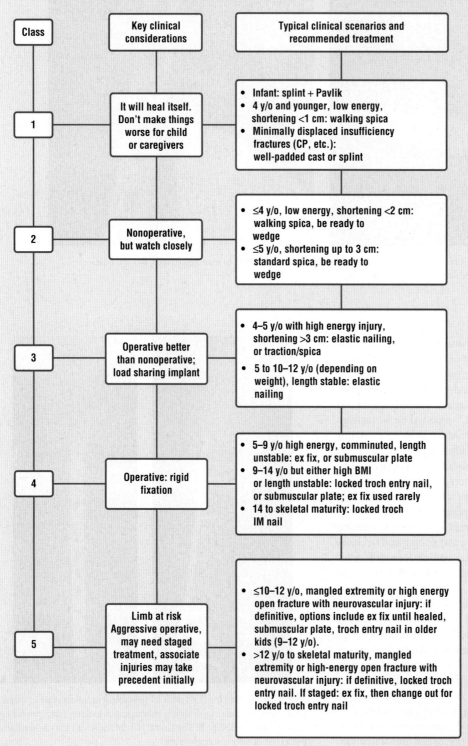

Class	Key clinical considerations	Typical clinical scenarios and recommended treatment
1	It will heal itself. Don't make things worse for child or caregivers	• Infant: splint + Pavlik • 4 y/o and younger, low energy, shortening <1 cm: walking spica • Minimally displaced insufficiency fractures (CP, etc.): well-padded cast or splint
2	Nonoperative, but watch closely	• ≤4 y/o, low energy, shortening <2 cm: walking spica, be ready to wedge • ≤5 y/o, shortening up to 3 cm: standard spica, be ready to wedge
3	Operative better than nonoperative; load sharing implant	• 4–5 y/o with high energy injury, shortening >3 cm: elastic nailing, or traction/spica • 5 to 10–12 y/o (depending on weight), length stable: elastic nailing
4	Operative: rigid fixation	• 5–9 y/o high energy, comminuted, length unstable: ex fix, or submuscular plate • 9–14 y/o but either high BMI or length unstable: locked troch entry nail, or submuscular plate; ex fix used rarely • 14 to skeletal maturity: locked troch IM nail
5	Limb at risk. Aggressive operative, may need staged treatment, associate injuries may take precedent initially	• ≤10–12 y/o, mangled extremity or high energy open fracture with neurovascular injury: if definitive, options include ex fix until healed, submuscular plate, troch entry nail in older kids (9–12 y/o). • >12 y/o to skeletal maturity, mangled extremity or high-energy open fracture with neurovascular injury: if definitive, locked troch entry nail. If staged: ex fix, then change out for locked troch entry nail

Algorithm 24-1. Authors' preferred treatment for femoral shaft fractures: a comprehensive decision-making system for pediatric femur fracture management.

MANAGEMENT OF EXPECTED ADVERSE OUTCOMES AND UNEXPECTED COMPLICATIONS RELATED TO FEMORAL SHAFT FRACTURES

Femoral Shaft Fractures:
COMMON ADVERSE OUTCOMES AND COMPLICATIONS

- Leg length discrepancy
- Angular deformity
- Rotational deformity
- Delayed union
- Nonunion
- Muscle weakness
- Infection
- Neurovascular injury
- Compartment syndrome

LEG LENGTH DISCREPANCY

The most common sequela after femoral shaft fractures in children is leg length discrepancy. The fractured femur may be initially short from overriding of the fragments at union; growth acceleration occurs to "make up" the difference, but often this acceleration continues and the injured leg ends up being longer. The potential for growth stimulation from femoral fractures has long been recognized, but the exact cause of this phenomenon is still unknown. Growth acceleration has been attributed to age, sex, fracture type, fracture level, handedness, and the amount of overriding of the fracture fragments. Age seems to be the most constant factor, but fractures in the proximal third of the femur and oblique comminuted fractures also have been associated with relatively greater growth acceleration.

Overgrowth after femoral fracture is most common in children 2 to 10 years of age. The average overgrowth is 0.9 cm, with a range of 0.4 to 2.5 cm.[170] Overgrowth occurs when the fracture is short, at length, or overpulled in traction at the time of healing. In general, overgrowth occurs most rapidly during the first 2 years after fracture and to a much lesser degree for the next year or so. Because the average overgrowth after femoral fracture is approximately 1 cm, shortening of 2 to 3 cm in the cast is the maximal acceptable amount.

Truesdell[186] first reported the phenomenon of overgrowth in 1921, and many researchers since have verified the existence of growth stimulation after fracture.[1,2,4,9,31,34,43,114,122,155] The relationship of the location of the fracture to growth is somewhat controversial. Staheli[177] and Malkawi et al.[114] reported that overgrowth was greatest if the fracture occurred in the proximal third of the femur, whereas Henry stated that the most overgrowth occurred in fractures in the distal third of the femur. Other investigators have found no relationship between fracture location and growth stimulation.[43,158,170] The relationship between fracture type and overgrowth also is controversial. In general, most researchers believe that no specific relationship exists between fracture type and overgrowth, but some have reported overgrowth to be more frequent after spiral, oblique, and comminuted fractures associated with greater trauma.

ANGULAR DEFORMITY

Some degree of angular deformity is frequent after femoral shaft fractures in children, but this usually remodels with growth. Angular remodeling occurs at the site of fracture, with appositional new bone formation in the concavity of the long bone. Differential physeal growth also occurs in response to diaphyseal angular deformity. Wallace and Hoffman[192] stated that 74% of the remodeling that occurs is physeal, and appositional remodeling at the fracture site occurs to a much lesser degree. However, this appears to be somewhat age dependent. It is clear that angular remodeling occurs best in the direction of motion at the adjacent joint.[192] That is, anterior and posterior remodeling in the femur occurs rapidly and with little residual deformity. In contrast, remodeling of a varus or valgus deformity occurs more slowly. The differential physeal growth in a varus or valgus direction in the distal femur causes compensatory deformity, which is usually insignificant. In severe varus bowing, however, a hypoplastic lateral condyle results, which may cause a distal femoral valgus deformity if the varus bow is corrected.

Guidelines for acceptable alignment vary widely. The range of acceptable anterior and posterior angulation varies from 30 to 40 degrees in children up to 2 years of age (Fig. 24-30), decreasing to 10 degrees in older children and adolescents. The range of acceptable varus and valgus angulation also becomes smaller with age. Varus angulation in infants and children should be limited to 10 to 15 degrees, although greater degrees of angulation may have a satisfactory outcome. Acceptable valgus angulation is 20 to 30 degrees in infants, 15 to 20 degrees in children up to 5 years of age, and 10 degrees in older children and adolescents. Compensation for deformity around the knee is limited, so guidelines for the distal femoral fractures should be stricter than proximal femoral fractures.

Late development of genu recurvatum deformity of the proximal tibia after femoral shaft fracture has been most often reported as a complication of traction pin or wire placement through or near the anterior aspect of the proximal tibial physis, excessive traction, pin track infection, or prolonged cast immobilization. However, proximal tibial growth arrest may complicate femoral shaft fracture, presumably as a result of occult injury.[78] Femoral pins are preferred for traction, but if tibial pins are required, the proximal anterior tibial physis must be avoided. Femoral traction pins should be placed 1 or 2 fingerbreadths proximal to the superior pole of the patella to avoid the distal femoral physis.

If significant angular deformity is present after fracture union, corrective osteotomy should be delayed for at least a year unless the deformity is severe enough to markedly impair function. This will allow determination of remodeling potential before deciding that surgical correction is necessary. The ideal osteotomy corrects the deformity at the site of fracture. In juvenile patients, however, metaphyseal osteotomy of the proximal or distal femur may be necessary. In adolescents with midshaft deformities, diaphyseal osteotomy and fixation with an interlocking intramedullary nail are often preferable.

Distal femoral angular malunion is being recognized after submuscular plating. Care in plate contouring and postoperative monitoring is recommended.

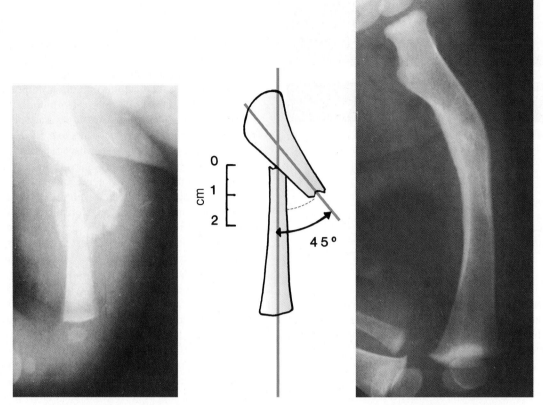

Figure 24-30. Remodeling potential of the femur during infancy. This infant sustained a femoral fracture during a breech delivery and was placed in a spica cast but with insufficient flexion of the hip. **Left:** At 3 weeks, union is evident with about 45 degrees of angulation in the sagittal plane and 1.5 cm of overriding. **Center:** Line drawing demonstrating true angulation. **Right:** Twelve months later the anterior angulation has reduced to a level such that it was not apparent to the family, and the shortening has reduced to less than 1 cm.

ROTATIONAL DEFORMITY

According to Verbeek,[188] rotational deformities of 10 degrees to more than 30 degrees occur in one-third of children after conservative treatment of femoral shaft fractures. Malkawi et al.[114] found asymptomatic rotational deformities of less than 10 degrees in two-thirds of their 31 patients. Salem and Keppler[166] noted a 47% incidence of torsional malunion ≥15 degrees in the patients they treated with elastic nails at one center in Germany. Torsional deformity usually is expressed as increased femoral anteversion on the fractured side compared with the opposite side, as demonstrated by physical examination; a difference of more than 10 degrees has been the criterion of significant deformity. However, Brouwer et al.[20] challenged this criterion, citing differences of 0 to 15 degrees in a control group of 100 normal volunteers. The accuracy of measurements from plain x-rays also has been disputed, and Norbeck et al.[142] suggested the use of computed tomographic (CT) scanning for greater accuracy.

Rotational remodeling in childhood femoral fractures is another controversy in the search for criteria on which to base therapeutic judgments. According to Davids[39] and Braten et al.,[19] up to 25 degrees of rotational malalignment at the time of healing of femoral fractures appears to be well tolerated in children. In their patients with more than 25 degrees

of rotational malalignment, however, deformity caused clinical complaints. Davids[39] found no spontaneous correction in his study of malunions based on CT measurements, but the length of follow-up is insufficient to state that no rotational remodeling occurs. Brouwer et al.[20] and others[14,63,144,188] reported slow rotational correction over time. Buchholz et al.[22] documented five children with increased femoral anteversion of 10 degrees or more after fracture healing in children between 3 and 6 years old. In three of five children there was full correction of the rotational deformity but the oldest of the children failed to correct spontaneously.

Certainly, in older adolescents, no significant rotational remodeling will occur. In infants and juveniles, some rotational deformity can be accepted[48] because either true rotational remodeling or functional adaptation allows resumption of normal gait. Up to 30 degrees of malrotation in the femur should result in no functional impairment unless there is pre-existing rotational malalignment. The goal, however, should be to reduce a rotational deformity to 10 degrees, based on alignment of the proximal and distal femur radiographically, interpretation of skin and soft tissue envelope alignment, and correct positioning within a cast, based on the muscle pull on the proximal fragment. The distal fragment should be lined up with the position of the proximal fragment determined by the muscles inserted upon it (see Fig. 24-2).

DELAYED UNION

Delayed union of femoral shaft fractures is uncommon in children. The rate of healing also is related to soft tissue injury and type of treatment. The time to fracture union in most children is rapid and age dependent. In infants, fracture can be healed in a 2 to 3 weeks. In children under 5 years of age, healing usually occurs in 4 to 6 weeks. In children 5 to 10 years of age, fracture healing is somewhat slower, requiring 8 to 10 weeks. Throughout adolescence, the time to healing continues to lengthen. By the age of 15 years, the mean time to healing is about 13 weeks, with a range from 10 to 15 weeks (Fig. 24-31). Application of an external fixation device appears to delay callus formation and slow the rate of healing. Flexible nailing allows some motion at the fracture site, promoting extensive callus formation. Bone grafting and internal fixation with either a compression plate or locked intramedullary nail is the usual treatment for delayed union in older children and adolescents. Delayed union of a femoral fracture treated with casting in a child 1 to 6 years of age is probably best treated by continuing cast immobilization until bridging callus forms or (rarely) by additional bone grafting.

NONUNION

Nonunions of pediatric femoral fractures are rare. They tend to occur in adolescents, in infected fractures, or in fractures with segmental bone loss or severe soft tissue loss. Tibial fractures are the most common source of pediatric nonunions; femoral fractures account for only 15% of nonunions in children. Even in segmental fractures with bone loss, young children may have sufficient osteogenic potential to fill in a significant fracture gap

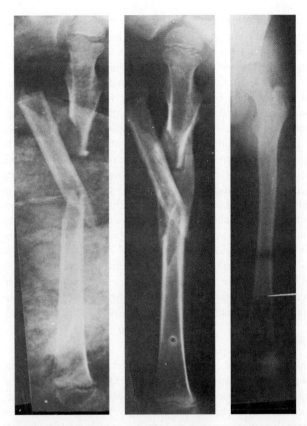

Figure 24-32. The effectiveness of remodeling of the femur in a child. **Left:** Comminuted fracture in an 8-year-old child managed with a femoral pin incorporated in a spica cast. The midfragment is markedly angulated. **Center:** Fracture after union 12 weeks later with filling in of the defect and early absorption of the protruding fragment. **Right:** Appearance at age 12 with only a minimal degree of irregularity of the upper femur remaining.

(Fig. 24-32).[126] For the rare femoral shaft nonunion in a child 5 to 10 years of age, bone grafting and plate-and-screw fixation have been traditional treatment methods, but more recently insertion of an interlocking intramedullary nail and bone grafting have been preferred, especially in children over 10 to 12 years of age. Aksoy et al.[3] reported a small series of nonunions in malunions salvaged with titanium elastic nails. Union was achieved in 6 to 9 months in most cases.

Robertson et al. reported the use of external fixators in 11 open femoral fractures. The time to union was delayed, but a satisfactory outcome occurred without subsequent procedures. This supports the belief that the rates of delayed union and nonunion are low in pediatric femoral fractures, because open fractures would have the highest rates of delayed union.

MUSCLE WEAKNESS

Weakness after femoral fracture has been described in the hip abductor musculature, quadriceps, and hamstrings, but persistent weakness in some or all of these muscle groups seldom causes a long-term functional problem. Hennrikus et al.[73] found that quadriceps strength was decreased in 30% of his patients and 18% had a significant decrease demonstrated by a one-leg hop test. Thigh atrophy of 1 cm was present in 42% of patients.

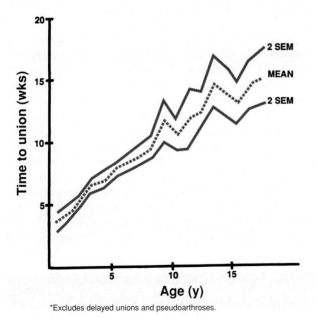

*Excludes delayed unions and pseudoarthroses.

Figure 24-31. Time required for union of femoral shaft fractures in childhood and adolescence. (Redrawn from Skak SV, Jensen TT. Femoral shaft fracture in 265 children. Log-normal correlation with age of speed of healing. *Acta Orthop Scand.* 1988;59(6):704–707, with permission.)

These deficits appeared to be primarily related to the degree of initial displacement of the fracture. Finsen et al. found hamstring and quadriceps deficits in patients with femoral shaft fractures treated with either rods or plates.

Damholt and Zdravkovic documented quadriceps weakness in approximately one-third of patients with femoral fractures, and Viljanto et al.[189] reported that this weakness was present when patients were treated operatively or nonoperatively. Biyani et al. found that hip abductor weakness was related to ipsilateral fracture magnitude, long intramedullary rods, and, to a lesser degree, heterotopic ossification from intramedullary rodding. Hedin and Larsson[67] found no significant weakness in any of 31 patients treated with external fixation for femoral fractures based on either Cybex testing or a one-leg hop test. They thought that the weakness seen in other studies may be related to prolonged immobilization.

Injury to the quadriceps muscle probably occurs at the time of femoral fracture, and long-term muscle deficits may persist in some patients regardless of treatment. Severe scarring and contracture of the quadriceps occasionally require quadricepsplasty.

INFECTION

Infection may rarely complicate a closed femoral shaft fracture, with hematogenous seeding of the hematoma and subsequent osteomyelitis. Fever is commonly associated with femoral fractures during the first week after injury, but persistent fever or fever that spikes exceedingly high may be an indication of infection. One should have a high index of suspicion for infection in type III open femur fractures. A series of 44 open femur fractures[82] reported no infection in type I and II fractures, but a 50% (5 of 10) of type III fractures developed osteomyelitis. Presumably this occurs because of the massive soft tissue damage accompanying this injury.

Pin track infections occasionally occur with the use of skeletal traction, but most are superficial infections that resolve with local wound care and antibiotic therapy. Occasionally, however, the infections may lead to osteomyelitis of the femoral metaphysis or a ring sequestrum that requires surgical debridement.

NEUROVASCULAR INJURY

Nerve and vascular injuries are uncommonly associated with femoral fractures in children.[163] An estimated 1.3% of femoral fractures in children are accompanied by vascular injury[163] such as intimal tears, total disruptions, or injuries resulting in the formation of pseudoaneurysms. Vascular injury occurs most frequently with displaced Salter–Harris physeal fractures of the distal femur or distal femoral metaphyseal fractures. If arteriography indicates that vascular repair is necessary after femoral shaft fracture, open reduction with internal fixation or external fixation of the fracture is usually recommended first to stabilize the fracture and prevent injury of the repair. Secondary limb ischemia also has been reported after the use of both skin and skeletal traction. Documentation of peripheral pulses at the time of presentation, as well as throughout treatment, is necessary.

Nerve abnormalities reported with femoral fractures in children include those caused by direct trauma to the sciatic or femoral nerve at the time of fracture and injuries to the peroneal nerve during treatment. Weiss et al.[193] reported peroneal nerve palsies in 4 of 110 children with femoral fractures treated with early 90/90 hip spica casting. They recommended extending the initial short leg portion of the cast above the knee to decrease tension on the peroneal nerve.

Riew et al.[160] reported eight nerve palsies in 35 consecutive patients treated with locked intramedullary rodding. The nerve injuries were associated with delay in treatment, preoperative shortening, and boot traction. Resolution occurred in less than 1 week in six of eight patients.

Many peroneal nerve deficits after pediatric femoral shaft fractures will resolve with time. In infants, however, the development of an early contracture of the Achilles tendon is more likely. Because of the rapid growth in younger children, this contracture can develop quite early; if peroneal nerve injury is suspected, an ankle-foot orthosis should be used until the peroneal nerve recovers. If peroneal, femoral, or sciatic nerve deficit is present at initial evaluation of a closed fracture, no exploration is indicated. If a nerve deficit occurs during reduction or treatment, the nerve should be explored. Persistent nerve loss without recovery over a 4- to 6-month period is an indication for exploration.

COMPARTMENT SYNDROME

Compartment syndromes of the thigh musculature are rare, but have been reported in patients with massive thigh swelling after femoral fracture and in patients treated with intramedullary rod fixation.[129] If massive swelling of thigh musculature occurs and pain is out of proportion to that expected from a femoral fracture, compartment pressure measurements should be obtained and decompression by fasciotomy should be considered. It is probable that some patients with quadriceps fibrosis[158] and quadriceps weakness[37] after femoral fracture had intracompartmental pressure phenomenon. Mathews et al.[117] reported two cases of compartment syndrome in the "well leg" occurring when the patient was positioned for femoral nailing in the hemilithotomy position. The fracture table has recently been a source of complications.[95] Vascular insufficiency related to Bryant traction may produce signs of compartment syndrome with muscle ischemia.[31] Janzing et al.[87] reported the occurrence of compartment syndrome using skin traction for treatment of femoral fractures. Skin traction has been associated with compartment syndrome in the lower leg in both the fractured and nonfractured sides. It is important to realize that in a traumatized limb, circumferential traction needs to be monitored closely and is contraindicated in the multiply injured or head-injured child. As noted in the spica cast section, several cases of leg compartment syndrome have been reported after spica cast treatment in younger children with femur fractures.

SPECIAL FRACTURES OF THE FEMORAL SHAFT

SUBTROCHANTERIC FRACTURES

Subtrochanteric fractures generally heal slowly, angulate into varus, and are more prone to overgrowth. These fractures offer a challenge, as the bone available between the fracture site and the femoral neck limits internal fixation options. In younger children, traction and casting can be successful.[41] Three weeks of traction is usually necessary, and the surgeon should place a good valgus mold at the fracture site, and monitor the fracture closely in the first 2 weeks after casting. When the patient returns for follow-up and the subtrochanteric fracture has slipped into varus malangulation, the cast can be wedged in clinic or casting can be abandoned for another method. Parents should be warned that loss of reduction in the cast is quite common, and wedging in clinic is a routine step in management. An external fixation strategy can be quite successful if there is satisfactory room proximally to place pins. Once there is satisfactory callus (about 6 weeks), the fixator can be removed and the weight bearing allowed in a walking spica (long leg cast with a pelvic band—place a valgus mold to stabilize fracture in the first few weeks after external fixator removal). Flexible nailing can be used, with a proximal and distal entry strategy (Fig. 24-33). A pitfall in this fracture is thinking the proximal fragment is too short to use flexible IM nails on the AP radiograph because the proximal fragment is pulled into flexion by the unopposed psoas muscle. Pombo and Shilt[151] reported a series of 13 children, averaging of 8 years old with subtrochanteric fractures, treated with flexible nailing. Results were excellent or satisfactory in all cases. Submuscular plating can also produce satisfactory results.[86] In adolescents, there is insufficient experience with this fracture to determine at what age intramedullary fixation with a reconstruction-type nail and an angled transfixion screw into the femoral neck is indicated. Antegrade intramedullary nail systems place significant holes in the upper femoral neck and should be avoided. Unlike subtrochanteric fractures in adults, nonunions are rare in children with any treatment method.

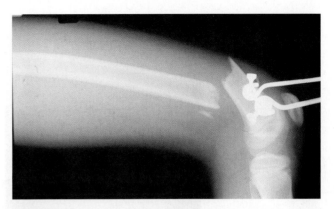

Figure 24-34. It is difficult to treat distal femoral shaft fractures in traction. The muscle forces around the knee often result in significant flexion at the fracture site.

SUPRACONDYLAR FRACTURES

Supracondylar fractures represent as many as 12% of femoral shaft fractures[175] and are difficult to treat because the gastrocnemius muscle inserts just above the femoral condyles and pulls the distal fragment into a position of extension (Fig. 24-34),[61] making alignment difficult (see Fig. 24-2). The traditional methods of casting and single-pin traction may be satisfactory in young children (Fig. 24-35). As mentioned in the external fixation section above, supracondylar fractures through a benign lesion are safely and efficiently treated with a brief period (4 to 6 weeks) of external fixation (Fig. 24-36), followed by a walking cast until the callus is solid and the pin sites are healed. In other cases, internal fixation is preferable, either with submuscular plating (Figs. 24-27 and 24-37) and fully threaded cancellous screws (if there is sufficient metaphyseal length) or with crossed smooth K-wires transfixing the fracture from the epiphysis to the metaphysis, as described for distal femoral physeal separations. If there is sufficient metaphyseal length, flexible nailing can be used, so long as fixation is satisfactory. The flexible nails can be either placed antegrade as originally described, or a retrograde if there is satisfactory distal bone for fixation near the nail entry site. Biomechanically, retrograde insertion is superior.[124] Pathologic fractures in this area are common, and an underlying lesion should always be sought.

OPEN FEMORAL FRACTURES

Open femoral fractures are uncommon in children because of the large soft tissue compartment around the femur. Proper wound care, debridement, stabilization, and antibiotic therapy are required to reduce the chance of infection.[61] In a study by Hutchins et al.,[82] 70% of children with open femoral fractures had associated injuries and 90% were automobile related. The average time to healing was 17 weeks, and 50% of the Gustilo type III injuries developed osteomyelitis.

External fixation of open femoral shaft fractures simplifies wound care and allows early mobilization. The configuration of the external fixator is determined by the child's size and the fracture pattern. Generally, monolateral half-pin frames are

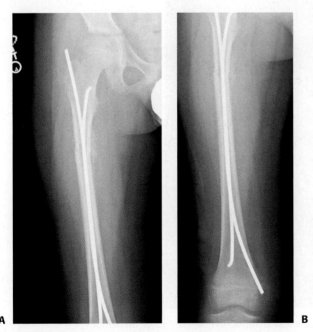

Figure 24-33. A, B: The combination of anterograde and retrograde titanium elastic nail insertion is a good solution for the proximal femur fracture.

(text continues on page 954)

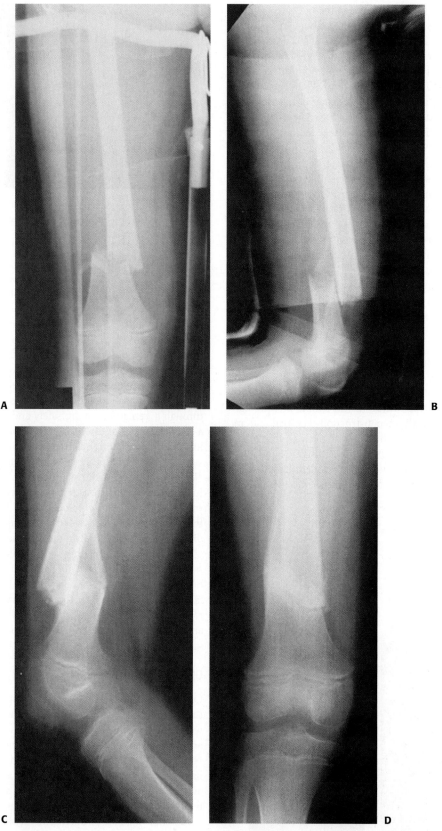

Figure 24-35. A: This 6-year-old patient sustained an unstable supracondylar fracture of the femur. **B:** The fracture was managed with immediate spica casting with the knee in 90 degrees of flexion, mandatory in such a case to prevent posterior angulation. Bayonet apposition, as shown in this figure (**C:** lateral and **D:** AP) is acceptable in a child of this age.

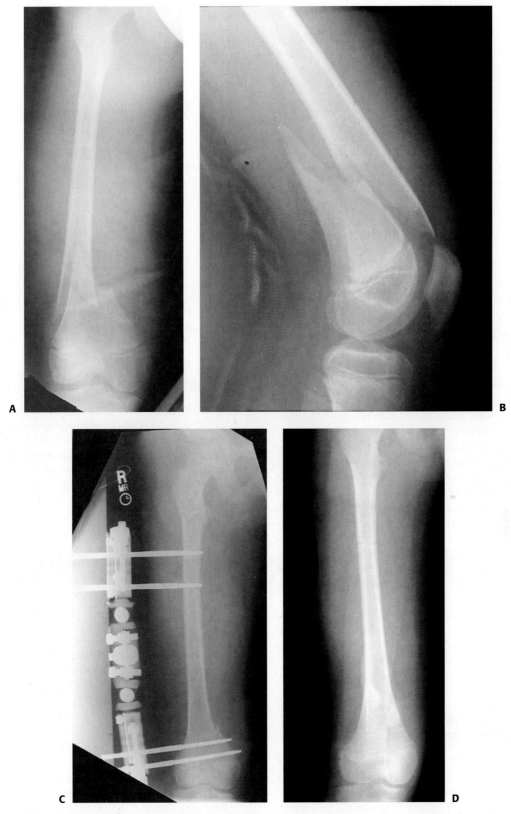

Figure 24-36. AP (**A**) and lateral (**B**) radiographs showing a fracture at the junction of the distal femoral metaphysis and diaphysis. **C:** The fractures reduced into near-anatomic alignment and an external fixator was used to control the distal fragment. **D:** The fixator was removed 8 weeks after injury, and after a brief period of weight bearing is tolerated a long leg cast, the fracture has healed in anatomic alignment with no shortening.

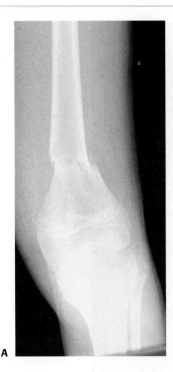
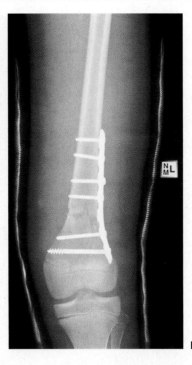

Figure 24-37. Preoperative (**A**) and postoperative (**B**) x-rays showing a fracture at the junction of the distal femoral metaphysis and diaphysis treated with plate fixation.

satisfactory, but thin-wire circular frames may be necessary if bone loss is extensive. External fixation provides good fracture control, but, as always, family cooperation is required to manage pin and fixator care.

Plate fixation also allows early mobilization as well as anatomic reduction of the femoral fracture. Wound care and treatment of other injuries are made easier in children with multiple traumas. However, this is an invasive technique with the potential for infection and additional injury to the already traumatized soft tissues in the area of the fracture. In emergency situations, plate fixation or intramedullary fixation may be used for Gustilo–Anderson type I and II fractures; type III fractures in older adolescents are better suited for external fixation or intramedullary nailing. Plate breakage can occur if bone grafting is not used for severe medial cortex comminution.

In older adolescents, submuscular plating or trochanteric entry nailing is often the optimal treatment choice. Closed nailing after irrigation and drainage of the fracture allows early mobilization and easy wound care in patients with Gustilo–Anderson type I, II, IIIA, and IIIB injuries, but the risk of osteonecrosis must be recognized.

FEMORAL FRACTURES IN PATIENTS WITH METABOLIC OR NEUROMUSCULAR DISORDERS

For patients with osteogenesis imperfecta who have potential for ambulation, surgical treatment with Rush, Bailey–Dubow, or Fassier rods is recommended for repeated fractures or angular deformity. Cast immobilization is minimized in patients with myelomeningocele or cerebral palsy, because of the frequency of osteoporosis and refracture in these patients. If possible, existing leg braces are modified for treatment of the femoral fracture. In nonambulatory patients, a simple pillow splint is used.

FLOATING KNEE INJURIES

These rare injuries occur when ipsilateral fractures of the femoral and tibial shafts leave the knee joint "floating" without distal or proximal bony attachments. They are high-velocity injuries, usually resulting from collision between a child pedestrian or cyclist and a motor vehicle. Most children with floating knee injuries have multiple-system trauma, including severe soft tissue damage, open fractures, and head, chest, or abdominal injuries.

Except in very young children, it is usually best to fix both fractures. If both fractures are open, external fixation of both the tibial and femoral fractures may be appropriate. If immediate mobilization is necessary, fixation of both fractures with external fixation, intramedullary nails, compression plates, or any combination of these may be indicated.

Letts et al.[105] described five patterns of ipsilateral tibial and femoral fractures and made treatment recommendations based on those patterns. Because of the high prevalence of complications after closed treatment, Bohn and Durbin[16] recommended open or closed reduction and internal fixation of the femoral fracture in older children. Arslan et al.[7] evaluated the treatment of the "floating knee" in 29 consecutive cases, finding that those treated operatively had a shorter hospital stay, decreased time to weight bearing, and fewer complications than those managed with splinting casting or traction. Arslan et al.[7] demonstrated that open knee fracture rather than ligamentous injury was a risk factor for poor outcome and that angulation was a predictor of future compromise of function.

Bohn and Durbin[16] reported that of 19 patients with floating knee injuries, at long-term follow-up 11 had limb length discrepancy secondary to either overgrowth of the bone after the fracture or premature closure of the ipsilateral physis (seven patients), genu valgum associated with fracture of the proximal tibial metaphysis (three patients), or physeal arrest (one patient).

Four patients had late diagnosis of ligamentous laxity of the knee that required operation. Other complications included peroneal nerve palsy, infection, nonunion, malunion, and refracture.

FRACTURES IN THE MULTIPLE-SYSTEM TRAUMA PATIENT

In a study of 387 previously healthy children with femoral fractures, the authors evaluated the effect of stabilization on pulmonary function. Patients with severe head trauma or cervical spine trauma are at greatest risk for pulmonary complications. Timing of treatment of femoral fractures appears to not affect the prevalence of pulmonary complications in children. Mendelson et al.[125] similarly showed no effect of timing of femoral fixation on long-term outcome but early fracture fixation did decrease hospital stay without increasing the risk of central nervous system or pulmonary complications.

Annotated References

Reference	Annotation
Beaty JH, Austin SM, Warner WC, et al. Interlocking intramedullary nailing of femoral-shaft fractures in adolescents: Preliminary results and complications. *J Pediatr Orthop.* 1994;14(2):178–183.	31 femoral-shaft fractures in 30 patients were treated with interlocking intramedullary nails. Two patients had overgrowth of >2.5 cm; none had angular or rotational malunions. One patient developed asymptomatic segmental avascular necrosis of the femoral head, which was not seen on radiographs until 15 months after injury. This study established that intramedullary nailing is a reasonable alternative for the treatment of isolated femoral-shaft fractures in older adolescents and in younger adolescents with multiple trauma, and noted the possible complication of AVN.
Crosby SN Jr., Kim EJ, Koehler DM, et al. Twenty-year experience with rigid intramedullary nailing of femoral shaft fractures in skeletally immature patients. *J Bone Joint Surg Am.* 2014;96(13):1080–1089.	Debate exists over the safety of rigid intramedullary nailing of femoral shaft fractures in skeletally immature patients. Among the 246 fractures, 24 complications (9.8%) occurred. At the time of the latest follow-up, 1.7% (4 of 241 patients) reported pain. The average Nonarthritic Hip Score was 92.4 points (range, 51–100 points), and 100% of patients reported satisfaction with their treatment. This large study confirmed that rigid intramedullary nailing is an effective technique for treatment of femoral shaft fractures in pediatric patients with an acceptable rate of complications.
Czertak DJ, Hennrikus WL. The treatment of pediatric femur fractures with early 90-90 spica casting. *J Pediatr Orthop.* 1999;19(2):229–232.	23 consecutive children younger than 6 years with a closed femoral shaft fracture stemming from low-energy trauma were treated with an early spica cast. Average shortening of the fracture at the time of cast removal was 1.0 cm (range, 0.1–2.1 cm). Final patient examinations were performed 18–24 months after the fracture. Overgrowth averaged 1.1 cm in the femur (range, 0.5–1.9 cm). Limb lengths in each patient were within 1 cm of the contralateral limb when measured by scanogram and by blocks. This study helped popularize "immediate spica casting" for toddlers with low energy fractures.
Edvardsen P, Syversen SM. Overgrowth of the femur after fracture of the shaft in childhood. *J Bone Joint Surg Br.* 1976;58(3):339–342.	This study beautifully documented the expected overgrowth after femoral shaft fracture. 26 children conservatively treated for fracture of the femoral shaft have been reviewed with regard to differences in limb length 7 to 10 years after the injury. Nearly two-thirds of the patients had overgrowth of the femur of 10 mm or more. Shortening of 15 to 20 mm at the fracture site was well compensated for by accelerated growth. Growth acceleration seemed to take place during the healing period and the difference at the end of healing was permanent. Overgrowth was promoted by comminuted and long oblique fractures and by overriding of the fracture ends, but was not influenced by the age at fracture, the duration of treatment or the level of fracture of the shaft. Growth of the tibia was not affected by the femoral fracture.
Flynn JM, Curatolo E. Pediatric femoral shaft fractures: a system for decision making. *Instr Course Lect.* 2015;64:453–460.	To determine which treatment option is best for a specific fracture type in a specific patient, pediatric femoral shaft fractures can be divided into five classes: (1) fractures that will heal with limited intervention; (2) fractures that should be treated without surgery, but must be watched closely; (3) fractures that benefit from surgical intervention with load-sharing implants; (4) fractures that may benefit from surgical intervention with rigid fixation; and (5) fractures in a patient with a limb at risk and associated injuries that require initial treatment precedence. This is currently the most useful classification and treatment for pediatric femoral shaft fractures.

Annotated References

Reference	Annotation
Flynn JM, Garner MR, Jones KJ, et al. The treatment of low-energy femoral shaft fractures: a prospective study comparing the "Walking Spica" with the traditional spica cast. *J Bone Joint Surg Am.* 2011;93(23):2196–2202.	This prospective cohort trial comparing walking and traditional hip spica casting showed that the walking hip spica cast gave similar orthopaedic outcomes with a much lower care burden for the family, and established walking spica as the standard treatment of low-energy fractures in children 1–4 yrs/o.
Flynn JM, Luedtke LM, Ganley TJ, et al. Comparison of titanium elastic nails with traction and a spica cast to treat femoral fractures in children. *J Bone Joint Surg Am.* 2004;86-A(4):770–777.	The results of this prospective study supported the empiric observations and published results of retrospective series indicating that a child in whom a femoral fracture is treated with titanium elastic nails achieves recovery milestones significantly faster than a child treated with traction and a spica cast. The complication rate associated with nailing compares favorably with that associated with traction and application of a spica cast. This study gave further support to TEN as centers were moving away for traction and casting in the early 21st century.
Heinrich SD, Drvaric DM, Darr K, et al. The operative stabilization of pediatric diaphyseal femur fractures with flexible intramedullary nails: A prospective analysis. *J Pediatr Orthop.* 1994;14(4):501–507.	78 diaphyseal femur fractures in 77 children were stabilized with flexible intramedullary nails. The patients ranged in age from 2 + 9 to 18 years. There were four unscheduled reoperations, but no major complications; all fractures united. The results obtained using flexible intramedullary nails for the stabilization of select pediatric diaphyseal femur fractures are comparable to nonoperative methods of treatment, but with less disruption to family life and a shorter hospitalization. This is one of the earliest and most important reports on what has become the standard of care for most femur fractures in children 5–12 yrs/o.
Hughes BF, Sponseller PD, Thompson JD. Pediatric femur fractures: effects of spica cast treatment on family and community. *J Pediatr Orthop.* 1995;15(4):457–460.	23 consecutive children with isolated closed femur fractures treated with early spica casts were studied to determine the impact of this treatment on family, school, and other support systems. Mobility was identified by families as the major problem. In families with two working parents, a mean of 3 weeks' time off work was needed. None of the children was accepted into school in cast. Mean time to independent walking was 5 days and to running, 25 days; skills returned faster in younger children. All aspects of spica treatment were easier for preschool children. This study added to the evidence that spica casting was very challenging for families and for school-aged children, and accelerated the trend towards operative management.
Kanlic EM, Anglen JO, Smith DG, et al. Advantages of submuscular bridge plating for complex pediatric femur fractures. *Clin Orthop Relat Res.* 2004;426:244–251.	The authors investigated whether a minimally invasive submuscular bridge plating technique provides stability for early functional treatment (without protective casting or bracing) and predictable healing. They showed that the technique offered the advantage of adequate stability for early functional treatment and predictable healing with maintenance of length and alignment for all pediatric femoral shaft fractures. This was one of the earliest and best series of submuscular plating, and brought it into the list of treatment options, especially for higher energy, length-unstable fractures.
Ligier JN, Metaizeau JP, Prevot J, et al. Elastic stable intramedullary nailing of femoral shaft fractures in children. *J Bone Joint Surg Br.* 1988;70(1):74–77.	This is the first report from the center that popularized TEN worldwide. They showed that complications were minimal, the most common being minor skin ulceration caused by the ends of the rods. A surprising feature was the low incidence of growth changes, with a mean lengthening of only 1.2 mm after an average follow-up of 22 months. Compared with conservative treatment, ESIN obviates the need for prolonged bed rest and is thus particularly advantageous for treating children.
Moroz LA, Launay F, Kocher MS, et al. Titanium elastic nailing of fractures of the femur in children. Predictors of complications and poor outcome. *J Bone Joint Surg Br.* 2006;88(10):1361–1366.	Between 1996 and 2003, 6 institutions in the United States and France contributed a consecutive series of 234 fractures of the femur in 229 children which were treated by titanium elastic nailing. There was a statistically significant relationship ($p = 0.003$) between age and outcome, and the odds ratio for poor outcome was 3.86 for children aged 11 years and older compared with those below this age. The difference between the weight of children with a poor outcome and those with an excellent or satisfactory outcome was statistically significant (54 kg vs. 39 kg; $p = 0.003$). A poor outcome was five times more likely in children who weighed more than 49 kg. This paper refined the age and weight indications for TEN.

REFERENCES

1. Aitken AP. Overgrowth of the femoral shaft following fracture in children. *Am J Surg.* 1948;49(1):147–148.
2. Aitken AP, Blackett CW, Cincotti JJ. Overgrowth of the femoral shaft following fracture in childhood. *J Bone Joint Surg Am.* 1939;21(2):334–338.
3. Aksoy MC, Caglar O, Ayvaz M, et al. Treatment of complicated pediatric femoral fractures with titanium elastic nail. *J Pediatr Orthop.* 2008;17(1):7–10.
4. Anderson M, Green WT. Lengths of the femur and the tibia: norms derived from orthoroentgenograms of children from five years of age until epiphyseal closure. *Am J Dis Child.* 1948;75(3):279–290.
5. Aronson DD, Singer RM, Higgins RF. Skeletal traction for fractures of the femoral shaft in children. A long-term study. *J Bone Joint Surg Am.* 1987;69(9):1435–1439.
6. Aronson J, Tursky EA. External fixation of femur fractures in children. *J Pediatr Orthop.* 1992;12(2):157–163.
7. Arslan H, Kapukaya A, Kesemenli C, et al. Floating knee in children. *J Pediatr Orthop.* 2003;23(4):458–463.
8. Baldwin K, Pandya N, Wolfgruber H, et al. Femur fractures in the pediatric population: abuse or accidental trauma? *Clin Orthop Relat Res.* 2011;469(3):798–804.
9. Barfod B, Christensen J. Fractures of the femoral shaft in children with special reference to subsequent overgrowth. *Acta Chir Scand.* 1959;116(3):235–250.
10. Bar-On E, Sagiv S, Porat S. External fixation or flexible intramedullary nailing for femoral shaft fractures in children. A prospective, randomised study. *J Bone Joint Surg Br.* 1997;79(6):975–978.
11. Beals RK, Tufts E. Fractured femur in infancy: the role of child abuse. *J Pediatr Orthop.* 1983;3(5):583–586.
12. Beaty JH, Austin SM, Warner WC, et al. Interlocking intramedullary nailing of femoral-shaft fractures in adolescents: preliminary results and complications. *J Pediatr Orthop.* 1994;14(2):178–183.
13. Bennett FS, Zinar DM, Kilgus DJ. Ipsilateral hip and femoral shaft fractures. *Clin Orthop Relat Res.* 1993;296:168–177.
14. Benum P, Ertresvag K, Hoiseth K. Torsion deformities after traction treatment of femoral fractures in children. *Acta Orthop Scand.* 1979;50(1):87–91.
15. Blakemore LC, Loder RT, Hensinger RN. Role of intentional abuse in children 1 to 5 years old with isolated femoral shaft fractures. *J Pediatr Orthop.* 1996;16(5):585–588.
16. Bohn WW, Durbin RA. Ipsilateral fractures of the femur and tibia in children and adolescents. *J Bone Joint Surg Am.* 1991;73(3):429–439.
17. Bopst L, Reinberg O, Lutz N. Femur fracture in preschool children: experience with flexible intramedullary nailing in 72 children. *J Pediatr Orthop.* 2007;27(3):299–303.
18. Bourdelat D. Fracture of the femoral shaft in children: advantages of the descending medullary nailing. *J Pediatr Orthop.* 1996;5(2):110–114.
19. Braten M, Terjesen T, Rossvoll I. Torsional deformity after intramedullary nailing of femoral shaft fractures. Measurement of anteversion angles in 110 patients. *J Bone Joint Surg Br.* 1993;75(5):799–803.
20. Brouwer KJ, Molenaar JC, van Linge B. Rotational deformities after femoral shaft fractures in childhood. A retrospective study 27–32 years after the accident. *Acta Orthop Scand.* 1981;52(1):81–89.
21. Bryant T. *The Practice of Surgery.* Philadelphia, PA: Galaxy Publishing; 1873.
22. Buchholz IM, Bolhuis HW, Broker FH, et al. Overgrowth and correction of rotational deformity in 12 femoral shaft fractures in 3-6-year-old children treated with an external fixator. *Acta Orthop Scand.* 2002;73(2):170–174.
23. Buford D Jr., Christensen K, Weatherall P. Intramedullary nailing of femoral fractures in adolescents. *Clin Orthop Relat Res.* 1998;350:85–89.
24. Burks RT, Sutherland DH. Stress fracture of the femoral shaft in children: report of two cases and discussion. *J Pediatr Orthop.* 1984;4(5):614–616.
25. Cannon SR, Pool CJ. Traumatic separation of the proximal femoral epiphysis and fracture of the mid-shaft of the ipsilateral femur in a child. A case report and review of the literature. *Injury.* 1983;15(3):156–158.
26. Carey TP, Galpin RD. Flexible intramedullary nail fixation of pediatric femoral fractures. *Clin Orthop Relat Res.* 1996;332:110–118.
27. Carmichael KD, Bynum J, Goucher N. Rates of refracture associated with external fixation in pediatric femur fractures. *Am J Orthop (Belle Mead NJ).* 2005;34(9):439–444; discussion 444.
28. Cassinelli EH, Young B, Vogt M, et al. Spica cast application in the emergency room for select pediatric femur fractures. *J Orthop Trauma.* 2005;19(10):709–716.
29. Chung SM. The arterial supply of the developing proximal end of the human femur. *J Bone Joint Surg Am.* 1976;58(7):961–970.
30. Ciarallo L, Fleisher G. Femoral fractures: are children at risk for significant blood loss? *Pediatr Emerg Care.* 1996;12(5):343–346.
31. Clark MW, D'Ambrosia RD, Roberts JM. Equinus contracture following Bryant's traction. *Orthopedics.* 1978;1(4):311–312.
32. Coffey C, Haley K, Hayes J, et al. The risk of child abuse in infants and toddlers with lower extremity injuries. *J Pediatr Surg.* 2005;40(1):120–123.
33. Cole WH. Results of treatment of fractured femurs in children with special reference to Bryant's overhead traction. *Arch Surg.* 1922;5(3):702–716.
34. Cole WH. Compensatory lengthening of the femur in children after fracture. *Ann Surg.* 1925;82(4):609–616.
35. Coyte PC, Bronskill SE, Hirji ZZ, et al. Economic evaluation of 2 treatments for pediatric femoral shaft fractures. *Clin Orthop Relat Res.* 1997;336:205–215.
36. Crosby SN Jr., Kim EJ, Koehler DM, et al. Twenty-year experience with rigid intramedullary nailing of femoral shaft fractures in skeletally immature patients. *J Bone Joint Surg Am.* 2014;96(13):1080–1089.
37. Czertak DJ, Hennrikus WL. The treatment of pediatric femur fractures with early 90-90 spica casting. *J Pediatr Orthop.* 1999;19(2):229–232.
38. Daly KE, Calvert PT. Accidental femoral fracture in infants. *Injury.* 1991;22(4):337–338.
39. Davids JR. Rotational deformity and remodeling after fracture of the femur in children. *Clin Orthop Relat Res.* 1994;302:27–35.
40. Davis TJ, Topping RE, Blanco JS. External fixation of pediatric femoral fractures. *Clin Orthop Relat Res.* 1995;318:191–198.
41. DeLee JC, Clanton TO, Rockwood CA Jr. Closed treatment of subtrochanteric fractures of the femur in a modified cast-brace. *J Bone Joint Surg Am.* 1981;63(5):773–779.
42. de Sanctis N, Gambardella A, Pempinello C, et al. The use of external fixators in femur fractures in children. *J Pediatr Orthop.* 1996;16(5):613–620.
43. Edvardsen P, Syversen SM. Overgrowth of the femur after fracture of the shaft in childhood. *J Bone Joint Surg Br.* 1976;58(3):339–342.
44. Epps HR, Molenaar E, O'Connor DP. Immediate single-leg spica cast for pediatric femoral diaphysis fractures. *J Pediatr Orthop.* 2006;26(4):491–496.
45. Evanoff M, Strong ML, MacIntosh R. External fixation maintained until fracture consolidation in the skeletally immature. *J Pediatr Orthop.* 1993;13(1):98–101.
46. Fein LH, Pankovich AM, Spero CM, et al. Closed flexible intramedullary nailing of adolescent femoral shaft fractures. *J Orthop Trauma.* 1989;3(2):133–141.
47. Ferguson J, Nicol RO. Early spica treatment of pediatric femoral shaft fractures. *J Pediatr Orthop.* 2000;20(2):189–192.
48. Ferry AM, Edgar MS Jr. Modified Bryant's traction. *J Bone Joint Surg Am.* 1966;48(3):533–536.
49. Flynn JM, Curatolo E. Pediatric femoral shaft fractures: a system for decision making. *Instr Course Lect.* 2015;64:453–460.
50. Flynn JM, Garner MR, Jones KJ, et al. The treatment of low-energy femoral shaft fractures: a prospective study comparing the "Walking Spica" with the traditional spica cast. *J Bone Joint Surg Am.* 2011;93(23):2196–2202.
51. Flynn JM, Hresko T, Reynolds RA, et al. Titanium elastic nails for pediatric femur fractures: a multicenter study of early results with analysis of complications. *J Pediatr Orthop.* 2001;21(1):4–8.
52. Flynn JM, Luedtke LM, Ganley TJ, et al. Comparison of titanium elastic nails with traction and a spica cast to treat femoral fractures in children. *J Bone Joint Surg Am.* 2004;86-A(4):770–777.
53. Flynn JM, Schwend RM. Management of pediatric femoral shaft fractures. *J Am Acad Orthop Surg.* 2004;12(5):347–359.
54. Frick KB, Mahar AT, Lee SS, et al. Biomechanical analysis of antegrade and retrograde flexible intramedullary nail fixation of pediatric femoral fractures using a synthetic bone model. *J Pediatr Orthop.* 2004;24(2):167–171.
55. Galpin RD, Willis RB, Sabano N. Intramedullary nailing of pediatric femoral fractures. *J Pediatr Orthop.* 1994;14(2):184–189.
56. Gordon JE, Swenning TA, Burd TA, et al. Proximal femoral radiographic changes after lateral transtrochanteric intramedullary nail placement in children. *J Bone Joint Surg Am.* 2003;85-A(7):1295–1301.
57. Gregory P, Pevny T, Teague D. Early complications with external fixation of pediatric femoral shaft fractures. *J Orthop Trauma.* 1996;10(3):191–198.
58. Gregory P, Sullivan JA, Herndon WA. Adolescent femoral shaft fractures: rigid versus flexible nails. *Orthopedics.* 1995;18(7):645–649.
59. Gross RH, Davidson R, Sullivan JA, et al. Cast brace management of the femoral shaft fracture in children and young adults. *J Pediatr Orthop.* 1983;3(5):572–582.
60. Gross RH, Stranger M. Causative factors responsible for femoral fractures in infants and young children. *J Pediatr Orthop.* 1983;3(3):341–343.
61. Gustilo RB. Current concepts in the management of open fractures. *Instr Course Lect.* 1987;36:359–366.
62. Gwyn DT, Olney BW, Dart BR, et al. Rotational control of various pediatric femur fractures stabilized with titanium elastic intramedullary nails. *J Pediatr Orthop.* 2004;24(2):172–177.
63. Hagglund G, Hansson LI, Norman O. Correction by growth of rotational deformity after femoral fracture in children. *Acta Orthop Scand.* 1983;54(6):858–861.
64. Hajek PD, Bicknell HR Jr., Bronson WE, et al. The use of one compared with two distal screws in the treatment of femoral shaft fractures with interlocking intramedullary nailing. A clinical and biomechanical analysis. *J Bone Joint Surg Am.* 1993;75(4):519–525.
65. Hedequist D, Bishop J, Hresko T. Locking plate fixation for pediatric femur fractures. *J Pediatr Orthop.* 2008;28(1):6–9.
66. Hedequist DJ, Sink E. Technical aspects of bridge plating for pediatric femur fractures. *J Orthop Trauma.* 2005;19(4):276–279.
67. Hedin H, Larsson S. Muscle strength in children treated for displaced femoral fractures by external fixation: 31 patients compared with 31 matched controls. *Acta Orthop Scand.* 2003;74(3):305–311.
68. Hedlund R, Lindgren U. The incidence of femoral shaft fractures in children and adolescents. *J Pediatr Orthop.* 1986;6(1):47–50.
69. Heideken J, Svensson T, Blomqvist P, et al. Incidence and trends in femur shaft fractures in Swedish children between 1987 and 2005. *J Pediatr Orthop.* 2011;31(5):512–519.
70. Heinrich SD, Drvaric D, Darr K, et al. Stabilization of pediatric diaphyseal femur fractures with flexible intramedullary nails (a technique paper). *J Orthop Trauma.* 1992;6(4):452–459.
71. Heinrich SD, Drvaric DM, Darr K, et al. The operative stabilization of pediatric diaphyseal femur fractures with flexible intramedullary nails: a prospective analysis. *J Pediatr Orthop.* 1994;14(4):501–507.
72. Henderson J, Goldacre MJ, Fairweather JM, et al. Conditions accounting for substantial time spent in hospital in children aged 1–14 years. *Arch Dis Child.* 1992;67(1):83–86.
73. Hennrikus WL, Kasser JR, Rand F, et al. The function of the quadriceps muscle after a fracture of the femur in patients who are less than seventeen years old. *J Bone Joint Surg Am.* 1993;75(4):508–513.
74. Herscovici D Jr., Scott DM, Behrens F, et al. The use of Ender nails in femoral shaft fractures: what are the remaining indications? *J Orthop Trauma.* 1992;6(3):314–317.
75. Hinton RY, Lincoln A, Crockett MM, et al. Fractures of the femoral shaft in children. Incidence, mechanisms, and sociodemographic risk factors. *J Bone Joint Surg Am.* 1999;81(4):500–509.

76. Ho CA, Skaggs DL, Tang CW, et al. Use of flexible intramedullary nails in pediatric femur fractures. *J Pediatr Orthop.* 2006;26(4):497–504.

77. Hosalkar HS, Pandya NK, Cho RH, et al. Intramedullary nailing of pediatric femoral shaft fracture. *J Am Acad Orthop Surg.* 2011;19(8):472–481.

78. Hresko MT, Kasser JR. Physeal arrest about the knee associated with non-physeal fractures in the lower extremity. *J Bone Joint Surg Am.* 1989;71(5):698–703.

79. Hughes BF, Sponseller PD, Thompson JD. Pediatric femur fractures: effects of spica cast treatment on family and community. *J Pediatr Orthop.* 1995;15(4):457–460.

80. Hull JB, Sanderson PL, Rickman M, et al. External fixation of children's fractures: use of the Orthofix Dynamic Axial Fixator. *J Pediatr Orthop.* 1997;6(3):203–206.

81. Humberger FW, Eyring EJ. Proximal tibial 90-90 traction in treatment of children with femoral-shaft fractures. *J Bone Joint Surg Am.* 1969;51(3):499–504.

82. Hutchins CM, Sponseller PD, Sturm P, et al. Open femur fractures in children: treatment, complications, and results. *J Pediatr Orthop.* 2000;20(2):183–188.

83. Illgen R 2nd, Rodgers WB, Hresko MT, et al. Femur fractures in children: treatment with early sitting spica casting. *J Pediatr Orthop.* 1998;18(4):481–487.

84. Infante AF Jr., Albert MC, Jennings WB, et al. Immediate hip spica casting for femur fractures in pediatric patients. A review of 175 patients. *Clin Orthop Relat Res.* 2000;376:106–112.

85. Irani RN, Nicholson JT, Chung SM. Long-term results in the treatment of femoral-shaft fractures in young children by immediate spica immobilization. *J Bone Joint Surg Am.* 1976;58(7):945–951.

86. Ireland DC, Fisher RL. Subtrochanteric fractures of the femur in children. *Clin Orthop Relat Res.* 1975;110:157–166.

87. Janzing H, Broos P, Rommens P. Compartment syndrome as a complication of skin traction in children with femoral fractures. *J Trauma.* 1996;41(1):156–158.

88. Johnson AW, Weiss CB Jr., Wheeler DL. Stress fractures of the femoral shaft in athletes–more common than expected. A new clinical test. *Am J Sports Med.* 1994;22(2):248–256.

89. Kanlic E, Cruz M. Current concepts in pediatric femur fracture treatment. *Orthopedics.* 2007;30(12):1015–1019.

90. Kanlic EM, Anglen JO, Smith DG, et al. Advantages of submuscular bridge plating for complex pediatric femur fractures. *Clin Orthop Relat Res.* 2004;426:244–251.

91. Karaoglu S, Baktir A, Tuncel M, et al. Closed Ender nailing of adolescent femoral shaft fractures. *Injury.* 1994;25(8):501–506.

92. Katz JF. Spontaneous fractures in paraplegic children. *J Bone Joint Surg Am.* 1953;35-A(1):220–226.

93. Kaweblum M, Lehman WB, Grant AD, et al. Avascular necrosis of the femoral head as sequela of fracture of the greater trochanter. A case report and review of the literature. *Clin Orthop Relat Res.* 1993;294:193–195.

94. Keeler KA, Dart B, Luhmann SJ, et al. Antegrade intramedullary nailing of pediatric femoral fractures using an interlocking pediatric femoral nail and a lateral trochanteric entry point. *J Pediatr Orthop.* 2009;29(4):345–351.

95. Kelly BA, Naqvi M, Rademacher ES, et al. Fracture table application for pediatric femur fractures: incidence and risk factors associated with adverse outcomes. *J Pediatr Orthop.* 2017;37(6):e353–e356.

96. Kirby RM, Winquist RA, Hansen ST Jr. Femoral shaft fractures in adolescents: a comparison between traction plus cast treatment and closed intramedullary nailing. *J Pediatr Orthop.* 1981;1(2):193–197.

97. Kocher M. American Academy of Orthopaedic Surgeons Specialty Day. 2004.

98. Kocher MS, Sink EL, Blasier RD, et al. Treatment of pediatric diaphyseal femur fractures. *J Am Acad Orthop Surg.* 2009;17(11):718–725.

99. Kong H, Sabharwal S. External fixation for closed pediatric femoral shaft fractures: where are we now? *Clin Orthop Relat Res.* 2014;472(12):3814–3822.

100. Krettek C, Haas N, Walker J, et al. Treatment of femoral shaft fractures in children by external fixation. *Injury.* 1991;22(4):263–266.

101. Landin LA. Fracture patterns in children: analysis of 8,682 fractures with special reference to incidence, etiology and secular changes in a Swedish urban population 1950–1979. *Acta Orthop Scand Supp.* 1983;202:1–109.

102. Large TM, Frick SL. Compartment syndrome of the leg after treatment of a femoral fracture with an early sitting spica cast. A report of two cases. *J Bone Joint Surg Am.* 2003;85-A(11):2207–2210.

103. Lascombes P, Haumont T, Journeau P. Use and abuse of flexible intramedullary nailing in children and adolescents. *J Pediatr Orthop.* 2006;26(6):827–834.

104. Lee SS, Mahar AT, Newton PO. Ender nail fixation of pediatric femur fractures: a biomechanical analysis. *J Pediatr Orthop.* 2001;21(4):442–445.

105. Letts M, Vincent N, Gouw G. The "floating knee" in children. *J Bone Joint Surg Br.* 1986;68(3):442–446.

106. Leu D, Sargent MC, Ain MC, et al. Spica casting for pediatric femoral fractures. A prospective, randomized controlled study of single-leg versus double-leg spica casts. *J Bone Joint Surg Am.* 2012;94(14):1259–1264.

107. Li Y, Hedequist DJ. Submuscular plating of pediatric femur fracture. *J Am Acad Orthop Surg.* 2012;20(9):596–603.

108. Ligier JN, Metaizeau JP, Prevot J, et al. Elastic stable intramedullary nailing of femoral shaft fractures in children. *J Bone Joint Surg Br.* 1988;70(1):74–77.

109. Loder RT. Pediatric polytrauma: orthopaedic care and hospital course. *J Orthop Trauma.* 1987;1(1):48–54.

110. Loder RT, O'Donnell PW, Feinberg JR. Epidemiology and mechanisms of femur fractures in children. *J Pediatr Orthop.* 2006;26(5):561–566.

111. Luhmann SJ, Schootman M, Schoenecker PL, et al. Complications of titanium elastic nails for pediatric femoral shaft fractures. *J Pediatr Orthop.* 2003;23(4):443–447.

112. Lynch JM, Gardner MJ, Gains B. Hemodynamic significance of pediatric femur fractures. *J Pediatr Surg.* 1996;31(10):1358–1361.

113. Mahajan J1, Hennrikus W, Piazza B. Overgrowth after femoral shaft fractures in infants treated with a Pavlik harness. *J Pediatr Orthop B.* 2016;25(1):7–10.

114. Malkawi H, Shannak A, Hadidi S. Remodeling after femoral shaft fractures in children treated by the modified blount method. *J Pediatr Orthop.* 1986;6(4):421–429.

115. Mann DC, Weddington J, Davenport K. Closed Ender nailing of femoral shaft fractures in adolescents. *J Pediatr Orthop.* 1986;6(6):651–655.

116. Mansour AA 3rd, Wilmoth JC, Mansour AS, et al. Immediate spica casting of pediatric femoral fractures in the operating room versus the emergency department: comparison of reduction, complications, and hospital charges. *J Pediatr Orthop.* 2010;30(8):813–817.

117. Mathews PV, Perry JJ, Murray PC. Compartment syndrome of the well leg as a result of the hemilithotomy position: a report of two cases and review of literature. *J Orthop Trauma.* 2001;15(8):580–583.

118. Matzkin EG, Smith EL, Wilson A, et al. External fixation of pediatric femur fractures with cortical contact. *Am J Orthop (Belle Mead NJ).* 2006;35(11):498–501.

119. Mazda K, Khairouni A, Pennecot GF, et al. Closed flexible intramedullary nailing of the femoral shaft fractures in children. *J Pediatr Orthop.* 1997;6(3):198–202.

120. McCarthy RE. A method for early spica cast application in treatment of pediatric femoral shaft fractures. *J Pediatr Orthop.* 1986;6(1):89–91.

121. McGraw JJ, Gregory SK. Ender nails: an alternative for intramedullary fixation of femoral shaft fractures in children and adolescents. *South Med J.* 1997;90(7):694–696.

122. Meals RA. Overgrowth of the femur following fractures in children: influence of handedness. *J Bone Joint Surg Am.* 1979;61(3):381–384.

123. Meaney JE, Carty H. Femoral stress fractures in children. *Skeletal Radiol.* 1992;21(3):173–176.

124. Mehlman CT, Nemeth NM, Glos DL. Antegrade versus retrograde titanium elastic nail fixation of pediatric distal-third femoral-shaft fractures: a mechanical study. *J Orthop Trauma.* 2006;20(9):608–612.

125. Mendelson SA, Dominick TS, Tyler-Kabara E, et al. Early versus late femoral fracture stabilization in multiply injured pediatric patients with closed head injury. *J Pediatr Orthop.* 2001;21(5):594–599.

126. Mesko JW, DeRosa GP, Lindseth RE. Segmental femur loss in children. *J Pediatr Orthop.* 1985;5(4):471–474.

127. Mileski RA, Garvin KL, Huurman WW. Avascular necrosis of the femoral head after closed intramedullary shortening in an adolescent. *J Pediatr Orthop.* 1995;15(1):24–26.

128. Miller ME, Bramlett KW, Kissell EU, et al. Improved treatment of femoral shaft fractures in children. The "pontoon" 90-90 spica cast. *Clin Orthop Relat Res.* 1987;219:140–146.

129. Miller DS, Markin L, Grossman E. Ischemic fibrosis of the lower extremity in children. *Am J Surg.* 1952;84(3):317–322.

130. Miner T, Carroll KL. Outcomes of external fixation of pediatric femoral shaft fractures. *J Pediatr Orthop.* 2000;20(3):405–410.

131. Momberger N, Stevens P, Smith J, et al. Intramedullary nailing of femoral fractures in adolescents. *J Pediatr Orthop.* 2000;20(4):482–484.

132. Mooney JF. The use of 'damage control orthopedics' techniques in children with segmental open femur fractures. *J Pediatr Orthop.* 2012;21(5):400–403.

133. Moroz LA, Launay F, Kocher MS, et al. Titanium elastic nailing of fractures of the femur in children. Predictors of complications and poor outcome. *J Bone Joint Surg Br.* 2006;88(10):1361–1366.

134. Morris S, Cassidy N, Stephens M, et al. Birth-associated femoral fractures: incidence and outcome. *J Pediatr Orthop.* 2002;22(1):27–30.

135. Morshed S, Humphrey M, Corrales LA, et al. Retention of flexible intramedullary nails following treatment of pediatric femur fractures. *Arch Orthop Traum Surg.* 2007;127(7):509–514.

136. Mubarak SJ, Frick S, Sink E, et al. Volkmann contracture and compartment syndromes after femur fractures in children treated with 90/90 spica casts. *J Pediatr Orthop.* 2006;26(5):567–572.

137. Murphy R, Kelly DM, Moisan A, et al. Transverse fractures of the femoral shaft are a better predictor of nonaccidental trauma in young children than spiral fractures are. *J Bone Joint Surg Am.* 2015;97(2):106–111.

138. Naranje SM, Stewart MG, Kelly DM, et al. Changes in the treatment of pediatric femoral fractures: 15-year trends from United States Kids' Inpatient Database (KID) 1997 to 2012. *J Pediatr Orthop.* 2016;36(7):e81–e85.

139. Narayanan UG, Hyman JE, Wainwright AM, et al. Complications of elastic stable intramedullary nail fixation of pediatric femoral fractures, and how to avoid them. *J Pediatr Orthop.* 2004;24(4):363–369.

140. Newton PO, Mubarak SJ. Financial aspects of femoral shaft fracture treatment in children and adolescents. *J Pediatr Orthop.* 1994;14(4):508–512.

141. Nicholson JT, Foster RM, Heath RD. Bryant's traction; a provocative cause of circulatory complications. *JAMA.* 1955;157(5):415–418.

142. Norbeck DE Jr., Asselmeier M, Pinzur MS. Torsional malunion of a femur fracture: diagnosis and treatment. *Orthop Rev.* 1990;19(7):625–629.

143. Nork SE, Hoffinger SA. Skeletal traction versus external fixation for pediatric femoral shaft fractures: a comparison of hospital costs and charges. *J Orthop Trauma.* 1998;12(8):563–568.

144. Oberhammer J. Degree and frequency of rotational deformities after infant femoral fractures and their spontaneous correction. *Arch Orthop Traum Surg.* 1980;97(4):249–255.

145. Oetgen ME, Blatz AM, Matthews A. Impact of clinical practice guideline on the treatment of pediatric femoral fractures in a pediatric hospital. *J Bone Joint Surg Am.* 2015;97(20):1641–1646.

146. O'Malley DE, Mazur JM, Cummings RJ. Femoral head avascular necrosis associated with intramedullary nailing in an adolescent. *J Pediatr Orthop.* 1995;15(1):21–23.

147. Ostrum RF, DiCicco J, Lakatos R, et al. Retrograde intramedullary nailing of femoral diaphyseal fractures. *J Orthop Trauma.* 1998;12(7):464–468.

148. Ozdemir HM, Yensel U, Senaran H, et al. Immediate percutaneous intramedullary fixation and functional bracing for the treatment of pediatric femoral shaft fracture. *J Pediatr Orthop.* 2003;23(4):453–457.

149. Pate O, Hedequist D, Leong N, et al. Implant removal after submuscular plating for pediatric femur fractures. *J Pediatr Orthop.* 2009;29(7):709–712.

150. Podeszwa DA, Mooney JF 3rd, Cramer KE, et al. Comparison of Pavlik harness application and immediate spica casting for femur fractures in infants. *J Pediatr Orthop.* 2004;24(5):460–462.

151. Pombo MW, Shilt JS. The definition and treatment of pediatric subtrochanteric femur fractures with titanium elastic nails. *J Pediatr Orthop.* 2006;26(3):364–370.

152. Porat S, Milgrom C, Nyska M, et al. Femoral fracture treatment in head-injured children: use of external fixation. *J Trauma*. 1986;26(1):81–84.
153. Pott P. *Some Few General Remarks on Fractures and Dislocations*. London: Howes; 1769.
154. Probe R, Lindsey RW, Hadley NA, et al. Refracture of adolescent femoral shaft fractures: a complication of external fixation. A report of two cases. *J Pediatr Orthop*. 1993;13(1):102–105.
155. Raney EM, Ogden JA, Grogan DP. Premature greater trochanteric epiphysiodesis secondary to intramedullary femoral rodding. *J Pediatr Orthop*. 1993;13(4):516–520.
156. Rathjen KE, Riccio AI, De La Garza D. Stainless steel flexible intramedullary fixation of unstable femoral shaft fractures in children. *J Pediatr Orthop*. 2007;27(4):432–441.
157. Reeves RB, Ballard RI, Hughes JL. Internal fixation versus traction and casting of adolescent femoral shaft fractures. *J Pediatr Orthop*. 1990;10(5):592–595.
158. Reynolds DA. Growth changes in fractured long-bones: a study of 126 children. *J Bone Joint Surg Br*. 1981;63-B(1):83–88.
159. Ricci WM, Bellabarba C, Evanoff B, et al. Retrograde versus antegrade nailing of femoral shaft fractures. *J Orthop Trauma*. 2001;15(3):161–169.
160. Riew KD, Sturm PF, Rosenbaum D, et al. Neurologic complications of pediatric femoral nailing. *J Pediatr Orthop*. 1996;16(5):606–612.
161. Roaten JD, Kelly DM, Yellin JL, et al. Pediatric femoral shaft fractures: a multicenter review of the AAOS clinical practice guidelines before and after 2009 [Epub ahead of print April 10, 2017]. *J Pediatr Orthop*. doi: 10.1097/BPO.0000000000000982.
162. Rohde RS, Mendelson SA, Grudziak JS. Acute synovitis of the knee resulting from intra-articular knee penetration as a complication of flexible intramedullary nailing of pediatric femur fractures: report of two cases. *J Pediatr Orthop*. 2003;23(5):635–638.
163. Rosental JJ, Gaspar MR, Gjerdrum TC, et al. Vascular injuries associated with fractures of the femur. *Arch Surg*. 1975;110(5):494–499.
164. Ryan JR. 90-90 skeletal femoral traction for femoral shaft fractures in children. *J Trauma*. 1981;21(1):46–48.
165. Sagan ML, Datta JC, Olney BW, et al. Residual deformity after treatment of pediatric femur fractures with flexible titanium nails. *J Pediatr Orthop*. 2010;30(7):638–643.
166. Salem KH, Keppler P. Limb geometry after elastic stable nailing for pediatric femoral fractures. *J Bone Joint Surg Am*. 2010;92(6):1409–1417.
167. Schenck RC Jr. *Basic Histomorphology and Physiology of Skeletal Growth*. New York, NY: Springer-Verlag; 1980.
168. Shaha JS, Cage JM, Black SR, et al. Redefining optimal nail to medullary canal diameter ratio in stainless steel flexible intramedullary nailing of pediatric femur fractures. *J Pediatr Orthop*. 2017;37(7):e398–e402.
169. Shaha J, Cage JM, Black S, et al. Flexible intramedullary nails for femur fractures in pediatric patients heavier than 100 pounds. *J Pediatr Orthop*. 2018;38(2):88–93.
170. Shapiro F. Fractures of the femoral shaft in children. The overgrowth phenomenon. *Acta Orthop Scand*. 1981;52(6):649–655.
171. Sink EL, Faro F, Polousky J, et al. Decreased complications of pediatric femur fractures with a change in management. *J Pediatr Orthop*. 2010;30(7):633–637.
172. Sink EL, Gralla J, Repine M. Complications of pediatric femur fractures treated with titanium elastic nails: a comparison of fracture types. *J Pediatr Orthop*. 2005;25(5):577–580.
173. Sink EL, Hedequist D, Morgan SJ, et al. Results and technique of unstable pediatric femoral fractures treated with submuscular bridge plating. *J Pediatr Orthop*. 2006;26(2):177–181.
174. Skaggs DL, Leet AI, Money MD, et al. Secondary fractures associated with external fixation in pediatric femur fractures. *J Pediatr Orthop*. 1999;19(5):582–586.
175. Smith NC, Parker D, McNicol D. Supracondylar fractures of the femur in children. *J Pediatr Orthop*. 2001;21(5):600–603.
176. Sola J, Schoenecker PL, Gordon JE. External fixation of femoral shaft fractures in children: enhanced stability with the use of an auxiliary pin. *J Pediatr Orthop*. 1999;19(5):587–591.
177. Staheli LT. Femoral and tibial growth following femoral shaft fracture in childhood. *Clin Orthop Relat Res*. 1967;55:159–163.
178. Stannard JP, Christensen KP, Wilkins KE. Femur fractures in infants: a new therapeutic approach. *J Pediatr Orthop*. 1995;15(4):461–466.
179. Stans AA, Morrissy RT, Renwick SE. Femoral shaft fracture treatment in patients age 6 to 16 years. *J Pediatr Orthop*. 1999;19(2):222–228.
180. Thometz JG, Lamdan R. Osteonecrosis of the femoral head after intramedullary nailing of a fracture of the femoral shaft in an adolescent. A case report. *J Bone Joint Surg Am*. 1995;77(9):1423–1426.
181. Thompson JD, Buehler KC, Sponseller PD, et al. Shortening in femoral shaft fractures in children treated with spica cast. *Clin Orthop Relat Res*. 1997;338:74–78.
182. Timmerman LA, Rab GT. Intramedullary nailing of femoral shaft fractures in adolescents. *J Orthop Trauma*. 1993;7(4):331–337.
183. Tolo VT. External fixation in multiply injured children. *Orthop Clin North Am*. 1990;21(2):393–400.
184. Toren A, Goshen E, Katz M, et al. Bilateral femoral stress fractures in a child due to in-line (roller) skating. *Acta Paediatr*. 1997;86(3):332–333.
185. Townsend DR, Hoffinger S. Intramedullary nailing of femoral shaft fractures in children via the trochanter tip. *Clin Orthop Relat Res*. 2000;376:113–118.
186. Truesdell ED. Inequality of the lower extremities following fracture of the shaft of the femur in children. *Ann Surg*. 1921;74(4):498–500.
187. Vangsness CT Jr., DeCampos J, Merritt PO, et al. Meniscal injury associated with femoral shaft fractures. An arthroscopic evaluation of incidence. *J Bone Joint Surg Br*. 1993;75(2):207–209.
188. Verbeek HO. Does rotation deformity, following femur shaft fracture, correct during growth? *Reconstr Surg Traumatol*. 1979;17:75–81.
189. Viljanto J, Kiviluoto H, Paananen M. Remodelling after femoral shaft fracture in children. *Acta Chir Scand*. 1975;141(5):360–365.
190. Volpon JB, Perina MM, Okubo R, et al. Biomechanical performance of flexible intramedullary nails with end caps tested in distal segmental defects of pediatric femur models. *J Pediatr Orthop*. 2012;32(5):461–466.
191. Wall EJ, Jain V, Vora V, et al. Complications of titanium and stainless steel elastic nail fixation of pediatric femoral fractures. *J Bone Joint Surg Am*. 2008;90(6):1305–1313.
192. Wallace ME, Hoffman EB. Remodelling of angular deformity after femoral shaft fractures in children. *J Bone Joint Surg Br*. 1992;74(5):765–769.
193. Weiss AP, Schenck RC Jr., Sponseller PD, et al. Peroneal nerve palsy after early cast application for femoral fractures in children. *J Pediatr Orthop*. 1992;12(1):25–28.
194. Winquist RA, Hansen ST Jr., Clawson DK. Closed intramedullary nailing of femoral fractures. A report of five hundred and twenty cases. *J Bone Joint Surg Am*. 1984;66(4):529–539.
195. Wood JN, Fakeye O, Mondestin V, et al. Prevalence of abuse among young children with femur fractures: a systematic review. *BMC Pediatr*. 2014;14:169.
196. Ziv I, Blackburn N, Rang M. Femoral intramedullary nailing in the growing child. *J Trauma*. 1984;24(5):432–434.

25

Fractures of the Distal Femoral Physis

Lindsay Andras and Brian G. Smith

INTRODUCTION TO FRACTURES OF THE DISTAL FEMORAL PHYSIS

Distal femoral physeal injuries are uncommon, accounting for fewer than 2% of all physeal injuries.[39,51,65] However, complications requiring additional surgery occur after approximately 40% to 60% of these injuries.[2,24,29,36,49,72,83,84] The most common complication is growth disturbance of the distal femur resulting in angular deformity and/or shortening. In one meta-analysis of the published literature from 1950 to 2007 that included 564 fractures, 52% of fractures resulted in a growth disturbance.[7] This complication has been reported in patients of all ages regardless of the mechanism of injury, type of fracture, anatomic reduction of the fracture, and the type of treatment.[2,24,29,36,49,83,84] In addition to growth complications, knee stiffness, ligamentous disruption, neurovascular injuries, and compartment syndrome may occur as a result of these injuries.[24,29,72,81,84] Although the prognosis is better for very young children and nondisplaced fractures, complications may occur after any distal femoral physeal injury. Careful clinical assessment, complete diagnostic imaging, anatomic reduction, and secure immobilization or fixation to maintain reduction are necessary to ensure the best possible outcomes. Close follow-up at regular 6-month intervals after fracture healing until skeletal maturity is recommended to allow for early detection and treatment of clinically significant growth disturbances.

MECHANISMS OF INJURY OF FRACTURES OF THE DISTAL FEMORAL PHYSIS

Most distal femoral physeal fractures are the result of high-energy mechanisms, such as motor vehicle or sports-related trauma, and occur in older children and adolescents. Children between the ages of 2 and 11 years are less likely to sustain these fractures compared to adolescents, or even infants.[72]

Infants and Toddlers

Neonates are susceptible to distal femoral physeal fractures from birth trauma. Factors that predispose the newborn to this injury include breech presentation, macrosomia, difficult vaginal delivery, and rapid labor and delivery.[41] This injury has been also reported after delivery by cesarean section.[37] Child abuse should be suspected in infants and toddlers when a small peripheral metaphyseal fragment of bone, also called a "corner fracture," or the "classic metaphyseal lesion," is identified in association with widening of the distal femoral physis on radiographs of the femur or knee (Fig. 25-1).[47] This radiographic finding is pathognomonic

for child abuse. If this radiographic sign is identified, regardless of the reported mechanism of injury, the child should be carefully examined for other signs of mistreatment; a skeletal survey is obtained to identify other skeletal injuries and an immediate referral to your institution's child protection team and local child welfare services must be initiated.

Pathologic Fractures

Underlying conditions such as neuromuscular disorders, joint contractures, or nutritional deficiencies may predispose some children, regardless of age, for separation of the distal femoral epiphysis.[3–5,50,62] Like other pathologic fractures, distal femoral physeal separations that occur in children with underlying conditions typically result from low-energy mechanisms, such as inadvertent twisting of the limb during transferring from a bed or stretching during physical therapy. Nonambulatory children, such as children with cerebral palsy, are particularly susceptible to pathologic fractures due to disuse osteopenia. Ambulatory children with spina bifida may develop epiphysiolysis, or a chronic separation of the distal femoral physis, and be unaware of it because of altered sensation. Salter–Harris fractures of the distal femur have been reported during manipulation of the knee under anesthesia in children who had developed knee contractures secondary to arthrofibrosis after treatment of displaced tibial eminence fractures.[87]

Biomechanics of Injury

In the adolescent with open growth plates about the knee, the most common mechanism of fracture of the distal femoral

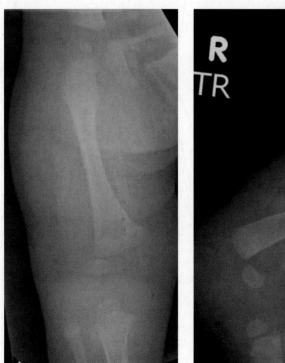
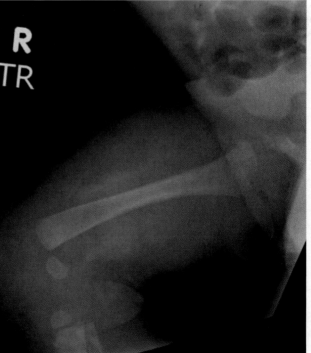

Figure 25-1. A 2-month-old female presenting with leg swelling. Radiographs revealed displaced Salter–Harris I fracture of the distal femur (**A** and **B**).

(continues)

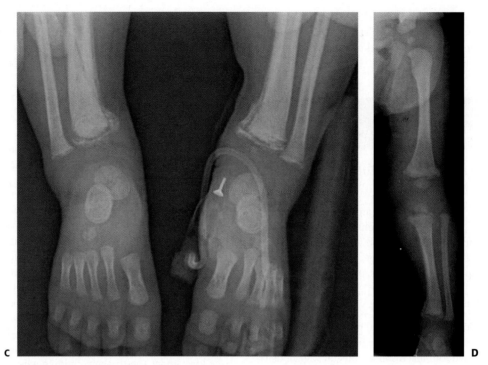

C

D

Figure 25-1. (*Continued*) Skeletal survey revealed numerous other fractures in various stages of healing consistent with nonaccidental trauma (**C** and **D**).

physis is a varus or valgus stress across the knee joint from a direct blow or buckling while landing from a jump or fall from a height. In most cases, this medially or laterally directed force is coupled with a torsional moment from direct application of force to the foot, or more commonly, from twisting of the knee on the planted foot. In an animal model, the physis is least able to resist torsional forces.[14] Knee hyperextension or hyperflexion forces result in sagittal plane displacement. The combination of forces applied to the physis, however, determines the direction of displacement of the distal fragment.

Loading the limb to failure across the immature knee is more likely to lead to physeal disruption due to tensile stresses that are transmitted through the ligaments to the adjacent physis than it is to disruption of the major knee ligaments.[25] Varus or valgus forces (Fig. 25-2A) create tension on one side of the physis and compression on the opposite side. The result is the disruption of the periosteum, which may become entrapped between the epiphysis and the metaphysis, and the perichondrial ring on the tension side, followed by a fracture plane that begins in the hypertrophic zone and proceeds in an irregular manner through the physis.[14] In adults, a similar mechanism of injury is more likely to cause ligamentous disruption rather than bone failure because ligaments of the mature knee are less able to withstand extreme tensile forces compared to the bone of the adult distal femur and proximal tibia (Fig. 25-2B).

INJURIES ASSOCIATED WITH FRACTURES OF THE DISTAL FEMORAL PHYSIS

Because many of these injuries are the result of high-energy mechanisms such as traffic accidents and motor sports, associated visceral injuries occur in approximately 5% of patients.[24]

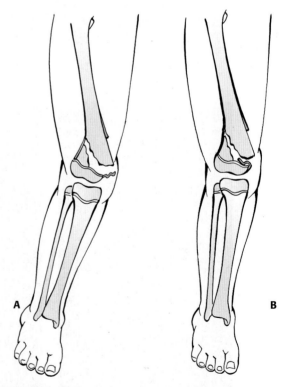

A

B

Figure 25-2. A: In a skeletally immature patient, valgus force at the knee is more likely to cause a physeal fracture of the distal femur than a medial collateral ligament tear, an injury that occurs in adults. **B:** With correction of the valgus deformity, periosteum may become entrapped. (Reprinted with permission from Skaggs DL, Flynn JF. Trauma about the knee, tibia, and foot. In: Skaggs DL, Flynn JF, eds. *Staying Out of Trouble in Pediatric Orthopaedics*. 1st ed. Philadelphia, PA: Lippincott Williams & Wilkins; 2006.)

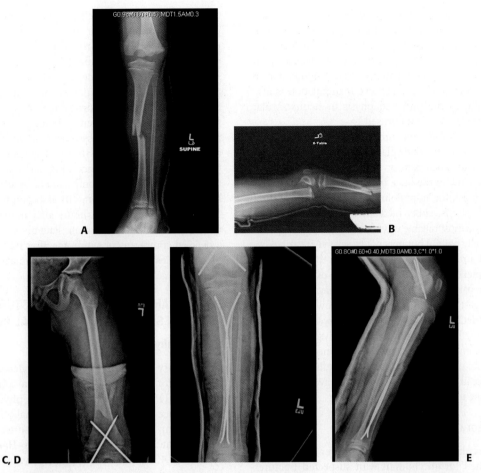

Figure 25-3. A 7-year-old girl struck by a car sustained this closed injury while crossing the street. Radiographs (**A,** AP and **B,** lat) reveal an anteriorly displaced distal femoral physeal separation and a tibial shaft fracture. Upon admission she had no pulse in the extremity. She underwent emergency open reduction and fixation of the distal femur and IM nail fixation of the tibia (**C–E**). Her pulses returned to normal after femur reduction. She did not develop a compartment syndrome.

Other musculoskeletal injuries are seen in association with distal femoral physeal fractures in 10% to 15% of patients.[24,84] Other long bone fractures, as well as pelvic and spine fractures, must be ruled out, especially if the mechanism of injury is high-energy motor trauma (Fig. 25-3). Knee ligament disruption, however, is the most common concomitant musculoskeletal injury. Knee instability is diagnosed in 8% to 37% of patients[10,24] and is typically diagnosed after fracture healing with the initiation of rehabilitation and return to activities. Salter–Harris type III fractures of the medial femoral condyle are most frequently associated with anterior cruciate ligament injuries.[15,53,69,86] Open fractures and vascular injuries are uncommon associated injuries, occurring in about 3% of patients. Peroneal nerve injury occurs in about 2% to 7% of patients with displaced fractures.[9,24]

SIGNS AND SYMPTOMS OF FRACTURES OF THE DISTAL FEMORAL PHYSIS

Presentation

Emergency department assessment for children who are victims of high-energy trauma with a suspected distal femoral physeal separation should be initially evaluated by the trauma team to identify potential life-threatening injuries, to evaluate the ABCs, and to initiate resuscitation protocols if indicated. On the initial survey, head trauma, thoracoabdominal injuries, unstable spine and pelvic fractures, and limb-threatening extremity injuries are the priorities. After stabilization of the cardiovascular status, a thorough secondary survey should focus on the extremities. Long-bone fractures and ligamentous injuries of the extremities are identified with a careful orthopedic examination of all four extremities. Although severe injuries may occur in association with fractures of the distal femoral physis, this fracture, however, occurs as an isolated injury in most patients.

For patients with displaced distal femoral physeal fractures, the diagnosis may be obvious. Patients typically describe severe pain, giving way of the limb and obvious knee deformity after a sports injury, motor vehicle accident, or other high-energy mechanism and are unable to walk or bear weight on the injured limb. On examination, visible limb malalignment, severe swelling, and often ecchymosis at the apex of the knee deformity are identified. In fractures with severe displacement, the skin at the apex may be tented or puckered from protrusion of the metaphyseal distal femur through the periosteum and quadriceps muscle into the dermis. Hematoma may be palpable beneath the skin. Abrasions or laceration of the overlying soft tissues may be a clue to the mechanism of injury or to an open fracture. Assessment of knee range of motion and ligament stability is not possible in most cases with obvious displacement because of pain and the poor reliability of the examination in the face of fracture instability. Aggressive manipulation is also potentially harmful to the fractured physis or neurovascular structures that are already compromised.

Patients with nondisplaced fractures are more difficult to diagnose. Many children with nondisplaced distal femoral physeal fractures present with knee pain or mild knee swelling after a twisting injury or blow to the knee but are able to bear weight, albeit with often a painful limp. Point tenderness at the level of the distal femoral physis, either medially or laterally about the knee, is perhaps the most reliable way to detect this injury. Range of motion is typically painful but may not be severely restricted in all cases, and fracture crepitus is absent because the periosteum is not fully disrupted. Varus/valgus stress testing of the knee ligaments is usually painful and, in some cases, may reveal subtle movement or suggest instability. The examiner, however, must be mindful that a skeletally immature patient with point tenderness at the physis is more likely to have sustained a physeal fracture of the distal femur, compared to disruption of the medial or lateral collateral ligaments of the knee. Therefore, forceful or repeated stress testing of the knee in these cases should be avoided to minimize trauma to the injured physis.

Motor and Sensory Testing

Careful neurovascular examination of the lower leg and foot must be performed for all children with suspected fractures of the distal femoral physis, especially for those with obvious limb deformity. Complete motor and sensory testing of the distal limb is necessary to identify injury of the sciatic nerve and its branches, the tibial and common peroneal nerves. Because the peroneal nerve is injured in about 2% of patients with displaced fractures[9] and is the most commonly injured nerve related to this fracture,[24] it is especially important that anterior (deep branch) and lateral (superficial branch) compartment muscle function and lower leg sensation be carefully documented. This nerve injury is typically a neurapraxia, the result of stretching from anterior or medial displacement of the distal femoral epiphysis.

Vascular Assessment

Although vascular injuries are rare after fractures of the distal femoral physis,[24,49,72,84] the vascular status must also be evaluated carefully. The distal pulses are palpated in the foot and ankle and other signs of adequate perfusion are evaluated. These other signs include assessment of capillary refill, skin temperature, and signs of venous insufficiency such as distal swelling or cyanosis. Doppler ultrasound and measurement of ankle–brachial indices may be useful for detecting less obvious vascular injury when pulses and other signs are equivocal. Laceration, intimal tear, and thrombosis in the popliteal artery may occur by direct injury to the artery by the distal end of the metaphysis when the epiphysis is displaced anteriorly during a hyperextension injury.[9,24,75] Because anteriorly displaced

fractures have an increased risk of neurovascular damage in general compared to other directions of displacement,[20,81] the patient must be particularly suspicious for a vascular injury with obvious hyperextension deformity of the knee.

Compartment syndrome after distal femoral physeal fracture is rare but in one series occurred in 1.2% of patients.[24] Signs of compartment syndrome in the lower leg such as severe swelling, tense compartments, increasing use of analgesics or anxiety, and pain with passive motion and other examination abnormalities consistent with the diagnosis are also evaluated. Compartmental pressure recordings should be obtained if there are clinical findings of compartment syndrome of the lower leg. Compartment syndrome in association with this fracture is more likely to manifest hours after injury; however, not at the time of initial presentation. Patients at risk for developing a delayed compartment syndrome after fracture are those with other injuries of the lower leg, such as tibial shaft fractures, and those with compromised vascularity.[24]

IMAGING AND OTHER DIAGNOSTIC STUDIES FOR FRACTURES OF THE DISTAL FEMORAL PHYSIS

Radiography

High-quality orthogonal radiographic views of the femur and knee are for diagnosing distal femoral physeal separations (Table 25-1). On the AP radiographic, physeal widening and the presence of a fracture line proximally in the metaphysis or distally in the epiphysis allows the surgeon to differentiate between the four most common Salter–Harris types, that is, types 1 to 4. In addition, epiphyseal varus (also called apex lateral angulation) or valgus (also called apex medial angulation) and medial or lateral translation in the coronal plane are determined on the AP view. The lateral projection defines the amount of angulation and translation of the epiphysis in the sagittal plane. The anteriorly displaced epiphysis is usually tilted so that the distal articular surface faces anteriorly. This direction of displacement is alternatively called hyperextension of the epiphysis or apex posterior angulation. The posteriorly displaced epiphysis is tilted downward so that the distal articular surface faces the popliteal fossa, sometimes described as hyperflexion of the epiphysis or apex anterior angulation. Minor degrees of displacement may be difficult to measure on plain films unless the x-ray projection is precisely in line with the plane of fracture. Even small amounts of displacement are significant.[36,49] Rotational malalignment of the distal fragment relative to the proximal fragment may be identified on either view and is dramatic in some cases with severe displacement.

Diagnosis of minimally displaced distal femoral physeal fractures is challenging. Because the physis is normally radiolucent, injury is typically identified because of physeal widening, epiphyseal displacement, or metaphyseal bone injury suggestive of a fracture. Without obvious radiographic abnormalities, nondisplaced Salter–Harris type I or III fracture without separation can be easily overlooked.[5,73,86] Oblique views of the distal femur may reveal an occult fracture through the epiphysis or metaphysis. In the past, stress views of the distal femur were recommended for patients with negative radiographs who

TABLE 25-1. Imaging Studies in the Evaluation of Distal Femoral Physeal Fractures

Study	Indications	Limitations
Standard radiographs	First study, often sufficient	May miss nondisplaced Salter–Harris type I or III fractures or underestimate fracture displacement
Computed tomography (CT)	Best defines fracture pattern and amount of displacement Useful for planning surgery, especially for metaphyseal comminution	Poor cartilage visualization. Increased radiation exposure Less useful than MRI in evaluating for occult Salter–Harris type I or III fractures
Magnetic resonance imaging (MRI)	Evaluation of occult Salter–Harris type I fracture, especially in infants with little epiphyseal ossification Identifies associated soft tissue injuries, especially with Salter–Harris type III fractures	Availability, cost, duration of procedure Fracture geometry less clear than with CT scans
Stress views	Differentiate occult Salter–Harris fracture from ligament injury	Painful, muscle spasm may not permit opening of fracture if patient awake. Potentially harmful to physis
Contralateral radiographs	Infants, or to assess physeal width Follow-up to compare growth	Usually not helpful in acute fractures
Ultrasonography, arthrography	Infants to assess swelling and displacement of epiphysis	Not useful after infancy

have an effusion or tenderness localized to the physis.[79] However, it is our practice to forego stress radiographs because they are painful to the patient and may damage the already compromised physis. Presumptive Salter–Harris I fractures are then either immobilized for 1 to 2 weeks and reexamined or are further evaluated with MRI.[53,79,82,86]

Magnetic Resonance Imaging

MRI is the most commonly used advanced imaging study for evaluating traumatic knee injuries in children and adolescents. The primary utility of MRI is to identify acute knee injuries when the examination and radiographs are nondiagnostic or to confirm diagnostic suspicions. In one large MRI study of 315 adolescents with acute traumatic knee injuries, physeal injuries of the distal femur were diagnosed in 7 patients with negative plain radiographs.[18] MRI also facilitates identification of knee ligament tears, meniscal pathology, and osteochondral fractures that may occur concomitantly with distal femoral physeal fractures,[53] both in the acute setting and after fracture healing. MR arteriography is one method of evaluating vascular anatomy and flow in patients with an abnormal vascular examination in association with displaced distal femoral physeal fractures.

Computed Tomography

Computed tomography (CT) scan is recommended for all patients with Salter–Harris III and IV fractures diagnosed on plain radiographs. In one study, CT identified fracture displacement and comminution that was not recognized on plain radiographs of the knee. The authors encouraged its use for evaluation of these fractures to identify displacement, define fracture geometry, and plan surgical fixation.[45] CT may also be useful to identify fractures and displacement in cases where the plain radiographs are negative but the examination is suspicious for a distal femoral physeal fracture.

SPECIAL SITUATIONS OF FRACTURES OF THE DISTAL FEMORAL PHYSIS

Neonate

Separation of the distal femoral epiphysis in a neonate is particularly difficult to diagnose on initial x-rays unless there is displacement, because only the center of the epiphysis is ossified at birth. This ossification center is in line with the axis of the femoral shaft on both AP and lateral views in normal infants. Any degree of malalignment of the ossification center from the shaft should raise suspicion for this fracture. Comparison views of the opposite knee and other modalities may also be helpful to identify its presence in neonates when radiographs of the affected leg are equivocal. MRI, performed under anesthesia, is another commonly used diagnostic imaging study that may help to identify a separation of the unossified femoral epiphysis.[89]

Unique to the neonate is the use of ultrasonography[35] to evaluate distal femoral physeal separation. Typically used to evaluate the immature hip for developmental dysplasia of the hip, diagnostic ultrasound imaging may also be used to evaluate the cartilaginous distal femur in a young child with incomplete ossification of the distal femoral epiphysis. Although this study is safe and readily available, it is unfamiliar to many technicians and radiologists, making its reliability questionable unless performed by an experienced team. This modality may be used not only to diagnose injuries but also to guide reduction. Knee arthrography, another option for evaluating the immature distal femoral epiphysis for possible disruption, is primarily used to facilitate reduction and fixation in the operating room.

One should remember to consider infection in a neonate with a painful or immobile limb.

Physeal Arrest

An effective method for determining the viability of the physis after healing of a traumatic injury is MRI performed with fat-suppressed three-dimensional spoiled gradient-recalled echo sequences.[22] Impending growth disturbance can be identified early with this MRI[22,26] technique and MRI can be used to map the extent of physeal bony bar formation to determine if excision is an option for treatment.[22,48] Although CT may also be used to map the location and area of physeal bars, it is out preference to use MRI because it does not expose the child to radiation and evaluates the quality of the physeal cartilage adjacent to the bar, a possible predictor of the success of physeal excision.

CLASSIFICATION OF FRACTURES OF THE DISTAL FEMORAL PHYSIS

Salter–Harris Classification

Salter–Harris Type	Energy Required	Risk of Physeal Arrest
1	Mild to moderate	Low
2	Moderate	Moderate
3	Significant	High
4	Significant	High
5	Significant	High
6	Moderate	Unknown

Direction of Displacement	Risks
Anterior	Vascular injury
Posterior	Nerve injury
Medial/Lateral	Neurovascular injury

Magnitude of Displacement	Risks
>50% of diameter of metaphysis	Higher rate of complications

Age at Fracture	Prognosis
Under age 2	Good
2–11	Fair to Poor
12 and above	Fair to Poor

Several types of classification schemes have been used to describe fractures of the distal each physis, each with some merit because of the information that its use provides to the surgeon. The Salter–Harris classification[75] is the most widely used classification scheme (Fig. 25-4). This familiar classification system, based on plain radiographs, is useful for the description of the types of physeal fractures of the distal femur. As opposed to its application to other physeal fractures, however, the Salter–Harris scheme is not as reliable in predicting the risk of growth disturbance as it relates to the fracture types.[24,49] For many physeal fractures in other anatomic sites, risk of growth disturbance is smaller after type I and II fractures and higher after types III

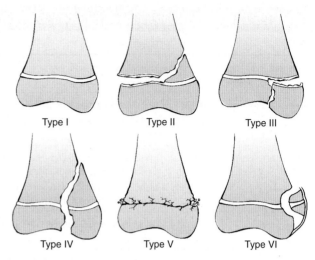

Figure 25-4. The Salter–Harris classification of fractures involving the distal femoral physis.

and IV. Distal femoral physeal fractures, however, are at risk for significant growth disturbance regardless of type.[7,49,83] This classification scheme is useful for treatment planning and is also a good indicator of the mechanism of injury.[20]

Salter–Harris I Fractures

The Salter–Harris type I pattern is a fracture that traverses the distal femoral physis, without extension either proximally into the metaphysis or distally into the epiphysis or knee joint (Fig. 25-5). Anatomically, this fracture cleaves the physis predominately across the physeal zones of cell hypertrophy and provisional calcification. Because of the undulation of the distal femoral physis, likely evolutionarily developed to increase the stability of the physeal plate when subject to shear stress, most distal femoral physeal fractures do not propagate cleanly across these zones but instead also extend into the germinal zones of the physis. This encroachment of the fracture line into cartilage precursor cells is likely the explanation for increased rates of growth disturbance after Salter–Harris I and II fracture types.

Although this fracture pattern may be seen in any age group of skeletally immature patients, it occurs more frequently in infants, the result of birth trauma or abuse, and in adolescents with sports-related trauma. Many Salter–Harris I fractures are nondisplaced and may go undetected. Sometimes, the diagnosis is made only in retrospect, after subperiosteal new bone formation occurs along the adjacent metaphysis, evident on follow-up radiographs 10 to 14 days after injury or by MRI. When displacement is present before the age of 2 years, it usually occurs in the sagittal plane. Approximately 15% of physeal fractures of the distal femur are Salter–Harris type I fractures.[7]

Salter–Harris II Fractures

The Salter–Harris type II pattern is the most common type of separation of the distal femoral epiphysis (Figs. 25-6 and 25-7). This pattern is characterized by a fracture line that extends through the physis incompletely and then exits proximally via

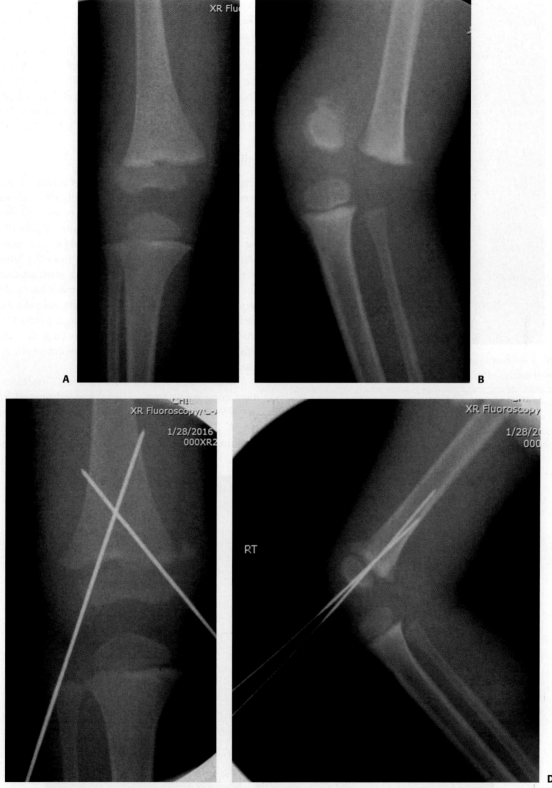

Figure 25-5. Preoperative (**A,B**) and postoperative (**C,D**) radiographs of a 2.5-year-old boy with Salter–Harris I right distal femur fracture, treated with closed reduction and percutaneous pinning. Pins are separated widely at fracture site to provide more stability.

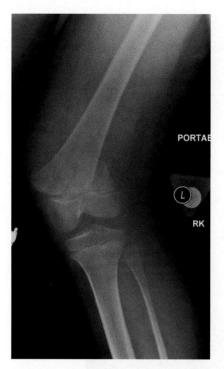

Figure 25-6. A 10-year-old male who was hit by a car and sustained this Salter–Harris II fracture of the distal femur. Patient was very petite so the fracture was reduced and stabilized with K-wires which were removed promptly at 4 weeks to decrease risk of infection. Follow-up radiographs 2 years later showed no evidence of growth disturbance. However, given the lateral location of the metaphyseal spike if the patient had developed a growth arrest a varus malalignment would have resulted.

an oblique extension of the fracture line through the metaphysis. The metaphyseal corner that remains attached to the epiphysis is called the Thurston Holland fragment. Although the direction of displacement varies, typically the direction of displacement is also the location of the metaphyseal fragment because the metaphyseal spike occurs on the side of compression forces. This fracture type may also be seen in children of all ages but is more common in adolescents. Slightly more than half (57%) of all distal femoral physeal fractures are Salter–Harris II fractures.[7]

Salter–Harris III Fractures

The Salter–Harris type III injury has a fracture line that traverses part of the physis then exits distally, with extension of the fracture line vertically across the physis, epiphysis, and its articular surface (Fig. 25-8). Most Salter–Harris III injuries of the distal femur traverse the medial physis and extend into the joint, separating the medial condyle from the lateral condyle of the distal femur. These injuries are often produced by valgus stress across the knee, the same mechanism of injury that produces medial collateral and cruciate ligament disruption in skeletally mature patients may have an associated injury to the cruciate ligaments.[15,66] This fracture occurs most frequently in older children and adolescents and comprises about 10% of all distal femoral physeal fractures.[7]

Nondisplaced Salter–Harris III and IV fractures and other more complex patterns of distal femoral physeal fracture may not always be detectable or fully delineated on plain radiographs, requiring MRI or CT to identify.[44,52,53,57] It has been hypothesized that the Salter–Harris type III fracture, seen mostly

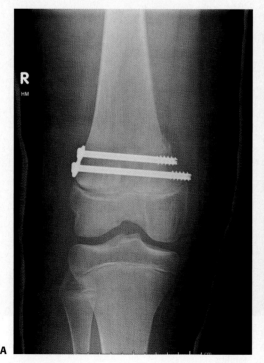
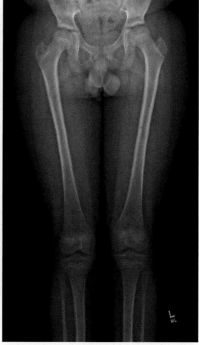

Figure 25-7 A 15-year-old male with right Salter–Harris II fracture after a bike accident. Fracture was stabilized with two cannulated screws using a washer for additional compression (**A**). Patient is currently being monitored to look for any evidence of growth arrest (**B**). Given the fracture pattern, if this were to occur, we would expect developing valgus malalignment (in contrast to the example in Fig. 25–6).

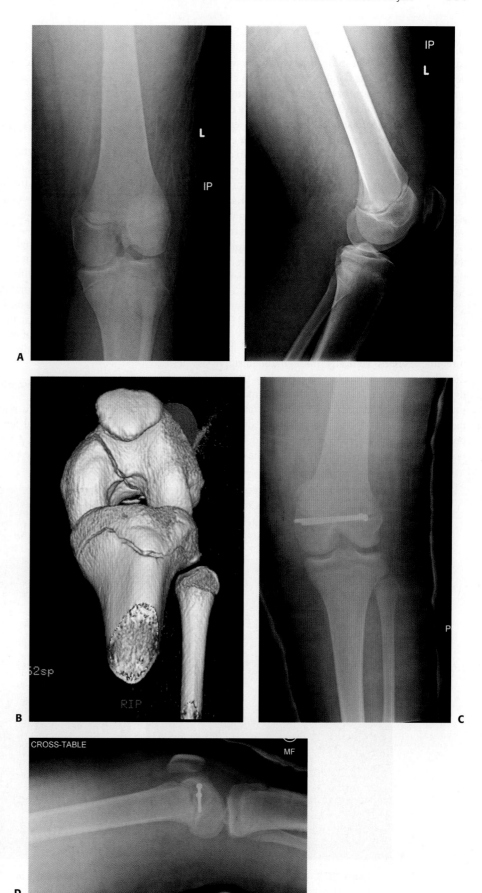

Figure 25-8. 15-year-old male with left Salter Harris III fracture shown in AP and lateral radiographs (**A**)and also visualized on CT (**B**). Although in the AP view the screws appear to be at the level of the physis (**C**), it is clearly visualized on the lateral that they are below this level (**D**), highlighting the undulating nature the distal femur physis.

in older children and adolescents, may occur as a consequence of the progression of closure of the distal femoral physis. This pattern of fracture occurs near skeletal maturity when the central portion of the distal femoral physis begins to close before the medial and lateral parts of the physis, similar to a juvenile Tillaux fracture of the distal tibia.[53] Occasionally, a type III fracture may occur in the coronal plane of the distal femoral condyle, more commonly the medial femoral condyle, similar to the "Hoffa fracture" of the posterior condyle seen in adults.[44,57] This fracture is difficult to diagnose with standard x-rays[73] and is also challenging to reduce and fix. A triplane fracture of the distal femur, a fracture that appears as a Salter–Harris I injury in the sagittal plane and a Salter–Harris III fracture in the coronal and sagittal planes, has also been described.[52] This triplane fracture is not completely analogous to the classic triplane fracture of the ankle, however, because, while the fracture line extends in three dimensions about the physis, the distal femoral physis is completely open.

Salter–Harris IV Fractures

In Salter–Harris type IV injuries of the distal femur, the fracture line extends vertically through the metaphysis, across the physis, ultimately extending through the epiphysis and its articular surface (Fig. 25-9). It is at times difficult to distinguish between Salter–Harris III and IV fractures because the metaphyseal fragment may be small and difficult to identify on plain radiographs. Salter–Harris III and IV fractures likely occur from similar mechanisms and in the same age ranges,

with both presenting management challenges that require anatomic realignment of the joint line and physis to minimize risk of growth disturbance. Of fractures of the distal femoral physis, this fracture type is seen slightly more frequently than type III fractures, accounting for about 12% of fractures.[7]

Salter–Harris V Fractures

When initial radiographs of the distal femur are normal but subsequent imaging months after the traumatic injury identify a growth arrest, this fracture is classified as a Salter–Harris V.[80] It is hypothesized that compression forces across the physis causes damage to the cartilage-producing cells in the growth plate but no epiphyseal displacement. Axial loading of the limb, such as from a fall from a height, is considered the classic mechanism of injury. It is important to bear in mind, however, that premature growth arrest also may occur in association with nonphyseal fractures of the femoral and tibial shafts.[8,33,56,77] MRI may identify bone contusion on both sides of the growth plate after a traumatic injury that may be a harbinger to its occurrence.[77] Approximately 3% of physeal separations of the distal femur are Salter–Harris V fractures.

Salter–Harris VI Fractures

Rang[60,71] proposed a sixth type of Salter–Harris fracture that applies to the distal femur in children and adolescents with open growth plates. A type VI injury is an avulsion fracture of the periphery of the physis, resulting in an osteocartilaginous

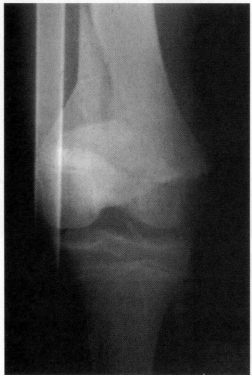
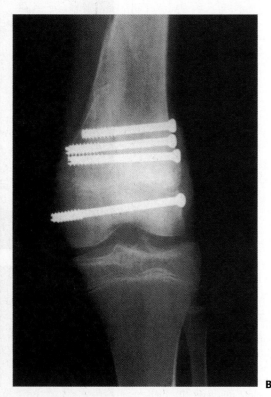

Figure 25-9. A: Comminuted Salter–Harris type IV fracture of the distal femur in a 14-year-old boy involved in a motor vehicle accident. **B:** Six months after open reduction and internal fixation with cannulated screws in the metaphysis and epiphysis.

fragment comprising a portion of the perichondrial ring of the physis as well as small pieces of metaphyseal and epiphyseal bone. These may occur at many different anatomic sites but are seen most commonly about the physes of the distal fibula, distal femur, and distal tibia.[32] The mechanism of distal femur injury is typically an indirect force such as varus stress that causes avulsion of the fragment from partial detachment of the proximal lateral collateral ligament, often resulting in no displacement of the epiphysis. Alternatively, open injuries that abrade or skeletonize the area around the physis or loss of a peripheral portion of the physis, such as occurs from lawnmower injuries or motor vehicle trauma, and burns around the physis are other possible mechanisms. This injury is not included in many large series of physeal fractures of the femur and is exceedingly rare. In one series of 29,878 children's fractures, only 36 were identified as Salter–Harris VI injuries.[32]

Classification by Displacement

Several authors have evaluated direction and magnitude of displacement to predict final outcome.[2,36,49,84] Direction of displacement may guide treatment but does not predict the frequency of poor outcomes.[2,36,81] Anterior displacement of the epiphysis, or apex posterior angulation, resulting from violent hyperextension of the knee is associated with an increased risk of neurovascular damage.[20,81] Peroneal nerve injury may occur with significant medial or lateral displacement of the epiphysis. Otherwise, direction of displacement has not been shown to correlate with other complications such as angular deformity, growth disturbance, or loss of motion.

By contrast, the magnitude of displacement has been shown to be predictive of complications.[2,36,84] The critical amount of displacement that is associated with worsening outcomes varies but, generally, displaced fractures of all Salter–Harris types are more likely to develop complications compared to nondisplaced fractures. In one study, fractures with displacement of greater than 50% of the transverse diameter of the distal femoral metaphysis on either radiographic view were more likely to develop growth complications compared to less displaced fractures.[84] Others have determined that displacement of more than one-third of bone width correlates with more frequent

complications.[2,36,49,84] Fractures without bony contact between the fragments and those with metaphyseal comminution,[36] both radiographic indicators of high-energy trauma, have also been correlated with an increased risk of complications.

Classification by Age

Age at the time of injury also correlates with the frequency and severity of complications.[72] Distal femoral epiphyseal fractures in children aged 2 to 11 years typically result from high-energy mechanisms and have a poorer prognosis compared to fractures in children younger than 2 years of age or older than 11 years.[24,72] Separations of the distal femoral epiphysis before the age of 2 years generally have satisfactory outcomes,[72,84] possibly because epiphyseal undulations and the central peak are not as prominent in infants (Fig. 25-10A), allowing fractures to occur with less force and less damage to germinal cells and their blood supply.[58] In adolescents, low-energy sports injuries are the most frequent cause of epiphyseal separation. Because children in this age group have little growth remaining, the consequences of growth disturbance, should this complication occur, are often trivial. In juveniles and adolescents, the fracture may pass through the central prominence and lead to central growth arrest because of interference with vascularity in this region or because of the fracture plane exiting and reentering the central physis (Fig. 25-10B).[58,72,82]

OUTCOME MEASURES FOR FRACTURES OF THE DISTAL FEMORAL PHYSIS

In the largest published series[2,24,84] outcomes of distal femoral physeal fractures are determined by clinical assessment and radiographic parameters at follow-up. The primary clinical factors are the resulting neurovascular status of the affected limb and the range of motion of the knee. Secondarily, knee stability is assessed by subjective reporting of symptoms of instability and objective clinical stress testing of the knee ligaments. No study reported knee scores or the results of instrumented tests of knee ligament laxity.

Radiographic assessment of the injured limb is utilized in most studies to assess fracture healing, to identify physeal bar

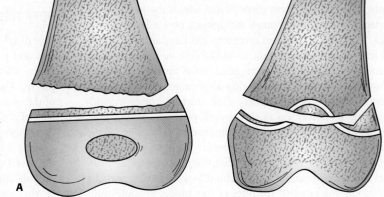

Figure 25-10. A: Distal femoral physeal separation prior to the age of 2 years may not disrupt growth because the physis is flat. **B:** After the age of 2 years, a central ridge and four quadrants of undulation develop in the distal femur. Fractures in this age group are more likely to cross multiple planes of bone and cartilage.

formation, to measure angular deformity about the knee, and to assess for leg-length discrepancies that may result from a growth disturbance. Fracture healing is determined subjectively by identifying fracture line bridging as well as clinical signs of healing. Physeal bar formation may be identified on plain radiographs but also is assessed by MRI or CT scan. Angular deformity is determined by measuring angulation of the fracture fragments or the tibiofemoral angle. Although limb-length discrepancy may be determined clinically, bilateral lower extremity scanograms, obtained by the Bell–Thompson method or by CT scanning, are utilized to assess the true LLD.

PATHOANATOMY AND APPLIED ANATOMY RELATING TO FRACTURES OF THE DISTAL FEMORAL PHYSIS

OSSIFICATION AND GROWTH

The epiphysis of the distal femur is the first epiphysis to ossify and is present at birth, appearing as a small round bony structure distal to and in line with the axis of the metaphysis. This epiphyseal ossification center is the only radiographic sign of the larger cartilaginous anlagen of the distal femur. With maturation, the bony distal epiphysis enlarges as the cartilage model ossifies and becomes bicondylar, at times appearing irregular along the distal articular surface as ossification proceeds. From birth to skeletal maturity, the distal femoral physis contributes 70% of the growth of the femur and 37% of the growth of the lower extremity. The annual rate of growth is approximately three-eighths of an inch or 9 to 10 mm. The growth of the distal femur, like the physes of other long bones, ceases at a mean skeletal age of 14 years in girls and 16 years in boys, with a wide range of variability.[1,88]

PHYSEAL ANATOMY

At birth, the distal femoral physis is flat, or planar, making this physis in infants the least stable compared to other age groups. With maturation, the physis assumes an undulating and more convoluted shape.[46] By the age of 2 to 3 years, the physis develops an intercondylar groove, or central prominence, as well as sulci that traverse medial and lateral proximal to each condyle. This configuration effectively divides the physis into four quadrants, each with concave surfaces that match the four convex surfaces of the distal femoral metaphysis over a large surface area. The complex physeal geometry and large area of the distal femoral physis contribute to its stability by better resisting shear and torsional forces compared to the smaller, flat physes of infants. The perichondral ring also circumferentially reinforces the physis at its periphery. This structure, combined with the some reinforcement of the physeal periphery by the knee ligaments, provides additional resistance to disruption of the physis.[17,55] During adolescence, however, the perichondrial ring becomes thinner. It is hypothesized that this change contributes to relative weakening of the distal femoral physis, partially explaining the fact that fractures of this physis in adolescents

are more frequent and generally occur from lower-energy mechanisms compared to children of 2 to 11 years of age.

The irregular configuration of the physis, while contributing to stability, however, also is an important factor in the high incidence of growth disturbance from these fractures. Fracture lines, instead of cleanly traversing the hypertrophic zone and area of provisional calcification, extend through multiple regions of the physis and damage germinal cells regardless of fracture type.[72] In addition, during reduction of displaced fractures, epiphyseal ridges may grind against the metaphyseal projections and further damage cartilage-producing resting cells. Minimizing contact and shear across the physis during reduction is preferable to improve the chances of normal growth after injury. Reductions in the operating room with muscle-relaxing agents, use of traction during reduction, avoiding a tourniquet which can tighten muscles, and limiting the number of closed manipulation attempts before converting to open reduction are some techniques that are generally recommended.

BONY ANATOMY

Proximal to the medial border of the medial condyle, a small area of the metaphysis of the distal femur widens abruptly, forming the adductor tubercle. The lateral metaphysis, by contrast, flares only minimally at the proximal part of the lateral condyle, forming the lateral epicondyle. The distal femur is divided into two discrete condyles at the level of the knee joint, separated by the intercondylar notch. Nearly the entire distal femur is covered by hyaline cartilage for articulation with the proximal tibia. The anterior, or patellar, surface just proximal to the intercondylar notch, has a shallow midline concavity to accommodate the longitudinal convex ridge of the undersurface of the patella. Posteriorly, the distal femur contacts the tibial cartilage as the knee flexes. The posterior condyles, projections of the femoral condyles posteriorly, contain this cartilage that extends on either side of the intercondylar notch and nearly to the posterior margin of the physis.

The distal femur has well-defined normal anatomical alignment parameters. The mechanical axis of the femur is formed by a line between the centers of the hip and knee joints (Fig. 25-11). A line tangential to the distal surfaces of the two condyles (the joint line) is in approximately 3 degrees of valgus relative to the mechanical axis. The longitudinal axis of the diaphysis of the femur inclines medially in a distal direction at an angle of 6 degrees relative to the mechanical axis.[34]

SOFT TISSUE ANATOMY

The distal femoral physis is completely extrasynovial. Anteriorly and posteriorly, the synovial membrane and joint capsule of the knee attach to the femoral epiphysis just distal to the physis. The suprapatellar pouch, however, is a ballooning out of the synovium that extends proximally over the anterior surface of the metaphysis. On the medial and lateral surfaces of the epiphysis, the proximal attachment of the synovium and capsule is distal to the physis and separated from the physis by the insertions of the collateral ligaments. The strong posterior capsule and all of the major ligaments of the knee are attached to the epiphysis distal to the physis. Varus/valgus-directed

NEUROVASCULAR ANATOMY

Arterial Anatomy

The popliteal artery runs along the posterior surface of the distal femur, separated from it by only a thin layer of fat.[19] Directly proximal to the femoral condyles, this artery sends off transverse branches medially and laterally, called the medial and lateral superior geniculate arteries, along the surface of the distal femoral metaphysis beneath the overlying muscles which they supply. The popliteal artery then continues distally, adjacent to the posterior capsule of the knee joint between the femoral condyles. At this level, the middle geniculate artery branches from it anteriorly to the posterior surface of the epiphysis, providing the primary blood supply to the distal femoral epiphysis and the physis. The distal femoral epiphysis, however, receives its blood supply from a rich anastomosis of vessels. Because of this, osteonecrosis of this epiphysis is exceedingly rare, occurring only in situations where distal femoral epiphysis is completely stripped of its soft tissue attachments. Since the popliteal artery and its branches course along the posterior distal femur, it is especially vulnerable to injury because of contact with the distal femoral metaphysis from hyperextension injuries of the knee with anterior displacement of the epiphysis. While tenting of the artery causing occlusion and arterial spasm are the most common reasons for vascular abnormalities related to distal femoral physeal fractures, intimal injury and laceration may also occur.

Nerve Supply

The sciatic nerve, extending from the upper thigh, divides into the common peroneal and tibial nerves just proximal to the popliteal space. The peroneal nerve then descends posteriorly, between the biceps femoris muscle and the lateral head of the gastrocnemius muscle, to a point just distal to the head of the fibula. The peroneal nerve then changes course, wrapping around the proximal fibula to enter the anterior compartment of the lower leg, where it divides into the deep and superficial branches. The common peroneal nerve's course between muscles protects it from direct injury from fracture ends. This nerve, however, because of limited excursion due to its anteriorly directed course around the fibular head, is susceptible to injury from stretch. Neurapraxia, and even axonotmesis of the common peroneal nerve, results most commonly from fractures with severe anterior displacement and medial translation (varus displacement).[81] The tibial nerve, coursing through the popliteal space adjacent to the popliteal artery, enters the calf along the arch of the soleus muscle. This nerve is vulnerable to injury from mechanisms that are similar to those that cause injury to the popliteal artery, although clinically tibial nerve injury is rare.

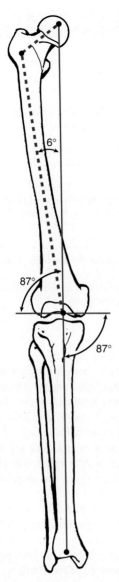

Figure 25-11. The mechanical and anatomic axis of the lower extremity. Note that the knee joint is in a mean of 3 degrees of valgus. The femoral shaft intersects the transverse plane of the distal femoral articular surface at an angle of 87 degrees.

forces that would cause collateral ligament disruption in adults often result in physeal separations in children and adolescents because the tensile strength of the ligaments is greater than that of the physis. The anterior and posterior cruciate ligaments originate in the upward-sloping roof of the intercondylar notch distal to the physis. Compression and tension forces can be transmitted across the extended knee to the epiphysis of the femur by taut ligaments. The medial and lateral heads of the gastrocnemius muscles originate from the distal femur proximal to the joint capsule and physis. Although forces generated by the gastrocnemius are probably not a major factor that contributes to fractures of the distal femoral physis, pull of the muscles may be a deforming force for metaphyseal fractures of the distal femur.

TREATMENT OPTIONS FOR FRACTURES OF THE DISTAL FEMORAL PHYSIS

Distal femoral physeal fractures in children and adolescents are challenging fractures that require careful preoperative evaluation and assessment of the injury including both physical and

TABLE 25-2. Methods of Treatment for Distal Femoral Physeal Fractures

Treatment	Pros	Cons	Indications
Closed reduction and immobilization	Avoids anesthesia	High risk of loss of reduction	Nondisplaced, stable fractures
Closed reduction and screw fixation	Minimal dissection	Only in reducible fractures	Reducible Salter–Harris type II fractures Nondisplaced Salter–Harris type III and IV fractures
Closed reduction and smooth pinning	Minimal dissection	Pins may lead to joint infection or require later removal	Reducible Salter–Harris type I fractures, and Salter–Harris type II fractures with small metaphyseal fragment
Open reduction and screws and/or pins	Anatomic reduction	Stiffness	Irreducible Salter–Harris type I and II fractures, displaced Salter–Harris type III and IV fractures
External fixation	Allows soft tissue access	Pin site (joint) infection	Severe soft tissue injury
Rigid plate crossing physis	Rigid fixation	Can stop future growth when spans physis	Adolescents near the end of growth. Severe injuries with growth disturbance inevitable Possible temporary fixation with extraperiosteal locked plating removed soon after union

radiographic examinations so as to devise an appropriate treatment plan (Table 25-2). The treatment principles for these injuries can be summarized as follows:

1. Restore the anatomy without iatrogenically compromising the distal femoral physis.
2. Stabilize the fracture in the position of anatomic reduction.

The surgeon must keep in mind that by definition there has already been an injury to the physis and further damage to the physis by repeated or forceful manipulations may contribute to one of the complications of this injury, premature physeal closure. Closed reduction of these injuries must be done gently, preferably under either under IV sedation or general anesthesia, so that this reduction be accomplished easily with minimal force. Once the reduction has been achieved, maintaining it has been shown to be vitally important for influencing outcome (as redisplaced fractures tend to have poor prognosis and higher complication rates).[7,84] Treatment is also guided by the Salter–Harris type. Salter–Harris types III and IV are intra-articular and require an anatomic reduction to minimize the potential for future arthritis and degenerative joint disease. Therefore these fractures are most commonly treated with open reduction and internal fixation to restore anatomic integrity of the joint surface. The ultimate goals of treatment are to maintain anatomic alignment of the lower extremity, preserve range of motion in the knee joint, and not disturb ongoing growth of the distal femoral physis.[68]

NONOPERATIVE TREATMENT OF FRACTURES OF THE DISTAL FEMORAL PHYSIS

Nondisplaced or minimally displaced distal femoral physeal fractures, especially Salter–Harris type I or II fractures, may be treated with, a gentle closed reduction and immobilization in a cast. Conceivably even a Salter–Harris type III or IV fracture that was completely nondisplaced could also be managed in this manner. The treating surgeon must be cognizant of the fact that displacement may have been far greater at the time of injury than the injury radiographs depict. At the time of the injury, the periosteum and/or resilience of the child's bone as well as reduction at the site of injury may have occurred, rendering the acute trauma or injury films to be either non- or minimally displaced.[68] Evidence of considerable soft tissue injury such as swelling, ecchymosis, and/or other skin changes may also be an indication that the fracture was more displaced at the time of injury.

If minimal force is required to perform a reduction, most series indicate that these fractures can still be successfully managed in this manner. This technique of a closed reduction and immobilization in a long-leg cast has been performed primarily in minimally or nondisplaced Salter–Harris type I and II fractures.

Careful assessment of stability of the fracture by the surgeon is crucial to having a successful outcome with closed reduction and manipulation. In a recent study of 82 patients immobilized in a long-leg cast, 36% had redisplacement in the first 2 weeks including 3 patients in a series of 29 immobilized with a hip spica cast.[24] Of the 32 patients that displaced in a cast in this study, only 8 were successfully remanipulated. Closed reduction and casting is never the best definitive treatment for displaced or unstable distal femoral physeal fractures because of the significant risk of fracture redisplacement.[2] Persistent widening after provisional reduction may reflect interposed periosteum and lead to reduction less than anatomic and more likely to redisplace.[68] Some believe that periosteal interposition may theoretically place the physis at increased risk for closure,[76] but there is very little evidence to support this opinion. Anatomic reduction is always the goal with these injuries and if an adequate reduction cannot be obtained by closed means, alternative methods of treatment must be utilized. In general, with nonoperative treatment the risk of redisplacement of these fractures is high, and the risk of growth disturbance is high, so only truly nondisplaced fractures are generally treated nonoperatively.

OPERATIVE TREATMENT OF FRACTURES OF THE DISTAL FEMORAL PHYSIS

Displaced distal femoral physeal fractures with more than 2 mm of malalignment typically require reduction and surgical stabilization with internal fixation. The overriding principle regarding reduction maneuvers is to avoid further injury to the physis (Fig. 25-12). Most authors recommend that the reductions be done with the patient relaxed with muscle relaxants or under general anesthesia. However, the so-called gentle reduction does not preclude the possibility of growth arrest, as has been noted by Thomson et al.[84] The technique of reduction relies on assessment of the fracture pattern. In a general sense, the concave side of the fracture would be gently manipulated to realign it with the long axis or shaft of the femur, essentially closing down the convexity of the fracture. The periosteum is typically intact on the concave side of the injury. For example, the periosteum on the side of the Thurston Holland fragment for Salter–Harris type II fractures is usually intact, but disrupted on the convex side of the fracture. Periosteal interposition at the fracture site is a frequent occurrence in these fractures and necessitates careful assessment of the postreduction imaging and anatomy.

For a Salter–Harris type II fracture that is displaced into valgus alignment such as the epiphysis is displaced laterally and there is a lateral Thurston Holland fragment of metaphysis attached to the epiphysis, the reduction maneuver would involve gentle longitudinal traction often with the knee flexed slightly and counter pressure applied over the distal medial femur while the epiphyseal portion of the fracture is gently guided back in place. Reduction is 90% traction and 10% manipulation to minimize iatrogenic trauma to the physis. More challenging reductions occur in the sagittal plain when the epiphysis is displaced either anteriorly or posteriorly. Anteriorly displaced physeal fractures generally require some level of knee flexion to achieve reduction. In all reductions, generally longitudinal traction is the first force applied followed by the gentle manipulation of the epiphysis back into place starting with counterpressure on the proximal segment in an opposite direction. For a displaced epiphysis that is anterior, holding the fracture reduced may require a significant amount of knee flexion, which especially in a swollen knee, which may not be advisable from a neurovascular standpoint. Fractures like these may require internal stabilization with pins simply to be able to splint the knee in slight flexion. Some authors recommend aspiration of the knee or the hematoma that may be present especially in Salter–Harris type III or IV fractures prior to closed reduction maneuvers. Various reports indicate redisplacement of reduced fractures in a cast of 30% or higher such that there has been a tendency for internal stabilization with implants for displaced fractures.[84] A recent report indicated that internal fixation is the preferred method of treatment for all displaced injuries.[2]

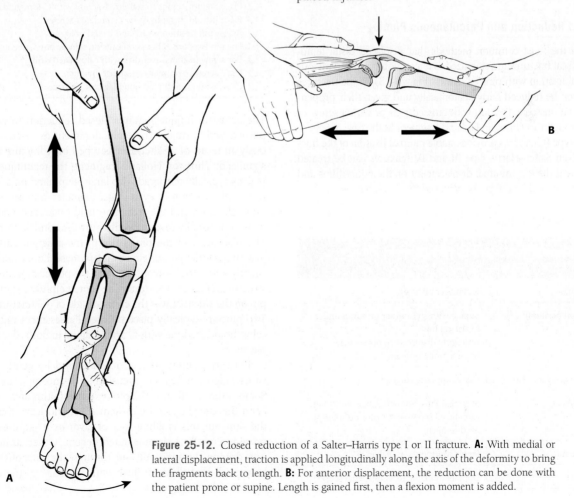

Figure 25-12. Closed reduction of a Salter–Harris type I or II fracture. **A:** With medial or lateral displacement, traction is applied longitudinally along the axis of the deformity to bring the fragments back to length. **B:** For anterior displacement, the reduction can be done with the patient prone or supine. Length is gained first, then a flexion moment is added.

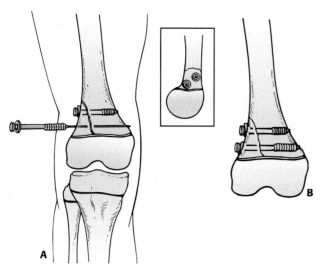

Figure 25-13. Screw fixation following closed or open reduction of Salter–Harris type II fracture with a large metaphyseal fragment. **A:** When using cannulated screws, place both guidewires before screw placement to avoid rotation of the fragment while drilling or inserting screw. Screw threads should be past the fracture site to enable compression. Washers help increase compression. Screws may be placed anterior and posterior to each other, which is particularly helpful when trying to fit multiple screws in a small metaphyseal fragment. **B:** This form of fixation is locally "rigid," but must be protected with long-leg immobilization.

Closed Reduction and Percutaneous Pinning

One of the most common methods that displaced distal femoral physeal fractures are stabilized is a technique of percutaneous internal fixation with pins or screws (Fig. 25-13). These fractures can often be reduced fairly anatomically and given their propensity to be unstable, fixation with crossed pins or with a screw or two through the Thurston Holland fragment in the case of Salter–Harris type II fractures provides stable internal fixation of the fracture. Even Salter–Harris type III and IV fractures can be treated this way if there is minimal displacement on the injury films and an anatomic reduction can be achieved by closed means.

Preoperative Planning

Closed Reduction and Percutaneous Pinning: PREOPERATIVE PLANNING CHECKLIST	
OR table	❑ Radiolucent flat-top
Position/positioning aids	❑ Supine with soft bolster or bump under ipsilateral hip
	❑ Anteriorly displaced epiphysis may require prone position
Fluoroscopy location	❑ C-arm opposite surgeon
Equipment	❑ Steinman Pins, Smooth; Large and small cannulated screw sets, major ortho set if need to open
Tourniquet	❑ Sterile tourniquet available
(Other)	❑ Doppler available to assess pedal pulses

Preoperative planning and room setup for percutaneous pinning would involve the use of a radiolucent table although a traction-type table is usually not necessary. Obviously, imaging must be available, as well as the appropriate instrumentation, typically cannulated large fragment screws and smooth Steinmann pins. Muscle relaxation of the patient provided by the anesthesiology team is especially helpful before initiating reduction maneuvers. Neurovascular status of the extremity should be checked routinely both before and after reduction maneuvers.

Positioning

At times, reduction is facilitated by placing a bump under the patient's thigh. In the case of flexion or extension-type physeal displacement, these injuries may actually be managed in a prone position.

Technique

✔ Closed Reduction and Percutaneous Pinning: KEY SURGICAL STEPS
❑ Assure adequate positioning and set-up with radiolucent table and C-arm
❑ Obtain closed reduction as anatomic as possible
❑ Verify reduction with imaging
❑ Stabilize reduction
❑ Place Steinman pins to stabilize fracture with C-arm guidance
❑ Place pins in metaphysis for cannulated screws
❑ Assess pin position on AP and lateral images
❑ For pin fixation, either bend outside skin or bury subcutaneously
❑ For screw fixation, over drill with cannulated drill
❑ Place screws over pins to stabilize fracture
❑ Close wounds and place long-leg cast or brace

The actual technique requires closed reduction to be accomplished with virtually anatomic alignment as discussed previously. In terms of a Salter–Harris type I or II fracture without a significant Thurston Holland fragment, the technique involves placing typically retrograde two large Steinmann pins. These are frequently 3.2-mm or even larger diameter smooth pins. With x-ray guidance and the reduction held by an assistant, a small incision is usually made laterally over the condyle in midpoint. The placement of the pin is not in the articular cartilage but just off the articular margin in the epiphyseal bone and directed slightly anteriorly to avoid injury to the posterior neurovascular structures (Fig. 25-14). It may be more helpful to start with the pin on the side that was the concave side of the fracture pattern. Two pins are typically placed. Careful assessment radiographically should be done with C-arm imaging in both AP and lateral planes.

Fracture stability may also be assessed by gently applying varus, valgus, or flexion–extension force once pins are in place. Some authors will leave the pins external in this area. Some will bend them slightly and cut them short and leave them under the skin but this is falling out of favor as it requires another procedure with no demonstrated benefit. Other authors advocate driving the pins out and through the metaphysis of the bone such that they are flush with the edge of the epiphysis

(text continues on page 979)

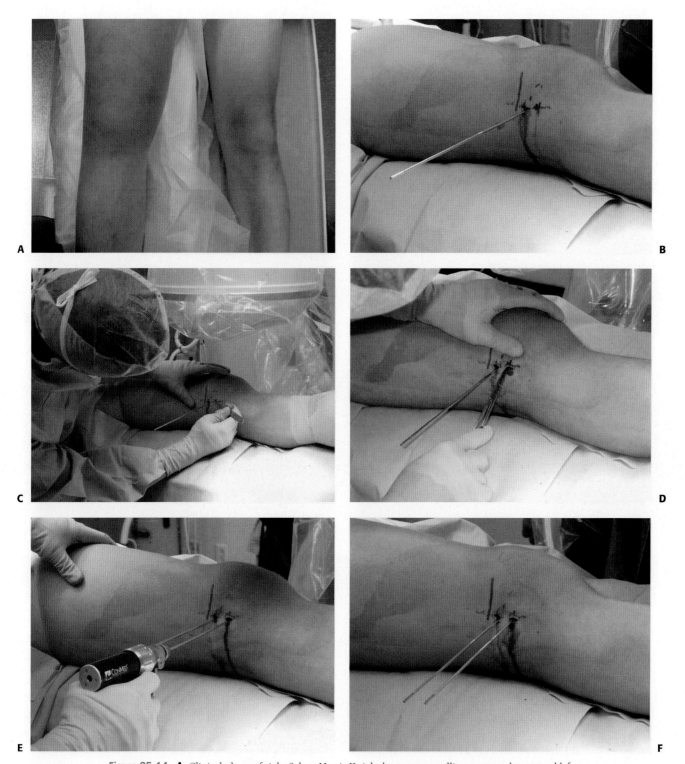

Figure 25-14. A: Clinical photo of right Salter–Harris II right knee; note swelling compared to normal left knee. **B:** Photo of knee showing guide pin for cannulated screw in place in Thurston Holland fragment. Vertical line marks cephalad extent of TH fragment. Smaller line marks the physis. **C:** Preparing entry site for second guide pin with C-arm guidance. **D:** Using a hemostat to spread IT band and periosteum and to create path to distal femur for pin placement. **E:** Placing guide pin parallel to original pin. **F:** Two pins in distal femur, parallel and verified in good position with C-arm.

(continues)

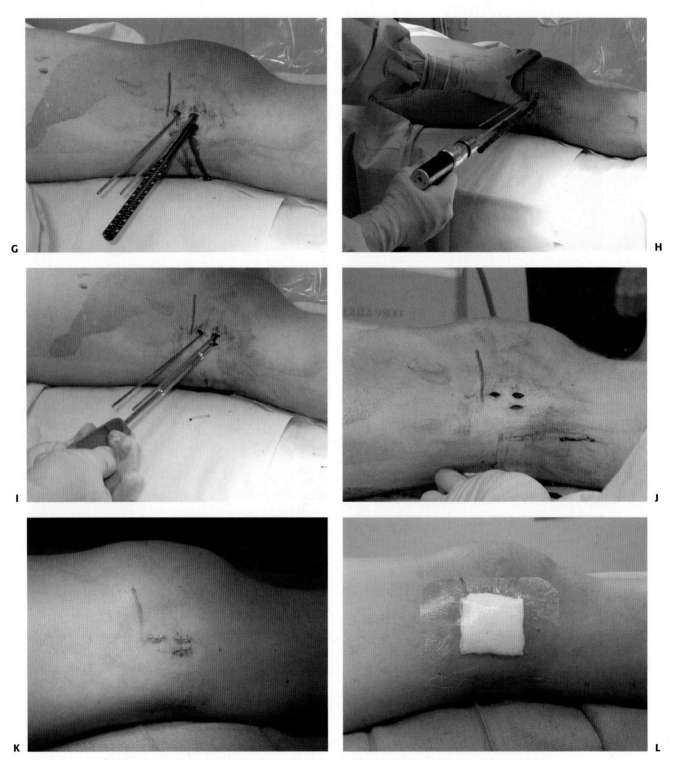

Figure 25-14. (*Continued*) **G:** Measuring depth of guide pin to determine screw length. Note a third pin was added. **H:** Drilling over guide pin: Note that far cortex does not need to be drilled. **I:** Placing cannulated cancellous screw. **J:** Appearance after screws are placed. **K:** Appearance after wound closure. **L:** Dressing in place.

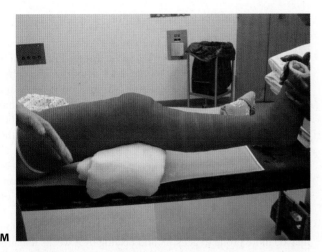

Figure 25-14. (*Continued*) **M:** Final cast in place.

at the entry site and bend them externally above the knee. One concern with external pins in this area is the issue that the joint itself could be contaminated since the pins are essentially intra-articular, hence the reason some surgeons drive the pins proximally to exit through the metaphysis.[68] Starting the pins proximally in the metaphysis and placing them across the fracture in an antegrade fashion and ending them in the subchondral bone of the epiphysis is becoming more popular in some centers to minimize pin tract infections that could communicate with the joint. Typically patients are immobilized in a fiberglass long-leg cast with the knee gently flexed or a brace if there is sufficient fracture stability, patient compliance, and a long enough femur to provide immobilization of the knee.

Postoperative Care

Distal femoral physeal fractures heal readily and are healed within 4 weeks, at which point pins may be removed. Touch-down weight bearing in the cast may be allowed in the last week or two prior to pin removal. Often a splint or hinged knee brace is used for a few weeks to facilitate regaining range of motion of the knee with increasing weight bearing, such that most patients are able to bear weight fully about 6 weeks postoperatively. Pin removal at 4 weeks may be done in the office if the pins are external or as a day surgery procedure if they were buried beneath the skin. It is important to stress that intra-articular pins should not be left in place for >4 weeks as this may lead to a septic joint, and infection should always be considered with any increasing discomfort, fevers, drainage, etc. The patients are instructed to work on quad strengthening and active range of motion of the knee often facilitated by physical therapy.

Screw Fixation

The technique for stabilizing a Salter–Harris type II fracture with a significant metaphyseal fragment again involves performing a gentle closed reduction under anesthesia. A small incision is then made in the metaphysis over the Thurston Holland fragment, which typically is either on the medial or lateral aspect of the distal femur. The guide pins from the cannulated

screw systems are used to help stabilize the fracture. Typically, only drilling the outer cortex is necessary, and one or two 6.5 or larger screws are used to stabilize the fracture fragment. Care must be taken to ensure that the screws do not approach or cross the physis. In general, screws are placed in a manner that is parallel to the distal femoral physis. The surgeon should consider use of washers as the metaphyseal bone is weak in this area. Again assessment of fracture stability by gentle stress with the hardware in and secure is helpful to ensure that internal fixation is adequate in providing optimum stability. Postoperative treatment would be the same with typically long-leg casting for 4 weeks. Screw removal is at the discretion of the family and surgeon at a convenient time in the future. Occasionally, the Thurston Holland permits only one screw to be placed. These fractures may be unstable enough that one screw is insufficient to provide adequate internal fixation. It is not uncommon that a single screw in a Salter–Harris II fracture may be supplemented with a Steinmann pin in the fashion described for percutaneous pinning. If one Steinmann pin is to be used, it would ideally enter on the side opposite the entry of the screw to provide stability of the fracture.

Closed Reduction and Screw Fixation of Salter–Harris III and IV Fractures

Minimally displaced Salter–Harris III fractures may also be managed with percutaneous reduction and screw fixation. The use of reduction bone forceps or clamps may be helpful in closing down a gap or diastasis of the condyles. Again, careful and accurate assessment of intraoperative imaging is essential to ascertain whether the reduction is adequate for percutaneous technique versus an open reduction.

Screw placement in a Salter–Harris III or IV fracture may be done in the epiphysis with x-ray guidance using a cannulated screw system. Care must be taken not to place the screws too distal in the epiphysis such that they would impinge on the intercondylar notch of the femur, and this should be assessed with intraoperative notch views if there is any question. Two screws are typically placed, one more anterior and one more posterior, to stabilize a Salter–Harris III fracture internally. A Salter–Harris IV fracture may have a metaphyseal fragment that is sufficiently large enough to be stabilized with a screw. The epiphyseal portion or the Salter–Harris IV fracture can then be stabilized by another screw (Fig. 25-15).

Challenges or problems with the technique of a closed reduction and internal fixation with pins or screws include an inadequate reduction that may be secondary to periosteal interposition. As mentioned, the periosteum is often torn on the convex side so an incomplete reduction that has still a wide physis on the convex side may need to be opened on that side to extract the periosteum to ensure an adequate, stable, and anatomic reduction. Interposed periosteum has been shown experimentally to increase the risk of growth disturbance.[67] In addition, when trying to utilize this technique for Salter–Harris type III or IV fractures, if the articular surface cannot be well aligned or if there is comminution present, an open approach would be necessary. Likewise, comminution of the metaphysis may make screw fixation of a Thurston Holland fragment

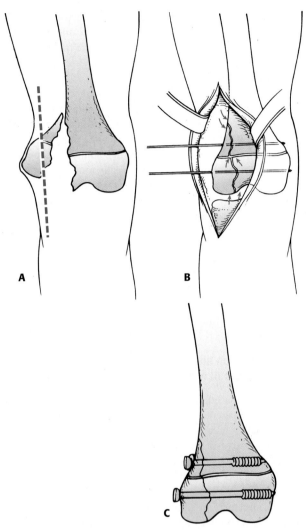

Figure 25-15. Open reduction of displaced lateral Salter–Harris type IV fracture of the distal femur. **A:** A longitudinal skin incision is made anteriorly on the knee at the location of the intra-articular fracture or in the midline if fracture severity raises concern of needing a total knee replacement in the future. **B:** Alignment of joint and physis are used to judge reduction. Guidewires for cannulated screws placed above and below physis, parallel to physis. **C:** Screws inserted in compression with washer on metaphyseal fragment. Washer is optional in epiphyseal fragment if later prominence is of more concern than need for additional compression.

difficult, necessitating that some Salter–Harris type II fractures be fixed internally in a stable configuration with transphyseal pins and not screws. The technique of using transphyseal pins to stabilize distal femoral physeal fractures requires the use of smooth pins to minimize injury to the physis. A recent article looked specifically at the issue of physeal injury and subsequent growth arrest to determine if the pins could possibly be the culprit causing the arrest.[27] The conclusion of this work was that the pins themselves were not the primary cause of the subsequent physeal arrest or growth disturbance. This potential for physeal arrest varied with increasing severity based on the Salter–Harris classification and percutaneous smooth pins were not statistically associated with the growth arrest.[27]

Open Reduction and Internal Fixation

Open reduction and internal fixation is necessary for all irreducible distal femoral physeal fractures. Irreducible fractures may have interposed periosteum on the side of the open physis or the convex side of the fracture. An incision is necessary over that area, whether it is medial or lateral; even in sagittal plane displacements, typically the incision is still on the medial or lateral aspect. The periosteum is carefully removed from the physis and care is taken to avoid causing any more injury to the physis by surgical instruments or retractors.[68] Evacuation of organized hematoma is helpful to achieve anatomic reduction. Internal fixation may proceed accordingly with either pins or screws as warranted.

Fractures that undergo open reduction and internal fixation may be more prone to get stiff, and healing by 4 weeks remains the norm, with early mobilization of the knee recommended starting at about 4 weeks.

Other Means of Fixation

The use of external fixators in open fractures of the knee involving the distal femoral physis may be a helpful means of managing severe soft tissue trauma and injuries, especially temporarily as in damage control for the multi-trauma patient. Typically one or even two half pins from an external fixation frame may be placed in the epiphysis of the fracture with two pins placed in the femoral shaft. Salter–Harris type III and IV fractures may be somewhat more difficult to manage with the external fixation technique and increase the risk of a septic joint. Fixation across the knee may be necessary.

Another means of fixation is a plate spanning the physis. A recent paper from France described good outcomes with this technique.[36] The plates were removed at a relatively early interval to minimize any growth disturbance and screw insertion and placement occurred so as to avoid the physis. Absorbable screws have also been used in some of these patients. There is little current literature on this technique.

In Salter–Harris type III and IV fractures, arthroscopically aided reduction of the fracture may be helpful in somewhat minimally displaced fractures to ensure an anatomic reduction of the joint line and articular cartilage.[43] In addition, visualization of the knee joint, whether with arthroscopy or at the time of arthrotomy, permits assessment for other associated injuries such as ligamentous injuries or meniscal injuries.

Most authors recommend dealing with intra-articular ligamentous injuries later after the fracture has healed. Peripheral tears of the meniscus may be repaired primarily at the time of an operative open reduction. As in most current protocols for ACL reconstruction, resolution of the acute phase swelling (and in this case fracture healing and rehabilitation) would be accomplished prior to consideration of ACL reconstruction.

For those fractures associated with vascular injuries, typically full and rapid reduction of the fracture and stabilization is necessary. If there is still a vascular compromise of the leg, the orthopedic surgical team may consider compartment pressure monitoring and/or fasciotomies as warranted while the vascular team is evaluating the need for intervention for an occluded artery.[68]

Authors' Preferred Treatment of Fractures of the Distal Femoral Physis (Algorithm 25-1)

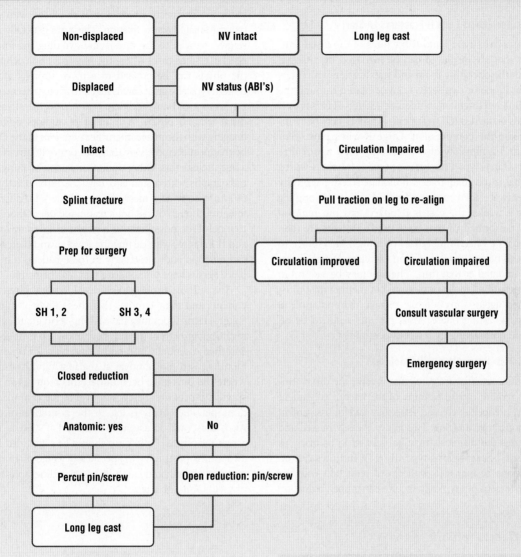

Algorithm 25-1. Authors' preferred treatment of physeal fractures of the distal femur.

The management of these fractures is focused on minimizing further injury or trauma to the physis, especially with reduction maneuvers. Displaced fracture reduction must be done easily, gently, and in a relaxed patient. Often the fractures reduce with longitudinal traction and a little medial or lateral pressure; aim at 90% traction and 10% manipulation. Repeated forceful reductions must be avoided to minimize potential iatrogenic injury to the physis. Treatment principles really are based on the Salter–Harris classification as well as the amount and degree of displacement. The authors have a very low threshold for operative stabilization of these fractures with pins or screws as needed.

For truly nondisplaced fractures regardless of Salter–Harris type, the authors are comfortable with a well-molded long-leg cast. In children with certain body types, especially obese patients that are relatively short stature, cast immobilization may not provide fracture stability. Treatment must be individualized to the specific patient and consideration given to the possibility that casting may not adequately stabilize a nondisplaced fracture. The treating surgeon must recall that what appears nondisplaced on radiographs in the emergency room may have displaced and returned to normal anatomic positioning at the time of injury, and not lulled into a false sense of fracture stability for "nondisplaced" fractures. CT is generally recommended to assess for displacement.

Should cast immobilization be elected as a treatment option for nondisplaced fractures, seeing the patient back in the office and obtaining the x-rays within 4 to 5 days is recommended to ensure that the fracture reduction is maintained or to identify loss of anatomic position as early as possible. Literature indicates that loss of reduction and reduction of fractures is associated with a higher incidence of physeal growth arrest, but accepting a malalignment is also less than ideal for the patient's functional outcome.

Displaced Salter–Harris I and II Fractures LA Start

Many Salter–Harris type I and II fractures of the distal femoral physis that are displaced can be managed by a closed reduction in the operating room and stabilization with internal fixation. If one or two screws can be placed through the Thurston Holland fragment to stabilize a Salter–Harris type II fracture, this is the desired treatment. Washers may be helpful to increase the compression. Large K-wires pins (generally 2.4 to 3.2 mm) are also commonly used to stabilize both Salter–Harris type I fractures or type II fractures with a fragment that is too small to accommodate screws. Typically these patients are then managed with 4 weeks of long-leg casting. At 4 weeks, the cast is removed and pin removal is typically performed (if pins were used). Patients are then transitioned to a knee immobilizer or hinged knee brace to allow them to begin range of motion exercises. Weight bearing is also initiated at that time. Therapy may be helpful to assist with regaining range of motion, but the therapist must be cautioned against any forcible passive manipulation in the early post-casting phase. Most patients seem to be off crutches and ambulating by 8 weeks postinjury.

Displaced Salter–Harris III and IV Fractures

Displaced intra-articular fractures that involve the distal femoral physis require careful scrutiny of the fracture alignment and pattern preoperatively and especially careful assessment of the intraoperative imaging. This injury is easily missed and in some series the diagnosis may be delayed in as many as 39% of cases.[63] Salter–Harris type III or IV fractures can on some occasions be managed with closed reduction with the use of bone forceps but typically require either open reduction

with an arthrotomy or arthroscopic assistance to ensure anatomic restoration of the articular cartilage. Once an anatomic reduction has been achieved, it is stabilized with percutaneous cannulated screw fixation. These are generally epiphyseal screws, parallel to the physis and avoiding the intercondylar notch. In some cases where the physis is approaching closure, the physis can be crossed to achieve stronger stabilization, though typically great care is taken to avoid placement near the physis to avoid any additional trauma to the already injured distal femoral physis. A number of authors point out that imaging with the image intensifier or C-arm in the OR may not be the most accurate way to assess postoperative reduction in a fracture like this. Other options include obtaining hard copy radiographs with a standard machine intraoperatively or use of arthroscopy as a means to assess the joint alignment and integrity, though this is not a technique the authors have used routinely. The postoperative regimen is the same as for type I and II fractures with casting for 4 weeks and then initiation of early motion and particularly in these patients a hinged knee brace versus knee immobilizer may also be helpful.

The authors explain to all distal femoral physeal fracture patients and their families that these physeal injuries of all Salter–Harris types may have a long-term guarded prognosis regarding growth of the physis. Follow-up is done at 1 week and then essentially at monthly intervals for the first several months; with pin removal at the first month visit. In cases where the pins have been buried this requires an additional surgical procedure. Screw removal of the cannulated screws done percutaneously is left to the discretion of the family. Also, these are occasionally removed if MRI is needed to assess the physis. Follow-up should be scheduled at 3, 6 and 12 months postinjury to specifically assess alignment of the extremity length and carefully assess radiographs for signs of physeal injury or arrest.

Potential Pitfalls and Preventive Measures

Repair of Distal Femoral Physeal Fractures: PITFALLS AND PREVENTION	
Pitfall	**Prevention**
• Missed diagnosis	• Immobilize and reexamine if uncertain, or MRI • Be cognizant of nondisplaced injury in infants, pathologic conditions, polytrauma, or unresponsive patients
• Inadequate reduction	• Skeptically examine intraoperative radiographs • Low threshold for opening if concern for inadequate reduction, gapping from periosteum
• Unrecognized vascular injury	• Thorough neurologic exam • Prompt reduction of the fracture if concern regarding vascular status • Involvement of vascular team if perfusion doesn't normalize with fracture reduction
• Loss of reduction	• Pin or screw fixation for all fractures that require reduction • Radiographs at 5–7 days postinjury • High long-leg cast with molding proximally or spica cast
• Growth disturbance	• Minimize trauma at reduction • Follow-up at 6, 12, and possibly 24 months with full-length radiographs of both lower extremities
• Knee joint instability	• Check ligaments when fracture stabilized or healed • Consider MRI, especially for type III fractures
• Stiffness	• Avoid prolonged immobilization • Remove casts in 4 weeks and apply knee immobilizer with gentle range of motion in most cases. Avoid aggressive manipulation because of risk of additional injury

Reduction Malalignment (Poor Reduction or Loss of Reduction)

Often displacement in distal femoral physeal fractures can be significant. In an operating room with muscle relaxation, reduction can often be accomplished without significant force by simply placing traction on the leg and guiding the epiphysis back into position. Traction should be considered the most important component of this reduction as it is imperative to avoid additional trauma to the already injured physis. Some surgeons prefer use of a fracture table for reduction though the authors preference is a standard radiolucent table as well as in some cases a radiolucent triangle for assistance with the reduction. Careful assessment both clinically and radiographically of leg alignment and fracture reduction needs to be done to ensure that as anatomically as possible a reduction is achieved. If the fracture remains malaligned in either the coronal or sagittal plane may persist and require subsequent late constructive surgery as well as create additional risk for growth arrest. It is especially critical to accurately assess imaging in the operating room to ensure that physeal widening, which may be subtle, is not present.

Interposed periosteum may cause physeal widening and block a more anatomic reduction as well as contribute to fracture instability that could lead to loss of reduction in a casted patient postoperatively. The surgeon should have a low threshold to make an incision and inspect the fracture to ensure there is no soft tissue impeding reduction in cases that may look less than anatomically reduced.

When a loss of reduction of what was thought to be a stable nondisplaced fracture in a cast is noted, the patient should be expeditiously returned to the operating room and anatomic alignment reestablished. Once an adequate reduction has been achieved, internal fixation in the form of pins or screws is needed to maintain the alignment.

If the fracture is more than 10 to 14 days old, healing may have already occurred along the physis, and manipulation at this point may cause iatrogenic damage to the physis, so closed reduction is no longer an option.

Reduction in Cases of Vascular Injury

Distal femoral physeal injuries require significant trauma to be sustained by the extremity to cause displacement of the physis. With that amount of force or pressure other associated injuries may occur. Displaced fractures in particular must be carefully assessed for neurovascular status at the time of injury in the emergency room. For Salter–Harris type II distal femoral physeal fractures that displace the epiphysis anteriorly, the distal portion of the femoral artery or popliteal artery is at risk from the distal end of the segment of the femur. Careful assessment of the pulses and circulation to the foot are essential. In patients with a documented vascular compromise or white foot, this reduction and surgery is an operative emergency and careful assessment postoperatively for return of vascular status is necessary. Consultation with the vascular surgical team is often necessary if concerns of vascular status remain postreduction. Vascular imaging may be needed to assess circulation if pulses are still diminished following reduction and stabilization of the distal femoral physeal fracture. Likewise some of these patients

may sustain such injury to the leg that a compartment syndrome could ensue, so careful monitoring of the compartments by clinical examination or if needed by compartment pressure measurements may be necessary.

Septic Knee

The literature substantiates that infection and in fact septic knee arthritis may result from pins left externally that are placed in a retrograde manner in the epiphysis on either side of the knee joint. Consequently the authors recommend that this pins are either removed no later than 4 weeks post op. Alternatively, a technique described by Blasier[12] places the pins retrograde across the physis and advances them up through the skin proximal to the knee joint. The pins left are flush with edge of the condyle or epiphysis distally. The areas can be closed and the pins are external above the knee joint. In the event of a septic joint the patient is returned to the operating room for irrigation and debridement. The pins may have to be left in if the fracture is not sufficiently healed at least 4 weeks postinjury. Appropriate antibiotic treatment and surgical wound management are necessary in these cases of an infection, especially in the first few weeks following the injury.

MANAGEMENT OF EXPECTED ADVERSE OUTCOMES AND UNEXPECTED COMPLICATIONS

Fractures of the Distal Femoral Physis: COMMON ADVERSE OUTCOMES AND COMPLICATIONS

- Loss of reduction
- Vascular injury
- Peroneal nerve injury
- Ligamentous injury
- Knee stiffness
- Growth disturbance
- Physeal arrest

In the immediate postoperative period, loss of reduction and neurovascular injuries are important complications. In follow-up, the most common complications of distal femoral physeal fractures include knee ligament injury, growth disturbances of the distal femur, neurovascular complications from the fracture, and persistent knee stiffness (Table 25-3).

LOSS OF REDUCTION

Redisplacement after closed reduction of distal femoral physeal separations has been reported in 30% to 70% of patients immobilized in a long-leg cast.[24,29,72,84] Placement of a hip spica cast may reduce this loss of reduction to as low as 10%.[24] Multiple attempts at initial closed reduction, and late reduction after injury or after a failed first attempt at reduction, are potentially damaging to the physis and may increase the risk of growth disturbance.[71] In one experimental rat model, risk of physeal injury was similar for fractures reduced after the equivalent of 7 human days. After 10 days, however, manipulation of physeal fractures led to diaphyseal fractures because of the degree of

TABLE 25-3. Complications of Fractures of the Distal Femoral Physis

	Number of Patients	Ligamentous Injury (%)	Neurovascular Problems (%)	Angular Deformity (%)	Shortening (%)	Stiffness (%)
Stephens and Louns[83]	20	25	5	25	40	25
Lombardo and Harvey[49]	34	23	3	33	35	33
Czitrom et al.[20]	41 22	0	2.5	41	14% clinical 58% radiographic	
Riseborough et al.[7(a)]	133[a]		4	25	55	23
Thomson et al.[84]	30	Two anterior cruciate ligament injuries		18	47	18
Eid and Hafez[24]	151	8% symptomatic 14% asymptomatic	10	51	38	29
Ilharreborde et al.[36(b)]	20	0		55	40	25
Arkader et al.[2]	73		1	12	12	4

[a]Series contains referred patients and may not represent true incidence.
[b]Salter–Harris type II fractures only.

physeal healing.[23] Based on the experimental evidence and clinical experience, it is reasonable to attempt manipulation, or repeat manipulation, of physeal fractures up to 10 days after injury. After 10 days, however, open reduction may be required to reestablish alignment and risk of physeal arrest may be increased. For children with more than 2 years of growth remaining who have Salter–Harris I and II fractures, observation for remodeling may be more prudent, depending on the degree of deformity. Osteotomy of the femur may be performed later if remodeling is incomplete. Older children with type I and II fractures are best treated with open reduction and fixation possibly combined with epiphysiodesis of the uninjured distal femur. For patients of all ages who present late after sustaining displaced Salter–Harris type III and IV fractures, open reduction is recommended as soon as possible to restore articular surface.[54]

NEUROVASCULAR ABNORMALITIES

Vascular Injury

Vascular injuries are possible but uncommon with this fracture, with most series reporting no vascular injuries.[24,49,72,84] Trauma to the popliteal artery may be caused by trauma from the distal end of the metaphysis and occurs most commonly from fractures caused by forced knee hyperextension resulting in anterior displacement of the epiphysis.[9,24,75] In the emergency department, clinical signs of vascular impairment should prompt the surgeon to perform emergency reduction of the fracture. It is our preference to perform the reduction in the operating room but, in situations when a delay of treatment in the operating room is expected, reduction of the gross deformity and splinting of the fracture is a reasonable course of action. Arteriography is not indicted prior to reduction of the fracture.

In the operating room, the fracture is reduced and stabilized first. If vascular examination is normal after reduction, as evidenced by return of distal pulses, normal capillary refill,

and symmetric ankle–brachial indices, the limb is splinted or casted with cut-outs to allow serial evaluation of the pulses easily and the child is admitted for observation. Because intimal injuries of the artery and thrombosis may occur in a delayed fashion, the child's vascular status is monitored closely for 24 hours or so after surgery for signs of worsening vascular status and compartment syndrome. Arteriography is sometimes utilized during the observation period to assess patients with distal perfusion and some abnormality of vascularity, such as diminished pulses, and for those with a worsening of vascular status after reduction and pinning.

If, after reduction and fixation in the operating room, distal perfusion does not return within 15 to 20 minutes, the time course over which vessel spasm typically recovers, immediate exploration of the vessel by a vascular surgeon is indicated. Although ischemia time may be increased when prolonged fracture stabilization is performed first, manipulation of the fracture after vascular surgery may compromise the repair. Arteriography is indicated only if the fracture has occurred in association with an ipsilateral pelvic fracture or another more proximal leg injury to localize the site of vascular injury. In most cases, thrombectomy and direct vessel repair or bypass of the injury with a vein graft are necessary to restore flow. If ischemia time exceeds 6 to 8 hours, four-compartment fasciotomies of the lower leg are done prophylactically in conjunction with the vascular repair to minimize the effects of reperfusion and treat prophylactically compartment syndrome of the calf.

Peroneal Nerve Injury

The peroneal nerve is the most frequently injured nerve after distal physeal separations.[24] It is injured primarily from traction, the result of anteromedial displacement most commonly, but may also be damaged from direct trauma as well. Most peroneal nerve injuries are neurapraxias that spontaneously recover within 6 to 12 weeks of injury.[24,81] Persistent neurologic deficit 3 months after fracture warrants electromyographic examination. If the conduction time is prolonged and fibrillation or denervation is present in distal muscles, exploration and microneural reanastomosis or resection of any neuroma may be indicated. Open injuries that result in peroneal nerve transection are best treated with repair or nerve grafting as early as possible after injury based on the child's condition and the status of the soft tissues about the nerve laceration. An ankle–foot orthosis is typically prescribed for patients with peroneal nerve injuries to facilitate rehabilitation and is discontinued after nerve recovery.

LIGAMENTOUS INJURIES

Symptomatic knee joint instability has been reported in 8% to 40% of patients with distal femoral physeal fractures.[10,24] Although these ligament injuries occur at the time of initial trauma, most are not identified until after the fracture has healed and rehabilitation has been initiated. The anterior cruciate ligament is most commonly disrupted, especially after Salter–Harris type III fractures of the medial femoral condyle.[15,53,69,86] Collateral ligament and posterior cruciate ligament disruptions and meniscal injuries may also occur after these fractures but are less common.

Difficulty with stairs, pain or swelling with activities and episodes of giving way, or knee buckling are typical presenting complaints indicative of knee. The physical examination may identify knee stiffness, signs of ligament instability, and joint line tenderness. Early diagnosis of injuries to the ligaments or menisci can facilitate earlier management[10] but, in many cases, the symptoms related to recovery from the fracture make identifying these other injuries challenging. A high index of suspicion is needed to diagnose associated ligamentous and meniscal injuries. When suspected, an MRI of the knee after healing of the fracture is the best way to delineate these injuries. Meniscal surgery, especially repair, is ideally done soon after fracture healing to facilitate rehabilitation. Knee ligament reconstruction is best done after knee range of motion has been restored and other factors are taken into account including the degree of instability, the child's age, and level of activity.

KNEE STIFFNESS

Limitation of knee motion after separation of the distal femoral epiphysis is seen in as many as one-third of the patients after fracture healing. This complication is the result of several factors including, intra-articular adhesions, capsular contracture, and muscle contractures, most notably the hamstrings and quadriceps. Initial treatment consists of active and active-assistive range-of-motion exercises. Drop-out casts and dynamic bracing may be of benefit for some with persistent stiffness. For patients with persistent stiffness and loss of functional range of motion despite nonsurgical treatments, surgical interventions may be utilized to restore mobility. Gentle knee manipulation under anesthesia is sometimes useful but is associated with the risk of periarticular fractures of the knee.[17] Surgical release of contractures and adhesions, followed by continuous passive motion, is most reliable for regaining motion.[78]

GROWTH DISTURBANCE

The most common complication of distal femoral epiphyseal fractures is growth disturbance. This complication is manifested clinically by the development of angular deformity in cases where the physeal injury is incomplete (Fig. 25-16), shortening of the limb after injuries that result in complete arrest, or, as in some cases, both angulation and limb shortening. In one

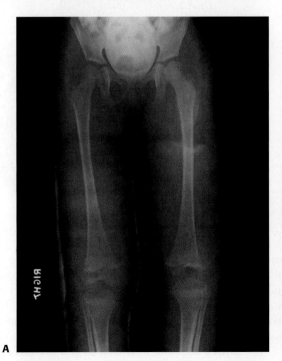
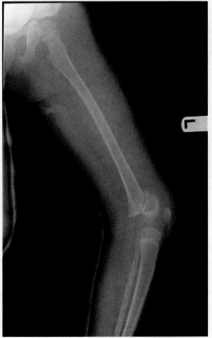

Figure 25-16. An 8-year-old girl struck by a car while on bicycle. Initial AP (**A**) and lateral (**B**) radiographs reveal displaced physeal fracture of the distal femur.

(continues)

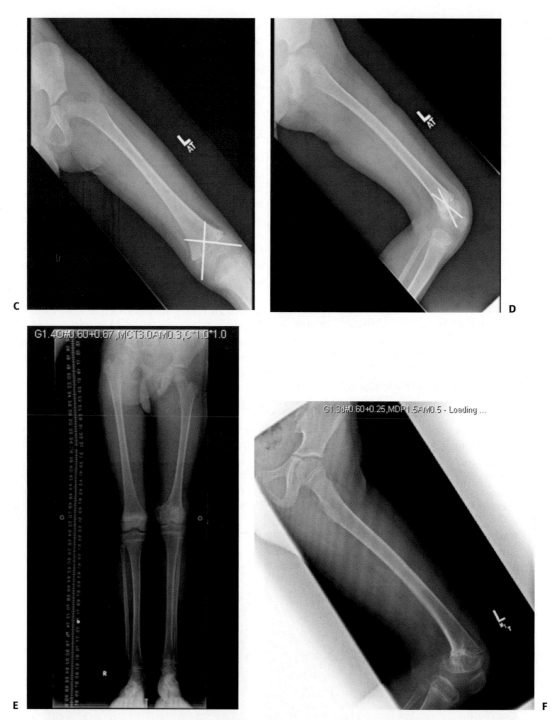

Figure 25-16. (*Continued*) **C, D:** She underwent closed reduction and pinning. **E, F:** Four years later she has angular deformity and shortening from asymmetric growth arrest.

meta-analysis of case series reported from 1950 to 2007 that included 564 fractures, 52% of fractures resulted in a growth disturbance.[7] Although Salter–Harris type I and II fractures in other areas of the body usually have a low risk of growth arrest, these Salter–Harris fractures in the distal femur are also at risk for premature physeal closure (Fig. 25-17). Of the most common Salter–Harris types, growth abnormalities are seen in 36% of type I fractures, 58% of type II fractures, 49% of type III fractures, and 64% of type IV fractures. Displaced distal femoral

physeal fractures are four times more likely to develop growth arrest compared to nondisplaced fractures. Growth disturbance is uncommon in patients younger than 2 years of age who sustain these injuries, possibly because of the flat shape of the physis in this age group[72] which reduces the damage of physeal cartilage precursor cells. Older children who have more than 2 years of growth remaining are at highest risk for this complication and are most likely to have clinically significant deformities resulting from physeal arrest.[72] Although adolescents

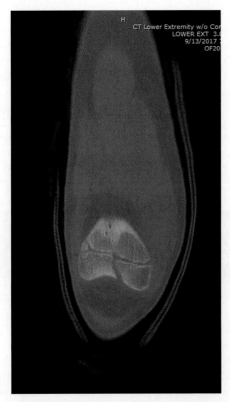

Figure 25-17. CT scan further elucidating a displaced Salter Harris III fracture.

frequently sustain this fracture and may develop growth complications, the clinical consequences of growth arrest are not as severe, compared to patients between the ages of 2 and 12 years. Increased growth arrest is also seen more commonly in patients who had surgery for these fractures, particularly if transphyseal fixation was used.[2]

Diagnosing Growth Arrest

The distal femur grows approximately 1 cm a year, consequently, growth arrest is typically evident by 6 months after distal femoral epiphyseal fracture healing. In some cases, however, incomplete cessation of growth, or even angular deformity, may not be evident clinically for 12 to 18 months after injury. Subtle radiographic clues are also appreciable 4 to 6 months of injury in many cases. Follow-up radiographs after fracture healing should be carefully scrutinized to determine if the physeal line is reconstituted and that Park–Harris growth arrest lines are running parallel to the physis on both AP and lateral views. Growth arrest lines develop when there is a temporary slowing of growth during periods of malnutrition, trauma, chemotherapy, or alcohol consumption, among other things.[28,30,59,61] The normal longitudinal orientation of the zone of provisional calcification becomes dense and interconnected, forming a transverse line in the metaphysis. After growth resumes, this dense layer moves away from the physis and is visible on radiographs as a radiodense line of bone in the metaphysis.[59] If the line is growing symmetrically away from the physis, then normal growth has resumed. Failure of a Park–Harris line to appear

is evidence suggestive of premature growth arrest. An oblique Park–Harris line that converges toward the physis indicates asymmetrical growth caused by a bone bridge across the physis that is preventing growth of one side of the physis and will lead to angular deformity.

Full-length standing x-rays of both lower extremities may also be a clue to help determine if growth disturbance has occurred. It is our practice to obtain standing radiographs of the lower extremities as soon as possible following the initial injury to document the leg-length difference and limb alignment at baseline for these children. Imaging is then repeated at approximately 6-month intervals so that any leg-length difference or change in angulation may be identified. Bilateral lower extremity scanograms and CT scanograms are also useful for measuring leg-length discrepancies but drawbacks compared to full-length radiographs include inability to assess the mechanical axis and increased radiation exposure, respectively.[74] If growth disturbance is suspected, MRI or CT is utilized to determine its extent; screw removal is typically done before imaging to improve the quality of imaging by eliminating the scatter effect of the metal. Physeal growth arrest is best detected by fat-suppressed three-dimensional spoiled gradient-recalled echo sequence MRI technique and may identify abnormalities as early as 2 months after injury.[22]

Treatment of Physeal Arrest

Early recognition and management of progressive angulation can reduce the need for osteotomy if the diagnosis is made before a clinically significant deformity develops by excising the physeal bar to allow resumption of normal growth. After deformity has developed, however, an osteotomy is generally required whether bar excision is performed or not. The bar is typically located across the portion of the physis that was directly injured. Physeal bars may arise after any fracture type but are most common after type II, III, and IV fractures. When asymmetric growth follows a type II separation, the portion of the physis protected by the Thurston Holland fragment is usually spared, as opposed to the growth inhibition in the portion separated from the metaphyseal fragment. For fractures with a medial metaphyseal spike, the resultant deformity is more likely to be valgus because of lateral growth arrest, whereas the opposite is true for fractures with a lateral metaphyseal spike. For type III and IV fractures, the physeal bar is usually centered on the site of the physis that was traversed by the fracture line.

Excision is generally recommended for posttraumatic physeal bars that constitute less than 50% of the total cross-sectional area of the distal femoral physis in children with a small degree of angulation and at least 2 years of growth remaining.[40,64] In one series, resumption of normal growth was seen in 80% of patients whereas others have reported lower success rates, with growth restoration seen in only 25% to 50% of patients.[11,16,31,90] Due to the unpredictable bar excision may be unreliable, it may be more prudent to perform ipsilateral hemiepiphysiodesis combined with contralateral distal femoral epiphysiodesis for patients who have mild angulation and less than 3 to 4 cm of growth remaining in the injured physis, a scenario most commonly encountered in older children and adolescents with less than 2 years of growth potential. For children with more than 4 cm of growth remaining, physeal bar excision is attempted for those bars that encompass less than 50% of the physis because the combination of ipsilateral hemiepiphysiodesis and contralateral epiphysiodesis results in unacceptable loss of overall height. For older children and adolescents with physeal bars that already have significant angulation distal femoral osteotomy may be done at the time of bilateral distal femoral physeal ablation surgery. Physeal bar excision in combination with distal femoral osteotomy may also be considered for those younger children who are candidates for bar resection and have angulation that exceeds 15 to 20 degrees.[40,42,64] If physeal bar excision fails to restore growth, or limb-length discrepancy is severe at the time of diagnosis of the growth disturbance, limb lengthening and other reconstructive procedures are options to consider based on the projected growth remaining and the limb-length difference.

COMPLETE PHYSEAL ARREST WITH LEG-LENGTH DISCREPANCY

Limb-length discrepancy is a frequently reported complication of distal femoral physeal fractures[2,24,36,72,84] but only 22% of patients with distal femoral physeal fractures have leg-length discrepancies measuring greater than 1.5 cm (Fig. 25-18).[7] This is the case because many fractures occur in older children and

adolescents with limited growth remaining at the time of injury. The treatment strategy varies, depending on the projected amount of discrepancy. Because the decision for treatment must often be made at the time of diagnosis of the complete arrest, methods of predicting the ultimate leg-length discrepancy that do not require serial measurements, such as the Paley or Menelaus methods, are utilized. Immediate contralateral distal femoral epiphysiodesis is indicated for older children and adolescents with projected discrepancies greater than 2 to 2.5 cm. For children with discrepancies that are projected to be larger than 2.5 cm, planning for limb lengthening is initiated.

SUMMARY, CONTROVERSIES, AND FUTURE DIRECTIONS RELATED TO FRACTURES OF THE DISTAL FEMORAL PHYSIS

Distal femoral physeal fractures, although relatively uncommon injuries, are prone to complications and require attentive diagnostic, operative, and postoperative management. They can result from both low- and high-energy mechanisms. Acutely, patient evaluation must focus on identifying possible associated injuries and the neurovascular status of the affected limb. Peroneal nerve and popliteal artery injuries, and compartment

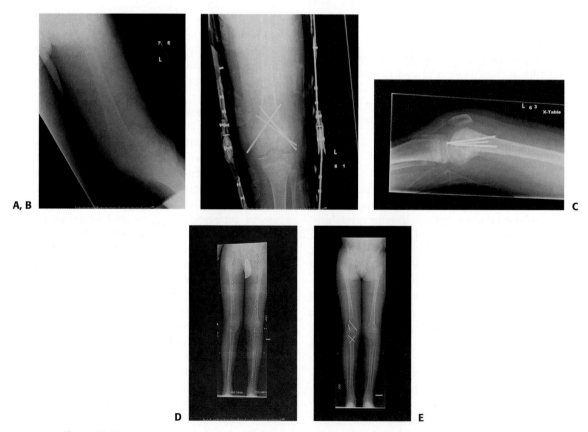

Figure 25-18 A 13-year-old boy fell off a wall. He sustained a comminuted fracture of the distal femur (**A**) with superficial abrasions over his leg and underwent closed reduction and fixation with smooth wires (**B** and **C**). Eighteen months later he has an LLD of about 2 cm. After a discussion with the family, screw epiphysiodeses of the femur and tibia were done (**D**). At 1-year follow-up he has nearly equal leg lengths (**E**).

syndrome of the leg may occur, especially in patients with high-energy mechanisms. Radiographs and CT scan are utilized to fully delineate the fracture pattern and to guide treatment. Most Salter–Harris I and II fractures may be treated with closed reduction and fixation with smooth wires or screws. Salter–Harris III and IV fractures frequently require open reduction and fixation to ensure anatomic alignment of the joint line and physis. Growth disturbances are the most common complication related to distal femoral physeal fractures and are seen in approximately half of the patients resulting in either angular deformities or leg-length discrepancies. Displaced fractures, regardless of Salter–Harris type, are prone to growth disturbances. Other complications of these injuries include ligamentous knee injuries, peroneal nerve palsies, and knee stiffness.

Some important issues regarding physeal fractures of the distal femur require clarification and warrant future study. The diagnosis of physeal separations in the face of negative radiographs by stress radiographs of the distal femur remains somewhat controversial. In a past era when open repair of medial collateral ligament injuries were performed, distinguishing physeal separations from ligament tears by stress views was important for making expedient treatment decisions.[28] Iatrogenic worsening of physeal injury, however, is a concern when performing this diagnostic test. Now, because initial treatment is similar for both injuries, specifically immobilization and not surgery, and with the increasing use of MRI to evaluate acute knee injuries, stress views are no longer routinely utilized for children and adolescents with possible physeal separations with few exceptions.

The best method of advanced imaging for displaced fractures is another area of controversy. For intra-articular fractures, some[45] have recommended the routine use of CT scan as part of the preoperative evaluation to help delineate the fracture pattern and to plan fixation. Others prefer MRI for these injuries, trading some diminution of bone details for the ability to diagnose chondral, meniscal, and ligament injuries.[53,82] In the acute setting, the best choice of imaging studies is unclear. The surgeon must weigh the pros and cons of each modality, taking into consideration, among other concerns, the availability of each of the modalities in the emergency setting, the radiation risk of CT, and familiarity with interpretation of MRI for fracture assessment. Further study on this topic is needed to optimize decision making.

Despite advanced imaging methods of fracture evaluation and modern surgical techniques for management of displaced fractures, complications, particularly growth disturbance affect approximately half of patients with this injury. Research for this injury must focus on the methods that diminish the incidence of growth disruption and restore growth when arrest occurs. The use of stem cells, cartilage cell regeneration, and other novel techniques are being investigated to address the problem of growth arrest after physeal injuries, including those of the distal femoral physis in children.[21,38,70,91]

Annotated References

Reference	Annotation
Arkader A, Warner WC Jr, Horn BD, et al. Predicting the outcome of physeal fractures of the distal femur. *J Pediatr Orthop.* 2007;27(6):703–708.	Series of 73 patients that showed both presence of displacement and Salter–Harris classification to be predictive of outcome. Degree and direction of displacement did not correlate with outcomes.
Basener CJ, Mehlman CT, DiPasquale TG. Growth disturbance after distal femoral growth plate fractures in children: a meta-analysis. *J Orthop Trauma.* 2009;23(9):663–667.	Meta-analysis with >500 fractures and overall rate of growth disturbance of 52%.
Brone LA, Wroble RR. Salter-Harris type III fracture of the medial femoral condyle associated with an anterior cruciate ligament tear. Report of three cases and review of the literature. *Am J Sports Med.* 1998;26(4):581–586.	Reports on a series of patients with Salter–Harris III fractures of the medial femoral condyle and associated ACL tears which were treated in a staged fashion, with ligament reconstruction performed at a second operation.
Broughton NS, Dickens DR, Cole WG, et al. Epiphyseolysis for partial growth plate arrest. Results after four years or at maturity. *J Bone Joint Surg Br.* 1989;71(1):13–16.	13 children treated with epiphysiodesis for growth arrest and there were no complications from the procedure. 8 of these had improvement or resolution of their alignment, while 5/13 underwent additional surgery.
Egol KA, Karunakar M, Phieffer L, et al. Early versus late reduction of a physeal fracture in an animal model. *J Pediatr Orthop.* 2002;22(2):208–211.	Animal model demonstrating that the smallest angular deformity developed in physeal fractures that were immediately reduced.
Garrett BR, Hoffman EB, Carrara H. The effect of percutaneous pin fixation in the treatment of distal femoral physeal fractures. *J Bone Joint Surg Br.* 2011;93(5):689–694.	55 Patients showed no association between percutaneous placement of smooth pins across the physis and growth arrest.
Khoshhal KI, Kiefer GN. Physeal bridge resection. *J Am Acad Orthop Surg.* 2005;13(1):47–58.	Discuss techniques and future research directions for resection of physeal bars.
Lippert WC, Owens RF, Wall EJ. Salter-Harris type III fractures of the distal femur: plain radiographs can be deceptive. *J Pediatr Orthop.* 2010;30(6):598–605.	Demonstrated increased displacement of fracture on CT scan and MRI compared to plain radiographs.

REFERENCES

1. Anderson M, Green WT, Messner MB. Growth and predictions of growth in the lower extremities. *J Bone Joint Surg Am.* 1963;45-A:1–14.
2. Arkader A, Warner WC Jr, Horn BD, et al. Predicting the outcome of physeal fractures of the distal femur. *J Pediatr Orthop.* 2007;27(6):703–708.
3. Aroojis AJ, Gajjar SM, Johari AN. Epiphyseal separations in spastic cerebral palsy. *J Pediatr Orthop B.* 2007;16(3):170–174.
4. Aroojis AJ, Johari AN. Epiphyseal separations after neonatal osteomyelitis and septic arthritis. *J Pediatr Orthop.* 2000;20(4):544–549.
5. Banagale RC, Kuhns LR. Traumatic separation of the distal femoral epiphysis in the newborn. *J Pediatr Orthop.* 1983;3(3):396–398.
6. Barmada A, Gaynor T, Mubarak SJ. Premature physeal closure following distal tibia physeal fractures: a new radiographic predictor. *J Pediatr Orthop.* 2003;23(6):733–739.
7. Basener CJ, Mehlman CT, DiPasquale TG. Growth disturbance after distal femoral growth plate fractures in children: a meta-analysis. *J Orthop Trauma.* 2009;23(9):663–667.
8. Beals RK. Premature closure of the physis following diaphyseal fractures. *J Pediatr Orthop.* 1990;10(6):717–720.
9. Beaty JH, Kumar A. Fractures about the knee in children. *J Bone Joint Surg Am.* 1994;76(12):1870–1880.
10. Bertin KC, Goble EM. Ligament injuries associated with physeal fractures about the knee. *Clin Orthop Relat Res.* 1983;(177):188–195.
11. Birch JG. Surgical treatment of physeal bar resection. In: Eilert RE, ed. *Instructional Course Lectures.* Rosemont, IL: American Academy of Orthopaedic Surgeons; 1992:445–450.
12. Blasier RD. Distal femoral physeal fractures. In: Sam W.Wiesel, ed. *Operative Techniques in Orthopaedic Surgery.* Philadelphia, PA: Lippincott Williams & Wilkins; 2011:1116–1121.
13. Braten M, Helland P, Myhre HO, et al. 11 femoral fractures with vascular injury: good outcome with early vascular repair and internal fixation. *Acta Orthop Scand.* 1996;67(2):161–164.
14. Bright RW, Burstein AH, Elmore SM. Epiphyseal-plate cartilage. A biomechanical and histological analysis of failure modes. *J Bone Joint Surg Am.* 1974;56(4):688–703.
15. Brone LA, Wroble RR. Salter-Harris type III fracture of the medial femoral condyle associated with an anterior cruciate ligament tear. Report of three cases and review of the literature. *Am J Sports Med.* 1998;26(4):581–586.
16. Broughton NS, Dickens DR, Cole WG, et al. Epiphyseolysis for partial growth plate arrest. Results after four years or at maturity. *J Bone Joint Surg Br.* 1989;71(1):13–16.
17. Chung SM, Batterman SC, Brighton CT. Shear strength of the human femoral capital epiphyseal plate. *J Bone Joint Surg Am.* 1976;58(1):94–103.
18. Close BJ, Strouse PJ. MR of physeal fractures of the adolescent knee. *Pediatr Radiol.* 2000;30(11):756–762.
19. Crock HV. *An Atlas of Vascular Anatomy of the Skeleton and Spinal Cord.* London: Martin Dunitz; 1996.
20. Czitrom AA, Salter RB, Willis RB. Fractures involving the distal epiphyseal plate of the femur. *Intl Orthop.* 1981;4(4):269–277.
21. Dahl WJ, Silva S, Vanderhave KL. Distal femoral physeal fixation: are smooth pins really safe? *J Pediatr Orthop.* 2014;34(2):134–138.
22. Ecklund K, Jaramillo D. Patterns of premature physeal arrest: MR imaging of 111 children. *Am J Roentgenol.* 2002;178(4):967–972.
23. Egol KA, Karunakar M, Phieffer L, et al. Early versus late reduction of a physeal fracture in an animal model. *J Pediatr Orthop.* 2002;22(2):208–211.
24. Eid AM, Hafez MA. Traumatic injuries of the distal femoral physis: A retrospective study on 151 cases. *Injury.* 2002;33(3):251–255.
25. El-Zawawy HB, Silva MJ, Sandell LJ, et al. Ligamentous versus physeal failure in murine medial collateral ligament biomechanical testing. *J Biomech.* 2005;38(4):703–706.
26. Gabel GT, Peterson HA, Berquist TH. Premature partial physeal arrest: Diagnosis by magnetic resonance imaging in two cases. *Clin Orthop Relat Res.* 1991;(272):242–247.
27. Garrett BR, Hoffman EB, Carrara H. The effect of percutaneous pin fixation in the treatment of distal femoral physeal fractures. *J Bone Joint Surg Br.* 2011;93(5):689–694.
28. González-Reimers E, Perez-Ramirez A, Santolaria-Fernandez F, et al. Association of Harris lines and shorter stature with ethanol consumption during growth. *Alcohol.* 2007;41(7):511–515.
29. Graham JM, Gross RH. Distal femoral physeal problem fractures. *Clin Orthop Relat Res.* 1990;(255):51–53.
30. Harris HA. The growth of the long bones in childhood with special reference to certain bony striations of the metaphysis and to the role of vitamins. *Arch Int Med.* 1926;38:785–806.
31. Hasler CC, Foster BK. Secondary tethers after physeal bar excision. A common source of failure? *Clin Orthop Relat Res.* 2002;(405):242–249.
32. Havranek P, Pesl T. Salter (Rang) type 6 physeal injury. *Eur J Pediatr Surg.* 2010;20(3):174–177.
33. Hresko MT, Kasser JR. Physeal arrest about the knee associated with non-physeal fractures in the lower extremity. *J Bone Joint Surg Am.* 1989;71(5):698–703.
34. Hsu RW, Himeno S, Coventry MB, et al. Normal axial alignment of the lower extremity and load-bearing distribution at the knee. *Clin Orthop Relat Res.* 1990;(255):215–227.
35. Hübner U, Schlicht W, Outzen S, et al. Ultrasound in the diagnosis of fractures in children. *J Bone Joint Surg Br.* 2000;82(8):1170–1173.
36. Ilharreborde B, Raquillet C, Morel E, et al. Long-term prognosis of Salter-Harris type 2 injuries of the distal femoral physis. *J Pediatr Orthop B.* 2006;15(6):433–438.
37. Jain R, Bielski RJ. Fracture of lower femoral epiphysis in an infant at birth: A rare obstetrical injury. *J Perinatol.* 2001;21(8):550–552.
38. Jie Q, Hu Y, Yang L, et al. Prevention of growth arrest by fibrin interposition into physeal injury. *J Pediatr Orthop B.* 2010;19(2):201–206.
39. Kawamoto K, Kim WC, Tsuchida Y, et al. Incidence of physeal injuries in Japanese children. *J Pediatr Orthop B.* 2006;15(2):126–130.
40. Khoshhal KI, Kiefer GN. Physeal bridge resection. *J Am Acad Orthop Surg.* 2005;13(1):47–58.
41. Krosin MY, Lincoln TL. Traumatic distal femoral physeal fracture in a neonate treated with open reduction and pinning. *J Pediatr Orthop.* 2009;29(5):445–448.
42. Langenskiöld A. Surgical treatment of partial closure of the growth plate. *J Pediatr Orthop.* 1981;1(1):3–11.
43. Lee YS, Jung YB, Ahn JH, et al. Arthroscopic assisted reduction and internal fixation of lateral femoral epiphyseal injury in an adolescent soccer player: report of one case. *Knee Surg Sports Traumatol Arthrosc.* 2007;15(6):744–746.
44. Lewis SL, Pozo JL, Muirhead-Allwood WF. Coronal fractures of the lateral femoral condyle. *J Bone Joint Surg Br.* 1989;71(1):118–120.
45. Lippert WC, Owens RF, Wall EJ. Salter-Harris type III fractures of the distal femur: plain radiographs can be deceptive. *J Pediatr Orthop.* 2010;30(6):598–605.
46. Lippiello L, Bass R, Connolly JF. Stereological study of the developing distal femoral growth plate. *J Orthop Res.* 1989;7(6):868–875.
47. Loder RT, Bookout C. Fracture patterns in battered children. *J Orthop Trauma.* 1991;5(4):428–433.
48. Loder RT, Swinford AE, Kuhns LR. The use of helical computed tomographic scan to assess bony physeal bridges. *J Pediatr Orthop.* 1977;17(3):356–359.
49. Lombardo SJ, Harvey JP Jr. Fractures of the distal femoral epiphyses. Factors influencing prognosis: a review of thirty-four cases. *J Bone Joint Surg Am.* 1977;59(6):742–751.
50. Mangurten HH, Puppala B, Knuth A. Neonatal distal femoral physeal fracture requiring closed reduction and pinning. *J Perinatol.* 2005;25(3):216–219.
51. Mann DC, Rajmaira S. Distribution of physeal and nonphyseal fractures in 2,650 long-bone fractures in children aged 0–16 years. *J Pediatr Orthop.* 1990;10(6):713–716.
52. Masquijo JJ, Allende V. Triplane fracture of the distal femur: a case report. *J Pediatr Orthop.* 2011;31(5):e60–e63.
53. McKissick RC, Gilley JS, DeLee JC. Salter-Harris Type III fractures of the medial distal femoral physis—a fracture pattern related to the closure of the growth plate: report of 3 cases and discussion of pathogenesis. *Am J Sports Med.* 2008;36(3):572–576.
54. Meyers MC, Calvo RD, Sterling JC, et al. Delayed treatment of a malreduced distal femoral epiphyseal plate fracture. *Med Sci Sports Exerc.* 1992;24(12):1311–1315.
55. Morscher E. Strength and morphology of growth cartilage under hormonal influence of puberty. Animal experiments and clinical study on the etiology of local growth disorders during puberty. *Reconstr Surg Traumatol.* 1968;10:3–104.
56. Navascués JA, González-López JL, López-Valverde S, et al. Premature physeal closure after tibial diaphyseal fractures in adolescents. *J Pediatr Orthop.* 2000;20(2):193–196.
57. Nork SE, Segina DN, Aflatoon K, et al. The association between supracondylar-intercondylar distal femoral fractures and coronal plane fractures. *J Bone Joint Surg Am.* 2005;87(3):564–569.
58. Ogden JA. Injury to the growth mechanisms of the immature skeleton. *Skeletal Radiol.* 1981;6(4):237–253.
59. Ogden JA. Growth slowdown and arrest lines. *J Pediatr Orthop.* 1984;4(4):409–415.
60. Ogden JA. Distal femoral epiphyseal injuries. In: Ogden JA, ed. *Skeletal Injury in the Child.* New York, NY: Springer; 2000:896–912.
61. Park EA. The imprinting of nutritional disturbances on the growing bone. *Pediatrics.* 1964;33(Suppl):815–862.
62. Parsch K. Origin and treatment of fractures in spina bifida. *Eur J Pediatr Surg.* 1991;1(5):298–305.
63. Pennock AT, Ellis HB, Willimon SC, et al. Intra-articular Physeal Fractures of the Distal Femur: A Frequently Missed Diagnosis in Adolescent Athletes. *Orthop J Sports Med.* 2017;5(10):2325967117731567.
64. Peterson HA. Partial growth plate arrest and its treatment. *J Pediatr Orthop.* 1984;4(2):246–258.
65. Peterson HA, Madhok R, Benson JT, et al. Physeal fractures: Part 1. Epidemiology in Olmsted County, Minnesota, 1979–1988. *J Pediatr Orthop.* 1994;14(4):423–430.
66. Petrin M, Weber E, Stauffer UG. Interposition of periosteum in joint fractures in adolescents; comparison of operative and conservative treatment (author's transl). *Z Kinderchir.* 1981;33(1):84–88.
67. Phieffer LS, Meyer RA Jr, Gruber HE, et al. Effect of interposed periosteum in an animal physeal fracture model. *Clin Orthop Relat Res.* 2000;(376):15–25.
68. Price CT, Herrara-Soto JA. Extra-articular fractures of the knee. In: Beaty JH, ed. *Rockwood and Wilkins Children's Fractures.* 7th ed. Philadelphia, PA: Wolters Kluwer/Lippincott Williams & Wilkins; 2010.
69. Rafee A, Kumar A, Shah SV. Salter-Harris type III fracture of the lateral femoral condyle with a ruptured posterior cruciate ligament: an uncommon injury pattern. *Arch Orthop Trauma Surg.* 2007;127(1):29–31.
70. Rajagopal K, Dutt V, Manickam AS, et al. Chondrocyte source for cartilage regeneration in an immature animal: Is iliac apophysis a good alternative? *Indian J Orthop.* 2012;46(4):402–406.
71. Rang M, Wenger DR. The physis and skeletal injury. In: Wenger DR, Pring ME, eds. *Rang's Children's Fractures.* Philadelphia, PA: Lippincott Williams & Wilkins; 2005:11–25.
72. Riseborough EJ, Barrett IR, Shapiro F. Growth disturbances following distal femoral physeal fracture-separations. *J Bone Joint Surg Am.* 1983;65(7):885–893.
73. Sabharwal S, Henry P, Behrens F. Two cases of missed Salter-Harris III coronal plane fracture of the lateral femoral condyle. *Am J Orthop.* 2008;37(2):100–103.
74. Sabharwal S, Zhao C, McKeon JJ, et al. Computed radiographic measurement of limblength discrepancy. Full-length standing anteroposterior radiograph compared with scanogram. *J Bone Joint Surg Am.* 2006;88(10):2243–2251.
75. Salter R, Harris WR. Injuries involving the epiphysial plate. *J Bone Joint Surg Am.* 1963;45(3):587–622.
76. Segal LS, Shrader MW. Periosteal entrapment in distal femoral physeal fractures: Harbinger for premature physeal arrest? *Acta Orthop Belg.* 2011;77(5):684–690.

77. Sferopoulos NK. Type V physeal injury. *J Trauma.* 2007;63(6):E121–E123.
78. Simonian PT, Staheli LT. Periarticular fractures after manipulation for knee contractures in children. *J Pediatr Orthop.* 1995;15(3):288–291.
79. Simpson WC Jr, Fardon DF. Obscure distal femoral epiphyseal injury. *South Med J.* 1976;69(10):1338–1340.
80. Skak SV. A case of partial physeal closure following compression injury. *Arch Orthop Trauma Surg.* 1989;108(3):185–188.
81. Sloboda JF, Benfanti PL, McGuigan JJ, et al. Distal femoral physeal fractures and peroneal palsy: outcome and review of the literature. *Am J Orthop (Belle Mead NJ).* 2007;36(3):E43–E45.
82. Stanitski CL. Stress view radiographs of the skeletally immature knee: a different view. *J Pediatr Orthop.* 2002;24(3):342.
83. Stephens DC, Louns DS. Traumatic separation of the distal femoral epiphyseal cartilage. *J Bone Joint Surg Am.* 1974;56(7):1383–1390.
84. Thomson JD, Stricker SJ, Williams MM. Fractures of the distal femoral epiphyseal plate. *J Pediatr Orthop.* 1995;15(4):474–478.
85. Tolo VT. External skeletal fixation for children's fractures. *J Pediatr Orthop.* 1983;3(4):435–442.
86. Torg JS, Pavlov H, Morris VB. Salter-Harris type-III fracture of the medial femoral condyle occurring in the adolescent athlete. *J Bone Joint Surg Am.* 1981;63(4):586–591.
87. Vander Have KL, Ganley TJ, Kocher MS, et al. Arthrofibrosis after surgical fixation of tibial eminence fractures in children and adolescents. *Am J Sports Med.* 2010;38(2):298–301.
88. Westh R, Menelaus M. A simple calculation for the timing of epiphyseal arrest: a further report. *J Bone Joint Surg Br.* 1981;63-(1):117–119.
89. White PG, Mah JY, Friedman L. Magnetic resonance imaging in acute physeal injuries. *Skeletal Radiol.* 1994;23(8):627–631.
90. Williamson RV, Staheli LT. Partial physeal growth arrest: treatment by bridge resection and fat interposition. *J Pediatr Orthop.* 1990;10(6):769–776.
91. Xian CJ, Foster BK. Repair of injured articular and growth plate cartilage using mesenchymal stem cells and chondrogenic gene therapy. *Curr Stem Cell Res Ther.* 2006;1(2):213–229.

26

Proximal Tibial Physeal Fractures

Benjamin J. Shore and Eric W. Edmonds

INTRODUCTION TO PROXIMAL TIBIAL PHYSEAL FRACTURES

Fractures of the proximal tibia physis require a significant amount of force, and therefore these injuries account for less than 1% of all physeal injuries.[31,44] Contrasting the distal femur discussed in the previous chapter, the proximal tibial physis has intrinsic varus–valgus and side-to-side translational stability because of the collateral ligaments and the lateral fibular buttress.[10] Although potentially problematiqc regarding an apophyseal fracture of the tibial tubercle, the metaphyseal overhang of the tubercle can provide anterior–posterior translational support.

An avulsion fracture of the tibial tuberosity is uncommon, accounting for less than 1% of all epiphyseal injuries and approximately 3% of all proximal tibial fractures.[6,31,44] Most fractures concerning the proximal tibial physis result in anterior, anterolateral, and anteromedial epiphysis displacement relative to the metaphysis caused by the anatomic stability mentioned above.[52] In the rare fracture with posterior displacement, the epiphysis and tubercle apophysis are displaced as a single unit.[37] Fractures of the proximal tibial metaphysis usually occur in children aged 3 to 6 years, and may be complete or greenstick. In contrast, the tibial tubercle fracture is most commonly sustained by adolescents.[33] The most critical features of proximal tibial physeal fractures are proximity to the popliteal artery and possible development of compartment syndrome associated with fracture displacement.

ASSESSMENT OF PROXIMAL TIBIAL PHYSEAL FRACTURES

MECHANISMS OF INJURY OF PROXIMAL TIBIAL PHYSEAL FRACTURES

These injuries require a significant amount of force to propagate a proximal tibial physis fracture, most often motor vehicle

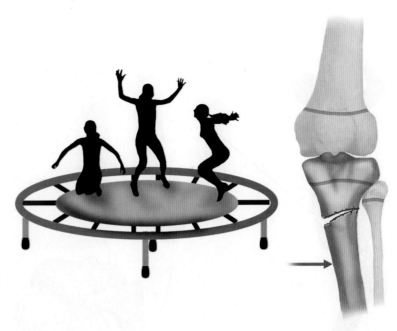

Figure 26-1. Jumping on the trampoline is a common mechanism for young children to sustain valgus and varus fractures of the proximal tibia.

trauma, sports injuries, or other events such as lawn mower accidents. However, Salter–Harris type II fractures have been reported in child abuse cases and Salter–Harris I fractures have been reported in arthrogrypotic children undergoing physical therapy stretching.[16,56]

Despite the fact that most purely physeal fractures displace anteriorly, a hyperextension force can result in the metaphyseal portion of the tibia displacing posteriorly toward the popliteal artery, which can result in vascular compromise. Valgus stress can open the physis medially with the fibula acting as a lateral resistance force (Fig. 26-1).[61] Rarely, a flexion force can cause a Salter–Harris type II or III fracture, which has a similar injury pattern to that of tibial tubercle avulsion injuries.

Tibial tubercle apophyseal fractures are more frequently the result of jumping activities, with the two most common reported being: (1) a strong quadriceps contraction during knee extension associated with jumping and (2) rapid passive flexion of the knee against the contracting quadriceps while landing (Fig. 26-2).[6,11,12,23,32,33,37,43] Moreover, tibial tuberosity fractures are reported almost exclusively in adolescent boys who tend to have greater quadriceps strength and may overcome the stability of the apophysis with a violent contraction of the muscle.[6,8,11,12,23,30,32,33,37] Because the proximal tibial physis closes from posterior to anterior, the fracture pattern depends on the amount of physeal closure present at the time of injury, as well as the degree of knee flexion.[47] When the injury occurs with the knee in either full extension or up to 30 degrees of flexion, avulsion of the tibial tubercle without fracture of the epiphysis will result; with greater than 30 degrees of flexion, avulsion of both the tibial tubercle and proximal tibial epiphysis occur where the majority are type III.[28]

INJURIES ASSOCIATED WITH PROXIMAL TIBIAL PHYSEAL FRACTURES

Although the proximal tibial physis and the tibial tubercle apophysis are intimately associated with each other, fractures of the two locations have a unique set of associated injuries. The proximal physis fracture is at risk for ligamentous, vascular, and neurologic injury; whereas, the tubercle apophyseal fractures are at particular risk for compartment syndrome.

Ligamentous injuries and internal derangement of the knee joint may occur during Salter–Harris III and IV proximal tibial physeal injuries in 40% of patients.[46] Associated injuries such as meniscal tears, cruciate ligament laxity, patellar or quadriceps tendon avulsions and compartment syndrome have been reported with tibial tubercle fractures.[7,19,40,45,60] However, in a recent systematic review of tibial tubercle fractures, low rates of tendon avulsion (2%), meniscal tears (2%), and cruciate ligament laxity (1%) was reported.[47]

Vascular compromise in proximal tibial physeal fractures can be devastating, but they are uncommon in isolated tubercle injuries.[10,52,62] The popliteal artery is tethered by its major branches near the posterior surface of the proximal tibial epiphysis. The posterior tibial branch passes under the arching fibers of the soleus. The anterior tibial artery travels anteriorly over an aperture above the proximal border of the interosseous membrane. A hyperextension injury that results in posterior displacement of the proximal tibial metaphysis may stretch and tear the tethered popliteal artery (Fig. 26-3). Even a minimally displaced fracture at presentation may have had significant displacement at the time of injury, and should therefore be monitored for vascular injury.[57] Diagnostic workup of these fractures does not mandate routine angiography as long vascular status is monitored during the initial 24 to 48 hours.

Regarding vascular injuries, the tibial tubercle avulsion fractures are at risk for bleeding of the anterior tibial recurrent artery (which traverses the base of the tubercle) into the anterior compartment. Rather than resulting in direct ischemia, this vascular compromise is associated with indirect ischemia through the development of compartment syndrome.[41]

A peroneal neuropathy may also be associated with a fracture of the proximal tibial physis, but it will often undergo spontaneous resolution of symptoms.

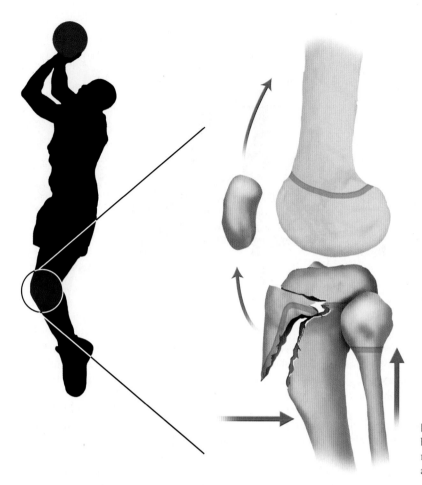

Figure 26-2. The tibial tubercle is commonly fractured because of the maximum generated force of the quadriceps contracture during jumping, primarily in male adolescents.

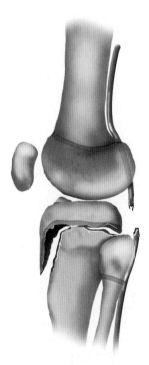

Figure 26-3. Tethering of the popliteal artery by the more distal tibial artery creates a situation wherein posterior metaphyseal tibia displacement can rupture the artery.

SIGNS AND SYMPTOMS OF PROXIMAL TIBIAL PHYSEAL FRACTURES

Physical examination of children with either a proximal physis or tubercle apophysis fracture may not be dissimilar. An important and sensitive finding is an inability to actively fully extend the knee in most displaced fractures. Pain, knee effusion, and a hemarthrosis will often be present in both. Limb deformity may or may not be present in either fracture type, and hamstring spasm may limit knee extension on examination.

The physeal injuries will have pain over the tibial physis distal to the joint line, in contrast to the tubercle injuries that will hurt directly anteriorly. Sometimes, the tubercle fractures will have a freely movable osseous fragment palpated subcutaneously between the proximal tibia and the femoral condyles, and may result in skin tenting; whereas, in the physeal fractures, the proximal metaphysis of the tibia is displaced posteriorly creating a concavity that can be palpated anteriorly at the level of the tibial tubercle. A valgus deformity suggests medial displacement of the metaphysis.

Careful physical examination with special attention to the aforementioned associated injuries should be performed at the time of initial assessment. Ischemia caused by disruption of the popliteal artery or secondary to compartment syndrome should not be missed on clinical examination. Asymmetric perfusion and pallor compared to the contralateral limb and distal pain should be recognized for potential signs of vascular compromise. Pulses should be assessed and compartments should be assessed by palpation, examination of sensation, and stretch testing of the anterior compartment through passive and active toe motion.

When the proximal end of the metaphysis protrudes under the subcutaneous tissues on the medial aspect of the knee, a tear of the distal end of the medial collateral ligament should be suspected in association with a physeal fracture. The presence of patella alta may represent either severity of tubercle displacement or concomitant rupture of the patella tendon. With a small avulsion, the child may be able to extend the knee actively through intact retinacular tissue, but active extension is impaired with larger injuries.

IMAGING AND OTHER DIAGNOSTIC STUDIES FOR PROXIMAL TIBIAL PHYSEAL FRACTURES

In proximal tibial physeal fractures, plain radiographs are the mainstay of evaluation, but nondisplaced physeal fractures may not be visible. Associated hemarthrosis can sometimes be the only indication of fracture and is primarily recognized by identifying an obliteration of the fat planes (predominately the loss of a crisp posterior border to the quadriceps tendon in mild-to moderate-sized hemarthrosis) (Fig. 26-4), or an increased

separation of the patella from the distal femur on lateral views in patients with severe hemarthrosis. Occasionally, relatively nondisplaced physeal fractures may have small Thurstan Holland fragments extending into the metaphysis. Often, fracture lines may only be visible on oblique view radiographs. At other times the metaphyseal fragments can be quite large (Fig. 26-5). Stress views can often differentiate a proximal tibial physeal fracture from a ligament injury, but there is potential risk for physeal injury and increased pain in a clinical setting when performing these x-rays. In young children (between the ages of 2 and 5 years) measurement of the anterior tilt angle of the proximal tibial physis on the lateral is helpful to diagnose fractures not otherwise appreciated.[55] When uncertain of the diagnosis, an MRI can distinguish between physeal fractures and ligament injuries in a safe, accurate, and more comfortable fashion than stress radiographs (Fig. 26-6).[54] Moreover, CT scans can define the bony injury better than MRI or plain film and is often helpful to define intra-articular involvement and determine treatment for Salter–Harris type III, IV, and complex tibial tubercle fractures (Fig. 26-7).

The standard method of identifying tibial tubercle fractures is via the lateral plain radiograph; however, more severe injuries should warrant advanced diagnostic imaging to help identify articular disruption and internal derangement that is often seen in these fracture patterns. Although, most patients with tibial

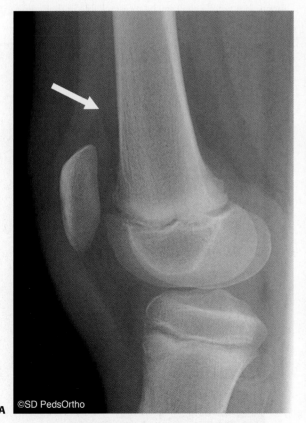
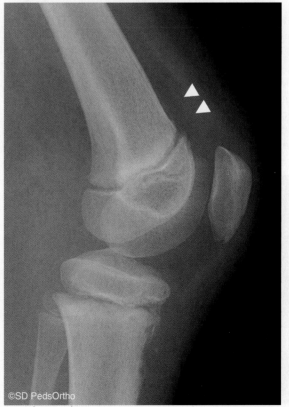

Figure 26-4. Often the only radiographic evidence of a physeal fracture may be a joint effusion, as seen in this lateral of a minimally displaced tibial tubercle fracture. **A:** Unaffected knee, right side, with *arrow* demonstrating normal crisp posterior border to the quadriceps tendon. **B:** Mild effusion with disruption of fat planes, *arrowheads* highlighting obliterated planes due to hemarthrosis.

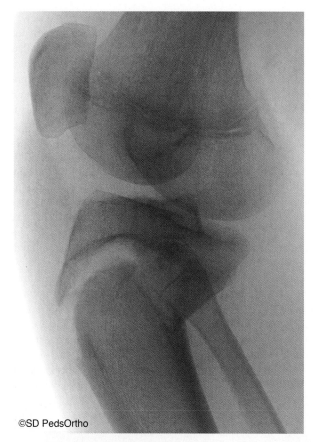

©SD PedsOrtho

Figure 26-5. Displaced fracture of the proximal tibial physis with a large posterior metaphyseal Thurstan Holland fragment, as well as an anterior conjoined tibial tubercle fragment.

tubercle fractures are adolescents (with developed secondary ossification of the tibial tubercle), fractures may occur in the more immature child and be seen merely has a small fleck of bone on plain film (Fig. 26-8). In order to improve the utility of diagnostic plain film, the lateral projection view should be done

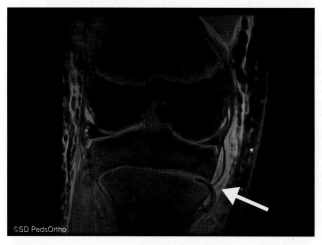

©SD PedsOrtho

Figure 26-6. MRI images can assist in differentiating physeal injuries from ligament ruptures. This coronal image demonstrates a proximal tibial physeal fracture with evidence of entrapped medical collateral ligament (MCL) fibers (*arrow*) limiting reduction.

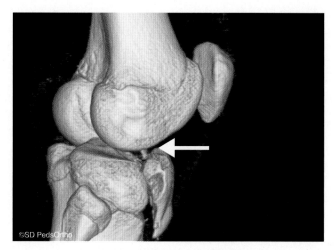

©SD PedsOrtho

Figure 26-7. Both 3D and standard CT images can help define fracture patterns that involve the joint surface to guide appropriate treatment. This 3D reconstruction demonstrates a tibial tubercle fracture with mild comminution at the joint surface (*arrow*).

with the tibia rotated slightly internal to bring the slightly lateral tubercle perpendicular to the x-ray cassette.

With regard to the tibial tubercle, it is important to remember that normal ossification may progress from more than one secondary center of ossification. Contralateral films may be helpful to distinguish normal ossification versus minimally displaced fragments, but patella alta may be more reliable in that comparison.

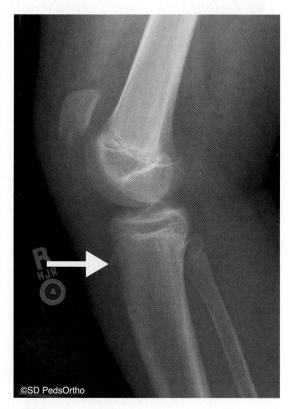

©SD PedsOrtho

Figure 26-8. Young children may only have evidence of a small fleck (*arrow*) to represent an otherwise larger cartilaginous fracture of the tibial tubercle.

CLASSIFICATION OF PROXIMAL TIBIAL PHYSEAL FRACTURES

Metaphyseal Fracture Patterns	
Direction of Injury	**Resultant Fracture Pattern**
• Valgus	• Medial-sided displacement
• Varus	• Lateral-sided displacement
• Hyperextension	• Posterior displacement

Tibial Tubercle Fracture Patterns	
Fracture Type	**Description**
• Type I	• Apophyseal injuries at the patellar tendon insertion (displaced/nondisplaced)
• Type II	• Apophyseal/epiphyseal injuries without intra-articular extension (displaced/nondisplaced)
• Type III	• Apophyseal/epiphyseal injuries with intra-articular extension (displaced/nondisplaced)
• Type IV	• Fracture of the entire proximal tibia, +/– posterior Thurstan Holland fragment (displaced/nondisplaced)
• Type V	• No fracture, pure avulsion injury of the patellar tendon

Proximal tibial physeal fractures are most commonly described using the Salter–Harris classification scheme that denotes the direction of fracture propagation relative to the growth plate. Age and mechanism of injury can dictate fracture location (Figs. 26-9 and 26-10).[33] Watson-Jones[58] described three types of avulsion fractures of the tibial tubercle, with subsequent modifications by Ogden and associates[37,38] who noted that the degree of displacement depends on the severity of injury to adjacent soft tissue attachments. Ryu[48] and Inoue[27] proposed a type IV fracture in which the physeal separation occurs through the tibial tuberosity and extends posteriorly into the horizontal tibial physis.

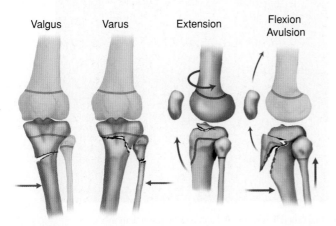

Figure 26-9. All proximal tibial physeal fractures can be classified based on the mechanism of injury: Varus/valgus, extension, and flexion avulsion injuries.

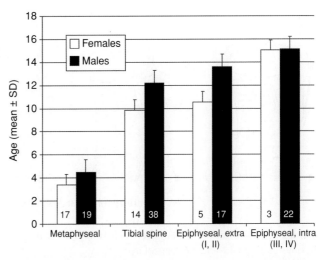

Figure 26-10. Bar graph representing the change in fracture patterns seen with increasing age.

Pace et al.[39] and Aerts et al.[1] have described modified surgical management techniques associated with these type IV fractures. A recent study delineating a three-dimensional classification of tibial tubercle fractures, highlights the risk for associated pathology when considering surgical fixation.[40] Pretell-Mazzini et al.[47] performed a systematic review of the literature surrounding tibial tubercle fractures and summarized the Ogden classification into the following five groups, where within each group the fracture can be displaced, nondisplaced, or comminuted: Type I fractures involved the tibial apophysis, where the patellar tendon inserts, type II fractures involved the apophysis and the epiphysis without intra-articular extension, type III fractures are similar to type II fracture with intra-articular extension, type IV fractures involved the entire proximal tibial physis and the fracture can exist posterior inferiorly creating an equivalent Thurstan Holland fragment, and finally type V injuries are not really fractures but pure avulsion injuries (Fig. 26-11).

OUTCOME MEASURES FOR PROXIMAL TIBIAL PHYSEAL FRACTURES

There are no specific outcome scores or tools validated for proximal tibial physeal fractures; however, most studies have used plain radiographs to determine healing and a few have utilized return to sports for functional outcomes.

PATHOANATOMY AND APPLIED ANATOMY RELATING TO PROXIMAL TIBIAL PHYSEAL FRACTURES

Present at birth, the ossific nucleus of the proximal tibial epiphysis lies central in the cartilaginous anlage. Usually singular, it can occasionally have two ossification centers, not including the universal secondary center of ossification of the tubercle that appears between 9 and 14 years of age. Closure of the proximal tibial physis and union between the epiphysis and tubercle

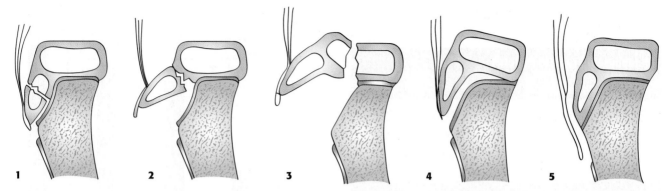

Figure 26-11. A Modified Ogden classification of tibial tubercle fractures.

centers occurs commonly in girls between 10 and 15 years and in boys between 11 and 17 years of age.

The development of the tibial tubercle has been further defined by Ehrenborg.[18] After birth is the cartilaginous stage that exists prior to development of the secondary ossification center and persists until the age of 9 years in girls and age of 10 years in boys. This is followed by the apophyseal stage, in which the ossification center appears in the tongue of cartilage that drapes over the anterior tibial metaphysis. The epiphyseal stage is marked by the tubercle and epiphyseal bony union, and this is followed by the final bony stage, wherein the proximal tibia becomes fully ossified. There is evidence that closure of the physis follows a predictable pattern.[5,17,21,37,40,51,53] In the sagittal plane, the proximal tibial physis has been shown to close in a posterior to anterior direction, with subsequent progression of closure toward the tubercle apophysis which is closing in a proximal to distal direction, simultaneously. In the coronal planes, the proximal tibial physis is closing in a medial to lateral direction; whereas, in the axial plane, the tibia is closing in a posteromedial to anterolateral direction.

The anatomy of the collateral ligaments provides some protection from epiphyseal disruption. The superficial portion of the medial collateral ligament extends distal to the physis inserting into the medial metaphysis, therefore acting as a medial buttress. The lateral collateral ligament inserts on the proximal pole of the fibula, and this entire lateral construct acts like a lateral buttress. Anteriorly, the patellar ligament attaches to the secondary ossification center of the tibial tuberosity that is draped over the metaphysis serving as a constraint to posterior displacement. The terminal insertion of the powerful quadriceps at the boundary between the secondary ossification centers of the tubercle and the proximal tibial epiphysis places the tubercle at risk for isolated or combined avulsion fractures. This risk is minimal until adolescence when the quadriceps mechanism is matured because some fibers of the patella tendon extend distal to the apophysis into the anterior aspect of the upper tibial diaphysis. Therefore, it is important to recognize that these adolescent avulsions often have extensive soft tissue damage that extends down the anterior diaphysis of the tibia (Fig. 26-12). The distal portion of the popliteal artery lies close to the posterior aspect of the proximal tibia.

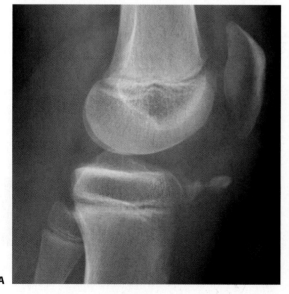
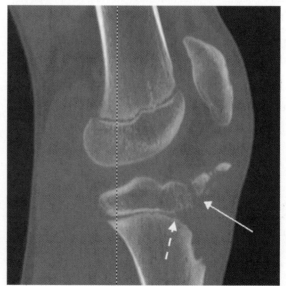

Figure 26-12. Example case with open reduction of the tibial tubercle fracture. **A:** Lateral radiograph demonstrating displaced tibial tubercle that does not extend into the join (Modified Ogden type 2). **B:** Sagittal CT scan that highlights that although this fracture does not involve the joint (*solid arrow*), it does involve the proximal tibial physis (*broken arrow*).

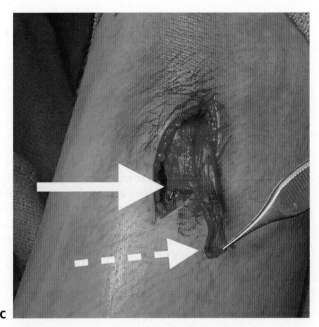

C

Figure 26-12. (*Continued*) **C:** Intraoperative photograph demonstrating that patella tendon fibers (*broken arrow*) extend greater than 2 cm distal to the fracture fragment (*solid arrow*), highlighting the soft tissue disruption that occurs. (Used with permission of the Children's Orthopaedic Center, Los Angeles.)

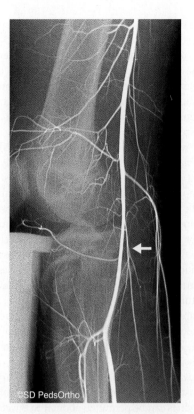

Figure 26-13. Arteriogram after a proximal tibial physeal fracture. Even with minimal displacement, note the construction of the popliteal artery (*arrow*).

Firm connective tissue septa hold the vessel against the knee capsule placing it at risk for injury during proximal tibia physeal fractures (Fig. 26-13). The lateral inferior geniculate artery crosses the surface of the popliteus muscle, anterior to the lateral head of the gastrocnemius, and turns forward underneath the lateral collateral ligament. The medial inferior geniculate artery passes along the proximal border of the popliteus muscle, anterior to the medial head of the gastrocnemius, and extends anterior along the medial aspect of the proximal tibia. The popliteal artery divides into the anterior tibial and posterior tibial branches beneath the arch of the soleus muscle. Much of the blood supply to the proximal tibial epiphysis is derived from an anastomosis between these geniculate arteries.[14,24] The tibial tubercle receives its main blood supply from a plexus of arteries behind the patellar ligament at the level of the attachment to the tibial tubercle.[14] This vascular anastomosis arises from the anterior tibial recurrent artery and may be torn with this fracture.[41,60] Several small branches extend down into the secondary ossification center. A smaller part of the blood supply enters the superficial surface of the tubercle from adjacent periosteal vessels.

TREATMENT OPTIONS FOR PROXIMAL TIBIAL PHYSEAL FRACTURES

NONOPERATIVE TREATMENT OF PROXIMAL TIBIAL PHYSEAL FRACTURES

None, or minimally displaced fractures can often be treated with closed reduction. If there is any displacement requiring

manipulation for closed reduction this is best done under anesthesia. One should have a low threshold for operative fixation.

Regarding tubercle reductions, a persistent gap between the distal end of the tubercle and the adjacent metaphysis may indicate an interposed flap of periosteum.[12,23] Minimally displaced, small avulsion fragments have been treated successfully with immobilization in a cylinder cast or long-leg cast with the knee fully extended.[11,12,32,37]

Indications/Contraindications

Nonoperative Treatment of Proximal Tibial Physeal Fractures: INDICATIONS AND CONTRAINDICATIONS	
Indications	**Relative Contraindications**
• No to minimal displacement	• Displacement • Joint involvement • Compartment syndrome • Open fracture • Floating knee

Closed Reduction of Proximal Tibial Tubercle and Physeal Fractures

Traction during the reduction maneuver will reduce the risk of physeal damage. There is little reason to re-create the deformity during reduction, and doing so may injure the physis. Prior to closed reduction, a tense knee effusion may be aspirated using sterile technique followed by an injection of 2 to 5 mL of either 0.5% bupivacaine, or 0.2% ropivacaine to relieve pain and augment the reduction attempt. However, many children will not tolerate this method of anesthesia and either moderate conscious sedation or general anesthesia should be employed, to ensure adequate muscle relaxation and protection of the physis with closed reduction.

Patients with a nondisplaced (2 mm or less) and stable proximal tibial epiphyseal fractures can be simply placed in a long-leg cast generally in full extension if that best reduces the fracture. Appropriate padding is important and thick (1/2 in) foam may be placed either along the popliteal fossa or on the bony prominences to protect the skin. The cast may be either univalved or bivalved to permit swelling. Almost universally, the child is then admitted to the hospital for observation and gentle elevation to monitor for the possibility of vascular injury and compartment syndrome, even in seemingly minimally displaced fractures.

Radiographs should be obtained at the time of reduction and cast placement to confirm appropriate alignment of the fracture. Future films should include both the AP and lateral x-rays at 1 week post-reduction to confirm maintenance of reduction. The cast may be removed 4 to 6 weeks after injury if the fracture demonstrates radiographic and clinical union. Return to normal activities can be permitted about 4 to 8 weeks following cast removal.

OPERATIVE TREATMENT OF PROXIMAL TIBIAL PHYSEAL FRACTURES

Indications/Contraindications

Fractures that are reducible via closed methods, but unstable, may be stabilized with crossing percutaneous smooth pins or screws. Fractures that cannot be anatomically reduced require open reduction for removal of soft tissue interposition (entrapped pes anserinus and periosteum have been reported).[13,56,61] Another relative indication for open reduction and internal fixation is to facilitate wound management when a vascular repair is necessary.

Open reduction is also indicated for all type III displaced injuries with intra-articular extension.[6,11,12,23,32,35,38] Residual displacement greater than 2 to 3 mm may lead to an extensor lag and quadriceps weakness.

Closed Reduction and Percutaneous Fixation

Preoperative Planning

✔ Closed Reduction and Percutaneous Pinning of Proximal Tibial Physeal Fractures: PREOPERATIVE PLANNING CHECKLIST	
OR table	☐ Radiolucent, preferably without metallic side bars
Position/positioning aids	☐ Assistant for counter traction, bump under operative leg to facilitate easy cross-table lateral fluoroscopy
Fluoroscopy location	☐ Opposite to surgeon and back table
Equipment	☐ C-arm, smooth pins, unopened trays for open reduction
Tourniquet	☐ Nonsterile ☐ May not need to inflate, unless surgery converted to open reduction, can tether quadriceps inhibiting anatomic reduction

If the reduction is performed in the emergency department but the fracture is deemed unstable, then a temporary splint should be placed and plans to move to the operating room should be made. However, if the initial attempt was undertaken in the operating room and the fracture was deemed unstable, then percutaneous pinning could be done immediately.

Positioning

The patient should be placed supine on a radiolucent table. A bolster under the ipsilateral buttocks helps keep the patella facing anteriorly and can be helpful for imaging during the procedure. A bump under the ankle makes lateral imaging easier and can aid in reduction, or an assistant can elevate the leg for lateral imaging. The surgeon stands on the ipsilateral side of the table. The C-arm comes in from the contralateral side, the image screen is positioned so the surgeon does not have to turn their head away from the field to see the screen, and the back table should be positioned behind the surgeon.

Surgical Approach

If an anatomic reduction is achieved, smooth K-wires are usually sufficient for fixation of the epiphyseal fragment and minimizes the risk of iatrogenic growth plate injury. One can use K-wires for the tibial tuberosity but screws are stronger and closing the apophyseal growth plate near the end of growth is not a concern. Pin size choice will depend on the size of the tibia, but usually range from a 0.062-in pin to a 2.5-mm pin in bigger children. One should consider leaving the pins extra articular, coming out distally, to help prevent a septic joint from a pin tract infection (Fig. 26-14).

Technique

✔ Closed Reduction and Percutaneous Pinning of Proximal Tibial Physeal Fractures: KEY SURGICAL STEPS
☐ Closed reduction of the fracture with C-arm guidance • Pin placement ☐ For smooth pin placement, bend and cut pins to be pulled at 4 weeks postoperatively ☐ For cannulated screws, close stab incisions with suture ☐ Place dressing and apply long-leg cast in full extension

Occasionally, for large Thurstan Holland fragments, a percutaneous compression screw may be placed to secure the fracture.

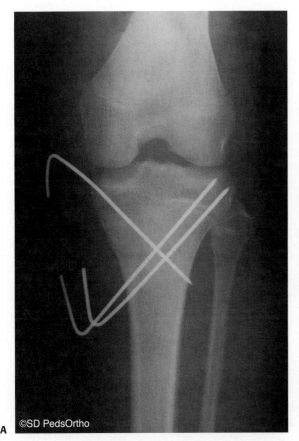
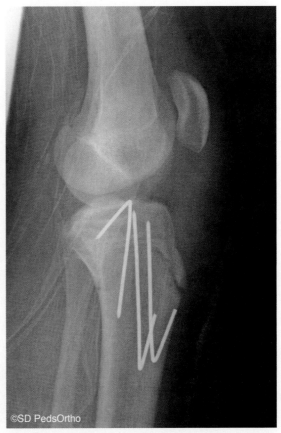

©SD PedsOrtho   ©SD PedsOrtho

A   B

Figure 26-14. A modified Ogden type IV tibial tubercle fracture, or Salter–Harris type II (with posterior metaphyseal fragment and tibial tubercle fracture). **A:** AP radiograph demonstrating cross-pin technique. **B:** Lateral radiograph demonstrating anatomic reduction with fixation.

Rather than using the cross-pin technique, or in conjunction with that technique, a small stab incision can be made directly over the fragment after reduction. Fluoroscopy guidance is then utilized to place the guide pin from a cannulated screw system, being sure not to violate the physis or the apophysis anteriorly. Length is measured, the proximal cortex drilled, and the screw is inserted and secured into place with fluoroscopy. If a bicortical purchase can be achieved, then that is optimal. Yet, cancellous screws can be utilized if the width of the tibial metaphysis exceeds the screw options (Fig. 26-15).

For the extra-articular tibial tubercle fragments a choice between the smooth pin (Fig. 26-16) and the screw (Fig. 26-17) can be made but the technique is the same. These fractures will often have soft tissue interposition and conversion to open reduction is common.

Fluoroscopy can confirm the reduction is anatomic. Even with open reduction an anatomically reduced fragment has some space between the osseous tubercle and the tibia, so a lateral image of the contralateral leg may help evaluate the reduction. While smooth K-wires may be preferable if there is lots of growth expected, cannulated screws provide more strength. There is no need to violate the posterior cortex of the tibia, which could harm neurovascular structures.

Open Reduction and Internal Fixation

Preoperative Planning

✔ **ORIF of Proximal Tibial Physeal Fractures:** PREOPERATIVE PLANNING CHECKLIST	
OR table	☐ Radiolucent, preferably without metallic side bars
Position/ positioning aids	☐ Assistant for counter-traction, bump under operative leg to facilitate easy cross-table lateral fluoroscopy
Fluoroscopy location	☐ Opposite to operative limb, surgeon, and back table
Equipment	☐ C-arm, smooth pins, trays for open reduction including a cannulated compression screw system (4.0 to 6.5 mm sizes available)
Tourniquet	☐ Nonsterile ☐ May not need to inflate, unless surgery converted to open reduction, can tether quadriceps inhibiting anatomic reduction
Other	☐ Confirm vascular status prior to surgery, and have sterile Doppler available

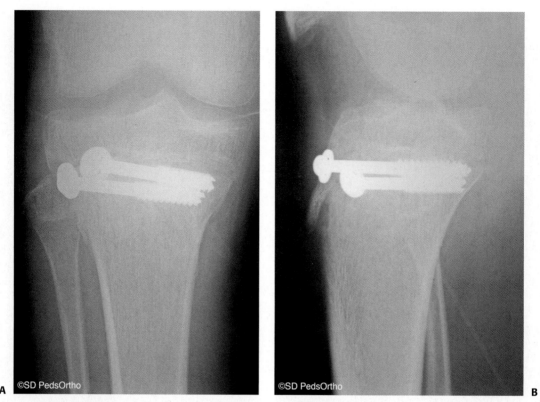

Figure 26-15. Salter–Harris type II proximal tibial physis fracture with two cannulated, partially threaded cancellous screws in the Thurstan Holland fragment. **A:** AP radiograph. **B:** Lateral radiograph.

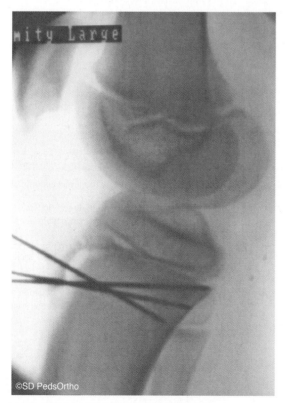

Figure 26-16. Intraoperative lateral fluoroscopy image demonstrating multiple smooth pin fixation of a tubercle fracture.

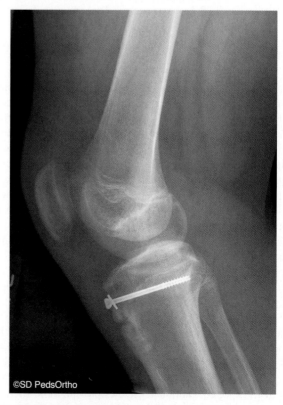

Figure 26-17. Postoperative lateral radiograph with single compression screw and washer fixation of an extra-articular tibial tubercle fracture.

A CT scan can help define if there is intra-articular involvement. If there is, one should plan on for either open or arthroscopic visualization of the joint surface. Have cannulated screws available, 4.0 to 6.5 mm for most cases.

Positioning

The patient should be placed supine on a radiolucent table. A bolster under the ipsilateral buttocks helps keep the patella facing anteriorly and can be helpful for imaging during the procedure. A bump under the knee or ankle makes lateral imaging easier, or an assistant can elevate the leg for lateral imaging. The surgeon stands on the ipsilateral side of the table. The C-arm comes in from the contralateral side, the image screen is positioned so the surgeon does not have to turn their head away from the field to see the screen, and the back table should be positioned behind the surgeon.

Surgical Approach

A longitudinal incision just lateral to the tibial tubercle (rather than directly over it) to minimize the potential for scar discomfort over the prominent bone. It may extend proximally into the joint if the articular surface is to be evaluated open, and may extend distally a bit for an anterior compartment release and replace avulsed extensor mechanism tissue. Care should be taken not to score or further damage the physis at the perichondral ring of LaCroix during the approach (Fig. 26-18). Often the extent of soft tissue disruption extends past the middle of the tibial diaphysis and an adequate incision is necessary to facilitate appropriate exposure. There are no vascular or neurologic structures at risk during this approach. A tourniquet is usually not needed, and may need to be released if it is hindering reduction of a displaced fracture caused by constriction of the quadriceps muscle.

Technique

> ### ✓ ORIF of Proximal Tibial Physeal Fractures: KEY SURGICAL STEPS
>
> ☐ Just lateral to the tibial tubercle exposure of proximal tibia
>   • If vascular repair needed consider medial approach to combine fracture reduction and vascular repair through a single incision
> ☐ Hematoma debridement and identification of all fracture components (fragment, fracture bed, physis, soft tissue injury, joint injury)
> ☐ Isolated tibial tubercle fractures are directly reduced with straight knee. Type IV fractures involving the entire physis may require traction and some leverage (90% traction, 10% leverage)
> ☐ Utilize C-arm fluoroscopy and place tentative smooth wire fixation or guidewires for cannulated screws
> ☐ Consider release of fascia off lateral tibia to release anterior compartment
> ☐ Closure of incision
> ☐ Cast application (long-leg or cylinder) in near full extension

After performing the anterior approach, the fracture bed is carefully cleared of debris such as fracture hematoma and an assessment is taken of the entire fracture personality. For example, a periosteal flap (from the diaphysis) is frequently entrapped in the fracture blocking an anatomic reduction.[12,23] Isolated tibial tubercle fractures are directly reduced with straight knee. Type IV fractures involving the entire physis may require traction and some leverage (90% traction, 10% leverage). For type II and III fractures screws should not violate the epiphysis (Fig. 26-19).

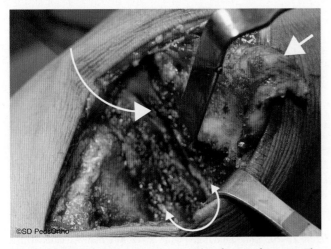

Figure 26-18. Intraoperative photograph of a C fracture. The patella is to the upper right and foot the lower left, with the physis (*curved arrow*) and fracture bed (*double-headed arrow*). There is evidence of a large periosteal avulsion attached to the tubercle fragment (*arrowhead*).

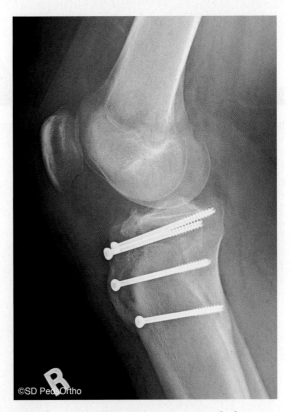

Figure 26-19. Lateral radiograph demonstrating multiple compression screw fixation of a Salter–Harris type IV proximal tibial physeal fracture.

For large epiphyseal fragments in type IV fractures smooth K-wires are usually sufficient for fixation of the epiphyseal fragment and minimize the risk of iatrogenic growth plate injury. Pin size choice will depend on the size of the tibia, but usually range from a 0.062-in pin to a 2.5-mm pin in bigger children. One should consider leaving the pins extra articular, coming out distally, to help prevent a septic joint from a pin tract infection.

For tibial tubercle fractures reduction is performed with the knee straight. Fluoroscopy can confirm the reduction is anatomic. Even with open reduction an anatomically reduced fragment has some space between the osseous tubercle and the tibia, so a lateral image of the contralateral leg may help evaluate the reduction. While smooth K-wires may be preferable if there is lots of growth expected, cannulated screws provide more strength. There is no need to violate the posterior cortex of the tibia with wires or screws, which could harm neurovascular structures. Historically many surgeons used large screws with washers, which usually required later removal due to prominence. Our preference is to use multiple 4.5-mm screws without washers when possible. A longitudinal splitting incision of the patella tendon allows the 4.5-mm heads to be buried in soft tissue. It is important to avoid splitting the bone, especially small fragments. Drilling the fracture fragment with a drill the size of the root diameter of the screw helps prevent this. A partially threaded screw placed first will provide compression. After that fully threaded screws will supplement the fixation (Fig. 26-20).

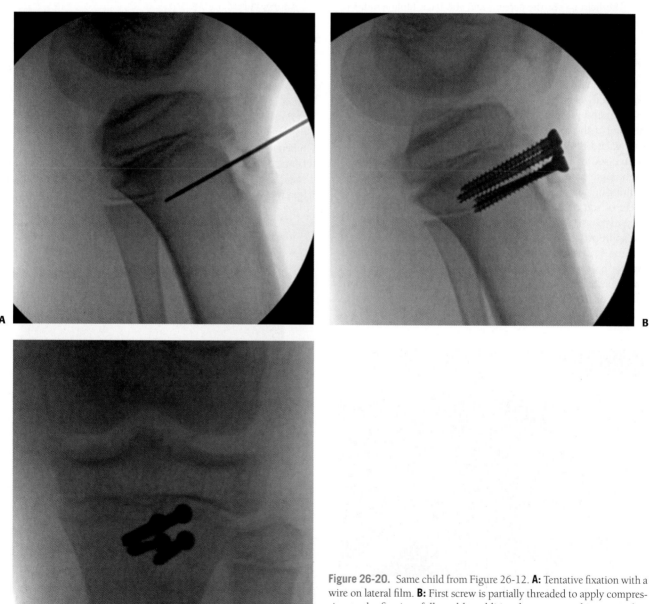

Figure 26-20. Same child from Figure 26-12. **A:** Tentative fixation with a wire on lateral film. **B:** First screw is partially threaded to apply compression to the fixation, followed by additional screws to achieve complete fixation of all the fragments on lateral view (**C**) and on anteroposterior radiographs. (Used with permission of the Children's Orthopaedic Center, Los Angeles.)

Authors' Preferred Treatment for Proximal Tibial Physeal Fractures (Algorithm 26-1)

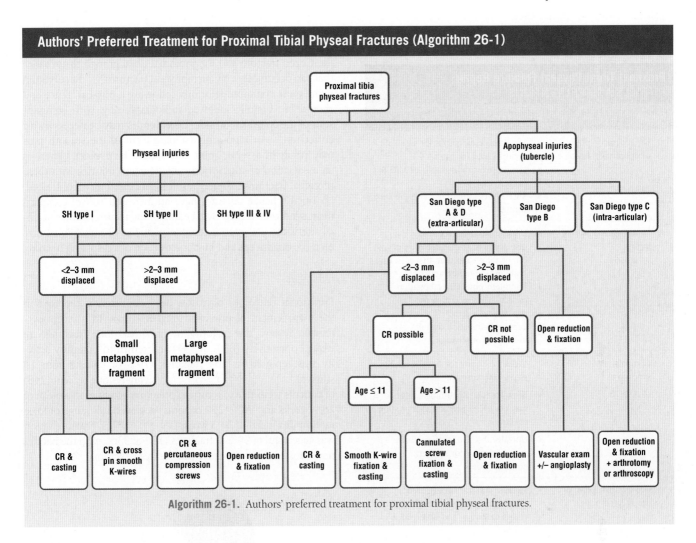

Algorithm 26-1. Authors' preferred treatment for proximal tibial physeal fractures.

Screw fixation can be used when the Thurstan Holland fragment is large enough to support this type of fixation. Alternatively, for tibial tubercle fractures, a tension band can be passed around the fragment or through the patellar ligament and fixed through a drill hole across the anterior tibia distal to the attachment of the tuberosity. This technique may be indicated in cases of a Soft-tissue avulsion, or if the bony fragments are too small or comminuted for fixation with K-wires or screws. A variation of these fractures that are similar to patella sleeve avulsions with small pieces of metaphyseal bone described by Davidson and Letts.[15] The wire is driven around the proximal pole of the patella or through a drill hole in the distal pole and then looped distally through a cannulated cortical screw or drill hole that is inserted across the anterior tibia distal to the patellar tendon insertion. Davidson and Letts[15] recommended fixation of these injuries with small cancellous screws and heavy nonabsorbable sutures to repair the torn retinaculum and periosteum. Tension band wiring has even been reported as a first-line method to facilitate rapid rehabilitation in athletes.[35]

Postoperative Care

The cast should be either univalved, bivalved, or have foam padding to permit swelling. Almost universally, the child is then admitted to the hospital for observation and gentle elevation to monitor for the high incidence of vascular injury and compartment syndrome. Shorter periods of immobilization may be used in younger adolescents if fixation is secure. For larger fragments that are securely fixed with two or more screws, a hinged knee brace can be substituted for cast immobilization. Range of motion and quadriceps strengthening are initiated 6 weeks following injury for these patients. For patients with small bone fragments or tenuous fixation casting and protective bracing may be longer.

Radiographs should be obtained at the time of reduction and cast placement to confirm appropriate alignment of the fracture. Future films should include both the AP and lateral x-rays at 1 week postreduction to confirm maintenance of reduction. The cast may be removed 4 to 6 weeks after injury if the fracture demonstrates radiographic and clinical union. Hinged Brace may be used for additional weeks. Return to normal activities can be permitted about 12 weeks following injury. Physis checks should be done between 4 and 6 months postoperatively via plain radiographs.

Potential Pitfalls and Preventive Measures
for Proximal Tibial Physeal Fractures

Proximal Tibial Physeal Fracture Repair: PITFALLS AND PREVENTIONS	
Pitfall	**Prevention**
• Unrecognized physeal or apophyseal fracture	• Scrutinize radiographs for signs of nondisplaced fractures • Obtain stress radiographs or MRI to confirm diagnosis • MCL injuries are unusual in the very young
• Unrecognized arterial injury	• Understand that maximal displacement at the time of injury can be far greater than that seen on static resting radiograph • Thorough physical examination particularly concerning the circulatory system • Repeat examination during in-hospital observation
• Compartment syndrome	• Vigilance during the first 24 hours to assess compartment status • Be aware that a neurologic injury may confound physical examination results • Univalve, bivalve, or place foam in cast to allow for swelling postreduction
• Growth disruption of the affected physis	• Metaphyseal fractures (Cozen injuries) may autocorrect the valgus deformity and observation is warranted • Recurvatum is the most common (especially following tubercle injuries) and may require surgical intervention
• Intra-articular pin placement	• May result in septic arthritis and should be avoided, try to place pins in a retrograde fashion from metaphysis to epiphysis
• Tourniquet utilization in tubercle fractures can hinder reduction	• Releasing the tourniquet, and thereby the quadriceps muscle, will assist in the reduction of tubercle fractures

With open physes, children with knee trauma, or those with polytrauma should have their radiographs scrutinized for nondisplaced proximal tibial fractures.[20,50] Overnight observation in the hospital is recommended for all fractures of the proximal tibia because of the risk of vascular injury or development of compartment syndrome. All casts should be at least univalved during early immobilization, and repeated compartment assessments must be performed and documented (Fig. 26-21). Arterial injuries can go unrecognized, especially in "minimally" displaced fractures, since the full displacement at time of injury is not known. Nondisplaced fractures can be misdiagnosed as

medial collateral ligament injuries.[59] Stress radiographs, or preferably an MRI can assist in correct diagnosis. Be cognoscente of the Cozen fracture and the proximal tibial growth disturbance that can occur following metaphyseal fractures.[26,34] Recurvatum is the most common deformity following a physeal injury and should be carefully followed radiographically, with comparisons of the contralateral side. Osteotomies may be necessary for correction.[42] An intra-articular placement of the smooth pins may result in a septic joint and should be avoided. There is an association of anterior cruciate ligament injuries with these proximal fractures that may result in late instability if untreated.

Tibial tubercle fractures have an increased risk of compartment syndrome caused by bleeding of the recurrent anterior tibial artery into the anterior compartment. Use of a tourniquet may bind the quadriceps and hinder reduction of a displaced fracture.

Outcomes

Functional outcomes have not been consistently reported in the management of proximal tibial fractures. In a recent systematic review, the majority of proximal tibial fractures are treated operatively (88% of 334) and return to preinjury activity was reported in 264 fractures (79% of patient from 19 studies).[2,3,6,7,9,11,12,19,22,25,28,29,32,35–38,45,60] Ninety-four percent (248) of patients were able to return to preinjury activities in a mean of 28.9 weeks and 98% (250 patients) achieved full range of knee motion in a mean of 22.3 weeks.[6,9,19,25,28,29,36,45,63] Fracture union was successful in 99% of fractures (334 of 336), with the painful nonunion fragments treated with delayed excision.[28,60]

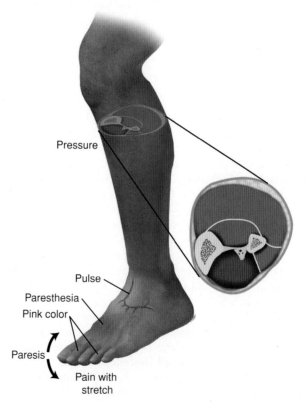

Figure 26-21. Physical examination findings in the setting of compartment syndrome.

In reviewing the literature, the overall complication rate in the management of tibial tubercle fractures is 28% (95 of 336 fractures). However, the most common complication is related to hardware irritation and bursitis (56%), followed by tenderness or prominence of tibial tubercle (18%).[47]

Injuries to the proximal tibia physis—are subject to limb shortening or angulation from subsequent growth arrest (Fig. 26-22). Any of the fracture patterns mentioned above can result in this particular complication; and, as with any physeal (or apophyseal) fracture, an anatomic reduction with fixation reduces but does not eliminate the risk of growth disturbance.[49] If a partial or complete growth arrest is diagnosed, there is limited recourse. Surgery can be done to limit deformity progression via epiphysiodesis or excision of an epiphyseal bar depending on estimations of remaining

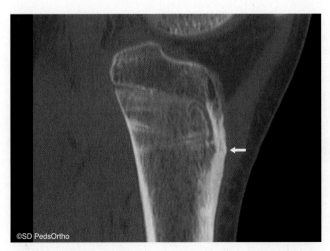

Figure 26-22. Sagittal CT scan 1 year after reduction and smooth wire fixation of a 12-year-old tibial tubercle fracture with subsequent physeal bar formation (*arrow*) and developing genu recurvatum.

growth and location of the arrest within the physis (Fig. 26-23). Therefore, frequent radiographic follow-up is important to achieve early recognition of the growth arrest and thereby limit the extent of disturbance through early intervention. As a reminder, the proximal tibia grows longitudinally at a mean rate of 6 mm per year. And the mean age of physeal closure at the proximal tibia is 14 years old in girls and 16 years old in boys. If angular growth disturbances are identified late, then an osteotomy can be done to correct the deformity. Even recurvatum following a tibial tubercle fracture can be corrected with an osteotomy.[42]

Compartment syndrome may occur following any proximal tibial physeal fracture caused by either a mechanical blockage of the vascular structures by a displaced fracture, damage to the popliteal artery, or tearing of the anterior tibial recurrent vessels that bleed into the anterior compartment.[41,60] It is important to recognize that even a minimally displaced fracture at the time of presentation, may have injured one of these vessels at the moment of fracturing. Furthermore, even minimal posterior displacement of the metaphysis can obstruct popliteal blood flow since that vessel is tethered against the bone by soft tissues and the distal anterior tibial artery.[10] Vigilant monitoring is recommended for all patients with proximal tibial physis or displaced tibial tuberosity avulsion fractures. Prophylactic anterior compartment fasciotomy should be considered at the time of open reduction because of the high risk associated with these fractures.[6]

Bursitis over prominent implants is common, especially for tibial tubercle fractures.[2,47,60] Countersinking the screw heads may not always be possible without risking fracture of the tuberosity fragment; however, 4.0 or 4.5 screw heads without washers can usually sink below the level of the patella tendon fibers without complication. Fixation with small screws or use of a tension band construct may be good alternatives, but fixation of these fractures should not be sacrificed for a potential risk of bursitis since the pull of the quadriceps muscle can displace fixed fractures. Families should be consulted that approximately 50% of patients may require a secondary procedure for implant removal after successful union of the fracture.

Less frequently, there have been reports of symptomatic knee instability, primarily in children sustaining Salter–Harris type III and IV proximal tibial injuries.[4,46] Refracture has also been reported for tibial tubercle fractures.[6,60] This was seen in two children, one after a rapid return to sports (4 weeks after injury) and one wherein a transverse proximal tibial fracture occurred 7 months postoperatively at the level of the retained screws. There is one report of arthrofibrosis and persistent loss of motion of 25 degrees in a Salter–Harris type III fracture at almost 2 years post-injury.[12] Finally, even a thrombophlebitis has been reported in the literature.[34]

SUMMARY OF PROXIMAL TIBIAL PHYSEAL FRACTURES

Fractures of the proximal tibial physis may be relatively uncommon, but they can result in deleterious consequences if poorly managed. Unrecognized compartment syndrome or arterial injury would be devastating to a young limb.

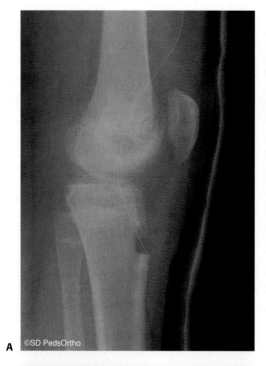
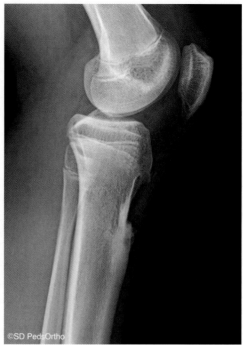
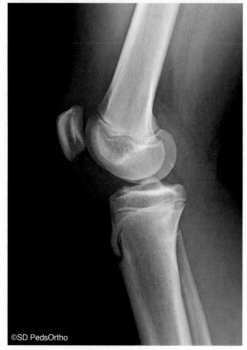

Figure 26-23. Same child as in Figure 26-22, after physeal bar excision and fat graft placement to correct deformity. **A:** Lateral radiograph showing initial postcorrective surgery. Three years after corrective surgery, the operated limb had 7 degrees of persistent recurvatum (**B**) compared to contralateral limb (**C**), but more than 2.5 cm of uninhibited longitudinal growth.

Annotated References

Reference	Annotation
Mubarak SJ, Kim JR, Edmonds EW, et al. Classification of proximal tibial fractures in children. *J Child Orthop.* 2009;3(3):191–197.	Retrospective study of 135 proximal tibia fractures over an 8-year period. The authors developed a new classification system which reflects the direction of force and fracture pattern
Ogden JA, Tross RB, Murphy MJ. Fractures of the tibial tuberosity in adolescents. *J Bone Joint Surg Am.* 1980;62(2):205–215.	This retrospective review reports 15 adolescent physeal fractures. In this paper the authors modified the existing Watson-Jones classification into the Ogden classification creating fracture subtypes based on displacement and comminution.

Annotated References

Reference	Annotation
Pace L, McCulloch, Momoh E, et al. Operatively treated type IV tibial tubercle apoplyseal fractures. *J Pediatr Orthop.* 2013;33(8):791–796.	24 Operatively treated Ogden Type IV tibial tubercle fractures were reviewed in 23 patients. This retrospective review discusses the management and complications associated with Type IV variant injuries. In this article the authors advocate for plate and screw fixation for the Type IV B tibial tubercle fractures.
Pandya N, Edmonds EW, Roocroft JH, et al. Tibial tubercle fractures: complications, classification, and the need for intra-articular assessment. *J Pediatr Orthop.* 2012;32(8)749–759.	This retrospective review of 41 operatively treated tibial tubercle fractures introduces a 4-part classification system which helps guide physicians regarding surgical management. The authors advocate preoperative CT/MRI to help identify intra-articular pathology that is often missed on plain radiographs.
Pretell-Mazzini J, Kelly DM, Sawyer JR, et al. Outcomes and complications of tibial tubercle fractures in pediatric patients: A systematic review of the literature. *J Pediatr Orthop.* 2016;36(5):440–446.	This systematic review reports on 23 eligible articles reporting on the management of tibial tubercle fractures for a review of 336 fractures. This is the most comprehensive review in the literature. This paper reviews the functional outcome, complications, and methods of treatment for tibial tubercle fractures. In addition, this paper attempts to synthesize the classification systems which have been previously published and reported on.
Ryu RK, Debenham JO. An unusual avulsion fracture of the proximal tibial epiphysis. Case report and proposed addition to the Watson-Jones classification. *Clin Orthop Relat Res.* 1985;(194):181–184.	A case report which makes modification to the Watson-Jones/Ogden tibial tubercle classification by adding Type IV which are tubercle fractures which extend into the posterior cortex of the tibia.

REFERENCES

1. Aerts BR, Ten Brinke B, Jakma TS, et al. Classification of proximal tibial epiphysis fractures in children: four clinical cases. *Injury.* 2015;46(8):1680–1683.
2. Ares-Rodriguez O, Seijas R, Nunez-Pereira S, et al. Type III fracture of the anterior tibial tuberosity in adolescents: two case reports. *Eur J Orthop Surg Traumatol.* 2008;18(5):399–403.
3. Balmat P, Vichard P, Pem R. The treatment of avulsion fractures of the tibial tuberosity in adolescent athletes. *Sports Med.* 1990;9(5):311–316.
4. Bertin KC, Goble EM. Ligament injuries associated with physeal fractures about the knee. *Clin Orthop Relat Res.* 1983;(177):188–195.
5. Blanks RH, Lester DK, Shaw BA. Flexion-type Salter II fracture of the proximal tibia. Proposed mechanism of injury and two case studies. *Clin Orthop Relat Res.* 1994;(301):256–259.
6. Bolesta MJ, Fitch RD. Tibial tubercle avulsions. *J Pediatr Orthop.* 1986;6(2):186–192.
7. Brey JM, Conoley J, Canale ST, et al. Tibial tuberosity fractures in adolescents: is a posterior metaphyseal fracture component a predictor of complications? *J Pediatr Orthop.* 2012;32(6):561–566.
8. Bright RW, Burstein AH, Elmore SM. Epiphyseal-plate cartilage: a biomechanical and histological analysis of failure modes. *J Bone Joint Surg Am.* 1974;56(4):688–703.
9. Buhari SA, Singh S, Wong HP, et al. Tibial tuberosity fractures in adolescents. *Singapore Med J.* 1993;34(5):421–424.
10. Burkhart SS, Peterson HA. Fractures of the proximal tibial epiphysis. *J Bone Joint Surg Am.* 1979;61(7):996–1002.
11. Chow SP, Lam JJ, Leong JC. Fracture of the tibial tubercle in the adolescent. *J Bone Joint Surg Br.* 1990;72(2):231–234.
12. Christie MJ, Dvonch VM. Tibial tuberosity avulsion fracture in adolescents. *J Pediatr Orthop.* 1981;1(4):391–394.
13. Ciszewski WA, Buschmann WR, Rudolph CN. Irreducible fracture of the proximal tibial physis in an adolescent. *Orthop Rev.* 1989;18(8):891–893.
14. Crock H. *An Atlas of Vascular Anatomy of the Skeleton and Spinal Cord.* London: Martin Dunitz; 1996.
15. Davidson D, Letts M. Partial sleeve fractures of the tibia in children: an unusual fracture pattern. *J Pediatr Orthop.* 2002;22(1):36–40.
16. Diamond LS, Alegado R. Perinatal fractures in arthrogryposis multiplex congenita. *J Pediatr Orthop.* 1981;1(2):189–192.
17. Dvonch VM, Bunch WH. Pattern of closure of the proximal femoral and tibial epiphyses in man. *J Pediatr Orthop.* 1983;3(4):498–501.
18. Ehrenborg G. The Osgood-Schlatter lesion: a clinical study of 170 cases. *Acta Chir Scand.* 1962;124:89–105.
19. Frey S, Hosalkar H, Cameron DB, et al. Tibial tuberosity fractures in adolescents. *J Child Orthop.* 2008;2(6):469–474.
20. Gupta SP, Agarwal A. Concomitant double epiphyseal injuries of the tibia with vascular compromise: a case report. *J Orthop Sci.* 2004;9(5):526–528.
21. Haines RW, Mohiuddin A, Okpa FI, et al. The sites of early epiphysial union in the limb girdles and major long bones of man. *J Anat.* 1967;101(Pt 4):823–831.
22. Hajdu S, Kaltenecker G, Schwendenwein E, et al. Apophyseal injuries of the proximal tibial tubercle. *Int Orthop.* 2000;24(5):279–281.
23. Hand WL, Hand CR, Dunn AW. Avulsion fractures of the tibial tubercle. *J Bone Joint Surg Am.* 1971;53(8):1579–1583.

24. Hannouche D, Duparc F, Beaufils P. The arterial vascularization of the lateral tibial condyle: anatomy and surgical applications. *Surg Radiol Anat.* 2006;28(1):38–45.
25. Howarth WR, Gottschalk HP, Hosalkar HS. Tibial tubercle fractures in children with intra-articular involvement: surgical tips for technical ease. *J Child Orthop.* 2011;5(6):465–470.
26. Hresko MT, Kasser JR. Physeal arrest about the knee associated with non-physeal fractures in the lower extremity. *J Bone Joint Surg Am.* 1989;71(5):698–703.
27. Inoue G, Kuboyama K, Shido T. Avulsion fractures of the proximal tibial epiphysis. *Br J Sports Med.* 1991;25(1):52–56.
28. Jakoi A, Freidl M, Old A, et al. Tibial tubercle avulsion fractures in adolescent basketball players. *Orthopedics.* 2012;35(8):692–696.
29. Levi JH, Coleman CR. Fracture of the tibial tubercle. *Am J Sports Med.* 1976;4(6):254–263.
30. Maffulli N, Grewal R. Avulsion of the tibial tuberosity: muscles too strong for a growth plate. *Clin J Sport Med.* 1997;7(2):129–132, discussion 132–133.
31. Mann DC, Rajmaira S. Distribution of physeal and nonphyseal fractures in 2,650 long-bone fractures in children aged 0–16 years. *J Pediatr Orthop.* 1990;10(6):713–716.
32. Mosier SM, Stanitski CL. Acute tibial tubercle avulsion fractures. *J Pediatr Orthop.* 2004;24(2):181–184.
33. Mubarak SJ, Kim JR, Edmonds EW, et al. Classification of proximal tibial fractures in children. *J Child Orthop.* 2009;3(3):191–197.
34. Navascues JA, Gonzalez-Lopez JL, Lopez-Valverde S, et al. Premature physeal closure after tibial diaphyseal fractures in adolescents. *J Pediatr Orthop.* 2000;20(2):193–196.
35. Nikiforidis PA, Babis GC, Triantafillopoulos IK, et al. Avulsion fractures of the tibial tuberosity in adolescent athletes treated by internal fixation and tension band wiring. *Knee Surg Sports Traumatol Arthrosc.* 2004;12(4):271–276.
36. Nimityongskul P, Montague WL, Anderson LD. Avulsion fracture of the tibial tuberosity in late adolescence. *J Trauma.* 1988;28(4):505–509.
37. Ogden JA, Southwick WO. Osgood-Schlatter's disease and tibial tuberosity development. *Clin Orthop Relat Res.* 1976;(116):180–189.
38. Ogden JA, Tross RB, Murphy MJ. Fractures of the tibial tuberosity in adolescents. *J Bone Joint Surg Am.* 1980;62(2):205–215.
39. Pace JL, McCulloch PC, Momoh EO, et al. Operatively treated type IV tibial tubercle apophyseal fractures. *J Pediatr Orthop.* 2013;33(8):791–796.
40. Pandya NK, Edmonds EW, Roocroft JH, et al. Tibial tubercle fractures: complications, classification, and the need for intra-articular assessment. *J Pediatr Orthop.* 2012;32(8):749–759.
41. Pape JM, Goulet JA, Hensinger RN. Compartment syndrome complicating tibial tubercle avulsion. *Clin Orthop Relat Res.* 1993;(295):201–204.
42. Pappas AM, Anas P, Toczylowski HM Jr. Asymmetrical arrest of the proximal tibial physis and genu recurvatum deformity. *J Bone Joint Surg Am.* 1984;66(4):575–581.
43. Pesl T, Havranek P. Acute tibial tubercle avulsion fractures in children: selective use of the closed reduction and internal fixation method. *J Child Orthop.* 2008;2(5):353–356.
44. Peterson HA, Madhok R, Benson JT, et al. Physeal fractures: Part 1. Epidemiology in Olmsted County, Minnesota, 1979–1988. *J Pediatr Orthop.* 1994;14(4):423–430.
45. Polakoff DR, Bucholz RW, Ogden JA. Tension band wiring of displaced tibial tuberosity fractures in adolescents. *Clin Orthop Relat Res.* 1986;(209):161–165.
46. Poulsen TD, Skak SV, Jensen TT. Epiphyseal fractures of the proximal tibia. *Injury.* 1989;20(2):111–113.
47. Pretell-Mazzini J, Kelly DM, Sawyer JR, et al. Outcomes and complications of tibial tubercle fractures in pediatric patients: a systematic review of the literature. *J Pediatr Orthop.* 2016;36(5):440–446.

48. Ryu RK, Debenham JO. An unusual avulsion fracture of the proximal tibial epiphysis. Case report and proposed addition to the Watson-Jones classification. *Clin Orthop Relat Res.* 1985;(194):181–184.
49. Salter R. Injuries involving the epiphyseal plate. *J Bone Joint Surg Am.* 1963;45:587.
50. Sferopoulos NK, Rafailidis D, Traios S, et al. Avulsion fractures of the lateral tibial condyle in children. *Injury.* 2006;37(1):57–60.
51. Shapiro F. *Developmental Bone Biology.* San Diego, CA: Academic Press; 2001.
52. Shelton WR, Canale ST. Fractures of the tibia through the proximal tibial epiphyseal cartilage. *J Bone Joint Surg Am.* 1979;61(2):167–173.
53. Smith JW. The structure and stress relations of fibrous epiphysial plates. *J Anat.* 1962;96:209–225.
54. Stanitski CL. Stress view radiographs of the skeletally immature knee: a different view. *J Pediatr Orthop.* 2004;24(3):342.
55. Stranzinger E, Leidolt L, Eich G, et al. The anterior tilt angle of the proximal tibia epiphyseal plate: a significant radiological finding in young children with trampoline fractures. *Eur J Radiol.* 2014;83(8):1433–1436.
56. Thompson GH, Gesler JW. Proximal tibial epiphyseal fracture in an infant. *J Pediatr Orthop.* 1984;4(1):114–117.
57. Tjoumakaris FP, Wells L. Popliteal artery transection complicating a non-displaced proximal tibial epiphysis fracture. *Orthopedics.* 2007;30(10):876–877.
58. Watson-Jones R, Wilson JN, eds. *Fractures and Joint Injuries.* New York: Churchill Livingstone; 1976.
59. Welch P, Wynne G. Proximal tibial epiphyseal fracture separation. *J Bone Joint Surg Am.* 1963;45(4):782–784.
60. Wiss DA, Schilz JL, Zionts L. Type III fractures of the tibial tubercle in adolescents. *J Orthop Trauma.* 1991;5(4):475–479.
61. Wood KB, Bradley JP, Ward WT. Pes anserinus interposition in a proximal tibial physeal fracture. A case report. *Clin Orthop Relat Res.* 1991;(264):239–242.
62. Wozasek GE, Moser KD, Haller H, et al. Trauma involving the proximal tibial epiphysis. *Arch Orthop Trauma Surg.* 1991;110(6):301–306.
63. Zrig M, Annabi H, Ammari T, et al. Acute tibial tubercle avulsion fractures in the sporting adolescent. *Arch Orthop Trauma Surg.* 2008;128(12):1437–1442.

27

Intra-Articular Injuries of the Knee

Dennis E. Kramer and Mininder S. Kocher

Fractures of the Tibial Spine (Intercondylar Eminence)

INTRODUCTION TO FRACTURES OF THE TIBIAL SPINE

Fractures of the tibial spine occur because of a chondroepiphyseal avulsion of the anterior cruciate ligament (ACL) insertion on the anteromedial tibial spine.[295,403] Tibial spine fractures were once thought to be the pediatric equivalent of midsubstance ACL tears in adults,[36,42,76,141,172,195,309,397,400] though recent evidence suggests that the relative incidence of ACL tears in children may be increasing,[347] and that tibial spine fractures in some adult populations may be more common than previously appreciated.[96,189]

Avulsion fracture of the tibial spine is a relatively uncommon injury in children: Skak et al.[355] reported that it occurred in 3 per 100,000 children each year. The most common causes of these fractures are bicycle accidents and athletic activities.[265]

Historically, a variety of treatment options have been reported, however, modern treatment is based specifically on fracture type. Nondisplaced fractures and hinged fractures which are able to be closed reduced can be treated without surgery. Displaced fractures which are not able to be reduced require open or arthroscopic reduction with internal fixation.

The prognosis for closed treatment of nondisplaced and reduced tibial spine fractures and for operative treatment of displaced fractures is good. Most series report healing with an excellent functional outcome despite some residual knee laxity.[33,36,42,181,197,239,259,274,278,359,397,400] Potential complications include nonunion, malunion, arthrofibrosis, residual knee laxity, and growth disturbance.[33,36,42,181,197,259,274,278,359,383,397,400]

ASSESSMENT OF FRACTURES OF THE TIBIAL SPINE

MECHANISMS OF INJURY FOR FRACTURES OF THE TIBIAL SPINE

Historically, the most common mechanism of tibial spine fracture in children has been a fall from a bicycle.[265,322] However, with increased participation in youth sports at earlier ages and at higher competitive levels, tibial spine fractures resulting from sporting activities are being seen with increased frequency. The most common biomechanical scenario leading to tibial spine fracture is forced valgus and external rotation of the tibia, although tibial spine avulsion fractures can also occur from hyperflexion, hyperextension, or tibial internal rotation. As with ACL injury, tibial spine fractures in sports may result from both contact and noncontact injuries.

A tibial spine fracture is actually a chondroepiphyseal avulsion of a fragment of the anteromedial tibial spine from the rest of the central proximal tibial epiphysis. In a cadaver study by Roberts and Lovell,[321,322] fracture of the anterior intercondylar spine was simulated by oblique osteotomy beneath the spine and traction on the ACL. In each specimen, the displaced fragment could be reduced into its bed by extension of the knee. In adults, the same stress might cause an isolated tear of the ACL, but in children the incompletely ossified tibial spine is generally weaker to tensile stress than the ligament, so failure occurs through the cancellous bone beneath the subchondral bone of the tibial spine. In addition, loading conditions may result in differential injury patterns. In experimental models, midsubstance ACL injuries tend to occur under rapid loading rates, whereas tibial spine avulsion fractures tend to occur under slower loading rates.[295,403]

Intercondylar notch morphology may also influence injury patterns. In a retrospective case-control study of 25 skeletally immature patients with tibial spine fractures compared to 25 age- and sex-matched skeletally immature patients with midsubstance ACL injuries, Kocher et al.[201] found narrower intercondylar notches in those patients sustaining midsubstance ACL injuries.

INJURIES ASSOCIATED WITH FRACTURES OF THE TIBIAL SPINE

Associated intra-articular injuries are relatively uncommon. Although Shea et al.[346] identified bone bruises in 18 of 20 MRI studies in children with tibial spine fractures, in a series of 80 skeletally immature patients who underwent surgical fixation of tibial spine fractures Kocher et al. found no intra-articular chondral injuries. Associated meniscal tears (Fig. 27-1) have been reported in 0%[168] to 40% of MRI studies. A recent prospective study reported meniscal injuries in 20/54, 37% of consecutive patients who underwent surgical treatment for tibial spine fractures.[115] Higher age, advanced tanner stage, and pubescence were significantly associated with an accompanying meniscal injury and 90% of these injuries involved the lateral meniscus.[115] Associated collateral ligament injury or proximal

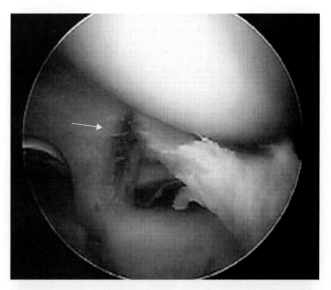

Figure 27-1. Longitudinal meniscus tear (*white arrow*) associated with tibial spine fracture.

ACL avulsion is uncommon, but has been described in case reports.[150,323] There is one published series of 21 tibial spine fractures associated with tibial plateau fractures, but the mean age was 20.8 years, with no reporting of age range or inclusion of pediatric patients.[96]

SIGNS AND SYMPTOMS OF FRACTURES OF THE TIBIAL SPINE

Patients typically present with a painful, swollen knee after an acute traumatic event. They are usually unable to bear weight on their affected extremity. On physical examination, there is often a large hemarthrosis because of the intra-articular fracture and limited motion due to pain, swelling, and occasionally mechanical impingement of the fragment in the intercondylar notch. Sagittal plane laxity is often present, but the contralateral knee should be assessed for physiologic laxity. Gentle stress testing should be performed to detect any tear of the medial collateral ligament (MCL) or lateral collateral ligament (LCL) or physeal fracture of the distal femur or proximal tibia.

Patients with late malunion of a displaced tibial spine fracture may lack full extension because of a mechanical bony block, and/or have increased knee laxity, with a positive Lachman and pivot-shift examination.

IMAGING AND OTHER DIAGNOSTIC STUDIES FOR FRACTURES OF THE TIBIAL SPINE

AP and lateral knee radiographs typically demonstrate the fracture, which is often seen best on the lateral view. The lateral radiograph is most useful in fracture classification. Radiographs should be carefully scrutinized, as the avulsed fragment may be mostly nonossified cartilage with only a small, thin ossified portion visible on the lateral view.

To guide treatment, important information to ascertain from the radiographs includes the fracture classification (Meyers and McKeever type, see below), amount of displacement, size of the

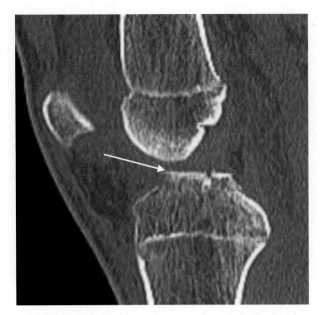

Figure 27-2. Sagittal CT cut showing a minimally displaced tibial spine fracture (*white arrow*) that can be treated conservatively without surgery as the majority of the ACL insertion on the tibia is reduced. (Kramer DE, Yen YM. Kocher MS Ch. 117 Tibial Spine Fractures. In Scott WN (ed.). *Insall & Scott Surgery of the Knee,* 6th Edition. Philadelphia: Elsevier 2017. ISBN 9780323400466.)

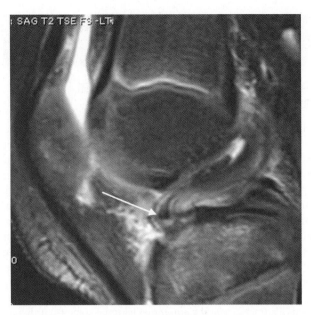

Figure 27-3. Sagittal T2 MRI showing a displaced McKeever Type III tibial spine fracture (*white arrow*) that requires surgical reduction and fixation. (Kramer DE, Yen YM. Kocher MS Ch. 117 Tibial Spine Fractures. In Scott WN (ed.). *Insall & Scott Surgery of the Knee,* 6th Edition. Philadelphia: Elsevier 2017. ISBN 9780323400466.)

fracture fragment, comminution of the fracture fragment, and status of the physes. Bone age radiographs may be obtained for patients around the time of skeletal maturity, if transphyseal screw fixation is being considered. In cases where displacement is unclear, a computerized tomography (CT) scan can be obtained (Fig. 27-2). If the majority of the ACL insertion on the tibia is intact, a nondisplaced, the fracture can be treated without surgery.

MRI is not required in the diagnosis and management of tibial spine fractures in children, particularly because operative cases typically undergo a thorough diagnostic arthroscopy to assess for possible concurrent intra-articular knee injuries, such as meniscal tears, but MRI may be helpful to confirm the diagnosis in cases with a very thin ossified portion of the avulsed fragment or evaluate for suspected associated injuries (Fig. 27-3).[168,217,346]

CLASSIFICATION OF FRACTURES OF THE TIBIAL SPINE

Fractures of the Tibial Spine:
MEYERS AND MCKEEVER CLASSIFICATION

- Type I: minimal displacement of the fragment from the rest of the proximal tibial epiphysis

- Type II: displacement of the anterior third to half of the avulsed fragment, which is lifted upward but remains hinged on its posterior border in contact with the proximal tibial epiphysis

- Type III: complete separation of the avulsed fragment from the proximal tibial epiphysis, with upward displacement and rotation

The classification system of Meyers and McKeever,[265] which is based on the degree of displacement of the tibial spine

fragment, continues to be widely used to classify fractures and guide treatment (Fig. 27-4). Radiographs of these fracture types are shown in Figure 27-5. The interobserver reliability between type I and type II/III fractures is good; however, differentiation between type II and III fractures may be difficult.[201]

Zaricznyj[412] further classified a type IV fracture to describe comminution of the tibial spine fragment.

OUTCOME MEASURES FOR FRACTURES OF THE TIBIAL SPINE

Although healing of the fracture on radiographs is important in determining timing for return to activities, the most important long-term outcome measures used to assess the results of tibial spine fracture fixation include functional knee scores, such as the Pedi-IKDC[207] and Lysholm[358] knee scores, and a patient's ability to make a full return to activities of daily life and sports activities, which can be assessed using the Marx or Tegner activity scores.[253] Asymmetry in the Lachman examination is not uncommon,[36,397] even after anatomic fixation of fractures, but has not been shown to correlate with symptomatic instability or long-term clinic results.

PATHOANATOMY AND APPLIED ANATOMY RELATING TO FRACTURE OF THE TIBIAL SPINE

The intercondylar spine is that part of the tibial plateau lying between the anterior poles of the menisci. It is triangular, with the base of the triangle running along the anterior border of the

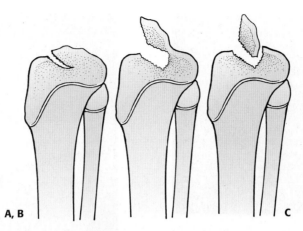

Figure 27-4. Classification of tibial spine fractures. **A:** Type I—minimal displacement. **B:** Type II—hinged posteriorly. **C:** Type III—complete separation.

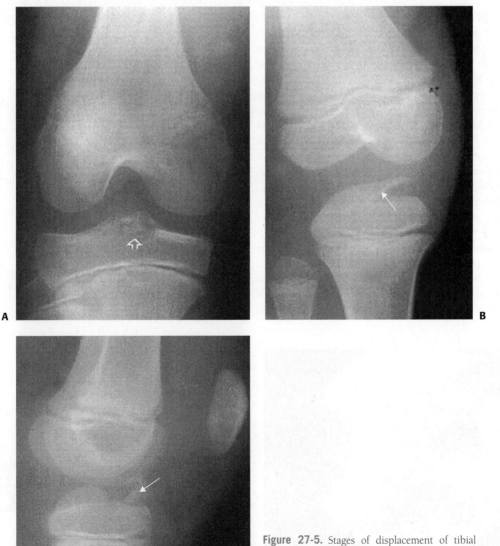

Figure 27-5. Stages of displacement of tibial spine fractures. **A:** Type I fracture (*white arrow*), minimal displacement (*open arrow*). **B:** Type II fracture (*white arrow*), posterior hinge intact. **C:** Type III fracture (*white arrow*), complete displacement and proximal migration.

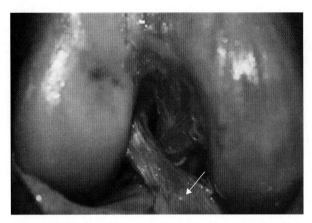

Figure 27-6. Anterior cruciate ligament insertion on the tibial spine (*white arrow*).

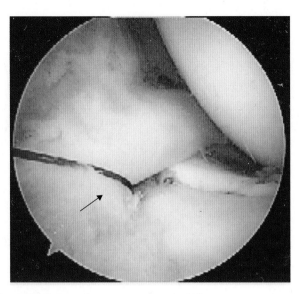

Figure 27-8. Retraction of an entrapped anterior horn medial meniscus using a retaining suture (*black arrow*).

proximal tibia. In the immature skeleton, the proximal surface of the spine is covered entirely with cartilage. The ACL attaches in the interspinous region of the spine and just anteriorly to the tibial spines, with separate slips anteriorly and laterally as well (Fig. 27-6). The ligament originates off the posterior margin of the lateral aspect of the intercondylar notch. The anterior horn of the lateral meniscus is typically attached in the region of the tibial intercondylar spine just adjacent to the ACL insertion. In 12 patients with displaced tibial spine fractures which did not reduce closed, Lowe et al.[240] reported that the anterior horn of the lateral meniscus consistently remained attached to the tibial spine fracture fragment. The posterior cruciate ligament (PCL) originates off the medial aspect of the intercondylar notch and inserts on the posterior aspect of the proximal tibia, distal to the joint line.

Meniscal or intermeniscal ligament entrapment under the displaced tibial spine fragment has been reported and may be a rationale for considering arthroscopic or open reduction in displaced tibial spine fractures (Fig. 27-7).[60,71,111,202] Meniscal entrapment prevents anatomic reduction of the tibial spine

fragment, which may result in increase of a block to extension and/or eventual anterior laxity.[141,172,397] Furthermore, meniscal entrapment itself may cause knee pain after fracture healing.[71] Falstie-Jensen and Sondergard Petersen,[111] Burstein et al.,[60] and Chandler and Miller[71] have all reported cases of meniscal incarceration-blocking reduction of type II or III tibial spine fractures in children. The prevalence of meniscal entrapment in tibial spine fractures may be common for displaced fractures. Although the anterior horn of the lateral meniscus may remain attached to the tibial spine fracture fragment, it may instead remain attached to the intermeniscal ligament, generating a soft tissue complex that may become incarcerated between the elevated bony or cartilaginous fracture fragment and its underlying bony bed. In a consecutive series of 80 skeletally immature patients who underwent surgical fixation of hinged or displaced tibial spine fractures which did not reduce in extension, Kocher et al.[202] found entrapment of the anterior horn medial meniscus ($n = 36$), intermeniscal ligament ($n = 6$), or anterior horn lateral meniscus ($n = 1$) in 26% (6/23) of hinged (type II) fractures and 65% (37/57) of displaced (type III) fractures. The entrapped meniscus can typically be extracted with an arthroscopic probe and retracted with a retaining suture (Fig. 27-8).

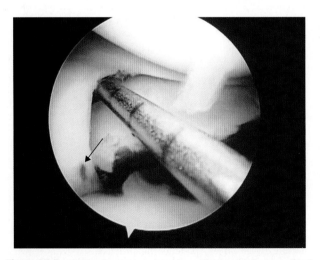

Figure 27-7. Meniscal entrapment under a tibial spine fracture (*black arrow*).

TREATMENT OPTIONS OF FRACTURES OF THE TIBIAL SPINE

Treatment options include cast immobilization,[274] closed reduction with immobilization,[398,400] open reduction with immobilization,[274] open reduction with internal fixation,[278,] arthroscopic reduction with immobilization,[259] arthroscopic reduction with suture fixation,[158,181] or suture mattress technique,[247] and arthroscopic reduction with wire,[33] screw

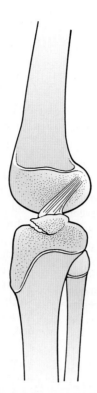

Figure 27-9. Reduction of type II tibial fracture with knee in 10 to 20 degrees of flexion.

fixation,[42] percutaneous K-wire fixation,[122,157] anchor fixation,[386] suture button fixation,[17] or bioabsorbable implant fixation.[275,342] Studies of the biomechanical strength of internal fixation suggest similar fixation strength between bioabsorbable and metallic internal fixation,[245] nonabsorbable and absorbable suture fixation,[233] inconsistent strength with suture anchor fixation[17] and increased fixation strength of suture fixation over internal fixation,[55,105] with advocates of both bioabsorbable implant fixation and suture techniques emphasizing the advantage of avoiding subsequent hardware removal procedures.[247,405]

NONOPERATIVE TREATMENT OF FRACTURE OF THE TIBIAL SPINE

Indications/Contraindications

Nonoperative Treatment of Fractures of the Tibial Spine: INDICATIONS AND CONTRAINDICATIONS	
Indications	**Relative Contraindications**
• Type I (nondisplaced) fractures	• Type III fractures
• Anatomic reduction of type II (hinged) fractures	• Persistent/recurrent displacement of type II fractures

Closed treatment is typically utilized for type I fractures and for type II fractures that successfully reduce with closed maneuvers.

Techniques

Closed reduction is usually performed with placement of the knee in full extension or 20 to 30 degrees of flexion. Aspiration of the intra-articular fracture hematoma, with or without the intra-articular injection of a short-acting local anesthetic, has historically been utilized prior to reduction, but is not required for a successful reduction and is performed less commonly today. Radiographs, most importantly the lateral view, are obtained to assess adequacy of reduction. If the proximal fracture fragment includes bony segments of the medial or lateral tibial plateau, extension may affect a reduction through pressure applied by medial or lateral femoral condyle (LFC) congruence (Fig. 27-9). Fractures confined within the intercondylar notch, however, are unlikely to reduce in this manner. Portions of the ACL are tight in all knee flexion positions; therefore there may not be any one position that eliminates the traction effect of the ACL on the fragment. Interposition of the anterior horn medial meniscus or intermeniscal ligament may further block reduction.

Outcomes

Closed reduction can be successful for some type II fractures, but is infrequently successful in type III fractures. While Bakalim and Wilppula[30] reported successful closed reduction in 10 patients, and Meyers and McKeever[266] recommended cast immobilization with the knee in 20 degrees of flexion for all type I and II fractures, Kocher et al.[202] reported successful closed reduction in only 50% of type II fractures (26/49). However, no type III fractures were able to be close reduced (0/57), in their series, and Meyers and McKeever[266] similarly recommended open reduction or arthroscopic treatment for all type III fractures. Smillie[356] suggested that closed reduction by hyperextension can be accomplished only with a large fragment.

OPERATIVE TREATMENT OF FRACTURE OF THE TIBIAL SPINE

Indications/Contraindications

Arthroscopic or open reduction with internal fixation of all type III fractures and type II fractures which do not reduce has been advocated for a variety of reasons, including concern over meniscal entrapment under the fractured tibial spine preventing anatomic closed reduction,[60,71,111] the potential for instability and loss of extension associated with closed reduction and immobilization,[141,172] the ability to evaluate and treat associated intra-articular meniscal or osteochondral injuries with surgery, and the opportunity for early mobilization following fixation. For displaced fractures, Wiley and Baxter[397] found a correlation between fracture displacement at healing with knee laxity and functional outcome.

Arthroscopic Reduction and Internal Fixation With Epiphyseal Cannulated Screws

Preoperative Planning

> ✔ **Arthroscopic Reduction and Internal Fixation of Tibial Spine Fractures With Epiphyseal Cannulated Screws:**
> PREOPERATIVE PLANNING CHECKLIST

OR table	☐ Standard table with lateral thigh post
Position/positioning aids	☐ Supine
Fluoroscopy location	☐ From operative side, perpendicular to table
Equipment	☐ Knee arthroscopy setup, 3.5- or 4-mm cannulated screw system (partially threaded)
Tourniquet	☐ Nonsterile

Technique

> ✔ **Arthroscopic Reduction and Internal Fixation of Tibial Spine Fractures With Epiphyseal Cannulated Screws:**
> KEY SURGICAL STEPS
>
> ☐ Flush hemarthrosis from knee prior to diagnostic arthroscopy
> ☐ Diagnostic arthroscopy (assess menisci)
> ☐ Fat pad debridement to improve visualization
> ☐ Debride fracture edges (underside of spine fragment and underlying fracture bed) with motorized shaver and/or curette
> ☐ Reduce spine fragment (retract intermeniscal ligament and/or meniscal anterior horn[s] if interposed) with tagging suture or probe through accessory transpatellar portal

> ☐ Maintain reduction with cannulated screw guidewire (appropriate vector usually requires start point medial or lateral to proximal patella)
> ☐ Assess reduction and measure optimal guidewire length with fluoroscopy
> ☐ Advance screw over guidewire to achieve fixation (screw tip should be proximal to physis)
> ☐ Repeat guidewire/screw steps for second screw if required

General anesthesia is typically used. The patient is positioned supine on the operating room table. A lateral breakaway post is used. Alternatively, a circumferential post can be used. A standard arthroscope is used in most patients. A small (2.7-mm) arthroscope is used in younger children. An arthroscopic fluid pump is used at 35 Torr. A tourniquet is routinely used. Standard anteromedial and anterolateral portals are used. Prior to insertion of the arthroscope through the arthroscopic cannula in the anterolateral portal, the large hemarthrosis should be evacuated, and use of up to 2 to 3 L of fluid for repetitive flushing of the joint prior to initiation of the diagnostic arthroscopy should be considered to optimize arthroscopic visualization. An accessory superomedial or superolateral portal can be later developed for guidewire and screw insertion.

A thorough diagnostic arthroscopic examination of the patellofemoral joint, medial compartment, and lateral compartment are essential to evaluate for concomitant injuries. Usually, some anterior fat pad must be excised with an arthroscopic shaver for complete visualization of the intercondylar spine fragment. Entrapped medial meniscus or intermeniscal ligament is extracted with an arthroscopic probe and retracted with a retention suture (see Fig. 27-7). The base of the tibial spine fragment is elevated (Fig. 27-10A) and the fracture bed debrided with an arthroscopic shaver or hand curette (Fig. 27-10B). Anatomic reduction is obtained using an arthroscopic probe or microfracture pick with the knee in 30 to 90 degrees of flexion (Fig. 27-10C). Cannulated guidewires can be placed through portals just off the superomedial or superolateral border of the patella, using a spinal needle to determine the optimal inferiorly directed vector for fracture fixation and taking care to avoid injury to the chondral surfaces adjacent to the intercondylar notch. The guidewires are placed into the intercondylar spine at the base of the ACL. Fluoroscopic assistance is utilized to confirm anatomic reduction, to guide correct wire orientation, and to avoid guidewire protrusion across the proximal tibial physis. A cannulated drill is used over the guidewires, taking care to drill the entire depth of the proximal fragment, but avoiding plunging through the proximal tibial physis. One or two screws are placed, based on the size of the tibial spine fragment (Fig. 27-10D). Partially threaded 3.5-mm diameter screws (Fig. 27-10E) are used in children and either 4- or 4.5-mm diameter screws are used in adolescents. The knee is brought through a range of motion (ROM) to ensure rigid fixation without fracture displacement and to evaluate for impingement of the screw head(s) in extension.

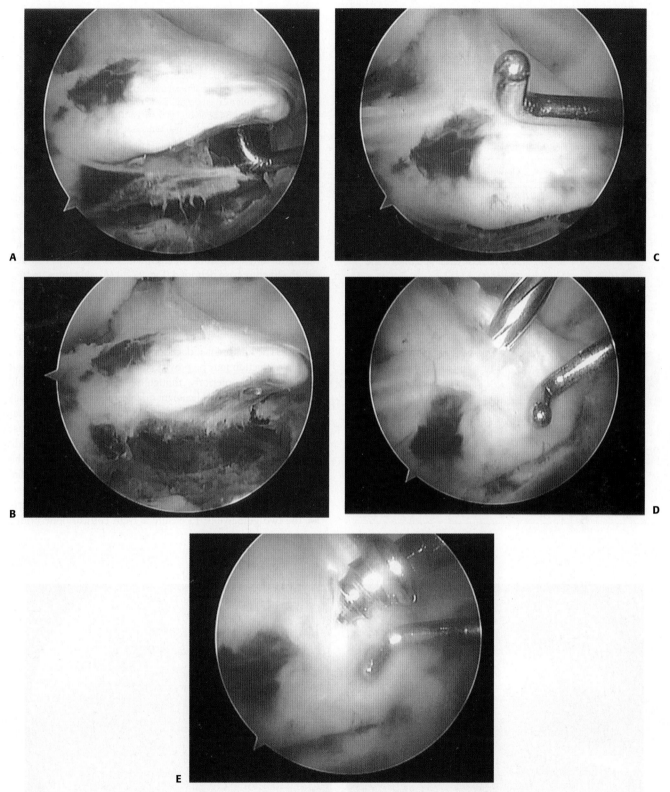

Figure 27-10. Arthroscopic reduction and cannulated screw internal fixation of a displaced tibial spine fracture. **A:** Elevation of the tibial spine fragment. **B:** Debridement of the fracture bed. **C:** Reduction of the tibial spine. **D:** Drilling over the cannulated screw guidewire. **E:** Cannulated screw fixation.

Arthroscopic Reduction and Internal Fixation With Suture

Preoperative Planning

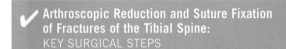

✔ Arthroscopic Reduction and Suture Fixation of Fractures of the Tibial Spine: PREOPERATIVE PLANNING CHECKLIST	
OR table	☐ Standard table with lateral thigh post
Position/positioning aids	☐ Supine
Fluoroscopy location	☐ Optional
Equipment	☐ Knee arthroscopy setup, ACL tibial guide with <3-mm guidewire (but not reamer), suture passing devices (to advance through ACL at level of footprint *and* to retrieve through <3-mm tibial tunnels), repair suture (no. 2 size or greater)
Tourniquet	☐ Nonsterile

Technique

✔ Arthroscopic Reduction and Suture Fixation of Fractures of the Tibial Spine: KEY SURGICAL STEPS
☐ Flush hemarthrosis from knee prior to diagnostic arthroscopy
☐ Diagnostic arthroscopy (assess menisci)
☐ Debride fat pad
☐ Debride fracture edges (underside of spine fragment and underlying fracture bed) with motorized shaver and/or curette. Consider removing excess bone from tibial side of fragment to allow for slight overreduction of spine fragment and account for ligamentous stretch of ACL fibers

☐ Reduce spine fragment (retract intermeniscal ligament and/or meniscal anterior horn[s] if interposed with tagging suture or probe through accessory transpatellar portal)
☐ Pass repair sutures through base of ACL at level of tibial footprint (one anterior, one posterior to maximize fixation/repair stability)
☐ Through a new proximal tibial incision, create two tibial tunnels (<3 mm) with ACL guide/guidewire on either side of fragment with 1-cm cortical bone bridge between tunnel starting points
☐ Pull trans-ACL sutures through tunnels using suture passer device
☐ Optimize reduction, tie sutures over bone bridge on maximum tension

Arthroscopic setup and examination is similar to the technique described for epiphyseal screw fixation. Accessory superomedial and superolateral portals are not used, though an accessory transpatellar working portal may be considered to facilitate fracture reduction and suture management. The fracture is elevated and the fracture base debrided (Fig. 27-11A) using tiny curettes. The authors typically remove some excess bone from the tibial side of the fracture site to allow for slight overreduction of the tibial spine fragment which may account for the intrinsic ACL fiber stretch injury which can occur at the time of tibial spine fracture. The fracture is reduced, or slightly overreduced and an optimal reduction may be provisionally maintained with a small K-wire directed inferiorly, though reduction of a previously entrapped intermeniscal ligament or anterior meniscal horn over the anterior aspect of the fragment often maintains the reduction adequately and the K-wire can interfere with suture passage through the base of the ACL. Two superiorly directed guide pins, approximately 2.7 mm in size, are then placed using the tibial ACL guide system from a small incision made just medial to the tibial tubercle and distal to the proximal tibial physis (Fig. 27-11B). Care is taken to create separate starting points for the two guidewires, to ensure a 1-cm cortical bone bridge

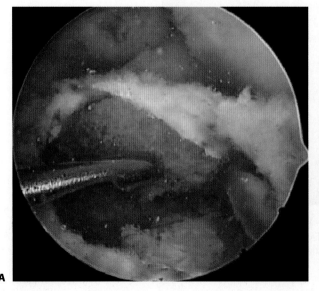
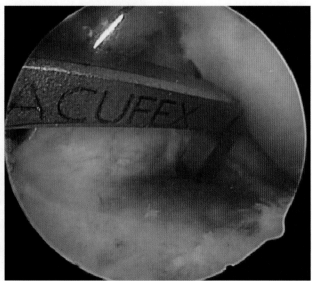

Figure 27-11. A: Preparation of the tibial spine fracture site with debridement of fibrinous clot using a curette. **B:** An ACL drill guide is used to plan tunnel placement.

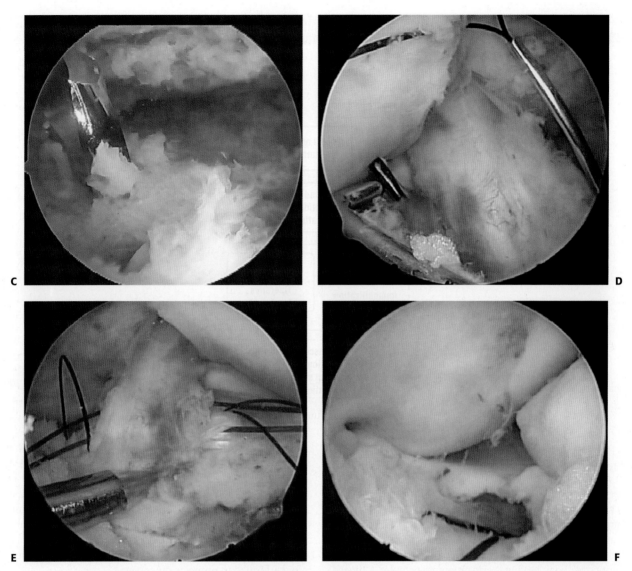

Figure 27-11. (*Continued*) **C:** The medial guide pin is drilled retrograde into the medial aspects of the tibial fracture site. **D:** Suture retrievers are passed separately through the medial and lateral tunnel. **E:** A curved suture passer is used to pass a suture through the retrievers and the base of the ACL. **F:** The suture retrievers are pulled distally to pull each end of the suture through the corresponding tibial tunnel and the fracture is slightly overreduced following suture fixation. (Kramer DE, Yen YM. Kocher MS Ch. 117 Tibial Spine Fractures. In Scott WN (ed.). *Insall & Scott Surgery of the Knee,* 6th Edition. Philadelphia: Elsevier 2017. ISBN 9780323400466.)

between the tibial tunnels for later suture tying, and to place the intra-articular exit points through either side of the base of the intercondylar spine fragment (Fig. 27-11C) right along the fracture line. Either suture passing devices or small wire loops (smaller than 2.7 mm in diameter) are then placed up the tibial tunnels, toward the medial and lateral sides of the base of the tibial spine fragment (Fig. 27-11D). At this point, a suture passing device is used to pass a suture through the medial wire loop, across the posterior aspect of the base of the ACL/tibial spine fragment and back out through the lateral wire loop. This process can be facilitated with the use of a transpatellar tendon portal to retrieve the suture. A second suture is then typically placed in the same direction through the medial wire loop, across the anterior base of the ACL/tibial spine fragment and out through the lateral wire loop (Fig. 27-11E). Once both sutures have been passed, these transtibial wire loops then pull the suture ends out through the inferior incision, and the sutures are tied down onto the tibia over the bony bridge, using arthroscopic assessment to confirm maintenance of the optimal reduction (Fig. 27-11F). Two or more ACL repair sutures are typically utilized so as to space the position of the "suture bridge" over a large segment of the ACL footprint and improve rotational stability of the fragment. Both absorbable and non–absorbable-braided sutures may be utilized for the ACL repair sutures as studies have not shown a difference,[338] and there are no published reports of complications associated with growth disturbance secondary to the bony bridging or prolonged nonabsorbable suture retention through the small transtibial guidewire tracts.

Authors' Preferred Treatment of Fractures of the Tibial Spine (Algorithm 27-1)

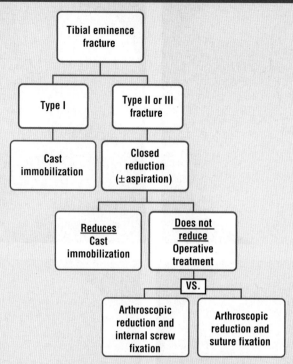

Algorithm 27-1. Authors' preferred treatment of tibial spine fractures in children.

Type I fractures are treated with a locked hinged knee brace in an older child or adolescent or long-leg cast immobilization in a younger child, applied in full extension (0 degrees), to prevent loss of reduction and a flexion contracture, which is generally harder to treat than loss of flexion. The patient and family are cautioned to elevate the leg to avoid swelling. Radiographs are repeated in 1 to 2 weeks to ensure that the fragment has not displaced. The cast/brace is removed 4 to 6 weeks after injury once bony healing is evident on radiographs. A hinged knee brace is then used and physical therapy initiated to regain motion and strength. Patients are typically allowed to return to sports 3 to 4 months after injury if they demonstrate fracture healing and adequate motion and strength.

Type II fractures are usually treated with a gentle attempt at closed reduction with simple knee extension. Aspiration of hematoma and injection of local anesthetic under sterile conditions may be considered if the patient is in severe pain, but is not required for a successful reduction and not typically utilized at our institution. Radiographs are taken to assess reduction, though if dynamic fluoroscopy is being

used, assessment of reduction should also be performed at 20 degrees of flexion and casted in the optimal position. If the fragment is reduced, closed management then can be initiated and follow-up radiographs are performed at 1 and 2 weeks postreduction to ensure maintenance of reduction. Length of casting and postcasting management is similar to type I fractures. If the fracture does not reduce anatomically or if the fracture later displaces, operative treatment should be performed to optimize outcomes.

Type III fractures may be treated with attempted closed reduction; however this is usually unsuccessful, and we favor primary operative treatment in the absence of significant medical comorbidities or surgical contraindications. The author's preferred operative treatment is arthroscopic reduction and internal fixation. However, open reduction through a medial parapatellar incision can also be performed per surgeon preference/experience, or if arthroscopic visualization is difficult. The author's preferred fixation is epiphyseal cannulated screws if the fragment is large or suture fixation if the fragment is small or comminuted.

Postoperative Care

Postoperatively, patients are placed in a postoperative hinged knee brace and maintained touch-down weight bearing for 6 weeks postoperatively. Motion is restricted to 0 to 30 degrees for the first 2 weeks, 0 to 60 degrees for the next 2 weeks, and then 0 to 90 for weeks 4 to 6, with full ROM after 6 weeks, provided early radiographic healing is seen. The brace is kept

locked in extension at night for the first 6 weeks to prevent a flexion contracture. Radiographs are obtained at each postoperative visit to evaluate maintenance of reduction and fracture healing (Fig. 27-12). Cast immobilization for 4 weeks postoperatively may be considered in younger children if there is concern for inability to comply with protected weight bearing and brace immobilization. Early initiation of physical therapy is routinely utilized to optimize motion, strength, and sports-specific

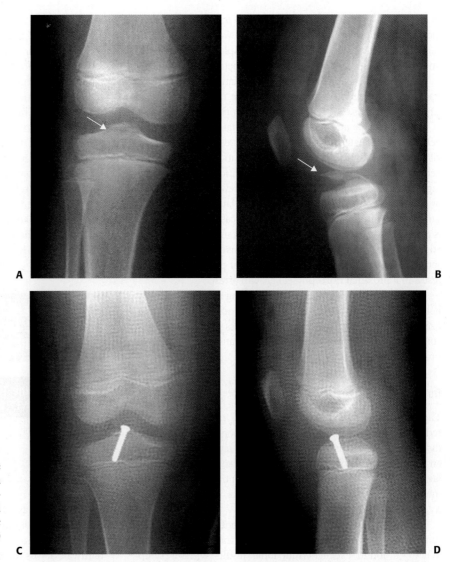

Figure 27-12. Type III tibial spine fracture in an 11-year-old male child treated with arthroscopic reduction and 3.5-mm cannulated screw fixation. Preoperative AP (**A**) and lateral (**B**) radiographs showing fracture (*white arrow*). Postoperative AP (**C**) and lateral (**D**) radiographs.

training. Patients are typically allowed to return to sports at 12 to 16 weeks postoperatively, depending on knee function. Screws are not routinely removed. Functional ACL bracing is utilized if there is residual knee laxity.

Potential Pitfalls and Preventive Measures

Repair of Fractures of the Tibial Spine:
POTENTIAL PITFALLS AND PREVENTIONS

Pitfall	Prevention
• Failure/loss of reduction of type II	• Ensure cast is in full extension • Obtain MRI if meniscal/intermeniscal interposition is suspected • Follow X-rays closely (5–7 days and 12–14 days postreduction) • Consider surgical intervention
• Inadequate visualization during arthroscopy	• Before starting arthroscopy, flush hemarthrosis until arthroscopy fluid clear • Make sure fat pad debridement is adequate
• Comminution of spine fragments during attempted screw fixation (or upon initial assessment)	• Use suture fixation instead of screw fixation
• Growth disturbance with screw fixation	• Multiple fluoroscopic views to ensure no physeal screw penetration
• Postoperative arthrofibrosis	• Ensure adequate fixation to allow early ROM • Immobilize in extension at night to avoid loss of extension

In the closed management of tibial spine fractures, follow-up radiographs must be obtained at 1 and 2 weeks postinjury to verify maintenance of reduction. Late displacement and malunion can occur, particularly for type II fractures.

During arthroscopic reduction and fixation of tibial spine fractures, arthroscopic visualization can be difficult unless the large hematoma is evacuated and flushed prior to introduction of the arthroscope and the large inflamed fat pad is adequately debrided. Adequate inflow and outflow is essential for proper visualization. Careful attention to preparation of the fracture bed is important to provide optimal conditions for bony healing. Attempted epiphyseal cannulated screw fixation of small or comminuted tibial spine fragments can fail as the screw may further comminute the fragment. In these cases, suture fixation is generally a better method. If epiphyseal cannulated screw fixation is used, fluoroscopy is necessary to ensure that the drill or screw does not traverse the proximal tibial physis, which may result in a proximal tibial physeal growth arrest.

Early mobilization and nighttime bracing in full extension is helpful to avoid arthrofibrosis which can occur with immobilization. However, in younger children (less than 7 years old), compliance with protected weight bearing and brace use can be problematic.

Outcomes

The prognosis for closed treatment of nondisplaced and reduced tibial spine fractures and for operative treatment of displaced fractures is good. Most series report healing with an excellent functional outcome despite some residual knee laxity.[33,36,42,181,197,259,274,278,359,376,397,400] Potential complications include nonunion, malunion, arthrofibrosis, residual knee laxity, and growth disturbance.[33,36,42,181,197,259,274,278,359,380,397,400]

Mild residual knee laxity is seen frequently, even after anatomic reduction and healing of tibial spine fractures. Baxter and Wiley[36,397] found excellent functional results without symptomatic instability in 17 pediatric knees with displaced tibial spine fractures, despite a positive Lachman examination in 51% of patients and increased mean instrumented knee laxity of 3.5 mm. After ORIF of type III fractures in 13 pediatric knees, Smith[359] identified patient-reported instability in only two patients, despite a positive Lachman examination in 87% of patients. In a group of 50 children after closed or open treatment, Willis et al.[400] found excellent clinical results despite a positive Lachman examination in 64% of patients and instrumented knee laxity of 3.5 mm for type II fractures and 4.5 mm for type III fractures. Similarly, Janarv et al.[172] and Kocher et al.[197] found excellent functional results despite persistent laxity even in anatomically healed fractures. More recent long-term follow-up studies have replicated these findings.[67,376] Despite four patients demonstrating signs, but no symptoms, of instability, Tudisco et al.[376] recently reported good results in 13 of 14 knees followed for a mean of 29 years postinjury, with the one suboptimal result reported in a type III fracture treated nonoperatively.

Persistent laxity despite anatomic reduction and healing of tibial spine fractures in children is likely related to plastic deformation of the collagenous fibers of the ACL occurring in association with tibial spine fracture. At the time of tibial spine fixation, the ACL often appears hemorrhagic within its sheath, but grossly intact and in continuity. In a primate animal model, Noyes et al.[295] found frequent elongation and disruption of ligament architecture despite gross ligament continuity in experimentally produced tibial spine fractures at both slow and fast loading rates. This persistent anteroposterior laxity despite anatomic reduction may be avoided by countersinking the tibial spine fragment within the epiphysis at the time of reduction and fixation. Later ACL injury after previous tibial spine fracture may be more common than previously thought. A recently reported case series of 101 patients over a 20-year period reported a 19% rate of delayed ACL reconstruction (ACL-R) in patients who had a prior tibial spine fracture.[272] Patients who were older at the time of tibial spine fracture were more likely to require ACL-R in the future.

MANAGEMENT OF EXPECTED ADVERSE OUTCOMES AND UNEXPECTED COMPLICATIONS IN FRACTURE OF THE TIBIAL SPINE

Fractures of the Tibial Spine:
COMMON ADVERSE OUTCOMES AND COMPLICATIONS

- Arthrofibrosis
- Nonunion
- Malunion
- ACL laxity

Poor results may occur after spine fractures associated with unrecognized injuries of the collateral ligaments or complications from associated physeal fracture.[264,359,369] In addition, hardware across the proximal tibial physis may result in growth disturbance with recurvatum deformity or shortening.[280]

Malunion of type II and III fractures may cause mechanical impingement of the knee during full extension (Fig. 27-13).[123] For symptomatic patients, this can be corrected by either osteotomy of the fragment and fixation in a more recessed, anatomic position or excision of the manumitted fragment with anatomic suture repair of the ACL to its bony footprint. Alternatively, excision of the fragment and ACL-R can be considered in adults and older adolescents.

Nonunion of type II and III tibial spine fractures treated closed can usually be managed by arthroscopic or open reduction with internal fixation.[188,238,383] Technically, debridement of the fracture bed and the fracture fragment to fresh, bleeding bone is essential to optimize bony healing. Bone graft may be required in cases of chronic nonunion. Similarly to management of malunions described above, excision of the fragment and ACL-R can alternatively be considered in adults and older adolescents, and may be preferable, given the increasingly favorable reports of outcomes of pediatric ACL-R techniques.

Stiffness and arthrofibrosis can be a challenging problem after both nonoperative and operative management of

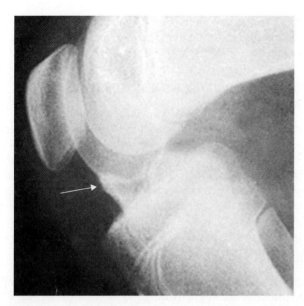

Figure 27-13. Lateral radiograph of a malunited displaced fracture of the intercondylar spine of the tibia (*white arrow*) with an extension block.

tibial spine fractures. The milieu of a major traumatic intra-articular injury, a large hemarthrosis, and immobilization can predispose to arthrofibrosis. Vander Have et al. reported on 20 cases of arthrofibrosis out of 205 patients (10%) from 4 institutions over a 10-year period who had undergone surgical intervention for tibial spine fracture, as well as 12 additional cases referred from other institutions. Of the 32 total cases, 25 (78%) had been immobilized for 4 to 6 weeks postoperatively without motion, and 24 (75%) required additional operative treatment within 6 months to address debilitating loss of knee motion.[380] The authors concluded that for fractures that undergo fixation, early mobilization utilizing physical therapy can minimize the risk of arthrofibrosis, an approach supported by subsequent analyses.[308] If stiffness is detected, dynamic splinting and aggressive physical therapy can be employed during the first 3 months from fracture.[300] If significant stiffness remains after 3 months from fracture, patients should be managed with manipulation under anesthesia, but only in conjunction with arthroscopic lyses of adhesions, an approach shown to be successful in resolving the stiffness in majority of cases.[380] Overly vigorous manipulation should be avoided to avert iatrogenic proximal tibial or distal femoral physeal fracture, which may lead to growth arrest or deformity requiring further treatment.[380]

Osteochondral Fractures

INTRODUCTION TO OSTEOCHONDRAL FRACTURES

Osteochondral fractures in skeletally immature patients are more common than once thought. They are typically associated with acute lateral patellar dislocations. The most common locations for these fractures are the inferior aspect of the patellar median ridge, the inferior medial patellar facet, or the lateral aspect of the LFC (Fig. 27-14). The osteochondral fracture fragments may range from small incidental loose bodies to large portions of the articular surface.

The diagnosis can be difficult to make because even a large osteochondral fragment may contain only a small ossified portion that is visible on plain radiographs. MRI has therefore emerged as having a critical role in identifying associated osteochondral fractures or chondral-only fragments in cases of traumatic patellar dislocation. Acute osteochondral fractures must be differentiated from acute chondral injuries, which do not involve subchondral bone, and osteochondritis dissecans (OCD),[117,203] which is most often a repetitive overuse lesion of the subchondral bone, which may result in a nonhealing stress fracture that can progress to separation of the overlying chondral fragment.

Treatment of acute osteochondral fractures includes removal of small loose bodies and fixation of larger osteochondral fragments. In cases associated with an acute patellar dislocation, patellar stabilization procedures such as lateral retinacular release, medial retinacular repair, medial patellofemoral ligament (MPFL) repair, or primary reconstruction may be performed adjunctively.

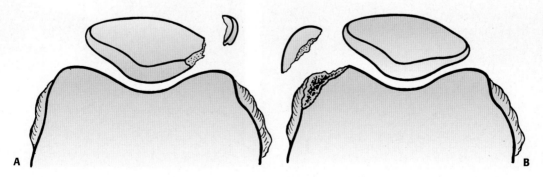

Figure 27-14. Osteochondral fractures associated with dislocation of the right patella. **A:** Medial facet. **B:** Lateral femoral condyle.

ASSESSMENT OF OSTEOCHONDRAL FRACTURES

MECHANISMS OF INJURY FOR OSTEOCHONDRAL FRACTURES

There are two primary mechanisms for production of an osteochondral fracture.[11,49,112,116,185,255,288,365] First, a direct blow to the knee with a shearing force applied to either the medial or LFC can create an osteochondral fracture. The second mechanism involves a flexion-rotation injury of the knee in which an internal rotation force is placed on a fixed foot, usually coupled with a strong quadriceps contraction. The subsequent contact between the tibia and femur or patella and LFC causes the fracture. This latter contact mechanism occurs during an acute patellar dislocation. When the patella dislocates laterally, the medial retinaculum and the associated MPFL tears, while the extensor mechanism still applies significant compressive forces as the patella shears laterally across the LFC. The medial border of the patella then temporarily becomes impacted on the prominent edge of the LFC before it slides back tangentially over the surface of the LFC because of pull of the quadriceps. Either the dislocation or the relocation phase of this injury can cause an osteochondral fracture to the LFC, the medial facet of the patella, or both (Fig. 27-15). Interestingly, osteochondral fractures are relatively uncommon in the setting of chronic, recurrent patellar subluxations or dislocations. In these situations, the laxity of the medial knee tissues and decreased compressive forces between the patella and the LFC prevent development of excessive shear forces. With more acute or traumatic dislocations, even if a frank osteochondral fracture does not occur, bone bruising is generally seen on MRI on both the patella and LFC, and chondral injuries, such as fissuring of the articular surface of the medial facet and median ridge, are also common.[187,291,293]

Most patients give a history of a twisting injury consistent with acute patellar dislocation, but a few report a direct blow to the lateral or medial femoral condyle, accounting for a shear injury. The prevalence of osteochondral fractures associated with acute patella dislocation ranges from 19% to 50% in the literature.[11,49,112,255,288,293,365]

INJURIES ASSOCIATED WITH OSTEOCHONDRAL FRACTURES

As described above, common injuries associated with osteochondral fractures caused by an acute patellar dislocation include MPFL tear and bone bruises or impaction injuries to the LFC and medial aspect of the patella. Other osteochondral fractures may occur in association with severe cruciate or collateral ligament tears, especially in the setting of a knee dislocation.

SIGNS AND SYMPTOMS OF OSTEOCHONDRAL FRACTURES

Acutely, osteochondral fractures present with severe pain, swelling, and difficulty in weight bearing.[9,35,103,132,152,163,175,185,232,288,297,325,326,356,362,401,402] If the osteochondral fracture is associated with an acute patellar dislocation, there is often tenderness to palpation over the medial patella and lateral aspect of the LFC, though medial femoral condylar tenderness may also be exhibited, either from a femoral-sided tear of the MPFL from the adductor tubercle region or because of a partial MCL sprain, which is not uncommon in association with patellar dislocation. The patient will usually resist attempts to flex or extend the knee and may hold the knee in 15 to 20 degrees of flexion for comfort. Typically there is a large hemarthrosis in the knee. The large hemarthrosis is due to an intra-articular fracture of the highly vascular subchondral bone. Joint aspiration may reveal fatty globules or a supernatant layer of fat if allowed to stand for 15 minutes indicating an intra-articular fracture. Similarly, fluid–fluid levels may be seen on MRI, from the separation of fat and blood. Patients who present in a delayed fashion after injury, may complain of loose-body type symptoms such as intermittent locking or catching of the knee associated with a knee effusion.

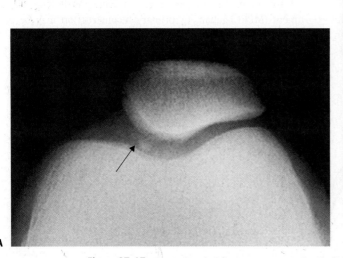

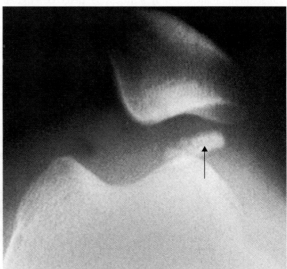

A

B

Figure 27-15. Osteochondral fractures associated with dislocation of the patella. **A:** Medial facet of patella (*black arrow*). **B:** Lateral femoral condyle (*black arrow*).

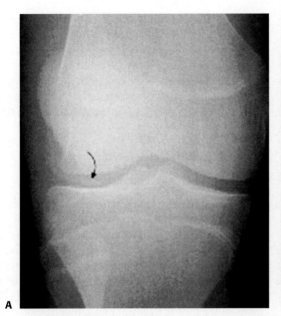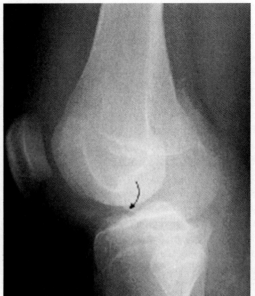

Figure 27-16. Osteochondral fracture of lateral femoral condyle after patellar dislocation. **A:** Fragment seen in lateral joint space (*black arrow*). **B:** Lateral view (*black arrow*).

IMAGING AND OTHER DIAGNOSTIC STUDIES FOR OSTEOCHONDRAL FRACTURES

Radiographic assessment of a possible osteochondral fracture should begin with anteroposterior, lateral, and skyline plain radiographs. However, a roentgenographic diagnosis can be difficult because even a large osteochondral fragment may contain only a small ossified portion that is visible on plain radiographs. A tunnel view may help locate a fragment in the region of the intercondylar notch. Because the osteochondral fragment may be difficult to see on plain radiographs, radiographs should be carefully assessed for even the smallest ossified fragment (Fig. 27-16).

Matelic et al.[255] report that standard radiographs failed to identify the osteochondral fracture in 36% of children who had an osteochondral fracture found during arthroscopy. For this reason, MRI is recommended in most cases, due to the importance of identifying a possible osteochondral fracture despite negative radiographs[54,196,340,396] or a large chondral fragment. Osteochondral fractures usually occur in the setting of an acute traumatic patellar dislocation in a patient with a large hemarthrosis, whereas ligamentously lax patients with chronic, recurrent, atraumatic patellar instability are less likely to sustain osteochondral fractures. A high-riding patella may also have a protective effect against associated intra-articular osteochondral fractures. Patients with an Insall index >1.3 have a decreased chance of sustaining an osteochondral fracture compared with patients who have an Insall index within normal limits.[54]

CLASSIFICATION OF OSTEOCHONDRAL FRACTURES

The classification of osteochondral fractures of the knee is based on the site, the type, and the mechanism of injury. The classification outlined in Table 27-1 is based on the descriptions of osteochondral fractures by Kennedy[185] and Smillie.[356]

OUTCOME MEASURES FOR OSTEOCHONDRAL FRACTURES

Healing of osteochondral fractures must be followed closely with radiographs, were applicable, as healing is the most important predictor of outcome. For fixation of osteochondral fractures with minimal subchondral bone or purely chondral fractures, follow-up MRI may be necessary to determine healing. Once healed, standard outcome measures, such as functional knee metrics (the Pedi-IKDC[207] and Lysholm[358] knee scores), can be used to assess the results and, paired with the Marx or Tegner activity scores,[253] ascertain a patient's ability to make a full return to activities of daily life and sports activities.

PATHOANATOMY AND APPLIED ANATOMY RELATING TO OSTEOCHONDRAL FRACTURES

The patella tracks in the trochlear groove between the medial and LFCs during flexion and extension of the knee.[132,163] With increasing knee flexion, the contact area on the articular surface

TABLE 27-1. Mechanism of Osteochondral Fractures

Site	Mechanism
Medial femoral condyle	Direct blow (fall)
	Compression and rotation (tibiofemoral)
Lateral condyle	Direct blow (kick)
	Compression and rotation (tibiofemoral)
	Acute patellar dislocation
Patella (medial margin)	Acute patellar dislocation

of the patella moves from the distal to the proximal aspect of the articular surface of the patella. Between 90 and 135 degrees of flexion, the patella glides into the intercondylar notch between the femoral condyles. The two primary areas of contact are the medial patellar facet with the medial femoral condyle and the superolateral quadrant of the lateral patellar facet with the LFC. Soft tissue support for the patellofemoral joint includes the quadriceps muscle, the MPFL, the patellar tendon, and the vastus medialis and lateralis muscles.

Dislocation of the patella may tear the medial retinaculum and MPFL, but the rest of the quadriceps muscle–patellar ligament complex continues to apply significant compression forces as the patella dislocates laterally. These forces are believed to cause fracture of the medial patellar facet, the LFC articular rim, or both (see Fig. 27-14).[184,185,295–297,323,324,326] Osteochondral fractures are uncommon with chronic recurrent subluxation or dislocation of the patella because of relative laxity of the medial retinaculum and lesser compressive forces on the patella and the LFC.

A histopathologic study by Flachsmann et al.[116] helps to explain the occurrence of osteochondral fractures in the skeletally immature at an ultrastructural level. They noted that in the joint of a juvenile, interdigitating fingers of uncalcified cartilage penetrate deep into the subchondral bone providing a relatively strong bond between the articular cartilage and the subchondral bone. In the adult, the articular cartilage is bonded to the subchondral bone by the well-defined calcified cartilage layer, the cement line. When shear stress is applied to the juvenile joint, the forces are transmitted into the subchondral bone by the interdigitating cartilage with the resultant bending forces causing the open pore structure of the trabecular bone to fail. In mature tissue, the plane of failure occurs between the deep and calcified layers of the cartilage, the tidemark, leaving the osteochondral junction undisturbed. Although the juvenile and adult tissue patterns are different, they both provide adequate fracture toughness to the osteochondral region. As the tissue transitions, however, from the juvenile to the adult pattern during adolescence, the fracture toughness is lost. The calcified cartilage layer is only partially formed and the interdigitating cartilage fingers are progressively replaced with calcified matrix. Consequently, the interface between the articular cartilage and the subchondral bone becomes a zone of potential weakness in the joint which may explain why osteochondral fractures are seen frequently in adolescents and young adults.

TREATMENT OPTIONS FOR OSTEOCHONDRAL FRACTURES

NONOPERATIVE TREATMENT OF OSTEOCHONDRAL FRACTURES

Nonoperative treatment of osteochondral fractures is reserved for small fragments, 5 mm or less, that have failed to cause or are unlikely to cause mechanical symptoms typically associated with a loose body. Each osteochondral fracture is unique so treatment

should be individualized, based on a patient's age and activity level, the size, location and status of the injured osteochondral fragment, and the degree of surrounding injury. However, as general principles, the larger the osteochondral fragment, the more bone attached to the fragment, and the more central the weight-bearing zone from which the fragment detached, the more the treating surgeon should consider an attempt at refixation.

OPERATIVE TREATMENT OF OSTEOCHONDRAL FRACTURES

Indications/Contraindications

The recommended management of acute osteochondral fractures of the knee is either surgical removal of the fragment or fixation of the fragment, depending on its size and the quality of the tissue.[195,202] In patients with an osteochondral fracture after acute patellar dislocation, concomitant repair of the medial retinaculum and MPFL, either at the patellar or femoral insertion sites of the ligament, or through an intrasubstance imbrications, at the time of fragment excision or fixation, may decrease the risk of recurrent patellar instability,[5,65,325] though there is conflicting evidence whether this repair improves the ultimate redislocation rate.[75,289,290,302]

Fixation

If the lesion is large (≥5 mm), easily accessible, involves a weight-bearing area, and has adequate subchondral bone attached to the chondral surface then fixation should be considered.[185,356,362,401,402]

Preoperative Planning

✔ Fixation of Osteochondral Fractures: PREOPERATIVE PLANNING CHECKLIST	
OR table	☐ If fluoroscopy planned, radiolucent table
Position/positioning aids	☐ Supine
Fluoroscopy location	☐ Nonoperative side, perpendicular to table
Equipment	☐ Small K-wires, bioabsorbable pins/tacks/screws, headless compression screws
	☐ instruments to assist with potential need for arthrotomy: retractors, etc.
Tourniquet	☐ Nonsterile

Technique

✔ Fixation of Osteochondral Fractures: KEY SURGICAL STEPS
☐ Diagnostic arthroscopy to retrieve loose body, assess viability, and assess fracture bed and feasibility of fixation
☐ If optimal fixation is achievable through arthroscopic means (rare), skip below arthrotomy step

- ❑ Arthrotomy (medial parapatellar or lateral parapatellar or directly over the donor site) to optimize access to fracture bed; if donor site on patella, make arthrotomy long enough to ensure adequate eversion of patella. If donor site on femoral condyles consider knee flexion to center donor site at level of incision
- ❑ Debride/prepare fracture bed and fragment
- ❑ Reduce fragment, provisionally fix with small K-wire
- ❑ Fixation with bioabsorbable pins, tacks, or screws or headless metal compression screws (reserved for larger fragments with adequate bone)
- ❑ Repair arthrotomy (taking care not to overtension to avoid increasing patellofemoral contact forces)

Fixation can be performed via arthroscopy or arthrotomy. Fixation options include K-wires, cannulated or solid metal screws, variable pitch headless screws, or bioabsorbable pins,[73,129,390] tacks, or screws, which have recently increased in popularity and have the advantage of not requiring implant removal.[99] For metal implants, hardware removal is typically performed after fracture healing, though headless compression screws may be buried beneath the superficial level of the cartilage and may be retained.[232] Traditionally, purely chondral

fragments with no subchondral bone attached were previously not considered amenable to refixation, because of concerns regarding poor healing capacity. However, new reports have suggested that large chondral-only fragments may be able to heal in children or adolescents if early refixation is pursued.[110,281,377] Fixation can also be successful in the setting of a chronic osteochondral fracture fragment if done correctly and should be considered in chronic cases meeting the above criteria if tissue quality is good.[107] In these cases there is often some overgrowth and swelling of the osteochondral fragment that may require careful trimming by the surgeon in order to get an anatomic reduction.

Removal of Fragments

If the osteochondral fracture fragment is small (<5 mm), damaged, has minimal subchondral bone or has fractured from a non–weight-bearing region of the knee, removal of loose bodies is typically recommended.[9,175,225,326] The fragment's crater should be debrided to stable edges and the underlying subchondral bone should be perforated through marrow stimulation techniques to encourage fibrocartilage formation.[225]

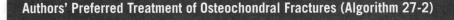

Authors' Preferred Treatment of Osteochondral Fractures (Algorithm 27-2)

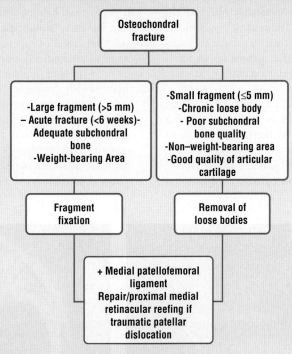

Algorithm 27-2. Authors' preferred treatment of osteochondral fracture in children.

In patients with an acute, traumatic patellar dislocation with a large hemarthrosis, MRI is performed, even if initial radiographs do not clearly show any associated osteochondral fracture. If MRI does not reveal any associated osteochondral fracture or any large chondral fragments, these patients are treated with a brief (1 to 2 weeks) period with a hinged

knee brace locked in extension for ambulation with crutches for comfort and weight bearing and ROM as tolerated, followed by use of a soft, lateral-stabilizing patellofemoral brace and physical therapy emphasizing patellar mobilization, straight-leg raises, progressive resistance exercises, and vastus medialis obliquus (VMO) strengthening. Routine diagnostic arthroscopy and MPFL repair are not performed on these patients without osteochondral fractures. Patients are allowed to return to sports 6 to 12 weeks after dislocation depending on their progress with rehabilitation, with use of the lateral-stabilizing brace during sports recommended for those who feel it helps limit pain or apprehension.

Patients with small (≤5 mm) osteochondral fractures or small chondral shear fragments, damaged fragments, and fractures involving non–weight-bearing areas are treated with arthroscopic removal of loose bodies. Occasionally, a patient may be seen more than 4 weeks following the initial injury with radiologic evidence of a small loose body but no symptoms; in such instances, arthroscopy may be deferred unless the patient develops mechanical symptoms. If arthroscopy is pursued for a small osteochondral fracture, the fragment's crater is debrided to stable edges to prevent further loose bodies from developing and the underlying subchondral bone should be perforated with marrow stimulation techniques, such as microfracture, to encourage fibrocartilage formation. Lateral retinacular release with medial retinacular/patellofemoral ligament repair is performed adjunctively in cases of traumatic patellofemoral dislocation to decrease the risk of recurrent patellofemoral instability.

Primary MPFL repair may be performed on either the patellar or femoral insertion sites if the site of the tear is clearly appreciated on MRI or intraoperatively. Alternatively, imbrication, a pants-over-vest advancement, or removal of a small elliptical segment of retinacular tissue followed by side-to-side repair are all effective options for an intrasubstance MPFL tear or diffuse attenuation of the retinacular tissue.

Patients with large (>5 mm) osteochondral fractures where the chondral surface remains in good condition and the osteochondral fragment can be anatomically reduced back to the native donor site, or selected large purely chondral fragments with intact chondral surfaces which involve large weight-bearing areas, are treated with an attempt at fragment fixation. At times, the fragments can be very large, involving nearly the entire weight-bearing surface of the medial patellar facet (Fig. 27-17) or LFC (Fig. 27-18). Medial patellar facet osteochondral fractures can be fixed through an open lateral retinacular release by manually tilting the patella (see Fig. 27-17) or a medial parapatellar arthrotomy, which allows for tensioning of the medial retinacular repair during closure. LFC osteochondral fractures typically require a lateral parapatellar arthrotomy for fragment fixation (see Fig. 27-18). Z-shaped knee retractors are helpful for exposure and the knee is flexed or extended to optimize visualization of the fracture bed. The osteochondral fracture fragment and the fracture bed are debrided of fibrous tissue to healthy bone. The donor site edges should be cleared of all fibrinous debris and tested for stability using a tiny curette. The subchondral bone of the donor site may be perforated at this step to initiate bleeding prior to fragment reduction. The fragment is then reduced anatomically. At times the osteochondral fragment will have swelled and be larger than the donor site and may require trimming with a sharp knife or overcuretting of the donor site to achieve an anatomic reduction. For osteochondral fragments with large thick areas of subchondral bone, countersunk cannulated screws (3, 3.5, or 4.5 mm) or Herbert screws are often preferable for fixation, compared to bioabsorbable tacks or screws, because of the strength of fixation which allows for fragment compression and early mobilization. For osteochondral fragments with thin layers of subchondral bone, bioabsorbable tacks or screws are routinely employed for fixation which obviates the need for later implant removal (Fig. 27-19).[212] Because chondral-only fragments will have no subchondral bone upon which to compress metal screws, bioabsorbable tacks or a suture-based repair are preferred techniques.[110] Lateral retinacular release with medial retinacular/patellofemoral ligament repair is often performed adjunctively in cases of traumatic patellofemoral dislocation to decrease the risk of recurrent patellofemoral instability.

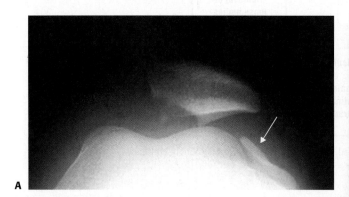
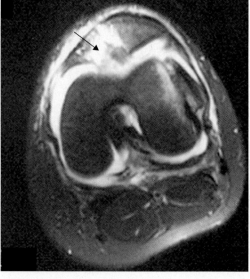

Figure 27-17. Fixation of a medial patellar facet osteochondral fracture in an adolescent male athlete. **A:** Skyline radiograph demonstrating a fracture of the medial patellar facet with the fragment in the lateral recess (*white arrow*). **B:** Axial MRI demonstrating medial facet fracture and loose fragment (*black arrow*).

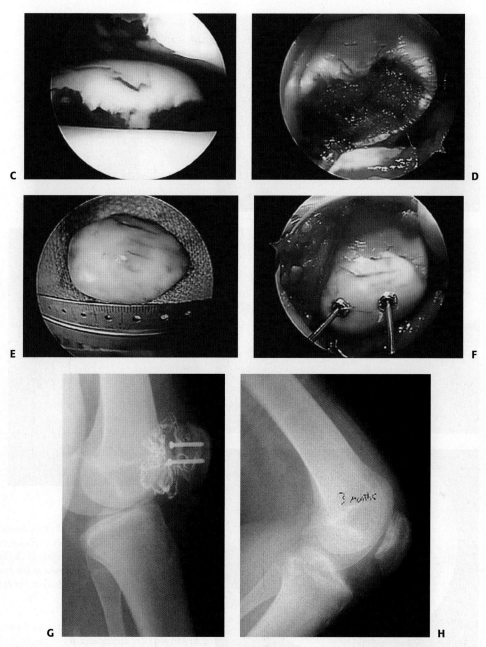

Figure 27-17. (*Continued*) **C:** Arthroscopic view of osteochondral fragment in the lateral recess. **D:** Open view of patella. **E:** Open view of osteochondral fragment. **F:** Open view of reduction and cannulated screw fixation of medial patellar facet. **G:** Intraoperative lateral radiograph after fracture fixation. **H:** Lateral radiograph 3 months after fracture fixation and 6 weeks after screw removal demonstrating healing.

Postoperative Care

Postoperatively, patients treated by excision of the fragment can begin ROM exercises immediately. Crutches may be necessary in the immediate postoperative period but patients can progress to weight bearing as tolerated. For weight-bearing lesions of the femoral condyles in which a microfracture/marrow stimulation technique was employed, weight bearing may be delayed and continuous passive motion (CPM) of the knee may be employed to aid with healing of the fibrocartilage.

Following osteochondral or chondral fragment fixation, patients are treated with touch-down weight bearing in a postoperative brace until fracture healing. ROM when not weight bearing is allowed from 0 to 30 degrees for the first 2 weeks, followed by 0 to 90 degrees until fracture healing. Healing typically occurs between 6 and 12 weeks postoperatively, and confirmation with follow-up MRI may be utilized if necessary although is not routinely employed (Fig. 27-20).[213] If metal screw fixation was utilized, second look arthroscopy is performed at a later date to confirm fragment healing, remove hardware, and assess the integrity of the articular surface. Return to athletic activities is permitted when full ROM is recovered and strength is symmetric.

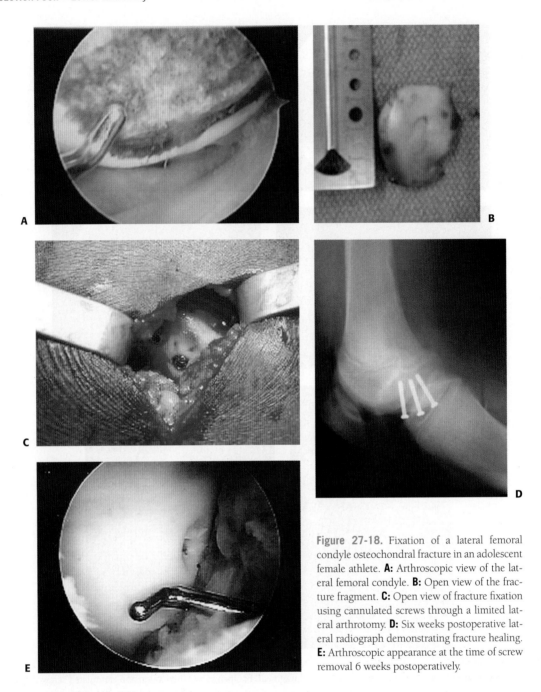

Figure 27-18. Fixation of a lateral femoral condyle osteochondral fracture in an adolescent female athlete. **A:** Arthroscopic view of the lateral femoral condyle. **B:** Open view of the fracture fragment. **C:** Open view of fracture fixation using cannulated screws through a limited lateral arthrotomy. **D:** Six weeks postoperative lateral radiograph demonstrating fracture healing. **E:** Arthroscopic appearance at the time of screw removal 6 weeks postoperatively.

Potential Pitfalls and Preventative Measures of Osteochondral Fractures

Repair of Osteochondral Fractures: POTENTIAL PITFALLS AND PREVENTIONS	
Pitfall	**Prevention**
• Further fragmentation of fracture fragment	• Extend portal incisions adequately for removal
	• Arthroscopically position fragment in gutter/anterior recess near arthrotomy site; retrieve only after full arthrotomy
• Fragment does not fit in bed	• Plan surgery for <7 days postinjury to prevent excessive swelling of fragment
	• Trim fragment cartilage to fit bed
	• Remove more bone from the donor site as needed to achieve anatomic reduction
• Inadequate fixation	• When possible, achieve at least two points of fixation for rotational stability
• Growth disruption	• In skeletally immature patients, implants should be short enough to avoid physeal trauma during fixation

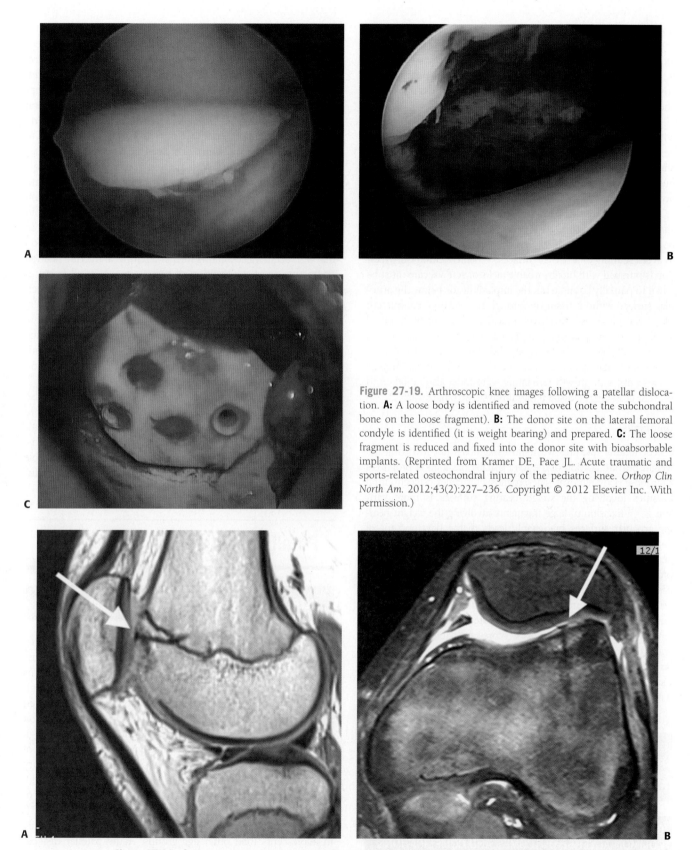

Figure 27-19. Arthroscopic knee images following a patellar dislocation. **A:** A loose body is identified and removed (note the subchondral bone on the loose fragment). **B:** The donor site on the lateral femoral condyle is identified (it is weight bearing) and prepared. **C:** The loose fragment is reduced and fixed into the donor site with bioabsorbable implants. (Reprinted from Kramer DE, Pace JL. Acute traumatic and sports-related osteochondral injury of the pediatric knee. *Orthop Clin North Am.* 2012;43(2):227–236. Copyright © 2012 Elsevier Inc. With permission.)

Figure 27-20. A: Postoperative T1 sagittal MRI. **B:** Postoperative proton density axial MRI both showing the bioabsorbable implant across an osteochondral fracture of the lateral trochlea (*white arrows*). (Reprinted by permission from Kramer DE, Yen YM, Simoni MK, et al. Surgical management of osteochondritis dissecans lesions of the patella and trochlea in the pediatric and adolescent population. *Am J Sports Med.* 2015;43(3):654–662. Copyright © 2015 SAGE Publications.)

An important pitfall to avoid is the failure to diagnose osteo-chondral fractures associated with acute, traumatic patellar dis-locations. Radiographs should be scrutinized for small osseous fragments, and MRI should be obtained in cases despite neg-ative radiographs with a clinical suspicion for possible osteo-chondral fracture.

In cases of arthroscopic removal of loose bodies associated with acute, traumatic patellar dislocation, consideration should be given to repair of the medial structures (medial retinaculum and MPFL) to decrease the risk of recurrent patellar instability, but with care taken not to overtension the medial tissues, so as not to excessively increase patellofemoral contact forces.[373]

In cases of osteochondral fracture fixation, adequate fixation should be obtained to allow for early motion. Screw heads must be countersunk or headless, variable pitch screws may be used to avoid scuffing of articular surfaces. When chondral-only fixa-tion is pursued with bioabsorbable tacks or screws, care must be taken to partially countersink the implant heads below the artic-ular surface without fissuring through the cartilage completely. Moreover, close postoperative clinical monitoring of crepitus, swelling, or new pain must be maintained, with consideration of serial MR imaging if necessary, because of risk of potential back out of the implants not seen on radiographs. In children or adolescents with growth remaining, care must also be taken to prevent crossing the distal femoral physis with hardware.

Outcomes

Osteochondral fractures with small fragments not involving the weight-bearing portion of the joint usually has a good prognosis after loose body removal. The prognosis for larger osteochondral fractures involving the weight-bearing surfaces is more vari-able.[129,337] Excision of large fragments involving the weight-bear-ing articular surfaces predictably leads to the development of degenerative changes.[16] Fracture fixation resulting in fragment healing with a congruous articular surface offers the best long-term prognosis; however even these cases may develop crepitus, stiff-ness, and degenerative changes. In a recent series of patients with osteochondral fractures in association with acute patellar disloca-tions, patients with osteochondral fractures of the weight-bearing femoral condyles had lower IKDC scores at final follow-up com-pared to those patients with non–weight-bearing lesions or patel-lar lesions.[340] Recently reported results of chondral-only fragment fixation have been favorable, but only small series or case reports with short-term follow-up have emerged.[110,281,377]

MANAGEMENT OF EXPECTED ADVERSE OUTCOMES AND UNEXPECTED COMPLICATIONS OF OSTEOCHONDRAL FRACTURES

Osteochondral Fractures:
COMMON ADVERSE OUTCOMES AND COMPLICATIONS

- Arthrofibrosis
- Loss of fixation/nonunion
- Osteoarthritis/focal chondral degeneration

Among the most common and concerning complications after both excision of loose bodies and fracture fixation is recurrent patellar instability with the possibility of further osteochondral injury. Although studies have suggested that concomitant MPFL repair decreases the risk of recurrent instability,[35,325] this concept remains controversial.[65,75,289,290,302] Stiffness is also a common complication following patellofemoral dislocation, particularly after fracture fixation. Adequate internal fixation is necessary to allow for early motion, which decreases the risk of arthrofibrosis. Stiffness may be treated with aggressive therapy and dynamic splinting during the first 3 to 4 months after injury.[300] Beyond this time frame, arthroscopic lysis of adhesions and manipulation under anesthesia is typically required, with care taken to avoid distal femoral physeal injury through excessive manipulation in skeletally immature patients. Nonunion after fragment fixation may also occur, necessitating further attempts at fracture fixation or fracture excision. Excision of larger osteochondral fractures involving the weight-bearing articular surfaces requires associ-ated chondral resurfacing, such as marrow stimulation proce-dures (microfracture), osteochondral grafting (mosaicplasty), or autologous chondrocyte implantation,[41,44,311,366] all of which may be more technically challenging, with somewhat less opti-mal outcomes, when performed for the patellofemoral joint, compared with the tibiofemoral articular surfaces.[113,130,151,246] Complications related to implants for fracture fixation may also occur. Proud screw heads may scuff articular surfaces. Prior to reabsorption, bioabsorbable implants may also scuff the carti-lage, and over time may be associated with reactive synovitis, sterile effusions, or fragmentation. In addition, bioabsorbable implants can loosen and break off over time causing a large effu-sion and mechanical loose-body type symptoms.

Patellar Dislocation

INTRODUCTION TO PATELLAR DISLOCATION

Patellar instability events are relatively common in adolescents. These episodes can range from an acute, traumatic patellar dis-location to chronic, recurrent patellar subluxations in patients with ligamentous laxity. The age- and sex-adjusted annual inci-dence of first time lateral patellar dislocation has been estimated at 23.2 per 100,000 person-years with a mean age at dislocation of 21.4 ± 9.9 years and 55% occurring in females.[334] For high school athletes, a recent study noted an overall injury rate of 1.95 per 100,000 athletic exposures (AEs). The highest injury rates were noted for girls' gymnastics (6.19 per 100,000 AEs), boys' football (4.10), and boys' wrestling (3.45) with the rate of injury was higher in competition (3.72) than practice (1.34).[271]

Acute, traumatic patellar dislocation occurs more commonly in adolescents than other age groups. Acute patellar disloca-tions in younger children usually occur in the context of under-lying patellofemoral dysplasia. Chronic, atraumatic, recurrent patellofemoral instability occurs most frequently in adolescent females, often with underlying laxity and risk factors related to abnormal coronal and rotational lower extremity alignment, such as genu valgum, femoral anteversion, and external tibial torsion.

Acute, traumatic patellar dislocations without associated osteochondral fracture are primarily treated with a short period of immobilization followed by patellofemoral bracing and rehabilitation. Acute, traumatic patellar dislocations with osteochondral fractures are treated as discussed in the previous section, with removal of loose bodies or fracture fixation followed by a patellar stabilization procedure. Chronic, recurrent, atraumatic patellofemoral instability is typically treated with patellofemoral bracing, and rehabilitation, with surgery reserved for symptomatic failures of above management. Recurrent patellofemoral instability which has been recalcitrant to nonoperative treatment can be managed with a variety of proximal and distal realignment procedures.

ASSESSMENT OF PATELLAR DISLOCATION

MECHANISMS OF INJURY FOR PATELLAR DISLOCATION

Patellar dislocations usually occur because of a flexion-rotation injury of the knee in which an internal rotation force is placed on a fixed foot, usually coupled with a strong quadriceps contraction. As the patella dislocates, the medial retinaculum and MPFL tear but the remaining quadriceps muscle–patellar ligament complex still applies significant compressive forces as the patella dislocates laterally and slides across the LFC. This primary injury mechanism, or the subsequent reduction of the patella medially back over the lateral edge of the lateral condyle, may result in associated osteochondral fracture. Reduction of the patella may occur spontaneously as the patient simply extends the knee after a fall or may require forced manual reduction, often with the need for sedation to allow for quadriceps muscle relaxation.

Less commonly, patellar dislocation can be caused by a direct blow to the medial aspect of the patella. Patellar dislocations are more likely to be caused by falls, or during the course of gymnastics, dancing, cheerleading, cutting, and pivoting sports. Along with cruciate or collateral ligament tear and meniscal injury, acute patellar dislocation should be considered in the evaluation of all knee injuries in adolescents and young adults.

INJURIES ASSOCIATED WITH PATELLAR DISLOCATION

Recent MRI evidence suggests a predictable constellation of findings in conjunction with patellar dislocation: MPFL injury either at the patellar attachment site (more common in adolescents), femoral attachment site, or both[27,114]; VMO edema in most patients; and osteochondral fracture in about one-third of patients, most of which shear off of the medial patellar facet, but more rarely may be from the LFC.[339] Whereas acute patellar dislocation is more commonly associated with trauma or severe twisting injuries of the knee, chronic patellar subluxation is associated with lower-energy mechanisms, is more common in children with ligamentous laxity or hypermobility syndromes, and has a lower frequency of significant intra-articular knee injuries.

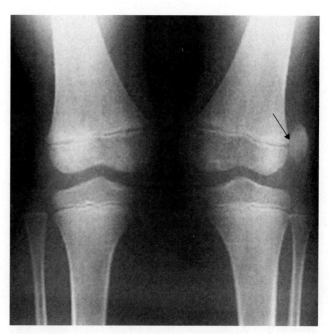

Figure 27-21. Acute dislocation of the left patella (*black arrow*) in a 6-year-old boy.

SIGNS AND SYMPTOMS OF PATELLAR DISLOCATION

Patients with an acute, traumatic patellar dislocation often give a history of a twisting injury. Patients may remember feeling or seeing the patella in a laterally displaced position. Most acute patellar dislocations spontaneously reduce or reduce with incidental knee extension. It is more unusual to see a patient with a patellar dislocation which is unreduced (Fig. 27-21). Patients may report a "pop" associated with dislocation and a second "pop" associated with spontaneous reduction.

Symptoms include diffuse peripatellar tenderness and pain with any attempt passively to displace the patella. Patients may have a positive lateral apprehension test with lateral translation of the patella. A defect may be palpable in the medial attachment of the VMO to the patella if the medial retinaculum is completely avulsed. Although often difficult to differentiate from diffuse tenderness throughout a swollen knee joint, the sites of greatest focal tenderness usually include the medial aspect of the patella (either from a chondral or bony contusion), the medial epicondyle (due to tearing of the femoral attachment of the MPFL), and lateral aspect of the LFC just proximal to the joint line (due to bony contusion). Hemorrhage into the joint may cause hemarthrosis, and severe hemarthrosis should suggest the possibility of an osteochondral fracture.[325] All knee ligaments should be carefully evaluated because the mechanism of patellar dislocation may cause associated ligamentous injuries, such as ACL or MCL tear.

IMAGING AND OTHER DIAGNOSTIC STUDIES FOR PATELLAR DISLOCATION

Radiographs after acute dislocation are obtained primarily to detect any associated osteochondral fracture. Occasionally, an osteochondral fragment from the medial aspect of the patella or the LFC is visible on the anteroposterior or lateral view.

A "patellar," "skyline," or "sunrise" view is difficult to obtain in a child after acute dislocation because the required flexed positioning of the knee causes pain, but should be attempted if possible. In a recent report, the "sliver sign," an intra-articular linear or curvilinear ossific density representing an osteochondral fragment, was seen on 19% of 219 cases of patellar dislocation, 8 of which were visible on a patellar view only.[145] Rarely, stress radiographs may be obtained for evaluation of suspected physeal fracture or ligamentous injury. In the setting of an acute patellar dislocation or recurrent dislocation with severe knee swelling, MRI has emerged as the gold standard of radiologic evaluation, because of its ability to detect the constellation of injuries associated with patellar dislocations, such as chondral shear injuries, cruciate or collateral ligament tears, and severe disruption of the medial retinaculum and MPFL. Moreover, the three-dimensional axial imaging of MRI allows for optimal assessment and quantification of the severity of potential risk factors for recurrence, such as patellar dysplasia (e.g., Wiberg classification),[283] trochlear dysplasia (e.g., Dejour classification),[23,91,312,375] patella alta (e.g., Salvatti–Insall ratio or Blackburne–Peel ratio),[166,167] lateral patellar displacement (e.g., congruence angle),[263] patellar tilt (e.g., lateral patellofemoral angle),[222] and femorotibial alignment at the level of the knee joint (e.g., tibial tubercle-trochlear groove distance [TT-TG]).[31,32,134] In patients assessed to have significant femoral anteversion or abnormal tibial torsion, use of newer MRI-sequencing protocols which additionally incorporate several slices of both the femoral neck and distal tibia in the scout views may be helpful for a formal version analysis to understand if an abnormal femoral and/or tibial rotational profile represents a contributing etiologic factor in the dislocation that may benefit from specific surgical procedures, such as derotational osteotomy.

CLASSIFICATION OF PATELLAR DISLOCATION

There is no universally agreed upon classification system for patellar instability. Previously, Dejour et al.[92] classified patellar instability into three types based on the number of dislocations and degree of anatomic abnormalities. Chotel et al.[72] proposed a more detailed classification system consisting of five clinical patterns based on age at presentation with ages ranging from birth to adolescents. Most recently Parikh and Lykissas[303] proposed a comprehensive classification system which divided patellar instability into four types (Table 27-2) to include all forms of instability seen in adolescents (types 1 and 2) and young children (types 3 and 4). Although medial patellar dislocation or subluxation is exceedingly rare, it has been described in association with a medially directed direct blow or following overzealous lateral release.[162]

OUTCOME MEASURES FOR PATELLAR DISLOCATION

The rate or occurrence of redislocation after operative or nonoperative treatment of patellar dislocation is the most basic assessment of treatment success. However, standard outcome measures, such as functional knee metrics (the Pedi-IKDC[207] and Lysholm[358] knee scores), should also be used to assess the results and, paired with the Marx or Tegner activity scores,[253] ascertain a patient's ability to make a full return to activities of

TABLE 27-2. Classification of Patellar Instability

Type I	First patellar dislocation
A	With osteochondral fracture
B	Without osteochondral fracture
Type II	Recurrent patellar instability (most common pattern)
A	Recurrent patellar subluxation
B	Recurrent (>2) patellar dislocation
Type III	Dislocatable patella
A	Passive patellar dislocation
B	Habitual patellar dislocation—in flexion or extension
Type IV	Dislocated patella
A	Reducible
B	Irreducible

Reprinted from Parikh SN, Lykissas MG. Classification of lateral patellar instability in children and adolescents. *Orthop Clin North Am.* 2016;47(1):145–152. Copyright © 2016 Elsevier Inc. With permission.

daily life and sports activities. The mean IKDC score for children and adolescents with a patellar instability episode has been reported to be approximately 50.[329]

PATHOANATOMY AND APPLIED ANATOMY RELATING TO PATELLAR DISLOCATIONS

The patella is a sesamoid bone in the quadriceps mechanism. As the insertion site of all muscle components of the quadriceps complex, it serves biomechanically to provide an extension moment during ROM of the knee joint. The trochlear shape of the distal femur stabilizes the patella as it tracks through an ROM. The hyaline cartilage of the patella is the thickest in the body.

At 20 degrees of knee flexion, the inferior pole of the patella contacts a relatively small area of the femoral groove. With further flexion, the contact area moves superiorly and increases in size. The medial facet of the patella comes in contact with the femoral groove only when flexion reaches 90 to 130 degrees.

The average adult trochlear femoral groove height is 5.2 mm and LFC height is 3.4 mm. The patellar articular cartilage is 6 to 7 mm in its thickest region, the thickest articular cartilage in the body, and is a reflection of the joint's inherent incongruity. The normal lateral alignment of the patella is checked by the medial quadriceps expansion and focal thickening of the capsule in the areas of the MPFL and medial meniscopatellar ligament.[95] Dynamic stability depends on muscle forces, primarily the quadriceps and hamstrings acting through an elegant lower extremity articulated lever system that creates and modulates forces during gait. The quadriceps blends with the joint capsule to provide a combination of dynamic and static balance. Tightness or laxity of any of the factors involved with maintenance of the balance leads to varying levels of instability. Desio et al.[95] using a cadaveric serial cutting model, found that the MPFL provided 60% of the resistance to lateral patellar translation at 20 degrees of knee flexion. If the deficit produced by attenuation of the medial vectors after acute dislocation is not eliminated, patellofemoral balance is lost, resulting in feelings of giving way and recurrent dislocation.

The quadriceps mechanism is aligned in a slightly valgus position in relation to the patellar tendon. This alignment can be approximated by a line drawn from the anterosuperior iliac spine to the center of the patella. The force of the patellar tendon is indicated by a line drawn from the center of the patella to the tibial tubercle. The angle formed by these two lines is called the *quadriceps angle* or *Q angle* (Fig. 27-22). As this angle increases, the pull of the extensor mechanism tends to sublux the patella laterally. Recurrent patellar dislocation is most likely associated with some congenital or developmental deficiency of the extensor mechanism, such as patellofemoral dysplasia, deficiency of the VMO, or an increased Q angle with malalignment of the quadriceps–patellar tendon complex. However, although the Q angle can be difficult to measure clinically, the increasing use of MRI in patients with patellar dislocation has generated heightened interest in, and application of, the TT-TG distance, which many consider an imaging equivalent of the Q angle. When significantly elevated above the normal value of approximately 13 mm—a common threshold for "abnormal" is 20 mm—the TT-TG has been shown to be a risk factor for both primary and recurrent patellar dislocation in adults, adolescents, and children. Recent studies have shown that TT-TG distances change with age in the pediatric population[97] and newer patellar instability ratios have been proposed including the TT-TG/TW (axial trochlear width) and TT-TG/PW (axial patellar width) which attempt to predict recurrent instability based on patient-specific anatomy.[64]

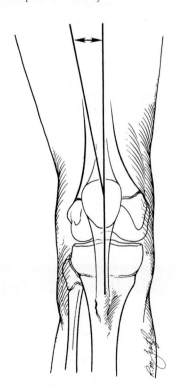

Figure 27-22. The Q angle. Normal valgus alignment of the quadriceps mechanism: Line drawn from the anterosuperior iliac spine to center of the patella, line drawn from center of the patella to tibial spine.

TREATMENT OPTIONS FOR PATELLAR DISLOCATION

NONOPERATIVE TREATMENT OF PATELLAR DISLOCATION

Indications/Contraindications

Nonoperative Treatment of Patellar Dislocations: INDICATIONS AND CONTRAINDICATIONS	
Indications	**Relative Contraindications**
• Primary patellar dislocation	• Osteochondral fracture/loose body >5 mm seen on X-ray or MRI
• Repeat patellar dislocation with few/no risk factors for recurrence	• Recurrent patellar dislocation with underlying/anatomic risk factors for recurrence

Most acute patellar dislocations in children reduce spontaneously; if they do not, reduction usually can be easily performed. Surgery is typically not indicated for primary acute patellar dislocations in children without associated loose bodies or osteochondral injuries.[35,220] Most patellar dislocations are treated nonoperatively with immobilization in extension, followed by patellofemoral bracing and rehabilitation focused on regaining normal ROM and strengthening of the quadriceps, particularly the VMO.

Technique

After appropriate sedation, reduction is achieved by flexing the hip to relax the quadriceps muscle, gradually extending the knee, and gently pushing the patella medially back into its normal position. Gentle reduction should be emphasized to avoid the risk of osteochondral fracture associated with patellar relocation.

Outcomes

The prognosis following patellar dislocations in children, when not associated with osteochondral injury, is generally good with success rates with regard to avoid redislocation placed at around 60% to 70%. Patients with a younger age at first dislocation and trochlear dysplasia are at higher risk for recurrent instability.[230,231] Cash and Hughston[68] noted 75% satisfactory results after nonoperative treatment in carefully selected patients.

Recurrent patellar dislocations with associated osteochondral injuries can lead to osteoarthritis of the patellofemoral joint. A recent study found that experiencing a patellar dislocation increases the likelihood of development of patellofemoral arthritis, with an adjusted odds ratio of 3.2.[78]

OPERATIVE TREATMENT OF PATELLAR DISLOCATION

Indications/Contraindications

Surgical repair may be considered if the VMO and/or MPFL is completely avulsed from the medial aspect of the patella, leaving a large, palpable soft tissue gap, and severely lateralized patella. If osteochondral fracture has occurred, arthroscopy/arthrotomy is indicated for removal or repair of an osteochondral loose body, as discussed in the previous section. The importance of performing a concurrent MPFL "repair" is controversial, but an MPFL tightening procedure, sometimes referred to as a "reefing," "imbrication," or "medial retinaculum plasty" procedure, with or without a lateral retinacular "release," which generally involves a longitudinal division of the tissue over the length of the patella, or lateral retinacular lengthening procedure, is still favored by many authors.[65,75,243,289,290,302]

Recurrent instability of the patella that has been recalcitrant to nonoperative treatment is typically managed through one of various proximal and/or distal patellofemoral realignment procedures. Proximal realignment options include isolated or combination procedures, including lateral retinacular release or lateral retinacular z-lengthening,[69] medial retinacular plication, reefing, or MPFL reconstruction using semitendinosus autograft, or, more commonly, allograft.[4,37,48,58,59,74,83,89,100,261,292,324]

Preoperative Planning

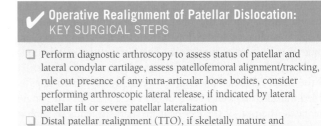

✔ Operative Realignment of Patellar Dislocation: PREOPERATIVE PLANNING CHECKLIST

OR table	☐ If fluoroscopy planned, radiolucent table
Position/positioning aids	☐ Supine
Fluoroscopy location	☐ Nonoperative side, perpendicular to table
Equipment	☐ If osteochondral fragment fixation planned), small K-wires, bioabsorbable pins/tacks/screws, headless compression screws
Tourniquet	☐ Nonsterile

Positioning

Arthroscopy is generally pursued prior to any open treatment related to patellar dislocation, so a standard arthroscopy setup should be used. However, for both arthroscopic and open techniques, most of the surgery is performed with the knee in full extension. If osteochondral fragment fixation is planned, a bump for both the knee and ankle are helpful to elevate the entire leg and facilitate true lateral X-rays, if necessary.

Operative Realignment of Patellar Dislocation

Surgical Approach and Technique

✔ Operative Realignment of Patellar Dislocation: KEY SURGICAL STEPS

☐ Perform diagnostic arthroscopy to assess status of patellar and lateral condylar cartilage, assess patellofemoral alignment/tracking, rule out presence of any intra-articular loose bodies, consider performing arthroscopic lateral release, if indicated by lateral patellar tilt or severe patellar lateralization

☐ Distal patellar realignment (TTO), if skeletally mature and indicated by elevated TT-TG

☐ Proximal patellar realignment (proximal medial reefing) versus MPFL reconstruction

The most common distal realignment approach in skeletally mature patients is the TTO, which may involve straight medialization of the tubercle (the Elmslie–Trillat procedure),[375] straight anteriorization (the Maquet procedure),[250] or a combination anteromedialization (an "AMZ," or the Fulkerson osteotomy).[121] However, these are contraindicated in patients with an open tibial tubercle apophysis because of the risk of a growth arrest, which can result in recurvatum deformity. In cases of significant patella alta, some authors have additionally proposed distalization of the tibial tubercle, with and without patellar tendon tenodesis, designed to shorten the tendon.[92,256] In skeletally immature patients, Galeazzi semitendinosus tenodesis[28,136] or the Roux–Goldthwait reconstruction[251,286] are distal realignment soft tissue procedures that have been traditionally utilized, though more recent studies have suggested that outcomes of these procedures may be less favorable than historically reported.[28,136,286] These perspectives have further stimulated interest in MPFL reconstruction techniques in skeletally immature children. However, there remains controversy about the appropriate technique and location of fixation of the graft on the femoral side, in part because of conflicting data on the true anatomic MPFL attachment relative to the distal femoral physis and how this relationship changes over time.[101,187,344] Literature detailing significant complications associated with MPFL reconstruction have emerged,[261,286,372,373] including inaccurate or inappropriate femoral fixation, making this an evolving topic with imprecise indications.[29] Other studies have supported MPFL reconstruction with attention to proper technique as a safe and effective procedure in adolescents with an open distal femoral physis.[284]

Authors' Preferred Treatment of Patellar Dislocation (Algorithm 27-3)

Most acute patellar dislocations in children without osteochondral fracture are treated by closed methods with satisfactory results. A knee immobilizer is generally used for approximately 2 weeks. Patients are allowed full weight bearing as tolerated. After immobilization, the patient is placed in a patellofemoral brace with a lateral bolster. Physical therapy is begun, emphasizing straight-leg raises, progressive resistance exercises, patellar mobilization, and vastus medialis strengthening. Patients are allowed to return to sports 6 to 12 weeks after injury, depending on their patellofemoral mechanics and progress with rehabilitation.

Acute surgical intervention for first time patellar dislocations is indicated most commonly for an associated osteochondral fracture. Removal of loose bodies for fragments

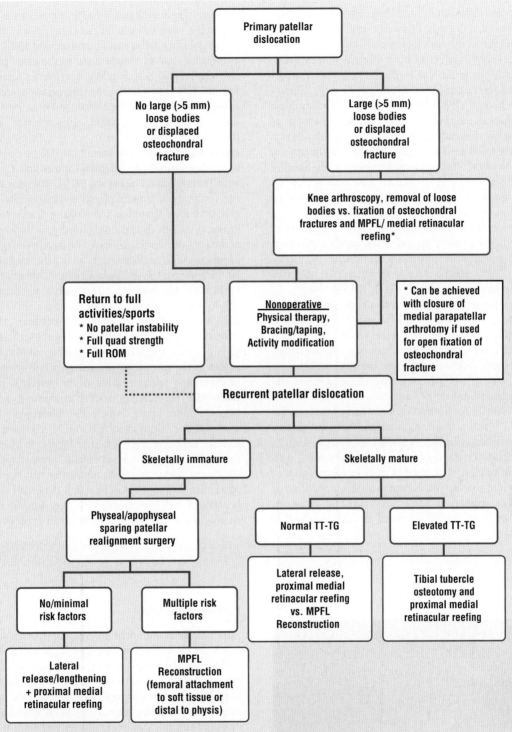

Algorithm 27-3. Authors' preferred treatment of patellar dislocations in children and adolescents.

≤5 mm or fracture fixation for larger fragments is performed as described previously. Adjunctive medial retinacular/MPFL reefing, either through excision of an elliptical segment (usually 1 cm wide, 2 cm long) of attenuated medial parapatellar retinacular tissue, or through a pants-over-vest advancement, is typically also performed to reduce the risk

of recurrent patellar instability, with or without lateral retinacular release or lengthening, depending on the tightness of the lateral patellar restraints.

Chronic patellar subluxation or dislocation is most common in adolescents, especially females. Several risk factors have been identified in children likely to have chronic subluxation or dislocation, including age younger than 16 years, abnormal Q angle, significant genu valgum, radiographic evidence of dysplasia of the patella or trochlea, LFC hypoplasia, femoral anteversion or external tibial torsion, significant atrophy of the VMO, connective tissue disorders predisposing to hypermobility of the patella (e.g., Ehlers–Danlos syndrome), elevated TT-TG distance, and multiple previous dislocations (Fig. 27-23).[13,51] Initial treatment of chronic patellar subluxation or dislocation in adolescents is immobilization followed by aggressive physical therapy for rehabilitation of the VMO and quadriceps muscles. Surgical intervention is warranted in children who do not respond to this treatment regimen and continue to have subluxation or dislocation episodes.[45,221] For the rare patient with minimal risk factors for recurrence or only minor, but recurrent symptomatic subluxation episodes, an isolated proximal soft tissue realignment procedure, consisting of medial retinaculum/MPFL reefing with lateral retinacular release or lengthening, may be considered (Fig. 27-24A).

If subluxation or dislocation persists despite this less invasive approach, or in patients with recurrent instability and multiple underlying risk factors (such as young age, trochlear dysplasia, elevated Q angles, hypermobility, and lateralized TT-TG distances), a more significant proximal realignment procedure or more complex combinations of proximal and distal realignment procedures are indicated. MPFL reconstruction allows for reconstitution of a robust medial patellar checkrein[37,58,89] and is indicated in patients with attenuation of medial retinacular tissues. A tendinous allograft such as a semitendinosis or gracilis tendon is generally used, with either suture fixation of an appropriately tensioned graft to the femoral and patellar periosteum in younger children, or suture anchor fixation in adolescents, utilizing intraoperative fluoroscopy to place the femoral anchor just distal to the distal femoral physis. Small (≤5 mm), short (≤20 mm), transverse bone tunnels may also be drilled under fluoroscopic guidance at the patellar and femoral MPFL attachment sites (being sure to remain distal to the distal femoral physis), using small biocomposite interference screws for graft fixation. It is important for the surgeon to ensure MPFL graft isometry and appropriate tension prior to establishing the insertion points during MPFL reconstruction. The goal of the reconstructed MPFL is to act as a check-rein from lateral patellar translation at knee ROM 0 to 30 degrees without increasing medial patellofemoral forces and to not tighten with knee flexion. Placing the MPFL insertion point proximal to the distal femoral physis will cause tightening of the graft with knee flexion and block knee flexion as the patient grows. A growth modulating/guided growth procedure such as medial hemi-epiphysiodesis with small plate may be added in patients with combined significant genu valgum and patellar instability in the setting of significant growth remaining.

In skeletally *mature* patients with a significantly abnormal Q angle or elevated TT-TG distance, TTO in conjunction with proximal realignment procedures is preferred. Tubercle medialization with the Elmslie–Trillat procedure (Fig. 27-24C) is effective in improving patellofemoral kinematics in the coronal plane, though a Fulkerson osteotomy incorporating anteriorization of the patella is preferred in cases with pre-existing patellar chondrosis or significant osteochondral injury which has undergone fixation or microfracture. Combined TTO/MPFL reconstruction procedures may give the greatest reduction in risk of redislocation, but represents a maximally invasive approach with significant operative times, increasing risk of stiffness and other complications. More research is needed to justify the benefits of MPFL reconstruction over simpler medial retinacular tightening procedures in conjunction with TTO.

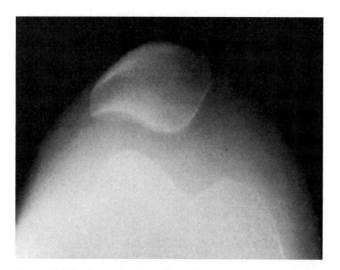

Figure 27-23. Chronic lateral patellar subluxation in a 13-year-old girl.

Postoperative Care

After patellar realignment procedures, patients are treated with touch-down weight bearing in a postoperative brace for 2 weeks. ROM when not weight bearing is limited to 0 to 30 degrees for the first 2 weeks. Patients may begin weight bearing as tolerated after 2 weeks, but only with the hinged knee brace locked in extension. When not ambulating, ROM is advanced to 0 to 60 degrees from post-op weeks 2 to 4 and from 0 to 90 degrees from post-op weeks 4 to 6. Weight bearing may be limited in patients who underwent a TTO procedure until radiographic evidence of healing which typically occurs at approximately 6 weeks postoperatively. At 6 weeks, the brace is unlocked when ambulating and discontinued by week 8, with weight-bearing strengthening exercises initiated. Straight ahead running is allowed around 3 months post-op, with advancement to agility and sports-specific exercises as indicated. Return to athletic activities is permitted when full ROM is recovered, strength is symmetric, and the knee feels stable with agility exercises.

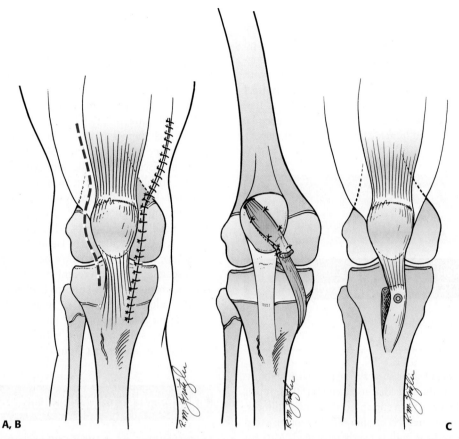

Figure 27-24. Surgical technique for the treatment of chronic patellar subluxation or dislocation. **A:** Lateral retinacular release and medial imbrication. **B:** Semitendinosus tenodesis. **C:** Elmslie–Trillat procedure.

Potential Pitfalls and Preventive Measures

Repair of Patellar Dislocation: POTENTIAL PITFALLS AND PREVENTIONS	
Pitfall	**Prevention**
• Unrecognized osteochondral fractures or chondral injuries	• Careful and detailed diagnostic arthroscopy to assess for chondral injuries in expected locations at start of patellar stabilization procedure
• Overconstraint of the knee blocking flexion following MPFL reconstruction	• Ensure graft isometry and appropriate tension prior to establishing insertion points during MPFL reconstruction so MPFL acts as a medial "check-rein" at knee ROM 0–30 without increasing medial patellofemoral forces and does not tighten with knee flexion
• Patellar fracture from patellar fixation of MPFL graft	• Avoid using long tunnels (>20 mm), large-diameter tunnels (>5 mm), oblique tunnels, complete transpatellar tunnels, or multiple tunnels

Unrecognized associated osteochondral fractures may present later as loose bodies. Unrecognized associated ligamentous injury can present later as knee instability. Aggressive nonoperative treatment should be pursued for cases of patellofemoral instability before considering surgical management, and MRI should be obtained for all patellar dislocation patients, particularly primary episodes, to evaluate for associated injuries and underlying anatomic risk factors, such as patellofemoral dysplasia. Overzealous and injudicious use of lateral retinacular release may result in iatrogenic medial patellar instability. For MPFL reconstruction procedures, while there are conflicting reports about the appropriate degrees of knee flexion at which MPFL tensioning and fixation should be pursued, ranging from 30 to 90 degrees,[4,5,12,38,59,74,83,235,261,285,324,413] graft isometry and assessment of tension through a wide ROM is indicated to avoid increasing patellar contact forces.[38,261] Fluoroscopy is indicated if short patellar and/or femoral bone tunnels are drilled for graft placement, with bioabsorbable or biocomposite interference screw fixation. We recommend against long tunnels (>20 mm), large-diameter tunnels (>5 mm), oblique tunnels, complete transpatellar tunnels, or multiple tunnels, to avoid subsequent patellar fracture in this young, active, athletic patient population.

Outcomes

A variety of surgical approaches are associated with relatively low rates of redislocation and good short-term knee scores in both adults and children.[4,29,65,299,413] Studies on MPFL reconstruction in an isolated pediatric population are rare. Nelitz et al.[284] reported on anatomic MPFL reconstruction in 21 consecutive children of mean age 12.2 years (range 10.3 to 13.9 years).

At mean 2.8-year follow-up no recurrent dislocations occurred, Kujala scores were improved but two patients with high-grade trochlear dysplasia still had a positive apprehension sign and Tegner activity scores did not improve.[284] Another study suggested that MPFL reconstruction in children was associated with consistently improved patellar height indices to within normal childhood ranges.[109] However, one recent study suggests that longer-term knee scores and satisfaction in children may be slightly lower than presumed from the low redislocation rates.[242]

MANAGEMENT OF EXPECTED ADVERSE OUTCOMES AND UNEXPECTED COMPLICATION OF PATELLAR DISLOCATION

Patellar Dislocation:
COMMON ADVERSE OUTCOMES AND COMPLICATIONS

- Arthrofibrosis
- Patellar subluxation/instability
- Patellar redislocation

Complications may occur after surgery for patellar instability. Lateral release alone without medial retinaculum/MPFL repair may not adequately prevent recurrent dislocation. Stiffness, with lack of knee flexion, may occur after MPFL reconstruction or Galeazzi tenodesis, if the graft is overly tensioned. A recent report noted at 16% rate of complications following MPFL reconstruction in 179 knees in a young patient population.[304] Complications included recurrent lateral patellar instability (8 patients), knee motion stiffness with flexion deficits (8 patients), patellar fractures (6 patients), and patellofemoral arthrosis/pain (5 patients). Eighteen of 38 (47%) complications were secondary to technical factors and were considered preventable and female sex and bilateral MPFL reconstructions were risk factors associated with postoperative complications.[304] After TTO, nonunion, hardware failure, neurovascular injury, and compartment syndrome have been reported.

Meniscal Injuries

INTRODUCTION TO MENISCAL INJURIES

Meniscal injuries in the pediatric athlete are being seen with increased frequency[19,47,61,77,118,180,192,195,200,249,260,270,276,294,331,379,387,406,411] Meniscal disorders include meniscal tears, discoid meniscus, and meniscal cysts. The exact incidence of meniscal injuries in children and adolescents is unknown, but is known to increase with age within this subpopulation.[88] The increased size, weight and speed of adolescents along with increased athletic demands lead to higher-energy injuries and an increase in intra-articular knee injuries. Meniscal injuries under the age of 10 are rare, unless associated with a discoid meniscus.[3,40,82,98,147,164,177,178,183,194,202,282,287,306,310,317,327,336,357,367,368,382,391]

Meniscal injury patterns differ in children compared to adults. It is estimated that longitudinal tears comprise 50% to 90% of meniscal tears in children and adolescents.[195] Bucket-handle displaced tears are not uncommon (see Fig. 27-1). Also in these age groups, meniscal injuries are commonly associated with ACL injuries.[66,106,202,249]

Although there is limited data on the subject, one report suggests that the incidence of medial meniscal tears is greater than lateral meniscal tears in the adolescent age group.[364] A recent series[332] involving a high rate of meniscus repairs performed with ACL-R in children with open physes conversely showed a significantly higher rate of lateral meniscal tears compared with medial meniscus tears. There also appears to be a relatively increased incidence of lateral tears in the preadolescent age group, which may in part be because of the existence of lateral discoid menisci.[195] A recent cross-sectional study compared assessed meniscal injury patterns in children mean age 13 compared to adolescents mean age 16 and found that children had a higher incidence of discoid meniscal tears, lower BMI, and meniscal tears not associated with ligamentous injuries (28% vs. 51% in the adolescent group).[349]

ASSESSMENT OF MENISCAL INJURIES

MECHANISMS OF INJURY FOR MENISCAL INJURIES

Injury to the nondiscoid meniscus is virtually always traumatic in nature in children and adolescents. Multiple studies have shown that between 80% and 90% of meniscal injuries in children and adolescents are sustained during sports activities.[3,138,139,249,364] These numbers may be lower in the preadolescent age group. Meniscal tears most commonly occur with cutting, pivoting and twisting motions, such as those performed frequently during football, soccer, and basketball. The mechanism involves rotation of the condyles relative to the tibial plateau, as the flexed knee moves toward extension. This rotational force with the knee partially flexed causes the condyle to force the menisci toward the center of the joint, leading to injury.

INJURIES ASSOCIATED WITH MENISCAL INJURIES

Twisting mechanisms may also cause associated ligamentous injuries, and ACL injuries are commonly associated with both medial and lateral meniscal tears in adolescents. Combined cruciate and meniscal injuries may also be associated with chondral injuries to the knee. Chronic meniscal pathology may also be associated with degenerative chondral changes, cyst formation, or congenital anomalies.[118]

SIGNS AND SYMPTOMS OF MENISCAL INJURIES

Pain and swelling at the knee joint line are the most common complaints of a patient with a meniscal tear. Other complaints include mechanical symptoms such as snapping, popping, clicking, catching, or locking. A bucket-handle tear that is displaced into the intercondylar notch may present with a locked knee or a knee unable to fully extend.

The differential diagnosis of acute meniscal tear in the pediatric patient includes other conditions that may result in a traumatic effusion, such as a ligamentous injury, osteochondral fracture, chondral injury, or patellofemoral dislocation. In addition, conditions causing pain at or adjacent to the joint line must be distinguished from meniscal tears, such as plica syndrome, iliotibial friction band syndrome, OCD, and bone bruises.[195]

The diagnosis of meniscal tear in children and adolescents can be difficult to make. Because of the diversity of pathology and the difficulty of examination in children, diagnostic accuracy of clinical examination for meniscus tear has been previously reported to be as low as 29% to 59%.[195,196] An accurate history may be difficult to obtain in a very young child. The older the patient, the more likely a history of specific injury. Pain is reported by approximately 85% of patients, predominantly in the area of the affected joint line. More than half of patients report giving way and swelling of the knee joint.

The most common physical examination signs, similar to adults, are joint line tenderness, pain with hyperflexion and/or hyperextension, and effusion.[19,260] However, some patients may have minimal findings on physical examination. McMurray's test may be helpful in the diagnosis of a subacute or chronic lesion, but with acute injury the knee may be too painful to allow these maneuvers.[84] The classic McMurray test may be of little value in the younger age group whose tears are peripheral and not degenerative posterior horn lesions.[195] Two recent studies, by examiners with pediatric sports medicine experience have shown the diagnostic accuracy of clinical examination to be 86.3% and 93.5% overall.[196,363]

IMAGING AND OTHER DIAGNOSTIC STUDIES FOR MENISCAL INJURIES

Routine radiographs are obtained primarily to rule out a fracture, OCD lesion, or other bony sources of knee pain.

MRI is the gold standard method for evaluating meniscal injuries in children. MRI accuracy rates reportedly range from 45% to 90% in the diagnosis of meniscal tears.[53,169,313] Kocher et al.[196] showed that for medial meniscal tears the sensitivity and specificity for MRI diagnosis were 79% and 92%, respectively.[196] For lateral meniscal tears, these numbers were 67% and 83%, respectively.

However, MRI should not be used indiscriminately as a screening procedure, because of significant limitations of the technique in this age group.[52,218,313,371] The sensitivity and specificity of MRI decrease in younger children compared to older adolescents.[196,363] In recent studies that compared the diagnostic accuracy of physical examination versus MRI, clinical examination rates were equivalent or superior to MRI.[196,363]

Normal MRI signal changes exist in the posterior horn of the medial and lateral meniscus in children and adolescents.[193,196,363] These signal changes do not extend to the superior or inferior articular surfaces of the meniscus and likely represent vascular developmental changes and can be easily mistaken for tears by inexperienced radiologists or clinicians.[195] When interpreting an MRI of the developing knee, care must be taken to identify a meniscal tear only when linear signal changes extend to the

articular surface. As with any test, clinical correlation is mandatory before treatment decisions are made.

CLASSIFICATION OF MENISCAL INJURIES

Classification is generally descriptive in nature and is based on the meniscus involved (medial vs. lateral), the location of the tear (posterior horn, body/pars intermedia, anterior horn), the chronicity of the tear (acute [<6 weeks], chronic [>6 weeks]), and the tear pattern (vertical/longitudinal, bucket-handle, horizontal cleavage, transverse/radial, or complex) (Fig. 27-25). Other important factors include site of the tear (outer/peripheral third, middle third, inner/central third), stability or involvement of the anterior or posterior horn attachment sites of the meniscus, and associated ligamentous and chondral injuries.

OUTCOME MEASURES FOR MENISCAL INJURIES

Tear recurrence or failure to heal a meniscus tear following repair is the most significant predictor of treatment success. Symptoms from retear generally warrant revision repair or, if the recurrent tear is not repairable, partial meniscectomy. On a longer-term basis, standard outcome measures, such as functional knee metrics (the Pedi-IKDC[207] and Lysholm[358] knee scores), should be used to assess results and paired with the Marx or Tegner activity scores[253] to ascertain a patient's ability to make a full return to activities of daily life and sports activities, which are the dual goals of surgery.

PATHOANATOMY AND APPLIED ANATOMY RELATING TO MENISCAL INJURIES

The menisci become clearly defined by as early as 8 weeks of embryologic development.[183] By week 14, they assume the normal mature anatomic relationships. At no point during their embryology are the menisci discoid in morphology.[183] Thus, the discoid meniscus represents an anatomic variant, not a vestigial remnant. The developmental vasculature of the menisci has been studied extensively by Clark and Ogden.[77] The blood supply arises from the periphery and supplies the entire meniscus. This vascular pattern persists through birth. During postpartum development, the vasculature begins to recede and by as early as the ninth month, the central third is avascular. This decrease in vasculature continues until approximately age 10, when the menisci attain their adult vascular pattern. Injection dye studies by Arnoczky and Warren[24] have shown that only the peripheral 10% to 30% of the medial and 10% to 25% of the lateral meniscus receive vascular nourishment. Importantly, the anterior and posterior horns have improved vascularity, compared with the body, or pars intermedia, of both the medial and lateral meniscus.[24]

The medial meniscus is C shaped. The posterior horn is larger in anterior–posterior width than the anterior horn. The medial meniscus covers approximately 50% of the medial tibial plateau. The medial meniscus is attached firmly to the medial joint capsule through the meniscotibial or coronary ligaments. There is a discrete capsular thickening at the level of the meniscal body which constitutes the deep MCL. The inferior surface is flat and

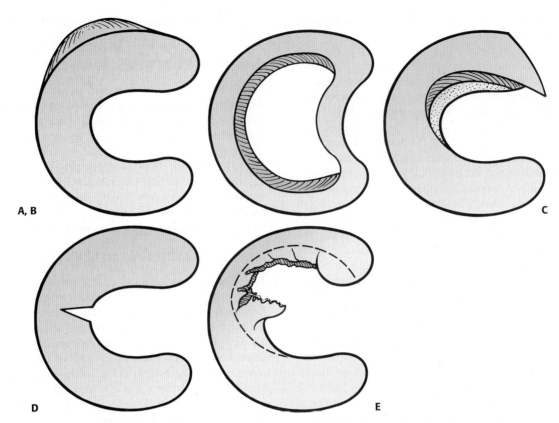

Figure 27-25. Meniscal tears in adolescents. **A:** Peripheral. **B:** Bucket handle. **C:** Horizontal cleavage. **D:** Transverse. **E:** Complex.

the superior surface concave so that the meniscus conforms to its respective tibial and femoral articulations. To maintain this conforming relationship, the medial meniscus translates 2.5 mm posteriorly on the tibia as the femoral condyle rolls backward during knee flexion.[138,139]

The lateral meniscus is more circular in shape and covers a larger portion, approximately 70%, of the lateral tibial plateau. The lateral meniscus is more loosely connected to the lateral joint capsule. There are no attachments in the area of the popliteal hiatus and the fibular collateral ligament does not attach to the lateral meniscus. Accessory meniscofemoral ligaments exist in up to one-third of cases. These arise from the posterior meniscus. If a discrete meniscofemoral ligament inserts anterior to the PCL it is known as the ligament of Humphrey, and if it inserts posterior to the PCL, the ligament of Wrisberg. Because of the lack of restraining forces, the lateral meniscus is able to translate four times as much as the medial meniscus, approximately 9 to 11 mm on the tibia with knee flexion. Both menisci are attached anteriorly via the anterior transverse meniscal ligament as well as the anterior roots.[138,139] Recent cadaveric research has more specifically documented the consistent anatomy of the posterior root attachments of the medial and lateral menisci in relation to common arthroscopic landmarks (Fig. 27-26).[174]

The meniscal blood supply arises from the superior, inferior, medial, and lateral geniculate arteries. These vessels form a perimeniscal synovial plexus. It is believed that the central two-thirds of the meniscus receive its nutrition through diffusion and mechanical pumping.

The menisci are composed primarily of type I collagen, accounting for 60% to 70% of its dry weight. Lesser amounts of types II, III, and VI collagen are also present. The collagen fibers are oriented primarily in a circumferential pattern, parallel with the long access of the meniscus.[138,139] There are also radial, oblique, and vertically oriented fibers in organized layers. Proteoglycans and glycoproteins are present, but in smaller concentrations than in articular cartilage.

A number of investigations have established the deleterious consequences of total and even partial meniscectomy on the chronic health of the articular cartilage.[3,106,195,249,260,317,319,379,382,391,406] Nowhere are these principles more important than in children and adolescents, in whom the long-term effects of meniscectomy will be magnified by higher activity levels and simple longevity.

It is now realized that the menisci actually have a number of different functions. The menisci serve to increase contact area and congruency of the femoral tibial articulation. This allows the menisci to participate in load sharing and reduces the contact stresses across the knee joint. It is estimated that the menisci transmit up to 50% to 70% of the load in extension and 85% of the load in 90 degrees of flexion.[6] Baratz et al.[34] showed that after total meniscectomy articular contact areas at a point in time may decrease by 75% and contact stresses on the involved areas increase by 235%. They also documented the deleterious effects of partial meniscectomy, demonstrating that contact stresses increase in proportion to the amount of meniscus removed. Excision of small bucket-handle tears of the medial meniscus

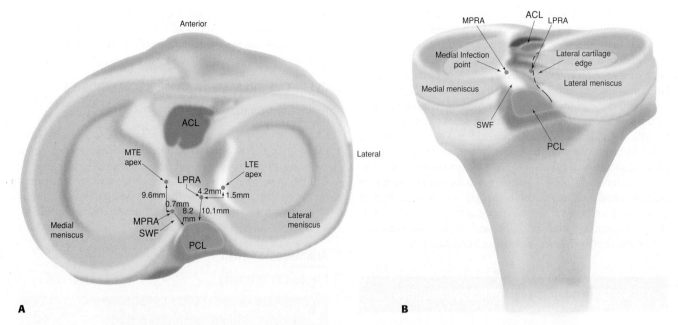

Figure 27-26. Illustration demonstrating the medial and lateral meniscal posterior root attachments and relevant arthroscopically pertinent anatomy (right knee). **A:** Superior view and (**B**) posterior view. ACL, anterior cruciate ligament bundle attachments; LPRA, lateral meniscus posterior root attachment; LTE, lateral tibial eminence; MPRA, medial meniscus posterior root attachment; MTE, medial tibial eminence; PCL, posterior cruciate ligament bundle attachments; SWF, shiny white fibers of posterior horn of medial meniscus. (Reprinted with permission from Johannsen AM, Civitarese DM, Padalecki JR, et al. Qualitative and quantitative anatomic analysis of the posterior root attachments of the medial and lateral menisci. *Am J Sports Med.* 2012;40(10):2342–2347. Copyright © 2012 SAGE Publications.)

increased contact stress by 65%, and resection of 75% of the posterior horn increased contact stresses equivalent to that after total meniscectomy.[34] Repair of meniscal tears, by either arthroscopic or open techniques, reduced the contact stresses to normal. Multiple other studies have corroborated these findings, illustrating the mechanical importance of the meniscus.[138,139]

Meniscal tissue is about ½ as stiff as articular cartilage, allowing it to participate in shock absorption as well. Shock absorption capacity in the normal knee is 20% higher than in the meniscectomized knee.[229,260] The menisci also have a role in joint stability. In the ACL-deficient knee the posterior horn of the medial meniscus plays a very important passive stabilizing role. In the ACL-deficient knee, medial meniscectomy leads to a 58% increase in anterior translation at 90 degrees of flexion.[229,352] Given the presence of neural elements within their substance, it is also theorized that the menisci may have a role in proprioception.

DISCOID LATERAL MENISCUS

Lateral meniscal tears may be seen in association with an underlying discoid lateral meniscus, particularly in younger children. The discoid lateral meniscus represents an anatomic variant of meniscal morphology. The incidence is thought to be 3% to 5% in the general population[98,178,195] and slightly higher in Asian populations.[98,178,195] Interestingly, OCD has been described associated with discoid lateral meniscus, both before and after saucerization.[46,90,149] Discoid morphology almost exclusively occurs within the lateral meniscus, but medial discoid menisci have been described in various case reports.[98,178,195] Although the

incidence of bilateral abnormality has been reported to be as high as 20%,[40,310,357] routine screening on the contralateral knee is not indicated as part of treatment of a discoid lateral meniscus, because of the high rates of asymptomatic cases not requiring intervention. A recent study[307] comparing cases of bilateral discoid menisci to those with unilateral discoid demonstrated that the bilateral cases required treatment at an average age 2 years younger than the unilateral cases, but that unilateral cases were more likely to have tearing than bilateral cases.[307] Discoid menisci are classified based on the system of Watanabe et al.[392]: Complete morphology (type I), incomplete morphology (type II), and any morphology that lacks peripheral attachments (type III). One recent study proposed a more complex classification scheme that incorporates description of the presence and location of instability, paired with morphology.[131] Although often synonymous with the so-called "snapping knee syndrome," discoid lateral menisci may manifest in a variety of ways. Symptoms are often related to the type of discoid present, peripheral stability of the meniscus, and the presence or absence of an associated meniscal tear.[98,178,287,327] Stable discoid menisci without associated tears will often remain asymptomatic, identified only as incidental findings during MRI or arthroscopy.[191] Unstable discoid menisci are more commonly present in younger children and often produce the so-called "snapping knee syndrome." In such instances, a painless and palpable, audible or visible snap is produced with knee ROM, especially near terminal extension. Discoid menisci with posterior instability and a redundant anterior segment may limit knee extension.[408] In children with stable discoid lateral menisci, symptoms often present when an associated tear is present. Unlike acute meniscal tears, such symptoms may present insidiously without significant previous trauma. Signs and symptoms of a meniscal tear may exist, including pain, swelling, catching, locking, and limited motion. On physical examination, there may be joint line tenderness, popping, limited motion, effusion, terminal motion pain, and positive provocative tests (McMurray test). Degenerative horizontal cleavage tears are the most common type of tear seen in this condition, reported in the largest series to occur in 58% to 98% of symptomatic discoid menisci.[40,310] One study showed that Wrisberg types were more likely to require treatment complete discoids, which in turn were more likely to require treatment than incomplete discoids.[307] Instability of a discoid meniscus may be more common than previously thought, with rates as high as 77% in a recent series[131] demonstrating anterior instability to be the most common form (53%), followed by posterior instability (16%) and combined anterior/posterior instability (6%).

TREATMENT OPTIONS FOR MENISCAL INJURIES

NONOPERATIVE TREATMENT OF MENISCAL INJURIES

Indications/Contraindications

Nonoperative Treatment of Meniscal Injuries:
INDICATIONS AND CONTRAINDICATIONS

Indications	Relative Contraindications
• Incidentally noted discoid meniscus with or without pathology	• Symptomatic tears • Tear which cause a loss of knee extension
• Small, nondisplaced, asymptomatic peripheral, vertical/longitudinal tears	• Symptomatic tears • Large tears ≥1 cm • Radial/flap tears, complex patterns

Incidentally noted discoid menisci with or without intrasubstance tearing should be managed nonoperatively. When discoid meniscal tears are symptomatic or block knee extension, surgical intervention should be considered. Some small (<1 cm), stable nondisplaced meniscal tears in the peripheral vascular region of the meniscus may heal nonoperatively or may become asymptomatic.[138,139,195] These can often be seen in the setting of ACL-R at which time they can be carefully probed to assess stability and need for repair.

Technique

Nonoperative treatment of acute meniscal injuries usually consists of rehabilitation of the injured knee with the avoidance of pivoting and sports for 12 weeks, with protection of weight bearing for 4 to 6 weeks to minimize shear forces across the healing meniscus.

Outcomes

As there has been a general evolution to more proactive treatment of meniscus tears, particularly in younger populations, there is sparse literature related to successful nonoperative treatment of meniscus tears. However, Weiss et al.[395] showed that few patients in a series of 80 with "stable" longitudinal, vertical meniscus tears required surgery or were symptomatic at a minimum of 2-year follow-up.

OPERATIVE TREATMENT OF MENISCAL INJURIES

Indications/Contraindications

Due to their larger size and often repairable tear patterns, the majority of meniscal tears in pediatric patients benefit from surgical treatment with an attempt at meniscal repair.[138,139,195] Arthroscopic management is standard, with either partial meniscectomy using motorized shavers and baskets (when tear is deemed irreparable) or meniscal repairs using outside-in, all-inside, or inside-out techniques.[86,138,139]

Arthroscopic Repair

Preoperative Planning

✔ Arthroscopic Repair of Meniscal Injuries:
PREOPERATIVE PLANNING CHECKLIST

OR table	☐ Standard
Position/positioning aids	☐ Supine, lateral thigh post (especially for medial meniscal tears)
Equipment	☐ Arthroscopy setup, inside-out meniscus repair cannulas, two meniscus repair sutures, all-inside meniscus repair implants
Tourniquet	☐ Nonsterile, thigh

Positioning

Supine positioning is used, with a nonsterile tourniquet placed on the operative thigh, and a lateral thigh post, which is particularly useful for application of valgus knee stress to access the posterior horn of the medial meniscus in appropriate tears.

Surgical Approach and Technique

✔ Arthroscopic Repair Meniscal Injuries:
KEY SURGICAL STEPS

- ☐ Diagnostic arthroscopy, assess position/pattern/size of tear
- ☐ For irreparable tears (radial/parrot beak flap/complex/degenerative), perform partial meniscectomy
  - • Use basket/punch instruments to trim torn portion, preserving as much of intact meniscus as possible
  - • Smooth transition zones between native/meniscectomized tissue
- ☐ For repairable tears, reduce any displaced portions to anatomic position
  - • Use meniscal rasp, shaver to freshen edges of meniscal tissue and/or peripheral capsular to stimulate healed
  - • Place meniscus repair sutures (preferably in vertical mattress pattern, inside-out)
  - • For posterior horn, select all-inside approach versus inside-out with mini-open protection of posterior structures
  - • Root repairs may require transtibial bone tunnels
- ☐ Assess stability of repaired meniscus

The historical treatment of a torn meniscus had been meniscectomy, but numerous reports[3,22,47,106,159,192,195,215,249,260,317,319,371,379,382,391,406] indicating the poor long-term results of meniscectomy in children have made this less common. Up to 60% to 75% of patients may have degenerative changes after meniscectomy. As a clear principle, as much of the meniscus should be preserved as possible, especially in the pediatric population which has a better healing potential and more significant long-term consequences.

The exact meniscal injury and potential for repair can be determined arthroscopically to help formulate treatment plans. In general, peripheral tears, which are most common in children, and longitudinal/vertical tears are good candidates for repair, with success rates of up to 90% reported.[85,148,153,252,276]

Although it was believed that longitudinal meniscal tears could heal if communication with peripheral blood supply existed, it was not until the work of Arnoczky et al.[25] in the 1980s that meniscal repairs were popularized, based on documentation of the meniscal blood supply. They believed that tears within 3 mm of the meniscosynovial junction were vascularized, and ones more than 5 mm away were avascular unless bleeding was seen at surgery. Children and adolescents may have greater healing potential for meniscal repair. In children and adolescents, repair of tears in the middle third zone typically heal as well,[85,148,153,252,276] making repair of both red–red and red–white zone tears the standard of care for vertical tears in this young population. Horizontal cleavage tears, transverse/radial tears, parrot beak or flap tears extending from the central third, and complex or degenerative tears most often should undergo partial meniscectomy, taking care to preserve as much meniscal tissue as possible. Occasionally, a complete radial tear will occur in a child, which would require a total or subtotal meniscectomy if treated with debridement. In these instances, side-to-side repair of the peripheral two-thirds of the torn meniscus with multiple nonabsorbable sutures should be trialed, at times in conjunction with partial debridement of the most central edges

(white–white zone) of the tear, which may not heal due to diminished vascularity. Newer techniques for repair of radial tears have recently been described and studied.[277] Similarly, if unstable meniscal root tears are encountered, surgical repair using a transtibial approach should be considered.[219] Repair of these tears have only been studied in adults and repair in children should take into account the potential presence of an open proximal tibial physis. The stability of the peripheral attachments should always be assessed meticulously with a probe, both before and after any meniscal interventions, to ensure there are no concomitant peripheral tears or underlying instability warranting repair. Familiarity with the arthroscopic appearance of normal meniscal mobility, and the differences between the medial and lateral side, is critical to the success of this assessment.

TREATMENT OPTIONS FOR DISCOID LATERAL MENISCUS

Several treatment options exist if the diagnosis of a discoid lateral meniscus is confirmed. For asymptomatic discoid lateral menisci, even if found incidentally on arthroscopy, no treatment is indicated. For stable, complete, or incomplete discoid menisci, partial meniscectomy, "saucerization," is the treatment of choice (Fig. 27-27). If meniscal instability with detachment is also identified during the arthroscopic examination, meniscal repair should be performed.[211] Historically, complete meniscectomy via open or arthroscopic means was suggested for such lesions, but has been clearly associated with poor long-term results and early degenerative changes,[3,8,106,146,195,227,249,260,298,317,319,379,382,406] so is contraindicated. Although there may be a rare instance where salvage of a degenerative or torn discoid meniscus may seem unobtainable, better arthroscopic technology and techniques have made meniscal preservation the ideal treatment through saucerization and repair.[2]

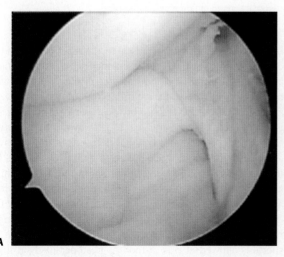 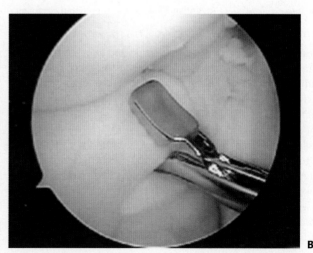

Figure 27-27. Discoid lateral meniscus saucerization. **A:** Complete type discoid lateral meniscus extending into the intercondylar notch. **B:** Excision of the central portion of the discoid meniscus.

(continues)

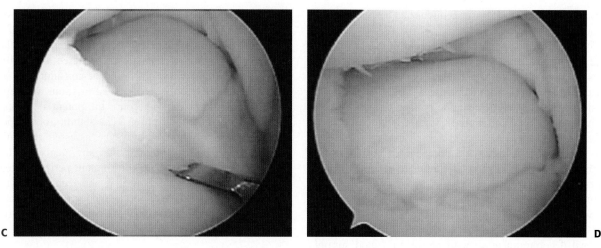

Figure 27-27. (*Continued*) **C:** Excision of the anterior portion of the discoid meniscus. **D:** Appearance after saucerization.

Authors' Preferred Treatment of Meniscal Injuries (Algorithm 27-4)

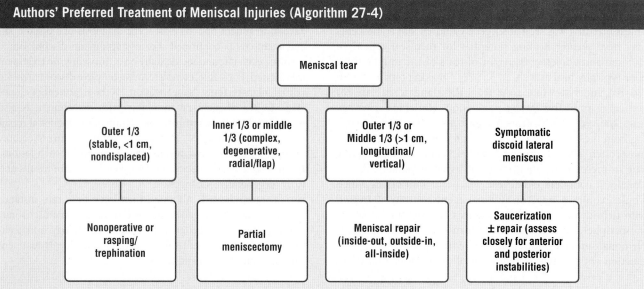

Algorithm 27-4. Authors' preferred treatment of meniscal tears in children and adolescents.

Treatment is based on size, site, shape and stability of the tear, acuity of the lesion, and knee stability. In a stable knee with an acute, arthroscopically documented outer third peripheral tear that is less than 1 cm long and cannot be displaced more than 3 mm, the tear may be allowed to heal. For a similarly sized tear in a chronic setting, we arthroscopically rasp or trephinate the interface between the meniscal edges and perform a repair. Protected weight bearing and limitation of flexion beyond 90 degrees is prescribed for 4 to 6 weeks following meniscal repair. Healing can be assessed based on physical examination. Return to sports and activities is based on the absence of physical examination findings and adequate rehabilitation, usually at 3 to 4 months postoperatively with a small tear.

For larger tears involving the outer third or middle third, which are longitudinal with an intact inner segment that can

be reduced anatomically, meniscal repair is performed. In the chronic setting, rasping of the fragment edge, trephination, and use of a fibrin clot may enhance healing. Patients who undergo meniscal repair are protected postoperatively to allow for meniscal healing. Our postoperative protocol for isolated meniscal repair involves touch-down weight bearing for 6 weeks postoperatively. ROM is restricted from 0 to 30 degrees for the first 2 weeks followed by 0 to 90 degrees for the next 6 weeks. Progressive mobilization and strengthening are pursued from 6 to 12 weeks, and sports-specific therapy and agility exercises are initiated at 3 months under the direction of a physical therapist, provided sufficient strength has been achieved for dynamic knee stability. Return to sports is allowed at 3 to 5 months postoperatively, if there is full ROM, near-symmetric strength, no symptoms (pain, swelling, locking), and resolution of physical examination

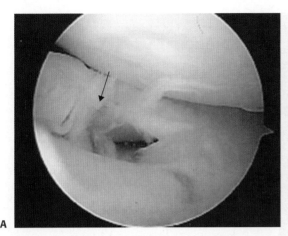 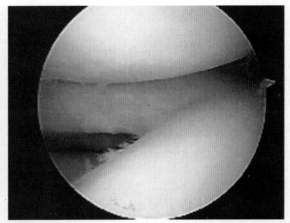

Figure 27-28. Complex inner third tear of the meniscus (**A**) treated with partial meniscectomy (**B**).

findings (joint line tenderness, McMurray maneuvers, terminal range joint line pain). Follow-up MRI is performed only in patients with persistent symptoms or concerning physical examination findings. Partial meniscectomy is performed for irreparable tears involving the inner third or middle third tears that are macerated, horizontal, degenerative, or complex. Care should be taken to preserve as much tissue as possible (Fig. 27-28). With horizontal tears, the smaller of the two leaves is resected back to a stable remnant. Rehabilitation after partial meniscectomy includes weight bearing as tolerated with crutches for comfort, ROM, and strengthening. Return to sports and activities is based on the absence of physical examination findings and adequate rehabilitation, usually at 2 to 3 months postoperatively. Patients who have undergone complete or near-total meniscectomy, should be followed long-term and periodically into young adulthood, to assess the possible development of degenerative changes. Weight-bearing radiographs in slight flexion to measure any compromise in the joint space represent a standard monitoring approach. In symptomatic patients or those with loss of joint space or degenerative changes, such as early osteophytes, meniscal transplant with an allograft meniscus or synthetic scaffold transplant procedure may be considered.[209]

In children and adolescents, the emphasis should be on meniscal repair over meniscectomy whenever possible because of greater healing potential in this age group, the long life span of these patients, the poor results of total and near-total meniscectomy, and the lack of reassuring longer-term results of partial meniscectomy. Meniscal repair techniques include inside-out techniques, outside-in techniques, all-inside techniques and transtibial tunnel techniques for repair of root tears. Outside-in techniques can be useful for anterior horn medial or lateral meniscal tears. For body and posterior horn tears, the traditional technique of meniscal repair has been inside-out repair with vertical or horizontal sutures (Fig. 27-29). Zone-specific cannulae are helpful to direct the small caliber, flexible suture needles to the appropriate position to avoid neurovascular structures. In addition, we frequently make an incision posteromedially or posterolaterally to retrieve the suture needles and tie the sutures onto the joint capsule, thus protecting the saphenous nerve and vein medially and the peroneal nerve laterally. Newer all-inside devices have made the technique of meniscal repair more efficient, but a lack of longer-term studies makes the relative effectiveness unknown (Fig. 27-30). In addition, reports of articular cartilage damage from the heads of bioabsorbable

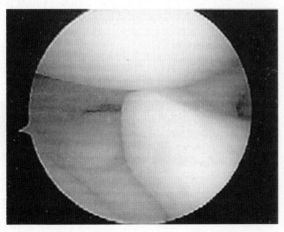 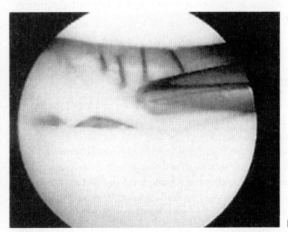

Figure 27-29. Longitudinal middle third tear of the meniscus (**A**) treated with inside-out meniscal repair (**B**).

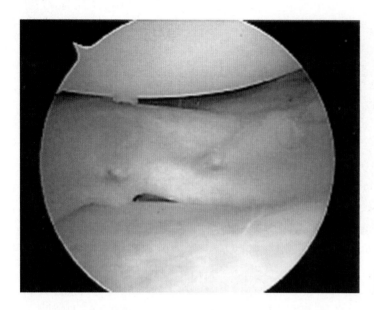

Figure 27-30. Longitudinal tear of the outer third of the posterior horn meniscus treated with all-inside fixation devices.

arrows and darts exist,[138,139] and these devices may cause slightly more trauma to the meniscal tissue than repair needles upon entry. Finally, the available devices may extend too far through the capsule in smaller pediatric knees, with potential for neurovascular injury. We prefer more recent all-inside suture devices with a low profile in the joint, and at times will utilize these for posterior horn tears in adolescent knees or the posterior horn portion of larger tears, with repair of the body through inside-out techniques. In place of a larger posterior incision, a smaller, portal-sized lateral or medial incision may be made, with retrieval of the percutaneous suture ends at the level of the capsule with a small curved clamp or arthroscopic probe. An arthroscopic knot pusher may be helpful to position the knots deep to these incisions, directly at their exit point through the capsule, to maintain optimal tightness of the repair suture. For smaller tears without substantial displacement, all-inside techniques are often used alone, whereas larger tears with displacement such as displaced bucket-handle tears will be addressed with an incision to safely accommodate all-inside technique throughout or in the above described "hybrid" manner with both all-inside (posterior horn) and inside-out (meniscal body) sutures.

Bucket-handle displaced tears with a locked knee are treated urgently to allow for reduction and meniscal repair, restore full knee ROM and to avoid further injury to the meniscus. Meniscal tears in association with ACL injuries are usually treated with meniscal repair concurrent with ACL-R. ACL-R is essential to provide a stable environment for meniscal healing and prevention of further meniscal tears. Moreover, healing rates are higher with concurrent ACL-R than with isolated meniscal repair, perhaps because of the healing environment of the associated postoperative hemarthrosis from the bone tunnels. For meniscal repair in association with ACL-R, return to sports is dictated by the ACL-R, usually at 6 months postoperatively.

Meniscal root tears are rarely encountered in the pediatric population. Meniscal extrusion on MRI may be a sign of a potential meniscal root injury. When unstable root tears are identified, we prefer reduction and repair using with a small single transtibial tunnel and tying the repair sutures over a suture button device. This tunnel typically passes through the center of the proximal tibial physis and thus a single tunnel/smaller size is preferred. Newer suture passing instruments have been developed to facilitate suture passage through the displaced meniscal root.

Postoperative Care

A variety of rehabilitation approaches may be employed in association with meniscus repair, with individualization of the regimen, depending on the severity of the tear and nature of the repair. Smaller tears that are discovered incidentally or well approximated by one or two repair sutures in association with ACL-R may allow for normal weight bearing and advancement of ROM as those protocols not involving meniscus repair. However, given that most tears in children are larger and involve a number of inside-out repair sutures, the standard protocol involves protection of weight bearing for 6 weeks with crutches and limiting ROM to 0 to 90 degrees.

Potential Pitfalls and Preventive Measures

Repair of Meniscal Injuries:
POTENTIAL PITFALLS AND PREVENTIONS

Pitfall	Prevention
• Posteromedial (saphenous nerve) or posterolateral (peroneal) nerve injury with inside-out repair of posterior horn	• Incision to achieve adequate retraction/protection of structures (assistant must see posterior capsule)

• Popliteal artery injury with all-inside repair of posterior horn	• Cut protective cannula to appropriate length for size of patient (especially in pediatric knee) • Direct cannula/device in appropriate vector to avoid central third of posterior knee
• Chondral injury to medial femoral condyle or lateral femoral condyle	• For tight medial compartment, consider trephination of MCL to open joint space, with postoperative bracing • For tight lateral compartment, elevation of foot in figure-four position

Several technical pitfalls exist during meniscal repair. During inside-out meniscal repair of the posterior horn, a posterolateral incision should be made for lateral meniscus repair to avoid iatrogenic injury to the peroneal nerve and a posteromedial incision should be made for medial meniscus repair to avoid iatrogenic injury to the saphenous vein or nerve. During all-inside repair with meniscal repair devices, consideration must be given to the size of the implant relative to the pediatric knee. Implants that protrude too far may injure neurovascular structures or cause local irritation or cysts. Implants that are high-profile or protrude, may damage the articular surface of the femoral condyle. Sterile effusions and synovitis may occur with bioabsorbable implants.

Outcomes

The prognosis after complete or near-total meniscectomy is poor with numerous reports[3,22,47,106,159,192,195,215,249,260,317,319,371,379,382,385,406] indicating poor long-term results with degenerative changes. The prognosis of meniscus repair in appropriately selected cases is good. Noyes and Barber-Westin looked at meniscal tears extending into the avascular zone in patients younger than 20 years old.[294,330] Skeletal maturity had been reached in 88%. Their success rate in this group was 75%. Despite these historical improved results with concomitant ACL-R, a recent study in children[216] reported a 26% failure rate in meniscal repair with ACL-R, with risk factors for failure being complex or bucket-handle tears. Johnson et al.[176] showed a 76% healing rate at an average follow-up of greater than 10 years in a population that averaged 20 years old at the time of surgery. Factors that have been shown to correlate with increased healing of meniscal repairs include: younger age, peripheral tears, repairs of the lateral meniscus, concomitant ACL-R, time from injury to surgery of less than 8 weeks, and tear length of less than 2.5 cm.[1,62,66,106,138,139,176] One series of 25 meniscal tears in children[214] demonstrated that healing rates of lateral and meniscal repairs were comparably high, with a mean Lysholm score of 95, regardless of zone or pattern, but that recurrent tears are more likely to occur in the body of the meniscus than the anterior or posterior horn. A recent case-control study on surgical treatment on meniscal pathology in 324 knees in children and adolescents showed a 13% rate of reoperation with higher rates seen following initial attempt at meniscal repair (18%), and in children with open physes and a bucket-handle tear (46%).[350]

Treatment of discoid meniscal tears with saucerization and repair has shown good mid- to long-term results over time with satisfactory clinical outcomes and preserved knee function although early degenerative changes are common.[7,228,409] Smaller meniscal width and greater severity of meniscal extrusion on postoperative MRI correlate with increased degenerative changes over time.[407] Promising short-term outcomes following allograft meniscal transplantation have been reported in adults and selected high school athletes with improved knee outcome measures, high rates of return to sports and reduced progression of radiographic arthrosis[70,226] although to date published reports on meniscal transplantation in the pediatric population remain rare.[209]

MANAGEMENT OF EXPECTED ADVERSE OUTCOMES AND UNEXPECTED COMPLICATIONS IN MENISCAL INJURIES

Meniscal Injuries:
COMMON ADVERSE OUTCOMES AND COMPLICATIONS

- Failure to heal/retear of meniscus repair
- Neurovascular injury (saphenous nerve, peroneal nerve, popliteal artery)

Complications after either arthroscopic or open repair may include hemorrhage, infection, persistent effusion, stiffness, and nerve injury. Both the popliteal artery and inferior geniculate branches are close to the posterior capsule and are easily lacerated. Postoperative infection should be suspected if swelling or pain persists with an elevated temperature. Swelling is best treated with external compression dressings, and stiffness is best prevented by appropriate postoperative rehabilitation.

Ligament Injuries

INTRODUCTION TO LIGAMENT INJURIES

Ligamentous injuries of the knee in children and adolescents were once considered rare.[80,318] Tibial spine avulsion fractures were considered the pediatric ACL injury equivalent.[197,201,202,318] However, major ligamentous injuries are being seen with increased frequency and have received increased attention.[10,14,18,20,26,39,43,50,56,57,76,94,103,108,120,135,142,144,156,171,178,179,190,204,205,210,236,237,241,254,257,258,267,268,273,276,305,314,348,353,361,364,378,388] The increased frequency of diagnosis of knee ligament injuries in children is likely related to increased participation in youth sports at higher competitive levels, the advent of arthroscopy and MRI, and an increased awareness of injuries in this age group.

ACL injury has been reported in 10% to 65% of pediatric knees with acute traumatic hemarthroses in series ranging from

35 to 138 patients.[196,241,364,378] Stanitski[363] reported 70 children and adolescents with acute traumatic knee hemarthroses; arthroscopic examination revealed ACL injuries in 47% of those 7 to 12 years of age and in 65% of those 13 to 18 years of age.

Injury patterns in the skeletally immature knee are dependent on the loading conditions and the developmental anatomy. Fractures of the epiphyses or physes about the knee are more common than ligamentous injuries alone. Historical literature suggested that isolated knee ligament injury in children younger than 14 years of age was rare because of the relative strength of the ligaments compared to the physes.[102,179,257] However, a recent report investigating rates of pediatric knee injuries presenting to a large children's hospital emergency room suggested that over a 12-year period, the rate of tibial spine fractures increased by 1%, whereas cases of ACL tears had increased by 11%.[333] The inherent ligamentous laxity in children also may offer some protection against ligament injury, but this decreases as the adolescent approaches skeletal maturity. Faster loading conditions favor ligamentous injuries, whereas slower loading conditions favor fracture. Narrowing of the intercondylar notch during skeletal development may also predispose to ligamentous injury.[201] Fractures and ligamentous injuries may also occur concurrently.

Management of ligamentous injuries, particularly ACL injuries in skeletally immature patients, is controversial. Nonreconstructive treatment of complete tears typically results in recurrent functional instability with risk of injury to meniscal and articular cartilage. A variety of reconstructive techniques have been utilized, including physeal-sparing, partial transphyseal, and transphyseal methods using various grafts. Conventional adult ACL-R techniques risk potential iatrogenic growth disturbance due to physeal violation. Growth disturbances after ACL-R in skeletally immature patients have been reported.

ASSESSMENT OF LIGAMENT INJURIES

MECHANISMS OF INJURY FOR LIGAMENT INJURIES

The mechanism of ligamentous injury varies with the child's age. In younger children, ligamentous injury is often associated with significant polytrauma. In contrast, adolescents are more likely to sustain ligamentous injury during contact sports or sports that require "cutting" maneuvers while running.[355] Older adolescents may describe the knee as buckling or moving or jumping out of place and can usually relate the location and severity of their pain as well as the time between injury and onset of pain and swelling. Rapid intra-articular effusion within 2 hours of injury suggests hemarthrosis, most commonly from injury to the ACL. The most common mechanism in adolescents is abduction, flexion, and internal rotation of the femur on the tibia occurring during athletic competition when the weight-bearing extremity is struck from the lateral side.

Isolated injury of the LCL is rare in children, but a direct blow to the medial aspect of the knee may tear the LCL, usually with avulsion from the fibula or a physeal injury through the distal femur.[165] MCL injuries are very common in young athletic adults but do also occur in children and adolescents and typically result from a direct lateral blow to the knee or a pivoting activity that produces a valgus moment across the joint.[320,345] They are most commonly purely ligamentous injuries although bony avulsions do occur. Isolated injuries of the ACL or PCL are more common.[161,165,257] Disruption of the ACL with minimal injury to other supporting structures may be caused by hyperextension, marked internal rotation of the tibia on the femur, and pure deceleration. In contrast, isolated injury of the PCL most often is caused by a direct blow to the front of the tibia with the knee in flexion. The most extensive description of PCL injuries in children to date recently demonstrated that the majority of these injuries are sustained during sports, with less common causes including falls from height, trampoline injuries, and motor vehicle accidents.[206]

INJURIES ASSOCIATED WITH LIGAMENT INJURIES

Common injuries associated with ACL tear include meniscus injuries (lateral more commonly than medial, in the acute setting), and MCL tears. MCL injuries are commonly seen with patellar dislocation events both of which may be caused by a valgus moment across the knee.[316] Posterolateral corner and PCL injuries frequently occur in conjunction with each other. Complete and partial knee dislocations may have a variety of patterns of associated injuries, as described above.

SIGNS AND SYMPTOMS OF LIGAMENT INJURIES

In general, acute knee hemarthrosis suggests rupture of a cruciate ligament, an osteochondral fracture, a peripheral tear in the vascular portion of a meniscus, or a tear in the deep portion of the joint capsule.[84,87] The absence of hemarthrosis is not, however, an indication of a less severe ligament injury, because with complete disruption, the blood in the knee joint may escape into the soft tissues rather than distend the joint. Palpation of the collateral ligaments and their bony origins and insertions should locate tenderness at the site of the ligament injury. A defect in the collateral ligaments often can be felt if the MCL is avulsed from its insertion on the tibia or if the LCL is avulsed from the fibular head. If the neurovascular status is normal, stability should be evaluated by varus/valgus stress testing, which may be done immediately after injury in cooperative adolescents but can be more difficult in younger ages or those with significant pain. Beginning the examination by testing the uninjured knee often calms patients and makes them more cooperative; it also establishes a baseline for assessing the ligamentous stability of the injured knee as knee laxity varies during childhood.[154] Valgus and varus stress testing of the MCL and LCL should be done at both 20 degrees of flexion and full extension, which may demonstrate gross instability if there is cruciate ligament rupture as well (Fig. 27-31).

The anterior drawer test, as described by Slocum, is the classic maneuver for testing the stability of the ACL (Fig. 27-32). The Lachman and pivot-shift tests, however, are considered more sensitive for evaluating ACL injury when the examination can be done in a relaxed, cooperative adolescent, but may be confounded if there is significant guarding. The posterior drawer test (Fig. 27-33), quad active test, and assessment of the posterior sag sign are the key maneuvers for evaluation of the integrity of the PCL.

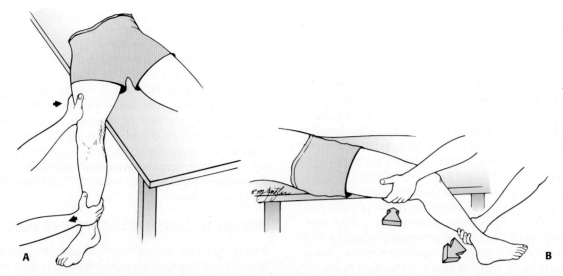

Figure 27-31. Valgus stress test of medial collateral ligament. Extremity is abducted off table, knee is flexed to 20 degrees, and valgus stress is applied. **A:** Frontal view. **B:** Lateral view.

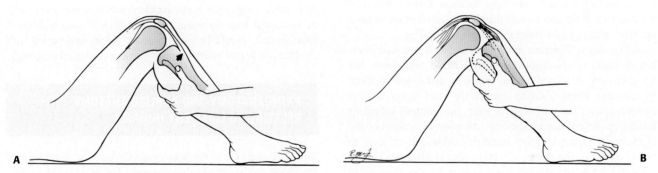

Figure 27-32. Anterior drawer test of anterior cruciate ligament. Foot is positioned in internal, external, and neutral rotation during examination. With anterior cruciate insufficiency, an anterior force (**A**) displaces the tibia forward (**B**).

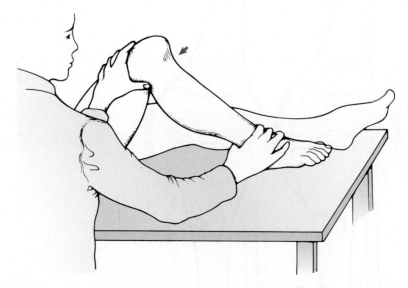

Figure 27-33. Posterior cruciate ligament injury. Note posterior sagging of the tibia with posterior cruciate injury.

IMAGING AND OTHER DIAGNOSTIC STUDIES FOR LIGAMENT INJURIES

Anteroposterior and lateral radiographs are obtained when any ligament injury of the knee is suspected in children. The radiographs are carefully inspected for evidence of occult epiphyseal or physeal fractures or bony avulsions. The intercondylar notch, especially, is inspected to detect a tibial spine fracture. Occasionally, a small fragment of bone avulsed from the medial femur or proximal tibia indicates injury to the MCL. Similarly, avulsion of a small fragment of bone from the proximal fibular epiphysis or the lateral aspect of the distal femur may indicate LCL injury.

MRI is frequently used to further delineate ligamentous injuries in the knee. MRI should be used to confirm an uncertain diagnosis or to gain further information that may affect treatment. Conventional MRI can give information regarding MCL injury, LCL injury, ACL injury, PCL injury, posterolateral corner injury, bone bruising, chondral injury, and meniscal injury.

CLASSIFICATION OF LIGAMENT INJURIES

Classification of knee ligament injuries is based on the severity of the injury, the specific anatomic location of the injury, and the direction of the subsequent instability caused by an isolated ligament injury or combination of ligament injuries.

A first-degree ligament sprain is a tear of a minimal number of fibers of the ligament with localized tenderness but no instability. A second-degree sprain is disruption of more ligamentous fibers, causing asymmetry with stress testing, compared with the contralateral knee, but minimal or minor instability. A third-degree sprain is complete disruption of the ligament, resulting in gross instability. Although difficult to assess clinically, the degree of sprain also is determined with collateral ligaments during stress testing by the amount of separation of the joint surfaces: First-degree sprain, 5 mm or less (normal/baseline); second-degree sprain, 5 to 10 mm; and third-degree sprain, more than 10 mm.

The anatomic classification of knee ligament injuries (femoral attachment avulsion, midsubstance/interstitial tear, or tibial attachment avulsion) describes the exact location of the disruption,[119] whether in the MCL (Fig. 27-34), ACL, LCL (Fig. 27-35), or PCL. Finally, the instability of the knee joint caused by the ligament disruption may be classified as having one-plane instability (simple or straight), rotary instability (anteromedial, anterolateral, posterolateral, or posteromedial), or combined instability (anterolateral–posterolateral, anterolateral–anteromedial, or anteromedial–posteromedial),[160,354] which may be helpful in planning treatment.

OUTCOME MEASURES FOR LIGAMENT INJURIES

Even though retear of a reconstructed ligament, particularly the ACL, is a well-described phenomenon that can occur even without any technical error or oversight in rehabilitation, it remains the most important assessment of outcome. However, for athletes, particularly elite athletes, return to sports and the ability to play at the previous level of competition may be important metrics as well. On a longer-term basis, standard outcome measures, such as functional knee measures (the Pedi-IKDC[207] and Lysholm[358] knee scores), should be used to assess results and paired with the Marx or Tegner activity scores[253] to assess surgical outcomes.

PATHOANATOMY AND APPLIED ANATOMY RELATING TO LIGAMENT INJURIES

The MCL and LCL of the knee originate from the distal femoral epiphysis and insert into the proximal tibial and fibular epiphyses, respectively, except for the superficial portion of the MCL,

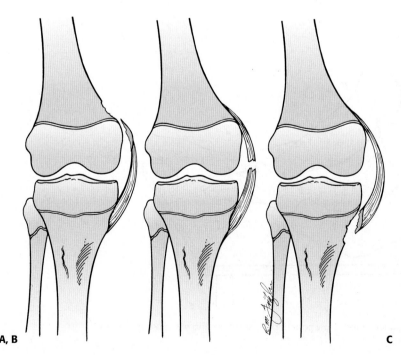

A, B

C

Figure 27-34. Medial collateral ligament injury. **A:** Femoral origin. **B:** Middle portion. **C:** Tibial insertion.

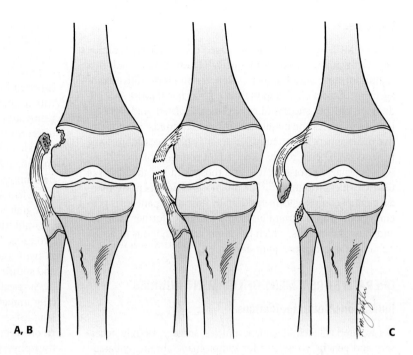

Figure 27-35. Lateral collateral ligament injury. **A:** Femoral origin. **B:** Middle portion. **C:** Fibular insertion.

A, B   **C**

which inserts into the proximal tibial metaphysis distal to the physis (Fig. 27-36). In children, these ligaments are generally stronger than the physes, and significant tensile stresses usually produce epiphyseal or physeal fractures rather than ligamentous injury. The ACL originates from the posterolateral intercondylar notch and inserts into the tibia slightly anterior to the intercondylar spine. The ACL in children has collagen fibers continuous with the perichondrium of the tibial epiphyseal cartilage; in adults, the ligament inserts directly into the proximal tibia by way of Sharpey fibers. This anatomic difference probably accounts for the fact that fracture of the anterior tibial spine occurs more

frequently in children than does ACL injury. The PCL originates from the anteromedial aspect of the intercondylar notch and attaches on the posterior aspect of the proximal tibial epiphysis.

TREATMENT OPTIONS FOR LIGAMENT INJURIES

NONOPERATIVE TREATMENT OF LIGAMENT INJURIES

Isolated collateral ligament injuries are usually successfully treated with bracing and rehabilitation.[320] Isolated ligamentous PCL injuries are typically managed with bracing and rehabilitation as well. Partial ACL tears with a negative pivot-shift test may also be managed conservatively.

Indications/Contraindications

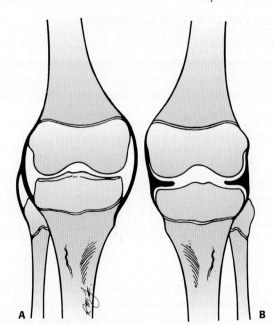

Figure 27-36. Anatomy of medial and collateral ligaments of the knee in the adolescent. **A:** Superficial origins and insertions. **B:** Capsular and meniscal attachments.

Nonoperative Treatment of Ligament Injuries: INDICATIONS AND CONTRAINDICATIONS	
Indications	**Relative Contraindications**
• Partial ACL tear (<50% fibers, negative pivot-shift test, younger child)	• >50% tear, positive pivot shift, older adolescent • Symptomatic instability • Associated injury requiring operative treatment with prolonged rehabilitation regimen and maximum knee stability (e.g., meniscus repair)
• Primary (midsubstance) PCL tear	• Complete bony avulsion injury of footprint
• Partial/incomplete LCL/ PCL injury	• Symptomatic instability despite prolonged PT regimen (quad strengthening)

Outcomes

Isolated MCL injuries that are managed conservatively typically heal well without prolonged sequella, although may result in a significant time out of sports.[320] Reports on conservative management of isolated LCL/posterolateral corner injuries in children are rare but successful management isolated grade III LCL injuries in professional athletes has been reported.[63] Nonoperative management of partial ACL tears may be successful in some patients, with better results expected for younger children, those with a negative pivot-shift test, and those with less than 50% of the ACL fibers ruptured.[204] The prognosis of nonoperative management of complete tears in skeletally immature patients is generally poor, with recurrent instability leading to further meniscal and chondral injuries, which has implications in terms of development of degenerative joint disease.[10,135,171,223,258,268,273,314]

OPERATIVE TREATMENT OF LIGAMENT INJURIES

Indications/Contraindications

For isolated collateral ligament injuries, surgery is rarely necessary and generally reserved for symptomatic chronic collateral ligament deficiency. Acute collateral ligament injuries with large bony avulsions with significant displacement are rare and acute repair may be considered in these situations in the setting of marked knee instability.[389] Combined injury patterns are treated on an individual basis based on ligaments involved and degree of instability. For example, combined ACL/MCL injuries can be successfully managed with ACL-R and nonoperative management of the MCL injury.[335]

The general approach to complete ACL ruptures in skeletally immature children has evolved, and has been the source of considerable controversy. Nonoperative management of complete tears in skeletally immature patients, which may include functional bracing, physical therapy, and activity modification, generally has a poor prognosis, with recurrent instability leading to further meniscal and chondral injuries which has implications in terms of development of degenerative joint disease.[10,135,171,258,268,273,314]

Conventional surgical reconstruction techniques risk potential iatrogenic growth disturbance due to physeal violation. Cases of growth disturbance have been reported in animal models[103,104,142,156,173,341,360] and clinical series.[205,210,236] Animal models have demonstrated mixed results regarding growth disturbances from soft tissue grafts across the physes.

A recent radiologic study[410] investigated 43 pubertal skeletally immature patients who underwent transphyseal ACL-R with metaphyseal fixation of quadruple hamstring autograft. The authors identified MRI evidence of focal bone bridges within or adjacent to the femoral or tibial tunnels in 12% of patients. Although no gross growth disturbances were perceived clinically, premature physeal closure was identified radiologically in two of the patients, all of whom had less than 3 years of growth remaining, by bone age assessment. These data, derived from bone tunnels with cross-sectional areas all under 3% of that of the physes (significantly lower than the threshold previously identified by Janarv et al.,[173]) underscore the potential adverse sequelae of transphyseal techniques in younger patients with more significant growth remaining).

Despite these published basic science and radiologic data, clinical reports of growth deformity after ACL-R remain relatively sparse. Kocher et al.[205] reported an additional 15 cases of growth disturbances gleaned from a questionnaire of expert experience, including 8 cases of distal femoral valgus deformity with an arrest of the lateral distal femoral physis, 3 cases of tibial recurvatum with an arrest of the tibial tubercle apophysis, 2 cases of genu valgum without arrest because of a lateral extra-articular tether, and 2 cases of leg-length discrepancy (one shortening and one overgrowth). Associated risk factors for disturbance or deformity included fixation hardware placed across the lateral distal femoral physis in three cases, bone plugs of a patellar tendon graft across the distal femoral physis in three cases, large (12-mm) tunnels in two cases, lateral extra-articular tenodesis in two cases, fixation hardware across the tibial tubercle apophysis in two cases, of the over-the-top femoral position in one case, and suturing near the tibial tubercle apophysis in one case.

Surgical techniques to address ACL insufficiency in skeletally immature patients include primary repair, extra-articular tenodesis, transphyseal reconstruction, partial transphyseal reconstruction, and physeal-sparing reconstruction. Partial transphyseal reconstructions violate only one physis with a tunnel through the proximal tibial physis and over-the-top positioning on the femur or a tunnel through the distal femoral physis with an epiphyseal tunnel in the tibia.[18,50,144] A variety of physeal-sparing reconstructions have been described to avoid tunnels across either the distal femoral or proximal tibial physis.[14,57,94,143,190,198,199,224,267,305,378]

In prepubescent patients, physeal-sparing techniques have been described that use hamstrings tendons under the intermeniscal ligament and over-the-top on the femur, through all-epiphyseal femoral and tibial tunnels, and with a femoral epiphyseal staple.[14,57,94,143,190,198,199,267,305,378]

IT Band Physeal-Sparing ACL Reconstruction

Preoperative Planning

✔ IT Band Physeal-Sparing ACL Reconstruction: PREOPERATIVE PLANNING CHECKLIST	
OR table	❑ Standard
Position/positioning aids	❑ Lateral thigh post
Equipment	❑ Meniscotome/closed tendon stripper ❑ Extra long curved snap ❑ Curved rasp
Tourniquet	❑ Nonsterile, thigh

Positioning

Standard positioning for arthroscopy is utilized, though some surgeons prefer a circumferential knee holder or standard table placed in "the ACL position," which involves a small amount of Trendelenburg angulation to the table, with the foot of the table dropped to the floor, with the contralateral knee in a well-leg holder or hanging free as well.

Surgical Approaches and Technique

The procedure is performed under general anesthesia, with or without a femoral nerve block for regional anesthesia. The child is positioned supine on the operating table with a pneumatic tourniquet about the upper thigh which is used routinely. Examination under anesthesia is performed to confirm ACL insufficiency.

First, the iliotibial band graft is obtained. An incision of approximately 6 cm is made obliquely from the lateral joint line to the superior border of the iliotibial band (Fig. 27-37A). Proximally, the iliotibial band is separated from subcutaneous tissue using a periosteal elevator under the skin of the lateral thigh. The anterior and posterior borders of the iliotibial band are incised and the incisions carried proximally under the skin using curved meniscotomes (see Fig. 27-37A). The iliotibial band is detached proximally under the skin using a curved meniscotome or an open tendon stripper. Alternatively, a separate incision can be made at the upper thigh to release the iliotibial band. The iliotibial band is left attached distally at Gerdy's tubercle. Dissection is performed distally to separate the iliotibial band from the joint capsule and from the lateral patellar retinaculum (Fig. 27-37B). The free proximal end of the iliotibial band is then tubularized with a no. 2 high-tensile strength braided suture with a whip stitch construct.

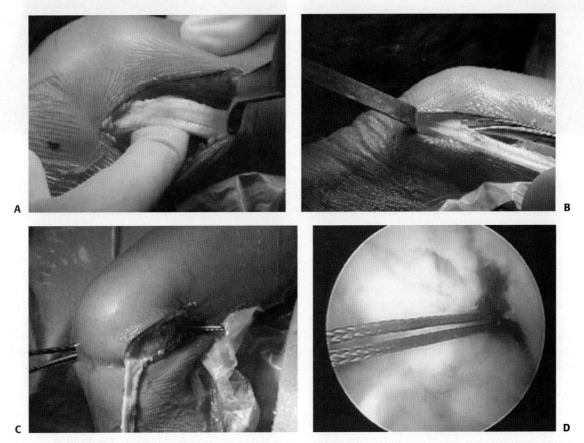

Figure 27-37. Technique of physeal-sparing combined intra-articular and extra-articular anterior cruciate ligament reconstruction using iliotibial band. **A:** The iliotibial band is harvested through an oblique lateral knee incision. **B:** The iliotibial band graft is detached proximally, left attached distally, and dissected free from the lateral patellar retinaculum. **C:** The iliotibial band graft is brought through the knee using a full-length clamp placed from the anteromedial portal through the over-the-top position into the lateral incision. **D:** The graft is then brought through the over-the-top position.

(continues)

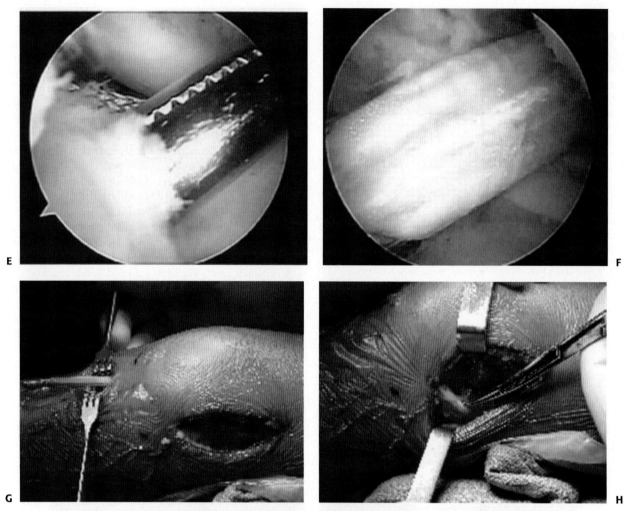

Figure 27-37. (*Continued*) **E:** A clamp is placed from a proximal medial leg incision under the intermeniscal ligament. A groove is made in the anteromedial tibial epiphysis using a rasp. **F:** The graft is brought through the knee in the over-the-top position and under the intermeniscal ligament. **G:** The graft is brought out the proximal medial leg incision. **H:** It is sutured to the intermuscular septum and periosteum of the lateral femoral condyle through the lateral knee incision and it is sutured in a trough to the periosteum of the proximal medial tibial metaphysis.

Arthroscopy of the knee is then performed through standard anterolateral viewing and anteromedial working portals. Management of meniscal injury or chondral injury is performed if present. The over-the-top position on the femur and the over-the-front position under the intermeniscal ligament are identified. Minimal notchplasty is performed to avoid iatrogenic injury to the perichondrial ring of the distal femoral physis which is in very close proximity to the over-the-top position.[39] The free end of the iliotibial band graft is brought through the over-the-top position using a full-length clamp (Fig. 27-37C) or a two-incision rear-entry guide (Fig. 27-38) and out the anteromedial portal (Fig. 27-37D).

A second incision of approximately 4.5 cm is made over the proximal medial tibia in the region of the pes anserinus insertion. Dissection is carried through the subcutaneous tissue to the periosteum. A curved clamp is advanced extraperiosteally from this incision proximally along the anterior proximal tibial cortex into the joint under the intermeniscal ligament (Fig. 27-37E). A small groove is made in the anteromedial proximal tibial epiphysis under the intermeniscal ligament using a curved rat-tail rasp to bring the iliotibial band placement more posterior and allow for future intra-articular biologic tendon-to-bone healing. The free end of the iliotibial band is then brought through the joint (Fig. 27-37F), under the intermeniscal ligament in the anteromedial epiphyseal groove, and out the medial tibial incision (Fig. 27-37G). The band is secured on the femoral side through the lateral incision with the knee at 70 to 90 degrees flexion using figure-of-eight sutures to the periosteum of the LFC to effect an extra-articular reconstruction (Fig. 27-37H). The tibial side is then fixed through the medial incision with the knee flexed 30 degrees and tension

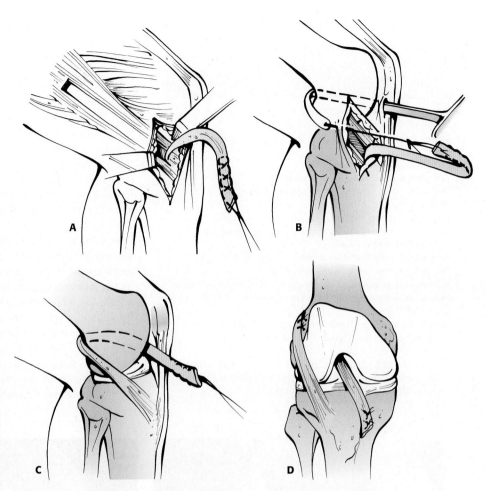

Figure 27-38. Physeal-sparing, combined intra-articular and extra-articular reconstruction utilizing autogenous iliotibial band for prepubescents. **A:** The iliotibial band graft is harvested free proximally and left attached to Gerdy tubercle distally. **B:** The graft is brought through the knee in the over-the-top position posteriorly. **C:** The graft is brought through the knee and under the intermeniscal ligament anteriorly. **D:** Resulting intra-articular and extra-articular reconstruction.

applied to the graft. Within the medial tibial incision, the periosteum is divided and a trough is made in the proximal tibial medial metaphyseal cortex. The graft is sutured to the periosteum on either side of the trough with no. 2 braided figure-of-eight sutures (see Fig. 27-38).

Postoperatively, the patient is maintained touch-down weight bearing for 6 weeks. ROM may be progressed slowly in 2-week intervals but generally is limited from 0 to 90 degrees for the first 6 weeks, followed by progressive full ROM. A CPM and cryotherapy are used for 2 weeks postoperatively. A protective postoperative brace is used for 6 weeks postoperatively, after which the rehabilitation regimen progresses to more advanced strengthening exercises from 6 to 12 weeks postoperatively, straight ahead running in the brace at around 3 months postoperatively, agility exercises around 4 to 5 months postoperatively, and return to sports around 6 months postoperatively, provided sufficient quad and hamstring strength have been achieved.

Physeal Respecting Transphyseal ACL Reconstruction

Preoperative Planning

For adolescent patients with growth remaining who have a complete ACL tear, we perform transphyseal ACL-R with autogenous hamstrings tendons with fixation away from the physes.[208] The procedure is performed under general anesthesia

as an ambulatory outpatient procedure, unless there are specific concerns about pain control or underlying medical conditions, in which case overnight observation can be pursued.

✔ Physeal Respecting Transphyseal ACL Reconstruction: PREOPERATIVE PLANNING CHECKLIST	
OR table	☐ Standard
Position/positioning aids	☐ Lateral thigh post
Equipment	☐ ACL drilling guide system, interference screws, suspensory fixation
Tourniquet	☐ Nonsterile, thigh

Positioning

Standard positioning for arthroscopy is utilized, though some surgeons prefer a circumferential knee holder or standard table placed in "the ACL position," which involves a small amount of Trendelenburg angulation to the table, with the foot of the table dropped to the floor, with the contralateral knee in a well-leg holder or hanging free as well.

Surgical Approaches and Technique

> ✔ **Physeal Respecting Transphyseal ACL Reconstruction:**
> KEY SURGICAL STEPS

- ❏ If positive Lachman/pivot-shift tests on examination under anesthesia, proceed to hamstring harvest
- ❏ Prepare tendons at back table, size and secure with suspensory button fixation
- ❏ Perform diagnostic arthroscopy
- ❏ Perform minimal notchplasty as needed
- ❏ Drill tibial tunnel keeping starting point on tibia medial to avoid tibial tubercle apophysis
- ❏ Drill femoral tunnel at femoral ACL insertion point using transtibial over the top guide or similar technique to ensure a 1–2 mm back wall is present
- ❏ Keep reamed tibial and femoral tunnels "small" (8–9 mm)
- ❏ Pass graft through tunnels using passing suture
- ❏ Achieve femoral fixation using suspensory suture button technique to avoid implants across the distal femoral physis
- ❏ Cycle graft
- ❏ Secure graft to tibia with interference screw with knee at 30 degrees of flexion and posterior drawer force held across tibia
- ❏ Use shorter length tibial screw for tibial fixation to avoid implants across proximal tibial physis or use a post and spiked washer to keep fixation distal to proximal tibial physis

The patient is positioned supine on the operating table with a pneumatic tourniquet about the upper thigh which is not used routinely. Examination under anesthesia is performed to confirm ACL insufficiency.

First, the hamstrings tendons are harvested. If the diagnosis is in doubt, arthroscopy can be performed first to confirm ACL tear. A 3-cm incision is made over the palpable pes anserinus tendons on the medial side of the upper tibia (Fig. 27-39A). Dissection is carried through skin to the sartorius fascia. Care is taken to protect superficial sensory nerves. The sartorius tendon is incised longitudinally and the gracilis and semitendinosus tendons are identified. The tendons are dissected free distally and their free ends whip-stitched with a no. 2 braided suture. They are dissected proximally using sharp and blunt dissection. Fibrous bands to the medial head of gastrocnemius should be identified and released. A closed tendon stripper is used to dissect the tendons free proximally. Alternatively, the tendons can be left attached distally, and an open tendon stripper used to release the tendons proximally. The tendons are taken to the back table, where excess muscle is removed and the remaining ends are whip-stitched with additional no. 2 sutures. The tendons are folded over a suspensory fixation button. The graft diameter is sized and the graft is placed under tension.

Arthroscopy of the knee is then performed through standard anterolateral viewing and anteromedial working portals.

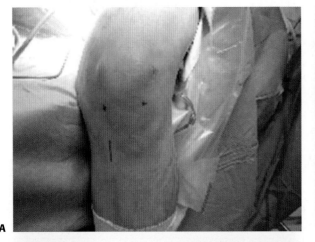

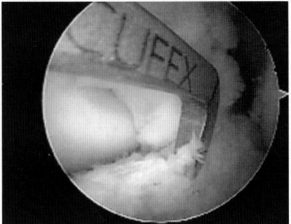

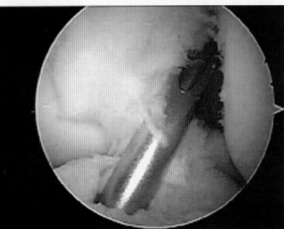

Figure 27-39. Transphyseal reconstruction with autogenous hamstrings for adolescents with growth remaining. **A:** The gracilis and semitendinosus tendons are harvested through an incision over the proximal medial tibia. **B:** The tibial guide is used to drill the tibial tunnel. **C:** The transtibial over-the-top offset guide is used to drill the femoral tunnel.

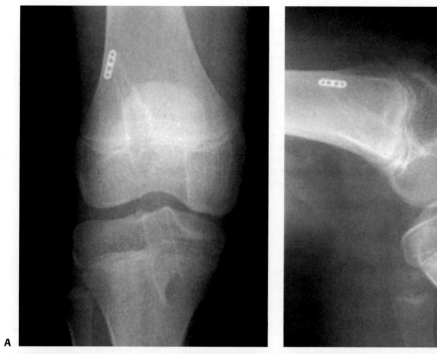

Figure 27-40. Transphyseal reconstruction with autogenous hamstrings for adolescents with growth remaining. Postoperative anteroposterior (**A**) and lateral (**B**) radiographs.

Management of meniscal injury or chondral injury is performed if present. The over-the-top position on the femur is identified. Minimal notchplasty may be performed if notably stenotic. A tibial tunnel guide (set at 55 degrees) is used through the antero-medial portal (Fig. 27-39B). A guidewire is drilled through the hamstrings harvest incision into the posterior aspect of the ACL tibial footprint. The guidewire entry point on the tibia should be kept medial to avoid injury to the tibial tubercle apophysis. The guidewire is reamed with the appropriate diameter reamer. Excess soft tissue at the tibial tunnel is excised to avoid arthrofibrosis or a "cyclops lesion."[170] The transtibial over-the-top guide of the appropriate offset to ensure a 1- or 2-mm back wall is used to pass the femoral guide pin (Fig. 27-39C). Slight over-drilling to accommodate the diameter of the suspensory fixation button is completed, then full diameter reaming up to the lateral femoral cortex to accommodate the graft. The graft is then pulled into the joint using the tagging sutures placed on the slotted end of the guidewire, and graft is advanced into optimal position via the suspensory fixation system of choice. The knee is then extended to ensure no graft impingement. The knee is then cycled approximately 10 times with tension applied to the graft. The graft is fixed on the tibial side with the knee in 20 to 30 degrees of flexion, tension applied to the graft, and a posterior force placed on the tibia. On the tibial side, the graft is either fixed with a soft tissue interference screw if there is adequate tunnel distance below the physis to ensure metaphyseal placement of the screw or with a post and spiked washer. Fluoroscopy can be used to ensure that the fixation is away from the physes. Postoperative radiographs are shown in Figure 27-40.

Postoperatively, the patient is maintained partial weight bearing for 2 weeks. ROM is limited from 0 to 90 degrees for the first 2 weeks, followed by progressive full ROM. A CPM from 0 to 90 degrees and cryotherapy are used for 2 weeks postoperatively. A protective postoperative brace is used for 6 weeks postoperatively.

Authors' Preferred Treatment of Ligament Injuries (Algorithms 27-5, 27-6, 27-7, 27-8, and 27-9)

Medial Collateral Ligament (Algorithm 27-5)

Isolated grade I or II sprains of the MCL are treated with a hinged knee brace for 1 to 3 weeks, with a shorter course of crutches for comfort. Return to athletic activities is allowed when a full, painless ROM is achieved and the patient can run and cut without pain. Isolated complete (grade III) disruption of the MCL can be treated with 6 weeks of immobilization in a hinged knee brace followed by formal physical therapy focused on rehabilitation of the quadriceps muscles and knee motion, provided this is an isolated injury. The physician must ensure that there is no associated injury to the ACL before pursuing nonoperative treatment for a grade III MCL injury. Grade III disruptions of the MCL in adolescents associated with injury of the ACL are usually treated with ACL-R without formal MCL repair, but medial stability must be gently assessed during the examination under anesthesia prior to the ACL-R procedure, which should be delayed at least 4 to 6 weeks following injury to ensure

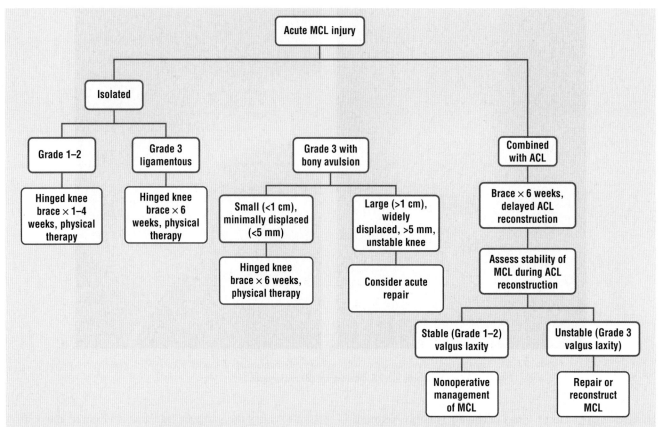

Algorithm 27-5. Authors' preferred treatment of medial cruciate ligament injuries.

resolution of the inflammatory phase of injury, resolution of full ROM, and adequate time for early MCL healing. While some authors do not routinely employ hinged knee bracing following ACL-R, in the presence of an MCL tear, we recommend protecting the MCL with a hinged knee brace to complete the collateral ligament's healing process in the early postoperative period. Surgical treatment of isolated MCL injuries is rarely, if ever necessary. Acute repair could be considered in the setting of a large, widely displaced bony avulsion with significant associated knee instability or chronic reconstruction may be considered in the setting of symptomatic chronic valgus instability.

Anterior Cruciate Ligament (Algorithm 27-6)

The overall goal of treatment of ACL rupture is reestablishment of a functional knee without progressive intra-articular damage or predisposition to premature osteoarthrosis. All skeletally immature patients (i.e., those with open physes) are not the same. Some have a tremendous amount of growth remaining, whereas others are essentially done growing. The consequences of growth disturbance in the former group would be severe, requiring osteotomy and/or limb lengthening. However, the consequences of growth disturbance in the latter group would be minimal.

When treating a skeletally immature athlete with an ACL injury, we divide patients into three groups: preadolescents, adolescents with significant growth remaining, and

older adolescents with closing physes. Patients are classified based upon skeletal age and physiologic age via Tanner staging. Skeletal age can be determined from an anteroposterior radiograph of the left hand and wrist as per the atlas of Greulich et al.[140] Alternatively, skeletal age can be estimated from knee radiographs as per the atlas of Pyle and Hoerr.[315] Physiologic age is established using the Tanner staging system (Table 27-3).[370] In the office, the patient can be informally staged by questioning. In the operating room, after the induction of anesthesia, Tanner staging can be confirmed.

For prepubescent patients, we perform a physeal-sparing, combined intra-articular and extra-articular reconstruction utilizing autogenous iliotibial band (see Fig. 27-38).[198,199] This procedure is a modification of the combined intra-articular and extra-articular reconstruction described by MacIntosh and Darby.[244] Our rationale for use of this technique is to provide knee stability and improve function in prepubescent skeletally immature patients with complete intrasubstance ACL injuries while avoiding the risk of iatrogenic growth disturbance by violating the distal femoral and/or proximal tibial physes. In our opinion, the consequences of potential iatrogenic growth disturbance caused by transphyseal reconstruction in these young patients are prohibitive, and the outcomes of this physeal-sparing technique[198] are comparable or superior to many series of adult-type reconstructions. Moreover, in a recent cadaveric kinematics study, Kennedy et al.[184] demonstrated that the iliotibial band physeal-sparing

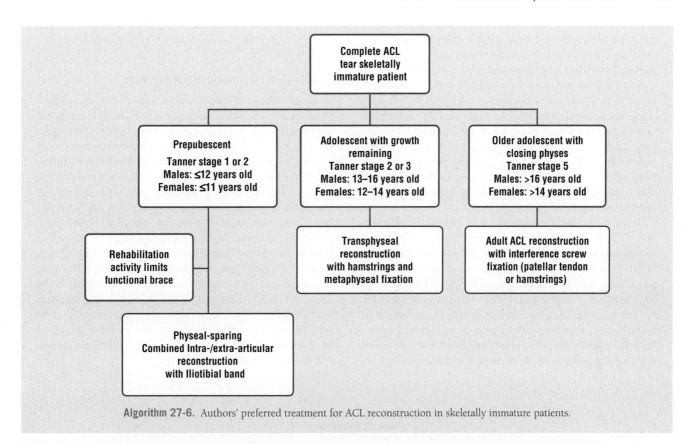

Algorithm 27-6. Authors' preferred treatment for ACL reconstruction in skeletally immature patients.

TABLE 27-3. Tanner Staging Classification of Secondary Sexual Characteristics

Tanner Stage		Male	Female
Stage 1 (Prepubertal)	Growth Development	5–6 cm/yr Testes <4 mL or <2.5 cm No pubic hair	5–6 cm/yr No breast development No pubic hair
Stage 2	Growth Development	5–6 cm/yr Testes 4 mL or 2.5–3.2 cm Minimal pubic hair at base of penis	7–8 cm/yr Breast buds Minimal pubic hair on labia
Stage 3	Growth Development	7–8 cm/yr Testes 12 mL or 3.6 cm Pubic hair over pubis Voice changes Muscle mass increases	8 cm/yr Elevation of breast; areolae enlarge Pubic hair of mons pubis Axillary hair Acne
Stage 4	Growth Development	10 cm/yr Testes 4.1–4.5 cm Pubic hair as adult Axillary hair Acne	7 cm/yr Areolae enlarge Pubic hair as adult
Stage 5	Growth Development	No growth Testes as adult Pubic hair as adult Facial hair as adult Mature physique	No growth Adult breast contour Pubic hair as adult
Other		Peak height velocity: 13.5 yrs	Adrenarche: 6–8 yrs Menarche: 12.7 yrs Peak height velocity: 11.5 yrs

construct better restored both anterior–posterior and rotational stability than the all-epiphyseal and transphyseal over-the-top reconstruction techniques.

In adolescent patients with significant growth remaining, we perform a "physeal respecting" transphyseal ACL-R with autogenous hamstrings tendons with smaller centralized tunnels and suspensory fixation on the femur while avoiding bone plugs or fixation across physes.[208] In older adolescent patients approaching skeletal maturity, we perform conventional adult ACL-R with interference screw fixation using either autogenous central third patellar tendon or autogenous hamstrings.

In skeletally immature patients as in adult patients, acute ACL-R is not performed within the first 3 weeks after injury to minimize the risk of arthrofibrosis. Prereconstructive rehabilitation is performed to regain ROM, decrease swelling, and resolve the reflex inhibition of the quadriceps. Rarely, consideration of staged ACL-R may be given in some cases if there is a displaced, bucket-handle tear of the meniscus that requires extensive repair to protect the meniscal repair from the early mobilization prescribed by ACL-R. Skeletally immature patients must be emotionally mature enough to actively participate in the extensive rehabilitation required after ACL-R.

Lateral Collateral Ligament (Algorithm 27-7)

Grade III injuries of the LCL are extremely rare in children. Occasionally, the lateral capsular sign[404] is seen on radiographs obtained for evaluation of knee injury. Most often, the LCL is avulsed from the proximal fibular epiphysis, with or without a cortical fleck fragment, as proximal and midsubstance tears are uncommon. This injury is treated in the same manner as injury to the MCL. For isolated grade III injuries, a 6-week period of immobilization in a hinged knee brace is recommended. For the rare case of an isolated LCL posterolateral corner injury associated with a large, displaced bony avulsion in an unstable knee, acute repair may be considered.[389] If ACL injury is associated with minor LCL injury, treatment is as described above for combined injuries of the MCL and ACL. In the setting of a complete LCL avulsion with complete ACL tear, repair of the LCL, in conjunction with ACL-R is pursued, usually between 2 and 4 weeks, so as to optimize the healing potential of the collateral ligament without undue risk of arthrofibrosis.

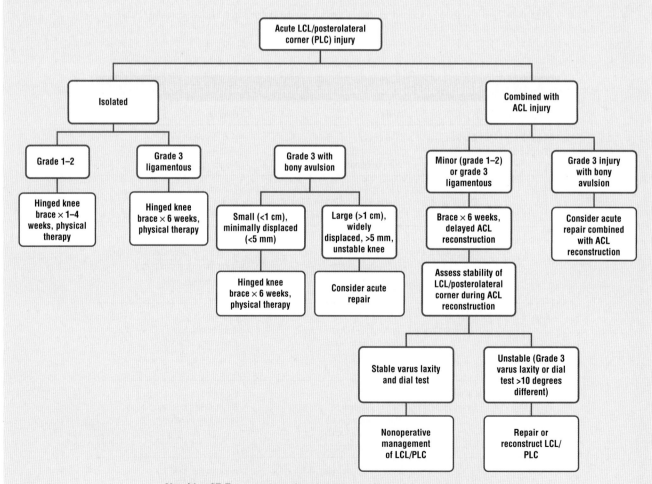

Algorithm 27-7. Authors' preferred treatment of lateral cruciate ligament injuries.

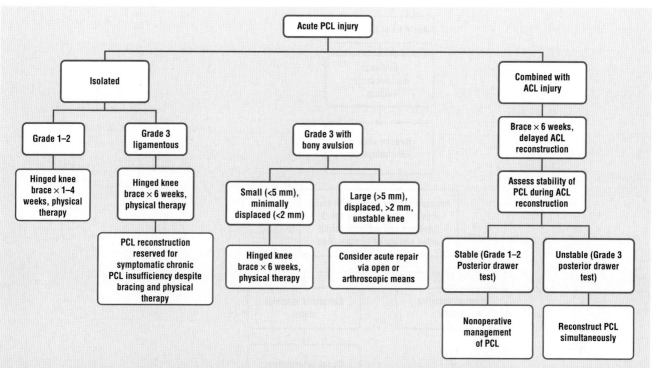

Algorithm 27-8. Authors' preferred treatment of posterior cruciate ligament injuries.

Posterior Cruciate Ligament (Algorithm 27-8)

In general, PCL injuries have traditionally been considered quite rare in children, with most case reports describing a bony avulsion injury.[133,328,374] Kocher et al.[206] recently described a series of 26 knees in patients 18 or younger with PCL injuries, 15 of which underwent surgery for gross instability secondary to either a partial tear ($n = 1$, 7%), a complete ligamentous tear ($n = 4$, 27%), or an osteochondral avulsion fragment from either the tibial or femoral footprint ($n = 10$, 67%). Of note, 53% of the operative cohort had a concomitant ligamentous injury, and 60% had concomitant meniscal tear.

For skeletally immature patients with isolated, purely ligamentous injuries we treat nonoperatively with bracing and physical therapy focusing on quadriceps strengthening. For displaced bony avulsions similar to tibial spine fractures we prefer acute repair. Bony avulsions off the femoral insertion can be treated with arthroscopic repair using bone tunnels and suture fixation, similar to tibial spine techniques, being careful to avoid the distal femoral physis. Bony avulsions off the tibia can be challenging to access and treat arthroscopically. When possible we perform arthroscopic-assisted repair of avulsions through small bony tunnels, with the limbs of suture tied over a cortical bone bridge, similar to the technique described above for tibial spine fractures. In many cases we favor a formal open posteromedial approach for these injuries with direct repair of the avulsed tibial fragment back to its donor bed, with suture or screw fixation, being cautious to avoid implants across the proximal tibial

physis. For skeletally mature adolescents with symptomatic chronic PCL insufficiency we will perform a PCL reconstruction with adult-based techniques, generally with an Achilles allograft.

For combined ACL/PCL injuries we typically treat the PCL injury nonoperatively with bracing for 6 weeks prior to ACL-R. We then assess the stability of the PCL intraoperatively during ACL-R and simultaneously reconstruct the PCL in the setting of chronic grade 3 laxity to posterior drawer testing.

Knee Dislocation (Algorithm 27-9)

Acute dislocations of the knee are uncommon in children because the forces required to produce dislocation are more likely to fracture the distal femoral or proximal tibial epiphysis.[125] Acute knee dislocation usually involves major injuries of associated soft tissues and ligaments and often neurovascular injuries. Injuries typically occur in older skeletally mature adolescents from high-energy trauma, such as motor vehicle injuries, pedestrian versus motor vehicle injury, bicycle versus motor vehicle injury, trampoline injuries, and high-energy contact sports.

Adequate follow-up studies of acute knee dislocations in children younger than 10 years of age are few,[93] and most information has been obtained from reports of knee dislocations in adults. Because of the potential for associated vascular injury, acute knee dislocations in children may be emergent situations. The dislocation causes obvious deformity about the knee. With anterior dislocation, the tibia is

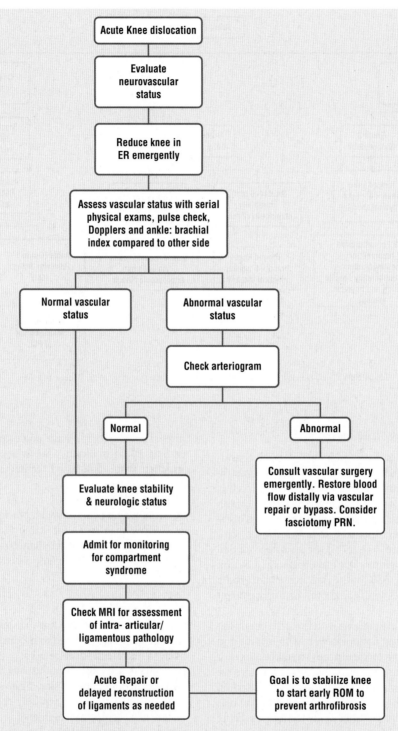

Algorithm 27-9. Authors' preferred treatment of knee dislocation.

prominent in an abnormal anterior position (Fig. 27-41). With posterior dislocation, the femoral condyles are abnormally prominent anteriorly.

After the dislocation is reduced, the stability of the knee should be evaluated with gentle stress testing. For isolated anterior or posterior dislocations, the integrity of the collateral ligaments should be carefully evaluated. Some knees may spontaneously reduce after dislocation or reduce with manipulation of the leg for transport.

The neurovascular status of the extremity should be carefully evaluated both before and after reduction, especially the dorsalis pedis and posterior tibial pulses and

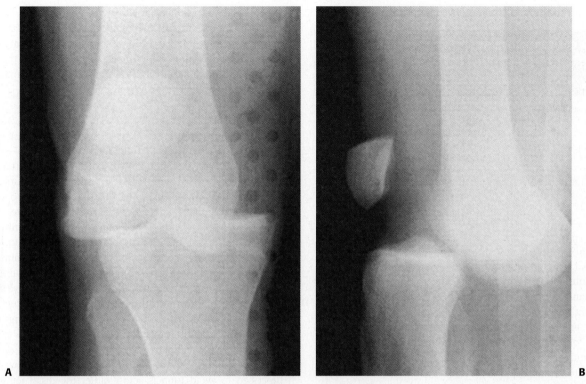

Figure 27-41. Anteromedial dislocation of the knee in a 14-year-old girl. **A:** AP X-ray. **B:** Lateral X-ray.

peroneal nerve function. There is increasing evidence supporting the diagnostic and prognostic value of the ankle–brachial index,[269] which may be positive (<0.9) because of significant vascular injury, despite normal pulses and Doppler. Any abnormal vascular findings, either before or after reduction, require arteriography, which may be done in the operating room to facilitate rapid transition to repair. Popliteal artery laceration or intimal tear may occur in 20% to 35% of cases.[81,93,125,137,186] Abnormalities in the sensory or motor function of the foot and distribution of the peroneal nerve function should be noted. Peroneal nerve injury has been reported in 16% to 40% of cases.[81,93,125,137,186] MRI is usually performed to assess the integrity of the cruciate and collateral ligaments, the posterolateral and posteromedial corners, the menisci, and the articular surfaces.

Knee dislocation usually occurs with disruption of both cruciate ligaments. With direct anterior or posterior dislocation, the collateral ligaments and the soft tissues may be retained because the femoral condyles are stripped out of their capsular and collateral ligament attachments, and when reduced slip back inside them. Associated medial displacement is often accompanied by LCL disruption. Associated lateral displacement is often accompanied by MCL disruption. Knee dislocations in adolescents have been associated with tibial spine fractures, osteochondral fractures of the femur or tibia, meniscal injuries, and peroneal nerve injuries.[81]

Treatment of knee dislocations includes both acute and delayed reconstructive management. Acutely, the knee is reduced under anesthesia. If emergent vascular surgery is performed, fasciotomies are usually also performed. However, ligamentous reconstruction is typically delayed. The knee is braced with protected weight bearing and limited motion, or occasionally application of external fixation is warranted to protect the vascular repair.

Reconstruction may be delayed approximately 2 to 4 weeks after injury, depending on the pattern. Primary ligament repairs become more difficult after this period of time because of scarring and lack of definition of tissues. Reconstructions may be staged or performed in a single multiligamentous knee procedure. Surgery often combines arthroscopic and open techniques. General principles include ligament repair for collateral ligament injuries, ligament reconstruction for midsubstance cruciate ligament injuries, and meniscal repair. Allograft tissue is often used because of the multiligamentous nature of the injury and the need to minimize tourniquet time and any additional knee trauma that would come from graft harvesting. Postoperatively, prolonged immobilization should be avoided because of the substantial risk of stiffness after knee dislocation surgery. Limited motion in a hinged knee brace and protected weight bearing are utilized, followed by mobilization and strengthening.

Potential Pitfalls and Preventive Measures

Repair of Ligament Injuries:
POTENTIAL PITFALLS AND PREVENTIONS

Pitfall	Prevention
• Growth disturbance	• Assess bone age accurately • Use soft tissue graft • Avoid transphyseal fixation/screw placement
• ACL retear	• Ensure adequate postoperative rehab, optimization of dynamic knee stability • Avoid allograft tissue

If a family wishes to pursue nonoperative treatment of complete ACL tears in children and adolescents, sufficient counseling must be performed so that the patient and the family understand the relative risks and benefits of nonoperative treatment versus ACL-R. In such instances, compliance with bracing and activity restriction must be monitored. Careful regular follow-up is necessary to evaluate for instability episodes and further meniscal/chondral injury. Should further meniscal or chondral injury occurs, ACL-R should be reemphasized, because of the risk of degenerative joint disease associated with injury episodes.

Pitfalls to avoid with the physeal-sparing iliotibial band reconstruction in prepubescents include harvesting a short graft insufficient to reach the medial tibial incision, difficulty passing the graft through the posterior joint capsule, and difficulty passing the graft under the intermeniscal ligament. Pitfalls to avoid with the transphyseal hamstrings reconstruction in adolescents with growth remaining include amputation of the hamstring grafts, poor tunnel placement, and graft impingement.

Based on the 15 cases of growth disturbance after ACL-R in skeletally immature patients that we reported, we recommend careful attention to technical details during ACL-R in skeletally immature patients, particularly the avoidance of fixation hardware across the lateral distal femoral epiphyseal plate.[205] Care should also be taken to avoid injury to the vulnerable tibial tubercle apophysis.[201,343] Given the cases of growth disturbances associated with transphyseal placement of patellar tendon graft bone blocks, we recommend the use of soft tissue grafts. Large tunnels should likely be avoided as likelihood of arrest is associated with greater violation of epiphyseal plate cross-sectional area. The reported cases and growing anecdotal evidence of genu valgum without arrest associated with lateral extra-articular tenodesis raise additional concerns about the effect of tension on physeal growth. Finally, care should be taken to avoid dissection or notching around the posterolateral aspect of the physis during over-the-top nonphyseal femoral placement to avoid potential injury to the very close perichondrial ring and subsequent deformity.[201]

Outcomes

The prognosis of ACL-R depends on the surgical procedure. Several case series exist regarding ACL-R in skeletally immature patients. However, most series are small and variably report the

patients' skeletal age and growth remaining. Primary ligament repair[76,108] and extra-articular tenodesis alone[135,258] have had poor results in children and adolescents, similar to adults. Transphyseal reconstructions with tunnels that violate both the distal femoral and proximal tibial physes have been performed with hamstrings autograft, patellar tendon autograft, and allograft tissue.[10,20,26,103,120,254,258,348,353,361,388] These anatomic ACL-R procedures have high success rates as in adult patients, however risk injury to the physis, particularly in prepubescent patients. However, those adolescents in the intermediate group—pubescent patients with still open growth plates—in whom transphyseal tunnels are used with "physeal-respecting" principles, are unlikely to have any risk of growth disturbance. In one follow-up outcome study of 61 knees in 59 skeletally immature Tanner stage 3 adolescents with growth remaining (mean chronologic age: 14.7 years old, range: 11.6 to 16.9 years old) who underwent transphyseal reconstruction with autogenous hamstrings graft and metaphyseal fixation, reported a revision rate of 3% with excellent functional outcome, return to competitive sports, and no cases of growth disturbance.[208] Other more recent studies have suggested that the rate of graft retear following ACL-R in this young patient population is much higher (10% to 20%) with younger age correlating with higher retear rates.[155,393]

A variety of physeal-sparing reconstructions have been described to avoid tunnels across either the distal femoral or proximal tibial physis.[14,57,94,143,190,267,305,378] In general these procedures are nonanatomic and may have some persistent knee laxity. However they avoid physeal violation, and rates of graft rupture, persistent or recurrent instability have generally been low. In a follow-up outcome study of 44 skeletally immature prepubescent children who were Tanner stage 1 or 2 (mean chronologic age: 10.3 years old; range: 3.6 to 14 years old) who underwent the physeal-sparing combined intra-articular and extra-articular ACL-R technique using autogenous iliotibial band that we describe above, we found a revision ACL-R rate of 4.5% with excellent functional outcome, return to competitive sports, and no cases of growth disturbance.[198,199] A more recent study on physeal sparing iliotibial band ACL reconstructions in 22 patients with a minimum of 3-year follow-up had a 14% rate of graft retearing requiring revision reconstruction.[399] Anderson[14,15] described a more anatomic physeal-sparing reconstruction in prepubescent children by utilizing carefully placed epiphyseal femoral and tibial tunnels with an autogenous hamstrings graft and epiphyseal fixation (Fig. 27-42). In 12 skeletally immature patients with mean age 13.3 years old (SD: 1.4), he found excellent functional outcome without growth disturbance. Other authors have reported similar successful results with this all-epiphyseal technique in the skeletally immature population.[79]

As interest in ACL-R techniques in skeletally immature patients has increased, however, the concept of transphyseal tunnel creation across open physes has remained controversial, as some authors contend that soft tissue graft placement without hardware across tunnels eliminates the risk of growth disturbance,[127,182,301,384] a notion supported by some animal models.[262] A recent report followed skeletally immature patients with serial long-leg radiographs at 6 and 12 months postoperatively following transphyseal ACL-R and identified four cases of growth disturbances.[351] One meta-analysis of 55 original studies assessed results

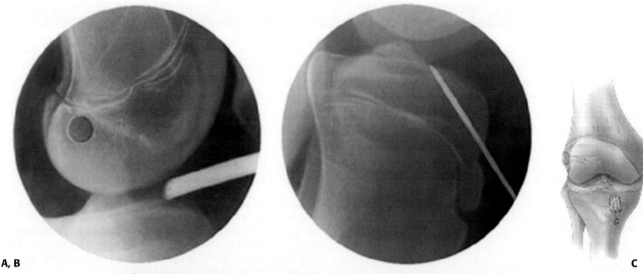

A, B   **C**

Figure 27-42. Physeal-sparing epiphyseal ACL reconstruction with autogenous hamstrings for prepubescents with growth remaining. **A:** Femoral tunnel placement within the epiphysis. **B:** Tibial tunnel placement within the epiphysis. **C:** Appearance after epiphyseal graft fixation.

in 935 patients with a median age of 13 at mean follow-up of 40 months, concluding that risk of angular deformity or leg-length discrepancy was 1.8%, and was actually lower in transphyseal transosseous reconstruction than physeal-sparing transosseous reconstruction, perhaps because of the more parallel orientation of the tunnels relative to the physis in the latter technique.

The risk of osteoarthritis following ACL-R in adolescents remains high. A recent report noted that in patients who were adolescents at the time of ACL-R there was significantly more radiographically visible osteoarthritic changes in their operated knee than in their noninvolved contralateral knee at 10 to 20 years following their reconstruction.[248]

Complications after ligament injury in children are similar to adults: arthrofibrosis,[296] persistent instability, unrecognized concomitant injury, infection, graft failure, neurovascular injury, deep venous thrombosis, and donor site morbidity. Graft failure is the most common complication and younger age at surgery is a major risk factor.[155,393,394] Typically revision ACL-R is the recommended treatment with use of autograft when possible. BTB autograft reconstruction would be the recommended graft choice if prior hamstring autograft failure occurred after skeletal maturity. Deep venous thromboses are rare but have been reported following ACL-R in adolescents.[279] Prompt diagnosis using ultrasound and appropriate treatment with anti-coagulation is recommended for these patients. A recent study of 933 ACL-R cases in children and adolescents with a mean age of 15 showed an arthrofibrosis rate of 8.3%, with older age (16 to 18 years), female age, concurrent meniscal repair, and patellar tendon autograft representing risk factors for arthrofibrosis requiring treatment. Although arthroscopic lysis of adhesions and manipulation under anesthesia were effective in improving ROM in this series of patients, 20% complained of some persistent pain at 6.3 years of mean follow-up. Dynamic splinting remains a viable option in this group of patients.[300]

In skeletally immature patients, despite continued controversy, growth disturbance can occur from iatrogenic physeal injury and remains important area of continued research.

Annotated References

Reference	Annotation
Clark CR, Ogden JA. Development of the menisci of the human knee joint. Morphological changes and their potential role in childhood meniscal injury. *J Bone Joint Surg Am.* 1983;65(4):538–547.	A description of the developmental vasculature of the menisci.

Annotated References

Reference	Annotation
Fairbank TJ. Knee joint changes after meniscectomy. *J Bone Joint Surg Br.* 1948;30B(4):664–670.	The first long-term follow-up study of patients after total meniscectomy which demonstrated that degenerative changes followed meniscectomy in a substantial proportion of patients.
Flachsmann R, Broom ND, Hardy AE, et al. Why is the adolescent joint particularly susceptible to osteochondral shear fracture?. *Clin Orthop Relat Res.* 2000;381:212–221.	A histopathologic study which helps to explain the occurrence of osteochondral fractures in the skeletally immature at an ultrastructural level.
Fulkerson J, Becker GJ, Meaney JA, et al. Anteromedial tibial tubercle transfer without bone graft. *Am J Sports Med.* 1990;18(5):490–496.	A description of the anteromedialization "Fulkerson" osteotomy for the treatment of patellar instability.
Kocher MS, Micheli LJ, Gerbino P, et al. Tibial eminence fractures in children: prevalence of meniscal entrapment. *Am J Sports Med.* 2003;31(3):404–407.	In a consecutive series of 80 skeletally immature patients who underwent surgical fixation of hinged or displaced tibial spine fractures which did not reduce in extension, Kocher et al.[202] found entrapment of the anterior horn medial meniscus ($n = 36$), intermeniscal ligament ($n = 6$), or anterior horn lateral meniscus ($n = 1$) in 26% (6/23) of hinged (type II) fractures and 65% (37/57) of displaced (type III) fractures.
Kocher MS, Saxon HS, Hovis WD, et al. Management and complications of anterior cruciate ligament injuries in skeletally immature patients: Survey of the Herodicus Society and The ACL Study Group. *J Pediatr Orthop.* 2002;22(4):452–457.	The authors report 15 cases of growth disturbances following ACL reconstruction gleaned from a questionnaire of expert experience. Associated risk factors included fixation hardware or bone plugs placed across the lateral distal femoral physis, large (12-mm) tunnels, lateral extra-articular tenodesis, fixation hardware across the tibial tubercle apophysis, over-the-top femoral position, and suturing near the tibial tubercle apophysis.
Kocher MS, Smith JT, Iversen MD, et al. Reliability, validity, and responsiveness of a modified International Knee Documentation Committee Subjective Knee Form (Pedi-IKDC) in children with knee disorders. *Am J Sports Med.* 2011;39(5):933–939.	Validation of a pediatric-specific questionnaire for knee symptoms—the Pedi-IKDC.
Lewallen LW, McIntosh AL, Dahm DL. Predictors of recurrent instability after acute patellofemoral dislocation in pediatric and adolescent patients. *Am J Sports Med.* 2013;41(3):575–581.	This article reports on the importance of young age and trochlear dysplasia as risk factors for recurrent instability following patellar dislocations in young patients.
Meyers MH, McKeever FM. Fracture of the intercondylar eminence of the tibia. *J Bone Joint Surg Am.* 1970;52:1677–1684.	Origin of classification system for tibial spine fractures.
Mitchell JJ, Mayo MH, Axibal DP, et al. Delayed anterior cruciate ligament reconstruction in young patients with previous anterior tibial spine fractures. *Am J Sports Med.* 2016;44(8):2047–2056.	A recently reported case series of 101 patients over a 20-year period reported a 19% rate of delayed ACL reconstruction in patients who had a prior tibial spine fracture. Patients who were older at the time of tibial spine fracture were more likely to require ACL reconstruction in the future.
Pressman AE, Letts RM, Jarvis JG. Anterior cruciate ligament tears in children: An analysis of operative versus nonoperative treatment. *J Pediatr Orthop.* 1997;17(4):505–511.	The authors report when comparing the results of operative versus nonoperative management of complete ACL injuries in adolescents, those managed by ACL reconstruction had less instability, higher activity and return to sports levels, and lower rates of subsequent reinjury and meniscal tears.

REFERENCES

1. Accadbled F, Cassard X, Sales de Gauzy J, et al. Meniscal tears in children and adolescents: results of operative treatment. *J Pediatr Orthop B.* 2007;16(1):56–60.
2. Adachi N, Ochi M, Uchio Y, et al. Torn discoid lateral meniscus treated using partial central meniscectomy and suture of the peripheral tear. *Arthroscopy.* 2004;20(5):536–542.
3. Aglietti P, Bertini FA, Buzzi R, et al. Arthroscopic meniscectomy for discoid lateral meniscus in children and adolescents: 10-year follow-up. *Am J Knee Surg.* 1999;12(2):83–87.
4. Ahmad CS, Brown GD, Stein BS. The docking technique for medial patellofemoral ligament reconstruction: Surgical technique and clinical outcome. *Am J Sports Med.* 2009;37(10):2021–2027.
5. Ahmad CS, Stein BE, Matuz D, et al. Immediate surgical repair of the medial patellar stabilizers for acute patellar dislocation. A review of eight cases. *Am J Sports Med.* 2000;28(6):804–810.
6. Ahmed AM, Burke DL. In-vitro measurement of static pressure distribution in synovial joints—Part I: Tibial surface of the knee. *J Biomech Eng.* 1983;105(3):216–225.
7. Ahn JH, Kim KI, Wang JH, et al. Long-term results of arthroscopic reshaping for symptomatic discoid lateral meniscus in children. *Arthroscopy.* 2015;31(5):867–873.
8. Ahn JH, Lee SH, Yoo JC, et al. Arthroscopic partial meniscectomy with repair of the peripheral tear for symptomatic discoid lateral meniscus in children: results of minimum 2 years of follow-up. *Arthroscopy.* 2008;24(8):888–898.
9. Aichroth PM. Osteochondral fractures and osteochondritis dissecans in sportsmen's knee injuries (Abstract). *J Bone Joint Surg Br.* 1977;59:108.
10. Aichroth PM, Patel DV, Zorrilla P. The natural history and treatment of rupture of the anterior cruciate ligament in children and adolescents. A prospective review. *J Bone Joint Surg Br.* 2002;84(1):38–41.
11. Alleyne KR, Galloway MT. Management of osteochondral injuries of the knee. *Clin Sports Med.* 2001;20(2):343–364.
12. Amis AA, Firer P, Mountney J, et al. Anatomy and biomechanics of the medial patellofemoral ligament. *Knee.* 2003;10(3):215–220.

13. Amis AA. Current concepts on anatomy and biomechanics of patellar stability. *Sports Med Arthrosc Rev.* 2007;15:48–56.
14. Anderson AF. Transepiphyseal replacement of the anterior cruciate ligament in skeletally immature patients. A preliminary report. *J Bone Joint Surg Am.* 2003;85-A(7):1255–1263.
15. Anderson AF. Transepiphyseal replacement of the anterior cruciate ligament using quadruple hamstring grafts in skeletally immature patients. *J Bone Joint Surg Am.* 2004;86-A Suppl 1(Pt 2):201–209.
16. Anderson AF, Pagnani MJ. Osteochondritis dissecans of the femoral condyles. Long-term results of excision of the fragment. *Am J Sports Med.* 1997;25(6):830–834.
17. Anderson CN, Nyman JS, McCullough KA, et al. Biomechanical evaluation of physeal-sparing fixation methods in tibial eminence fractures. *Am J Sports Med.* 2013;41(7):1586–1594.
18. Andrews M, Noyes FR, Barber-Westin SD. Anterior cruciate ligament allograft reconstruction in the skeletally immature athlete. *Am J Sports Med.* 1994;22(1):48–54.
19. Andrish JT. Meniscal injuries in children and adolescents: diagnosis and management. *J Am Acad Orthop Surg.* 1996;4(5):231–237.
20. Angel KR, Hall DJ. The role of arthroscopy in children and adolescents. *Arthroscopy.* 1989;5(3):192–196.
21. Anstey DE, Heyworth BE, Price MD, et al. Effect of timing of ACL reconstruction in surgery and development of meniscal and chondral lesions. *Phys Sportsmed.* 2012;40(1):36–40.
22. Appel H. Late results after meniscectomy in the knee joint. A clinical and roentgenologic follow-up investigation. *Acta Orthop Scand Suppl.* 1970;133:1–111.
23. Arendt EA, Dejour D. Patella instability: building bridges across the ocean a historic review. *Knee Surg Sports Traumatol Arthrosc.* 2013;21(2):279–293.
24. Arnoczky SP, Warren RF. Microvasculature of the human meniscus. *Am J Sports Med.* 1982;10(2):90–95.
25. Arnoczky SP, Warren RF, Spivak JM. Meniscal repair using an exogenous fibrin clot. An experimental study in dogs. *J Bone Joint Surg Am.* 1988;70(8):1209–1217.
26. Aronowitz ER, Ganley TJ, Goode JR, et al. Anterior cruciate ligament reconstruction in adolescents with open physes. *Am J Sports Med.* 2000;28(2):168–175.
27. Askenberger M, Arendt EA, Ekström W, et al. Medial patellofemoral ligament injuries in children with first-time lateral patellar dislocations: a magnetic resonance imaging and arthroscopic study. *Am J Sports Med.* 2016;44(1):152–158.
28. Aulisa AG, Falciglia F, Giordano M, et al. Galeazzi's modified technique for recurrent patella dislocation in skeletally immature patients. *J Orthop Sci.* 2012;17(2):148–155.
29. Baier C, Springorum HR, Beckmann J, et al. Treatment of patellar instability in children and adolescents. *Orthopade.* 2011;40(10):868–870, 872–874, 876.
30. Bakalim G, Wilppula E. Closed treatment of fracture of the tibial spines. *Injury.* 1974;5(3):210–212.
31. Balcarek P, Jung K, Frosch KH, et al. Value of the tibial tuberosity-trochlear groove distance in patellar instability in the young athlete. *Am J Sports Med.* 2011;39(8):1756–1761.
32. Balcarek P, Walde TA, Frosch S, et al. Patellar dislocations in children, adolescents and adults: a comparative MRI study of medial patellofemoral ligament injury patterns and trochlear groove anatomy. *Eur J Radiol.* 2011;79(3):415–420.
33. Bale RS, Banks AJ. Arthroscopically guided Kirschner wire fixation for fractures of the intercondylar eminence of the tibia. *J R Coll Surg Edinb.* 1995;40(4):260–262.
34. Baratz ME, Fu FH, Mengato R. Meniscal tears: the effect of meniscectomy and of repair on intraarticular contact areas and stress in the human knee. A preliminary report. *Am J Sports Med.* 1986;14(4):270–275.
35. Bassett FH. Acute dislocation of the patella, osteochondral fractures, and injuries to the extensor mechanism of the knee. *Instr Course Lect.* 1976;25:40–49.
36. Baxter MP, Wiley JJ. Fractures of the tibial spine in children. An evaluation of knee stability. *J Bone Joint Surg Br.* 1988;70(2):228–230.
37. Beasley LS, Vidal AF. Traumatic patellar dislocation in children and adolescents: treatment update and literature review. *Curr Opin Pediatr.* 2004;16(1):29–36.
38. Beck P, Brown NA, Greis PE, et al. Patellofemoral contact pressures and lateral patellar translation after medial patellofemoral ligament reconstruction. *Am J Sports Med.* 2007;35(9):1557–1563.
39. Behr CT, Potter HG, Paletta GA Jr. The relationship of the femoral origin of the anterior cruciate ligament and the distal femoral physeal plate in the skeletally immature knee. An anatomic study. *Am J Sports Med.* 2001;29(6):781–787.
40. Bellier G, Dupont JY, Larrain M, et al. Lateral discoid menisci in children. *Arthroscopy.* 1989;5(1):52–56.
41. Bentley G, Biant LC, Carrington RW, et al. A prospective, randomised comparison of autologous chondrocyte implantation versus mosaicplasty for osteochondral defects in the knee. *J Bone Joint Surg Br.* 2003;85(2):223–230.
42. Berg EE. Pediatric tibial eminence fractures: arthroscopic cannulated screw fixation. *Arthroscopy.* 1995;11(3):328–331.
43. Bergstrom R, Gillquist J, Lysholm J, et al. Arthroscopy of the knee in children. *J Pediatr Orthop.* 1984;4(5):542–545.
44. Berlet GC, Mascia A, Miniaci A. Treatment of unstable osteochondritis dissecans lesions of the knee using autogenous osteochondral grafts (mosaicplasty). *Arthroscopy.* 1999;15(3):312–316.
45. Betz RR, Magill JT, 3rd, Lonergan RP. The percutaneous lateral retinacular release. *Am J Sports Med.* 1987;15(5):477–482.
46. Beyzadeoglu T, Gokce A, Bekler H. Osteochondritis dissecans of the medial femoral condyle associated with malformation of the menisci. *Orthopedics.* 2008;31(5):504.
47. Bhaduri T, Glass A. Meniscectomy in children. *Injury.* 1972;3(3):176–178.
48. Bicos J, Fulkerson JP, Amis A. Current concepts review: the medial patellofemoral ligament. *Am J Sports Med.* 2007;35(3):484–492.
49. Birk GT, DeLee JC. Osteochondral injuries. Clinical findings. *Clin Sports Med.* 2001;20(2):279–286.
50. Bisson LJ, Wickiewicz T, Levinson M, et al. ACL reconstruction in children with open physes. *Orthopedics.* 1998;21(6):659–663.
51. Boden B, Pearsall AW, Garrett WE Jr, et al. Patellofemoral instability: evaluation and management. *J Am Acad Orthop Surg.* 1997;5(1):47–57.
52. Boden SD, Davis DO, Dina TS, et al. A prospective and blinded investigation of magnetic resonance imaging of the knee. Abnormal findings in asymptomatic subjects. *Clin Orthop Relat Res.* 1992;(282):177–185.
53. Boger D, Kingston S. MRI of the normal knee. *Am J Knee Surg.* 1988;1:99–103.
54. Bohndorf K. Imaging of acute injuries of the articular surfaces (chondral, osteochondral and subchondral fractures). *Skeletal Radiol.* 1999;28(10):545–560.
55. Bong MR, Romero A, Kubiak E, et al. Suture versus screw fixation of displaced tibial eminence fractures: a biomechanical comparison. *Arthroscopy.* 2005;21(10):1172–1176.
56. Bradley GW, Shives TC, Samuelson KM. Ligament injuries in the knees of children. *J Bone Joint Surg Am.* 1979;61(4):588–591.
57. Brief LP. Anterior cruciate ligament reconstruction without drill holes. *Arthroscopy.* 1991;7(4):350–357.
58. Brown GD, Ahmad CS. Combined medial patellofemoral ligament and medial patellotibial ligament reconstruction in skeletally immature patients. *J Knee Surg.* 2008;21(4):328–332.
59. Buckens CF, Saris DB. Reconstruction of the medial patellofemoral ligament for treatment of patellofemoral instability: a systematic review. *Am J Sports Med.* 2010;38(1):181–188.
60. Burstein DB, Viola A, Fulkerson JP. Entrapment of the medial meniscus in a fracture of the tibial eminence. *Arthroscopy.* 1988;4(1):47–50.
61. Busch MT, Fernandez MD, Aarons C. Partial tears of the anterior cruciate ligament in children and adolescents. *Clin Sports Med.* 2011;30(4):743–750.
62. Buseck MS, Noyes FR. Arthroscopic evaluation of meniscal repairs after anterior cruciate ligament reconstruction and immediate motion. *Am J Sports Med.* 1991;19(5):489–494.
63. Bushnell BD, Bitting SS, Crain JM, et al. Treatment of magnetic resonance imaging-documented isolated grade III lateral collateral ligament injuries in National Football League athletes. *Am J Sports Med.* 2010;38(1):86–91.
64. Camp CL, Heidenreich MJ, Dahm DL, et al. Individualizing the tibial tubercle-trochlear groove distance: patellar instability ratios that predict recurrent instability. *Am J Sports Med.* 2016;44(2):393–399.
65. Camp CL, Krych AJ, Dahm DL, et al. Medial patellofemoral ligament repair for recurrent patellar dislocation. *Am J Sports Med.* 2010;38(11):2248–2254.
66. Cannon WD Jr, Vittori JM. The incidence of healing in arthroscopic meniscal repairs in anterior cruciate ligament-reconstructed knees versus stable knees. *Am J Sports Med.* 1992;20(2):176–181.
67. Casalonga A, Bourelle S, Chalencon F, et al. Tibial intercondylar eminence fractures in children: the long-term perspective. *Orthop Traumatol Surg Res.* 2010;96(5):525–530.
68. Cash JD, Hughston JC. Treatment of acute patellar dislocation. *Am J Sports Med.* 1988;16(3):244–249.
69. Ceder LC, Larson RL. Z-plasty lateral retinacular release for the treatment of patellar compression syndrome. *Clin Orthop Relat Res.* 1979;(144):110–113.
70. Chalmers PN, Karas V, Sherman SL, et al. Return to high-level sport after meniscal allograft transplantation. *Arthroscopy.* 2013;29(3):539–544.
71. Chandler JT, Miller TK. Tibial eminence fracture with meniscal entrapment. *Arthroscopy.* 1995;11(4):499–502.
72. Chotel F, Bérard J, Raux S. Patellar instability in children and adolescents. *Orthop Traumatol Surg Res.* 2014;100(1 Suppl):S125–S137.
73. Chotel F, Knorr G, Simian E, et al. Knee osteochondral fractures in skeletally immature patients: French multicenter study. *Orthop Traumatol Surg Res.* 2011;97(8 Suppl):S154–S159.
74. Christiansen SE, Jacobsen BW, Lund B, et al. Reconstruction of the medial patellofemoral ligament with gracilis tendon autograft in transverse patellar drill holes. *Arthroscopy.* 2008;24(1):82–87.
75. Christiansen SE, Jakobsen BW, Lund B, et al. Isolated repair of the medial patellofemoral ligament in primary dislocation of the patella: a prospective randomized study. *Arthroscopy.* 2008;24(8):881–887.
76. Clanton TO, DeLee JC, Sanders B, et al. Knee ligament injuries in children. *J Bone Joint Surg Am.* 1979;61(8):1195–1201.
77. Clark CR, Ogden JA. Development of the menisci of the human knee joint. Morphological changes and their potential role in childhood meniscal injury. *J Bone Joint Surg Am.* 1983;65(4):538–547.
78. Conchie H, Clark D, Metcalfe A, et al. Adolescent knee pain and patellar dislocations are associated with patellofemoral osteoarthritis in adulthood: a case control study. *Knee.* 2016;23(4):708–711.
79. Cordasco FA, Mayer SW, Green DW. All-inside, all-epiphyseal anterior cruciate ligament reconstruction in skeletally immature athletes: return to sport, incidence of second surgery, and 2-year clinical outcomes. *Am J Sports Med.* 2017;45(4):856–863.
80. Crawford AH. Fractures about the knee in children. *Orthop Clin North Am.* 1976;7(3):639–656.
81. Dart CH Jr, Braitman HE. Popliteal artery injury following fracture or dislocation at the knee. Diagnosis and management. *Arch Surg.* 1977;112(8):969–973.
82. Dashefsky JH. Discoid lateral meniscus in three members of a family. Case reports. *J Bone Joint Surg Am.* 1971;53(6):1208–1210.
83. Davis DK, Fithian DC. Techniques of medial retinacular repair and reconstruction. *Clin Orthop Relat Res.* 2002;(402):38–52.
84. DeHaven KE. Diagnosis of acute knee injuries with hemarthrosis. *Am J Sports Med.* 1980;8(1):9–14.
85. DeHaven KE. Meniscus repair in the athlete. *Clin Orthop Relat Res.* 1985;(198):31–35.
86. DeHaven KE, Arnoczky SP. Meniscus repair: basic science, indications for repair, and open repair. *Instr Course Lect.* 1994;43:65–76.
87. DeHaven KE, Collins HR. Diagnosis of internal derangements of the knee. The role of arthroscopy. *J Bone Joint Surg Am.* 1975;57(6):802–810.
88. DeHaven KE, Lintner DM. Athletic injuries: comparison by age, sport, and gender. *Am J Sports Med.* 1986;14(3):218–224.
89. Deie M, Ochi M, Sumen Y, et al. Reconstruction of the medial patellofemoral ligament for the treatment of habitual or recurrent dislocation of the patella in children. *J Bone Joint Surg Br.* 2003;85(6):887–890.

90. Deie M, Ochi M, Sumen Y, et al. Relationship between osteochondritis dissecans of the lateral femoral condyle and lateral menisci types. *J Pediatr Orthop.* 2006;26(1):79–82.

91. Dejour H, Goutallier D, Furioli J. Unbalanced patella. X–Criticism of therapeutic methods and indications. *Rev Chir Orthop Reparatrice Appar Mot.* 1980;66(4):238–244.

92. Dejour H, Walch G, Nove-Josserand L, et al. Factors of patellar instability: an anatomic radiographic study. *Knee Surg Sports Traumatol Arthrosc.* 1994;2(1):19–26.

93. DeLee JC. Complete dislocation of the knee in a 9-year-old. *Contemp Orthop.* 1979;1:29–32.

94. DeLee JC, Curtis R. Anterior cruciate ligament insufficiency in children. *Clin Orthop Relat Res.* 1983;(172):112–118.

95. Desio SM, Burks RT, Bachus KN. Soft tissue restraints to lateral patellar translation in the human knee. *Am J Sports Med.* 1998;26(1):59–65.

96. Di Caprio F, Buda R, Ghermandi R, et al. Combined arthroscopic treatment of tibial plateau and intercondylar eminence avulsion fractures. *J Bone Joint Surg Am.* 2010;92(Suppl 2):161–169.

97. Dickens AJ, Morrell NT, Doering A, et al. Tibial tubercle-trochlear groove distance: defining normal in a pediatric population. *J Bone Joint Surg Am.* 2014;96(4):318–324.

98. Dickhaut SC, DeLee JC. The discoid lateral-meniscus syndrome. *J Bone Joint Surg Am.* 1982;64(7):1068–1073.

99. Dines JS, Fealy S, Potter HG, et al. Outcomes of osteochondral lesions of the knee repaired with a bioabsorbable device. *Arthroscopy.* 2008;24(1):62–68.

100. Drez D, Edwards TB, Williams CS. Results of medial patellofemoral ligament reconstruction in the treatment of patellar dislocation. *Arthroscopy.* 2001;17(3):298–306.

101. Düppe K, Gustavsson N, Edmonds EW. Developmental morphology in childhood patellar instability: age-dependent differences on magnetic resonance imaging. *J Pediatr Orthop.* 2016;36(8):870–876.

102. Eady JL, Cardenas CD, Sopa D. Avulsion of the femoral attachment of the anterior cruciate ligament in a seven-year-old child. A case report. *J Bone Joint Surg Am.* 1982;64:1376–1378.

103. Edwards PH, Grana WA. Anterior cruciate ligament reconstruction in the immature athlete: long-term results of intra-articular reconstruction. *Am J Knee Surg.* 2001;14(4):232–237.

104. Edwards TB, Greene CC, Baratta RV, et al. The effect of placing a tensioned graft across open growth plates. A gross and histologic analysis. *J Bone Joint Surg Am.* 2001;83-A(5):725–734.

105. Eggers AK, Becker C, Weimann A, et al. Biomechanical evaluation of different fixation methods for tibial eminence fractures. *Am J Sports Med.* 2007;35(3):404–410.

106. Eggli S, Wegmuller H, Kosina J, et al. Long-term results of arthroscopic meniscal repair. An analysis of isolated tears. *Am J Sports Med.* 1995;23(6):715–720.

107. Enea D, Busilacchi A, Cecconi S, et al. Late-diagnosed large osteochondral fracture of the lateral femoral condyle in an adolescent: a case report. *J Pediatr Orthop B.* 2013;22(4):344–349.

108. Engebretsen L, Steffen K, Bahr R, et al. The International Olympic Committee Consensus statement on age determination in high-level young athletes. *Br J Sports Med.* 2010;44(7):476–484.

109. Fabricant PD, Ladenhauf HN, Salvati EA, et al. Medial patellofemoral ligament (MPFL) reconstruction improves radiographic measures of patella alta in children. *Knee.* 2014;21(6):1180–1184.

110. Fabricant PD, Yen YM, Kramer DE, et al. Fixation of chondral-only shear fractures of the knee in pediatric and adolescent athletes. *J Pediatr Orthop.* 2017;37(2):156.

111. Falstie-Jensen S, Sondergard Petersen PE. Incarceration of the meniscus in fractures of the intercondylar eminence of the tibia in children. *Injury.* 1984;15(4):236–238.

112. Farmer JM, Martin DF, Boles CA, et al. Chondral and osteochondral injuries. Diagnosis and management. *Clin Sports Med.* 2001;20(2):299–320.

113. Farr J. Autologous chondrocyte implantation improves patellofemoral cartilage treatment outcomes. *Clin Orthop Relat Res.* 2007;463:187–194.

114. Felus J, Kowalczyk B. Age-related differences in medial patellofemoral ligament injury patterns in traumatic patellar dislocation: case series of 50 surgically treated children and adolescents. *Am J Sports Med.* 2012;40(10):2357–2364.

115. Feucht MJ, Brucker PU, Camathias C, et al. Meniscal injuries in children and adolescents undergoing surgical treatment for tibial eminence fractures. *Knee Surg Sports Traumatol Arthrosc.* 2017;25(2):445–453.

116. Flachsmann R, Broom ND, Hardy AE, et al. Why is the adolescent joint particularly susceptible to osteochondral shear fracture?. *Clin Orthop Relat Res.* 2000;381:212–221.

117. Flynn JM, Kocher MS, Ganley TJ. Osteochondritis dissecans of the knee. *J Pediatr Orthop.* 2004;24(4):434–443.

118. Fowler PJ. Meniscal lesions in the adolescent: the role of arthroscopy in the management of adolescent knee problems. In: Kennedy JC, ed. *The Injured Adolescent Knee.* Baltimore, MD: Williams & Wilkins; 1979:43–76.

119. Fowler PJ. The classification and early diagnosis of knee joint instability. *Clin Orthop Relat Res.* 1980;(147):15–21.

120. Fuchs R, Wheatley W, Uribe JW, et al. Intra-articular anterior cruciate ligament reconstruction using patellar tendon allograft in the skeletally immature patient. *Arthroscopy.* 2002;18(8):824–828.

121. Fulkerson JP, Becker GJ, Meaney JA, et al. Anteromedial tibial tubercle transfer without bone graft. *Am J Sports Med.* 1990;18(5):490–496.

122. Furlan D, Pogorelic Z, Biocic M, et al. Pediatric tibial eminence fractures: arthroscopic treatment using K-wire. *Scand J Surg.* 2010;99(1):38–44.

123. Fyfe IS, Jackson JP. Tibial intercondylar fractures in children: a review of the classification and the treatment of mal-union. *Injury.* 1981;13(2):165–169.

124. Garcia A, Neer CS, 2nd. Isolated fractures of the intercondylar eminence of the tibia. *Am J Surg.* 1958;95(4):593–598.

125. Gartland JJ, Benner JH. Traumatic dislocations in the lower extremity in children. *Orthop Clin North Am.* 1976;7(3):687–700.

126. Gaulrapp HM, Haus J. Intraarticular stabilization after anterior cruciate ligament tear in children and adolescents: results 6 years after surgery. *Knee Surg Sports Traumatol Arthrosc.* 2006;14(5):417–424.

127. Gebhard F, Ellermann A, Hoffmann F, et al. Multicenter-study of operative treatment of intraligamentous tears of the anterior cruciate ligament in children and adolescents: comparison of four different techniques. *Knee Surg Sports Traumatol Arthrosc.* 2006;14(9):797–803.

128. Gelb HJ, Glasgow SG, Sapega AA, et al. Magnetic resonance imaging of knee disorders. Clinical value and cost-effectiveness in a sports medicine practice. *Am J Sports Med.* 1996;24(1):99–103.

129. Gkiokas A, Morassi LG, Kohl S, et al. Bioabsorbable pins for treatment of osteochondral fractures of the knee after acute patella dislocation in children and young adolescents. *Adv Orthop.* 2012;2012:249687.

130. Gobbi A, Kon E, Berruto M, et al. Patellofemoral full-thickness chondral defects treated with second-generation autologous chondrocyte implantation: results at 5 years' follow-up. *Am J Sports Med.* 2009;37(6):1083–1092.

131. Good CR, Green DW, Griffith MH, et al. Arthroscopic treatment of symptomatic discoid meniscus in children: classification, technique, and results. *Arthroscopy.* 2007;23(2):157–163.

132. Goodfellow J, Hungerford DS, Zindel M. Patellofemoral joint mechanics and pathology. 1. Functional anatomy of the patellofemoral joint. *J Bone Joint Surg Br.* 1976;58:287–290.

133. Goodrich A, Ballard A. Posterior cruciate ligament avulsion associated with ipsilateral femur fracture in a 10-year-old child. *J Trauma.* 1988;28(9):1393–1396.

134. Goutallier D, Bernageau J, Lecudonnec B. The measurement of the tibial tuberosity. Patella groove distanced technique and results (author's transl). *Rev Chir Orthop Reparatrice Appar Mot.* 1978;64(5):423–428.

135. Graf BK, Lange RH, Fujisaki CK, et al. Anterior cruciate ligament tears in skeletally immature patients: meniscal pathology at presentation and after attempted conservative treatment. *Arthroscopy.* 1992;8(2):229–233.

136. Grannatt K, Heyworth BE, Ogunwole O, et al. Galeazzi semitendinosus tenodesis for patellofemoral instability in skeletally immature patients. *J Pediatr Orthop.* 2012;32(6):621–625.

137. Green NE, Allen BL. Vascular injuries associated with dislocation of the knee. *J Bone Joint Surg Am.* 1977;59(2):236–239.

138. Greis PE, Bardana DD, Holmstrom MC, et al. Meniscal injury: I. Basic science and evaluation. *J Am Acad Orthop Surg.* 2002;10(3):168–176.

139. Greis PE, Holmstrom MC, Bardana DD, et al. Meniscal injury: II. Management. *J Am Acad Orthop Surg.* 2002;10(3):177–187.

140. Greulich WW, Pyle SI, Todd TW. *Radiographic Atlas of Skeletal Development of the Hand and Wrist.* Stanford, CA: Stanford University Press; 1959.

141. Gronkvist H, Hirsch G, Johansson L. Fracture of the anterior tibial spine in children. *J Pediatr Orthop.* 1984;4(4):465–468.

142. Guzzanti V, Falciglia F, Gigante A, et al. The effect of intra-articular ACL reconstruction on the growth plates of rabbits. *J Bone Joint Surg Br.* 1994;76(6):960–963.

143. Guzzanti V, Falciglia F, Stanitski CL. Physeal-sparing intraarticular anterior cruciate ligament reconstruction in preadolescents. *Am J Sports Med.* 2003;31(6):949–953.

144. Guzzanti V, Falciglia F, Stanitski CL. Preoperative evaluation and anterior cruciate ligament reconstruction technique for skeletally immature patients in Tanner stages 2 and 3. *Am J Sports Med.* 2003;31(6):941–948.

145. Haas JP, Collins MS, Stuart MJ. The "sliver sign": a specific radiographic sign of acute lateral patellar dislocation. *Skeletal Radiol.* 2012;41(5):595–601.

146. Habata T, Uematsu K, Kasanami R, et al. Long-term clinical and radiographic follow-up of total resection for discoid lateral meniscus. *Arthroscopy.* 2006;22(12):1339–1343.

147. Hamada M, Shino K, Kawano K, et al. Usefulness of magnetic resonance imaging for detecting intrasubstance tear and/or degeneration of lateral discoid meniscus. *Arthroscopy.* 1994;10(6):645–653.

148. Hamberg P, Gillquist J, Lysholm J. Suture of new and old peripheral meniscus tears. *J Bone Joint Surg Am.* 1983;65(2):193–197.

149. Hashimoto Y, Yoshida G, Tomihara T, et al. Bilateral osteochondritis dissecans of the lateral femoral condyle following bilateral total removal of lateral discoid meniscus: a case report. *Arch Orthop Trauma Surg.* 2008;128(11):1265–1268.

150. Hayes JM, Masear VR. Avulsion fracture of the tibial eminence associated with severe medial ligamentous injury in an adolescent. A case report and literature review. *Am J Sports Med.* 1984;12(4):330–333.

151. Henderson IJ, Lavigne P. Periosteal autologous chondrocyte implantation for patellar chondral defect in patients with normal and abnormal patellar tracking. *Knee.* 2006;13(4):274–279.

152. Henderson N, Houghton GR. Osteochondral fractures of the knee in children. In: Houghton GR, Thompson GH, eds. *Problematic Musculoskeletal Injuries in Children.* London: Butterworths; 1983.

153. Henning CE, Lynch MA, Clark JR. Vascularity for healing of meniscus repairs. *Arthroscopy.* 1987;3(1):13–18.

154. Hinton RY, Rivera VR, Pautz MJ, et al. Ligamentous laxity of the knee during childhood and adolescence. *J Pediatr Orthop.* 2008;28(2):184–187.

155. Ho B, Edmonds EW, Chambers HG, et al. Risk factors for early ACL reconstruction failure in pediatric and adolescent patients: a review of 561 cases. *J Pediatr Orthop.* 2018;38:388–392.

156. Houle JB, Letts M, Yang J. Effects of a tensioned tendon graft in a bone tunnel across the rabbit physis. *Clin Orthop Relat Res.* 2001;391:275–281.

157. Hua GJ, Liu YP, Xu PR, et al. Arthroscopic minimally invasive treatment of tibial intercondylar eminence fractures in children. *Zhongguo Gu Shang.* 2011;24(9):723–725.

158. Huang TW, Hsu KY, Cheng CY, et al. Arthroscopic suture fixation of tibial eminence avulsion fractures. *Arthroscopy.* 2008;24(11):1232–1238.

159. Huckell JR. Is meniscectomy a benign procedure?. A long-term follow-up study. *Can J Surg.* 1965;8:254–260.

160. Hughston JC, Andrews JR, Cross MJ, et al. Classification of knee ligament instabilities. Part I. The medial compartment and cruciate ligaments. *J Bone Joint Surg Am.* 1976;58(2):159–172.

161. Hughston JC, Bowden JA, Andrews JR, et al. Acute tears of the posterior cruciate ligament. Results of operative treatment. *J Bone Joint Surg Am.* 1980;62(3):438–450.

162. Hughston JC, Deese M. Medial subluxation of the patella as a complication of lateral retinacular release. *Am J Sports Med.* 1988;16(4):383–388.

163. Hungerford DS, Barry M. Biomechanics of the patellofemoral joint. *Clin Orthop Relat Res.* 1979;(144):9–15.

164. Ikeuchi H. Arthroscopic treatment of the discoid lateral meniscus. Technique and long-term results. *Clin Orthop Relat Res.* 1982;(167):19–28.

165. Indelicato PA, Hermansdorfer J, Huegel M. Nonoperative management of complete tears of the medial collateral ligament of the knee in intercollegiate football players. *Clin Orthop Relat Res.* 1990;(256):174–177.

166. Insall J, Goldberg V, Salvati E. Recurrent dislocation and the high-riding patella. *Clin Orthop Relat Res.* 1972;88:67–69.

167. Insall J, Salvati E. Patella position in the normal knee joint. *Radiology.* 1971;101(1):101–104.

168. Ishibashi Y, Tsuda E, Sasaki T, et al. Magnetic resonance imaging AIDS in detecting concomitant injuries in patients with tibial spine fractures. *Clin Orthop Relat Res.* 2005;(434):207–212.

169. Jackson DW, Jennings LD, Maywood RM, et al. Magnetic resonance imaging of the knee. *Am J Sports Med.* 1988;16:29–38.

170. Jackson DW, Schaefer RK. Cyclops syndrome: loss of extension following intra-articular anterior cruciate ligament reconstruction. *Arthroscopy.* 1990;6(3):171–178.

171. Janarv PM, Nystrom A, Werner S, et al. Anterior cruciate ligament injuries in skeletally immature patients. *J Pediatr Orthop.* 1996;16(5):673–677.

172. Janarv PM, Westblad P, Johansson C, et al. Long-term follow-up of anterior tibial spine fractures in children. *J Pediatr Orthop.* 1995;15(1):63–68.

173. Janarv PM, Wikstrom B, Hirsch G. The influence of transphyseal drilling and tendon grafting on bone growth: an experimental study in the rabbit. *J Pediatr Orthop.* 1998;18(2):149–154.

174. Johannsen AM, Civitarese DM, Padalecki JR, et al. Qualitative and quantitative anatomic analysis of the posterior root attachments of the medial and lateral menisci. *Am J Sports Med.* 2012;40(10):2342–2347.

175. Johnson EW Jr, McLeod TL. Osteochondral fragments of the distal end of the femur fixed with bone pegs: report of two cases. *J Bone Joint Surg Am.* 1977;59(5):677–679.

176. Johnson MJ, Lucas GL, Dusek JK, et al. Isolated arthroscopic meniscal repair: a long-term outcome study (more than 10 years). *Am J Sports Med.* 1999;27(1):44–49.

177. Johnson RG, Simmons EH. Discoid medical meniscus. *Clin Orthop Relat Res.* 1982;(167):176–179.

178. Jordan MR. Lateral meniscal variants: evaluation and treatment. *J Am Acad Orthop Surg.* 1996;4(4):191–200.

179. Joseph KN, Fogrund H. Traumatic rupture of the medial ligament of the knee in a 4-year-old boy. *J Bone Joint Surg Am.* 1978;60:402–403.

180. Juhl M, Boe S. Arthroscopy in children, with special emphasis on meniscal lesions. *Injury.* 1986;17(3):171–173.

181. Jung YB, Yum JK, Koo BH. A new method for arthroscopic treatment of tibial eminence fractures with eyed Steinmann pins. *Arthroscopy.* 1999;15(6):672–675.

182. Kaeding CC, Flanigan D, Donaldson C. Surgical techniques and outcomes after anterior cruciate ligament reconstruction in preadolescent patients. *Arthroscopy.* 2010;26(11):1530–1538.

183. Kaplan EB. Discoid lateral meniscus of the knee joint; nature, mechanism, and operative treatment. *J Bone Joint Surg Am.* 1957;39-A(1):77–87.

184. Kennedy A, Coughlin DG, Metzger MF, et al. Biomechanical evaluation of pediatric anterior cruciate ligament reconstruction techniques. *Am J Sports Med.* 2011;39(5):964–971.

185. Kennedy JC. *The Injured Adolescent Knee.* Baltimore, MD: Williams & Wilkins; 1979.

186. Kennedy JC. Complete dislocation of the knee joint. *J Bone Joint Surg Am.* 1963;45:889–904.

187. Kepler CK, Bogner EA, Hammoud S, et al. Zone of injury of the medial patellofemoral ligament after acute patellar dislocation in children and adolescents. *Am J Sports Med.* 2011;39(7):1444–1449.

188. Keys GW, Walters J. Nonunion of intercondylar eminence fracture of the tibia. *J Trauma.* 1988;28(6):870–871.

189. Kieser DC, Gwynne-Jones D, Dreyer S. Displaced tibial intercondylar eminence fractures. *J Orthop Surg (Hong Kong).* 2011;19(3):292–296.

190. Kim SH, Ha KI, Ahn JH, et al. Anterior cruciate ligament reconstruction in the young patient without violation of the epiphyseal plate. *Arthroscopy.* 1999;15(7):792–795.

191. Kim YG, Ihn JC, Park SK, et al. An arthroscopic analysis of lateral meniscal variants and a comparison with MRI findings. *Knee Surg Sports Traumatol Arthrosc.* 2006;14(1):20–26.

192. King AG. Meniscal lesions in children and adolescents: a review of the pathology and clinical presentation. *Injury.* 1983;15(2):105–108.

193. King SJ, Carty HM, Brady O. Magnetic resonance imaging of knee injuries in children. *Pediatr Radiol.* 1996;26(4):287–290.

194. Klingele KE, Kocher MS, Hresko MT, et al. Discoid lateral meniscus: prevalence of peripheral rim instability. *J Pediatr Orthop.* 2004;24(1):79–82.

195. Kocher M, Micheli LJ. The pediatric knee: evaluation and treatment. In: Insall JN, Scott WN, eds. *Surgery of the Knee.* 3rd ed. New York: Churchill-Livingstone; 2001:1356–1397.

196. Kocher MS, DiCanzio J, Zurakowski D, et al. Diagnostic performance of clinical examination and selective magnetic resonance imaging in the evaluation of intraarticular knee disorders in children and adolescents. *Am J Sports Med.* 2001;29(3):292–296.

197. Kocher MS, Foreman ES, Micheli LJ. Laxity and functional outcome after arthroscopic reduction and internal fixation of displaced tibial spine fractures in children. *Arthroscopy.* 2003;19(10):1085–1090.

198. Kocher MS, Garg S, Micheli LJ. Physeal sparing reconstruction of the anterior cruciate ligament in skeletally immature prepubescent children and adolescents. *J Bone Joint Surg Am.* 2005;87(11):2371–2379.

199. Kocher MS, Garg S, Micheli LJ. Physeal sparing reconstruction of the anterior cruciate ligament in skeletally immature prepubescent children and adolescents. Surgical technique. *J Bone Joint Surg Am.* 2006;88(suppl 1 pt 2):283–293.

200. Kocher MS, Klingele K, Rassman SO. Meniscal disorders: normal, discoid, and cysts. *Orthop Clin North Am.* 2003;34(3):329–340.

201. Kocher MS, Mandiga R, Klingele K, et al. Anterior cruciate ligament injury versus tibial spine fracture in the skeletally immature knee: a comparison of skeletal maturation and notch width index. *J Pediatr Orthop.* 2004;24(2):185–188.

202. Kocher MS, Micheli LJ, Gerbino P, et al. Tibial eminence fractures in children: prevalence of meniscal entrapment. *Am J Sports Med.* 2003;31(3):404–407.

203. Kocher MS, Micheli LJ, Yaniv M, et al. Functional and radiographic outcome of juvenile osteochondritis dissecans of the knee treated with transarticular arthroscopic drilling. *Am J Sports Med.* 2001;29(5):562–566.

204. Kocher MS, Micheli LJ, Zurakowski D, et al. Partial tears of the anterior cruciate ligament in children and adolescents. *Am J Sports Med.* 2002;30(5):697–703.

205. Kocher MS, Saxon HS, Hovis WD, et al. Management and complications of anterior cruciate ligament injuries in skeletally immature patients: survey of the Herodicus Society and The ACL Study Group. *J Pediatr Orthop.* 2002;22(4):452–457.

206. Kocher MS, Shore B, Nasreddine AY, et al. Treatment of posterior cruciate ligament injuries in pediatric and adolescent patients. *J Pediatr Orthop.* 2012;32(6):553–560.

207. Kocher MS, Smith JT, Iversen MD, et al. Reliability, validity, and responsiveness of a modified International Knee Documentation Committee Subjective Knee Form (Pedi-IKDC) in children with knee disorders. *Am J Sports Med.* 2011;39(5):933–939.

208. Kocher MS, Smith JT, Zoric BJ, et al. Transphyseal anterior cruciate ligament reconstruction in skeletally immature pubescent adolescents. *J Bone Joint Surg Am.* 2007;89(12):2632–2639.

209. Kocher MS, Tepolt FA, Vavken P. Meniscus transplantation in skeletally immature patients. *J Pediatr Orthop B.* 2016;25(4):343–348.

210. Koman JD, Sanders JO. Valgus deformity after reconstruction of the anterior cruciate ligament in a skeletally immature patient. A case report. *J Bone Joint Surg Am.* 1999;81(5):711–715.

211. Kramer DE, Micheli LJ. Meniscal tears and discoid meniscus in children: diagnosis and treatment. *J Am Acad Orthop Surg.* 2009;17(11):698–707.

212. Kramer DE, Pace JL. Acute traumatic and sports-related osteochondral injury of the pediatric knee. *Orthop Clin North Am.* 2012;43(2):227–236, vi.

213. Kramer DE, Yen YM, Simoni MK, et al. Surgical management of osteochondritis dissecans lesions of the patella and trochlea in the pediatric and adolescent population. *Am J Sports Med.* 2015;43(3):654–662.

214. Kraus T, Heidari N, Svehlik M, et al. Outcome of repaired unstable meniscal tears in children and adolescents. *Acta Orthop.* 2012;83(3):261–266.

215. Krause WR, Pope MH, Johnson RJ, et al. Mechanical changes in the knee after meniscectomy. *J Bone Joint Surg Am.* 1976;58(5):599–604.

216. Krych AJ, Pitts RT, Dajani KA, et al. Surgical repair of meniscal tears with concomitant anterior cruciate ligament reconstruction in patients 18 years and younger. *Am J Sports Med.* 2010;38(5):976–982.

217. Lafrance RM, Giordano B, Goldblatt J, et al. Pediatric tibial eminence fractures: evaluation and management. *J Am Acad Orthop Surg.* 2010;18(7):395–405.

218. LaPrade RF, Burnett QM, 2nd, Veenstra MA, et al. The prevalence of abnormal magnetic resonance imaging findings in asymptomatic knees. With correlation of magnetic resonance imaging to arthroscopic findings in symptomatic knees. *Am J Sports Med.* 1994;22(6):739–745.

219. LaPrade RF, Matheny LM, Moulton SG, et al. Posterior meniscal root repairs: outcomes of an anatomic transtibial pull-out technique. *Am J Sports Med.* 2017;45(4):884–891.

220. Larsen E, Lauridsen F. Conservative treatment of patellar dislocations. Influence of evident factors on the tendency to redislocation and the therapeutic result. *Clin Orthop Relat Res.* 1982;(171):131–136.

221. Larson RL. The unstable patella in the adolescent and preadolescent. *Orthop Rev.* 1985;14:156–162.

222. Laurin CA, Levesque HP, Dussault R, et al. The abnormal lateral patellofemoral angle: a diagnostic roentgenographic sign of recurrent patellar subluxation. *J Bone Joint Surg Am.* 1978;60(1):55–60.

223. Lawrence JT, Argawal N, Ganley TJ. Degeneration of the knee joint in skeletally immature patients with a diagnosis of an anterior cruciate ligament tear: is there harm in delay of treatment?. *Am J Sports Med.* 2011;39(12):2582–2587.

224. Lawrence JT, Bowers AL, Belding J, et al. All-epiphyseal anterior cruciate ligament reconstruction in skeletally immature patients. *Clin Orthop Relat Res.* 2010;468(7):1971–1977.

225. Lee BJ, Christino MA, Daniels AH, et al. Adolescent patellar osteochondral fracture following patellar dislocation. *Knee Surg Sports Traumatol Arthrosc.* 2013; 21(8):1856–1861.

226. Lee BS, Bin SI, Kim JM. Articular cartilage degenerates after subtotal/total lateral meniscectomy but radiographic arthrosis progression is reduced after meniscal transplantation. *Am J Sports Med.* 2016;44(1):159–165.

227. Lee DH, Kim TH, Kim JM, et al. Results of subtotal/total or partial meniscectomy for discoid lateral meniscus in children. *Arthroscopy.* 2009;25(5):496–503.

228. Lee YS, Teo SH, Ahn JH, et al. Systematic review of the long-term surgical outcomes of discoid lateral meniscus. *Arthroscopy.* 2017;33:1884–1895.

229. Levy IM, Torzilli PA, Warren RF. The effect of medial meniscectomy on anterior-posterior motion of the knee. *J Bone Joint Surg AM.* 1982;64:883–888.

230. Lewallen L, McIntosh A, Dahm D. First-time patellofemoral dislocation: risk factors for recurrent instability. *J Knee Surg.* 2015;28(4):303–309.

231. Lewallen LW, McIntosh AL, Dahm DL. Predictors of recurrent instability after acute patellofemoral dislocation in pediatric and adolescent patients. *Am J Sports Med.* 2013;41(3):575–581.

232. Lewis PL, Foster BK. Herbert screw fixation of osteochondral fractures about the knee. *Aust N Z J Surg.* 1990;60(7):511–513.

233. Liao W, Li Z, Zhang H, et al. Arthroscopic fixation of tibial eminence fractures: a clinical comparative study of nonabsorbable sutures versus absorbable suture anchors. *Arthroscopy.* 2016;32(8):1639–1650.

234. Liddle AD, Imbuldeniya AM, Hunt DM. Transphyseal reconstruction of the anterior cruciate ligament in prepubescent children. *J Bone Joint Surg Br.* 2008;90(10):1317–1322.

235. Lind M, Jakobsen BW, Lund B, et al. Reconstruction of the medial patellofemoral ligament for treatment of patellar instability. *Acta Orthop.* 2008;79(3):354–360.

236. Lipscomb AB, Anderson AF. Tears of the anterior cruciate ligament in adolescents. *J Bone Joint Surg Am.* 1986;68(1):19–28.

237. Lo IK, Kirkley A, Fowler PJ, et al. The outcome of operatively treated anterior cruciate ligament disruptions in the skeletally immature child. *Arthroscopy.* 1997;13(5):627–634.

238. Lombardo SJ. Avulsion of a fibrous union of the intercondylar eminence of the tibia. A case report. *J Bone Joint Surg Am.* 1994;76(10):1565–1568.

239. Louis ML, Guillaume JM, Launay F, et al. Surgical management of type II tibial intercondylar eminence fractures in children. *J Pediatr Orthop B.* 2008;17(5):231–235.

240. Lowe J, Chaimsky G, Freedman A, et al. The anatomy of tibial eminence fractures: arthroscopic observations following failed closed reduction. *J Bone Joint Surg Am.* 2002;84-A(11):1933–1938.

241. Luhmann SJ. Acute traumatic knee effusions in children and adolescents. *J Pediatr Orthop.* 2003;23(2):199–202.

242. Luhmann SJ, O'Donnell JC, Fuhrhop S. Outcomes after patellar realignment surgery for recurrent patellar instability dislocations: a minimum 3-year follow-up study of children and adolescents. *J Pediatr Orthop.* 2011;31(1):65–71.

243. Ma LF, Wang CH, Chen BC, et al. Medial patellar retinaculum plasty versus medial capsule reefing for patellar dislocation in children and adolescents. *Arch Orthop Trauma Surg.* 2012;132(12):1773–1780.

244. MacIntosh DL, Darby DT. Lateral substitution reconstruction in proceedings and reports of universities, colleges, councils, and associations. *J Bone Joint Surg Br.* 1976;58:142.

245. Mahar AT, Duncan D, Oka R, et al. Biomechanical comparison of four different fixation techniques for pediatric tibial eminence avulsion fractures. *J Pediatr Orthop.* 2008;28(2):159–162.

246. Mandelbaum BR, Browne JE, Fu F, et al. Articular cartilage lesions of the knee. *Am J Sports Med.* 1998;26(6):853–861.

247. Mann MA, Desy NM, Martineau PA. A new procedure for tibial spine avulsion fracture fixation. *Knee Surg Sports Traumatol Arthrosc.* 2012;20(12):2395–2398.

248. Månsson O, Sernert N, Rostgard-Christensen L, et al. Long-term clinical and radiographic results after delayed anterior cruciate ligament reconstruction in adolescents. *Am J Sports Med.* 2015;43(1):138–145.

249. Manzione M, Pizzutillo PD, Peoples AB, et al. Meniscectomy in children: a long-term follow-up study. *Am J Sports Med.* 1983;11(3):111–115.

250. Maquet P. Advancement of the tibial tuberosity. *Clin Orthop Relat Res.* 1976;(115):225–230.

251. Marsh JS, Daigneault JP, Sethi P, et al. Treatment of recurrent patellar instability with a modification of the Roux-Goldthwait Technique. *J Pediatr Orthop.* 2006;26(4):461–465.

252. Marshall SC. Combined arthroscopic/open repair of meniscal injuries. *Contemp Orthop.* 1987;14(6):15–24.

253. Marx RG, Jones EC, Allen AA, et al. Reliability, validity, and responsiveness of four knee outcome scales for athletic patients. *J Bone Joint Surg Am.* 2001;83-A(10):1459–1469.

254. Matava MJ, Brown CD. Osteochondritis dissecans of the patella: arthroscopic fixation with bioabsorbable pins. *Arthroscopy.* 1997;13(1):124–128.

255. Matelic TM, Aronsson DD, Boyd DW Jr, et al. Acute hemarthrosis of the knee in children. *Am J Sports Med.* 1995;23(6):668–671.

256. Mayer C, Magnussen RA, Servien E, et al. Patellar tendon tenodesis in association with tibial tubercle distalization for the treatment of episodic patellar dislocation with patella alta. *Am J Sports Med.* 2012;40(2):346–351.

257. Mayer PJ, Micheli LJ. Avulsion of the femoral attachment of the posterior cruciate ligament in an eleven-year-old boy. Case report. *J Bone Joint Surg Am.* 1979;61:431–432.

258. McCarroll JR, Shelbourne KD, Porter DA, et al. Patellar tendon graft reconstruction for midsubstance anterior cruciate ligament rupture in junior high school athletes. An algorithm for management. *Am J Sports Med.* 1994;22(4):478–484.

259. McLennan JG. The role of arthroscopic surgery in the treatment of fractures of the intercondylar eminence of the tibia. *J Bone Joint Surg Br.* 1982;64(4):477–480.

260. Medlar RC, Mandiberg JJ, Lyne ED. Meniscectomies in children. Report of long-term results (mean, 8.3 years) of 26 children. *Am J Sports Med.* 1980;8(2):87–92.

261. Melegari TM, Parks BG, Matthews LS. Patellofemoral contact area and pressure after medial patellofemoral ligament reconstruction. *Am J Sports Med.* 2008;36(4):747–752.

262. Meller R, Kendoff D, Hankemeier S, et al. Hindlimb growth after a transphyseal reconstruction of the anterior cruciate ligament: a study in skeletally immature sheep with wide-open physes. *Am J Sports Med.* 2008;36(12):2437–2443.

263. Merchant AC, Mercer RL, Jacobsen RH, et al. Roentgenographic analysis of patellofemoral congruence. *J Bone Joint Surg Am.* 1974;56(7):1391–1396.

264. Meyers MH. Isolated avulsion of the tibial attachment of the posterior cruciate ligament of the knee. *J Bone Joint Surg Am.* 1975;57(5):669–672.

265. Meyers MH, McKeever FM. Fracture of the intercondylar eminence of the tibia. *J Bone Joint Surg Am.* 1959;41-A(2):209–220; discussion 220–222.

266. Meyers MH, McKeever FM. Fracture of the intercondylar eminence of the tibia. *J Bone Joint Surg Am.* 1970;52:1677–1684.

267. Micheli LJ, Rask B, Gerberg L. Anterior cruciate ligament reconstruction in patients who are prepubescent. *Clin Orthop Relat Res.* 1999;(364):40–47.

268. Millett PJ, Willis AA, Warren RF. Associated injuries in pediatric and adolescent anterior cruciate ligament tears: does a delay in treatment increase the risk of meniscal tear? *Arthroscopy.* 2002;18(9):955–959.

269. Mills WJ, Barei DP, McNair P. The value of the ankle-brachial index for diagnosing arterial injury after knee dislocation: a prospective study. *J Trauma.* 2004;56(6):1261–1265.

270. Mintzer CM, Richmond JC, Taylor J. Meniscal repair in the young athlete. *Am J Sports Med.* 1998;26(5):630–633.

271. Mitchell J, Magnussen RA, Collins CL, et al. Epidemiology of patellofemoral instability injuries among high school athletes in the United States. *Am J Sports Med.* 2015;43(7):1676–1682.

272. Mitchell JJ, Mayo MH, Axibal DP, et al. Delayed anterior cruciate ligament reconstruction in young patients with previous anterior tibial spine fractures. *Am J Sports Med.* 2016;44(8):2047–2056.

273. Mizuta H, Kubota K, Shiraishi M, et al. The conservative treatment of complete tears of the anterior cruciate ligament in skeletally immature patients. *J Bone Joint Surg Br.* 1995;77(6):890–894.

274. Molander ML, Wallin G, Wikstad I. Fracture of the intercondylar eminence of the tibia: a review of 35 patients. *J Bone Joint Surg Br.* 1981;63-B(1):89–91.

275. Momaya AM, Read C, Steirer M, et al. Outcomes after arthroscopic fixation of tibial eminence fractures with bioabsorbable nails in skeletally immature patients. *J Pediatr Orthop B.* 2018;27:8–12.

276. Morrissy RT, Eubanks RG, Park JP, et al. Arthroscopy of the knee in children. *Clin Orthop Relat Res.* 1982;(162):103–107.

277. Moulton SG, Bhatia S, Civitarese DM, et al. Surgical techniques and outcomes of repairing meniscal radial tears: a systematic review. *Arthroscopy.* 2016;32(9):1919–1925.

278. Mulhall KJ, Dowdall J, Grannell M, et al. Tibial spine fractures: an analysis of outcome in surgically treated type III injuries. *Injury.* 1999;30(4):289–292.

279. Murphy RF, Heyworth B, Kramer D, et al. Symptomatic venous thromboembolism after adolescent knee arthroscopy. *J Pediatr Orthop.* 2016. [Epub ahead of print] PMID: 27861210

280. Mylle J, Reynders P, Broos P. Transepiphysial fixation of anterior cruciate avulsion in a child. Report of a complication and review of the literature. *Arch Orthop Trauma Surg.* 1993;112(2):101–103.

281. Nakamura N, Horibe S, Iwahashi T, et al. Healing of a chondral fragment of the knee in an adolescent after internal fixation. A case report. *J Bone Joint Surg Am.* 2004;86-A(12):2741–2746.

282. Nathan PA, Cole SC. Discoid meniscus. A clinical and pathologic study. *Clin Orthop Relat Res.* 1969;64:107–113.

283. Nebel G, Lingg G. The Wiberg Forms of Patellae—are they disposing to early arthrosis? (author's transl). *Radiologe.* 1981;21(2):101–103.

284. Nelitz M, Dreyhaupt J, Reichel H, et al. Anatomic reconstruction of the medial patellofemoral ligament in children and adolescents with open growth plates: surgical technique and clinical outcome. *Am J Sports Med.* 2013;41(1):58–63.

285. Nelitz M, Reichel H, Dornacher D, et al. Anatomical reconstruction of the medial patellofemoral ligament in children with open growth-plates. *Arch Orthop Trauma Surg.* 2012;132(11):1647–1651.

286. Nelitz M, Theile M, Dornacher D, et al. Analysis of failed surgery for patellar instability in children with open growth plates. *Knee Surg Sports Traumatol Arthrosc.* 2012;20(5):822–828.

287. Neuschwander DC, Drez D Jr, Finney TP. Lateral meniscal variant with absence of the posterior coronary ligament. *J Bone Joint Surg Am.* 1992;74(8):1186–1190.

288. Nietosvaara Y, Aalto K, Kallio PE. Acute patellar dislocation in children: incidence and associated osteochondral fractures. *J Pediatr Orthop.* 1994;14(4):513–515.

289. Nikku R, Nietosvaara Y, Aalto K, et al. Operative treatment of primary patellar dislocation does not improve medium-term outcome: a 7-year follow-up report and risk analysis of 127 randomized patients. *Acta Orthop.* 2005;76(5):699–704.

290. Nikku R, Nietosvaara Y, Kallio PE, et al. Operative versus closed treatment of primary dislocation of the patella. Similar 2-year results in 125 randomized patients. *Acta Orthop Scand.* 1997;68(5):419–423.

291. Nomura E, Horiuchi Y, Inoue M. Correlation of MR imaging findings and open exploration of medial patellofemoral ligament injuries in acute patellar dislocations. *Knee.* 2002;9(2):139–143.

292. Nomura E, Inoue M, Kobayashi S. Long-term follow-up and knee osteoarthritis change after medial patellofemoral ligament reconstruction for recurrent patellar dislocation. *Am J Sports Med.* 2007;35(11):1851–1858.

293. Nomura E, Inoue M, Kurimura M. Chondral and osteochondral injuries associated with acute patellar dislocation. *Arthroscopy.* 2003;19(7):717–721.

294. Noyes FR, Barber-Westin SD. Arthroscopic repair of meniscal tears extending into the avascular zone in patients younger than twenty years of age. *Am J Sports Med.* 2002;30(4):589–600.

295. Noyes FR, DeLucas JL, Torvik PJ. Biomechanics of anterior cruciate ligament failure: An analysis of strain-rate sensitivity and mechanisms of failure in primates. *J Bone Joint Surg Am.* 1974;56(2):236–253.

296. Nwachukwu BU, McFeely ED, Nasreddine A, et al. Arthrofibrosis after anterior cruciate ligament reconstruction in children and adolescents. *J Pediatr Orthop.* 2011;31(8):811–817.

297. Ogden J. *Skeletal Injury in the Child.* 2nd ed. Philadelphia, PA: Lea & Febiger; 1989.

298. Okazaki K, Miura H, Matsuda S, et al. Arthroscopic resection of the discoid lateral meniscus: long-term follow-up for 16 years. *Arthroscopy.* 2006;22(9):967–971.

299. Oliva F, Ronga M, Longo UG, et al. The 3-in-1 procedure for recurrent dislocation of the patella in skeletally immature children and adolescents. *Am J Sports Med.* 2009;37(9):1814–1820.

300. Pace JL, Nasreddine AY, Simoni M, et al. Dynamic splinting in children and adolescents with stiffness after knee surgery. *J Pediatr Orthop.* 2018;38:38–43.

301. Paletta JG Jr. Special considerations. Anterior cruciate ligament reconstruction in the skeletally immature. *Orthop Clin North Am.* 2003;34(1):65–77.

302. Palmu S, Kallio PE, Donell ST, et al. Acute patellar dislocation in children and adolescents: a randomized clinical trial. *J Bone Joint Surg Am.* 2008;90(3):463–470.

303. Parikh SN, Lykissas MG. Classification of lateral patellar instability in children and adolescents. *Orthop Clin North Am.* 2016;47(1):145–152.

304. Parikh SN, Nathan ST, Wall EJ, et al. Complications of medial patellofemoral ligament reconstruction in young patients. *Am J Sports Med.* 2013;41(5):1030–1038.

305. Parker AW, Drez D Jr, Cooper JL. Anterior cruciate ligament injuries in patients with open physes. *Am J Sports Med.* 1994;22(1):44–47.

306. Patel D, Dimakopoulos P, Denoncourt P. Bucket handle tear of a discoid medial meniscus. Arthroscopic diagnosis—partial excision. A case report. *Orthopedics.* 1986;9(4):607–608.

307. Patel NM, Cody SR, Ganley TJ. Symptomatic bilateral discoid menisci in children: a comparison with unilaterally symptomatic patients. *J Pediatr Orthop.* 2012;32(1):5–8.

308. Patel NM, Park MJ, Sampson NR, et al. Tibial eminence fractures in children: earlier posttreatment mobilization results in improved outcomes. *J Pediatr Orthop.* 2012;32(2):139–144.

309. Pellacci F, Mignani G, Valdiserri L. Fractures of the intercondylar eminence of the tibia in children. *Ital J Orthop Traumatol.* 1986;12(4):441–446.

310. Pellacci F, Montanari G, Prosperi P, et al. Lateral discoid meniscus: treatment and results. *Arthroscopy.* 1992;8(4):526–530.

311. Peterson L, Minas T, Brittberg M, et al. Treatment of osteochondritis dissecans of the knee with autologous chondrocyte transplantation: results at two to ten years. *J Bone Joint Surg Am.* 2003;85-A(suppl 2):17–24.

312. Pfirrmann CW, Zanetti M, Romero J, et al. Femoral trochlear dysplasia: MR findings. *Radiology.* 2000;216:858–864.

313. Polly DW Jr, Callaghan JJ, Sikes RA, et al. The accuracy of selective magnetic resonance imaging compared with the findings of arthroscopy of the knee. *J Bone Joint Surg Am.* 1988;70(2):192–198.

314. Pressman AE, Letts RM, Jarvis JG. Anterior cruciate ligament tears in children: an analysis of operative versus nonoperative treatment. *J Pediatr Orthop.* 1997;17(4):505–511.

315. Pyle SI, Hoerr NL. *A Radiographic Standard of Reference the Growing Knee.* Springfield: Charles Thomas; 1969.

316. Quinlan JF, Farrelly C, Kelly G, et al. Co-existent medial collateral ligament injury seen following transient patellar dislocation: observations at magnetic resonance imaging. *Br J Sports Med.* 2010;44(6):411–414.

317. Raber DA, Friederich NF, Hefti F. Discoid lateral meniscus in children. Long-term follow-up after total meniscectomy. *J Bone Joint Surg Am.* 1998;80(11):1579–1586.

318. Rang M. *Children's Fractures.* 2nd ed. Philadelphia, PA: Lippincott; 1983.

319. Rangger C, Klestil T, Gloetzer W, et al. Osteoarthritis after arthroscopic partial meniscectomy. *Am J Sports Med.* 1995;23(2):240–244.

320. Roach CJ, Haley CA, Cameron KL, et al. The epidemiology of medial collateral ligament sprains in young athletes. *Am J Sports Med.* 2014;42(5):1103–1109.

321. Roberts JM. Fractures of the condyles of the tibia. An anatomical and clinical end-result study of one hundred cases. *J Bone Joint Surg Am.* 1968;50(8):1505–1521.

322. Meyers MH, McKeever FM. Fractures of the intercondylar eminence of the tibia. *J Bone Joint Surg Am.* 1970;52:1677–1684.

323. Robinson SC, Driscoll SE. Simultaneous osteochondral avulsion of the femoral and tibial insertions of the anterior cruciate ligament. Report of a case in a thirteen-year-old boy. *J Bone Joint Surg Am.* 1981;63(8):1342–1343.

324. Ronga M, Oliva F, Giuseppe Longo U, et al. Isolated medial patellofemoral ligament reconstruction for recurrent patellar dislocation. *Am J Sports Med.* 2009;37(9):1735–1742.

325. Rorabeck CH, Bobechko WP. Acute dislocation of the patella with osteochondral fracture: a review of eighteen cases. *J Bone Joint Surg Br.* 1976;58(2):237–240.

326. Rosenberg NJ. Osteochondral fractures of the lateral femoral condyle. *J Bone Joint Surg Am.* 1964;46:1013–1026.

327. Rosenberg TD, Paulos LE, Parker RD, et al. Discoid lateral meniscus: case report of arthroscopic attachment of a symptomatic Wrisberg-ligament type. *Arthroscopy.* 1987;3(4):277–282.

328. Ross AC, Chesterman PJ. Isolated avulsion of the tibial attachment of the posterior cruciate ligament in childhood. *J Bone Joint Surg Br.* 1986;68(5):747.

329. Rothermich MA, Nepple JJ, Raup VT, et al. A Comparative analysis of international knee documentation committee scores for common pediatric and adolescent knee injuries. *J Pediatr Orthop.* 2016;36(3):274–277.

330. Rubman MH, Noyes FR, Barber-Westin SD. Arthroscopic repair of meniscal tears that extend into the avascular zone. A review of 198 single and complex tears. *Am J Sports Med.* 1998;26(1):87–95.

331. Saddawi ND, Hoffman BK. Tear of the attachment of a normal medial meniscus of the knee in a four-year-old-child. A case report. *J Bone Joint Surg Am.* 1970;52(4):809–811.

332. Samora WP, 3rd, Palmer R, Klingele KE. Meniscal pathology associated with acute anterior cruciate ligament tears in patients with open physes. *J Pediatr Orthop.* 2011;31(3):272–276.

333. Sampson NR, Beck NA, Baldwin KD, et al. Knee injuries in children and adolescents: has there been an increase in ACL and meniscus tears in recent years?. In: *Presented at the 2011 American Academy of Pediatrics National Conference and Exhibition.* Boston, MA:15–18(Abstract 14815).

334. Sanders TL, Pareek A, Hewett TE, et al. Incidence of first-time lateral patellar dislocation: a 21-year population-based study. *Sports Health.* 2018;10:146–151.

335. Sankar WN, Wells L, Sennett BJ, et al. Combined anterior cruciate ligament and medial collateral ligament injuries in adolescents. *J Pediatr Orthop.* 2006;26(6):733–736.

336. Schlonsky J, Eyring EJ. Lateral meniscus tears in young children. *Clin Orthop Relat Res.* 1973;(97):117–118.

337. Schmal H, Strohm PC, Niemeyer P, et al. Fractures of the patella in children and adolescents. *Acta Orthop Belg.* 2010;76(5):644–650.

338. Schneppendahl J, Thelen S, Twehues S, et al. The use of biodegradable sutures for the fixation of tibial eminence fractures in children: a comparison using PDS II, Vicryl and FiberWire. *J Pediatr Orthop.* 2013;33(4):409–414.

339. Seeley M, Bowman KF, Walsh C, et al. Magnetic resonance imaging of acute patellar dislocation in children: patterns of injury and risk factors for recurrence. *J Pediatr Orthop.* 2012;32(2):145–155.

340. Seeley MA, Knesek M, Vanderhave KL. Osteochondral injury after acute patellar dislocation in children and adolescents. *J Pediatr Orthop.* 2013;33(5):511–518.

341. Seil R, Pape D, Kohn D. The risk of growth changes during transphyseal drilling in sheep with open physes. *Arthroscopy.* 2008;24(7):824–833.

342. Sharma A, Lakshmanan P, Peehal J, et al. An analysis of different types of surgical fixation for avulsion fractures of the anterior tibial spine. *Acta Orthop Belg.* 2008;74(1):90–97.

343. Shea KG, Apel PJ, Pfeiffer RP, et al. The anatomy of the proximal tibia in pediatric and adolescent patients: implications for ACL reconstruction and prevention of physeal arrest. *Knee Surg Sports Traumatol Arthrosc.* 2007;15(4):320–327.

344. Shea KG, Grimm NL, Belzer J, et al. The relation of the femoral physis and the medial patellofemoral ligament. *Arthroscopy.* 2010;26(8):1083–1087.

345. Shea KG, Grimm NL, Ewing CK, et al. Youth sports anterior cruciate ligament and knee injury epidemiology: who is getting injured? In what sports? When?. *Clin Sports Med.* 2011;30(4):691–706.

346. Shea KG, Grimm NL, Laor T, et al. Bone bruises and meniscal tears on MRI in skeletally immature children with tibial eminence fractures. *J Pediatr Orthop.* 2011;31(2):150–152.

347. Shea KG, Pfeiffer R, Wang JH, et al. Anterior cruciate ligament injury in pediatric and adolescent soccer players: an analysis of insurance data. *J Pediatr Orthop.* 2004;24(6):623–628.

348. Shelbourne KD, Gray T, Wiley BV. Results of transphyseal anterior cruciate ligament reconstruction using patellar tendon autograft in tanner stage 3 or 4 adolescents with clearly open growth plates. *Am J Sports Med.* 2004;32(5):1218–1222.

349. Shieh A, Bastrom T, Roocroft J, et al. Meniscus tear patterns in relation to skeletal immaturity: children versus adolescents. *Am J Sports Med.* 2013;41(12):2779–2783.

350. Shieh AK, Edmonds EW, Pennock AT. Revision meniscal surgery in children and adolescents: risk factors and mechanisms for failure and subsequent management. *Am J Sports Med.* 2016;44(4):838–843.

351. Shifflett GD, Green DW, Widmann RF, et al. Growth arrest following ACL reconstruction with hamstring autograft in skeletally immature patients: a review of 4 cases. *J Pediatr Orthop.* 2016;36(4):355–361.

352. Shoemaker SC, Markolf KL. The role of the meniscus in the anterior-posterior stability of the loaded anterior cruciate-deficient knee. Effects of partial versus total excision. *J Bone Joint Surg Am.* 1986;68(1):71–79.

353. Simonian PT, Metcalf MH, Larson RV. Anterior cruciate ligament injuries in the skeletally immature patient. *Am J Orthop (Belle Mead NJ).* 1999;28(11):624–628.

354. Sisk T. Knee injuries. In: AH C, ed. *Campbell's Operative Orthopaedics.* Vol. 3. 7th ed. St. Louis, MO: CV Mosby; 1987:2336–2338.

355. Skak SV, Jensen TT, Poulsen TD, et al. Epidemiology of knee injuries in children. *Acta Orthop Scand.* 1987;58(1):78–81.

356. Smillie I. *Injuries of the Knee Joint.* Edinburgh: Churchill-Livingstone; 1978.

357. Smillie IS. The congenital discoid meniscus. *J Bone Joint Surg Br.* 1948;30B(4):671–682.

358. Smith HJ, Richardson JB, Tennant A. Modification and validation of the Lysholm Knee Scale to assess articular cartilage damage. *Osteoarthritis Cartilage.* 2009;17(1):53–58.

359. Smith JB. Knee instability after fractures of the intercondylar eminence of the tibia. *J Pediatr Orthop.* 1984;4(4):462–464.

360. Stadelmaier DM, Arnoczky SP, Dodds J, et al. The effect of drilling and soft tissue grafting across open growth plates. A histologic study. *Am J Sports Med.* 1995;23(4):431–435.

361. Stanitski CL. Anterior cruciate ligament injury in the skeletally immature patient: diagnosis and treatment. *J Am Acad Orthop Surg.* 1995;3(3):146–158.

362. Stanitski CL. Patellar instability in the school-age athlete. *Instr Course Lect.* 1998;47:345–350.

363. Stanitski CL. Correlation of arthroscopic and clinical examinations with magnetic resonance imaging findings of injured knees in children and adolescents. *Am J Sports Med.* 1998;26(1):2–6.

364. Stanitski CL, Harvell JC, Fu F. Observations on acute knee hemarthrosis in children and adolescents. *J Pediatr Orthop.* 1993;13(4):506–510.

365. Stanitski CL, Paletta GA Jr. Articular cartilage injury with acute patellar dislocation in adolescents. Arthroscopic and radiographic correlation. *Am J Sports Med.* 1998;26(1):52–55.

366. Steadman JR, Briggs KK, Rodrigo JJ, et al. Outcomes of microfracture for traumatic chondral defects of the knee: average 11-year follow-up. *Arthroscopy.* 2003;19(5):477–484.

367. Stilli S, Reggiani LM, Muccioli GM, et al. Arthroscopic treatment for symptomatic discoid lateral meniscus during childhood. *Knee Surg Sports Traumatol Arthrosc.* 2011;19(8):1337–1342.

368. Sugawara O, Miyatsu M, Yamashita I, et al. Problems with repeated arthroscopic surgery in the discoid meniscus. *Arthroscopy.* 1991;7(1):68–71.

369. Sullivan DJ, Dines DM, Hershon SJ, et al. Natural history of a type III fracture of the intercondylar eminence of the tibia in an adult. A case report. *Am J Sports Med.* 1989;17(1):132–133.

370. Tanner JM, Whitehouse RH. Clinical longitudinal standards for height, weight, height velocity, weight velocity, and stages of puberty. *Arch Dis Child.* 1976;51(3):170–179.

371. Tapper EM, Hoover NW. Late results after meniscectomy. *J Bone Joint Surg Am.* 1969;51(3):517–526 passim.

372. Thaunat M, Erasmus PJ. Recurrent patellar dislocation after medial patellofemoral ligament reconstruction. *Knee Surg Sports Traumatol Arthrosc.* 2008;16(1):40–43.

373. Thaunat M, Erasmus PJ. Management of overtight medial patellofemoral ligament reconstruction. *Knee Surg Sports Traumatol Arthrosc.* 2009;17(5):480–483.

374. Torisu T. Isolated avulsion fracture of the tibial attachment of the posterior cruciate ligament. *J Bone Joint Surg Am.* 1977;59(1):68–72.

375. Trillat A, Dejour H, Couette A. Diagnosis and treatment of recurrent dislocations of the patella. *Rev Chir Orthop Reparatrice Appar Mot.* 1964;50:813–824.

376. Tudisco C, Giovarruscio R, Febo A, et al. Intercondylar eminence avulsion fracture in children: long-term follow-up of 14 cases at the end of skeletal growth. *J Pediatr Orthop B.* 2010;19(5):403–408.

377. Uchida R, Toritsuka Y, Yoneda K, et al. Chondral fragment of the lateral femoral trochlea of the knee in adolescents. *Knee.* 2012;19(5):719–723.

378. Vahasarja V, Kinnuen P, Serlo W. Arthroscopy of the acute traumatic knee in children. Prospective study of 138 cases. *Acta Orthop Scand.* 1993;64(5):580–582.

379. Vahvanen V, Aalto K. Meniscectomy in children. *Acta Orthop Scand.* 1979;50(6 pt 2):791–795.

380. Vander Have KL, Ganley TJ, Kocher MS, et al. Arthrofibrosis after surgical fixation of tibial eminence fractures in children and adolescents. *Am J Sports Med.* 2010;38(2):298–301.

381. Vanderhave KL, Moravek JE, Sekiya JK, et al. Meniscus tears in the young athlete: results of arthroscopic repair. *J Pediatr Orthop.* 2011;31(5):496–500.

382. Vandermeer RD, Cunningham FK. Arthroscopic treatment of the discoid lateral meniscus: results of long-term follow-up. *Arthroscopy.* 1989;5(2):101–109.

383. Vargas B, Lutz N, Dutoit M, et al. Nonunion after fracture of the anterior tibial spine: case report and review of the literature. *J Pediatr Orthop B.* 2009;18(2):90–92.

384. Vavken P, Murray MM. Treating anterior cruciate ligament tears in skeletally immature patients. *Arthroscopy.* 2011;27(5):704–716.

385. Vedi V, Williams A, Tennant SJ, et al. Meniscal movement. An in-vivo study using dynamic MRI. *J Bone Joint Surg Br.* 1999;81(1):37–41.

386. Vega JR, Irribarra LA, Baar AK, et al. Arthroscopic fixation of displaced tibial eminence fractures: a new growth plate-sparing method. *Arthroscopy.* 2008;24(11):1239–1243.

387. Volk H, Smith FM. "Bucket-handle" tear of the medial meniscus in a 5-year-old boy. *J Bone Joint Surg Am.* 1953;35:234–236.

388. Volpi P, Galli M, Bait C, et al. Surgical treatment of anterior cruciate ligament injuries in adolescents using double-looped semitendinosus and gracilis tendons: supraepiphysary femoral and tibial fixation. *Arthroscopy.* 2004;20(4):447–449.

389. von Heideken J, Mikkelsson C, Boström Windhamre H, et al. Acute injuries to the posterolateral corner of the knee in children: a case series of 6 patients. *Am J Sports Med.* 2011;39(10):2199–2205.

390. Walsh SJ, Boyle MJ, Morganti V. Large osteochondral fractures of the lateral femoral condyle in the adolescent: outcome of bioabsorbable pin fixation. *J Bone Joint Surg Am.* 2008;90(7):1473–1478.

391. Washington ER, 3rd, Root L, Liener UC. Discoid lateral meniscus in children. Long-term follow-up after excision. *J Bone Joint Surg Am.* 1995;77(9):1357–1361.

392. Watanabe M, Takada S, Ikeuchi H. *Atlas of Arthroscopy.* Tokyo: Igaku-Shoin; 1969.

393. Webster KE, Feller JA. Exploring the high reinjury rate in younger patients undergoing anterior cruciate ligament reconstruction. *Am J Sports Med.* 2016;44(11):2827–2832.

394. Webster KE, Feller JA, Leigh WB, et al. Younger patients are at increased risk for graft rupture and contralateral injury after anterior cruciate ligament reconstruction. *Am J Sports Med.* 2014;42(3):641–647.

395. Weiss CB, Lundberg M, Hamberg P, et al. Non-operative treatment of meniscal tears. *J Bone Joint Surg Am.* 1989;71(6):811–822.

396. Wessel LM, Scholz S, Rusch M, et al. Hemarthrosis after trauma to the pediatric knee joint: what is the value of magnetic resonance imaging in the diagnostic algorithm?. *J Pediatr Orthop.* 2001;21(3):338–342.

397. Wiley JJ, Baxter MP. Tibial spine fractures in children. *Clin Orthop Relat Res.* 1990;(255):54–60.

398. Wilfinger C, Castellani C, Raith J, et al. Nonoperative treatment of tibial spine fractures in children-38 patients with a minimum follow-up of 1 year. *J Orthop Trauma.* 2009;23(7):519–524.

399. Willimon SC, Jones CR, Herzog MM, et al. Micheli anterior cruciate ligament reconstruction in skeletally immature youths: a retrospective case series with a mean 3-year follow-up. *Am J Sports Med.* 2015;43(12):2974–2981.

400. Willis RB, Blokker C, Stoll TM, et al. Long-term follow-up of anterior tibial eminence fractures. *J Pediatr Orthop.* 1993;13(3):361–364.

401. Wombwell JH, Nunley JA. Compressive fixation of osteochondritis dissecans fragments with Herbert screws. *J Orthop Trauma.* 1987;1(1):74–77.

402. Woo R, Busch M. Management of patellar instability in children. *Oper Tech Sports Med.* 1998;6:247–258.

403. Woo SL, Hollis JM, Adams DJ, et al. Tensile properties of the human femur-anterior cruciate ligament-tibia complex. The effects of specimen age and orientation. *Am J Sports Med.* 1991;19(3):217–225.

404. Woods GW, Stanley RF, Tullos HS. Lateral capsular sign: x-ray clue to a significant knee instability. *Am J Sports Med.* 1979;7(1):27–33.

405. Wouters DB, De Graaf JS, Hemmer PH, et al. The arthroscopic treatment of displaced tibial spine fractures in children and adolescents using Meniscus Arrows®. *Knee Surg Sports Traumatol Arthrosc.* 2011;19(5):736–739.

406. Wroble RR, Henderson RC, Campion ER, et al. Meniscectomy in children and adolescents. A long-term follow-up study. *Clin Orthop Relat Res.* 1992;(279):180–189.

407. Yamasaki S, Hashimoto Y, Takigami J, et al. Risk factors associated with knee joint degeneration after arthroscopic reshaping for juvenile discoid lateral meniscus. *Am J Sports Med.* 2017;45(3):570–577.

408. Yoo WJ, Jang WY, Park MS, et al. Arthroscopic treatment for symptomatic discoid meniscus in children: midterm outcomes and prognostic factors. *Arthroscopy.* 2015;31(12):2327–2334.

409. Yoo WJ, Choi IH, Chung CY, et al. Discoid lateral meniscus in children: limited knee extension and meniscal instability in the posterior segment. *J Pediatr Orthop.* 2008;28(5):544–548.

410. Yoo WJ, Kocher MS, Micheli LJ. Growth plate disturbance after transphyseal reconstruction of the anterior cruciate ligament in skeletally immature adolescent patients: an MR imaging study. *J Pediatr Orthop.* 2011;31(6):691–696.

411. Zaman M, Leonard MA. Meniscectomy in children: results in 59 knees. *Injury.* 1981;12(5):425–428.

412. Zaricznyj B. Avulsion fracture of the tibial eminence: treatment by open reduction and pinning. *J Bone Joint Surg Am.* 1977;59(8):1111–1114.

413. Zhao J, Huangfu X, He Y, et al. Recurrent patellar dislocation in adolescents: medial retinaculum plication versus vastus medialis plasty. *Am J Sports Med.* 2012;40(1):123–132.

28

Fractures of the Shaft of the Tibia and Fibula

Christine Ann Ho and James F. Mooney

Fractures of the Shaft of the Tibia and Fibula

INTRODUCTION TO FRACTURES OF THE SHAFT OF THE TIBIA AND FIBULA

The true incidence of tibia/fibula fractures in pediatric patients is unknown. The most recent North American data are derived from a review of a national US injury database reported by Naranje et al. in 2016.[107] The authors found that fractures of the tibial/fibular shaft are the second most common long bone fractures in children, after forearm fractures, with an annual occurrence of 11 per 1,000 children over the course of childhood.[107] In addition, fractures of tibia and fibula are the second most frequent injuries among pediatric orthopedic trauma admissions (21.5%), after femur fractures.[38] The peak incidence occurs in children between the ages of 10 and 14 years[107] with an approximate 2:1 ratio of males to females injured.[38,73]

Seventy percent of pediatric tibial fractures are isolated injuries; ipsilateral fibular fractures occur with 30% of tibial fractures.[21,157] These fractures can be incomplete (torus, greenstick) or complete. Shannak reviewed 117 pediatric tibia fractures in 1988 and found that 51% occurred in the distal third, and 39% in the middle third.[134] In that study, 35% of pediatric tibial fractures were oblique, 32% comminuted, 20% transverse, and 13% spiral.[134] Isolated spiral or short oblique tibia fractures (often minimally or nondisplaced) in children less than 3 to 4 years of age constitute a unique fracture type often termed a "toddler's fracture."

ASSESSMENT OF FRACTURES OF THE SHAFT OF THE TIBIA AND FIBULA

MECHANISMS OF INJURY FOR FRACTURES OF THE SHAFT OF THE TIBIA AND FIBULA

Rotational forces result in oblique or spiral fractures, and are responsible for approximately 80% of all tibial fractures that present without an associated fibular fracture.[21,99,134] Most tibial fractures in children of 4 to 14 years of age are the result of sporting or traffic accidents.[21,99,134] In addition, the tibia is one of the most commonly fractured long bones in abused children.[85] Approximately 11% to 26% of all abused children with a long bone injury have a fractured tibia.[82,94,118] The vast majority of tibia fracture in children and adolescents, regardless of mechanism, are closed injuries.

INJURIES ASSOCIATED WITH FRACTURES OF THE SHAFT OF THE TIBIA AND FIBULA

Concomitant fractures of the ankle and foot are the most common injuries associated with fractures of the tibia and fibula, followed by humeral, femoral, and radial/ulnar fractures.[19] In a 1994 report, the average Injury Severity Score of a child with a tibial fracture was 10 (range, 0 to 45) with an average hospital stay of 6.5 days (range, 1 to 50 days).[19] There have been no updates of this information in the recent English literature. Isolated fibular fractures are fairly uncommon in children, and in the majority of cases are the result of a direct blow to the area of the fracture.[58,146]

CLASSIFICATION OF FRACTURES OF THE SHAFT OF THE TIBIA AND FIBULA

Nonphyseal injuries of the tibia and the fibula can be classified into three major categories based on the combination of bones fractured and the location of the injuries. These include fractures of the proximal or distal tibial metaphysis, and those involving the diaphyseal region.

PATHOANATOMY AND APPLIED ANATOMY OF FRACTURES OF THE SHAFT OF THE TIBIA AND FIBULA

BONY STRUCTURE OF THE TIBIA AND FIBULA

The tibia ("flute") is the second largest bone in the body. There are two concave condyles at the proximal aspect of the tibia. The medial condyle is larger, deeper, and narrower than the lateral condyle. An elevated process, the tibial tubercle, located anteriorly between the two condyles, is the site of attachment of the patellar tendon. The shaft of the tibia is the shape of a prism, with a broad proximal extent that decreases in size until the distal third, where it gradually increases again in size. The tibial crest is prominent anteromedially from the tibial tubercle to the tibial plafond and is subcutaneous without overlying musculature.[48]

TABLE 28-1. Muscle Origins and Insertions on the Tibia

Muscle	Origin or Insertion
Semimembranosus	Inserts on the inner tuberosity of the proximal tibia
Tibialis anterior, EDL, biceps femoris	Attach to lateral condyle of the tibia
Sartorius, gracilis, semitendinosus	Insert on the proximal medial surface of the tibial metaphysis
Tibialis anterior	Arises on the lateral surface of the tibial diaphysis
Popliteus, soleus, FDL, tibialis posterior	Attaches to the posterior diaphysis of the tibia
Patellar tendon	Inserts into the tibial tubercle
Tensor fascia lata	Attaches to Gerdy tubercle, the lateral aspect of the proximal tibial metaphysis
Secondary slip of the tensor fascia lata	Occasionally inserts into the tibial tubercle

The tibia develops from three ossification centers: One in the shaft and one each in the proximal and distal epiphysis. The tibial diaphysis begins to ossify at 7 weeks of gestation and ossification expands proximally and distally. The proximal epiphyseal center appears shortly after birth and unites with the shaft as the growth plate closes between 14 and 16 years of age. The distal epiphyseal ossification center appears in the second year of life, and the distal tibial physis closes between 14 and 15 years of age. Average age of growth plate closure varies between male and females. Additional ossification centers are found occasionally in the medial malleolus and in the tibial tubercle.[48] The tibia articulates with the condyles of the femur proximally, with the fibula at the knee and the ankle, and with the talus distally.[46] Twelve muscles have either their origin or insertion on the tibia (Table 28-1).

The fibula articulates with the tibia and the talus. The fibular diaphysis ossifies at approximately 8 weeks of gestation. The distal fibular ossification center becomes visible at approximately 2 years of age, in most patients, and the proximal secondary ossification center generally appears at 4 years. The distal fibular physis closes completely by approximately 16 years; the proximal physis closes later, between the ages of 15 and 18 years.[48] Nine muscles have either their origin or insertion on the fibula (Table 28-2).[48]

VASCULAR ANATOMY OF THE TIBIA AND FIBULA

The popliteal artery descends vertically and posteriorly between the condyles of the femur, and passes between the medial and lateral heads of the gastrocnemius muscle. It ends at the distal border of the popliteus muscle, where it divides into the anterior and posterior tibial arteries. The anterior

TABLE 28-2.   Muscle Origins and Insertions on the Fibula

Muscle	Origin or Insertion
Soleus, FHL	Arise from the posterior aspect of the fibular diaphysis
Peroneus longus, peroneus brevis	Arise from the lateral aspect of the fibular diaphysis
Biceps femoris, soleus, peroneus longus	Attach to the head of the fibula
Extensor digitorum longus, peroneus tertius, extensor hallucis longus	Attach to the anterior surface of the fibular shaft
Tibialis posterior	Arise from the medial aspect of the fibular diaphysis

tibial artery passes between the tibia and the fibula over the proximal aspect of the intraosseous membrane, enters the anterior compartment of the lower leg, and divides into a series of smaller branches. The posterior tibial artery divides several centimeters distal to this point, giving rise to the peroneal artery (Fig. 28-1).[48]

NEURAL ANATOMY OF THE TIBIA AND FIBULA

The posterior tibial nerve runs adjacent and posterior to the popliteal artery in the popliteal fossa, and then enters the deep posterior compartment of the leg. This nerve provides innervation to the muscles of the deep posterior compartment

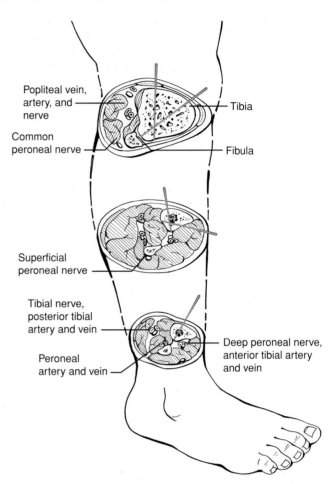

Figure 28-2. Fibroosseous compartments of the leg.

and sensation to the plantar aspect of the foot. The common peroneal nerve passes laterally around the proximal neck of the fibula. It divides into deep and superficial branches, and then passes into the anterior and the lateral compartments of the lower leg, respectively. Each branch innervates the muscles within its compartment. The deep peroneal nerve provides sensation to the first web space. The superficial branch is responsible for sensation across the dorsal and lateral aspects of the foot.

FASCIAL COMPARTMENTS

The lower leg has four fascial compartments (Fig. 28-2). The anterior compartment contains the extensor digitorum longus, the extensor hallucis longus, and the tibialis anterior muscles; the anterior tibial artery and deep peroneal nerve run in this compartment. The lateral compartment contains the peroneus longus and brevis muscles. The superficial peroneal nerve runs through this compartment. The superficial posterior compartment contains the soleus and gastrocnemius muscles. The deep posterior compartment contains the flexor digitorum longus, the flexor hallucis longus, and the tibialis posterior muscles. The posterior tibial artery, peroneal artery, and posterior tibial nerve run in this compartment.[48]

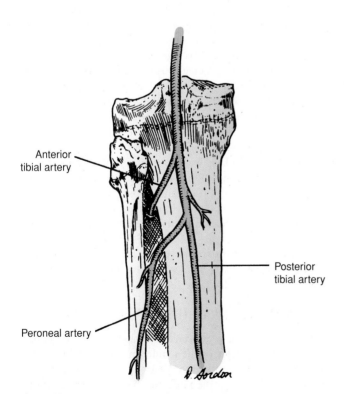

Figure 28-1. Vascular anatomy of the proximal tibia.

Fractures of the Proximal Tibial Metaphysis

INTRODUCTION TO FRACTURES OF THE PROXIMAL TIBIAL METAPHYSIS

Proximal tibial fractures are the least common nonphyseal tibial fractures in children.[4] Greater attention is given to the sequelae of pediatric proximal tibial metaphyseal fractures than to the management of the acute injury itself. The peak incidence for proximal tibia metaphyseal fractures is between the ages of 3 and 6 years.[104] The most common mechanism of injury is a low-energy force applied to the lateral aspect of the extended knee either directly or indirectly through axial loading. The cortex of the medial tibial metaphysis fails in tension, often resulting in an incomplete greenstick fracture. Compression (torus) and complete fractures can occur in this area, but are less common. The fibula generally escapes injury, although plastic deformation may occur.[24,71,75,81,150,156,161] As a child matures, physeal fractures are seen more commonly in the proximal tibia due to the relative weakness of the physis compared to maturing cortical bone.

ASSESSMENT OF FRACTURES OF THE PROXIMAL TIBIAL METAPHYSIS

MECHANISM OF INJURY OF PROXIMAL TIBIAL METAPHYSIS FRACTURES

Pediatric proximal tibial metaphyseal fractures most commonly occur secondary to valgus force, followed by varus, then extension, and finally flexion. An axial load on an extended knee, such as during trampoline-related activities, is a common mechanism for the valgus fractures. Varus metaphyseal fractures are rarer; it is hypothesized that the proximal fibula may act as a protective buttress on the lateral tibial metaphysis.[104]

INJURIES ASSOCIATED WITH FRACTURES OF THE PROXIMAL TIBIAL METAPHYSIS

Unlike physeal proximal tibial fractures, there are few associated injuries that occur in conjunction with proximal tibial metaphyseal fractures. Completely displaced metaphyseal fractures may be associated with injury to the popliteal artery, but this is an uncommon scenario in this younger age group.

SIGNS AND SYMPTOMS OF FRACTURES OF THE PROXIMAL TIBIAL METAPHYSIS

Children with proximal tibia metaphyseal fractures present with pain, swelling, and tenderness in the region of the fracture. Motion of the knee causes moderate pain, and in most cases the child will not walk. Crepitance is seldom identified on physical examination, particularly if the fracture is incomplete.

IMAGING AND OTHER DIAGNOSTIC STUDIES FOR FRACTURES OF THE PROXIMAL TIBIAL METAPHYSIS

Orthogonal plain radiographs of the affected tibia are sufficient to diagnose proximal tibial metaphyseal fractures in most cases. Radiographs usually demonstrate a complete or greenstick fracture of the proximal tibial metaphysis. The medial aspect of the fracture often is widened, producing a valgus deformity of the proximal tibia. Subtle fractures from a purely axial load may not be visualized on radiographs, but an increase in the anterior tilt angle of the proximal tibial physis (an anterior slope of the tibial plateau) may be detected on the lateral radiograph, and may serve as indirect evidence of a fracture (Fig. 28-3).[147]

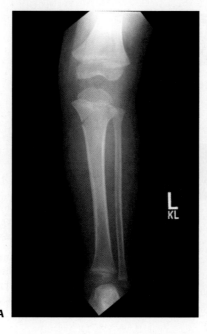
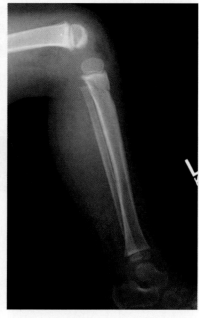

Figure 28-3. Anteroposterior (**A**) and lateral (**B**) radiographs of the proximal tibial metaphyseal fracture with an intact fibula in a 3-year-old child. Note the subtle increased anterior angle of the proximal tibial physis,

A   B

CLASSIFICATION OF FRACTURES OF THE PROXIMAL TIBIAL METAPHYSIS

There is no commonly accepted comprehensive classification system for pediatric proximal tibial fractures. Typically, these fractures are described by the predominant deformity in the coronal plane (varus, valgus, complete).

OUTCOME MEASURES FOR FRACTURES OF THE PROXIMAL TIBIAL METAPHYSIS

There are no commonly used outcome measures for fractures of the proximal tibial metaphysis.

PATHOANATOMY AND APPLIED ANATOMY RELATED TO PROXIMAL TIBIAL METAPHYSIS FRACTURES

The popliteal artery, popliteal vein, and tibial nerve vein lie in close proximity to the posterior proximal tibia. As the popliteal artery exits the distal popliteus muscle, it divides into the anterior and posterior tibial arteries. The anterior tibial artery pierces the interosseous membrane at the level of the fibular neck and joins the deep peroneal nerve in the anterior compartment of the leg. The tibial nerve lies adjacent and to the posterior tibial artery in the deep posterior compartment of the leg. The common peroneal nerve lies just posterior and deep to the inserting tendon of the biceps femoris and courses anteriorly at the level of the fibular neck, where it divides into the deep and superficial peroneal nerves. Open approaches to the proximal tibia are rarely needed to remove interposed tissue, and when performed are most safely done from the medial side to avoid the neurovascular structures and to access the pes anserinus if repair is needed.

TREATMENT OPTIONS FOR FRACTURES OF THE PROXIMAL TIBIAL METAPHYSIS

NONOPERATIVE TREATMENT OF FRACTURES OF THE PROXIMAL TIBIAL METAPHYSIS

Indications/Contraindications

Nonoperative Treatment of Fractures of the Proximal Tibial Metaphysis:
INDICATIONS AND CONTRAINDICATIONS

Indications
• Nondisplaced closed fractures
• Displaced closed fractures amenable to closed reduction

Contraindications
• Open fractures
• Body habitus unamenable to long-leg cast treatment
• Failure to attain or maintain adequate closed reduction in a cast

Casting

Nondisplaced proximal tibial metaphyseal fractures can be treated with an appropriately padded long-leg cast for 4 to 6 weeks until there is radiographic healing, the fracture is nontender, and the patient can bear weight comfortably. As many of these fractures occur in younger children who may have limited verbal skills, care must be taken to place sufficient cast padding in areas of bony prominence, and to mold the cast so as to minimize the risk of slippage. This level of attention to detail will aid in limiting skin breakdown and irritation, such as over the calcaneal tuberosity. In a standard medial metaphyseal fracture, a varus mold should be applied as the fracture tends to go into valgus over time. This is one of the only situations in orthopedics in which starting off in varus is a good thing.

Displaced proximal tibial metaphyseal fractures are treated with closed manipulation under sedation or general anesthesia. Fluoroscopy is useful to verify anatomic reduction. A slight varus mold in the cast is preferred to anticipate the postfracture tibial valgus that may occur. While a long-leg cast in flexion may help to prevent weightbearing, it is often easier to mold, manipulate, and radiographically visualize the fracture with a long-leg cast in a position closer to full extension. Most of these transverse fractures are stable enough to permit weightbearing as tolerated (Fig. 28-4).

OPERATIVE TREATMENT OF PROXIMAL TIBIAL METAPHYSIS FRACTURES

Indications/Contraindications

In rare cases, an acceptable closed reduction cannot be attained or maintained, and an open reduction is required. This may

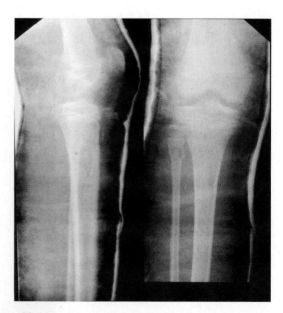

Figure 28-4. Anteroposterior and lateral radiographs of the proximal tibia and distal femur in a child who sustained a nondisplaced fracture of the proximal tibial and fibular metaphysis. The knee is casted in extension which facilitates accurate measurements of fracture alignment.

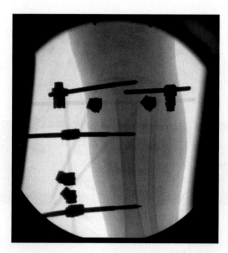

Figure 28-5. Anteroposterior radiograph of a 3-year-old female with a severe closed head injury, ipsilateral femur, and proximal tibia metaphyseal fractures. The tibia fracture was stabilized with a modified uniplanar external fixator.

be secondary to interposition of soft tissue in the fracture site, usually on the medial side. In such a situation, a standard approach to the anteromedial proximal tibia may be required to facilitate removal and fracture reduction. The pes anserinus insertion may also be repaired through this approach if necessary. Occasionally, a larger adolescent child may have a body habitus that precludes successful cast treatment, or severe swelling also may also exclude circumferential casting as a safe treatment option.

Percutaneous fixation with smooth pins or an external fixator may be required in extremely uncommon cases. Pin placement should avoid physeal violation and knee joint penetration if possible. Retrograde insertion of smooth crossed pins may be technically easier than an antegrade approach, and careful dissection should be used to avoid injury to the deep peroneal nerve and anterior tibial artery on the lateral entry point. Stabilization with pins or external fixation is often useful in polytrauma patients or those with extensive associated soft tissue injuries (Fig. 28-5).

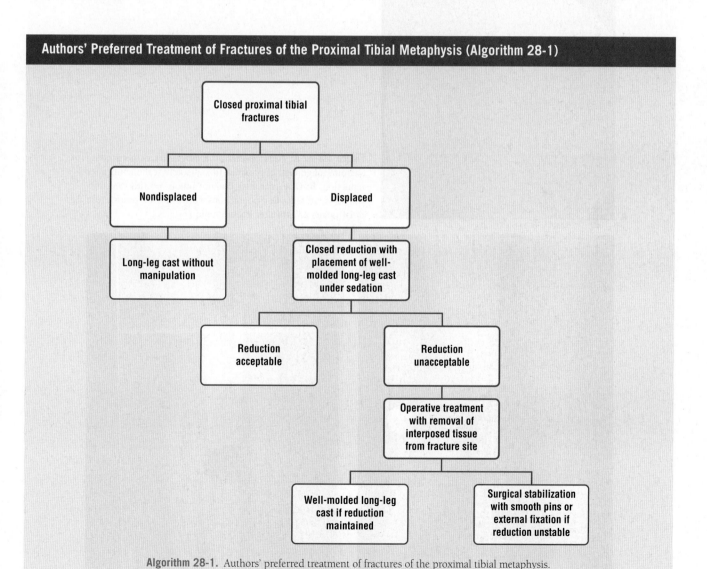

Authors' Preferred Treatment of Fractures of the Proximal Tibial Metaphysis (Algorithm 28-1)

Algorithm 28-1. Authors' preferred treatment of fractures of the proximal tibial metaphysis.

Postoperative Care

After surgical intervention, a period of limited weight bearing is recommended for most patients without stable fixation. These fractures may have slightly prolonged healing due to soft tissue stripping and may require lengthier immobilization. Smooth pins may be protected under a sterile dressing and cast until removal. External fixator pins should be cleansed with dilute saline/hydrogen peroxide solution twice a day, or as per the treating surgeon's external fixator care protocol. Fractures stabilized with isolated cast treatment require regular weekly follow-up visits and radiographs to verify maintenance of the reduction. If there is loss of reduction, cast wedging or repeat reduction efforts may be indicated. In most cases, immobilization is required for approximately 4 to 6 weeks after injury. Weight bearing and discontinuation of cast treatment or pins may occur when there is visible callus

and the fracture is nontender to palpation. The child may return to regular activities after recovery of normal knee and ankle range of motion. Long-term follow-up with forewarning to the family of the possibility of progressive tibial deformity is mandatory.

MANAGEMENT OF EXPECTED ADVERSE OUTCOMES AND UNEXPECTED COMPLICATIONS RELATED TO FRACTURES OF THE PROXIMAL TIBIAL METAPHYSIS

The most recognized late sequela of a proximal tibial metaphyseal fracture is development of a progressive valgus deformity (Fig. 28-6A,B). When the child initially presents for

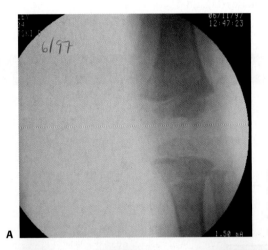

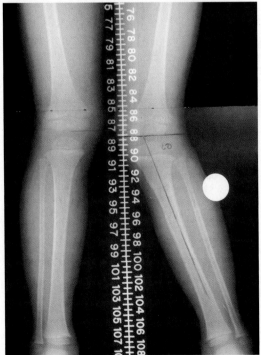

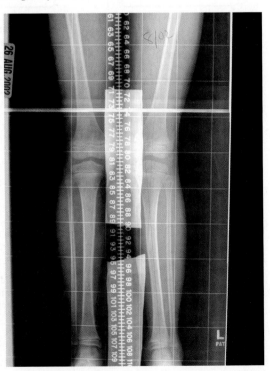

Figure 28-6. A: Anteroposterior radiographs demonstrating anatomic alignment of proximal tibia metaphyseal fracture after reduction. **B:** One year after fracture union, postfracture tibia valgus is present. **C:** Spontaneous correction of postfracture tibial valgus 2 years after fracture union.

treatment of a tibia fracture at risk of developing genu valgum, it is crucial that the possibility of this unpredictable postfracture problem is discussed with the family. Parents should be counseled at the time of initial treatment about this possibility and the need for monitoring and serial radiographs after the fracture is healed.

In 1953, Cozen[24] was the first to report valgus deformity following a proximal tibial metaphyseal fracture. He described four patients with valgus deformities after fractures in this area. In two cases, the valgus was present at the time of cast removal, suggesting loss of reduction as a potential cause of the deformity. In the other two patients the tibia valga developed gradually during subsequent growth of the patient. Since that time, multiple other investigators[8,71,75,150,156] have reported development of tibia valga, even in fractures without any significant malalignment at the time of initial treatment. Nenopoulos reported a 90% incidence of progressive tibial valgus deformity in patients with minimally or nondisplaced proximal tibia metaphyseal fractures.[109] Robert et al.[126] analyzed 25 patients with proximal tibial fractures. Twelve children with a greenstick or a complete fracture developed valgus deformities, whereas no child with a torus fracture developed a deformity. Altered growth at the distal tibial physis appeared to compensate for the proximal tibia valga in three children. Corrective osteotomies were performed in four children. The valgus deformity recurred in two of these four children, and two had iatrogenic compartment syndromes.

Many theories have been proposed to explain the development of a valgus deformity after a proximal tibial metaphyseal fracture (Table 28-3).

While even appropriate operative and nonoperative treatment may still result in development of posttraumatic tibial valgus, several preventative measures have been proposed.

TABLE 28-3. Proposed Etiologies of Post-Fracture Tibia Valga in Proximal Tibial Metaphyseal Fractures

Overgrowth of medial proximal tibial callus or medial physis[150]
- Entrapped medial periosteum leads to increase in physeal growth[128]
- Increased vascular flow to medial proximal physis with asymmetric physeal response[75]
  - Bone scans demonstrating increased tracer uptake in medial physis months after fracture[161]
  - Increase in medial collateral geniculate vascularity[112]

Growth arrest of the lateral proximal tibial physis[43,81]

Inadequate reduction or loss of reduction[140,161]

Interposed soft tissue (medial collateral ligament/pes anserinus/periosteum) leading to medial gapping and a valgus deformity

Loss of tethering effect of pes anserinus tendon plate on medial physis leading to medial physeal overgrowth and hemichonrodiastasis[6,27,29,158,164]

Tethering effect of fibula

Early weight bearing producing developmental valgus[123]

Exploration of the fracture, followed by removal and repair of any in-folded periosteum that forms the foundation of the pes anserinus tendon plate, has been suggested as an approach that may decrease the risk of a developmental valgus deformity, but there is little data to support this approach. Houghton and Rooker demonstrated that division of the periosteum around the medial half of the proximal tibia in rabbits induced a valgus deformity and hypothesized that the increasing valgus angulation was due to a mechanical release of the restraints that the periosteum imposes on activity of the physis.[67]

Development of tibia valga has been reported to occur after simple excision of a bone graft from the proximal tibial metaphysis,[150] proximal tibial osteotomy,[71] and osteomyelitis of the proximal tibial metaphysis.[150] Tibia valga deformity can occur after healing of a nondisplaced fracture, and can recur after corrective tibial osteotomy, further supporting the premise that asymmetric physeal growth is the cause of most posttraumatic tibia valga deformities.[161]

The natural history of postfracture proximal tibia valga is one of slow progression of the deformity, followed by gradual restoration of normal alignment over time. The deformity usually is apparent by 6 months post injury, and may progress for up to 18 to 24 months. Zionts and MacEwen[162] followed seven children with progressive valgus deformities of the tibia for an average of 39 months after metaphyseal fractures. Most of the deformity developed during the first year after injury, but angulation continued at a slower rate for up to 17 months after injury. Six of their seven patients had spontaneous clinical corrections. At an average of 39 months follow-up, all children had less than a 10-degree deformity. Long-term follow-up (average, 15 years) of these same seven patients revealed spontaneous correction of metaphyseal–diaphyseal and mechanical tibiofemoral angles with the mechanical axis remaining lateral to the center of the knee joint.[152] Cincinnati Sportmedicine and Orthopaedic Center knee scores were excellent in five patients and fair in two patients, one who had tibial osteotomy due to lateral knee pain. America Orthopaedic Foot and Ankle Society ankle scores were excellent in three patients and good in four.

A child with a posttraumatic valgus deformity should be followed until adequate spontaneous correction occurs. This may take 18 to 36 months (Fig. 28-6C). Bracing does not alter the natural history of posttraumatic tibia valga and is not recommended.[70] Surgical intervention may be indicated in patients more than 18 months post injury with a mechanical axis deviation greater than 10 degrees as a result of tibial valgus. Tibial osteotomies are not recommended in patients with postfracture valgus if they have significant growth remaining because of the possibility of recurrent valgus or other potential complications (Fig. 28-7). Instead, guided growth with temporary mechanical tethering (hemiepiphysiodesis) of the proximal medial tibial physis can restore alignment gradually without the risks of osteotomy. Hemiepiphysiodesis may be accomplished through a variety of methods utilizing staples, screws, or tension band plate and screw devices (Fig. 28-8).[100,145] Because the valgus deformity is often associated with some element of overgrowth, a contralateral shoe lift of appropriate size may make the deformity appear less apparent.[113,126,145,150]

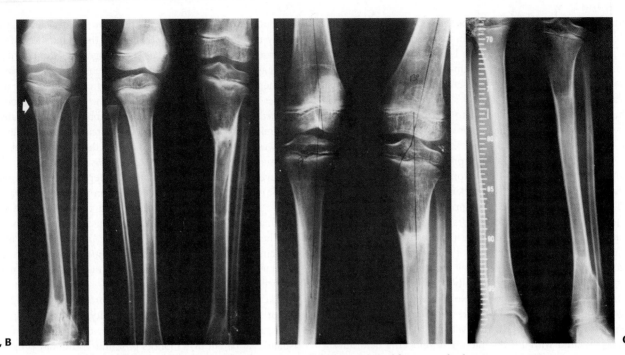

A, B   C, D

Figure 28-7. Developmental valgus after a proximal tibial metaphyseal fracture and subsequent corrective osteotomy. **A:** Radiograph taken 6 months after a fracture of the proximal tibia. The injury was nondisplaced. The scar from the initial proximal metaphyseal fracture is still seen (*arrow*). This child developed a moderate valgus deformity of the tibia within 6 months of fracture. **B:** A proximal tibial corrective osteotomy was performed. **C:** Two months postoperatively, the osteotomy was healed and the deformity corrected. **D:** Five months later, there was a recurrent valgus deformity of 13 degrees. (Courtesy of John J.J. Gugenheim, MD.)

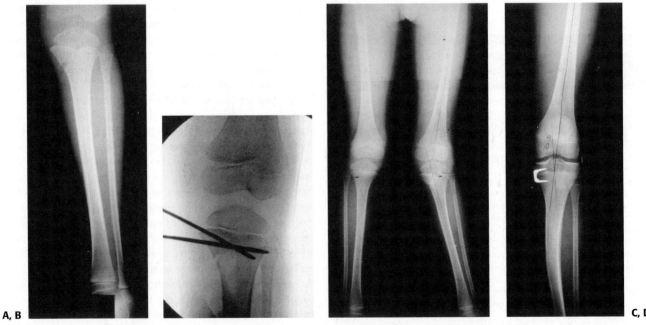

A, B   C, D

Figure 28-8. A: Anteroposterior image of a Salter–Harris type II fracture of the proximal tibia. Notice the valgus alignment. **B:** This fracture was treated with percutaneous pin fixation after reduction. **C:** This patient developed tibia valga over a period of approximately 2 years following the injury. **D:** A medial proximal tibial hemiepiphysiodesis using a staple was performed.

Diaphyseal Fractures of the Tibia and Fibula

INTRODUCTION TO DIAPHYSEAL FRACTURES OF THE TIBIA AND FIBULA

Fractures of the tibial/fibular shaft may occur in children of any age, and may be caused by a variety of mechanisms, ranging from a low-energy fall to a high-energy motor vehicle accident. While most closed pediatric diaphyseal tibia fractures are treated successfully with nonoperative methods, fractures with significant displacement, soft tissue injury, or open injuries, may be more commonly treated with surgical management.

ASSESSMENT OF DIAPHYSEAL FRACTURES OF THE TIBIA AND FIBULA

MECHANISMS OF INJURY FOR DIAPHYSEAL FRACTURES OF THE TIBIA AND FIBULA

Most tibial fractures in children under 11 years of age are caused by torsional forces and occur in the distal third of the tibial diaphysis. These oblique and spiral fractures occur when the body rotates above a foot that is in a fixed position on the ground. The fracture line generally initiates in the distal anteromedial aspect of the bone and propagates proximally in a posterolateral direction.

If there is not an associated fibula fracture, the intact fibula prevents significant shortening of the tibia; however, varus angulation develops in approximately 60% of isolated tibial fractures within the first 2 weeks after injury (Fig. 28-9).[159] In such cases, forces generated by contraction of the long flexor muscles of the lower leg are converted into an angular moment by the intact fibula increasing the risk of varus malalignment (see Fig. 28-9C). Isolated transverse and comminuted fractures of the tibia are caused most commonly by direct trauma. Transverse fractures of the tibia with an intact fibula generally are stable, and seldom displace significantly.[18,76] Comminuted or segmental tibial fractures with an intact fibula tend to drift into varus alignment similar to oblique and spiral fractures.[18,76,159]

INJURIES ASSOCIATED WITH DIAPHYSEAL FRACTURES OF THE TIBIA AND FIBULA

Approximately 30% of pediatric tibial diaphyseal fractures have an associated fibular fracture.[157,159] The fibular fracture may be either complete or incomplete with some element of plastic deformation. A diaphyseal tibia fracture with an associated displaced fracture of the fibula often tends toward valgus angulation because of the action of the muscles in the anterolateral aspect of the leg and the lack of an intact lateral strut (Fig. 28-10). Any fibular injury must be identified and corrected to minimize the risk of recurrence of angulation after reduction (Fig. 28-11).

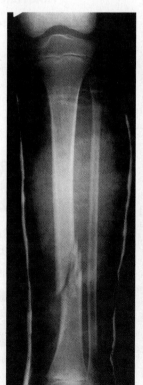
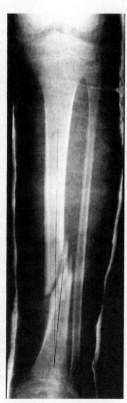
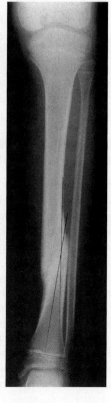

Figure 28-9. Anteroposterior radiograph of a distal one-third tibial fracture without concomitant fibular fracture in a 10-year-old child. **A:** The alignment in the coronal plane is acceptable (note that the proximal and distal tibial growth physes are parallel). **B:** A varus angulation developed within the first 2 weeks after injury. **C:** A 10-degree varus angulation was present after union.   **A, B**   **C**

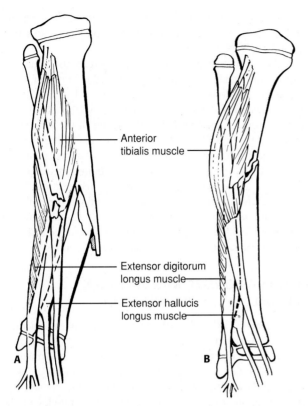

Figure 28-10. A: Fractures involving the middle third of the tibia and fibula may shift into a valgus alignment because of the activity of the muscles in the anterior and the lateral compartments of the lower leg. **B:** Fracture of the middle tibia without an associated fibular fracture tends to shift into varus because of the force created by the anterior compartment musculature of the lower leg and the tethering effect of the intact fibula.

An isolated fracture of the fibular shaft is rare in children, and results most commonly from a direct blow to the lateral aspect of the leg. Most isolated fractures of the fibular shaft are nondisplaced and heal quickly with symptomatic care and immobilization (Fig. 28-12). As with any fracture, the joints above and below must be examined to evaluate for any ipsilateral injuries, such as a subtle concomitant transitional ankle fracture.[78]

SIGNS AND SYMPTOMS OF DIAPHYSEAL FRACTURES OF THE TIBIA AND FIBULA

The signs and symptoms associated with tibial and fibular diaphyseal fractures vary with the severity of the injury and the mechanism by which the fractures were produced. Pain is the most common symptom. Children with fractures of the tibia or fibula have swelling at the fracture site, and the area is tender to palpation. Almost all children with any type of tibia fracture will refuse to bear weight on the injured limb. If there is significant fracture displacement, a bony defect or prominence may be palpable. Immediate neurologic impairment is rare except with fibular neck fractures causing injury to the adjacent common peroneal nerve.

Although arterial disruption is uncommon in pediatric tibial and fibular diaphyseal fractures, both dorsalis pedis and the posterior tibial pulses should be assessed, and a Doppler examination should be performed if the pulses are not palpable,

or are asymmetric with the contralateral limb. Capillary refill, sensation, and pain response patterns, particularly pain with passive motion, should be monitored. Concomitant soft tissue injuries must be evaluated carefully. Bone and soft tissue injuries associated with open fractures should be treated aggressively to reduce the risk of late complications.

IMAGING AND OTHER DIAGNOSTIC STUDIES OF DIAPHYSEAL FRACTURES OF THE TIBIA AND FIBULA

Anteroposterior and lateral radiographs that include the knee and ankle joints should be obtained whenever a tibial and/or fibular shaft fracture is/are suspected. Though uncommon, tibial shaft fractures may occur in combination with transitional fractures involving the distal tibial metaphysis, and as such, close evaluation of the ankle radiographs is essential (Fig. 28-13). Comparison views of the uninvolved leg are rarely indicated. Children with suspected fractures not apparent on the initial radiographs may need treatment with supportive splinting or casting to control symptoms associated with the injuries. Periosteal new bone formation evident on plain radiographs obtained 10 to 14 days after injury confirms the diagnosis in most cases.

CLASSIFICATION OF DIAPHYSEAL FRACTURES OF THE TIBIA AND FIBULA

There is no commonly used pediatric classification system for tibia/fibular shaft fractures. Fractures are generally described based on location, fracture pattern, the direction of displacement, whether the fibula is intact, and the presence of an open injury.

OUTCOME MEASURES FOR DIAPHYSEAL FRACTURES OF THE TIBIA AND FIBULA

While there are no specific outcome measures for pediatric diaphyseal tibia and fibula fractures, the Titanium Elastic Nail (TEN) outcome scoring system (Table 28-4), initially proposed for use in pediatric femur fractures treated with TENs,[36] may be used to assess results after treatment of pediatric tibia fractures with flexible intramedullary fixation.[59,117,131] In addition, the Pediatric Outcome Data Collection Instrument (PODCI) may be used to assess functional recovery after pediatric injuries.[129]

> **TREATMENT OPTIONS FOR DIAPHYSEAL FRACTURES OF THE TIBIA AND FIBULA**

NONOPERATIVE TREATMENT OF DIAPHYSEAL FRACTURES OF THE TIBIA AND FIBULA

Indications/Contraindications

> **Nonoperative Treatment of Diaphyseal Fractures of Tibia and Fibula:** INDICATIONS AND CONTRAINDICATIONS[61]

Indications
- Nondisplaced closed fractures
- Displaced closed fractures amenable to closed reduction

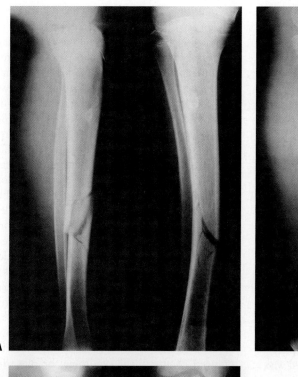

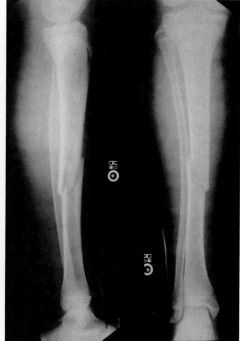

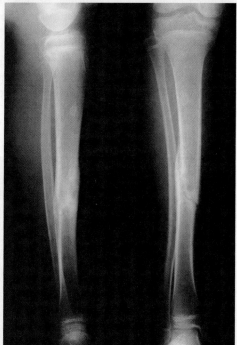

Figure 28-11. A: Anteroposterior and lateral radiograph of the lower leg in a 12-year-old child showing a comminuted tibial fracture with a concomitant plastic deformation of the fibula. Note the valgus alignment of the tibia. **B:** This patient had a closed manipulation and casting correcting the valgus alignment in the tibia and partially correcting the plastic deformation of the fibula. **C:** At union, there is an anatomic alignment of the tibia with a mild residual plastic deformation of the fibula.

Cast Immobilization

Most uncomplicated pediatric diaphyseal tibial shaft factures, with/or without associated fibular shaft fractures, can be managed with closed manipulation and casting. Displaced fractures should be managed with reduction under appropriate sedation, using fluoroscopic assistance when available. This can be done in the emergency room or in the operating room depending on the availability of sedation and fluoroscopy. An experienced assistant is extremely helpful. A reduction plan should be made before

Contraindications (Relative)
- Open fractures
- Body habitus unamenable to long-leg cast treatment
- Severe swelling with concern for compartment syndrome
- Segmental fractures
- Polytrauma
- Floating knee
- Failure to attain or maintain adequate closed reduction in a cast (Absolute)

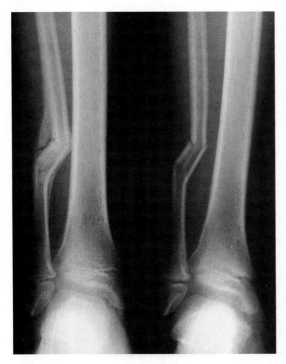

Figure 28-12. Distal one-third fibular fracture in an 8-year-old who was struck on the lateral side of the leg (*right*). There is moderate new bone formation 6 weeks after injury (*left*).

fracture pattern and alignment. The cast material is taken to the inferior aspect of the patella anteriorly and to a point 2 cm distal to the popliteal flexion crease posteriorly. It may be best to use plaster for the initial cast because of its ability to conform to the contour of the leg and the ease with which it can be manipulated while setting. The alignment of the fracture is reassessed after the short-leg cast has been applied, and the cast is then extended to the mid-thigh with the knee flexed. Others believe it is safer to apply a long-leg cast at first, to avoid the proximal edges of the short cast causing skin problems. Most children with complete, unstable diaphyseal tibial fractures are placed into a bent-knee (45-degree) long-leg cast to control rotation at the fracture site and to assist in maintaining non–weight-bearing status during the initial healing phase. The child's ankle initially may be left in some plantarflexion (20 degrees for fractures of the middle and distal thirds, 10 degrees for fractures of the proximal third) to prevent generation of apex posterior angulation (recurvatum) at the fracture site. In a child, there is little risk of developing a permanent equinus contracture, as any initial plantarflexion can be corrected at a cast change once the fracture becomes more stable. In the face of any significant swelling, regardless of the cast material used, consideration should be given to univalved or bivalved cast splitting so as to minimize the risk of cast-induced compartment syndrome, or place foam under the Webril to allow for swelling. After casting, strong consideration should be given to hospital admission for elevation and neurovascular monitoring, especially in higher-energy injuries with significant fracture displacement and/or initial swelling. Note that it is not critical to have anatomic alignment at this time, as the cast may be wedged at 7 to 14 days after some healing, and decreased swelling has taken place.

manipulation based on review of the deforming forces associated with the specific fracture pattern. In most cases, a short-leg cast is applied with the foot in the appropriate position and either a varus or valgus mold at the fracture site, depending on the

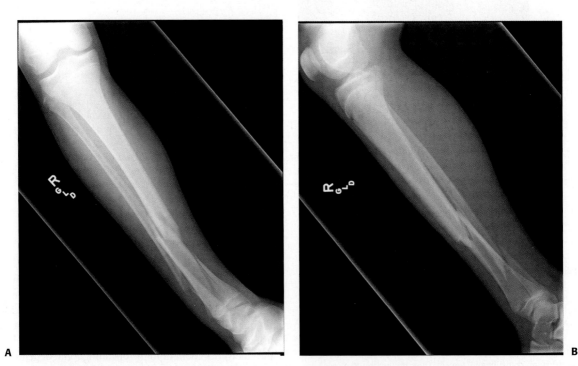

Figure 28-13. A, B: Anteroposterior and lateral radiographs of an adolescent patient with a tibial shaft fracture.

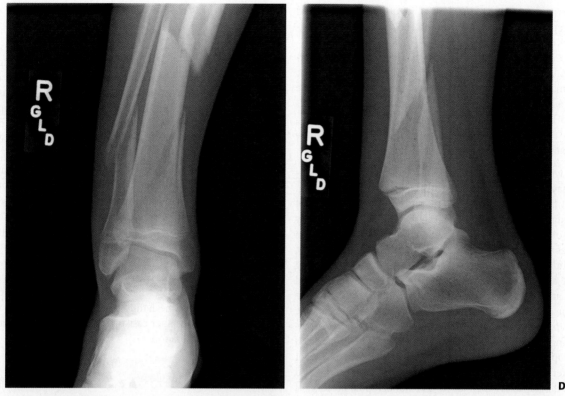

Figure 28-13. (*Continued*) **C, D:** Dedicated anteroposterior, and lateral views of the ankle demonstrate an associated Salter–Harris II distal tibia fracture.

It is important to have a discussion with the family at the initiation of care that cast treatment of tibial fractures, especially in adolescent patients, may be lengthy, will require frequent clinical and radiographic follow-up, and may need further intervention to maintain alignment. The radiographic position of the fracture should be checked weekly during the first 3 weeks after the cast has been applied. Muscle atrophy and a reduction in soft-tissue swelling may cause the fracture to drift into unacceptable alignment. Cast wedging may be performed in an attempt to improve alignment, and in some cases a second cast application with remanipulation of the fracture under sedation or anesthesia may be necessary to obtain acceptable alignment. Acceptable position is somewhat controversial and varies based on patient age as well as location and direction of the deformity.[33] Remodeling of angular deformity is limited in the tibia. No absolute numbers exist, but the following general guidelines may be beneficial in decision making (Table 28-5):

- Varus and valgus deformity in the upper and midshaft tibia remodel slowly, if at all. Up to 10 degrees of deformity can be accepted in patients less than 8 years old, and a little more than 5 degrees of angulation in those older than 8 years of age.

TABLE 28-4. TEN Outcome Scoring

	Excellent Result	Satisfactory Result	Poor Result
Leg-length inequality	<1.0 cm	<2.0 cm	>2.0 cm
Malalignment	5°	10°	>10°
Pain	None	None	Present
Complication	None	Minor and resolved	Major/lasting morbidity

Reprinted with permission from Flynn JM, Hresko T, Reynolds RA, et al. Titanium elastic nails for pediatric femur fractures: a multicenter study of early results with analysis of complications. *J Pediatr Orthop.* 2001;21(1):4–8.

TABLE 28-5. Acceptable Alignment of a Pediatric Diaphyseal Tibial Fracture

Patient Age	<8 Years	≥8 Years
Valgus	5 degrees	5 degrees
Varus	10 degrees	5 degrees
Angulation anterior	10 degrees	5 degrees
Posterior angulation	5 degrees	0 degrees
Shortening	10 mm	5 mm
Rotation	5 degrees	5 degrees

- Moderate translation of the shaft of the tibia in a young child is acceptable, whereas in an adolescent, at least 50% apposition is recommended.
- Up to 10 degrees of apex anterior angulation may be tolerated, although remodeling is slow.
- Minimal apex posterior angulation (recurvatum) may be accepted.
- Up to 1 cm of shortening is acceptable.

Cast Wedging

Patients with a loss of fracture reduction and unacceptable angulation may benefit from repeated manipulation of the fracture. This can be attempted in the clinic setting through the use of cast "wedging." Fracture alignment in the cast can be altered by creation of a closing wedge, an opening wedge, or a combination of wedges without the need for repeated sedation. Unfortunately, this technique is labor intensive and has become something of a lost art. The location for wedge placement is determined by evaluating the child's leg radiographically, and marking the midpoint of the tibial fracture on the outside of the cast. One should approach wedging similar to using the center of rotation of angulation (CORA) in lower extremity reconstruction. If fluoroscopy is not available, a series of paper clips are placed at 2-cm intervals on the surface of the cast and anteroposterior and lateral radiographs are then taken. The radiographic position of the paper clips will help define the location of the fracture and the site most suitable for placement of the wedge.

Opening Wedge Technique

The side of the cast opposite the apex of the fracture is cut perpendicular to the long axis of the bone. A small segment of the cast is left intact directly over the apex of the malaligned fracture (~25%). A cast spreader is used to spread the cast open in a controlled manner. Pre-made and measured plastic shims (Fig. 28-14) or a stack of tongue depressors of the appropriate size are placed into the open segment to maintain the distraction of the site, and the cast is wrapped with new casting material after the alignment has been assessed radiographically (Fig. 28-15). It is imperative that the edges of any shims or wedging material added do not protrude into the cast padding or cause pressure on the underlying skin. This wedging technique effectively lengthens the tibia while correcting the malalignment (Fig. 28-16).

After any cast wedging, especially early after injury when there may be residual leg swelling, it is recommended to observe the patient for a period of time to be certain that signs and symptoms of compartment syndrome do not develop. Cast wedging may be somewhat painful, but any discomfort should subside quickly. The family should be alerted that if increasing pain develops after cast wedging, the patient should return urgently for evaluation.

Closing Wedge Technique

Closing wedge technique is generally not recommended as it shortens the fracture and can pinch soft tissues.

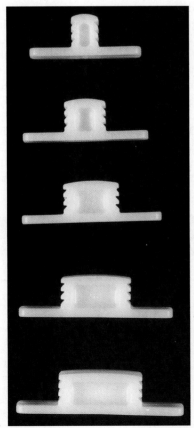
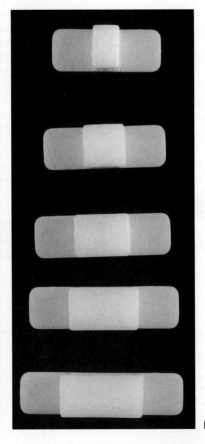

Figure 28-14. A, B: Blocks used to hold casts open after wedge corrections of malaligned fractures. The wings on the blocks prevent the blocks from migrating toward the skin.

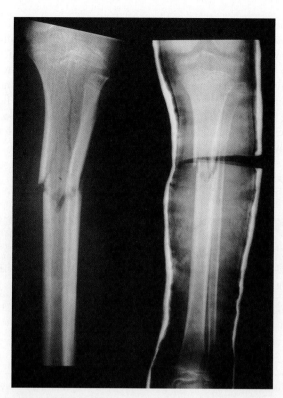

Figure 28-15. Comminuted fracture of the tibia and fibula in a 12-year-old boy struck by a car (**left**). Notice the extension of the fracture into the metaphysis from the diaphyseal injury. The fracture is in a valgus alignment. The fracture could not be maintained in an acceptable alignment. The cast was wedged with excellent result (**right**).

Outcomes of Nonoperative Treatment of Diaphyseal Fractures of the Tibia and Fibula

The length of immobilization varies with the child's age and the type of fracture. Hoaglund and States[63] reported that in 43 closed fractures in children, the average time in a cast was 2.5 months (range, 1.5 to 5.5 months). Prolonged immobilization (>3 months) may be necessary for some fractures, especially in the adolescent population.[62]

Rates of success of cast treatment of pediatric tibial fractures range from 60% to 96%.[62,83] The wide variation in success may be related to the level of experience in the art of casting and resources available in clinic to mold and wedge casts. The need for a cast wedge or cast change to maintain alignment occurred in 21% of a series of adolescent patients, but nonoperative management has been found to be safe and effective in treating 96% of closed pediatric tibial fractures.[62,79]

Few children with a tibial fracture require extensive rehabilitation beyond basic crutch or walker training. Most children limp with an out-toeing rotation gait on the involved extremity for several weeks to a month after the cast is removed. This is secondary to muscle weakness, joint stiffness, and a tendency to circumduct the limb during swing phase, rather than malalignment or malrotation of the fracture. As the muscle atrophy and weakness resolve, the limp improves. Knee range-of-motion exercises and quadriceps strengthening may be useful in an older child progressing from a bent-knee cast to weight bearing on a short-leg cast. The child may return to sports when the fracture is healed and the patient has regained strength and function comparable to that of the uninjured leg.

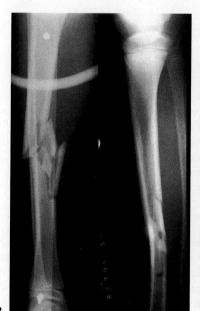
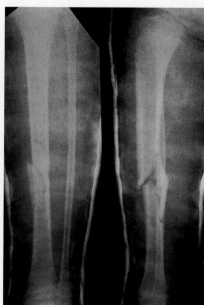
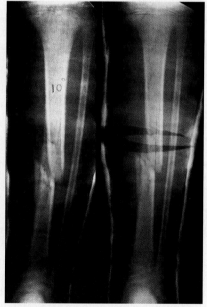

A, B

C

Figure 28-16. A: Anteroposterior and lateral tibial radiographs of an 11-year-old boy who was struck by an automobile, sustaining a markedly comminuted tibial fracture without concomitant fibular fracture. **B:** Despite the comminution, length and alignment were maintained in a cast. **C:** The patient's fracture shifted into a varus malalignment that measured 10 degrees (**right**). The cast was wedged, resulting in the reestablishment of an acceptable coronal alignment (**left**).

(continues)

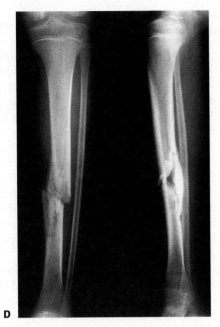

Figure 28-16. (*Continued*) **D:** The patient's fracture healed without malunion.

OPERATIVE TREATMENT OF DIAPHYSEAL FRACTURES OF THE TIBIA AND FIBULA

Indications/Contraindications

Surgical Stabilization of Diaphyseal Tibia Fractures:
INDICATIONS

Absolute Indications
• Failure to attain or maintain adequate closed reduction

Relative Indications
• Open fracture
   • Fracture associated with significant soft tissue injury
   • Fracture associated with compartment syndrome
   • Floating knee
• Segmental Fractures
   • Fracture associated with closed head injury and/or polytrauma
• Fractures in large, obese children that may be difficult to control in a cast
• Patients for whom external circumferential immobilization may be contraindicated

Historically, operative treatment has been recommended infrequently for tibial shaft fractures in children. In 1980, Weber et al.[157] reported that only 29 (4.5%) of 638 pediatric tibial fractures in their study required surgical intervention. However, there has been increasing interest in surgical stabilization, particularly for unstable closed tibial shaft fractures as well as open fractures or those with associated soft tissue injuries. The current relative indications for operative treatment include open fractures, most fractures with an associated compartment syndrome, some fractures in children with spasticity (head injury or cerebral palsy), fractures in which open treatment facilitates nursing care (floating knee, multiple long

bone fractures, multiple system injuries), and unstable fractures in which adequate alignment cannot be either attained or maintained (see Table 28-3).[7,15,27,34,39,50,68,80] Common methods of fixation for tibial fractures undergoing operative treatment include percutaneous metallic pins, bioabsorbable pins,[13] external fixation,[1,28,105] and plates with screws; the use of flexible intramedullary titanium or stainless steel nails or, in some cases, intramedullary Steinmann pins, is becoming increasingly common.[40,45,47,89,105,111,124,130,153]

Flexible Intramedullary Nails

Preoperative Planning

✔ **Flexible Intramedullary Nailing of Diaphyseal Tibial Fractures:** PREOPERATIVE PLANNING CHECKLIST	
OR table	☐ Radiolucent
Position/positioning aids	☐ Supine ☐ Bump under the ipsilateral hip to rotate leg to neutral ☐ Folded blankets or foam positioner (ramp or wedge)
Fluoroscopy location	☐ Contralateral side of operative extremity
Equipment	☐ Flexible nail implants and instrumentation (commercially available) ☐ Femoral distractor available or adequate assistance for intraoperative traction
Tourniquet	☐ Nonsterile at thigh level but do not elevate unless necessary
(Other)	☐ Preoperative antibiotics ☐ General anesthesia with adequate muscle relaxation

Positioning

The patient is positioned supine on a radiolucent table with a bump under the ipsilateral hip to maintain the leg in neutral rotation. Additional soft tissue bumps or commercially available foam ramps or triangles are also helpful to elevate and stabilize the operative leg above the nonoperative leg, and to assist in obtaining lateral fluoroscopy images. Fluoroscopy is positioned perpendicular to the limb adjacent to the contralateral extremity.

Surgical Approach

Intramedullary fixation is performed most commonly in children using stainless steel or titanium elastic nails. In most cases, the implants are placed in a proximal to distal fashion from medial and lateral proximal insertion points, although there are reports of successful management with insertion of two implants through a single insertion site.[23] Retrograde fixation through the medial malleolus may be used in rare instances because of soft tissue injuries about the planned proximal insertion sites or very proximal shaft fractures that preclude proximal entry points. When performing flexible nail fixation, fluoroscopy is used to localize the medial and lateral entry points for the

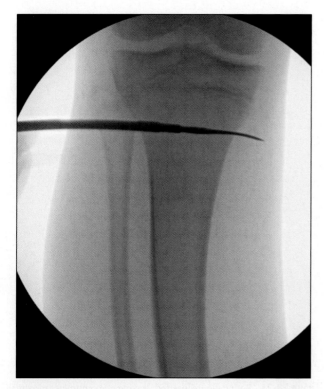

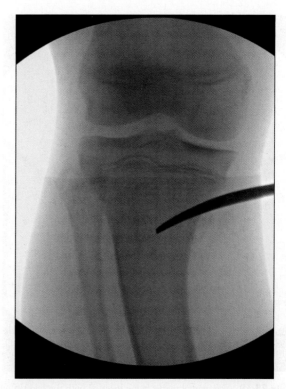

Figure 28-17. Fluoroscopy is used to localize the entry point for placement of medial and lateral elastic nails.

Figure 28-18. After entering the cortex, the awl is directed distally in the metaphysis.

elastic nails at the level of the tibial tubercle (Fig. 28-17). The skin incision must extend proximally 2 to 3 cm to prevent skin injury during insertion of nails. Medially, the bony entry point is easily found due to its subcutaneous nature. Laterally, dissection proceeds through the anterolateral musculature down to bone. Dissection should be limited distally and posteriorly so as to avoid the branches of the peroneal nerve. Care must be taken to avoid injury to the proximal tibial physes, including the tibial tubercle apophysis.

Technique

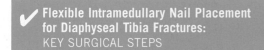

Flexible Intramedullary Nail Placement for Diaphyseal Tibia Fractures:
KEY SURGICAL STEPS

☐ Pre-select size of flexible nails based on canal size at isthmus
☐ Supine position with ipsilateral bump on a radiolucent table
☐ Prep extremity toes-to-thigh tourniquet
☐ Have adequate soft blanket bumps or knee triangle available
☐ Medial and lateral proximal tibial incisions—do not violate periochondral ring
☐ Distal aspect of incision at the point of proposed nail insertion sites
   • Starting holes medially and laterally at, or just proximal to, the level of tibial tubercle. Use drill or awl
☐ Contour flexible nails to allow maximum balanced spread at the level of the fracture site
☐ Pass nails to fracture site. Reduce fracture with traction and manipulation
☐ Pass nails into distal metaphysis. Ensure fracture does not distract
   • Check lateral view on C-arm. Rotate nails as necessary to minimize possible recurvatum deformity

Selection of nail diameter should be based on a target of 60% to 80% total canal fill at the isthmus. Two nails of equal diameter and identical material should be selected; placement of differently sized nails or nail of different metallurgy will lead to unbalanced fixation. Care should be taken to ensure that the entry points are distal enough to avoid the physes. Either an awl or a power drill may be used to enter the intramedullary canal. The drill should be at least 1 mm larger than the selected nail. Begin the drill or awl perpendicular to the long axis of the tibia until the cortex is engaged. The drill or awl should then be directed distally bevel the starting site so as to facilitate insertion of the nail into the canal (Fig. 28-18). The opposite cortex should not be violated with the drill or awl.

Many commercially available nails have a "ski tip" or spatulated end. Keeping the rounded portion of the end against the far cortex prevents perforation during nail insertion (Fig. 28-19). Once the nails are advanced to the level of the fracture site, the fracture is reduced, and one nail is advanced just past the fracture. The second nail is then advanced across the fracture site before both nails are driven farther into the distal fragment (Fig. 28-20). Alternatively, one nail may be advanced all the way, then the surgeon may start placing the second nail. Each nail is then advanced to a point approximately 1 cm proximal to the desired final distal position (Fig. 28-21). The nails are cut as close to the bone as possible, then a tamp is used to advance the nails to their final position, taking care to stay proximal to the distal tibia physis (Fig. 28-22). If removal of the nails is anticipated after healing, leave enough length of flexible nail to simplify future retrieval. External splinting or short leg casting is commonly used to supplement stability.

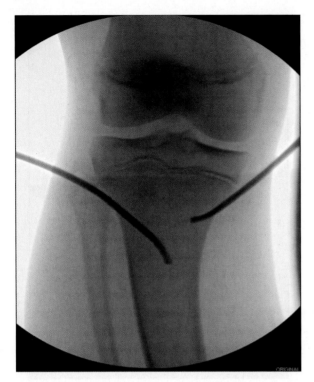

Figure 28-19. The medial nail is being inserted with the "ski tip" end rotated so that perpendicular to the entry site. The already inserted lateral nail has been rotated 180 degrees so that the rounded portion can glide along the far cortex during advancement.

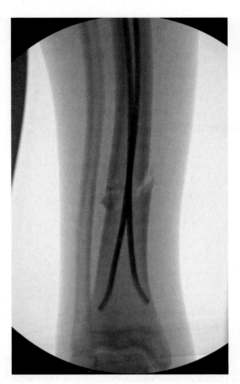

Figure 28-21. Both nails are inserted, leaving one centimeter proximal to the physis.

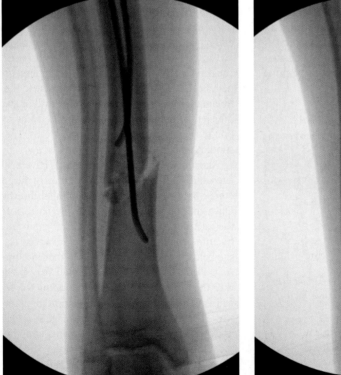

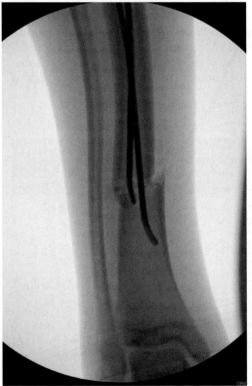

Figure 28-20. A: The medial nail is carefully inserted across the fracture site. **B:** The lateral nail is rotated to allow passage across the fracture site, then will be derotated to direct the tip laterally into the distal fragment.

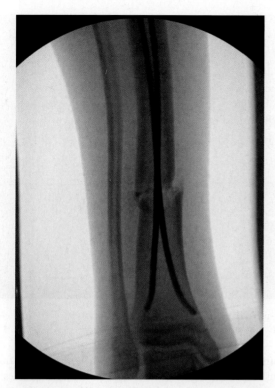

Figure 28-22. Nails have been cut close to the skin at the proximal entry point, then a tamp used to seat the distal end, taking care to not violate to the physis.

External Fixation

Preoperative Planning

✔ External Fixation of Diaphyseal Tibia Fractures: PREOPERATIVE PLANNING CHECKLIST	
OR table	❑ Radiolucent
Position/positioning aids	❑ Supine ❑ Bump under the ipsilateral hip to rotate leg to neutral ❑ Folded blankets or foam positioner (ramp or wedge) to allow slight knee flexion
Fluoroscopy location	❑ Ipsilateral side of operative extremity
Equipment	❑ Large external fixator set
Tourniquet	❑ Nonsterile at thigh level but do not inflate unless necessary
(Other)	❑ Preoperative antibiotics ❑ General anesthesia with adequate muscle relaxation

Positioning

Positioning is identical to positioning for flexible nail placement, but the fluoroscopy unit should be positioned on the ipsilateral side of the injured extremity. This is done so as to allow placement of the external fixation pins with a minimum of obstruction by the unit itself.

Surgical Approach

Knowledge of cross-sectional anatomy is crucial for safe placement of external fixation devices. The anteromedial subcutaneous border of the tibia is safest for placement of unilateral fixation pins. In addition, the lack of soft tissue coverage minimizes soft tissue movement around the pins, and thereby limits the risk of pin track infections.

Safe zones for half-pin fixation (see Fig. 28-2).

- Proximal tibia—Distal to the tibial tuberosity, over the oblique medial subcutaneous tibia shaft
- Middle tibia—Medial subcutaneous tibia shaft. The anterior tibial artery/vein and deep peroneal nerve lie along the posterolateral border of the tibia, and care should be taken that pin insertion does not violate the neurovascular bundle
- Distal tibia—Medial subcutaneous tibia. Anterior placement will jeopardize the anterior tibial artery and vein.

Technique

✔ Unilateral External Fixator for Diaphyseal Tibia Fractures: KEY SURGICAL STEPS
❑ Planned pin insertion sites marked at the level of the skin in the safe zones
❑ Two pins inserted in each of the proximal and distal fragments

❑ Conventional pins
  • Pre-drill both cortices through a trocar
  • Insert pins through a drill sleeve by hand, engage both cortices so that the pin is threaded into the far cortex but not protruding excessively

❑ Self-drilling pins/Schanz screws
  • Insert pins through a drill sleeve, advance until pin reaches the far cortex
  • Advance by hand until tip of the pin engages the inside of the far cortex

❑ Connect the two pins of each main fragment to a rod via pin-to-rod clamps
❑ Loosely connect the two rods with a third rod using rod-to-rod clamps
❑ Manually reduce the fracture and verify under fluoroscopy
❑ Tighten the rod-to-rod clamps and reconfirm reduction with fluoroscopy
❑ Add additional rods if extra stability is needed
❑ Note: In cases without use of rod-to-rod clamps, the proximal and distal-most pins are placed first to establish fracture length and then attached to a single longitudinal rod. Intermediate pins are then placed and attached to the rod. A second bar can be added to form a more rigid "double-stack" construct if desired

The most versatile and most widely available external fixation device for pediatric tibial fractures is a unilateral frame. The technique is identical to placement of a monolateral external fixator for adult tibia fractures, except for the care taken to not violate the physes, and pins are rarely placed proximal to the tibial tubercle. The unilateral frame is easy to apply and allows minor corrections in angular alignment and length. Secondary pins can be used for added support (Fig. 28-23); these are connected to the standard pins or the body of the external fixation device. This allows control of segmental fragments as needed.

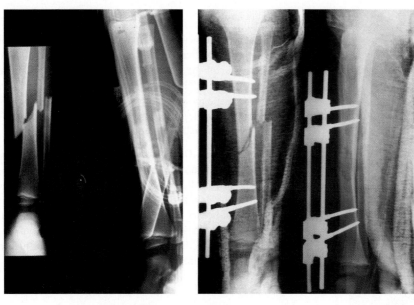
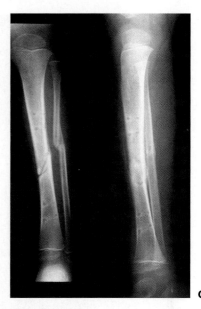

A, B   C

Figure 28-23. A, B: Type II open fracture of the tibia in a 5-year-old boy treated with debridement, unilateral external fixation, and split-thickness skin graft. **C:** Four months after removal of the external fixation.

Fracture reduction tools can be applied to the pin clamps to assist in manipulating the fracture. A small-pin or thin-wire circular frame may be indicated for complicated fractures adjacent to the joint. Unilateral frames may be placed to span an adjacent joint so as to use ligamentotaxis as an indirect reduction method to establish and maintain alignment (Fig. 28-24). An anterior frame allows for rubber bands rather than second metatarsal half-pins to prevent equinus (Fig. 28-25). While medial frames are sometimes easiest for the surgeon to apply, they may lead to

months of discomfort for the patients when they hit the frame against the other leg when walking or sleeping. If frames are placed in two parts, with the proximal and distal part connected by a separate bar (Fig. 28-26) later minor adjustments are much easier than when all pins are connected by straight bars.

Unusual fracture patterns, such as periphyseal fractures, fractures with significant bone or soft tissue loss, or fracture with delayed presentation, are appropriate candidates for multiplanar or circular external fixation.[69]

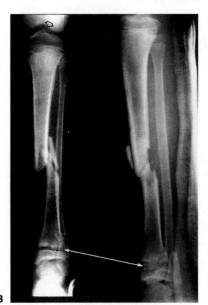
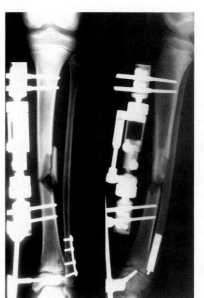
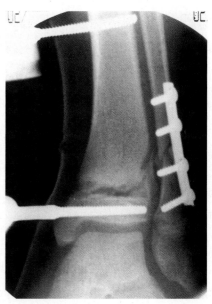

A, B   C

Figure 28-24. A: Anteroposterior and lateral radiographs of the tibia of a 12-year-old boy who was struck by a car. This child sustained a grade IIIB open middle one-third tibial fracture, a Salter–Harris type II fracture of the distal tibial physis with associated distal fibular fracture (*closed arrows*), and a tibial eminence fracture (*open arrow*). **B:** Irrigation and debridement and application of an external fixation device were performed. **C:** The fracture of distal tibial physis was stabilized with a supplemental pin attached to the external fixation device. Open reduction and internal fixation of the fibula was performed to enhance the stability of the external fixator in the distal tibia.

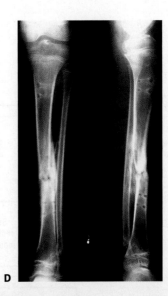

Figure 28-24. (*Continued*) **D:** Anteroposterior and lateral radiographs of the tibia approximately 9 months after injury demonstrate healing of the tibial eminence fracture, the comminuted middle one-third tibial fracture, and the distal tibial physeal fracture. The distal tibial physis remains open at this time.

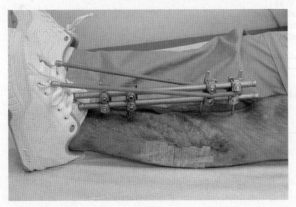

Figure 28-25. An anterior frame allows for rubber bands to prevent equinus, but care must be taken to ensure ankle dorsiflexion is not limited by the frame. (Used with permission by the Children's Orthopaedic Center, Los Angeles.)

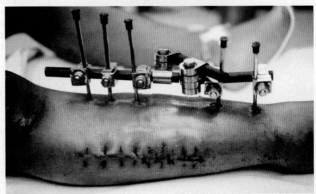

Figure 28-26. An external fixator with pins in the proximal and distal fragment independently mobile makes later adjustments much easier than if all pins are connected to a straight rod. (Used with permission by the Children's Orthopaedic Center, Los Angeles.)

Authors' Preferred Treatment of Closed Diaphyseal Fractures (Algorithm 28-2)

Simple pediatric diaphyseal tibial fractures unite quickly in most cases, and cast immobilization can be used without affecting the long-term range of motion of the knee and the ankle. A bent-knee, long-leg cast provides maximal comfort to the patient and controls rotation of the fracture fragments. The cast should be bivalved initially to limit the effect of any swelling. Children with nondisplaced or minimally displaced fractures that do not require manipulation generally are not admitted to the hospital. Children with more extensive injuries should be admitted for neurovascular observation and instruction in wheelchair, crutch, or walker use.

Significantly displaced fractures disrupt the surrounding soft tissues and produce a large hematoma in the fascial compartments of the lower leg. Circulation, sensation, and both active and passive movement of the toes should be monitored carefully after injury. The child should be admitted to the hospital, and reduction should be performed with adequate sedation and fluoroscopy if available. Most fractures are casted after reduction, and the cast may be bivalved or split to allow room for swelling. The limb should be kept elevated for 48 to 72 hours after injury to minimize swelling. The fracture should be evaluated clinically and radiographically within a week of initial manipulation to verify maintenance of the reduction. The cast can be wedged to correct minor alignment problems. Significant loss of alignment requires repeat reduction with adequate anesthesia and/or utilization of a more rigid fixation method. The long-leg cast may be changed to a short-leg, weight-bearing cast or a removable boot at 4 to 6 weeks after injury. In some cases, children over 11 years of age may transitioned to a patellar tendon-bearing cast after removal of the long-leg cast in an effort to maintain immobilization of the fracture, while limiting the potential for significant knee stiffness.[132] Weight-bearing immobilization is

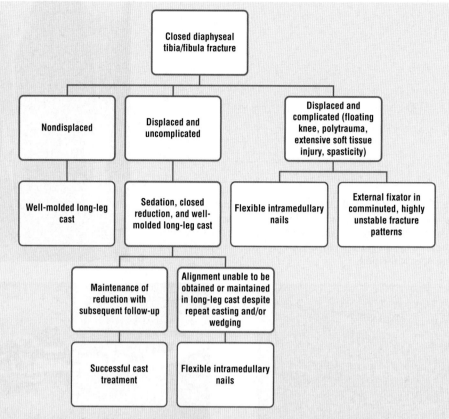

Algorithm 28-2. Authors' preferred treatment of closed diaphyseal fractures.

maintained until sufficient callus is evident and the fracture is nontender to palpation.

Fractures in patients with complicating factors—including spasticity, a floating knee, multiple long-bone fractures, an associated transitional ankle fracture, extensive soft tissue damage, multiple system injuries, or an inability to obtain or maintain an acceptable reduction—should be stabilized with a more rigid fixation method, such as external fixation or flexible intramedullary nails (Figs. 28-27 and 28-28). It is the authors' preference to use either stainless steel or titanium flexible intramedullary nails, if at all possible, in these situations. In closed fractures, external fixation is reserved for comminuted or highly unstable fracture patterns or damage control in multi-trauma.

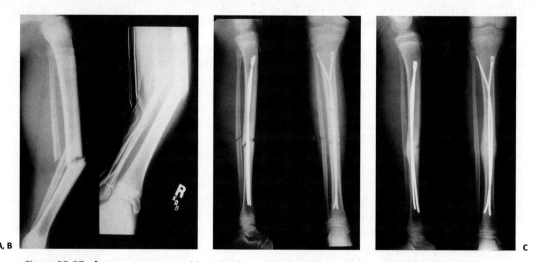

A, B   C

Figure 28-27. A: Anteroposterior and lateral radiographs of a 12-year-old who was involved in a motor vehicle accident sustaining a grade I open middle one-third tibial and fibular fractures. **B:** This injury was treated with intramedullary nail fixation. **C:** At union, the patient has an anatomic alignment and no evidence of a growth disturbance.

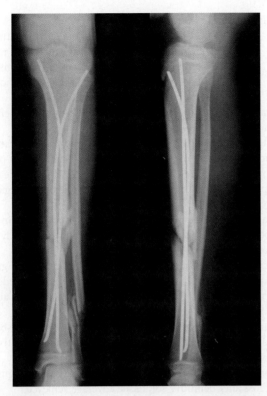

Figure 28-28. Anteroposterior radiograph of a 14-year-old who was involved in a motor vehicle accident sustaining a distal one-third tibial fracture and comminuted distal fibular fracture. This was stabilized with titanium elastic nails.

Postoperative Care

Despite surgical stabilization, many pediatric tibia fractures still require some level of external stabilization such as a cast.[44,131] Weightbearing is dependent on the pattern of fracture and stability of fixation. In general, weightbearing is allowed by 6 weeks post-injury if adequate callus is observed and the fracture is nontender.

For patients treated with external fixation, a posterior splint may be applied to help prevent the patient from developing an equinus contracture. This splint should be easy to remove for pin care and dressing changes of any associated soft tissue injury. Splinting to maintain position of the ankle and foot can be avoided by external fixation, be it unilateral or circular, to the forefoot. Routine pin care with dilute saline/hydrogen peroxide solution once or twice daily is instituted postoperative day #1.

Potential Pitfalls and Preventive Measures

Diaphyseal Fractures of the Tibia/Fibula: SURGICAL PITFALLS AND PREVENTIONS

Pitfall	Prevention
Flexible Intramedullary Nails	
• Inability to pass nails	• Pre-bend gentle curve (10 degrees) at leading end of nail
	• Decrease nail diameter
• Penetration of opposite cortex	• Orient smooth curved end of "ski tip" to bounce off opposite cortex
• Inability to reduce fracture	• Femoral distractor or qualified assistant to maintain traction
	• Open reduction
	• Anesthetic muscle relaxation
• Inability to maintain alignment after nails passed	• Contour nails for maximum spread at level of fracture
	• Balanced fixation with nails of similar size and material
External Fixation	
• Lack of stability after fixation	• Add more pins or bars
	• Plate the fibula
• Early loosening of pins	• Careful insertion technique to avoid heat necrosis
• Pin track infections	• Small skin incisions to release tension around pins and wires
	• Daily pin cleaning
• Development of delayed or pending nonunion	• Dynamize the fixator frame, increase weightbearing

Outcomes

Treatment of closed diaphyseal pediatric tibial shaft fractures remains controversial. Marengo et al. reported retrospectively on 80 closed, displaced tibial shaft fractures with intact fibulas, with 26 tibias treated by flexible intramedullary nailing and 54 tibias treated with closed reduction and casting.[95] While the surgically treated fractures had more initial displacement than those treated closed, valgus and procurvatum deformities were statistically significantly improved from injury radiographs in the flexible nailing group. In addition the small numerical differences between the surgical and casting groups were not clinically significant; however the immobilization time was significantly shorter in the surgical group. The only complication in this series was a fracture that displaced in the cast and was converted to flexible intramedullary nails.

Kubiak et al.[89] compared the use of titanium flexible nails with external fixation in a mixed group of patients with open and closed tibial fractures. Although the groups were not matched and were reviewed retrospectively, the authors reported a clinically significant decrease in time to union with titanium nails compared to external fixation. Gordon et al.[46] retrospectively reviewed 60 pediatric patients with open or closed tibial shaft fractures managed with flexible nails. They found an 18% complication rate; the most common complication was delayed union. In this study, those patients with delayed time to union tended to be older (mean age 14.1 years) versus the mean age of the study population (11.7 years). Srivastava et al.[143] reviewed a mixed group of 24 patients with open or closed tibial shaft fractures managed with titanium nails. All patients went on to union at an average of 20.4 weeks. The total complication rate was 20%, including two patients with mild sagittal plane malunions at final follow-up.

In contrast to femoral shaft fractures, studies have failed to find poorer outcomes in regard to malunion rate or time to union in use of intramedullary flexible nails in the older, heavier pediatric patient population,[44,95] although severity of injury for these patients may be higher.[5] Pandya et al. reported a 20% rate of compartment syndrome after flexible nailing of 31 pediatric closed and open tibia fractures.[120] In this series, 83% of children who were 50 kg or greater developed compartment syndrome. Overall, the authors found that pediatric patients who developed compartment syndrome after IM nailing were heavier (53 kg vs. 39 kg), were more likely to present with a neurologic injury, and more likely to have comminuted tibia fractures.[120] Despite the rising popularity of surgical stabilization, the advantages of flexible nailing over casting of pediatric tibia fractures are still unclear.[61]

Open reduction, internal fixation of pediatric tibial fractures has been demonstrated to have statistically significantly increased rates of anatomic reduction, lower rates of subsequent surgery, but longer surgical times and higher rates of wound complications when compared to flexible nailing.[122] However, both methods have high rates of union and return to activity.

There are little data that look at the outcomes of pediatric tibia fractures managed with various types of external fixation. However, when Shore et al. compared use of unilateral versus multiplanar external fixation for pediatric tibia fractures, they found no significant difference in cost or complications.[136]

There are some older pediatric patients who may be best managed with reamed or unreamed rigid tibial nails, as one would a skeletally mature adult patient. There are no reports in the literature that look specifically at which skeletal age this would be considered acceptable, and at which age the possible risk of injury to the proximal tibial physis is completely acceptable. However, the authors generally reserve these "adult style" devices for patients with a bone age of 15 years or greater, or with a radiographically closed, or closing, proximal tibial physis. Families should be warned that there is a high rate of knee pain following such tibial nails.

Open Tibial Fractures

INTRODUCTION TO OPEN TIBIAL FRACTURES

Most open tibial fractures in children involve the diaphyseal region and are treated similarly to comparable injuries in adults. In addition, these fractures and associated soft tissue injuries are classified utilizing the Gustilo and Anderson System.[53] Most open fractures of the tibia result from high-velocity/high-energy injuries.[127]

TREATMENT OPTIONS FOR OPEN TIBIAL FRACTURES

Management principles for open tibial fractures include the following:

- Initiation of appropriate antibiotic therapy immediately.

- Timely debridement and irrigation[121]
  - Consideration may be given to nonoperative treatment with irrigation and debridement in the emergency room and administration of antibiotics in select, noncontaminated, low-energy grade I open fractures,[11,42] although studies supporting this practice are underpowered.
- Fracture reduction followed by stabilization with either internal or external devices.
- Intraoperative angiography (after rapid fracture stabilization) and management of possible elevation of compartment pressures when sufficiency of the vascular perfusion is unclear.
- Open wound treatment with loose gauze packing or negative pressure dressing.[28,102]
- Staged debridement of necrotic soft tissue and bone in the operating room as needed until the wounds are ready for closure or coverage.
- Delayed closure, application of a split-thickness skin graft, or use of delayed local or free vascularized flaps as needed.
- Acute shortening when soft tissues and vascular status allow in fractures with segmental bone loss.[90]
- Cancellous bone grafting (autologous or allograft) for bone defects or delayed union after maturation of soft tissue coverage.
- Bone transport or limb lengthening in patients with segmental loss after definitive soft tissue coverage achieved.[90]

These principles are similar to those used in adult patients. However, there is evidence that differences exist between pediatric and adult fracture patients. As such, the principles of treatment for open tibial fractures in adults are altered somewhat by the unique characteristics of the pediatric skeleton. These differences include the following[7,27,45,52,142]:

- Comparable soft tissue and bony injuries heal more reliably in children than in adults, particularly in patients less than 11 years of age.[74]
- Devitalized uncontaminated bone that can be covered with soft tissue can incorporate into the fracture callus, and in some cases may be left within the wound.
- External fixation can be maintained, when necessary, until fracture consolidation with fewer concerns about delayed or nonunion than in adults.
- Retained periosteum can regenerate bone, even after segmental bone loss in younger children.
- After thorough irrigation and debridement, many uncontaminated grade I open wounds may be closed primarily without an increased risk of infection.[65,106]
- Casts may be used for definitive stabilization in select stable open tibia fractures.[20,25,65,106]

OPERATIVE TREATMENT OF OPEN TIBIAL FRACTURES

Preoperative Planning

When surgical stabilization is planned, preoperative planning for open tibia fractures is similar to the previously described techniques for flexible intramedullary nailing or external fixation of closed tibia fractures. As with all open fractures, a thorough debridement of devitalized tissue and copious irrigation with sterile saline is necessary. Adequate soft tissue coverage is a mandatory part of operative treatment of these injuries, and early involvement with appropriate teams, such as plastic surgery or microsurgery specialists, is crucial to the management strategy.

Technique

Open tibial fractures of any grade should have a thorough and expedient irrigation and debridement of the wound, although there is evidence that infection rate is similar in injuries managed at less than 6 hours after injury and those treated later.[138] There are some recent data that emergency department irrigation and debridement with administration of antibiotics may be appropriate for some simple, uncontaminated grade I open fractures.[11,42] However, the patient numbers in these studies are too small to draw meaningful conclusions. The patient's tetanus status must be determined, and prophylaxis should be administered as indicated. Appropriate intravenous antibiotic treatment is initiated as soon as possible and maintained as required based on the severity of the open fracture.

In those fractures requiring formal operative debridement, the soft tissue wounds should be extended to be certain that the area is cleansed and debrided of all nonviable tissue and foreign material. If in doubt of tissue viability, especially in younger children, leave the tissue in place and reevaluate later. Children heal much better than adults. Devitalized bone may be left in place if it is clean and can be covered by soft tissue, and this is determined on a case-by-case basis. The operative wound

extension may be closed along with the open segment in clean grade I injuries. The traumatic wound should be allowed to heal by secondary intention if there is moderate contamination after irrigation and debridement. Patients with uncomplicated grade I fractures can be placed in a splint or a cast, or simple smooth pin fixation will prevent displacement of the fracture (Fig. 28-29). Use of this limited fixation does not preclude supplemental splinting or casting. Wounds associated with grade II and III fractures are debrided of devitalized tissue and foreign material. Most children with grade II and all children with grade III wounds require more rigid fracture stabilization which aids in soft tissue coverage (Fig. 28-30). External fixation or intramedullary nails may be used at the surgeon's discretion based on fracture stability and personal experience. More rigid fixation limits the need for significant external splinting, thereby allowing better access for wound care and sequential compartment evaluation as needed.

Delayed primary closure can be performed if the wound is clean and does not involve significant skin and muscle loss. In such cases, it is imperative that closure under tension is avoided. Negative pressure dressings have been widely adopted in many trauma centers, are convenient to use and some evidence suggests they have beneficial effects on soft tissues such as less need for flap coverage[28] and decreased infection rate.[56] Flap coverage was associated with a decreased rate of infection in a review of the literature of 54 grade IIIB tibial shaft fractures in children.[41] Definitive options include a wide variety of local rotational or pedicled myocutaneous flaps. Vascularized free

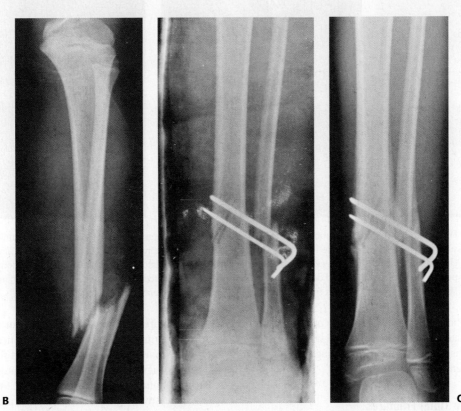

A, B   **C**

Figure 28-29. A: Anteroposterior radiograph of a grade I open distal one-third tibial fracture in a 7-year-old child. **B:** Two percutaneous pins were used to stabilize this fracture after irrigation and debridement. **C:** Good fracture callus was present and the pins were removed 4 weeks after injury.

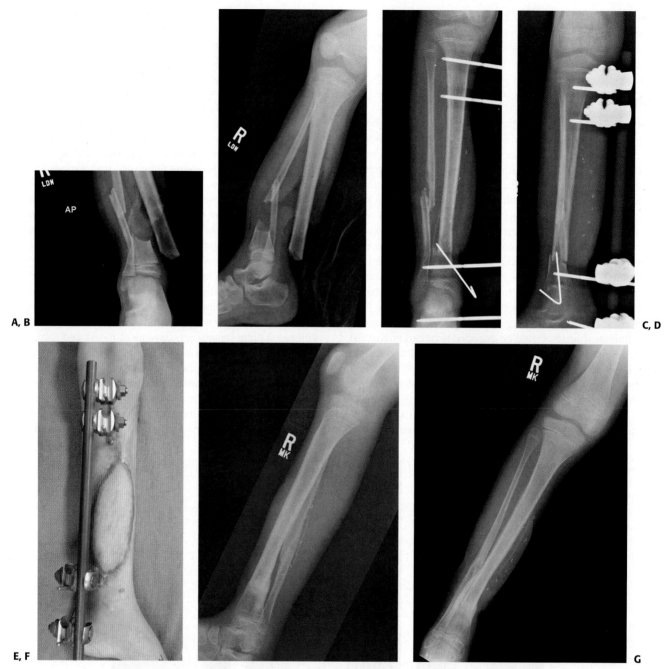

Figure 28-30. A and **B:** Anteroposterior and lateral radiographs of a grade IIIB open tibia/fibula fractures sustained by a 9-year-old male in an agricultural accident. **C–E:** Anteroposterior/lateral radiographs, and clinical image of a patient 8 weeks after placement of spanning monolateral external fixator with additional percutaneous pin fixation, and delayed coverage with anterior thigh free flap. **F** and **G:** Anteroposterior and lateral radiographs of a patient 9 months post injury. Patient had excellent clinical result.

flaps are viable options in cases for which no other method of closure is appropriate. In cases with segmental bone loss as well as significant soft tissue injury, acute shortening with plans for subsequent lengthening has been successful.[90]

Outcomes of Open Tibial Fractures

Kreder and Armstrong[88] found an average time to union of 5.4 months (range, 1.5 to 24.8 months) in a series of 56 open tibial fractures in 55 children. The factor with the most effect on union time was the age of the patient. Grimard et al.[52] reported that the age of the patient and the grade of the fracture were significantly associated with union time. Blasier and Barnes[14] found that children under 12 years of age required less aggressive surgical treatment and healed more rapidly than older children. They also found that younger children were more resistant to infection and had fewer complications than older children.

Buckley et al.[20] reported on 41 children with 42 open fractures of the tibia (18 grade II, 6 grade IIIA, 4 grade IIIB, and 2 grade IIIC). Twenty-two (52%) of the fractures were comminuted. All wounds were irrigated and debrided, and antibiotics were administered for at least 48 hours. Twenty-two fractures were treated with reduction and cast application, and 20 with external fixation. Three children had early infections, and one of these patients developed late osteomyelitis. All infections had resolved at final reported follow-up. The average time to union was 5 months (range, 2 to 21 months), and was directly proportional to the severity of the soft tissue injury. Fracture pattern also had an effect on time to union. Segmental bone loss, infection, and the use of an external fixation device were associated with delayed union. Four angular malunions of more than 10 degrees occurred, three of which spontaneously corrected. Four children had more than 1 cm of overgrowth.

In a series of 40 open lower extremity diaphyseal fractures in 35 children, Cramer et al.[25] reported 22 tibial fractures (1 grade I, 10 grade II, and 11 grade III). External fixation was used for 15 fractures, casting for 5, and internal fixation for 2. Two children required early amputation, 4 required soft tissue flap coverage, and 13 children had skin grafts. Two additional children with initially closed injuries required fasciotomy for compartment syndrome and were included in the group of open tibial fractures. Ten of the 24 injuries healed within 24 weeks. Five children required bone grafting before healing.

Hope and Cole[65] reported the results of open tibial fractures in 92 children (22 grade I, 51 grade II, and 19 grade III). Irrigation and debridement were performed on admission, intravenous (IV) antibiotics were given for 48 hours, and tetanus prophylaxis was administered when necessary. Primary closure was performed in 51 children, and 41 traumatic wounds were left open. Eighteen soft tissue injuries healed secondarily, and 23 required either a split thickness skin graft or a tissue flap. Sixty-five (71%) of the 92 fractures were reduced and immobilized in an above-the-knee plaster cast. External fixation was used for unstable fractures, injuries with significant soft tissue loss, and fractures in patients with multiple system injuries. Early complications of open tibial fractures in these children were comparable with those in adults. Primary closure did not increase the risk of infection if the wound was small and uncontaminated. At reevaluation 1.5 to 9.8 years after injury, the authors found that 50% of the patients complained of pain at the fracture site; 23% reported decreased abilities to participate in sports, joint stiffness, and cosmetic defects; and 64% had leg-length inequalities. Levy et al.[92] found comparable late sequelae after open tibial fractures in children, including a 25% prevalence of nightmares surrounding the events of the accident. Blasier and Barnes[14] and Song et al.[142] found that most late complications associated with pediatric open tibial fractures occurred in children over the age 12 and 11 years, respectively.

Skaggs et al.[139] reviewed their experience with open tibial fractures and found no increased incidence of infection in patients initially debrided more than 6 hours after injury when compared to children treated similarly less than 6 hours after fracture. However, it appears that fractures with more severe soft tissue injuries were more likely to receive more expedient treatment, thereby complicating the analysis. This apparent selection bias in some ways limits the overall usefulness of the study.

Most recently, in a 2017 report of pediatric open tibia fractures, Nandra et al. reported on 61 pediatric open tibial fractures with a mean age of 9 years, who were treated with a variety of fixation and wound management methods.[106] Increasing Gustilo-Anderson classification and age greater than 12 years of age were statistically associated with longer union time. Two of the three deep infections occurred in patients who underwent open plate fixation. Nine patients required revision of their monolateral external fixator to a multiplanar fixator due to delayed union or unacceptable alignment.

Some published reports highlight concerns about the use of external fixators in open tibia fractures in pediatric patients. Myers et al.[105] reviewed 31 consecutive high-energy tibia fractures in children treated with external fixation. Nineteen of the fractures were open, with mean follow-up of 15 months. The authors found a high rate of complications in this patient population, including delayed union (particularly in patients of at least 12 years of age), malunion, leg-length discrepancy, and pin tract infections. However, Monsell et al. reported no nonunions and no complications in a group of 10 pediatric patients with open diaphyseal tibia fractures managed with a programmable circular external fixator. In addition, they had no patients with deep infection, nor were there any cases of refracture after fixator removal.[101]

When comparing a cohort of 14 patients who underwent immediate intramedullary flexible nailing of open tibial shaft to a group of 12 patients having flexible nailing of closed tibial shaft fractures, Pandya and Edmonds reported similar low wound and infectious complications, although bone healing was delayed in patients with Gustilo 2 or 3 injuries.[119] Compartment syndrome risk was high in both groups (open = 14%, closed = 17%), and systemic complications were noted in two patients with closed head injuries. To date, there are no published studies which directly and prospectively compare the use of flexible intramedullary nails with external fixation for open pediatric tibial shaft fractures.

While used infrequently, plating of pediatric tibia fractures has been reported. One series of 14 open pediatric tibial fractures treated with limited-contact places in minimally invasive percutaneous osteosynthesis reported mean union time of 18 weeks (range, 11 to 32 weeks) and no infections.[116] Supracutaneous plates with locking screws in lieu of traditional external fixation has also been described.[125]

The vast majority of the literature addressing the subject of soft tissue coverage for open tibia fractures involves adult patients, and they may be relevant to the skeletally mature, but less relevant to young children with better healing potential.

Multiple authors have reported on the use of negative pressure dressings in the management of soft tissue injuries in pediatric patients. Dedmond et al.[28] reviewed the Wake Forest experience with negative pressure dressings in pediatric patients with type III open tibia fractures. They found that use of this device decreased the need for free tissue transfer to obtain coverage in this patient population. When focusing on the rate of infection, Halvorson et al.[56] found that use of negative pressure dressings in the management of open fractures, including open tibia fractures, appeared to be safe and effective when compared to historical controls. A recent literature review of adults with open tibial fractures concluded negative pressure dressings applied immediately after the first debridement, seems to be an optimal bridge to the final reconstruction up to 7 days.[22] It has been our experience that negative pressure dressings have little downside other than skin irritation and may be used to speed up healing by secondary intention.

MANAGEMENT OF EXPECTED ADVERSE OUTCOMES AND UNEXPECTED COMPLICATIONS RELATED TO DIAPHYSEAL FRACTURES OF THE TIBIA AND FIBULA

It is uncommon to have poor outcomes or complications related to nonoperative treatment of closed tibial shaft fractures, as long as the appropriate radiographic follow-up and need for subsequent cast adjustment is respected. The majority of complications in pediatric tibial shaft fractures are most related to open fractures.

Diaphyseal Fractures of the Tibia and Fibula:
COMMON ADVERSE OUTCOMES AND COMPLICATIONS

- Compartment syndrome
- Vascular injuries
- Infection
- Angular deformity
- Malrotation
- Leg-length discrepancy
- Anterior tibial physeal closure
- Delayed union and nonunion

COMPARTMENT SYNDROME

Compartment syndrome may occur after any type of tibia fracture, ranging from a seemingly minor closed injury to a severe, comminuted fracture. In addition, it is important to remember that compartment syndrome may occur in the face of significant soft tissue injury associated with extensively open fractures, as well as with closed injuries and after tibia fracture stabilization. Shore et al. reported an 11.6% incidence of compartment syndrome in 216 tibial shaft fractures; multivariable predictors included 14 years of age and older and motor vehicle accidents.[137] Compartment syndrome rates after flexible nailing of pediatric tibial fractures range from 2% to 20% and may be associated with larger, obese children.[44,120] However, these cohorts included open tibia fractures, which sustained higher-energy injuries that were potentially more displaced with more soft tissue injury and therefore more biased toward complications.

Diagnosis

Close observation and elevation of these affected limb, whether the fracture was treated with casting or surgical stabilization, is necessary in all patients with displaced tibia fractures. It is crucial to monitor soft tissue swelling, pain escalation, and

neurovascular examinations. In pediatric patients, this should be carefully scrutinized for the first 24 to 48 hours after treatment. Patients with a compartment syndrome often complain of pain out of proportion to the apparent severity of the injury. Increasing pain, often noted as continually increasing analgesic requirements, is the most important early sign of potential compartment syndrome in children.[6] In addition, pain with passive range of motion appears to be an early and strong clinical finding. Hyperesthesia, motor deficits, and decreased pulses are late changes and denote significant tissue injury. These signs occur only after the ischemia has been well established and the injury is permanent.[77,158] Late complications of untreated lower extremity compartment syndrome include clawed toes, dorsal bunion, and limited subtalar motion secondary to necrosis and subsequent fibrous contracture of the muscles originating in the deep posterior compartment.[77]

Treatment

Any cast or splint should be bivalved, split or otherwise loosened, and the cast padding divided, in a patient with increased or increasing pain associated with treatment of a tibia fracture. If, after removal of all encircling wraps, there is no relief, compartment syndrome should be considered. Compartment pressures may be obtained, but in most cases pediatric patients with clinical findings consistent with elevated pressures should undergo surgical release. Any child who has objective or subjective evidence of a compartment syndrome should undergo an emergent fasciotomy. Although, there is some controversy in the literature, if compartmental pressure monitoring is utilized, symptomatic patients with compartment pressures greater than 30 mm Hg may benefit from fasciotomy.[72,144,158]

The two-incision technique is used most widely for fasciotomies, although a single incision, perifibular release is favored at some centers (Fig. 28-31).[97,98] The fascia surrounding each compartment of concern should be opened widely. The wounds are left open and delayed primary closure is performed when possible. Negative pressure wound dressings may be of benefit in the management of fasciotomy wounds before closure or coverage. Split thickness skin grafting of the wounds may be necessary in some cases. Fibulectomy has been recommended by some authors as a method by which all compartments can be released through a single approach. Most literature does not support its use, and this procedure should not be performed in skeletally immature patients due to the risk of potential proximal migration of the distal fibular remnant and resulting ankle valgus. Long-term ankle valgus may result in ankle instability, gait impairment, and potentially problematic limb length discrepancy.

In a long-term review of patients from the Children's Hospital of Philadelphia, Flynn et al. found that most children with lower extremity compartment syndrome, including those associated with tibia fractures, had good or excellent clinical results. This appeared to be true even in those patients with long time periods from injury to fasciotomy.[35] Shore et al. reported that full functional recovery was achieved in 92% of patients with tibial compartment syndrome, and there was one below knee amputation in their cohort of 25 cases.[137]

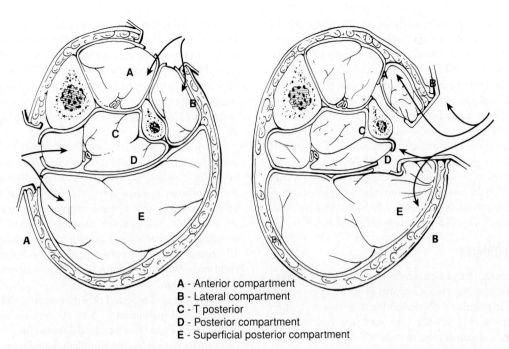

A - Anterior compartment
B - Lateral compartment
C - T posterior
D - Posterior compartment
E - Superficial posterior compartment

Figure 28-31. A: Decompressive fasciotomies through a two-incision approach. The anterior lateral incision allows decompression of the anterior and lateral compartments. The medial incision allows decompression of the superficial posterior and the deep posterior compartments. **B:** A one-incision decompression fasciotomy can be performed through a lateral approach that allows a dissection of all four compartments.

VASCULAR INJURIES

Vascular injuries associated with tibial fractures are uncommon in children; however, when they do occur, the sequelae can be devastating. In an evaluation of 14 patients with lower extremity fractures and concomitant vascular injuries, Allen et al.[2] noted that only three children returned to normal function. One factor leading to a poor outcome was a delay in diagnosis. Evaluation for vascular compromise is imperative in all children with tibial fractures.

The displaced proximal tibial metaphyseal fracture is the pattern of injury most frequently associated with vascular injury, and often involves the anterior tibial artery as it passes between the fibula and the tibia into the anterior compartment.[54,64] The anterior tibial artery may be injured with distal tibial fractures, as the vessel may be injured if the distal fragment translates posteriorly. Posterior tibial artery injuries are rare, except in fractures associated with crushing or shearing caused by accidents involving heavy machinery, or those secondary to gunshot wounds involving the lower leg and ankle region.

Vascular injuries have been reported in approximately 5% of children with open tibial fractures. Arterial injuries associated with open tibial fractures include those to the popliteal artery, the posterior tibial artery, the anterior tibial artery, and the peroneal artery. Amputation rates as high as 79% have been reported with grade IIIC fractures. Isolated anterior tibial and peroneal artery injuries generally have a good prognosis, whereas injuries of the posterior tibial and popliteal arteries have much less satisfactory prognoses, and more commonly require vascular repairs or reconstructions.[2,54,64] Patients with open tibial fractures and vascular disruption may benefit from temporary arterial, and possibly venous, shunting before the bony reconstruction is performed. This approach allows meticulous debridement and repair of the fracture, while maintaining limb perfusion until the primary vascular repair is performed.[39] However, in most cases, rapid fracture stabilization, usually using external fixation, can be performed before vascular reconstruction without the need for temporary shunts.

INFECTION

The risk of infection in treatment of pediatric tibial diaphyseal fractures is mainly isolated to open tibial shaft fractures and is at highest risk in those with grade III injuries.[138] The best treatment is prevention with timely intravenous antibiotic administration, timely irrigation and debridement, repeated debridements as needed, and early soft tissue coverage. Surgical stabilization of the fracture protects that soft tissue and can reduce infection risk.

Prolonged wound healing, continued drainage, delayed fracture union, and hardware failure may all be signs of infection. Laboratory values may be normal in low grade, chronic infections, and intraoperative bone biopsy and culture are sometimes needed to establish the diagnosis of osteomyelitis. As in any treatment of osteomyelitis, initial surgical treatment includes debridement of involved bone and nonviable soft tissue as well as removal of any loose or broken retained implants. A spanning external fixator device placed through noninfected areas maintains bony stabilization to allow fracture healing in cases of nonunion. Antibiotics are tailored to intraoperative bony culture results, and soft tissue coverage options include local wound care, negative pressure dressings, skin grafts, or local or free soft tissue flaps.

Ostermann et al. reported 115 grade II and 239 grade III tibial fractures in a series of 1,085 open fractures. All patients were treated with early broad-spectrum antibiotics, serial debridements, and the application of an external fixation device. Tobramycin-impregnated polymethylmethacrylate (PMMA) was placed into the wounds, and dressings were changed every 48 to 72 hours until the wounds spontaneously closed, underwent delayed primary closure, or received flap coverage. No infections occurred in grade I fractures; approximately 3% of grade II fractures and 8% of grade III fractures developed infections. No infections occurred in patients who had the wound closed within 8 days of injury. On the basis of these and other analyses, it is now recommended that wounds associated with open tibial fractures be covered within 7 days of injury whenever possible.[114,154]

ANGULAR DEFORMITY

Spontaneous correction of significant axial displacement after a diaphyseal fracture of a child's forearm or femur is common. Remodeling of an angulated tibial shaft fracture, however, often is often incomplete (Fig. 28-32).[16] As such, the goal of treatment should be to obtain as close to anatomic alignment as possible. Swaan and Oppers[148] evaluated 86 children treated for

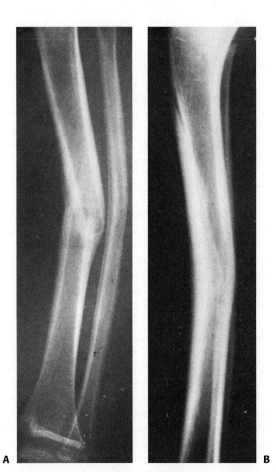

Figure 28-32. A 4-year 2-month-old child with a middle one-third transverse tibial fracture and a plastically deformed fibular fracture. **A:** Lateral view shows 20-degree posterior angulation. **B:** The deformity is still 15 degrees 4 years after the injury.

fractures of the tibia. The original angulation of the fracture was measured on radiographs in the sagittal and frontal projections. Girls 1 to 8 years of age and boys 1 to 10 years of age demonstrated moderate spontaneous correction of residual angulation after union. In girls 9 to 12 years of age and boys 11 to 12 years of age, approximately 50% of the angulation was corrected. No more than 25% of the deformity was corrected in children over 13 years of age.

Bennek and Steinert[12] found that recurvatum malunion of more than 10 degrees did not correct completely. In this study, 26 of 28 children with varus or valgus deformities at union had significant residual angular deformities at follow-up. Valgus deformities had a worse outcome because the tibiotalar joint was left in a relatively unstable position. Weber et al.[157] demonstrated that a fracture with varus malalignment of 5 to 13 degrees completely corrected at the level of the physis. Most children with valgus deformities of 5 to 7 degrees did not have a full correction.

Hansen et al.[58] reported on 102 pediatric tibial fractures, 25 of which had malunions of 4 to 19 degrees. Residual angular malunions ranged from 3 to 19 degrees at final follow-up, without a single patient having complete remodeling and correction. The spontaneous correction was approximately 13.5% of the total deformity. Shannak[134] reviewed the results of treatment of 117 children with tibial shaft fractures treated with closed reduction and long-leg casts. Multiplanar deformities did not remodel as completely as those in a single plane. The least correction occurred in apex posterior angulated fractures, followed by fractures with valgus malalignment (Fig. 28-33). Spontaneous remodeling of malunited tibial fractures in children appears to be limited to the first 18 months after fracture.[31,58]

MALROTATION

Rotational malalignment of the tibia does not correct spontaneously with remodeling and should be avoided.[58] A computerized tomographic (CT) evaluation of tibial rotation can be performed if there is any question about the rotational alignment of the fracture that is not evident on clinical examination.

Rotational malunion of more than 20 to 30 degrees may produce functional impairment and may necessitate a subsequent derotational osteotomy of the tibia, though this is quite rare. Most commonly, derotational osteotomy of the tibia is performed in the supramalleolar aspect of the distal tibia. The fibula may be left intact, particularly for planned derotation of less than 30 degrees. Maintaining continuity of the fibula adds stability and limits the possibility of introducing an iatrogenic angular deformity to the distal tibia.

LEG-LENGTH DISCREPANCY

Hyperemia associated with fracture repair may stimulate the physes in the involved leg, producing growth acceleration, particularly in younger children. Tibial growth acceleration after fracture is less than that seen after femoral fractures in children of comparable ages. Shannak[134] showed that the average growth acceleration of a child's tibia after fracture is approximately 4.5 mm. Comminuted fractures appear to have the greatest risk of accelerated growth and overgrowth.

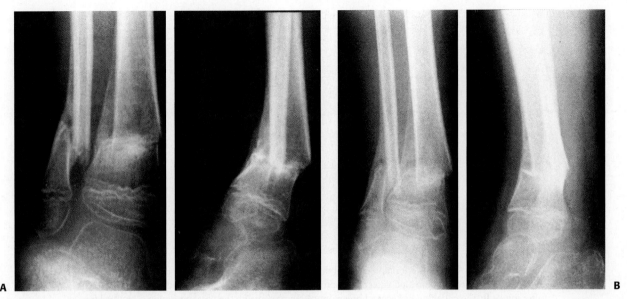

Figure 28-33. A: Anteroposterior and lateral radiographs 2 months after injury in a 6-year-old boy reveal a valgus and anterior malunion at the fracture. **B:** One year later, the child still has a moderate valgus and anterior malalignment of the distal fractured segment. This malalignment produced painful hyperextension of the knee at heel strike during ambulation.

Swaan and Oppers[148] reported that young children have a greater chance for overgrowth than older children. Accelerated growth after tibial fracture generally occurs in children under 10 years of age, whereas older children may have a mild growth inhibition associated with the fracture.[58] The amount of fracture shortening also has an effect on growth stimulation. Fractures with significant shortening have more physeal growth after fracture union than injuries without shortening at union.[99] The presence of angulation at union does not appear to affect the amount of overgrowth.[50]

Anterior Tibial Physeal Closure

Morton and Starr[103] reported closure of the anterior proximal tibial physis after fracture in two children. Both patients sustained a comminuted fracture of the tibial diaphysis without a concomitant injury of the knee. The fractures were reduced and stabilized with Kirschner wires reportedly placed distal to the tibial tubercle. A genu recurvatum deformity developed after premature closure of the anterior physis. Smillie[141] reported one child who had an open tibial fracture complicated by a second fracture involving the supracondylar aspect of the femur. This patient also developed a recurvatum deformity secondary to closure of the anterior proximal tibial physis. At present, no universally acceptable explanation can be given for this phenomenon.

Patients have demonstrated apparently iatrogenic closure after placement of a proximal tibial traction pin, the application of pins and plaster, and after application of an external fixation device. Some children may have an undiagnosed injury of the tibial physis at the time of the ipsilateral tibial diaphyseal fracture.[84] Regardless of etiology, premature closure of the physis produces a progressive recurvatum deformity and loss of

the normal anterior to posterior slope of the proximal tibia as the child grows. Management may require surgical intervention including proximal tibial osteotomy with all the inherent risks and potential complications of that procedure.

NONUNION/DELAYED UNION

Nonunions and delayed unions are rare in pediatric patients with lower-energy, closed fractures. Achieving adequate fracture stability is of utmost importance in prevention of delayed healing, regardless of method employed. Inadequate immobilization or noncompliance with weight-bearing restrictions that allows patterned micro- or macromotion may slow the rate of healing and lead to delayed or nonunion. Fractures treated with flexible nailing must have some compression and motion at the fracture site. As such, use of stiffer and larger diameter nails may limit necessary micromotion, or may introduce distraction at the fracture site which may slow fracture healing. The use of an external fixation device may be associated with increased time to union in some patients, particularly those with open fractures resulting from high-energy injury.[47,93,105] In patients treated with external fixation, care must be taken to advance weight bearing appropriately and to dynamize the fixator frame as soon as possible to maximize bone healing. In patients with a suspected delayed union or nonunion, a 1-cm fibulectomy will allow increased compression at the delayed union or nonunion site with weight bearing and often will induce healing (Fig. 28-34).

In any pediatric long bone fracture that exhibits delayed healing, infection must be ruled out. With a proven aseptic nonunion, treatment is targeted to the type of nonunion, hypertrophic or atrophic. Hypertrophic nonunions have a failure of stability, and callus debridements, additional fixation or

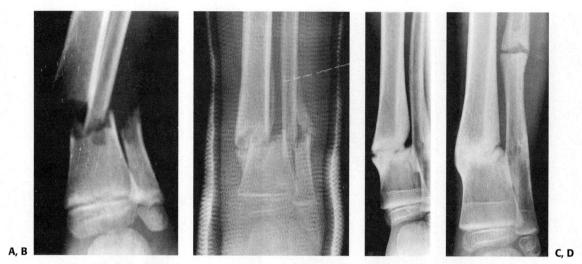

Figure 28-34. A: Anteroposterior radiograph of the distal tibia and fibula in a 5-year-old boy with an open fracture. **B:** Early callus formation is seen 1 month after injury. **C:** The tibia has failed to unite 10 months after injury. **D:** The patient underwent a fibulectomy 4 cm proximal to the tibial nonunion. The tibial fracture united 8 weeks after surgery.

revision of existing fixation, and protected weightbearing help to achieve union. Atrophic nonunions are uncommon in pediatric patients unless there is severe soft tissue and bony loss at the time of injury. Posterolateral bone grafting is an excellent technique to produce union in children (Fig. 28-35). Avascular bone may require resection, bone grafting (autograft or vascularized bone graft), or even bone transport. Adolescents near skeletal maturity with a delayed or nonunion of the tibia can be managed with a reamed intramedullary nail, concomitant fibular osteotomy, and correction of any angulation at the nonunion site as necessary (Fig. 28-36). Addressing soft tissue coverage with vascularized tissue flaps can improve vascular perfusion to the area of the delayed or non-union.

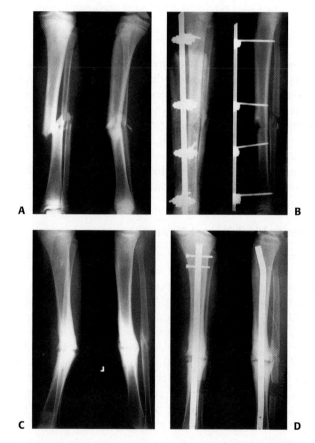

Figure 28-36. A: Anteroposterior and lateral radiographs of a 14-year-old adolescent who was struck by a car, sustaining a grade IIIB open fracture of the tibia. **B:** Anteroposterior and lateral radiographs of the tibia after irrigation and debridement, and application of an external fixation device. **C:** The patient developed a nonunion at the tibia, which progressively deformed into an unacceptable varus alignment. **D:** The nonunion was treated with a fibular osteotomy followed by a closed angular correction of the deformity and internal fixation with a reamed intramedullary nail.

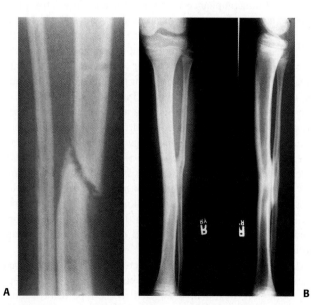

Figure 28-35. A: Nonunion of an open tibial fracture. **B:** After posterolateral tibial bone graft.

Fractures of the Distal Tibial Metaphysis

INTRODUCTION TO FRACTURES OF THE DISTAL TIBIAL METAPHYSIS

Fractures of the distal tibial metaphysis are uncommon injuries in children, with an incidence between 0.35% and 0.45% of all pediatric fractures.[31,57]

MECHANISM OF INJURY FOR DISTAL TIBIAL METAPHYSIS FRACTURES

Distal tibial metaphyseal fractures are often greenstick injuries resulting from increased compressive forces along the anterior tibial cortex. This fracture often occurs secondary to an axial load on a dorsiflexed foot. The anterior cortex is impacted while the posterior cortex is displaced under tension, with a tear of the overlying periosteum. A combined valgus and recurvatum deformity may occur, which can be corrected with reducing the fracture with the ankle in plantarflexion (Fig. 28-37).

TREATMENT OPTIONS FOR FRACTURES OF THE DISTAL TIBIAL METAPHYSIS

NONOPERATIVE TREATMENT OF FRACTURES OF THE DISTAL TIBIAL METAPHYSIS

Reduction of these injuries should be performed with adequate sedation and maintained with a long-leg cast. In cases in which the fracture has displaced or angulated into recurvatum, the foot should be left in moderate plantarflexion to minimize the risk of apex posterior angulation at the fracture site. The foot is brought up to neutral after 3 to 4 weeks, and a short-leg walking cast is applied. Nondisplaced fractures can be immobilized in either a short- or long-leg cast at the surgeon's discretion.

OPERATIVE TREATMENT OF FRACTURES OF THE DISTAL TIBIAL METAPHYSIS

Unstable, displaced fractures can be treated with closed reduction and percutaneous pins[17] (Fig. 28-38), antegrade flexible nails,[9,26,135] open reduction and internal fixation, or percutaneous plating[96] (Fig. 28-39) with good reported results for all techniques. Open reduction and internal fixation of an associated distal fibula fracture may limit the risk of malalignment in an unstable distal tibia fracture. The surgical technique for management of these fractures with flexible nails is essentially identical to that described previously for diaphyseal tibia fractures.

Special Fractures

TODDLER'S FRACTURES

INTRODUCTION TO TODDLER'S FRACTURES

Seemingly minor episodes involving young children that result in external rotation of the foot with the knee in a fixed position may produce a spiral fracture of the tibia without a concomitant fibular fracture. This entity is most frequently termed

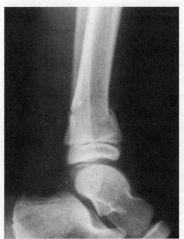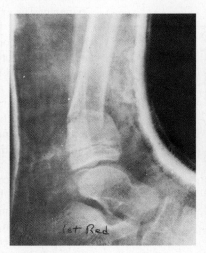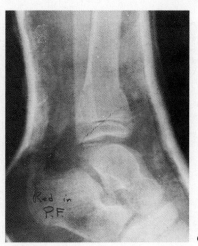

Figure 28-37. A: Fracture of the distal tibia in a 7-year-old child. The lateral radiograph demonstrates a mild recurvatum deformity. **B:** The ankle was initially immobilized in an ankle neutral position, producing an increased recurvatum deformity. The cast was removed and the ankle remanipulated into plantarflexion to reduce the deformity. **C:** The ankle was then immobilized in plantar flexion, which is the proper position for this type of fracture.

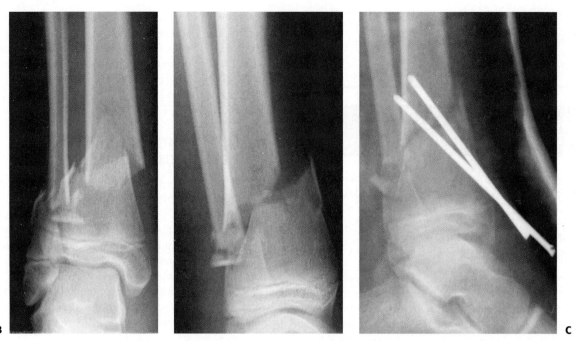

Figure 28-38. A, B: Unstable distal metadiaphyseal fractures of the tibia and fibula in a 15-year-old girl. **C:** This fracture was stabilized with percutaneous pins because of marked swelling and fracture instability.

a "toddler's fracture" (Fig. 28-40). This fracture pattern was first reported by Dunbar et al.[32] in 1964. The traumatic episode often is unwitnessed by the parent or adult caretaker,[115] Common examples of this include injuries occurring when a child sustains a low-energy fall or attempts to extricate his/her foot from between the uprights of a playpen or crib. Most children with this injury are under 6 years of age, and in one study the average age was 27 months. Sixty-three of 76 such fractures reported by Dunbar et al.[32] were in children under 2.5 years of age. Occasionally, a child may sustain a toddler's fracture in a fall from a height.[151] Oudjhane et al.[115] analyzed

the radiographs of 500 acutely limping toddlers and identified 100 in whom a fracture was the etiology of the gait disturbance. The most common site of fracture was the distal metaphysis of the tibia.

ASSESSMENT OF TODDLER'S FRACTURES

The physical findings in a patient with a possible toddler's fracture are often subtle. The child typically presents with a history of a new-onset limp or refusal to bear weight on the limb. The examination should begin with an evaluation of the uninvolved side, as this serves as a control for the symptomatic extremity. The examination begins at the hip and proceeds to the thigh, knee, lower leg, ankle, and foot. It is important to note areas of point tenderness, any increase in local or systemic temperature, and any swelling or bruising of the leg.[151] In those patients in whom the examination appears to point to the lower leg as the source of the problem, plain radiographs should be obtained. The requested images should include radiographs of the tibia and fibula obtained in the anteroposterior, lateral, and internal rotation oblique projections. The internally rotated oblique view may be the only view that will demonstrate an acute nondisplaced toddler's fracture. Occasionally, fluoroscopy may be beneficial in the identification of subtle fractures, but is rarely available in the office setting. In cases in which initial radiographs are negative, but the history and examination are consistent with diagnosis of a toddler's fracture, treatment immobilization is indicated.[55,58] In these cases, follow-up radiographs will often demonstrate periosteal new bone formation approximately 10 to 14 days after injury (Fig. 28-41).

Technetium radionuclide bone scans can assist in the diagnosis of unapparent fractures, but are rarely utilized due to the

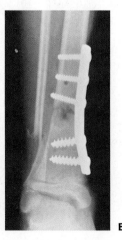

Figure 28-39. A: Anteroposterior radiograph of a distal one-third tibial and fibular fractures in a 9-year-old girl with a closed head injury and severe spasticity. The initial reduction in a cast could not be maintained. **B:** Open reduction and internal fixation with a medial plate was used to achieve and maintain the alignment.

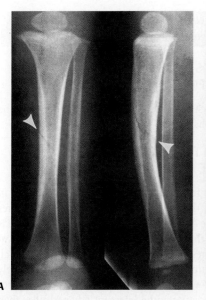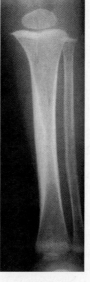

Figure 28-40. A: Anteroposterior and lateral radiographs of an 18-month-old child who presented with refusal to bear weight on her leg. Note the spiral middle one-third "toddler's" fracture (*arrow heads*). **B:** This fracture healed uneventfully after 4 weeks of immobilization in a cast.

amount of radiation. MRI can also be used, but the risk of sedation or anesthesia may not be warranted.

TREATMENT OF TODDLER'S FRACTURES

As these fractures are inherently stable, a child with a toddler's fracture may be immobilized in a long-leg cast, short-leg cast, or a walking boot for approximately 3 to 4 weeks at the discretion of the treating physician. The fracture is stable, and the patient may bear weight on the cast, splint or boot when comfortable. Bauer and Lovejoy reported a statistically significant earlier return to weight bearing for patients in a boot compared to a short leg cast (2.5 weeks vs. 2.8 weeks), but found that nearly all patients in their cohort of 192 toddlers resumed full weightbearing by 4 weeks, regardless of immobilization type.[10]

FLOATING KNEE

INTRODUCTION TO FLOATING KNEE

Although uncommon in children, significant trauma can cause ipsilateral fractures involving both the tibia and the femur. The term "floating knee" describes the flail knee joint resulting from

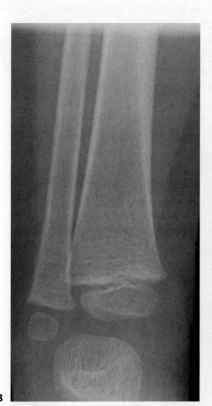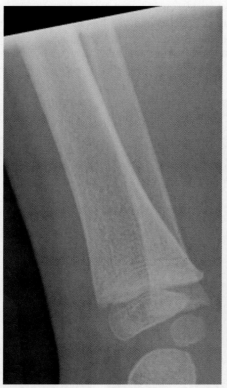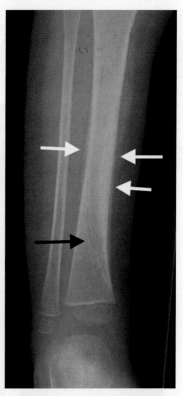

Figure 28-41. A, B: Anteroposterior and lateral radiographs of a 27-month-old refusing to bear weight at presentation are negative. **C:** 3 weeks later, an anterioposterior radiograph demonstrates the fracture line (*black arrow*) and periosteal bone formation (*white arrows*), confirming the diagnosis of a toddlers fractures. (Used with permission by the Children's Orthopaedic Center, Los Angeles.)

fractures of the shaft or metaphyseal region of the ipsilateral femur and tibia.[3,91] The most common mechanism of trauma resulting in this injury pattern involves either a pedestrian or cyclist struck by an automobile.[16,91]

TREATMENT OF FLOATING KNEE

In the past, these injuries often were treated with traction and casting. The extent of the injuries often left permanent functional deficits, including malunion, limb-length discrepancy, and knee stiffness when not managed aggressively.[16]

Today most children with ipsilateral tibia and femoral fractures are treated with operative stabilization of the femur and either cast immobilization after closed reduction or operative fixation of the tibia.[160] In pediatric patients, multiple treatment combinations can be utilized to care for a patient with floating knee injury. For example, the femoral fracture can be stabilized with a unilateral external fixator, plate and screw constructs, or some form of intramedullary fixation. Patients near skeletal maturity may be candidates for proximal lateral entry reamed femoral nails, although the other options remain viable as well. Plate fixation, either open or percutaneous, is useful for fractures in the subtrochanteric or supracondylar area of the femur in adolescents, although external fixation may be useful in these areas as well. In most cases, the tibial fracture is reduced and stabilized after the femoral fracture has been stabilized. Closed tibial fractures in these situations may be treated with cast immobilization or operative intervention. Open tibial fractures associated with an ipsilateral femoral fracture should be stabilized with an external fixator or flexible intramedullary nails whenever possible (Fig. 28-42). Stable fixation of both fractures allows early range of motion of the knee, earlier weight bearing, and improves overall function.[160]

STRESS FRACTURES OF THE TIBIA AND FIBULA

INTRODUCTION TO STRESS FRACTURES OF THE TIBIA AND FIBULA

Numerous reports of stress fractures involving the tibia and the fibula have been published.[29,149]

ASSESSMENT AND TREATMENT OF STRESS FRACTURES OF THE TIBIA AND FIBULA

The pattern of stress fractures in children differs from that in adults.[29,30] In adults, the fibula is involved in stress fractures twice as often as the tibia; in pediatric patients, the tibia is affected more often than the fibula (Fig. 28-43). The prevalence of stress fractures in boys and girls appears to be equal, although stress fractures have been reported to be increasingly common in females with eating disorders.[108] These injuries typically occur in pediatric and adolescent athletes older than 10 years of age, and have a history of insidious onset of pain that worsens with sporting activities.[49,155]

Stress fractures occur when the repetitive force applied to a bone is exceeded by the bone's capacity to withstand it. Initially, osteoclastic tunnel formation increases. These tunnels normally fill with mature bone. With continued force, cortical reabsorption accelerates. Woven bone is produced to splint the weakened cortex. However, this bone is disorganized and does not have the strength of the bone it replaces. A fracture occurs when bone reabsorption outstrips bone production. When the offending force is reduced or eliminated, bone production exceeds bone reabsorption. This produces

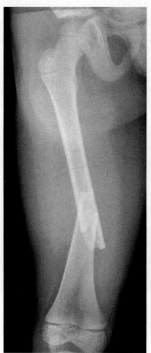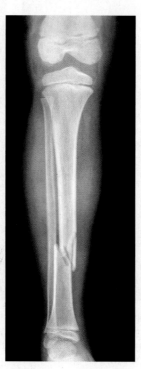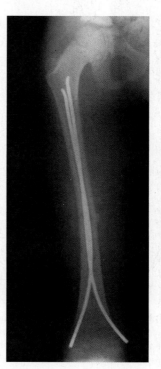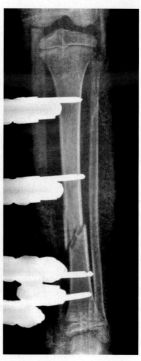

A, B

C, D

Figure 28-42. A, B: Floating knee injury in a 7-year-old boy. **C:** Femoral fracture was fixed with flexible intramedullary nails. **D:** Tibial fracture was stabilized with external fixation.

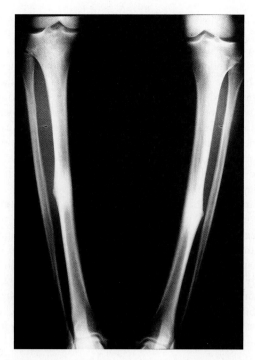

Figure 28-43. Bilateral midtibial stress fractures in an adolescent with genu varus.

cortical and endosteal widening with dense repair bone that later remodels to mature bone.[115]

A child with a tibial stress fracture usually has an insidious onset of symptoms.[29,133] There is evidence of local tenderness that worsens with activity. The pain tends to be worse in the day, particularly during activities, and improves at night and with rest. The knee and the ankle have full range of motion. Usually, there is minimal, if any, swelling at the fracture site.[29,66,86]

Initial radiographs may be normal. Radiographic changes consistent with a stress fracture generally become evident approximately 2 weeks after the onset of symptoms.[29] Radiographic findings consistent with fracture repair can manifest in one of three ways: Localized periosteal new bone formation, endosteal thickening, or, rarely, a radiolucent cortical fracture line (Fig. 28-44).[29,30,86,133]

In cases in which the plain radiographs are normal, MRI may be helpful. Magnetic resonance imaging (MRI)[66,86] shows a localized band of very low signal intensity continuous with the cortex. These MR findings can be diagnostic for a stress fracture, and will differentiate such lesions from malignancy, thereby obviating the need for biopsy. CT rarely demonstrates the fracture line, but often delineates increased marrow density, endosteal and periosteal new bone formation, and may show soft tissue edema within the area of concern.

Tibia Stress Fractures

The most common location for a tibial stress fracture is in the proximal third.[37] The child normally has a limp of gradual onset with no history of a specific injury. The pain is described as dull, occurring in the calf near the upper end of the tibia on its medial aspect, and occasionally is bilateral. Physical findings include local tenderness on one or both sides of the tibial crest with a varying degree of swelling.

The treatment of a child with a stress fracture of the tibia begins with activity modification. An active child can rest in a prefabricated walking boot for 4 to 6 weeks followed by gradual increase in activity.[110] Nonunions of stress fractures of the tibia have been described. Green et al.[49] reported six nonunions, each in the middle third of the tibia. Three of these nonunions were in children. Two required excision of the nonunion site with iliac crest bone grafting. The third was treated by electromagnetic stimulation. In cases of stress fractures involving female athletes with dietary, nutritional, and menstrual irregularities, collaboration between pediatric orthopedists, primary care physicians, endocrinologists, and nutritionist is recommended.[60]

Fibula Stress Fractures

Pediatric fibular stress fractures normally occur between the ages of 2 and 8 years.[51,87] The fractures are normally localized to the distal third of the fibula. The child presents with a limp and may complain of pain. Swelling normally is not present. The obvious bony mass commonly seen in a stress fracture of the fibula in an adult is rarely seen in a comparable fracture in a child.

Often the earliest plain radiographic sign of a stress fracture of the fibula is the presence of "eggshell" callus along the shaft of the fibula. The fracture itself cannot always be seen because the periosteal callus may obscure the changes in the narrow canal. MRI can help to identify stress fractures before the presence of radiographic changes. Radionuclide bone imaging is rarely used because of radiation.

The differential diagnosis includes sarcoma of bone, osteomyelitis, and a soft tissue injury without accompanying bony injury. A careful history, physical examination, laboratory

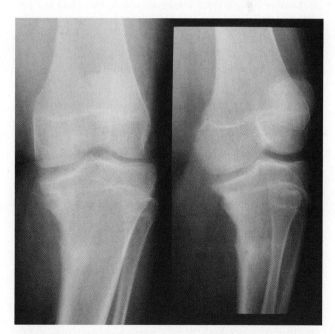

Figure 28-44. Anteroposterior and lateral radiographs of the knee of a 15-year-old with adolescent onset tibia vara. Note the posteromedial stress fracture.

workup, and use of necessary radiographic imaging can usually allow differentiation of a stress fracture from infection or neoplasm.[155] Once a diagnosis of a fibular stress fracture is made, treatment is similar to that used in tibial injuries.

SUMMARY, CONTROVERSIES, AND FUTURE DIRECTIONS RELATED TO PEDIATRIC TIBIAL SHAFT FRACTURES

Tibia fractures are extremely common injuries in all pediatric age groups. While the risk of potential complications does exist, the vast majority of tibia fractures, regardless of anatomic location within the bone, heal without difficulty, and cause few long-term functional deficits. Tibia fractures that pose particular concerns, either due to potential problems with management of the acute fracture or secondary to secondary to delayed complications, include proximal tibial metaphyseal fractures and open fractures of the diaphyseal region.

Despite the ubiquitous nature of tibia fractures, few controversies exist regarding diagnosis or management, and direct care of most tibia fractures has changed little over time. The area of greatest change has been the increasing use of flexible nails, with or without external immobilization, in the care of diaphyseal and metadiaphyseal fractures. Similarly, the overwhelming use of closed cast treatment for the same fractures has diminished, and the art of cast management/wedging has decreased as well over time. The standard of the long-leg cast for tibia fractures may be going the way of the spica cast for many femur fractures. Especially for diaphyseal fractures in older pediatric patients, the long-leg cast is being replaced by flexible intramedullary nails, due to the relative conveniences that they offer to the patient, family and physician.

Change in the management of pediatric tibia fractures in the future seems inevitable, and it will most likely mirror approaches to care for other pediatric fractures. An increasing number of diaphyseal tibia fractures will receive surgical treatment, most likely with some form of "growth plate friendly" intramedullary fixation, particularly in older children and adolescents. However, closed treatment with cast immobilization will remain the primary method of care for the vast majority of tibia fractures in younger children for the immediate future.

Annotated References

Reference	Annotation
Buckley SL, Smith G, Sponseller PD, et al. Open fractures of the tibia in children. *J Bone Joint Surg Am*. 1990;72(10):1462–1469.	Report of single-center experience with operative management of open tibia fractures in children. The incidences of compartment syndrome, vascular injury, infection, and delayed unions were similar when compared to the adult literature with open injuries.
Flynn JM, Bashyal RK, Yeger-McKeever M, et al. Acute compartment syndrome of the leg in children: Diagnosis and outcome. *J Bone Joint Surg Am*. 2011;93:937–941.	Large two-center study that reviewed a 17-year experience with acute compartment of the leg in children. Despite often lengthy delays in time to treatment, most children with compartment syndrome had acceptable results after surgical management.
Gordon JE, Gregush RV, Schoenecker PL, et al. Complications after titanium elastic nailing of pediatric tibial fractures. *J Pediatr Orthop*. 2007;27(4):442–446.	Single-center, retrospective review of 60 diaphyseal tibia fractures in children treated with intramedullary fixation. While complications were low, 11% of patients demonstrated delayed or nonunions.
Kinney MC, Nagle D, Bastrom T, et al. Operative versus conservative management of displaced tibial shaft fractures in adolescents. *J Pediatr Orthop*. 2016;36(7):661–666.	Outcomes were similar in patients treated originally with both closed and operative treatments. Predictors of failure of closed reduction included initial fracture displacement and presence of a fibula fracture.
Naranje SM, Erali RA, Warner WC, et al. Epidemiology of pediatric fractures presenting to emergency departments in the United States. *J Pediatr Orthop*. 2016;36(4):e45–48.	The most recent epidemiologic data on pediatric fractures in the United States. Generated from a review of the 2010 national Electronic Surveillance System database.
Rinker B, Valerio IL, Stewart DH, et al. Microvascular free flap reconstruction in pediatric lower extremity trauma: a 10-year review. *Plat Reconstr Surg*. 2005;115(6):1618–1624.	Review of 28 flaps placed due to lower extremity trauma in 26 patients over a 10-year period. Patients receiving free-flap coverage within 7 days of injury had a statistically lower rate of complications than those having a longer time period to soft tissue coverage.
Shore BJ, Glotzbecker MP, Zurakowski D, et al. Acute compartment syndrome in children and teenagers with tibial shaft fractures; incidence and multivariate risk factors. *J Orthop Trauma*. 2013;27(11):616–621.	Single-center review of the incidence of ACS in pediatric patients with tibia fractures. The incidence was much higher than previously reported in the literature, and associated with patient age >14 years old and when the injury was secondary to an MVA.
Tuten HR, Keeler KA, Gabos PG, et al. Posttraumatic tibia valga in children. A long-term follow-up note. *J Bone Joint Surg Am*. 1999;81(6):799–810.	A small case series with long-term mean follow-up of 15 years that documents spontaneous resolution of the post-Cozen fracture deformity, and provides the basis for a period of watchful observation in these patients.

REFERENCES

1. Al-Sayyad MJ. Taylor Spatial Frame in the treatment of pediatric and adolescent tibial shaft fractures. *J Pediatr Orthop.* 2006;26(2):164–170.
2. Allen MJ, Nash JR, Ioannidies TT, et al. Major vascular injuries associated with orthopaedic injuries to the lower limb. *Ann R Coll Surg Engl.* 1984;66(2):101–104.
3. Arslan H, Kapukaya A, Kesemenli C, et al. Floating knee in children. *J Pediatr Orthop.* 2003;23(4):458–463.
4. Aslani H, Tabrizi A, Sadighi A, et al. Treatment of open pediatric tibial fractures by external fixation versus flexible intramedullary nailing: A comparative study. *Arch Trauma Res.* 2013;2(3):108–112.
5. Backstrom IC, MacLennan PA, Sawyer JR, et al. Pediatric obesity and traumatic lower-extremity long-bone fracture outcomes. *J Trauma Acute Care Surg.* 2012; 73(4):966–971.
6. Bae DS, Kadiyala RK, Waters PM. Acute compartment syndrome in children: contemporary diagnosis, treatment, and outcome. *J Pediatr Orthop.* 2001;21(5):680–688.
7. Bartlett CS, 3rd, Weiner LS, Yang EC. Treatment of type II and type III open tibia fractures in children. *J Orthop Trauma.* 1997;11(5):357–362.
8. Bassey LO. Valgus deformity following proximal metaphyseal fractures in children: Experiences in the African tropics. *J Trauma.* 1990;30(1):102–107.
9. Bauer J, Hirzinger C, Metzger R. Quadruple ESIN (Elastic Stable Intramedullary Nailing): Modified Treatment in Pediatric Distal Tibial Fractures. *J Pediatr Orthop.* 2017;37(2):e100–e103.
10. Bauer JM, Lovejoy SA. Toddler's fractures: Time to weight-bear with regard to immobilization type and radiographic monitoring. *J Pediatr Orthop.* 2017.
11. Bazzi AA, Brooks JT, Jain A, et al. Is nonoperative treatment of pediatric type I open fractures safe and effective? *J Child Orthop.* 2014;8(6):467–471.
12. Bennek J, Steinert V. [Bone development after abnormal healing of lower leg shaft fractures in children]. *Zentralbl Chir.* 1966;91(17):633–639.
13. Benz G, Kallieris D, Seebock T, et al. Bioresorbable pins and screws in paediatric traumatology. *Eur J Pediatr Surg* 1994;4(2):103–107.
14. Blasier RD, Barnes CL. Age as a prognostic factor in open tibial fractures in children. *Clin Orthop Relat Res.* 1996(331):261–264.
15. Blick SS, Brumback RJ, Poka A, et al. Compartment syndrome in open tibial fractures. *J Bone Joint Surg Am.* 1986;68(9):1348–1353.
16. Bohn WW, Durbin RA. Ipsilateral fractures of the femur and tibia in children and adolescents. *J Bone Joint Surg Am.* 1991;73(3):429–439.
17. Brantley J, Majumdar A, Jobe JT, et al. A biomechanical comparison of pin configurations used for percutaneous pinning of distal tibia fractures in children. *Iowa Orthop J.* 2016;36:133–137.
18. Briggs TW, Orr MM, Lightowler CD. Isolated tibial fractures in children. *Injury.* 1992;23(5):308–310.
19. Buckley SL, Gotschall C, Robertson W, Jr., et al. The relationships of skeletal injuries with trauma score, injury severity score, length of hospital stay, hospital charges, and mortality in children admitted to a regional pediatric trauma center. *J Pediatr Orthop.* 1994;14(4):449–453.
20. Buckley SL, Smith G, Sponseller PD, et al. Open fractures of the tibia in children. *J Bone Joint Surg Am.* 1990;72(10):1462–1469.
21. Cheng JC, Shen WY. Limb fracture pattern in different pediatric age groups: A study of 3,350 children. *J Orthop Trauma.* 1993;7(1):15–22.
22. Cherubino M, Valdatta L, Tos P, et al. Role of negative pressure therapy as damage control in soft tissue reconstruction for open tibial fractures. *J Reconstr Microsurg.* 2017;33(S 01):S08–S13.
23. Coury JG, Lum ZC, O'Neill NP, et al. Single incision pediatric flexible intramedullary tibial nailing. *J Orthop.* 2017;14(3):394–397.
24. Cozen L. Fracture of the proximal portion of the tibia in children followed by valgus deformity. *Surg Gynecol Obstet.* 1953;97(2):183–188.
25. Cramer KE, Limbird TJ, Green NE. Open fractures of the diaphysis of the lower extremity in children. Treatment, results, and complications. *J Bone Joint Surg Am.* 1992;74(2):218–232.
26. Cravino M, Canavese F, De Rosa V, et al. Outcome of displaced distal tibial metaphyseal fractures in children between 6 and 15 years of age treated by elastic stable intramedullary nails. *Eur J Orthop Surg Traumatol.* 2014;24(8):1603–1608.
27. Cullen MC, Roy DR, Crawford AH, et al. Open fracture of the tibia in children. *J Bone Joint Surg Am.* 1996;78(7):1039–1047.
28. Dedmond BT, Kortesis B, Punger K, et al. Subatmospheric pressure dressings in the temporary treatment of soft tissue injuries associated with type III open tibial shaft fractures in children. *J Pediatr Orthop.* 2006;26(6):728–732.
29. Devas MB. Stress fractures in children. *J Bone Joint Surg Br.* 1963;45:528–541.
30. Devas MB, Sweetnam R. Stress fractures of the fibula; a review of fifty cases in athletes. *J Bone Joint Surg Br.* 1956;38-b(4):818–829.
31. Domzalski ME, Lipton GE, Lee D, et al. Fractures of the distal tibial metaphysis in children: Patterns of injury and results of treatment. *J Pediatr Orthop.* 2006;26(2):171–176.
32. Dunbar JS, Owen HF, Nogrady MB, et al. Obscure tibial fracture of infants—The toddler's fracture. *J Can Assoc Radiol.* 1964;15:136–144.
33. Dwyer AJ, John B, Krishen M, et al. Remodeling of tibial fractures in children younger than 12 years. *Orthopedics.* 2007;30(5):393–396.
34. Evanoff M, Strong ML, MacIntosh R. External fixation maintained until fracture consolidation in the skeletally immature. *J Pediatr Orthop.* 1993;13(1):98–101.
35. Flynn JM, Bashyal RK, Yeger-McKeever M, et al. Acute traumatic compartment syndrome of the leg in children: Diagnosis and outcome. *J Bone Joint Surg Am.* 2011; 93(10):937–941.
36. Flynn JM, Hresko T, Reynolds RA, et al. Titanium elastic nails for pediatric femur fractures: A multicenter study of early results with analysis of complications. *J Pediatr Orthop.* 2001;21(1):4–8.
37. Fottner A, Baur-Melnyk A, Birkenmaier C, et al. Stress fractures presenting as tumours: A retrospective analysis of 22 cases. *Int Orthop.* 2009;33(2):489–492.
38. Galano GJ, Vitale MA, Kessler MW, et al. The most frequent traumatic orthopaedic injuries from a national pediatric inpatient population. *J Pediatr Orthop.* 2005; 25(1):39–44.
39. Gates JD. The management of combined skeletal and arterial injuries of the lower extremity. *Am J Orthop (Belle Mead NJ).* 1995;24(9):674–680.
40. Gicquel P, Giacomelli MC, Basic B, et al. Problems of operative and non-operative treatment and healing in tibial fractures. *Injury.* 2005;36(Suppl 1):A44–A50.
41. Glass GE, Pearse M, Nanchahal J. The ortho-plastic management of Gustilo grade IIIB fractures of the tibia in children: A systematic review of the literature. *Injury.* 2009;40(8):876–879.
42. Godfrey J, Choi PD, Shabtai L, et al. Management of pediatric type I open fractures in the emergency department or operating room: A multicenter perspective. *J Pediatr Orthop.* 2017.
43. Goff CW. *Surgical Treatment of Unequal Extremities.* Springfield, IL: Charles C. Thomas; 1960.
44. Goodbody CM, Lee RJ, Flynn JM, et al. Titanium elastic nailing for pediatric tibia fractures: Do older, heavier kids do worse? *J Pediatr Orthop.* 2016;36(5):472–477.
45. Goodwin RC, Gaynor T, Mahar A, et al. Intramedullary flexible nail fixation of unstable pediatric tibial diaphyseal fractures. *J Pediatr Orthop.* 2005;25(5):570–576.
46. Gordon JE, Gregush RV, Schoenecker PL, et al. Complications after titanium elastic nailing of pediatric tibial fractures. *J Pediatr Orthop.* 2007;27(4):442–446.
47. Gordon JE, Schoenecker PL, Oda JE, et al. A comparison of monolateral and circular external fixation of unstable diaphyseal tibial fractures in children. *J Pediatr Orthop B.* 2003;12(5):338–345.
48. Gray H. *Anatomy: Descriptive and Surgical.* New York: Bounty Books; 1977.
49. Green NE, Rogers RA, Lipscomb AB. Nonunions of stress fractures of the tibia. *Am J Sports Med.* 1985;13(3):171–176.
50. Greiff J, Bergmann F. Growth disturbance following fracture of the tibia in children. *Acta Orthop Scand.* 1980;51(2):315–320.
51. Griffiths AL. Fatigue fracture of the fibula in childhood. *Arch Dis Child.* 1952; 27(136):552–557.
52. Grimard G, Naudie D, Laberge LC, et al. Open fractures of the tibia in children. *Clinical Orthop Relat Res.* 1996(332):62–70.
53. Gustilo RB, Anderson JT. Prevention of infection in the treatment of one thousand and twenty-five open fractures of long bones: Retrospective and prospective analyses. *J Bone Joint Surg Am.* 1976;58(4):453–458.
54. Haas LM, Staple TW. Arterial injuries associated with fractures of the proximal tibia following blunt trauma. *South Med J.* 1969;62(12):1439–1448.
55. Halsey MF, Finzel KC, Carrion WV, et al. Toddler's fracture: Presumptive diagnosis and treatment. *J Pediatr Orthop.* 2001;21(2):152–156.
56. Halvorson J, Jinnah R, Kulp B, et al. Use of vacuum-assisted closure in pediatric open fractures with a focus on the rate of infection. *Orthopedics.* 2011;34(7):e256–e260.
57. Hanlon CR, Estes WL, Jr. Fractures in childhood, a statistical analysis. *Am J Surg.* 1954;87(3):312–323.
58. Hansen BA, Greiff J, Bergmann F. Fractures of the tibia in children. *Acta Orthop Scand.* 1976;47(4):448–453.
59. Heo J, Oh CW, Park KH, et al. Elastic nailing of tibia shaft fractures in young children up to 10 years of age. *Injury.* 2016;47(4):832–836.
60. Heyworth BE, Green DW. Lower extremity stress fractures in pediatric and adolescent athletes. *Curr Opin Pediatr.* 2008;20(1):58–61.
61. Ho CA. Tibia shaft fractures in adolescents: How and when can they be managed successfully with cast treatment? *J Pediatr Orthop.* 2016;36(Suppl 1):S15–S18.
62. Ho CA, Dammann G, Podeszwa DA, et al. Tibial shaft fractures in adolescents: Analysis of cast treatment successes and failures. *J Pediatr Orthop B.* 2015;24(2):114–117.
63. Hoaglund FT, States JD. Factors influencing the rate of healing in tibial shaft fractures. *Surg Gynecol Obstet.* 1967;124(1):71–76.
64. Hoover NW. Injuries of the popliteal artery associated with fractures and dislocations. *Surg Clin North Am.* 1961;41:1099–1112.
65. Hope PG, Cole WG. Open fractures of the tibia in children. *J Bone Joint Surg Br.* 1992;74(4):546–553.
66. Horev G, Korenreich L, Ziv N, et al. The enigma of stress fractures in the pediatric age: Clarification or confusion through the new imaging modalities. *Pediatr Radiol.* 1990;20(6):469–471.
67. Houghton GR, Rooker GD. The role of the periosteum in the growth of long bones. An experimental study in the rabbit. *J Bone Joint Surg Br.* 1979;61-b(2):218–220.
68. Hull JB, Sanderson PL, Rickman M, et al. External fixation of children's fractures: Use of the orthofix dynamic axial fixator. *J Pediatr Orthop B.* 1997;6(3):203–206.
69. Iobst CA. Hexapod external fixation of Tibia fractures in children. *J Pediatr Orthop.* 2016;36(Suppl 1):S24–S28.
70. Ippolito E, Pentimalli G. Post-traumatic valgus deformity of the knee in proximal tibial metaphyseal fractures in children. *Ital J Orthop Traumatol.* 1984;10(1):103–108.
71. Jackson DW, Cozen L. Genu valgum as a complication of proximal tibial metaphyseal fractures in children. *J Bone Joint Surg Am.* 1971;53(8):1571–1578.
72. Janzing HM, Broos PL. Routine monitoring of compartment pressure in patients with tibial fractures: Beware of overtreatment! *Injury.* 2001;32(5):415–421.
73. Joeris A, Lutz N, Wicki B, et al. An epidemiological evaluation of pediatric long bone fractures—a retrospective cohort study of 2716 patients from two Swiss tertiary pediatric hospitals. *BMC pediatrics.* 2014;14:314.
74. Jones BG, Duncan RD. Open tibial fractures in children under 13 years of age—10 years experience. *Injury.* 2003;34(10):776–780.
75. Jordan SE, Alonso JE, Cook FF. The etiology of valgus angulation after metaphyseal fractures of the tibia in children. *J Pediatr Orthop.* 1987;7(4):450–457.
76. Karlsson MK, Nilsson BE, Obrant KJ. Fracture incidence after tibial shaft fractures. A 30-year follow-up study. *Clin Orthop Relat Res.* 1993(287):87–89.
77. Karlstrom G, Lonnerholm T, Olerud S. Cavus deformity of the foot after fracture of the tibial shaft. *J Bone Joint Surg Am.* 1975;57(7):893–900.

78. Karrholm J, Hansson LI, Svensson K. Incidence of tibio-fibular shaft and ankle fractures in children. *J Pediatr Orthop*. 1982;2(4):386–396.
79. Kattan JM, Leathers MP, Barad JH, et al. The effectiveness of cast wedging for the treatment of pediatric fractures. *J Pediatr Orthop B*. 2014;23(6):566–571.
80. Katzman SS, Dickson K. Determining the prognosis for limb salvage in major vascular injuries with associated open tibial fractures. *Orthop Rev*. 1992;21(2):195–199.
81. Keret D, Harcke HT, Bowen JR. Tibia valga after fracture: Documentation of mechanism. *Arch Orthop Trauma Surg*. 1991;110(4):216–219.
82. King J, Diefendorf D, Apthorp J, et al. Analysis of 429 fractures in 189 battered children. *J Pediatr Orthop*. 1988;8(5):585–589.
83. Kinney MC, Nagle D, Bastrom T, et al. Operative versus conservative management of displaced tibial shaft fracture in adolescents. *J Pediatr Orthop*. 2016;36(7):661–666.
84. Knight JL. Genu recurvatum deformity secondary to partial proximal tibial epiphyseal arrest: Case report. *Am J Knee Surg*. 1998;11(2):111–115.
85. Kocher MS, Kasser JR. Orthopaedic aspects of child abuse. *J Am Acad Orthop Surg*. 2000;8(1):10–20.
86. Kozlowski K, Azouz M, Barrett IR, et al. Midshaft tibial stress fractures in children (report of four cases). *Australas Radiol*. 1992;36(2):131–134.
87. Kozlowski K, Urbonaviciene A. Stress fractures of the fibula in the first few years of life (report of six cases). *Australas Radiol*. 1996;40(3):261–263.
88. Kreder HJ, Armstrong P. A review of open tibia fractures in children. *J Pediatr Orthop*. 1995;15(4):482–488.
89. Kubiak EN, Egol KA, Scher D, et al. Operative treatment of tibial fractures in children: Are elastic stable intramedullary nails an improvement over external fixation? *J Bone Joint Surg Am*. 2005;87(8):1761–1768.
90. Laine JC, Cherkashin A, Samchukov M, et al. The management of soft tissue and bone loss in type IIIB and IIIC pediatric open tibia fractures. *J Pediatr Orthop*. 2016; 36(5):453–458.
91. Letts M, Vincent N, Gouw G. The "floating knee" in children. *J Bone Joint Surg Br*. 1986;68(3):442–446.
92. Levy AS, Wetzler M, Lewars M, et al. The orthopedic and social outcome of open tibia fractures in children. *Orthopedics*. 1997;20(7):593–598.
93. Liow RY, Montgomery RJ. Treatment of established and anticipated nonunion of the tibia in childhood. *J Pediatr Orthop*. 2002;22(6):754–760.
94. Loder RT, Bookout C. Fracture patterns in battered children. *J Orthop Trauma*. 1991;5(4):428–433.
95. Marengo L, Paonessa M, Andreacchio A, et al. Displaced tibia shaft fractures in children treated by elastic stable intramedullary nailing: Results and complications in children weighing 50 kg (110 lb) or more. *Eur J Orthop Surg Traumatol*. 2016; 26(3):311–317.
96. Masquijo JJ. Percutaneous plating of distal tibial fractures in children and adolescents. *J Pediatr Orthop B*. 2014;23(3):207–211.
97. Matsen FA, 3rd, Clawson DK. The deep posterior compartmental syndrome of the leg. *J Bone Joint Surg Am*. 1975;57(1):34–39.
98. Matsen FA, 3rd, Winquist RA, Krugmire RB, Jr. Diagnosis and management of compartmental syndromes. *J Bone Joint Surg Am*. 1980;62(2):286–291.
99. Mellick LB, Reesor K, Demers D, et al. Tibial fractures of young children. *Pediatr Emerg Care*. 1988;4(2):97–101.
100. Metaizeau JP, Wong-Chung J, Bertrand H, et al. Percutaneous epiphysiodesis using transphyseal screws (PETS). *J Pediatr Orthop*. 1998;18(3):363–369.
101. Monsell FP, Howells NR, Lawniczak D, et al. High-energy open tibial fractures in children: Treatment with a programmable circular external fixator. *J Bone Joint Surg Br*. 2012;94(7):989–993.
102. Mooney JF, 3rd, Argenta LC, Marks MW, et al. Treatment of soft tissue defects in pediatric patients using the V.A.C. system. *Clin Orthop Relat Res*. 2000(376):26–31.
103. Morton KS, Starr DE. Closure of the anterior portion of the upper tibial epiphysis as a complication of tibial-shaft fracture. *J Bone Joint Surg Am*. 1964;46:570–574.
104. Mubarak SJ, Kim JR, Edmonds EW, et al. Classification of proximal tibial fractures in children. *J Child Orthop*. 2009;3(3):191–197.
105. Myers SH, Spiegel D, Flynn JM. External fixation of high-energy tibia fractures. *J Pediatr Orthop*. 2007;27(5):537–539.
106. Nandra RS, Wu F, Gaffey A, et al. The management of open tibial fractures in children: A retrospective case series of eight years' experience of 61 cases at a paediatric specialist centre. *Bone Joint J*. 2017;99-b(4):544–553.
107. Naranje SM, Erali RA, Warner WC, Jr., et al. Epidemiology of pediatric fractures presenting to emergency departments in the United States. *J Pediatr Orthop*. 2016;36(4):e45–e48.
108. Nattiv A. Stress fractures and bone health in track and field athletes. *J Sci Med Sport*. 2000;3(3):268–279.
109. Nenopoulos S, Vrettakos A, Chaftikis N, et al. The effect of proximal tibial fractures on the limb axis in children. *Acta Orthop Belg*. 2007;73(3):345–353.
110. Niemeyer P, Weinberg A, Schmitt H, et al. Stress fractures in adolescent competitive athletes with open physis. *Knee Surg Sports Traumatol Arthrosc*. 2006;14(8):771–777.
111. O'Brien T, Weisman DS, Ronchetti P, et al. Flexible titanium nailing for the treatment of the unstable pediatric tibial fracture. *J Pediatr Orthop*. 2004;24(6):601–609.
112. Ogden JA. *Tibia and Fibula*. Philadelphia, PA: Lea & Febiger; 1982.
113. Ogden JA, Ogden DA, Pugh L, et al. Tibia valga after proximal metaphyseal fractures in childhood: A normal biologic response. *J Pediatr Orthop*. 1995;15(4):489–494.
114. Ostermann PA, Henry SL, Seligson D. Timing of wound closure in severe compound fractures. *Orthopedics*. 1994;17(5):397–399.
115. Oudjhane K, Newman B, Oh KS, et al. Occult fractures in preschool children. *J Trauma*. 1988;28(6):858–860.
116. Ozkul E, Gem M, Arslan H, et al. Minimally invasive plate osteosynthesis in open pediatric tibial fractures. *J Pediatr Orthop*. 2016;36(4):416–422.
117. Ozkul E, Gem M, Arslan H, et al. How safe is titanium elastic nail application in the surgical treatment of tibia fractures in children? *Acta Orthop Belg*. 2014;80(1):76–81.
118. Pandya NK, Baldwin K, Wolfgruber H, et al. Child abuse and orthopaedic injury patterns: Analysis at a level I pediatric trauma center. *J Pediatr Orthop*. 2009;29(6):618–625.
119. Pandya NK, Edmonds EW. Immediate intramedullary flexible nailing of open pediatric tibial shaft fractures. *J Pediatr Orthop*. 2012;32(8):770–776.
120. Pandya NK, Edmonds EW, Mubarak SJ. The incidence of compartment syndrome after flexible nailing of pediatric tibial shaft fractures. *J Child Orthop*. 2011; 5(6):439–447.
121. Patzakis MJ, Wilkins J, Moore TM. Use of antibiotics in open tibial fractures. *Clin Orthop Relat Res*. 1983;(178):31–35.
122. Pennock AT, Bastrom TP, Upasani VV. Elastic intramedullary nailing versus open reduction internal fixation of pediatric tibial shaft fractures. *J Pediatr Orthop*. 2017; 37(7):e403–e408.
123. Pollen AG. *Fractures and Dislocation in Children*. Baltimore, MD: Williams & Wilkins; 1973.
124. Qidwai SA. Intramedullary Kirschner wiring for tibia fractures in children. *J Pediatr Orthop*. 2001;21(3):294–297.
125. Radhakrishna VN, Madhuri V. Management of pediatric open tibia fractures with supracutaneous locked plates. *J Pediatr Orthop B*. 2017;27(1):13–16.
126. Robert M, Khouri N, Carlioz H, et al. Fractures of the proximal tibial metaphysis in children: Review of a series of 25 cases. *J Pediatr Orthop*. 1987;7(4):444–449.
127. Robertson P, Karol LA, Rab GT. Open fractures of the tibia and femur in children. *J Pediatr Orthop*. 1996;16(5):621–626.
128. Rooker GD, Salter RB. *Prevention of valgus deformity following fracture of the proximal metaphysis of the tibia in children. Paper presented at: British Orthopaedic Association1980*; Canterbury, England.
129. Sabatini CS, Curtis TA, Mahan ST. Patient-based outcomes after tibia fracture in children and adolescents. *Open Orthop J*. 2014;8:41–48.
130. Salem KH, Lindemann I, Keppler P. Flexible intramedullary nailing in pediatric lower limb fractures. *J Pediatr Orthop*. 2006;26(4):505–509.
131. Sankar WN, Jones KJ, David Horn B, et al. Titanium elastic nails for pediatric tibial shaft fractures. *J Child Orthop*. 2007;1(5):281–286.
132. Sarmiento A. A functional below-the-knee cast for tibial fractures. *J Bone Joint Surg Am*. 1967;49(5):855–875.
133. Savoca CJ. Stress fractures. A classification of the earliest radiographic signs. *Radiology*. 1971;100(3):519–524.
134. Shannak AO. Tibial fractures in children: Follow-up study. *J Pediatr Orthop*. 1988;8(3):306–310.
135. Shen K, Cai H, Wang Z, et al. Elastic stable intramedullary nailing for severely displaced distal tibial fractures in children. *Medicine*. 2016;95(39):e4980.
136. Shore BJ, DiMauro JP, Spence DD, et al. Uniplanar versus Taylor spatial frame external fixation for pediatric diaphyseal tibia fractures: A comparison of cost and complications. *J Pediatr Orthop*. 2016;36(8):821–828.
137. Shore BJ, Glotzbecker MP, Zurakowski D, et al. Acute compartment syndrome in children and teenagers with tibial shaft fractures: Incidence and multivariable risk factors. *J Orthop Trauma*. 2013;27(11):616–621.
138. Skaggs DL, Friend L, Alman B, et al. The effect of surgical delay on acute infection following 554 open fractures in children. *J Bone Joint Surg Am*. 2005;87(1):8–12.
139. Skaggs DL, Kautz SM, Kay RM, et al. Effect of delay of surgical treatment on rate of infection in open fractures in children. *J Pediatr Orthop*. 2000;20(1):19–22.
140. Skak SV. Valgus deformity following proximal tibial metaphyseal fracture in children. *Acta Orthop Scand*. 1982;53(1):141–147.
141. Smillie IS. *Injuries of the Knee Joint*. 2nd ed. Baltimore, MD: Williams & Wilkins; 1951.
142. Song KM, Sangeorzan B, Benirschke S, et al. Open fractures of the tibia in children. *J Pediatr Orthop*. 1996;16(5):635–639.
143. Srivastava AK, Mehlman CT, Wall EJ, et al. Elastic stable intramedullary nailing of tibial shaft fractures in children. *J Pediatr Orthop*. 2008;28(2):152–158.
144. Staudt JM, Smeulders MJ, van der Horst CM. Normal compartment pressures of the lower leg in children. *J Bone Joint Surg Br*. 2008;90(2):215–219.
145. Steel HH, Sandrow RE, Sullivan PD. Complications of tibial osteotomy in children for genu varum or valgum. Evidence that neurological changes are due to ischemia. *J Bone Joint Surg Am*. 1971;53(8):1629–1635.
146. Stevens PM. Guided growth for angular correction: A preliminary series using a tension band plate. *J Pediatr Orthop*. 2007;27(3):253–259.
147. Stranzinger E, Leidolt L, Eich G, et al. The anterior tilt angle of the proximal tibia epiphyseal plate: A significant radiological finding in young children with trampoline fractures. *Eur J Radiol*. 2014;83(8):1433–1436.
148. Swaan JW, Oppers VM. Crural fractures in children. A study of the incidence of changes of the axial position and of enhanced longitudinal growth of the tibia after the healing of crural fractures. *Arch Chir Neerl*. 1971;23(4):259–272.
149. Taunton JE, Clement DB, Webber D. Lower extremity stress fractures in athletes. *Phys Sportsmed*. 1981;9(1):77–86.
150. Taylor SL. Tibial overgrowth: A cause of genu valgum. *J Bone Joint Surg Am*. 1963; 45:659.
151. Tenenbein M, Reed MH, Black GB. The toddler's fracture revisited. *Am J Emerg Med*. 1990;8(3):208–211.
152. Tuten HR, Keeler KA, Gabos PG, et al. Posttraumatic tibia valga in children. A long-term follow-up note. *J Bone Joint Surg Am*. 1999;81(6):799–810.
153. Vallamshetla VR, De Silva U, Bache CE, et al. Flexible intramedullary nails for unstable fractures of the tibia in children. An eight-year experience. *J Bone Joint Surg Br*. 2006;88(4):536–540.
154. van der Werken C, Meeuwis JD, Oostvogel HJ. The simple fix: External fixation of displaced isolated tibial fractures. *Injury*. 1993;24(1):46–48.
155. Walker RN, Green NE, Spindler KP. Stress fractures in skeletally immature patients. *J Pediatr Orthop*. 1996;16(5):578–584.

156. Weber BG. Fibrous interposition causing valgus deformity after fracture of the upper tibial metaphysis in children. *J Bone Joint Surg Br*. 1977;59(3):290–292.

157. Weber BG, Brunner C, Freuner F. *Treatment of Fractures in Children and Adolescents*. Berlin: Springer-Verlag; 1980.

158. Whitesides TE, Haney TC, Morimoto K, et al. Tissue pressure measurements as a determinant for the need of fasciotomy. *Clin Orthop Relat Res*. 1975(113):43–51.

159. Yang JP, Letts RM. Isolated fractures of the tibia with intact fibula in children: A review of 95 patients. *J Pediatr Orthop*. 1997;17(3):347–351.

160. Yue JJ, Churchill RS, Cooperman DR, et al. The floating knee in the pediatric patient. Nonoperative versus operative stabilization. *Clin Orthop Relat Res*. 2000(376):124–136.

161. Zionts LE, Harcke HT, Brooks KM, et al. Posttraumatic tibia valga: A case demonstrating asymmetric activity at the proximal growth plate on technetium bone scan. *J Pediatr Orthop*. 1987;7(4):458–462.

162. Zionts LE, MacEwen GD. Spontaneous improvement of post-traumatic tibia valga. *J Bone Joint Surg Am*. 1986;68(5):680–687.

29

Ankle Fractures

Kevin G. Shea and Steven L. Frick

Ankle Fractures

INTRODUCTION TO ANKLE FRACTURES

Injuries to the distal tibial and fibular physes are generally reported to account for 25% to 38% of all physeal fractures,[79,155] second in frequency only to distal radial physeal fractures[142]; however, Peterson et al.[143] reported that phalangeal physeal fractures were most common, followed by physeal injuries of the radius and ankle. In skeletally immature individuals, physeal ankle fractures are slightly more common than fractures of the tibial or fibular diaphysis,[120] and these fractures are a common cause of hospital admission in children.[44]

Participation in sports is associated with a significant number of ankle injuries, including sprains and fractures. Up to 58% of physeal ankle fractures occur during sports activities[65,197] and account for 10% to 40% of all injuries to skeletally immature athletes.[132,137,159,182] Physeal ankle fractures are more common in males than in females in some studies.[178] Other studies have

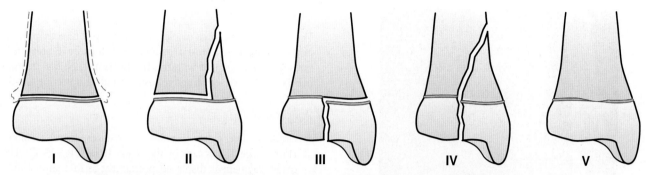

Figure 29-1. Salter–Harris anatomic classification as applied to injuries of the distal tibial epiphysis. This can also be applied to the distal fibula. This system has the highest interobserver reproducibility and is recommended for communication among care providers who have not seen radiographs.

demonstrated that ankle injuries may be more likely in young female soccer athletes compared with males.[106] Fractures of the ankle are associated with the following sports activities: Trampolines,[170] scooters,[119] soccer,[106] basketball,[48] skating,[131] and downhill skiing.[14] Increased BMI is also a risk factor for ankle injury in the skeletally immature.[198]

In addition to sports, higher-energy trauma is associated with a significant number of distal tibia and fibular fractures in children. These fractures occur in approximately 10% to 20% of trauma patients presenting to the emergency room.[14] Tibial physeal fractures are most common between the ages of 8 and 15 years, and fibular fractures are most common between 8 and 14 years of age.[178]

ASSESSMENT OF ANKLE FRACTURES

CLASSIFICATIONS AND MECHANISMS OF INJURY FOR ANKLE FRACTURE

There is no generally accepted fracture classification for ankle fractures in children that predicts outcome and directs treatment. Fracture classifications are usually based upon anatomy[2,135,141,178] or mechanism-of-injury descriptions.[4,10,103] Anatomical classifications distinguish fractures based on the regions of the metaphysis, physis, and epiphysis. Mechanism-of-injury classifications incorporate the forces, which produce the fracture and the anatomic position of the foot and ankle that existed at the time of the injury.

Since its description, the Salter–Harris classification system has been widely used to describe the anatomic features of fractures associated with open physes. This straightforward anatomic classification (Fig. 29-1) has five distinct categories, which can be applied to most periarticular regions.

Injury classifications based upon the mechanism of injury may have some advantages. The description of the injury includes the anatomic deformity and the forces that produced the injury. An understanding of these forces can facilitate reduction of a displaced fracture. Advanced imaging techniques that allow for comprehensive three-dimensional visualization of the fracture anatomy also facilitate surgical planning and reduction techniques.

Both anatomical and mechanism-of-injury classifications can provide useful information for determining appropriate treatment. The prognoses for growth and deformity have been predicted on the basis of both types of classification.[89,90,178] A theoretical advantage of mechanism-of-injury classifications is that identification of the force producing the injury might give even more information about the possible development of growth arrest than anatomical classifications.

Ideally, classification systems should have high inter- and intraobserver agreement. Thomsen et al.[187] studied the reproducibility of the Lauge-Hansen (mechanism-of-injury) and Weber (anatomical) classifications in a series of adult ankle fractures. After all investigators in the study had received a tutorial on both systems and their application, they were asked to classify 94 fractures. On the first attempt, only the Weber classification produced an acceptable level of interobserver agreement. On a second attempt, the Weber classification and most of the Lauge-Hansen classification achieved an acceptable level of interobserver agreement. These authors concluded that all fracture classification systems should have demonstrably acceptable interobserver agreement rates before they are adopted, an argument made even more forcefully in an editorial by Burstein.[29] Vahvanen and Aalto[189] compared their ability to classify 310 ankle fractures in children with the Weber, Lauge-Hansen, and Salter–Harris classifications. They found that they were "largely unsuccessful" using the Weber and Lauge-Hansen classifications, but could easily classify the fractures using the Salter–Harris system. We thus recommend using the Salter–Harris classification when assessing ankle fractures, and especially when communicating to others who have not seen x-rays (Fig. 29-2).

Dias and Tachdjian,[51] who modified the Lauge-Hansen classification based on their review of 71 fractures (Fig. 29-3). Their original classification (1978) consisted of four types in which the first word refers to the position of the foot at the time of injury and the second word refers to the force that produces the injury.

Other fracture types were subsequently added, including axial compression, juvenile Tillaux, triplane, and other physeal injuries by Tachdjian.[183] Syndesmosis injuries have also been recently described.[46] "Axial compression injury" describes the mechanism of injury but not the position of the foot. Juvenile Tillaux and triplane fractures are called transitional fractures as they occur when the physis is transitioning from open to closed, and are believed to be caused by external rotation.[158] The final category, "other physeal injuries," includes diverse injuries, many of which have no specific mechanism of injury.

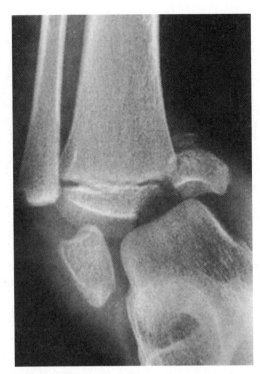

Figure 29-2. Comminuted Salter–Harris type IV fracture of the distal tibia and displaced Salter–Harris type I fracture of the distal fibula produced by an inversion (shearing) mechanism in a 10-year-old girl.

Dias–Tachdjian Classification of Ankle Fracture in Children

Supination–Inversion

- Grade I: The adduction or inversion force avulses the distal fibular epiphysis (Salter–Harris type I or II fracture). Occasionally, the fracture is transepiphyseal; rarely, the lateral ligaments fail (see Fig. 29-3).
- Grade II (Fig. 29-4): Further inversion produces a tibial fracture, usually a Salter–Harris type III or IV and rarely a Salter–Harris type I or II injury, or the fracture passes through the medial malleolus below the physis (Fig. 29-5).

Supination–Plantarflexion

The plantarflexion force displaces the epiphysis directly posteriorly, resulting in a Salter–Harris type I or II fracture. Fibular fractures were not reported with this mechanism. The tibial fracture may be difficult to see on anteroposterior radiographs (Fig. 29-6).

Supination–External Rotation

- Grade I: The external rotation force results in a Salter–Harris type II fracture of the distal tibia (Fig. 29-7). The distal fragment is displaced posteriorly, as in a supination–plantarflexion injury, but the Thurstan-Holland fragment is visible on the anteroposterior radiographs, with the fracture line extending proximally and medially.
- Grade II: With further external rotation, a spiral fracture of the fibula is produced, running from anteroinferior to posterosuperior (Fig. 29-8).

Pronation–Eversion–External Rotation

A Salter–Harris type I or II fracture of the distal tibia occurs simultaneously with a transverse fibular fracture. The distal tibial fragment is displaced laterally and the Thurstan-Holland fragment, when present, is lateral or posterolateral (Fig. 29-9). Less frequently, a transepiphyseal fracture occurs through the medial malleolus (Salter–Harris type II).

Axial Compression

This results in a Salter–Harris type V injury of the distal tibial physis. Initial radiographs usually show no abnormality, and the diagnosis is established when growth arrest is demonstrated on follow-up radiographs.

Transitional Fractures of the Distal Tibia and Fibula

Because the distal tibial physis closes in an asymmetric pattern over a period of about 18 months, injuries sustained during this period can produce fracture patterns that are not seen in younger children with completely open physes.[116] This group of fractures has been labeled "transitional" fractures because they occur

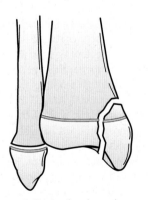 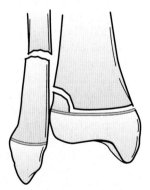 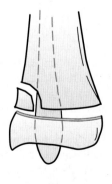 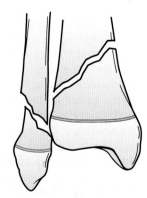

A. Supination–inversion B. Pronation–eversion external rotation C. Supination–plantarflexion D. Supination–external rotation

Figure 29-3. Dias–Tachdjian classification of physeal injuries of the distal tibia and fibula.

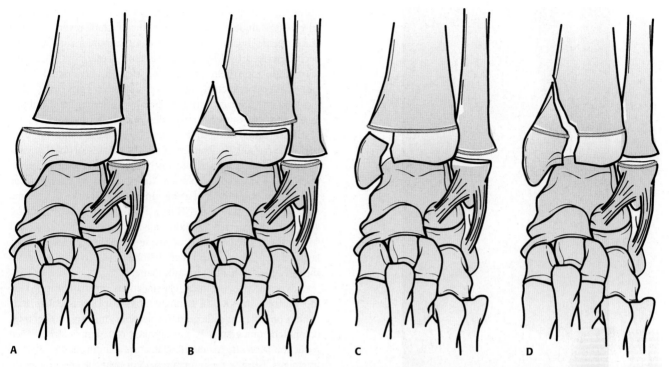

Figure 29-4. Variants of grade II supination–inversion injuries (Dias–Tachdjian classification). **A:** Salter–Harris type I fracture of the distal tibia and fibula. **B:** Salter–Harris type I fracture of the fibula, Salter–Harris type II tibial fracture. **C:** Salter–Harris type I fibular fracture, Salter–Harris type III tibial fracture. **D:** Salter–Harris type I fibular fracture, Salter–Harris type IV tibial fracture.

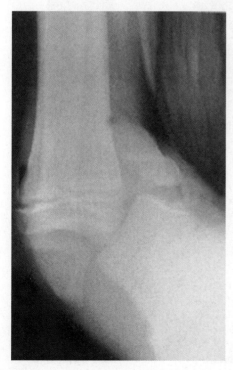

Figure 29-5. Severe supination–inversion injury with displaced fracture of the medial malleolus distal to the physis of the tibia.

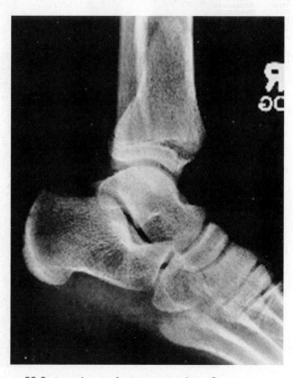

Figure 29-6. Lateral view of a supination–plantarflexion injury.

during the transition from a skeletally immature ankle to a skeletally mature ankle. Such fractures, which include juvenile Tillaux and "triplane" fractures with two to four fracture fragments, have been described by Kleiger and Mankin,[100] Marmor,[121] Cooperman et al.,[41] Kärrholm et al.,[88] and Denton and Fischer.[49] The adolescent pilon fracture has been described by Letts et al.[109] The incisural fracture has been described by Cummings and Hahn.[47] Syndesmosis injuries have been described by Cummings.[46]

Classification of these fractures is even more confusing than that of other distal tibial fractures. Advocates of mechanism-of-injury systems agree that most juvenile Tillaux and triplane fractures are caused by external rotation, but they disagree as to the position of the foot at the time of the injury.[50,51,148] Some authors[50] classify juvenile Tillaux fractures as stage I injuries, with further external rotation causing triplane fractures, and still further external rotation causing stage II injuries with fibular fracture. Others emphasize the extent of physeal closure as the only determinant of fracture pattern.[40]

Advocates of anatomical classifications are handicapped by the different anatomical configurations triplane fractures may exhibit on different radiograph projections, making tomography, computed tomography (CT) scanning, or examination at open reduction necessary to determine fracture anatomy and number of fragments. Because these fractures occur near the end of growth, growth disturbance is rare. Anatomical classification is, therefore, more useful for descriptive purposes than for prognosis.

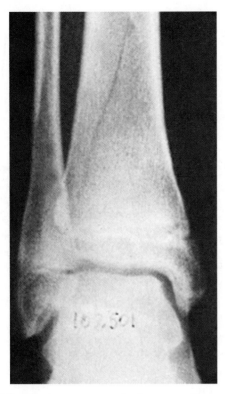

Figure 29-7. Stage I supination–external rotation injury in a 10-year-old child; the Salter–Harris type II fracture begins laterally.

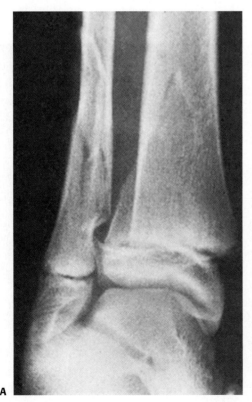
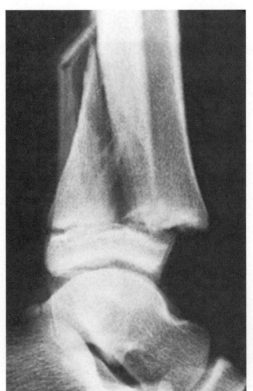

Figure 29-8. Stage II supination–external rotation injury. **A:** Oblique fibular fracture also is visible on anteroposterior view. **B:** Lateral view shows the posterior metaphyseal fragment and posterior displacement.

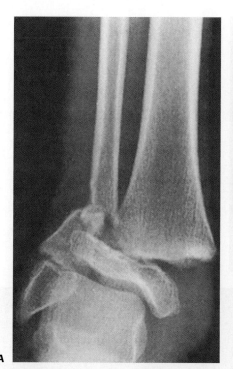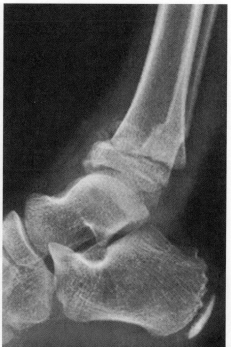

Figure 29-9. A: According to the Dias–Tachdjian classification, this injury in a 12-year-old boy would be considered a pronation–eversion–external rotation injury resulting in a Salter–Harris type II fracture of the distal tibia and a transverse fibular fracture. **B:** The anterior displacement of the epiphysis, visible on the lateral view, however, makes external rotation an unlikely component of the mechanism of injury; the mechanism is more likely pronation–dorsiflexion.

Juvenile Tillaux Fracture of the Distal Tibia and Fibula

The juvenile Tillaux fracture is a Salter–Harris type III fracture involving the anterolateral distal tibia. The portion of the physis not involved in the fracture is closed (Fig. 29-10).

Triplane Fracture of the Distal Tibia and Fibula

A group of fractures that have in common the appearance of a Salter–Harris type III fracture on the anteroposterior radiographs

and of a Salter–Harris type II fracture on the lateral radiographs (Fig. 29-11A,B). CT scans can be very helpful to understand the complex anatomy of these fractures (Fig. 29.11C–E).[11,44,99] Ipsilateral triplane and diaphyseal fractures have been reported, and one of the fractures can be missed if adequate images are not obtained.[11,44,82]

Adolescent Pilon Fractures of the Distal Tibia and Fibula

The pediatric/adolescent pilon fracture[109] is defined as a fracture of the "tibial plafond with articular and physeal involvement, variable

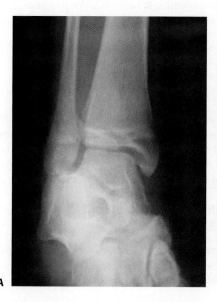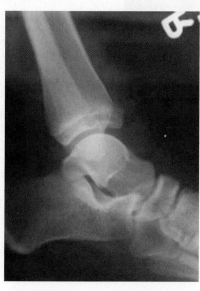

Figure 29-10. A: Anteroposterior radiograph of Salter–Harris type III/juvenile Tillaux fracture. **B:** Lateral radiograph of Salter–Harris type III/juvenile Tillaux fracture.

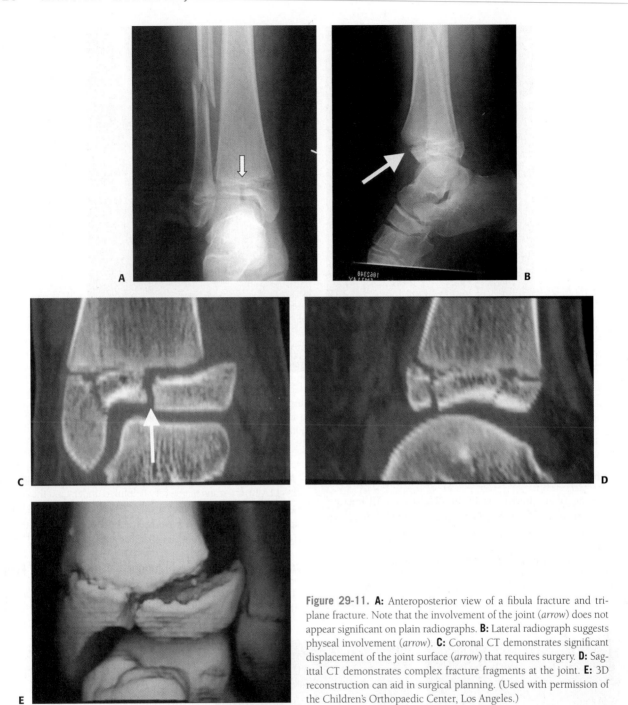

Figure 29-11. A: Anteroposterior view of a fibula fracture and triplane fracture. Note that the involvement of the joint (*arrow*) does not appear significant on plain radiographs. **B:** Lateral radiograph suggests physeal involvement (*arrow*). **C:** Coronal CT demonstrates significant displacement of the joint surface (*arrow*) that requires surgery. **D:** Sagittal CT demonstrates complex fracture fragments at the joint. **E:** 3D reconstruction can aid in surgical planning. (Used with permission of the Children's Orthopaedic Center, Los Angeles.)

talar and fibular involvement, variable comminution, and greater than 5 mm of displacement" (Fig. 29-12). Based upon a small number of cases, Letts et al. developed a three-part classification system. Type I fractures have minimal comminution and no physeal displacement. Type II fractures have marked comminution and less than 5 mm of physeal displacement. Type III fractures have marked comminution and more than 5 mm of physeal displacement.

Incisura Fractures of the Distal Tibia and Fibula

Incisural fractures are fractures that resemble Tillaux on standard radiographs, but the size of the fragment is smaller than that typically seen with the Tillaux fractures (Fig. 29-13).[47] On the CT scan, this fracture does not extend to the anterior cortex of the distal tibia (Fig. 29-14). The mechanism of injury may be an avulsion of the fragment by the interosseous ligament. This may be a variant of an adult tibiofibular diastasis injury.

SYNDESMOSIS INJURIES OF THE DISTAL TIBIAL AND FIBULAR FRACTURES

The authors have seen syndesmosis injuries in young patients. These have been associated with fractures of the distal fibula, Tillaux injuries, Salter–Harris I fractures, and proximal fibula

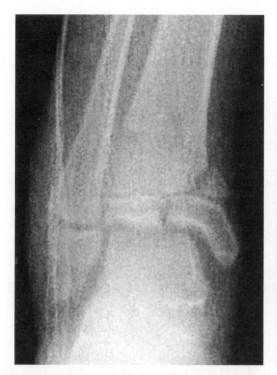

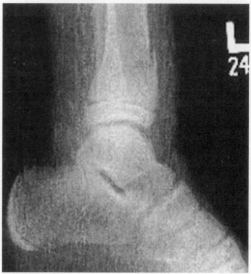

Figure 29-12. Anteroposterior and lateral radiographs of a pilon fracture in an adolescent.

fractures (Figs. 29-15 to 29-17). These fractures are probably rare and there is very limited literature on this injury.[140]

STRESS FRACTURES OF THE DISTAL TIBIA AND FIBULA

Stress fractures can occur in the distal tibial metaphyseal area (Fig. 29-18), or through the distal fibular physis (Fig. 29-19). These patients may present with warmth, swelling, and pain around the metaphyseal or physeal regions. In our experience,

these injuries are more common in gymnasts, ice skaters, and running/endurance athletes. We have seen stress fractures through the distal fibular physeal scar in running athletes.

SIGNS AND SYMPTOMS OF DISTAL TIBIAL AND FIBULAR FRACTURES

Patients with significantly displaced fractures have severe pain and obvious deformity. The position of the foot relative to the

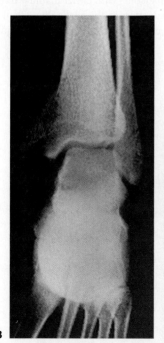

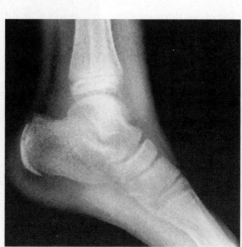

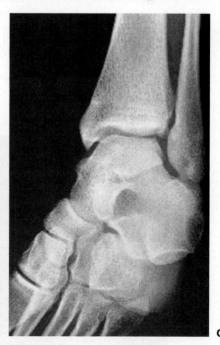

A, B   C

Figure 29-13. Anteroposterior (**A**), lateral (**B**), and oblique (**C**) views of the ankle demonstrating an apparent small juvenile Tillaux fracture in a 14-year-old girl.

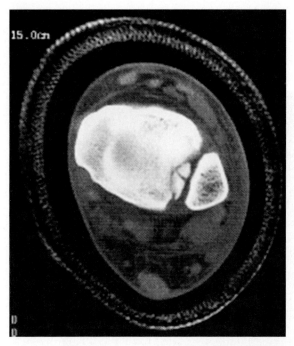

Figure 29-14. Incisural fracture: CT scan at the level of the tibiotalar joint demonstrates that the fracture fragment does not include the attachment of the anterior-inferior tibiofibular ligament.

leg may provide important information about the mechanism of injury (Fig. 29-20) and should be considered in planning reduction. The status of the skin, pulses, and sensory and motor function should be determined and recorded. Tenderness, swelling, and deformity in the ipsilateral leg and foot should be noted. In patients with tibial shaft fractures, the ankle should be carefully evaluated clinically and radiographically.

Although compartment syndromes are rare, they do occur in these locations.[43,127] If patients are admitted to the hospital,

discussion with the nursing staff about signs and symptoms of compartment syndrome is important. If patients are treated as outpatients, the patient and family should be informed about the possibility of compartment syndrome and instructed to return to the hospital for evaluation if problems with pain control develop.

EVALUATION FOR OTHER INJURIES

In low-energy ankle fractures, or those that occur during sports and play activity, other injuries are uncommon. In cases of higher-energy trauma such as motor vehicle/pedestrian accidents, the possibility of other injuries needs to be considered. A thorough physical evaluation to identify occult injuries is important. Some injuries can be missed, and ongoing awareness of this possibility is important during the hospitalization for more significant injuries.

IMAGING AND OTHER DIAGNOSTIC STUDIES FOR DISTAL TIBIAL AND FIBULAR FRACTURES

Patients with nondisplaced or minimally displaced ankle fractures often have no deformity, minimal swelling, and moderate pain. Because of their benign clinical appearance, such fractures may be easily missed if radiographs are not obtained. Petit et al.[145] reviewed 2,470 radiographs from pediatric emergency rooms, demonstrating abnormal radiographic findings in 9%. Guidelines known as the Ottawa Ankle Rules have been established for adults to determine which injuries require radiographs.[181] The Ottawa Ankle Rules have also been evaluated in children over the age of 5. These rules appear to be a reliable tool to exclude fractures in children greater than 5 years of age presenting with ankle and midfoot injuries and may significantly decrease x-ray use with a low likelihood of missing a fracture.[53] The indications for radiographs according to the guidelines are complaints of pain near a malleolus with either inability to bear weight or tenderness to palpation at the malleolus. Chande[38] prospectively studied 71 children with acute ankle injuries

Figure 29-15. A: Syndesmosis injury with distal fibula fracture. Radiographs with comparison of right and left sides. Note the widening of the medial clear space and the syndesmosis. **B:** Use of two percutaneously placed cannulated screws to reduce the syndesmosis.

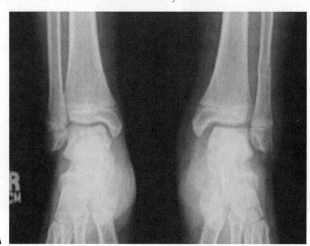

A

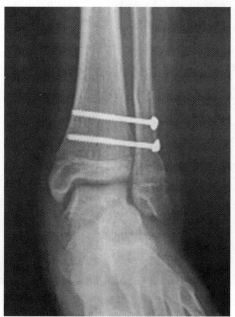

B

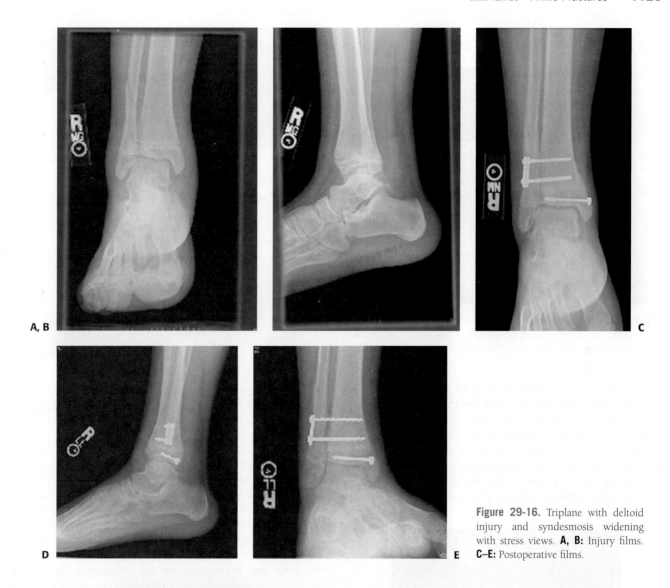

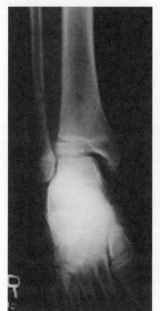

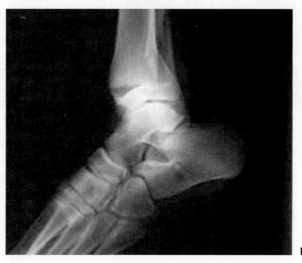

Figure 29-16. Triplane with deltoid injury and syndesmosis widening with stress views. **A, B:** Injury films. **C–E:** Postoperative films.

Figure 29-17. A, B: Deltoid and possible syndesmosis injury associated with triplane fracture pattern.

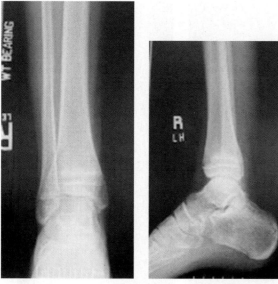

Figure 29-18. Distal tibia stress fracture. A 15-year-old male with 6 weeks of pain while running cross-country. Anteroposterior radiograph shows callus formation in the distal tibia metaphysis.

to determine if these guidelines could be applied to pediatric patients with ankle injuries. It was determined that if radiographs were obtained only in children with tenderness over the malleoli, and inability to bear weight, a 25% reduction in radiographic examinations could be achieved without missing any fractures. The physical examination should focus upon physeal areas of the tibia and fibula, when evaluating ankle injuries, to determine if radiographs are necessary. Interpretation of

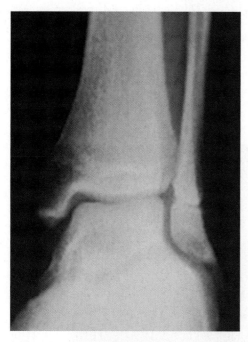

Figure 29-19. Stress fracture of distal fibula. A 16-year-old male with 6 weeks of pain while running track. Anteroposterior radiograph shows widened physis. The clinical examination shows point tenderness over the fibular physis.

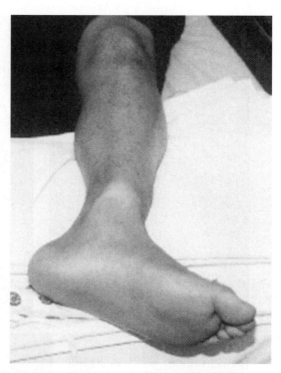

Figure 29-20. Severe clinical deformity in a 14-year-old boy with an ankle fracture. It is obvious without radiographs that internal rotation will be needed to reduce this fracture.

radiographs should focus upon signs of physeal injury, including soft tissue swelling in these regions.

For patients with obvious deformities, anteroposterior, mortise, and lateral radiographs centered over the ankle may provide sufficient information to plan treatment. Although obtaining views of the joint above and below is recommended for most fractures, obtaining a film centered over the mid-tibia to include the knee and ankle joints on the radiographs significantly decreases the quality of ankle views and is not recommended.

For patients without obvious deformities, a high-quality mortise view of the ankle is essential in addition to anteroposterior and lateral views. On a standard anteroposterior view, the lateral portion of the distal tibial physis is usually partially obscured by the distal fibula. The vertical component of a triplane or Tillaux fracture can be hidden behind the overlying fibular cortical shadow.[108] A study by Vangsness et al.[190] found that diagnostic accuracy was essentially equal when using anteroposterior, lateral, and mortise views compared with using only mortise and lateral views. Therefore, if only two views are to be obtained, the anteroposterior view may be omitted and lateral and mortise views obtained.

Haraguchi et al.[71] described two special views designed to detect avulsion fractures from the lateral malleolus that are not visible on routine views, and to distinguish whether they represent avulsions of the anterior tibiofibular ligament or the calcaneofibular ligament attachments. The anterior tibiofibular ligament view is made by positioning the foot in 45 degrees of plantarflexion and elevating the medial border of the foot 15 degrees. The calcaneofibular ligament view is obtained by rotating the leg 45 degrees inward.

Stress views are occasionally recommended historically to rule out ligamentous instability, but the authors see only rare indications for stress radiography in skeletally immature patients. The discomfort of stress views in an acute injury can be avoided by using other imaging options, such as magnetic resonance imaging (MRI). Stress views under anesthesia (regional and/or general) may be appropriate in some cases. This approach can allow for painless evaluation of the injured ankle with intra-operative comparison to the un-injured ankle.

Bozic et al.[24] studied the age at which the radiographic appearance of the incisura fibularis, tibiofibular clear space, and tibiofibular overlap develops in children. The purpose of their study was to facilitate the diagnosis of distal tibiofibular syndesmotic injury in children. They found that the incisura became detectable at a mean age of 8.2 years for girls and 11.2 years for boys. The mean age at which tibiofibular overlap appeared on the AP view was 5 years for both sexes; on the mortise view, it was 10 years for girls and 16 years for boys. The range of clear space measurements in normal children was 2 to 8 mm, with 23% of children having a clear space greater than 6 mm—a distance considered abnormal in adults.

CT is useful in the evaluation of intra-articular fractures, especially juvenile Tillaux and triplane fractures (Fig. 29-21).[6,11,27,44,59,86,99] Transverse images are obtained with thin cuts localized to the joint, and high-quality reconstructions can be produced in the coronal and sagittal planes without repositioning the ankle. Three-dimensional CT reconstructions may add further useful information, and readily available software packages allow easy production of such images (Fig. 29-22). These images can assist with minimally invasive approaches, the use of percutaneous reduction clamps, and positioning of fixation screws.

MRI may be useful in the evaluation of complex fractures of the distal tibia and ankle in patients with open physes. Smith et al.[177] found that of four patients with acute (3 to 10 days) physeal injuries, MRI showed that three had more severe fractures than indicated on plain films (Fig. 29-23). Early MRI studies (3 to 17 weeks after injury) not only added information about the pattern of physeal disruption but also supplied early information about the possibility of growth abnormality. MRI has been reported to be occasionally helpful in the identification of osteochondral injuries to the joint surfaces in children with ankle fractures.[98] Although these injuries may be more common in adult fractures, we believe that these types of injuries are rare in younger patients.

Carey et al.[32] obtained MRI studies on 14 patients with known or suspected growth plate injury. The MRI detected 5 radiographically occult fractures in the 14 patients, changed the Salter–Harris classification in 2 cases, and resulted in a change in treatment plan in 5 of the 14 patients studied. These studies would seem to contradict an earlier study by Petit et al.[144] that showed only 1 patient in a series of 29 patients in whom MRI revealed a diagnosis different from that made on plain films. Iwinska-Zelder et al.[81] found that the MRI changed

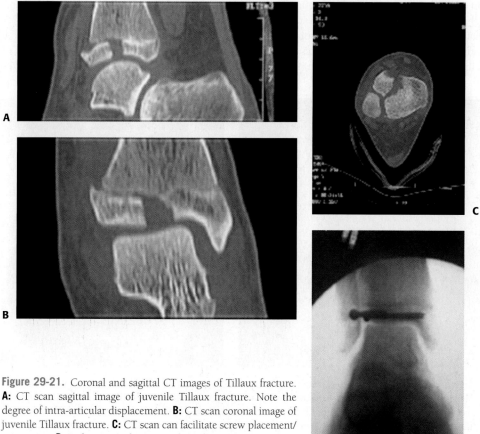

Figure 29-21. Coronal and sagittal CT images of Tillaux fracture. **A:** CT scan sagittal image of juvenile Tillaux fracture. Note the degree of intra-articular displacement. **B:** CT scan coronal image of juvenile Tillaux fracture. **C:** CT scan can facilitate screw placement/ orientation. **D:** Reduction with intraepiphyseal screws.

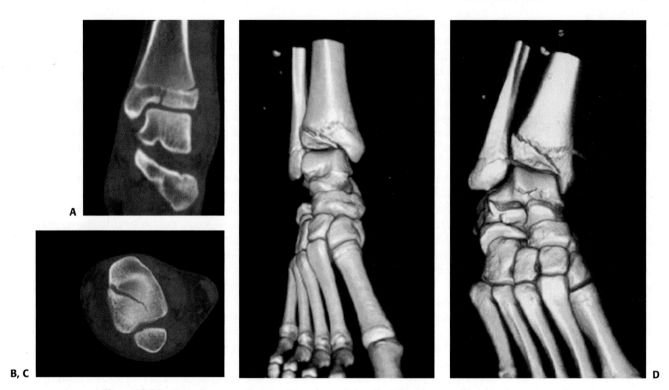

Figure 29-22. Three-dimensional CT reconstruction of juvenile Tillaux fracture. **A:** Coronal CT image of minimally displaced juvenile Tillaux fracture. **B:** Sagittal CT image of minimally displaced juvenile Tillaux fracture. **C, D:** Three-dimensional reconstruction of juvenile Tillaux fracture.

the management in 4 of 10 patients with ankle fractures seen on plain radiographs. Siffert et al.[173] found the MRI identified physeal injuries that were not identified by plain radiographs. At this time, the indications for MRI in the evaluation of ankle fractures in skeletally immature patients are still being defined, but this imaging modality may be a more sensitive tool for identification of minimally displaced or more complex injuries.[11] In a recent prospective study of skeletally immature patients with clinically diagnosed Salter I fractures of the distal fibula, none of the 18 patients imaged by MRI had evidence of physeal

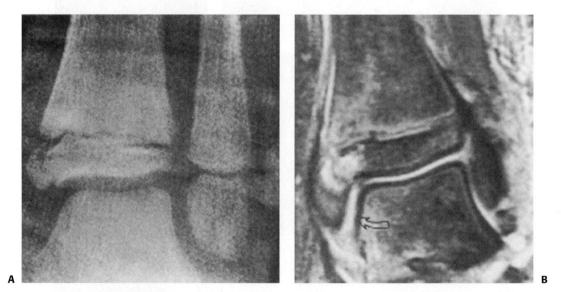

Figure 29-23. A: Follow-up radiograph of a 7-year-old boy 1 week after an initially nondisplaced Salter–Harris type III fracture from a supination–inversion injury of the distal tibia. **B:** Because of the incomplete ossification of this area and concern that the fracture might have displaced, MRI was performed. Note that the distance between the medial malleolus and the talus is greater than the distance between the talus and the distal tibia or lateral malleolus, confirming displacement of the fracture.

injury. The patients had a mean age of 8 years, and over 70% had evidence of ligamentous sprain on MRI. This questions the principle that the physis is the weak link in the musculoskeletal system in this age group.[21] If physeal arrest occurs, MRI scans are useful for mapping physeal bars.[62,73]

The use of ultrasound to detect radiographically occult fractures may be used for pediatric ankle fractures.[174]

Pitfalls in Diagnosis

A number of accessory ossification centers and normal anatomical variations may cause confusion in the interpretation of plain films of the ankle (Fig. 29-24). In a group of 100 children between the ages of 6 and 12 years, Powell found accessory ossification centers on the medial side (os subtibiale) in 20% and on the lateral side (os subfibulare) in 1%. If they are asymptomatic on clinical examination, these ossification centers are of little concern, but tenderness localized to them may indicate an injury. Stress views to determine motion of the fragments or MRI scanning may occasionally be considered if an injury to an accessory ossification center is suspected.

Clefts in the lateral side of the tibial epiphysis may simulate juvenile Tillaux fractures, and clefts in the medial side may simulate Salter–Harris type III fractures.[95] The presence of these clefts on radiographs of a child with an ankle injury may result in overtreatment if they are misdiagnosed as a fracture. Conversely, attributing a painful irregularity in these areas to anatomical variation may lead to undertreatment (Fig. 29-25).

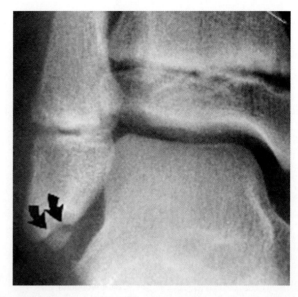

Figure 29-24. Secondary ossification center in the lateral malleolus (*arrows*) of a 10-year-old girl. Note the smooth border of the fibula and the ossification center. She also has a secondary ossification center in the medial malleolus.

Other anatomical variations include a bump on the distal fibula that simulates a torus fracture and an apparent offset of the distal fibular epiphysis that simulates a fracture. These radiographic findings should be correlated with physical examination

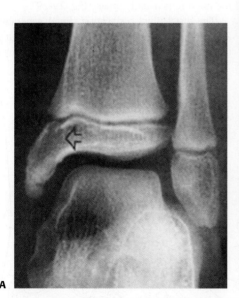 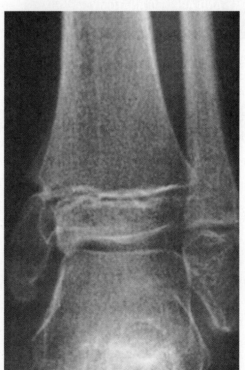

A **B**

Figure 29-25. A: Mortise view of the ankle of a 10-year-old girl who had slight swelling and tenderness at the medial malleolus after an "ankle sprain." The ossicle at the tip of the medial malleolus was correctly identified as an os subtibiale. A subtle line extending from the medial physis to just distal to the medial tibial plafond (*arrow*) was also believed to be an anatomic variant. **B:** Four weeks after injury, soreness persisted and radiographs clearly demonstrated a displaced Salter–Harris type III fracture.

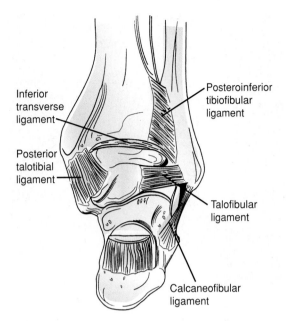

Figure 29-26. Posterior view of the distal tibia and fibula and the ligaments making up the ankle mortise.

findings of focal swelling and point tenderness that correspond with the imaging in the diagnosis of skeletal injury.

PATHOANATOMY AND APPLIED ANATOMY RELATING TO ANKLE FRACTURES

The ankle joint closely approximates a hinge joint. It is the articulation between the talus and the ankle mortise, which is a syndesmosis consisting of the distal tibial articular surface, the medial malleolus, and the distal fibula or lateral malleolus.

Four ligamentous structures bind the distal tibia and fibula into the ankle mortise (Fig. 29-26). The anterior and posterior-inferior tibiofibular ligaments course inferiorly from the anterior and posterior surfaces of the distal lateral tibia to the anterior and posterior surfaces of the lateral malleolus. The anterior ligament is important in the pathomechanics of "transitional" ankle fractures. Just anterior to the posterior-inferior tibiofibular ligament is the broad, thick inferior transverse ligament, which extends down from the lateral malleolus along the posterior border of the articular surface of the tibia, almost to the medial malleolus. This ligament serves as a part of the articular surface for the talus. Between the anterior and posterior-inferior tibiofibular ligaments, the tibia and fibula are bound by the interosseous ligament, which is continuous with the interosseous membrane above. This ligament may be important in the pathomechanics of what we have termed incisural fractures.

On the medial side of the ankle, the talus is bound to the ankle mortise by the deltoid ligament (Fig. 29-27). This ligament arises from the medial malleolus and divides into superficial and deep layers. Three parts of the superficial layer are identified by their attachments: Tibionavicular, calcaneotibial, and posterior talotibial ligaments. The deep layer is known as the anterior talotibial ligament, again reflecting its insertion and origin. On the lateral side, the anterior and posterior talofibular ligament, with the calcaneofibular ligaments, make up the lateral collateral ligament (Fig. 29-28).

In children, all medial and lateral ligaments originate distal to the tibial or fibular physis. Because the ligaments are often stronger than the physes, physeal fractures have generally been viewed as more common than ligamentous injuries in children. Advanced imaging studies have shown that the rate of ankle fractures compared to ligamentous injuries is variable,[57] and this is likely dependent on multiple factors such as the mechanism of injury, rate of force application, relative strength of the physis, and age of the patient. When distal tibia and fibular fragments are displaced together, the syndesmosis at the level of the fracture is usually intact (Fig. 29-29).

The distal tibial ossification center generally appears at 6 to 24 months of age. Its malleolar extension begins to form around the age of 7 or 8 years and is mature or complete at the age of

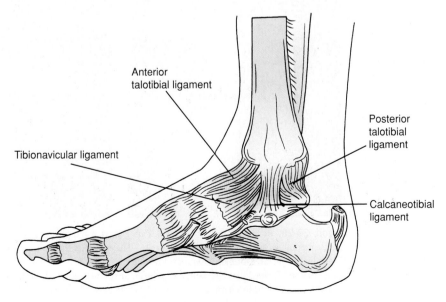

Figure 29-27. Medial view of the ankle demonstrating the components of the deltoid ligament.

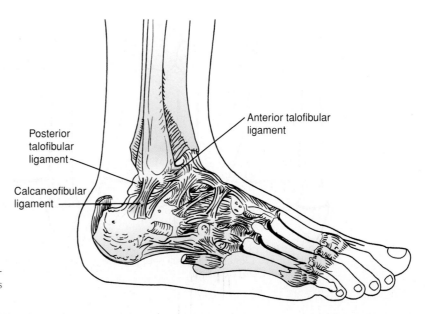

Posterior talofibular ligament

Anterior talofibular ligament

Calcaneofibular ligament

Figure 29-28. Lateral view of the ankle demonstrating the anterior and posterior talofibular ligaments and the calcaneofibular ligament.

10 years. The medial malleolus develops as an elongation of the distal tibia ossific nucleus, although in 20% of cases, this may originate from a separate ossification center, the os tibial. This can be mistaken as a fracture.[93] The physis usually closes around the age of 15 years in girls and 17 years in boys. This process takes approximately 18 months and occurs first in the central part of the physis, extending next to the medial side, and finally ending laterally. This asymmetric closure sequence is an important anatomical feature of the growing ankle and is responsible for certain fracture patterns in adolescents, especially transitional fractures (Fig. 29-30).

The distal fibular ossification center appears around the ages of 9 to 24 months. This physis is located at the level of the ankle joint initially, and moves distally with growth.[91,196] Closure of this physis generally follows closure of the distal tibial physis by 12 to 24 months.

The locations of the sensory nerves are important anatomic landmarks, as surgical exposures should aim to protect these structures. The superficial peroneal nerve branches may be most vulnerable around the ankle, especially during arthroscopic and arthrotomy approaches for triplane and Tillaux fractures.[12] This

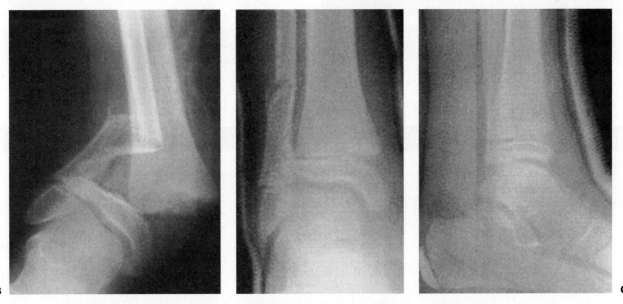

A, B   C

Figure 29-29. A: Pronation–external rotation injury resulting in a Salter–Harris type I fracture of the distal tibial physis. Note that despite this severe displacement, the relationship between the distal epiphysis of the tibia and distal fibula is preserved, and widening of the syndesmosis between the tibia and fibula is not present in this region. **B, C:** Anteroposterior and lateral radiographs demonstrate satisfactory closed reduction.

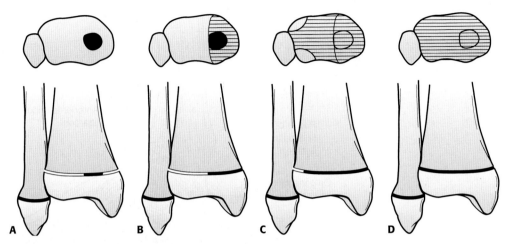

Figure 29-30. Closure of the distal tibial physis begins centrally (**A**), extends medially (**B**), and then laterally (**C**) before final closure (**D**).

is important when arthroscopic and percutaneous reduction techniques are employed for fracture treatment.

TREATMENT OPTIONS FOR ANKLE FRACTURES

For current treatment options, see Table 29-1.

NONOPERATIVE TREATMENT OF ANKLE FRACTURES

Indications/Contraindications

Nonoperative Treatment of Ankle Fractures: INDICATIONS AND CONTRAINDICATIONS	
Indications	**Contraindications**
• Nondisplaced, stable fracture patterns • Stable, minimally displaced fracture patterns	• Significant intra-articular displacement or step off of articular surface, more than 2 mm • Unstable fracture patterns • Significant fracture displacement

Appropriate treatment of ankle fractures in children depends on the location of the fracture, the degree of displacement, and the age of the child (Table 29-1). Nondisplaced fractures may be simply immobilized. A recent randomized clinical trial for minimally displaced low-risk ankle fractures compared a fiberglass posterior splint to a removable ankle stirrup brace. This study demonstrated good outcomes in both groups.[7] Closed reduction and cast immobilization may be appropriate for displaced fractures; if the closed reduction cannot be maintained with casting, skeletal fixation may be necessary. If closed reduction is not possible, open reduction may be indicated, followed by internal fixation or cast immobilization.

The anatomic type of the fracture (usually defined by the Salter–Harris classification), the mechanism of injury, and the amount of displacement of the fragments are important considerations. When the articular surface is disrupted, the amount of articular step-off or separation must be measured. The neurologic and vascular status of the limb or the status of the skin may require emergency treatment of the fracture and associated problems. The general health of the patient and the time since injury must also be considered.

TABLE 29-1. Current Treatment Options

Fracture	Options	Pros	Cons
Distal tibia physis	Above-knee vs. below-knee cast	Below-knee casts may allow for less knee stiffness and muscle atrophy of the thigh	For fractures with potential for displacement, the below-knee cast may increase the risk of displacement.
	Local anesthesia with sedation vs. general anesthesia (closed reduction of fractures)	Local anesthesia techniques combined with sedation in the ER may be less expensive, and allow for early reduction	Guidelines for sedation techniques must follow guidelines established by the American Society of Anesthesiologists, and adequate facilities and personnel may not be available in all emergency rooms.
	Minimally invasive approaches (including arthroscopic assistance) vs. traditional open surgical exposures	Arthroscopic-assisted procedures may allow for smaller incisions, and better assessment of articular reductions than open exposures	Additional equipment and OR staffing requirements for arthroscopy are necessary. Surgeon experience with arthroscopy may be more limited.
	Bioabsorbable vs. metal implants	Bioabsorbable devices do not require removal, and subsequent imaging studies (CT, MRI) are not affected by these implants	First-generation implants have a higher risk of local inflammation, and the quality of fixation may be less secure.

OPERATIVE TREATMENT OF ANKLE FRACTURES

Preoperative Planning

Operative treatment is indicated for open fractures or injuries with severe soft tissue injury, when there is displacement of the articular surface, or when acceptable position and alignment cannot be maintained with closed methods.

✔ Operative Repair of Ankle Fractures: PREOPERATIVE PLANNING CHECKLIST	
OR table	❏ Radiolucent component can be valuable. Confirm that the fracture can be easily seen prior to prepping and draping the patient's fracture site.
Position/positioning aids	❏ Allowing the ankle to be moved off the table to the side, can allow easy access for C-arm evaluation. In some cases, a bump can be placed behind the hip on the injured side, to allow for the ankle to be positioned with more, rather than less inward rotation.
Fluoroscopy location	❏ Best location may be just off to the side of the patient, as they are positioned on the table. This allows the ankle to be moved off the side of the table, to allow easy visualization with the C-arm. We find that use of the mini C-arm has many advantages over the larger C-arm, including: lower radiation dose, easy maneuverability, does not require additional OR staff to operate, etc.
Equipment	❏ Appropriate orthopedic reduction tools, including large and medium bone reduction clamps, dental picks, excellent lighting source, cannulated screw systems, etc. Headlights may be valuable in some cases.
Tourniquet	❏ Use may be optional, depending on surgeon preference. Clear visualization of the fracture planes may be enhanced by use of the tourniquet.

Advanced Imaging Studies

CT has replaced tomograms and gives better bone resolution than MRI for intra-articular fractures. For intra-articular and multi-fragmented fracture patterns, CT can help plan reduction and fixation techniques. High-resolution scans with three-dimensional reconstructions provide excellent anatomic detail. For minimally invasive approaches using percutaneous screw fixation, these images can be used to plan small incisions and for precise screw placement during surgery. The CT scan can also facilitate percutaneous placement of clamps, to allow for compression perpendicular to the plane of the fracture. A clear preoperative evaluation should determine optimal screw position and orientation, and these images should also be available during the procedure to assist with screw placement.

OPEN REDUCTION AND INTERNAL FIXATION OF ANKLE FRACTURES

Technique

✔ ORIF of Ankle Fractures: KEY SURGICAL STEPS
❏ Expose ankle fracture using x-rays and/or CT scans to plan incision placement
❏ Review anatomy of all superficial nerve branches about the ankle
❏ Apply arthroscopic ankle distractor if appropriate
❏ Preserve soft tissue attachments as much as possible
❏ Reduce and provisionally stabilize joint
❏ Reduce physis and metaphysis as appropriate
❏ Plate fixation may be necessary to maintain the reduction
❏ Use the C-arm to confirm length, location of the implants

Expose ankle fracture that allows for exposure/reduction of the metaphyseal, epiphyseal, and intra-articular portion as necessary. Use of CT and x-rays is invaluable for planning incision placement. Review the anatomy of all superficial nerve branches about the ankle, to avoid inadvertent nerve injury and secondary neuroma formation. Apply arthroscopic ankle distractor across ankle joint if traction may facilitate reduction, visualization of the fracture. In many cases, minimal fracture exposure is necessary. In some cases, more extensive exposure is valuable, to help with reduction. Preserve soft tissue attachments as much as possible, to avoid injury to bone vascularity. In some cases, contralateral ankle x-rays may be obtained of the opposite ankle from the C-arm, to help guide reduction of the injured side. Keep these images readily available to help with reduction. Because of the importance of intra-articular surface reduction, prioritize reduction of joint surface. Joint reduction may be obtained and enhanced with strategic bone clamp placement. Provisional stabilization may be obtained with K-wires. K-wires from cannulated screw systems may be placed, and some of these K-wires may be used for placement of cannulated screws over the wires. In some cases, cannulated screws can be placed over washers, to enhance compression across the fracture planes, and minimize the penetration of screws into the relatively soft epiphyseal and metaphyseal bone.

Reduce physis and metaphysis as appropriate. Use of K-wires and cannulated screws can facilitate and maintain reduction. In some cases, placement of K-wires may be used as a "joystick" and a reduction tool to help with anatomic reduction of a displaced fragment. When possible, use of smooth K-wires across the physis may be necessary to maintain reduction. Smooth wires may be less likely to cause physeal arrest. In some cases, screws may be placed across the physis that is approaching closure, including juvenile plafond fractures and transitional fracture patterns. Plate fixation may be necessary in some cases, to help the reduction on the fibula, and in some cases, on the tibial side as well. Use the C-arm to confirm length, location of the implants. A preoperative CT scan can be used to help plan placement of all screws, as well as allow the surgeon to plan for the appropriate screw length, and thread length. Optimized screw and thread length can improve compression of fractures. During screw, K-wire placement, be vigilant about surrounding neurovascular structures. If these devices penetrate too deeply, can injure these structures. Remain

Figure 29-31. Ankle arthroscopy. **A:** Arthroscopic view of fracture gap in distal tibia articular surface. **B:** Arthroscopic view of fracture gap in distal tibial articular surface after reduction.

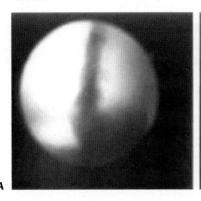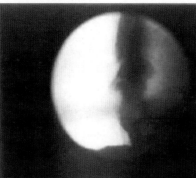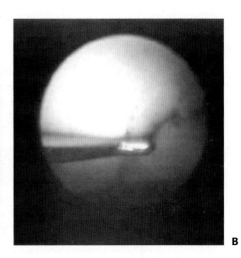

A   B

vigilant for the possibility of compartment syndrome, as this may occur after ankle fracture in children.

Arthroscopy

The use of arthroscopy can facilitate minimally invasive procedures, and also be a tool to help guide reduction during open procedures using larger incisions. Several clinical series document the effectiveness of arthroscopic assistance for Tillaux fractures[83,124,138] and triplane fractures.[80,83] The joint surfaces can be readily visualized through small incisions, avoiding the need for a larger arthrotomy. Even in cases where an arthrotomy is used, the scope can be utilized either with or without fluid to visualize the reduction of the fragments (Fig. 29-31). The fluid of the arthroscopy pump can also be used to wash out the fracture site, increasing visualization during reduction. Avoidance of high pump pressure will minimize the risks of soft tissue infiltration.

Different size scopes are available, including 2.8 and 4.5 mm. We prefer to use smaller-diameter scopes, especially in younger patients. The smaller scope has a smaller field of view, but this does not seem to be much of a disadvantage for viewing the displaced cartilage surfaces. The smaller scope also delivers less

fluid to the joint, which may require additional time to clean the hematoma from the joint and fracture, but has a lower risk of causing soft tissue infiltration around the joint.

Fluoroscopy

The small C-arm unit will also assist with minimally invasive approaches. This can be easily rotated to allow for AP, oblique, or lateral views. If the ankle distractor is used, position the foot and distractor to allow easy access by the C-arm (Fig. 29-32).

Ankle Distraction

Use of the ankle distractor (normally used for arthroscopy procedures) can assist with reduction of displaced extra-articular fractures, such as Salter–Harris type I or II patterns. When combined with the relaxation of general anesthesia, a few minutes of distraction across the physis can facilitate reduction. The distraction across the fracture may increase the likelihood that the first attempt at reduction will be successful; this may reduce the trauma to the physis during the reduction, perhaps reducing the risk of physeal arrest. Juvenile Tillaux and triplane fracture

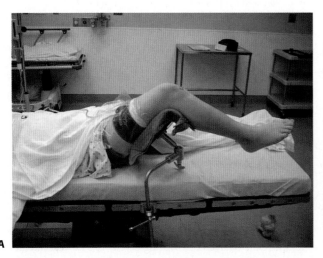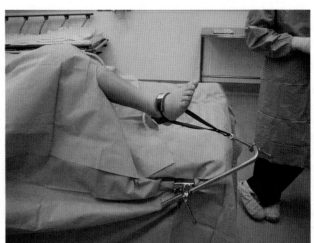

A   B

Figure 29-32. Use of ankle distractor. **A:** Thigh positioner to allow for ankle distractor. **B:** Sterile ankle distractor in place.

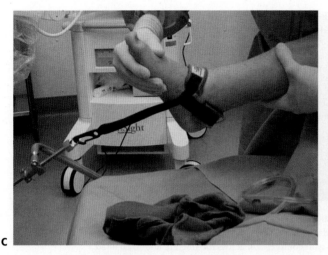
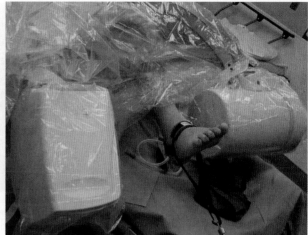

C   **D**

Figure 29-32. (*Continued*) **C:** Distractor can remain in place during reduction maneuvers. **D:** C-arm can be brought into the field to evaluate the reduction.

reduction can also be facilitated with ankle distraction, and this will also facilitate arthroscopic ankle visualization. The ankle distractor obviates the need to have the surgeon pull manually for several minutes. The surgeon can then focus on the application of other forces, such as rotation or varus/valgus to facilitate fracture reduction. Although skeletal traction using a calcaneal pin is an option,[35] we prefer to use an ankle strap and special distractor routinely used for arthroscopy (Arthrex, Naples, Florida). The ankle distractor can be positioned to allow for anteroposterior and lateral mini C-arm images (see Fig. 29-32).

Percutaneous Clamps

Precise placement of clamps can facilitate the reduction of fractures. Careful study of imaging studies, especially CT scans, can guide precise placement of clamps to provide maximal compression across fracture planes. Forces normal or near normal to the fracture planes are ideal. Care should be taken during placement, to prevent injury to neurologic and vascular structures, including sensory nerves. The skin can be divided, and then

deeper dissection through the subcutaneous tissues can be performed with a hemostat. The hemostat is used to bluntly distract the tissues away from the skin portal, and then advanced to the bone surface. The tips of the clamp can now be placed with minimal risk to neurovascular structures. The clamp can be compressed, to facilitate reduction of triplane and Tillaux fractures (Figs. 29-33 and 29-34).

Implants

Different implants are available for fixation of ankle fractures. Smooth pins have the advantage that they do not place a threaded tip across the physis, therefore reducing the risk of iatrogenic physeal arrest. The main disadvantage of smooth pins is that they do not allow for compression. These pins can also migrate through bone, and into soft tissues. Bending the ends at the surface of the skin to prevent migration is important. These pins should be removed early, as soon as the fracture stability is adequate. In most cases, we remove the pins between 14 and 21 days after surgery. Careful management of the pin–skin

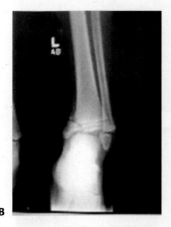
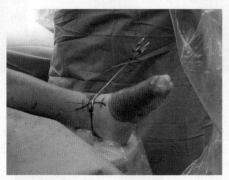
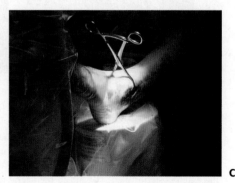

A, B   **C**

Figure 29-33. A: Anteroposterior view of displaced Salter–Harris type I fibula fracture and Salter–Harris type IV intra-articular medial malleolus fracture. **B:** Use of percutaneous clamps to facilitate reduction of medial malleolus fracture. **C:** Use of percutaneous clamps to facilitate reduction.

(continues)

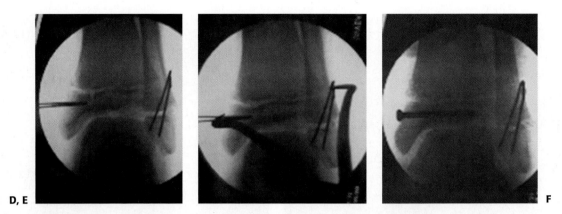

D, E   **F**

Figure 29-33. (*Continued*) **D:** Use of two pins as "joysticks" to guide reduction of the displaced medial malleolus fracture. **E:** Use of percutaneous clamps to facilitate reduction and compression across the epiphyseal fracture. **F:** Use of percutaneous epiphyseal screws to gain compression across the fracture and to facilitate reduction.

interface with dressings that limit motion is believed to lower the risk of pin inflammation and infection.

In most physeal injuries, the use of screws or threaded devices across the physis should be avoided when possible. In some cases, a screw implant may be necessary to cross a physis, to maintain an articular reduction. The adequacy of reduction of the joint surface is probably more important than the physis. In patients approaching skeletal maturity, the use of screw

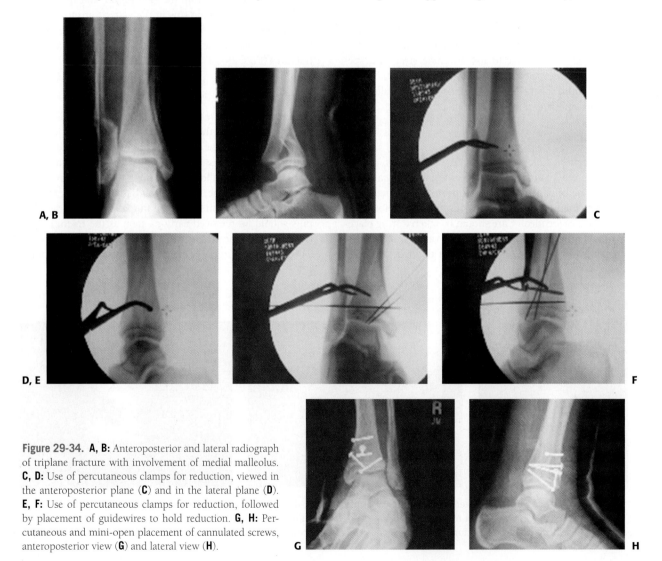

A, B   **C**

D, E   **F**

G   **H**

Figure 29-34. A, B: Anteroposterior and lateral radiograph of triplane fracture with involvement of medial malleolus. **C, D:** Use of percutaneous clamps for reduction, viewed in the anteroposterior plane (**C**) and in the lateral plane (**D**). **E, F:** Use of percutaneous clamps for reduction, followed by placement of guidewires to hold reduction. **G, H:** Percutaneous and mini-open placement of cannulated screws, anteroposterior view (**G**) and lateral view (**H**).

implants across a physis that is approaching closure is probably a reasonable choice, especially in case where compression and/or stability are important, such as juvenile Tillaux fractures (Fig. 29-35).

Distal Tibial Fractures

Salter–Harris Type I and II Fractures

Cast immobilization is sufficient treatment for nondisplaced Salter–Harris type I fractures of the distal tibia. A below-knee cast worn for 3 to 4 weeks may suffice, with the first 1 to 2 weeks limited to nonweight bearing. An above-knee cast may also be used, although this may not be necessary as these fractures are usually very stable. In very active patients who may

not comply with activity/weight-bearing restrictions, this type of cast may be an advantage. After cast removal, use of a removable leg/ankle walking boot may be used, followed by a therapy program in older patients or those trying to return to competitive sports at an earlier time. In our experience, formal supervised therapy is not necessary in younger patients. The normal activity of these children is usually sufficient therapy.

Most displaced fractures can be treated with closed reduction and cast immobilization. An above-knee non–weight-bearing cast is preferable initially, as this should reduce the risk of displacement after reduction, although no evidence clearly supports above-knee compared to below-knee casts. These casts may be changed to a short-leg walking cast or removable walking boot at 3 to 4 weeks. These fractures can displace

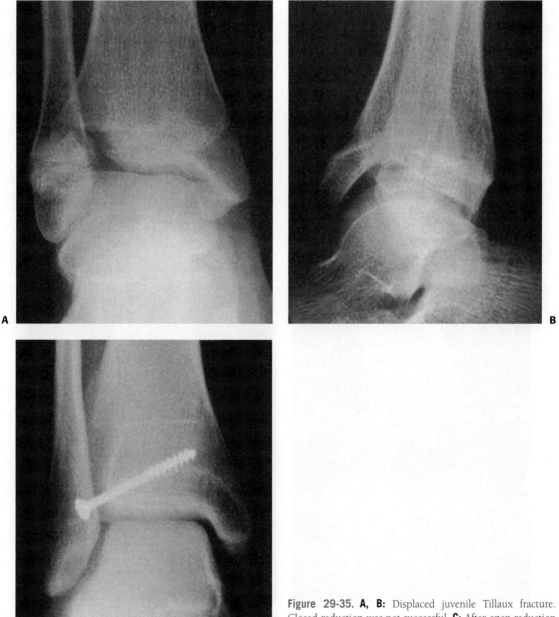

Figure 29-35. A, B: Displaced juvenile Tillaux fracture. Closed reduction was not successful. **C:** After open reduction with internal fixation with a small fragment screw.

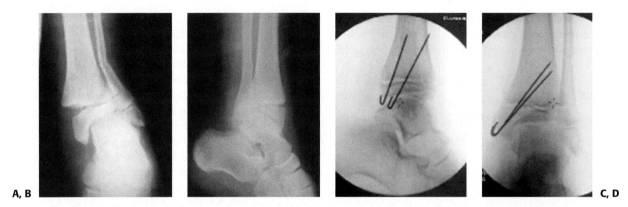

A, B   **C, D**

Figure 29-36. A, B: Displaced distal tibial Salter–Harris type II fracture, with distal diaphyseal fibula fracture. **C, D:** Fracture treated with closed reduction and internal fixation.

in the first 1 to 2 weeks postoperatively, and close follow-up with radiographic surveillance for this is necessary. One of the authors (KS) frequently places one or two K-wires at the time of closed reduction, to prevent displacement after reduction under anesthesia (Fig. 29-36). These pins are usually removed in the clinic 2 to 3 weeks after placement. Under these circumstances, a below-knee cast can be used.

Salter–Harris Type II Fractures

Salter–Harris type II fractures can be caused by any of the four mechanisms of injury described by Dias and Giegerich.[50] In the series of Spiegel et al.,[178] Salter–Harris type II fractures were the most common injuries (44.8%). In addition to the direction of displacement of the distal tibial epiphysis and the nature of any associated fibular fracture, the location of the Thurstan-Holland fragment is helpful in determining the mechanism of injury; for example, a lateral fragment indicates a pronation–eversion–external rotation injury; a posteromedial fragment, a

supination–external rotation injury; and a posterior fragment, a supination–plantarflexion injury (Fig. 29-37).

Nondisplaced fractures can be treated with cast immobilization usually with an above-knee cast for 3 to 4 weeks, followed by a below-knee walking cast or removable cast/walking boot for another 3 to 4 weeks.

Although most authors agree that closed reduction of significantly displaced Salter–Harris type II ankle fracture should be attempted, opinions differ as to what degree of residual displacement or angulation is unacceptable and requires open reduction. Based on follow-up of 33 Salter–Harris type II ankle fractures, Carothers and Crenshaw[33] concluded that "accurate reposition of the displaced epiphysis at the expense of forced or repeated manipulation or operative intervention is not indicated since spontaneous realignment of the ankle occurs even late in the growing period." They found no residual angulation at follow-up in patients who had up to 12 degrees of tilt after reduction, even in patients as old as 13 years of age at the time of injury. Spiegel et al.,[178] however, reported complications at

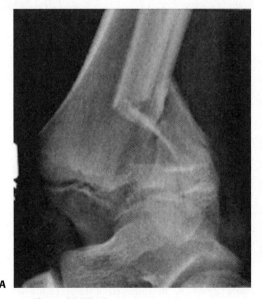
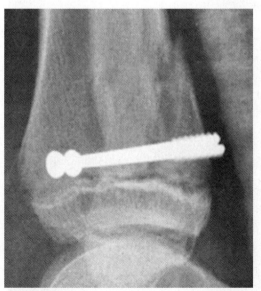

A   **B**

Figure 29-37. A: Severe plantarflexion injury with severe swelling of the ankle and foot; the reduction obtained was unstable. **B:** The reduction was stabilized by two transmetaphyseal screws placed percutaneously.

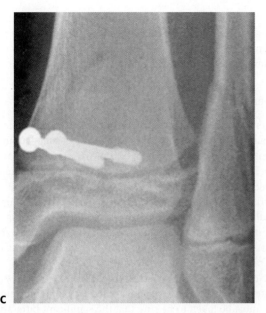

Figure 29-37. (*Continued*) **C:** Anteroposterior view confirms an anatomic reduction.

follow-up in 11 of 16 patients with Salter–Harris type II ankle fractures. Because 6 of these 11 patients had angular deformities that were attributed to lack of adequate reduction of the fracture, Spiegel et al. recommend "precise anatomical reduction."

Barmada et al.[6] reviewed a series of Salter–Harris type I and II fractures. In patients with more than 3 mm of physeal widening, the risk of premature physeal closure was 60%, compared with 17% in patients with less than 3 mm of physeal

widening. Although they were unable to demonstrate a significant decrease in partial physeal arrest in those treated with surgery, they recommended open reduction and removal of the entrapped periosteal flap. A subsequent study at the same institution recommended avoiding open reduction if gross deformity was not present, as patients treated with open reduction for entrapped periosteum did not have lower rates of premature physeal closure. Leary et al.[104] studied 15 distal tibia fractures with premature physeal closure, and found residual gap and number of reduction attempts did not predict early closure, but initial displacement did. The literature on the value of open reduction and removal of interposed periosteum to lower the incidence of premature physeal closure is conflicted in these fractures, and it is likely that multiple variables are involved (energy of initial injury, amount of displacement, number of reduction attempts, age of patient).

Incomplete reduction is frequently caused by interposition of soft tissue between the fracture fragments. Grace[67] reported three patients in whom the interposed soft tissue included the neurovascular bundle, resulting in circulatory embarrassment when closed reduction was attempted. In this situation, open reduction and extraction of the soft tissue obviously is required. As noted above, a less definitive indication for open reduction is interposition of the periosteum, which causes physeal widening with no or minimal angulation. Good results have been reported after open reduction and extraction of the periosteal flap (Fig. 29-38).[96] It is not clear that failure to extract the periosteum in such cases results in physeal arrest sufficient to warrant operative treatment. Wattenbarger et al.[193] and Phieffer et al.[147] have attempted to determine the relationship between physeal bar formation and interposed periosteum, although at this time it is unclear if the periosteal flap increases the risk of physeal arrest.

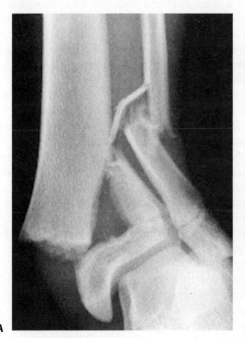
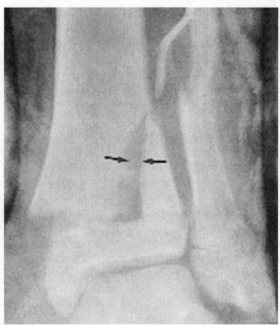

Figure 29-38. A: Severely displaced pronation–eversion–external rotation injury. **B:** Closed reduction was unsuccessful, and a valgus tilt of the ankle mortise was noted. At surgery, soft tissue was interposed laterally (*arrows*).

(*continues*)

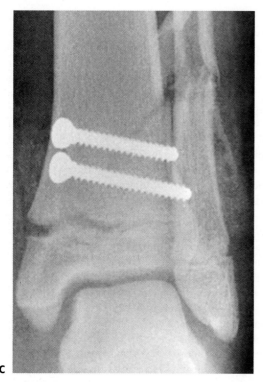

C

Figure 29-38. (*Continued*) **C:** Reduction completed and stabilized with two cancellous screws placed above the physis.

Because of risk of iatrogenic damage to the distal tibial physis during closed reduction, many authors recommend the use of general anesthesia with adequate muscle relaxation for children with Salter–Harris type II distal tibial fractures. However, no study has compared the frequency of growth abnormalities in patients with these fractures reduced under sedation and local analgesia to those with fractures reduced with the use of general anesthesia. One of the authors (KS) uses general anesthesia, and an arthroscopic ankle distractor to distract the fracture before reduction, with the theoretical advantage of reducing the risk of physeal damage during the reduction maneuver (see Fig. 29-32).

When closed reductions are not performed under general anesthesia, they are usually done under IV sedation. Alioto et al.[2a] demonstrated significantly improved pain relief with hematoma block for ankle fractures in a study comparing patients treated with IV sedation to patients receiving hematoma block.[49] Intravenous regional anesthesia or Bier block has also been reported to be effective for pain relief in lower extremity injuries.[105]

One advantage of reduction in the operating room with general anesthesia is the ease with which percutaneous pins can be placed to maintain reduction of the fractures. It is the experience of one of the authors that Salter–Harris I and II fractures will occasionally displace after closed reduction and above-knee casting. If there is any concern about redisplacement or stability after closed reduction under general anesthesia, smooth pins can be placed.

Surgeons using regional block anesthesia within the first 2 to 3 days after the fracture should consider the potential for compartment syndrome. In fractures that have a higher risk of compartment syndrome, regional anesthesia, especially peripheral nerve blocks with longer-acting agents, might delay the recognition of a compartment syndrome.[128]

Salter–Harris Type III and IV Fractures

Salter–Harris type III and IV fractures are discussed together because the mechanism of injury is the same (supination–inversion) and their treatment and prognosis are similar. Juvenile Tillaux and triplane fractures are considered separately. In the series of Spiegel et al.[178] 24.1% of the fractures were Salter–Harris type III injuries and 1.4% were type IV. These injuries are usually produced by the medial corner of the talus being driven into the junction of the distal tibial articular surface and the medial malleolus. As the talus shears off the medial malleolus, the physis may also be damaged (Fig. 29-39).

Nondisplaced Salter–Harris types III and IV fractures can be treated with below-knee or above-knee cast immobilization, but care must be taken to be sure that the significant intra-articular displacement is not present. Radiographs frequently underestimate the degree of intra-articular involvement and step-off of the articular surfaces. CT imaging may be necessary to fully appreciate the degree of displacement. We recommend any time there is a question of joint involvement of an ankle fracture that a CT, preferably with 3D reconstructions is obtained. Follow-up radiographs and/or CT scans in the first 2 weeks may also be necessary to confirm that no displacement occurs after casting.

Salter–Harris type III fractures of the medial malleolus have a high risk of physeal arrest. One study suggested that the rate of physeal arrest could be reduced by the use of open reduction and internal fixation.[93,102] Luhmann et al.[115] have recently studied a series of medial malleolar fractures with growth disturbance following treatment, and recommend anatomic reduction as fractures with as little as 2 mm of step-off went on to premature physeal closure. Others have also emphasized the importance of anatomic reduction and early treatment to reduce the risk of physeal arrest.[146]

Based upon principles of fracture treatment in adults, displaced intra-articular fractures are treated with as anatomical a reduction as possible. Studies in children confirming the importance of articular reduction to within 2 mm are few, although most recommend anatomic articular reduction in displaced fractures involving the articular surface. Failure to obtain anatomical reduction may result in articular incongruity and posttraumatic arthritis, which often becomes symptomatic 5 to 8 years after skeletal maturity.[36] The risk of growth arrest has also been linked to the adequacy of reduction, although the literature is still unclear if anatomic reduction reduces the risk of physeal arrest (Fig. 29-40).[169] Some recent series suggest early anatomic reduction is associated with a lower risk of physeal arrest.[169] Closed reduction may be attempted but is likely to succeed only in minimally displaced fractures. If closed reduction is obtained, it can be maintained with a cast or with percutaneous pins or screws supplemented by a cast.

If anatomical reduction cannot be obtained by closed methods, open reduction and internal fixation or mini-open arthroscopic reduction should be carried out. Lintecum and

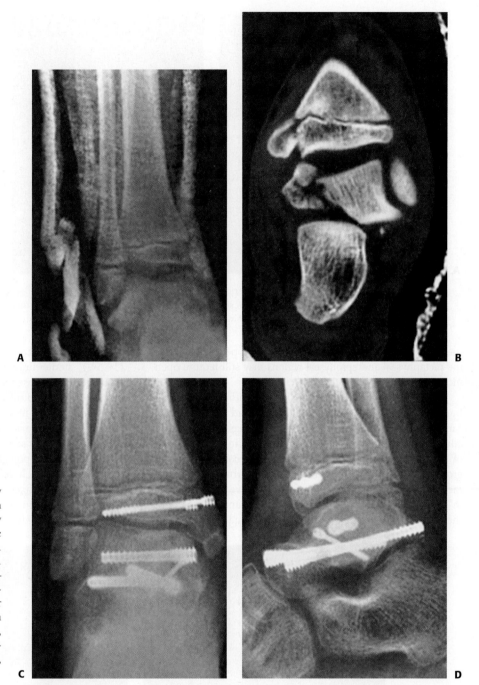

Figure 29-39. A: Severe ankle injury sustained by an 8-year-old involved in a car accident. The anteroposterior view in the splint does not clearly show the Salter–Harris type IV fracture of the tibia. The dome of the talus appears abnormal. **B:** CT scan shows the displaced Salter–Harris type IV fracture of the medial malleolus and a severe displaced intra-articular fracture of the body of the talus. **C, D:** Open reduction of both fractures was performed, and Herbert screws were used for internal fixation. (Courtesy of Armen Kelikian, MD.)

Blasier[111] described a technique of open reduction achieved through a limited exposure of the fracture with the incision centered over the fracture site combined with percutaneous cannulated screw fixation. This technique was performed on 13 patients—8 Salter–Harris IV fractures, 4 Salter–Harris III fractures, and 1 triplane fracture. The authors reported one growth arrest at follow-up averaging 12 months. Beaty and Linton[8] reported a Salter–Harris type III fracture with an intra-articular fragment; these fractures require open reduction for inspection of the joint to ensure that no osteochondral fragments are impeding reduction. Arthroscopic evaluation of the joint may also be an option. Internal fixation devices should be inserted

within the epiphysis, parallel to the physis in patients with greater than 2 years of growth remaining, and should avoid entering ankle joint (see Figs. 29-21 and 29-41).

Arthroscopic-assisted fixation of fractures with intra-articular involvement has been described by several centers. Jennings et al.[83] presented a series of five triplane and one Tillaux fractures treated with arthroscopic assistance. The outcome was excellent for fracture reduction and ankle function. Kaya et al.[94] review 10 patients with juvenile Tillaux fractures treated with arthroscopic assistance, demonstrating excellent reduction and clinical outcomes.[138] One of the primary advantages of arthroscopic fixation is that it allows for visualization of

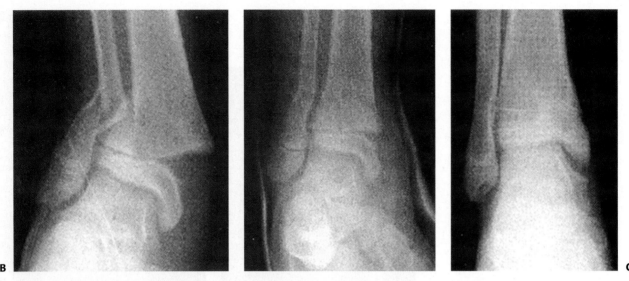

Figure 29-40. A: Anteroposterior view of a patient with a pronation–eversion–external rotation fracture. **B:** Postreduction view shows residual gapping of physis suggesting periosteal interposition. **C:** Anteroposterior view obtained for a new injury (medial malleolar fracture) shows premature closure of the physis.

the articular surfaces, although the need for open reduction of the metaphyseal and epiphyseal regions may still require open incisions.

Options for internal fixation include smooth K-wires, small fragment cortical and cancellous screws, and 3- and 4-mm cannulated screws (Fig. 29-42). Several reports[10,19,28] have advocated the use of absorbable pins for internal fixation of ankle fractures. Benz et al.[9] reported no complications or growth abnormalities after the use of absorbable pins with metal screw supplementation for fixation of five ankle fractures in patients between the ages of 5 and 13 years. In reports of the use of absorbable pins without supplemental metal fixation

in adults,[16,50,61,77] complications have included displacement (14.5%), sterile fluid accumulation requiring incision and drainage (8.1%), pseudarthrosis (8%), distal tibiofibular synostosis (3.8%), and infection (1.6%). Bucholz et al.[28] reported few complications in a series of fractures in adults fixed with absorbable screws made of polylactide and suggested that complications in earlier series might be related to the fact that those pins were made of polyglycolide. A report in 1993 by Böstman et al.[19] however, included few complications in a series of fractures in children fixed with polyglycolide pins. A follow-up report by Rokkanen et al.[157] in 1996 reported 3.6% infection and 3.7% failure of fixation.

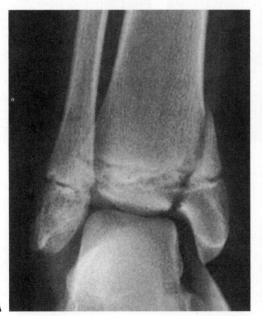
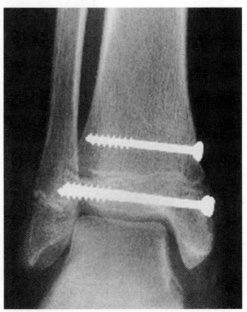

Figure 29-41. A: Grade II supination–inversion injury in a 12-year-old girl, resulting in a displaced Salter–Harris type IV fracture of the distal tibia and a nondisplaced Salter–Harris type I fracture of the distal fibula. **B:** After anatomic open reduction and stable internal fixation.

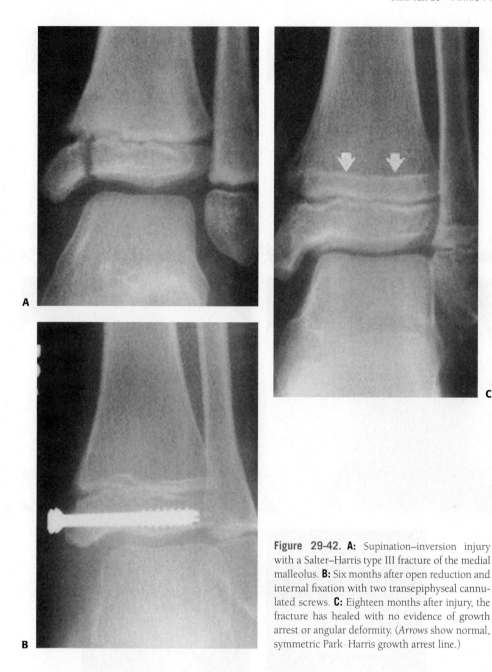

Figure 29-42. A: Supination–inversion injury with a Salter–Harris type III fracture of the medial malleolus. **B:** Six months after open reduction and internal fixation with two transepiphyseal cannulated screws. **C:** Eighteen months after injury, the fracture has healed with no evidence of growth arrest or angular deformity. (*Arrows* show normal, symmetric Park–Harris growth arrest line.)

The main advantage of absorbable pins and screws is that hardware removal is avoided. Böstman compared the cost-effectiveness of absorbable implants in 994 patients treated with absorbable implants to 1,173 patients treated with metallic implants. To be cost-effective, the hardware removal rates required were calculated to range from 19% for metacarpal fractures to 54% for trimalleolar fractures.[17] At this time, the indications for absorbable pins remain unclear.

Recent studies in the adult literature suggest second-generation bioabsorbable screws have lower complication rates, and their use may be increasing.[149,176] Additional studies in adult patients using ultrasound and MRI have not detected deleterious effects on healing with newer screw designs.[70,121] The presence of the physis, and the low-grade inflammation that

may accompany the dissolution of these implants, however, may increase the risk of physeal arrest, and additional studies in adult and pediatric patients will be necessary to confirm the effectiveness and safety of these devices.[92]

Open Reduction and Internal Fixation of Salter–Harris Type III or IV Fracture of the Distal Tibia

The patient is placed supine on an operating table that is radiolucent at the lower extremity. For a minimally displaced Salter III fracture of the medial malleolus closed reduction with percutaneous screws may be sufficient, but we have a low threshold for a small incision over the anteromedial joint to verify joint congruity after reduction (Fig. 29-43).

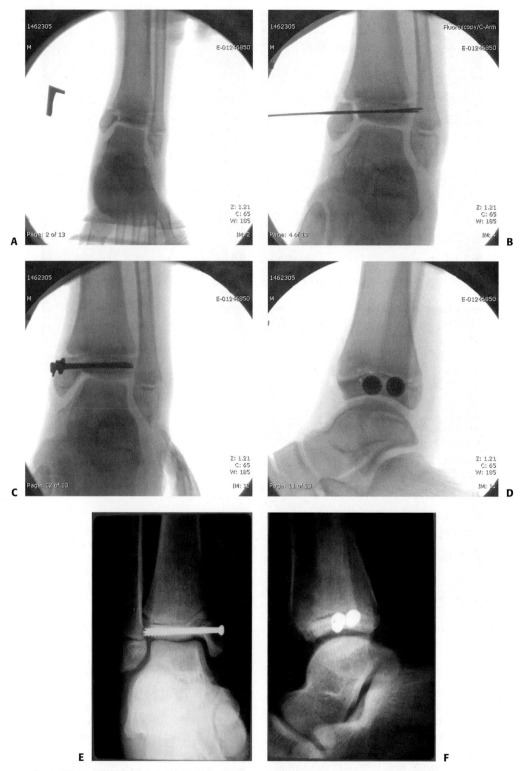

Figure 29-43. A: Medial malleolus fracture. **B:** Two parallel threaded pins from a cannulated screw system are placed across the fracture site. **C:** As the screws are compressed, the fracture is reduced. An arthrogram, arthroscope, or direct visualization can confirm anatomic joint reduction. Washers help prevent the screw heads from entering the bone, and maximize compressive force. **D:** Lateral view confirms good position of screws. Note that particular care must be taken with screw placement. **E:** In a different patient, the screws look acceptable in the AP plane. **F:** In the lateral plane, however, it is evident that one screw is in the joint. This is unacceptable and must be revised. Because of the curve of the distal tibia in the sagittal plane, this view is essential before the patient leaves the operating room. (Used with permission of the Children's Orthopaedic Center, Los Angeles.)

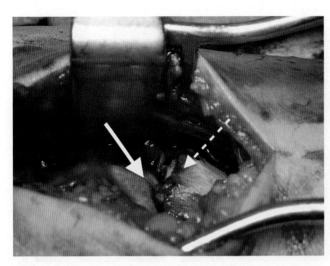

Figure 29-44. Displaced medial malleolus fracture. *Dashed arrow* shows the distal tibial metaphysis. *Solid arrow* shows the interposed periosteum. Usually a smaller incision is adequate for removal of periosteum and fracture reduction. (Used with permission of the Children's Orthopaedic Center, Los Angeles.)

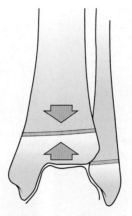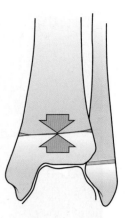

Figure 29-45. Compression-type injury of the tibial physis. Early physeal arrest can cause leg-length discrepancy.

Periosteum often flips into this fracture, preventing an anatomic reduction. This can usually be removed with a very small incision and a skin hook (Fig. 29-44).

The incision should allow visualization of the joint surface at the fracture site, and may be vertical or diagonal depending on the nature of the fracture. The saphenous vein may be identified, dissected free, and retracted depending on the size of the incision. The fracture site is identified, and an anteromedial capsulotomy of the ankle joint is performed. The fracture surfaces are exposed and gently cleaned with irrigation and forceps (curettage is not used).

For Salter–Harris type IV fractures, the periosteum may be elevated several millimeters from the metaphyseal fracture edges. The epiphyseal edges and joint surfaces are examined through the arthrotomy. The perichondral ring should not be elevated from the physis. For Salter–Harris type III fractures, the reduction is evaluated by checking the joint surface and epiphyseal fracture edges through the arthrotomy. The epiphyseal fragment is grasped with a small towel clip or reduction forceps, and the fracture is reduced. Internal fixation is performed under direct vision and fluoroscopic control. It is important to view both the lateral and anteroposterior projections because of the curved shape of the distal tibial articular surface. If the fragment is large enough, 4-mm cannulated lag screws are inserted through the epiphyseal fragment; if the fragment is too small for screws, smooth K-wires are used. The reduction and the position of the internal fixation are checked through the arthrotomy. In fractures with a significant Thurstan-Holland fragment, a metaphyseal screw may be used if a gap exists after the epiphyseal screws are inserted. After reduction of the tibial fracture, an associated Salter–Harris type I or II fibular fracture usually reduces and is stable. If it is not, closed reduction and fixation with percutaneous oblique smooth K-wires are performed.

The patient is kept nonweight bearing for 3 weeks, and then the cast is changed to a below-knee walking cast, which is worn for an additional 3 weeks. Frequent follow-up evaluations (every 3 to 6 months for the first year and yearly thereafter until normal growth resumes) are necessary to detect growth abnormalities.

Salter–Harris Type V Fractures

Salter–Harris type V fractures of the ankle are believed to be caused by severe axial compression and crushing of the physis (Fig. 29-45). As originally described, these injuries are not usually associated with significant displacement of the epiphysis relative to the metaphysis, which make diagnosis of acute injury impossible from plain radiographs; the diagnosis can only be made on follow-up radiographs when premature physeal closure is evident (Fig. 29-46).

Spiegel et al.[178] have designated comminuted fractures that are otherwise unclassifiable as Salter–Harris type V injuries.

The incidence of Salter–Harris type V ankle fractures is difficult to establish because of the difficulty of diagnosing acute injuries. Spiegel et al.[178] included two type V fractures in their series, but both were comminuted fractures rather than the classic crush injury without initial radiographic abnormality.

Because of the uncertain nature of this injury, no specific treatment recommendations have been formulated. Treatment is usually directed primarily toward the sequelae of growth arrest that invariably follows Salter–Harris type V fractures. Perhaps more sophisticated scanning techniques will eventually allow identification and localization of areas of physeal injury so that irreparable damaged cells can be removed and replaced with interposition materials to prevent growth problems, but at present this diagnosis is made only several months after injury.

Other Fractures of the Distal Tibia

Accessory ossification centers of the distal tibia (os subtibiale) and distal fibula (os fibulare) are common and may be injured. Treatment usually consists of cast immobilization for 3 to 4 weeks. Ogden and Lee[136] reported good results after cast immobilization in 26 of 27 patients with injuries involving the medial side of the tibia; only one patient required surgery. In contrast, 5 to 11 patients with injuries involving the lateral side had persistent symptoms that required excision.

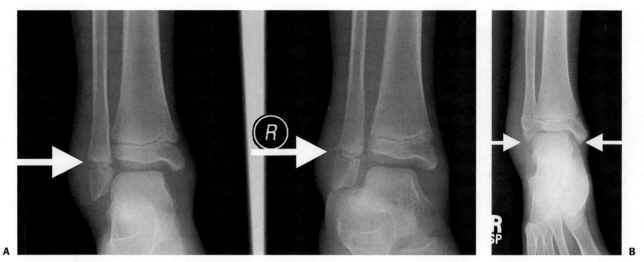

Figure 29-46. A: An 8-year-old girl had a minimally displaced fracture of the distal. This could be classified as a Salter II fracture as there is a very small metaphyseal piece present. Note the normal relative lengths of the lateral malleolus, more distal than the medial malleolus. *Arrow* shows distal fibular physis in normal position at level of ankle joint. **B:** Three years later at age 11, a complete growth arrest is noted. The tips of the lateral malleolus and medial malleolus (*arrows*) are at the same level. (Used with permission of the Children's Orthopaedic Center, Los Angeles.)

Injuries to the perichondral ring of the distal tibial and fibular physes, with physeal disruption, have been described.[74] Most of these injuries are caused by skiving of the bone by machinery such as lawn mowers. They may result in growth arrest or retardation and in angular deformities.

Juvenile Tillaux Fractures

This fracture is the adolescent counterpart of the fracture in adults described by the French surgeon Tillaux. It occurs when with external rotation of the foot, the anterior-inferior tibiofibular ligament through its attachments to the anterolateral tibia, avulses a fragment of bone corresponding to the portion of the distal tibial physis that is still open (Fig. 29-47). In the series of Spiegel et al.[178] these fractures occurred in 2.9% of patients.

Tillaux fractures may be isolated injuries or may be associated with ipsilateral tibial shaft fractures.[42] The fibula usually prevents marked displacement of the fracture and clinical deformity is generally absent. Swelling is usually slight, and local tenderness is at the anterior lateral joint line, in contrast to ankle sprains where the tenderness tends to be below the level of the ankle joint.

A mortise view is essential to see the distal tibial epiphysis unobstructed by the fibula (Fig. 29-48). Steinlauf et al.[179] reported a patient in whom the Tillaux fragment became entrapped between the distal tibia and fibula producing apparent diastasis of the ankle joint. To allow measurement of displacement from plain films, the radiograph beam would have to be directly in line with the fracture site, which makes CT confirmation of reduction desired after all closed reductions of these fractures.

Both below-knee and above-knee casts have been used for immobilization of nondisplaced juvenile Tillaux and triplane fractures. Fractures with more than 2 mm of displacement, especially those associated with articular incongruity, may be best treated with closed or open reduction.[44,94] Closed reduction is attempted by internally rotating the foot and applying direct pressure over the anterolateral tibia. If necessary, percutaneous pins can be used for stabilization of the reduction. If closed reduction is not successful, open reduction or percutaneous reduction with arthroscopic assistance may be needed. Occasionally, percutaneously inserted pins can be used to manipulate the displaced fragment into anatomical position and then advanced to fix the fragment in place.[167] Screw fixation within

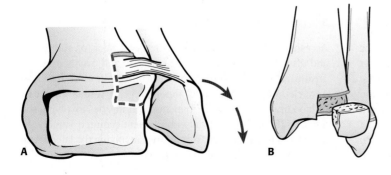

Figure 29-47. Juvenile Tillaux fracture. Mechanism of injury: The anteroinferior tibiofibular ligament avulses a fragment of the lateral epiphysis (**A**) corresponding to the portion of the physis that is still open (**B**).

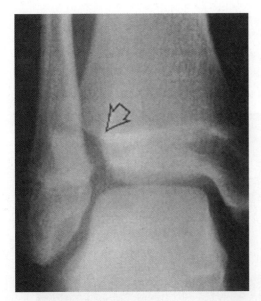

Figure 29-48. Anteroposterior mortise view of a 14-year-old who sustained a juvenile Tillaux fracture.

the epiphysis is usually the preferred fixation method (see Figs. 29-21, 29-32 and 29-33).

Triplane Fracture

Kärrholm notes that Gerner-Smidt in 1963 described triplane and Tillaux fractures as different stages of the same injury.[87] In 1957, Johnson and Fahl[84] described a triplane fracture in their report of 27 physeal ankle injuries and reported that they had seen 10 such fractures. Despite these earlier reports, the nature of triplane fractures was not appreciated until Marmor's[121] report in 1970 of an irreducible ankle fracture that at surgery was found to consist of three parts (Fig. 29-49). Two years after Marmor's report, Lynn[116] reported two additional such fractures and coined the term triplane fracture. He described the fracture as consisting of three major fragments: (1) the anterolateral quadrant of the distal tibial epiphysis, (2) the medial and posterior portions of the epiphysis in addition to a posterior metaphyseal spike, and (3) the tibial metaphysis. Cooperman et al.,[41]

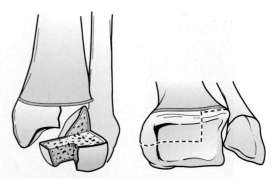

Figure 29-50. Anatomy of a two-part lateral triplane fracture (left ankle). Note the large posterolateral epiphyseal fragment with its posterior metaphyseal fragment. The anterior portion of the medial malleolus remains intact.

however, in their 1978 report of 15 such fractures concluded that, based on tomographic studies, most were two-part fractures produced by external rotation (Fig. 29-50). Variations in fracture patterns were attributed to the extent of physeal closure at the time of injury. Kärrholm et al.[88] reported that CT evaluation of four adolescents with triplane fractures confirmed the existence of two-part and three-part fractures and also revealed four-part fractures (Fig. 29-51).

El-Karef et al.[55] studied 21 triplane fractures, identifying 19 as lateral triplane variants, and 2 as medial variants. Twelve were two-part fractures, six were three-part fractures, and three were four-part fractures.

Von Laer[191] described a subgroup of two-part and three-part triplane fractures in which the fracture line on the anteroposterior radiographs did not extend into the ankle joint but into the medial malleolus instead (Fig. 29-52). Shin et al.[171] reported five patients with intramalleolar triplane variants. They divided these into three types: Type I, an intramalleolar intra-articular fracture; type II, an intramalleolar, intra-articular fracture outside the weight-bearing surface; and type III, an intramalleolar, extra-articular fracture (Fig. 29-53). These authors found that CT scans with three-dimensional reconstruction were helpful in determining displacement and deciding if surgery is indicated.

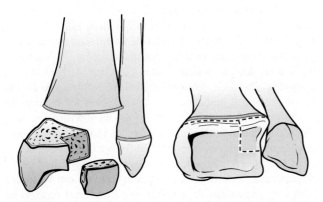

Figure 29-49. Anatomy of a three-part lateral triplane fracture (left ankle). Note the large epiphyseal fragment with its metaphyseal component and the smaller anterolateral epiphyseal fragment.

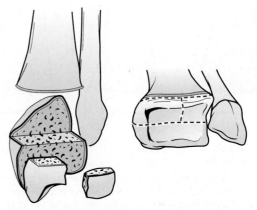

Figure 29-51. Anatomy of a four-part lateral triplane fracture (left ankle). The anterior epiphysis has split into two fragments, and the posterior epiphysis is the larger fragment with its metaphyseal component.

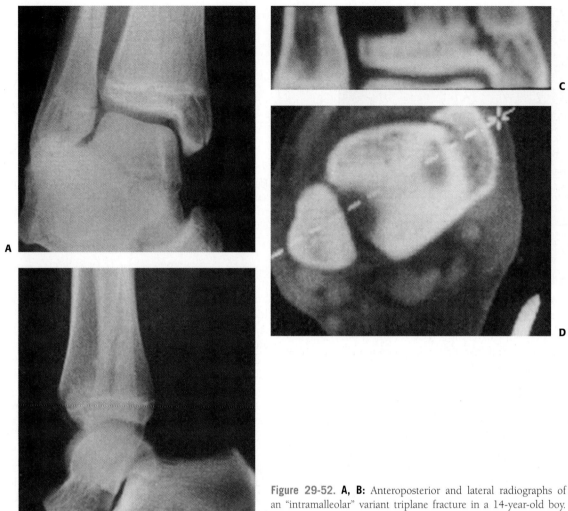

Figure 29-52. A, B: Anteroposterior and lateral radiographs of an "intramalleolar" variant triplane fracture in a 14-year-old boy. **C, D:** CT scans demonstrate extra-articular nature of the fracture.

In the series of Spiegel et al.[178] 7.3% were triplane fractures. Kärrholm[89] reviewed 209 triplane fracture patients and found the mean age at the time of injury was 14.8 for boys and 12.8 for girls. This type of injury did not occur in children younger than

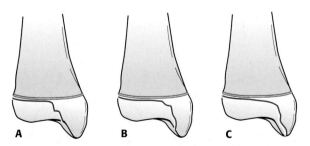

Figure 29-53. Schematic drawing of the immature distal tibial physis demonstrating types I, II, and III intramalleolar triplane fractures. **A:** Type I intramalleolar, intra-articular fracture at the junction of the tibial plafond and the medial malleolus. **B:** Type II intramalleolar, intra-articular fracture outside the weight-bearing zone of the tibial plafond. **C:** Type III intramalleolar, extra-articular fracture. (Adapted with permission from Shin AY, Moran ME, Wenger DR. Intramalleolar triplane fractures of the distal tibial epiphysis. *J Pediatr Orthop.* 1997;17(3):352–355.)

10 or older than 16.7 years. The incidence is higher in males than females.[168] Patients with triplane fractures may have completely open physes. Swelling is usually more severe than with Tillaux fractures, and deformity may be more severe, especially if the fibula is also fractured. Radiographic views should include anteroposterior, lateral, and mortise views. Rapariz et al.[151] found that 48% of triplane fractures were associated with fibular fracture and 8.5% were associated with ipsilateral tibial shaft fracture. Healy et al.[75] reported a triplane fracture associated with a proximal fibula fracture and syndesmotic injury (Maisonneuve equivalent). Failure to detect such injury may lead to chronic instability. Therefore, tenderness proximal to the ankle should be sought and if found may be an indication for radiographs of the proximal leg. CT scans may also be essential for more detailed evaluation of the articular surface and the fracture anatomy, in more complex cases (Fig. 29-54; see Fig. 29-11).

Nondisplaced triplane fractures, those with less than 2 mm of displacement, as well as extra-articular fractures can be treated with cast immobilization with the foot in internal rotation for lateral fractures and in eversion for medial fractures, but this should be defined on CT scan, not radiographs alone. These are rotational injuries, so the ability of a well-molded below-knee

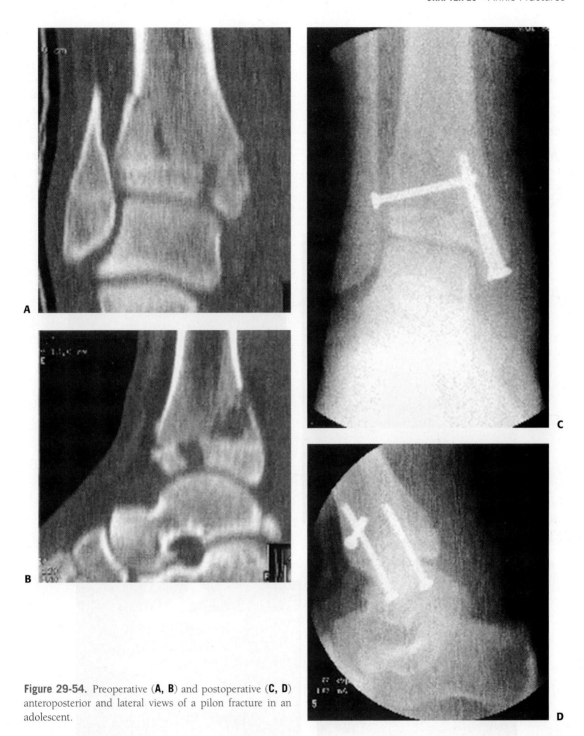

Figure 29-54. Preoperative (**A, B**) and postoperative (**C, D**) anteroposterior and lateral views of a pilon fracture in an adolescent.

cast to maintain the reduction is questioned by some; a comparative study of below-knee and above-knee casts has not been done. Fractures with more than 2 mm of displacement (65% of the injuries in Kärrholm's series) require reduction; this may be attempted in the emergency department or in the operating room with the use of general anesthesia. Closed reduction of lateral triplane fractures is attempted by internally rotating the foot. Based on the mechanism of injury, the most logical maneuver for reduction of medial triplane fractures is abduction. If closed reduction is shown to be adequate by image intensification a cast is applied or percutaneous screws are inserted for fixation if necessary.

Well-placed percutaneous screws will prevent secondary displacement in a cast, and may make follow-up radiographs and clinical visits less frequent. If closed reduction is done, a postreduction CT scan of the ankle joint in the cast is usually necessary to confirm adequate reduction. If closed reduction is unsuccessful, open reduction is required. This can be accomplished through an anterolateral approach for lateral triplane fractures or through an anteromedial approach for medial triplane fractures. Additional incisions may be necessary for adequate exposure.

The use of well-placed percutaneous clamps and arthroscopic assistance may help with the reduction and minimize the need for incisions. Careful review of the CT scans can help guide percutaneous clamp and screw placement that improves the biomechanics of clamp reduction and screw placement.[86] Care should be taken to avoid injury to neurologic and vascular structures during clamp or percutaneous screw placement.

Open Reduction of Triplane Fracture

The patient is placed supine on a radiolucent operating table with padded elevation behind the hip on the affected side. The surgical approach depends on the fracture anatomy as determined by the preoperative CT scan, and can vary greatly. A two-part medial triplane fracture can be approached through a hockey-stick anteromedial incision. The fracture fragments are irrigated to remove debris, and any interposed periosteum is removed. The fracture is reduced, and reduction is confirmed by direct observation through an anteromedial arthrotomy and by image intensification. Two 4-mm cancellous screws are inserted from medial to lateral or from anterior to posterior or both, depending on the fracture pattern (Fig. 29-55). Anterior-to-posterior screw placement may require an additional antero-lateral incision or the screws may be inserted percutaneously. Arthroscopic-assisted techniques, with the use of percutaneous clamps and screws may also be used (see Fig. 29-34).

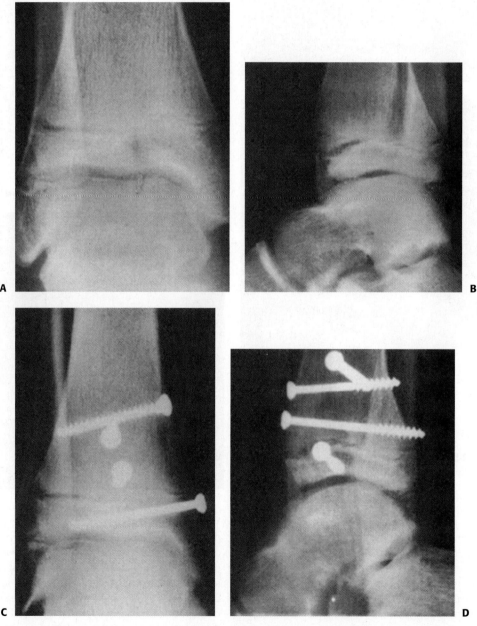

Figure 29-55. Irreducible three-part triplane fracture in a 13-year-old girl. **A:** Crush injury to medial malleolus and distal tibia metaphysis. **B:** The percutaneous pins can be used to manipulate the fracture. **C, D:** After open reduction with internal fixation. Note anterior-to-posterior and medial-to-lateral screw placement that avoids the physis.

For two-part lateral triplane fractures, these can be approached with a hockey-stick anterolateral approach. The fracture is reduced and stabilized with two screws placed from lateral to medial or from anterior to posterior or both, and reduction is confirmed through direct observation and by image intensification. In addition to open techniques, arthroscopic-assisted techniques with the use of percutaneous clamps and screws may also be used (see Fig. 29-34).

Fractures with three or more parts may occasionally require more exposure for reduction and internal fixation. If the fibula is fractured, posterior exposure of the tibial fracture can be readily obtained by detaching the anterior and posterior-inferior tibiofibular ligaments and turning down the distal fibula on the lateral collateral ligament (Fig. 29-56). If the fibula is not fractured, a fibular osteotomy may be needed in very rare circumstances for adequate visualization of the articular surface. Careful dissection is necessary to avoid iatrogenic fractures through the physis of the fibula. Medial exposure is obtained through an anteromedial or posteromedial incision. Reduction and internal fixation are carried out in a stepwise fashion. For typical three-part fractures, the Salter–Harris type II fracture may be reduced first by provisional fixation to the distal tibia through the metaphyseal fragment. Usually, the Salter–Harris type III fragment can then be reduced and provisionally fixed to the stabilized type II fragment (Fig. 29-57). Occasionally, the order of reduction and fixation should be reversed. Fractures with four or more fragments require additional steps, but

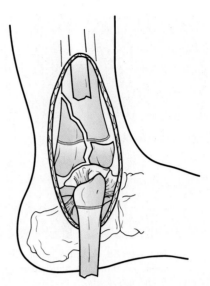

Figure 29-56. Transfibular approach to a complex triplane fracture.

fixation of the Salter–Harris type II or IV fragment through the metaphysis to the distal tibia is usually best performed first. This step can be followed by fixation of the Salter–Harris type III fragment or fragments (Fig. 29-58). After reduction, reliable patients may be treated with immobilization in a short-leg, non–weight-bearing cast for 3 to 4 weeks. At 3 to 4 weeks, they

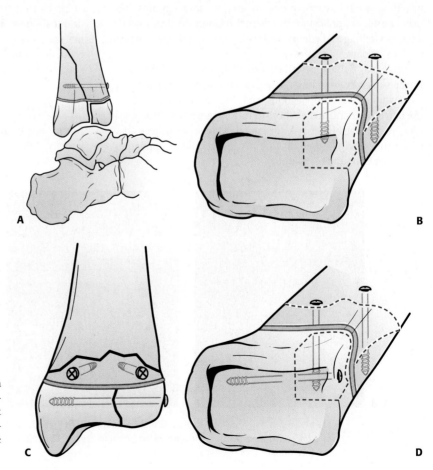

Figure 29-57. Open reduction with internal fixation of a three-part lateral triplane fracture. **A, B:** Reduction and fixation of the Salter–Harris type II fragment to the metaphysis. **C, D:** Reduction and internal fixation of the Salter–Harris type III fragment to the Salter–Harris type II fragment.

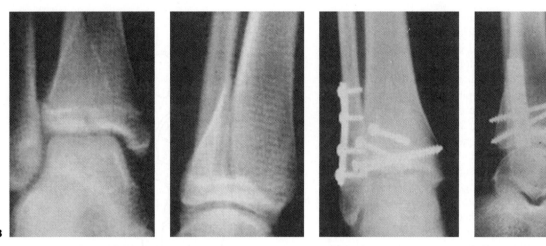

A, B   **C, D**

Figure 29-58. A, B: Irreducible three-part lateral triplane fracture in a 14-year-old boy. **C, D:** After open reduction through a transfibular approach and internal fixation with anterior-to-posterior and lateral-to-medial screws.

may be converted to a weight-bearing cast or walking boot for an additional 3 to 4 weeks.

Pilon Fractures

Although these fractures are relatively rare in young patients, they can be associated with severe soft tissue swelling. Similar to the treatment in adults with these injuries, management of the soft tissues is critical to prevent complications of skin loss, infection, wound healing problems, etc.[54,185] Initial approaches may consist of application of external fixation, or dressings to address swelling and edema, with delay in surgical intervention for 5 to 15 days (Fig. 29-59).[54]

Letts et al.[109] have described a small series of pilon fractures in the skeletally immature. The patients in this series did not have wound/skin complications, and only 2/8 developed postoperative osteoarthritis at short-term follow-up. As these fractures may be at higher risk for complications, we believe that treatment principles used in adult patients should be applied to this patient population as well.[5,13,107,109,139,154]

Syndesmosis Injuries

Several publications have described triplane fracture in association with a syndesmosis injury.[46] These have been associated with the following fracture patterns: Distal fibula, Salter I and II, triplane, and Tillaux. Medial joint space widening may be an important anatomic factor to evaluate during treatment of external rotation mechanism injuries, and this should improve after surgical treatment.[66] During surgical treatment of pediatric/adolescent ankle fractures, evaluation for syndesmosis injuries should probably be performed in a manner similar to the treatment of adult fractures. Syndesmosis reduction and fixation may be necessary (see Fig. 29-15), in some cases.

Open Fractures and Lawn Mower Injuries

Severe open ankle fractures are often produced by high-velocity motor vehicular accidents or lawn mower injuries (Fig. 29-60).[68,74] Approximately 25,000 lawn mower injuries

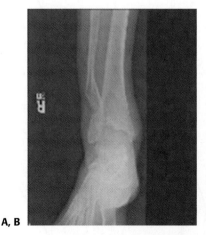
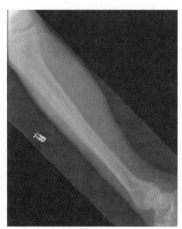
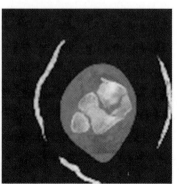

A, B   **C**

Figure 29-59. Pilon fracture treated with spatial frame. **A, B:** Preoperative anteroposterior and lateral view of adolescent pilon fracture with depressed articular region. **C:** Axial CT scan showing comminution of articular surface.

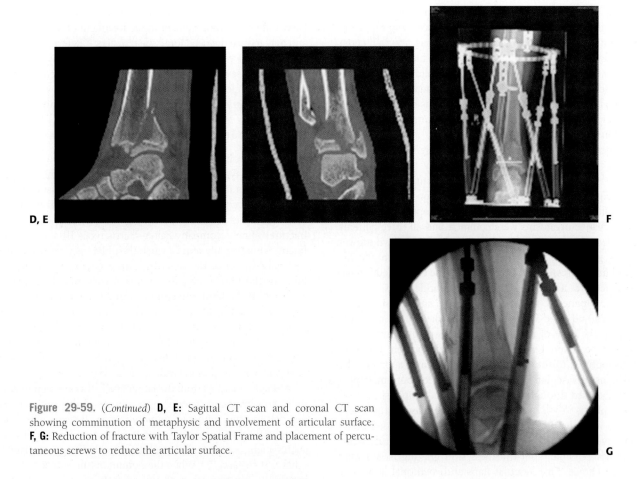

Figure 29-59. (*Continued*) **D, E:** Sagittal CT scan and coronal CT scan showing comminution of metaphysic and involvement of articular surface. **F, G:** Reduction of fracture with Taylor Spatial Frame and placement of percutaneous screws to reduce the articular surface.

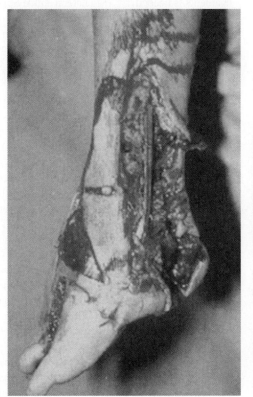

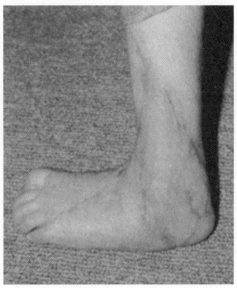

Figure 29-60. **A:** Severe lawn mower injury in a 5-year-old boy. **B:** One year after initial treatment with debridement, free flap, and skin graft coverage.

occur each year, 20% of which are in children. Ride-on mowers produce the most severe injuries, requiring more surgical procedures and resulting in more functional limitations.[1,3,52,161,192] Loder et al.[112] reviewed 144 children injured by lawn mowers. The average age at the time of injury was 7 years. The child was a bystander in 84 cases. Sixty-seven children required amputation. Soft tissue infection occurred in 8 of 118 and osteomyelitis in 6 of 117.

Principles of treatment are the same as in adults: Copious irrigation and debridement, tetanus toxoid, and intravenous antibiotics. Gaglani et al.[63] reported the bacteriologic findings in three children with infections secondary to lawn mower injuries. They found that organisms infecting the wounds were frequently different than those found on initial debridement, calling into question the value of intraoperative cultures. Gram-negative organisms were common and all three patients were infected with fungi as well. In children with lawn mower injuries, grass, dirt, and debris are pushed and blown into the wound under pressure, and removal of these embedded foreign objects requires meticulous mechanical debridement.

In most patients, the articular surface and physis should be aligned and fixed with smooth pins that do not cross the physis at the time of initial treatment. Exposed physeal surfaces can be covered with local fat to help prevent union of the metaphysis to the epiphysis. An external fixator may be used if neurovascular structures are injured, but small pins should be used through the metaphysis and epiphysis, avoiding the physis.[78,85,114,152,160] Wound closure may be a problem in cases with significant soft tissue injury and exposed bone. Skin coverage with local tissue is ideal; but if local coverage is not possible, split-thickness skin grafting is generally the next choice. Free vascular flaps and rotational flaps may be required for adequate coverage, although the necessity for flap coverage has decreased with the widespread use of vacuum-assisted closure techniques. Klein et al.[101] reported two cases that had associated vascular injury precluding such flaps, that were covered successfully with local advancement flaps made possible by multiple relaxing incisions. Mooney et al.[126] reported cross-extremity flaps for such cases. They found external fixation for linkage of the lower extremities during the procedure to be valuable. After fixation removal, range of motion returned readily.

Vosburgh et al.[192] reported 33 patients with lawn mower injuries to the foot and ankle. They found that the most severe injuries were to the posterior plantar aspect of the foot and ankle. Of their patients, five required split-thickness skin grafts and one vascularized flap for soft tissue coverage. Two ultimately required Syme amputation. Four of the patients had complete disruption of the Achilles tendon. Three had no repair or reconstruction of the triceps surae tendon, and one had delayed reconstruction 3 months after injury. Vosburgh et al.[192] speculate that dense scarring in the posterior ankle results in a "physiologic tendon" and that extensive reconstructive surgery is not always necessary for satisfactory function. Boyer et al.[23] reported a patient with deltoid ligament loss because of a severe grinding injury that was reconstructed with a free plantaris tendon graft. Soft tissue coverage was achieved using a free muscle transfer. Rinker et al.[153] have also described the use of soft tissue transfer to assist pediatric patients with severe soft tissue loss.

The development of vacuum-assisted closure devices has been a dramatic improvement in the treatment of these injuries, and may reduce the need for tissue transfers.[76] Referral to centers with experience with these treatment protocols may be necessary for these severe injuries. Our experience with the use of vacuum-assisted closure devices in high-energy trauma with severe soft tissue injury has shown very good results for limb salvage.

Distal Fibula Fractures

Fractures involving the fibular physis are most commonly Salter–Harris type I or II fractures that are caused by a supination–inversion injury. Isolated fibular fractures are usually minimally displaced and can be treated with immobilization in a below-knee cast for 3 to 4 weeks. Significantly displaced fibular fractures often accompany Salter–Harris types III and IV tibial fractures and usually reduce when the tibial fracture is reduced. Internal fixation of the tibial fracture generally results in stability of the fibular fracture such that cast immobilization is sufficient. If the fibular fracture is unstable after reduction and fixation of the tibial fracture, fixation with a smooth intramedullary or obliquely inserted Kirschner wire is recommended (see Fig. 29-33). In older adolescents in whom growth is not a consideration, an intramedullary rod, screw, or plate-and-screw device may be used as in adults (Fig. 29-61).

Avulsion fractures from the lateral malleolus are seen in children with inversion "sprain" type injuries to the ankle. These may fail to unite with cast immobilization. Patients with such nonunions may have pain without associated instability. In such patients simple excision of the ununited fragment usually relieves their pain.[49,72] When the nonunions are associated with instability, reconstruction of one or more of the lateral ankle ligaments is needed.[25,26] (See Lateral Ankle Sprains.)

Avulsion fracture of the accessory ossification centers of the distal fibula (os subfibulare) is also common. In the series report by Ogden and Lee,[136] 5 of 11 patients with injuries treated with casting had persistent symptoms and required excision.

Lateral Ankle Sprains

In 1984, Vahvanen[189a] published a prospective study of 559 children who presented with severe supination injuries or sprains of the ankle.[194] Forty patients, 28 boys and 12 girls, with an average age of 12 years (range 5 to 14 years) were surgically explored. The indications for surgery included swelling, pain over the anterior talofibular ligament, limp, clinical instability, and when visible, a displaced avulsion fracture. Such fractures were visible radiographically in only 8 patients but were found at surgery in 19. Thirty-six ankles were found to have injury of the anterior talofibular ligament at surgery. Only 16 of these had either a positive lateral or anterior drawer stress test. At follow-up all patients were pain free and none complained of instability. Based upon the incidence of residual disability after such injuries in adults reported in the literature (21% to 58%), these authors suggested primary surgical repair may be indicated in some cases. In our clinical experience, acute surgical repair of ankle sprains is very rarely indicated in the skeletally immature.

In cases with residual laxity and associated symptoms, delayed surgical repair may be necessary in older patients.

Figure 29-61. A: Salter–Harris type II fracture of the distal fibula in a 15-year-old. **B:** Lateral view shows the fibular metaphyseal fragment (*arrow*). Considerable soft tissue swelling was noted in the medial aspect of the ankle. **C:** Stress films showed complete disruption of the deltoid ligament. **D:** The fibular fracture was fixed with a cannulated screw; the deltoid ligament was not repaired.

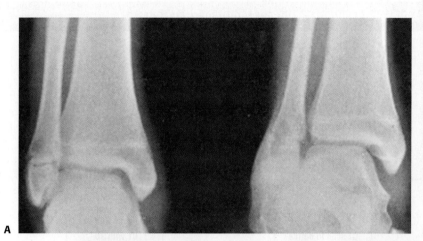
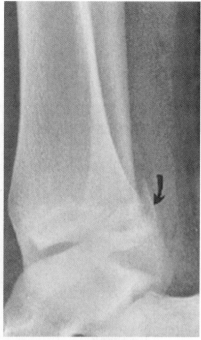
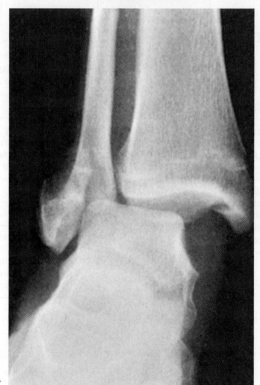
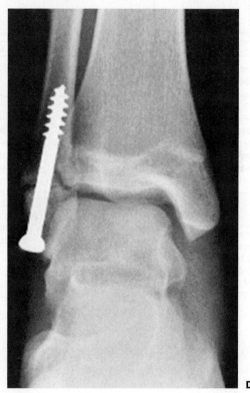

Busconi and Pappas[31] reported 60 skeletally immature children with chronic ankle pain and instability. Fifty of these children responded to rehabilitation, but 10 had persistent symptoms. Although three of these patients' initial radiographs were within normal limits, all patients with persistent symptoms eventually were found to have ununited osteochondral fractures of the fibular epiphysis. All 10 patients with persistent symptoms were treated with excision of the ununited osteochondral fracture and a Broström reconstruction of the lateral collateral ligament. All were able to return to activities and none reported further pain or instability.

Ankle Dislocations

Nusem et al.[133] reported a 12-year-old girl who was seen with a posterior dislocation of the ankle without associated fracture.

This was a closed injury and resulted from forced inversion of a maximally plantarflexed foot. The dislocation was reduced under IV sedation and the ankle immobilized in a short-leg cast for 5 weeks. The patient was asymptomatic at follow-up 4 years after injury. The inversion stress views at that time revealed only a three-degree increase laxity compared to the uninjured side. The anterior drawer sign was negative. There was no evidence of avascular necrosis of the talus on follow-up radiographs. Mazur et al.[122] have also reported ankle dislocation without a fracture in a pediatric patient.

Authors' Preferred Treatment of Distal Tibial and Fibular Fractures (Algorithm 29-1)

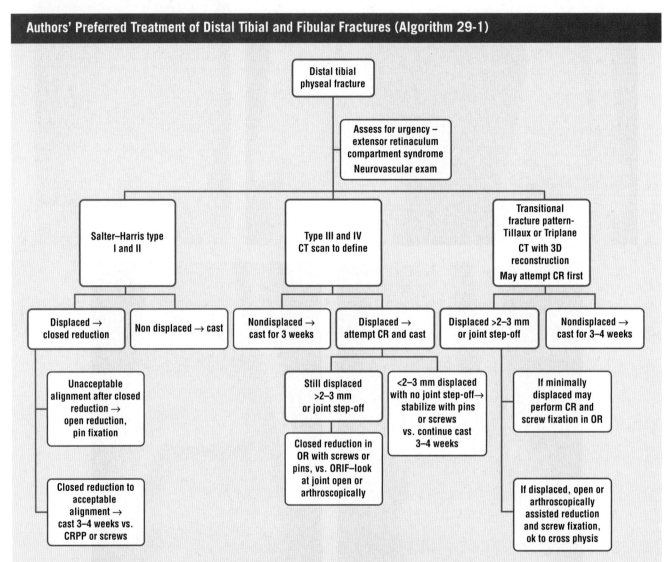

Algorithm 29-1. Treatment of distal tibial and fibular fractures.

Salter–Harris Type I and II Fractures of the Distal Tibia

We prefer to treat nondisplaced Salter–Harris type I and II fractures initially with immobilization using either an above-knee or below-knee cast dependent on patient characteristics. Nonweight bearing is continued until 2 to 4 weeks post-injury, when the cast is changed to a below-knee walking cast or walking boot which is worn for an additional 2 to 3 weeks. Follow-up radiographs are obtained every 6 months for 1 to 2 years or until a Park–Harris growth arrest line parallel to the physis is visible and there is no evidence of physeal deformity.

For displaced fractures in children with at least 3 years of growth remaining, our objective is to obtain no more than 10 to 15 degrees of plantar tilt for posteriorly displaced fractures, 5 to 10 degrees of valgus for laterally displaced fractures, and 0 degrees of varus for medially displaced fractures (Fig. 29-62). Studies in the adult literature suggest that minor alteration in alignment of the ankle joint may have significant effect on tibiotalar contact pressures.[93,186,188] If there is a question about the ability to remodel the fracture, it is probably best to perform a reduction. For children with 2 years or less of growth remaining, the amount of acceptable angulation is reduced to 5 degrees or less. We recognize that all of the recommendations about acceptable alignment are based on clinical experience and judgment, and none have been rigorously studied.

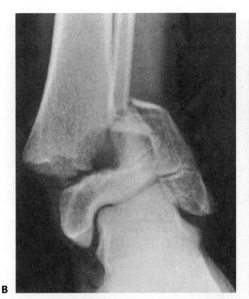
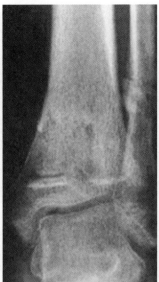
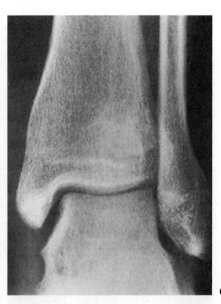

A, B   **C**

Figure 29-62. A: Displaced pronation–eversion–external rotation fracture of the distal tibia in a 12-year-old boy was treated with closed reduction and cast immobilization. **B:** After cast removal, a 10-degree valgus tilt was present. **C:** At maturity, the deformity has completely resolved.

If resources are available, we may attempt reduction of markedly displaced fractures with the use of general anesthesia with good muscle relaxation and image intensifier control. The use of an ankle distractor can facilitate distraction across the fracture, and may facilitate reduction (see Fig. 29-32). In children with mildly displaced fractures, especially if anesthesia is not going to be available for many hours, an attempt at gentle closed reduction under a hematoma block supplemented as needed by well-monitored intravenous sedation is a good option. Many emergency rooms are well equipped and have adequate staff to perform appropriate and safe sedation for treatment of fractures and dislocation. This approach may allow for more timely treatment, especially if operating room access is limited. Once adequately reduced, the fractures are usually stable and a long-leg cast can be used for immobilization. Rarely, for markedly unstable fractures or severe soft tissue injuries that require multiple debridements, percutaneous screws are used when the Thurstan-Holland fragment is large enough to accept screw fixation. When the fragment is too small, smooth wire fixation across the physis is the only alternative. Repeated attempts at closed manipulation of these fractures may increase the risk of growth abnormality and should be avoided. In patients with fractures that are not seen until 7 to 10 days after injury, residual displacement is probably best accepted, unless significant deformity or angulation is present. If growth does not sufficiently correct malunion, corrective osteotomy can be performed later.

Open reduction of these fractures is occasionally indicated. The exception usually has been pronation–eversion–external rotation fractures with interposed soft tissue, which may include lateral and posterior displacement. For cases that have undergone an attempt at closed reduction, close inspection of the medial physis should be performed with image intensification. In some cases, the medial physeal space will appear abnormally widened, which may suggest incarceration of a large flap of periosteum in the physis. If alignment is satisfactory these can be treated nonoperatively. For malaligned fractures, a small anteromedial incision is made and any interposed soft tissues, such as periosteum or tendons, are extracted. Even though reduction is usually stable, we generally use internal fixation. Fixation options include screw fixation through both the metaphyseal and epiphyseal fragments, avoiding fixation across the physis if possible (Fig. 29-63). Percutaneous smooth pins can also be placed from the medial malleolus, oriented proximally to engage the metaphysis (Figs. 29-31 and 29-64).

Salter–Harris Types III and IV Fractures of the Distal Tibia

Treatment of nondisplaced Salter–Harris type III and IV fractures is the same as for nondisplaced type I and II fractures with three modifications. First, after casting, the alignment is confirmed with a CT scan and/or radiographs. Second, these patients are examined more frequently (once a week) for the first 2 to 3 weeks after cast application to ensure that the fragments do not become displaced. Third, these patients are examined every 6 to 12 months after cast removal for 24 to 36 months to detect any growth abnormality.

Fractures with 2 mm or more of displacement after the best possible closed reduction may be treated with open reduction and internal fixation with anatomical alignment of the physis and intra-articular fracture fragments.

For minimally displaced fractures, closed reduction is attempted in the emergency room or the operating room,

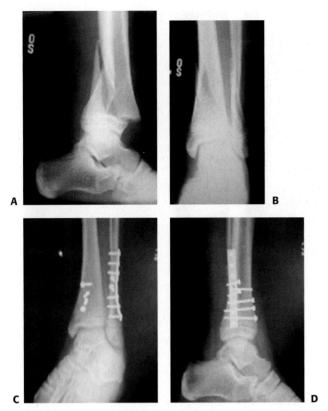

Figure 29-63. Salter–Harris type II distal tibial fracture with fibular fracture. **A:** Lateral view. **B:** Anteroposterior view. **C, D:** After percutaneous placement of tibial screws and plating of fibular fracture.

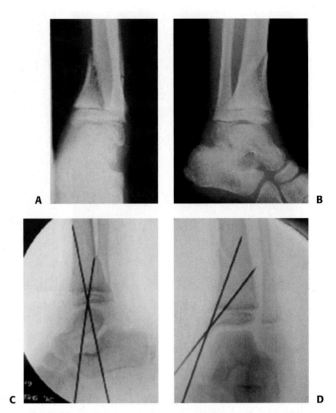

Figure 29-64. Salter–Harris type II distal tibial fracture with fibular fracture. **A:** Anteroposterior view. **B:** Lateral view. **C, D:** Percutaneous placement of K-wires.

depending on local resources and practices. Reduction may be attempted by applying longitudinal traction to the foot, followed by eversion of the foot and direct digital pressure over the medial malleolus. If image intensification confirms anatomical reduction, but the fracture is unstable, the fracture may be fixed with two percutaneous smooth wires placed in the epiphysis parallel to the physis. Reduction is confirmed by a short, continuous fluoroscopic examination. Percutaneous clamp placement may also facilitate reduction in some of these cases. Cannulated screws can be inserted if the epiphysis is large enough. For fractures that are seen more than 7 to 14 days after injury, we may accept up to 2 mm of displacement without attempting closed or open reduction. Reliable patients whose fractures are fixed with pins and/or screws may be immobilized in below-knee casts. Above-knee casts are used for other patients.

In cases where arthroscopic assistance is used, the visualization of the ankle joint can also assist with the evaluation of reduction. In some cases, the fractures may still have a small gap present with the articular surface, but the presence of step-off or intra-articular incongruity can be clearly evaluated with the scope visualization of the articular surface. It has been our experience that the C-arm views may show excellent reduction of the subchondral bone of the articular surface, and the arthroscopic or open views may show that the cartilage surfaces are not as well reduced as one would expect based upon these radiographic images. Arthrogram is helpful if open or arthroscopic visualization is not done.

Fractures with more than 2 mm of displacement or step-off should be reduced, regardless of whether the fracture is acute or not. Closed reduction can be attempted, but these fractures typically require open reduction, arthroscopic-assisted reduction, or mini-open reduction with arthroscopic assistance. Occasionally, primary debridement of callus and soft tissue back to normal-appearing physis and fat grafting has been successful for fractures that are more than 2 weeks old.

For fractures stabilized with internal fixation, below-knee casts may be used. If there is concern about fracture stability, above-knee casts can be used.

Salter–Harris Type V Fractures of the Distal Tibia

These injuries are quite rare. The risk of physeal arrest is thought to be quite high for this injury pattern, because of direct damage of the germinal layer of the physis.[93] A pure Salter V fracture is not identified until months after the injury.

The prognosis for this injury is poor, and treatment is usually focused upon treating the complications of angular deformity and/or physeal arrest.[93]

Juvenile Tillaux Fractures

For nondisplaced fractures and fractures displaced less than 2 mm, we prefer immobilization in an above-knee cast with the knee flexed 30 degrees and the foot neutral or internally rotated. If the position appears acceptable on plain films, CT scanning in the transverse plane with coronal and sagittal reconstructions may be used to confirm acceptable reduction. For fractures with more than 2 mm of initial displacement, manipulation may be attempted by internal rotation of the foot and application of direct pressure over the anterolateral joint line. If reduction is not obtained with this maneuver, reduction can be attempted by dorsiflexing the pronated foot and then internally rotating the foot.[118] If successful reduction is obtained, percutaneous fixation (screws or pins) can be placed with C-arm guidance. Percutaneous clamps can be used to obtain and hold reduction during screw placement. If there are questions about the adequacy of reduction, this can be confirmed by use of an arthrotomy or ankle arthroscope.

In cases in which the reduction is not ideal, there are several options. Schlesinger and Wedge[167] have described a technique using percutaneous manipulation of a Tillaux fragment with a Steinmann pin.[93] Small Kirschner wires or the threaded tip wires from a cannulated screw set can be inserted into the Tillaux fragment under fluoroscopic control, to act as a "joystick" to reduce the fracture (Fig. 29-65). Ideally, one or both of these pins can then be passed across the fracture site after reduction has been obtained if the guidewire is carefully placed initially, and the cannulated screw can then be placed over the pins (Figs. 29-66 and 29-67). As there is no meaningful growth present in most patients who get Tillaux fractures, crossing the growth plate with a screw is acceptable, and may help in fracture reduction (see Fig. 29-35).

If reduction is not successful, open reduction is performed. The patient is placed in a supine position, and a

vertical incision is placed over the fracture. A small incision is made, perhaps 2 to 3 cm, to allow for visualization. The fracture plane is identified, and direct pressure or clamps can be applied to maintain the reduction. A guidewire from the cannulated screw system (a 4-mm cannulated system usually works well in this age group) is placed, followed by placement of the screw.

A short-leg, non–weight-bearing cast or boot is worn for 3 weeks, followed by a weight-bearing cast or walking boot for another 3 weeks.

Triplane Fractures

For nondisplaced or minimally displaced (less than 2 mm) fractures, we prefer immobilization in a long-leg cast with the knee flexed 30 to 40 degrees. The position of the foot is determined by whether the fracture is lateral (internal rotation) or medial (eversion). A CT scan may be obtained after reduction and casting to document adequate reduction. Plain films or CT scans are obtained approximately 7 days after cast application to verify that displacement has not recurred. At 3 to 4 weeks, the cast is changed to a below-knee walking cast or walking boot, which is worn another 3 to 4 weeks.

The ability to reduce fractures in the ER with appropriate conscious sedation varies among institutions. For institutions that have such capabilities, fracture reduction can be attempted in the ER. For fractures with more than 2 mm of displacement, an attempt closed reduction with sedation in the emergency department is warranted. An above-knee cast is applied. If plain radiographs show satisfactory reduction, a CT scan is obtained. If reduction is acceptable, treatment is the same as for nondisplaced fractures.

If the reduction is unacceptable, closed reduction is attempted in the operating room with the use of general

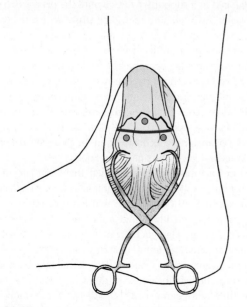

Figure 29-65. Technique for reduction of a Salter–Harris type IV fracture of the distal tibia.

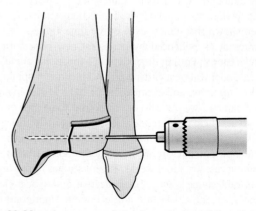

Figure 29-66. Advancement of pin after reduction of juvenile Tillaux fracture.

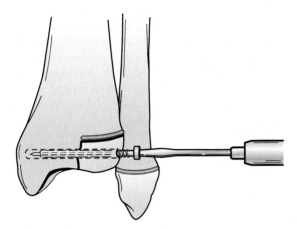

Figure 29-67. Percutaneous insertion of 4-mm cannulated screw over pin that has been advanced into the medial distal tibia after reduction of the juvenile Tillaux fracture fragment.

anesthesia. If fluoroscopy shows an acceptable reduction, percutaneous screws are inserted, avoiding the physis, and a short-leg cast is applied. If closed reduction is unacceptable, open reduction or mini-open reduction with the use of percutaneous clamps is performed. Preoperative CT scanning may be helpful for evaluating the position of the fracture fragments in the anteroposterior and lateral planes and for determining the appropriate skin incisions, percutaneous clamp placements, and screw location.

Fractures Involving the Distal Fibula

It is at times difficult to differentiate between a nondisplaced Salter fracture of the distal fibula and a sprain of the talofibular ligaments. A recent study of children with ankle injuries with MRI suggests the incidence of a Salter fracture of the distal fibula is 3%.[22] A careful physical examination can help differentiate between a fracture and a sprain. A sprain should have maximal tenderness over the ligaments, anterior to the distal fibula, while a fracture should have maximal tenderness on the bone, which is often best palpated from a posterior approach to avoid overlap with the anterior ligament pain and help differentiate the two. However, a few days old after the injury generalized swelling and pain can make localization more challenging. If one is confident that maximal tenderness is directly on the growth plate, treatment for a fracture should be initiated even in the setting of negative radiographs. When an examination is carried out by an orthopedic surgeon who feels there is bony tenderness, it has been shown that almost 20% of the time a physeal fracture is present as evidenced by periosteal new bone formation weeks later.[164] Putting the patient in a functional ankle splint or cast boot will treat either a physeal fracture or sprain, with follow-up x-rays and examination in 10 to 14 helping to differentiate the two. An MRI or ultrasound at the time of injury could also help differentiate a physeal fracture from a sprain.

We usually treat radiologically confirmed nondisplaced fibular physeal fractures with immobilization in a below-knee walking cast for 3 to 4 weeks. Recent studies found use of a removable ankle brace to be as effective, and to be preferable from a patient satisfaction and economic standpoint when compared to fiberglass posterior splints.[7,22] Closed reduction

of displaced Salter–Harris types I and II fibular fractures, is usually successful. In cases where reduction is unsuccessful, one may accept up to 50% displacement without problems at long-term follow-up, especially in those with 3 to 4 years of growth remaining. Acceptance of this displacement may be more reasonable in young patients with significant remodeling potential, although in older patients, displaced fractures may have more effect on ankle function, and more anatomic reduction may be advantageous. Dias and Giegerich,[50] however, reported a patient with a symptomatic spike that required excision after incomplete reduction.

Lateral Ankle Sprains and Lateral Ligament Avulsion Injuries

The diagnosis of an ankle sprain is less common in younger patients, although recognition of ankle sprain injuries in children is becoming more common with advanced imaging using ultrasound and MRI. If the pain can be localized to the ligaments, and there is no pain over the distal fibular physis, then ankle sprain is the likely diagnosis. The authors prefer functional treatment for ankle sprains, allowing weight bearing as tolerated in a supportive device until the patient is pain free (typically 3 weeks), and then progressive return to activities. Very severe ankle sprains are offered casting for 1 week which seems to significantly relieve pain. Elevation is also very important for pain relief over the first few days. Surgical treatment is reserved for those patients who develop late symptoms. Chronic pain and instability can occur in young patients, especially adolescents. In these cases, a Broström-type reconstruction[26] may be appropriate, although Letts et al.[110] have described nonanatomic reconstruction in younger patients (Evans, Watson–Jones, Chrisman, and Snook).

Avulsion fractures can be identified that originate from the distal fibula, and special radiographic views may facilitate diagnosis (Fig. 29-68).[71] These avulsion-type injuries can lead to symptoms, and a high index of suspicion is important in younger patients. Haraguchi et al.[71] evaluated a series of severe ankle sprains, and found that 26% had evidence of distal fibular avulsion injury. Children and adults over 40 years of age had the highest incidence of this injury. Patients were treated with weight-bearing casts for 3 to 4 weeks. Nonoperative treatment yielded satisfactory results in this series.

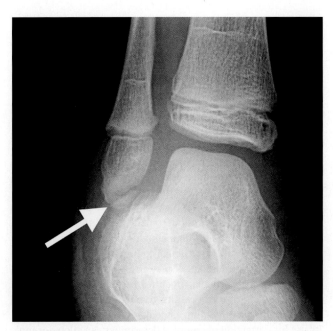

Figure 29-68. Fibula avulsion fracture in a 7-year-old. (Used with permission of the Children's Orthopaedic Center, Los Angeles.)

Postoperative Care and Rehabilitation

Usually a below-knee cast is worn during the last 2 to 3 weeks of immobilization, and weight bearing to tolerance is allowed during this time. After immobilization is discontinued, ankle range-of-motion exercises and strengthening exercises are begun. Protective splinting or bracing is usually not required after cast removal. Running is restricted until the patient demonstrates an essentially full, painless range of ankle and foot motion and can walk without a limp. Running progresses from jogging to more strenuous running and jumping as soreness and endurance dictate. For athletes, unrestricted running and jumping ability should be achieved before returning to sports. Protective measures such as taping or functional bracing may be beneficial for return to sports.

Younger patients with physeal ankle fractures recover quickly and require little or no formal physical therapy. For this reason, and because of compliance considerations, fractures treated with internal fixation are usually protected with below-knee casting instead of starting an early range-of-motion program in a removable splint. In older patients who may have a higher risk of arthrofibrosis, we may start early motion in a removable boot, and have them start a formal supervised physical therapy program.

Potential Pitfalls and Preventive Measures

Ankle Fractures:
SURGICAL PITFALLS AND PREVENTIONS

Pitfall	Prevention
Procedure Name	
• Arthrofibrosis	• Prevention—early ROM. Fractures heal more rapidly in young patients, and early ROM and weight bearing is usually possible

• Nonunion, Malunion	• This is very rare in younger patients, and anatomic reduction will reduce this risk
• Physeal arrest	• This complication is rarely related to surgical technique—it is usually a direct complication from the severe trauma to the physis which occurs at the time of the fracture. Counsel patients and families about this ahead of time, and let them know that close follow-up, and even surgery may be necessary to address growth plate arrests.
• Weakness, delayed recovery	• In more severe injuries, physical therapy may be a valuable tool to help with weakness, delayed recovery. Many of these patients recover well without formal physical therapy programs, especially low-energy, minimally displaced injuries

MANAGEMENT OF EXPECTED ADVERSE OUTCOMES AND UNEXPECTED COMPLICATIONS OF DISTAL TIBIAL AND FIBULAR FRACTURES

Ankle Fractures:
COMMON ADVERSE OUTCOMES AND COMPLICATIONS

- Delayed union and nonunion
- Deformity secondary to malunion
- Physeal arrest or growth disturbance
- Medial malleolus overgrowth
- Arthritis
- Chondrolysis
- Osteonecrosis of the distal tibial epiphysis
- Compartment syndrome
- Osteochondral defects
- Synostosis
- Reflex sympathetic dystrophy/complex regional pain syndrome
- Osteopenia

DELAYED UNION AND NONUNION

Delayed union and nonunion are extremely rare after distal tibial physeal fractures (Fig. 29-69). Dias and Giegerich[50] reported one patient with a delayed union and one patient with a previous physeal bar excision who had a nonunion that healed after open reduction, internal fixation, and bone grafting. Siffert and Arkin[173] reported nonunion in a patient with avascular necrosis of the distal tibial epiphysis. We have seen two younger patients with Salter–Harris type III fractures that appeared to be progressing to nonunion. Because neither patient had any complaints of pain nor any evidence of progressive displacement of the fracture and stress views showed no instability, no treatment was undertaken. Both fractures eventually united. We have seen one patient with a nonunion after open reduction and internal fixation in whom pin fixation and cast immobilization were discontinued prematurely. The fracture healed after repeat open reduction and internal fixation.

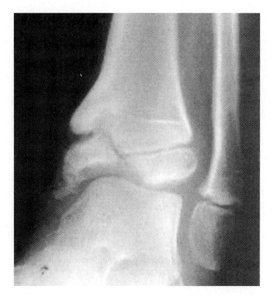

Figure 29-69. Complex nonunion of a Salter–Harris type III fracture of the medial malleolus in an 8-year-old boy. Note that the distal tibial epiphysis is in valgus, whereas the talus is in varus. (Courtesy of Brent Broztman, MD.)

Nonunion of a fracture of the fibular epiphysis has been reported by Mirmiran and Schuberth.[125] This was treated successfully with open reduction and internal fixation.

DEFORMITY SECONDARY TO MALUNION

Malunion usually occurs after triplane fractures that are either incompletely reduced or are initially immobilized in below-knee casts. It has also been reported after Salter–Harris type I and II injuries. Phan et al.[146a] reported an increase in the outward foot progression angle in children following transitional fractures, but it is not known if perhaps an outwardly rotated foot predisposes one to these fractures. Derotational osteotomy may be performed for extra-articular fractures if discomfort and stiffness occur. Guille et al.[69] reported a rotational malunion of lateral malleolar fracture that lead to a stress fracture of the distal fibula that went on to delayed union. Their patient improved after correction of the malrotated distal fibula and bone grafting of the delayed union site.

Takakura et al.[184] described successful open wedge osteotomy for varus deformity in nine patients. Scheffer and Peterson[165] recommend opening wedge osteotomy when the angular deformity is 25 degrees or less and the limb length discrepancy is or will be 25 mm or less at maturity. Preoperative planning should include templating the various types of osteotomies to determine which technique will maintain the proper mechanical alignment of the tibia and ankle joint and will not make the malleoli unduly prominent. Osteotomy is not recommended for malunion of intra-articular fractures because it cannot correct the joint incongruity that results from malunion (Fig. 29-70).

The use of the three-dimensional frames continues to evolve. Its use for correction of complex deformities can allow for multiplanar corrections, including rotation, length, and angular deformity.[58,172] Another option to treat secondary deformity is the use of "guided growth," the use of medial malleolar screws or medial stapling devices.[180]

PHYSEAL ARREST OR GROWTH DISTURBANCE

Deformity caused by growth arrest usually occurs after Salter–Harris types III and IV fractures in which a physeal bar develops at the fracture site, leading to varus deformity that progresses with continued growth. Spiegel et al.[178] reported growth problems in 9 of 66 patients with Salter–Harris type II fractures.

Earlier reports[33,45,64] attributed the development of physeal bars to crushing of the physis at the time of injury, but more

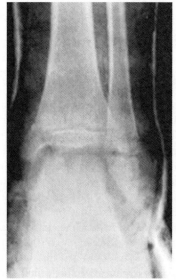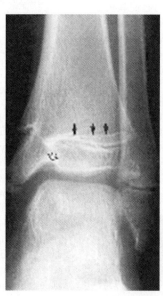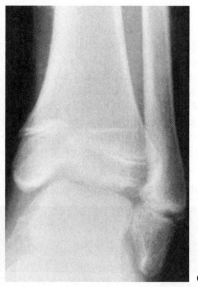

A, B   C

Figure 29-70. A: This apparently nondisplaced medial malleolar fracture in an 11-year-old boy was treated with immobilization in a long-leg cast. **B:** Fourteen months after injury, there is a clear medial osseous bridge and asymmetric growth of the Park–Harris growth arrest lines (*black arrows*). Note the early inhibition of growth on the subchondral surface of the fracture (*open arrow*). **C:** Five years after injury, the varus deformity has increased significantly and fibular overgrowth is apparent.

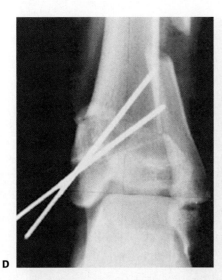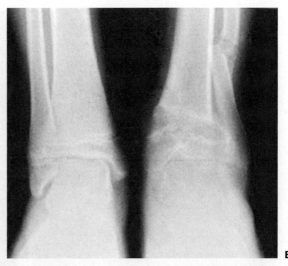

Figure 29-70. (*Continued*) **D:** The deformity was treated with a medial opening-wedge osteotomy of the tibia, an osteotomy of the fibula, and epiphysiodesis of the most lateral portion of the tibial physis and fibula. **E:** Three months after surgery, the osteotomies are healed and the varus deformity is corrected; the joint surface remains irregular. (Courtesy of Earl A. Stanley Jr, MD.)

recent reports[84,102] discount this explanation and claim that with anatomical reduction (open reduction and internal fixation if needed), the incidence of physeal bar formation can be decreased. The validity of this claim is difficult to determine from published reports. One problem is the small numbers of patients in all series, and the even smaller numbers within each group in each series. Another problem is the age of the patients in operative and nonoperative groups in the various series; for example, many children reported to do well with a particular treatment method and have so little growth remaining that treatment may have had little or no effect on growth.

A recent study by Rohmiller et al.[156] analyzed the outcome of 91 Salter–Harris I and II fractures of the distal tibia. They identified premature physeal closure in 40%. This series identified a trend toward increased premature physeal closure in fractures that had worse displacement after reduction. They recommended operative reduction to restore anatomic alignment, to reduce the risk of premature physeal closure.

Kling et al.[102] reported physeal bars in two of five patients treated nonoperatively and in none of three patients treated operatively in children 10 years of age and younger. In another series of 65 physeal ankle fractures, Kling[102] concluded that the frequency of growth-related deformities could be reduced by open reduction and internal fixation of Salter–Harris III and IV fractures.

However, in one of the authors experience with eight patients (prior author), two of five treated operatively developed physeal bars, whereas none of the three patients treated nonoperatively had physeal bars. This supports the conclusion of Cass and Peterson,[34] Ogden,[135] and others that growth problems after these injuries may not always be prevented by open reduction and internal fixation. Open reduction of displaced Salter–Harris type III and IV ankle fractures would seem advisable to restore joint congruity, regardless of whether growth potential can be preserved.

Harris growth lines have been reported to be reliable predictors of growth abnormality.[79] The use of MRI and/or CT scan may assist with evaluation of physeal bars. Spontaneous resolution of physeal bars has been reported[20,37] but is rare. Excision of small bony bars, particularly those on the periphery after restores normal growth (Fig. 29-71). Large bars may require osteotomy.

Kärrholm et al.[91] reported on eight children with growth arrest of the distal tibial and/or fibular physis. Distal fibular physeal arrest could lead to either progressive ankle valgus (Fig. 29-72; see Fig. 29-46) or an otherwise normal ankle.

They found that continued fibular growth with complete arrest of tibial growth was usually compensated by proximal migration of the fibula so that varus deformity did not occur.

Because the amount of growth remaining in the distal tibial physis is small (approximately 0.25 in per year) in most older patients with these injuries, the amount of leg-length discrepancy resulting from complete growth arrest tends to be relatively small. Treatment may be required if the anticipated discrepancy is projected to be clinically significant.

Imaging techniques to identify physeal arrest and bars include plane radiographs, computerized tomography, and MRI. CT scans can be useful for clear delineation of the bony anatomy, especially in cases in which surgical intervention is necessary. Recent studies have also used MRI scans.[62,113,163] Although the resolution capability is more limited, the avoidance of ionizing radiation is a theoretical advantage of MRI scans over CT scans, in some areas of the body, but a limited cut CT scan of a distal tibia should not have a dangerous dose of radiation.

MEDIAL MALLEOLUS OVERGROWTH

Overgrowth of the medial malleolus has been reported after fractures of the distal tibia metaphysis and epiphysis. A recent series of 83 patients with fractures in this region demonstrated 2 patients with medial malleolus overgrowth. In both cases, there was no evidence of functional impairment.[130]

ARTHRITIS

Epiphyseal ankle fractures that do not extend into the joint have a low risk of posttraumatic arthritis, but injuries that extend into the joint may produce this complication. Caterini et al.[36]

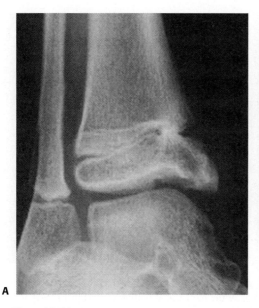
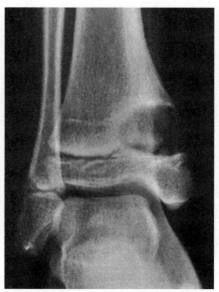

Figure 29-71. A: One year after open reduction and internal fixation of a Salter–Harris type III fracture of the distal tibia in a 7-year-old boy, varus deformity has been caused by a physeal bar. **B:** Two years after excision of the physeal bar and insertion of cranioplast, satisfactory growth has resumed and the deformity has resolved.

found that 8 of 68 (12%) patients had pain and stiffness that began from 5 to 8 years after skeletal maturity. Ertl et al.[56] found that at 36 months to 13 years after injury only 8 of 15 patients evaluated were asymptomatic.

Ramsey and Hamilton[150] demonstrated in a cadaver study that 1 mm of lateral talar displacement decreases tibiotalar contact area by 42%, which greatly increases the stress on this weight-bearing joint. More recently, Michelson et al.[123] reported that a cadaver study using unconstrained specimens suggested that some lateral talar displacement occurs with normal weight bearing. Because of their findings, they questioned the current criterion of 2 mm of displacement for unstable ankle fractures. However, the results of Ramsey and Hamilton's study correlate well with other studies

that have shown increased symptoms in patients in whom more than 2 mm of displacement was accepted.[36,107]

Implant removal after fracture surgery remains controversial, and the indications for removal are not well defined in the literature.[30] Charlton et al.[39] have demonstrated that the periepiphyseal or subchondral screws may alter the joint contact pressures about the ankle. After removal of the screws from the subchondral bone, the contact pressure is normalized. For hardware in the subchondral bone, Charlton's study suggests that implant removal of transepiphyseal screws may be appropriate, but there is not clinical data to support or refute this.

CHONDROLYSIS

Chondrolysis is a rare complication of adolescent ankle fractures.[15,162] Treatment options include therapy, nonsteroidal anti-inflammatories, etc. Recent clinical studies have evaluated the effects of joint distraction for posttraumatic chondrolysis, although experience with this technique in young patients is very limited.[162]

COMPARTMENT SYNDROME

This complication is discussed in detail in Chapter 5. Fractures of the distal tibia and ankle joint are infrequently associated with compartment syndromes.[43,127]

OSTEOCHONDRAL DEFECTS

Osteochondral injuries, primarily of the talus, are increasingly recognized after ankle injury in adults and the skeletally immature.[117,134,166] MRI may play a role in identification of treatment of these injuries.[11]

SYNOSTOSIS

Posttraumatic tibiofibular synostosis is a rare complication of fractures in this region. This can lead to growth disturbance,

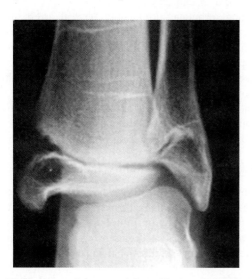

Figure 29-72. Valgus deformity of the ankle, lateral displacement of the talus with widening of the joint medially, and severe shortening of the fibula after early physeal arrest in a child who sustained an ankle injury at 6 years of age. (Courtesy of James Roach, MD.)

including angular deformity and lower extremity length discrepancy.[129,196] Synostosis in this area alters the normal pattern of movement between the tibia and fibula, and has been associated with pain in some patients. In a small clinical series, Frick et al.[60] demonstrated symptoms of pain, prominence of the fibula, and ankle deformity in 5/8 patients with this synostosis. In this series, the normal growth pattern of distal migration of the fibula was altered, resulting in decreased distances between the proximal physes of the tibia and fibula, and proximal positioning of the distal fibula with respect to the distal tibia. Munjal et al.[129] demonstrated successful synostosis excision in a 7-year-old patient, which lead to normalization of the ankle joint at 16 months after surgery.

REFLEX SYMPATHETIC DYSTROPHY/COMPLEX REGIONAL PAIN SYNDROME

Reflex sympathetic dystrophy or complex regional pain syndrome occasionally develops after ankle injuries, and is treated initially with an intensive formal physical therapy regimen that encourages range of motion and weight bearing.[93,196] For patients who do not respond quickly to such a program, physical therapy in association with regional anesthesia interventions may be considered.[196] Referral to chronic pain clinic/specialist may be appropriate in some of these cases.

SUMMARY, CONTROVERSIES, AND FUTURE DIRECTIONS RELATED TO ANKLE FRACTURES

Many questions remain unanswered about the optimal treatment of ankle fractures in skeletally immature patients and will have to be answered with clinical trials. The relationship between physeal displacement and the development of subsequent physeal arrest is still unclear. Interposition of periosteum in the fracture may play a role in physeal arrest, although this has not been clarified in animal models or clinical trials. Recent studies in the adult literature have suggested that minimally angular deformities about the distal tibia can have pronounced effects on the tibiotalar contact pressures.[93,186,188] The limits of fracture remodeling and the magnitude of acceptable deformity in growing children are still not well defined in the literature.

Advanced imaging techniques have improved our understanding of these fractures, and may play an increasing role in the use of computer-aided reduction techniques and other forms of minimally invasive surgery. CT scanning requires ionizing radiation, but provides high resolution model reconstruction. In addition, recent studies utilizing advanced imaging have cast doubt on the commonly accepted principle that the physis is always weaker than ankle ligaments. It appears that ankle sprain injuries are more common than previously believed, and are often misdiagnosed as Salter I fractures of the distal fibula.

The use of cultured chondrocytes and gene therapy may eventually play a role in the treatment of these fractures, either to prevent or treat a physeal arrest.[98] The surgical treatment of physeal bars to restore normal growth remains unsuccessful in a substantial percentage of cases, and further understanding of the basic mechanisms controlling physeal growth may help us develop more successful strategies.

ACKNOWLEDGMENTS

The authors and editors wish to acknowledge Drs. Luciano Dias and Jay Cummings for the past contributions to this chapter.

Annotated References

Reference	Annotation
Chande VT. Decision rules for roentgenography of children with acute ankle injuries. *Arch Pediatr Adolesc Med.* 1995;149:255–258.	Application of the Ottawa Ankle Rules in children were successful at limiting radiographs and not missing fractures.
Cooperman DR, Spiegel PG, Laros GS. Tibial fractures involving the ankle in children. The so-called triplane epiphyseal fracture. *J Bone Joint Surg Am.* 1978;60:1040–1046.	Classic article describing the triplane fracture (sagittal, transverse, coronal) in 6% of 237 epiphyseal ankle fractures. Level of Evidence: IV
Ertl JP, Barrack RL, Alexander AH, et al. Triplane fracture of the distal tibial epiphysis. Long-term follow-up. *J Bone Joint Surg Am.* 1988;70:967–976.	23 patients with triplane fracture were followed for a minimum of 18 months. Residual displacement of the fracture of more than 2 mm predicted a suboptimal result, however some patients with anatomic reduction had early degenerative arthritis and ankle symptoms. Computed tomography was helpful in delineating the fracture pattern and degree of displacement. Level of Evidence: IV
Hynes D, O'Brien T. Growth disturbance lines after injury of the distal tibial physis. Their significance in prognosis. *J Bone Joint Surg Br.* 1988;70:231–233.	Radiographs from 26 patients with distal tibial physis oh fractures were reviewed to characterize the timing and appearance of growth slowdown lines. A parallel line typically seen in the first 6 to 12 weeks following fracture, moving away from the physis is predictive of return of normal growth without angular deformity. Level of Evidence: IV

Annotated References

Reference	Annotation
Kling TF Jr, Bright RW, Hensinger RN. Distal tibial physeal fractures in children that may require open reduction. *J Bone Joint Surg Am.* 1984;66:647–657.	Case series demonstrating that growth disturbances are common following Salter–Harris type III and type IV fractures of the distal tibia, and that anatomic reduction of the physis decreases the incidence of growth disturbance. Level of Evidence: III
Mubarak SJ. Extensor retinaculum syndrome of the ankle after injury to the distal tibial physis. *J Bone Joint Surg Br.* 2002;84:11–14.	6 patients presented after distal tibial physeal injury with severe pain and swelling, anesthesia in the web space of the great toe and weakness of the toe extensors. Pain with passive flexion was present. Compartment syndrome was diagnosed and can exist beneath the superior extensor retinaculum of the ankle, and is treated by release of the superior extensor retinaculum with fracture fixation. Level of Evidence: IV
Ogden JA, Lee J. Accessory ossification patterns and injuries of the malleoli. *J Pediatr Orthop.* 1990;10:306–316.	This article reviews the normal growth and development of the ossification centers of the distal tibia and distal fibula. Differentiation between normal accessory ossification centers and avulsion fractures can be difficult. Radiographic and histologic samples are presented. Level of Evidence: IV
Phieffer LS, Meyer RA Jr, Gruber HE, et al. Effect of interposed periosteum in an animal physeal fracture model. *Clin Orthop Relat Res.* 2000:15–25.	This animal model studies the effect of interposed periosteum on physeal fracture healing. Interposition of periosteum in a physeal fracture model resulted in small histologic bar formation and a small increase in leg-length discrepancy compared to fracture alone.
Spiegel PG, Cooperman DR, Laros GS. Epiphyseal fractures of the distal ends of the tibia and fibula. A retrospective study of two hundred and thirty-seven cases in children. *J Bone Joint Surg Am.* 1978;60:1046–1050.	237 fractures of the distal end of the tibia and or fibula. 32% complication rate, highest in patients with Salter–Harris type III and type IV tibial fractures with more than 2 mm of displacement. Complications correlated with type of fracture, severity of displacement/comminution, and adequacy of reduction. Level of Evidence: IV

REFERENCES

1. Adler P. *Ride on Mower Hazard Analysis 1987–1990.* Washington, DC: Directorate for Epidemiology, USA Consumer Product Safety Commission; 1993:1–65.
2. Aitken AP, Magill HK. Fractures involving the distal femoral epiphyseal cartilage. *J Bone Joint Surg Am.* 1952;34:96–108.
2a. Alioto RJ, Furia JP, Marquardt JD. Hematoma block for ankle fractures: a safe and efficacious technique for manipulations. *J Orthop Trauma.* 1995;9(2):113–116.
3. Alonso JE, Sanchez FL. Lawn mower injuries in children: a preventable impairment. *J Pediatr Orthop.* 1995;15:83–89.
4. Ashhurst APC, Bromer RS. Classification and mechanism of fractures of the leg bones involving the ankle. *Arch Surg.* 1992;4:51–129.
5. Assal M, Ray A, Stern R. The extensible approach for the operative treatment of high-energy pilon fractures: surgical technique and soft-tissue healing. *J Orthop Trauma.* 2007;21:198–206.
6. Barmada A, Gaynor T, Mubarak SJ. Premature physeal closure following distal tibia physeal fractures: a new radiographic predictor. *J Pediatr Orthop.* 2003;23:733–739.
7. Barnett PL, Lee MH, Oh L, et al. Functional outcome after air-stirrup ankle brace or fiberglass backslab for pediatric low-risk ankle fractures: a randomized observer-blinded controlled trial. *Pediatr Emerg Care.* 2012;28:745–749.
8. Beaty JH, Linton RC. Medial malleolar fracture in a child. A case report. *J Bone Joint Surg Am.* 1988;70:1254–1255.
9. Benz G, Kallieris D, Seebock T, et al. Bioresorbable pins and screws in paediatric traumatology. *Eur J Pediatr Surg.* 1994;4:103–107.
10. Bishop PA. Fractures and epiphyseal separation fractures of the ankle: Classification of 332 cases according to mechanism of their production. *AJR Am J Roentgenol.* 1932;28:49–67.
11. Blackburn EW, Aronsson DD, Rubright JH, et al. Ankle fractures in children. *J Bone Joint Surg Am.* 2012;94:1234–1244.
12. Blair JM, Botte MJ. Surgical anatomy of the superficial peroneal nerve in the ankle and foot. *Clin Orthop Relat Res.* 1994;305:229–238.
13. Blauth M, Bastian L, Krettek C, et al. Surgical options for the treatment of severe tibial pilon fractures: a study of three techniques. *J Orthop Trauma.* 2001;15:153–160.
14. Blitzer CM, Johnson RJ, Ettlinger CF, Aggeborn K. Downhill skiing injuries in children. *Am J Sports Med.* 1984;12:142–147.
15. Bojescul JA, Wilson G, Taylor DC. Idiopathic chondrolysis of the ankle. *Arthroscopy.* 2005;21:224–227.
16. Böstman OM. Distal tibiofibular synostosis after malleolar fractures treated using absorbable implants. *Foot Ankle.* 1993;14:38–43.
17. Böstman OM. Metallic or absorbable fracture fixation devices. A cost minimization analysis. *Clin Orthop Relat Res.* 1996;329:233–239.
18. Böstman O, Hirvensalo E, Vainionpaa S, et al. Degradable polyglycolide rods for the internal fixation of displaced bimalleolar fractures. *Int Orthop.* 1990;14:1–8.
19. Böstman O, Mäkelä EA, Södergård J, et al. Absorbable polyglycolide pins in internal fixation of fractures in children. *J Pediatr Orthop.* 1993;13:242–245.
20. Bostock SH, Peach BG. Spontaneous resolution of an osseous bridge affecting the distal tibial epiphysis. *J Bone Joint Surg Br.* 1996;78:662–663.
21. Boutis K, Narayanan UG, Dong FF, et al. Magnetic resonance imaging of clinically suspected Salter-Harris I fracture of the distal fibula. *Injury.* 2010;41:852–856.
22. Boutis K, Plint A, Stimec J, et al. Radiograph-negative lateral ankle injuries in children: occult growth plate fracture or sprain? *JAMA Pediatr.* 2016;170(1):e154114.
23. Boyer MI, Bowen V, Weiler P. Reconstruction of a severe grinding injury to the medial malleolus and the deltoid ligament of the ankle using a free plantaris tendon graft and vascularized gracilis free muscle transfer: case report. *J Trauma.* 1994;36:454–457.
24. Bozic KJ, Jaramillo D, DiCanzio J, et al. Radiographic appearance of the normal distal tibiofibular syndesmosis in children. *J Pediatr Orthop.* 1999;19:14–21.
25. Broström L. Sprained ankles. V. Treatment and prognosis in recent ligament ruptures. *Acta Chir Scand.* 1966;132:537–550.
26. Broström L. Sprained ankles. VI. Surgical treatment of "chronic" ligament ruptures. *Acta Chir Scand.* 1966;132:551–565.
27. Brown SD, Kasser JR, Zurakowski D, et al. Analysis of 51 tibial triplane fractures using CT with multiplanar reconstruction. *AJR Am J Roentgenol.* 2004;183:1489–1495.
28. Bucholz RW, Henry S, Henley MB. Fixation with bioabsorbable screws for the treatment of fractures of the ankle. *J Bone Joint Surg Am.* 1994;76:319–324.
29. Burstein AH. Fracture classification systems: do they work and are they useful? *J Bone Joint Surg Am.* 1993;75:1743–1744.
30. Busam ML, Esther RJ, Obremskey WT. Hardware removal: indications and expectations. *J Am Acad Orthop Surg.* 2006;14:113–120.
31. Busconi BD, Pappas AM. Chronic, painful ankle instability in skeletally immature athletes. Ununited osteochondral fractures of the distal fibula. *Am J Sports Med.* 1996;24:647–651.
32. Carey J, Spence L, Blickman H, et al. MRI of pediatric growth plate injury: correlation with plain film radiographs and clinical outcome. *Skeletal Radiol.* 1998;27:250–255.
33. Carothers CO, Crenshaw AH. Clinical significance of a classification of epiphyseal injuries at the ankle. *Am J Surg.* 1955;89:879–889.
34. Cass JR, Peterson HA. Salter-Harris Type-IV injuries of the distal tibial epiphyseal growth plate, with emphasis on those involving the medial malleolus. *J Bone Joint Surg Am.* 1983;65:1059–1070.
35. Casteleyn PP, Handelberg F. Distraction for ankle arthroscopy. *Arthroscopy.* 1995;11:633–634.
36. Caterini R, Farsetti P, Ippolito E. Long-term followup of physeal injury to the ankle. *Foot Ankle.* 1991;11:372–383.
37. Chadwick CJ. Spontaneous resolution of varus deformity at the ankle following adduction injury of the distal tibial epiphysis. A case report. *J Bone Joint Surg Am.* 1982;64:774–776.

38. Chande VT. Decision rules for roentgenography of children with acute ankle injuries. *Arch Pediatr Adolesc Med.* 1995;149:255–258.
39. Charlton M, Costello R, Mooney JF, 3rd, et al. Ankle joint biomechanics following transepiphyseal screw fixation of the distal tibia. *J Pediatr Orthop.* 2005;25:635–640.
40. Clement DA, Worlock PH. Triplane fracture of the distal tibia. A variant in cases with an open growth plate. *J Bone Joint Surg Br.* 1987;69:412–415.
41. Cooperman DR, Spiegel PG, Laros GS. Epiphyseal fractures of the distal ends of the tibia and fibula. A retrospective study of two hundred and thirty-seven cases in children. *J Bone Joint Surg Am.* 1978;60:1046–1050.
42. Cox PJ, Clarke NM. Juvenile Tillaux fracture of the ankle associated with a tibial shaft fracture: a unique combination. *Injury.* 1996;27:221–222.
43. Cox G, Thambapillay S, Templeton PA. Compartment syndrome with an isolated Salter Harris II fracture of the distal tibia. *J Orthop Trauma.* 2008;22:148–150.
44. Crawford AH. Triplane and Tillaux fractures: is a 2 mm residual gap acceptable? *J Pediatr Orthop.* 2012;32(Suppl 1):S69–S73.
45. Crenshaw AH. Injuries of the distal tibial epiphysis. *Clin Orthop Relat Res.* 1965;41:98–107.
46. Cummings RJ. Triplane ankle fracture with deltoid ligament tear and syndesmotic disruption. *J Child Orthop.* 2008;2:11–14.
47. Cummings RJ, Hahn GA Jr. The incisural fracture. *Foot Ankle Int.* 2004;25:132–135.
48. Damore DT, Metzl JD, Ramundo M, et al. Patterns in childhood sports injury. *Pediatr Emerg Care.* 2003;19:65–67.
49. Denton JR, Fischer SJ. The medial triplane fracture: report of an unusual injury. *J Trauma.* 1981;21:991–995.
50. Dias LS, Giegerich CR. Fractures of the distal tibial epiphysis in adolescence. *J Bone Joint Surg Am.* 1983;65:438–444.
51. Dias LS, Tachdjian MO. Physeal injuries of the ankle in children: classification. *Clin Orthop Relat Res.* 1978;136:230–233.
52. Dormans JP, Azzoni M, Davidson RS, et al. Major lower extremity lawn mower injuries in children. *J Pediatr Orthop.* 1995;15:78–82.
53. Dowling S, Spooner CH, Liang Y, et al. Accuracy of Ottawa Ankle Rules to exclude fractures of the ankle and midfoot in children: a meta-analysis. *Acad Emerg Med.* 2009;16:277–287.
54. Dunbar RP, Barei DP, Kubiak EN, et al. Early limited internal fixation of diaphyseal extensions in select pilon fractures: upgrading AO/OTA type C fractures to AO/OTA type B. *J Orthop Trauma.* 2008;22:426–429.
55. El-Karef E, Sadek HI, Nairn DS, et al. Triplane fracture of the distal tibia. *Injury.* 2000;31:729–736.
56. Ertl JP, Barrack RL, Alexander AH, et al. Triplane fracture of the distal tibial epiphysis. Long-term follow-up. *J Bone Joint Surg Am.* 1988;70:967–976.
57. Farley FA, Kuhns L, Jacobson JA, et al. Ultrasound examination of ankle injuries in children. *J Pediatr Orthop.* 2001;21:604–607.
58. Feldman DS, Shin SS, Madan S, et al. Correction of tibial malunion and nonunion with six-axis analysis deformity correction using the Taylor Spatial Frame. *J Orthop Trauma.* 2003;17:549–554.
59. Feldman F, Singson RD, Rosenberg ZS, et al. Distal tibial triplane fractures: diagnosis with CT. *Radiology.* 1987;164:429–435.
60. Frick SL, Shoemaker S, Mubarak S. Altered fibular growth patterns after tibiofibular synostosis in children. *J Bone Joint Surg Am.* 2001;83(2):247–254.
61. Frokjaer J, Moller BN. Biodegradable fixation of ankle fractures. Complications in a prospective study of 25 cases. *Acta Orthop Scand.* 1992;63:434–436.
62. Gabel GT, Peterson HA, Berquist TH. Premature partial physeal arrest. Diagnosis by magnetic resonance imaging in two cases. *Clin Orthop Relat Res.* 1991;272:242–247.
63. Gaglani MJ, Friedman J, Hawkins EP, Campbell JR. Infections complicating lawn mower injuries in children. *Pediatr Infect Dis J.* 1996;15:452–455.
64. Gill GG, Abott LO. Varus deformity of ankle following injury to distal epiphyseal cartilage of tibia in growing children. *Surg Gynecol Obstet.* 1941;72:659–666.
65. Goldberg VM, Aadalen R. Distal tibial epiphyseal injuries: the role of athletics in 53 cases. *Am J Sports Med.* 1978;6:263–268.
66. Gourineni P, Gupta A. Medial joint space widening of the ankle in displaced Tillaux and Triplane fractures in children. *J Orthop Trauma.* 2011;25:608–611.
67. Grace DL. Irreducible fracture-separations of the distal tibial epiphysis. *J Bone Joint Surg Br.* 1983;65:160–162.
68. Grosfeld JL, Morse TS, Eyring EJ. Lawn mower injuries in children. *Arch Surg.* 1970;100:582–583.
69. Guille JT, Lipton GE, Bowen JR, et al. Delayed union following stress fracture of the distal fibula secondary to rotational malunion of lateral malleolar fracture. *Am J Orthop (Belle Mead NJ).* 1997;26:442–445.
70. Handolin L, Kiljunen V, Arnala I, et al. Effect of ultrasound therapy on bone healing of lateral malleolar fractures of the ankle joint fixed with bioabsorbable screws. *J Orthop Sci.* 2005;10:391–395.
71. Haraguchi N, Kato F, Hayashi H. New radiographic projections for avulsion fractures of the lateral malleolus. *J Bone Joint Surg Br.* 1998;80:684–688.
72. Haramati N, Roye DP, Adler PA, et al. Non-union of pediatric fibula fractures: easy to overlook, painful to ignore. *Pediatr Radiol.* 1994;24:248–250.
73. Havranek P, Lizler J. Magnetic resonance imaging in the evaluation of partial growth arrest after physeal injuries in children. *J Bone Joint Surg Am.* 1991;73:1234–1241.
74. Havranek P, Pesl T. Salter (Rang) type 6 physeal injury. *Eur J Pediatr Surg.* 2010;20:174–177.
75. Healy WA, 3rd, Starkweather KD, Meyer J, Teplitz GA. Triplane fracture associated with a proximal third fibula fracture. *Am J Orthop (Belle Mead NJ).* 1996;25:449–451.
76. Herscovici D Jr, Sanders RW, Scaduto JM, et al. Vacuum-assisted wound closure (VAC therapy) for the management of patients with high-energy soft tissue injuries. *J Orthop Trauma.* 2003;17:683–688.
77. Hirvensalo E. Fracture fixation with biodegradable rods. Forty-one cases of severe ankle fractures. *Acta Orthop Scand.* 1989;60:601–606.
78. Horowitz JH, Nichter LS, Kenney JG, et al. Lawnmower injuries in children: lower extremity reconstruction. *J Trauma.* 1985;25:1138–1146.
79. Hynes D, O'Brien T. Growth disturbance lines after injury of the distal tibial physis. Their significance in prognosis. *J Bone Joint Surg Br.* 1988;70:231–233.
80. Imade S, Takao M, Nishi H, et al. Arthroscopy-assisted reduction and percutaneous fixation for triplane fracture of the distal tibia. *Arthroscopy.* 2004;20:e123–e128.
81. Iwinska-Zelder J, Schmidt S, Ishaque N, et al. [Epiphyseal injuries of the distal tibia. Does MRI provide useful additional information?]. *Radiologe.* 1999;39:25–29.
82. Jarvis JG, Miyanji F. The complex triplane fracture: ipsilateral tibial shaft and distal triplane fracture. *J Trauma.* 2001;51:714–716.
83. Jennings MM, Lagaay P, Schuberth JM. Arthroscopic assisted fixation of juvenile intra-articular epiphyseal ankle fractures. *J Foot Ankle Surg.* 2007;46:376–386.
84. Johnson EW Jr, Fahl JC. Fractures involving the distal epiphysis of the tibia and fibula in children. *Am J Surg.* 1957;93:778–781.
85. Johnstone BR, Bennett CS. Lawn mower injuries in children. *Aust N Z J Surg.* 1989;59:713–718.
86. Jones S, Phillips N, Ali F, et al. Triplane fractures of the distal tibia requiring open reduction and internal fixation. Pre-operative planning using computed tomography. *Injury.* 2003;34:293–298.
87. Kärrholm J. The triplane fracture: four years of follow-up of 21 cases and review of the literature. *J Pediatr Orthop B.* 1997;6:91–102.
88. Kärrholm J, Hansson LI, Laurin S. Computed tomography of intraarticular supination–eversion fractures of the ankle in adolescents. *J Pediatr Orthop.* 1981;1:181–187.
89. Kärrholm J, Hansson LI, Laurin S. Supination–eversion injuries of the ankle in children: a retrospective study of radiographic classification and treatment. *J Pediatr Orthop.* 1982;2:147–159.
90. Kärrholm J, Hansson LI, Laurin S. Pronation injuries of the ankle in children. Retrospective study of radiographical classification and treatment. *Acta Orthop Scand.* 1983;54:1–17.
91. Kärrholm J, Hansson LI, Selvik G. Changes in tibiofibular relationships due to growth disturbances after ankle fractures in children. *J Bone Joint Surg Am.* 1984;66:1198–1210.
92. Kaukonen JP, Lamberg T, Korkala O, et al. Fixation of syndesmotic ruptures in 38 patients with a malleolar fracture: a randomized study comparing a metallic and a bioabsorbable screw. *J Orthop Trauma.* 2005;19:392–395.
93. Kay RM, Matthys GA. Pediatric ankle fractures: evaluation and treatment. *J Am Acad Orthop Surg.* 2001;9:268–278.
94. Kaya A, Altay T, Ozturk H, et al. Open reduction and internal fixation in displaced juvenile Tillaux fractures. *Injury.* 2007;38:201–205.
95. Keats TE. *Atlas of Normal Roentgen Variants That May Simulate Disease.* 5th ed. St Louis, MO: Year Book; 1992.
96. Keats TE. Fractures of the ankle and foot. In: Drennan JC, ed. *The Child's Foot and Ankle.* New York: Raven Press; 1992.
97. Kerr R, Forrester DM, Kingston S. Magnetic resonance imaging of foot and ankle trauma. *Orthop Clin North Am.* 1990;21:591–601.
98. Khoshhal KI, Kiefer GN. Physeal bridge resection. *J Am Acad Orthop Surg.* 2005;13:47–58.
99. Kim JR, Song KH, Song KJ, et al. Treatment outcomes of triplane and Tillaux fractures of the ankle in adolescence. *Clin Orthop Surg.* 2010;2:34–38.
100. Kleiger B, Mankin HJ. Fracture of the lateral portion of the distal tibial epiphysis. *J Bone Joint Surg Am.* 1964;46:25–32.
101. Klein DM, Caligiuri DA, Katzman BM. Local-advancement soft-tissue coverage in a child with ipsilateral grade IIIB open tibial and ankle fractures. *J Orthop Trauma.* 1996;10:577–580.
102. Kling TF Jr, Bright RW, Hensinger RN. Distal tibial physeal fractures in children that may require open reduction. *J Bone Joint Surg Am.* 1984;66:647–657.
103. Lange-Hansen N. Fractures of the ankle. II. Combined experimental-surgical and experimental-roetgenologic investigations. *Arch Surg.* 1950:60;957–985.
104. Leary JT, Handling M, Talerico M, et al. Physeal fractures of the distal tibia: predictive factors of premature physeal closure and growth arrest. *J Pediatr Orthop.* 2009;29:356–361.
105. Lehman WL, Jones WW. Intravenous lidocaine for anesthesia in the lower extremity. A prospective study. *J Bone Joint Surg Am.* 1984;66:1056–1060.
106. Leininger RE, Knox CL, Comstock RD. Epidemiology of 1.6 million pediatric soccer-related injuries presenting to US emergency departments from 1990 to 2003. *Am J Sports Med.* 2007;35:288–293.
107. Lerner A, Stein H. Hybrid thin wire external fixation: an effective, minimally invasive, modular surgical tool for the stabilization of periarticular fractures. *Orthopedics.* 2004;27:59–62.
108. Letts RM. The hidden adolescent ankle fracture. *J Pediatr Orthop.* 1982;2:161–164.
109. Letts M, Davidson D, McCaffrey M. The adolescent pilon fracture: management and outcome. *J Pediatr Orthop.* 2001;21:20–26.
110. Letts M, Davidson D, Mukhtar I. Surgical management of chronic lateral ankle instability in adolescents. *J Pediatr Orthop.* 2003;23:392–397.
111. Lintecum N, Blasier RD. Direct reduction with indirect fixation of distal tibial physeal fractures: a report of a technique. *J Pediatr Orthop.* 1996;16:107–112.
112. Loder RT, Brown KL, Zaleske DJ, et al. Extremity lawn-mower injuries in children: report by the Research Committee of the Pediatric Orthopaedic Society of North America. *J Pediatr Orthop.* 1997;17:360–369.
113. Lohman M, Kivisaari A, Vehmas T, et al. MRI in the assessment of growth arrest. *Pediatr Radiol.* 2002;32:41–45.
114. Love SM, Grogan DP, Ogden JA. Lawn-mower injuries in children. *J Orthop Trauma.* 1988;2:94–101.
115. Luhmann SJ, Oda JE, O'Donnell J, et al. An analysis of suboptimal outcomes of medial malleolus fractures in skeletally immature children. *Am J Orthop (Belle Mead NJ).* 2012;41:113–116.
116. Lynn MD. The triplane distal tibial epiphyseal fracture. *Clin Orthop Relat Res.* 1972;86:187–190.
117. Malanga GA, Ramirez-Del Toro JA. Common injuries of the foot and ankle in the child and adolescent athlete. *Phys Med Rehabil Clin N Am.* 2008;19:347–371, ix.
118. Manderson EL, Ollivierre CO. Closed anatomic reduction of a juvenile Tillaux fracture by dorsiflexion of the ankle. A case report. *Clin Orthop Relat Res.* 1992:262–266.

119. Mankovsky AB, Mendoza-Sagaon M, Cardinaux C, et al. Evaluation of scooter-related injuries in children. *J Pediatr Surg.* 2002;37:755–759.

120. Mann DC, Rajmaira S. Distribution of physeal and nonphyseal fractures in 2,650 long-bone fractures in children aged 0–16 years. *J Pediatr Orthop.* 1990;10:713–716.

121. Marmor L. An unusual fracture of the tibial epiphysis. *Clin Orthop Relat Res.* 1970;73:132–135.

122. Mazur JM, Loveless EA, Cummings RJ. Ankle dislocation without fracture in a child. *Am J Orthop (Belle Mead NJ).* 2007;36:E138–E140.

123. Michelson JD, Clarke HJ, Jinnah RH. The effect of loading on tibiotalar alignment in cadaver ankles. *Foot Ankle.* 1990;10:280–284.

124. Miller MD. Arthroscopically assisted reduction and fixation of an adult Tillaux fracture of the ankle. *Arthroscopy.* 1997;13:117–119.

125. Mirmiran R, Schuberth JM. Non union of an epiphyseal fibular fracture in a pediatric patient. *J Foot Ankle Surg.* 2006;45:410–412.

126. Mooney JF, 3rd, DeFranzo A, Marks MW. Use of cross-extremity flaps stabilized with external fixation in severe pediatric foot and ankle trauma: an alternative to free tissue transfer. *J Pediatr Orthop.* 1998;18:26–30.

127. Mubarak SJ. Extensor retinaculum syndrome of the ankle after injury to the distal tibial physis. *J Bone Joint Surg Br.* 2002;84:11–14.

128. Mubarak SJ, Wilton NC. Compartment syndromes and epidural analgesia. *J Pediatr Orthop.* 1997;17:282–284.

129. Munjal K, Kishan S, Sabharwal S. Posttraumatic pediatric distal tibiofibular synostosis: a case report. *Foot Ankle Int.* 2004;25:429–433.

130. Nenopoulos SP, Papavasiliou VA, Papavasiliou AV. Outcome of physeal and epiphyseal injuries of the distal tibia with intra-articular involvement. *J Pediatr Orthop.* 2005;25:518–522.

131. Nguyen D, Letts M. In-line skating injuries in children: a 10-year review. *J Pediatr Orthop.* 2001;21:613–618.

132. Nilsson S, Roaas A. Soccer injuries in adolescents. *Am J Sports Med.* 1978;6:358–361.

133. Nusem I, Ezra E, Wientroub S. Closed posterior dislocation of the ankle without associated fracture in a child. *J Trauma.* 1999;46:350–351.

134. O'Loughlin PF, Heyworth BE, Kennedy JG. Current concepts in the diagnosis and treatment of osteochondral lesions of the ankle. *Am J Sports Med.* 2010;38:392–404.

135. Ogden JA. *Skeletal Injury in the Child.* Philadelphia, PA: Lea & Febiger; 1982.

136. Ogden JA, Lee J. Accessory ossification patterns and injuries of the malleoli. *J Pediatr Orthop.* 1990;10:306–316.

137. Orava S, Saarela J. Exertion injuries to young athletes: a follow-up research of orthopaedic problems of young track and field athletes. *Am J Sports Med.* 1978;6:68–74.

138. Panagopoulos A, van Niekerk L. Arthroscopic assisted reduction and fixation of a juvenile Tillaux fracture. *Knee Surg Sports Traumatol Arthrosc.* 2007;15:415–417.

139. Papadokostakis G, Kontakis G, Giannoudis P, et al. External fixation devices in the treatment of fractures of the tibial plafond: a systematic review of the literature. *J Bone Joint Surg Br.* 2008;90:1–6.

140. Pesl T, Havranek P. Rare injuries to the distal tibiofibular joint in children. *Eur J Pediatr Surg.* 2006;16:255–259.

141. Peterson HA. Physeal fractures: Part 3. Classification. *J Pediatr Orthop.* 1994;14:439–448.

142. Peterson CA, Peterson HA. Analysis of the incidence of injuries to the epiphyseal growth plate. *J Trauma.* 1972;12:275–281.

143. Peterson HA, Madhok R, Benson JT, et al. Physeal fractures: Part 1. Epidemiology in Olmsted County, Minnesota, 1979–1988. *J Pediatr Orthop.* 1994;14:423–430.

144. Petit P, Panuel M, Faure F, et al. Acute fracture of the distal tibial physis: role of gradient-echo MR imaging versus plain film examination. *AJR Am J Roentgenol.* 1996;166:1203–1206.

145. Petit P, Sapin C, Henry G, et al. Rate of abnormal osteoarticular radiographic findings in pediatric patients. *AJR Am J Roentgenol.* 2001;176:987–990.

146. Petratos DV, Kokkinakis M, Ballas EG, et al. Prognostic factors for premature growth plate arrest as a complication of the surgical treatment of fractures of the medial malleolus in children. *Bone Joint J.* 2013;95-B:419–423.

146a. Phan VC, Wroten E, Yngve D. Foot progression angle after distal tibial physeal fractures. *J Pediatr Orthop.* 2002;22(1):31–35.

147. Phieffer LS, Meyer RA Jr, Gruber HE, et al. Effect of interposed periosteum in an animal physeal fracture model. *Clin Orthop Relat Res.* 2000;376:15–25.

148. Pollen AG. Fractures involving the epiphyseal plate. *Reconstr Surg Traumatol.* 1979;17:25–39.

149. Raikin SM, Ching AC. Bioabsorbable fixation in foot and ankle. *Foot Ankle Clin.* 2005;10:667–684, ix.

150. Ramsey PL, Hamilton W. Changes in tibiotalar area of contact caused by lateral talar shift. *J Bone Joint Surg Am.* 1976;58:356–357.

151. Rapariz JM, Ocete G, Gonzalez-Herranz P, et al. Distal tibial triplane fractures: long-term follow-up. *J Pediatr Orthop.* 1996;16:113–118.

152. Reff RB. The use of external fixation devices in the management of severe lower-extremity trauma and pelvic injuries in children. *Clin Orthop Relat Res.* 1984;188:21–33.

153. Rinker B, Amspacher JC, Wilson PC, et al. Subatmospheric pressure dressing as a bridge to free tissue transfer in the treatment of open tibia fractures. *Plast Reconstr Surg.* 2008;121:1664–1673.

154. Ristiniemi J. External fixation of tibial pilon fractures and fracture healing. *Acta Orthop Suppl.* 2007;78(3):5–34.

155. Rogers LF. The radiography of epiphyseal injuries. *Radiology.* 1970;96:289–299.

156. Rohmiller MT, Gaynor TP, Pawelek J, et al. Salter-Harris I and II fractures of the distal tibia: does mechanism of injury relate to premature physeal closure? *J Pediatr Orthop.* 2006;26:322–328.

157. Rokkanen P, Bostman O, Vainionpaa S, et al. Absorbable devices in the fixation of fractures. *J Trauma.* 1996;40:S123–S127.

158. Rosenbaum AJ, DiPreta JA, Uhl RL. Review of distal tibial epiphyseal transitional fractures. *Orthopedics.* 2012;35:1046–1049.

159. Roser LA, Clawson DK. Football injuries in the very young athlete. *Clin Orthop Relat Res.* 1970;69:219–223.

160. Ross PM, Schwentker EP, Bryan H. Mutilating lawn mower injuries in children. *JAMA.* 1976;236:480–481.

161. Rougraff BT, Kernek CB. Lawn mower injury resulting in Chopart amputation in a young child. *Orthopedics.* 1996;19:689–691.

162. Sabharwal S, Schwechter EM. Five-year followup of ankle joint distraction for post-traumatic chondrolysis in an adolescent: a case report. *Foot Ankle Int.* 2007;28:942–948.

163. Sailhan F, Chotel F, Guibal AL, et al. Three-dimensional MR imaging in the assessment of physeal growth arrest. *Eur Radiol.* 2004;14:1600–1608.

164. Sankar WN, Chen J, Kay R, et al. Incidence of occult fracture in children with acute ankle injuries. *J Pediatr Orthop.* 2008;28:500–501.

165. Scheffer MM, Peterson HA. Opening-wedge osteotomy for angular deformities of long bones in children. *J Bone Joint Surg Am.* 1994;76:325–334.

166. Schenck RC Jr, Goodnight JM. Osteochondritis dissecans. *J Bone Joint Surg Am.* 1996;78:439–456.

167. Schlesinger I, Wedge JH. Percutaneous reduction and fixation of displaced juvenile Tillaux fractures: a new surgical technique. *J Pediatr Orthop.* 1993;13:389–391.

168. Schnetzler KA, Hoernschemeyer D. The pediatric triplane ankle fracture. *J Am Acad Orthop Surg.* 2007;15:738–747.

169. Schurz M, Binder H, Platzer P, et al. Physeal injuries of the distal tibia: long-term results in 376 patients. *Int Orthop.* 2010;34:547–552.

170. Shankar A, Williams K, Ryan M. Trampoline-related injury in children. *Pediatr Emerg Care.* 2006;22:644–646.

171. Shin AY, Moran ME, Wenger DR. Intramalleolar triplane fractures of the distal tibial epiphysis. *J Pediatr Orthop.* 1997;17:352–355.

172. Siapkara A, Nordin L, Hill RA. Spatial frame correction of anterior growth arrest of the proximal tibia: report of three cases. *J Pediatr Orthop B.* 2008;17:61–64.

173. Siffert RS, Arkin AM. Post-traumatic aseptic necrosis of the distal tibial epiphysis; report of a case. *J Bone Joint Surg Am.* 1950;32-A:691–694.

174. Simanovsky N, Lamdan R, Hiller N, et al. Sonographic detection of radiographically occult fractures in pediatric ankle and wrist injuries. *J Pediatr Orthop.* 2009;29:142–145.

175. Singleton TJ, Cobb M. High fibular fracture in association with triplane fracture: reexamining this unique pediatric fracture pattern. *J Foot Ankle Surg.* 2010;49:491–494.

176. Sinisaari IP, Luthje PM, Mikkonen RH. Ruptured tibio-fibular syndesmosis: comparison study of metallic to bioabsorbable fixation. *Foot Ankle Int.* 2002;23:744–748.

177. Smith BG, Rand F, Jaramillo D, et al. Early MR imaging of lower-extremity physeal fracture-separations: a preliminary report. *J Pediatr Orthop.* 1994;14:526–533.

178. Spiegel PG, Cooperman DR, Laros GS. Epiphyseal fractures of the distal ends of the tibia and fibula. A retrospective study of two hundred and thirty-seven cases in children. *J Bone Joint Surg Am.* 1978;60:1046–1050.

179. Steinlauf SD, Stricker SJ, Hulen CA. Juvenile Tillaux fracture simulating syndesmosis separation: a case report. *Foot Ankle Int.* 1998;19:332–335.

180. Stevens PM, Kennedy JM, Hung M. Guided growth for ankle valgus. *J Pediatr Orthop.* 2011;31:878–883.

181. Stiell IG, Greenberg GH, McKnight RD, et al. A study to develop clinical decision rules for the use of radiography in acute ankle injuries. *Ann Emerg Med.* 1992;21:384–390.

182. Sullivan JA, Gross RH, Grana WA, et al. Evaluation of injuries in youth soccer. *Am J Sports Med.* 1980;8:325–327.

183. Tachdjian MO. *The Child's Foot.* Philadelphia, PA: WB Saunders; 1985.

184. Takakura Y, Takaoka T, Tanaka Y, et al. Results of opening-wedge osteotomy for the treatment of a post-traumatic varus deformity of the ankle. *J Bone Joint Surg Am.* 1998;80:213–218.

185. Tarkin IS, Clare MP, Marcantonio A, et al. An update on the management of high-energy pilon fractures. *Injury.* 2008;39:142–154.

186. Tarr RR, Resnick CT, Wagner KS, et al. Changes in tibiotalar joint contact areas following experimentally induced tibial angular deformities. *Clin Orthop Relat Res.* 1985;199:72–80.

187. Thomsen NO, Overgaard S, Olsen LH, et al. Observer variation in the radiographic classification of ankle fractures. *J Bone Joint Surg Br.* 1991;73:676–678.

188. Ting AJ, Tarr RR, Sarmiento A, et al. The role of subtalar motion and ankle contact pressure changes from angular deformities of the tibia. *Foot Ankle.* 1987;7:290–299.

189. Vahvanen V, Aalto K. Classification of ankle fractures in children. *Arch Orthop Trauma Surg.* 1980;97:1–5.

189a. Vahvanen V, Westerlund M, Nikku R. Lateral ligament injury of the ankle in children. Follow-up results of primary surgical treatment. *Acta Orthop Scand.* 1984;55(1):21–25.

190. Vangsness CT Jr, Carter V, Hunt T, et al. Radiographic diagnosis of ankle fractures: are three views necessary? *Foot Ankle Int.* 1994;15:172–174.

191. von Laer L. Classification, diagnosis, and treatment of transitional fractures of the distal part of the tibia. *J Bone Joint Surg Am.* 1985;67:687–698.

192. Vosburgh CL, Gruel CR, Herndon WA, et al. Lawn mower injuries of the pediatric foot and ankle: observations on prevention and management. *J Pediatr Orthop.* 1995;15:504–509.

193. Wattenbarger JM, Gruber HE, Phieffer LS. Physeal fractures, part I: histologic features of bone, cartilage, and bar formation in a small animal model. *J Pediatr Orthop.* 2002;22:703–709.

194. Whipple TL, Martin DR, McIntyre LF, et al. Arthroscopic treatment of triplane fractures of the ankle. *Arthroscopy.* 1993;9:456–463.

195. Wilder RT, Berde CB, Wolohan M, et al. Reflex sympathetic dystrophy in children. Clinical characteristics and follow-up of seventy patients. *J Bone Joint Surg Am.* 1992;74:910–919.

196. Wuerz TH, Gurd DP. Pediatric physeal ankle fracture. *J Am Acad Orthop Surg.* 2013;21:234–244.

197. Zaricznyj B, Shattuck LJ, Mast TA, et al. Sports-related injuries in school-aged children. *Am J Sports Med.* 1980;8:318–324.

198. Zonfrillo MR, Seiden JA, House EM, et al. The association of overweight and ankle injuries in children. *Ambul Pediatr.* 2008;8:66–69.

30

Fractures, Dislocations, and Other Injuries of the Foot

Amy L. McIntosh and Haemish Crawford

Fractures and Dislocations of the Foot

INTRODUCTION TO FRACTURES AND DISLOCATIONS OF THE FOOT

Trauma to the pediatric foot has been traditionally treated non-operatively by orthopedic surgeons.[16,141] The dogma existed that the bones of the foot were predominantly cartilaginous and would remodel as the child matures. Few, if any, long-term studies exist to measure the outcomes of these treatments.

Children are now involved in sports and activities of greater physical intensity that leads to more complex fractures and dislocations.[4,40,44,136] It is not uncommon for young children to be competing in motocross, extreme skiing, go-karting, and rock climbing.[4,165] Professional sport has brought about more intense training and greater expectations from the child, the parent, and the coach. Physicians may feel pressure that injuries need to be treated "quicker" and rehabilitation time decreased. These expectations should not get in the way of treating the child's foot injury in the best possible way.

As the child grows into a young adult, the largely cartilaginous foot becomes ossified and fracture and dislocation patterns change. Ogden[126] showed that the cartilaginous bones were elastic, absorbing, and dissipating the energy from the trauma differently than the adult foot, which resulted in different fracture patterns. The management algorithms for the adolescent foot are therefore quite different from the infant's foot; however, the exact age at which this occurs needs to be individualized for each patient. The amount of fracture angulation and joint line displacement to accept is one of the real challenges in treating the skeletally immature foot. Some complex fractures of the talus and calcaneus in adolescents are in fact best internally fixed according to the principles used to treat adult trauma.

An in-depth knowledge of the anatomy of the growing foot is helpful as the variable ossification centers, apophyses, and physes make fracture recognition difficult. Most of the papers quoted in this chapter are level IV (uncontrolled case series) or level V (expert consensus). One of the problems with pediatric foot and ankle research is that long follow-up intervals are necessary to validate treatments. There are no pediatric outcome scores for children's foot trauma, so prediction of outcome is dependent on orthopedic first principles of anatomic reduction, union, and effective rehabilitation. Long-term retrospective studies also have the difficulty of locating children treated decades earlier and, therefore, the follow-up rate is low.

ANATOMY OF THE GROWING FOOT

The child's foot is different from the adult foot in that the bones are largely cartilaginous until adolescence. Although the mechanisms of injury are similar, the resulting fracture is usually less severe in the child as the energy of the injury is dissipated by the elasticity of the cartilage. The cartilage also makes interpretation of imaging more difficult and fractures may not be appreciated on plain radiograph. Computed tomography (CT) and magnetic resonance imaging (MRI) scans assist in clarification of anatomy and identification of fractures. The remodeling potential of cartilage allows some displacement and angulation of fractures to be accepted in children, whereas in adults it may be unacceptable.

Secondary areas of ossification, accessory bones, and growth plates also make fracture recognition more difficult. The appearance of the ossification centers are summarized in Figure 30-1.[5] The calcaneus and talus are usually ossified at birth and the cuboid ossification center usually becomes evident shortly after.[157] The navicular does not develop its primary ossification center until the child is around 3 years of age. Figure 30-2 shows the accessory ossicles and sesamoid bones in the foot which can also be confused with fractures especially if they are bipartite or if the accessory bones are closely adhered. It is useful clinically to radiograph the opposite foot if any doubt exists as to what may be normal or pathologic.

MECHANISMS OF INJURY AND ASSESSMENT OF FRACTURES AND DISLOCATIONS OF THE FOOT

The history provided by the patient is not always accurate in childhood trauma. Often, other children or adults who

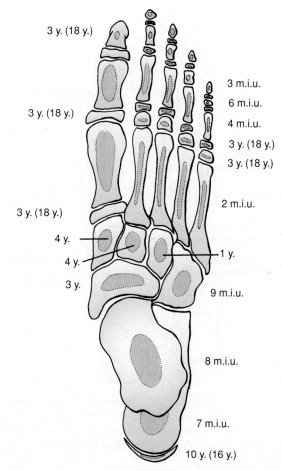

Figure 30-1. Appearance and fusion times of foot ossification centers, with figures in parentheses indicating the time of fusion of the primary and secondary ossification centers (y., years; m.i.u., months in utero). (From Aitken JT, Joseph J, Causey G, et al. *A Manual of Human Anatomy.* 2nd ed. London: E & S Livingstone; 1966:80, with permission.)

witnessed the accident can give a more accurate account than the patient. The degree of force, the speed and height of the fall, and the way the foot is twisted all help predict the degree of displacement or severity of the injury. Additionally, the ability to weight bear, degree of instability, and the location of the pain are important to ascertain.

Careful examination of the foot often will guide the surgeon to the site of injury. The child frequently complains of the whole foot "hurting"; however, systematic palpation helps localize the most painful site. Appropriate radiographs can then be obtained. Bruising and swelling will also help predict the injury pattern. Isolated bruising on the sole of the midfoot often overlies a subtle Lisfranc injury whereas excessive dorsal swelling may predict a more severe fracture–dislocation.[145] In a crush injury, the possibility of increased compartment pressures should be considered.

Multiple injuries must also be ruled out via a complete secondary survey. For example, bilateral calcaneus fractures following a fall may be associated with a tibial fracture or spinal column injury.

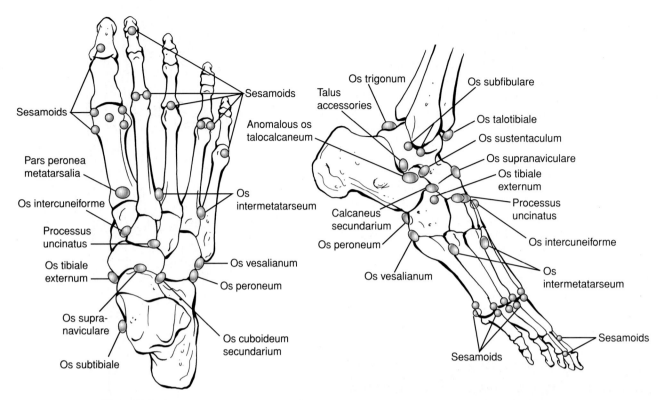

Figure 30-2. Diagrammatic representation of accessory ossicles and sesamoid bones about the foot and ankle. Note that the sesamoid bones can be bipartite and that accessory ossicles can be multicentric. (From Traughber PD. Imaging of the foot and ankle. In: Coughlin MJ, Mann RA. *Surgery of the Foot and Ankle.* 7th ed. St. Louis, MO: Mosby; 1999.)

Talar Fractures

INTRODUCTION TO TALAR FRACTURES

Fractures of the talus are very rare in children and adolescents.[37,124] Talus fractures most commonly occur through the neck and occasionally the body. Although rare, talus fractures are important to recognize because of the possible complication of avascular necrosis (AVN), which can occur because of the precarious blood supply. The majority of talus fractures in children can be treated with cast immobilization whereas displaced fractures in adolescents need to be treated operatively similar to an adult fracture.

ASSESSMENT OF TALAR FRACTURES

MECHANISMS OF INJURY FOR TALAR FRACTURES

A fall from a height is a common mechanism of injury causing talar fractures.[79,98,111,167] The foot is forcibly dorsiflexed and the neck of the talus impinges against the anterior lip of the distal tibia. This shear force usually results in a vertical or slightly

oblique fracture line at the junction of the body and neck of the talus. When dorsiflexion is combined with supination of the foot, impingement occurs more medially and the medial malleolus may be fractured as well. With displaced fractures, the subtalar joint may become subluxed. The talus can also be fractured with crushing injuries, and open fractures are well described in lawnmower accidents.[124] Fractures of the lateral process of the talus have been described recently in snowboarding accidents where the mechanism appears to be forced dorsiflexion and inversion of the ankle.[95]

INJURIES ASSOCIATED WITH TALAR FRACTURES

The force required to fracture a child's talus is almost twice that required to fracture the other ankle and tarsal bones.[131] Therefore, other injuries often coexist with talus fractures. A number of studies have found fractures of the calcaneus, malleoli, tibia, and lumbar spine in the presence of a talus fracture.[20,26,65,127,128] Hawkins,[65] in his study of adult talus fractures, found 64% of the patients had an associated musculoskeletal injury.

SIGNS AND SYMPTOMS OF TALAR FRACTURES

Other foot fractures and dislocations can present similarly to talus fractures. The ankle and foot are swollen and the foot is usually held plantarflexed. Because of this soft tissue swelling, the foot needs to be examined closely for increased compartment pressure. As with all fractures, the soft tissues need to be inspected for any puncture wounds, abrasions, or fracture blisters as these are important in determining the management of the patient.

There may be less swelling so careful palpation around the talus is needed to detect the source of the pain. Once the foot has been clinically assessed, the appropriate radiographic investigations can be performed.

IMAGING AND OTHER DIAGNOSTIC STUDIES FOR TALAR FRACTURES

The routine radiographs for a fractured talus include an anteroposterior (AP), lateral, and oblique views. Canale and Kelly[26] have described a pronated oblique view of the talus which may demonstrate the fracture more clearly. The fractures are not always easy to see in young children, as the talus is largely cartilaginous until the second decade.[111] The cartilage anlage often leads to an underestimation of fracture displacement. Some authors have even suggested the use of MRI to show the morphology better in children less than 10 years old.[124,174]

Once the fracture is identified, a CT scan can be useful in assessing the fracture plane, comminution, degree of displacement, and any other associated foot or ankle fractures. This study is particularly useful when pain prohibits the full range of radiographs mentioned above to be taken. If an open reduction is planned, the CT scan will also aid in the preoperative planning.

CLASSIFICATION OF TALAR FRACTURES

Fractures of the talus can be classified as occurring either in the body or the neck. Some authors suggest classifying talar fractures

based on the age of the patient as children less than 6 years of age generally have a better prognosis.[111] Hawkins[65] described an x-ray classification to define the different types of fractures of the talar neck and used it to predict the risk of AVN (Fig. 30-3).

Hawkins Classification Talar Fractures	
Type	**Description**
I	• Undisplaced talar neck fracture
II	• Displaced talar neck fracture with subtalar subluxation or dislocation
III	• Displaced fracture of the talar neck with dislocation of both the subtalar and ankle joints

FRACTURES OF THE TALAR NECK

Most talar fractures in children are of the talar neck. The Hawkins classification (see Fig. 30-3) was developed so it could be used to predict if the talus would become avascular because of the disruption of the tenuous blood supply. Canale and Kelly[26] later modified the classification (see Fig. 30-3) to include a type IV injury in which there is subluxation or dislocation of the ankle, subtalar, and talonavicular joints. In the adult literature, the majority of talar fractures are types II and III.[26,65] This classification has been used to help predict the type of treatment required and the outcome one can expect (Table 30-1).

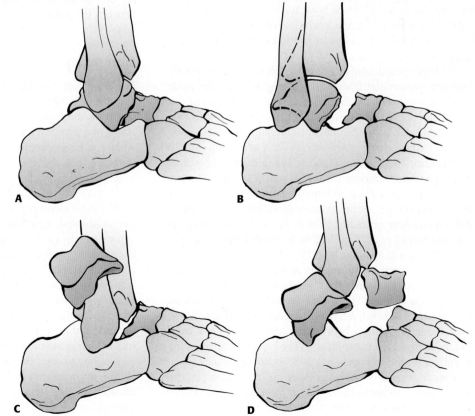

Figure 30-3. Hawkins classification of talar neck fractures (see text for details). **A:** Type I, nondisplaced fracture of the talar neck. **B:** Type II, displaced talar neck fracture with subluxation or dislocation of the subtalar joint. **C:** Type III, displaced talar neck fracture with associated dislocation of the talar body from both the subtalar and tibiotalar joints. **D:** Type IV, as suggested by Canale and Kelly, displaced talar neck fracture with an associated dislocation of the talar body from subtalar and tibiotalar joints and dislocation of the head and neck fragment from the talonavicular joint. (Reprinted with permission from Canale ST, Kelly FB Jr. Fractures of the neck of the talus: Long-term evaluation of seventy-one cases. *J Bone Joint Surg Am.* 1978;60(2):143–156.)

TABLE 30-1. Hawkins Classification of Talar Neck Fractures

Type	Description	Treatment	Affect on Blood Supply[a]	Osteonecrosis Rate (%)
Type I	Stable, undisplaced vertical fracture through talar neck.	8 weeks in cast, 4 weeks in CAM cast.	Theoretical damage to only one vessel entering talar neck.	0–10
Type II	Displaced fracture with subtalar joint subluxation or dislocation; normal ankle joint.	Immediate closed reduction.[b] A near anatomic reduction delays surgical treatment.	Two of three blood supply vessels lost: Neck vessel and one entering the tarsal canal.	20–50
Type III	Same as type II but with subluxation or dislocation of both the ankle and subtalar joint.	Direct to operating room for combined anteromedial and anterolateral surgical approach (see text).	All three sources of blood affected.	80–100
Type IV	Very rare; basically a type III with talonavicular joint displacement.	Same as type III.	Not related to blood supply.	100

CAM, controlled active motion.

[a]See text for further details of blood supply to the talus.

[b]Reduction maneuver: Maximal plantarflexion and foot traction to realign head and body in sagittal plane. Varus/valgus with or without supination/pronation stress realigns neck in coronal plane.

PATHOANATOMY AND APPLIED ANATOMY RELATED TO TALAR NECK FRACTURES

The talus is composed of three parts: the body, neck, and head. Ossification starts from one center that appears in the sixth intrauterine month. The talus ossification process starts in the head and neck and proceeds in a retrograde direction toward the subchondral bone of the body. Approximately two-thirds of the talar body is articular cartilage with just a small area of bare bone on the neck where the bone receives its nutrient blood supply. There are no tendon insertions into the talus. The stability is provided by the capsular and ligamentous attachments to the surrounding bones.

The superior articular surface of the talus is wider anteriorly than it is posteriorly. Traditional teaching suggests the ankle should generally be immobilized in neutral dorsiflexion so this widest part of the talus is engaged in the ankle mortise to help prevent an equinus contracture. This technique is of less importance in younger children who are less likely to develop equinus contractures. The lateral wall of the superior articular surface curves posteriorly whereas the medial wall is straight. The two walls converge posteriorly to form the posterior tubercle of the talus. Often, there is a separate ossification center (os trigonum) that appears here on radiographs at 11 to 13 years of age in boys and 8 to 10 years of age in girls. It usually fuses to the talus 1 year after it appears (Fig. 30-4).[113]

The short neck of the talus is medially deviated approximately 10 to 44 degrees and plantarflexed between 5 and 50 degrees in relation to the axis of the body.[56] Beneath the talar neck is the tarsal canal, a funnel-shaped area that contains the anastomotic ring formed between the artery of the tarsal canal and the artery of the tarsal sinus.[118] The broad interosseous ligament joining the calcaneus and talus is also within the canal.

The tarsal canal is conical in shape and runs from posteromedial (apex) to anterolateral where the base of the cone is known as the sinus tarsi (Fig. 30-5).

The lateral process of the talus is a large wedge-shaped process that is covered in articular cartilage. It articulates with the fibula superiorly and laterally and with the subtalar joint inferiorly. The lateral talocalcaneal ligament is attached to the most distal part of the process.[64,66]

The head of the talus is entirely cartilaginous, convex, and articulates with the concave surface of the navicular. The undersurface of the talus is comprised of three articulating surfaces for the calcaneus: the posterior, middle, and anterior facet. Between the posterior and middle facets is a transverse groove which forms the roof of the tarsal canal.

Blood Supply

The blood supply of the talus has been extensively studied.[9,62,118] The nutrient arteries are derived from the three major vessels that cross the ankle joint: posterior tibial artery, anterior tibial artery, and peroneal artery (Fig. 30-6). Branches of these three vessels perforate circumferentially the short talar neck, which is the only part of the talus denude of articular cartilage. A fracture in this area can disrupt this intricate anastomosis of vessels and leads to AVN of the body of the talus.

The main blood supply to the talus is through the artery of the tarsal canal, which branches off the posterior tibial artery approximately 1 cm proximal to the origin of the medial and lateral plantar arteries. It passes between flexor digitorum longus and flexor hallucis longus before entering the tarsal canal where it anastomoses with the artery of the tarsal sinus. Before entering the canal, the artery of the tarsal canal gives off a deltoid branch that penetrates the deltoid ligament and supplies the medial third of the talar body.[57] A dorsal vessel of the deltoid branch anastomoses with the medial branch of the dorsalis pedis artery to enter the talar neck.

The second source of blood supply is from the anterior tibial artery and its terminal extension, the dorsalis pedis artery. Multiple vessels from these arteries penetrate the dorsal neck of

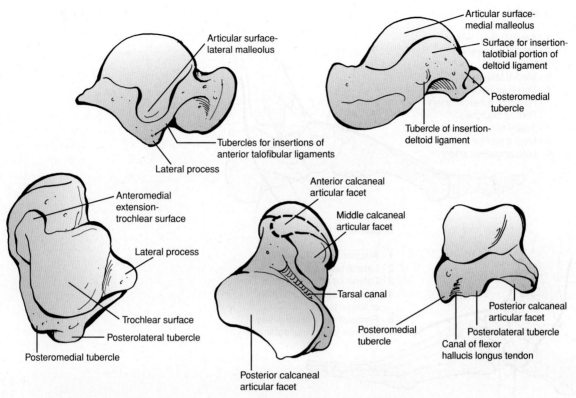

Figure 30-4. Anatomic details of the talus are important when correlating high-definition imaging, such as CT scans, with normal anatomy for the purposes of fracture management decision making.

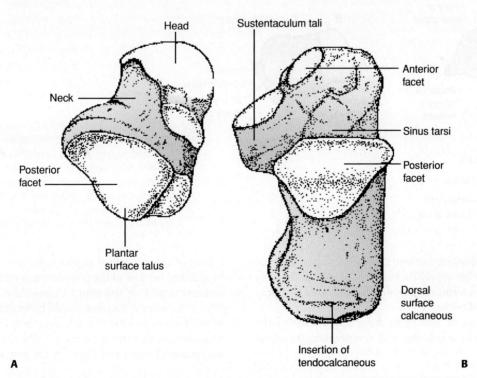

Figure 30-5. Subtalar joint opened such that the medial borders of the joint face each other. **A:** Plantar surface of the talus, which articulates with the dorsal surface of the calcaneus. Note the extensive area of the talus that is articular cartilage. **B:** Dorsal surface of the calcaneus with the articular facets occupying the anterior half of the calcaneus. (Reprinted with permission from Sammarco GJ. Anatomy. In: Helal B, Rowley D, Cracchiolo AC, et al., eds. *Surgery of Disorders of the Foot and Ankle.* 1st ed. Philadelphia, PA: Lippincott-Raven; 1996.)

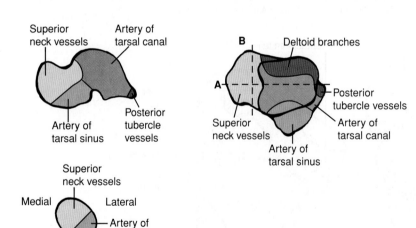

A. Medial

1 - Anterior tibial artery
2 - Medial recurrent
tarsal artery
3 - Medial talar artery
4 - Posterior tibial artery
5 - Posterior tubercle artery
6 - Deltoid branches
7 - Artery of tarsal canal
8 - Medial plantar artery
9 - Lateral plantar artery

B. Lateral

1 - Anterior tibial artery
2 - Lateral talar artery
3 - Lateral tarsal artery
4 - Posterior recurrent branch
of lateral tarsal
6 - Perforating peroneal artery
7 - Anterior lateral malleolar artery

Superior neck vessels
Artery of tarsal canal
Artery of tarsal sinus
Posterior tubercle vessels

Deltoid branches
Superior neck vessels
Posterior tubercle vessels
Artery of tarsal canal
Artery of tarsal sinus

Superior neck vessels
Medial   Lateral
Artery of tarsal sinus

Figure 30-6. Arterial blood supply to the talus. Medial blood supply (**A**) and lateral blood supply (**B**). Dorsal view with sagittal cut through length (*a*) of talus and transverse cut through neck of talus (*b*). (Reprinted by permission from Gelberman RH, Mortensen WW. The arterial anatomy of the talus. *Foot Ankle.* 1983;4(2): 64–72. Copyright © 1983 SAGE Publications.)

the talus. The third source of blood supply is from the peroneal artery. Small branches supply the posterior process of the talus and a larger branch forms the artery of the sinus tarsi to supply the lateral aspect of the talus.

Within the capsular and ligamentous attachments to the talus there are small vessels that also contribute to the blood supply.[130]

TREATMENT OPTIONS FOR FRACTURES OF THE TALAR NECK

The treatment of talar fractures is based on the severity of the fracture and the age of the child. The Hawkins classification system is useful in directing the treatment. In a child less than

8 years of age, a less than perfect reduction of the fracture can be accepted because of the remodeling potential,[79,98,111] and the outcome in patients less than 12 years old is favorable in most cases.[48] Adolescent fractures should be treated the same way as an adult injury. In a recent series, complications following pediatric talus fracture treatment were correlated with high-energy mechanism of injury and displacement requiring reduction.[167]

Nonoperative Treatment

Hawkins Type I Fractures

Undisplaced fractures of the talar neck can be treated for 6 to 8 weeks of nonweight bearing in a below-knee cast. The child can then start taking full weight if the fracture has healed radiographically. Canale and Kelly[26] accepted 5 mm of displacement and 5 degrees of angulation of the talar neck in their series.

Hawkins Type II Fractures

A displaced or severely angulated talar neck fracture usually presents with significant soft tissue swelling and pain. This makes management more difficult than type I injuries. Achieving adequate radiographs to assess the degree of displacement is difficult without sedation. The distal fragment of the neck is usually displaced dorsally and medially.

The fracture and subluxation of the subtalar joint should be reduced under general anesthesia, most often by gentle plantarflexion and pronation of the foot. If a stable reduction is achieved, a well-molded below-knee cast can be applied with the foot in plantarflexion. This initial cast is changed to a more neutral position at 4 weeks and then removed 8 weeks following fracture reduction. Postoperative serial radiographs or a CT scan should be performed as the fracture position may be lost when the soft tissue swelling subsides. If the fracture is unstable after reduction, percutaneous Kirschner wire (K-wire) fixation is useful to hold the fracture. Two K-wires can be passed through a small dorsomedial incision and across the fracture. The incision should be on the medial side of extensor hallucis longus to avoid damage to the tibial vessels. Although the amount of residual displacement or angulation acceptable is not clearly defined, it may be better to accept a few millimeters of offset and up to 10 degrees of angulation rather than perform an open reduction and risk devascularizing the talus further.

Hawkins Type III Fractures

These fractures are a result of a serious injury and require urgent surgery to openly reduce and internally fix the talus.

Operative Treatment of Talar Fractures

Surgical Approaches

There are three surgical approaches to the fractured talar neck: posterolateral, anteromedial, and anterolateral. The decision on the approach depends on the condition of the soft tissues and the familiarity of the approach by the surgeon. Occasionally, more than one approach is required if adequate reduction cannot be achieved. It is preferable to use the posterolateral approach as this causes less potential disruption to the blood supply; however, direct visualization of the talar neck is not possible. The timing of the open reduction of these fractures is somewhat controversial. With such a tenuous blood supply, one would think that urgent reduction and internal fixation is indicated. Lindvall et al.[104] compared the results of surgery within 6 hours to delayed surgery in 26 fractures of the talus in adult patients and found no significant difference in outcome. One can conclude, that the severity of the injury, the quality of the reduction, and the surgical outcomes had a bigger influence on long-term outcome than if the surgery was fixed emergently or delayed (greater than 12 hours).

Posterolateral Approach

This approach is commonly used to internally fixate fractures of the talar neck once it has been reduced. The patient is positioned supine so the other approaches can be utilized if necessary. The incision is made just lateral to the Achilles tendon. Blunt dissection is then carried out down to the joint capsule avoiding damage to the sural nerve. The posterior joint capsule can then be opened if not already torn by the injury and the posterior process of the talus can be identified. If possible, two partially threaded cannulated 4.5- or 6.5-mm screws can be used to provide compression across the fracture. It is preferable to use titanium screws which are MRI compatible to allow investigation of AVN during fracture healing if necessary. If only one screw is used, a separate K-wire should also be passed across the fracture for rotational stability. These posterior screws are more stable biomechanically than anterior screws (Fig. 30-7).[167]

Anteromedial Approach

This approach is useful to visualize the talar neck and directly reduce the fracture. Often, there is comminution of the medial wall of the neck which makes restoring length difficult. With the patient supine, the incision is made from just anterior to the medial malleolus and directly distally down the midfoot. Deeper dissection is carried out medial to the tibialis anterior and the extensor hallucis longus tendons. The dissection down to the capsule is in the interval between the tibialis anterior and tibialis posterior tendons. This approach avoids damage to the deltoid branch of the posterior tibial artery and the medial

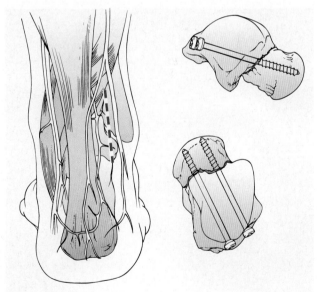

Figure 30-7. Posterolateral approach to the talus. Incision is based lateral to the Achilles tendon. The Achilles tendon and flexor hallucis longus are reflected medially. The posterolateral talar tubercle is the starting point for the guide pin. **Right:** Screws are directed in line with the long axis of the neck of the talus in a plantar-medial direction such that the distal threads of the screw are all in the distal fragment (talar head), beyond the fracture line to allow for compression. Combinations of two screws or one screw and one smooth pin are determined by size and anatomy. (From Adelaar RS. Complex fractures of the talus. *Instr Course Lect.* 1997;46:323–338, with permission.)

branches of the anterior tibial artery. This approach is potentially less harmful to the blood supply of the talus when compared to the anterolateral approach.[3]

Anterolateral Approach

One advantage of this approach is that it permits excellent exposure of the lateral talar neck, which is not usually comminuted allowing anatomic reduction. The approach also gives good access to the subtalar joint. The disadvantage to this approach is that it may disrupt the blood supply more than the other approaches. The incision starts at the tip of the lateral malleolus and extends to the base of the fourth metatarsal. Care must be taken to avoid damaging the sural nerve with deeper dissection. In the base of the incision is the artery of the sinus tarsi which should be visualized if possible.

Following open reduction and internal fixation (ORIF) of talar neck fractures, the foot is placed in a non–weight-bearing below-knee cast for 6 to 8 weeks. Radiographs are then taken to assess fracture healing and the presence or absence of the Hawkins sign. If the subchondral lucent line is present, one can assume there is adequate blood supply to the body of the talus and osteonecrosis is unlikely to occur. If the fracture has also healed, the child can start progressive weight bearing as tolerated. The absence of a subchondral lucency during healing should alert the surgeon to the possible development of osteonecrosis (Fig. 30-8). The patient should continue to be nonweight bearing until the lucency is present. If it is still not present 3 months postinjury, an MRI scan should be performed

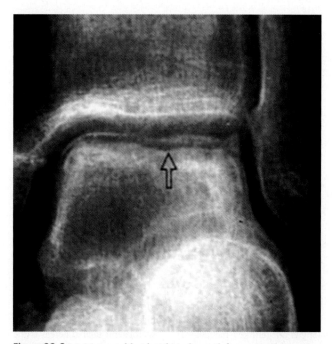

Figure 30-8. A 14-year-old girl with a talar neck fracture and a positive Hawkins sign (*arrow*). Disuse osteoporosis leads to halo-like image of the talus on the AP view denoting adequate talar dome vascularization; if there had been no blood supply, there would be no blood flow to loose calcium. If this happens, the dome of the talus would become denser and more radio-opaque than the surrounding bones that are undergoing diffuse osteoporosis.

which will assess the vascularity more accurately.[67] The use of titanium screws in the open reduction makes this possible. The decision on the amount of weight bearing in the presence of altered blood supply to the talus is not clear. AVN of the talus often takes 18 months to 2 years to revascularize so it would be impractical, if not impossible, to keep a child nonweight bearing for this period in the hope it will prevent premature collapse of the body.

FRACTURES OF THE TALAR BODY AND DOME

Fractures of the talar body are less common than of the neck, representing 29% and 45% of talus pediatric talus fractures in two recent series.[79,167] In 1977, Sneppen et al.[168] described a classification system based on the anatomic position of the fracture in the talus. This was later modified by DeLee[42] and the result is a five-part classification.

Sneppen Classification System of Talar Body Fractures	
Grade	**Fracture Type**
1	• Transchondral/osteochondral
2	• Coronal, sagittal, or horizontal shear
3	• Posterior tubercle
4	• Lateral process
5	• Crush fracture

Undisplaced fractures can be treated in a non–weight-bearing below-knee cast for 6 to 8 weeks until the fracture is healed and the outcome is excellent. Undisplaced intra-articular fractures can be treated in the same way; however, serial radiographs must be taken to confirm displacement does not occur. Anatomic reduction of displaced fractures has been recommended because residual displacement of the articular surfaces leads to degenerative osteoarthritis.[97]

FRACTURES OF THE LATERAL PROCESS OF THE TALAR BODY

Fractures of the lateral process of the talus are uncommon in adults and children, and a high level of suspicion is required if the diagnosis is to be made. The lateral process is a wedge-shaped prominence that forms almost the whole lateral wall of the talus. The mechanism of injury is a forced dorsiflexion injury with inversion of the foot.[64] The talocalcaneal ligament may avulse the lateral process.

Isolated fractures of the lateral process of the talus are often not recognized on the initial radiographs.[64,66,112] Wu et al.[189] found that 42% of fractures were missed initially in their series of lateral process fractures. The lateral process is best visualized

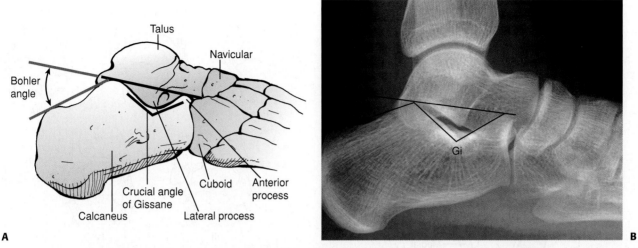

Figure 30-9. Diagrammatic (**A**) and radiographic (**B**) depictions of the crucial angle of Gissane (Gi) and the Bohler (Bo) angles. The Bohler angle is more frequently used for decision making regarding fracture management. For measuring the Bohler angle, the landmarks on the lateral radiograph of the calcaneus are the anterior and posterior facets and the superior margin of the calcaneal tuberosity.

on the mortise view so the fibula is not overlying it. On the lateral radiograph, the lateral process is seen just superior to the angle of Gissane.[66] This is the angle between a line drawn along the lateral border of posterior facet and a line drawn along the anterior process (Fig. 30-9). If there is persistent pain laterally around the ankle following an inversion ankle injury, one should have a high suspicion for a lateral process fracture or an osteochondral injury. If not clearly seen on the plain films, a CT scan should be performed to assess the talus and rule out any other coexisting fractures.[85,123]

The incidence of this rare injury is increasing because of the increased popularity of snowboarding.[85,95,122] Kirkpatrick et al.[87] reviewed 3,213 snowboarding injuries and found an unusually high incidence of lateral process fractures, representing 13.5% of all snowboarding foot and ankle injuries.

The treatment of nondisplaced fractures of the lateral process is with a non–weight-bearing cast for 6 to 8 weeks. Displaced fractures are best treated with ORIF; however, the degree of displacement that is acceptable in a child is not clearly defined. What may be more important is the congruity of the joint surface of the talus. A step or gap in the articular surface of more than 2 to 3 mm may be useful criteria as to when to open reduce the fracture. The fracture can be held with one 3.5-mm partially threaded cancellous screw inserted from lateral to medial perpendicular to the fracture line. A below-knee cast is then worn for 6 weeks.[64,66,95,173]

FRACTURES OF THE OSTEOCHONDRAL SURFACE OF THE TALUS

Damage to the osteochondral surface of the talus can be caused by direct trauma or may be caused by an underlying osteochondral lesion (osteochondritis dissecans [OCD]) that may have been present for some time and has been made symptomatic by

the injury. The pathogenesis and etiology of OCD are controversial; however, most authors report preceding trauma as a cause of the defects (Canale and Bedding[25] 80%, Letts et al.[99] 79%, Higuera et al.[70] 63%, and Perumal et al.[131] 47%). Medial lesions are usually deeper and cup shaped compared to the thinner "wafer" type lateral lesions. Lateral lesions are more often associated with trauma and more symptomatic than medial lesions. It is postulated that medial lesions may be caused by repetitive microtrauma.[25,26] Berndt and Harty,[12] in 1959, used freshly amputated legs to biomechanically reproduce injuries to the ankle and observe the injuries inflicted. They showed that the anterolateral talus hits the medial aspect of the fibula with dorsiflexion and inversion and that plantarflexion and inversion caused posteromedial osteochondral lesions (Fig. 30-10).

The initial radiographs following an ankle injury in a child should be closely assessed for an osteochondral injury. If pain and swelling persist for over 2 months after an "ankle sprain," then further investigations should be carried out to look for an osteochondral lesion, which will initially be a further radiograph series. However, an MRI scan is often more useful at this stage to look for an osteochondral lesion as a small percentage are purely cartilaginous. Some consider an MRI arthrogram useful in further determining whether the fragment is detached as occasionally the arthrographic contrast can be seen deep to the osteochondral lesion. The bone scan has largely been superseded by the MRI scan in the diagnosis and assessment of these lesions. The bone scan is useful, however, when it is not clear if the pain in the child's ankle is coming from the osteochondral lesion or some other pathology. A normal bone scan in the presence of a stage I or II osteochondral lesion may indicate a soft tissue lesion as being a source of the pain.

Mechanical symptoms of locking and catching are not as common as one would think but can occur with these lesions if the loose fragment becomes trapped within the joint. The pain seems to be related to the synovitis and effusion that develops secondary to the uneven articular surface. On examination, the

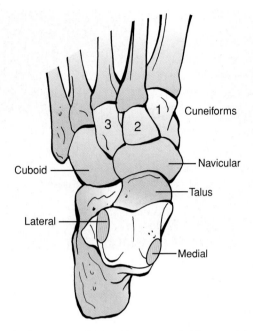

Figure 30-10. Typical positions of osteochondral lesions of the talus. Berndt and Harty[12] found that of 201 osteochondral lesions in adults 56% were on the medial side and 44% on the lateral side. Letts et al. found medial lesions in 79% of 24 children, lateral lesions in 21%, and central lesions in 1%. (Reprinted with permission from Letts M, Davidson D, Ahmer A. Osteochondritis dissecans of the talus in children. *J Pediatr Orthop.* 2003;23(5):617–625.)

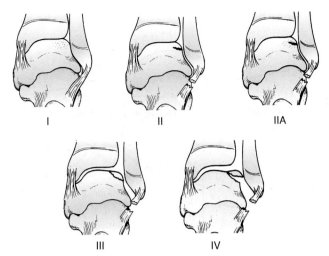

Figure 30-11. Adaptation of the Berndt and Harty[12] (1959) classification of osteochondral injuries of the talus by Anderson et al.[8] Stage I is identified only by MRI scanning, which demonstrates trabecular compression of subchondral bone; stage II lesions have incomplete separation of the osteochondral fragment from the talus. If a subchondral cyst also is present, the lesion is designated stage IIa. Stage III lesions occur when the fragment is no longer attached to the talus but is undisplaced. Stage IV indicates both complete detachment and displacement. (Reprinted with permission from Alexander IF, Chrichton KI, Grattan-Smith Y, et al. Osteochondral fractures of the dome of the talus. *J Bone Joint Surg Am.* 1989;71(8):1143–1152.)

ankle is slightly swollen and can be painful on passive movement as the loose fragment passes under the tibia. With plantarflexion of the foot, the anterolateral talus can be palpated directly and a lesion here can be painful on direct pressure.

CLASSIFICATION OF FRACTURES OF THE OSTEOCHONDRAL SURFACE OF THE TALUS

Fractures of the Osteochondral Surface of the Talus: BERNDT AND HENRY CLASSIFICATION

- Stage I: Subchondral trabecular compression fracture (not seen radiographically)
- Stage II: Incomplete separation of an osteochondral fragment
- Stage III: The osteochondral fragment is unattached but undisplaced
- Stage IV: A displaced osteochondral fragment

Berndt and Harty[12] classified osteochondral fractures of the talar dome into four stages based on radiographic criteria (Fig. 30-11).

Anderson et al.[8] modified this classification after correlating clinical findings with radiographs and MRI scans. They described the stage I lesion as not visible on plain radiographs but visible on an MRI scan. They also introduced a stage IIa lesion, which is an undisplaced osteochondral lesion with a subchondral cyst adjacent to the floor of the lesion. Anderson et al.[8] felt a stage IIa lesion should be treated surgically

whereas a stage II lesion can initially be treated nonoperatively (Fig. 30-12).

A further classification was proposed by Pritsch et al.[138] in 1986 based on the arthroscopic appearance of the articular cartilage. The quality of the articular cartilage was placed into one of three grades:

Grade I: Intact, firm, and shiny articular cartilage
Grade II: Intact but soft articular cartilage
Grade III: Frayed articular cartilage

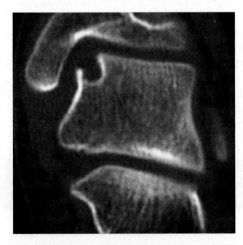

Figure 30-12. This CT scan clearly shows a well-circumscribed cyst at the base of a stage II osteochondral lesion. This would be classified by Anderson et al.[8] as a stage IIa lesion.

They used this classification to determine which lesions should be treated with activity modification (grade I), who should have arthroscopic drilling (grade II), and finally which patients require arthroscopic curettage and microfracture (grade III).

TREATMENT OPTIONS FOR OSTEOCHONDRAL FRACTURES OF THE TALUS

The treatment of osteochondral lesions of the talus in children is challenging. Only a few papers purely address this condition in children,[69,97,129] and the rest of the literature is a combination of adult and childhood lesions. It is important to distinguish between an acute osteochondral fracture and a chronic osteochondral lesion as the two may require different treatment strategies.

To enable thorough assessment, these patients need to be followed up for a minimum of 2 years as it takes this long for the lesion to become radiographically healed despite the child often being clinically normal.[129]

Nonoperative Treatment

Most authors agree that the primary treatment of stage I and stage II lesions is nonoperative.[12,69,97,129] The symptomatic patient can be immobilized for 6 weeks in a below-knee walking cast or a Cam walker (Fig. 30-13). This usually relieves the acute symptoms; over the next 6 weeks, the patient has activity modification maintaining a pain-free range of movement. This allows the fracture to heal before returning to active sports. Higuera et al.[70] treated their stage III lesions nonoperatively as well and all seven patients had good outcomes.

Operative Treatment

The outcomes of surgery for osteochondral fractures of the talus are controversial. It is hard to compare results between authors as they have often used different outcome measures. Some authors use pain as their primary outcome[97] whereas others also consider radiologic healing. The long-term outcome of an asymptomatic subchondral lucency in the talar body is unknown. In some series, the patients have had arthrotomies[97] whereas others had arthroscopic debridement.[129] The staging of

the lesions are also subject to interobserver variability.[97] With modern ankle arthroscopy equipment and newer surgical techniques, ankle arthroscopy has become the primary surgical treatment for both medial and lateral lesions of the talar dome. The anterolateral lesions are more accessible; however, with good ankle distraction and different portal placement posteromedial lesions are accessible, as well.

Recently, Perumal et al.[131] reviewed 31 patients with a juvenile OCD and a minimum of 6-month follow-up. They recommended nonoperative treatment with an ankle brace and activity modification for 6 months in most cases. Only 16% of the lesions healed radiographically in that timeframe. If pain continues after this time and the lesion is still present, further immobilization and activity modification is recommended. They recommend arthroscopic surgery for patients with type II lesions who are not prepared to modify their activities longer than 6 months, and patients with type III lateral lesions, and all stage IV lesions. Thirteen of the 31 patients were treated surgically.

Arthroscopic treatment options include:

- Drilling the lesion (antegrade or retrograde)[86]
- Curettage and microfracture
- Internal fixation with bioabsorbable nails
- Bone grafting and internal fixation

In stage II lesions with intact articular cartilage, Kumai et al.[90] showed excellent results drilling through the lesion into the subchondral bone. The authors also found that in skeletally immature patients, there may be an increased tendency for the lesion to heal when compared to the adult patients. Retrograde drilling can be performed using specific tip directed instrumentation. This approach avoids damage to the articular cartilage and may prevent fragmentation of a small lesion. Access to a posteromedial lesion can be difficult. One approach is to use a transmalleolar portal after drilling a 3.5-mm drill through the medial malleolus or to use a posteromedial portal, taking care to avoid damaging the neurovascular bundle.

Curettage and microfracture is a very effective, relatively straightforward procedure. It is particularly useful in small stage III and stage IV lesions where the fragment is too small to internally fix or there is no subchondral bone on the lesion

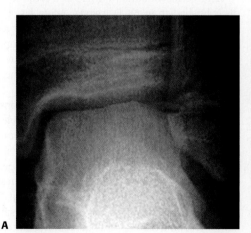 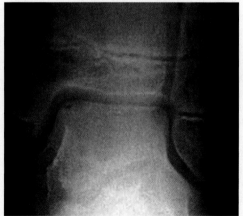

Figure 30-13. A: Anterolateral stage III osteochondral lesion that was treated by arthroscopic excision and microfracture. **B:** Posteromedial stage II osteochondral lesion that was treated successfully nonoperatively.

for healing. The articular cartilage is debrided back to stable tissue and the subchondral bone is curettaged until bleeding occurs. Either a microfracture pick or 2-mm drill is then used in the subchondral bone. Anderson et al.[8] would suggest this treatment for all stage IIa lesions where a subchondral cyst is present.

Internal fixation with or without bone grafting is a difficult procedure for the inexperienced arthroscopist. It is preferable to use absorbable pegs or nails rather than metallic implants. In large stage III and IV acute osteochondral lesions, this is probably the treatment of choice rather than excising the fragment.

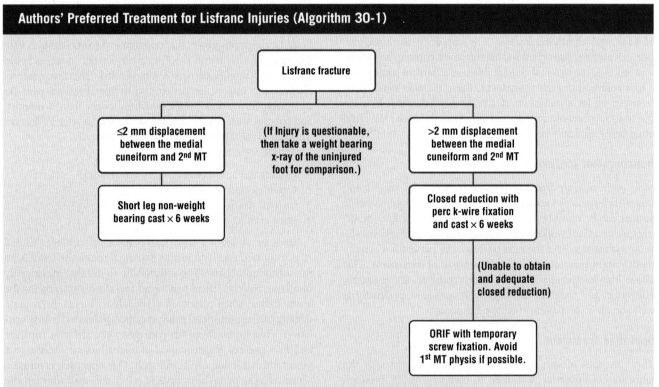

Authors' Preferred Treatment for Lisfranc Injuries (Algorithm 30-1)

Algorithm 30-1. Authors' preferred treatment for Lisfranc injuries.

For simple undisplaced fractures, a below-knee nonwalking cast is applied for 6 weeks.

Displaced lateral process fractures need to be anatomically reduced especially if they are intra-articular and there is 2 to 3 mm of incongruity in the joint surface. A lateral approach is used and a single compression screw inserted across the fracture. The foot is immobilized in a below-knee cast for 6 weeks.

Displaced talar neck fractures should be operated on as soon as possible. If the fracture can be reduced closed, the author prefers a posterolateral approach to insert the compression screws as this helps preserve the tenuous blood supply (see Fig. 30-7). These screws are best inserted through this open approach so an accurate starting point can be found and neurovascular structures protected. The author has no hesitation to use an anteromedial approach as well to help with fracture reduction before inserting the screws. Through this approach, the neck fragment can be stabilized while the screws are being compressed and anatomic fracture reduction can be seen. Usually, two 4.5-mm partially

threaded titanium screws are used depending on the size of the talus and degree of fragmentation. The titanium screws allow MRI postoperatively if osteonecrosis is suspected.

Acute osteochondral injuries need to be recognized and distinguished from OCD lesions. Acute lesions should be repaired after assessing the amount of bone present on the lesion. This can be initially assessed arthrocopically but is repaired through an arthrotomy depending on the position on the talus. The author prefers to repair the lesion with dissolvable nails.

The author treats types I to III OCD lesions nonoperatively for 6 months. Initially, the child or adolescent wears a Cam walker for 4 to 6 weeks to help the symptoms settle and then an elastic ankle support and activity modification. If symptoms persist, the author performs a repeat MRI scan and, if the staging has worsened, proceeds to an arthroscopic debridement and microfracture or stabilization. For patients with displaced fragments on presentation (stage IV), the author recommends arthroscopic removal and microfracture or repair if possible.

MANAGEMENT OF EXPECTED ADVERSE OUTCOMES AND UNEXPECTED COMPLICATIONS RELATED TO TALAR FRACTURES

Osteonecrosis of the talus is the most serious complication of talus fractures. It has been reported in a number of large series of predominantly adult patients.[26,65] Osteonecrosis of the body of the talus occurs when the blood supply has been disrupted by a fracture of the talar neck. The result is necrosis of the talar dome and possible collapse of the articular surface. Hawkins[65] described the presence of a subchondral lucent line, the "Hawkins sign," as prognostic of a good outcome as it indicates adequate blood flow to the talar body. The absence of the sign on a 6- to 8-week radiograph implies there is inadequate blood supply and osteonecrosis may evolve. In adults, a negative Hawkins sign has been found to be highly sensitive but not specific for future development of AVN.[174]

In adults, the incidence of osteonecrosis seems directly related to the Hawkins classification type. Hawkins[65] showed that type I fractures had a 0% to 10% AVN rate, type II fractures a 20% to 50% AVN rate, type III an 80% to 100% AVN rate, and all type IV fractures develop AVN. Canale and Kelly[26] had similar long-term results.

Osteonecrosis has also been seen in pediatric talus fractures, with multiple authors reporting cases of talus AVN.[98,111,140,173] The Hawkins sign was described in adults, and Ogden[126] suggests this sign may not be as reliable in the cartilaginous talar dome of a child. The rate of AVN after pediatric talus fractures is uncertain, with recent series ranging from 0% to 20%.[48,79] More recently, a series of 25 pediatric talus fractures reported no cases of AVN a final follow up in patients less than 12 years old. This finding suggests that, while case reports exist of AVN in young patients,[140,173] the outcome can be expected to be favorable in patients younger than 12 years old who have sustained a talus fracture.[48]

The dilemma for the treating surgeon is what to advise the patient regarding weight bearing when the Hawkins sign is not present by 8 weeks. Some of the above series report AVN occurring 6 months after the injury and not resolving for many years. There does not appear to be any series comparing outcomes in patients who bear weight over this period and those who do not. If the Hawkins sign is not present, it is advisable to perform an MRI scan at 3 months to establish if AVN is present or not.[67,171] If present, it may be advisable to encourage the child to avoid impact activities to prevent collapse rather than have a prolonged period of nonweight bearing.

Calcaneal Fractures

INTRODUCTION TO CALCANEAL FRACTURES

Fractures of the calcaneus are rare in children with an incidence of only 1 in 100,000 fractures.[182] The treatment of these fractures has historically been nonoperative, relying on the largely cartilaginous bone to remodel with time. The majority of fractures in children are extra-articular[117] whereas in older children the fracture pattern resembles those in adults. Children appear to have more coexisting lower limb fractures than adults but fewer fractures of the axial skeleton.[156]

Calcaneal fractures in young children are often missed or are diagnosed late. At the other end of the spectrum, the adolescent patient has often had a major fall and has a displaced intra-articular fracture. This older age group should be treated like the adult population with ORIF restoring the joint congruity and calcaneal height and width. The challenge for the surgeon is at what age and what degree of displacement is this more aggressive treatment indicated in a group of patients traditionally treated nonoperatively.

ASSESSMENT OF CALCANEAL FRACTURES

MECHANISMS OF INJURY FOR CALCANEAL FRACTURES

By far the most common mechanism of injury is a fall from a height.[19,75,134] The axial load drives the talus into the calcaneus resulting in the fracture. The degree of comminution appears to be less in children even though they often fall from greater heights than adults.[20] Wiley and Profitt[186] found that in young children, the fall was usually less than 4 ft and in children older than 10 years the fall was greater than 14 ft. They noted that the minor falls in the younger children often resulted in undisplaced fractures that were diagnosed late.

In Schmidt and Weiner's[161] review of pediatric calcaneal fractures they found that children less than 14 years of age predominantly had extra-articular fractures, hypothesizing that the calcaneus in this age bracket absorbs the compression force rather than dissipating it through the joint. This finding is supported by More et al.,[117] who found 78% extra-articular fractures in their series of pediatric calcaneus fractures.

Vehicle-related injuries were the second biggest cause of calcaneal fractures in both Schmidt and Weiner[161] and Wiley and Profitt's reviews.[186] Fractures of the calcaneus can also occur in major crush injuries when compartment syndrome may coexist and open fractures are common in lawnmower injuries.

SIGNS AND SYMPTOMS OF CALCANEAL FRACTURES

Any child who has fallen from a height and landed on their feet should be examined carefully for a calcaneal fracture. Associated injuries should also be evaluated with a thorough secondary survey, especially of the lower limbs and spine.

The foot will often be extremely swollen with bruising around the heel and dorsum of the foot. Symptoms and signs of compartment syndrome, including excessive pain, pallor, paresthesia, and pulselessness should be assessed. In more subtle injuries, careful palpation is necessary to elucidate areas of pain which may disclose an underlying undisplaced fracture.

Many calcaneal fractures in children are initially missed and diagnosed late. Often, the fracture line is not evident on the initial radiographs. Inokuchi et al.[76] reported that 44% of fractures in their series were initially missed, as were 55% of those reported by Schantz and Rasmussen[158] and 44% of those reported by Wiley and Profitt.[186]

A differential diagnosis must be kept in mind for other causes of heel pain in a child. These include Sever disease, osteomyelitis, a unicameral bone cyst, or a stress fracture.[126]

INJURIES ASSOCIATED WITH CALCANEAL FRACTURES

Schmidt and Weiner[161] reviewed 56 children with calcaneal fractures and found a number of associated injuries. These included fractures of the lumbar spine, lower limb fractures, a pelvic fracture, and upper extremity fractures. These other skeletal injuries were more frequent in children over 13 years of age. Associated lower limb fractures occurred twice as frequently as in adults; however, injuries to the axial skeleton occurred half as often as in adults. Wiley and Profitt,[186] however, only had two patients with accompanying significant injuries in their series of 32 pediatric calcaneal fractures.

IMAGING AND OTHER DIAGNOSTIC STUDIES FOR CALCANEAL FRACTURES

Radiography

Calcaneal fractures in children are often not diagnosed initially as the radiographic findings are usually more subtle than in adults.[87,110,156,166,182] Subsequent radiographs at 2 weeks often show the fracture line. The majority of these fractures are extra-articular.[156]

The standard views for a suspected calcaneal fracture are posteroanterior, lateral, and axial views. The posteroanterior view shows the calcaneocuboid and talonavicular joints well. The lateral view is excellent at showing the congruity of the posterior articular facet and allows calculation of Bohler angle (see Fig. 30-9). The axial view demonstrates the tuberosity, the body, the sustentaculum tali, and the posterior facet of the calcaneus. Oblique views are also useful and will show a fracture of the anterior process more clearly (Fig. 30-14).[142] The oblique views also define the subtalar joint well and, thus, are very useful in identifying intra-articular fractures. Broden views can also be taken that look at the posterior facet of the calcaneus. These are taken with the leg internally rotated 40 degrees and the x-ray beam angled between 15 and 40 degrees toward the head.[18] This image is a difficult radiograph for the technicians to master and almost the same information can be achieved by ordering a mortise view of the ankle to look at the posterior facet of the subtalar joint.

The lateral view is useful for measuring the Bohler angle, which is the angle between a line drawn from the highest point of the anterior process to the highest point of the posterior facet and a line drawn tangential to the highest point of the calcaneal tuberosity. The normal value in an adult is between 20 and 40 degrees. In a child, the angle is slightly less than in an adult, which may be caused by the incomplete ossification of the calcaneus. It is advisable to perform a lateral radiograph of the contralateral calcaneus to use as a comparison rather than accept the absolute value of Bohler angle. The child's calcaneus does not resemble that of an adult until after 10 years of age.[73,124,174] Another angle which is not easy to measure is "the crucial angle of Gissane," which is the angle formed by two strong cortical

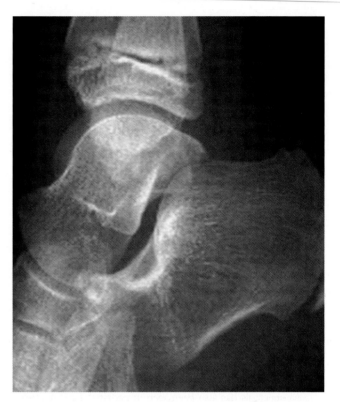

Figure 30-14. Fracture of the anterior process of the calcaneus.

struts seen on the lateral radiograph. One runs along the lateral margin of the posterior facet and the other runs up to the anterior process of the calcaneus. This angle ranges from 95 to 105 degrees (see Fig. 30-9).[51]

When reviewing radiographs of children's feet, it is always important to be cognizant of the ossification centers and accessory bones within the growing foot, which often are confused with fractures (see Figs. 30-1 and 30-2).[27] The os calcis is the earliest tarsal bone to ossify with the primary ossification center appearing in the third intrauterine month. The secondary ossification center appears around 6 to 8 years and is the crescentic epiphysis seen posteriorly. This epiphysis fuses to the body of the calcaneus between 14 and 16 years of age.

The use of a technetium-labeled bone scan in diagnosing calcaneal fractures is uncommon with the ready availability of MRI scans. The bone scan has been used to evaluate a nonlocalized painful limp in a toddler. However, often clinical judgment and radiographic follow-up are sufficient in the diagnosis of pain following trauma, making a bone scan unnecessary.[159]

Computed Tomography

CT scanning has evolved as the best method to evaluate the fractured calcaneus. Not only does it clearly show the fracture lines and altered anatomy, but also reveals injuries to adjacent bones. Sanders et al.[156] have used CT scans to develop a classification system that is particularly useful in the preoperative planning of open reduction of these fractures. The primary and secondary fracture lines are identified and the degree of comminution and position of the fragments is more accurately seen than in the radiographs. The primary fracture line usually runs obliquely from plantar medial to dorsolateral exiting the posterior facet. Secondary fracture lines that develop off this primary line are also seen and their pattern determines the classification of the fracture (Fig. 30-15). The CT scan also allows a three-dimensional reconstruction which can be useful in preoperative planning.

Buckingham et al.[20] and Ogden[126] reviewed 9 patients with 10 calcaneal fractures and performed CT scans on all of them. They found the fracture patterns in these adolescents (average 13.4 years old) to be very similar to those found in adults. They did find less comminution in children than in adults, even though the children reportedly had fallen from greater heights.

MRI scans are largely unnecessary. They can be useful in young children when the calcaneus is still largely cartilaginous and a fracture is not seen on plain films or CT.

CLASSIFICATION OF CALCANEAL FRACTURES

Children's calcaneal fractures were traditionally classified according to their adult counterparts using the Essex-Lopresti[52] and Letournel[98] classifications. Schmidt and Weiner[161] reviewed 62 calcaneal fractures in children and compared them to the adult literature.[147] They used the classification systems of Essex-Lopresti[52] and Chapman and Galway[32] and added a new fracture type (type VI) to develop a classification for pediatric calcaneal fractures which is in routine use today (Fig. 30-16).

For adolescent fractures, it is probably more appropriate to use the Sanders classification.[152] This is an adult classification system that was developed after reviewing the CT scans on 120 cases preoperatively and at minimum 1-year follow-up. The follow-up CT scans were correlated with the clinical outcome scores to help validate the classification system used.

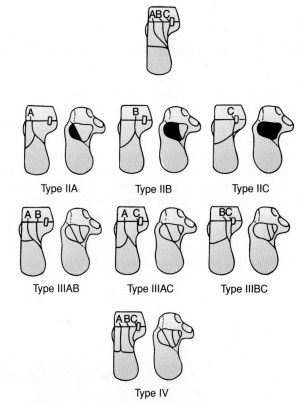

Figure 30-15. Sanders CT-based classification of intra-articular fractures of the calcaneus in adults. (Reprinted with permission from Sanders R. Intraarticular fractures of the calcaneus: Present state of the art. *J Orthop Trauma.* 1992;6(2):252–265.)

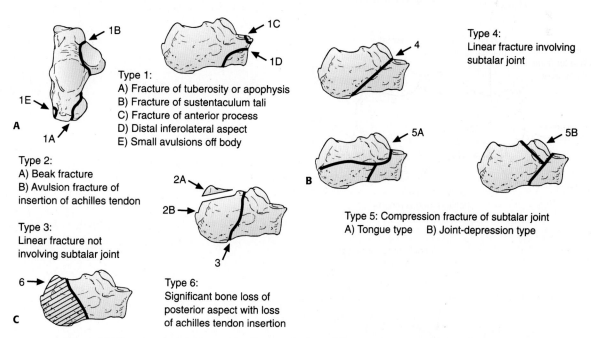

Figure 30-16. Schmidt and Weiner classification of calcaneal fracture patterns in children. **A:** Extra-articular fractures. **B:** Intra-articular fractures. **C:** Type VI fracture pattern with significant bone loss, soft tissue injury, and loss of Achilles tendon insertion. (Reprinted with permission from Schmidt TL, Weiner DS. Calcaneus fractures in children: An evaluation of the nature of injury in 56 children. *Clin Orthop Relat Res.* 1982;171:150–155.)

PATHOANATOMY AND APPLIED ANATOMY RELATING TO CALCANEAL FRACTURES

The calcaneus is the largest tarsal bone and has an unusual shape. It has three articular facets (anterior, middle, and posterior) on the superior surface where it articulates with the talus to form the subtalar joint (see Fig. 30-5). Anteriorly there is a saddle-shaped articular surface for the cuboid. The posterior facet is the largest facet and is slightly convex. The middle facet is anterior and medial to the posterior facet, lying on the sustentaculum tali. It is concave like the anterior facet with which it is often contiguous. Between the middle and posterior facets lies the calcaneal groove, which forms the inferior wall of the sinus tarsi. Posteriorly, the tendoachilles inserts into the tuberosity of the calcaneus, which is the entire area behind the posterior facet. On the lateral surface of the calcaneus are two shallow grooves with a small ridge in between (the peroneal trochlea). The peroneus longus and brevis run either side of this trochlea. The medial side is concave and is structurally stronger than the lateral side. The sustentaculum tali projects from the medial wall and supports the middle articular facet on its surface. The tendon of flexor hallucis longus runs on the undersurface of the sustentaculum. On the plantar surface are the medial and lateral processes, which represent the origin of the abductor hallucis and abductor digiti minimi muscles, respectively (Fig. 30-17).

Secondary ossification occurs in the calcaneal apophysis between the ages of 6 and 10 years. Inflammation in the apophysis around this age causes heel pain and is referred to as Sever disease.

The use of CT scans has defined the surgical anatomy of the calcaneus to help make treatment decisions. The coronal views show the important posterior facet and the sustentaculum tali and the height and width of the heel. The position of the peroneal tendons and flexor hallucis tendon can also be seen. The sagittal

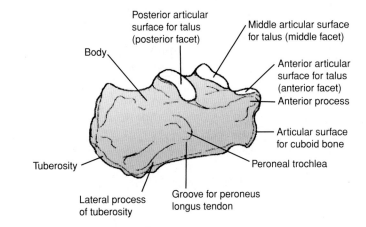

A

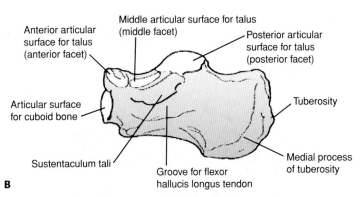

B

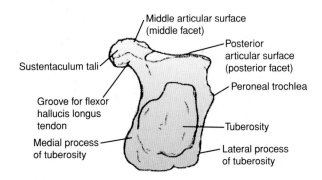

C

Figure 30-17. Anatomic details of various angles of the calcaneus including lateral (**A**), medial (**B**), and coronal (**C**) views through the level of the sustentaculum tali, which correlate with the CT scan view important in reconstruction of the posterior facet.

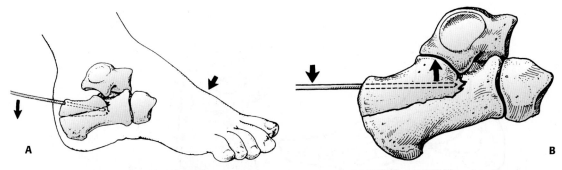

Figure 30-18. Percutaneous reduction technique for tongue-type fractures of the calcaneus, as described by Essex-Lopresti.[51] This technique remains an alternative to conservative treatment and open reduction with internal fixation of displaced, tongue-type fractures. **A:** A pin is inserted into the tongue fragment and used as a joystick to manipulate the fragment into better position, usually with a downward force on the pin and the forefoot (plantarflexion). **B:** After reduction, the pin is driven across the fracture to maintain reduction. (Redrawn with permission from Tornetta A III. The Essex-Lopresti reduction for calcaneal fractures revisited. *J Orthop Trauma.* 1998;12(7):469–473.)

views provide additional information about the posterior facet and also show the anterior process well. The axial views visualize the calcaneocuboid joint well, the anterior-inferior aspect of the posterior facet, and the sustentaculum tali. This information can be used in planning the reconstruction of the calcaneus.[149,150]

TREATMENT OPTIONS FOR CALCANEAL FRACTURES

Calcaneal fractures in growing children are usually less severe than in the adult population and often do well with nonoperative treatment.[19,75] In adolescents, fracture patterns are often similar to adults and require ORIF. The challenge to the orthopedic surgeon is to recognize the patient that requires this treatment. There is a degree of remodeling that will take place in the child and hence the amount of growth remaining, degree of ossification, and difference in morphology from the contralateral side all should be considered in making treatment decisions.

Extra-articular fractures of the calcaneus can be treated by cast immobilization for 6 weeks. The child can start weight bearing in this cast when comfortable and can be changed to a Cam walker for the final few weeks.[19,75]

Tongue-type fractures can be treated nonoperatively if the posterior gap is less than 1 cm and the Achilles tendon has not been significantly shortened by bringing the fragment up proximally. Occasionally, the technique described by Essex-Lopresti[52] for percutaneous reduction of tongue-type fractures (Fig. 30-18) is useful.

ORIF is reserved for the intra-articular fractures with displacement of the fragments and depression of the joint surfaces. These fractures occur almost exclusively in the adolescent patient where the ossification process is complete. The adult literature abounds with indications for internal fixation, surgical approaches, rehabilitation, complications, and outcome measures (Fig. 30-19).[10,149,152] These series only have a few adolescent fractures among them, and therefore it is difficult to draw any conclusions specifically about children's calcaneal fractures. The literature on the management of displaced intra-articular

fractures in children is somewhat conflicting in the indications for surgery. Schantz and Rasmussen[158] reported on the outcome of displaced intra-articular fractures in children less than 15 years old treated nonoperatively. The majority of the patients had a good outcome; however, four complained of pain an average of 12 years after injury.[154] Brunet[19] asserts that the outcome does not correlate to the severity of the fracture in young patients, which is likely due to the remodeling potential of the calcaneus in this age group. Mora et al.[119] also concluded that open reduction may be suitable only for severely displaced fractures in adolescents. The difficulty is defining the age or maturity of the patient that may predict a poor outcome if the fracture is left unreduced. Using validated quality-of-life scales 2 to 8 years after surgery, Buckley et al.[21] found that younger patients (adults under the age of 30 years) who had operative treatment had better gait satisfaction scores than those who did not have surgery. Allmacher et al.[6] questioned whether short-term or intermediate results of displaced intra-articular calcaneal fractures can predict long-term functional outcome. Using validated outcome instruments, they studied adult patients treated nonoperatively and found that nonoperative treatment often led to pain and loss of function, which increased in the second decade after injury.

Good results have been reported with open reduction internal fixation has been used to treat displaced, intra-articular closed calcaneus fractures in older children, mean ages 11.5 to 13 years old.[132,134] In these studies, only one incisional breakdown was reported in 35 patients, which was successfully treated with wet-to-dry dressings and oral antibiotics. Ceccarelli[28] found that skeletally mature children with displaced intra-articular fractures had better clinical and radiologic outcomes if treated by open reduction rather than nonoperatively. Is there any other important take-home message from this paper that would help a surgeon decide who would benefit from open reduction? Buckingham et al.[20] reviewed 10 adolescent patients and reported good or excellent outcomes in 8 patients. They had no wound complications and the motion was hardly affected in seven patients.

The surgery for these fractures is technically demanding, and, if the treating surgeon is not experienced with the approach, the child is best referred to a colleague who is.

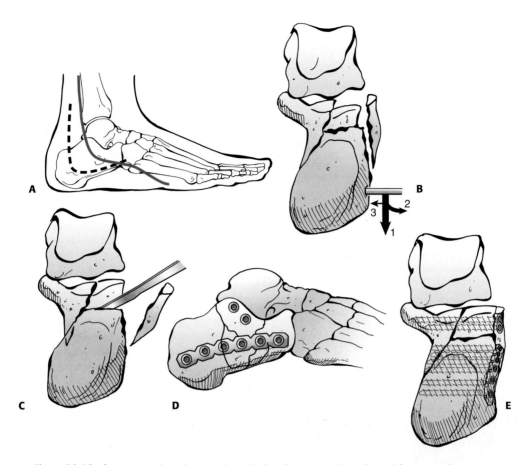

Figure 30-19. A: Lateral L-shaped approach to displaced intra-articular calcaneal fractures. The incision (*dashed line*) is laterally based, with the proximal arm approximately half the distance from the fibula to the posterior border of the foot and the distal arm halfway from the tip of the fibula to the sole of the foot. The sural nerve is illustrated. A full-thickness, subperiosteal flap exposes the entire lateral calcaneus. **B:** Reduction maneuvers 1, 2, and 3 (*densest arrow indicates greatest displacement*) with a Schanz screw are used to pull the tuberosity down and allow access to disimpact the posterior facet (**C**) after the lateral wall of the calcaneus is levered open. The posterior facet is then reduced anatomically, held provisionally with K-wires, and then fixed with two partially threaded cancellous screws (outside of plate) into the sustentaculum tali. Lateral view (**D**) of reduced calcaneus and axial view (**E**) of reduced fracture with hardware. (Redrawn with permission from Benirschke SK, Sangeorzan BJ. Extraarticular fractures of the foot: Surgical management of calcaneal fractures [Review]. *Clin Orthop Relat Res.* 1993;292:128–134.)

Authors' Preferred Treatment for Calcaneal Fractures (Algorithm 30-2)

The key decision in treating children's calcaneal fractures is which require surgical intervention. Almost all closed fractures in children less than 10 years of age can be treated nonoperatively because of the remodeling potential, which includes intra-articular fractures that are displaced.

Extra-articular fractures of the calcaneus can be treated by nonoperative means with a below-knee cast for 6 weeks. Weight bearing in the cast can start after 2 to 3 weeks as the patient becomes more comfortable.

Undisplaced intra-articular fractures can also be treated in a below-knee cast. In this group of patients, it is advisable for them to be nonweight bearing for 6 weeks or until the fracture is healed to prevent further displacement.

Adolescent patients with displaced intra-articular fractures are best treated by ORIF (see Figs. 30-19 and 30-20). Prior to surgery, a thorough assessment of the skin needs to be performed. Surgery should be delayed to allow swelling to subside and fracture blisters to resolve, which will decrease some of the wound complications seen after open fixation of adult calcaneal fractures. An important point in performing this surgery is to maintain thick skin flaps, restore joint congruity, use specialized calcaneal plates, and be prepared to bone graft the defect. An outline of the surgical technique is in Table 30-2.

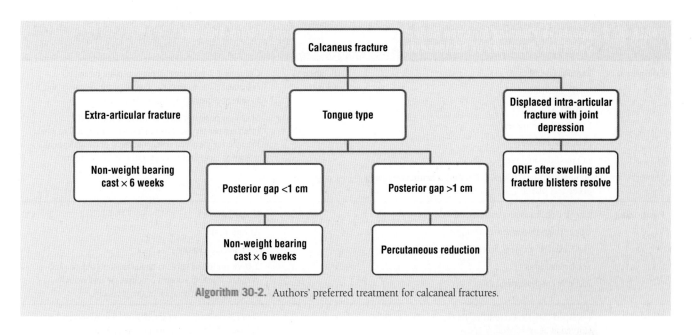

Algorithm 30-2. Authors' preferred treatment for calcaneal fractures.

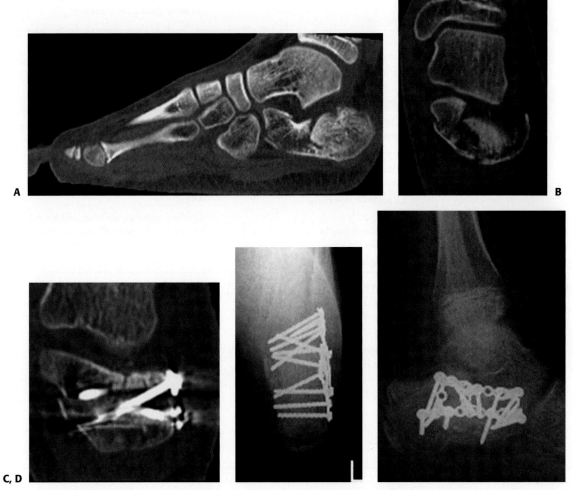

Figure 30-20. Intra-articular depressed fracture of the calcaneus in a 13-year-old boy. **A:** Preoperative sagittal CT shows the depression of the posterior facet into the body of the calcaneus. **B:** Coronal CT shows the displacement of the fracture fragments. **C:** Postoperative CT scans are useful at checking the fracture reduction and length and position of the screws. **D, E:** Postoperative radiographs confirm restoration of the Bohler angle.

TABLE 30-2. Operative Planning for Open Reduction and Internal Fixation of Intra-Articular Calcaneal Fractures in Adolescents

Equipment	Radiolucent table Image Intensifier K-wires with driver Lambotte osteotomes Periosteal elevators AO modular foot set Synthes calcaneal plates, 2.7-mm reconstruction plates, H cervical plates	Fixation Closure	Contour 2.7-mm reconstruction plate or an AO calcaneal plate to the lateral wall of the os calcis and fix to anterior process and the posterior tuber Maintain posterior facet reduction with two interfragmentary screws angled well inferiorly to avoid the inferiorly curved medial surface of the calcaneal posterior facet and to engage the sustentaculum
Positioning	Lateral decubitus on contralateral side Upper thigh pneumatic tourniquet Hip flexed 45 degrees, knee flexed 90 degrees Seattle cushions Radiolucent operating table		Irrigation Always drain Two-layered closure 2-0 Vicryl to the subcutaneous tissues (Interrupted vertical. Place all sutures on clips, tie individually commencing at the apex of the incision)
Incision	L-shaped incision (Letournel, Regazzoni, Bernirschke) Curved at apex Proximal extent 3-cm cephalad to tip of fibula anterior to lateral border of Achilles tendon Distal extent tip of base of fifth metatarsal		Skin closure with interrupted 3-0 Nylon All-gower Donati sutures (all placed on clips and then tied individually commencing at the apex moving symmetrically to the proximal and distal extent of the wound holding multiple sutures to maintain even tension)
Exposure	Blunt dissection with scissors proximally to identify the short saphenous vein and sural nerve Sharp dissection with no. 15 blade direct to lateral wall of os calcaneus Subperiosteal reflection with scalpel Sharp dissection and reflection of peroneal tendons and attachment of calcaneofibular ligament dorsally Keep dorsal to the muscle belly of abductor digiti minimi Protect peroneal tendons with baby Hoffmann retractors when exposing the anterior process and calcaneocuboid joint Elevate flap dorsally to expose the posterior facet of the talus and sinus tarsi Maintain flap anteriorly with K-wires placed into the body and neck of the talus and the fibula Deflate tourniquet when exposure complete	Dressings Postoperative	Gelnet dressing Well-padded below-knee popliteal joint back slab supporting toes Elevation on two pillows IV antibiotics CT scan to check reduction and exclude screw malposition Remove drain when drainage is less than 10 mL over an 8-hr period Review wound for hematoma and skin viability within 48 hrs Continue splintage, elevation, and restricted mobility non–weight-bearing until sutures removed 14–18 days postsurgery
Reduction	Place Schanz pin in inferior aspect of posterior tuber Reduce fracture by traction on the Schanz pin displacing posterior tuber inferiorly and thence medially Reflect lateral wall laterally if necessary Reduce anterior process first, then posterior facet, and finally restore alignment of the os calcis by confirming reduction and alignment of the crucial angle Thus reduce anterior to posterior, medial to lateral, and dorsal to plantar Provisional reduction maintained with multiple K-wires Reduction and alignment confirmed by screening with image intensifier		

Courtesy of Dr. Campbell ACL. *FRACS, Adult Foot and Ankle Surgeon*. Auckland City Hospital, New Zealand.

WOUND COMPLICATIONS

Wound dehiscence is the most common complication following open reduction of adult calcaneal fractures.[10,72,99,152]

Although reported to occur in up to 25% of adult fractures, the incidence is lower in children. Pickle et al.[136] had no wound problems in the six adolescents (age range: 11 to 16 years) they treated with ORIF. All the patients were treated with an extensile lateral approach an average of 10.5 days from the time of injury. The lower incidence in children reflects fewer risk factors in this group when compared to the adult population. Smoking, obesity, and diabetes can all contribute to wound problems.

Wound dehiscence can be decreased by meticulous closure of the incision. In adults, it has been shown that a two-layer closure is preferable to a single layer of sutures.[1,55] Wound dehiscence can occur from days to weeks after the surgery. The best initial treatment is immobilization to decrease tension on the wound edges, which is best accomplished by using a below-knee cast with a large window cut around the entire incision. This technique allows space for wound dressing changes and debridements as necessary. Oral antibiotics may be required if superficial infection is present. Once the wound is healed, gradual mobilization can be reinstated.

In serious deep wound infections, the patient will require rehospitalization, repeat surgical debridements, and intravenous antibiotics. Often, the use of a suction dressing (Vacuum Assisted Closure® [KCI Licensing, Inc., San Antonio, TX]) is advisable in recalcitrant wounds. This device has been shown to be safe and effective by Mooney et al.[118] for traumatic wounds in pediatric patients of all ages. Skin closure is usually not possible following such radical debridement. It is very helpful to consult with plastic surgeons early in the course of treatment as the patient often requires tissue transfer to cover the exposed metalware.

COMPLEX REGIONAL PAIN SYNDROME

This syndrome, previously known as reflex sympathetic dystrophy (RSD), is a devastating painful disorder that can occur following operative or nonoperative management of a calcaneal fracture or other foot trauma. The condition is usually diagnosed when there is severe pain present out of proportion to the severity of the injury following the acute phase of healing. The pain is difficult to control, even with narcotics. The child will not bear weight or even allow the foot to be examined. Light touch even by water may stimulate an unusual pain response. The foot clinically demonstrates the signs of autonomic dysfunction. There is often a grayish discoloration, cold clammy skin, and decreased hair growth. Through disuse of the foot, the calf will atrophy. If radiographs are taken, the bones of the foot may show patchy disuse osteopenia.

There is a marked preponderance of lower extremity cases in children compared to adults.[178] Sarrail et al.[157] reviewed RSD in 24 children and adolescents and found that 73% had foot or ankle injuries. Wilder et al.[183] reviewed 70 children (average age, 12.5 years) with RSD and 87% had injuries to the lower limb. Eighty-four percent of their patients were girls, and the average time from injury to a diagnosis of RSD was 12 months. Despite multidisciplinary treatments, 54% of patients still had persistent symptoms of RSD at 3 years after diagnosis. They emphasized that complex regional pain syndrome (CRPS) has a different disease course in children when compared with adults and needs to be treated appropriately. CRPS occurs most commonly in girls with the incidence peaking at or just before puberty.[178]

Most tertiary children's hospitals now have multidisciplinary pain teams that treat CRPS. These comprise a physician (anesthetist or pediatrician), a psychiatrist or clinical psychologist, a physiotherapist, and sometimes an occupational therapist. The child initially undergoes a multidisciplinary assessment that involves both schooling and social circumstances. The physiotherapist carries out a thorough functional assessment.

The treatment focuses on improving function and, therefore, extensive physiotherapy is performed initially. Analgesics need to be used to facilitate this treatment and include anti-inflammatory drugs, amitriptyline, and gabapentin. In severe cases, regional blocks can be used to control the pain. Children appear to respond to physiotherapy better than adults and they require less medication and invasive procedures. The recurrence rate of CRPS is higher in children, though do they respond well to the reinitiation of treatment.[178]

PERONEAL TENDONITIS/DISLOCATION

Peroneal tendon pain can occur in both the operated and nonoperated foot. Pain in the peroneal tendons on movement or direct palpation may indicate prominent underlying implants. Simply removing the offending screw or plate may help. Buckingham et al.[20] recommended the routine removal of implants in their series of adolescent calcaneal fractures as this resulted in improved symptoms in 6 of 8 patients.

The extensile L-shaped lateral incision has largely prevented the peroneal tendon subluxation that used to occur with the Kocher incision. Care has to be taken at the proximal and distal ends of this incision as the sural nerve can be damaged and a painful neuroma can develop.

In patients with calcaneal fractures treated nonoperatively, a displaced lateral wall can sublux or even dislocate the peroneal tendons. Lateral impingement pain can also result from the fragment coming in direct contact with the fibula.

Diagnostic local anesthetic injections have been useful in differentiating the cause of pain in the adult foot but its use in children is limited. However, it can be considered in adolescents.

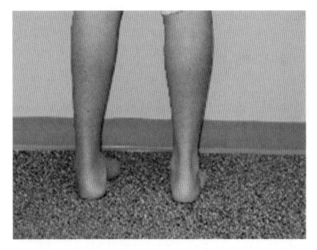

Figure 30-21. Posterior view demonstrating cavovarus deformity of the left foot. (Courtesy of Dr. Thomas Lee, MD.)

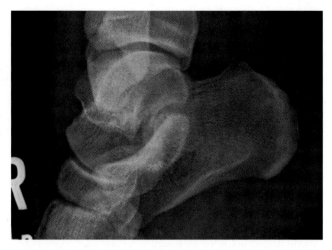

Figure 30-22. Lateral view showing subluxation of the subtalar joint.

Subtalar Dislocation

Subtalar dislocations (peritalar dislocation) occur infrequently and are particularly uncommon in children. They occur most often in young adult males. There are no series published on this condition in children; however, Dimentberg and Rosman[44] reported on five talonavicular dislocations.

A medial dislocation is the most common type (85%) and results from a forced inversion injury to the foot. The talonavicular and talocalcaneal ligaments rupture whereas the calcaneonavicular ligament stays intact. The result is that the bones of the foot dislocate medially whereas the talus remains in the ankle mortise (Fig. 30-21). The foot looks markedly deformed and the talar head can be palpated laterally. A lateral dislocation is caused by a forced eversion injury and results in a laterally displaced "flatfoot." Dougherty et al. presented a case report on this rare injury in a 19-month-old girl following a minor fall.[47]

Radiographs are difficult to interpret in this unusual injury (Figs. 30-22 and 30-23). The key is to look for the "empty navicular" where the talar head no longer articulates with it. A CT scan is useful to look for any associated fractures or osteochondral damage; however, it is probably more useful to perform this after a closed reduction to confirm anatomic alignment (Fig. 30-24).

The treatment for a closed subtalar dislocation is a reduction under general anesthesia. The knee should be flexed to relax the tendoachilles and then the deformity accentuated before a reduction is carried out. Usually, the reduction is stable and anatomic reduction can be confirmed by radiographs and CT

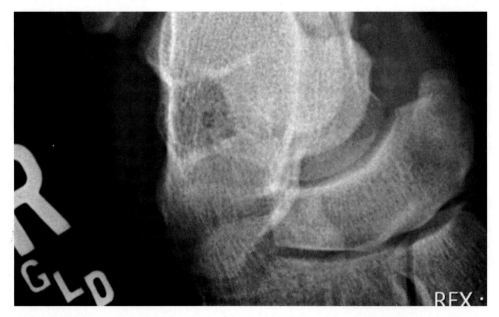

Figure 30-23. There is incongruity of the calcaneocuboid joint on the A/P x-ray associated with the subtalar subluxation.

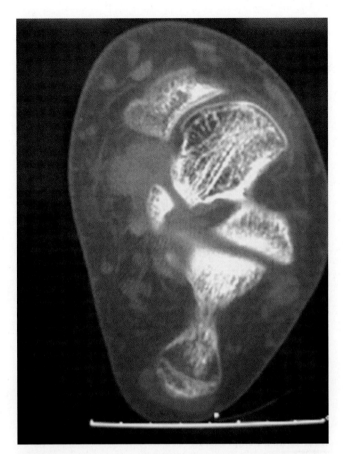

Figure 30-24. CT scan axial view shows marked talar head uncoverage ("ball is not in cup"). There is also significant incongruity of the subtalar joint. (Courtesy of Dr. Thomas Lee, MD.)

Isolated injuries to this area are rare and one needs to look for other associated fractures and dislocations.

Hosking and Hoffman[71a] reviewed four cases of midtarsal dislocations in children, and this is the only report in the literature of this injury in the pediatric age group. The children had an average age of 9.5 years, and the mechanism of injury was forced supination in three of the patients. They all had associated midtarsal injuries and presented with significant swelling. The key to making the diagnosis, which was delayed in three of the patients, was subluxation or dislocation of the calcaneocuboid joint on the lateral radiograph. The AP view only showed the dislocation in two patients and the oblique view showed it in one patient.

The dislocation can usually be reduced closed and held with percutaneous K-wires. If an anatomic reduction is not possible closed, then an open reduction must be performed.

A CT scan should be obtained to more clearly define the associated injuries to both the midtarsal bones and rest of the foot. One of the patients in Hosking and Hoffman's[71a] series had an ipsilateral tibial fracture. Therefore, associated injuries may be present due to the significant force required to cause a midfoot disruption in a child.

Isolated fractures of the mid tarsal bones are rare. The navicular, cuboid, and cuneiforms are usually fractured in association with a Chopart joint (talonavicular and calcaneocuboid) dislocation or a Lisfranc injury. The navicular has a number of conditions that can mimic a fracture. Between the ages of 2 and 5 years, the navicular can become avascular (Kohler disease) and cause pain and limp while the changes seen on radiograph can look similar to a fracture (Fig. 30-25). Likewise, an accessory navicular may mimic an avulsion fracture of the navicular tuberosity. These can be differentiated from a fracture as they

scan. The foot is immobilized until the child is comfortable enough to start gentle mobilizations. K-wire stabilization and 6 weeks of immobilization are necessary for unstable dislocations.

Occasionally, the subtalar dislocation is irreducible by closed means and has to be opened through an anteromedial approach. The bone or soft tissue (often the tibialis posterior tendon) is removed from the joint and the foot reduced.

Midtarsal Injuries

Fractures and dislocations of the navicular, cuboid, and cuneiforms are rare pediatric foot injuries. The midtarsal region extends from the calcaneocuboid and talonavicular joints (Chopart's joint) to the metatarsals. It includes the cuboid, navicular, and three cuneiform bones. These bones are interlinked by extremely strong ligaments especially on the plantar surface. The lateral side of the midfoot is more stable than the medial side. The shape of these small bones and strength of their ligaments help maintain the longitudinal and transverse arch of the foot. Disruption of this rigid anatomy therefore requires a large force especially in the cartilaginous bones of a child's foot.

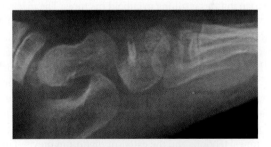

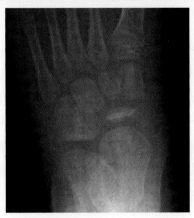

Figure 30-25. Kohler disease of the navicular that can occasionally be confused with a stress fracture.

have smooth, rounded edges and are usually symmetrical when a radiograph is taken of the other foot. Stress fractures of the navicular are also becoming an increasingly common problem as children and adolescents train more aggressively for competitions (see stress fractures of the foot). These stress fractures usually run in the sagittal plane in the middle third of the bone. They are often difficult to see on plain radiographs but are more easily seen on bone scans, CT, and MRI.

CUBOID FRACTURES

Cuboid fractures were considered a rare foot injury in children and were usually associated with other foot fractures. Recent literature, however, reveals that this fracture may occur more often than we thought and in isolation. Senaran et al.[163] reported on 28 consecutive cuboid fractures in preschool children from 1998 to 2004. They found most patients had an avoidance gait pattern and walked on the outside of their foot. They used the "nutcracker" maneuver to help diagnose the fracture. To perform this test, the heel is stabilized by the examiner and the forefoot is abducted. Pain in the lateral aspect of the foot indicates a cuboid fracture. The diagnosis was then confirmed on initial or subsequent radiographs. Initial radiographs did not demonstrate the fracture in 71% of cases. A below-knee cast or Cam walker was used for 2 to 3 weeks and all fractures healed without complications. Six patients had ipsilateral fractures in the tibia or foot.[158] Cuboid fractures have been classified by Weber and Locher[181] into distal impaction shear-type fractures (type 1) and burst fractures (type 2).

Ceroni et al.[30] reported on four female teenagers who had equestrian injuries resulting in cuboid fractures. The mechanism of the injury was a crush to the foot when the horse fell and abduction of the forefoot while it was still in the stirrup. All four cuboid fractures were associated with other midfoot fractures and the authors recommend CT scans for patients in this age group with a cuboid fracture. Two patients underwent surgical reconstruction and had good functional outcomes with return to sports. A lateral incision was used from the tip of the fibula to the base of the fifth metatarsal. The interval was developed between the peroneal tendons and the extensor digitorum brevis. The lateral column length was restored using an allograft block.[30]

Tarsometatarsal Injuries (Lisfranc Fracture–Dislocation)

INTRODUCTION TO TARSOMETATARSAL INJURIES

Tarsometatarsal (TMT) injuries, often referred to as a Lisfranc injury, are more common in adults than they are in children.[183] The degree of injury varies from a subtle disruption of the Lisfranc ligament to an extensive fracture–dislocation of the

forefoot. Subtle injury can be difficult to diagnose, and, if left untreated, can develop into a painful chronic problem.

Although mostly described as isolated case reports,[17,29,139] there are a few series reported in the literature.[22,71,181]

ASSESSMENT OF TARSOMETATARSAL INJURIES

MECHANISMS OF INJURY FOR TARSOMETATARSAL INJURIES

TMT injuries result from either a direct blow to the foot, usually secondary to a falling object, or by indirect forces, where there is forced plantarflexion of the forefoot combined with a rotational force (Fig. 30-26).[180,181] In a recent series, 61% were sports related.[71]

Traumatic Impact in the Tiptoe Position

This mechanism is an indirect injury where a load is applied to the foot while it is in the tiptoe position, such as when jumping to the ground and landing on the toes, producing acute plantarflexion at the TMT joint. The result is a TMT joint dislocation and usually a fracture at the base of the second metatarsal. Another example would be by putting the foot down suddenly to reduce speed while riding a bike.

Heel-to-Toe Compression

In this situation, the patient is in a kneeling position when the impact load strikes the heel, which is a direct compression type injury and usually results in lateral dislocation of the lesser metatarsals and fracture of the base of the second metatarsal.

The Fixed Forefoot

In this third mechanism, the child falls backward while the forefoot is fixed to the ground by a heavy weight. An example would be a fall backward while the foot is pinned under the wheel of a car. The patient's heel, which is resting on the ground, becomes the fulcrum for the forefoot injury.

In Wiley's[184] review of 18 patients with TMT joint injuries, 10 (56%) were a fall from a height in the "tiptoe" position, 3 (18%) suffered "heel-to-toe" compression, and 4 (22%) sustained a fall backward while their forefoot was pinned to the ground. One patient could not recall their mechanism of injury following a motorbike collision.

Atypical Lisfranc injuries have recently been reported in mini scooter injuries where the foot is planted to break speed. The resulting dorsiflexion, axial loading, and abduction cause the metatarsals to be impacted laterally. The result is a fracture of the base of the second metatarsal and a crush fracture of the cuboid.[13]

SIGNS AND SYMPTOMS OF TARSOMETATARSAL INJURIES

The diagnosis of these injuries may be difficult, and in adults as many as 20% of injuries are misdiagnosed or overlooked.[23] Some of the injuries are subtle and will present with minor

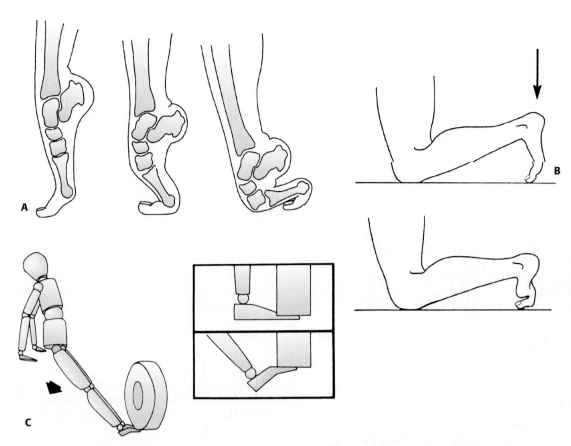

Figure 30-26. Mechanism of Lisfranc injuries. **A:** The most common mechanism of injury: Progression from the "tiptoe" position to complete collapse of the TMT joint. **B:** Plantarflexion injury: Direct heel-to-toe compression produces acute plantar flexion of the TMT joint. **C:** Backward fall with the forefoot pinned.

pain and swelling at the base of the first and second metatarsals. This finding can be accompanied by ecchymosis on the plantar aspect of the midfoot where the TMT ligaments have been torn (Fig. 30-27).[145] Gently abducting and pronating the forefoot while the hindfoot is held fixed with the other hand would indicate the injury,[120] though this would be quite painful acutely. Alternatively, the child can be asked to try and perform a single limb heel lift. Pain in the midfoot often implies a TMT joint injury. With significant trauma, there is greater ligamentous injury and the resulting swelling makes it difficult to recognize any bony anatomy. It is important to assess the foot for a compartment syndrome in such circumstances, particularly when the foot has been crushed as part of the mechanism of injury.

The examiner of any child's foot following trauma needs to have a high level of suspicion for a Lisfranc injury as they are uncommon and difficult to diagnose but can result in a poor outcome if left untreated.

CLASSIFICATION OF TARSOMETATARSAL INJURIES

Hardcastle et al.[64] developed a classification system based on the one developed by Quénu and Küss[140] in 1909 (Fig. 30-28).

- Type A: Total incongruity. There is total incongruity of the entire metatarsal joint in a single plane. This can be either coronal or sagittal or combined.

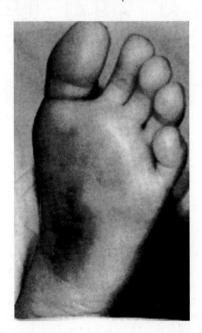

Figure 30-27. Plantar ecchymosis sign. Ecchymosis along the plantar aspect of the midfoot is an important clinical finding in subtle Lisfranc TMT injuries. (Reprinted with permission from Ross G, Cronin R, Hauzenblas J, et al. Plantar ecchymosis sign: A clinical aid to diagnosis of occult Lisfranc tarsometatarsal injuries. *J Orthop Trauma.* 1996;10(2):119–122.)

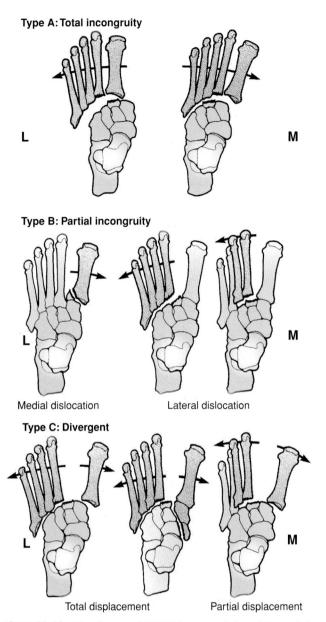

Type A: Total incongruity

L   M

Type B: Partial incongruity

L   M

Medial dislocation   Lateral dislocation

Type C: Divergent

L   M

Total displacement   Partial displacement

Figure 30-28. Classification of TMT dislocations. *L*, lateral; *M*, medial. (Redrawn from DeLee JC. Fractures and dislocations of the foot. In: Mann RA, Coughlin MJ. *Surgery of the Foot and Ankle.* 6th ed. St. Louis, MO: Mosby; 1993:1465–1703; Hardcastle PH, Reschauer R, Kutshca-Lissberg E, et al. Injuries to the tarsometatarsal joint. Incidence, classification, and treatment. *J Bone Joint Surg Br.* 1982;64(3):349–356.)

- Type B: Partial incongruity. Only partial incongruity of the joint is seen involving either medial displacement of the first metatarsal or lateral displacement to the four lateral metatarsals. The medial dislocation involves displacement of the first metatarsal from the first cuneiform because of disruption of the Lisfranc ligament or fracture at the base of the metatarsal, which remains attached to the ligament.
- Type C: Divergent pattern. The first metatarsal is displaced medially; any combination of the lateral four metatarsals may be displaced laterally. This is associated with partial or total incongruity.

This classification does not address the nondisplaced TMT joint injury, which can often be overlooked on initial assessment.

Most children's injuries are type B with minimal displacement, whereas types A and C are rare.[63,137,181]

IMAGING AND OTHER DIAGNOSTIC STUDIES FOR TARSOMETATARSAL INJURIES

The initial x-ray evaluation includes AP, lateral, and oblique views of the foot. These should be performed weight bearing if possible to stress the joint complex.

On the AP radiograph, the lateral border of the first metatarsal should be in line with the lateral border of the medial cuneiform and the medial border of the second metatarsal should line up with the medial border of the middle cuneiform. On the oblique radiograph, the medial border of the fourth metatarsal should be in line with the medial border of the cuboid. The examiner looks for a disruption in these lines. A recent radiographic review of pediatric feet non–weight-bearing AP views demonstrated normal relationships in the pediatric foot including an MT1 to MT2 distance of less than 3 mm and an MC to MT2 distance of less than 2 mm in children older than 6 years old (Fig. 30-29).[88] It is very useful to obtain a weight-bearing radiograph of the opposite foot for comparison (Fig. 30-30). When the radiographs appear normal or minimally displaced and a Lisfranc injury is still suspected, alternative imaging with CT or MRI scans is strongly recommended. The CT scan will

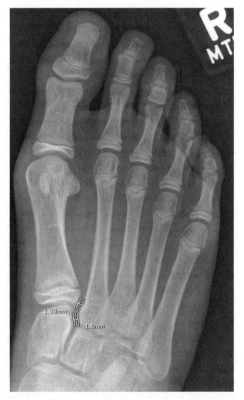

Figure 30-29. Measurement of the distance between the base of first metatarsal and second metatarsal (MT1-MT2 distance, measured at 1.88 mm in this image) and between the medial cuneiform and second metatarsal (MC-MT2 distance, measured at 1.8 mm in this image).

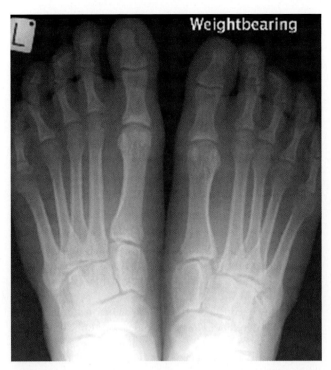

Figure 30-30. Weight-bearing radiographs show a subtle Lisfranc injury to the right foot. Weight-bearing radiographs are essential for diagnosis; using the opposite foot for comparison is also helpful.

often show a small avulsion fracture of the first TMT ligament and will show any other associated fractures in the foot.[59,93,105] The MRI scan can accurately visualize a partial tear or complete rupture of the first TMT ligament.[135]

A fracture of the base of the second metatarsal should alert the examiner to the possibility of a TMT dislocation, recognizing that these injuries can spontaneously reduce. Likewise, a cuboid fracture in combination with a fracture of the base of the second metatarsal is highly suspicious for a Lisfranc injury (Fig. 30-31). The figure legend says these two fractures are pathognomonic of a Lisfranc injury—need to be consistent here.

If weight-bearing radiographs are not possible, an abduction stress view can be obtained; however, in children these are difficult to obtain without general anesthesia. Bone scans may be helpful in the diagnosis of this injury when radiographs are normal, although they are not specific for the severity of the injury[61] and less useful than MRI or CT.

PATHOANATOMY AND APPLIED ANATOMY RELATING TO TARSOMETATARSAL INJURIES

The TMT joint complex comprises the TMT joints, the intertarsal joints, and the intermetatarsal joints. The area represents the apex of the longitudinal and transverse arches of the foot and therefore its structural integrity is crucial in maintaining normal foot function. At the same time, there needs to be enough motion between the joints to allow the transfer of weight evenly from the hindfoot to the forefoot during the walking cycle. This intricate relationship is achieved by the anatomy of the tarsal and metatarsal bones and the arrangement of the ligaments. These midfoot bones are trapezoidal in cross section with their base dorsal. This creates a "Roman arch" effect, which is structurally very strong and helps maintain the transverse arch in the midfoot. The TMT joint complex can be divided up into a medial column and a lateral column. The medial column is a continuation of the talus and navicular and includes the cuneiforms and the medial three metatarsals. The lateral column is a continuation of the calcaneus and comprises the cuboid and the fourth and fifth metatarsals which articulate with it. The medial column has far less mobility than the lateral column, reflecting the increased need for stability on the medial side of the foot to maintain the longitudinal arch. This stability is also provided by the second metatarsal, which is "keyed" into the step formed by the cuneiforms. This anatomy explains why the second metatarsal is usually fractured when a dislocation occurs across the TMT joint. The ligaments play a big role in maintaining stability medially and movement laterally, as well. The plantar ligaments are extremely strong compared to the weaker dorsal

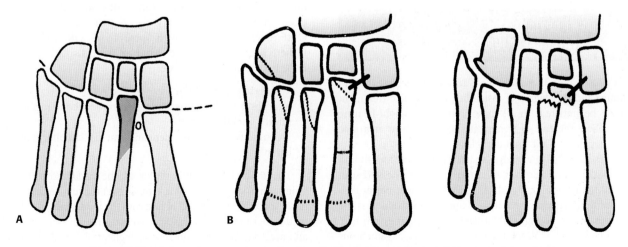

Figure 30-31. A: Second metatarsal is the "keystone" of the locking mechanism. **B:** Fractures of the cuboid and second metatarsal are pathognomonic signs of disruption of the TMT joints.

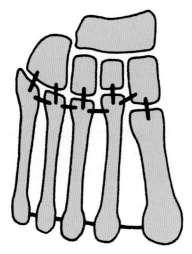

Figure 30-32. The ligamentous attachments at the TMT joints. There is only a flimsy connection between the bases of the first and second metatarsals (not illustrated). The second metatarsal is recessed and firmly anchored.

ligaments. The intermetatarsal ligaments help bind the lateral four metatarsals together but are absent between the first and second metatarsals. Instead, the second metatarsal is connected to the medial cuneiform by the Lisfranc ligament (medial interosseous ligament) (Fig. 30-32).

The dorsalis pedis artery crosses the cuneiforms before it courses between the first and second metatarsals to form the plantar arterial branch. The deep peroneal nerve travels beside the artery but continues on to supply sensation to the first web space. This neurovascular bundle can be damaged by the injury and care must be taken protect these structures when internally fixing these fracture–dislocations. The tibialis anterior tendon inserts into the base of the first metatarsal and medial cuneiform. The peroneous longus tendon inserts into the plantar surface of the base of the first metatarsal and acts as a flexor of this bone. Together, these two muscles and their tendon insertions give added stability to the medial column of the foot.

TREATMENT OPTIONS FOR TARSOMETATARSAL INJURIES

The key to treating these injuries is to recognize the extent of the injury and the degree of instability. Appropriate treatment can then be initiated. In all these injuries, a weight-bearing radiograph at the end of treatment should confirm anatomic congruency of the TMT joint complex.

When a clinical diagnosis of a "sprain" is made, the foot should be immobilized in a below-knee cast for 6 weeks. The MRI scan may confirm a partial tear of the first TMT ligament. Regardless this painful injury takes time to heal and immobilization is the best treatment. In young adult athletes, these injuries can take a long time to heal.[114] When there is complete intraligamentous rupture or an avulsion fracture of the first TMT ligament and no displacement of the joint surfaces, a below-knee cast for 6 weeks

is advised. Whether the patient should be weight bearing or not for the entire 6 weeks is debatable. Wiley[184] treated the children with undisplaced TMT joint injuries in his series with 3 to 4 weeks of immobilization with good results.

Displaced fractures of the TMT joint need to be anatomically reduced and stabilized. Myerson et al.[121] found that following a closed reduction greater than 2-mm displacement or a talometatarsal angle of greater than 15 degrees would lead to a poor outcome. A closed reduction is best carried out under a general anesthetic when the acute swelling has subsided. "Finger traps" can help with traction on the toes while the displaced metatarsals are manipulated into place. If a stable anatomic reduction is achieved clinically and this is confirmed radiologically, a well-molded below-knee cast can be applied. Radiographs in the cast should also be taken while the patient is under anesthesia to confirm the reduction has been held. The non–weight-bearing cast is worn for 6 weeks with radiographs taken at 1 and 2 weeks to confirm the fracture–dislocation has remained reduced.

If the closed reduction results in an anatomic reduction but the fragments are unstable, K-wire fixation is used to hold the alignment of the foot. Stout 0.062-in smooth K-wires should be used. Their placement is determined by the direction of displacement of the metatarsals and how many are involved. The most important wire is used to stabilize the second metatarsal to the medial cuneiform. Additional wires can be used between the first metatarsal and the medial cuneiform, and between the lesser metatarsals and their corresponding tarsal bones. A useful wire can also be passed from the first metatarsal to the second metatarsal. These K-wires are left bent over outside of the skin and are removed at 4 to 6 weeks when mobilization is initiated if the radiographs confirm healing. Again, full weight-bearing radiographs are necessary when comfort allows and after K-wire removal to confirm adequate stability. Wiley[184] used K-wire fixation in four patients. He removed these at 3 to 4 weeks and the alignment was maintained in all the children. There were some joint incongruities from intra-articular fractures that were not surgically addressed but they did not seem to alter the clinical outcome.

ORIF is rarely required for these fractures in younger children. However, in a recent series of 56 patients with a Lisfranc injury and mean age of 14.2 years, ORIF was used in 34% of cases. In this series, skeletally mature patients tended to have ORIF more than patients with open physes. ORIF is indicated if there is greater than 1 to 2 mm of joint displacement. The impediments to reduction are:

- Tibialis anterior tendon
- Interposition of fracture fragments in the second metatarsal-middle cuneiform joint
- Incongruity of the first metatarsal-medial cuneiform articulation[15]

The entire TMT joint complex can be visualized using two longitudinal incisions.[155] One is made over the first second metatarsal space and the second in line with the fourth metatarsal. The medial incision allows identification of the neurovascular bundle and access to the first and second metatarsal cuneiform joints. The lateral incision allows access to the lesser TMT joints. After anatomic reduction, the joints can held reduced with K-wires or

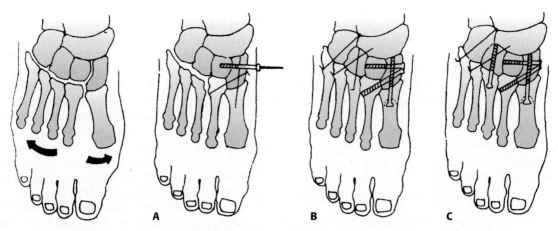

Figure 30-33. Sequence of repair for reduction and stabilization of TMT fracture–dislocations. **A:** Stabilization of the first ray by alignment of the metatarsal, medial cuneiform, and navicular. **B:** Stabilization of the Lisfranc ligament by accurate alignment of the second metatarsal to the medial cuneiform, as well as the medial and middle cuneiforms. **C:** Alignment and stabilization of the third through fifth metatarsal rays. Cannulated screws can be used instead of pins as needed for stability and compression. (Redrawn from Trevino SG, Kodros S. Controversies in tarsometatarsal injuries. *Orthop Clin North Am.* 1995;26:229–238.)

with 3.5-mm screws (Fig. 30-33). Small chondral defects can be excised and larger ones repaired. Care must be taken to avoid the proximal growth plate of the first metatarsal if screw fixation is used. The use of K-wire stabilization of the lesser metatarsals rather than screws as it is important to maintain the mobility in these joints long-term. Debate exists as to when to remove the

screws across these weight-bearing joints. In a child, it would seem appropriate to remove the screws once pain free weight bearing is established as the ligaments and bone would have healed by this stage and further displacement is unlikely. Leaving the screws in for longer than 3 months risks damage to the joint and possible screw breakage.

Authors' Preferred Treatment for Tarsometatarsal Injuries (Algorithm 30-3)

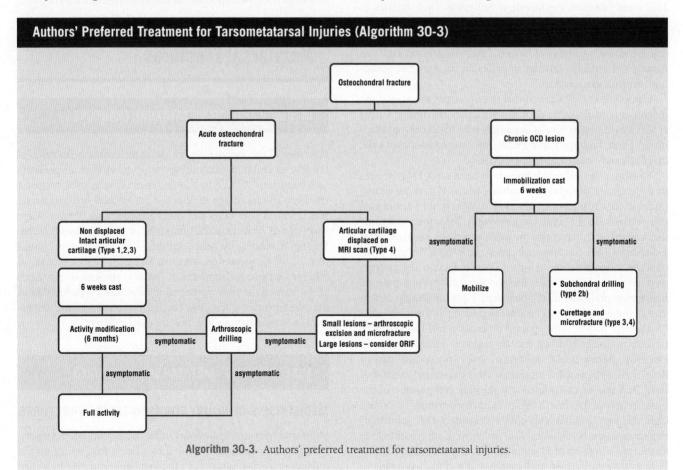

Algorithm 30-3. Authors' preferred treatment for tarsometatarsal injuries.

Most children have a type B TMT dislocation with minimal displacement. The most important step in treatment is confirming the diagnosis and treating them until the joint is stable. If any doubt exists, the author takes a comparable radiograph of the other foot. The author routinely orders a CT scan of the midfoot to assess the extent of the injury and to look for any associated injuries.

An injury with less than 1 to 2 mm of displacement is treated in a below-knee non–weight-bearing cast for 6 weeks. Weight-bearing radiographs are taken after removal of the cast to assess stability. These radiographs are repeated 6 weeks later once pain free weight bearing is achieved to confirm no further displacement.

If the TMT joint is displaced greater than 1 to 2 mm, then the author performs a closed reduction and routinely uses percutaneous K-wire fixation with image intensifier assistance. Although these injuries can be held with cast immobilization, the author prefers the assurance of knowing the fracture–dislocation is being held internally. This fixation is especially useful when the foot is very swollen and repeated assessments are necessary to rule out compartment syndrome. In the rare circumstance of an open reduction, the author prefers to use temporary screw fixation. These injuries are usually far more severe than a type B dislocation and the TMT joints are very unstable. After open reduction through two longitudinal incisions, 3.5-mm cortical screws are used to hold the reduction taking care to avoid the proximal growth plate of the first metatarsal. These screws are removed usually within a month of cast removal.

Regardless of the way the fracture–dislocation is treated, all these patients must be investigated at outpatient appointments with weight-bearing radiographs to confirm that the ligaments have healed and there is no residual subluxation.

MANAGEMENT OF EXPECTED ADVERSE OUTCOMES AND UNEXPECTED COMPLICATIONS RELATED TO COMPLICATIONS OF TARSOMETATARSAL INJURIES

The most common complication following TMT injuries is posttraumatic arthritis, which often occurs because the injury is "missed" and a subtle fracture–dislocation remains displaced. Another cause is a loss of reduction. Lastly, the trauma itself can damage the articular cartilage and, despite an anatomic reduction, arthritis can develop.

Hardcastle et al.[64] showed that the outcomes are poor if the diagnosis is made more than 6 weeks after the injury. Curtis et al.[38] found similar results in athletes who had a delayed diagnosis. These findings reinforce the importance of making the diagnosis early and treating appropriately.

Posttraumatic arthritis is known to occur after TMT injuries in a significant percentage of adults, which is best prevented by achieving an anatomic reduction.[120] Wiss et al.[188] performed gait analysis on 11 adult patients with TMT joint fracture–dislocations and found that no patient walked normally after a displaced TMT fracture–dislocation. In Wiley's[184] series of 18 children, none of whom required open reduction, 14 patients were asymptomatic 3 to 8 months postinjury. Four patients had minor persisting TMT joint pain 1 year following injury. Two of these patients had residual angulation at the injury site. One patient had an unrecognized dislocation and had not been treated; the other had not had an anatomic reduction due to extensive intra-articular fractures. One 16-year-old patient developed asymptomatic osteonecrosis of the second metatarsal head, and this was attributed to a possible compromise of the blood supply at the time of injury. Buoncristiani et al.[22] followed eight children (3 to 10 years old) with indirect TMT joint injuries treated in a below-knee cast. Seven were asymptomatic at an average follow-up of 32 months; one developed early degenerative changes on radiographs and had midfoot pain.

The treatment for painful TMT joint arthritis is arthrodesis if conservative care fails, which is extremely unusual in children. An arthrodesis often requires extensive soft tissue release to allow anatomic reduction of the joint and rigid internal fixation with screws. It is important not to fuse the lesser TMT joints if possible as mobility here is important for the long-term foot function.

Metatarsal Fractures

INTRODUCTION TO METATARSAL FRACTURES

Fractures of the metatarsals are the most common fractures of the foot in children, accounting for up to 60% of all pediatric foot fractures.[37,38,125,162] In a large series of metatarsal fractures, children 5 years of age or less had an isolated first metatarsal fracture in 51% of cases and children older than 5 years of age had isolated fifth metatarsal fractures in 55% of cases.[147a] This finding is echoed by other authors.[125,162] Owen et al. found that 7% of all metatarsal fractures and 20% of first metatarsal fractures were not diagnosed at initial consultation. Fractures of the base of the fifth metatarsal are discussed separately from the other metatarsal fractures because the anatomy, fracture patterns, and treatment indications are quite different.

ASSESSMENT OF METATARSAL FRACTURES

MECHANISMS OF INJURY FOR METATARSAL FRACTURES

Metatarsal fractures result from either a direct or indirect injury. Direct injuries are usually caused by a heavy load falling on the forefoot or a crush injury (i.e., the foot being run over by a car).

The metatarsals can be fractured anywhere along the shaft but typically they are fractured middiaphyseal. Indirect injuries are caused by axial loading or torsional forces and usually produce spiral fractures of the proximal shaft or neck of the metatarsal. Singer et al.[166] found in a recent study of 125 children that if the patient was less than 5 years of age, the most common mechanism was a fall from a height occurring within the home. In children older than 5 years of age, the most common mechanism occurred playing sports and on a level playing surface.

SIGNS AND SYMPTOMS OF METATARSAL FRACTURES

Direct injuries can result in significant swelling and bruising of the foot due to soft tissue injury as well as the metatarsal fractures. Careful evaluation for compartment syndrome should take place. An indirect injury usually has more subtle clinical findings and careful palpation will usually locate the site of the fracture. An infant with a metatarsal fracture due to an unwitnessed injury may present with minimal swelling but an inability to bear weight.

INJURIES ASSOCIATED WITH METATARSAL FRACTURES

Proximal fractures of the metatarsals are often associated with tarsal fractures or fracture–dislocations, which should be evaluated further with a CT scan. A fracture of the second metatarsal and a cuboid fracture are highly suggestive of a TMT joint dislocation rather than two isolated fractures. Singer et al.[166] found that the first and fifth metatarsals were more often isolated fractures, whereas if multiple metatarsals were fractured, they were always contiguous bones and involved the second, third, and fourth metatarsals.

IMAGING AND OTHER DIAGNOSTIC STUDIES FOR METATARSAL FRACTURES

Radiographic evaluation should consist of AP, lateral, and oblique views of the whole foot. The AP view often gives the impression that the fractures are minimally displaced; however, the lateral view can show significant plantar or dorsal displacement. Other associated fractures may be apparent on the plain radiographs and if any doubt exists, especially if there has been significant trauma, a CT scan of the entire foot is advised. In a young child, if a metatarsal fracture is suspected but not visible on the initial radiograph, a repeat film taken 10 to 14 days later often shows the fracture or early callus.

CLASSIFICATION OF METATARSAL FRACTURES

No classification system exists for fractures of the first through fourth metatarsals. Fractures of the fifth metatarsal are classified according to location (see section on fifth metatarsal treatment below).

TREATMENT OPTIONS FOR METATARSAL FRACTURES

Most metatarsal fractures in children can be treated nonoperatively in a below-knee cast. The child with a displaced fracture often needs to be admitted overnight for pain relief and observation for compartment syndrome. The initial treatment includes elevation for the severe swelling that coexists with the fractures. Immobilization may be performed by a well-padded cast, splint, or a Cam walker. Once the swelling subsides, a molded below-knee cast can be applied. Weight bearing can be initiated when pain allows, and the cast can usually be removed at 3 to 4 weeks at which time the patient can be transitioned to a Cam walker.

The acceptable amount of angulation or shortening in a child has not been determined. A closed reduction of the central metatarsals is indicated in an adult if there is more than 10 degrees angulation in the dorsal plain or more than 4 mm of translation in any plane.[160] These criteria may be appropriate for an older adolescent whose growth plates had closed but are far too stringent for a skeletally immature patient. If there is severe dorsal angulation of greater than 20 degrees or "tenting" of the skin and shortening of greater than 5 mm, then a closed reduction is indicated, which is best performed under a general anesthetic when the swelling has subsided. Finger traps have been advocated by some surgeons to help with traction while the metatarsals are manipulated. A below-knee cast can be molded on both the dorsal and plantar aspects of the foot; however, the need to allow for swelling suggests implants should be used to hold fracture reduction rather than molding of a cast. To accommodate the swelling, the cast can be applied with the ankle in slight equinus. When it is changed 2 weeks later, a neutral position can be obtained.

First metatarsal fractures need careful attention, especially in an adolescent patient. The first ray is important in maintaining the longitudinal arch of the foot. The position of the first metatarsal head in relation to the lesser metatarsal heads is also important. A closed reduction should be considered if there is greater than 10 degrees of dorsal angulation or any shortening of the first metatarsal. It is unusual to have angulation in the coronal plane if the second metatarsal is intact and transverse displacement is acceptable if there is no shortening.

If a closed reduction is performed, K-wire fixation is at times required. Intramedullary placement is difficult to perform without opening the fracture and passing the wires under direct vision. Small, dorsal, longitudinal incisions are made over the fracture sites and dissection is carefully carried out down to the fracture. The wire is drilled down the distal fragment to exit the plantar skin. The wire is then withdrawn enough to allow the fracture to be reduced, then the wire is driven retrograde across the fracture site and sufficiently far enough into the proximal fragment. Another technique is to hold fracture reduction by placing K-wires across the fractured metatarsal to an adjacent nonfractured metatarsal both proximal and distal to the fracture. The K-wire is cut and bent outside the skin to facilitate removal in the outpatient clinic 3 to 4 weeks later when the patient can be placed in a walking cast for 2 more weeks to allow fracture consolidation. This technique can also be used when an open reduction is required for an irreducible fracture or the fracture is open.

FRACTURES OF THE BASE OF THE FIFTH METATARSAL

Fractures of the fifth metatarsal are the most common metatarsal fracture in children, constituting almost 50% of all metatarsal

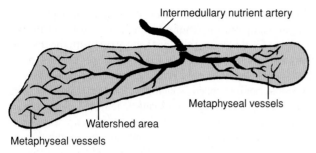

Figure 30-34. Blood supply of the proximal fifth metatarsal.

fractures in some series.[68,125,138,162] Traditionally, treatment has been based on the adult literature.

The fifth metatarsal has a number of tendinous insertions at its base. The peroneus brevis tendon inserts on the dorsal aspect of the tubercle and the peroneus tertius attaches on the dorsal aspect of the fifth metatarsal at the metaphyseal–diaphyseal junction. The strong plantar aponeurosis inserts into the plantar aspect of the tubercle at the base.

The nutrient artery enters the shaft of the fifth metatarsal medially at the junction of the proximal and middle thirds of the diaphysis and sends intraosseous branches proximally and distally (Fig. 30-34). Proximally within the bone are the metaphyseal vessels, and the small area where these overlap with the proximal vessels from the nutrient artery is known as the watershed area. This region corresponds with Zone 2 and fractures in this area have a higher rate delayed of union or nonunion in those close to maturity. The proximal apophyseal growth center of the fifth metatarsal can often be confused for a fracture. One series of diagnosed proximal fifth metatarsal fractures in children ages 7 to 16 years old found that 47% of these injuries were actually a misidentified growth center.[144] The apophyseal growth center (os vesalianum) has a longitudinal

orientation roughly parallel to the metatarsal shaft, which distinguishes it from a transverse orientated fracture (Fig. 30-35). The os vesalianum usually appears by age 9 years and unites with the metaphysis between ages 12 and 15 years (Fig. 30-36).

Classification

Fractures of the base of the fifth metatarsal are classified into one of three zones according to their location (Fig. 30-37). Zone 1 is the cancellous tuberosity, which includes the insertion of the peroneus brevis tendon, the abductor digiti minimi tendon, and the strong calcaneometatarsal ligament of the plantar fascia. Zone 2 is the distal aspect of the tuberosity where the dorsal and plantar ligamentous attachments to the fourth metatarsal attach. Zone 3 extends from distal to these ligamentous attachments to approximately the middiaphyseal area. Herrera-Soto et al.[69] classified fifth metatarsal fractures in a review of 103 children. They define a type I fracture as a "fleck" injury. A type II fracture is a tubercle fracture with an intra-articular extension. A type III fracture represents a fracture at the proximal diaphyseal region (Jones fracture).

Treatment

Traditionally, treatment has reflected the adult literature. Treatment of fractures of the base of the fifth metatarsal in children is determined primarily by the fracture zone, and, somewhat, by age.

Zone 1 Fractures

These injuries are usually traction-type injuries where the force from the peroneus brevis tendon and the pull from the plantar aponeurosis result in an avulsion fracture of the fifth metatarsal. Some authors suggest the fracture may be an avulsion at the origin of abductor digiti minimi.[83,143] Treatment involves a weight-bearing below-knee walking cast for 3 to

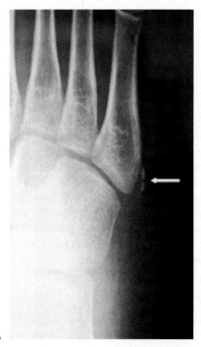

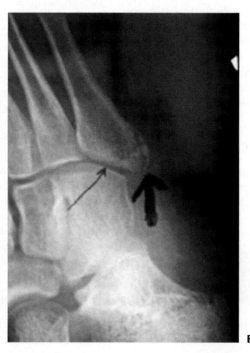

A   **B**

Figure 30-35. A: A normal apophysis of the base of the fifth metatarsal at the attachment of the peroneus brevis (*arrow*) in a 10-year-old girl. **B:** The *thicker arrow* points to the normal apophysis, which is roughly parallel to the metatarsal. The *thinner arrow* points toward a fracture, which is roughly perpendicular to metatarsal.

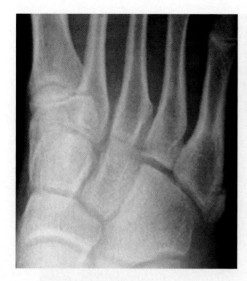

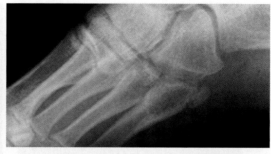

Figure 30-36. This 11-year-old girl had pain in her proximal fifth metatarsal after twisting her foot during physical education at school. No fracture was visible; however, her secondary ossification center is clearly seen running parallel to the shaft of the metatarsal.

6 weeks. Herrera-Soto et al.[69] found all 30 of their children with an extra-articular type 1 fracture treated in this way healed with good outcomes even if they were displaced. Undisplaced intra-articular tuberosity fractures also healed well in the series[68]; however, displaced (>2 mm) intra-articular fractures took significantly longer to heal. Radiographic union usually lags behind resolution of symptoms, and most patients are asymptomatic after 3 weeks.[68] This delay in radiographic union should not prevent the child returning to full activities as symptoms allow. Treatment with a Cam walker rather than a cast may be considered. Nonunion can occur but usually is asymptomatic.[39] Although operative fixation of acute tuberosity avulsions rarely is indicated, it may be considered for significant displacement (more than 3 mm) in young active patients who want to return to competitive sports sooner (Fig. 30-38).

Zone 2 Fractures

Zone 2 fractures include the Jones fracture, which is an oblique fracture in the watershed area at the proximal metaphyseal–diaphyseal junction. It typically occurs in adolescents and is thought to be caused by a combination of vertical loading and coronal shear forces at the junction of the stable proximal metaphysis and the mobile fifth metatarsal diaphysis. Frequently, these fractures are stress injuries, usually involving athletic adolescents who present with a traumatic event superimposed on prior symptoms.[24,36,81,82,92,148] Determining the duration of symptoms is important because chronic injuries are unlikely to respond to nonoperative treatment as well as acute

fractures. Critical radiographic analysis will show cortical sclerosis in the chronic injuries.

Acute injuries should be immobilized in a short-leg non–weight-bearing cast for 6 weeks. Serial radiographs and examinations are necessary to determine adequate healing. Further non–weight-bearing immobilization may be necessary if the fracture has not healed clinically and radiographically at 6 weeks. With evidence of callus and diminished tenderness, the patient can begin protected weight bearing in a hard-soled shoe or Cam walker for an additional 4 weeks. This protected weight bearing may prevent refracture.[68] In a series of adults successful healing in 14 of 15 patients treated with non–weight-bearing casts, whereas only 4 of 10 who were allowed to bear weight went on to union.[172] Herrera-Soto et al.[69] reported 15 fractures in this zone (type III) and found a higher rate of delayed union and refracture in patients over 13 years of age. They feel that primary internal fixation in this age group may be indicated.

For chronic zone 2 fractures with more than 3 months of symptoms, nonoperative management is unlikely to be successful. Nonetheless, it is worthwhile initially trying 6 weeks immobilization in a non–weight-bearing below-knee cast or brace. If this attempt fails, internal fixation is required. One technique is to insert an intramedullary screw from proximal to distal to stabilize the fracture site. A 4-mm cancellous screw is usually sufficient; however, in an older adolescent with a capacious intramedullary canal, a 6.5-mm cancellous screw may give better fixation and compression. It is beneficial to curette the intramedullary canal and use cancellous bone graft, which can be harvested from the distal tibia (Fig. 30-39).[94]

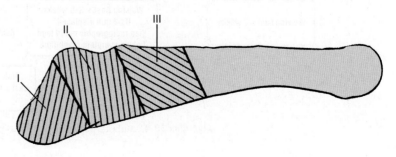

Figure 30-37. The three anatomic zones of the proximal fifth metatarsal.

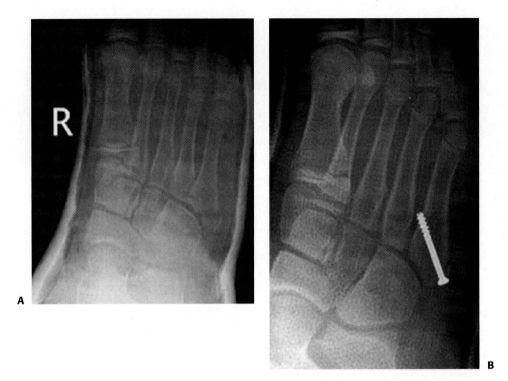

Figure 30-38. A: A 12-year-old boy who is a professional snowboarder with a displaced, intra-articular fifth metatarsal fracture. **B:** This was reduced open and internally fixed, which allowed him to compete 8 weeks after surgery.

Zone 3 Fractures

Zone 3 fractures are usually stress fractures in athletes. Acute fractures in this zone with no prodromal symptoms can be treated with a below-knee non–weight-bearing cast for 6 weeks followed by protective weight bearing for 4 weeks. In the more common scenario, involving pain with activity for several months, this period of casting is often unsuccessful but worth trying initially.

The stress fracture may heal clinically with 6 to 12 weeks of immobilization and radiographs will confirm the reconstitution of the medullary canal and fracture site less sclerosis. Electrical or ultrasound stimulation may be used. If the chronic stress fracture does not heal, surgical intervention is required similar to that in a zone 2 fracture outlined above. Some authors advocate a more aggressive open debridement of the fracture site with bone grafting before introducing the intramedullary screw.[137,172]

Authors' Preferred Treatment of Metatarsal Fractures (Algorithm 30-4)

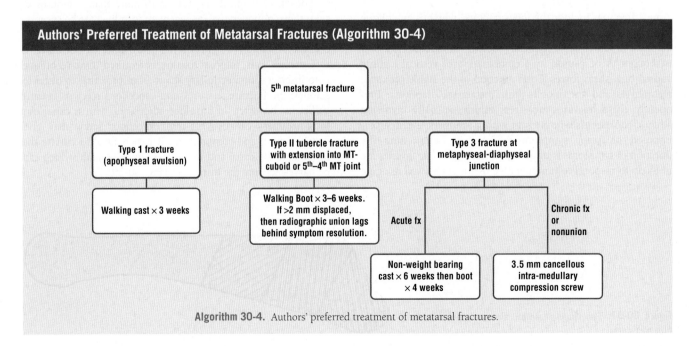

Algorithm 30-4. Authors' preferred treatment of metatarsal fractures.

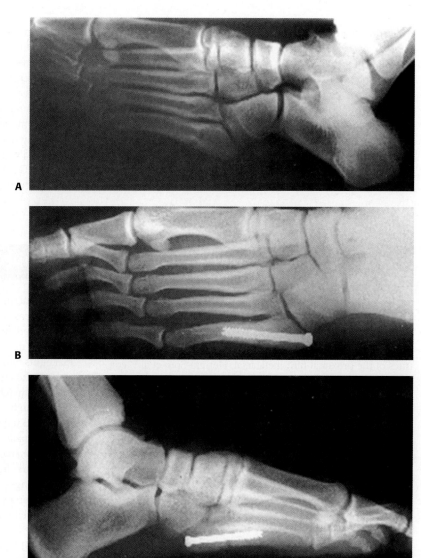

Figure 30-39. This 15-year-old high-level basketball player sustained a proximal fifth metatarsal fracture at the metaphyseal–diaphyseal junction. The patient chose intramedullary screw fixation because of his desire to return to sports as promptly as possible, lessen his time in immobilization, and lessen the risk of delayed union or nonunion. **A:** Radiograph at time of injury. **B, C:** After intramedullary screw fixation. (Courtesy of Keith S. Hechtman, MD.)

Lesser metatarsal fractures are usually treated nonoperatively in a below-knee walking cast for 3 to 4 weeks. Grossly displaced fractures in older children with greater than 20 degrees of dorsiflexion or more than 5 mm of shortening are treated with closed reduction under a general anesthetic and a well-molded below-knee cast. If the reduction is difficult, percutaneous K-wires are used for supplementary support. Except for open injuries, rarely is an open reduction through longitudinal incisions required.

A shortened or rotated distal fracture of the first or fifth metatarsal is treated by closed reduction and crossed K-wire fixation.

Proximal fifth metatarsal fractures present a more challenging problem. Treatment is determined by the location of the fracture in the bone and the age and activity level of the child. If inadequately treated, they can go on to a delayed or nonunion. For zone 1 fractures that are intra-articular and displaced greater than 3 to 4 mm, the author recommends

ORIF with a 3.5-mm partially threaded screw, especially if the child is involved in competitive sports, as this will allow an earlier return to sports. This fixation is perpendicular to the fracture line and gives maximum compression. The screw is inserted through a direct lateral approach. Care must be taken to identify and protect the sural nerve, which is usually directly under the incision. The peroneous brevis and peroneous tertius tendons are identified, and the area between them at their insertion into the proximal fifth metatarsal is a good starting point for the screw. The author prefers to insert a bicortical cannulated compression screw. This can either be a partially threaded cancellous screw or a fully threaded cortical screw. The fracture can usually be indirectly reduced and held with a K-wire. In difficult fracture patterns or in delayed presentations, the fracture line needs to be clearly seen and can be held reduced with a compression clamp.

The author treats zone 2 fractures (Jones fractures) with a non–weight-bearing cast for 6 weeks and then protected weight bearing in a moon-boot for 2 to 4 weeks as comfort allows. A study by Herrera-Soto et al.[69] showing poor results with this treatment in patients more than 13 years old indicates that primary internal fixation may be a better option in this age group. Acute zone 3 fractures are treated similarly, with perhaps earlier weightbearing if nondisplaced, or there are early signs of healing

Chronic fractures or nonunions should be treated with internal fixation. The author prefers to perform this with an intramedullary screw that compresses the fracture site. If a 3.5-mm cancellous screw does not achieve adequate internal fixation in the medullary canal, increase the diameter of the screw until it does. Often, a 4-mm malleolar screw is used. Sclerotic bone can be removed with a small curette down the medullary canal. If this is not possible, the fracture site should be debrided open with small osteotomes and rongeurs. Bone grafting is required for these chronic injuries and can be harvested from the distal tibia.

Grossly displaced shaft and distal metaphyseal fractures are treated with closed reduction and cast immobilization for 6 weeks. Occasionally, crossed K-wires are required.

MANAGEMENT OF EXPECTED ADVERSE OUTCOMES AND UNEXPECTED COMPLICATIONS RELATED TO METATARSAL FRACTURES

The most common complication of treating metatarsal fractures is nonunion, which is more common in zone 2 and zone 3 fractures of the proximal fifth metatarsal. Herrera-Soto et al.[69] concluded that pediatric fifth metatarsal fractures behaved similarly to adult fractures and can be treated the same. If a symptomatic nonunion develops and surgery is indicated, the procedure should include a thorough debridement of the sclerotic medullary canal, bone graft, and a strong appropriately sized compression screw across the fracture site.[58]

Phalangeal Injuries

INTRODUCTION TO PHALANGEAL INJURIES

Phalangeal fractures are common in children and may account for up to 18% of pediatric foot fractures.[37] Most toe injuries are treated by primary care physicians, so orthopedic surgeons only see the more severe fractures. Phalangeal fractures are the result of direct trauma by a falling object or indirect trauma when the unprotected toe is struck against a hard object (the so-called "stubbing"). The proximal phalanx is more commonly injured than the distal phalanges.

The toes must be closely examined for any break in the skin especially at the base of the nail as this may indicate an open Salter–Harris fracture with an associated nail bed injury. These compound injuries require a thorough debridement, repair of the nail bed, and often a single longitudinal K-wire to stabilize the fracture (Fig. 30-40). IV antibiotics should be given for 24 hours followed by 7 days of oral antibiotics. Nail bed injuries should be repaired as meticulously as in the hand with glue or sutures. A poorly repaired germinal matrix will cause abnormal nail growth and difficulty with shoe wear long after the fracture has healed.

TREATMENT OPTIONS FOR PHALANGEAL INJURIES

Closed fractures of the phalanges rarely require reduction and can be treated by simple "buddy strapping" to the adjacent toe and immediate mobilization. A hard-soled shoe or Cam walker may help minimize pain; however, crowding in the toe box may make this more uncomfortable than bare feet. An angulated toe in both the coronal and sagittal plane usually remodels well if the growth plate is still open. In adolescents, a percutaneous K-wire can be used if the fracture is grossly unstable and unable to be held reduced by strapping alone. This wire can be passed longitudinally through the tip of the affected toe or obliquely across the fracture. It is extremely unusual to get any growth disturbance from a smooth wire crossing the growth plate in the phalanges. These pins can be removed in clinic 4 to 6 weeks later. Laterally angulated fractures of the little toe sometimes need closed reduction before strapping them to the fourth toe.

NAIL BED INJURIES

✔ **Repair of Nail Bed Injuries:**
SURGICAL STEPS

- ☐ Use sterile tourniquet (glove)
- ☐ Remove the nail
- ☐ Thoroughly clean the nail bed gently
- ☐ Repair the nail bed with fine absorbable suture (6-0 or 7-0 rapid dissolving suture) or glue
- ☐ Protect the eponychial fold by replacing the nail or holding it open with another spacer
- ☐ Cover with sterile dressing and tape
- ☐ Leave dressing intact for 10 days then debulk dressing

Nail bed injuries to the toes should be treated similarly to those to the fingers. Failure to address the nail bed adequately can lead to abnormal nail growth and problems with shoewear (Fig. 30-41).

GREAT TOE FRACTURES

The great toe is injured by the same mechanisms as the lesser toes, with sports injury being a common etiology.[134] Standard AP and lateral radiographs are taken. It is useful to have the

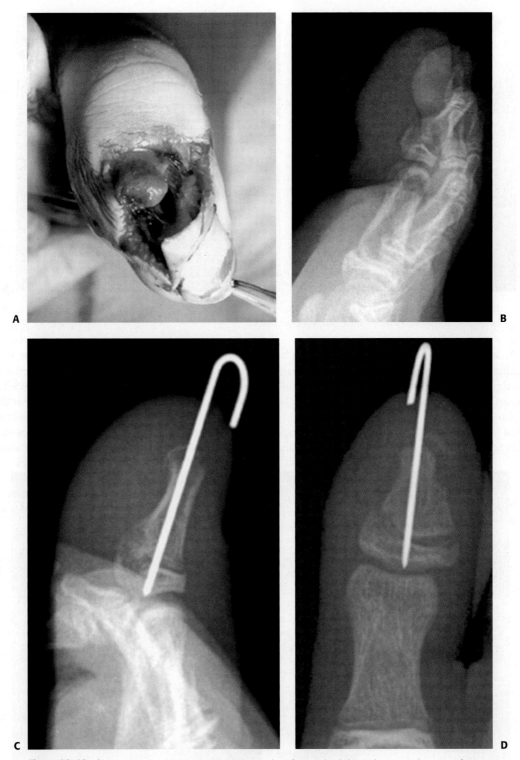

Figure 30-40. A: This 7-year-old boy "stubbed" his toe barefoot on his bike and sustained an open fracture of the tuft of the distal phalanx and associated laceration of the germinal matrix. **B:** Preoperative radiograph shows the small tuft fracture. **C, D:** The wound was thoroughly debrided, germinal matrix repaired, and a K-wire passed across the fracture to hold the fragment and soft tissues reduced.

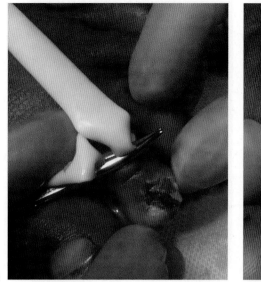
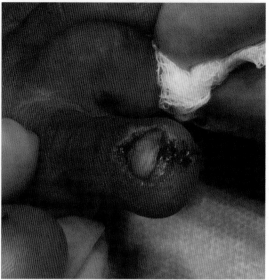

Figure 30-41. Second toe distal phalangeal fracture with nail bed split. **A:** Before repair of nail bed. **B:** Nail bed repaired with absorbable suture and nail glued back.

patient hold the lesser toes dorsiflexed with a small towel to maximize visualization on the lateral view. Intra-articular fractures of the proximal phalanx are more common in the great toe than the other toes. They are usually Salter–Harris type III or IV fractures (Fig. 30-42).

Most of these fractures can be managed with "buddy strapping" to the second toe. If greater than 25% of the joint surface is involved and there is displacement of more than 2 to 3 mm of the joint surface, reduction should be performed. Fracture reduction may be held by strapping to the second toe or a percutaneous K-wire. In the rare occasion that this is not successful, an open reduction can be performed either through a midlateral or dorsal incision. However, caution should be advised when pursuing open reduction of these injuries as

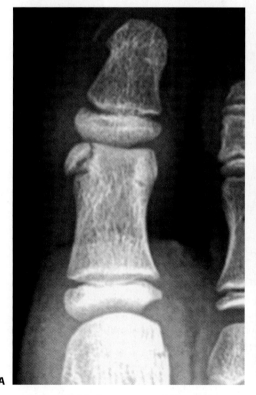
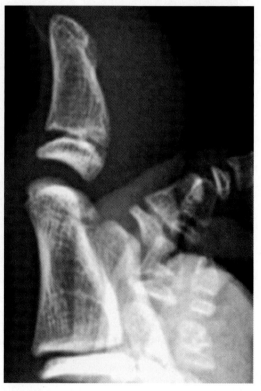

Figure 30-42. A: An 11-year-old boy with an intra-articular fracture of the proximal phalanx of the great toe. Successful treatment was achieved with simple buddy strapping. **B:** A lateral radiograph of the great toe is best taken with the lesser toes held flexed with a bandage.

Kramer et al.[89] reported significant complications in six out or nine patients treated with open reduction in their series. With diaphyseal fractures, axial alignment and rotation both need to be addressed with the closed reduction. Often, the clinical appearance of the toe following the reduction is more useful than the postreduction radiograph as the toe usually looks "fine" even though the radiograph shows malalignment.

Other Injuries to the Foot

LAWNMOWER AND OTHER MUTILATING INJURIES

There are approximately 9,400 lawnmower injuries a year in the United States affecting children 20 years or younger with an average age of 10.7 years.[175] These accidents occur with all types of lawnmowers; however, the most common and severe injuries involve a riding-mower.[92a,103,176] Seventy-two percent of children who have severe lawnmower injuries are bystanders.[46,176] Ross et al.,[150] however, had a higher number of children in their series who fell off the riding-mowers and were run over. Seventy-eight percent of all lawnmower accidents occur in boys.[175] Loder et al.[105] reviewed 235 children who had a traumatic amputation and found that these injuries are more common in the spring and summer. Garay et al[57a] recommended annual springtime "publicity campaigns" to remind the public of the dangers involved with lawnmowers during this peak time. With millions of dollars in new estimated annual burdens in prosthetic costs for children with amputations due to lawnmowers, the cost of a public relations campaign would likely be dwarfed in comparison. Children under the age of 14 years are most susceptible to injury with those under the age of 6 years having the greatest risk of death.[121] Hand injuries are the most common type (34.6%), followed by the leg (18.9%) and the foot (17.7%) (Fig. 30-43).[175]

The initial treatment for these children is thorough assessment of the injuries and appropriate resuscitation. Often, a large volume of blood has been lost. Once the child is stabilized, a secondary survey can be conducted to assess the extent of the injury to each limb. With regard to the foot, these injuries are mutilating and heavily contaminated with soil and grass. After inspection, the wound should be dressed and a firm bandage applied to prevent further bleeding. Antibiotics need to be administered as soon as possible and include a cephalosporin, aminoglycoside, and penicillin. The patient's tetanus status should be ascertained and tetanus prophylaxis administered if unknown.

The child then needs to be taken urgently to the operating room for the initial debridement. Considerable time should be spent meticulously removing foreign material. A water jet lavage system can be useful, but should be used with care as it can force debris further in to the soft tissue envelopes. Clearly devitalized tissue should be debrided. Questionable tissue should be left as there will be return trips to the operating room, and tissue in younger children especially may have remarkable recovery at times. It is useful to involve a plastic surgeon even at this initial surgery so they can see the extent of the damage

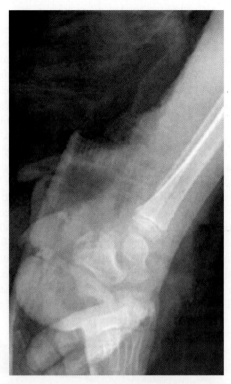

Figure 30-43. A 4-year-old boy with a severe lawnmower accident after being run over by the driver. There was extensive soft tissue loss and compound fractures to the foot. Despite multiple debridements, the leg was amputated below the knee.

and start planning for definitive coverage. The child will generally need at least three trips to the operating room and some cases many more.[46] These return trips should be every 24 to 48 hours depending on the state of the wound. Each debridement is important and should not be left to the most junior member of the surgical team. Every piece of viable skin is vital and may be the difference between a primary closure over an amputation stump or a skin graft or tissue transfer. There is no hurry to close the wound until the soft tissue and bone is completely free of foreign material and the tissues are well perfused. Shilt et al.[165] and many others have found the use of VAC safe and effective in managing of lawnmower injuries. Fractures need to be stabilized and initially external fixation is useful, which allows for further debridements and does not compromise later internal fixation once the soft tissue coverage has been determined.

Skin grafting or flap coverage of lawnmower injuries is required in approximately 50% of cases.[46] Unlike adults, split-thickness skin grafting can function very well on the weight-bearing surfaces in children.[46,176] When the soft tissue defect is large or there is exposed bone that would be better to preserve than excise, a free tissue transfer is helpful.[50,100] Lin et al.[103] reviewed 93 pediatric foot soft tissue defect microsurgical reconstructions. They reported excellent results with free musculocutaneous flaps or skin grafted muscle flaps. For plantar foot reconstructions, the musculocutaneous flaps had better results with fewer tropic ulcers and fewer resurfacing procedures. They also found that reconstruction of the tendons in the immediate setting led to fewer subsequent operations than staged tendon reconstructions.[103]

One of the problems with free flaps is their bulk and subsequent problems with shoe fitting. An alternative to a free muscle flap is a free fascial flap. A common one is the temporoparietal fascial flap.[33,41,167] This fascia is supplied by the superficial temporal artery which is a terminal branch of the external carotid. The graft can be as large as 12 × 14 cm. This varies with the age and size of the child. It is harvested through an incision within the hairline, which results in a cosmetic closure (Fig. 30-44A). The fascial flap can then be used to cover exposed bone and tendons in the foot (Fig. 30-44B–D). Split skin can then be grafted onto the fascia and any surrounding areas of full-thickness skin loss.

One of the most difficult decisions to make while treating these severe injuries is whether to salvage the affected part of the limb or amputate the questionable part. This decision is based largely on what the likely functional outcome will be and what effect prolonged treatments and hospitalizations will have on the child. Amputation rates vary between 16% and 78% in the literature.[7,46,176] A mangled extremity severity score (MESS) has been developed in adults to help surgeons make these decisions.[80] The MESS score was validated in children by Fagelman

et al.[53] However, they did not include fractures below the ankle. It is useful to ask for a colleague's advice when contemplating an amputation so the advantages and disadvantages can be discussed. If an amputation is performed, as much length of the bone should be preserved as possible, and transdiaphyseal amputation should generally be avoided to prevent problems with stump overgrowth.[2,104] The functional outcome for these patients is generally satisfactory. Vosburgh et al.[180] reviewed the functional outcome of 21 children with lawnmower accidents. They found that isolated forefoot injuries resulted in 88% of normal function compared to 72% of normal function in patients with injuries to the posterior and plantar aspects of their foot.

CRUSH INJURIES

Severe crush injuries to the foot in children are rare but the consequences of not recognizing the degree of injury can be devastating. The most common cause is the foot being run over

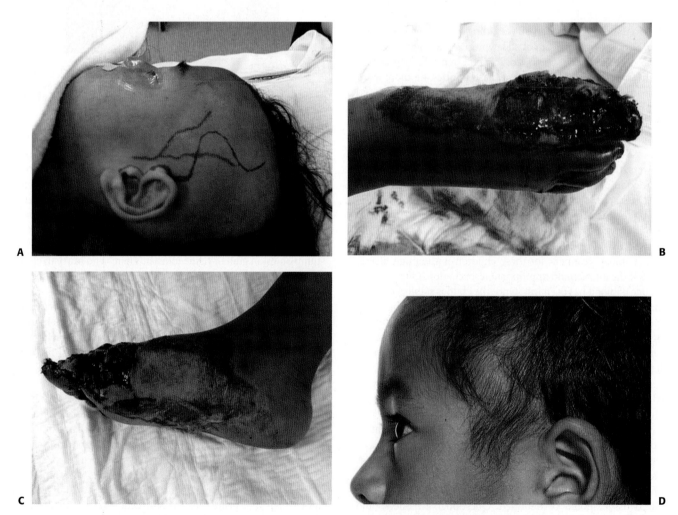

Figure 30-44. A: Temporoparietal fascia is harvested through the incision marked by the *green line. Red line* is markings of superficial temporal artery. **B, C:** Severe crush and degloving injury to the foot in a 6-year-old boy run over by a car **D:** The incision for harvesting the temporoparietal graft heals with an excellent cosmetic result.

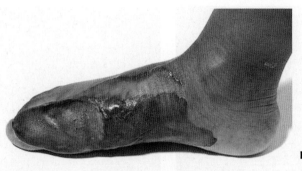

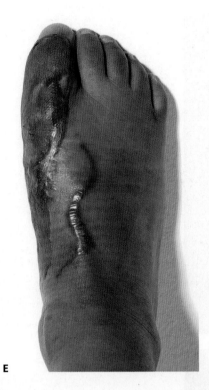

Figure 30-44. (*Continued*) **E, F:** The temporoparietal graft has healed with skin grafting to cover the defect. (Courtesy Dr. Jonathan Wheeler, Consultant Plastic Surgeon, Middlemore Hospital, Auckland, New Zealand.)

by a car tire resulting in both a crush and shearing force (see Fig. 30-44). An alternative injury would be a heavy weight falling on the foot.

The child presents with an extremely painful, tight foot usually with the skin intact. Shoes can be difficult to remove and they may need sedation first. Initial primary and secondary surveys need to be completed and then a thorough assessment of the foot undertaken.

It is important to continually assess the child for compartment syndrome and perform fasciotomies when indicated (see Compartment Syndrome below).

SESAMOID FRACTURES

There are a number of sesamoid bones in the foot. The most commonly symptomatic ones are the two within the plantar plate of the first metatarsophalangeal joint and in the flexor hallucis brevis tendons. These medial and lateral sesamoid bones functioning both shock absorption and as a fulcrum to improve the biomechanical function of the tendons to the first toe.

Acute sesamoid fractures are rare in children and diagnosis is difficult because of the variable anatomy of the medial and lateral sesamoid bones. They can have more than one ossification center which may not unite, resulting in a partite sesamoid. The incidence of partite sesamoids varies between 19% and 31%.[45,88] The incidence of a partite sesamoid is approximately 10 times higher in the medial sesamoid compared to the lateral one. The incidence of bilaterality varies between 25% and 85%.[35,77]

An acute fracture to the sesamoids is usually caused by a fall from a height onto the forefoot which may be associated with a forced dorsiflexion of the first metatarsal. The injury results in acute pain and swelling under the first metatarsal head and pain on first toe dorsiflexion. Common causes of sesamoid pain are stress fractures or inflammation of the sesamoid (sesamoiditis), which occurs from repetitive dorsiflexion of the great toe (e.g., in runners and dancers).

Radiographs need to be taken to help differentiate whether the condition is acute or chronic. Anteroposterior and lateral weight-bearing views coned on the sesamoids should be requested. A tangential view is also advisable (Fig. 30-45). An acute fracture will usually be transverse and have a "jagged" appearance with sharp corners. It is not widely displaced as the fragments are contained within the plantar plate. Wide displacement would represent a major disruption to the first metatarsophalangeal joint which would be obvious clinically. Another useful tip is that the sum of the fragment sizes should add up to the "normal sesamoid size." Two partite fragments are often much larger when combined than one would normally expect with a fracture. Radiographs of the opposite foot can be helpful for comparison. However with the variable incidence of bilaterality, a definitive diagnosis is not always possible.

Treatment for a closed injury with an intact planter plate is nonoperative. Immobilization in a below-knee plaster cast with a toe plate for 4 to 6 weeks is advisable. Alternatively a moot-boot with a midfoot ridge to unload the forefoot can be used. Transition from the cast into a stiff-soled shoe that continues to prevent dorsiflexion will give symptomatic relief. With stress fractures and sesamoiditis a longer period of immobilization may be necessary.

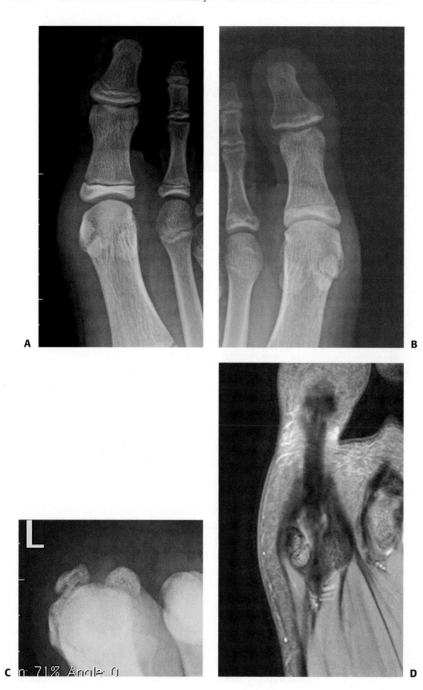

Figure 30-45. A: Medial sesamoid of the right foot appears fractured following a great toe injury. A radiograph of the left foot confirms a similar partite sesamoid that is asymptomatic. **B:** Asymptomatic partite patella in the contralateral uninjured foot. **C:** Tangential sesamoid views can be useful however in this case the radiograph does not show the transverse partite sesamoid. **D:** An MRI scan of the right foot 5 months after the injury for a different problem shows the partite medial sesamoid.

Surgical intervention is rarely required. If a symptomatic nonunion occurred this can be treated by open reduction and bone grafting which is technically difficult or by excision of the smaller of the two fragments. Either way care needs to be taken to avoid damage to the plantar plate.

COMPARTMENT SYNDROME

Compartment syndrome of the foot can occur in children with severe soft tissue injuries in the presence or absence of associated fractures.[165a] Most commonly, it occurs with severe crush injuries of the forefoot where there are multiple fractures and dislocations; however, it can occur without any fracture, such as the case of a car running over a foot causing crush and shear injury to soft tissue. The symptoms are not as obvious as they are in compartment syndrome of the forearm or leg, and increased pain with passive motion of the toes is not always present. There is significant pain from the injury itself, which often requires considerable amounts of pain relief. Pallor, pain on passive extension, paresthesia, and a dorsalis pedis pulse that is difficult to palpate likewise can be clinical signs in a large number of foot injuries. The clinician needs to have a high index of suspicion for a compartment syndrome and if any doubt exists, the compartment pressures should be measured or the child taken urgently to the operating room for a decompression of the foot.

Compartment pressure measurements are difficult to perform with invasive catheterization in an awake child with foot trauma. Often, the compartments need to be measured under a general anesthetic, so the child and parents need to be warned that the surgeon may proceed to a decompression. There are nine compartments in the foot, and it is difficult to confirm exact compartment location. It is important to measure the pressure in the calcaneal compartment as it appears to be the most sensitive.[109] When a pressure of greater than 30 mm Hg is measured in any compartment, a fasciotomy should be performed.[109,119] It may be more accurate to use a measurement that takes into account the patient's blood pressure. In adults, the threshold is a measured pressure that is less than 30 mm Hg below the patient's diastolic blood pressure.[108]

There are nine fascial compartments in the foot that contain the intrinsic muscles and short plantar flexors. All the compartments should be released during a decompression regardless of the clinical findings or compartment measurements. The most thorough way to achieve this is by using the three incision technique (Fig. 30-46).[119] Two dorsal longitudinal incisions are made in line with the second and fourth metatarsals. Dissection is then carried out through the interosseous compartments and fascia to enable decompression of the deep plantar compartments. Puncturing the fascia and spreading with a hemostat is effective and safe. The lateral compartment is decompressed through the incision over the fourth metatarsal by dissecting deep to the fifth metatarsal. A medial incision is made along the arch of the foot as far posterior as the medial malleolus. This incision allows decompression of the medial compartment and a more thorough decompression of the deep compartments. It also allows decompression of the tarsal tunnel. Dissection is carried out on both the dorsal and plantar surfaces of the abductor hallucis muscle, freeing it from both the plantar fascia and bony attachments. Care must be taken to avoid damaging the lateral plantar nerve and vessels which lie on the quadrates plantae muscle. The deep compartments can now be easily released under direct vision. These three incisions are usually well placed to help with fracture reduction and K-wiring to stabilize the foot at the same time as the decompression. The wounds should be left open initially and closed 5 to 7 days later. Often, one of the wounds will require split-skin grafting.

Although uncommon in children, late sequelae of missed compartment syndrome can lead to disability including claw toe deformity, paresthesia, cavus deformity, stiffness, and

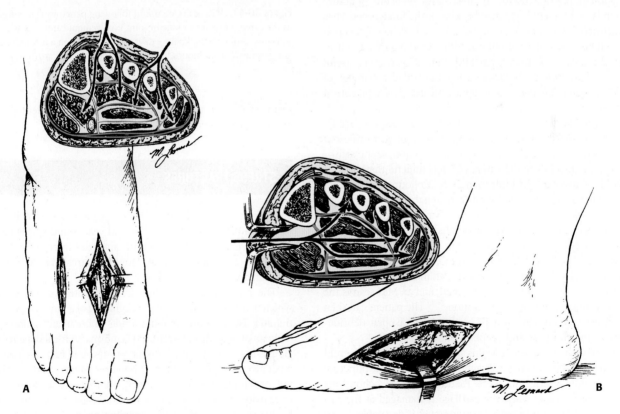

Figure 30-46. Surgical approaches for fasciotomy of the foot. **A:** The dorsal approach is made through an incision over the second and fourth metatarsal shafts and is more suitable for injuries of the forefoot or midfoot. **B:** The medial approach is more suitable for injuries of the hindfoot, with the incision extending from the base of the first metatarsal to the medial malleolus. A tarsal tunnel release can be done through this incision. (Reprinted by permission from Myerson MS. Experimental decompression of the fascial compartments of the foot: The basis for fasciotomy in acute compartment syndromes. *Foot Ankle.* 1988;8(6):308–314. Copyright © 1988 SAGE Publications.)

residual pain.[14,168] While compartment syndrome of the foot in adults is sometimes observed initially with later tendon releases if needed, there has not been a similar experience reported in the growing child.

PUNCTURE WOUNDS

Puncture wounds to the foot are extremely common in children and frequently treated by primary care physicians or in the emergency department. Most injuries can be treated by simply removing the offending foreign body, irrigating the entry site, giving tetanus prophylaxis if required, and a short course of oral antibiotics. It is important to carefully assess the foreign body that is removed to make sure a small part of it has not been retained in the foot. Often, the patient will bring the offending foreign body with them if it broke off or came out spontaneously. The depth of penetration should also be assessed by looking at the length of the foreign object as well as the point of entry. This approach may help predict if a joint or tendon sheath has been penetrated. The amount of contamination can also help determine if an open debridement is necessary and the length of administration of antibiotics.

Radiographs are useful in most cases of acute puncture wounds as a foreign body may be seen. If the foreign body has punctured a joint, air may be seen as well. When a retained foreign body is suspected but not seen on radiograph, an ultrasound scan can be useful. An MRI scan is even more useful at identifying foreign bodies and has the added advantage of showing secondary changes of septic arthritis or osteomyelitis if the puncture wound is chronic (Fig. 30-47).

If a patient with a treated puncture wound does not rapidly improve clinically, further investigation is required to rule out a retained foreign body, deep soft tissue infection, septic arthritis, or osteomyelitis. Eidelman et al.[49] recommend that patients who have an established infection 24 to 36 hours after a puncture wound should be admitted to hospital for IV antibiotics. In their series of 80 children with puncture wounds, a delay in diagnosis or presentation was associated with deep infection.[48] The most common organism causing deep infections in their study was *Staphylococcus aureus* and Group A *Streptococcus*. A complete blood count, erythrocyte sedimentation rate, and C-reactive protein should be performed, and an MRI scan is the most accurate radiologic investigation.[74,90] The patient can then be treated accordingly with IV antibiotics and open debridement of the entry site and deeper tissues.

Septic arthritis or osteomyelitis should be suspected if a child presents with foot pain and swelling following a nail puncture wound while wearing sneakers. Pseudomonas osteochondritis is thought to occur when the cartilage is damaged at the initial injury.[54] The source of the pseudomonas is debatable. Some authors have postulated that it is from the sneakers.[53,91] The patient should be admitted to hospital. A thorough debridement of the affected soft tissues, cartilage, and bone should be carried out. IV antibiotics are administered often for 5 to 7 days or until the infection has clearly resolved.[76,78] The long-term sequelae of pain, growth arrests, chronic osteomyelitis, and

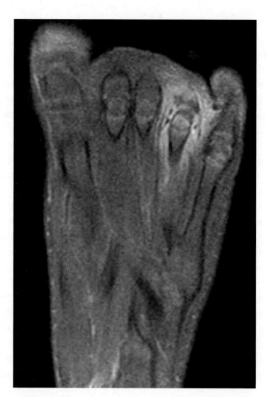

Figure 30-47. MRI scans are useful following penetrating foot injuries as the extent of the soft tissue or joint involvement can be clearly seen. This 6-year-old boy had pain 4 days after standing on a nail in barefeet, and despite oral antibiotics he had developed a septic arthritis.

recurrence make this an important infection to identify early and treat aggressively.

STRESS FRACTURES

Stress fractures in children are becoming more common because of overtraining in youth athletics and year-round sports participation.[31] The tibia, fibula, femur, and pars interarticularis are the areas commonly affected. However, stress fractures in the foot can also occur.[34,43,60,186]

The predominant symptom is "pain with weight bearing," which usually coincides with the beginning of an intense period of training. The repetitive training results in bone fatigue and eventual partial or complete fracture. The normal cortical bone remodeling is accelerated and resorption occurs at a faster rate than the reparative process resulting in bone weakening and inevitable microfracture. Therefore, treatment attempts to break this cycle by activity modification and protected weight bearing to prevent further fracture and allow the reparative process to "catch up."

Patients with stress fractures in the foot present with pain on weight bearing and often no history of any particular causative injury. A thorough history of their training regimen is essential, particularly any increases or changes in technique, playing surface, or footwear. On examination, there is point tenderness but minimal swelling. Radiographs taken early in the process are often normal but later can show periosteal layering of new bone on the cortex and osteolysis at the fracture site. Bone scans are often more sensitive initially and a three-phase technetium bone scan is helpful when the radiographs are normal in the first 2 to 3 weeks after the onset of symptoms.[49] MRI has been shown to identify stress fractures before radiographic changes are evident, and, in a prospective study of collegiate basketball players, MRI demonstrated marrow edema even before stress fractures were clinically evident.[107]

As well as concentrating on the fracture, the patient should be assessed for any conditions that could predispose to stress fractures. These conditions include metabolic bone diseases, amenorrhea, eating disorders, and incorrect training techniques. A cause may be as simple as a change in footwear that has led to increased stress in a particular bone in the foot.

The second metatarsal is the most common bone in the foot to get a stress fracture, which often occurs at the neck of the metatarsal at the junction of the mobile shaft and rigid metaphysis. Treatment involves rest and partial weight bearing in a moon-boot for 4 to 6 weeks. It is best to avoid a cast as during this time the athlete can maintain physical fitness with swimming, deep water running, and exercycling. A gradual return to activity can be restarted when radiographs confirm adequate healing and the symptoms have abated, which often takes 8 to 12 weeks. Stress fractures of the navicular are disabling and difficult to treat. They occur most commonly in basketball players, hurdlers, and runners.[115] Bennell and Bruckner[11] reviewed 18 large studies of stress fractures and found that the incidence of navicular stress fractures can range between 0% and 28.6% of injuries among track and field athletes. These fractures are thought to arise because of overuse and the reduced vascularity that can exist in the central third of the navicular. They are difficult to diagnose and one needs to have a high level of suspicion as with any other stress fracture. The fracture is often diagnosed by MRI, and if this is positive in the region of the navicular, a CT scan is very helpful in delineating the stress response from an acute injury. The fracture line on CT, and if present on radiograph, is vertically orientated in the middle third of the bone. Most of these fractures heal with rest and protective weight bearing. However, some do go on to delayed or nonunion. The treatment for a painful nonunion is ORIF with autogenous bone grafting. The average time for the return to activity following a navicular stress fracture in athletes is 5.6 months.[84] Stress fractures of the base of the fifth metatarsal usually occur in zone 2 or 3 and their treatment is discussed earlier in the chapter under the section fractures of the fifth metatarsal base.

Stress fractures can also occur in the cuboid, calcaneus, and sesamoid bones of the foot.

Annotated References

Reference	Annotation
Dougherty CP, Nebergall RW, Caskey PM. Lateral subtalar dislocation in a 19-month-old female. *Am J Orthop.* 2003;32(12):598–600.	A case report of a lateral subtalar dislocation in a 19-month-old female after a minor fall. Review of the literature reveals no prior report of this injury in a patient of this age. This case illustrates the importance of thoroughly examining the pediatric patient. When fracture is not diagnosed and a child refuses to use the affected extremity, examination to rule out occult fracture or dislocation must be included. Level of Evidence: V
Eberl R, Singer G, Schalamon J, et al. Fractures of the talus—differences between children and adolescents. *J Trauma.* 2010;68:126–130.	From 1990 to 2005, 24 patients (18 males, 6 females) presented with 25 fractures of the talus. The medical records were reviewed retrospectively. Follow-up was performed by radiographical grading, and the functional outcome was measured using the Foot-Function-Index. Adolescents present with more severe fractures of the talus compared with children younger than 12 years. In addition, we did not observe persistent osteonecrosis in patients younger than 12 years old, and the outcome is favorable in most cases irrespective of the mode of treatment. Level of Evidence: IV
Hill JF, Heyworth BE, Lierhaus A, et al. Lisfranc injuries in children and adolescents. *J Pediatr Orthop B.* 2017;26(2):159–163.	Fifty-six children treated for bony or ligamentous Lisfranc injuries over a 12-year period were reviewed. Overall, 51% of fractures and 82% of sprains were sports related ($P = 0.03$). A total of 34% of the cohort underwent open reduction internal fixation, which was more common among patients with closed physes (67%). Full weight bearing was allowed in open reduction internal fixation patients at a mean of 14.5 weeks, compared to 6.5 weeks in the nonoperative group. Complications were rare (4%) and included physeal arrest in one patient and a broken, retained implant in one patient. Level of Evidence: IV
Kamphuis SJ, Meijs CM, Kleinveld CM, et al. Talar fractures in children: A possible injury after go-karting accidents. *J Foot Ankle Surg.* 2015;54(6):1206–1212.	This is a case series that describes six talar fractures in four patients that resulted from go-karting accidents. Talar fractures caused severe damage to the tibiotalar joint, talocalcaneal or subtalar joint, and the talonavicular joint. This damage leads to complications such as avascular necrosis, arthritis, nonunion, delayed union, and neuropraxia, which have the potential to cause long-term disability in a child. Level of Evidence: V.

Annotated References

Reference	Annotation
Knijnenberg LM, Dingemans SA, Terra MP, et al. Radiographic anatomy of the pediatric Lisfranc joint. *J Pediatr Orthop*. 2016. Sep 3. [Epub ahead of print].	Foot radiographs without traumatic injury taken between August 2014 and February 2015 in patients younger than 18 years were reviewed. Using a non–weight-bearing anteroposterior view of the foot the distance between the base of metatarsal 1 and metatarsal 2 (MT1-MT2) and the distance between the medial cuneiform (MC) and the base of metatarsal 2 (MC-MT2) were measured. Median normal values were calculated per age. In the analysis were 243 patients. The distance between the base of MT1-MT2 was constant below 3 mm. Measurements for both MT1-MT2 and MC-MT2 distance approached adult values at the age of 6. Level of Evidence: III.
Kramer DE, Mahan ST, Hresko MT. Displaced Intra-articular Fractures of the Great Toe in Children: Intervene With Caution! *J Pediatr Orthop*. 2014;34(2):144–149.	Seven boys and three girls with a mean age of 12.6 years (range, 8.7 to 15.7 years) were identified. The mechanism of injury was a direct blow from a stubbed toe (eight cases) or a dropped object onto the foot (two cases). There were seven intra-articular fractures of the proximal phalanx base, four of which occurred in the setting of an open physis. Mean fracture displacement was 4.4 mm. Open reduction was necessary in nine cases, with K-wire fixation used in nine cases. Median follow-up was 50.5 months (range, 11 to 123 months). Seven fractures healed at a mean of 7.9 weeks. Nine patients returned to full activity without limitation at latest follow-up. Six patients had significant complications: two underwent revision open reduction internal fixation (one for postoperative redisplacement and the other for painful nonunion), one suffered a refracture, one developed posttraumatic arthritis requiring interphalangeal joint fusion, one developed an asymptomatic fibrous nonunion with avascular necrosis of the fragment, and one had K-wire migration necessitating early surgical removal. Conclusions: Intra-articular fractures of the great toe primarily occur in adolescents after direct impact injuries. The most common location was the proximal phalangeal base. There is a high complication rate after surgical intervention, although most patients were asymptomatic at latest follow-up. Level of Evidence: IV
Petit CJ, Lee BM, Kasser JR, et al. Operative treatment of intraarticular calcaneal fractures in the pediatric population. *J Pediatr Orthop*. 2007;27(8):856–862.	Children with closed displaced intra-articular calcaneal fractures treated with open reduction internal fixation at Boston Children were reviewed at an average of 67 months postoperatively. Fourteen fractures in 13 patients who met the inclusion criteria were treated with open reduction internal fixation. We found seven tongue-type and seven joint depression-type fractures based on the Essex-Lopresti classification. Based on the Sanders classification, we found nine type II (two-part) fractures and five type III (three-part) fractures. The average preoperative and postoperative Bohler angles were 11.8 and 28.4 degrees (P < 0.0001), respectively. The average subjective AOFAS hindfoot score was 64 of a possible 68 points. Of 14 fractures, 13 were fixed with a buttressing plate laterally. One patient was fixed with a single 3.5-mm cortical screw and had the lowest AOFAS hindfoot score. Four minor complications in three patients were encountered. Level of Evidence: IV
Petnehazy T, Schalamon J, Hartwig C, et al. Fractures of the hallux in children. *Foot Ankle Int*. 2015;36:60–63.	Three hundred seventeen patients (mean age = 11.7 years; range, 1 to 18 years; 65% males) sustained a fracture of the hallux. Most accidents (28%) occurred at sports facilities, and soccer was the most common cause of a fracture of the hallux (28%). Closed injuries were diagnosed in 92% of the patients; 8% of the children presented with open fractures. In 144 children, the growth plate was affected. Fifty-nine patients presented with diaphyseal fractures, 42 patients with osseous avulsions, and 40 patients with fractures of the distal part of the phalanx. Nineteen children had incomplete and 13 patients comminuted fractures. The vast majority of the children (86%) were treated conservatively. Operative interventions were required in 14% of the patients. Good outcome was achieved in both conservatively and operatively treated patients. Level of Evidence: IV

Annotated References

Reference	Annotation
Riccardi G, Riccardi D, Marcarelli M, et al. Extremely proximal fractures of the fifth metatarsal in the developmental age. *Foot Ankle Int.* 2011;32(5):S526–S532.	Between 2001 and 2003, the radiographs of 481 patients (558 ft) between 6 months and 16 years that were diagnosed with a proximal fifth metatarsal fracture were reviewed. The x-rays were evaluated for the presence and morphology of the growth nucleus of the base of the fifth metatarsal in the 7- to 16-year age group because this is the time interval in which the nucleus becomes visible radiographically. They identified the nucleus of the base of the fifth metatarsal in 115 patients for a total of 132 ft. A fracture of the fifth metatarsal was found in 12.8%. A misdiagnosis had been made in 47%. Misdiagnosis was strictly related to the presence of the growth nucleus of the apophysis except two cases where an accessory bone was present. Level of Evidence: IV
Smith JT, Curtis TA, Spencer S, et al. Complications of Talus Fractures in Children. *J Pediatr Orthop.* 2010;30(8):749–757.	This study included 29 children with talus fractures sustained between 1999 and 2008 at an average age of 13.5 years (range, 1.2 to 17.8 years). Avascular necrosis occurred in two patients (7%), arthrosis in five (17%), delayed union in one (3%), neurapraxia in two (7%), infection in zero, and the need for further surgery in three (10%). Both high-energy mechanism and fracture displacement corresponded to a greater number of posttraumatic complications. The number and severity of talus fractures increased in older children. Level of Evidence: IV
Talkhani S, Reidy D, Fogarty E, et al. Avascular necrosis of the talus after a minimally displaced neck of talus fracture in a 6 year old child. *Injury.* 2000;31(1):63–65.	Case report of ANV after a nondisplaced talar neck fracture in a 6-year-old child. Level of Evidence: V
Tezval M, Dumont C, Stürmer KM. Prognostic reliability of the Hawkins sign in fractures of the talus. *J Orthop Trauma.* 2007;(8):538–543.	Between January 1995 and December 2000, a total of 41 patients (13 females, 28 males) with displaced talar fractures were operated on. Thirty-four patients with a mean age of 35 years (range 12 to 60 years) were followed for more than 36 months (range 36 to 52 months). The prognostic reliability of the Hawkins sign was studied in 31 of these patients using a two-by-two table. No Hawkins sign was found in the five patients who developed avascular necrosis (AVN) of the talus. In the remaining 26 patients who did not develop AVN, a positive (full) Hawkins sign was observed 11 times, a partially positive Hawkins sign 4 times, and a negative Hawkins sign 11 times. The Hawkins sign thus showed a sensitivity of 100% and a specificity of 57.7%. The Hawkins sign (if present) appeared between the sixth and the ninth week after trauma. The Hawkins sign is a good indicator of talus vascularity following fracture. If a full or partial positive Hawkins sign is detected, it is unlikely that AVN will develop at a later stage after injury. Level of Evidence: IV
Wu Y, Jiang H, Wang B. Fracture of the lateral process of the talus in children: A kind of ankle injury with frequently missed diagnosis. *J Pediatr Orthop.* 2016;36(3):289–293.	From March 2011 to October 2013, 12 children with lateral process fracture of the talus were treated. The age at the time of injury ranged from 8 to 13 years. Concomitant injuries included undisplaced calcaneus fractures in one case and distal fibula epiphysis injury in one case. Seven of the cases were initially diagnosed in our department, and the diagnosis was missed in five cases. The missed diagnosis rate was 42%. All patients were followed up for 18 months on an average. Follow-up radiographs did not show avascular necrosis of the talus, nonunion, and malunion in any patient. The mean AOFAS hindfoot score was 96 points. The clinical result was found to be excellent in ten patients, good in one patient, and fair in one patient (the success rate was 92%). The lateral process of talus fracture is a frequently missed injury. Level of Evidence: IV

REFERENCES

1. Abidi NA, Dhawan S, Gruen GS, et al. Wound-healing risk factors after open reduction and internal fixation of calcaneal fractures. *Foot Ankle Int.* 1998;19(12):856–861.
2. Abraham E, Pellicore RJ, Hamilton RC, et al. Stump overgrowth in juvenile amputees. *J Pediatr Orthop.* 1986;6(1):66–71.
3. Adelaar RS. Complex fractures of the talus. *Instr Course Lect.* 1997;46:323–338.
4. Adirim TA, Cheng TL. Overview of injuries in the young athlete. *Sports Med.* 2003;33(1):75–81.
5. Aitken AP. Fractures of the os calcis—treatment by closed reduction. *Clin Orthop Relat Res.* 1963;30:67–75.
6. Allmacher DH, Galles KS, Marsh JL. Intra-articular calcaneal fractures treated nonoperatively and followed sequentially for 2 decades. *J Orthop Trauma.* 2006; 20(7):464–469.

7. Alonso JE, Sanchez FL. Lawn mower injuries in children: A preventable impairment. *J Pediatr Orthop.* 1995;15(1):83–89.
8. Anderson IF, Crichton KJ, Grattan-Smith T, et al. Osteochondral fractures of the dome of the talus. *J Bone Joint Surg Am.* 1989;71(8):1143–1152.
9. Aquino MD, Aquino L, Aquino JM. Talar neck fractures: A review of vascular supply and classification. *J Foot Surg.* 1986;25(3):188–193.
10. Benirschke SK, Kramer PA. Wound healing complications in closed and open calcaneal fractures. *J Orthop Trauma.* 2004;18(1):1–6.
11. Bennell KL, Brukner PD. Epidemiology and site specificity of stress fractures. *Clin Sports Med.* 1997;16(2):179–196.
12. Berndt AL, Harty M. Transchondral fractures (osteochondritis dissecans) of the talus. *J Bone Joint Surg Am.* 1959;41(6):988–1028.
13. Bibbo C, Davis WH, Anderson RB. Midfoot injury in children related to mini scooters. *Pediatr Emerg Care.* 2003;19(1):6–9.
14. Bibbo C, Lin SS, Cunningham FJ. Acute traumatic compartment syndrome of the foot in children. *Pediatr Emerg Care.* 2000;16(4):244–248.
15. Blair WF. Irreducible tarsometatarsal fracture-dislocation. *J Trauma.* 1981;21(11):988–990.
16. Blount W. Injuries of the foot. In: Beaty JH, Kasser JR, eds. *Fractures in Children.* Philadelphia, PA: Williams and Wilkins; 1955:195–196.
17. Bonnel F, Barthelemy M. Injuries of Lisfranc's joint: Severe sprains, dislocations, fractures. Study of 39 personal cases and biomechanical classification. *J Chir (Paris).* 1976;111(5–6):573–592.
18. Broden B. Roentgen examination of the subtaloid joint in fractures of the calcaneus. *Acta Radiol.* 1949;31(1):85–91.
19. Brunet JA. Calcaneal fractures in children. Long-term results of treatment. *J Bone Joint Surg Br.* 2000;82(2):211–216.
20. Buckingham R, Jackson M, Atkins R. Calcaneal fractures in adolescents. CT classification and results of operative treatment. *Injury.* 2003;34(6):454–459.
21. Buckley R, O'Brien J, McCormack R. *Personal Gait Satisfaction of Patients with Displaced Intraarticular Calcaneal Fractures: A 2- to 8-Year Follow-Up. Poster Presentation 2770 in Orthopaedic Trauma Association Annual Meeting:* Salt Lake City, Utah; October 2003.
22. Buoncristiani AM, Manos RE, Mills WJ. Plantar-flexion tarsometatarsal joint injuries in children. *J Pediatr Orthop.* 2001;21(3):324–327.
23. Burroughs KE, Reimer CD, Fields KB. Lisfranc injury of the foot: A commonly missed diagnosis. *Am Fam Physician.* 1998;58(1):118–124.
24. Byrd T. Jones fracture: Relearning an old injury. *South Med J.* 1992;85(7):748–750.
25. Canale ST, Belding RH. Osteochondral lesions of the talus. *J Bone Joint Surg Am.* 1980;62(1):97–102.
26. Canale ST, Kelly FB Jr. Fractures of the neck of the talus. Long-term evaluation of 71 cases. *J Bone Joint Surg Am.* 1978;60(2):143–156.
27. Carroll N. Fractures and dislocations of the tarsal bones. In: Letts RM, ed. *Management of Pediatric Fractures.* New York: Churchill Livingstone; 1994.
28. Ceccarelli F, Faldini C, Piras F, et al. Surgical versus nonsurgical treatment of calcaneal fractures in children: A long-term results comparative study. *Foot Ankle Int.* 2000;21(10):825–832.
29. Cehner J. Fractures of the tarsal bones, metatarsals, and toes. In: Weber B, Brunner C, Freuler F, eds. *Treatment of Fractures in Children and Adolescents.* New York: Springer-Verlag; 1980.
30. Ceroni D, De Rosa V, De Coulon G, et al. Cuboid nutcracker fracture due to horseback riding in children: Case series and review of the literature. *J Pediatr Orthop.* 2007;27(5):557–561.
31. Chambers HG. Ankle and foot disorders in skeletally immature athletes. *Orthop Clin North Am.* 2003;34(3):445–459.
32. Chapman H, Galway H. Os calcis fractures in childhood. *J Bone Joint Surg.* 1977;59B:510.
33. Cheney ML, Varvares MA, Nadol JB. The temporoparietal fascial flap in head and neck reconstruction. *Arch Otolaryngol Head Neck Surg.* 1993;119:618–623.
34. Childress H. March fracture in a 7-year-old boy. *J Bone Joint Surg Am.* 1946;28:877.
35. Chisis D, Peyser A, Milgram C. Bone scintigraphy in the assessment of hallucial sesamoids. *Foot Ankle Int.* 1995;16:291–294.
36. Craigen MA, Clarke NM. Bilateral "Jones" fractures of the fifth metatarsal following relapse of talipes equinovarus. *Injury.* 1996;27(8):599–601.
37. Crawford A. Fractures and dislocations of the foot and ankle. In: Green NE, ed. *Skeletal Trauma in Children.* Philadelphia, PA: WB Saunders; 1994:449–516.
38. Curtis MJ, Myerson M, Szura B. Tarsometatarsal joint injuries in the athlete. *Am J Sports Med.* 1993;21(4):497–502.
39. Dameron TB Jr. Fractures of the proximal fifth metatarsal: Selecting the best treatment option. *J Am Acad Orthop Surg.* 1995;3(2):110–114.
40. Damore DT, Metzl JD, Ramundo M, et al. Patterns in childhood sports injury. *Pediatr Emerg Care.* 2003;19(2):65–67.
41. David SK, Cheney ML. An anatomic study of the temporoparietal fascia flap. *Arch Otolaryngol Head and Neck Surgery.* 1995;121(10):1153–1156.
42. DeLee J. Fracture and dislocations of the foot. In: Mann RA, ed. *Surgery of the Foot and Ankle.* St. Louis, MO: Mosby; 1993.
43. Devas MB. Stress fractures in children. *J Bone Joint Surg Br.* 1963;45:528–541.
44. Dimentberg R, Rosman M. Peritalar dislocations in children. *J Pediatr Orthop.* 1993;13(1):89–93.
45. Dobas DC, Silvers MD: The frequency of the partite sesamoids of the first metatarsophalangeal joint. *J Am Podiatr Assoc.* 1977;67:880–882.
46. Dormans JP, Azzoni M, Davidson RS, et al. Major lower extremity lawn mower injuries in children. *J Pediatr Orthop.* 1995;15(1):78–82.
47. Dougherty CP, Nebergall RW, Caskey PM. Lateral subtalar dislocation in a 19-month-old female. *Am J Orthop.* 2003;32(12):598–600.
48. Eberl R, Singer G, Schalamon J, et al. Fractures of the talus—differences between children and adolescents. *J Trauma.* 2010;68:126–130.
49. Eidelman M, Bialik V, Miller Y, et al. Plantar puncture wounds in children: Analysis of 80 hospitalized patients and late sequelae. *Isr Med Assoc J.* 2003;5(4):268–271.
50. Englaro EE, Gelfand MJ, Paltiel HJ. Bone scintigraphy in preschool children with lower extremity pain of unknown origin. *J Nucl Med.* 1992;33(3):351–354.
51. Erdmann D, Lee B, Roberts CD, et al. Management of lawnmower injuries to the lower extremity in children and adolescents. *Ann Plast Surg.* 2000;45(6):595–600.
52. Essex-Lopresti P. The mechanism, reduction technique, and results in fractures of the os calcis. *Br J Surg.* 1952;39:395–419.
53. Fagelman MF, Epps HR, Rang M. Mangled extremity severity score in children. *J Pediatr Orthop.* 2002;22(2):182–184.
54. Fisher MC, Goldsmith JF, Gilligan PH. Sneakers as a source of Pseudomonas aeruginosa in children with osteomyelitis following puncture wounds. *J Pediatr.* 1985;106(4):607–609.
55. Fitzgerald RH Jr, Cowan JD. Puncture wounds of the foot. *Orthop Clin North Am.* 1975;6(4):965–972.
56. Folk JW, Starr AJ, Early JS. Early wound complications of operative treatment of calcaneus fractures: Analysis of 190 fractures. *J Orthop Trauma.* 1999;13(5):369–372.
57. Fortin PT, Balazsy JE. Talus fractures: Evaluation and treatment. *J Am Acad Orthop Surg.* 2001;9(2):114–127.
57a. Garay M, Hennrikus WL, Hess J, et al. Lawnmowers versus children: the devastation continues. *Clin Orthop Relat Res.* 2017;475(4):950–956.
58. Gelberman RH, Mortensen WW. The arterial anatomy of the talus. *Foot Ankle.* 1983;4(2):64–72.
59. Glasgow MT, Naranja RJ Jr, Glasgow SG, et al. Analysis of failed surgical management of fractures of the base of the fifth metatarsal distal to the tuberosity: The Jones fracture. *Foot Ankle Int.* 1996;17(8):449–457.
60. Goiney RC, Connell DG, Nichols DM. CT evaluation of tarsometatarsal fracture-dislocation injuries. *AJR Am J Roentgenol.* 1985;144(5):985–990.
61. Griffin LY. Common sports injuries of the foot and ankle seen in children and adolescents. *Orthop Clin North Am.* 1994;25(1):83–93.
62. Groshar D, Alperson M, Mendes DG, et al. Bone scintigraphy findings in Lisfranc joint injury. *Foot Ankle Int.* 1995;16(11):710–711.
63. Haliburton RA, Sullivan CR, Kelly PJ, et al. The extraosseous and intraosseous blood supply of the talus. *J Bone Joint Surg Am.* 1958;40-A(5):1115–1120.
64. Hardcastle PH, Reschauer R, Kutshca-Lissberg E, et al. Injuries to the tarsometatarsal joint. Incidence, classification, and treatment. *J Bone Joint Surg Br.* 1982;64(3):349–356.
65. Hawkins LG. Fracture of the lateral process of the talus. *J Bone Joint Surg Am.* 1965;47:1170–1175.
66. Hawkins LG. Fractures of the neck of the talus. *J Bone Joint Surg Am.* 1970;52(5):991–1002.
67. Heckman JD, McLean MR. Fractures of the lateral process of the talus. *Clin Orthop Relat Res.* 1985;199:108–113.
68. Henderson RC. Posttraumatic necrosis of the talus: The Hawkins sign versus magnetic resonance imaging. *J Orthop Trauma.* 1991;5(1):96–99.
69. Herrera-Soto JA, Scherb M, Duffy MF, et al. Fractures of the fifth metatarsal in children and adolescents. *J Pediatr Orthop.* 2007;27(4):427–431.
70. Higuera J, Laguna R, Peral M, et al. Osteochondritis dissecans of the talus during childhood and adolescence. *J Pediatr Orthop.* 1998;18(3):328–332.
71. Hill JF, Heyworth BE, Lierhaus A, et al. Lisfranc injuries in children and adolescents. *J Pediatr Orthop B.* 2017;26(2):159–163.
71a. Hosking KV, Hoffman EB. Midtarsal dislocations in children. *J Pediatr Orthop.* 1999;19(5):592–595.
72. Howard CB, Benson MK. The ossific nuclei and the cartilage anlage of the talus and calcaneum. *J Bone Joint Surg Br.* 1992;74(4):620–623.
73. Howard JL, Buckley R, McCormack R, et al. Complications following management of displaced intra-articular calcaneal fractures: A prospective randomized trial comparing open reduction internal fixation with nonoperative management. *J Orthop Trauma.* 2003;17(4):241–249.
74. Hubbard AM, Meyer JS, Davidson RS, et al. Relationship between the ossification center and cartilaginous anlage in the normal hindfoot in children: Study with MR imaging. *AJR Am J Roentgenol.* 1993;161(4):849–853.
75. Imoisili MA, Bonwit AM, Bulas DI. Toothpick puncture injuries of the foot in children. *Pediatr Infect Dis J.* 2004;23(1):80–82.
76. Inokuchi S, Usami N, Hiraishi E, et al. Calcaneal fractures in children. *J Pediatr Orthop.* 1998;18(4):469–474.
77. Jacobs RF, McCarthy RE, Elser JM. Pseudomonas osteochondritis complicating puncture wounds of the foot in children: A 10-year evaluation. *J Infect Dis.* 1989;160(4):657–661.
78. Jahss MH. The sesamoids of the hallux. *Clin Orthop.* 1981;157:88–97.
79. Jarvis JG, Skipper J. Pseudomonas osteochondritis complicating puncture wounds in children. *J Pediatr Orthop.* 1994;14(6):755–759.
80. Jensen I, Wester JU, Rasmussen F, et al. Prognosis of fracture of the talus in children. 21 (7- to 34-)-year follow-up of 14 cases. *Acta Orthop Scand.* 1994;65(4):398–400.
81. Johansen K, Daines M, Howey T, et al. Objective criteria accurately predict amputation following lower extremity trauma. *J Trauma.* 1990;30(5):568–572; discussion 572–573.
82. Josefsson PO, Karlsson M, Redlund-Johnell I, et al. Closed treatment of Jones fracture. Good results in 40 cases after 11–26 years. *Acta Orthop Scand.* 1994;65(5):545–547.
83. Josefsson PO, Karlsson M, Redlund-Johnell I, et al. Jones fracture. Surgical versus nonsurgical treatment. *Clin Orthop Relat Res.* 1994;299:252–255.
84. Kamphuis SJ, Meijs CM, Kleinveld S, et al. Talar fractures in children: A possible injury after go-karting accidents. *J Foot Ankle Surg.* 2015; 54(6):1206–1212.
85. Kewenter Y. Die sesambienedes 1. Metatarsophalangealgelenks des menschen. *Acta Orthop Scand.* 1936;(suppl 2):1–113.
86. Khan KM, Fuller PJ, Brukner PD, et al. Outcome of conservative and surgical management of navicular stress fracture in athletes. Eighty-six cases proven with computerized tomography. *Am J Sports Med.* 1992;20(6):657–666.
87. Kirkpatrick DP, Hunter RE, Janes PC, et al. The snowboarder's foot and ankle. *Am J Sports Med.* 1998;26(2):271–277.

88. Knijnenberg LM, Dingemans SA, Terra MP, et al. Radiographic anatomy of the pediatric lisfranc joint. *J Pediatr Orthop*. 2016.

89. Kramer DE, Mahan ST, Hresko MT. Displaced intra-articular fractures of the great toe in children: Intervene with caution! *J Pediatr Orthop*. 2014;34(2):144–149.

90. Kumai T, Takakura Y, Higashiyama I, et al. Arthroscopic drilling for the treatment of osteochondral lesions of the talus. *J Bone Joint Surg Am*. 1999;81(9):1229–1235.

91. Laliotis N, Pennie BH, Carty H, et al. Toddler's fracture of the calcaneum. *Injury*. 1993;24(3):169–170.

92. Lau LS, Bin G, Jaovisidua S, et al. Cost effectiveness of magnetic resonance imaging in diagnosing Pseudomonas aeruginosa infection after puncture wound. *J Foot Ankle Surg*. 1997;36(1):36–43.

92a. Lau ST, Lee YH, Hess DJ, et al. Lawnmower injuries in children: a 10-year experience. *Pediatr Surg Int*. 2006;22(3):209–214.

93. Laughlin TJ, Armstrong DG, Caporusso J, et al. Soft tissue and bone infections from puncture wounds in children. *West J Med*. 1997;166(2):126–128.

94. Lawrence SJ, Botte MJ. Jones' fractures and related fractures of the proximal fifth metatarsal. *Foot Ankle*. 1993;14(6):358–365.

95. Leenen LP, van der Werken C. Fracture-dislocations of the tarsometatarsal joint, a combined anatomical and computed tomographic study. *Injury*. 1992;23(1):51–55.

96. Lehman RC, Torg JS, Pavlov H, et al. Fractures of the base of the fifth metatarsal distal to the tuberosity: A review. *Foot Ankle*. 1987;7(4):245–252.

97. Leibner ED, Simanovsky N, Abu-Sneinah K, et al. Fractures of the lateral process of the talus in children. *J Pediatr Orthop B*. 2001;10(1):68–72.

98. Letournel E. Open treatment of acute calcaneal fractures. *Clin Orthop Relat Res*. 1993;290:60–67.

99. Letts M, Davidson D, Ahmer A. Osteochondritis dissecans of the talus in children. *J Pediatr Orthop*. 2003;23(5):617–625.

100. Letts RM, Gibeault D. Fractures of the neck of the talus in children. *Foot Ankle*. 1980;1(2):74–77.

101. Levin LS, Nunley JA. The management of soft-tissue problems associated with calcaneal fractures. *Clin Orthop Relat Res*. 1993;290:151–156.

102. Lickstein LH, Bentz ML. Reconstruction of pediatric foot and ankle trauma. *J Craniofac Surg*. 2003;14(4):559–565.

103. Lin CH, Mardini S, Wei FC, et al. Free flap reconstruction of foot and ankle defects in pediatric patients: Long-term outcome in 91 cases. *Plast Reconstr Surg*. 2006;117(7):2478–2487.

104. Lindvall E, Haidukewych G, DiPasquale T, et al. Open reduction and stable fixation of isolated, displaced talar neck and body fractures. *J Bone Joint Surg Am*. 2004;86-A(10):2229–2234.

105. Loder RT. Demographics of traumatic amputations in children. Implications for prevention strategies. *J Bone Joint Surg Am*. 2004;86-A(5):923–928.

106. Love SM, Grogan DP, Ogden JA. Lawnmower injuries in children. *J Orthop Trauma*. 1988;2(2):94–101.

107. Lu J, Ebraheim NA, Skie M, et al. Radiographic and computed tomographic evaluation of Lisfranc dislocation: A cadaver study. *Foot Ankle Int*. 1997;18(6):351–355.

108. Main BJ, Jowett RL. Injuries of the midtarsal joint. *J Bone Joint Surg Br*. 1975;57(1):89–97.

109. Major NM. Role of MRI in prevention of metatarsal stress fractures in collegiate basketball players. *AJR Am J Roentgenol*. 2006;186(1):255–258.

110. Manoli A 2nd. Compartment syndromes of the foot: Current concepts. *Foot Ankle*. 1990;10(6):330–334.

111. Manoli A, Fakhouri A, Weber T. Compartmental catheterization and fasciotomy of the foot. *Operative Tech Orthop*. 1992;2:203–210.

112. Matteri RE, Frymoyer JW. Fracture of the calcaneus in young children. Report of three cases. *J Bone Joint Surg Am*. 1973;55(5):1091–1094.

113. Mazel C, Rigault P, Padovani JP, et al. [Fractures of the talus in children. Apropos of 23 cases]. *Rev Chir Orthop Reparatrice Appar Mot*. 1986;72(3):183–195.

114. McCrory P, Bladin C. Fractures of the lateral process of the talus: A clinical review. "Snowboarder's ankle." *Clin J Sport Med*. 1996;6(2):124–128.

115. McDougall A. The os trigonum. *J Bone Joint Surg Br*. 1955;37-B(2):257–265.

116. Meyer SA, Callaghan JJ, Albright JP, et al. Midfoot sprains in collegiate football players. *Am J Sports Med*. 1994;22(3):392–401.

117. Monteleone GP Jr. Stress fractures in the athlete. *Orthop Clin North Am*. 1995;26(3):423–432.

118. Mooney JF 3rd, Argenta LC, Marks MW, et al. Treatment of soft tissue defects in pediatric patients using the V.A.C. system. *Clin Orthop Relat Res*. 2000;376:26–31.

119. Mora S, Thordorson DB, Zionts LE, et al. Pediatric calcaneal fractures. *Foot Ankle Int*. 2001;22(6):471–477.

120. Mulfinger GL, Trueta J. The blood supply of the talus. *J Bone Joint Surg Br*. 1970;52(1):160–167.

121. Myerson MS. Experimental decompression of the fascial compartments of the foot—the basis for fasciotomy in acute compartment syndromes. *Foot Ankle*. 1988;8(6):308–314.

122. Myerson MS, Fisher RT, Burgess AR, et al. Fracture dislocations of the tarsometatarsal joints: End results correlated with pathology and treatment. *Foot Ankle*. 1986;6(5):225–242.

123. Newman R, Miles R. *Hazard Analysis: Injuries Associated with Riding Type Mowers*. Washington, DC: U.S.C.P.S. Commission; 1981.

124. Nicholas R, Hadley J, Paul C, et al. "Snowboarder's fracture": Fracture of the lateral process of the talus. *J Am Board Fam Pract*. 1994;7(2):130–133.

125. Noble J, Royle SG. Fracture of the lateral process of the talus: Computed tomographic scan diagnosis. *Br J Sports Med*. 1992;26(4):245–246.

126. Ogden J. The foot. In: Ogden J, ed. *Skeletal Injury in the Child*. New York: Springer Verlag; 2000.

127. Owen RJ, Hickey FG, Finlay DB. A study of metatarsal fractures in children. *Injury*. 1995;26(8):537–538.

128. Paccola C, Kunioka C. Bifid calcaneus. *The Foot*. 1991;1:49–50.

129. Pennal GF. Fractures of the talus. *Clin Orthop Relat Res*. 1963;30:53–63.

130. Penny JN, Davis LA. Fractures and fracture-dislocations of the neck of the talus. *J Trauma*. 1980;20(12):1029–1037.

131. Perumal V, Wall E, Babekir N. Juvenile osteochondritis dissecans of the talus. *J Pediatr Orthop*. 2007;27(7):821–825.

132. Peterson L, Goldie IF. The arterial supply of the talus. A study on the relationship to experimental talar fractures. *Acta Orthop Scand*. 1975;46(6):1026–1034.

133. Peterson L, Romanus B, Dahlberg E. Fracture of the collum tali—an experimental study. *J Biomech*. 1976;9(4):277–279.

134. Petit CJ, Lee BM, Kasser JR, et al. Operative treatment of intraarticular calcaneal fractures in the pediatric population. *J Pediatr Orthop*. 2007;27(8):856–862.

135. Petnehazy T, Schalamon J, Hartwig C, et al. Fractures of the hallux in children. *Foot Ankle Int*. 2015;36:60–63.

136. Pickle A, Benaroch TE, Guy P, et al. Clinical outcome of pediatric calcaneal fractures treated with open reduction and internal fixation. *J Pediatr Orthop*. 2004;24(2):178–180.

137. Potter HG, Deland JT, Gusmar PB, et al. Magnetic resonance imaging of the Lisfranc ligament of the foot. *Foot Ankle Int*. 1998;19(7):438–446.

138. Pritsch M, Horoshovski H, Farine I. Arthroscopic treatment of osteochondral lesions of the talus. *J Bone Joint Surg Am*. 1986;68(6):862–865.

139. Purvis JM, Burke RG. Recreational injuries in children: Incidence and prevention. *J Am Acad Orthop Surg*. 2001;9(6):365–374.

140. Quénu E, Küss G. Étude sur les luxations du metataese (luxations métatarsotariennes) du diastasis entre le 1er et la 2e metatarsien. *Rev Chir Orthop Reparatrice Appar Mot*. 1909;39:281–336.

141. Quill GE Jr. Fractures of the proximal fifth metatarsal. *Orthop Clin North Am*. 1995;26(2):353–361.

142. Rainaut J, Cedard C, D'Hour J. Tarso-metatarsal luxations. *Rev Chir Orthop Reparatrice Appar Mot*. 1966;52:449–462.

143. Rammelt S, Zwipp H, Gavlik JM. Avascular necrosis after minimally displaced talus fracture in a child. *Foot Ankle Int*. 2000;21(12):1030–1036.

144. Rang M. The foot. In: Rang M, ed. *Children's Fractures*. 2nd ed. Philadelphia, PA: JB Lippincott; 1974.

145. Rasmussen F, Schantz K. Radiologic aspects of calcaneal fractures in childhood and adolescence. *Acta Radiol Diagn (Stockh)*. 1986;27(5):575–580.

146. Riccardi G, Riccardi D, Marcarelli M, et al. Extremely proximal fractures of the fifth metatarsal in the developmental age. *Foot Ankle Int*. 2011;32(5):526–532.

147. Richli WR, Rosenthal DI. Avulsion fracture of the fifth metatarsal: Experimental study of pathomechanics. *AJR Am J Roentgenol*. 1984;143(4):889–891.

147a. Robertson NB, Roocroft JH, Edmonds EW. Childhood metatarsal shaft fractures: treatment outcomes and relative indications for surgical intervention. *J Child Orthop*. 2012;6(2):125–129.

148. Rosenberg GA, Patterson BM. Tarsometatarsal (Lisfranc's) fracture-dislocation. *Am J Orthop*. 1995;(suppl):7–16.

149. Ross G, Cronin R, Hauzenblas J, et al. Plantar ecchymosis sign: A clinical aid to diagnosis of occult Lisfranc tarsometatarsal injuries. *J Orthop Trauma*. 1996;10(2):119–122.

150. Ross PM, Schwentker EP, Bryan H. Mutilating lawnmower injuries in children. *JAMA*. 1976;236(5):480–481.

151. Rowe C, Sakellarides H. Fractures of the os calcis, a long-term follow-up study of 146 patients. *JAMA*. 1963;184:920.

152. Sammarco GJ. The Jones fracture. *Instr Course Lect*. 1993;42:201–205.

153. Sanders R. Intra-articular fractures of the calcaneus: Present state of the art. *J Orthop Trauma*. 1992;6(2):252–265.

154. Sanders R. Fractures and fracture-dislocations of the calcaneus. In: Coughlin M, Mann R, eds. *Surgery of the Foot and Ankle*. 7th ed. St. Louis, MO: Mosby; 1999.

155. Sanders R. Displaced intra-articular fractures of the calcaneus. *J Bone Joint Surg Am*. 2000;82(2):225–250.

156. Sanders R, Fortin P, DiPasquale T, et al. Operative treatment in 120 displaced intraarticular calcaneal fractures. Results using a prognostic computed tomography scan. *Clin Orthop Relat Res*. 1993;290:87–95.

157. Sarrail R, Launay F, Marez M. Reflex dystrophy in children and adolescents. *J Bone Joint Surg Br*. 2004;86(suppl):23.

158. Schantz K, Rasmussen F. Good prognosis after calcaneal fracture in childhood. *Acta Orthop Scand*. 1988;59(5):560–563.

159. Schindler A, Mason DE, Nanni JA. Occult fracture of the calcaneus in toddlers. *J Pediatr Orthop*. 1996;16(2):201–205.

160. Schenck RC Jr, Heckman JD. Fractures and dislocations of the forefoot: Operative and nonoperative treatment. *J Am Acad Orthop Surg*. 1995;3(2):70–78.

161. Schmidt TL, Weiner DS. Calcaneal fractures in children. An evaluation of the nature of the injury in 56 children. *Clin Orthop Relat Res*. 1982;171:150–155.

162. Schopfner C, Coin C. Effect of weight-bearing on the appearance and development of the secondary calcaneal epiphysis. *Radiology*. 1968;86:201–206.

163. Senaran H, Mason D, De Pellegrin M. Cuboid fractures in preschool children. *J Pediatr Orthop*. 2006;26(6):741–744.

164. Shereff MJ. Fractures of the forefoot. *Instr Course Lect*. 1990;39:133–140.

165. Shilt JS, Yoder JS, Manuck TA, et al. Role of vacuum-assisted closure in the treatment of pediatric lawnmower injuries. *J Pediatr Orthop*. 2004;24(5):482–487.

165a. Silas SI, Herzenberg JE, Myerson MS, et al. Compartment syndrome of the foot in children. *J Bone Joint Surg Am*. 1995;77(3):356–361.

166. Singer G, Cichocki M, Schalamon J, et al. A study of metatarsal fractures in children. *J Bone Joint Surg Am*. 2008;90(4):772–776.

167. Smith JT, Curtis TA, Spencer S, et al. Complications of talus fractures in children. *J Pediatr Orthop*. 2010;30(8):749–757.

168. Sneppen O, Christensen SB, Krogsoe O, et al. Fracture of the body of the talus. *Acta Orthop Scand*. 1977;48(3):317–324.

169. Stanitski CL. Pediatric and adolescent sports injuries. *Clin Sports Med*. 1997;16(4):613–633.

170. Starshak RJ, Simons GW, Sty JR. Occult fracture of the calcaneus—another toddler's fracture. *Pediatr Radiol.* 1984;14(1):37–40.

171. Swanson TV, Bray TJ, Holmes GB Jr. Fractures of the talar neck. A mechanical study of fixation. *J Bone Joint Surg Am.* 1992;74(4):544–551.

172. Swoboda B, Scola E, Zwipp H. [Surgical treatment and late results of foot compartment syndrome]. *Unfallchirurg.* 1991;94(5):262–266.

173. Talkhani S, Reidy D, Fogarty E, et al. Avascular necrosis of the talus after a minimally displaced neck of talus fracture in a 6 year old child. *Injury.* 2000;31(1):63–65.

174. Tezval M, Dumont C, Stürmer KM. Prognostic reliability of the Hawkins sign in fractures of the talus. *J Orthop Trauma.* 2007;(8):538–543.

175. Thordarson DB, Triffon MJ, Terk MR. Magnetic resonance imaging to detect avascular necrosis after open reduction and internal fixation of talar neck fractures. *Foot Ankle Int.* 1996;17(12):742–747.

176. Torg JS, Balduini FC, Zelko RR, et al. Fractures of the base of the fifth metatarsal distal to the tuberosity. Classification and guidelines for nonsurgical and surgical management. *J Bone Joint Surg Am.* 1984;66(2):209–214.

177. Tucker DJ, Feder JM, Boylan JP. Fractures of the lateral process of the talus: Two case reports and a comprehensive literature review. *Foot Ankle Int.* 1998;19(9):641–646.

178. Vanderwilde R, Staheli LT, Chew DE, et al. Measurements on radiographs of the foot in normal infants and children. *J Bone Joint Surg Am.* 1988;70(3):407–415.

179. Vollman D, Smith GA. Epidemiology of lawnmower-related injuries to children in the United States, 1990–2004. *Pediatrics.* 2006;118(2):e273–e278.

180. Vosburgh CL, Gruel CR, Herndon WA, et al. Lawnmower injuries of the pediatric foot and ankle: Observations on prevention and management. *J Pediatr Orthop.* 1995;15(4):504–509.

181. Weber M, Locher S. Reconstruction of the cuboid in compression fractures: Short to midterm results in 12 patients. *Foot Ankle Int.* 2002;23(11):1008–1013.

182. Wilder RT. Management of pediatric patients with complex regional pain syndrome. *Clin J Pain.* 2006;22(5):443–448.

183. Wilder RT, Berde CB, Wolohan M, et al. Reflex sympathetic dystrophy in children. Clinical characteristics and follow-up of 70 patients. *J Bone Joint Surg Am.* 1992;74(6):910–919.

184. Wiley JJ. The mechanism of tarsometatarsal joint injuries. *J Bone Joint Surg Br.* 1971;53(3):474–482.

185. Wiley JJ. Tarsometatarsal joint injuries in children. *J Pediatr Orthop.* 1981;1(3):255–260.

186. Wiley JJ, Profitt A. Fractures of the os calcis in children. *Clin Orthop Relat Res.* 1984;188:131–138.

187. Wilson DW. Injuries of the tarsometatarsal joints. Etiology, classification, and results of treatment. *J Bone Joint Surg Br.* 1972;54(4):677–686.

188. Wiss DA, Kull DM, Perry J. Lisfranc fracture-dislocations of the foot: A clinical-kinesiological study. *J Orthop Trauma.* 1987;1(4):267–274.

189. Wu Y, Jiang H, Wang B. Fracture of the lateral process of the talus in children: A kind of ankle injury with frequently missed diagnosis. *J Pediatr Orthop.* 2016;36(3):289–293.

190. Yngve D. Stress fractures in the pediatric athlete. In: Sullivan J, Grana W, eds. *The Pediatric Athlete.* Park Ridge, IL: American Academy of Orthopaedic Surgeons; 1990:235–240.

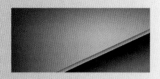

Index

Page numbers followed by an *f* indicate figures; page numbers followed by a *t* indicate tables.